P9-DXM-751

Brief Contents

Clinical Nursing Skills & Techniques

8th Edition

Anne Griffin Perry, RN, MSN, EdD, FAAN
Associate Dean and Professor
School of Nursing
Southern Illinois University—Edwardsville
Edwardsville, Illinois

Patricia A. Potter, RN, MSN, PhD, FAAN
Director of Research, Patient Care Services
Barnes-Jewish Hospital
St. Louis, Missouri

Wendy R. Ostendorf, RN, MS, EdD, CNE
Associate Professor of Nursing
Neumann University
Aston, Pennsylvania

ELSEVIER

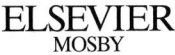

3251 Riverport Lane
St. Louis, Missouri 63043

CLINICAL NURSING SKILLS & TECHNIQUES   ISBN 978-0-323-08383-6

Notices

Knowledge and best practice in this field are constantly changing. As new research and experience broaden our understanding, changes in research methods, professional practices, or medical treatment may become necessary.

Practitioners and researchers must always rely on their own experience and knowledge in evaluating and using any information, methods, compounds, or experiments described herein. In using such information or methods they should be mindful of their own safety and the safety of others, including parties for whom they have a professional responsibility.

With respect to any drug or pharmaceutical products identified, readers are advised to check the most current information provided (i) on procedures featured or (ii) by the manufacturer of each product to be administered, to verify the recommended dose or formula, the method and duration of administration, and contraindications. It is the responsibility of practitioners, relying on their own experience and knowledge of their patients, to make diagnoses, to determine dosages and the best treatment for each individual patient, and to take all appropriate safety precautions.

To the fullest extent of the law, neither the Publisher nor the authors, contributors, or editors, assume any liability for any injury and/or damage to persons or property as a matter of products liability, negligence or otherwise, or from any use or operation of any methods, products, instructions, or ideas contained in the material herein.

International Standard Book Number: 978-0-323-08383-6

Senior Content Strategist: Tamara Myers
Managing Editor: Jean Sims Fornango
Publishing Services Manager: Deborah L. Vogel
Senior Project Manager: Jodi M. Willard
Design Direction: Brian Salisbury

Printed in Canada

Last digit is the print number: 9 8 7 6 5 4

As always, this book is dedicated to my children. To be their mother brings more joy, honor, and sense of pride than I could ever imagine. They and their loved ones are truly my shining stars. As they grow, things change, and I now dedicate this book to:

My daughter, Rebecca Lacey Perry Bryan, her husband, Robert Donald Bryan, their three daughters Cora Elizabeth Bryan, Amalie Mary Bryan, and Noelle Anne Bryan, and their son Shepherd Charles Bryan; and to my son, Horace Mitchell "Mitch" Perry and his partner Samuel Jacob Cox.

Anne G. Perry

I wish to dedicate this new edition of our text to the incredible friends, work colleagues, and scholars I have been so fortunate to associate with throughout my career.

Patricia A. Potter

For my husband, who believes in me, even when I do not believe in myself.

Wendy R. Ostendorf

About the Authors

ANNE GRIFFIN PERRY, RN, MSN, EdD, FAAN

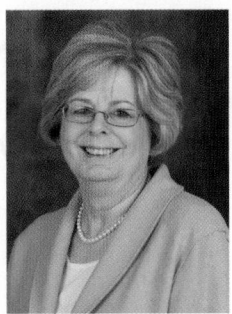

Dr. Anne G. Perry, Professor and Associate Dean for Academic Programs at Southern Illinois University—Edwardsville, is a Fellow in the American Academy of Nursing. She received her BSN from the University of Michigan, her MSN from Saint Louis University, and her EdD from Southern Illinois University—Edwardsville. Dr. Perry is a prolific and influential author and speaker. Her work includes four major textbooks (*Basic Nursing*, *Fundamentals of Nursing*, *Nursing Interventions and Clinical Skills*, and *Clinical Nursing Skills and Techniques*), 24 journal articles, 10 abstracts, and 12 nursing research and education grants. She has presented more than 50 papers at conferences across the United States. She has acted as an editorial board member of numerous journals (*Journal of Nursing Measurement*, *Intensive Care Medicine*, *AACN Clinical Issues*, and *Perspectives in Respiratory Nursing*), and she was one of a few key consultants on *Mosby's Nursing Skills Videos*, and *Mosby's Nursing Skills Online*. Dr. Perry currently serves on the NANDA board of directors and on the advisory board for Louis and Clark Community College School of Nursing.

Dr. Perry has been involved in the front lines of nursing education since 1973, first as an instructor and then through various roles of leadership at Saint Louis University Hospital and School of Nursing and now at Southern Illinois University—Edwardsville. As a clinician and researcher, Dr. Perry's contributions to pulmonary nursing and nursing language development involve both research and policy making. She has investigated and published findings regarding topics that include weaning from mechanical ventilation, uses of the therapeutic intervention scoring system, critical care, and validation of nursing diagnoses.

PATRICIA A. POTTER, RN, MSN, PhD, FAAN

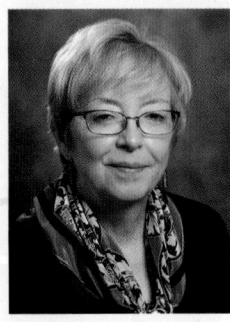

Dr. Patricia Potter received her BSN at the University of Washington in Seattle, and her MSN and PhD at Saint Louis University in St. Louis, Missouri. A groundbreaking author for more than 25 years, her work includes four major textbooks (*Basic Nursing*, *Fundamentals of Nursing*, *Nursing Interventions and Clinical Skills*, and *Clinical Nursing Skills and Techniques*) and more than 20 journal articles. She has been an unceasing advocate of evidence-based practice and quality improvement in her roles as administrator, educator and, more recently, director of research.

Dr. Potter has devoted a lifetime to nursing education, practice, and research. She spent a decade teaching at Barnes Hospital School of Nursing and Saint Louis University. She entered into a variety of managerial and administrative roles, ultimately becoming the director of nursing practice at Barnes-Jewish Hospital. In that capacity she sharpened her interest in the development of nursing practice standards and the measurement of patient outcomes in defining nursing practice. Her most recent passion has been in the area of nursing research, specifically cancer family caregiving, the cancer patient symptom experience, and the effects of compassion fatigue on nurses. Dr. Potter is currently a director of research for patient care services at Barnes-Jewish Hospital.

WENDY R. OSTENDORF, RN, MS, EdD, CNE

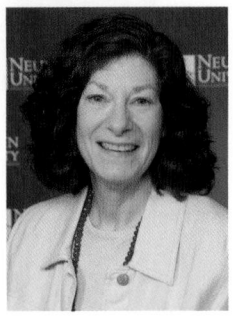

Dr. Wendy R. Ostendorf received her BSN from Villanova University, her MS from the University of Delaware, and her EdD from the University of Sarasota. She currently serves as an associate professor of nursing in the Division of Nursing and Health Sciences at Neumann University in Aston, Pennsylvania. She has contributed more than 20 chapters to multiple nursing textbooks and has served as section editor for two major textbooks *Nursing Interventions and Clinical Skills*, and *Clinical Nursing Skills and Techniques*. She has presented more than 25 papers at conferences at the local, national, and international levels.

Professionally, Dr. Ostendorf has a diverse background in pediatric and adult critical care. She has taught at the undergraduate and graduate level for 30 years. With decades of practice as a clinician, her educational experiences have influenced her teaching philosophy and perceptions of the nursing profession. Dr. Ostendorf's current interests include the history and image of nursing as it has been represented in film, which she has developed into an undergraduate nursing course.

Contributors

Nicole Bartow, RN, MSN
Instructor/Director of the Essig Clinical Simulation Center
Sinclair School of Nursing
University of Missouri
Columbia, Missouri

Aurelie Chinn, RN, MSN
Academic Nursing Skills Specialist/Simulation Technician/
    Instructor
Associate Degree Nursing Program
Cabrillo College
Aptos, California

Janice C. Colwell, RN, MSN, CWOCN, FAAN
Advanced Practice Nurse
University of Chicago, Department of Surgery
Chicago, Illinois

Charlene Compher, PhD, RD, CNSC, LDN, FADA
Associate Professor of Nutrition Science
University of Pennsylvania School of Nursing
Philadelphia, Pennsylvania

Kelly Jo Cone, RN, PhD, CNE
Professor, Graduate Program
Saint Francis Medical Center College of Nursing
Peoria, Illinois

Pamela A. Cupec, RN, MS, ONC, CRRN, ACM
Senior Professional Case Manager
University of Pittsburgh Medical Center—Passavant
Pittsburgh, Pennsylvania

Ruth M. Curchoe, RN, MSN, CIC
Infection Prevention Consulting
Hilton, New York

Jane Fellows, MSN, RN, CWOCN
Wound/Ostomy CNS
Duke University Health System
Durham, North Carolina

Susan Jane Fetzer, RN, BSN, MSN, MBA, PhD
Associate Professor
College of Health and Human Services
University of New Hampshire
Durham, New Hampshire

Cathy E. Flasar, MSN, APRN
Family Nurse Practitioner (FNP)
American Society for Pain Management Nurses
St. Louis, Missouri

Kathleen Gerhart-Gibson, MSN, RN, CCRN
Nursing Instructor
School of Nursing
Neumann University
Aston, Pennsylvania

Roberta L. Harrison, PhD, RN, CRRN
Assistant Professor
School of Nursing
Southern Illinois University—Edwardsville
Edwardsville, Illinois

Lori Klingman, MSN, RN
Faculty
Ohio Valley Hospital School of Nursing
McKees Rocks, Pennsylvania

Nancy Laplante, PhD, RN
Assistant Professor
School of Nursing
Neumann University
Aston, Pennsylvania

Nelda K. Martin, RN, CCNS, ANP-BC
Clinical Nurse Specialist/Adult Nurse Practitioner
Barnes-Jewish Hospital, Heart and Vascular Program
St. Louis, Missouri

Kristin L. Mauk, PhD, DNP, RN, CRRN, GCNS-BC, GNP-BC, FAAN
Professor of Nursing and Kreft Endowed Chair
School of Nursing
Valparaiso University
Valparaiso, Indiana

Pamela L. Ostby, RN, MSN, OCN®
Affiliate Assistant Professor
Goldfarb School of Nursing
Barnes-Jewish College
St. Louis, Missouri

Jeanne Marie Papa, MBE, MSN, ACNP-BC, CCRN
Professor of Nursing
Neumann University
Aston, Pennsylvania

Jacqueline Raybuck Saleeby, PhD, RN, BCCS
Associate Professor, Nursing
School of Health Professions
Maryville University
St. Louis, Missouri

Phyllis Ann Schiavone, MSN, CRNP
Nurse Practitioner
Hospital of the University of Pennsylvania
Philadelphia, Pennsylvania

Lois Schick, MN, MBA, CPAN, CAPA
Perianesthesia Consultant & Per Diem Bedside Nurse
Exempla Lutheran Medical Center
Wheat Ridge, Colorado

Paula Ann Stangeland, PhD, RN, CRRN
Assistant Professor
University of Texas Medical Branch School of Nursing
Galveston, Texas

E. Bradley Strecker, RN, PhD
Associate Professor
Program Director Accelerated BSN Program
MidAmerica Nazarene University
Olathe, Kansas

Virginia Strootman, RN MS CRNI
Vice President of Clinical Services
Specialty Pharmacy Nursing Network, Inc.
Sarasota, Florida

Donna L. Thompson, MSN, CRNP, FNP-BC, CCCN
Nurse Practitioner—Continence Specialist
Urology Health Specialist
Drexel Hills, Pennsylvania

Pamela E. Windle, MS, RN, NE-BC, CPAN, CAPA, FAAN
Nurse Manager
St. Luke's Episcopal Hospital
Houston, Texas

Terry L. Wood, PhD, RN, CNE
Assistant Clinical Professor
Southern Illinois University—Edwardsville
Edwardsville, Illinois

Patricia H. Worthington, MSN, RN, CNSC
Nutritional Support Clinical Specialist
Thomas Jefferson University Hospital, Department of Nursing
Philadelphia, Pennsylvania

Rita Wunderlich, MSN, PhD
Assistant Professor
Goldfarb School of Nursing
Barnes-Jewish College
St. Louis, Missouri

Valeria J. Yancey, PhD, RN, HNC, CHPN
Associate Professor
School of Nursing
Southern Illinois University—Edwardsville
Edwardsville, Illinois

CONTRIBUTORS TO PREVIOUS EDITIONS

We would like to acknowledge the following people who contributed to previous editions of *Clinical Nursing Skills & Techniques*.

Jeannette Adams, PhD, MSN, APRN, CRNI
Della Aridge, RN, MSN
Elizabeth A. Ayello, PhD, MS, BSN, RN, CS, CWOCN
Sylvia K. Baird, BSN, MM
Margaret Benz, RN, MSN, CSANP
Barbara J. Berger, MSN, RN
Lyndal Guenther Brand, RN, BSN, MSN
Peggy Breckinridge, RN, BSN, MSN, FNP
Victoria M. Brown, RN, BSN, MSN, PhD
Gina Bufe, RN, BSN, MSN(R), PhD, CS
Gale Carli, MSN, MHed, BSN, RN
Ellen Carson, PhD
Maureen Carty, MSN, OCN
Mary F. Clarke, MA, RN
Janice C. Colwell, RN, MS, CWOCN
Kelly Jo Cone, RN, BSN, MS, PhD, CNE
Dorothy McDonnell Cooke, RN, PhD
Eileen Costantinou, RN, BSN, MSN
Sheila A. Cunningham, RN, BSN, MSN
Ruth Curchoe, RN, MSN, CIC
Rick Daniels, RN, BSN, MSN, PhD
Mardell Davis, RN, MSN, CETN
Carolyn Ruppel d'Avis, RN, BSN, MSN
Patricia A. Dettenmeier, RN, BSN, MSN(R), CCRN
Wanda Cleveland Dubuisson, BSN, MN
Sharon J. Edwards, RN, MSN, PhD
Martha E. Elkin, RN, MSN
Deborah Oldenburg Erickson, RN, BSN, MSN
Debra Farrell, BSN, CNOR
Linda Fasciani, RN, BSN, MSN
Jane Fellows, RN, MSN, CWOCN
Susan Jane Fetzer, RN, BA, BSN, MSN, MBA, PhD

Cathy Flasar, MSN, APRN, BC, FNP
Marlene S. Foreman, BSN, MN, RNCS
Carol P. Fray, RN, MA
Leah W. Frederick, RN, MS, CIC
Paula Goldberg, RN, MS, MSN
Thelma Halberstadt, EdD, MS, BS, RN
Amy Hall, PhD, MS, BSN, RN
Linda C. Haynes, PhD, RN
Diane Hildwein, RN, BC, MA
Maureen B. Huhmann, MS, RD
Nancy C. Jackson, RN, BSN, MSN, CCRN
Ruth L. Jilka, RD, CDE
Teresa M. Johnson, RN, MSN, CCRN
Judith Ann Kilpatrick, RN, DNSC
Carl Kirton, RN, BSN, MA, CCRN, ACRN, ANP
Lori Klingman, MSN, RN
Marilee Kuhrik, RN, MSN, PhD
Nancy S. Kuhrik, RN, MSN, PhD
Diane M. Kyle, RN, BSN, MS
Nancy Laplante, PhD, RN
Louise K. Leitao, RN(c), BSN, MA
Gail B. Lewis, RN, MSN
Ruth Ludwick, PhD, MSN, BSN, RNC, CNS
Mary Kay Macheca, MSN(R), RN, CS, ANP, CDE
Jill Feldman Malen, RN, MS, NS, ANP
Mary K. Mantese, RN, MSN
Elizabeth Mantych, RN, MSN
Tina Marrelli, MSN, MA, RN
Nelda K. Martin, APRN, BC, CCNS, ANP
Mary Mercer, RN, MSN
Rita Mertig, MS, BSN, RNC, CNS
Norma Metheny, PhD, MSN, BSN, FAAN
Mary Dee Miller, RN, BSN, MS, CIC
Sharon M.J. Muhs, MSN, RN

Kathleen Mulryan, RN, BSN, MSN
Lynne M. Murphy, RN, MSN
Elaine K. Neel, RN, BSN, MSN
Meghan G. Noble, PhD, RN
Marsha Evans Orr, RN, BS, MS, CS
Dula F. Pacquiao, EdD, RN, CTN
Sharon Phelps, RN, BSN, MS
Catherine A. Robinson, BA, RN
Judith Roos, RN, MSN
Mary Jane Ruhland, MSN, RN, BC
Jan Rumfelt, RNC, MSN, EdD
Jacqueline Raybuck Saleeby, PhD, RN, CS
Linette M. Sarti, RN, BSN, CNOR
Kelly M. Schwartz, RN, BSN
April Sieh, RN, BSN, MSN
Marlene Smith, RN, BSN, M.Ed.
Julie S. Snyder, MSN, RNC
Laura Sofield, MSN, APRN, BC
Sharon Souter, MSN, BSN
Martha A. Spies, RN, MSN
Patricia A. Stockert, RN, BSN, MS, PhD
Sandra Ann Szekely, RN, BSN
Lynn Tier, RN, MSN, LNC
Nancy Tomaselli, RN, MSN, CS, CRNP, CWOCN, CLNC
Riva Touger-Decker, PhD, RD, FADA
Anne Falsone Vaughan, MSN, BSN, CCRN
Cynthia Vishy, RN, BSN
Pamela Becker Weilitz, MSN(R), RN, CS, ANP
Joan Domigan Wentz, MSN, RN
Laurel Wiersema, RN, MSN
Terry L. Wood, PhD, RN
Rita Wunderlich, PhD (Cand.), MSN(R), CCRN
Rhonda Yancey, BSN, RN
Valerie Yancey, PhD, RN, HNC, CHPN

Reviewers

Faisal Aboul-Enein, PhD, RN
Clinical Coordinator
Institute of Health Sciences
Texas Women's University
Houston, Texas

Janet J. Adams, MSN, RT(R), RN
Nursing Instructor
Southeast Missouri State University
Cape Girardeau, Missouri

Michelle Aebersold, PhD, RN
Clinical Assistant Professor
Lead Faculty—Clinical Learning Center
University of Michigan School of Nursing
Ann Arbor, Michigan

Patricia N. Allen, MSN, APRN
Clinical Assistant Professor
Indiana University
Bloomington, Indiana

Jocelyn Anderson, RN, MN
Coordinator, Nursing Skills Lab
Health Sciences, Education & Wellness Institute
Bellevue College
Bellevue, Washington

Marty Bachman, PhD, RN, CNS, CNE
Nursing Program Director, Department Chair
Front Range Community College—Larimer Campus
Larimer, Colorado

Nakia C. Best, MSN, RN
Clinical Assistant Professor
University of North Carolina School of Nursing
Chapel Hill, North Carolina

Patricia C. Buchsel, RN, MSN, OCN©, FAAN
Clinical Instructor
Seattle University College of Nursing
Seattle, Washington

Lauren G. Cline, MN, RN
Clinical Nurse Educator, Clinical Instructor
University of Washington School of Nursing
Seattle, Washington

Patricia Conley, MSN, RN
Staff Nurse, Progressive Cardio-Pulmonary Care Unit
Research Medical Center
Kansas City, Missouri

Jessica Doolen, RN, MSN, FNP-C, CNE
Lecturer/Clinical Instructor
School of Nursing
University of Nevada
Las Vegas, Nevada

Yvette Egan, RN, BSN, MS
Clinical Assistant Professor
School of Nursing
University of Wisconsin
Madison, Wisconsin

Kelli M. Fuller, DNP, ANP-BC
Instructor
Goldfarb School of Nursing
Barnes-Jewish College
St. Louis, Missouri

Margaret Gingrich, MSN, CRNP
Professor of Nursing
Harrisburg Area Community College
Harrisburg, Pennsylvania

Jacqueline Guhde, MSN, RN, CNS
Senior Instructor
The University of Akron
Akron, Ohio

Carolyn Hosking, RN, BN, MSN
Nursing Lecturer
Thompson River University
Williams Lake, British Columbia, Canada

Brenda L. Hoskins, DNP, ARNP, GNP-BC, FAANP
Associate Clinical Professor
College of Nursing
University of Iowa
Grinnell, Iowa

Helena Jermalovic, RN, BSN, MSN
Assistant Professor
University of Alaska, Anchorage
Anchorage, Alaska

Mary Ann Jessee, MSN, RN
Assistant Professor
Vanderbilt University School of Nursing
Nashville, Tennessee

Barbara Kaplan, RN, MSN
Instructor, Coordinator Evans Center for Caring Skills
Nell Hodgson Woodruff School of Nursing
Emory University
Atlanta, Georgia

Christina D. Keller, RN, MSN
Instructor, Radford University Clinical Simulation Center
Radford University
Radford, Virginia

Sharon C. Kelly, BSN, RN
Coordinator of Nursing Skills Laboratory
Spokane Community College
Spokane, Washington

Patricia Ketcham, RN, MSN
Director of Nursing Laboratories
Oakland University
Rochester, Michigan

Laura M. Logan, MSN, RN
Clinical Instructor
Stephen F. Austin State University
Nacogdoches, Texas

Diana R. Mager, DNP, RN-BC
Assistant Professor
Fairfield University
Fairfield, Connecticut

Sheila Matye, MSN, RN, RNC-NIC, CNE
Associate Clinical Professor
College of Nursing
Montana State University
Bozeman, Montana

Angela McConachie, RN, DNP, FNP-C
Instructor
Goldfarb School of Nursing
Barnes-Jewish College
St. Louis, Missouri

Jean Mills, MS, RN, BC
Clinical Instructor, Department of Biobehavioral Health Science
University of Illinois College of Nursing
Urbana, Illinois

Cynthia Muldar, RNC, MS, MSN, CNP
Associate Professor
University of South Dakota
Sioux Falls, South Dakota

Rebecca Otten, RN, EdD
Coordinator, Prelicensure Programs
California State University—Fullerton
Fullerton, California

Susan Porterfield, PhD, MSN, MS, BSN, BS, FNP-C
NP Coordinator/Assistant Professor
Florida State University
Tallahassee, Florida

Cherie Rebar, PhD, MBA, RN, FNP
Associate Director, Division of Nursing
Chair, AS & BSN Nursing Programs
Associate Professor
Kettering College
Kettering, Ohio

Jill Reed, MSN, APRN-C
Nursing Instructor
University of Nebraska Medical Center
College of Nursing
Kearny, Nebraska

Jennifer Richardson, RN, MSN
Nursing Instructor
Santa Rosa Junior College
Santa Rosa, California

Kellie J. Richardson, RN, MSN
Instructor
Kilgore Associate Degree Nursing Program
Kilgore College
Kilgore, Texas

Angela Stone Schmidt, RN, MNSc, PhD
Director of Graduate Programs
Associate Professor of Nursing
College of Nursing and Health Professions
Arkansas State University
Jonesboro, Arkansas

Debra Lee Sevello, RNP, MSN
Assistant Professor of Nursing
Rhode Island College
Providence, Rhode Island

Gale Sewell, RN, MSN, CNE
Assistant Professor of Nursing
Indiana Wesleyan University
Marion, Indiana

Cindy Sheppard, MSN, RN, APN-BC
Associate Professor of Nursing
Schoolcraft College
Lavonia, Michigan

Sara Smith, RNC-OB, MSN/ED
Nursing Laboratory Coordinator
University of Hawaii—Hilo School of Nursing
Hilo, Hawaii

Lori Stephens, MN, RN
Clinical Faculty—Nursing
Skagit Valley College
Mount Vernon, Washington

Susan Thompson, RN, BSN, BSL, MFS
Clinical Assistant Professor
College of Nursing & Health Innovation
Arizona State University
Phoenix, Arizona

Lynn Lear Tier, MSN, RN, LNC
Associate Professor of Nursing
Learning Center Coordinator
Florida College of Health Sciences, School of Nursing
Orlando, Florida

Susan A. Wheaton, RN, BSN, MSN
LRC Director/Lecturer/Clinical Instructor
University of Maine
Orono, Maine

Janet Willis, RN, BSN, MS
Professor of Nursing
Harrisburg Area Community College
Harrisburg, Pennsylvania

Jill Witte, MSN, FNP-C
Advanced Practice Nurse Practitioner
American Academy of Nurse Practitioners
Adjunct Faculty, Bellin College
Green Bay, Wisconsin

Aimee Woda, PhD(c), RN, BC
Clinical and Laboratory Instructor
Marquette University
Milwaukee, Wisconsin

Lea Wood, MSN, RN
Coordinator, Instructional Lab
Sinclair School of Nursing
University of Missouri
Columbia, Missouri

Jean Yockey, MSN, PhD
Associate Professor
School of Health Sciences: Nursing, Health Affairs
University of South Dakota
Vermillion, South Dakota

Melody Ziobro, MS, RN
Assistant Professor
School of Nursing
Morrisville State College
Morrisville, New York

Damien Zsiros, MSN, RN, CNE, CRNP
Nursing Instructor
Pennsylvania State University, Fayette Campus
Uniontown, Pennsylvania

CLINICAL REVIEWERS

Carol Bauer, MSN, ANP-BC, OCN, CWOCN
Wound, Ostomy and Continence Nurse Practitioner
Karmanos Cancer Center
Detroit, Michigan

Phyllis Bonham, PhD, MSN, RN, CWOCN, DPNAP, FAAN
Wound, Ostomy and Continence Nurse
Director, Wound Care Education Program
Medical University of South Carolina
Charleston, South Carolina

Rosemary Kates, RN, MSN, APRN-BC, CWOCN
Nurse Practitioner—Surgery
Lourdes Medical Association—Surgical Division
Our Lady of Lourdes Medical Center
Camden, New Jersey

Keith D. Lamb, RCP, RRT
Specialist, Surgical Critical Care/Trauma
Christiana Care Health Systems
Newark, Delaware

Elizabeth M. Lyman, MSN, RN, CNSC
Senior Program Coordinator for the Nutrition Support Team
Children's Mercy Hospitals and Clinics
Kansas City, Missouri

Susan L. Maditz, MSN, RN, CWOCN
Wound, Ostomy, and Continence Nurse Clinician
West Virginia University Healthcare
Morgantown, West Virginia

Manju Maliakal, MSN, CMSRN
RN, Administrative Supervisor
Baylor Medical Center at Carrollton
Carrollton, Texas

Angie Sims, RN, CRNI, OCN
Assistant Head Nurse IV Therapy
Providence Portland Medical Center
Portland, Oregon

Marion F. Winkler, PhD, RD, CNSD
Surgical Nutrition Specialist and Associate Professor of Surgery
Rhode Island Hospital and Alpert Medical School
Brown University
Providence, Rhode Island

Preface to the Student

Numerous features are built into this text to help you identify key pieces of information and study more efficiently. Additional study tools and review questions may be found on the companion Evolve site: http://evolve.elsevier.com/Perry/skills

Evolve media resources are available for every chapter.

Key Terms call attention to critical terminology.

Objectives highlight key information to follow.

22

Parenteral Medications

MEDIA RESOURCES
- evolve http://evolve.elsevier.com/Perry/skills
- Review Questions
- Video Clips
- Audio Glossary
- NSO Nursing Skills Online

KEY TERMS

Adverse reaction	Compatibility	Induration	Parenteral
Air embolus	Continuous subcutaneous	Infiltration	Phlebitis
Allergic reaction	infusion (CSQI or CSCI)	Infusion	Piggyback infusion
Ampule	Diluent	Injection	Saline lock
Anaphylactic reaction	Extravasation	Intradermal (ID) injection	Subcutaneous injection
Aqueous	Hematemesis	Intramuscular (IM) injection	Vial
Aspirate	Hematuria	Intravenous (IV) injection	Volume-control
Blunt-tip vial access cannula	Hypodermoclysis	Medication administration	administration set (Volutrol)
Bolus	Incompatibility	record (MAR)	Z-track method

OBJECTIVES

Mastery of content in this chapter will enable the nurse to:
- Correctly prepare injectable medications from a vial and an ampule.
- Identify advantages, disadvantages, and risks of administering medications by each injection route.
- Evaluate the effectiveness and outcomes of administering medications by each injection route.
- Explain the importance of selecting the proper-size syringe and needle for an injection.
- Discuss factors to consider when selecting injection sites.
- Discuss ways to promote patient comfort while administering an injection.
- Correctly administer intradermal, subcutaneous, and intramuscular injections.
- Compare the risks of three different intravenous routes.
- Correctly administer an intravenous infusion by intravenous piggyback, intermittent infusion, or bolus through a hanging intravenous line or saline lock.
- Initiate, maintain, and discontinue a continuous subcutaneous infusion.

STEP	RATIONALE
c Inject medication slowly. Normally you feel resistance. If not, needle is too deep; remove and begin again.	Slow injection minimizes discomfort at site. Dermal layer is tight and does not expand easily when you inject solution.

Clinical Decision Point *It is not necessary to aspirate because dermis is relatively avascular.*

d While injecting medication, note that small bleb (approximately 6 mm [¼ inch]) resembling mosquito bite appears on skin surface (see illustration).	Bleb indicates that you deposited medication in dermis.
e After withdrawing needle, apply alcohol swab or gauze gently over site.	Do not massage site. Apply bandage if needed.
15 Help patient to comfortable position.	Gives patient sense of well-being.
16 Discard uncapped needle or needle enclosed in safety shield and attached syringe in puncture- and leak-proof receptacle.	Prevents injury to patients and health care personnel. Recapping needles increases risk for a needlestick injury (OSHA, 2012).
17 Remove gloves and perform hand hygiene.	Reduces transmission of microorganisms.
18 Stay with patient for several minutes and observe for any allergic reactions.	Dyspnea, wheezing, and circulatory collapse are signs of severe anaphylactic reaction.

STEP 14b   Intradermal needle tip inserted into dermis.

STEP 14d   Injection creates small bleb.

EVALUATION

1 Return to room in 15 to 30 minutes and ask if patient feels any acute pain, burning, numbness, or tingling at injection site.	Continued discomfort could indicate injury to underlying tissues.
2 Ask patient to discuss implications of skin testing and signs of hypersensitivity.	Patient's ability to recognize signs of skin testing helps to ensure timely reporting of results.

3   Inspect bleb. *Optional:* Use skin pencil and draw circle around perimeter of injection site. Read TB test site at 48 to 72 hours; look for induration (hard, dense, raised area) of skin around injection site of:
  • 15 mm or more in patients with no known risk factors for tuberculosis.
  • 10 mm or more in patients who are recent immigrants; injection drug users; residents and employees of high-risk settings; patients with certain chronic illnesses; children less than 4 years of age; and infants, children, and adolescents exposed to high-risk adults.
	Determines if reaction to antigen occurs; indication positive for TB or tested allergens.
	
	Degree of reaction varies based on patient condition.
	Site must be read at various intervals to determine test results. Pencil marks make site easy to find. You determine results of skin testing at various times, based on type of medication used or type of skin testing completed. Manufacturer directions determine when to read test results.

Clinical Decision Points highlight points to consider when performing skills to ensure effective outcomes and promote safety.

Extensive illustrations demonstrate step-by-step procedures for more thorough understanding.

Quick Response codes may be scanned to link to video clips directly from the text page.

STEP	RATIONALE
8 Dispose of supplies in puncture- and leak-proof container.	Prevents accidental needlesticks (OSHA, 2012).
9 Remove gloves and perform hand hygiene.	Reduces transmission of microorganisms.
10 Stay with patient for several minutes and observe for any allergic reactions.	Dyspnea, wheezing, and circulatory collapse are signs of severe anaphylactic reaction.

EVALUATION

1 Observe patient for signs or symptoms of adverse reaction.	IV medications act rapidly.
2 During infusion periodically check infusion rate and condition of IV site.	IV must remain patent for proper drug administration. Infiltration of IV site requires discontinuing infusion.
3 Ask patient to explain purpose and side effects of medication.	Evaluates patient's understanding of instruction.

Unexpected Outcomes

1 Patient develops adverse or allergic reaction to medication.

2 Medication does not infuse over established time frame.

3 IV site shows signs of infiltration or phlebitis (see Chapter 28).

Related Interventions

- Stop medication infusion immediately.
- Follow agency policy or guidelines for appropriate response to allergic reaction (e.g., administration of antihistamine such as diphenhydramine [Benadryl] or epinephrine) and reporting of adverse medication reactions.
- Notify patient's health care provider of adverse effects immediately.
- Add allergy information to patient record per agency policy.
- Determine reason (e.g., improper calculation of flow rate, poor positioning of IV needle at insertion site, infiltration).
- Take corrective action as indicated.
- Stop IV infusion and discontinue access device.
- Treat IV site as indicated by agency policy.
- Insert new IV catheter if therapy continues.
- For infiltration determine how harmful IV medication is to subcutaneous tissue. Provide IV extravasation care (e.g., injecting phentolamine [Regitine] around IV infiltration site) as indicated by agency policy or consult pharmacist to determine appropriate follow-up care.

Recording and Reporting

- Immediately record medication, dose, route, infusion rate, and date and time administered on MAR or computer printout. Include initials or signature.
- Record volume of fluid in medication bag or Volutrol on intake and output (I&O) form.
- Report any adverse reactions to patient's health care provider.

Special Considerations

Teaching

- Review all IV medications with patient and significant others, including why patient is receiving the medication and potential adverse effects, including allergic responses.
- Teach patient and/or significant others not to alter the ordered rate of infusion without consulting the prescriber. IV medications need to be infused at a specified rate to achieve their desired effect and avoid adverse effects.
- Teach patient and/or significant others to report any adverse effects immediately.

Pediatric

- Infants and young children are more vulnerable to alterations in fluid balance and do not adjust quickly to changes in fluid

balance. Therefore, to assess fluid balance, monitor I&O carefully when infusing IV medications (Hockenberry and Wilson, 2011).

Gerontologic

- Altered pharmacokinetics of medications and the effects of polypharmacy place older adults at risk for medication toxicity. Carefully monitor the response of older adults to IV medications (Touhy and Jett, 2010).
- Older adults are at risk for developing fluid volume overload and require careful assessment for signs of overload and heart failure.

Home Care

- Patients or significant others who administer IV medications at home require education about the steps of medication administration. The patient or significant other needs to perform several return demonstrations of IV medication administration before performing this skill independently. In addition, patients and significant others need to know signs of IV medication administration complications such as phlebitis and infiltration and what to do for any problems.

Unexpected Outcomes/Related Interventions help you anticipate problems and respond appropriately.

Recording and Reporting guidelines for each skill detail what to document and report.

Special Considerations indicate special teaching considerations, as well as procedure modifications needed for pediatric, gerontologic, and home care populations.

NSO icon links to online course lessons.

Home Care

- Self-administration of an IM injection is difficult, especially in the vastus lateralis. Teach a significant other to identify and administer injections in this site.
- Instruct adult patients who require frequent injections to apply EMLA cream to the injection site before administration.
- Patients need instruction in safe disposal of syringes and needles (see Skill 22-3, Home Care Considerations).
- See Skill 41-1 for information about modifying safety risks in the home.

SKILL 22-5   Administering Medications by Intravenous Bolus

 IV Medication Administration Module I Lesson 4

In the past nurses often mixed medications into large volumes of intravenous (IV) fluids (500 to 1000 mL). However, today's safety standards and evidence-based practice no longer support this practice on a routine basis (Infusion Nurses Society [INS], 2011; ISMP, 2011; TJC, 2012). Many patient safety risks such as incorrect calculation, poor aseptic technique, incorrect labeling, pump programming errors, lack of medication knowledge, and mix-up with another medication occur when nurses have to prepare medications in IV containers on patient care units. There are a number of current best practices for preparation and administration of IV medication (Box 22-4).

An IV bolus is one method of medication administration currently practiced on patient care units. It introduces a concentrated dose of a medication directly into a vein by way of an existing IV access. An IV bolus or "push" usually requires small volumes of fluid, which is an advantage for patients who are at risk for fluid

overload. Administering medications by IV bolus is common in emergencies when you need to deliver a fast-acting medication quickly. Because these medications act quickly, it is essential that you monitor patients closely for adverse reactions. Agencies have policies and procedures that identify the medications that nurses are allowed to administer by IV push and other IV routes. These policies are based on the medication, compatibility and availability of staff, and type of monitoring equipment available. There are advantages and disadvantages to administering IV push medications (Box 22-5).

The IV bolus is a dangerous method to administer medications because it allows no time to correct errors. Administering an IV push medication too quickly can cause death. Therefore be very careful in calculating the correct amount of the medication to give. In addition, a bolus may cause direct irritation to the lining of blood vessels; thus always confirm placement of the IV catheter or needle. Never give an IV bolus if the insertion site appears edematous or reddened or if the IV fluids do not flow at the ordered rate. Accidental injection of some medications into tissues surrounding a vein can cause pain, sloughing of tissues, and abscesses.

Verify the rate of administration of IV push medication using agency guidelines or a medication reference manual. The Institute for Safe Medication Practices (ISMP, 2011) has identified the

BOX 22-4   Best Practices for Administration of Intravenous Solutions and Medications

- Use standardized concentrations and dosages of medication.
- Use standardized procedures for ordering, preparing, and administering intravenous (IV) medications.
- Administer solutions and medications prepared and dispensed from the pharmacy or as commercially prepared when possible.
- Never prepare high-alert medications (e.g., heparin, dopamine, dobutamine, nitroglycerin, potassium, antibiotics, or magnesium) on a patient care unit.
- Use standardized infusion concentrations of "high-alert" medications.
- Optimize the storage of IV medications.
- Use the mnemonic CATS PRRR to help remember safety steps for administering IV medications: C, compatibilities; A, aseptic; T, tubing correct; S, site checked; P, pump safety first for right rate; R, release clamps; R, return and document patient (Billings & Kowalski, 2005).
- Standardized label practices. Bold patient name, generic drug, and patient-specific dose.
- Use technology such as intelligent-infusion devices, barcode medication administration, and electronic medication administration record.

Data from American Society of Health-System Pharmacists [ASHP]: Preventing patient harm, *Am J Health-Syst Pharm*; 65:2367, 2008; Infusion Nurses Society: Infusion nursing standards of practice, *J Intraven Nurs*; 2011; Institute for Safe Medication Practices (ISMP): Guidelines for standard available at http://www.ismp.org/tools/guidelines/, accessed July 2011; Institute for Safe Medication Practices: Designing a medication label for intravenous piggyback medications for inpatient use, 2011, available at http://www.ismp.org/tools/guidelines/labelformats/IVPB.asp, accessed July 5, 2012; The Joint Commission: National Patient Safety Goals, hospital accreditation program, www.jointcommission.org, accessed July

BOX 22-5   Advantages and Disadvantages of the Intravenous Push Method

Advantages	Disadvantages
• There is rapid onset of medication effects, which is useful in patients experiencing critical or emergent health problems. • Medications can be prepared quickly and given over a shorter time than by intravenous (IV) piggyback. • Doses of short-acting medications can be titrated based on a patient's needs and responses to the drug therapy. This is important for infants, children, and older patients. • Method provides a more accurate dose of medication delivered because no medication is left in intravenously.	• Not all medications can be delivered by IV push. • There is higher risk for infusion reactions; some are mild to severe because the medication action peaks quickly. • When giving medication quickly (e.g., less than 1 minute), there is very little opportunity to stop the injection if an adverse reaction occurs. • Risk for infiltration and phlebitis is increased, especially if a highly concentrated medication, a small peripheral vein, or a short venous access device is used. • Hypersensitivity reaction can cause an immediate or delayed systemic reaction to a medication, requiring supportive measures.

Mosby's Nursing Video Skills, Student Version, 4th edition contains 130 entirely new, high-definition video skills.

Preface to the Instructor

The evolution of technology and knowledge influences the way we teach clinical skills to nursing students and improves the quality of care possible for every patient. However, the foundation for success in performing nursing skills remains a competent, well-informed nurse who thinks critically and asks the right questions at the right time. That outcome is the driving factor behind this new edition.

In this eighth edition of *Clinical Nursing Skills & Techniques* we have adapted our headings to bring content relevant to the *Quality and Safety Education for Nurses* (QSEN) initiative to the forefront. You will now find sections on *Evidence-Based Practice, Patient-Centered Care, Safety,* and *Documentation and Collaboration,* making the related content even more visible. The opening chapter on *Using Evidence in Nursing Practice* prepares the student to understand and use the evidence-based practice information included in every chapter.

New content areas include **Communicating with a Cognitively Impaired Patient** (Skill 3-5), **Adverse Event/Incident Reporting** (Procedural Guideline 4-4), **Caring for Patients with Multidrug-Resistant Organisms (MDRO) and *Clostridium difficile*** (Procedural Guideline 7-1), and **Wheelchair Transfer Techniques** (Procedural Guideline 9-1). All other topics have been updated to the most recent standards in nursing practice.

Your students will find that *Clinical Nursing Skills & Techniques* provides a comprehensive resource that will serve them well through their nursing training and right into their clinical practice careers.

CLASSIC FEATURES

- **Over 200 basic, intermediate, and advanced nursing skills and procedures.**
- **Five-step nursing process** format provides a consistent presentation that helps students apply the process while learning each skill.
- **Skills and Procedures list, Objectives,** and **Key Terms** open each chapter.
- **Over 1200 full-color photos and drawings** help students master the material covered.
- **Evidence-Based Practice** in each chapter presents students with the newest scientific evidence for the procedures and protocols presented. Recent research findings are discussed, and their implications for patient care are explored.
- **Rationales** are given for steps within skills so students learn the *why* as well as the *how* of each skill. Rationales include citations from the current literature.
- **Clinical Decision Points** alert students to key steps that affect patient outcomes and help them modify care as needed to meet individual patient needs.

- **Recording and Reporting** sections follow the evaluation discussion and alert students to what information should be documented in each situation.
- **Delegation and Collaboration** defines communication within the patient care team and the nurse's responsibility when delegating to assistive personnel.
- **Unexpected Outcomes** and **Related Interventions** remind students to be alert for potential problems and help them determine appropriate nursing interventions.
- **Special Considerations** sections include additional considerations when performing the skill for specific populations of patients or in specific settings and may include:
  - **Teaching Considerations**
  - **Pediatric Considerations**
  - **Geriatric Considerations**
  - **Home Care Considerations**
- **Glossary** defines all key terms.

NEW TO THIS EDITION:

- **Quick Response codes** (scan with smartphone or tablet with camera to view video clips) on the text pages link video clips to the appropriate skill or procedure, allowing students to view the video immediately after reading the implementation section of the skill.
- **NSO icon** links text content with the new edition of *Nursing Skills Online,* which has been simultaneously revised with the textbook to provide completely coordinated information.
- **Patient-Centered Care** section in each chapter prepares nurses to recognize the importance of having patients partner in performing skills in a compassionate and coordinated way based on respect for patient's preferences, values, and needs (QSEN core competency).
- **Safety Guidelines** section in each chapter covers global recommendations on the safe execution of the particular skill set covered (QSEN core competency).
- **Expanded and improved end-of-chapter exercises** include a case study as well as review questions.
- **Additional review questions on Evolve** include a brand new set of unique questions for every chapter.
- **TEACH for RN** instructor manual helps you capitalize on the all new clinical material in the text, new skills video series, and online course. Additional case studies and discussion questions unique to the TEACH manual expand the in-class material available to you.
- For the first time, **an Image Collection is available** with *Clinical Nursing Skills & Techniques.*

Contents

Using Evidence in Nursing Practice

MEDIA RESOURCES

- **evolve** learning system http://evolve.elsevier.com/Perry/skills

  - Review Questions
  - Audio Glossary

KEY TERMS

Clinical guidelines
Evidence-based practice (EBP)
Hypothesis

Peer reviewed
PICOT question
Variable

OBJECTIVES

Mastery of content in this chapter will enable the nurse to:

- Define the key terms listed.
- Discuss how evidence improves the relevance and accuracy of nursing skills.
- Describe the six steps of evidence-based practice.
- Explain the components of a PICOT question.
- Discuss the process for evaluating evidence in the literature.

- Identify the elements to review when critiquing a scientific article.
- Discuss ways to apply evidence in nursing practice.
- Explain the importance of identifying outcomes in the evaluation of an evidence-based practice change.

Cathy works on a medical oncology unit where patients undergo chemotherapy and radiation for leukemia, lymphoma, and other forms of cancer. Because of their chemotherapy, many patients experience a drop in their platelet count and clotting factors, increasing their risk for bleeding. Cathy recently cared for a 42-year-old woman who fell while trying to get to the bathroom and hit her head against the bed frame, resulting in a serious intracranial bleed. Cathy discusses the situation with two nurse colleagues and asks, "How can we reduce the number of falls and injuries to our patients on the oncology unit?" The nurse specialist for the unit tells Cathy, "I heard about an approach to fall prevention on one of the surgical floors; it involves hourly rounding. Let's ask this question, *"In adult oncology patients, will the use of hourly rounding compared with the current fall prevention protocol affect the incidence of falls during hospitalization?"* Feeling frustrated that their existing fall prevention protocol was not effective in reducing falls, the group agrees that the question is the right one to search in the literature.

This clinical case study highlights how professional nurses address problems in their practice. Evidence-based practice (EBP) is a process of making informed decisions about the way you care for patients. It all begins with asking clinical questions. Clinical questions lead nurses like Cathy and her colleagues to find evidence from the research literature, quality improvement data, risk management trends, and the opinions of nurse experts. Nurses then apply the evidence to make relevant and informed changes in practice such as fall prevention in the case study.

There are elements of all nursing procedures within this textbook that are evidence based. For example, the length of time necessary to wash hands, the technique for determining the position of a feeding tube in the stomach, and the technique for giving an intramuscular injection are based on evidence. Clinical research led to the answers for how these nursing procedures should be performed. The use of such evidence in practice enables clinicians like Cathy to provide the highest quality of care to their patients and families. EBP requires nurses to always think about their practice, raise pertinent clinical questions, search for the evidence that pertains to their questions, apply relevant evidence in practice changes, and evaluate the outcomes.

A CASE FOR EVIDENCE

One of the key messages in the 2010 report of the Institute of Medicine (IOM), *The Future of Nursing: Leading Change, Advancing Health,* is for nurses to be full partners with physicians and other health care professionals in redesigning health care in the United States (IOM, 2010). Nursing is well positioned to lead change and advance health through the use of EBP, a process that makes nurses more autonomous in changing health care practices. The IOM recommends that nurses be accountable for their own contributions to delivering high-quality care and work collaboratively with leaders from other health professions. The EBP process is a perfect vehicle to achieve that aim.

EBP is a guide for making accurate, timely, and appropriate clinical decisions. It is an interdisciplinary process that results in applying the newest knowledge available in health care sciences to the bedside. It is important to translate best evidence into best practices at a patient's bedside. For example, using a sliding board to transfer a patient from bed to stretcher instead of lifting and using the research-based Braden scale to routinely assess a patient's risk for skin breakdown are examples of using evidence at the bedside. Evidence-based practice is a problem-solving approach to the delivery of health care that integrates the best evidence from scientific studies and patient care data along with clinicians' expertise and patient preferences and values (Melnyk et al., 2009). In this textbook you learn that use of evidence in nursing procedures or skills provides scientific guidelines for how to perform skills more effectively and improve patient outcomes.

As a professional nurse you need to stay informed and aware of the most current evidence. Typically new students diligently read their textbooks and assigned scientific articles. A good textbook incorporates current evidence into the practice guidelines and nursing skills at the time it is published. However, because a textbook relies on the scientific literature, a portion of the book can become outdated by the time it is published. Articles from nursing and the health care literature are available on almost any topic involving nursing practice. New research is reported every day. Although the scientific basis of nursing practice has grown, some practices are still not "research based" (based on findings from well-designed research studies) because findings are inconclusive or researchers have not yet studied the practices. For example, in the past nurses changed intravenous (IV) site dressings daily and applied antibiotic ointment to reduce the incidence of infection at a site. However, there was no evidence at the time to support this practice. IV care was based on tradition. Recent research has shown that topical antibiotics offer no benefit and daily dressing changes are not beneficial unless a dressing becomes soiled or compromised. In addition, a current standard of care is to cleanse an adult's IV site with chlorhexidine antiseptic solution, not antibiotic ointment (Infusion Nurses Society [INS], 2011). The challenge is to obtain the very best, most current information at the right time, when you need it for patient care.

The best evidence comes from well-designed, systematically conducted research studies found in scientific journals. Unfortunately much of that evidence does not reach the bedside. Many health care settings do not have a process to help staff adopt new evidence in practice. Nurses in practice settings, unlike educational settings, may not have easy access to databases for scientific literature. Instead they often care for patients on the basis of tradition, preferences, or convenience. Because there are often obstacles to research-based practice in clinical settings, it is important for administrators to provide a supportive environment and adequate facilitation of change. Researchers have found that implementation of EBP is enhanced when organization leaders commit to improving practices and there are links to management structures and processes to support change (VanDeusen et al., 2010).

Research evidence alone is often not enough to justify a change in practice (Melnyk et al., 2010). You must also use sources of evidence that include quality improvement and risk management data, infection control data, retrospective or concurrent chart review, and clinicians' expertise. Nonresearch-based evidence is very valuable to fully inform you of practice issues in your setting. But remember, it is important that you not rely on nonresearch-based evidence alone. Research-based evidence is more likely to be timely, accurate, and relevant. When you face a clinical problem, seek out all sources of evidence to find the best solution in caring for patients.

Even when you use the best evidence available, application and outcomes will differ based on your patients' values, preferences, concerns, and/or expectations. As a nurse you develop critical thinking skills to determine whether evidence is relevant and appropriate to your patients and to a clinical situation. For example, some research suggests that therapeutic massage is effective in promoting sleep and reducing fatigue in patients who undergo coronary artery bypass surgery (Nerbass et al., 2010). However, if you care for a patient from a culture in which touch is a taboo, the use of massage is inappropriate. Using your clinical expertise and considering patients' cultures, values, and preferences ensure that you apply new evidence in practice both ethically and appropriately. EBP requires good nursing judgment; it is not finding research evidence and applying it blindly.

STEPS OF EVIDENCE-BASED PRACTICE

The multistep EBP process requires a spirit of inquiry (i.e., an ongoing curiosity about the best evidence to make clinical decisions) (Melnyk et al., 2009). Using a step-by-step approach ensures that you will obtain the strongest available evidence to apply in patient care. With a spirit of inquiry in place, there are six steps of EBP (Melnyk and Fineout-Overholt, 2010):

1. Ask a clinical question.
2. Search for the most relevant and best evidence that applies to the question.
3. Critically appraise the evidence you gather.
4. Apply or integrate evidence along with your clinical expertise, patient preferences, and values in making a practice decision or change.
5. Evaluate the practice decision or change.
6. Communicate your results.

Ask the Clinical Question

Every day nurses perform interventions (e.g., changing dressings, giving medications, providing comfort measures) that stimulate questions such as, "Why do we use this approach?" or "Is there a better way?" Always think about your practice when caring for patients. Question what does not make sense to you and what you think needs clarification. It is also important to include colleagues from all disciplines to give their perception of the clinical problem or issue. As shown in the previous case study, think about a patient care problem or an area of interest that is time consuming, costly, or not logical. Often The Joint Commission (TJC) standards (e.g., the annual patient safety goals) spark questions for you to pose about your patients. Clinical questions often arise as a result of either a problem- or a knowledge-focus trigger. A problem-focused trigger develops as you care for a patient or notice a trend on a nursing unit. For example, a problem-focused trigger might arise while caring for an unconscious patient: "Which is the best anti-infective solution to use when giving oral care to unconscious patients?" Examples of problem-focused trends include the increase in number of pressure ulcers or incidence of urinary tract infections on a nursing unit. A knowledge-focused trigger arises when you ask a question regarding new information about a topic. For example, "What is the current evidence to reduce bloodstream infection in central venous catheters?" Important knowledge sources often include standards and practice guidelines available from national agencies such as the Agency for Healthcare Research and Quality (AHRQ), the Infusion Nurses Society (INS), and the American Association of Critical Care Nurses (AACN).

There are two types of clinical questions: background and foreground (Stillwell et al., 2010a; Nollan et al., 2010; Straus, 2011). A background question is broad and general. For example, "Which interventions are effective in reducing falls in oncology patients?" The answer to the question provides general knowledge about the problem or topic of interest. A background question has the advantage of allowing you to explore a vast array of options for your area of interest. In contrast, a foreground question is specific and relevant to a practice issue (Stillwell et al., 2010a). It is a question that must be asked to decide which of two interventions is likely the more effective in addressing a practice issue. For example, "In adult oncology patients, will the use of hourly rounding compared with a standard fall prevention protocol affect the incidence of falls?" When you ask a question and search the scientific literature, you do not want to read 100 articles to find the handful that are most helpful. This happens if you ask a background question. If you ask a foreground question, you are able to identify a few select articles that specifically address your practice question.

A foreground question is clearly worded when you use a PICOT format (Melnyk and Fineout-Overholt, 2010). Box 1-1 summarizes the five elements of a PICOT question. The key words of a PICOT question make it easier to search for evidence in the scientific literature. Examples of PICOT questions follow: *In abdominal surgery patients (P), does epidural analgesia (I) compared with patient-controlled analgesia (C) affect pain severity (O) in the first 48 hours after surgery? In oncology patients (P) does the use of a case management model (I) compared with a telephone call-back system (C) improve patient adherence to chemotherapy (O) during the first 3 months (T)?*

A well-designed PICOT question does not have to include all five elements. For example, a comparison intervention is not pertinent when a PICOT question is about meaning such as, "Do family caregivers (P) of hospice patients feel anxiety (O) when providing hands-on care? A time element is also not always required (Stillwell et al., 2010a). However, the elements of Population, an Intervention or issue of interest, and Outcome are essential for a well-designed PICOT question.

A clearly stated PICOT question helps to identify knowledge gaps for a specific clinical problem or situation. When you form well–thought-out questions, the type of evidence you lack for clinical practice becomes clearer when you search the literature. Examples of different knowledge gaps include the following:

- *Diagnosis*: Questions about the selection and interpretation of diagnostic tests. *Example*: Does the use of a disposable oral thermometer compared with an electronic oral thermometer measure body temperature accurately in a patient with an endotracheal tube?
- *Prognosis*: Questions about a patient's likely clinical outcome. *Example*: Is there a difference in the incidence of deep vein thrombosis in surgical patients wearing sequential compression stockings compared to those who wear elastic stockings?
- *Therapy*: Questions about the selection of the most beneficial treatments. *Example*: Which bowel regimen is most effective in relieving constipation caused by the administration of opioid therapy in oncology patients with chronic pain?
- *Prevention*: Questions about screening and prevention methods to reduce the risk of disease. *Example*: Does performance of a prostate-specific antigen (PSA) test in an older adult who is asymptomatic of prostate disease decrease his risk for mortality from prostate cancer?
- *Education*: Questions about best teaching strategies for colleagues, patients, or family members. *Example*: Is the use of visual aids compared with low-literacy teaching booklets more effective to educate low-literacy adults about therapeutic diets?
- *Meaning*: Questions that seek understanding of a phenomenon. *Example*: How do patients with cervical cancer perceive their quality of life?

Search for the Best Evidence

In the case study the nurse specialist conducts a literature search on the basis of the PICOT question. Key words from the question direct the search, including "falls," "cancer," "injury," "rounding," and "adult." The literature search results in four articles pertaining to risk factors for falls and outcomes from hourly rounding.

Once you have a clear and concise PICOT question, you are ready to search for evidence. Evidence exists in quality or performance improvement data, existing clinical practice guidelines, or computerized bibliographical databases. Do not hesitate to ask for help from faculty or expert nurses to find appropriate evidence. When you are assigned to a health care setting, consider using advanced practice nurses, staff educators, risk managers, and infection control nurses as resources.

When searching the scientific literature for evidence, seek the assistance of a medical librarian who knows the relevant databases (Box 1-2). A database is an electronic library of published scientific studies, including peer-reviewed research. A peer-reviewed article is one that has been evaluated by a panel of experts familiar with the topic or subject matter of the article. The librarian translates the elements of your PICOT question into the language or key

---

BOX 1-1 | Developing a PICOT Question

P = Patient population of interest
Identify your patients by age, gender, ethnicity, disease, or health problem.

I = Intervention or issue of interest
Which intervention do you think is worthwhile to use in practice (e.g., a treatment, diagnostic test, prognostic factor)?

C = Comparison intervention or issue of interest
Which standard of care or current intervention do you usually use now in practice?

O = Outcome
Which result do you wish to achieve or observe as a result of an intervention (e.g., change in patient's behavior, physical finding, change in patient's perception)?

T = Time
How long does it take for an intervention to achieve the outcome?

BOX 1-2	Searchable Scientific Literature Databases and Sources
CINAHL	Cumulative Index of Nursing and Allied Health Literature. Includes studies in nursing, allied health, and biomedicine http://www.cinahl.com
MEDLINE	Includes studies in medicine, nursing, dentistry, psychiatry, veterinary medicine, and allied health http://www.ncbi.nim.nih.gov
EMBASE	Biomedical and pharmaceutical studies http://www.embase.com
PsycINFO	Psychology and related health care disciplines http://www.apa.org/psycinfo
Cochrane Database of Systematic Reviews	Full text of regularly updated systematic reviews prepared by the Cochrane Collaboration; includes completed reviews and protocols http://www.cochrane.org/reviews
National Guidelines Clearinghouse	Repository for structured abstracts (summaries) about clinical guidelines and their development; also includes condensed version of guideline for viewing http://www.guideline.gov
PubMed	Health science library at the National Library of Medicine; offers free access to journal articles http://www.nlm.nih.gov

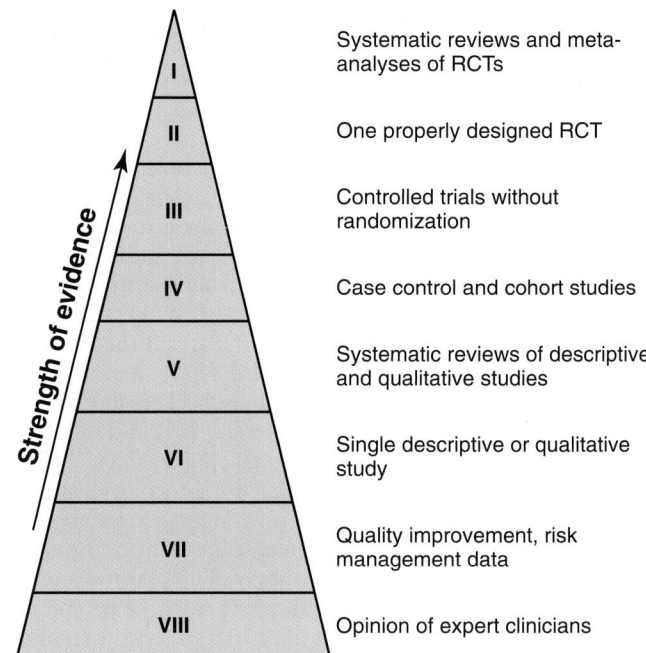

FIG 1-1   The evidence pyramid. *RCT,* Randomized controlled trial.

- I — Systematic reviews and meta-analyses of RCTs
- II — One properly designed RCT
- III — Controlled trials without randomization
- IV — Case control and cohort studies
- V — Systematic reviews of descriptive and qualitative studies
- VI — Single descriptive or qualitative study
- VII — Quality improvement, risk management data
- VIII — Opinion of expert clinicians

Strength of evidence

written, types of studies, or age of patients. This reduces the number of articles further to give you a more manageable number to review for your PICOT question (Stillwell et al., 2010b).

CINAHL, PubMed (which includes MEDLINE), and the Cochrane Database of Systematic Reviews are among the most comprehensive databases and represent the scientific knowledge base of health care (Melnyk and Fineout-Overholt, 2010). Some databases are available through vendors at a cost, some are free of charge, and some offer both options. Nursing students and nurses who work in academic medical centers usually have access to an institutional subscription through a vendor. One of the common vendors is OVID, which offers several different databases. Some databases such as PubMed are available free on the Internet. The Cochrane Database of Systematic Reviews is a valuable source of synthesized evidence (i.e., preappraised evidence). It includes the full text of regularly updated systematic reviews and protocols for reviews that are currently in progress. The National Guidelines Clearinghouse (NGC) is a database supported by the AHRQ. It contains clinical guidelines (i.e., systematically developed statements about a plan of care for a specific set of clinical circumstances involving a specific patient population). The NGC is a valuable source when you want to develop a plan of care for a patient.

The pyramid in Fig. 1-1 represents a hierarchy for rating available scientific evidence. It is important to learn about the types of studies to help you know which ones have the best scientific evidence. The strongest evidence is at the top of the pyramid; the weakest is at the bottom. You can use the rating scale of I to VIII when you later critique each article that you obtain in your search of the literature. Table 1-1 describes types of studies in the evidence hierarchy, beginning with the study at the top of the hierarchy, a systematic review.

If your PICOT question leads you to a systematic review, celebrate! A systematic review is the perfect answer to a PICOT question. Basically a researcher has asked the same PICOT question you have asked and then examined all of the well-designed relevant randomized controlled trials (RCTs) that ask the same question. A systematic review explains if the evidence for which you are searching exists and whether there is good cause to change

words that yield the best evidence search. For example, consider this PICOT question: "Does the use of computerized home instruction compared with a group class improve oncology patients' adherence to oral chemotherapy 3 months following treatment?" The key words include *oncology patient, computerized instruction, adherence,* and *chemotherapy*. A good librarian recommends using the indexing language or controlled vocabulary of the database that you are searching. This means that, by using the words that the database contains, you will likely have a more inclusive search (Stillwell et al., 2010b). In the previous example the word *oncology* might be entered instead as "cancer" to fit the database language. When conducting a search, you enter and manipulate the different key words until you get the combination that gives you the articles about your question that you want to read. When you enter a key word to search a database, be prepared for some confusion in the evidence that you obtain. The vocabulary within published articles is often vague. The word that you select sometimes has one meaning to one author and a very different meaning to another. Each key word generates a set of articles. For example, in the PubMed database *oncology patient* generates 122,000 articles, *adherence* generates 64,878 articles, and *chemotherapy* generates over 2 million articles. That's a lot of reading. In addition, you want to read only articles that address all three of the topics. If you combine the key terms of a search using the Boolean connector *and,* the combination of "oncology patient *and* chemotherapy *and* adherence" generates 274 articles. A librarian can also show you how to limit a search by categories such as the time frame during which the article was

TABLE 1-1	Types of Studies in the Evidence Hierarchy	
Study Type	**Description**	**Example**
Systematic review or meta-analysis	An author or panel of experts reviews the evidence from randomized controlled trials about a specific clinical question and summarizes the state of the science. In a meta-analysis, there is the addition of a statistical analysis that combines data from all studies.	35 studies were examined to evaluate the outcomes of case-managed, integrated home and community care services for older persons, including those with dementia. Evidence from RCTs showed that case management improves function and appropriate use of medications, increases use of community services, and reduces nursing home admission (Low,Yap, and Brodaty, 2011).
Randomized controlled trial (RCT)	A researcher tests an intervention against the usual standard of care. Participants are randomly assigned to either a control group (receives standard care) or a treatment group (receives the experimental intervention), with both measured on the same outcomes to see if there is a difference.	Researchers conducted an RCT among 125 critically ill patients receiving tube feedings. The study determined the effect of returning (treatment) or discarding gastric residual volume (GRV) on gastric emptying delays and feeding, electrolyte, and comfort outcomes. Findings showed a lower incidence and severity of delayed gastric emptying when GRV was returned. No significant differences were found for feeding delays, electrolyte imbalance, or changes in vital signs. The study findings support that the return of gastric content aspirated improved GRV management without increasing the risk for potential complications (Juvé-Udina et al., 2009).
Case control study	Researchers study one group of subjects with a certain condition (e.g., obesity) at the same time as another group of subjects who do not have the condition to determine if there is an association between the condition and predictor variables (e.g., exercise pattern, family history, history of depression).	In a historical case control, researchers studied a group of 19,951 children who had been admitted to an emergency department for asthma attacks. The researchers compared the effectiveness of the use of inhaled beta-agonists given via a metered-dose inhaler (MDI) with spacers versus the use of nebulizers. This was part of an evidence-based asthma pathway. The use of an MDI with spacer was effective in the management of acute asthma (Goh et al., 2010).
Descriptive study	Study describes the concepts under study. It sometimes examines the prevalence, magnitude, and/or characteristics of a concept.	A convenience sample of 100 patients and 100 unrelated family caregivers were surveyed to examine their perceptions of the caregiving skills they perform, the difficulty they experience in performing certain skills, and their associated learning needs (Potter et al., 2010).
Qualitative study	Study examines individuals' experiences with health problems or life experiences and the contexts in which the experiences occur.	Researchers asked 392 nurses to discuss a care episode from their practice. Cases describing patients with cancer involved nurses' use of powerful emotive language. The influence of patients' cancer experience affects nurses personally and professionally (Kendall, 2007).
Quality improvement data, risk management information	Data collected within a health care agency offer important trending information about clinical conditions and problems. Staff in the agency review the data periodically to identify problem areas and seek solutions.	Article reviews the results of a 2-year quality improvement campaign involving physicians and nurses at a teaching hospital to improve the identification and accurate documentation of pressure ulcers (Dahlstrom et al., 2011).
Clinical experts	Accessing clinical experts on a nursing unit is an excellent way to learn about current evidence. Clinical experts often write clinical articles on topics that require application of evidence in the literature.	Clinical article describes an evidence-based practice project. The practice change involved interventions, including a campaign to raise geriatric awareness, the creation of "falls tool boxes," education of staff and family, and implementation of a structured hourly patient rounds schedule (Murphy et al., 2008).

practice. In the Cochrane Library all entries include information on systematic reviews.

Individual RCTs have been the gold standard for research (Padian et al., 2010; Titler et al., 2001). An RCT is a formal experiment for testing therapies and establishing cause and effect. Historically few RCTs have been conducted in nursing, but this is changing. The nature of nursing causes researchers to ask questions that are not always answered best by an RCT. Nurses care for patients' responses to disease or health problems. For example, they assist patients with problems such as knowledge deficit, symptom management, and coping with psychological distress and with the problems in these areas that often occur simultaneously. An RCT cannot easily be designed to learn how patients handle such complex health problems.

More often you find articles in the nursing literature that involve controlled trials without randomization (i.e., descriptive studies). Even though these types of studies represent a lower level of evidence, if a study results in relevant findings, it helps you decide if your PICOT question can be answered.

The use of clinical experts is at the bottom of the evidence pyramid, but do not consider clinical experts a poor source of evidence. Expert clinicians frequently use evidence as they build their own practice, and they are rich sources of information for clinical problems.

Critique the Evidence

In the case study the nurses on the oncology unit conduct their unit-based practice committee (UPC) meeting. During the meeting Cathy and her colleagues decide that it is important to include key members of their interdisciplinary team (pharmacy and physical therapy). The UPC then reviews the articles carefully, using a rapid-appraisal checklist. After the group evaluates the articles for the strength of evidence and synthesizes the findings, they decide that there is evidence for implementing hourly rounding with focused patient assessment to prevent falls. The staff notes that one of the articles recommends hourly rounding during daytime hours and rounding every 2 hours during evening and night hours. Another article summarizes fall risks for patients in an acute care hospital and highlights factors to include in a nursing assessment such as medications (e.g., antihistamines, sedatives, analgesics, and antiemetics).

Once you have found research articles that address your PICOT question, the next step is to review the articles critically to determine if there is evidence that answers your question. It is important to use an approach that does not bog you down by reviewing every single element of each article. Melnyk et al. (2010) recommend the use of a rapid critical appraisal (RCA) that answers three important questions:

- What are the results of the study, and are they important?
- Are they valid?
- Will the results help you care for your patients?

Many organizations use an RCA checklist (Fig. 1-2) for recording article reviews. You begin an article review by determining if the research study was valid or conducted in a well-designed way. This

---

Example of a Rapid Critical Appraisal Form

- Why was the study done? (Is there a clear explanation of the study purpose?)

- Are the study findings valid?
    How were study participants chosen? How many were chosen?
    Are the study instruments valid and reliable?
    Does the research approach fit the purpose of the study?
    How were accuracy and completeness of data ensured?
    Do the study findings fit the data that were generated?

- What are the results of the study, and are they important?
    Yes
    No
    Unknown

- Is the finding from the study clearly identified?

- Are the results logical, consistent, and easy to follow?

- Are the results plausible and believable?

- How do the results fit with previous research in the area?

- Will the results help me in caring for my patients?

- Do the results apply to my patients?

- How would I use the findings in my practice?

- How would patient and family values be considered in applying these results?

- Do we have the resources to apply this in our practice setting?

FIG 1-2   Example of a rapid critical appraisal form. (*Adapted from Melnyk B, Fineout-Overholt E: Evidence-based practice in nursing and health care: a guide to best practice, Philadelphia, 2010, Lippincott Williams & Wilkin; Fineout-Overholt E et al: Evidence-based practice step by step: critical appraisal of the evidence, Part 1, AJN 110(7):47, 2010.*)

requires knowing the type of study using the evidence pyramid. For example, if you have an RCT to review, were subjects randomized? Does the sample of subjects appear to be large enough to test the intervention effectively? Were all subjects measured for the same outcomes? In contrast, if you read a qualitative study, did the researcher study a sufficient representation of subjects, and did the approach allow for a thorough and objective review of findings? As you read each article, you ask the second question: What are the results and were they important? If you have an RCT, you want to know if an intervention worked or not. If you have a descriptive study, is the information relevant to your PICOT question?

You might also choose to review a clinical article that explains a clinical practice topic relevant to your PICOT question. A clinical article is not rated for its level of evidence; but it can offer useful information, especially if you decide to implement a change related to the practice topic. To learn how to read research and clinical articles, know each of the common elements. This will help you decide if an article is complete and well explained. Articles should include the following elements:

- *Abstract*: A brief summary of the article that tells you if the article is research or clinically based. An abstract summarizes the purpose of the study or clinical topic, the major themes or findings, and the implications for nursing practice.
- *Introduction*: Contains information about the purpose of the article and the importance of the topic for the audience who reads it. The introduction usually contains brief supporting evidence as to why the topic is important from the author's point of view.

After reading the abstract and introduction, you will decide if you want to continue to read the entire article. You will know if the topic of the article is similar to your PICOT question or related closely enough to provide you useful information. Remember that the research question does not need to be the same as yours but close enough to offer useful information. If this is the case, continue to read the next elements of the article:

- *Literature review or background*: A good author offers a detailed background of the level of scientific or clinical information that exists about the topic of the article. The review offers an explanation about what led the author to conduct a study or report on a clinical topic. Perhaps the article itself does not address your PICOT question the way you desire but possibly leads you to other more useful articles. The literature review gives you a good idea of how past research led to the researcher's question.
- *Article narrative*: The "middle section" or narrative of an article differs according to the type of evidence-based article, either clinical or research (Melnyk and Fineout-Overholt, 2010). A clinical article describes a clinical topic, which often includes a description of a patient population, the nature of a certain disease or health problem, how it affects patients, and the appropriate nursing therapies. Clinical articles often describe how to use a therapy or new technology. A research article describes the conduct of a research study, including its purpose; how the study was designed; and the results. A narrative of a research article contains several standard subsections:
  - *Purpose statement*: Explains the focus or intent of a study. It identifies which concepts will be researched.
  - *Methods or design*: Explains how a research study is organized and conducted to answer the research question(s). This is where you learn the type of study (i.e., RCT, case control, or qualitative). You also learn how many subjects or persons are in a study. In health care studies subjects

---

BOX 1-3 | Common Statistical Terms

Sample Size: Number (n) of individuals in a study.

Significance: A measure that gives the likelihood that a finding or a result is caused by the intervention being tested and not by chance. Most researchers set the level of significance at a p value of 0.05 or 0.01. For example, if the effects of an intervention are significant at $p < 0.05$, it means that the likelihood of the effect occurring by chance is less than 5%; thus it is more likely that the intervention made a true difference.

Confidence interval (CI): The range (e.g., range of a mean score) in which clinicians can expect to get results if they present an intervention as it was in a study (Fineout-Overholt et al., 2010). The CI tells you the precision of a study. A 95% CI means that clinicians can be 95% confident that their findings will be within the range given in the study.

Effect size: When the effect of an intervention is statistically significant, it does not necessarily mean that it is big, important, or helpful in decision making. It simply means that you can be confident that there is a difference. An effect size greater than 0.05 is considered a large effect.

---

sometimes include patients, family members, or health care staff. The language in the methods section is sometimes confusing if it explains details about how the researcher designs the study to minimize bias so as to obtain the most accurate results possible. Use your faculty member as a resource to help interpret this section.

- *Results or conclusions*: Clinical and research articles have a summary section. In a clinical article the author explains the clinical implications for the topic. In a research article the author explains the results and whether a research question is answered. For example, in a qualitative study there is a thorough summary of the descriptive themes and ideas that arise from the researcher's analysis of data. A quantitative study includes a full description of the study subjects and a statistical analysis of findings. It is important to learn some of the common statistical terms (Box 1-3). A good author discusses limitations to a study in the results section. The information on limitations helps you decide if you want to use the evidence with your patients.
- *Clinical implications*: A research article includes a section that explains if the findings from the study have clinical implications. The researcher explains how to apply findings in a practice setting for the type of subjects studied.

As you critique each article, complete your RCA checklist. You may choose to rate each article by its level and strength of evidence, using the scale of I to VIII from the evidence pyramid (see Fig. 1-1). It also helps to review multiple articles with a group of colleagues involved in the EBP process. Each person can review a single article; then you can come together as a group to review your total findings. At that time you discuss the third important question: Will the results help you care for your patients?

Use critical thinking to consider the scientific rigor of the evidence and how well it answers your area of interest. Scientific rigor is the extent to which the findings of a study are valid, reliable, and relevant to a patient population of interest. Consider the evidence in light of your patients' concerns and preferences. Your review of articles offers a snapshot conclusion based on combined evidence about one focused topical area. As a clinician judge whether to use the evidence for a particular patient or group of patients who usually have complex medical histories and patterns of responses (Melnyk and Fineout-Overholt, 2010). Ethically always consider evidence that will benefit patients and do no harm. Decide if the evidence is relevant, is easily applicable in your setting of practice, and has the potential for improving patient outcomes.

Apply the Evidence

Based on their experience and a review of their unit fall index reports, the staff on the oncology unit know that patients on the unit fall during all hours of the day and night. The unit practice committee recommends starting a new hourly rounds program using a focused fall screening tool and nursing assessments for key fall risk factors. Registered nurses (RNs) will round on patients on all even hours and conduct focused assessments of fall risk factors such as weakness, pain, or the need to go to the bathroom. If a patient is found to be at high fall risk, the physical therapists will be asked to consult and assess patients' lower-extremity strength and overall balance. Pharmacy will place alerts on medication administration records so nurses can monitor patients receiving antihistamines before blood transfusions. Nursing assistive personnel (NAP) will round on odd hours and do follow-up observations to be sure that patients have their toileting needs met, are comfortable, and have no further needs. Each hour the nursing staff will inform patients that someone from the nursing team will return in an hour for another check. The unit practice committee plans to have a staff orientation and set a date for the start of the hourly rounding protocol.

After reviewing all of the evidence, you decide if it answers your PICOT question. If so, your next step is to implement a plan to apply evidence into practice. One important step for an individual or an interdisciplinary EBP committee to address is the resources needed for a practice change project. Are added costs or new equipment involved with a practice change? Do you have adequate staff to make the practice change work as planned? Do management and medical staff support you in the change? If the barriers to practice change are excessive, adopting a practice change can be difficult, if not impossible.

In the case study the oncology UPC involves other disciplines and their managers in planning their project. The committee forms a plan for implementing their hourly rounding protocol. There are key steps for applying evidence into practice:

1. Plan how to collect baseline data on the outcomes that will evaluate the effect of your practice change (e.g., the oncology nurses will be able to refer to fall index data collected during the 6 months before implementation of the protocol). The nurses will continue to collect the fall index and the fall-related injury rate once the new protocol begins.
   a. Know which outcomes to measure and how to collect them (e.g., to measure pain acuity use a self-report pain scale; to measure ambulation determine the distance a patient walks each time).
   b. Be sure that the outcomes are measurable. Use scales (e.g., Pain and Braden scales), physiologic measures (e.g., temperature, blood pressure, pulse oximetry), or survey tools.
   c. Choose outcomes that are not costly to collect. Use existing equipment if you can.
   d. Who will collect the data? It is usually best to limit the number of staff who collect data to ensure better accuracy

and consistency in measurement. Be sure that each person collects data the same way and accurately.
   e. Establish a way to record all data.
2. Test your practice change in a pilot project. This means that you implement the change in practice for a set period of time (e.g., 3 to 6 months). Consider how long it will take to show that your practice change made a difference (Poe and White, 2010). Apply evidence in a manner that integrates well with existing practice for all affected disciplines. Consider how you can introduce your practice change into existing policies, standards of care, and assessment or clinical protocols.
3. Involve all staff in the patient care area or unit where you work. An interdisciplinary approach brings together ideas from different perspectives. This is very important for creating a climate of EBP.
4. Be sure to educate all nurses or other staff who will be involved in the project before you begin implementation. Also keep them informed of the progress of the change.

The goal of any EBP change is to ensure the highest quality of care by using evidence that promotes the best outcomes (Poe and White, 2010). Proper planning is essential before implementing your practice change. Once you implement your intervention, monitor the project closely and consider how staff and patients are responding.

Evaluate the Practice Decision or Change

On the oncology unit the UPC made sure that outcome measures were in place when the protocol began. A fall index rate was collected monthly. The staff decided to add a monthly report of injuries from falls to the outcome data. Three months after implementing the protocol the medical oncology unit was cautiously optimistic. The average fall index for the unit dropped from 5.1 to 3.7, and the injury rate also dropped. The nurses observed a decline in patients' use of call lights, which was attributed to their knowing that nurses and assistive personnel would visit frequently. The UPC members surveyed nursing and physical therapy staff about the change and found that the majority were enthused and agreed that hourly rounding needed to be a routine part of their unit practice. The nursing staff is able to see that use of the protocol improves patient outcomes and gives them more time to coordinate care because of fewer distractions from patient calls.

After implementing a practice change, your next step is to evaluate the effect. You do this by analyzing the outcome data that you collect during the pilot project. Outcome evaluation tells you if your practice change improved conditions, created no change, or worsened conditions. For examples, after using a new, transparent IV dressing, the staff analyzed their audits, which included the incidence of dislodged IVs and the incidence and rating of phlebitis. Their findings showed reduction in the number of catheters that became dislodged and in onset and severity of phlebitis. After using a new approach to educating clinic patients about medications and administration schedules, follow-up phone calls to patients found an improved understanding of doses and times to administer. However, patients were not able to explain which side effects to expect. Once an evaluation is complete, you must decide to continue the EBP, make a revision, or discontinue the practice change. Analysis of an EBP change may require assistance from statisticians if you or your team members collect extensive data. Be sure to use reliable resources and be thorough in examining all data.

Communicating a Practice Change

Six months after starting the new fall prevention protocol, the fall index of the oncology unit continues to remain low. An added outcome is an improvement in patient satisfaction scores. Cathy submits the protocol for an abstract in the hospital publication, *Nursing Research Day*. Her abstract, "Using Evidence To Prevent Falls," is well accepted by her peers and becomes a standard for other nursing units in the hospital.

After applying evidence, it is important to communicate the change in practice and the results to nursing and other health care colleagues. This is true whether the results are successful or unsuccessful. There are many ways to communicate the outcomes of EBP: talking with a colleague, sharing results in staff meetings, presenting in workshops or seminars, submitting an abstract for a poster presentation, and publishing an article. As a professional you are responsible for communicating important information about nursing practice. Sharing evidence and the effects of any practice change motivates others within a health care setting and makes them excited about potential practice improvements on their work units. When you successfully adopt an EBP way of thinking, it becomes very natural to talk about available evidence and continue seeking solutions for problems in patient care.

IMPACT OF EVIDENCE-BASED PRACTICE ON NURSING

This chapter provides a brief introduction to EBP. Of all of the initiatives introduced in health care, EBP may be the most important. With the rapid, ongoing expansion of research knowledge in health care, it is essential to remain accountable by applying evidence in patient care. When evidence exists about ways to improve patient outcomes, it becomes important for that evidence to reach the bedside. Your patients expect nursing professionals to be informed and to use the safest and most appropriate interventions. Use of evidence enhances nursing, improving patients' perceptions of excellent nursing care.

? Critical Thinking Exercises

Maria Gonzalez is a 45-year-old Hispanic woman who is admitted to the hospital with inflammatory bowel disease, which she has had for 2 years. The disease is an inflammation of the intestines. As a result, Maria has a recurrence of bloody diarrhea, abdominal cramping, and a fever. During her hospital stay Maria receives IV fluids, corticosteroids, and antiinfective drugs. Jeanne is the nurse assigned to coordinate Maria's discharge home. Jeanne is concerned about Maria's diet at home and wonders how it might affect her disease, particularly the frequency of diarrhea. She learns that Maria eats three large meals a day with a diet high in carbohydrates. In consultation with her instructor, Jeanne asks if a low-carbohydrate diet might be best for Maria. The instructor suggests that Jeanne conduct a literature search to see what the most current evidence suggests.

1 Given this clinical case study, write the PICOT question that is the basis of Jeanne's inquiry.
2 The librarian helps Jeanne conduct a literature search. Among the articles located in the search is a systematic review. Explain why a systematic review is the best source of evidence.
3 One of the articles found by the librarian describes a study in which a researcher studied 45 patients with inflammatory bowel disease and 52 patients with normal intestinal function to determine if there is an association between frequency of diarrhea and ingestion of high-carbohydrate intake. Which type of study did this researcher conduct?

✓ REVIEW QUESTIONS

1 Place the steps of evidence-based practice in the correct order:
1 _____ Search the literature for evidence.
2 _____ Evaluate outcomes of the practice change.
3 _____ Communicate the findings.
4 _____ Apply evidence in making a practice change.
5 _____ Ask a PICOT question.
6 _____ Critique the available evidence.

2 A nurse is talking with colleagues and shares what she learned at a recent conference on wound care. She suggests that the group discuss which is the best antiinfective solution to use to clean infected incisions? Which type of trigger for a clinical question is this?
1 Problem-focused
2 Knowledge-focused
3 Peer-focused
4 PICOT-focused

3 Which question contains the primary components of a PICOT question?
1 Are oral steroids effective for female adults with adult-onset asthma?
2 Which steroid preparations are best for male teenagers with activity-induced asthma who play sports?
3 Does the use of inhalers improve bronchial air flow?
4 Does the use of medication via an inhaler versus a nebulizer affect oxygen saturation in asthmatic children?

4 A group of nurses on an obstetric unit are discussing the results of their patient satisfaction scores. They've noticed the scores dropping over the last 3 months. Their manager has expressed concern as to why the female patients do not think that nurses are responsive to their needs. The nurses decide to address the issue in their EBP committee where they will form a PICOT question. This scenario is an example of which type of trigger for an EBP question?
1 Administrative-focused
2 Knowledge-focused
3 Problem-focused
4 Time-focused

5 The nurses on the obstetric unit have identified a PICOT question to address the patient satisfaction problem, "Does hourly rounding improve female obstetric patients' perceptions of satisfaction with nursing care?" Place each element of the PICOT question in the correct category.
1 P _____
2 I _____
3 C _____
4 O _____
5 T _____

6   A nurse has developed a clinical question, "Do oncology patients feel hopelessness when experiencing side effects of chemotherapy?" Which type of research article should the nurse be sure to include in her search for evidence on this topic?

   1   Case study

   2   Systematic review

   3   Quality improvement project

   4   Qualitative study

7   A staff nurse is talking to a clinical nurse specialist on a surgical unit. The nurse specialist is helping the nurse identify the clinical question that interests her most. The nurse explains that she is interested in using guided imagery to help patients gain better pain relief. She believes that it would be most effective beginning 24 hours after surgery through discharge because pain would be less acute during that time frame. The nurse specialist asks the nurse which outcome she would want to achieve. What would be the nurse's best answer?

   1   Ability of patients to follow coaching while performing guided imagery

   2   Patients' reported level of pain severity

   3   The frequency patients ask for pain medication after surgery

   4   The time it takes to perform the guided imagery exercise

8   Which of the following is a background question?

   1   What is the most effective method for teaching patients with diabetes how to self-administer insulin?

   2   Does the use of chewing gum compared with NPO reduce postoperative ileus in a patient undergoing colon resection?

   3   Does a low-fat diet reduce incidence of postoperative nausea in patients undergoing colon resection?

   4   Does the use of demonstration versus viewing a DVD program affect the ability of patients with diabetes to self-administer insulin?

9   A UPC on a medicine unit is planning to pilot an EBP change. Which of the following steps would enhance involvement of all staff on the unit in the practice change? (Select all that apply.)

   1   Involve only nurses familiar with the practice issue.

   2   Educate all nurses or other staff who will be involved in the project before implementation.

   3   Keep all staff on the unit informed of the progress of the change.

   4   Include all staff involved in collecting outcome information.

10   A UPC is planning to adopt a new type of pulse oximeter to improve accuracy of measurement and reduce patient discomfort while wearing the device. Which resources should the committee consider before beginning a pilot evaluation of the oximeter? (Select all that apply.)

   1   The accuracy of the device

   2   Cost of the device

   3   Support from doctors for the change

   4   The patients' satisfaction with the device

REFERENCES

Dahlstrom M, et al: Improving identification and documentation of pressure at an urban academic hospital, *JT Comm J Qual Patient Saf* 37(3):123, 2011.

Fineout-Overholt E, et al: Evidence-based practice, step by step: critical appraisal of the evidence. Part II, *AJN* 110(9):41, 2010.

Goh AE, et al: Efficacy of metered-dose inhalers for children with acute asthma exacerbations, *Pediatric Pulmonol* 46(5):421, 2010.

Infusion Nurses Society: Infusion nursing standards of practice, *J Intraven Nurs* Jan/Feb:34(1S), 2011.

Institute of Medicine: *The future of nursing: leading change, advancing health*, Robert Wood Johnson Foundation Initiative on the Future of Nursing at the Institute of Medicine, October 5, 2010, available at http://www.iom.edu/Reports/2010/The-Future-of-Nursing-Leading-Change-Advancing-Health.aspx, accessed August 28, 2011.

Juvé-Udina ME, et al: To return or to discard? Randomised trial on gastric residual volume management, *Intensive Crit Care Nurs* 25(5):258, 2009. Epub July 16, 2009.

Kendall S: Witnessing tragedy: nurses' perceptions of caring for patients with cancer, *Int J Nurs Pract* 13(2):111, 2007.

Low LF, Yap MH, Brodaty H: A systematic review of different models of home and community care services for older persons, *BMC Health Serv Res* 11(1):93, 2011.

Melnyk BM, Fineout-Overholt E: *Evidence-based practice in nursing and healthcare: a guide to best practice*, ed 2, Philadelphia, 2010, Lippincott Williams & Wilkins.

Melnyk BM, et al: Igniting a spirit of inquiry: an essential foundation for evidence-based practice, *AJN* 109(11):49, 2009.

Melnyk BM, et al: The seven steps of evidence-based practice, *AJN* 110(1):51, 2010.

Murphy TH, et al: Falls prevention for elders in acute care: an evidence-based nursing practice initiative, *Crit Care Nurs Q* 31(1):33, 2008.

Nerbass FB, et al: Effects of massage therapy on sleep quality after coronary artery bypass graft surgery, *Clinics (Sao Paulo)* 65(11):1105, 2010.

Nollan R, et al: Asking compelling clinical questions. In Melnyk BM, Fineout-Overholt E, editors: *Evidence-based practice in nursing and health-care: a guide to best practice*, ed 2, Philadelphia, 2010, Lippincott Williams & Wilkins, p 25.

Padian N, et al: Weighing the gold standard: challenges in HIV prevention research, *AIDS* 24(5):621, 2010.

Poe SS, White KM: *Johns Hopkins nursing evidence-based practice: implementation and translation*, Indianapolis, 2010, Sigma Theta Tau International, p 164.

Potter P, et al: An analysis of educational and learning needs of cancer patients and unrelated family caregivers, *J Cancer Educ* 25(4):5382, 2010.

Stillwell SB, et al: Asking the clinical question: a key step in evidence-based practice, *AJN* 110(3):58, 2010a.

Stillwell SB, et al: Searching for the evidence, *AJN* 110(5):41, 2010b.

Straus SE: *Evidence-based medicine: how to practice and teach EBM*, ed 4, Edinburgh, 2011, Elsevier/Churchill Livingstone.

Titler MG, et al: The Iowa Model of Evidence-Based Practice to Promote Quality Care, *Crit Care Nurs Clin North Am* 13(4):497, 2001.

VanDeusen L, et al: Strengthening organizations to implement evidence-based clinical practices, *Health Care Manage Rev* 35(3):235, 2010.

Admitting, Transfer, and Discharge

MEDIA RESOURCES

- ℮volve http://evolve.elsevier.com/Perry/skills
  learning system

  - Review Questions
  - Audio Glossary

KEY TERMS

Advance directives
Condition of participation
Continuum of care
Discharge planning

Health Insurance Portability
 and Accountability Act
 (HIPAA)

Patient's rights
Patient Self-Determination
 Act

The Joint Commission
 (TJC)
Transitional care

OBJECTIVES

Mastery of content in this chapter will enable the nurse to:
- Describe a nurse's role in maintaining continuity of care through a patient's admission, transfer, and discharge from an acute care facility.
- Explain the purpose and importance of advance directives.

- Identify the ongoing needs of patients in the discharge planning process.
- Explain the role of a patient's family in the admission, transfer, or discharge process.

Patients entering the health care system have unique and individual health needs. It is important for patient care to be integrated across a variety of settings, services, health care practitioners, and care levels to maintain a continuum of care. The Joint Commission (TJC) (2012a) defines the continuum of care as matching an individual's ongoing needs with the appropriate level and type of medical, psychological, health, or social care or services within an organization or across multiple organizations. This continuum flows from preadmission to admission, throughout the acute care hospitalization as the discharge plan is developed, through care transition, and after hospitalization on discharge home or to another health care setting. Essential in promoting continuity of patient care is the need for transitional care. Transitional care consists of nursing actions implemented to ensure coordination and continuity of care for patients who are transferring between different care settings or care levels (McLeod and others, 2011).

A nurse plays a key role in coordinating resources for a patient's care from admission to discharge or from one level of care to the next. He or she identifies patients' ongoing health care needs and anticipates physical, psychological, and social deficits that have implications for resuming normal activities. In addition, a nurse involves family and significant others in a plan of care, provides health education, and assists in making health care resources available to patients. To separate the processes of admission and discharge is a critical error; the two are simultaneous and continuous. Discharge planning begins at the time of admission. Patients and families need to be involved in the planning and decision making. They also need to understand the implications of any health problems and the responsibilities for continued care either in the home or next level of care setting.

EVIDENCE-BASED PRACTICE

Evidence shows that effective communication is an essential component of the admission, transfer, and discharge of patients. Evidence also indicates that poor communication can lead to misunderstandings, clinical errors, and poor outcomes (Pope et al., 2008). Research shows that the development of admission, discharge, and transfer teams within both adult and pediatric facilities improves the emergency department (ED) admission process, patient care productivity, and nurse-patient satisfaction (Giangiulio et al., 2008). The keys to good communication include:
- Knowing when, how, and what to communicate regarding patient issues (Krautscheid, 2008).
- Patient comprehension of accurate, timely, complete, and unambiguous information from providers (TJC, 2012a).

- Concise and specific documentation of information.
- Use of a combination of verbal and written information to provide patient teaching.
- Use of computer-generated summaries of pertinent discharge information to improve patient care after discharge. Provide patients with copies of the pertinent information at time of discharge.
- Use of medication reconciliation to avoid medication errors such as omissions, duplications, dosing errors, or drug interactions (TJC, 2012a).
- Use of electronically reconciled medication lists to provide patients with a better understanding of medication administration instructions and potential adverse effects of the discharge medication.
- High-quality discharge teaching that improves a patient's readiness for discharge.
- Use of a discharge-planning checklist to help patients and family members consider practical aspects of being discharged home.

PATIENT-CENTERED CARE

Communication and culture function together, preserving tradition and influencing verbal and nonverbal expressions (Giger, 2013). Research demonstrates that patients may experience a decrease in safety, health outcomes, and quality of care based on their race, ethnicity, language, disability, and sexual orientation (TJC, 2011). When admitting, transferring, or discharging patients, it is important to understand their cultural beliefs and practices. Be aware of the cultural variables that will affect your patient and family assessment, approach to nursing care, and teaching during admission or discharge. Common cultural variations include perception of time or acceptance of bodily contact. For example, some cultures consider touch taboo, whereas others are highly tactile.

To promote effective communication and plan care, it is beneficial to learn about a patient's cultural background. Modify your communication approaches to meet a patient's cultural needs and ensure that he or she understands your communication. For example, schedule the admission, transfer, or discharge of Orthodox Jewish patients so they can begin observance of the Sabbath (sundown on Friday to sundown on Saturday) undisturbed.

Safety Guidelines

1. Identify whether a patient has a sensory or communication need.
2. Identify if a patient uses any assistive devices.
3. Screen all patients on admission to a health care setting for possible discharge needs to ensure that appropriate teaching is completed.
4. Include the patient, family, and relevant health care professionals early in planning to promote successful transition through the health care system.
5. Consider a patient's educational background, health literacy level, and ability to understand instructions.
6. Coordinate the health care providers who contribute to a patient's care needs to develop a plan of care for discharge to ensure a safe transition to home or an alternate care facility.
7. Assist other health care personnel in assessing appropriate resources needed as patient's transition through the health care system.

SKILL 2-1 Admitting Patients

A patient may enter the health care system in a variety of ways (e.g., hospital, clinic, or physician's or health care provider's office). The admission process is typically the first point of contact a patient has with a health care agency. There are common procedures for admitting patients to these settings (Box 2-1). Most patients enter the health care system through a scheduled admission process. However, some patients require emergency admission. For example, a patient admitted through the ED is often not able to undergo the same registration process that takes place in a hospital admission office. Family members usually provide pertinent information for the hospital records while the staff are caring for the patient. In contrast, an older-adult patient with self-care limitations undergoes extensive screening before being accepted as a nursing home resident.

Admission officers, secretaries, and technicians are the personnel involved in the preliminary admission process such as interviewing patients and reviewing information about insurance, demographic data, and agency procedures. Technicians usually collect routine specimens and perform screening procedures such as electrocardiograms (ECGs). A nurse performs the admission assessment.

Role of the Admission Personnel

The admission personnel initiate and maintain a courteous and professional relationship with patients while providing their safety, legal rights, and privacy. A private interview area gives patients and families a place to reveal important identifying information, including a patient's full legal name, age, birth date, address, next of kin, health care provider, religious preference, occupation, and type of insurance. If a patient does not speak English or has a severe hearing impairment, an interpreter assists during the admission procedure.

At this time the admission personnel secures an identification (ID) band legibly stating the patient's full legal name, hospital or agency number, health care provider, and birth date to the patient's wrist. Health care providers use the ID band to identify a patient when performing treatments or procedures. If a patient is unconscious, you cannot perform identification until family members arrive. Hospital staff provide a patient who has been a victim of

BOX 2-1	Common Procedures for Admission to the Health Care System

- Placement of patient in appropriate receiving area
- Explanation of patient's rights and elements of advance directives
- Orientation to relevant health care agency's policies and procedures
- Assessment of patient's health care problems and needs
- Preliminary testing and screening (specific for each agency and patient's condition)
- Development of an individualized plan of care
- Determination of patient's payment source for health care

crime with an anonymous name under the agency's "blackout" or "do not publish" procedure.

A patient's legal rights are met by instructing the patient or legal guardian to read the general consent form for treatment. During admission all patients receive information regarding their rights related to health care services. This information should be available in multiple languages and alternate formats (e.g., audio, visual, or written). In 1999 the Centers for Medicare and Medicaid Services (CMS) introduced a Patients' Rights Condition of Participation that all hospitals are required to meet to receive Medicare and Medicaid reimbursement. The condition requires hospitals to notify each patient of his or her rights (Box 2-2). Other regulatory agencies such as TJC also require agencies to provide for specific patient rights (Box 2-3). Each agency has policies and procedures describing a patient's rights and the role of the nurse in ensuring those rights.

The Patient Self-Determination Act, effective December 1, 1991, requires all Medicare- and Medicaid-recipient hospitals to provide patients with information about their right to accept or reject medical treatment. At the time of registration patients receive information about advance directives and are referred to appropriate resources if they want to discuss advance directives or receive help in completing an advance directive document (Box 2-4).

Patients must also receive information about the Health Insurance Portability and Accountability Act (HIPAA). HIPAA is a federal law finalized in 2003, designed to protect the privacy of patient health information and referred to as *protected health information (PHI)* (U.S. Department of Health and Human Services [USDHHS], 2003). Three key concepts of HIPAA are: (1) agencies are required to inform patients of the privacy rights they have and how the agency will handle their PHI; (2) the agency and the health care providers are to use or disclose a patient's PHI only for the purposes of treatment, payment, or health care operations; and (3) health care providers disclose only the minimum amount of PHI necessary, on a need-to-know basis, to accomplish the

---

BOX 2-2 | Patients' Rights Provided for by CMS

Code of Federal Regulations Title 42, Chapter IV, Part 482, Sec. 482.13 Condition of Participation: Patients' Rights

Standard 1: Notice of Rights
- A hospital must protect and promote each patient's rights.
- A hospital must inform each patient whenever possible or, when appropriate, the patient's representative of the patient's rights in advance of furnishing or discontinuing patient care.
- The hospital must have a process for prompt resolution of patient grievances and must inform each patient whom to contact to file a grievance.

Standard 2: Exercise of Rights
- The patient has the right to participate in the development and implementation of his or her plan of care.
- The patient or his or her representative has the right to make informed decisions regarding his or her care.
- The patient's rights include being informed of his or her health status, involved in care planning and treatment, and able to request or refuse treatment. This right must not be construed as a mechanism to demand the provision of treatment or services deemed medically unnecessary or inappropriate.
- The patient has the right to formulate advance directives and have hospital staff and practitioners who provide care in the hospital comply with these directives.
- The patient has the right to have a family member or representative of his or her choice and his or her own health care provider notified promptly of his or her admission to the hospital.

Standard 3: Privacy and Safety
- The patient has the right to personal privacy.
- The patient has the right to receive care in a safe setting.
- The patient has the right to be free from all forms of abuse or harassment.

Standard 4: Confidentiality of Patient Record
- The patient has the right to the confidentiality of his or her clinical records.
- The patient has the right to access information contained in his or her clinical records within a reasonable time frame.

Standard 5: Restraint or Seclusion
- The patient has the right to be free from physical or mental abuse and corporal punishment.
- The patient has the right to be free from restraints or seclusion of any form that are not medically necessary or are used as a means of coercion, discipline, convenience, or retaliation by staff. A restraint is any manual method or physical or mechanical device, material, or equipment attached or adjacent to the patient's body that he or she cannot easily remove that restricts freedom of movement or normal access to one's body. A drug used as a restraint is a medication used to control behavior or to restrict the patient's freedom of movement and is not a standard treatment for the patient's medical or psychiatric condition. Seclusion is the involuntary confinement of a patient alone in a room or area from which the patient is physically prevented from leaving.
- A restraint or seclusion can only be used if needed to improve the patient's well-being and less restrictive interventions have been determined to be ineffective.
- The use of a restraint or seclusion must be selected only when other less restrictive measures have been found to be ineffective to protect the patient or others from harm and in accordance with the order of a physician or other licensed independent practitioner.
- This order must never be written as a standing order or on an as-needed basis (i.e., prn). The order must be followed by consultation with the patient's treating physician, as soon as possible, if someone other than the patient's treating physician or health care provider ordered the restraint or seclusion.
- The use of a restraint or seclusion must be:
  - In accordance with a written modification to the patient's plan of care.
  - Implemented in the least restrictive manner possible.
  - In accordance with safe and appropriate restraining techniques.
  - Ended at the earliest possible time.
- The condition of the restrained or secluded patient must be assessed, monitored, and reevaluated continually.
- All staff who have direct patient contact must have ongoing education and training in the proper and safe use of restraints and seclusion.

Modified from Centers for Medicare and Medicaid Services: Medicare and Medicaid programs, hospital conditions of participation: patients' rights; final rule, *Fed Reg* 71(236):71426, 2009.
CMS, Centers for Medicare and Medicaid Services.

BOX 2-3	The Joint Commission Patients' Rights Standards

- Right to an appropriate level of care
- Right to receive safe care
- Respect for cultural values and religious beliefs
- Privacy
- Consent obtained for recording or filming made for purposes other than the identification, diagnosis, or treatment of patients
- Confidentiality of information
- Recognition and prevention of potential abuse situation
- Notification of unanticipated outcomes
- Involvement in care decisions
- Information on risks and benefits of investigational studies
- End-of-life care
- Advance directives
- Organ procurement
- A right to have advance directives and to have them followed
- Freedom from unnecessary restraints
- Informed consent for various procedures
- The right to refuse care
- The right to have their pain believed and relieved
- Communication with administration
- Education

From The Joint Commission: *Comprehensive accreditation manual for hospitals,* Chicago, 2012, The Joint Commission.

BOX 2-4	Advance Directives

- An advance directive is a document that gives a patient's directions about future medical care or designates another person(s) to make medical decisions if the individual loses decision-making capacity.
- An advance directive conveys the patient's choice in continuing medical care when the patient is unable to speak or make decisions.
- Advance directives may include a living will, power of attorney for health care, or notarized handwritten document.
- A copy of the document should be available in the patient's medical record. If not available, the substance of the advance directive should be documented in the medical record, and a family member should be asked to bring the advance directive to the hospital.
- The attending health care provider is notified of the patient's advance directive.
- Witnesses for an advance directive document should not be medical personnel, nor should they be related to the patient or heirs to the patient's estate. A social worker often fulfills this requirement.

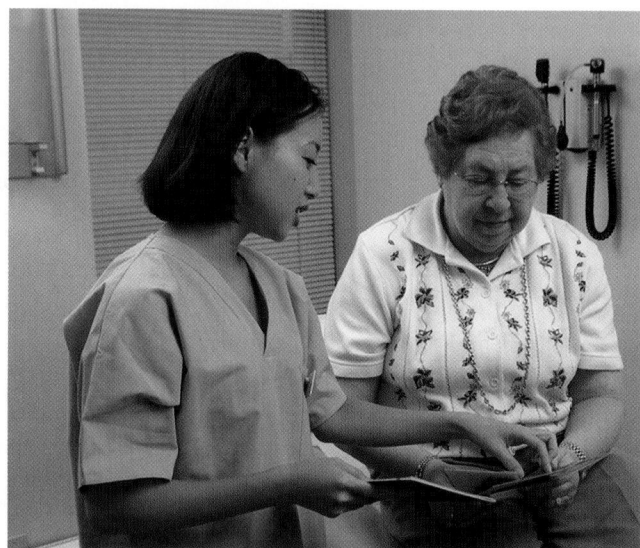

FIG 2-1   Nurse explains HIPPA regulations to patient.

purpose of the use. In addition to existing laws, new proposals include allowing patients to know who has accessed their information (USDHHS, 2011).

The HIPAA privacy regulations also give patients the right to access their records, request amendments to the PHI contained in their records, request restriction of certain uses or disclosures of their PHI, request that they be sent information at an alternative address or telephone number, and request an accounting of PHI disclosures (Fig. 2-1). Know your agency-specific policies and procedures related to HIPAA.

Role of the Nurse

On admission nurses complete a thorough nursing assessment, review any advance directives, and ensure that necessary diagnostic testing is completed. If patients were receiving health care before admission (e.g., home health care, long-term care), a nurse provides for continuity of care when a patient is admitted. Admitting

personnel consult with nursing staff to ensure that a patient's room assignment is based on the patient's condition, health care needs, developmental level, activity level, expected length of stay, and personal preferences. For example, the best room for an older patient who is acutely ill, at risk for falls, and receiving multiple treatments is one close to the nurses' station. The nurse identifies any known allergies and, if any exist, places an allergy band on the patient and properly documents the known allergies in the medical record.

When a patient is admitted through the ED, the nurse notifies the nursing division and reports on the patient's admission information, including his or her name; admitting physician or health care provider; chief complaint; and any treatments or testing completed and the outcome, diagnosis, and pertinent information related to the patient's condition (e.g., initial vital signs, allergies, level of consciousness, and intravenous [IV] fluid infusing). An escort takes the patient and family members to the nursing division and introduces them to the nurse assuming the patient's care. The ED nurse shares pertinent observations about the patient's behavior (e.g., anxiety, fear, or level of knowledge regarding need for health care) with the nursing staff to foster continuity of care and assist the patient and family in coping with a new environment and procedures.

Patients admitted on the morning of a surgical procedure or treatment are "same day" admissions. A nurse provides basic instructions about the purpose of the surgery or treatment, preparatory procedures, and postsurgical or posttreatment care. Admission and consent forms, diagnostic tests, patient teaching, and instructions are usually completed before the actual day of surgery. Nurses use a variety of resources such as classes, videotapes, information booklets, and calls to home for patient teaching.

Nurses are active in coordinating the initial admission process for all patients. A patient's condition influences the extent and type of admission activities. Always note the patient's level of fatigue and comfort. For example, when a critically ill patient reaches a hospital nursing division, he or she undergoes extensive examination and treatment procedures immediately. Little time is available for you to orient the patient and family to the division or learn of the patient's fears or concerns. When a patient enters a hospital for elective treatment, you have more time to prepare him or her psychologically for hospitalization. Early psychological preparation when the patient is still at home prepares patients for hospitalization.

Delegation and Collaboration

The skill of completing the nursing assessment during admission to a health care agency cannot be delegated to nursing assistive personnel (NAP). Do not delegate admission vital signs because a nurse must conduct the baseline assessment. The nurse directs the NAP to:

- Prepare the patient's room with equipment needed before admission.
- Gather and secure the patient's personal care items.
- Escort and orient the patient and family to the nursing unit.
- Collect ordered specimens.

Equipment

- ❏ Hospital gown
- ❏ Bedpan and urinal (if needed)
- ❏ Washbasin, bath towel, and washcloth
- ❏ Toiletry items (e.g., soap, toothpaste, hand lotion; *optional* in some hospitals)
- ❏ Facial tissues
- ❏ Water pitcher and drinking cup
- ❏ Kidney or emesis basin
- ❏ Disposable thermometer (see agency policy)
- ❏ Sphygmomanometer
- ❏ Stethoscope
- ❏ Pulse oximeter (*optional*)
- ❏ Documentation forms (see agency policy)

STEP	RATIONALE
ROOM PREPARATION	
1 Perform hand hygiene and prepare room equipment and furniture. Prepare bed by adjusting it to the lowest horizontal position if patient is ambulatory. Place bed in high position if patient is arriving by stretcher. Turn down top sheet and bedspread. Arrange room furniture for easy access to bed. Adjust lights, temperature, and ventilation.	Promotes patient's comfort by preventing delays during care. Proper position of bed lessens likelihood of patient fall during transfer and back injuries to staff assisting patient into bed.
2 Be sure that equipment is in working order. Assemble any special equipment (e.g., suction, oxygen supplies, or IV pole) in patient's room.	Prevents delays in delivering immediate treatment and provides for smooth transition between caregivers.
ASSESSMENT	
1 Greet patient and family cordially by name. Introduce yourself by name and job title; explain your responsibilities in patient's care.	Providing personalized care reduces anxiety about admission, clarifies staff roles, and expedites patient requests.
2 Identify patient using two identifiers (i.e., name and birthday or name and account number) according to agency policy. Compare identifiers with information on patient's identification bracelet.	Ensures correct patient. Complies with The Joint Commission standards and improves patient safety (2012b).
3 If patient does not speak English or has a severe hearing impairment, arrange for a translation service so you are able to conduct a nursing assessment.	Translation services are preferable to using family members to ensure correct translation of medical terminology.
4 Assess patient's general appearance, noting signs or symptoms of physical distress (see Chapter 6).	Provides baseline assessment.

Clinical Decision Point *If patient is having acute physical problems, postpone routine admission procedures until you meet his or her immediate needs. Complete a focused assessment at this point.*

5 Determine patient's ability to understand and implement health information by asking a health literacy question.	This supports patient's ability to understand information and allows you to use appropriate teaching methods such as the "teach back" method (TJC, 2011a).

STEP	RATIONALE
6 Assess patient's and family's psychological status by noting verbal and nonverbal behaviors and responses to greetings and explanations.	Anxiety influences how well patient adapts to a health care environment and retains instruction.
7 Assess vital signs (see Chapter 5) and height and weight (see Chapter 6).	Provides baseline measurement to compare future findings. Determines alterations from normal range.
8 Assess for fall risk using scale with grading criteria per agency policy. Consider patient's risk factors (e.g., neurologic disorders; history of previous fall; urinary urgency or incontinence; use of sedatives, antihypertensives, and analgesics; history of unsteady gait; use of assistive devices; history of orthostatic hypotension; memory deficits) (Kulik, 2011).	Provides data to determine patient's risk for injury and whether patient needs to be placed on fall precautions.
9 Have family or friends leave room unless patient wishes to have them assist with changing into a hospital gown or pajamas. Close door and curtains. Help patient undress and assist patient into comfortable position.	Provides for privacy and prepares patient for examination.
10 Obtain nursing history as soon as possible after patient's arrival to nursing division. Apply standards of nursing care adopted by hospital (e.g., functional health patterns). Data include:	Each patient is to have an admission assessment prepared by a registered nurse (RN) (TJC, 2012a). Each agency sets a time frame for completion of admission assessment (maximum time 24 hours).
a Patient's perception of illness and health care needs.	Establishes a baseline of patient's clinical status.
b Past medical history.	
c Presenting signs and symptoms and reason for hospitalization.	Identifies signs and symptoms in case the patient's condition deteriorates.
d Completion of a review of health status based on standards such as elimination, nutrition and metabolism, activity and exercise, self-concept, values and beliefs, cultural factors, social support, and cognitive function.	A comprehensive health history provides a holistic view of patient's health problems and response to those problems.
e Risk factors for illness.	Allows you to institute preventive care measures and educate patient about health promotion behaviors.
f History of allergies, including type of substance and a description of the reaction that patient has previously experienced.	Patients often have sensitivity to a drug or substance rather than a true allergy; this needs to be clarified. Specify all allergens to prevent accidental exposure.

Clinical Decision Point *Provide patient with allergy arm band listing allergies to foods, drugs, latex, or other substances; document allergies according to hospital policy.*

STEP	RATIONALE
g Detailed medication history, including prescribed, over-the-counter (OTC), and alternative therapies such as herbs and hormones.	Assesses potential for drug interactions and often explains patient's presenting signs and symptoms.
h Patient's knowledge of health problems and expectations of care.	Enables you to recognize and meet patient expectations when possible.
11 Conduct physical assessment of appropriate body systems (see Chapter 6). If not obtained in admitting, instruct patient to provide a urine specimen. Inform patient if collecting blood specimens or performing tests.	Provides objective data for identifying health problems. When unannounced procedures are performed, patients become anxious. Preparation of patient relieves anxiety.
12 Check health care providers' orders for treatment measures to initiate immediately.	Delay causes deterioration of patient's condition.
13 Orient patient to nursing division.	
a Introduce staff members who enter room. Always introduce patient by last name unless patient indicates otherwise.	Helps patient recognize caregivers. Shows respect for patient.
b Tell patient and family the name of the nurse manager in charge of the division and explain that person's role in solving problems.	Provides means for patient to communicate problems.
c Explain visiting hours and their purpose.	Provides knowledge and increases willingness to observe policy for visiting hours, which ensures that patient receives adequate rest.
d Discuss smoking policy and identify smoking areas for patient and family if available.	A hospital-wide smoking policy that prohibits the use of smoking materials throughout the hospital is required. Some hospitals may have a designated smoking area.

STEP	RATIONALE
e Demonstrate use of equipment (e.g., bed, over-bed table, lighting).	Patient's safety depends on patient understanding correct use of equipment.
f Show patient how to use nurse call light and position it in a convenient place. Have patient demonstrate use of light. Discuss with patient any specific fall risks and encourage him or her to ask for assistance when getting out of bed.	Ensures that patient knows how to call for assistance.
g Escort patient to bathroom (if able to ambulate).	Patient's safety depends in part on understanding how to use toilet facilities.

Clinical Decision Point *Ensure that patient knows how to call for assistance while in bathroom. (An emergency call light is usually in bathrooms.)*

h Explain hours for mealtime and nourishments to patient and family.	Family often wishes to visit during evening to help with meals.
i Describe services available (e.g., chaplain, beauty shop, activity therapy).	Offers patient options for making decisions.

NURSING DIAGNOSES

- Anxiety
- Deficient knowledge regarding hospital procedures and planned therapies
- Fear
- Ineffective coping, individual or family
- Powerlessness
- Risk for injury

Related factors are individualized based on patient's condition or needs.

PLANNING

1 Expected outcomes following completion of procedure:	
• Patient is able to explain purpose and schedule of planned treatments and procedures.	Understanding treatment plan gives patient a better sense of control and reduces anxiety about the unknown.
• Patient demonstrates how to call for nurse when assistance is needed.	Falls commonly occur when patients attempt to get out of bed without assistance.
• Patient is able to ambulate (if condition permits) in room free of obstacles.	Ensures patient safety and mobility in room.
• Patient can safely and efficiently use equipment in the room.	Equipment used in care of patient frequently poses hazards; assists in reducing some anxiety.
• Patient verbalizes understanding of smoking policy, visiting hours, mealtimes, and services available.	Knowledge of hospital policies assists patient in adapting to the health care environment.

IMPLEMENTATION

1 Complete patient medication reconciliation by checking home medication list for duplication, omission, or potential drug interactions with newly ordered medications. Update medication list based on health care provider's orders for treatment.	Medication reconciliation on admission helps to make sure that patient is taking the correct medications and avoid medication errors (TJC, 2012a).
2 Inform patient about procedures or treatments scheduled for the next shift or day (e.g., visits by health care provider or dietitian). These vary based on nature of patient's condition.	Patient has right to be informed of any scheduled procedures or treatments. Being able to anticipate planned therapies minimizes anxiety.
3 Complete learning needs assessment for patient and family.	Identifies patient's and family's educational needs and learning preferences.
4 Give patient and family chance to ask questions about procedures or therapies. (If patient is unresponsive or unable to understand, review with family.)	Provides opportunity to clarify expectations and misconceptions.
5 Collect valuables that patient chooses to keep at agency. Complete clothing and valuables listing sheet (see agency policy). Have patient or family member sign it. Place valuables in agency safe or send home with family.	Accounts for placement of valuables and prevents loss.
6 Ensure that patient and family have time together alone if desired.	Admission is often stressful and fatiguing. Allows time for decision making.
7 Be sure that call light is within easy reach and bed is in low position. (Check agency policy regarding use of side rails.)	Provides for patient's safety. Side rails enhance patient's ability to position in bed but are considered a restraint if they obstruct patient's ability to get out of bed when desired (TJC, 2012a).
8 Perform hand hygiene.	Reduces spread of microorganisms.

STEP	RATIONALE

EVALUATION

1 Have patient explain own fall risks, hospital policies, tests, and procedures through discussion and questions.	Patient demonstrates learning and understanding through feedback.
2 Have patient demonstrate use of call light.	Return demonstration confirms learning.
3 Monitor patient's ability to ambulate independently.	Provides data to judge patient's safety in ambulating without injury.
4 Check patient's room setup regularly.	Determines if care area is free of obstacles.

Unexpected Outcomes	Related Interventions
1 Patient denies understanding hospital policies or knowing purpose or schedule for tests and procedures.	• Schedule a follow-up session with patient. • Keep information focused and specific to patient's situation. Include family if helpful.
2 Patient becomes restless, expresses concerns, or displays tension in body movements.	• Give patient time to discuss fears and concerns. • Show caring and compassion so patient becomes willing to communicate openly.
3 Patient falls or is injured.	• Attend to patient's immediate physical needs, inform health care provider of the injury or fall, reassess patient's environment, alter care plan as needed, ensure that the environment is free of safety hazards, and complete incident report (see Chapter 13).

Recording and Reporting

- Record history and assessment findings in nurses' notes, electronic health record (EHR), or on appropriate forms. Begin to develop nursing plan of care. Confer with patient and family as needed.
- If patient has an advance directive, place copy in the medical record. In the absence of the actual advance directive, document the substance of the directive in the medical record (TJC, 2012a).
- Notify health care provider of patient's arrival; report any unusual findings. Secure admission orders if not previously provided.

Special Considerations
Teaching

- Explain to patient that a different nurse provides care on each shift. Explain time frame for how assignments are made.
- Teaching occurs throughout the admission process. Provide information regarding physical assessment findings, risks for falling, nature of patient's illness, planned diagnostic and treatment procedures, medications, and hospital routines. Do not begin a formal teaching plan until you have completed the assessment and developed a care plan.
- In an emergency situation or if patient is unable to perform aspects of his or her care, instruct family members in the rationale for any procedures and routines to be used in patient's care.

Pediatric

- Hospitalization is a major crisis for children who feel stress from separation, loss of control, bodily injury, and pain. Separation anxiety is most common from middle infancy throughout the toddler years, especially ages 16 to 30 months. Preschoolers are better able to tolerate brief periods of separation, but their protest behaviors are more subtle than those in younger children (e.g., refusal to eat, difficulty sleeping, withdrawing from others). School-age children are able to cope with separation but have an increased need for parental security and guidance (Hockenberry and Wilson, 2011). Explain the rooming-in and visiting policies of the agency. Allow and encourage parental involvement in the child's care. Allow parents to assist with routine care activities (e.g., bathing, eating) and when possible to remain with the child during procedures.
- Parental input during admission assessment is essential because they can provide input on the child's normal behavior and deviations caused by illness (Moorey, 2010).
- Incorporate the child's usual routines such as favorite food, bedtime practices, and toileting into the plan of care. Encourage the parent to bring a favorite toy, blanket, or other items to make child feel more comfortable in the unfamiliar setting.

Gerontologic

- Hospitalized older adults often experience functional declines such as new-onset incontinence, malnutrition, pressure ulcers, and falls. Interventions that retain functional status (e.g., physical therapy, nutrition consultation) include providing coordinated interdisciplinary care (Touhy and Jett, 2010).
- Patients who typically fall in the hospital are those who have been admitted recently and are unfamiliar with surroundings, have acute illness, take four or more medications, or have been relocated recently. Visual changes that occur with aging often lead to falls in hospitalized older-adult patients (Touhy and Jett, 2010).

SKILL 2-2 Transferring Patients

Patients transfer to different patient care units and agencies to receive alternate forms and levels of therapy and services and to have essential care continued closer to home. When patients transfer, you need to ensure continuity of nursing care and improve transitions across the continuum of care. The goal is to continue health care to avoid therapeutic interruptions or omissions that may hinder progress toward recovery. Collaborate early with health care providers and members of the interdisciplinary team to ensure efficient patient transfer with optimal patient outcomes. There is evidence that interprofessional teams provide more integrated care than individual providers, particularly for patients with complex physiological, psychological, and social needs (Blewett and others, 2009). Open collaboration and effective communication help to ensure that quality patient care is realized.

When transferring a patient from one patient care unit to another within an agency, it is important to complete the process without interrupting care activities when possible. When providing a "hand off" of a patient to another unit, it is essential that information about the patient's care, treatment, services, and current condition and any recent or anticipated changes are communicated accurately to meet patient safety goals (TJC, 2012a). Policies and procedures are usually similar throughout an agency. A nurse first provides a telephone report to the receiving nurse. This allows the receiving nurse to prepare for the patient (e.g., preparing the room and securing necessary equipment). As clinically appropriate, a nurse or technician accompanies the patient during transport, providing the receiving nurse with the patient's medical record; introducing the patient to the receiving nurse; and providing an updated report, including any changes in clinical status or plan of care.

In the Emergency Department (ED), when a patient is transferred from one agency to another, a nurse completes the transfer in compliance with the Emergency Medical Treatment and Labor Act (EMTALA) (CMS, 2011). EMTALA is a federal law intended to protect patients from being transferred against their wishes and thus defines how an appropriate facility-to-facility transfer is accomplished. An appropriate transfer includes:

- Informing the patient of the risks and benefits of the transfer.
- Obtaining the patient's written consent for transfer.
- Having the transferring hospital provide medical treatment within its capacity.
- Having available space and qualified personnel for treatment of the patient at the receiving agency and an agreement to accept transfer of the patient and provide treatment.
- Making copies of all relevant medical records, including a transfer form, sent by the transferring agency to the receiving facility.
- Transporting the patient using qualified personnel and transportation equipment (e.g., ambulance with advanced cardiac life support [ACLS] versus basic life support [BLS]).

Although this law primarily affects the ED, know EMTALA policies and transfer policies for inpatient transfers of the agency. Many agencies follow the same policies for all patient transfers.

Delegation and Collaboration

The skill of assessment and decision making conducted during transfers cannot be delegated to nursing assistive personnel (NAP). The nurse directs the NAP to:
- Assist the patient with dressing.
- Gather and secure the patient's personal belongings and any equipment that goes with the patient.
- Escort the patient to the nursing unit or transport area.

Equipment

❏ Transfer forms
❏ Copies of documents such as medical records, radiology films, laboratory test results (as appropriate)
❏ Special equipment as needed: wheelchair or stretcher, emesis basin, bedpan and urinal, oxygen tank and tubing, IV pole, cardiac monitor, and emergency medications

STEP	RATIONALE

ASSESSMENT

1 Obtain transfer order from sending health care provider. Order includes name of receiving agency (when applicable), receiving health care provider's name, and statement of patient's stability for transfer.	Health care provider is legally responsible for releasing patient from medical care and arranging for receiving health care provider. Patient has legal right to refuse transfer against medical advice.
2 In collaboration with health care provider and members of the interdisciplinary team, assess reason for patient's transfer (e.g., change in condition, services available at agency, patient or family preferences regarding patient's location).	Patient needs to have access to agency with best resources to meet health care needs. Health care provider determines patient's physical stability for transfer.
3 Identify patient using two identifiers (i.e., name and birthday or name and account number) according to agency policy. Compare identifiers with information on patient's identification bracelet.	Ensures correct patient. Complies with The Joint Commission standards and improves patient safety (TJC, 2012b).
4 Assess individuals at high risk for transitional care problems (e.g., older adults with multiple health issues, depression, non-English speakers, and low-income patients).	Identifying patients at risk for transitional care problems allows for better continuity of care and improved patient outcomes (Touhy and Jett, 2010). Patients may require consultation with needed resources (e.g., care manager, psychologist).

STEP	RATIONALE
5 Explain purpose of transfer thoroughly and provide time to discuss patient's and family's feelings about the change in care setting. As necessary, obtain patient's written consent to transfer. If patient is unable to consent, patient's family provides this consent.	Patients need to be informed of transfer plans in a timely manner (TJC, 2011). A patient requires adequate psychological preparation. In the event of a clinical emergency in which patient and patient's family are unable to consent, this consent is waived, and patient is transferred to a higher level of care based on the clinical judgment of the health care provider requesting the transfer.
6 Assess patient's current physical condition and determine method for transport. When transferring to new agency, assess method of transport to transferring vehicle (e.g., wheelchair or stretcher) (consult agency policy).	Patient's condition often changes quickly and influences stability for transfer and type of support needed during transport.

Clinical Decision Point *Determine if patient's status and safety require life-support equipment. Staff assisting with transfer needs training in life-support measures. When transporting to new agency, a vehicle equipped with life-support equipment is necessary.*

STEP	RATIONALE
7 Assess if patient requires pain relief or other medications for symptom management.	Ensures patient's comfort during transfer.
8 Ensure that staff have notified patient's family or significant others of transfer as desired by patient.	Provides adequate communication with family or significant others to assist with patient's emotional and psychological adjustment to the transfer (TJC, 2011).

NURSING DIAGNOSES

- Anxiety
- Deficient knowledge regarding transfer procedure
- Fear
- Pain, acute and chronic
- Powerlessness
- Relocation stress syndrome
- Risk for relocation stress syndrome

Related factors are individualized based on patient's condition or needs.

PLANNING

1 Expected outcomes following completion of procedure:	
• Patient's vital signs and physiologic status remain the same following transfer.	Treatments are planned so as not to interrupt physical support of patient during transfer.
• Patient incurs no injury during transport procedures.	Safety measures are successful in transferring patient from wheelchair or stretcher to transport vehicle.
• Patient or family explains purpose of transfer and procedure for transport.	Understanding provides patient with sense of control.
• Receiving nursing staff acquire and confirm written plan of care.	Ensures continuity of care.
• Patient socializes with family members, staff, and/or other residents.	Identifies that patient has not developed relocation stress syndrome.
2 Arrange for patient's transport to an agency by chosen vehicle (social worker involvement may be necessary).	Transfer needs to occur without delays so patient has access to all needed resources at all times.
3 When transfer is to a new agency, contact the agency and arrange for bed in appropriate setting. Confirm willingness of agency to accept patient (usually social worker or discharge coordinator completes).	Prevents delays when patient arrives at destination. Receiving hospital ensures that there is available space and qualified personnel to treat patients. Hospital also agrees in advance to transfer.

IMPLEMENTATION

1 Make sure that documentation in patient's record is complete with care plan that has individualized nursing care measures.	Accurate information is necessary for receiving agency to assume patient's care.
2 Complete nursing care transfer form according to agency policy. (When transfer is to a different nursing unit, entire medical record accompanies patient.)	Form summarizes patient's pertinent nursing care needs to ensure continuity of care and prevent unnecessary duplication of services.
3 Complete medication reconciliation per agency policy. Check patient's current orders against the most recent medication administration record and the original home medication list. Communicate updated medication list to next provider of care.	Ensures that patient receives correct medications at new facility and decreases medication errors (TJC, 2012a).
4 Have NAP gather patient's personal care items, clothing, and valuables. Check the entire room and all storage areas. Secure in suitcase or container.	Prevents loss of articles during transfer.

STEP	RATIONALE
5 Anticipate problems that patient frequently develops just before or during transfer. Perform necessary nursing therapies such as suctioning or changing a dressing.	Ensures patient's comfort and safety during transport.
6 Assist in transferring patient to stretcher or wheelchair using safe patient-handling techniques (see Chapter 9).	It is easier to move patient transported to outside agency by stretcher into transport vehicle.
7 Perform and document final assessment of patient's physical stability.	Minimizes risk of patient developing complications during transfer.

Clinical Decision Point *Priority assessment includes vital signs, clear airway, patency of IV lines and accuracy of infusion rate, and patient's level of consciousness.*

8 When transfer occurs to an outside agency, accompany patient to transport vehicle.	Ensures that medically qualified personnel are in attendance until patient leaves agency/unit.
9 Call receiving agency/unit and notify of impending transfer and patient's status (check agency policy).	Notification of nurse in charge or nurse assuming care of patient ensures better continuity of care at time of patient's arrival.

EVALUATION

1 During the final assessment compare data with the previous findings.	Determines if patient's condition is changing.
2 Inspect patient's alignment and positioning on stretcher/wheelchair.	Proper alignment and positioning reduce risk of an injury occurring during transport.
3 Ensure that equipment needed for transfer is functioning.	Equipment such as oxygen must last through transport for patient safety.
4 Confirm that patient understands transfer and procedures through discussion and questions.	Feedback helps to ensure learning.
5 Determine if receiving agency/nurse has questions about patient's care.	Provides for clear communication and continuity of care.
6 Evaluate patient for inappropriate behaviors (e.g., acting out, refusing medication).	Provides information about relocation adaptation.

Unexpected Outcomes
1 Patient's physical status deteriorates during preparation.

2 Patient sustains injury during transfer to wheelchair or stretcher.

3 Patient is confused or uncertain about transfer.
4 Receiving staff misinterpret directions for patient's care.

5 Patient will not socialize and demonstrates inappropriate behaviors.

Related Interventions
- Call health care provider immediately.
- Initiate necessary interventions to stabilize patient's condition.
- Stabilize patient and call health care provider.
- Complete incident (occurrence) report (see Chapter 4).
- Provide clarification or additional explanation.
- Sending agency has nurse or health care provider call to confirm that there are no questions regarding patient's care.
- Include patient in developing plan of care.
- Identify previous coping mechanisms.
- Ensure that all caregivers introduce themselves.

Recording and Reporting
- Nurse sending patient documents patient's status, including vital signs and other assessment findings, nursing plan of care, date and time of transfer, and method of transport.
- Nurse receiving patient documents patient's arrival at agency by recording date and time of arrival, reason for transfer, method of transport, patient's condition, and care provided at time of arrival.

Special Considerations
Teaching
- A transfer frequently creates anxiety for a patient and family members. Carefully repeat instructions about the transfer when patient and family are better able to understand your explanation. In this situation be sure to have patient restate any critical information.

Pediatric
- Children need their parents' comfort and security; thus make sure that parents are well informed. Involve older children in any discussion regarding transfers. Allow a parent to accompany the child in the transfer.

Gerontologic
- When transferring an older-adult patient to a new facility, relocation is stressful. Ensure that significant support persons are still accessible and that patient is thoroughly oriented to new surroundings. Also make sure that patient is able to take important memorabilia and has an opportunity to make decisions about care (Touhy and Jett, 2010).

Long-Term Care
- It is important that patients receive the level of services appropriate to their physical and mental health needs. Participation of social worker or discharge planner in transfer process ensures that transfer to a long-term care facility is appropriate.

- On patient's arrival at long-term care facility, complete a Resident Assessment Instrument (RAI). The RAI consists of the minimum data set (MDS), resident assessment protocols, and utilization guidelines specified in state operations guidelines (Touhy and Jett, 2010).

- Essential components of successful transfer to a long-term care facility are accurate communication of medication lists and advance directives. Possible use of a standardized transfer form can assist in accurate communication (LaMantia and others, 2010).

SKILL 2-3   Discharging Patients

Discharge planning facilitates the transition of a patient from a health care agency to the most independent level of care, whether that is home or another agency. The overall goal of discharge planning is to provide the most appropriate level and quality of care throughout all stages of a patient's illness. The discharge planning process is comprehensive and multidisciplinary, including all caregivers who are involved in the care of the patient. Every hospitalized patient requires discharge planning. The trend toward a shortened length of stay in the acute care setting makes discharge planning increasingly difficult, but all the more essential. The Joint Commission identifies the elements of a comprehensive discharge planning model (Box 2-5).

Development of a discharge plan with outcomes mutually accepted by a patient and caregivers and ongoing communication about its progress are essential (TJC, 2011, 2012a). Effective discharge planning can decrease hospital readmission and increase patient satisfaction (Rose and Haugen, 2010). The discharge process is simple or complex and occurs in three phases: acute, transitional, and continuing care. In the acute phase medical attention dominates discharge planning efforts. During the transitional phase the need for acute care is still present, but its urgency declines, and patients begin to address and plan for their future health care needs. In the continuing care phase patients are able to participate in planning and implementing continuing care activities needed after discharge.

The greatest challenge in effective discharge planning is communication. Communication issues are minimized when an organization has a discharge coordinator or case manager responsible for discharge planning. Staff members in these roles are responsible for thoroughly assessing a patient's health care needs at discharge, identifying available and needed resources, and linking the patient and family to the proper resources. Staff are also responsible for coordinating services (as appropriate) and following up on patients' progress after discharge.

Discharge from an agency is stressful for a patient and family. Before a patient is discharged, the patient and family need to know how to manage care in the home and what to expect in regard to any continuing physical problems. Without the necessary equipment and professional resources, a patient risks loss of rehabilitation gains made before discharge. Failure to understand restrictions or implications of health problems often causes a patient to develop complications. Poor discharge planning ignores a patient's needs within the home and increases the chance of the patient needing to reenter the health care system prematurely.

Delegation and Collaboration
The skill of assessment, care planning, and instruction included in discharging patients cannot be delegated to nursing assistive personnel (NAP). The nurse directs the NAP to:
- Gather and secure the patient's personal items and any supplies that accompany him or her.
- Transport the patient to the discharge transport vehicle.

Equipment
- ❏ Wheelchair or stretcher
- ❏ Discharge documentation forms (see agency policy)
- ❏ Patient instruction sheets
- ❏ Plastic bag for personal belongings

BOX 2-5	The Joint Commission Recommendations for Discharge Planning Process

- Address patient communication needs during discharge. This includes the patient's preferred language and any sensory or communication impairments.
- Ensure that language services are available during discharge for both patient and family members.
- Engage patients and families in discharge planning and instruction.
- Provide discharge instruction that meets patient needs.
  - Instruction may involve use of pictures, diagrams, or models to illustrate instruction.
  - Use discharge instruction that meets health literacy needs. Materials should be at fifth grade or lower reading level.
- Identify follow-up providers who can meet unique patient needs.
  - Create a list of follow-up providers that offer services and accommodations that meet the patient's communication, cultural, religious, mobility, and other needs.
  - Refer patients to appropriate care provider (e.g., community clinic).

Modified from The Joint Commission: *Advancing effective communication, cultural competence, and patient- and family-centered care: a roadmap for hospitals,* Oakbrook Terrace, 2011, The Joint Commission.

STEP	RATIONALE

ASSESSMENT

1 From time of admission, assess patient's discharge needs using nursing history and discussions with patient and health care provider. Use care plan to focus on ongoing assessments of patient's physical health, functional status, psychosocial support system, financial resources, health values, cultural and ethnic background, level of education, and barriers to care that are needed.

Planning for discharge begins at admission and continues throughout patient's stay in agency. Discharge planning interventions focus on helping patients achieve maximum functioning.

STEP	RATIONALE
2 Identify patient using two identifiers (e.g., name and birthday or name and account number) according to agency policy). Compare identifiers with information on patient's identification bracelet.	Ensures correct patient. Complies with The Joint Commission standards and improves patient safety (TJC, 2012a).
3 Assess patient's and family's need for health teaching related to how to perform home therapies, use of home medical equipment, restrictions resulting from health alterations, and possible complications.	Improves understanding of health care needs and ability to achieve self-care at home. Inclusion of family member in teaching sessions provides patient with available resource.
4 Assess for barriers to learning (e.g., fatigue, pain, lack of motivation).	Determines timing and approach to instruction. Different types of educational materials are effective with different individual learning styles. If printed material is to be used, be sure that material at proper reading level is available.
5 Assess for environmental factors within the home that interfere with self-care (e.g., size of rooms, doorway clearances, steps, bathroom facilities). (A home care nurse is usually available on referral to assist with assessment.)	Environmental factors within patient's home pose safety risks or problems for self-care. For example, throw rugs are a fall hazard for a patient discharged with crutches or a walker (see Chapter 41).
6 Collaborate with health care provider and interdisciplinary team (e.g., physical therapy) in assessing need for referral for skilled home care services or extended care facility.	Patients eligible for home care must be confined to home as a result of illness, are under a health care provider's care, and require skilled nursing care on an intermittent basis.
7 Assess patient's and family's perceptions of continued health care needs outside the hospital. Include an assessment of family caregivers' perceived ability to provide care to patient, including ability to adjust to demands of patient care, impact of care demands on their lives (e.g., providing hands-on care, preparing special diets), and potential ongoing nature of patient's needs.	Patients and family members often disagree on health care needs of patient after discharge. Identifying discrepancies early helps in more accurately developing the discharge plan. Family caregiving is a highly stressful experience. Family members who are not properly prepared for caregiving are frequently overwhelmed by patient's needs, which can lead to unnecessary hospital readmissions (Sobolewski, 2011).

Clinical Decision Point *It is often necessary to talk with patient and family separately to learn about true concerns or doubts.*

STEP	RATIONALE
8 Assess patient's acceptance of health problems and related restrictions.	Affects willingness to follow therapies and restrictions.
9 Consult other health care team members (e.g., dietitian, social worker) about anticipated needs after discharge. Make appropriate referrals in a timely manner.	Members of all health care disciplines collaborate to determine patient's needs and functional abilities.

NURSING DIAGNOSES

- Anxiety
- Caregiver role strain
- Deficient knowledge regarding home care restrictions

- Impaired home maintenance
- Interrupted family processes
- Relocation stress syndrome

- Self-care deficit: feeding, toileting, dressing/grooming, bathing/hygiene

Related factors are individualized based on patient's condition or needs.

PLANNING

1 Expected outcomes following completion of procedure:
- Patient or family caregiver explains how health care is to continue in home (or other facility), which treatments or medications patient needs, and when to seek medical attention for problems.

  Increases likelihood of care not being interrupted in home (or other facility).

- Patient is able to demonstrate self-care activities (or family member is able to administer care measures).

  Feedback ensures learning.

- Obstacles to patient's mobility and hazards to ambulation in home setting are removed.

  Patient is often physically weakened or has physical changes resulting from illness that predispose to injury.

STEP	RATIONALE

IMPLEMENTATION

1 Preparation before day of discharge:

  a Suggest ways to change physical arrangement of home to meet patient's needs (see Chapter 41).

Maintains patient's level of independence and ability to retain function within safe environment.

  b Provide patient and family with information about community health care resources (e.g., medical equipment companies, Meals on Wheels, adult day care). Referrals are usually made while patient is in hospital.

Community resources offer services that patient or family cannot provide.

  c Conduct teaching sessions with patient and family as soon as possible during hospitalization (e.g., signs and symptoms of complications, information regarding medications, use of medical equipment, follow-up care, diet, exercise, restrictions imposed by illness or surgery). Review and give patient discharge materials such as pamphlets, books, or multimedia resources. Refer patient to reliable and current resources on the Internet.

Gives patient opportunities to practice new skills, ask questions, and obtain necessary feedback to ensure learning.
A combination of written and verbal information is effective in improving patient satisfaction and knowledge (TJC, 2011).

  d Communicate patient's and family's response to teaching and proposed discharge plan to other health care team members.

Facilitates development of individualized discharge plan.

2 Procedure on day of discharge:

  a Let patient and family ask questions or discuss issues related to home care. A final opportunity to demonstrate learned skills is helpful.

Allows for final clarification of information previously discussed. Helps relieve anxiety.

  b Check health care provider's discharge orders for prescriptions, change in treatments, or need for special medical equipment. (Make sure that orders are written as early as possible.) Arrange for delivery and setup of equipment (e.g., hospital bed, oxygen) before patient arrives home.

Only a health care provider is able to authorize a discharge. Early check of orders permits nurse to attend to any last-minute treatments or procedures well before discharge.

  c Determine whether patient or family has arranged for transportation.

Patient's condition at discharge determines method of transport.

  d Provide privacy and assistance as patient dresses and packs all personal belongings. Check all closets and drawers for belongings. Obtain copy of valuables list signed by patient and have security or appropriate administrator deliver valuables to patient.

Prevents loss of personal items. Patient's signature verifies receipt of items and relieves nursing department of liability for losses.

  e Complete medication reconciliation per agency policy. Check discharge medication orders against the medication administration record and home medication list. Provide patient with prescriptions or pharmacy-dispensed medications ordered by health care provider. Offer a final review of information needed to facilitate safe medication self-administration.

Medication reconciliation decreases risk of medication errors and ensures that patient is receiving correct medication at home (TJC, 2012a). Review of drug information provides feedback to determine patient's success in learning about medications.

  f Provide information on follow-up appointments to health care provider's office. Provide phone number of unit.

Provides patient with contact for questions that arise after discharge. Ensures continuity of care to prevent rehospitalization.

  g Contact agency business office to determine whether patient needs to finalize arrangements for payment of bill. Arrange for patient or family to visit business office.

Source of concern for many patients is whether agency has accepted insurance or other payment forms.

  h Acquire utility cart to move patient's belongings. Obtain wheelchair for patient. Transport patients leaving by ambulance on ambulance stretchers.

Provides for safe transport.

  i Assist patient to wheelchair or stretcher using safe patient handling and transfer techniques (see Chapter 9). Escort patient to entrance of agency where source of transportation is waiting (see agency policy) (see illustrations). Lock wheelchair wheels. Assist patient in transferring into transport vehicle. Help place personal belongings in vehicle.

Prevents injury to nurse and patient. Agency policy requires escort to ensure patient's safe exit. Agency's liability ends once patient is safely in vehicle.

STEP	RATIONALE
j Return to division. Notify admitting or appropriate department of time of discharge. Notify housekeeping of need to clean patient's room.	Allows agency to prepare for admission of next patient.

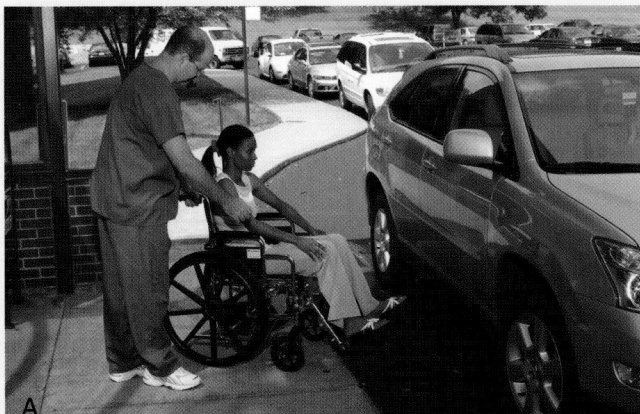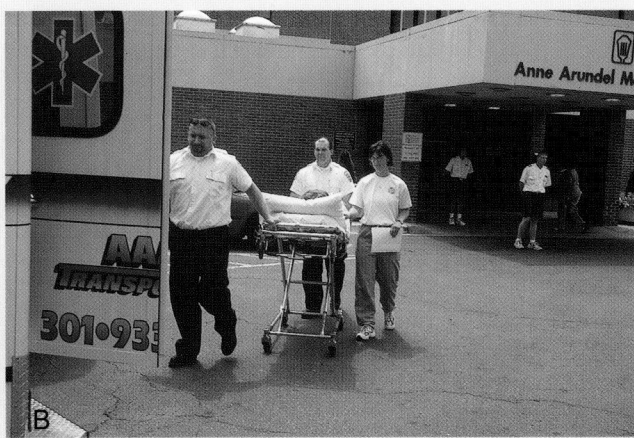

STEP 2i **A,** Nurse escorts patient to transport vehicle at time of discharge via a wheelchair. **B,** Many patients are discharged via stretcher.

EVALUATION

1 Ask patient or family member to describe nature of illness, treatment regimens, and physical signs or symptoms to be reported to a health care provider.	Measures patient's or family's learning.
2 Have patient or family member perform any treatments that will continue in the home.	Return demonstrations allow you to evaluate level of learning.
3 Home care nurse inspects home, identifies obstacles that pose risks for patient, and recommends revisions.	Provides continuity of care.

Unexpected Outcomes	Related Interventions
1 Patient or family is unable to explain self-care measures.	• Provide immediate clarification or offer additional instruction.
2 Patient or family demonstrates treatment measures incorrectly.	• Plan additional time to demonstrate treatment measures. • Ask patient to explain which aspect of procedure is difficult to perform and why. • If patient or family continues to be unable to correctly demonstrate treatment measures, request referral for home *care* services.
3 Environmental risks are still present in home.	• Reassess reason for changes not being implemented. • Home care nurse attempts to problem solve and seek appropriate solution.
4 Patient or family resists discharge plans and refuses assimilation of new roles needed for home care.	• Contact additional resources (e.g., social work, home care, pastoral care).
5 Patient refuses continued treatment and asks to leave the hospital before planned discharge.	• Talk with patient to determine reason for request to leave the hospital. Attempt to resolve the pressing issue for patient; involve family and social worker as appropriate. • Notify health care provider to talk with patient and explain the risks of leaving the hospital with unresolved health care needs and the benefits of continued treatment. • Inform patient that his or her health insurance provider may not pay for hospitalization as a result of leaving against medical advice (AMA). • Request that patient sign discharge AMA form documenting that he or she understands the risk involved in leaving. • Complete incident report and document thoroughly all communications/actions taken in attempt to have patient continue treatment (see Chapter 4).

Recording and Reporting

- Complete documentation of patient's discharge on discharge summary form (Box 2-6). Give patient a signed copy of form.
- Document unresolved problems and description of arrangements made for resolution in nurses' notes and electronic health record (EHR).
- Document patient's vital signs and status of health problems at time of discharge in nurses' notes and EHR.

BOX 2-6 | **Elements of a Written Discharge Summary Form**

- Mode of discharge: Ambulatory, wheelchair, stretcher
- Instructions for self-care activities: Activity, diet, medications, special treatments such as wound care, self-catheterization, tracheostomy care
- Reconciled list of discharge medications with dose, frequency, route, reasons for change in medication or for newly prescribed medications
- Signs and symptoms of complications or drug reactions for which to be observant
- Signs and symptoms that the patient should consider normal
- Correct settings for any equipment required
- Planned follow-up appointment at health care provider's office, clinic
- Name and contact information of health care provider and/or nursing unit
- Explanation of pertinent emergency procedures
- Patient's signature, showing understanding of instructions

Modified from Louden K: Creating a better discharge summary, *ACP Hospitalist* 3:1, 2009; National Quality Forum (NQF): *National voluntary consensus report, standards for public reporting of patient safety information: a consensus report,* Washington, DC, 2010, NQF.

Special Considerations
Teaching
- Assess patient's fatigue and pain levels before beginning any instruction. Keep focused on the important teaching topics to cover.

Pediatric
- Once family members have learned how to perform any necessary caregiver skills, have them assume care before child returns home. Many hospitals incorporate a trial period requiring family to manage care before child's discharge home (Hockenberry and Wilson, 2011).
- Discharge planning should be completed in partnership with children and parents. Over 80% of pediatric discharges are simple and do not require complex teaching or planning (Gibbens, 2010).

Gerontologic
- Older adults are interested in more information about community resources and social supports once discharged (Price, 2011).
- Older adults and their families often overestimate their ability to manage care after discharge. They also disagree about what postdischarge care includes. Make referrals to home care to address needs associated with functional decline and help prevent readmission to the hospital.

Home Care
- Assess availability and skill of primary family caregiver (e.g., spouse or friend): assess time availability, ability and willingness to give care, emotional and physical stamina, and knowledge of caregiving. Assess additional resources, including friends or neighbors who are available to help.
- Refer patients who meet the eligibility criteria to home care agencies for assistance.
- Inform patient or family member and patient's health care provider as to decision to accept or not accept patient for admission to home care agency.

⁇ Critical Thinking Exercises

Mrs. Hampton, a 68-year-old retired school teacher, is transferring from intensive care to your nursing unit following a cerebrovascular accident. She entered the ED 2 days ago with slurred speech and weakness of the right arm and leg. She has a history of primary hypertension, coronary artery disease, and type 2 diabetes mellitus. Her condition is stabilized. The intensive care nurse calls you to give a report on Mrs. Hampton. The nurse notes the admitting diagnosis, vital signs, pain level, and transferring health care provider's orders.

1 Which other information would you like to have about Mrs. Hampton?
2 The nurse arrives with Mrs. Hampton in a wheelchair; she is accompanied by her husband. Which interventions would you select to reduce Mr. and Mrs. Hampton's anxiety related to the transfer out of the intensive care unit?
3 Mr. Hampton states that his wife has an advance directive. What is the role of a nurse in understanding a patient's advance directive?
4 Mr. Hampton tells you that his wife is going home in a few days because she is doing so well. She will be going home using a walker. He says that he hopes he will be able to take care of her once she is at home. How do you respond to Mr. Hampton? Which interventions do you need to take before Mrs. Hampton's discharge?

✓ REVIEW QUESTIONS

1 In which of the following steps of the admission process can the admission personnel participate? (Select all that apply.)
  1 Explaining information about a patient's rights to health care services
  2 Attaching an ID band after verifying that the information is correct
  3 Reviewing the details of a patient's advance directive for clarity
  4 Explaining how HIPAA is enforced in the agency
  5 Printing a patient's allergies on the allergy band before attaching it to the patient
  6 Helping a patient know what is included in the basic admission process
2 Who is responsible for developing a patient's discharge plan?
  1 The primary nurse
  2 The medical social worker
  3 The nurse caring for the patient the longest
  4 The patient's health care team

3 Which statement *best* explains why it is essential to assess and document the clinical status of a patient immediately before transfer or at time of discharge?
  1 Increased reimbursement to the hospital occurs because of additional diagnosis codes.
  2 Potential changes in a patient's clinical needs may require nursing interventions to provide for patient safety during transport.
  3 Hospital documentation requirements could prevent transfer of a patient unless the information is current.
  4 The necessary information needs to be reflective of a discharge plan for visiting accrediting agencies.

4 A toddler is hospitalized for the first time. Which strategy is most effective to make the child feel more comfortable?
  1 Have the parents visit only sporadically so the toddler does not get upset.
  2 Have the child bring a favorite blanket for comfort.
  3 Ask the parents what time the toddler usually goes to bed.
  4 Find out the toddler's favorite foods and beverages.

5 You are caring for a hospitalized patient who requires transfer to a skilled nursing facility. Which of the following interventions *best* facilitates a referral to a skilled nursing facility?
  1 Providing teaching and instruction that supports the patient's continued independence
  2 Providing a variety of options for skilled care facilities to the patient and family
  3 Matching the services provided at the skilled care facility with the patient's needs
  4 Providing accurate information about the patient to the skilled care facility so nurses have a clear understanding of patient's needs

6 When completing an admission on a patient from a different culture, the nurse needs to:
  1 Speak slowly and clearly so the patient can understand the nurse.
  2 Respect the patient's health beliefs and customs.
  3 Get all information about the patient from the family members.
  4 Use common slang terms that the culture understands.

7 When a patient arrives on the nursing division for admission to his or her room, what is the first thing the nurse should do?
  1 Complete the admission assessment
  2 Orient the patient to the room
  3 Order all the patient's medication
  4 Complete all ordered diagnostic tests

8 You are caring for a patient in the ED who decides to leave without completion of his medical treatment. Which type of patient discharge should the nurse document?
  1 Against medical advice (AMA)
  2 Patient-initiated discharge (PID)
  3 Voluntary discharge (VD)
  4 Without physician or health care provider order (WPO)

9 _____ are nursing actions implemented to ensure coordination and continuity of care for patients who are transferring between different care settings or care levels.

10 When determining the health literacy of your patient before beginning discharge teaching, it is essential that the information is at which appropriate reading level?
  1 Sixth grade
  2 Tenth grade
  3 Fifth grade
  4 College level

REFERENCES

Blewett L and others: Improving geriatric transitional care through inter-professional care teams, *J Eval Clin Pract* 16:57, 2009.

Centers for Medicare and Medicaid Services: Chapter IV: Medicare and Medicaid Services, Department of Health and Human Services Centers, Part 482.43, Condition of participation, discharge planning, 2011, available at http://www.gpo.gov/fdsys/pkg/CFR-2011-title42-vol5/pdf/CFR-2011-title42-vol5-sec482-43.pdf, accessed August 28, 2012.

Giangiulio M and others: Initiation and evaluation of an admission, discharge, transfer (ADT) nursing program in a pediatric setting, *Issues Comprehensive Pediatr Nurs* 31:63, 2008.

Gibbens C: Nurse facilitated discharge for children and their families, *Paediatr Nurs* 22(1):14, 2010.

Giger JN: *Transcultural nursing: assessment and intervention*, ed 6, St Louis, 2013, Mosby.

Hockenberry MJ, Wilson D: *Wong's nursing care of infants and children*, ed 9, St Louis, 2011, Mosby.

Krautscheid L: Improving communication among healthcare providers: preparing student nurses for practice, *Int J Nurs Educ Scholarship* 5(1):10, 2008.

Kulik C: Components of a comprehensive fall risk assessment, *Am Nurs Today*, special supplement 6(2):6, 2011.

LaMantia M, et al: Interventions to improve transitional care between nursing homes and hospitals: a systematic review, *J Am Geriatr Soc* 58:77, 2010.

McLeod J, et al: Care transitions for older patients with musculoskeletal disorders: continuity from the providers' perspective, *Int J Integr Care* 18:1568, 2011.

Moorey S: Unplanned hospital admission: supporting children, young people, and their families, *Paediatr Nurs* 22(10):22, 2010.

Pope B, et al: Raising the SBAR: how better communication improves patient outcomes, *Nursing* 38(3):41, 2008.

Price B: How to map a patient's social support network, *Nurs Older People* 23(2):28, 2011.

Rose K, Haugen M: Discharge planning: your last chance to make a good impression, *MedSurg Nurs* 19(1):47, 2010.

Sobolewski S: The challenge of improving transitional care, *Home Healthc Nurse* 29(1):640, 2011.

The Joint Commission: *Advancing effective communication, cultural competence, and patient- and family-centered care: a roadmap for hospitals*, Oakbrook Terrace, 2011, The Commission.

The Joint Commission: *2012 Comprehensive accreditation manual for hospitals: the official handbook*, Chicago, Oakbrook Terrace, Ill, 2012a, The Commission.

The Joint Commission (TJC): *National Patient Safety Goals*, Oakbrook Terrace, Ill, 2012b, The Commission, available at http://www.jointcommission.org/standards_information/npsgs.aspx.

Touhy T, Jett K: *Ebersole and Hess' Gerontological nursing & healthy aging*, ed 3, St Louis, 2010, Mosby.

US Department of Health and Human Services: *Summary of the HIPAA privacy rule*, Washington, DC, 2003, Office for Civil Rights.

US Department of Health and Human Services: HIPAA privacy rule revisions on disclosures accounting, access reporting, *Fed Reg* 76:31426, 2011.

Communication

MEDIA RESOURCES

- **evolve** http://evolve.elsevier.com/Perry/skills
  learning system

  - Review Questions
  - Audio Glossary

KEY TERMS

Active listening	De-escalation	Paraphrasing	Termination phase
Cadence	Empathy	Reflecting	Therapeutic silence
Clarifying	Interviewing	Restating	Working phase
Comforting	Orientation phase	Summarizing	

OBJECTIVES

Mastery of content in this chapter will enable the nurse to:
- Identify guidelines to use in therapeutic communication.
- Explain the communication process.
- Identify the purposes of therapeutic communication, communication in various phases of the nurse-patient relationship, and special issues related to communication.

- Develop skills for therapeutic communication in various phases of the nurse-patient relationship.
- Develop therapeutic communication skills for communicating with anxious, angry, and depressed patients.
- Develop therapeutic communication skills for communication with cognitively impaired patients.

Effective communication positively influences nursing care. A nurse's responsibility to effectively communicate extends beyond the patient to include family members/significant others and members of the health care team. This chapter does not intend to give a complete introduction to the complicated process of communication. Rather the purpose is to provide a framework for you to develop therapeutic skills that are essential to the communication process.

Communication is an interaction between two or more persons that involves the exchange of information between a sender and a receiver (Fig. 3-1). It is an essential component of the human experience, involving the expression of emotions, ideas, and thoughts through verbal (words or written language) and nonverbal (behaviors) exchanges. Therapeutic communication is an application of the process of communication to promote the well-being of a patient.

Verbal communication includes both spoken and written words. To send an accurate message the sender of verbal communication needs to be aware of the tone, volume, and cadence (pace or rate) of his or her voice. In addition, he or she needs to be aware of cultural differences between sender

and receiver such as the use of dialect or slang. Other issues that the sender must consider with written communication include barriers such as the receiver's cognitive and visual impairments. In addition, consider the developmental perspectives of the receiver because these influence the method of communication used.

Nonverbal communication describes all behaviors that convey messages without the use of words. This type of communication includes body movement, physical appearance, personal space, and touch. As a nurse be aware of body language, which includes posture, body position, gestures, eye contact, facial expression, and movement (Fig. 3-2). For clarity make sure that nonverbal communication is consistent with the spoken word. When assessing a patient's needs, assess the nonverbal messages received from him or her and validate them. For example, if you observe a patient wringing her hands and sighing often, ask, "You seem anxious today. Is there anything on your mind?" You avoid problems in language behavior through the consistent use of clear, mutually understood verbal terminology and nonverbal gestures. To avoid misinterpretation of nonverbal cues, be aware of any cultural

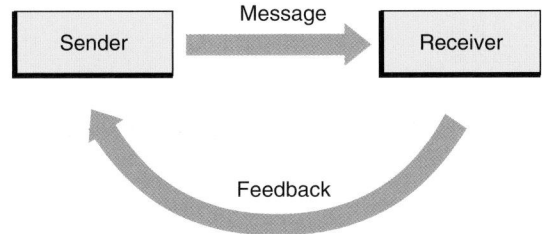

FIG 3-1   Communication is a two-way process.

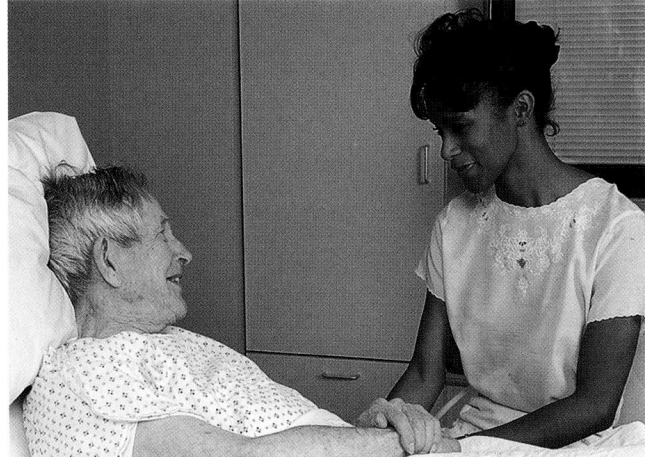

FIG 3-2   An open, relaxed posture conveys interest.

norms or values (e.g., eye contact) that patients may have (see Skill 3-1).

Therapeutic communication is essential for excellent nursing practice. Nurses use communication skills in caring for patients by providing information and comfort, promoting understanding, clarifying misinformation, assisting in developing plans of care, and facilitating wellness through patient teaching. The nurse-patient relationship promotes a connection, which is an essential component of the healing process.

EVIDENCE-BASED PRACTICE

Effective therapeutic communication with patients across the life span is essential for successful nursing practice. Research identifies the following health outcomes as a result of effective therapeutic communication: empowerment, control of chronic disease, satisfaction with care, and improved quality of life (Rohrer et al., 2008). Nurse researchers and clinicians have developed creative modes of communicating with patients. For example, when interacting with patients with severe communication impairments, nurses can use augmentative and assistive communication (AAC). These include use of unaided AAC techniques (e.g., hands, face, and/or feet) and manual sign language, pantomime, gestures, and eye-blink systems. Aided AAC techniques include use of picture books, alphabet books, and pencil and paper systems (Finke et al., 2008). The nurse must initially determine the best mode of communication for a particular patient. The goal of any AAC technique is for patients with complex communication needs to effectively engage in interactions with nurses, family members, and other members of the health care team. Recommendations made from these studies underscore the need for nurses to improve and increase their efforts to communicate with these patients; they

need to be creative in their use of strategies. Nurses should receive adequate training in use of these AAC strategies and understand the implications of communication impairment. Research demonstrates the importance of being persistent in trying to communicate with such patients; allow for sufficient time for a patient to respond and pay close attention to nonverbal responses. In addition, it is essential to maintain a quiet environment. The use of these strategies can facilitate a successful nurse-patient interaction.

Managing patients with behavioral and/or cognitive impairments requires communication skills to assess and redirect patients and modify any negative behaviors. Effective communication is essential to the quality of life and well-being of patients (Boschart, 2009). Research shows that use of specific behavior-management strategies effectively reduces agitation and improves interactions with patients having difficulty with comprehension.

- Use role play and emphasize empathy.
- Use problem-free conversations and support strategies to demonstrate concern for patients.
- Frame brief interventions in a positive manner.
- Use video training programs in teaching communication strategies to nurses who interact with patients who have communication difficulties (Miller, 2008).
- Use therapeutic communication techniques to de-escalate a patient's anxiety or anger.

Communicating effectively with children with visual impairments and other disabilities poses a challenge for nurses (Parker et al., 2008). These children often lack access to powerful visual nonverbal cues such as facial expressions and gestures. To improve children's communication skills use:

- Microswitch interventions (supportive speech-output programs).
- Multicomponent partner training (tactile sign language, touch cues).
- Dual communication boards.
- Object symbols and adult-directed prompting and reinforcement.

This study provides evidence that children with impairments can develop functional communication skills if they are given intensive, consistent communication interventions and a mechanism for self-expression (Parker et al., 2008).

PATIENT-CENTERED CARE

Patient-centered care improves communication, promotes patient involvement in care, creates a positive relationship with health care providers, and results in improved adherence to treatment regimens. This strategy respects patients' beliefs and values about health and illness, including those of culturally diverse patients. In addition, patient-centered care includes patients and significant others in collaboration with health care providers to make decisions related to wellness and illness care. Benefits include improved satisfaction with care, self-efficacy and empowerment to manage care, and quality of life (Murphy, 2011; Robinson et al., 2008; Tucker et al., 2011).

The Quality and Safety Education for Nurses (QSEN) initiative includes specific quality and safety outcomes that are required of nurses to practice safely and effectively in complex health care systems (McKeon et al., 2009). The American Association of Colleges of Nursing (AACN) has recommended that students learn these patient-centered care competencies through teaching strategies such as unfolding case studies and simulation. Computer-based simulation is a recommended strategy to teach safe clinical practice. A study that examined the effectiveness of computer-based simulation compared to traditional simulation in teaching patient-centered competencies for prelicensure nursing students found that students in both groups achieved similar competencies (McKeon et al., 2009).

Nurses face challenges when communicating with culturally and linguistically diverse patients. Effective communication between culturally diverse patients and nurses is essential to improving health outcomes. Furthermore, patient-centered care has been described as one approach to cultural competency education to guide health care providers to deliver respectful care that is responsive to patient preferences (Wilkerson et al., 2010). The following skills are necessary for using a patient-centered approach: the ability to elicit a patient's personal story, explore health beliefs and practices, and negotiate a health care management plan that is respectful of these preferences. In addition, it is also helpful to speak plainly; avoid mimicking a patient's accent or dialect. Understand that members of certain cultures use cultural phrases or slang common to their culture and this is not an indication they do not understand English.

When you communicate with patients of diverse cultures, an interpreter is sometimes necessary. A lack of attention to language barriers can lead to poor-quality communication and poor health outcomes (Bischoff and Hudelson, 2010). It is important to use trained medical interpreters rather than relying on bilingual colleagues or a patient's family or friends. The reliance on untrained interpreters has been associated with poor quality of health care and breaches of confidentiality. In the United States hospitals must follow requirements for providing culturally and linguistically appropriate health care to patients. When using an interpreter, address the patient and family directly; do not direct questions or comments to the interpreter. Take care to determine if the patient understood. Speak slowly in normal tones and avoid overly technical jargon or terms unique to a culture (Box 3-1). Adopting a flexible, respectful attitude that also communicates interest in the patient bridges any communication barriers that exist because of cultural differences between patient and caregiver.

Safety Guidelines

1 Listen to what and how a patient communicates, including content and verbal and nonverbal messages. Some patients express themselves clearly without difficulty. However, indirect and nonverbal cues communicate a patient's needs.

BOX 3-1 Special Approaches for Patients Who Speak Different Languages

- Use a caring tone of voice and facial expressions to help alleviate patients' fears and anxieties.
- Speak slowly and distinctly but not loudly.
- Use gestures, pictures, and role playing to help patients understand.
- Repeat a message in different ways if necessary.
- Be alert to and use words that a patient seems to understand and use them frequently.
- Keep messages simple and repeat them frequently.
- Avoid using medical terms that a patient may not understand.
- Use an appropriate language dictionary or have a medical interpreter or family member make flash cards to communicate key phrases.

From Giger J: *Transcultural nursing: assessment and interventions*, ed 6, St Louis, 2013, Mosby.

2 Know your attitudes toward the patient or situation. You need to be aware of your personal feelings to control how you communicate issues. Being unaware of personal feelings may lead to negative consequences in communication.

3 Control external factors in both the environmental setting (temperature of room, privacy issues) and the psychological setting (emotional state of the nurse and patient) that influence or hinder communication. When you are talking with a patient about his or her personal concerns, privacy is important. When teaching, try to have a family member/significant other present with whom to reinforce the content of the instruction. If a patient is experiencing subjective distress in the form of pain or anxiety, take measures to minimize these subjective experiences. Controlling noise level and interruptions is also important.

4 Establish and understand the purpose of interaction. This is an essential quality of effective communication. Without this quality communication is casual and superficial.

5 Guide the interaction, depending on the patient's condition and response. Patient needs remain the focus. For example, you establish that the purpose of the interaction is patient teaching; however, the patient just learned about the death of a loved one and expresses the need to talk about the death. You assist the patient by grieving first, remaining flexible and creative in the interaction.

SKILL 3-1 Establishing the Nurse-Patient Relationship

A therapeutic nurse-patient relationship is the foundation of nursing care and involves using patient-centered therapeutic communication skills. Communication is essential in nursing since effective communication among patients, families, and health care providers is central to quality care (Majerovitz et al., 2009). The primary goal of therapeutic communication for the nurse is to promote wellness and personal growth in patients. Therapeutic communication empowers patients to make decisions but differs from social communication in that it is patient centered and goal directed with limited disclosure from the professional.

Social communication involves equal opportunity for personal disclosure, and both participants seek to have personal needs met (Keltner et al., 2011). Nurses do not share intimate details of their personal lives with patients. However, they use personal self-disclosure (e.g., outside interests, thoughts about local news, experience as a nurse) cautiously in selected situations. Personal

self-disclosure is useful for the following goals: (1) to educate patients, (2) to build therapeutic alliances with patients, and (3) to encourage patients' independence (Fortinash and Holoday-Worret, 2008). For example, you share selected personal thoughts and life experiences with a patient to show that you understand what the patient is experiencing.

Skills essential to therapeutic communication include active listening, broad openings, humor, sharing perceptions, clarifying, focusing, informing, paraphrasing, reflecting, restating, summarizing, suggesting, using therapeutic silence, and using open-ended statements/questions. Most of these skills are defined with case illustrations identifying therapeutic and nontherapeutic examples of their use (Box 3-2). Paraphrasing is another skill that involves restating a patient's original message by transforming the message into your own words without losing the meaning. You achieve empathy in communication through the use of all the

BOX 3-2	Therapeutic Communication Techniques

Technique: Listening

Definition: An active process of receiving information and examining one's reaction to messages received

Example: Consider the cultural practice of your patient, maintain appropriate eye contact, and be receptive to nonverbal communications

Therapeutic Value: Nonverbally communicates nurse's interest and acceptance to patient

Nontherapeutic Threat: Failure to listen, interrupting patient

Technique: Broad Openings

Definition: Encouraging patient to select topics for discussion

Example: "What are you thinking about?"

Therapeutic Value: Indicates acceptance by nurse and value of patient's initiative

Nontherapeutic Threat: Domination of interaction by nurse; rejecting responses

Technique: Restating

Definition: Repeating main thought that patient has expressed

Example: "You say that your mother left you when you were 5 years old."

Therapeutic Value: Indicates that nurse is listening and validates, reinforces, or calls attention to something important that has been said

Nontherapeutic Threat: Lack of validation of nurse's interpretation of message; being judgmental; reassuring; defending

Technique: Clarification

Definition: Attempting to improve the nurses' understanding of words, vague ideas, or the patient's unclear thoughts or asking patient to explain what he or she means

Example: "I'm not sure what you mean. Could you tell me again?"

Therapeutic Value: Helps to clarify patient's feelings, ideas, and perceptions and provide an explicit correlation between them and the patient's actions

Nontherapeutic Threat: Failure to probe; assumed understanding

Technique: Reflection

Definition: Directing back to patient ideas, feelings, questions, or content

Example: "You're feeling tense and anxious, and it's related to a conversation you had with your sister last night?"

Therapeutic Value: Validates nurse's understanding of what patient is saying and signifies empathy, interest, and respect for patient

Nontherapeutic Threat: Stereotyping patient's responses, inappropriate timing of reflections; inappropriate depth of feeling of reflections; inappropriate to the cultural experience and educational level of the patient

Technique: Humor

Definition: Discharging energy through comic enjoyment of the imperfect

Example: "This gives a whole new meaning to 'Just relax.'"

Therapeutic Value: Can promote insight by making conscious repressed material, resolving paradoxes, tempering aggression, and revealing new options; is a socially acceptable form of sublimation

Nontherapeutic Threat: Indiscriminate use; belittling patient; screen to avoid therapeutic intimacy

Technique: Informing

Definition: Demonstrating skills or giving information

Example: "I think it would be helpful for you to know more about how your medication works."

Therapeutic Value: Helpful in patient education about relevant aspects of patient's well-being and self-care

Nontherapeutic Threat: Giving advice

Technique: Focusing

Definition: Asking questions or making statements that help patient expand on a topic of importance

Example: "I think it would be helpful if we talk more about your relationship with your father."

Therapeutic Value: Allows patient to discuss central issues related to problem and keeps communication process goal directed

Nontherapeutic Threat: Allowing abstractions and generalizations; changing topics

Technique: Sharing Perceptions

Definition: Asking patient to verify nurse's understanding of what patient is thinking or feeling

Example: "You're smiling, but I sense that you're really very angry with me."

Therapeutic Value: Conveys nurse's understanding to patient and has potential for clearing up confusing communication

Nontherapeutic Threat: Challenging patient; accepting literal responses; reassuring; testing; defending

Technique: Theme Identification

Definition: Clarifying underlying issues or problems experienced by patient that emerge repeatedly during nurse-patient relationship

Example: "I've noticed that in all the relationships that you've described you've been hurt or rejected by the man. Do you think this is an underlying issue?"

Therapeutic Value: Allows nurse to best promote patient's exploration and understanding of important problems

Nontherapeutic Threat: Giving advice; reassuring; disapproving

Technique: Silence

Definition: Using silence or nonverbal communication for a therapeutic reason

Example: Sitting with patient and nonverbally communicating interest and involvement

Therapeutic Value: Allows patient time to think and gain insights, slows the pace of the interaction, and encourages patient to initiate conversation while conveying nurse's support, understanding, and acceptance

Nontherapeutic Threat: Questioning patient: asking for "why" responses; failing to break a nontherapeutic silence

Technique: Suggesting

Definition: Presenting alternative ideas for patient's consideration relative to problem solving

Example: "Have you thought about responding to your boss in a different way when he raises that issue with you? For example, you could ask him whether a specific problem has occurred."

Therapeutic Value: Increases patient's perceived options or choices.

Nontherapeutic Threat: Giving advice, inappropriate timing; being judgmental

Modified from Keltner N et al: *Psychiatric nursing*, ed 6, St Louis, 2011, Mosby.

aforementioned skills. Empathy is being sensitive and understanding of a patient's feelings and communicating this understanding to the patient. It differs from sympathy in that sympathy is nonobjective and noncritical.

Barriers to therapeutic communication include giving an opinion, offering false reassurance, being defensive, showing approval or disapproval, stereotyping, and asking, "Why?" The use of "why" questions causes increased defensiveness in patients and hinders communication. The therapeutic nurse-patient relationship is goal directed, with a patient moving toward productive modes of interpersonal functioning. Three overlapping phases characterize the nurse-patient relationship: orientation, working, and termination. The orientation phase involves learning about the patient and any initial concerns and needs. During orientation you clarify your role and that of other health care providers, establish rapport with the patient, collect information, establish goals, and clarify misunderstandings. When the orientation phase is successful and the patient is ready, work toward effective goal attainment begins with the working phase of the nurse-patient relationship. The termination phase consists of evaluation and summary of progress toward prescribed goals. Prepare for termination generally at the beginning of a patient relationship. You must communicate effectively with patients throughout all three phases of the nurse-patient relationship.

Delegation and Collaboration

All health care providers must practice effective communication. The skill of establishing therapeutic communication cannot be delegated to nursing assistive personnel (NAP). The NAP observes and receives information from patients because of the length of time they are with patients. The nurse directs the NAP about:

- The proper way to interact verbally and nonverbally with select patients.
- Ways to arrange the environment to ensure privacy and confidentiality.
- Special considerations pertaining to communication with patients who are cognitively or sensorially impaired, older children, and anxious and potentially violent patients.

STEP	RATIONALE

ASSESSMENT

1 The first contact a nurse has with a patient occurs during the orientation phase. Address patient by name and introduce self and role on health care team ("Hello, my name is Sally Regan, and I am the registered nurse assigned to take care of you today. …") Use clear, specific communication (verbal and nonverbal) to provide information and clarify concerns.

Congruent verbal and nonverbal communication expresses warmth and respect and helps to establish rapport. Clear, specific communication decreases confusion and anxiety and improves the quality of health care (O'Halloran et al., 2009).

2 Assess the following behaviors: patient's needs, coping strategies, defenses, and adaptation styles.

Recurrent themes in patient's response help to identify problem areas related to health status (e.g., avoidance of questions, request for information, expression of a loss).

3 Determine patient's need to communicate (e.g., constant use of call light, crying, patient who does not understand an illness or who has just been admitted).

Patients in need of support, comfort, knowledge, or encouragement benefit from meaningful communication.

4 Assess reason patient needs health care.

Nature of illness affects patient's coping ability and effectiveness in communicating needs and concerns.

5 Assess factors about self and patient that normally influence communication: perceptions, values, and beliefs; emotions; sociocultural background; severity of illness; knowledge; age; verbal ability; roles and relationships; environmental setting; physical comfort or discomfort (see illustration).

Communication is a dynamic process influenced by interpersonal and intrapersonal processes. By assessing factors that influence communication, you can more accurately assess a patient's perception of health status (Rohrer et al., 2008).

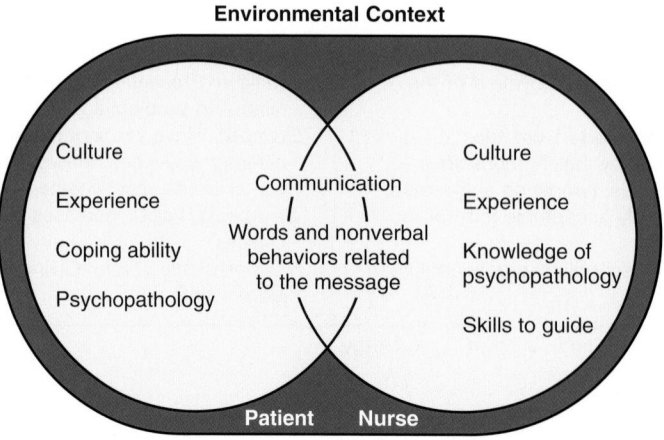

STEP 5   Essential and influencing variables of the therapeutic communication environment. *(Modified from Keltner N et al: Psychiatric nursing, ed 6, St Louis, 2011, Mosby.)*

STEP	RATIONALE

6 Assess personal barriers to communicating with patient (e.g., bias toward patient's condition, anxiety from inexperience).

Barriers prevent you from conveying empathy and caring and obtaining relevant assessment information.

7 Assess patient's language and ability to speak. Does patient have difficulty finding words or associating ideas with accurate word symbols? Does patient have difficulty with expression of language and/or reception of messages? What is patient's primary language?

Assessment determines need for special communication techniques (e.g., picture boards, aids such as a medical interpreter) (see illustration).

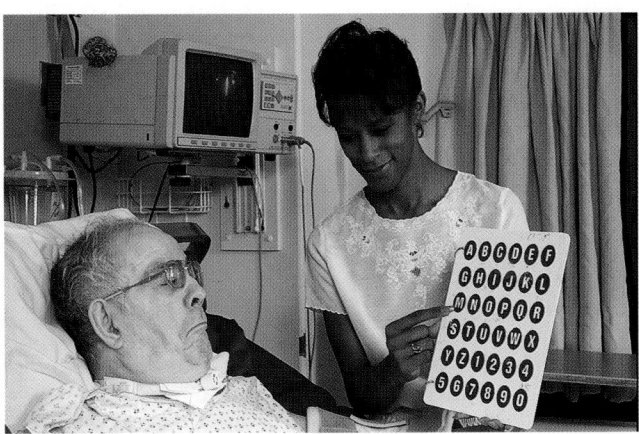

STEP 7   Communication tools for patient who cannot speak.

8 Assess patient's literacy level. Does he or she skip over uncommon or hard word, avoid asking questions, or have difficulty discussing concepts about illness? *Option:* use a standardized instrument such as the Rapid Estimate of Adult Literacy in Medicine (REALM) (Davis et al., 1993) or the Test of Functional Health Literacy in Adults (TOFHLA) (Parker et al., 1995).

Health literacy has a direct effect on health outcomes. Assessing patient's level of health literacy allows you to design more effective communication and teaching approaches.

9 Assess patient's ability to hear. Be sure that hearing aid is functional if worn. Be sure that patient hears and understands words (see Chapter 6).

Patients with hearing deficits require techniques to enhance hearing reception (e.g., speaking in normal tone, speaking so patient can see face).

10 Observe patient's pattern of communication and verbal or nonverbal behavior (e.g., gestures, tone of voice, eye contact).

Observation determines type of and manner of communication that you will use.

11 Assess resources available in selecting communication methods:

  a Review information in medical record and consider your past experience.

Relying totally on information from patient restricts the quality of interaction. Additional resources provide insight into best methods of communicating.

  b Consult with family, health care provider, and other health care team members concerning patient's condition, problems, and impressions.

Collaboration with health care team members facilitates your response to patient based on integration of knowledge. Seek information from family after patient approval. Patient privacy must be maintained.

12 Before initiating the working phase of nurse-patient relationship, assess patient's readiness to work toward goal attainment.

Patient's goals are identified and agreed on by effective communication skills such as restating and clarifying.

13 Consider when patient is due to be discharged or transferred from health care agency.

This allows you to anticipate the amount of time available to work with patient and when termination of relationship is to occur.

NURSING DIAGNOSES

- Anxiety
- Deficient knowledge
- Fear

- Impaired social interaction
- Impaired verbal communication
- Ineffective coping

- Noncompliance
- Readiness for enhanced decision making

Related factors are individualized based on patient's condition or needs.

STEP	RATIONALE

PLANNING

1 Expected outcomes following completion of procedure:

- Patient expresses ideas, fears, and concerns clearly and openly with relief of anxiety.
- Patient health care goals are identified and achieved.
- Patient verbalizes understanding of information communicated by nurse.

Once patients are able to talk directly about emotions, the focus is on coping more effectively with them (Keltner et al., 2011). Interaction remains patient focused.

This provides a means to build trust and develop a knowledge base for patient to make decisions.

2 Orientation phase

a Prepare by providing a warm and accepting environment, establishing trust, formulating individualized patient goals, considering time allocation, formulating initial questions, and mentally preparing to keep one's mind clear of other concerns or distractions.

Preparation is part of planned process that facilitates communication and interaction. Planning for orientation phase assists in identifying actual or potential problems, current health status, and experience. Without preparation, a risk exists of casual, nongoal-oriented communication.

b Prepare patient and environment physically: provide a quiet environment, maintain privacy, reduce distractions or interruptions, and take care of patient's physical needs (e.g., comfort or hygiene) before beginning discussion.

Taking care of basic needs promotes an environment for interaction and decreases patient distractions and interruptions.

3 Working phase

a Use open-ended questions to identify strategies to develop a realistic plan to meet identified health goals of patients (e.g., "Tell me about your goals for this hospitalization/visit to the health care agency").

Open-ended questions promote goal attainment and avoid risk of misinterpretation.

4 Termination phase

a Prepare by identifying methods of summarizing and synthesizing information pertinent for aftercare (e.g., "What are your plans for follow-up to maintain your health status?").

Effective communication by summarizing and synthesizing information reinforces behavior change.

IMPLEMENTATION

1 Orientation Phase: Establish the nurse-patient relationship.

a Create a climate of warmth and acceptance. Be aware of nonverbal cues, both sent and received. Provide comfort and support to patient.

This facilitates open exchange without fear or anxiety.

b Use appropriate nonverbal behaviors (e.g., good eye contact, open relaxed position, sitting eye level with patient [see Fig. 3-2]).

Appropriate nonverbal behaviors facilitate communication by providing a nonverbal message that shows interest in what patient has to say.

c Observe patient's nonverbal behaviors, including body language. If verbal behaviors do not match nonverbal behaviors, seek clarification from patient.

Congruence between patient's verbal and nonverbal behaviors ensures that you receive the correct message.

d Explain purpose of interaction when information is to be shared.

Information and explanation can decrease anxiety about the unknown.

e Use active listening.

Active listening conveys interest in the patient's needs, concerns, and problems; conveys empathy.

f Identify patient's expectations in seeking health care.

Identifying expectations conveys a level of interest in patient's needs.

g Interview patient about health status, lifestyle, support systems, patterns of health and illness, and strengths and limitations.

Interview facilitates a positive nurse-patient relationship and the development of trust, putting the patient at ease.

h Encourage patient to ask for clarification at any time during the communication.

This gives patient a sense of control and keeps channels of communication open.

i Use therapeutic communication techniques when interacting with patient (refer to Box 3-2).

Techniques establish a greater understanding of messages sent and received.

2 Working Phase: Set mutual goals.

a Use therapeutic communication skills such as restating, reflecting, and paraphrasing to identify and clarify strategies for attainment of mutually agreed-on goals.

For communication between nurse and patient to be effective, both need to possess the skills and knowledge required for participation within the communicative interaction (Finke et al., 2008).

b Discuss and prioritize problem areas.

A patient, nonjudgmental, supportive approach minimizes patient anxiety.

STEP	RATIONALE
c Provide information to patient and help him or her to express needs and feelings.	Patient is able to respond to help, develop workable solutions based on goals, and fully participate in a realistic plan for his or her well-being.
d Use questions carefully and appropriately. Ask one question at a time and allow sufficient time to answer. Use direct questions. Use open-ended statements as much as possible such as, "Tell me about how you are feeling today."	This helps patient to express self and allows you to obtain thorough information about patient's needs and concerns.

Clinical Decision Point *Avoid asking questions about information that may not yet have been disclosed to the patient (e.g., human immunodeficiency virus [HIV] status, diagnostic test results). Avoid asking "why" questions; this causes increased defensiveness in the patient and prevents communication.*

STEP	RATIONALE
e Avoid communication barriers.	Barriers result in a message not being received, being distorted, or not being understood.
3 Termination Phase: Communicate with the patient.	
a Use therapeutic communication skills to discuss discharge or termination issues and guide discussion related to specific patient changes in thoughts and behaviors.	Communication skills reinforce behaviors/skills learned during working phase of relationship.
b Summarize with patient what you discussed during interaction, including goal achievement.	Signals the close of interaction and allows you and patient to depart with the same idea. Provides a sense of closure and mutual understanding.

EVALUATION

1 Observe patient's verbal and nonverbal responses to your communication, noting his or her willingness to share information and concerns during orientation phase.	Verbal and nonverbal feedback reveals patient's interest and willingness to communicate and reflects patient's ability to form a therapeutic relationship.
2 Note your response to patient and patient's response to you. Reflect on effectiveness of therapeutic techniques used in establishing rapport with patient.	Sensitivity to one's ability in using therapeutic communication skills helps improve ability to adjust techniques when necessary.
3 During working phase evaluate patient's ability to work toward identified goals. Elicit feedback (verbal and nonverbal) to determine success of goal attainment. Evaluate patient's health status in relation to identified goals. Reevaluate and identify barriers if patient goals are not met.	Feedback is an essential step in evaluating new behaviors. Modifications are necessary if goals cannot be met.
4 During termination phase summarize and restate. Reinforce patient's strengths, outline issues still requiring work, and develop an action plan.	Evaluates patient progress in terms of attainment of mutually agreed-on goals.

Unexpected Outcomes	Related Interventions
1 Patient verbally and nonverbally expresses feelings of anxiety, fear, anger, confusion, distrust, and helplessness. Patient often responds to internal and external factors and cues.	• Reassess patient's level of anxiety, fear, and distrust. Attempt to determine the cause of anxiety or fear. • Repeat message to patient at a later time. • Determine influence affecting clear communication (e.g., cultural issues, literacy issues, physical limitations).
2 Feedback between nurse and patient reveals a lack of understanding and ineffective communication. Barriers to communication exist.	• Assess for and remove barriers to communication. • Repeat message using another approach if possible. • Consider cultural norms associated with eye contact, use of touch, personal space, and nonverbal behaviors. • Avoid using medical terms that patient does not understand.
3 Nurse's personal issues interfere with establishment of a therapeutic nurse-patient relationship.	• Appropriately adjust communication style (e.g., be nonjudgmental, patient, and understanding). • Use special approaches (gesture, pictures, role playing) for patients who have communication impairments.
4 Nurse is unable to acquire information about patient's ideas, fears, and concerns. Communication techniques do not promote patient's willingness to communicate openly. Trust is not established. Goals are not identified and therefore cannot be achieved.	• Use alternative communication techniques to promote patient's willingness to communicate openly. • Offer another professional with whom patient can talk to obtain necessary information.

Recording and Reporting

- Record in nurses' notes and electronic health record (EHR) the communication pertinent to patient's health, response to illness or therapies, and responses that demonstrate understanding or lack of understanding (include verbal and nonverbal cues).
- Report any relevant information obtained through patient's verbal and nonverbal behaviors to members of health care team.

Special Considerations

Teaching

- Use gestures, pictures, and role playing to help patient understand. Be alert to literacy status; determine if patient is able to access health information adequately. Be alert to words that patient seems to understand and use them frequently.
- Individualize patient teaching to meet patient needs. Always conduct teaching toward meeting patient's learning needs with consideration for his or her preferred methods for learning.

Pediatric

- Communicating with children requires an understanding of feelings and thought processes from the child's perspective (Hockenberry and Wilson, 2011).
- Use vocabulary that is familiar to the child, based on his or her level of understanding (age and developmental level). Try to be on same eye level as patient.

- Understand the child's cognitive, developmental, and functional level to select most appropriate communication techniques. Some age-appropriate communication techniques include storytelling and drawing (Hockenberry and Wilson, 2011).

Gerontologic

- Be aware of any cognitive or sensory impairment. Assess each patient individually and avoid stereotyping older adults who have cognitive or sensory impairments.
- It is important to understand the value of effective communication skills, history, and personality among older adults in terms of providing both human and therapeutic responses. Regression to earlier defenses is normal and adaptive with this population, particularly when facing illness.
- Make sure that older-adult patient with visual or hearing impairment uses assistive devices such as eyeglasses, large-print reading material, or hearing aids to assist in communication.

Home Care

- Identify primary family caregiver for patient and adapt techniques to assess level of understanding regarding his or her condition.
- Incorporate communication into patient's daily activities (e.g., bathing and dressing).

SKILL 3-2 Communicating with an Anxious Patient

Patients in the health care setting sometimes experience anxiety for a variety of reasons. A newly diagnosed illness, separation from loved ones, threat associated with diagnostic tests or surgical procedures, and expectations of life changes are just a few factors that cause anxiety. How successfully a patient copes with anxiety depends in part on previous experiences, the presence of other stressors, the significance of the event causing anxiety, and the availability of supportive resources. You can be a support to patients and help to decrease their anxiety through effective communication. Communication methods reviewed in this skill assist you in helping an anxious patient to clarify factors causing anxiety and cope more effectively. There are four stages of anxiety with corresponding behavioral manifestations: mild, moderate, severe, and panic (Box 3-3).

BOX 3-3	Behavioral Manifestations of Anxiety: Stages of Anxiety

Mild Anxiety
- Increased auditory and visual perception
- Increased awareness of relationships
- Increased alertness
- Able to problem solve

Moderate Anxiety
- Selective inattention
- Decreased perceptual field
- Focus only on relevant information
- Muscle tension; diaphoresis

Severe Anxiety
- Focus on fragmented details
- Headache, nausea, dizziness
- Unable to see connections between details
- Poor recall

Panic State of Anxiety
- Does not notice surroundings
- Feeling of terror
- Unable to cope with any problem

Delegation and Collaboration

The skill of communicating with an anxious patient cannot be delegated to nursing assistive personnel (NAP). The NAP may interact with anxious patients and must know how to respond and what to observe and report to the nurse. The nurse instructs the NAP about:

- The basic communication skills needed to interact verbally and nonverbally with anxious patients.
- The reason for a patient's anxiety.

STEP	RATIONALE

ASSESSMENT

1 Provide a brief, simple introduction; introduce yourself and explain purpose of interaction.	Anxiety limits amount of information patient can understand.
2 Assess for physical, behavioral, and verbal cues that indicate that patient is anxious such as dry mouth, sweaty palms, tone of voice, frequent use of call light, difficulty concentrating, wringing of hands, and statements such as, "I'm scared."	Anxiety interferes with usual manner of communication and thus interferes with patient's care and treatment. Extreme anxiety interferes with comprehension, attention, and problem-solving abilities.

STEP	RATIONALE
3 Assess for possible factors causing patient anxiety (e.g., hospitalization, unknown diagnosis, fatigue).	Understanding the source of anxiety assists in patient support and communication.
4 Assess factors influencing communication with patient (e.g., environment, timing, presence of others, values, experiences, need for personal space because of heightened anxiety).	Assessment helps to identify effective communication strategies.
5 Discuss with family members the possible causes of patient's anxiety.	Gathering information about patient from a family perspective is useful because family may provide new information or understanding of the situation (Keltner et al., 2011).

NURSING DIAGNOSES

- Anxiety
- Deficient knowledge
- Decisional conflict

- Fear
- Defensive coping
- Impaired social interaction

- Impaired verbal communication
- Ineffective coping

Related factors are individualized based on patient's condition or needs.

PLANNING

1 Expected outcomes following completion of procedure:	
• Patient will sense less anxiety during interactions with nurse.	Patient gains resources (e.g., use of deep-breathing exercises, guided imagery) to cope with stressor(s).
• Patient is able to discuss area of concern.	Communication techniques ease anxiety and allow patient to focus on problem.

Clinical Decision Point *First acknowledge and take care of anxious patient's physical and emotional discomfort but avoid dwelling on physical complaints. Focus on understanding patient, providing feedback and assisting in problem solving, and providing atmosphere of warmth and acceptance.*

2 Prepare for communication by considering the following: patient goals, time allocation, and resources.	Allows patient to establish rapport, achieve a sense of calm, and begin to analyze source of anxiety.
3 Recognize personal level of anxiety and consciously try to remain calm (breathe slowly and deeply, relax pelvic floor muscles). Be aware of nonverbal cues that indicate own anxiety (e.g., body language, posture, cadence of speech).	Your anxiety increases patient's anxiety.
4 Prepare a quiet, calm area, allowing ample personal space.	Decreasing stimuli has a calming effect. Invasion of personal space increases anxiety.

IMPLEMENTATION

1 Use appropriate nonverbal behaviors and active listening skills such as staying with patient at bedside and having a relaxed posture.	Nonverbal messages to patient express interest and help to alleviate anxiety.
2 Use appropriate verbal techniques that are clear and concise to respond to anxious patient. Use brief statements that acknowledge current state of feelings and provide direction to patient such as, "It seems to me that you're anxious" or "I notice that you seem anxious. Would you like to go to your room to rest?"	Appropriate techniques and statements provide reassurance and prevent further escalation of anxiety.
3 Help patient acquire alternative coping strategies such as progressive relaxation, slow deep-breathing exercises, and visual imagery (see Chapter 15).	Coping mechanisms provide foundation for effective communication so patient can explore causes of anxiety and steps to alleviate anxious feelings.
4 Provide necessary comfort measures.	Pain heightens patient's anxiety.

EVALUATION

1 Observe for continuing presence of physical signs and symptoms or behaviors reflecting anxiety.	Observation determines extent to which planned interaction relieved patient's anxiety.
2 Have patient discuss ways to cope with anxiety in the future and make decisions about own care.	This measures patient's ability to assume more health-promoting behavior.
3 Evaluate patient's ability to discuss factors causing anxiety.	This measures patient's ability to attend or focus on area of concern.

STEP	RATIONALE

Unexpected Outcomes

1 Physical signs and symptoms of anxiety continue. Your interaction has increased patient's anxiety; source of anxiety is not resolved.

2 Patient displays difficulty in decision making by avoiding your efforts at focusing discussion or is unable to discuss real concerns. Anxiety continues to prevent problem solving.

3 Anxiety continues to escalate.

Related Interventions

- Use refocusing or distraction skills such as relaxation or guided imagery to reduce anxiety (Fortinash and Holoday-Worret, 2008).

- Be clear and direct when communicating with patient to avoid misunderstanding.
- When used appropriately, touch helps control feelings of panic.

- Continue to use previous steps.
- Be very direct and clear when making requests. If patient needs to deal with stimulus causing anxiety, reintroduce when he or she is less anxious.
- Although touch is therapeutic, it requires individualized assessment of patient's anxiety level and need for personal space; some patients perceive this as threatening. When used appropriately, reassurance through human touch helps to control feelings of panic.
- As a last resort administer an antianxiety medication (per orders).

Recording and Reporting
- Record in nurses' notes and EHR cause of patient's anxiety and any exhibited signs and symptoms of behaviors.
- Report methods used to relieve anxiety and patient's response to ensure continuity of care between nurses.

Special Considerations
Teaching
- Teaching patient to identify possible sources of anxiety such as illness, hospitalization, knowledge deficits, or other known stressors gives patient knowledge of anxiety and increases his or her sense of control.
- Remember that patients and their family members who are under stress often require repeated explanations.

Pediatric
- Children often demonstrate anxiety through physical and behavioral signs but are unable to express anxiety verbally. Some children express anxiety through restless behavior, physical complaints, or behavioral regression. Note any changes in child's behavior that occur during illness or hospitalization (Hockenberry and Wilson, 2011).

Gerontologic
- Anxiety is one of the most common symptoms seen in older adults. Patients often become ritualistic and intent on

performing activities a certain way. Anxiety develops as a result of a specific event or a general pattern of change (e.g., decline in health) (Meiner, 2011).
- Manage anxiety based on patient's presenting behaviors with consideration of any cognitive/physical impairment.
- Psychosocial factors such as anxiety and confusion, lack of mobility, and spatial organization of a long-term care facility are factors that decrease social contacts, thus hindering communication with peers and health care providers. This leads to further feelings of isolation, boredom, and increased anxiety.
- Older adults who are socially isolated have multiple medical problems and are more likely to have anxious and/or depressive symptoms. In addition, they are less likely to seek care for these symptoms.

Home Care
- Manage anxiety based on patient's presenting behaviors with a consideration of any cognitive/physical impairment.
- Anticipation of a home care visit increases a patient's anxiety and leads to exacerbation of symptoms. Therefore some patients avoid home care visits (Fortinash and Holoday-Worret, 2008).

SKILL 3-3   Communicating with an Angry Patient

Anger is the common underlying factor associated with potential for violence. Patients become angry for a variety of reasons. Anger is often directly related to a patient's experience with illness, or it is associated with problems that existed before the patient entered the health care setting. In the health care setting you have frequent contact with a patient and thus often become the target of his or her anger. It is important for you to understand that in many cases a patient's ability to express anger is important to recovery. For example, when a patient has experienced a significant loss, anger becomes a means to help cope with grief. Some patients express anger toward their nurses, but the anger often hides a specific problem or concern. For example, a patient diagnosed as having cancer voices displeasure with the nurse's care instead of expressing a fear of dying.

Dealing with angry patients is very stressful. Anger often represents rejection or disapproval of your care. Your efforts at satisfying an angry patient's needs can result in a failure to meet the priorities of other patients. Allow patients to express anger openly and do not feel threatened by their words. However, do not allow a patient's anger to threaten or compromise care. Skills for communicating with an angry or a potentially violent patient allow you to help the patient dealing with anger constructively and refocus emotional energy toward effective problem solving. De-escalation skills are useful techniques that you can use to manage a potentially violent patient; these skills range from using nonthreatening verbal and nonverbal messages to safely disengaging and controlling the aggressor physically (Fortinash and Holoday-Worret, 2008).

Delegation and Collaboration

De-escalation is a skill that cannot be delegated to nursing assistive personnel (NAP). The nurse instructs the NAP about:

- The proper way to interact verbally and nonverbally with the angry patient.
- Their role as the nurse uses de-escalation techniques.
- Approaches that have been successful and unsuccessful in communicating with angry patients.

STEP	RATIONALE

ASSESSMENT

1 Observe for behaviors that indicate that the patient is angry (e.g., pacing, clenched fist, loud voice, throwing objects) and/or expressions that indicate anger (e.g., repeated questioning of nurse, not following requests, aggressive outbursts, threats).

Anger is a normal expression of frustration or response to feeling threatened. However, its expression often interferes with or blocks communication and interactions.

2 Assess factors that influence communication with the angry patient such as refusal to comply with treatment goals, use of sarcasm or hostile behavior, having a low frustration level, or being emotionally immature.

Assessment allows you to accurately evaluate the situation or patient experiences that block or facilitate communication.

3 Consider resources (e.g., health care team or family) available to assist in communicating with potentially violent patient.

This assists in clarifying cause and intervention required to deal with patient's anger.

4 Assess for underlying medical conditions that may potentially lead to violent behavior.

Patients with medical conditions such as traumatic brain injury, dementia, or drug/alcohol withdrawal may exhibit hostile, aggressive behaviors.

Clinical Decision Point *With some violent behaviors (e.g., physical aggression) you may not be able to de-escalate the situation. When this potential exists, know whom to call for assistance (e.g., trained psychology technicians, security staff). Personal safety is paramount.*

NURSING DIAGNOSES

- Anxiety
- Defensive coping
- Fear
- Impaired social interaction
- Impaired verbal communication
- Ineffective coping
- Risk for other-directed violence
- Risk for self-directed violence

Related factors are individualized based on patient's condition or needs.

PLANNING

1 Expected outcomes following completion of procedure:
  - Patient no longer exhibits verbal and nonverbal expressions of anger.

De-escalation techniques successfully allow patient to express anger in a constructive way.

2 Prepare for interaction with an angry patient:
  a Pause to collect own thoughts, feelings, and reactions.

Awareness and control of your reaction and responses facilitate more constructive interaction.

  b Determine what patient is saying.

Clarification of patient need or concern may help to de-escalate situation.

  c Attempt a calm, firm, assertive approach. Try to talk in comfortable, reassuring voice.

Approach tends to lessen patient's agitation and anger.

3 Prepare the environment to de-escalate a potentially violent patient:

Potentially violent patient needs to be in an environment with decreased stimuli and have protection from injury to self or against others.

Encourages patient's expression of anger rather than provokes it.

  a Encourage other people, particularly those who provoke anger, to leave room or area.

Avoids pressuring patient; helps to prevent injury if anger becomes out of control.

  b Maintain adequate distance.
  c Maintain open exit. Position self closest to door to facilitate escape from a potentially violent situation. Do not block exit so patient feels that escape is unattainable.

Prevents feeling of being trapped for both you and patient. Feeling trapped may cause a violent outburst. Safety of both parties is paramount.

  d When anger begins to disturb others, close door. This is particularly important when a patient becomes agitated.

Agitation and anxiety can spread to others. Some hospital rooms are equipped with security windows and cameras to allow for observation of patients.

Clinical Decision Point *Some patients are disruptive to one another, especially those who are hyperactive, intrusive, threatening, or exhibiting bizarre behaviors. For these patients, first try the least-restrictive measures before using more restrictive measures such as seclusion.*

STEP	RATIONALE
e Reduce disturbing factors in room (e.g., noise, drafts, inadequate lighting).	Reduces irritants that may heighten anger.
f Take care of patient's physical and emotional needs and discomforts (e.g., offer analgesic for pain).	Physical and emotional needs are often factors in patient's anger; sometimes patient is not aware of these needs.

IMPLEMENTATION

1 Responding to a potentially violent patient	
a Maintain nonthreatening verbal and nonverbal communication skills (e.g., use gestures that are slow and deliberate rather than sudden and abrupt).	Less chance of misinterpretation of message and less threatening. A relaxed atmosphere prevents further escalation. Creates climate of acceptance for patient.
b Use therapeutic silence and allow patient to vent feelings.	Often de-escalates anger. Anger expends emotional and physical energy; patient runs out of momentum and energy to maintain anger at high level.
c Answer questions as appropriate; if patient asks power-struggle type of question (challenging or confrontational type), redirect and set limits by giving clear, concise expectations. Inform patient of potential consequences without sounding threatening and follow through with consequences if patient does not change behaviors.	Setting limits on power-struggle questions provides structure and helps diffuse anger.
d If patient is making verbal threats to harm others, remain calm yet professional and continue to set limits on inappropriate behavior.	Angry patient loses ability to process information rationally and therefore may impulsively express anger through intimidation.

Clinical Decision Point *If imminent harm to another is present on discharge, notify proper authorities (e.g., nurse manager, security).*

e Maintain personal space and safety with patient who is making verbal threats of violence directed at others. Maintain nonthreatening position and nonverbal behavior, including body language, position, and cadence.	Avoiding sudden movements and loud tones prevents giving the appearance of an attack.

Clinical Decision Point *A potentially violent patient can be impulsive and explosive; therefore you need to keep personal safety skills in mind. In this case, avoid touch.*

f If patient appears to be calm and anger is defused, explore alternatives to situation or feelings of anger.	Processing with patient can prevent future explosive outbursts and teach patient effective ways of dealing with anger.

EVALUATION

1 Observe for continuing behaviors or verbal expressions of anger.	Indicates success of communication efforts.
2 Note patient's ability to answer questions and problem solve.	Determines whether anger has lessened so patient is able to focus on alternative coping skills.

Unexpected Outcomes

1 Patient continues to demonstrate nonverbal behaviors or verbal expression of anger or violence. You are unable to assist him or her in relieving source of anger or expressing anger openly without violent acts.

Related Interventions

- Reassess factors and remove or alter factors contributing to anger.
- Take charge with calm, firm directions. Give as-needed (prn) medications as ordered for agitation/escalating behaviors.
- Direct patient to a quiet area for a "time-out."
- Make sure that fellow staff members are available to assist if necessary.

Recording and Reporting

- Record in nurses' notes and EHR the cause of patient's anger (if determined), behaviors patient exhibits, de-escalation technique used, and patient's response to de-escalation efforts.
- Report technique used to de-escalate and patient's response to nurse in charge.

Special Considerations
Teaching

- Patients experiencing emotionally charged situations do not always comprehend instruction. Focus on understanding patient; providing feedback and assisting in problem solving; and providing an atmosphere of safety, warmth, and acceptance.

- Teaching patient to identify possible factors that contribute to angry outbursts such as inadequate coping skills, low frustration levels, illness, hospitalization, knowledge deficits, or other known stressors may give him or her a sense of control.
- Once anger has been de-escalated, teach patient new adaptive methods of coping with anger.

Pediatric
- Set limits for inappropriate behaviors exhibited by child such as a time-out. Apply such limits immediately because children tend to have less internal control over their own behaviors (Hockenberry and Wilson, 2011).

Gerontologic
- Patients who have cognitive impairments often exhibit tantrum-like behaviors in response to real or perceived frustration.

Use distraction techniques to remove cognitively impaired older-adult patient from disturbing stimuli or redirect patient to activity that is pleasurable (Meiner, 2011).

Home Care
- Personal safety for nurse against potentially violent patient or family member extends to all health care settings, including patient's home. You may be in a potentially dangerous situation while giving care to patient at home because you are without support from other staff members.
- Be aware of physical surroundings of home, including possible exits.
- If de-escalation does not occur and you believe your safety is threatened, call for assistance or remove yourself from the situation.

SKILL 3-4 Communicating with a Depressed Patient

Depression is a state of feelings that is more than just sadness. It is a common psychiatric condition that affects a person's ability to function in day-to-day activities. There are many symptoms of depression, the most common being apathy, feelings of sadness, fatigue, guilt, poor concentration, sleep disturbances, and suicidal thoughts. Depression results in both subjective and objective behaviors and patient reports of increased physical complaints (Box 3-4). Some patients report feeling anxious when depressed.

BOX 3-4	Symptoms of Depression
Common Symptoms	**Other Symptoms**
• Apathy	• Fatigue
• Sadness	• Thoughts of death
• Sleep disturbances	• Decreased libido
• Hopelessness	• Feeling inadequate
• Helplessness	• Psychomotor agitation
• Worthlessness	• Verbal berating of self
• Guilt	• Spontaneous crying
• Anger	• Dependency, passiveness

From Keltner N et al: *Psychiatric nursing*, ed 6, St Louis, 2011, Mosby.

Objective signs include decrease in performance of activities of daily living (ADLs) and decreased time spent in social activities (altered social interaction).

Many patients in acute care settings suffering from either acute or chronic health conditions have symptoms of depression. Some patients have been formally diagnosed and treated with medications and/or psychotherapy; others may not have been diagnosed and therefore have not been treated. Use the nursing process to develop nursing interventions, expected outcomes, and evaluation of these outcomes for patients with depression. The intervention strategies emphasize use of therapeutic communication techniques.

Delegation and Collaboration
The skill of communicating effectively with a depressed patient cannot be delegated to nursing assistive personnel (NAP). The nurse instructs the NAP about:
- The basic skills needed to interact verbally and nonverbally with the depressed patient.
- The possible causes and signs and symptoms of the patient's depression.

STEP	RATIONALE

ASSESSMENT

1 Assess for physical, behavioral, and verbal cues that indicate that patient is depressed such as feelings of sadness, tearfulness, difficulty concentrating, increase in reports of physical complaints, and statements such as, "I'm sad/depressed."

2 Assess for possible factors causing patient's depression (e.g., acute or chronic illness, personal vulnerability, recent loss).

3 Assess factors influencing communication with patient (e.g., environment, timing, presence of others, values, experiences, poor concentration).

4 Discuss possible causes of patient's depression with family members, including past history of the illness if necessary.

Depression interferes with usual manner of communication and thus with patient's care and treatment. If depression is severe, it interferes with comprehension, attention, and problem-solving abilities.

Patient's depressive state is sometimes unknown. Understanding the possible cause of depression assists in patient support and communication.

Understanding factors that influence communication helps you identify effective communication strategies.

Gathering information about patient from a family perspective is useful because family provides new information or understanding of the situation (Keltner et al., 2011).

STEP	RATIONALE

NURSING DIAGNOSES

- Decisional conflict
- Hopelessness
- Impaired social interaction
- Impaired verbal communication
- Ineffective coping
- Ineffective role performance
- Risk for self-directed violence
- Spiritual distress

Related factors are individualized based on patient's condition or needs.

PLANNING

1 Expected outcomes following completion of procedure:	
• Patient is able to discuss source of depression.	Patient is given resources to cope with feelings of depression.
• Patient is able to discuss ways to cope with depression.	
2 Prepare for communication by considering patient goals, time allocation, and resources.	Effective communication allows patient to establish rapport, achieve a sense of calm, and begin to analyze source(s) of depression.
3 Be aware of your nonverbal cues that affect communication with depressed patient (e.g., body language, posture, cadence of speech). Remain nonjudgmental.	Your personal feelings regarding depression may negatively affect interaction with patient.
4 Prepare environment physically by providing a quiet, calm area, allowing ample personal space.	Decreasing stimuli has a calming effect.
Invasion of personal space increases anxiety, thereby preventing communication with the depressed patient.

Clinical Decision Point *First acknowledge and take care of depressed patient's physical and emotional discomfort but avoid dwelling on physical complaints. Focus on understanding patient, providing feedback, and assisting in problem solving.*

IMPLEMENTATION

1 Provide brief, simple introduction; introduce yourself and explain purpose of interaction.	Symptoms associated with depression limit amount of information that patient can understand.
2 Accept patient as he or she is and focus on positive aspects of patient. Provide positive feedback.	Depressed patients often have low self-esteem. This approach helps to focus on their strengths.
3 Be honest and empathic.	Honesty and empathy facilitate the development of trust.
4 Use appropriate nonverbal behaviors and active listening skills such as staying with patient at bedside.	Nonverbal messages to patient express your interest and help to alleviate depressive symptoms.
5 Use appropriate verbal techniques that are clear and concise when responding to patient. Use observational statements that acknowledge current state of feelings and provide direction to patient.	Appropriate techniques and statements provide reassurance to depressed patient. Expresses empathy.
6 Use open-ended questions such as, "Tell me about how you're feeling" or "You seem sad. Tell me about your sadness."	Encourages patient to continue talking, facilitating an in-depth discussion of symptoms.
7 Reward small decisions and independent actions. When necessary, make decisions that patients are not ready to make. Present situations that require no decision making.	Depressed patients are often overly dependent and indecisive.
8 Respond to anger therapeutically; avoid becoming defensive or angry and encourage verbal expression of anger.	Some depressed patients are angry; understand that anger is a symptom of their depression. Verbal expression often reduces tension.
9 Provide necessary comfort measures.	Depressed patients often have multiple somatic complaints; address and adequately treat the physical complaints (e.g., pain, nausea).
10 Spend time with patient who is withdrawn.	This communicates patient's worth.
11 Ask patient about suicidal ideation and presence of a plan.	Depressed patients are at increased risk for suicide. Other risk factors include general medical conditions, hopelessness, male gender, and increased age. The more developed the plan, the greater the risk of suicide (Keltner et al., 2011).

STEP	RATIONALE

EVALUATION

1 Observe for continuing presence of physical signs and symptoms or behaviors reflecting depression.

Observation determines extent to which planned interaction relieved patient's depressive symptoms.

2 Have patient discuss ways to cope with depression in the future and make decisions about own care.

Discussion measures patient's ability to assume more health-promoting behavior.

3 Evaluate patient's ability to discuss factors causing depression.

Evaluation measures patient's ability to attend to or focus on area of concern.

Unexpected Outcomes

1 Depressive behaviors continue; interaction has been ineffective at relieving depressive symptoms.

2 Patient reports suicidal ideation with or without plan.

Related Interventions

- Continue to use therapeutic communication skills but try different techniques.

- Refer patient to mental health professional for consultation regarding use of pharmacologic agents and/or formal psychotherapy to treat depression.

- Refer patient to mental health professional for evaluation and possible admission to an inpatient psychiatric treatment facility.

Recording and Reporting

- Record in nurses' notes and EHR both objective and subjective behaviors (associated with depression) that patient is displaying and objective behaviors (associated with depression) observed by the nurse.
- Record and report methods used to improve these behaviors and patient's response.

Special Considerations
Teaching

- Teaching patient to identify possible sources of depression such as acute or chronic illness, personal vulnerability, ineffective coping, or other known stressors gives patient knowledge of depression and increases his or her sense of control over feelings of depression.
- Make teaching modifications with a consideration of impaired concentration and memory related to patient's depressed status (e.g., present a small amount of material at a time).

Pediatric

- Children often demonstrate symptoms of depression that differ from those of adults. They manifest depression through physical (increased somatic complaints) and behavioral signs (poor school performance, social isolation) and are often unable to express depression verbally. Some children express depression through restless behavior or behavioral regression. It is important to note any changes in child's behavior that occur during illness or hospitalization (Hockenberry and Wilson, 2011).

Gerontologic

- Depression among older adults is a major health concern. It is important to differentiate between depression and any underlying medical illness in this population because the symptoms sometimes overlap. In addition, suicide risk is increased in older adults because this age-group experiences multiple losses such as loss of health status, independence, and social support system and financial losses (Keltner et al., 2011).

Home Care

- Depression is often present in home care settings. Educate family caregivers about how to identify symptoms. Manage depression based on patient's presenting behaviors with a consideration of any cognitive/physical impairment.

SKILL 3-5 Communicating with a Cognitively Impaired Patient

Nurses must communicate with patients who have complex physical and psychological issues. Patients with cognitive impairments pose a challenge for nurses because these patients may have limited ability to communicate. The act of communicating and expressing oneself is affected by a person's ability; consequently patients with cognitive impairments may have a disability that negatively affects communication (McGhee, 2011). Different types of cognitive impairments include acute and chronic. Acute cognitive impairment or delirium is largely reversible and may be caused by conditions such as infection, polypharmacy, and metabolic changes. Once the cause is identified and treated, the patient's mental status returns to a baseline condition. Chronic types of cognitive impairments include dementia (Alzheimer's disease, vascular dementia, frontal-temporal dementia), traumatic brain injury, and HIV-related cognitive dysfunction. These are irreversible, and the cognitive decline may be progressive.

Cognitive impairments accompanied by communication deficits often hinder a patient's ability to initiate conversation. Since it is time-consuming to interact with these patients, they may be deprived of human contact, which leads to depression, detachment, and isolation. The patient's inability to participate in self-care results in inadequate care and frustration by the health care staff. Patients with cognitive impairments may be at risk for physical status changes such as infection, falls and injury, and poor nutrition. A lack of quality nurse-patient interaction and communication barriers negatively affect patient outcomes. A patient-centered approach stresses the uniqueness of each patient and his or her individuality when assessing the patient's ability to communicate. Communication is essential to everyday life, and the nurse needs to be creative in the way he or she interacts with patients with cognitive impairments to ensure that the messages are sent and received.

Delegation and Collaboration

The skill of communicating effectively with a cognitively impaired patient cannot be delegated to nursing assistive personnel (NAP). The nurse instructs the NAP about:

- The proper communication skills needed to interact verbally and nonverbally with the cognitively impaired patient.
- The possible causes and signs and symptoms of the patient's cognitive impairment.

STEP	RATIONALE
ASSESSMENT	
1 Assess for physical, behavioral, and verbal cues that indicate that a patient is cognitively impaired. Assess the orientation status of the patient (person, place, time) and perform a mini-mental examination (see Chapter 6).	If the patient is unable to think, speak, or understand, communication strategies need to be adjusted to communicate effectively.
2 Assess for possible factors causing patient's cognitive impairment (e.g., acute or chronic illness, fever, fluid and electrolyte imbalance, past history).	Patient's cognitive state is sometimes unknown to nurse. Understanding the possible cause of mental decline assists in patient support and communication.
3 Assess factors influencing communication with patient (e.g., environment, timing, presence of others, values, experiences, prior sensory loss, poor concentration).	Understanding factors that influence communication helps you to identify effective communication strategies.
4 You may need to discuss possible causes of patient's cognitive impairment with family members or caregivers, including current illness, treatment regimen, and past medical history.	Gathering information about patient from a family perspective is useful because family provides new information or understanding of the situation. It is important to establish patient's baseline mental status.

NURSING DIAGNOSES

- Acute confusion
- Decisional conflict
- Hopelessness
- Impaired social interaction
- Impaired verbal communication
- Ineffective coping
- Ineffective role performance
- Knowledge deficit

Related factors are individualized based on patient's condition or needs.

STEP	RATIONALE
PLANNING	
1 Expected outcomes following completion of procedure: • Patient is able to communicate needs to nurse.	Patient receives adequate resources to communicate effectively, given the limitations related to cognitive impairment.
2 Prepare for communication by considering type of cognitive impairment, communication impairments, time allocation, and resources.	Effective communication allows patient to establish rapport and have a quality nurse-patient interaction.
3 Be aware of your nonverbal cues that affect communication with the cognitively impaired patient (e.g., body language, posture, cadence of speech). Remain nonjudgmental.	Frustration in communication with patients with cognitive impairment may negatively affect interaction with patient.
4 Prepare environment physically by providing a quiet, calm area. Reduce distractions such as external noises.	Decreasing stimuli has a calming effect. Ensuring that the environment is quiet and free from distractions enhances the communication experience.
IMPLEMENTATION	
1 Approach patient from the front and face him or her when speaking.	This strategy ensures that patient both sees and hears you.
2 Provide brief, simple introduction; introduce yourself and explain purpose of interaction.	Symptoms associated with cognitive impairment limit amount of information that patient can understand.
3 Use appropriate nonverbal behaviors and active listening skills such as staying with patient at bedside or use of touch.	Nonverbal messages to patient express your interest and convey empathy. Use of touch may help with concentration and reassurance.
4 Use clear and concise verbal techniques to respond to patient. Use simple language and speak slowly; use short and simple sentences. Ask yes-or-no questions.	Appropriate techniques and statements provide reassurance to cognitively impaired patient.
5 Ask one question at a time and allow time for response. Avoid rushing patient.	This gives patient time to process the information and respond.
6 Repeat sentences using a steady voice and avoid being too quick to guess what the patient is trying to express.	Repetition allows time for patient to respond; it can be frustrating for patient if you misinterpret his or her message or pressure him or her to respond.

STEP	RATIONALE
7 Use augmentative and assistive communication (AAC) devices to facilitate communication such as pictogram grid, talking mats, objects.	Talking mats are communication aids that use picture symbols so the patient can place relevant images below a visual scale to indicate feelings (McGhee, 2011).
8 Provide assistive devices such as eyeglasses or hearing aids to help with communication.	Use of such devices facilitates clarity of communication experiences.
9 Do not argue with patient or correct him or her if mistakes are made.	Arguing can lead to increased frustration and agitation.
10 Maintain meaningful interactions with patients and use creative modes of communication based on patient's comfort level and abilities.	Superficial, brief human contact may lead to sense of isolation and detachment.

EVALUATION

1 Observe for clarity and understanding of messages sent and received.	Observation determines extent to which cognitively impaired patient is able to express self.
2 Observe verbal and nonverbal behaviors.	Observation reveals if patient is comfortable and needs have been met.

Unexpected Outcomes
1 Messages that are sent and received are not understood.

2 Patient becomes frustrated, and communication with nurse becomes more challenging.

Related Interventions
- Continue to use therapeutic communication skills when interacting with cognitively impaired patient. Be creative in using alternative strategies.
- Speak to patient as an adult and give time to process information. Use verbal and nonverbal methods to convey empathy with their frustration.
- Allow for periods of adequate rest; make frequent attempts to interact to minimize social isolation.

Recording and Reporting
- Record in nurses' notes and EHR both objective and subjective behaviors (associated with cognitive impairment) that patient is displaying and objective behaviors (associated with cognitive impairment) observed by the nurse.
- Record and report the methods used to communicate and patient's response.

Special Considerations
Teaching
- Teach patient to use various methods to communicate such as pictorial board or communication aids.
- Make teaching modifications with a consideration of impaired concentration and memory related to patient's cognitive status (e.g., present a small amount of material at a time; use simple and short phrases; repeat information as needed).

Pediatric
- Children may exhibit cognitive impairments because of metabolic or neurologic conditions that may be acute or chronic in duration. Communication strategies with children should take into consideration their developmental level. Use pictures and drawings for patients who are unable to read.

Gerontologic
- Many older adults have cognitive impairments. These impairments pose serious barriers to the reliability of the nurse's assessment of patients; therefore it is important to use effective verbal and nonverbal communication strategies. Poor communication can compromise care, leading to increased anxiety and frustration.

Home Care
- Manage care based on patient's presenting behaviors with a consideration of any cognitive/physical impairment. Include the family caregiver and friends in using effective communication strategies.

Critical Thinking Exercises

You are assigned to care for Mrs. Jones, an 84-year-old woman who was admitted to the hospital 2 days ago after falling at her son's home. She recently moved in with her son, her only child, following the sudden death of her husband. Her husband had been her primary caregiver since she was diagnosed with Alzheimer's disease 3 years ago. Neither her husband nor her son wanted to put her into a long-term care facility. She had emergency surgery to repair a fractured wrist. During shift report on a medical-surgical unit, the nurse tells you that the patient is withdrawn and confused. In addition, she has difficulty understanding verbal direction from the nursing staff.

1 Which steps are necessary to effectively communicate with a cognitively impaired patient?

When you approach the patient to perform an initial assessment, she is looking out the window and seems disoriented. She appears disheveled, and her lunch tray is untouched. You ask her if she needs assistance with ADLs such as bathing, dressing, and feeding, but you get a response that you cannot understand.

2 What should you do first to prepare to communicate with Mrs. Jones? Explain your choice(s).

You contact her son, who is her legal guardian; he tells you that he doesn't know his mother's baseline level of functioning because his father had been in denial about her mental decline and overall deterioration. The son does not know if she is capable of managing her own ADLs or needs assistance.

3 Describe strategies to use to determine Mrs. Jones' own sense of her ability to perform ADLs.

✓ REVIEW QUESTIONS

1 Which approach reflects an obstacle to effective nurse-patient communication?
   1 Discussing fears about a patient with members of the health care team
   2 Obtaining information about a critically ill patient from his or her family
   3 Admitting a mistake to a patient's family
   4 Avoiding issues that are uncomfortable for a patient

2 The nurse is caring for a postoperative patient who is still having pain despite analgesia administration. Which statement by the nurse best reflects therapeutic communication?
   1 "I think your doctor needs to know that you're still in pain."
   2 "What do you want me to do about your pain problem?"
   3 "When it comes to pain, your doctor tends to undermedicate his patients."
   4 "Your pain will be a lot better in the morning."

3 A patient recovering from a bilateral mastectomy for breast cancer tearfully tells the nurse that she is feeling depressed and worthless as a woman. Which communication phrase is not effective?
   1 "Many women have body image concerns after undergoing this surgery."
   2 "Tell me more about how you feel."
   3 "Why do you feel depressed and worthless?"
   4 "How long have you been feeling this way?"

4 Which initial approach would be best when working with an anxious patient?
   1 Tell the patient that everything he or she says will be kept private.
   2 Ask the patient what he or she believes is causing his or her anxiety.
   3 Watch the patient's behavior for the amount of anxiety being exhibited.
   4 Explain what the patient can expect in terms that he or she can understand.

5 A nurse is working with a potentially threatening patient. Which nursing intervention is most appropriate?
   1 Speaking clearly and slightly louder so the patient does not need the nurse to repeat what was said.
   2 Positioning himself or herself near the exit of the room to prevent being blocked by the patient.
   3 Bringing in other team members so the patient knows there are others to help him or her gain control.
   4 Asking the patient which comfort measures he or she uses when he or she becomes out of control.

6 A visitor from another country became ill and required hospitalization. He is having difficulty getting the staff to understand his needs. Which approach by the nurse demonstrates the most cultural sensitivity?
   1 Asking one of the patient's family members to help with the communication process
   2 Using good eye contact while speaking clearly with easily understood words
   3 Obtaining a medical interpreter to facilitate the communication process
   4 Touching the patient more often while assessing him to make him feel that the nurse cares about him

7 A patient is exhibiting signs and symptoms of anxiety. What should be the first step in establishing communication with him or her?
   1 Providing good personal hygiene
   2 Letting the patient make as many choices as possible
   3 Being nonjudgmental and accepting of feelings
   4 Exhibiting appropriate nonverbal behaviors and active listening skills

8 A nurse is working with an older adult with a cognitive impairment who is having a tantrum and acting hostile toward other patients in the dayroom. Which approach by the nurse is most appropriate to handle this situation?
   1 Asking three other staff members to help put the patient back to bed
   2 Using the patient's favorite crackers to distract him from the other patients
   3 Explaining to the patient how he will benefit by behaving better
   4 Asking the family how they managed the tantrums while the patient was still living at home

9 A patient recovering from a recent amputation of his foot because of diabetes has been very withdrawn and not sleeping or eating well. Which initial nursing intervention would be most effective to help him with his depression?
   1 Suggesting the use of antidepressant medication to his health care provider
   2 Spending time with the patient and telling him how lucky he is that he was able to keep most of his leg
   3 Talking with physical therapy about how soon he can be fitted for a prosthesis
   4 Encouraging the patient to talk about his feelings while allowing angry outbursts

10 The nurse is preparing to provide patient education. Which question is most appropriate for the nurse to ask?
   1 Are you ready to learn now?
   2 Can you use a computer?
   3 Is your family here to learn also?
   4 How do you best learn?

REFERENCES

Bischoff A, Hudelson P: Communicating with foreign language–speaking patients: is access to professional interpreters enough? *J Travel Med* 17(1):15, 2010.
Boschart V: A communication intervention for nursing staff in chronic care, *J Adv Nurs* 65(9):1823, 2009.
Davis TC, et al: Rapid estimate of adult literacy in medicine: a shortened screening instrument, *Fam Med* 25(6):391, 1993.
Finke E, et al: A systematic review of the effectiveness of nurse communication with patients with complex communication needs with a focus on the use of augmentative and alternative communication, *J Clin Nurs* 17:2102, 2008.
Fortinash K, Holoday-Worret P: *Psychiatric mental health nursing*, ed 4, St Louis, 2008, Mosby.
Hockenberry MJ, Wilson D: *Wong's nursing care of infants and children*, ed 9, St Louis, 2011, Mosby.
Keltner N, et al: *Psychiatric nursing*, ed 6, St Louis, 2011, Mosby.
Majerovitz J, et al: We're on the same side: improving communication between nursing home and family, *Health Commun* 24:12, 2009.
McGhee J: Effective communication with people who have dementia, *Nurs Stand* 25(25):40, 2011.
McKeon LM, et al: Developing patient-centered care competencies among prelicensure students using simulation, *J Nurs Educ* 48(12):711, 2009.
Meiner S: *Gerontologic nursing*, ed 4, St Louis, 2011, Mosby.
Miller C: Communication difficulties in hospitalized older adults with dementia: try these techniques to make communicating with patients easier and more effective, *Am J Nurs* 108(3):58, 2008.
Murphy J: Patient as the center of the health care universe: a closer look at patient-centered care, *Nurs Econ* 29(1):35, 2011.
O'Halloran R, et al: The number of patients with communication related impairments in acute hospital stroke units, *Int J Speech Lang Pathol* 11(6):438, 2009.
Parker A, et al: Evidence-based communication practices for children with visual impairments and additional disabilities: an examination of single-subject design studies, *J Vis Impair Blind* 102(9):540, 2008.
Parker RM, et al: The test of functional health literacy in adults: a new instrument for measuring patients' literacy skills, *J Gen Intern Med* 10(10):537, 1995.
Robinson J, et al: Patient-centered care and adherence: definitions and applications to improve outcomes, *J Am Acad Nurse Pract* 20:600, 2008.
Rohrer J, et al: Patient centeredness, self-rated health, and patient empowerment: should providers spend more time communicating with their patients? *J Eval Clin Pract* 14(4):548, 2008.
Tucker C, et al: Patient-centered culturally sensitive health care: model testing and refinement, *Health Psychol* 30(3):342, 2011.
Wilkerson L, et al: Assessing patient-centered care: one approach to health disparities education, *J Gen Intern Med* 25(suppl 2):86, 2010.

Documentation and Informatics

MEDIA RESOURCES

- evolve *learning system* http://evolve.elsevier.com/Perry/skills

  - Review Questions
  - Audio Glossary

KEY TERMS

Acuity systems	DAR	Incident report	SOAP
Case management	Documentation	Kardex	SOAPIE
Change-of-shift report	Documentation system	Objective data	Standardized care plan
Charting by exception (CBE)	Electronic health record	PIE	Subjective data
Critical/collaborative pathway	Flow sheet	Problem-oriented medical record (POMR)	Variance
	Focus charting		
	Hand-off	SBAR	

OBJECTIVES

Mastery of content in this chapter will enable the nurse to:
- List guidelines for effective communication and reporting.
- Describe measures to maintain confidentiality of patient information.
- Identify the purpose of the patient record.
- Describe the elements of a hand-off report and when it would be used.
- Discuss the role of computerization in documentation.
- Write a nurse's progress note using SOAP, SOAPIE, PIE, focus, and SBAR charting formats.

- Describe information found in a patient care profile and nursing Kardex.
- Accurately complete a nursing flow sheet.
- Explain guidelines used in documentation of home care and long-term care.
- Describe the role of critical pathways in multidisciplinary documentation.
- Complete an incident (adverse event) report accurately.

Nursing documentation is an essential and important component of health care delivery. Documentation is anything entered into a patient's electronic health record or written in a patient record. The Joint Commission's concern about communication errors in accredited health care organizations has led to continually updating goals to improve safety (TJC, 2012b). Nursing documentation ensures continuity of care, provides legal evidence, and evaluates patient outcomes. One of the challenges you will face is documenting quality patient care within the constraints imposed by regulations, limited resources, and finances. Your documentation provides a detailed account of a patient's plan of care, important assessment, and treatment, which must be an accurate and timely evaluation of information. Effective documentation ensures continuity of care, maintains standards, and reduces errors. The quality of documentation depends on your ability to communicate effectively in both the written and spoken word. Furthermore, technology now offers new tools to improve documentation and patient care. You are held accountable for the accuracy of documentation that is in the patient record, and this information is confidential and needs to be protected.

Accreditation agencies such as The Joint Commission specify guidelines for documentation and require health care agencies to monitor and evaluate patient outcomes and appropriateness of care. This evaluation process occurs through an audit of information that is documented in patient records. The Joint Commission provides requirements for documentation in their standards (TJC, 2012a).

ELECTRONIC HEALTH RECORDS

Comprehensive computer systems in health care delivery have unlimited potential for improving the accuracy, efficiency, and quality of documentation. Researchers estimate that only 12% of health care agencies have a basic electronic record (Kutney-Lee and Kelly, 2011). However, the traditional paper medical record is no longer meeting the needs of today's health care industry. Key information such as patient allergies, current medications, and treatment complications may be lost from one episode of care (e.g., hospitalization or clinic visit) to the next visit, or they may be illegible, thus risking a patient's safety (Green and Thomas, 2008). The electronic health record (EHR) is a longitudinal electronic record of patient health information generated by one or more encounters in a care delivery setting (HIMSS, 2011). The EHR provides access to a patient's health record information at the time and place that clinicians need it. The EHR improves patient care quality by displaying clinical information that is patient centered where it is needed in a timely manner. It can provide better information access for patients and health care providers (Murphy, 2010). By 2014 the EHR should be implemented nationwide. Beginning in 2014, incentive payments from the Centers for Medicare and Medicaid Services will begin to diminish and there will be no incentive payments after 2015 for agencies that cannot demonstrate meaningful use of an EHR (Reimer, 2011).

Although EHRs are the wave of the future, many agencies have computerized medical record systems. Computerized documentation has features that potentially can improve documentation accuracy, timeliness and completeness of data entry, and communication among health care disciplines (Burnes-Bolton et al., 2008). In addition, computerized documentation systems are designed to reduce errors and provide standardized care plans or treatment protocols. Such a system relies on many data collection components, including flow sheets, medication records, and clinical care summaries. Software programs allow quick access to assessment data, and information automatically transfers to different reports. New technology allows for the use of pen-based or voice recognition programs.

The transition to computerized documentation presents both opportunities and challenges to nurses and nurse managers (Fig. 4-1). The Security Rule of HIPAA (1996) provides standards for the protection of electronic health information. The successful implementation of a computerized documentation system requires preparation, involvement, and commitment of the entire nursing staff. Awareness of legal risks and confidentiality issues are important challenges in the transition from paper to computerized systems. Numerous nursing and medical professional organizations have developed guidelines and strategies for safe computer charting (Box 4-1).

EVIDENCE-BASED PRACTICE

Computer-based health care records, informatics, and implementation of the electronic patient record all have major implications for the practice of nursing, the documentation of nursing care, improving patient safety, and evidence-based practice (Cherry, 2011, Watkins et al., 2009). Computer-based documentation systems are integral to improving and documenting quality nursing care. This type of system maintains a continual record of care planned and/or provided to a patient by nurses and other members of the health care team that can be used for research and assess quality of documentation and patient care (Saranto and Kinnunen, 2009). The nursing process is the foundation for all care of the patient. Documenting care within the patient care plan communicates the care provided, standardizes care, and helps nurses to perform care that is evidence based (Fogelberg-Dahm, 2008). Making sound decisions during implementation of computerized systems is the key to long-term success (Stone and Yoder, 2012).

BOX 4-1	Use of Electronic Health Record

- Sign on to the electronic health record (EHR) using only your password.
- Never share passwords and keep your password private.
- Review assessment data, problems identified (nursing diagnoses), goals and expected outcomes, and interventions and patient responses during contact with each patient before data entry.
- Follow procedures for entering information in all appropriate program functions.
- Review previously documented entries with those that you enter, noting if there is significant change in patient's status. Report changes to patient's health care provider.
- Do not leave information about a patient displayed on a monitor where others can see it. Keep a log that accounts for every copy of a computerized file that you have generated from the system.
- Follow agency confidentiality procedures for documenting sensitive material such as diagnosis of human immunodeficiency virus (HIV) infection.
- Know and implement agency protocol to correct documentation errors.
- Never create, change, or delete records unless your agency provides you with this authority.
- Software systems have a system for backup files. If you inadvertently delete part of the permanent record, follow agency policy. It is necessary to type an explanation into the computer file with the date, time, and your initials, and submit an explanation in writing to your manager.
- Save information as documentation is completed.
- Protect printouts from computerized records. Shredding printouts and logging in the number of copies generated by each caregiver minimize duplicate records and protect the confidentiality of patient information.
- Sign off when you leave the computer.

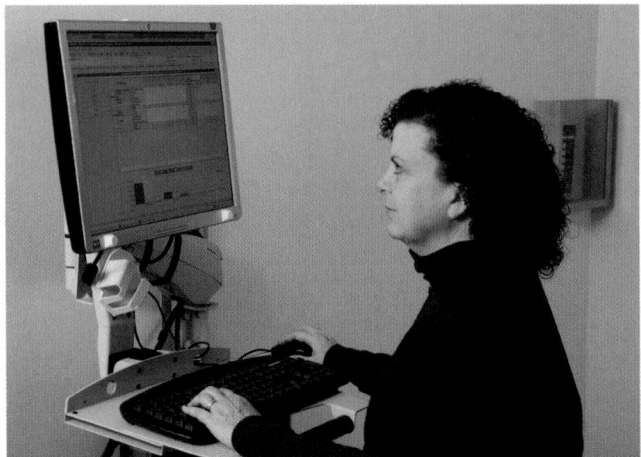

FIG 4-1   Computerized documentation provides many benefits.

- Try to ensure that all computer modules are available and implemented in a timely manner.
- Be sure that the system can be modified to meet the needs of different nursing specialties (e.g., emergency department, labor and delivery).
- Choose a system that flows in a manner that is similar to the paper flow pathway previously used.
- Is the new system interoperable with any existing systems?
- Is there high quality training and support available before, during, and after implementation?
- Can the nurses and other users access the data seamlessly and without difficulty?

CONFIDENTIALITY

All members of the health care team are legally and ethically obligated to keep patient information confidential. Do not discuss a patient's examinations, observations, conversations, or treatments with other patients or staff not involved in the patient's care, unless the patient grants permission. Patient records and computer screens are accessed only by persons caring for the patient and must be kept out of view of anyone not caring for him or her. Sometimes patients request copies of their records, and they have a right to read them. One exemption to information access involves patients with mental illness. These patients can be denied access if it could cause personal harm to their physical or mental health. Agencies have specific policies for controlling the manner in which records are shared; usually they require patients to provide written permission for the release of medical information.

The Health Insurance Portability and Accountability Act of 1996 (HIPAA) protects patients' private health information. HIPAA governs all areas of health information management (e.g., reimbursement, coding, security, and patient records) (USDHHS, 1999). Previously the rule required written consent for disclosure of all patient information. Under new regulations, to eliminate barriers that delay access to care, providers are only to notify patients of their privacy policy and make a reasonable effort to obtain written acknowledgment of this notification. As a result of this act, patients have more control over their personal health care information and who has access to this information.

When you are a student in a clinical setting, confidentiality and compliance with HIPAA legislation are part of professional practice. You review the medical record only for information needed to provide safe, efficient care. For example, when you are assigned to provide complete care for a patient, you need to review the current medical record and plan of care. However, do not share information with other classmates or access the medical records of other patients on the specific clinical area. To further maintain confidentiality and protect patient privacy, do not have patient identifiers (e.g., room number, date of birth, medical record number, or other identifiable demographic information) on written materials used in your student clinical practice and do not photocopy, cut, or paste any patient information from the electronic record.

STANDARDS

Current Joint Commission standards require that all patients who are admitted to a health care agency have an assessment of physical, psychosocial, environmental, self-care, patient education, and discharge planning needs (TJC, 2012a). The Joint Commission standards require documentation to be within the context of the nursing process, including evidence of patient and family teaching and discharge planning. Agency standards or policies often state the frequency of assessment; thus it is essential to know the standards of your health care organization.

The standards developed by The Joint Commission provide structure for health care organizations. Health care organizations are accountable to ensure adherence to documentation standards to protect the patient. Electronic records and information create complexities in information management and potential for error. The goal of information management is to support decision making and improve patient outcomes, therefore ensuring patient safety.

PATIENT-CENTERED CARE

The Joint Commission has recently released a roadmap of new standards that support care based on individual needs of the patient. Patient-centered care is care that is respectful to patient's values and beliefs. It includes culture, ethnicity, age, spiritual beliefs, spoken and written language, and patient literacy. It also identifies and addresses patient mobility and any precautions and safety risks of the patient (TJC, 2012a). Patient-centered care encourages active participation of a patient in all care decisions and questioning from patient and family. The patient role should no longer be passive but one of active, informed involvement that improves communication among patient, family, and the health care team. Effective communication that is patient centered increases patient safety (Carayon and Wood, 2009). Communication is individualized to a unique patient's needs gathered during admission to the hospital setting. Nurses continue to monitor for changes that may be needed in communication style across the patient's life span (TJC, 2012a).

MULTIDISCIPLINARY COMMUNICATION WITHIN THE HEALTH CARE TEAM

Patient care requires effective communication among the members of the health care team. Records and reports communicate specific information about a patient's health status and the interventions that all health care team members contribute toward improving his or her health. Multidisciplinary communication and documentation are necessary to provide more efficient and effective health care and improve patient outcomes.

A patient's record or chart is a confidential, permanent legal document containing information relevant to a patient's health care. Nurses and other health care providers record information about a patient's health care after each patient contact. The record is a continuing account of the patient's health status and needs, treatments delivered, results of diagnostic tests, and response to therapy.

Reports are oral, written, or audiotaped exchanges of information among caregivers (Fig. 4-2). Patient information may be received or reported verbally, by fax, or via paging system. Reports include information about a patient's clinical status, observations made about his or her behavior, data pertaining to diagnostic tests, and directions for changes in therapy. Common reports given by nurses include telephone reports, transfer reports, and adverse event reports (see Procedural Guideline 4-3).

Patient hand-off reports (see Procedural Guideline 4-1), a standardized approach to communication of patient information among caregivers, is being used by many health care organizations. A patient hand-off is not limited to nursing alone but can be interdisciplinary among all who provide care to the patient. Hand-off

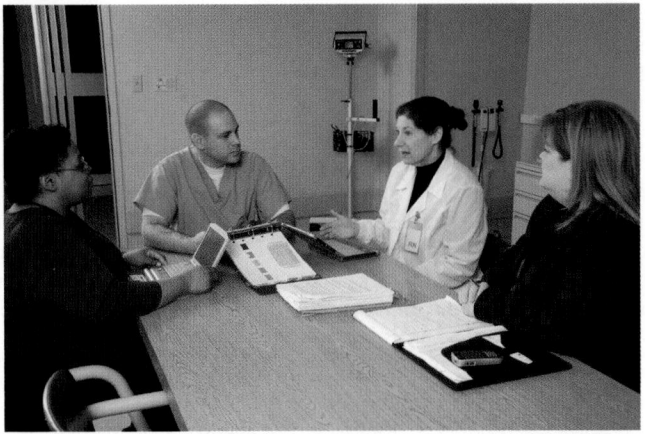

FIG 4-2 Communication among members of the health care team.

must occur during shift change or any time the patient changes caregivers (TJC, 2012a; 2012b). They are to be used by nurses for relief coverage for breaks, for shift report, when patients transfer to different departments for studies, or for transfer to a different level of care within a hospital. Hand-off is also used across the health care continuum when patients leave one health system for another. Effective hand-off allows for face-to-face communication when available, which allows the person receiving care of the patient the opportunity to ask questions. During a hand-off communication process the patient and patient information are transferred to the next caregiver. Acceptance of patient care information and the associated caregiver responsibilities are achieved through effective communication that is complete and accurate. For example, during hand-off the sender of the patient information initially presents the patient name, room number, age, gender diagnosis, medical history, discharge planning, and confidential information. This is followed by patient vital signs and clinical assessments, changes in clinical condition, medication review, fluid balance, and patient safety risk assessment factors. The patient is an active participant in the hand-off process. Once hand-off is completed, the receiver of the information is given an opportunity to ask questions and confirm understanding. Incomplete or comprehensive information can negatively affect a patient's safety. A comprehensive hand-off not only is information sharing but also is the acceptance and effective transfer of all patient authority and responsibility (Joint Commission Center for Transforming Healthcare, 2011; Runy, 2008).

When a nurse receives any information from a physician or health care provider by phone, he or she must ensure the accuracy and completeness of the information by writing it down and reading it back to the physician. When you accept a verbal order, telephone order, or critical test result, write down the order or critical test result as you hear it and then read it back to the individual who has given the order. By stating the information back, also called the *read-back*, to the individual giving the order or test result, you verify that the complete order or test result has been received and understood (NQF, 2011; TJC, 2011).

A nurse also communicates information through discussions or conferences among health care team members. For example, a discharge planning conference often involves members of all disciplines (i.e., nursing, medicine, social work, physical therapy, and dietary) who meet to discuss a patient's progress toward established discharge goals. A nurse needs to document this information in a patient's permanent record so all caregivers benefit from the information and plan the patient's care accordingly.

GUIDELINES FOR QUALITY DOCUMENTATION AND REPORTING

Quality documentation and reporting enhance efficient, safe, individualized patient care; you achieve this through the use of standard guidelines. Accurate documentation is one of the best defenses of legal claims associated with nursing care. Five common issues in malpractice caused by inadequate or incorrect documentation include (1) failing to document the correct time of events, (2) failing to record verbal orders or have them signed, (3) charting actions in advance to save time, (4) documenting incorrect data, and (5) failing to give a report or giving an incomplete report to an oncoming shift (Table 4-1).

To limit liability nursing documentation must clearly indicate that a nurse provided individualized, goal-directed nursing care to a patient based on the nursing assessment. The recorded information in a patient's record must describe exactly what happened to the patient. This is best achieved when you chart immediately after you have provided an intervention (Brown and King, 2008). Include all assessment findings, care plans, interventions, patient responses to interventions, and consultations/referrals in the medical record. Quality documentation and reporting must have the following characteristics: they must be factual, accurate, complete, current, and organized.

Factual

A record or report contains descriptive, objective information about what you see, hear, feel, and smell. An objective description is the result of direct observation and measurement such as "respiratory rate 20 and unlabored." Avoid terms such as *appears*, *seems*, or *apparently*, which are often subject to interpretation. For example, the description "the patient seems to be in pain" does not accurately communicate the facts to another caregiver. The phrase *seems* is not supported by any objective facts. Objective documentation needs to include your observations of patient behavior. For example, objective signs of pain include increased pulse rate, increased respiration, diaphoresis, or guarding a body part.

The only subjective data included in a record are what the patient actually verbalizes. Write subjective information with quotation marks, using the patient's exact words whenever possible. For example, you record, "Patients states, 'My stomach hurts.'" You also include complementary objective findings so the database is descriptive.

Accurate

The use of exact measurements in documentation establishes accuracy. For example, charting that an abdominal wound is "5 cm (2-inches) in length without redness, edema, or drainage" is more descriptive than "large wound healing well." It is essential to avoid unnecessary words and irrelevant details. For example, the fact that a patient is watching television is only necessary when this activity is significant to the patient's status and plan of care.

The Joint Commission requires health care organizations to standardize abbreviations, symbols, acronyms, and dose designations and establish a list of abbreviations that should never be used (TJC, 2012a). Use abbreviations carefully to avoid misinterpretation and minimize errors by spelling out confusing abbreviations. It is essential to know the abbreviation list of the agency in which you work and to use only the accepted abbreviations, symbols, and measures (e.g., metric) so all documentation is accurate and in compliance with standards. For example, the abbreviation for *every day* (*qd*) **is no longer used** (Box 4-2; see Chapter 20). If a treatment or medication is needed daily, the written order or

TABLE 4-1 | Legal Guidelines for Recording

Guidelines	Rationale	Correct Action
Do not erase, apply correction fluid, or scratch out errors made while recording.	Charting becomes illegible: it appears as if you were attempting to hide information or deface record.	Draw single line through error, write word *error* above it, and sign your name or initials. Then record note correctly. Check agency policy.
Do not write retaliatory or critical comments about patient or care by other health care professionals.	Statements can be used as evidence for nonprofessional behavior or poor quality of care.	Enter only objective descriptions of patient's behavior; use quotations for patient's comments.
Need to add additional patient information.	New information is acquired. Forgot to chart during a shift.	If additional information is to be added to an existing entry, write the date and time of the new entry on the next available space and mark it as an addendum (date and time of prior note). Write the current date and time in the next available space and mark it as a late entry (date and time/shift missed).
Correct all errors promptly.	Errors in recording can lead to errors in treatment.	Avoid rushing to complete charting; be sure that information is accurate.
Record all facts.	Record must be accurate and reliable.	Be certain that entry is factual; do not speculate or guess.
Do not leave blank spaces in nurses' notes.	Another person can add incorrect information in space.	Chart consecutively, line by line; if space is left, draw line horizontally through it and sign your name at end.
Record all entries legibly and in black ink.	Illegible entries can be misinterpreted, causing errors and lawsuits; ink cannot be erased; black ink is more legible when records are photocopied or transferred to microfilm.	Never erase entries or use correction fluid and never use pencil.
If order is questioned, record that you sought clarification.	If you perform an order known to be incorrect, you are just as liable for prosecution as the health care provider.	Do not record "physician made error." Instead, chart that "Dr. Smith was called to clarify order for analgesic."
Chart only for yourself.	You are accountable for information that you enter into chart.	Never chart for someone else. **Exception:** If caregiver has left unit for day and calls with information that needs to be documented, include the name of the source of information in the entry and that the information was provided via telephone.
Avoid using generalized, empty phrases such as "status unchanged" or "had good day."	Specific information about patient's condition or case can be deleted accidentally if information is too generalized.	Use complete, concise descriptions of care.
Begin each entry with time and end with your signature and title.	This guideline ensures that correct sequence of events is recorded; signature documents who is accountable for care delivered.	Do not wait until end of shift to record important changes that occurred several hours earlier; be sure to sign each entry.
For computer documentation keep your password to yourself.	Maintains security and confidentiality.	Once logged on to the computer, do not leave the computer screen unattended.

BOX 4-2 | Official "Do Not Use" Abbreviations

Do Not Use	Potential Problem	Use Instead
U, u (unit)	Mistaken for "0" (zero), the number "4" (four), or "cc"	Write "unit"
IU (International Unit)	Mistaken for IV (intravenous) or the number 10 (ten)	Write "International Unit"
Q.D., QD, q.d., qd (daily)	Mistaken for one another	Write "daily"
Q.O.D., QOD, q.o.d, qod (every other day)	Period after the Q mistaken for "I" and the "O" mistaken for "I"	Write "every other day"
Trailing zero (X.0 mg)	Decimal point is missed	Write X mg
Lack of leading zero (.X mg)		Write 0.X mg
MS	Can mean morphine sulfate or magnesium sulfate	Write "morphine sulfate"
MSO4 and MgSO4	Confused for one another	Write "magnesium sulfate"

TJC: *Facts about the official "Do Not Use" list,* available at http://www.jointcommission.org/facts_about_the_official_/, accessed February 1, 2012.

care plan should write out the word *"daily"* or *"every day."* The abbreviation *qd (every day)* can be misinterpreted to mean O.D. *(right eye)*.

Correct spelling demonstrates a level of competency and attention to detail. Many terms are easy to misinterpret because they sound similar (e.g., dysphagia or dysphasia and dram or gram). Some spelling errors result in serious treatment errors (e.g., the names of certain medications such as digitoxin and digoxin or morphine and Numorphan are similar and you need to transcribe them carefully to ensure that a patient receives the correct medication).

The Joint Commission standards (2012a) require that "all entries in medical records be dated and a method is established to identify the authors of entries." Therefore each entry in a patient's record ends with the caregiver's full name or initials and status. Sometimes you document interventions performed by another caregiver. For example, "Patient ambulated by Sue Smith, NA." As a nursing student you need to enter full name, student nurse abbreviation (e.g., SN, NS), and educational institution such as "David Jones, SN (student nurse), CTCC (Central Texas Community College)."

Records need to reflect accountability during the time frame of the entry, which you accomplish best when you chart your own observations and actions. The signature holds that nurse accountable for information recorded. If information was inadvertently omitted from the record, it is acceptable for nurses to ask colleagues to chart information after they leave work. The entry needs to clearly show what was done and by whom (e.g., "At 11 AM Sam Turner, RN, called and reported that at 8 AM Demerol 100 mg IM was administered to patient for abdominal pain"). The nurse recording the information then signs this entry.

Complete

The information within a recorded entry or a report must be complete, containing appropriate and essential information. Criteria for thorough communication exist for certain health problems or nursing activities (Table 4-2). Document entries in a patient's medical record and describe nursing care that you administer and the patient's response. For example:

> 1915 Patient verbalizes sharp, throbbing pain localized along lateral side of right ankle, beginning approximately 15 minutes ago after twisting his foot on the stairs. Patient rates pain as 7 on a scale of 0 to 10. Pain increased to an 8 with movement, relieved to a 6 with elevation. Pedal pulses equal bilaterally. Right ankle circumference 1 cm larger than left. Ice applied. Percocet 2 tabs by mouth given for pain.
>
> 1945 Patient states pain somewhat relieved following application of ice and rates pain as 6 on a scale of 0 to 10. Health care provider notified for new analgesic order. Lee Turno, RN.

You record routine activities such as vital signs, daily hygiene, and ambulation on graphic records and flow sheets. Changes in functional ability or status require more detailed documentation. For example, your patient was unable to move from the bed to the chair without shortness of breath and now is no longer short of breath during this transfer. This change warrants more than simply recording incidence of ambulation on a flow sheet. Instead describe specifically how the patient responded during the transfer.

Current

Current documentation includes making timely entries in a patient's record, which avoids omissions and delay in patient care (TJC, 2012a). To increase accuracy and decrease unnecessary duplication, many health care agencies locate medical records near

TABLE 4-2	Examples of Criteria for Reporting and Recording
Topic	**Criteria To Report or Record**
Assessment	
Subjective data	Description of episode/event in patient's words in quotation marks Clarify onset, location, description of condition (severity; duration; frequency; precipitating, aggravating, and relieving factors)
Patient behavior (e.g., anxiety, confusion, hostility)	Onset, behaviors exhibited, precipitating factors
Objective data (e.g., rash, tenderness, breath sounds)	Onset, location, description of condition (severity; duration; frequency; precipitating, aggravating, and relieving factors)
Nursing Interventions and Evaluation	
Treatments (e.g., enema, bath, dressing change)	Time administered, equipment used (if appropriate), patient's response (objective and subjective changes) compared to previous treatment (e.g., rated pain 2 on a scale of 0-10 during dressing change or "patient reported no abdominal cramping during enema")
Medication administration	Immediately after administration document: time medication given, dose, route, any preliminary assessment (e.g., pain level, vital signs), patient response or effect of medication (e.g., 1200 "Pain reported at 7 (scale 0-10). Tylenol 500 mg given PO." 1230: "Patient reports pain level 2 (scale 0-10) at 1330" or "Pruritus and hives developed over lower abdomen 1 hour after penicillin was given.")
Patient teaching	Information presented; method of instruction (e.g., discussion, demonstration, videotape, booklet); patient response, including questions and evidence of understanding such as return demonstration or change in behavior
Discharge planning	Measurable patient goals or expected outcomes, progress toward goals, need for referrals

a patient's bedside, which facilitate immediate documentation of care activities. Document the following activities or findings at the time of occurrence:

- Vital signs
- Pain assessment and evaluation
- Administration of medications and treatments
- Preparation for diagnostic tests or surgery
- Change in patient's status and who was notified
- Treatment for a sudden change in patient's status
- Patient response to intervention
- Admission, transfer, discharge, or death of a patient

Many health care agencies use military time, a 24-hour system that avoids misinterpretation of AM and PM times. The military clock ends with midnight at 2400 and begins 1 minute after midnight at 0001. For example, 1:00 PM is 1300 military time; 10:22 AM is 1022 military time. Fig. 4-3 compares military and civilian times.

Organized

You need to present written communication in logical order beginning with assessments, nursing interventions, and finally patient responses. Communication is more effective when it is clear, concise, and brief. Entries are more organized and clear if you make a list of what to include before beginning to record in the permanent legal record.

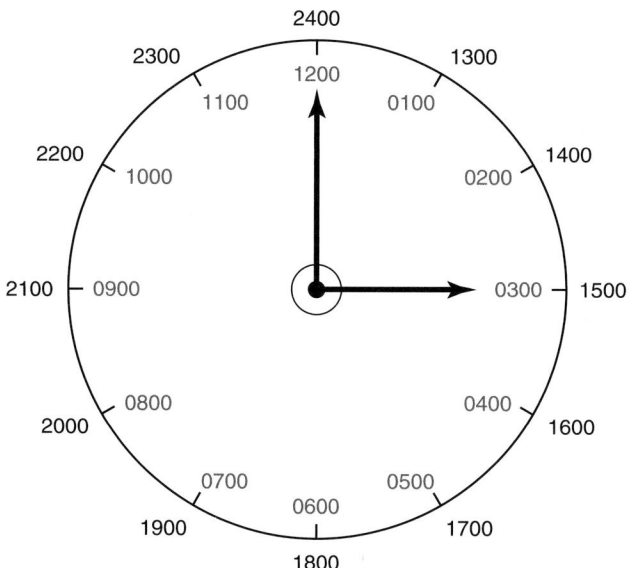

FIG 4-3 Military time clock. Instead of two 12-hour cycles, the military clock is one 24-hour time cycle (e.g., 3 PM is 1500 military time).

COMMON RECORD-KEEPING FORMS OR SCREENS

The patient chart or medical record contains evidence of a patient's health status. The chart includes a variety of forms or screens (as in the case of electronic records) to facilitate quick and comprehensive documentation. Use of these forms helps avoid duplication of information within the record.

Admission Nursing History Forms

A nurse completes a comprehensive nursing history form or screen to gather baseline assessment data when a patient is admitted to a nursing care unit. You use the admission data to form a plan of care and compare it to any changes in a patient's condition. The nursing history guides the admitting nurse through a complete assessment to identify relevant nursing diagnoses or problems for the patient's care plan. Each health care agency designs these forms or screens based on the standards of practice and philosophy of nursing care. Examples of information included in the nursing history are patient allergies, primary spoken/written language, advance directives, disabilities, and mobility/fall risk and medication reconciliation.

Flow Sheets and Graphic Records

Flow sheets and graphic records permit concise documentation of nursing information and patient data over time. They are especially useful for the documentation of routine observations or repeated specific measurements for a patient such as vital signs (see Chapter 6), intake and output, hygiene measures, medication administration (see Chapter 20), and pain assessment. Flow sheets use a format or system for entry of information, usually every 24 hours. (Fig. 4-4). When documenting a significant change that you

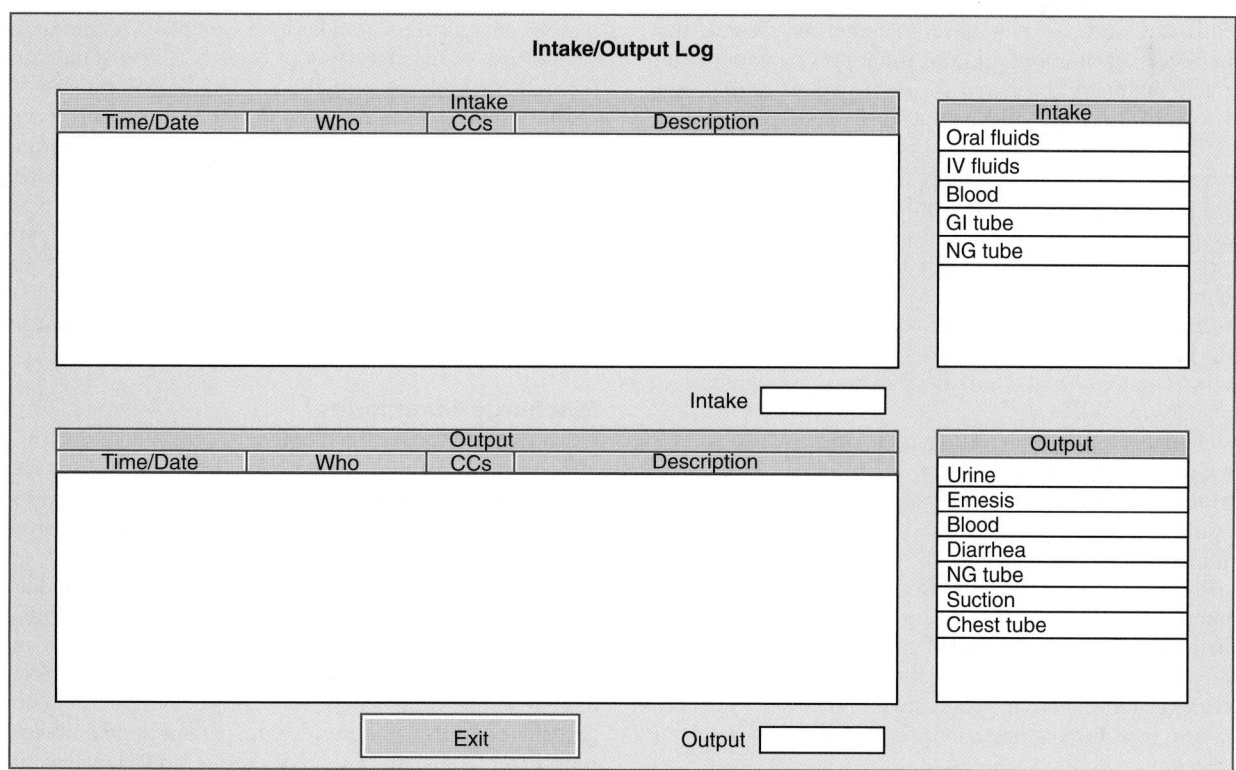

FIG 4-4 Graphic and intake-output record. Electronic version. (*Courtesy ER Choice, Irving, Texas.*)

recognize on a flow sheet, describe the change in the progress notes, including the patient's response to nursing interventions. For example, if a patient's blood pressure becomes dangerously low, record in the progress notes the blood pressure, relevant assessment such as pallor or dizziness, and any interventions to raise the blood pressure. Also include an evaluation of the interventions such as repeated blood pressures and relief of dizziness. Other health care providers such as nursing assistants may have the responsibility to document on nursing flow sheets or screens. Flow sheets and screens provide a quick, easy reference for the health care team members to assess a patient's status.

Patient Education Record

Patient teaching and education are essential nursing interventions. Many health care organizations have an education record that identifies a patient's knowledge base about his or her diagnosis, treatment, and medications. The goal of patient and family education is to promote health behavior and self-care by involving the patient and/or family in decisions, which improves health outcomes. Standards for patient education include assessment of needs, functional abilities, learning styles, and readiness to learn. You base patient education needs on the assessment and then teach patients about topics such as safe and effective use of medications, nutrition and dietary modifications, safe use of medical equipment, pain control, rehabilitative methods to promote and improve functional abilities, and self-care activities (TJC, 2012a). Hospitals provide educational materials for patients by handouts, many of which are accessed by the computer network in the hospital. When documenting on a patient teaching record, be specific about the information and/or skills taught, the patient's learning response, and information given to the patient.

Patient Care Summary or Kardex

Many health care agencies now have computerized systems that provide a concise set of information in the form of a patient care summary. This summary prints out for each patient during each shift. Data are updated automatically as new orders and nursing decisions enter the system.

In some health care settings a Kardex ("cardboard flip-over" file) kept at the nurses' station provides information for daily patient care needs. It has two parts: an activity and treatment section and a nursing care plan section. The updated information in both the patient summary and the Kardex eliminate the need for repeated referral to the chart for routine information throughout the day. The forms do not always become part of the permanent record. Information commonly found on the patient care summary or Kardex includes the following:

- Basic demographic data (e.g., age, religion)
- Primary medical diagnosis
- Current health care provider's orders (e.g., diet, activity, dressing changes)
- A nursing care plan
- Nursing orders or interventions (e.g., intake and output, comfort measures, teaching)
- Scheduled tests and procedures
- Safety precautions used in the patient's care
- Factors related to activities of daily living
- Nearest relative/guardian or person to contact in an emergency
- Emergency code status
- Allergies

Acuity Records

Many health care organizations use a patient acuity system as a method of determining the intensity of nursing care required for a group of patients. Acuity measurements for patients on a unit serve as a guide for determining staffing needs. An acuity recording system determines the hours of nursing care and number of staff required for a nursing unit.

Typically nurses enter acuity data into a computerized system in the morning. The administrative staff collects the acuity data electronically and use it to make appropriate staffing decisions. Acuity levels allow the nursing staff to compare patients with one another. For example, an acuity system might rate bathing patients from 1 to 5 (1 is totally dependent, 5 is independent); a patient returning from surgery who requires frequent monitoring and extensive care has an acuity level of 1. On the same continuum another patient awaiting discharge after a successful recovery from surgery has an acuity level of 5. Accurate acuity ratings justify the number and qualifications of staff needed to safely care for patients on a particular unit.

Standardized Care Plans

The trend among many health care organizations is to computerize care plans. These systems provide daily computer-generated care plans, which incorporate several nursing diagnoses or problems in a single care plan. These systems improve nursing documentation and facilitate high-quality care that is based on scientific evidence and proven experience (Fogelberg-Dahm, 2008). Standardized care plans are based on agency standards of nursing practice and are established guidelines used to care for patients with similar health problems. After completing a nursing assessment, you identify the patient's nursing diagnosis or health problem and select an appropriate standardized care plan for the patient medical record. You individualize it for each patient. Most standardized care plans allow for the addition of patient-specific outcomes and target dates for achieving these outcomes.

One advantage of standardized care plans is the establishment of evidence-based standards of care. By using standardized plans nurses learn to recognize the accepted requirements of care for patients. They also improve continuity of care among professional nurses. The Joint Commission supports the use of standardized care plans and no longer requires a written care plan for each patient.

One disadvantage of standardized care plans is an increased risk that the unique, individualized therapies needed by patients will go unrecognized. Standardized care plans do not replace your professional judgment and decision making. In addition, care plans need to be updated on a regular basis to ensure that content is current and appropriate.

Discharge Summaries

Discharge planning is a comprehensive process with emphasis placed on preparing a patient for discharge from a health care organization. Discharge planning, case management, and utilization review are all involved in patient care. A prospective payment system based on diagnosis-related groups (DRGs) encourages health care organizations to be more efficient and discharge a patient as soon as possible. Early hospital discharge improves hospital chances of full reimbursement. It is important to ensure that a patient's discharge results in desirable outcomes. You enhance discharge planning when you are responsive to changes in a patient's condition and involve the patient and family in the planning process (Bauer et al., 2009; Rose and Haugen, 2010). The discharge summary includes essential information for the patient, family, and health care organization (Box 4-3).

BOX 4-3 | **Discharge Summary Information**

- Use clear, concise descriptions in patient's own language.
- Provide step-by-step description of how to perform a procedure (e.g., home medication administration). Reinforce explanation with printed instructions for the patient to take home.
- Identify precautions to follow when performing self-care or administering medications.
- Review any restrictions that may relate to activities of daily living (e.g., bathing, ambulating, and driving).
- Review signs and symptoms of complications to report to health care provider.
- List names and phone numbers of health care providers and community resources for the patient to contact.
- Identify any unresolved problem, including plans for follow-up and continuous treatment.
- List actual time of discharge, mode of transportation, and who accompanied patient.

Discharge planning begins at admission and becomes a more prominent part of care as a patient gets closer to discharge. There must be evidence of the involvement of the patient and family members in the discharge planning process so the patient and family have the necessary information and resources to return home (Bauer et al., 2009; Rose and Haugen, 2010). The Joint Commission (2012b) has standards for patient and family education necessary for effective discharge planning. When a patient is discharged from a health care organization, the members of the health care team prepare a discharge summary. It provides important information relating to the patient's ongoing health problems and need for health care after discharge. Discharge planning achieves specific outcomes that include identifying patients with ongoing health needs, collaborating with other health care professions to determine level of care, matching patients with appropriate referrals and resources, and streamlining the transition to the next level of care (Rose and Haugen, 2010). Include in the discharge summary the reason for hospitalization; significant findings; current status of the patient; and the teaching plan that is given to the patient or family, home care, rehabilitation, or long-term care facility (TJC, 2012a). Discharge summaries make the summary concise and instructive. They emphasize previous learning by the patient and family and care that needs to continue in any restorative care setting.

CHARTING SYSTEMS

A variety of documentation systems (computerized and written) exist for recording patient information and progress. The documentation system selected by nursing reflects the philosophy of the health care organization. The same documentation system is used throughout a specific agency, but there are several acceptable methods for recording health care data.

Narrative Documentation

A nurse enters narrative documentation for recording nursing care and activities that cannot be thoroughly explained on flow sheets or other standardized screens or forms. Narrative charting uses a storylike format to document specific information about a patient's conditions and nursing care, usually presented in chronologic order. Narrative charting is useful in emergency situations when the time and order of events are important. Organize a narrative in a clear, concise way (e.g., by using the nursing process to order

the data). In many settings methods such as focus or SBAR charting has replaced narrative charting.

Problem-Oriented Medical Records

A problem-oriented medical record (POMR) is a structured method of documenting narratives that emphasizes a patient's problems. This method organizes data using the nursing process, which facilitates communication about patient needs. Data are organized by problem or diagnosis. Ideally all members of the health care team contribute to the list of identified patient problems. This approach assists in coordinating an individualized plan of care with the following sections: database, problem list, care plan, and progress notes.

Patient Database

A database contains all available information pertaining to a patient. This section is the foundation for identifying patient problems and planning care. The database remains active and current for each patient and is revised as new data become available.

Problem List

You develop a patient's problem list after analyzing his or her assessment data. The problem list includes the patient's physiologic, psychological, sociocultural, spiritual, developmental, and environmental needs. Identify and list priority problems in chronologic order to serve as an organizing guide for the patient's care. Add new problems as they are identified during the ongoing nursing assessment. When a problem is resolved, you record the date and draw a line through the problem and its number.

Nursing Care Plan

All disciplines involved in a patient's care contribute to the development of a plan of care for a specific problem. For example, for a patient having a nutritional deficit, a nurse recommends feeding approaches, and a registered dietitian recommends types of dietary supplements. Care plan standards require that a plan of care be developed for all patients on admission to a health care organization (TJC, 2012a). Generally these plans include nursing diagnoses, expected outcomes, and interventions.

Progress Notes

Health care team members use progress notes to monitor and record the progress of a patient's problem (Box 4-4). Narrative notes, flow sheets, and discharge summaries are formats used to document patient progress (see Procedural Guideline 4-2).

SBAR Documentation. Structured communication provides a model for data about a patient's condition. SBAR is a technique that provides a framework for communication among members of the health care team such as physicians when there is a change in patient's condition. You apply this method to both written and verbal communication. SBAR standardizes communication and improves the effectiveness of information (Dunsford, 2009). When a patient's condition changes, use the following SBAR mnemonic:

- **S:** Situation (Identify yourself, your unit, and the patient. State what is happening at the present time.)
- **B:** Background (Give patient's diagnosis, reason for admission. Explain the circumstances leading up to the situation.) Have patient's chart available when reporting.
- **A:** Assessment (Provide specific information [i.e., quantitative and qualitative data] as necessary. What do you think the problem is?)
- **R:** Recommendation (Explain what you need. Be clear and specific. What would you do to correct the problem?) Read back any verbal or telephone orders received following your recommendation.

BOX 4-4 | Formats for Recording Progress Notes

Narrative Note

Describes patient data in a narrative paragraph

Example:

Patient states, "I'm dreading this surgery because last time I had a terrible reaction to the anesthesia and such terrible pain when they made me get out of bed." Noted muscle tension and loud, agitated voice. Notified anesthesiologist, Dr. Martin, of patient's prior experience. Discussed alternatives for anesthesia and pain-control options. Stressed importance of activity for circulation/healing. Encouraged to keep nurses informed of pain level/need for medication and that pain may be present but manageable.

SBAR (Acronym for Situation, Background, Assessment, and Recommendation)

SBAR is a system of structured communication used to share information about a patient's condition.

Example:

S (Situation): Patient verbalized preoperative fears. Nurse noted muscle tension and loud, agitated voice.

B (Background): Patient fearful of surgery because of past experiences with anesthesia and pain.

A (Actions taken): Notified anesthesiologist, Dr. Martin, of patient's prior experience. Discussed alternatives for anesthesia and pain-control options. Stressed importance of activity for circulation/healing. Encouraged to keep nurses informed of pain level/need for medication and that pain may be present but manageable.

R (Recommendation): Assess pain level at least every 4 hours after surgery. Provide nonpharmacologic pain-management techniques, and administer medication as needed.

SOAP (Acronym for Subjective Data, Objective Data, Assessment, and Plan)

Usually based on a numbered list of problems or nursing diagnoses

Example:

S (Subjective data) (the patient's statements regarding the problem): Patient states, "I'm dreading this surgery because last time I had a terrible reaction to the anesthesia and such terrible pain when they made me get out of bed."

O (Objective data) (observations that support or are related to subjective data): Noted muscle tension and loud, agitated voice.

A (Assessment/Analysis) (conclusions reached based on data): Fear related to pain/anesthesia.

P (Plan) (the plan for dealing with the situation): Notified anesthesiologist, Dr. Martin, of patient's prior experience.

Discussed alternatives for anesthesia and pain-control options. Stressed importance of activity for circulation/healing. Encouraged to keep nurses informed of pain level/need for medication and that pain may be present but manageable.

PIE (Acronym for Problem, Intervention, and Evaluation)

Problem-oriented system in which progress notes are written based on a list of identified problems and detailed data may be entered by any member of the health care team

Example:

P (Problem): Patient states, "I'm dreading this surgery because last time I had a terrible reaction to the anesthesia and such terrible pain when they made me get out of bed." Noted muscle tension and loud, agitated voice.

I (Intervention): Notified anesthesiologist, Dr. Martin, of patient's prior experience. Discussed alternatives for anesthesia and pain-control options. Stressed importance of activity for circulation/healing. Encouraged to keep nurses informed of pain level/need for medication and that pain may be present but manageable.

E (Evaluation): Patient stated that she was "very relieved." Stated that she would tell the nurses about pain.

Focus or DAR Charting (Acronym for Data, Action, and Response)

A way to organize progress notes to make them more clear and organized

Example:

D (Data): Patient states, "I'm dreading this surgery because last time I had a terrible reaction to the anesthesia and such terrible pain when they made me get out of bed." Noted muscle tension and loud, agitated voice.

A (Nursing Action): Notified anesthesiologist, Dr. Martin, of patient's prior experience. Discussed alternatives for anesthesia and pain-control options. Stressed importance of activity for circulation/healing. Encouraged to keep nurses informed of pain level/need for medication and that pain may be present but manageable.

R (Patient Response): Patient stated that she was "very relieved." Stated understanding of the importance of informing the nurses about pain.

NOTE: Some agencies add *P (Plan)* and refer to this as DARP charting.

Example:

P (Plan): Assess pain level at least every 4 hours after surgery. Provide nonpharmacologic pain management techniques and administer medication as needed.

SBAR is a concrete approach for framing conversations, especially critical ones that require a nurse's immediate attention and action. It allows for an easy and focused way to set expectations for what the team will communicate. SBAR promotes the provision of safe, efficient, timely, and patient-centered communication (Chaboyer et al., 2010; Day, 2010).

SBAR can also be used for multiple forms of communication. It can be used for a brief targeted report (e.g., as a preprocedure or postprocedure report) or as a change-of-shift report as shown here (Pope et al., 2008; Thomas et al., 2009).

S Situation (admission date, chief complaint and diagnosis)

B Background (medical history, allergies, code status, isolation, significant interventions, pain management, responses to interventions, report of abnormal studies, who was notified, any interventions, intravenous [IV] access)

A Assessment (review of systems: neurologic, respiratory, cardiac, gastrointestinal, genitourinary, musculoskeletal, peripheral vascular, skin, hematologic, endocrine, and psychosocial; vital signs; pain assessment and goals; blood sugar and sliding scale coverage; fall risk)

R Recommendations (patient's daily goals, consultations, planned treatments, upcoming tests or surgery, discharge planning, and patient education

SOAP Documentation. One way to structure narrative notes to document patient progress is the SOAP format. SOAP is a mnemonic for the following:

S: Subjective data (patient statements about the problem)

O: Objective data (data that are measured and observed or related to subjective data)

A: Assessment/Analysis (conclusions based on the subjective and objective data)

P: Plan (what the caregiver plans to do)

Some agencies add an *I* and *E* (i.e., SOAPIE). The *I* stands for *intervention*, and the *E* represents *evaluation*. The logic for SOAP (IE) notes is similar to that of the nursing process: collect data about a patient's problems, draw conclusions, and develop a plan of care. Number each SOAP note and title it according to the problem on the list.

PIE Documentation. The PIE note format of documentation is similar to that of SOAP charting in its problem-oriented nature. However, it differs from the SOAP method in that PIE charting has a nursing origin, whereas SOAP originated from a medical model. PIE is a mnemonic for the following:

P Problem or nursing diagnosis for the patient

I Interventions or actions taken

E Evaluation of the outcomes of nursing interventions

The PIE format simplifies documentation by combining the care plan and progress note into one record. The PIE format differs from that of SOAP because there are no assessment data in the narrative note. Assessment data are included in documentation on the flow sheets of each shift. You number or label the PIE notes according to a patient's problems. Resolved problems are dropped from daily documentation after your review. Continuing problems are documented daily.

Focus Charting. Another narrative format is focus charting or DAR (data, action, response). One distinction of focus charting is that it places less importance on patient problems and focuses on patient concerns such as a sign or symptom, a condition, a nursing diagnosis, a behavior, a significant event, or a change in condition. Each entry includes data (both subjective and objective), actions or nursing interventions, and patient response (e.g., evaluation of effectiveness). Nurses need to broaden their thinking to include any patient concerns, not just problem areas, and to apply critical thinking. Focus charting saves time because it is easy for caregivers to understand, is adaptable to most health care settings, and enables all caregivers to track a patient's condition and progress.

Source Records

In a source record a patient's chart is organized so each discipline (i.e., nursing, medicine, social work, and respiratory therapy) has a separate section in which to record data. The advantage of a source record is that it is easy for caregivers to locate the proper section of the record in which to make entries.

A disadvantage of the source record is that information about a specific problem may be distributed throughout the record. For example, the nurse describes the character of a patient's fractured femur pain and use of repositioning and narcotic analgesia in the nurses' notes and electronic health record (EHR). The health care provider notes in a separate section of the record the patient's bone healing and the plan for casting or surgery. The results of x-ray examinations that show bone healing are in the radiology results section of the record. The method makes it difficult to find chronologic information about patient care or how the team is coordinating care to meet all of the patient's needs.

Charting by Exception

Charting by exception (CBE) is a system of documentation that aims to eliminate redundancy, makes documentation of routine care more concise, emphasizes abnormal findings, and identifies trends in clinical care. CBE is a shorthand method for documenting based on clearly defined standards of practice and predetermined criteria for nursing assessments and interventions. This system involves completing a flow sheet that incorporates standard assessment and intervention criteria by placing a check mark in the appropriate standard box on the flow sheet to indicate normal findings and routine interventions. You write a narrative nurse's note *only* when there is an exception to the established standard or abnormal data are present. Assessments are standardized on forms so all health care providers evaluate and document findings consistently (Fig. 4-5).

The presumption with CBE is that the nurse assessed the patient and all standards are met unless otherwise documented. Changes in a patient's condition require thorough and precise descriptions of what happened, actions taken, and patient response to treatment. Legal risks in using CBE include difficulty in proving safe care if nurses are not disciplined in documenting exceptions.

Case Management Plan and Critical Pathways

Case management is a delivery of care model that coordinates patient services to provide high-quality patient care experiences that are cost effective and provide optimal patient outcomes (Hospital Case Management, 2010; Park and Huber, 2009). Collaboration and communication are promoted in a multidisciplinary approach using critical or collaborative pathways for a specific disease or condition that is summarized into a standardized care plan. Case management plans incorporate standardized documents that include short care plans for the problem, key interventions, and expected outcomes for patients with a specific disease or condition (Fig. 4-6). These pathways provide the ideal sequence and timing of interventions for all members of the health care team. Use of critical pathways provides a resource for caregivers to ensure that clinical care is given with transparent accountability (Earle-Foley, 2011). The goal of a critical pathway is to improve the quality of care, reduce risks, increase patient satisfaction, and improve outcomes (Marchisio and others, 2009).

Case management programs use multidisciplinary plans of care summarized into critical pathways, which include key interventions and expected outcomes within an established time frame (see Fig. 4-6). Critical pathways are evidence based, and the assessment and monitoring, interventions, and expected outcomes are based on research and/or clinical evidence from the literature or the practice standards of the health care agency.

Critical pathways state the goals and important treatment interventions based on best practice and patient expectations by documenting, monitoring, and evaluating variances and providing resources and outcomes. Variances are unexpected occurrences, unmet goals, and interventions not specified within the critical pathway time frame and reflect a positive or negative change. A positive variance occurs when a patient progresses more rapidly than the case management plan expected (e.g., use of a Foley catheter is discontinued a day early). A negative variance occurs when the activities on the critical pathway do not happen as predicted or outcomes are unmet (e.g., oxygen therapy is necessary for a new-onset breathing problem). Your responsibility is to document the variance and include causative factors, actions taken, patient response, and outcomes. Over time the recurrence of similar variances lead the health care team to revise a critical pathway, particularly if it affects quality of care or length of stay.

STANDARDIZED LANGUAGE

Standardized language enhances use of accurate nursing diagnoses, increases effective nursing interventions, and improves patient outcomes (Müller-Staub, 2009). Nursing care is more effective and

BARNES-JEWISH HOSPITAL

Nursing Shift Assessment C-6

Requested by: CAROL

789651458 X
Collins, Phil

S.S.

Dr.

Unit: Bed:

Search Interval   From: 05-Dec-2009 at 07:00
                   To: 06-Dec-2009 at 14:51

Patient Assessment

		Monday 12/06 07:00
N/S	**NEUROSENSORY STANDARD** Alert and awake. If asleep awakens to name. Verbal appropriate, clear, and understandable. Swallows without coughing. Oriented to time, place, person and situation. Behavior is appropriate to situation. Moves all extremities well, ambulates with steady gait.	Within Normal Limits
RESP	**RESPIRATORY STANDARD** Respirations are even and unlabored. Nailbeds and mucous membranes are pink. Patent airway. Lung sounds clear to auscultation. No cough noted	Within Normal Limits
CARD	**CARDIOVASCULAR STANDARD** Regular palpable pulses. Skin pallor within patient's norm. Skin warm and dry. No edema.	Within Normal Limits
SKIN	**SKIN INTEGRITY STANDARD** Skin and mucous membranes intact without notable lesions or impaired integrity. Mucous membranes moist and pink. Braden Score greater than 17.	* Exception as noted below
	Braden Risk Assessment	Mobility: Slightly Limited (3) Sensory: Slightly Limited (3) Moisture: Occasionally Moist (3) Activity: Walks Occasionally (3) Nutrition: Adequate (3) Friction/Shear: Potential Problem (2) Total Score 17
	Casts, Splints, Braces Type: Fiberglass Cast Site: Right Lower Leg	Maintains correct anatomical position No pressure areas noted Distal extremity pink warm to touch Palpable distal pulse Capillary Refill <3 seconds Sensation normal Able to move distal phalanges.
	VASCULAR ACCESS STANDARD IV SITE: Site free of redness, swelling, pain, bleeding, drainage, IV patent, dressing occlusive and intact.	
NUTR	**NUTRITION STANDARD** Tolerating prescribed diet without nausea and vomiting. Eating at least 75% of each meal without difficulty. Feeds self.	Within normal limits
	Diet Type	Regular
GI	**GASTROINTESTINAL STANDARD** Abdomen soft. Bowel sounds active all 4 quadrants. No pain with palpation. Having bowel movements within patient's normal pattern, consistency, and color.	Within Normal Limits
GU	**GENITOURINARY STANDARD** Continent of urine. Urine clear and yellow to amber color.	Within Normal Limits
PSYCH	**PSYCHOSOCIAL STANDARD** Accepts situation and facial expressions are appropriate. family support available and patient receives visitors. Able to communicate without assistance.	Within Normal Limits
EDU	Health Status Teaching	
	Tests/Procedures/Therapies	
	Medication Teaching	
	Nutrition Teaching	
	Medical Equipment Teaching	
HMGT	Equipment	
Charted By		cl

Signatures:
cl   C. Logan, RN

Printed: 06-Dec-2009 at 14:51

FIG 4-5 Charting by exception—assessment form. When standards in far left column are not met, a detailed note explaining findings must be entered. (*Courtesy Barnes-Jewish Hospital, BJC Health System, St Louis, Mo.*)

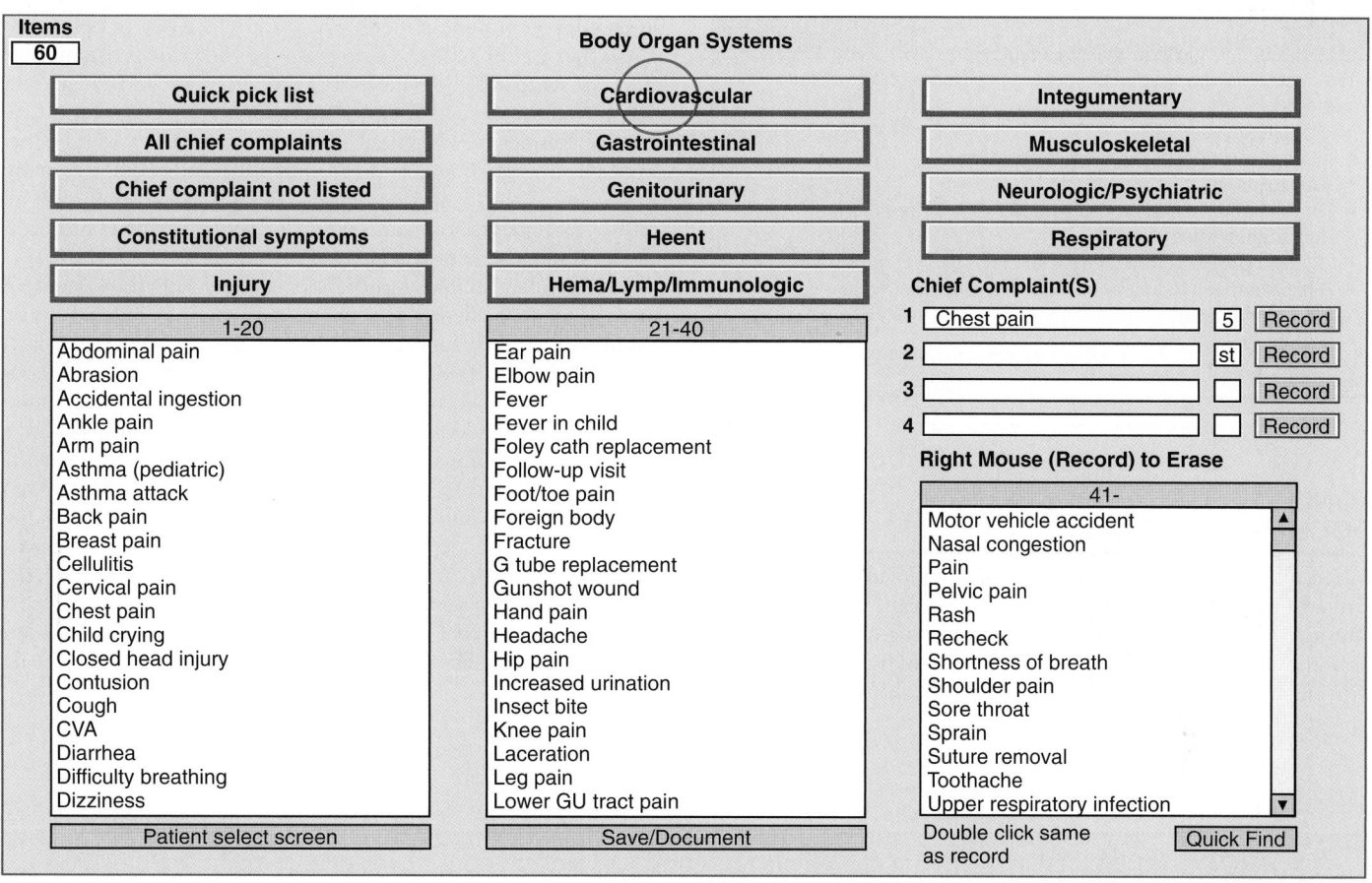

FIG 4-6 Electronic Documentation. Nursing record. (*Courtesy ER Choice, Irving, Tex.*)

appropriate to patient needs when nurses use the same language to identify patient problems and plan patient outcomes. Several classification systems provide standardized language. The North American Nursing Diagnosis Association (NANDA) International (NANDA-I) (2012) has established standardized nursing diagnoses to describe patients' responses to health problems. The Nursing Interventions Classification (NIC) provides a label name, definition, and list of activities that a nurse performs to complete an intervention (Center for Nursing and Clinical Effectiveness, 2011a). Use of this standardized language in documentation may prove useful to communicate patient care needs more clearly.

Another standard form of language being used throughout health care is patient outcomes. The Nursing Outcomes Classification (NOC) provides an outcome label, a definition, and a list of interventions that can result in the outcome (Center for Nursing and Clinical Effectiveness, 2011b). The use of outcomes is essential when evaluating the achievement of patient care goals and the appropriateness of patient interventions.

Outcome statements require a target date for completion and evaluation of a patient's progress toward achievement at specific intervals. Evaluation of progress determines if the patient's problem or diagnosis is resolved or if you need to revise or extend the plan. You individualize each outcome for the particular patient using specific measurement criteria. Such a process promotes continuity of care across the continuum of a patient's care and centers on the patient's and family's ability to restore, maintain, or improve the patient's health. The implementation of NANDA-I, NIC, and NOC nursing diagnoses, interventions, and outcomes can lead to higher quality of nursing diagnosis documentation, etiology-specific nursing interventions, and nursing-specific patient outcomes (Müller-Staub et al., 2008).

HOME CARE DOCUMENTATION

Home care continues to grow with shorter hospitalizations and increasing numbers of older adults requiring home care services. Medicare has specific guidelines for establishing eligibility for home care reimbursement. Skilled home nursing care is divided into six categories of practice: assessment, diagnosis, outcomes identification, planning, implementation, and evaluation of a care plan (Gorski, 2008). When you provide care in the home, documentation has different implications than in other areas of nursing. One primary difference is that the patient and family rather than the nurse witness the majority of care. In addition, documentation systems need to provide the entire health care team with the necessary information to work together effectively (Box 4-5). The documentation is both the quality control and the justification for reimbursement from Medicare, Medicaid, or private insurance companies. It is important to consistently document all of your services for reimbursement (e.g., direct skilled care, patient instructions, skilled observation, and evaluation visits) (TJC, 2012a).

Computerized patient records are evolving in the home care setting. The electronic health record will facilitate clarity, continuity of care, and comprehensiveness because of increased standardization of language (Gjevjon and Hellesø, 2010).

BOX 4-5 | Home Care Forms for Documentation

The usual forms used to document home care include the following:

- Patient assessment
- Referral source information/intake form
- Discipline-specific care plans
- Physician or health care provider's plan of treatment
- Medication sheet
- Clinical progress notes
- Miscellaneous (conference notes, verbal order forms, telephone calls)
- Discharge summary
- Reports to third-party payers

LONG-TERM HEALTH CARE DOCUMENTATION

Increasing numbers of older adults and disabled people in the United States require care in long-term health care agencies. Nursing personnel face documentation challenges much different from those in the acute care setting. Adding EHR documentation will enhance communication among the health care providers, along with improving patient safety and efficiency of delivery of care (Cherry et al., 2011). Changes in the Medicare program determine the standards and policies for reimbursement and documentation in long-term care. The federally mandated Long-Term Care Facility Resident Assessment Instrument provides standardized protocols for assessment and care planning and promotes quality improvement within and among agencies (Adams-Wendling et al., 2008). Documentation and coding of services will continue to impact reimbursement (Field and Gross, 2009).

Each resident in long-term care is assessed using the Long-Term Care Facility Resident Assessment Instrument mandated by the Omnibus Budget Reconciliation Act of 1989 (OBRA) and updated in 1998 (HCFA, 1998). A registered nurse is responsible for coordinating the plan of care. Documentation supports the assessment and planning process for patients using a multidisciplinary approach. Communication among health care providers, including nurses, social workers, recreational therapists, and dietitians, is essential in the documentation process. The fiscal support for long-term care residents depends on the justification of nursing care as demonstrated in sound documentation of the services rendered. The overall goal is a system of clinical documentation that identifies potential or actual problems and provides improved actions for each problem, which result in improved care for residents (Duda-Gardiner, 2010).

PROCEDURAL GUIDELINE 4-1 Giving a Hand-Off Report

In addition to written documentation, a nurse provides a change-of-shift report to the next nurse assuming responsibility for patient care. The purpose of the report is to provide continuity of care for the patient. The Joint Commission 2012 *National Patient Safety Goals* (2012b) for health care organizations standardize an approach to hand-off communication that includes opportunities to ask and respond to questions. Nurses give a hand-off report face-to-face, by audiotape recording, via telephone conversation, through a written report, in a computer format, or during "walking-planning" rounds at each patient's bedside. It is important to have some type of guidelines for reporting to avoid repetitive, irrelevant, and speculative communication (Chaboyer et al., 2010; Robert Wood Johnson Foundation, 2009). It is essential to schedule an opportunity for oncoming nurses to ask questions for clarification after listening to the report to prevent omissions in care and ensure that appropriate interventions continue. Regardless of the form of the hand-off report, you must maintain confidentiality.

Delegation and Collaboration

The skill of giving a hand-off report cannot be delegated to nursing assistive personnel (NAP). Licensed practical nurses (LPNs) may report on patients for whom they care directly. The nurse directs the NAP about what to report to the nurse (e.g., increased pain, changes in vital signs) so there can be assessment, validation, and reporting of any changes in the hand-off report.

Equipment

❑ Worksheets, patient care summary or nursing Kardex, nursing care plan, critical pathway, or multidisciplinary treatment plan
❑ Tape recorder (according to agency policy)

Procedural Steps

1 Develop an organized format for delivering report that provides a description of patient needs and problems.
2 Gather information from documentation sources, NAP report, or other relevant documents.

Clinical Decision Point *Report only relevant information to next shift to ensure staff's timely responsiveness.*

3 Prioritize information based on patient's needs and problems.
4 For each patient include:
   a *Background information:* Patient's name, gender, age, current primary reason for hospitalization, and brief history. Also include any known allergies, emergency code status (i.e., do not resuscitate [DNR]) and special needs as related to any physical challenges (e.g., blind, hearing deficit, amputee).
   b *Assessment data:* Provide objective observations and measurements made by the nurse during the shift. Describe patient's condition and emphasize any recent changes. Include any relevant information reported by patient, family, or health care team members such as laboratory data and diagnostic test results.
   c *Nursing diagnoses or patient problems:* State the nursing diagnoses or patient problem appropriate for patient. (Some agencies do not include nursing diagnoses in report.)
   d *Interventions, outcomes, and evaluation:* (Steps can be combined in a report.)
      (1) Describe therapies or treatments administered during shift and expected outcomes (e.g., medication changes, use of oxygen, referral visits). Specify how you

PROCEDURAL GUIDELINE 4-1   Giving a Hand-Off Report—cont'd

implemented interventions uniquely for this patient. Report on evaluation by explaining patient's response and whether outcomes are met. Do not explain basic steps of a procedure.

(2) Describe instructions or education given in the teaching plan and patient's/family's ability to demonstrate learning.

e *Family information*: Report on family visitation or involvement, specifically as it influenced patient. Explain if you included family members in care procedures or instruction.

f *Discharge plan*: Review patient's progress toward discharge during each change-of-shift report. Discuss education progress, communication with referral agencies, and family preparation for discharge. This plan also identifies roles and responsibilities of the multidisciplinary team and their follow-up visits.

g *Current priorities*: Clearly explain the priorities to which oncoming nurse must attend.

(1) Report significant clinical changes.

(2) Report on immediate treatment planned for any new admission.

(3) Explain status of activities for patients preparing for procedures and treatments.

(4) Describe current physical status of patients returning from diagnostic or operative procedures.

5 Ask staff from oncoming shift if they have any questions regarding information provided.

6 If using a tape recorder, periodically evaluate for clarity, organization, rate of speaking, and volume level.

PROCEDURAL GUIDELINE 4-2   Documenting Nurses' Progress Notes

A variety of forms and formats communicate information about a patient's health status and care. Accurate documentation reflects the quality of care and provides evidence of each health care team member's accountability in giving care. The purpose of a patient's record is to provide information for communication, education, assessment, research, financial billing, auditing, and legal documentation (Table 4-3).

Because the nursing process directs a nurse's approach to patient care, documentation needs to reflect this process. Nurses record assessment data, changes in a patient's condition, nursing interventions, and an evaluation of the patient's progress toward established outcomes. Prompt documentation of this data increases accuracy and promotes effective communication to all members of the health care team.

Progress notes provide a format for documenting a patient's health status and progress. You can use a variety of formats when writing notes, including SBAR, SOAP, SOAPIE, PIE, and DAR. All caregivers need to be able to read the progress note and have a clear picture of the problem, level of care required, and results of interventions. The nurse caring for the patient is responsible for writing and signing each progress note, which includes full name and title.

Delegation and Collaboration

The skill of documenting nurse progress notes cannot be delegated to nursing assistive personnel (NAP). The nurse instructs the NAP about:

- What repetitive care activities to document on flow sheets (e.g., vital signs, intake and output [I&O], routine care).
- What to report to the nurse (e.g., increased pain, changes in vital signs) so he or she can reassess, validate, and document any changes in the progress note.

Equipment

❑ Progress note form (written or electronic)
❑ Black pen

Procedural Steps

1 Review assessment data, problems identified, goals and expected outcomes, nursing interventions, and patient response during contact with each patient and before documentation.

2 Document patient information in the narrative format chosen by the health care agency.
Follow guidelines for charting to ensure quality documentation.

3 After each patient contact, identify information that needs to be documented. Consider:
a Abnormal findings.
b Changes in status.
c New problems identified.

4 Document in a timely fashion without leaving open spaces between notes and include date and time.

5 Using agency format, document in chronological order the following:
a Pertinent, factual, objective data
b Selected subjective data that validates or clarifies
c Nursing actions taken
d Patient responses to actions taken
e Additional plans needing to be implemented
f To whom information has been reported, including name and status

6 Sign progress note with full name or first initial and last name and status according to agency policy. Do not leave any open space between this note and the previously written note. Students are usually required to indicate their level of education and school affiliation.

7 Review previously documented entries with those that you enter, noting if there is significant change in the patient's status. Report any changes to the patient's health care provider.

TABLE 4-3	Purposes of Records

Purpose	Description
Communication	The record is a means for health care team members to communicate a patient's *needs* (e.g., individual therapies, patient education, discharge planning) and *progress* (e.g., response to therapies). Anyone reading the record should have a clear understanding of the plan of care.
Education	The record contains a variety of information, including medical and nursing diagnoses, signs and symptoms of disease, successful and unsuccessful therapies, diagnostic findings, and patient behaviors. Students of nursing, medicine, and other health-related disciplines use records as educational resources.
Assessment	Records provide data that nurses use to identify and support nursing diagnoses and plan proper interventions for care. Information from records adds to the nurse's own observations and assessment. Information in medical progress notes allows a nurse to anticipate the status of a patient and conduct an assessment that augments, validates, or confirms health care provider findings.
Research	Statistical data relating to the frequency of clinical disorders, complications, use of specific medical and nursing therapies, recovery from illness, and death can be gathered from patient records. Records describe characteristics of patient populations in a health care agency.
Financial billing	The medical record is a document that shows the extent to which hospitals should be reimbursed for services. For the agency to obtain full reimbursement, the record needs to show that all health care providers' orders were completed adequately and correctly, and it must reflect results of those orders.
Auditing and monitoring	A regular review of information in patient records gives a basis for evaluation of the quality and appropriateness of care provided in an agency. The Joint Commission (2012a) requires health care organizations to establish quality assessment and improvement programs to conduct objective, ongoing reviews of patient care. Review of records reveals information about the processes and outcomes of care.
Legal documentation	A medical record must be accurate because it is a legal document. In case of a lawsuit, the medical record, not the nursing care, is on trial. Nursing care may have been excellent; however, care not documented is care not done as far as a court of law is concerned.

PROCEDURAL GUIDELINE 4-3   Adverse Event/Incident Reporting

An incident or adverse event is any event not consistent with the routine operation of a health care unit or routine care of a patient. Examples include patient falls, needlestick injuries, medication errors, or a visitor becoming ill. The National Quality Forum (2011) identified a standardized list of preventable, serious adverse events that facilitate reporting of such events (Table 4-4). In 2011 the Institute of Medicine examined the safety of Health IT and its impact on patients (IOM, 2011). Included in this report was a recommendation that IT vendors should have a mandatory obligation to report adverse events, and users should voluntarily report these events. Completion of an occurrence report happens when there is actual or potential patient injury (near miss) that is not part of the patient record. Document in the patient's record an objective description of what you observed and follow-up actions taken without reference to the incident report/occurrence report. Reporting helps to identify high-risk trends in nursing care or daily unit operations that warrant correction. You complete the report even if an injury does not occur or is not apparent. The information from the reports helps nursing staff find solutions to prevent repeated incidents. The reports are an important part of the quality improvement program of a unit.

Adverse event/incident reports are important sources of data for enhancing understanding of underlying causes of events that, when analyzed, can improve patient safety (ASHRM, 2008).

Delegation and Collaboration

The skill of incident reporting cannot be delegated to nursing assistive personnel (NAP). The nurse directs the NAP to:
- Report to the nurse any event such as a fall, incorrect treatment, or adverse reaction.
- Report to the nurse any pertinent information about the incident so an incident report can be completed.

Equipment
- ❏ Incident report/occurrence report form or screen
- ❏ Black pen

Procedural Steps
1 Use clinical reasoning skills to systematically and carefully determine what was involved in the incident. Either report the event as witnessed or determine from NAP what specifically occurred. Record the exact sequence of events involved, including time and type of incident; injury to patient, nurse, or other staff; and observation of factors that possibly contributed to the event (e.g., wet floor discovered in area of patient fall). Notify risk management per agency protocol.

Clinical Decision Point *Prepare the report on any questionable event. Do not avoid reporting because you believe that punitive actions will occur if reports are filed.*

2 Assess extent of any injury to patient or others, including patient's subjective report and objective physical examination findings.
3 If the adverse event involves an injury, take steps to restore individual's safety such as stabilizing patient's position after a fall and assessing for further injuries.
4 When patient sustains an injury, call the health care provider immediately.
5 When visitor or staff member sustains an injury, refer to emergency department or appropriate treatment setting.
6 Complete incident report form.

Clinical Decision Point *Document on report form as quickly as possible. The closer to the event, the more accurate the recording. (NOTE: This also necessitates that staff readily know where incident forms are kept and which forms to use for patients, visitors, and staff.)*

TABLE 4-4	Examples of Serious Reportable Events Occurring Within a Health Care Agency
• Surgery or other invasive procedure performed on the wrong patient • Patient death or serious injury associated with use of restraints or bedrails • Patient death or serious injury associated with use or function of a device in patient care in which device is used or functions other than intended • Patient death or serious injury associated with a fall • Patient death or serious injury associated with electrical shock	• Unintended retention of foreign object in a patient after surgery or invasive procedure • Patient death or serious injury associated with elopement • Patient death or serious injury associated with medication error • Patient death or serious injury associated with unsafe administration of blood products • Stage 3 or 4 pressure ulcer acquired after admission to a health care agency

Data from National Quality Forum: *Serious reportable events in health care: a consensus report-2011 update*, Washington, DC, 2011, National Quality Forum.

PROCEDURAL GUIDELINE 4-3 Adverse Event/Incident Reporting—cont'd

a Record time of incident and describe exactly what occurred or was observed, using objective findings and observations. Use language that does not allow for subjective interpretation. Do not include personal opinions or feelings. Document victim's interpretation of incident by using quotes.

b Objectively describe patient's or staff member's condition when incident was discovered or observed.

c Describe measures taken by any caregivers at time of incident.

d Send completed report to designated department.

7 When patient is involved, document events of incident in patient's chart.
   a Do not duplicate all information from report.
   b Do not record that report was completed.
   c Only enter objective description of what happened.
   d Record any assessment and intervention activities initiated as a result of event.

8 File the report properly with the risk management department or designated persons.

Critical Thinking Exercises

You and the nursing assistive personnel (NAP) are caring for a 55-year-old woman with type 2 diabetes who is scheduled for an appendectomy that evening. Elements of her care include monitoring vital signs every 2 hours, pain assessment, preoperative preparation, and glucose monitoring every 4 hours.

1 Noting the four elements of care listed, list the elements for which documentation may be delegated to NAP.

2 As you correctly noted, documentation of preoperative preparation cannot be delegated. Because the NAP will be providing other aspects of care, which information do you need to include in a report to the NAP about pain assessment, glucose monitoring, and preoperative preparation?

3 When you assess a patient's pain, it is important that you record your findings. Select the method of recording used in your agency and do a sample recording of the pain assessment.

4 The NAP reports to you that a patient's vital signs are 90/50, pulse 110, respirations 24. The patient states that he "feels dizzy and sweaty" after walking. Using the SBAR technique, how would you communicate this information to the physician or health care provider?

5 You have just completed preoperative teaching for a patient who is having surgery tomorrow for a total hip replacement. How would you document a patient's understanding of the information in a narrative note?

REVIEW QUESTIONS

1 When documenting information in a narrative note, the nurse should: (Select all that apply.)
   1 Document data immediately after care or treatment.
   2 Record information provided by another nurse.
   3 Begin each new entry with the date and time.
   4 Draw a single line through an error entry.

2 Military time is frequently used to document care. If oral hygiene was performed at 4:00 PM, what time would it be if documented according to military time?
   1 0400
   2 1400
   3 1600
   4 2400

3 There are multiple types of narrative charting. Which components would be found in focus charting?
   1 Data-Action-Response
   2 Problem-Intervention-Evaluation
   3 Subjective-Objective-Assessment-Plan
   4 Subjective-Evaluation-Assessment-Plan-Implementation-Evaluation

4 There are four purposes for charting by exception. Which statement best explains one of these purposes?
   1 To identify a change in a patient's condition
   2 To identify a change in a patient's medical orders
   3 To identify trends in clinical care
   4 To identify trends in resource utilization

5 Change-of-shift report or hand-off is an important component of care. Which standardized form of communication is used for exchanging patient information during handoff?
   1 SOAP documentation
   2 PIE Documentation
   3 SBAR documentation
   4 Focus charting

6 A patient with a complex medical condition and an unusual family situation has just been admitted to the nursing unit. What type of documentation is most appropriate for documenting this critical situation?
   1 SBAR documentation
   2 Charting by exception
   3 Focus charting
   4 PIE documentation

7 The nurse is documenting the care delivered to his patients. The best documentation would contain which of the following characteristics?
1 The majority of the documentation provides subjective data.
2 The nurse's hunches are included in case a sudden change occurs in the patient's condition.
3 The documentation contains only objective data.
4 The documentation reflects individualized care based on assessment data.

8 During report the nurse refers to a critical pathway and notes that a positive variance has occurred with one of the patients. Which information provided by the nurse would support this statement?
1 A Foley catheter needed to be inserted because the patient couldn't void.
2 A patient's fever dropped dramatically and sooner than expected.
3 A patient had to be taken back to surgery
4 A patient's family has been visiting frequently.

9 Unexpected events occur in the health care arena. When would an incident report need to be completed?
1 When less than standard patient care has been provided
2 To document an injury to a patient or visitor
3 To identify potential risks in new treatments
4 To identify when an adverse situation almost occurred in care

10 After receiving a narcotic for pain, the patient's respirations drop to a dangerous but stable level. Which documentation statement regarding the situation is best?
1 "Too much morphine was given; being monitored frequently and is stable; family at bedside and has been told of situation."
2 "Incident report filed after patient received too much pain medication and had decreased respirations; is resting quietly; doctor notified."
3 "Dilaudid 1 mg IV. RR8, BP 100/68, P 70 afterward; being monitored q15 min—see graphic for VS; MD notified."
4 "Sleeping deeply and snoring after receiving narcotic IV; VS stable; nail beds pink, oxygen ready if needed; supervisor notified."

REFERENCES

Adams-Wendling L, et al: Strategies for translating the resident care plan into daily practice, *J Gerontol Nurs* 34(8):53, 2008.

American Society for Healthcare Risk Management (ASHRM): Data for safety: turning lessons learned into actionable knowledge. 2008, available at ASHRM.org, accessed July 23, 2011.

Bauer M, et al: Hospital discharge planning for frail older people and their family, *J Clin Nurs* 18:2539, 2009.

Brown A, King D: The science of documentation, *Dean's Notes: A Communication Service to Nursing School Deans, Administrators, and Faculty* 29(4):2, 2008.

Burnes-Bolton L, et al: Smart technology, enduring solutions, *J Healthc Inf Manag* 22(4):24, 2008.

Carayon P, Wood K: Patient safety. Chapter 3: The role of human factors and systems engineering, *Inf Knowll Systems Manager* 8:23, 2009.

Center for Nursing Classification and Clinical Effectiveness: Nursing Interventions Classification (NIC), 2011a, available at http://www.nursing.uiowa.edu/center-for-nursing-classification-and-clinical-effectiveness, accessed February 1, 2012.

Center for Nursing Classification and Clinical Effectiveness: Nursing Outcomes Classification (NOC), 2011b, available at http://www.nursing.uiowa.edu/center-for-nursing-classification-and-clinical-effectiveness, accessed February 1, 2012.

Chaboyer W, et al: Bedside nursing handover: a case study, *Int J Nurs Pract* 16:27, 2010.

Cherry B, et al: Experiences with electronic health records: early adopters in long-term care facilities, *Health Care Manag Rev* 36(3):265, 2011.

Day D: Keeping patients safe during intrahospital transport, *Crit Care Nurse* 30(4):18, 2010.

Duda-Gardiner S: Resident assessment protocol, care area assessment: are they really the same? *Long-Term Care Magazine* July 2010, p 26, available at http://www.ltlmagazine.com/article/resident-assessment-protocol-care-area-assessment, accessed February 1, 2012.

Dunsford J: Structured communication: improving patient safety with SBAR, *AWHONN* 13(5):385, 2009.

Earle-Foley: Evidenced-based practice: issues, paradigms, and future pathways, *Nurs Forum* 46(1):38, 2011.

Field C, Gross J: Transition to MDS 3.0: Now is the time to prepare staff for 2010 implementation. *Long-Term Care Magazine* September 2009, p 36, available at http://www.ltlmagazine.com/article/transition-mds-30, accessed February 2012.

Fogelberg-Dahm M: Nurses' experiences of and opinions about using standardized care plans in electronic health records—a questionnaire study, *J Clin Nurs* 17(16):2137, 2008.

Gjevjon E, Hellesø R: The quality of home care nurses' documentation in new electronic patient records, *J Clin Nurs* 19:100, 2010.

Gorski L: Implementing home health standards in clinical practice: an overview of the updated standards, *Home Healthcare Nurse* 26(5):309, 2008.

Green S, Thomas J: Interdisciplinary collaboration and the electronic medical record, *Pediatr Nurs* 34(2):225, 2008.

Health Care Financing Administration (HCFA): Long-term care facility resident assessment instrument (RAI) user's manual, Washington, DC, 1998, HCFA.

Healthcare Information and Management Systems Society: The electronic health record. 2011, available at http://himss.org/ASP/topics_ehr.asp, accessed February 1, 2012.

Hospital Case Management: A monthly update on hospital-based care planning, *AHC Media LLC* 18(6):81, 2010.

Institute of Medicine: Health IT and patient safety: building safer systems for better care, Washington, DC, 2011, IOM.

Joint Commission Center for Transforming Healthcare: Hand-off communications, Fact Sheet 9.29.2011, available at www.centerfortransformingcare.org, accessed February 1, 2012.

Kutney-Lee A, Kelly D: The effect of hospital electronic health record adoption on nurse-assessed quality of care and patient safety, *J Nurs Adm* 41(11):467, 2011.

Marchisio S, et al: Effect of introducing a care pathway to standardize treatment and nursing of schizophrenia, *Commun Mental Health J* 45:255, 2009.

Müller-Staub M: Evaluation of the implementation of nursing diagnoses, interventions and outcomes, *Int J Nurs Terminol Classif* 20(1):9, 2009.

Müller-Staub M, et al: Implementing nursing diagnostics effectively: cluster randomized trial, *J Adv Nurs* 63(3):291, 2008.

Murphy J: The journey to meaningful use of electronic health records, *Nurs Econ* 28(4):283, 2010.

NANDA International: Nursing diagnoses: definitions and classification 2012-2014. West Sussex, UK, 2012, Wiley Blackwell.

National Quality Forum: Serious reportable events in health care: a consensus report-2011 update. Washington, DC, 2011, National Quality Forum.

Park E, Huber D: Case management workforce in the United States, *J Nurs Scholarship* 41(2):175, 2009.

Pope B, et al: Raising the SBAR—How better communication improves patient outcomes, *Nursing* 38(3):41, 2008.

Reimer J: What is "meaningful use" when it comes to electronic health records, *JNSD* 27(3):157, 2011.

Robert Wood Johnson Foundation: *Charting nursing's future: addressing the quality and safety gap.* Part 1: *Case studies in transforming hospital nursing and building cultures of safety,* 2009, available at http://www.rwjf.org/pr/product.jsp?id=45629, accessed February 1, 2012.

Rose K, Haugen M: Discharge planning: your last chance to make a good impression, *Medsurg Nurs* 19(1):47, 2010.

Runy L: Patient handoffs: the pitfalls and solutions of transferring patients safely from one caregiver to another, *Hospitals and Health Networks* May 2008, p 1, available at http://www.hhnmag.com/hhnmag/gateFold/PDF/05_2008/5.08_hhn_gate.pdf, accessed February 1, 2012.

Saranto K, Kinnunen U: Evaluating nursing documentation-research designs and methods: systematic review, *J Adv Nurs* 65(3):464, 2009.

Stone A, Yoder L: Strategic considerations during electronic health record implementation, *J Nurs Adm* 42(4):299, 2012.

The Joint Commission (TJC): 2009 National patient safety goals, *Joint Commission Perspect* 28(7):12, 2011.

The Joint Commission (TJC): *2012 Comprehensive accreditation manual for hospitals: the official handbook,* Oakbrook Terrace, Ill, 2012, The Commission.

The Joint Commission (TJC): *National Patient Safety Goals,* Oakbrook Terrace, Ill, 2012, The Commission, available at http://www.jointcommission.org/standards_information/npsgs.aspx.

Thomas C, et al: The SBAR communication technique, *Nurse Educator* 34(4):176, 2009.

US Department of Health and Human Services (USDHHS): Standards for privacy of individuals, Health Insurance Portability and Accountability Act of 1996, 64 *Fed Reg* 60053 (1999), 45 CFR Part 160 and Subparts A and E of Part 164, available at http://www.hhs.gov/ocr/privacy/hipaa/administrative/privacyrule/index.html, accessed February 1, 2012.

Watkins T, et al: Terminology use in electronic health records: basic principles, *Urologic Nurs* 29(5):321, 2009.

Vital Signs

MEDIA RESOURCES

- **evolve** *learning system*   http://evolve.elsevier.com/Perry/skills
  - Review Questions
  - ▶ Video Clips
  - Audio Glossary

- Mosby's Nursing Video Skills, 4th edition
- **NSO** Nursing Skills Online

KEY TERMS

Afebrile	Dysrhythmia	Orthostatic hypotension	S_2
Antipyretic	Febrile	Oximetry	Sphygmomanometer
Apical pulse	Fever	Oxygen saturation	Systolic pressure
Axillary	Heatstroke	Postural hypotension	Tachycardia
Bradycardia	Hypertension	Premature ventricular	Tachypnea
Bradypnea	Hyperthermia	contraction (PVC)	Thermoregulation
Core temperature	Hypotension	Pulse deficit	Tympanic
Diastolic pressure	Hypothermia	Pyrexia	Vasoconstriction
Dyspnea	Orthopnea	S_1	Vasodilation

OBJECTIVES

Mastery of content in this chapter will enable the nurse to:
- Identify when it is appropriate to assess each vital sign.
- Accurately assess a patient's oral, rectal, axillary, tympanic membrane, and temporal artery temperatures.
- Correctly record vital signs.
- Describe factors that cause variations in body temperature, pulse, respirations, blood pressure, and oxygen saturation.
- Discuss factors in selecting temperature measurement sites.
- Accurately assess a patient's radial and apical pulses.
- Explain implications of a pulse deficit.
- Accurately assess a patient's respirations.

- Accurately measure a patient's blood pressure using techniques of auscultation and palpation.
- Discuss benefits and disadvantages of using an automatic blood pressure machine.
- Describe factors in selecting an extremity to measure blood pressure.
- Accurately assess a patient's oxygenation status using pulse oximetry.
- Identify ranges of acceptable vital sign values for infant, child, and adult.
- Appropriately delegate vital sign measurements to nursing assistive personnel.

Temperature, pulse, blood pressure, respirations and oxygen saturation are the most frequent measurements obtained by health care practitioners. These measurements indicate if the circulatory, pulmonary, neurological, and endocrine body systems are functioning normally. Because of their importance as indicators of the body's physiological status and response to physical, environmental, and psychological stressors, they are referred to as vital signs. Vital signs reveal sudden changes in a patient's condition, as well as changes that occur progressively over time. Any difference between a patient's normal baseline measurement and present vital signs may indicate the need for nursing therapies and necessary medical interventions.

Pain, a subjective symptom, is often referred to as a vital sign along with the other physiologic signs. Frequently pain is the symptom that leads patients to seek health care. For this reason assessment of a patient's pain status is critical to understanding his or her clinical status and progress. You will frequently perform assessment of a patient's level of comfort and pain with vital sign measurements (see Chapter 15).

Vital signs are included in a routine physical assessment (see Chapter 6). The nurse's findings aid in determining whether it is necessary to assess specific body systems more thoroughly. For example, during a routine vital sign measurement, the nurse notes an abnormal respiratory rate; he or she then auscultates lung sounds. Measurement of a single vital sign assesses a specific aspect of a patient's condition. For example, following administration of an antipyretic medication, a nurse measures the patient's temperature to evaluate the effects of a drug. Part of your clinical judgment involves deciding which vital sign to measure, when to obtain measurements, and the frequency of assessment (Box 5-1). Always obtain a baseline measurement of vital signs on first contact with a patient to provide a means for comparison with later vital sign measurements.

EVIDENCE-BASED PRACTICE

Automatic blood pressure machines are common in many agencies when frequent blood pressure assessment is necessary. When results of machines are compared to manual blood pressures obtained using a stethoscope and sphygmomanometer, the results are not the same (Heinemann et al., 2008). Both systolic and diastolic blood pressures are lower when measured electronically. The greatest difference occurs with diastolic values (Skirton et al., 2011).

It is important to limit use of automated blood pressure monitors to those that are independently validated and biannually calibrated. Calibrate blood pressure manometers (aneroid and automatic) twice each year against a mercury manometer and/or return to manufacturer for calibration and repair (Nelson et al., 2008). These units are quick and easy to use and provide a large digital display that gives a distinct reading.

- Use auscultatory devices to obtain blood pressure when a patient has cardiac dysrhythmias or unstable or low blood pressure (Skirton et al., 2011).
- Use electronic machines for screening blood pressures in normotensive patients.
- Use auscultatory devices to verify abnormal blood pressure measurements obtained with electronic machines, to manage hypertension, or following traumatic events (Skirton et al., 2011).

PATIENT-CENTERED CARE

Vital sign measurements require removing clothing or exposing areas considered inappropriate or offensive to patients from other cultures. You must be sensitive to each patient's need for privacy and observe cultural norms. When reporting findings, patients from cultures with paternalistic values rely on a male elder to receive information on their behalf.

- Provide privacy when performing apical pulse assessment, especially for traditional female patients and elders from Asian, Middle Eastern, Hispanic, and African cultures (Giger, 2013).
- Procedures that are normally noninvasive sometimes produce anxiety because of cultural variables of touch, privacy, and gender.
- Consult the health care provider and family decision maker regarding giving information to the patient about abnormal vital signs.
- Collectivistic cultures (e.g., Hispanics, Africans, and Asians) demonstrate their caring for ill members by protecting them from bad news about their health and well-being (Giger, 2013).

Safety Guidelines

1. A nurse caring for a patient is responsible for measuring vital signs. Nurses analyze vital signs to interpret their significance and make decisions about appropriate interventions.
2. Equipment must be clean, functional, properly calibrated, and appropriate for the patient's size, age, condition, and characteristics.
3. A nurse knows a patient's usual range of vital signs. His or her usual values may differ from the acceptable range for that age or physical state. They serve as a baseline for comparison with later findings; thus you detect changes in condition over time.
4. A nurse knows a patient's medical history, therapies, and prescribed medications. Some illnesses or treatments cause predictable vital sign changes. Most medications affect at least one of the vital signs.
5. Control or minimize environmental factors that affect vital signs. For example, assessing the patient's temperature in a warm, humid room may yield a value that is not a true indicator of the patient's condition.

BOX 5-1	When to Take Vital Signs

1. On admission to a health care agency
2. In a hospital or care facility on a routine schedule according to a health care provider's order or standards of practice of agency
3. When assessing patient during home care visits
4. Before, during, and after a surgical or invasive diagnostic procedure
5. Before, during, and after the administration of medications or application of therapies that affect cardiovascular, respiratory, or temperature-control functions
6. Before, during, and after a transfusion of any type of blood products
7. Before, during, and after nursing interventions influencing a vital sign (e.g., before and after patient previously on bed rest ambulates, before and after patient performs range-of-motion exercises)
8. When patient reports specific symptoms of physical distress (e.g., feeling "funny" or "different")
9. When patient's general physical condition changes (e.g., loss of consciousness, increased intensity of pain)

6 Use an organized, systematic (step-by-step) approach when taking vital signs ensures accuracy of findings.

7 Based on the patient's condition, collaborate with the health care provider to decide the minimum frequency of vital sign assessment for each patient. Following surgery or treatment intervention, measure vital signs more frequently to detect complications. In a clinic or outpatient setting take vital signs before the health care provider examines the patient and after any invasive procedures. As a patient's physical condition worsens, it is important to monitor the vital signs as often as every 5 to 15 minutes. You are responsible for judging whether more frequent assessments are necessary.

8 Analyze the results of vital sign measurements and incorporate all the clinical findings about a patient in determining nursing diagnoses. Do not interpret vital signs in isolation. You need to know related physical signs or symptoms and be aware of the patient's ongoing health status.

9 Verify, communicate, and document significant changes in vital signs. Baseline measurements allow a nurse to identify changes in vital signs. When vital signs appear abnormal, it helps to have another nurse repeat the measurement. Inform the health care provider when vital signs become abnormal and report any changes to the nurse in charge.

SKILL 5-1 Measuring Body Temperature

NSO *Vital Signs Module / Lessons 1 and 2*

 Video Clip

Body temperature is the difference between the amount of heat produced by body processes and the amount of heat lost to the external environment. The core temperature, or temperature of the deep body tissues, is under control of the hypothalamus and remains within a narrow range. Skin or body surface temperature rises and falls as the temperature of the surrounding environment changes, and it fluctuates dramatically.

The body tissues and cells function best within a relatively narrow temperature range, from 36° to 38° C (96.8° F to 100.4° F), but no single temperature is normal for all people. For healthy young adults the average oral temperature is 37° C (98.6° F). In clinical practice nurses learn the temperature range of individual patients. An acceptable temperature range for adults depends on age, gender, range of physical activity, hydration status, and state of health (Fig. 5-1).

Many factors affect body temperature, but physiologic and behavioral control mechanisms act to maintain a constant core temperature. For example, the mechanism of peripheral vasodilation increases blood flow to the skin, which increases the amount of heat radiated to the environment. Control mechanisms have failed when heat produced by the body is not equal to heat lost to the environment. For example, patients without sweat gland function are unable to tolerate warm temperatures because they cannot adequately cool themselves. Fever occurs when heat loss mechanisms are unable to keep pace with excess heat production, resulting in an abnormal rise in body temperature. When an individual has a febrile condition (i.e., pyrexia), initiate temperature-control measures such as controlling environmental temperatures, removing external coverings, and administering ordered antipyretics to achieve better temperature control.

The purpose of measuring body temperature is to obtain a representative average temperature of core body tissues. Average usual temperature varies, depending on the measurement site used. Research findings from numerous studies are contradictory; however, it is generally accepted that rectal temperatures are usually 0.5° C (0.9° F) higher than oral temperatures. Axillary and tympanic temperatures are usually 0.5° C (0.9° F) lower than oral temperatures. Sites reflecting core temperature are more reliable indicators of body temperature than sites reflecting surface temperatures (Mazerolle et al., 2011) (Box 5-2).

To ensure accurate temperature readings you need to measure each site correctly. Use the same site when repeated measurements are necessary or when comparing temperature measurements over time. Each site has advantages and disadvantages (Box 5-3). You need to determine the safest and most accurate site for the patient.

Several types of thermometers are commonly available to measure body temperature (Box 5-4). The mercury-in-glass thermometer, once the standard device found in the clinical setting, is now prohibited because of the potential mercury hazards. However,

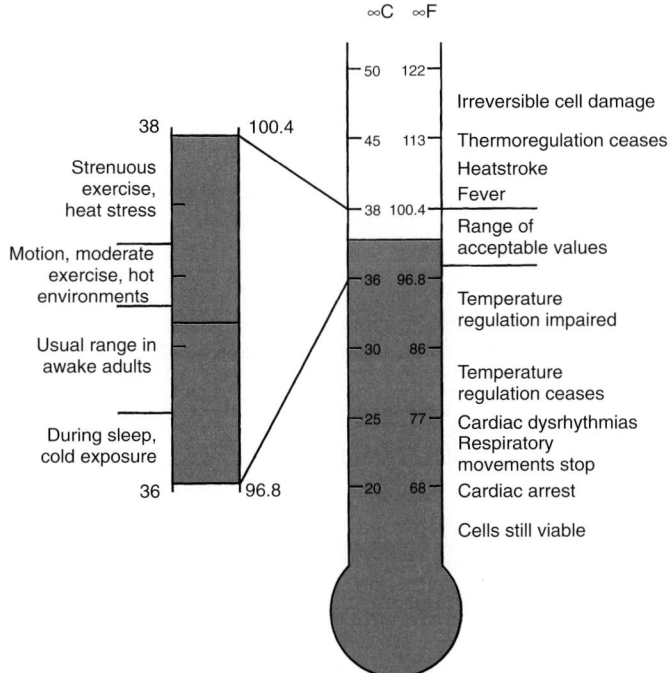

FIG 5-1 Ranges of normal temperature values and physiologic consequences of abnormal body temperature. (*Modified from Thibodeau GA, Patton KT: Anatomy and physiology, ed 7, St Louis, 2010, Mosby.*)

BOX 5-2	Core and Surface Temperature Measurement Sites

Core Site	Surface Site
• Rectum	• Skin
• Tympanic membrane	• Oral cavity
• Temporal artery	• Axilla
• Esophagus	
• Pulmonary artery	
• Urinary bladder	

BOX 5-3 | Advantages and Limitations of Select Temperature Measurement Sites

Oral
Advantages
- Easily accessible—requires no position change
- Comfortable for patient
- Provides accurate surface temperature reading
- Reflects rapid change in core temperature
- Reliable route to measure temperature for intubated patients

Limitations
- Causes delay in measurement if patient recently ingested hot/cold fluids or foods, chewed gum, or smoked
- Not used with patients who have had oral surgery or facial trauma or are unable to position in mouth, shaking chills, or history of seizures
- Not used with infants; small children; or confused, unconscious, or uncooperative patients
- Risk for body fluid exposure

Tympanic Membrane
Advantages
- Easily accessible site
- Obtained without disturbing, waking, or repositioning patient
- Used for patients with tachypnea without affecting breathing
- Provides accurate core reading because eardrum is close to hypothalamus; sensitive to core temperature changes
- Very rapid measurement (2 to 5 seconds)
- Unaffected by oral intake of food or fluids or smoking
- Used in newborns to reduce infant handling and heat loss

Limitations
- More variability of measurement than with other core temperature devices
- Requires removal of hearing aids before measurement
- Requires disposable sensor cover with only one size available
- Readings possibly distorted with otitis media and cerumen impaction
- Not used with patients who have had surgery of the ear or tympanic membrane
- Does not accurately measure core temperature changes during and after exercise
- Affected by ambient temperature devices such as incubators, radiant warmers, and facial fans
- Anatomy of ear canal makes it difficult to correctly position in neonates, infants, and children younger than 3 years of age
- Inaccuracies reported because of incorrect positioning of handheld unit

Rectal
Advantages
- Argued to be reliable when oral temperature cannot be obtained

Limitations
- Lags behind core temperature during rapid temperature changes
- Not used for patients with diarrhea or those who have had rectal surgery, rectal disorders, bleeding tendencies, or neutropenia

- Requires positioning and is often source of patient embarrassment and anxiety
- Risk for body fluid exposure
- Requires lubrication
- Not used for routine vital signs in newborns
- Readings influenced by impacted stool

Axilla
Advantages
- Safe and inexpensive
- Used with newborns and unconscious patients

Limitations
- Long measurement time
- Requires continuous positioning
- Measurement lags behind core temperature during rapid temperature changes
- Not recommended for detecting fever in infants and young children
- Requires exposure of thorax, which can result in temperature loss, especially in newborns
- Affected by exposure to the environment, including time it takes to place thermometer
- Underestimates core temperature

Skin
Advantages
- Inexpensive
- Provides continuous reading
- Safe and noninvasive
- Used for neonates

Limitations
- Measurement lags behind other sites during temperature changes, especially during hyperthermia
- Impaired adhesion from diaphoresis or sweat
- Affected by environmental temperature
- Cannot be used for patients with allergy to adhesive

Temporal Artery
Advantages
- Easy to access without position change
- Very rapid measurement
- Comfortable with no risk of injury to patient or nurse
- Eliminates need to disrobe or unbundle
- Can be used for premature infants, newborns, and children
- Reflects rapid change in core temperature
- Sensor cover not required

Limitations
- Inaccurate with head covering or hair on forehead
- Affected by skin moisture such as diaphoresis or sweating

mercury-in-glass thermometers are sometimes found in patients' homes.

Delegation and Collaboration
The skill of temperature measurement can be delegated to nursing assistive personnel (NAP). The nurse instructs the NAP by:

- Communicating the appropriate route, device, and frequency of temperature measurement.
- Explaining any precautions needed in positioning the patient for rectal temperature measurement.
- Reviewing the usual temperature values and significant changes to report to the nurse.

| BOX 5-4 | Types of Thermometers |

Electronic Thermometer (Fig. 5-2)
- Thermometer is a rechargeable battery-powered display unit with a thin wire cord and a temperature-processing probe covered by a disposable cover.
- Within 1 minute after placement, the thermometer displays a digital temperature reading.
- Separate probes are available for oral and axillary temperature measurement (blue tip) and rectal temperature measurement (red tip).

Tympanic Thermometer
- The probe consists of an otoscope-like speculum with an infrared sensor tip that detects heat radiated from the tympanic membrane of the ear (Fig. 5-3).
- Within seconds after placing in the ear canal and depressing the scan button, a digital reading appears on the display unit. A sound signals when the peak temperature has been measured.

Temporal Artery Thermometer
- An infrared scanner is swept across the forehead. If the patient is diaphoretic, also scan just behind the ear (Fig. 5-4).
- Within seconds after scanning, a digital reading appears on the display unit.

Chemical Dot Single-Use or Reusable Thermometer
- Thermometer consists of thin strips of plastic with a temperature sensor at one end and chemically impregnated dots formulated to change color at different temperatures (Fig. 5-5).
- Chemical dots on the thermometer change color to reflect temperature reading, usually within 60 seconds.
- It is useful for screening temperatures, especially in infants, during invasive procedures, for a patient on protective isolation, and in orally intubated critical care clients.
- It is not appropriate for monitoring fever in acutely ill clients or monitoring temperature therapies.
- It can be used at axillary or rectal site if covered by a plastic sheath with a placement time of 3 minutes.

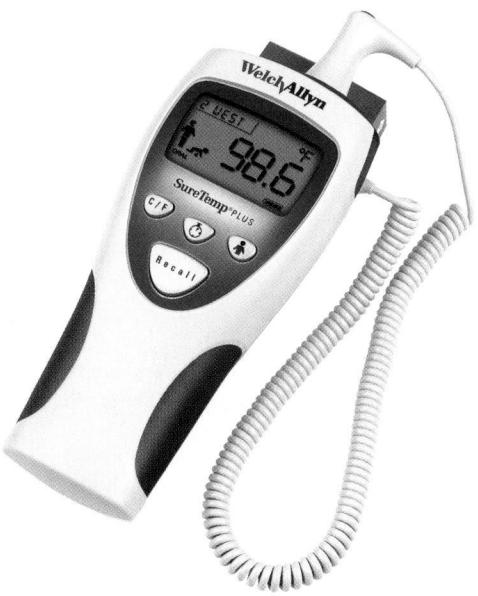

FIG 5-2   Electronic thermometer with disposable plastic probe cover. (*Photo courtesy Welch Allyn.*)

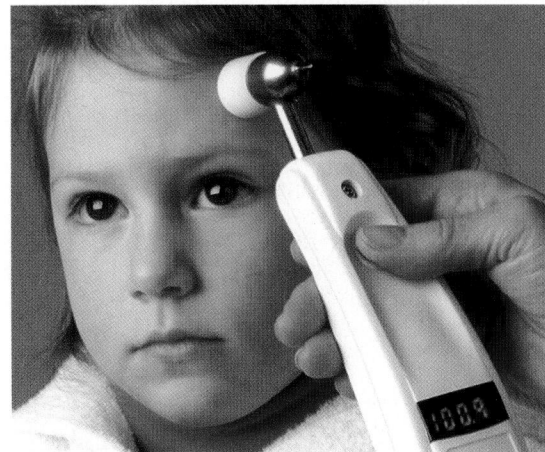

FIG 5-4   A temporal artery thermometer measures the heat from blood flowing through the superficial temporal artery. (*Photo courtesy Exergen.*)

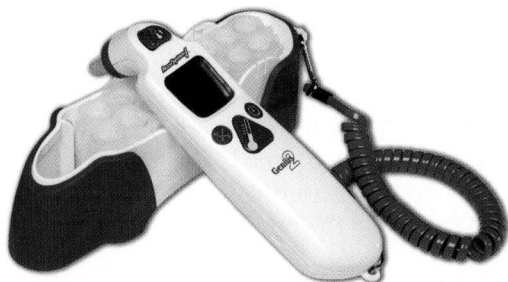

FIG 5-3   Tympanic membrane thermometer with disposable plastic probe cover. (*Copyright © Covidien. All rights reserved.*)

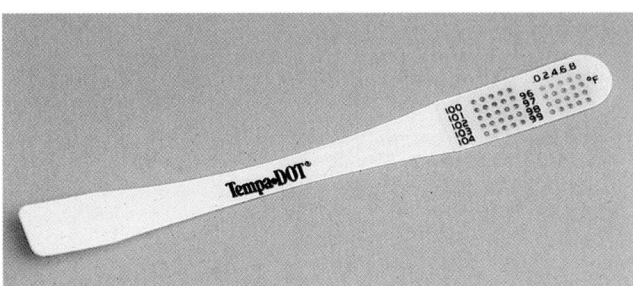

FIG 5-5   Chemical dot, disposable, single-use thermometer.

Equipment
- Thermometer (selected based on site used; see Box 5-3)
- Soft tissue or wipe
- Alcohol swab
- Water-soluble lubricant (for rectal measurements only)
- Pen and vital sign flow sheet, record form, or electronic health record (EHR)
- Clean gloves (optional), plastic thermometer sleeve, disposable probe or sensor cover
- Towel

STEP	RATIONALE

ASSESSMENT

1 Determine need to measure patient's body temperature:

  a Note patient's risks for temperature alterations:

    • Expected or diagnosed infection

    • Open wounds or burns

    • White blood cell count below $5000/mm^3$ or above $12,000/mm^3$

    • Immunosuppressive drug therapy

    • Injury to hypothalamus

    • Exposure to temperature extremes

    • Blood product infusion

    • Hypothermia or hyperthermia therapy

    • Postoperative status

> Certain conditions place patients at risk for temperature alterations and require more frequent temperature measurement and nursing assessment.

  b Assess for signs and symptoms that accompany temperature alteration:

    • *Hyperthermia*: Decreased skin turgor, dry mucous membranes; tachycardia; hypotension; decreased venous filling; concentrated urine

    • *Heatstroke*: Hot, dry skin; tachycardia; hypotension; excessive thirst; muscle cramps; visual disturbances; confusion or delirium

    • *Hypothermia*: Pale skin; skin cool or cold to touch; bradycardia and dysrhythmias; uncontrollable shivering; reduced level of consciousness; shallow respirations

> Physical signs and symptoms alert you to alterations in body temperature.

  c Assess for factors that normally influence temperature:

    • Age

> Allows nurse to accurately assess for presence and significance of temperature alteration.
>
> Older adults have a narrower range of temperature than younger adults.

Clinical Decision Point *No single temperature is normal for all people. A temperature within an acceptable range in an adult may reflect a fever in an older adult. Undeveloped temperature-control mechanisms in infants and children cause temperature to rise and fall rapidly (Davie and Amoore, 2010).*

    • Exercise

> Muscle activity increases metabolism, which increases heat production and raises temperature (Davie and Amoore, 2010).

    • Hormones

> Women have wider temperature fluctuations than men because of menstrual cycle hormonal changes, because body temperature varies during menopause, and because women have thicker layer of subcutaneous fat (Davie and Amoore, 2010).

    • Stress

> Stress elevates temperature.

    • Environmental temperature

> Infants and older adults are more sensitive to environmental temperature changes.

    • Medications

> Some drugs impair or promote sweating, vasoconstriction, or vasodilation or interfere with ability of hypothalamus to regulate temperature.

    • Daily fluctuations

> Body temperature normally changes 0.5° to 1° C (0.9° to 1.8° F) during a 24-hour period. Temperature is lowest during early morning. Most patients have maximum temperature elevation between 5 PM and 7 PM; temperature falls gradually during night.

2 Determine appropriate measurement site and device for patient (see Box 5-3). Use disposable thermometer for patient on isolation precautions.

> Determines if patient's status contraindicates selection of a specific method or site.

3 Determine previous baseline temperature and measurement site (if available) from patient's record.

> Allows nurse to assess for change in condition. Provides comparison with future temperature measurements.

4 Assess patient's knowledge of procedure.

> Encourages cooperation; minimizes risks and anxiety. Identifies teaching needs.

STEP	RATIONALE

NURSING DIAGNOSES

- Hyperthermia
- Hypothermia

- Ineffective thermoregulation

- Risk for imbalanced body temperature

Related factors are individualized based on patient's condition or needs.

PLANNING

1 Expected outcomes following completion of procedure:
- Body temperature is within acceptable range for patient's age-group.
- Body temperature returns to baseline range following therapies for abnormal temperature.

Thermoregulation is maintained.

Environmental factors that alter temperature are controlled.

2 Explain to patient the way you will measure temperature and importance of maintaining proper position until reading is complete.

Promotes patient cooperation and increases compliance. Patients are often curious about their temperatures and should be cautioned against prematurely removing thermometer to read results.

3 Collect and bring appropriate supplies to the patient's bedside.

Ensures an organized approach for body temperature measurement

4 Verify that patient has not had anything to eat or drink and not has chewed gum or smoked within the past 15 minutes of having oral temperature measured (Davie and Amoore, 2010).

Oral food and fluids, smoking, and gum can alter temperature measurement.

IMPLEMENTATION

1 Perform hand hygiene.

Reduces transmission of microorganisms.

2 Assist patient to comfortable position that provides easy access to temperature measurement site.

Ensures patient's comfort and accuracy of temperature reading.

3 Obtain temperature reading.

a **Assess oral temperature (electronic):**

(1) *Optional:* Apply clean gloves when there are respiratory secretions or facial or mouth wound drainage.

An oral probe cover is removable without physical contact.

(2) Remove thermometer pack from charging unit. Attach oral thermometer probe stem (blue tip) to thermometer unit. Grasp top of probe stem, being careful not to apply pressure on ejection button.

Charging provides battery power. Ejection button releases plastic cover from probe stem.

(3) Slide disposable plastic probe cover over thermometer probe stem until cover locks in place (see illustration).

Soft plastic cover will not break in patient's mouth and prevents transmission of microorganisms between patients.

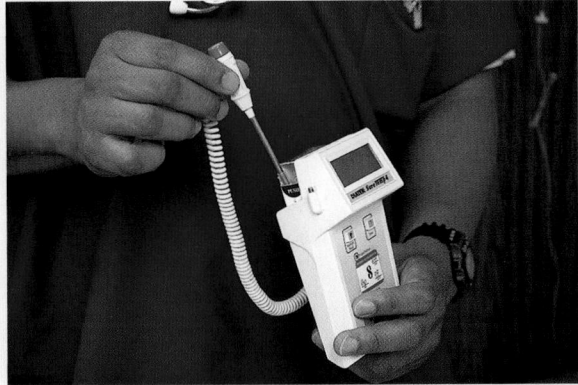

STEP 3a(3)   Nurse inserts electronic thermometer probe stem into probe cover. Cover snaps in place.

STEP	RATIONALE
(4) Ask patient to open mouth; gently place thermometer probe under tongue in posterior sublingual pocket lateral to center of lower jaw (see illustration).	Heat from superficial blood vessels in sublingual pocket produces temperature reading. With electronic thermometer temperatures in right and left posterior sublingual pocket are significantly higher than in area under front of tongue.

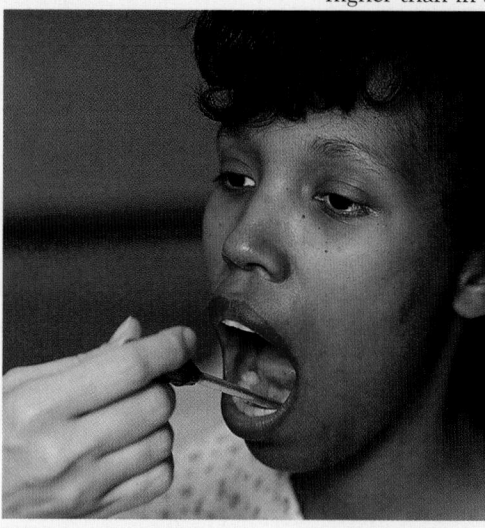

STEP 3a(4)   Probe under tongue in posterior sublingual pocket.

STEP	RATIONALE
(5) Ask patient to hold thermometer probe with lips closed.	Maintains proper position of thermometer during recording.
(6) Leave thermometer probe in place until audible signal indicates completion and patient's temperature appears on digital display; remove thermometer probe from under patient's tongue.	Probe must stay in place until signal occurs to ensure accurate reading.
(7) Push ejection button on thermometer probe stem to discard plastic probe cover into appropriate receptacle.	Reduces transmission of microorganisms.
(8) If wearing gloves, remove and dispose in appropriate receptacle and perform hand hygiene.	Reduces transmission of microorganisms.
(9) Return thermometer probe stem to storage position of thermometer unit.	Protects probe stem from damage. Returning thermometer probe stem automatically causes digital reading to disappear.
b Assess rectal temperature (electronic):	
(1) Draw curtain around bed and/or close room door. Assist patient to side-lying or Sims' position with upper leg flexed. Move aside bed linen to expose only anal area. Keep patient's upper body and lower extremities covered with sheet or blanket.	Maintains patient's privacy, minimizes embarrassment, and promotes comfort.
(2) Perform hand hygiene and apply clean gloves. Cleanse anal region when feces and/or secretions are present. Remove soiled gloves and reapply clean gloves.	Maintains standard precautions when exposed to items soiled with body fluids (e.g., feces).
(3) Remove thermometer pack from charging unit. Attach rectal thermometer probe stem (red tip) to thermometer unit. Grasp top of probe stem, being careful not to apply pressure on ejection button.	Ejection button releases plastic cover from probe stem.
(4) Slide disposable plastic probe cover over thermometer probe stem until cover locks in place.	Soft plastic probe cover prevents transmission of microorganisms between patients.
(5) Using a single use package, squeeze a liberal amount of lubricant on tissue. Dip probe cover of thermometer, blunt end, into lubricant, covering 2.5 to 3.5 cm (1 to 1½ inches) for adult.	Lubrication minimizes trauma to rectal mucosa during insertion. Tissue avoids contamination of remaining lubricant in container.
(6) With nondominant hand separate patient's buttocks to expose anus. Ask patient to breathe slowly and relax.	Fully exposes anus for thermometer insertion. Relaxes anal sphincter for easier thermometer insertion.
(7) Gently insert thermometer into anus in direction of umbilicus 3.5 cm (1½ inches) for adult. Do not force thermometer.	Ensures adequate exposure against blood vessels in rectal wall.
(8) If you feel resistance during insertion, withdraw immediately. Never force thermometer.	Prevents trauma to mucosa.

STEP	RATIONALE

Clinical Decision Point *If you cannot adequately insert thermometer into rectum or resistance is felt during insertion, remove thermometer and consider alternative method for obtaining temperature.*

(9) Once positioned, hold thermometer probe in place until audible signal indicates completion and patient's temperature appears on digital display; remove thermometer probe from anus (see illustration).

Probe must stay in place until signal occurs to ensure accurate reading.

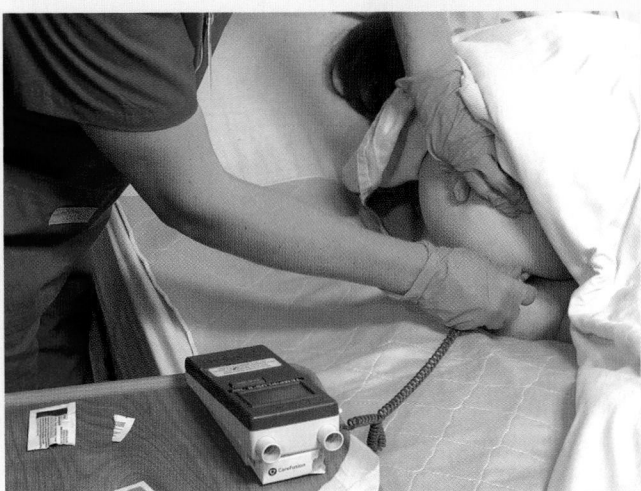

STEP 3b(9)   Probe inserted into anus.

(10) Push ejection button on thermometer stem to discard plastic probe cover into appropriate receptacle. Wipe probe stem with alcohol swab, paying particular attention to ridges where probe stem connects to probe.

Reduces transmission of microorganisms.

(11) Return thermometer stem to storage position of recording unit.

Protects probe stem from damage. Returning thermometer stem automatically causes digital reading to disappear.

(12) Wipe patient's anal area with soft tissue to remove lubricant or feces and discard tissue. Assist patient in assuming a comfortable position.

Provides for comfort and hygiene.

(13) Remove and dispose of gloves in appropriate receptacle. Perform hand hygiene.

Reduces transmission of microorganisms.

c Assess axillary temperature (electronic):

(1) Draw curtain around bed and/or close room door. Assist patient to supine or sitting position. Move clothing or gown away from shoulder and arm.

Maintains patient's privacy, minimizes embarrassment, and promotes comfort. Exposes axilla for correct thermometer probe placement.

(2) Remove thermometer pack from charging unit. Attach oral thermometer probe stem (blue tip) to thermometer unit. Grasp top of thermometer probe stem, being careful not to apply pressure on ejection button.

Charging provides battery power. Ejection button releases plastic cover from probe stem.

(3) Slide disposable plastic probe cover over thermometer stem until cover locks in place.

Soft plastic probe cover prevents transmission of microorganisms between patients.

STEP	RATIONALE

(4) Raise patient's arm away from torso. Inspect for skin lesions and excessive perspiration; if needed, dry axilla. Insert thermometer probe into center of axilla (see illustration), lower arm over probe, and place arm across patient's chest.

Maintains proper position of thermometer against blood vessels in axilla.

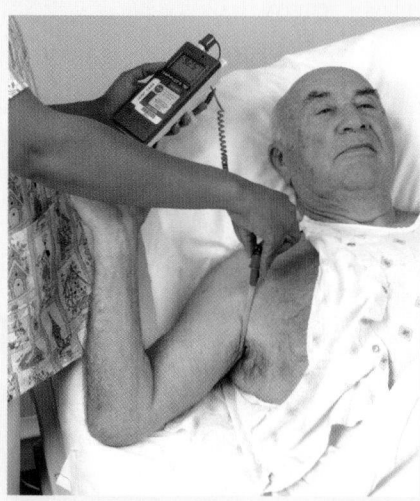

STEP 3c(4)   Place thermometer probe in axilla.

Clinical Decision Point *Do not use axilla if skin lesions are present because local temperature is sometimes altered and area may be painful to touch.*

(5) Once thermometer probe is positioned, hold it in place until audible signal indicates completion and patient's temperature appears on digital display; remove thermometer probe from axilla.

Thermometer probe must stay in place until signal occurs to ensure accurate reading.

(6) Push ejection button on thermometer stem to discard plastic probe cover into appropriate receptacle.

Reduces transmission of microorganisms.

(7) Return thermometer stem to storage position of recording unit.

Returning thermometer stem to storage position automatically causes digital reading to disappear. Protects stem from damage.

(8) Assist patient in assuming comfortable position, replacing linen or gown.

Restores comfort and sense of well-being.

(9) Perform hand hygiene.

Reduces transmission of microorganisms.

d Assess tympanic membrane temperature:

(1) Assist patient in assuming comfortable position with head turned toward side, away from you. If patient has been lying on one side, use upper ear. Obtain temperature from patient's right ear if you are right-handed. Obtain temperature from patient's left ear if you are left-handed.

Ensures comfort and facilitates exposure of auditory canal for accurate temperature measurement.
Heat trapped in ear facing down causes false-high temperature reading
The less acute the angle of approach, the better the probe seal.

(2) Note if there is an obvious presence of cerumen (earwax) in patient's ear canal.

Cerumen impedes the lens cover of speculum. Switch to other ear or select alternative measurement site.

(3) Remove thermometer handheld unit from charging base, being careful not to apply pressure to ejection button.

Charging base provides battery power. Removal of handheld unit from base prepares it to measure temperature. Ejection button releases plastic probe cover from thermometer tip.

(4) Slide disposable speculum cover over the otoscope-like lens tip until it locks in place. Be careful not to touch lens cover.

Soft plastic probe cover prevents transmission of microorganisms between patients. Lens cover should not have dust, fingerprints, or cerumen obstructing optical pathway.

(5) Insert speculum into ear canal following manufacturer instructions for tympanic probe positioning:

Correct positioning of probe with respect to ear canal allows maximal exposure of tympanic membrane.

STEP	RATIONALE

(a) Pull ear pinna backward, up, and out for an adult (see illustration). For children less than 3 years of age, pull pinna down and back, point covered probe toward midpoint between eyebrow and sideburns. For children older than 3 years, pull pinna up and back (Hockenberry and Wilson, 2011).

The ear tug straightens the external auditory canal, allowing maximum exposure of tympanic membrane and therefore correctly positioning speculum.

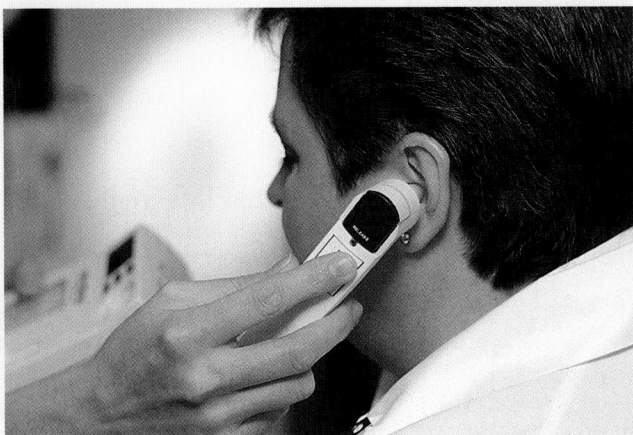

STEP 3d(5)(a)   Tympanic membrane thermometer with probe cover placed in patient's ear.

(b) Move thermometer in a figure-eight pattern.

Some manufacturers recommend movement of speculum tip in a figure-eight pattern that allows sensor to detect maximum tympanic membrane heat radiation.

(c) Fit speculum tip snug in canal, pointing toward the nose.

Gentle pressure seals ear canal from ambient air temperature, which alters readings as much as 2.8° C (5° F).

(6) Once positioned, press scan button on handheld unit. Leave speculum in place until audible signal indicates completion and patient's temperature appears on digital display.

Pressing scan button causes detection of infrared energy. The speculum tip must stay in place until signal occurs to ensure accurate reading.

(7) Carefully remove speculum from auditory meatus. Push ejection button on handheld unit to discard speculum cover into appropriate receptacle.

Reduces transmission of microorganisms. Automatically causes digital reading to disappear.

(8) If temperature is abnormal or second reading is necessary, replace probe cover and wait 2 minutes before repeating in same ear or repeat measurement in other ear. Consider an alternative temperature site or instrument.

Lens cover must be free of cerumen to maintain optical path. Time allows ear canal to regain usual temperature.

(9) Return handheld unit to thermometer base.

Protects sensor tip from damage.

(10) Help patient assume a comfortable position.

Restores comfort and sense of well-being.

(11) Perform hand hygiene.

Reduces transmission of microorganisms.

e Assess temporal artery temperature:

(1) Ensure that forehead is dry; dry with a towel if needed.

Moisture interferes with thermometer sensor.

(2) Place sensor firmly on patient's forehead.

Flush contact avoids measurement of ambient temperature.

(3) Press red scan button with your thumb. Slowly slide thermometer straight across forehead while keeping sensor flat and firmly on skin (see Fig. 5-4).

Thermometer continuously scans for highest temperature when scan button is depressed.

(4) If patient is diaphoretic, keeping scan button depressed, lift sensor after sweeping forehead and touch sensor on neck just behind the earlobe. Peak temperature occurs when clicking sound during scanning stops. Release scan button.

Sensor is cooled by diaphoresis, resulting in an inaccurate temperature. Area behind earlobe is less affected by diaphoresis.

(5) Gently clean sensor with alcohol swab and perform hand hygiene.

Prevents transmission of microorganisms.

4 Inform patient of temperature reading and record measurement.

Promotes participation in care and understanding of health status.

5 Return thermometer to charger.

Maintains battery charge of thermometer unit.

STEP	RATIONALE

EVALUATION

1 If you are assessing temperature for the first time, establish it as baseline if it is within acceptable range.

Used to compare future temperature measurements.

2 Compare temperature reading with patient's previous baseline and acceptable temperature range for patient's age-group.

Body temperature fluctuates within narrow range; comparison reveals presence of abnormality. Improper placement or movement of thermometer can cause inaccuracies. Second measurement confirms initial findings of abnormal body temperature.

3 If patient has fever, take temperature approximately 30 minutes after administering antipyretics and every 4 hours until temperature stabilizes.

Determines if temperature begins to fall in response to therapy.

Unexpected Outcomes

1 Patient has temperature 1° C (1.8° F) or more above usual range.

Related Interventions

- Initiate measures to lower body temperature:
  - Cool room environment (Thompson and Kagan, 2010).
  - Reduce external covering on patient's body to promote heat loss but do not induce shivering (Thompson and Kagan, 2010).
  - Keep clothing and bed linen dry.
  - Apply hypothermia blanket as ordered (see Chapter 40).
  - Limit physical activity and sources of emotional stress.
  - Administer antipyretics as ordered.
  - Increase fluid intake to at least 3 L daily (unless contraindicated).
  - Initiate measures to stimulate appetite and provide nutrients to meet increased energy needs.
  - Prevent or control spread of infection.
  - Provide wound care (see Chapter 38).
  - Perform pulmonary hygiene (see Chapter 24).
  - Promote adequate urinary elimination (see Chapter 33).

2 Patient has temperature 1° C (1.8° F) or more below usual range.

- Initiate measures to raise body temperature:
  - Apply warm blankets and, unless contraindicated, offer warm liquids.
  - Apply hyperthermia blankets if ordered (see Chapter 40).
  - Remove wet clothing or linen.

3 Unable to obtain temperature.

- Reassess correct placement of temperature probe or sensor.
- Choose alternative temperature measurement site.
- Obtain alternative temperature measurement device.

Recording and Reporting

- Record temperature and route on vital sign flow sheet, nurses' notes, or electronic health record (EHR).
- Report abnormal findings to nurse in charge or health care provider.

Special Considerations
Teaching

- Identify patient's ability to initiate preventive health measures and recognize alteration in body temperature. Educate patients and family members about measures to prevent body temperature alterations.
- Educate patients about risk factors for hypothermia and frostbite: fatigue; malnutrition; hypoxemia; cold, wet clothing; alcohol intoxication.
- Educate patients about risk factors for heatstroke: strenuous exercise in hot, humid weather; tight-fitting clothing in hot environments; exercising in poorly ventilated areas; sudden exposures to hot climates; poor fluid intake before, during, and after exercise.
- Educate patients regarding importance of taking and continuing antibiotics as directed until course of treatment for infection is completed.

Pediatric

- Infants and young children may lose more heat to the environment because of their increased body surface area/volume ratios.
- Critically ill children sometimes have cool skin but a high core temperature because of poor perfusion to the skin.
- Use axillary temperatures for screening purposes only; axillary temperature cannot be relied on to detect fever in infants and young children (Lim et al., 2008).
- Children may assume prone position for rectal temperature measurement.
- With children who cry or become restless, it is best to take temperature as the last vital sign.

Gerontologic

- The temperature of older adults is at the lower end of the acceptable temperature range: 36° C (96.8° F).
- Temperatures considered within normal range often reflect a fever in an older adult.
- Adults without teeth or older adults with poor muscle control may be unable to close their mouth tightly enough to obtain accurate oral temperature readings.
- Older adults are very sensitive to environmental temperature changes because their thermoregulatory systems are not as efficient (Ebersole et al., 2008).

- Oral temperature measurement is more reliable in older adults because cerumen tends to be drier and cilia become stiff, contributing to buildup of cerumen impaction, which interferes with accurate tympanic temperature measurement (Lu et al., 2009).
- A decrease in sweat gland reactivity in the older adult results in a higher threshold for sweating at high temperatures, which can lead to hyperthermia.
- With aging a loss of subcutaneous fat reduces the insulating capacity of the skin.
- Older adults are at high risk for hypothermia because of diminished sensation to cold, abnormal vasoconstrictor responses, and impaired shivering.

Home Care

- Assess temperature and ventilation of patient's environment to determine existence of any environmental conditions that influence patient's temperature.
- In the home some patients continue to use mercury-in-glass thermometers. Assess safe storage of these thermometers to protect from breakage and mercury spills. Educate patient and family caregiver on proper use of the thermometer, mercury hazards, and proper disposal of any mercury-containing devices. Suggest alternative temperature measurement devices for home use.

SKILL 5-2 Assessing Radial Pulse

NSO *Vital Signs Module / Lesson 3*

 Video Clip

The ejection of blood from the heart distends the walls of the aorta. Because of the force of the blood exiting the heart, aortic distention creates a pulse wave that travels rapidly toward the extremities. When the pulse wave reaches a peripheral artery, you can feel it by palpating the artery lightly against underlying bone or muscle. The pulse is the palpable bounding of the blood flow. The number of pulsing sensations occurring in 1 minute is the pulse rate.

Assessing the patient's peripheral pulse sites offers valuable data for determining the integrity of the cardiovascular system. An abnormally slow, rapid, or irregular pulse indicates the inability of the heart to deliver adequate blood to the body; a pulse deficit may be present (see Procedural Guideline 5-1). The strength or amplitude of a pulse reflects the volume of blood ejected against the arterial wall with each heart contraction. If the volume decreases, the pulse often becomes weak and difficult to palpate. In contrast, a full bounding pulse is an indication of increased volume.

The integrity of peripheral pulses indicates the status of blood perfusion to the area distributed by the pulse (Table 5-1). For example, assessment of the right femoral pulse determines whether blood flow to the right leg is adequate. If a peripheral pulse distal to an injured or treated area of an extremity feels weak on palpation, the volume of blood reaching tissues below the affected area may be inadequate, and surgical intervention may be necessary.

You can assess any artery for pulse rate, but the radial and carotid arteries are commonly used because they are easy to palpate (Fig. 5-6). When a patient's condition suddenly worsens, the carotid site is recommended for finding a pulse quickly. Assessment of other peripheral pulse sites such as the brachial or femoral artery is unnecessary when routinely obtaining vital signs. Other peripheral pulses are assessed when a complete physical (see Chapter 6) is conducted or when the radial artery is not available for assessment because of surgery, trauma, or impaired blood flow.

Delegation and Collaboration

The skill of radial pulse measurement can be delegated to nursing assistive personnel (NAP) if the patient's condition is stable. The skill cannot be delegated when the patient's condition is unstable

TABLE 5-1	Pulse Sites	
Site	**Location**	**Rationale for Selection**
Temporal	Over temporal bone of head, above and lateral to the eyebrow	Easily accessible site to assess pulse in children
Carotid	Along medial edge of sternocleidomastoid muscle in neck	Easily accessible site to assess character of peripheral pulse; used during physiologic shock or cardiac arrest when other sites are not palpable
Apical	Fourth to fifth intercostal space at left midclavicular line	Site used to auscultate apical pulse
Brachial	Groove between biceps and triceps muscles at antecubital fossa	Site used to auscultate upper-extremity blood pressure; assesses status of circulation to lower arm
Radial	Radial or thumb side of forearm at wrist	Common site to assess character of peripheral pulse; assesses status of circulation to hand
Ulnar	Ulnar side of forearm at the wrist	Site used to assess status of circulation to ulnar side of hand; used to perform Allen's test
Femoral	Below inguinal ligament, midway between symphysis pubis and anterior superior iliac spine	Site used to assess character of pulse during physiologic shock or cardiac arrest when other pulses are not palpable; assesses status of circulation to the leg
Popliteal	Behind knee in popliteal fossa	Site used to auscultate lower-extremity blood pressure; assesses status of circulation to lower leg
Posterior tibial	Inner side of each ankle, below medial malleolus	Site used to assess status of circulation to the foot
Dorsalis pedis	Along top of foot between extension tendons of great and first toe	Site used to assess status of circulation to the foot

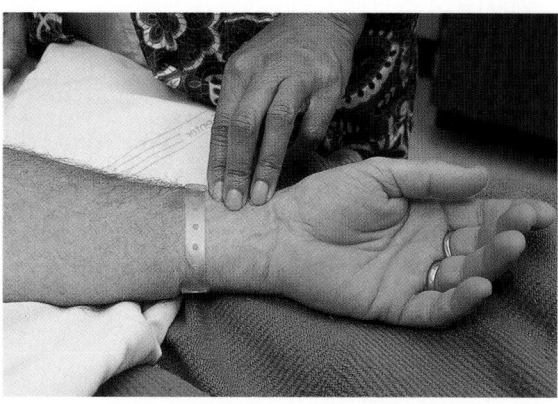

FIG 5-6 Palpating the radial pulse.

since the patient is at high risk for acute or serious cardiac problems or when the nurse is evaluating a response to a treatment or medication. The nurse instructs the NAP by:

- Communicating the appropriate site for pulse rate; frequency of measurement; and factors related to the patient history such as risk for abnormally slow, rapid, or irregular pulse.
- Reviewing patient's usual pulse rate and significant changes to report to the nurse.
- Reviewing the specific abnormalities to report to the nurse for further assessment.

Equipment
❑ Wristwatch with second hand or digital display
❑ Pen and vital sign flow sheet or electronic health record (EHR)

STEP	RATIONALE

ASSESSMENT

1 Determine need to assess radial pulse:

  a Assess for any risk factors for pulse alterations:
  - A history of heart disease
  - Cardiac dysrhythmia
  - Onset of sudden chest pain or acute pain from any site
  - Invasive cardiovascular diagnostic tests
  - Surgery
  - Sudden infusion of large volume of intravenous (IV) fluid
  - Internal or external hemorrhage
  - Administration of medications that alter cardiac function

  Certain conditions place patients at risk for pulse alterations. A history of peripheral vascular disease often alters pulse rate and quality.

  b Assess for signs and symptoms of altered cardiac function such as presence of dyspnea, fatigue, chest pain, orthopnea, syncope, palpitations, edema of dependent body parts, cyanosis, or pallor of skin (see Chapter 6).

  Physical signs and symptoms often indicate alteration in cardiac function, which affects radial pulse rate and rhythm.

  c Assess for signs and symptoms of peripheral vascular disease such as pale, cool extremities; thin, shiny skin with decreased hair growth; thickened nails.

  Physical signs and symptoms indicate alteration in local arterial blood flow.

  d Assess for factors that influence radial pulse rate and rhythm: age, exercise, position changes, fluid balance, medications, temperature, sympathetic stimulation (e.g., caffeine or nicotine).

  Can anticipate factors that alter pulse, ensuring accurate interpretation.
  Dysrythmics, cardiotonics, antihypertensives, vasodilators, and vasoconstrictors affect pulse rate and rhythm.

2 Determine patient's previous baseline pulse rate (if available) from patient's record.

  Allows you to assess for change in condition. Provides comparison with future pulse measurements.

NURSING DIAGNOSES

- Activity intolerance
- Decreased cardiac output
- Deficient fluid volume
- Ineffective peripheral tissue perfusion

Related factors are individualized based on patient's condition and needs.

PLANNING

1 Expected outcomes following completion of procedure:
  - Radial pulse is palpable, within usual range for patient's age.
  - Rhythm is regular.
  - Radial pulse is strong, firm, and elastic.

  Usual range for adults is 60 to 100 beats/min.
  Cardiac status is stable.
  Radial artery is patent.

2 Explain to patient that you will assess radial pulse rate (HR). Encourage patient to relax as much as possible. If he or she has been active, wait 5 to 10 minutes before assessing pulse. If patient has been smoking or ingesting caffeine, wait 15 minutes before assessing pulse.

  Anxiety, activity, caffeine, and smoking elevate heart rate. Assessing radial pulse rate at rest allows for objective comparison of values.

3 Collect appropriate equipment and bring to patient's bedside

  Ensures an organized approach for assessing a radial pulse.

STEP	RATIONALE

IMPLEMENTATION

1 Perform hand hygiene.
2 If necessary, draw curtain around bed and/or close door.
3 Assist patient with assuming a supine or sitting position.
4 If patient is supine, place his or her forearm straight alongside or across lower chest or upper abdomen with wrist extended straight (see illustration A). If sitting, bend patient's elbow 90 degrees and support lower arm on chair or on nurse's arm. Place tips of first two or middle three fingers of hand over groove along radial or thumb side of patient's inner wrist (see illustration B). Slightly extend or flex wrist with palm down until you note strongest pulse.

Reduces transmission of microorganisms.
Maintains privacy and minimizes embarrassment.
Provides easy access to pulse sites.
Fingertips are most sensitive parts of hand to palpate arterial pulsation. Nurse's thumb has pulsation that interferes with accuracy. Relaxed position of lower arm and extension of wrist permit full exposure of artery to palpation.

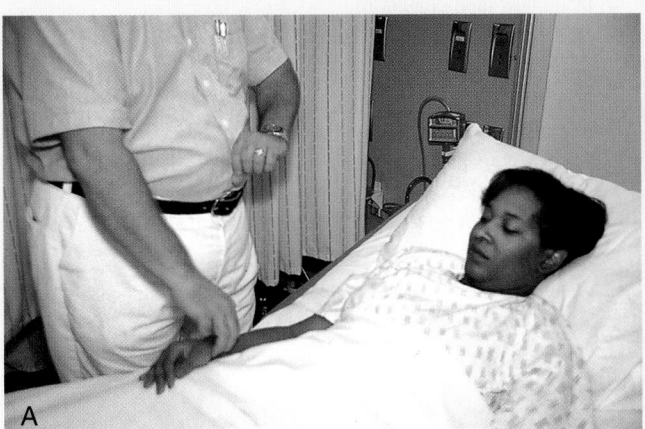
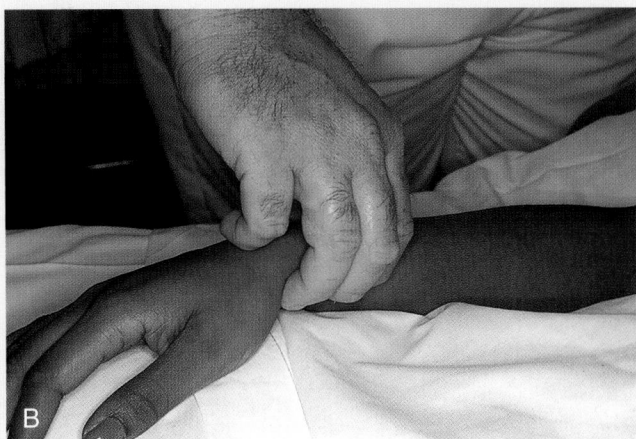

STEP 4 **A,** Pulse check with patient's forearm at side with wrist extended. **B,** Hand placement for pulse check.

5 Lightly compress against radius, obliterate pulse initially, and relax pressure so pulse becomes easily palpable.
6 Determine strength of pulse. Note whether thrust of vessel against fingertips is bounding (4+); full increased, strong (3+); expected (2+); barely palpable, diminished (1+); or absent, not palpable (0).
7 After palpating a regular pulse, look at watch second hand and begin to count rate. Count the first beat after the second hand hits the number on the dial; count as one, then two, and so on.
8 If pulse is regular, count rate for 30 seconds and multiply total by 2.
9 If pulse is irregular, count rate for a full 60 seconds. Assess frequency and pattern of irregularity.
10 When pulse is irregular, compare radial pulses bilaterally.

Pulse assessment is more accurate when using moderate pressure. Too much pressure occludes pulse and impairs blood flow.
Strength reflects volume of blood ejected against arterial wall with each heart contraction. Accurate description of strength improves communication among nurses and other health care providers.
Rate is determined accurately only after pulse has been palpated. Timing begins with zero. Count of one is first beat palpated after timing begins.

A 30-second count is accurate for rapid, slow, or regular pulse rates.

Inefficient contraction of heart fails to transmit pulse wave, resulting in irregular pulse. Longer time ensures accurate count.
A marked difference between pulses indicates that arterial flow is compromised to one extremity and nurse needs to take action.

Clinical Decision Point *If pulse is irregular, assess for pulse deficit (see Procedural Guideline 5-1), which may indicate alterations in heart function.*

11 Assist patient return to comfortable position.
12 Discuss findings with patient as needed.
13 Perform hand hygiene.

Promotes comfort and sense of well-being.
Promotes participation in care and understanding of health status.
Reduces transmission of microorganisms.

STEP	RATIONALE

EVALUATION

1 If assessing pulse for first time, establish radial pulse as baseline if it is within acceptable range.

Used to compare future pulse assessments.

2 Compare pulse rate and character with patient's previous baseline and acceptable range for patient's age.

Allows nurse to assess for change in patient's condition and presence of cardiac alteration.

Unexpected Outcomes

1 Patient has weak, thready, or difficult-to-palpate radial pulse.

Related Interventions

- Assess both radial pulses and compare findings.
- Observe for symptoms associated with ineffective tissue perfusion, including pallor and cool skin distal to weak pulse.
- Assess for swelling in surrounding tissues or any encumbrance (e.g., dressing or cast) that may impede blood flow.
- Obtain Doppler or ultrasound stethoscope to detect low-velocity blood flow (see Chapter 6).
- Have another nurse assess pulse.

2 An adult patient's pulse rate is more than 100 beats/min (tachycardia).

- Identify related data, including fever, pain, fear or anxiety, recent exercise, low blood pressure, blood loss, or inadequate oxygenation.
- Observe for signs and symptoms associated with abnormal cardiac function, including dyspnea, fatigue, chest pain, orthopnea, syncope, palpitations, edema of body parts, cyanosis, or pallor of the skin.

3 An adult patient's pulse rate is less than 60 beats/min (bradycardia).

- Auscultate the apical pulse (see Skill 5-3).
- Confer with health care provider and be prepared to order/obtain an electrocardiogram.

4 Patient has an irregular pulse.

- Auscultate apical pulse (see Skill 5-3).
- Assess for pulse deficit (see Procedural Guideline 5-1).

Recording and Reporting

- Record pulse rate and assessment site on vital sign flow sheet, nurses' notes, or EHR.
- Document measurement of pulse rate after administration of specific therapies in nurses' notes and EHR.
- Report abnormal findings to nurse in charge or health care provider.

Special Considerations

Teaching

- Patients taking certain prescribed cardiotonic or antidysrhythmic medications need to learn to assess their own pulse rates to detect side effects of medications. Patients undergoing cardiac rehabilitation need to learn to assess their own pulse rates to determine their response to exercise.
- Teach patients taking heart medications or starting a prescribed exercise regimen how to monitor carotid pulse rate.

Pediatric

- Radial artery is difficult to assess in an infant. Apical, femoral, or brachial pulse is best site for assessing pediatric heart rate and rhythm until 2 years of age.

- Children often have a sinus dysrhythmia, which is an irregular heartbeat that speeds up with inspiration and slows down with expiration.
- Breath holding in a child affects pulse rate.

Gerontologic

- Older adults have a reduced heart rate with exercise because of a decreased responsiveness to catecholamines.
- It takes longer for the heart rate to rise in the older adult to meet sudden increased demands that result from stress, illness, or excitement. Once elevated, the pulse rate of an older adult takes longer to return to normal resting rate (Ebersole et al., 2008).
- Peripheral vascular disease is more common among older adults, making radial pulse assessment difficult.

Home Care

- Patients taking certain prescribed cardiac medications should learn to assess their own pulse rates to detect side effects of medications.

SKILL 5-3 Assessing Apical Pulse

NSO *Vital Signs Module / Lesson 3*

 Video Clip

The apical pulse is the most reliable noninvasive way to assess cardiac function. The apical pulse rate is the assessment of the number and quality of apical sounds in 1 minute. Each apical pulse is the combination of two sounds, S_1 and S_2. S_1 is the sound of the tricuspid and mitral valves closing at the end of ventricular filling, just before systolic contraction begins. S_2 is the sound of the pulmonic and aortic valves closing at the end of the systolic contraction.

You use a stethoscope to auscultate sound waves of the apical pulse (Fig. 5-7). The stethoscope is a closed cylinder that amplifies sound waves as they reach the surface of the body. The five major parts of the stethoscope are the earpieces, binaurals, tubing, bell, and diaphragm.

The plastic or rubber earpieces should fit snugly and comfortably in your ears. Binaurals should be angled and strong enough so the earpieces stay firmly in place without causing discomfort. The earpieces follow the contour of the ear canal, pointing toward the face when the stethoscope is in place.

The polyvinyl tubing should be flexible and 30 to 45 cm (12 to 18 inches) in length; longer tubing decreases sound transmission. Stethoscopes can have one or two tubes. At the end of the tubing is the chest piece, consisting of a bell and diaphragm that you rotate into position, depending on which part you choose to use. To test, lightly tap to determine which side is functioning. Some stethoscopes have one chest piece that combines features of the bell and diaphragm. When you apply light pressure, the chest piece is a bell, whereas exerting more pressure converts the bell into a diaphragm.

The diaphragm is the larger, circular, flat-surfaced portion of the chest piece. It transmits high-pitched sounds created by high-velocity movement of air and blood. Position the diaphragm to make a tight seal against the patient's skin. Exert enough pressure to complete the seal, leaving a temporary red ring on the patient's skin after you remove the diaphragm.

The bell is the cone-shaped portion of the chest piece, usually surrounded by a rubber ring to avoid chilling the patient during placement. It transmits low-pitched sounds created by the low-velocity movement of blood. Hold the bell lightly against the skin for sound amplification.

Delegation and Collaboration

The skill of apical pulse measurement can be delegated to nursing assistive personnel (NAP) if the patient is stable and not at high risk for acute or serious cardiac problems. Often you measure the apical pulse when you suspect an irregularity in the radial pulse or when a patient's condition requires a more accurate assessment. In this situation pulse assessment cannot be delegated to NAP. When measurement of apical pulse is a routine practice, the nurse instructs the NAP by:

- Communicating the frequency of measurement and factors related to the patient history such as risk for abnormally slow, rapid, or irregular pulse.
- Reviewing patient's usual pulse values and the need to report any abnormalities in rate or rhythm to the nurse.

Equipment

- ❏ Stethoscope
- ❏ Wristwatch with second hand or digital display
- ❏ Pen and vital sign flow sheet or electronic health record (EHR)
- ❏ Alcohol swab

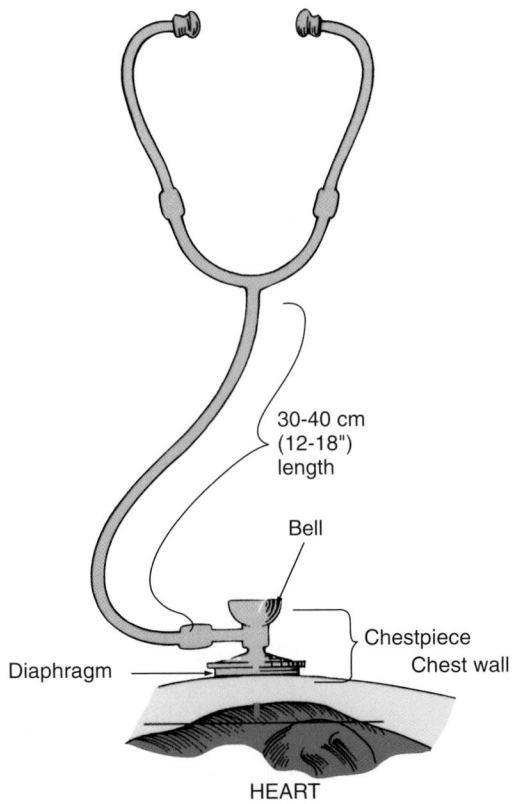

30-40 cm (12-18") length

Bell

Chestpiece
Chest wall

Diaphragm

HEART

FIG 5-7 Acoustic stethoscope.

STEP	RATIONALE

ASSESSMENT

1 Determine need to assess apical pulse:
  a Assess for any risk factors for apical pulse alteration:
  - Heart disease
  - Cardiac dysrhythmias
  - Onset of sudden chest pain or acute pain from any site
  - Invasive cardiovascular diagnostic tests
  - Surgery
  - Sudden infusion of large volume of intravenous (IV) fluid
  - Internal or external hemorrhage
  - Administration of medications that alter heart function

Certain conditions place patients at risk for pulse alterations.

  b Assess for signs and symptoms of altered cardiac function such as dyspnea, fatigue, chest pain, orthopnea, syncope, palpitations, edema of dependent body parts, cyanosis, or pallor of skin (see Chapter 6).

Physical signs and symptoms indicate alteration in cardiac output or stroke volume.

  c Assess for factors that normally influence apical pulse rate and rhythm:
  - Age

Allows you to anticipate factors that alter apical pulse, ensuring an accurate interpretation.
Infant's heart rate (HR) at birth ranges from 100 to 160 beats/min at rest; by age 2 pulse rate slows to 70 to 120 beats/min; by adolescence rate varies between 60 and 90 beats/min and remains so throughout adulthood (Hockenberry and Wilson, 2011).

  - Exercise

Physical activity increases HR; a well-conditioned patient may have a slower-than-usual resting HR that returns more quickly to resting rate after exercise.

  - Position changes

HR increases temporarily when changing from lying to sitting or standing position.

  - Medications

Antidysrhythmics, sympathomimetics, and cardiotonics affect rate and rhythm of pulse; large doses of narcotic analgesics can slow HR; general anesthetics slow HR; central nervous system stimulants such as caffeine can increase HR.

  - Temperature

Fever or exposure to warm environments increases HR; HR declines with hypothermia.

  - Sympathetic stimulation

Emotional stress, anxiety, or fear results in stimulation of the sympathetic nervous system, which increases HR.

2 Determine previous baseline apical rate (if available) from patient's record.

Allows nurse to assess for change in condition.

3 Determine any report of latex allergy. If patient has latex allergy, ensure that stethoscope is latex free.

Reduces risk of allergic reaction to stethoscope.

NURSING DIAGNOSES

- Activity intolerance
- Decreased cardiac output
- Ineffective peripheral tissue perfusion

Related factors are individualized based on patient's condition or needs.

PLANNING

1 Expected outcomes following completion of procedure:
  - Apical HR is within acceptable range.
  - Rhythm is regular.

Adults average 60 to 100 beats/min.
Cardiovascular status is stable.

2 Explain to patient that you will assess apical pulse rate. Encourage patient to relax and ask him or her not to speak. If patient has been active, wait 5 to 10 minutes before assessing pulse. If he or she has been smoking or ingesting caffeine, wait 15 minutes before assessing pulse.

Anxiety, activity, caffeine, and smoking elevate HR. Patient's voice interferes with nurse's ability to hear sound when measuring apical pulse. Assessing apical pulse rate at rest allows for objective comparison of values.

3 Collect and bring appropriate supplies to the patient's bedside.

Ensures an organized approach for assessing radial pulse.

STEP	RATIONALE

IMPLEMENTATION

1 Perform hand hygiene.

2 If necessary, draw curtain around bed and/or close door.

3 Assist patient to supine or sitting position. Move aside bed linen and gown to expose sternum and left side of chest.

4 Locate anatomic landmarks to identify point of maximal impulse (PMI), also called apical *impulse* (see Chapter 6). The heart is located behind and to left of sternum with base at top and apex at bottom. Find angle of Louis just below suprasternal notch between sternal body and manubrium; it feels like a bony prominence (see illustration A). Slip fingers down each side of angle to find second intercostal space (ICS) (see illustration B). Carefully move fingers down left side of sternum to fifth ICS and laterally to left midclavicular line (MCL) (see illustration C). A light tap felt within area 1 to 2.5 cm ($\frac{1}{2}$ to 1 inch) of PMI is reflected from apex of heart (see illustration D).

Reduces transmission of microorganisms.

Maintains privacy and minimizes embarrassment.

Exposes portion of chest wall for selection of auscultatory site.

Use of anatomic landmarks allows correct placement of stethoscope over apex of heart. This position enhances ability to hear heart sounds clearly. If unable to palpate PMI, reposition patient on left side. In the presence of serious heart disease, you may locate PMI to the left of the MCL or at the sixth ICS.

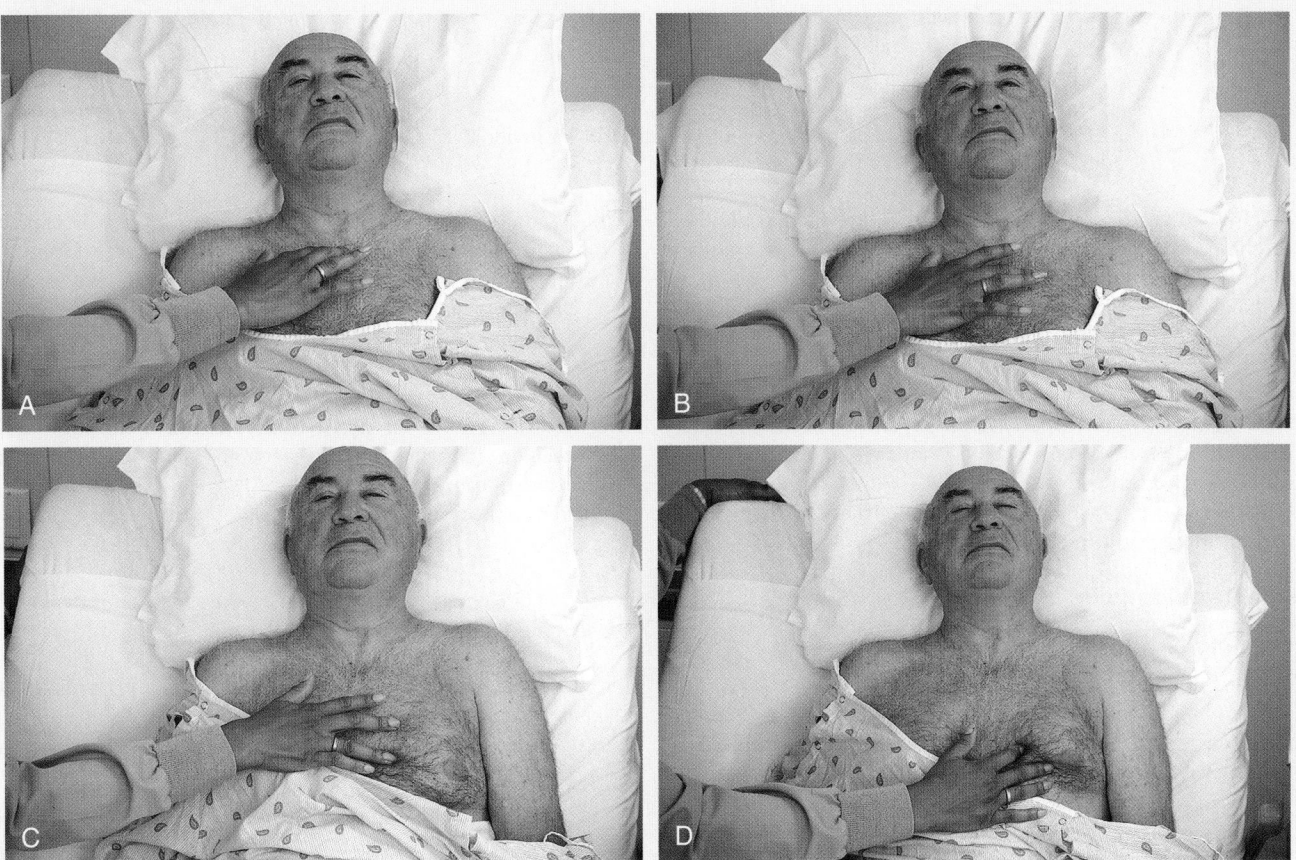

STEP 4 **A**, Nurse locates sternal notch. **B**, Nurse locates second intercostal space. **C**, Nurse locates fifth intercostal space. **D**, Nurse locates point of maximal impulse at fifth intercostal space at left midclavicular line.

5 Place diaphragm of stethoscope in palm of hand for 5 to 10 seconds.

Warming of metal or plastic diaphragm prevents patient from being startled and promotes comfort.

STEP	RATIONALE
6 Place diaphragm of stethoscope over PMI at fifth ICS, at left MCL, and auscultate for normal S_1 and S_2 heart sounds (heard as "lub-dub") (see illustrations).	Allow stethoscope tubing to extend straight without kinks that would distort sound transmission. Normal sounds S_1 and S_2 are high pitched and best heard with diaphragm.

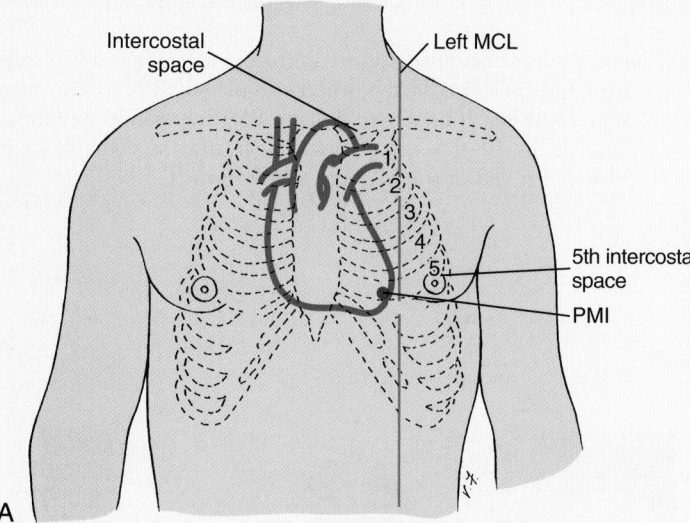

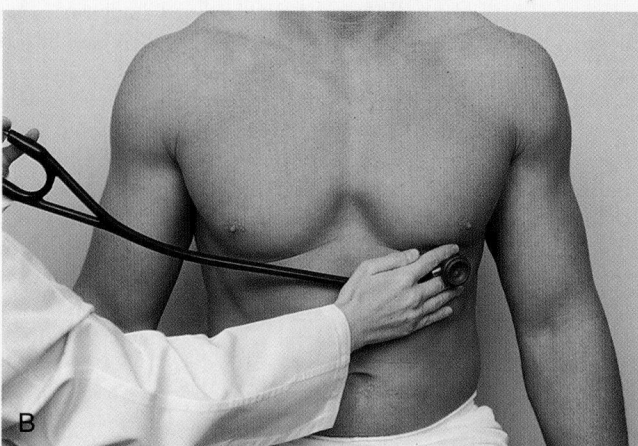

STEP 6   **A,** Location of point of maximal impulse (PMI) in adult. **B,** Listening to PMI in an adult.

7 When you hear S_1 and S_2 with regularity, use second hand of watch and begin to count rate: when sweep hand hits number on dial; start counting with zero, then one, two, and so on.	Apical rate is determined accurately only after you are able to auscultate sounds clearly. Timing begins with zero. Count of one is first sound auscultated after timing begins.
8 If apical rate is regular, count for 30 seconds and multiply by 2.	You can assess regular apical rate within 30 seconds.
9 If HR is irregular or patient is receiving cardiovascular medication, count for a full 1 minute (60 seconds).	Irregular rate is more accurately assessed when measured over longer interval.
10 Note regularity of any dysrhythmia (S_1 and S_2 occurring early or late after previous sequence of sounds) (e.g., every third or every fourth beat is skipped).	Regular occurrence of dysrhythmia within 1 minute indicates inefficient contraction of heart and potential alteration in cardiac output.
11 Replace patient's gown and bed linen; help him or her return to comfortable position.	Restores comfort and promotes sense of well-being.

Clinical Decision Point *If apical rate is abnormal or irregular, repeat measurement or have another nurse conduct measurement. Original measurement may be incorrect. Second measurement confirms initial findings of an abnormal HR.*

12 Discuss findings with patient as needed.	Promotes participation in care and understanding of health status.
13 Perform hand hygiene.	Reduces transmission of microorganisms.
14 Clean earpieces and diaphragm of stethoscope with alcohol swab routinely after each use.	Stethoscopes are frequently contaminated with microorganisms. Regular disinfection can control nosocomial infections.

EVALUATION

1 If assessing pulse for first time, establish apical rate as baseline if it is within an acceptable range.	Used to compare future pulse assessments.
2 Compare apical rate and character with patient's previous baseline and acceptable range of HR for patient's age.	Allows nurse to assess for change in patient's condition and for presence of cardiac alteration.

Unexpected Outcomes

1 An adult patient's apical pulse is greater than 100 beats/min (tachycardia).

2 Patient's apical pulse is less than 60 beats/min (bradycardia).

3 Patient's apical rhythm is irregular.

Related Interventions

- Identify related data, including fever, pain, fear or anxiety, recent exercise, low blood pressure, blood loss, or inadequate oxygenation.
- Observe for signs and symptoms associated with abnormal cardiac function, including dyspnea, fatigue, chest pain, orthopnea, syncope, palpitations, edema of body parts, cyanosis, or dizziness.

- Assess for factors that decrease HR such as digoxin and antiarrhythmic drugs.
- Observe for signs and symptoms associated with abnormal cardiac function, including dyspnea, fatigue, chest pain, orthopnea, syncope, palpitations, edema of body parts, cyanosis, or dizziness.
- Have another nurse assess apical pulse.
- Report findings to nurse in charge and/or health care provider. It may be necessary to withhold prescribed medications that alter HR until health care provider can evaluate need to alter dosage.

- Assess for pulse deficit (see Procedural Guideline 5-1).
- Report findings to nurse in charge and/or health care provider, who may order an electrocardiogram to detect cardiac conduction alteration.

Recording and Reporting

- Record apical pulse rate and rhythm on vital sign flow sheet, nurses' notes, or EHR.
- Document measurement of apical pulse rate after administration of specific therapies in appropriate area in EHR as per agency policy.
- If apical pulse not found at fifth ICS and left MCL, document location of PMI.
- Report abnormal findings to nurse in charge or health care provider.

Special Considerations

Teaching

- Teach caregivers of patients taking prescribed cardiotonic or antidysrhythmic medications how to assess apical pulse rates to detect side effects of medications.

Pediatric

- The PMI of an infant is usually located at the third to fourth ICS near the left sternal border.

- In infants and children younger than 2 years, an apical pulse is more reliable and is counted for 1 full minute because of possible irregularities in rhythm.
- Breath holding in an infant or child affects apical pulse rate.

Gerontologic

- The PMI is often difficult to palpate in some older adults because the anterior-posterior diameter of the chest increases with age and the heart becomes repositioned because of left ventricular enlargement.
- When assessing older adult women with sagging breast tissue, gently lift the breast tissue and place the stethoscope at the fifth ICS or the lower edge of the breast.
- Heart sounds are sometimes muffled or difficult to hear in older adults because of an increase in air space in the lungs.
- The older adult has a decreased HR at rest (Ebersole et al., 2008).

Home Care

- Assess home environment to determine which room affords a quiet environment for auscultation of apical rate.

PROCEDURAL GUIDELINE 5-1 Assessing Apical-Radial Pulse Deficit

The difference between pulses assessed from two different sites, or a pulse deficit, provides information about heart and blood vessel function. When a pulse deficit is assessed between the apical and radial pulses, the volume of blood ejected from the heart may be inadequate to meet the circulatory needs of the tissues, and intervention may be required. To assess for a pulse deficit, the nurse and a second health care provider assess a peripheral pulse rate and the apical pulse rate simultaneously and compare the measurements.

Delegation and Collaboration

The skill of assessing an apical-radial pulse deficit cannot be delegated to nursing assistive personnel (NAP) while the nurse assesses the apical pulse. Collaboration between the nurse and a second health provider is required.

Equipment

❏ Stethoscope
❏ Watch with second hand or digital display

Continued

PROCEDURAL GUIDELINE 5-1 Assessing Apical-Radial Pulse—cont'd

❏ Pen and vital sign flow sheet or electronic health record (EHR)
❏ Alcohol swab

Procedural Steps
1 Determine need to assess for pulse deficit. Irregular heart rate and signs and symptoms such as dyspnea, fatigue, chest pain, and palpitations may indicate abnormal cardiac function.
2 Perform hand hygiene.
3 Collect and bring appropriate supplies to the patient's bedside and draw curtain around bed and/or close door.
4 Explain to the patient that two people will be assessing heart function at the same time.
5 Assist patient to supine or sitting position. Move aside bed linen and gown to expose sternum and left side of chest.
6 Locate apical and radial pulse sites. Nurse auscultates apical pulse (see Skill 5-3) while second provider palpates radial pulse (see Skill 5-2).

7 Nurse begins pulse count by calling out loud when to begin counting pulses.
8 Each nurse completes a 60-second pulse count simultaneously. The count ends when the nurse states "stop." Sixty seconds is required when a discrepancy between pulse sites is expected or when the rhythm is irregular.
9 If the pulse count differs by more than 2, a pulse deficit exists. The pulse deficit reflects the number of ineffective cardiac contractions in 1 minute.
10 If a pulse deficit is noted, assess for other signs and symptoms of decreased cardiac output (see Chapter 6).
11 Discuss findings with patient as needed.
12 Perform hand hygiene.
13 Record apical pulse, radial pulse, and pulse deficit in nurses' notes and EHR. Inform the nurse in charge or health care provider of presence of a pulse deficit.

SKILL 5-4 Assessing Respirations

NSO *Vital Signs Module / Lesson 4*

Respiration is the exchange of oxygen (O_2) and carbon dioxide (CO_2) between cells of the body and the atmosphere. Three processes of respiration are: ventilation, mechanical movement of gases into and out of the lungs; diffusion, movement of oxygen and carbon dioxide between the alveoli and the red blood cells; and perfusion, distribution of red blood cells to and from the pulmonary capillaries. You assess ventilation by observing the rate, depth, and rhythm of respiratory movements. Accurate assessment of respiration depends on recognizing normal thoracic and abdominal movements. Normal breathing is both active and passive. On inspiration the diaphragm contracts, and the abdominal organs move down to increase the size of the chest cavity. At the same time the ribs and sternum lift outward to promote lung expansion. On expiration the diaphragm relaxes upward, and the ribs and sternum return to their relaxed position (Fig. 5-8). During quiet breathing the chest wall gently rises and falls. The body uses more energy during inspiration than during expiration. Expiration is an active process only during exercise, voluntary hyperventilation, and certain disease states.

Delegation and Collaboration
The skill of counting respirations can be delegated to nursing assistive personnel (NAP) unless the patient is considered unstable (i.e., complaints of dyspnea). The nurse instructs the NAP by:
• Communicating the frequency of measurement and factors related to patient history or risk for increased or decreased respiratory rate or irregular respirations.

 Video Clip

• Reviewing any unusual respiratory values and significant changes to report to the nurse.

Equipment
❏ Wristwatch with second hand or digital display
❏ Pen and vital sign flow sheet or electronic health record (EHR)

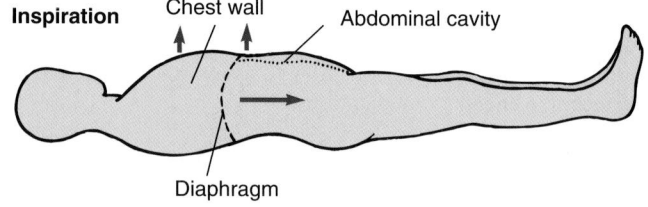

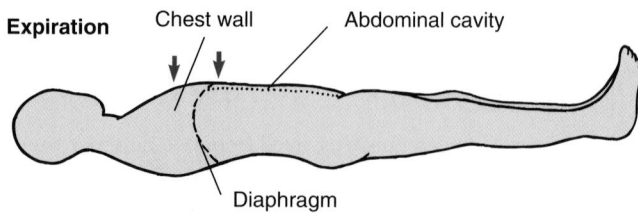

FIG 5-8 Diaphragmatic and chest wall movement during inspiration and expiration.

STEP	RATIONALE

ASSESSMENT

1 Determine need to assess patient's respirations:

a Assess for risk factors of respiratory alterations:

- Fever
- Pain and anxiety
- Diseases of chest wall or muscles
- Constrictive chest or abdominal dressings
- Presence of abdominal incisions
- Gastric distention
- Chronic pulmonary disease (emphysema, bronchitis, asthma)
- Traumatic injury to chest wall with or without collapse of underlying lung tissue
- Presence of a chest tube
- Respiratory infection (pneumonia, acute bronchitis)
- Pulmonary edema and emboli
- Head injury with damage to brainstem
- Anemia

Certain conditions place patient at risk for ventilatory alterations detected by changes in respiratory rate, depth, and rhythm.

b Assess for signs and symptoms of respiratory alterations such as the following:

- Bluish or cyanotic appearance of nail beds, lips, mucous membranes, and skin
- Restlessness, irritability, confusion, reduced level of consciousness
- Pain during inspiration
- Labored or difficult breathing
- Orthopnea
- Use of accessory muscles
- Adventitious breath sounds (see Chapter 6)
- Inability to breathe spontaneously
- Thick, frothy, blood-tinged, or copious sputum production

Physical signs and symptoms indicate alterations in respiratory status.

c Assess for factors that influence the character of respirations:

Allows you to anticipate factors that influence respirations, ensuring a more accurate interpretation.

- Exercise

Respirations increase in rate and depth to meet need for additional oxygen and rid body of carbon dioxide.

- Anxiety

Anxiety causes increase in respiration rate and depth because of sympathetic nervous system stimulation.

- Acute pain

Pain alters rate and rhythm of respirations; breathing becomes shallow. Patient inhibits or splints chest wall movement when pain is in area of chest or abdomen.

- Smoking

Chronic smoking changes pulmonary airways, resulting in an increased respiratory rate at rest when not smoking.

- Medications

Narcotic analgesics, general anesthetics, and sedative hypnotics depress rate and depth; amphetamines and cocaine increase rate and depth; bronchodilators cause dilation of airways, which ultimately slows respiratory rate.

- Body position

Standing or sitting erect promotes full ventilatory movement and lung expansion; stooped or slumped posture impairs ventilatory movement; lying flat prevents full chest expansion.

- Neurologic injury

Damage to the brainstem impairs the respiratory center and inhibits rate and rhythm.

- Hemoglobin function

Decreased hemoglobin levels lower amount of oxygen carried in blood, which results in increased respiratory rate to increase oxygen delivery. An increase in altitude lowers amount of saturated hemoglobin, which increases respiratory rate and depth.

STEP	RATIONALE

2 Assess pertinent laboratory values:
  a *Arterial blood gases (ABGs)*: Normal ranges (values vary slightly among agencies):
  • pH, 7.35 to 7.45
  • $PaCO_2$, 35 to 45 mm Hg
  • HCO_3, 22 to 28 mEq/L
  • PaO_2, 80 to 100 mm Hg
  • SaO_2, 95% to 100%
	ABG values measure arterial blood pH, partial pressure of oxygen and carbon dioxide, and arterial oxygen saturation, which reflect patient's oxygenation status.

b *Pulse oximetry (SpO₂)*: Normal $SpO_2 \geq$ 95%-100%; 90% is a red flag; anything less indicates hypoxemia (Valdez-Lowe et al., 2009) (see Procedural Guideline 5-3)	SpO_2 less than 85% is often accompanied by changes in respiratory rate, depth, and rhythm.

c *Complete blood count (CBC)*: Normal CBC for adults (values vary within agencies):
  • Hemoglobin: 14 to 18 g/100 mL, males; 12 to 16 g/100 mL, females
  • Hematocrit: 42% to 52%, males; 37% to 47%, females
  • Red blood cell count: 4.7 to 6.1 million/mm^3, males; 4.2 to 5.4 million/mm^3, females
	CBC measures red blood cell count; volume of red blood cells; and concentration of hemoglobin, which reflects patient's capacity to carry oxygen.

3 Determine previous baseline respiratory rate (if available) from patient's record.	Assesses for change in condition. Provides comparison with future respiratory measurements.

NURSING DIAGNOSES

• Activity intolerance	• Ineffective airway clearance	• Ineffective breathing pattern
• Impaired gas exchange	• Impaired spontaneous ventilation	

Related factors are individualized based on patient's condition or needs.

PLANNING

STEP	RATIONALE

1 Expected outcomes following completion of procedure:
  • Respiratory rate is within acceptable range.
  • Respirations are regular and of normal depth.
	Adults average 12 to 20 breaths/min.
	Respiratory status is stable.

2 If patient has been active, wait 5 to 10 minutes before assessing respirations.	Exercise increases respiratory rate and depth. Assessing respirations while patient is at rest allows for objective comparison of values.
3 Assess respirations after pulse measurement in adult.	Inconspicuous assessment of respirations immediately after pulse assessment prevents patient from consciously or unintentionally altering rate and depth of breathing.
4 Be sure that patient is in comfortable position, preferably sitting or lying with the head of the bed elevated 45 to 60 degrees.	Sitting erect promotes full ventilatory movement. Position of discomfort causes patient to breathe more rapidly.

Clinical Decision Point *Assess patients with difficulty breathing (dyspnea) such as those with heart failure or abdominal ascites or in late stages of pregnancy in the position of greatest comfort. Repositioning may increase the work of breathing, which increases respiratory rate.*

IMPLEMENTATION

STEP	RATIONALE
1 Draw curtain around bed and/or close door. Perform hand hygiene.	Maintains privacy. Prevents transmission of microorganisms.
2 Be sure that patient's chest is visible. If necessary, move bed linen or gown.	Ensures clear view of chest wall and abdominal movements.
3 Place patient's arm in relaxed position across abdomen or lower chest or place your hand directly over patient's upper abdomen.	A similar position used during pulse assessment allows respiratory rate assessment to be inconspicuous. Patient's or nurse's hand rises and falls during respiratory cycle.
4 Observe complete respiratory cycle (one inspiration and one expiration).	Rate is accurately determined only after nurse has viewed respiratory cycle.
5 After observing cycle, look at second hand of watch and begin to count rate: when sweep hand hits number on dial, begin time frame, counting one with first full respiratory cycle.	Timing begins with count of one. Respirations occur more slowly than pulse; thus timing does not begin with zero.

STEP	RATIONALE
6 If rhythm is regular, count number of respirations in 30 seconds and multiply by 2. If rhythm is irregular, less than 12, or greater than 20, count for 1 full minute.	Respiratory rate is equivalent to number of respirations per minute. Suspected irregularities require assessment for at least 1 minute (Box 5-5).
7 Note depth of respirations by observing degree of chest wall movement while counting rate. In addition, assess depth by palpating chest wall excursion or auscultating posterior thorax after you have counted rate (see Chapter 6). Describe depth as shallow, normal, or deep.	Character of ventilatory movement reveals specific disease states restricting volume of air from moving into and out of lungs.
8 Note rhythm of ventilatory cycle. Normal breathing is regular and uninterrupted. Do not confuse sighing with abnormal rhythm.	Character of ventilations reveals specific types of alterations. Periodically people unconsciously take single deep breaths or sighs to expand small airways prone to collapse.

Clinical Decision Point *Any irregular respiratory pattern or periods of apnea (cessation of respiration for several seconds) are symptoms of underlying disease in the adult, and you need to report this to the health care provider or nurse in charge. Further assessment and immediate intervention are often necessary.*

STEP	RATIONALE
9 Replace bed linen and patient's gown.	Restores comfort and promotes sense of well-being.
10 Perform hand hygiene.	Reduces transmission of microorganisms.
11 Discuss findings with patient as needed.	Promotes participation in care and understanding of health status.

EVALUATION

1 If assessing respirations for first time, establish rate, rhythm, and depth as baseline if within acceptable range.	Used to compare future respiratory assessment.
2 Compare respirations with patient's previous baseline and usual rate, rhythm, and depth.	Allows nurse to assess for changes in patient's condition and presence of respiratory alterations.
3 Correlate respiratory rate, depth, and rhythm with data obtained from pulse oximetry and ABG measurements if available.	Evaluation of ventilation, perfusion, and diffusion are interrelated.

BOX 5-5 | Alterations in Breathing Pattern

Alteration	Description
Apnea	Respirations cease for several seconds. Persistent cessation results in respiratory arrest.
Biot's respiration	Irregular respirations vary in depth and are interrupted by periods of apnea.
Bradypnea	Rate of breathing is regular but abnormally slow (fewer than 12 breaths/min).
Cheyne-Stokes respiration	Respiratory rate and depth are irregular, characterized by alternating periods of apnea and hyperventilation. Respiratory cycle begins with slow, shallow breaths that gradually increase to abnormal rate and depth. The pattern reverses; breathing slows and becomes shallow, climaxing in apnea before respiration resumes.
Hyperpnea	Respirations are increased in depth; occurs normally during exercise.
Hyperventilation	Rate and depth of respirations increase. Hypocarbia, an abnormally low level of carbon dioxide in the blood, may occur.
Hypoventilation	Respiratory rate is abnormally low; depth of ventilation may be depressed. Hypercarbia, an abnormally elevated level of carbon dioxide in the blood, may occur.
Kussmaul's respiration	Respirations are abnormally rapid and deep but regular; common in diabetic ketoacidosis.
Tachypnea	Rate of breathing is regular but abnormally rapid (more than 20 breaths/min).

Unexpected Outcomes

1 Patient's respiratory rate is below 12 breaths/minute (bradypnea) or above 20 breaths/minute (tachypnea). Breathing pattern is sometimes irregular (see Box 5-5). Depth of respirations is increased or decreased. Patient complains of feeling short of breath.

2 Patient demonstrates Kussmaul's, Cheyne-Stokes, or Biot's respirations (see Box 5-5).

Related Interventions

- Assess for related factors, including obstructed airway, abnormal breath sounds, productive cough, restlessness, anxiety, and confusion (see Chapter 6).
- Assist patient to supported sitting position (semi- or high-Fowler's) unless contraindicated.
- Provide oxygen as ordered (see Chapter 23).
- Assess for environmental factors that influence patient's respiratory rate such as secondhand smoke, poor ventilation, or gas fumes.
- Notify health care provider or nurse in charge if alteration continues.
- Notify health care provider for additional evaluation and possible medical intervention.

Recording and Reporting

- Record respiratory rate on vital sign flow sheet, nurses' notes, or EHR.
- Record abnormal depth and rhythm in appropriate area in nurses' notes and EHR.
- Document measurement of respiratory rate after administration of specific therapies in nurses' notes and EHR.
- Record type and amount of oxygen therapy, if used, in nurses' notes and EHR.
- Report abnormal findings to nurse in charge or health care provider.

Special Considerations

Teaching

- Patients who demonstrate decreased ventilation often benefit from learning deep breathing and coughing exercises.
- Instruct family caregiver to contact home care nurse or health care provider if unusual fluctuations in respiratory rate occur.

Pediatric

- Assess respiratory rates before other vital signs or assessments if you are able to view movement of chest wall or abdomen. This allows assessment of rate and rhythm before child becomes anxious because of stranger anxiety or fear of other assessment procedures.
- Average respiratory rate (breaths per minute) for newborns is 30 to 60; infant (6 months to 1 year) is 30; toddler (2 years) is

25 to 32; and child from 3 to 12 years is 20 (Hockenberry and Wilson, 2011).
- Children up to age 7 breathe abdominally; thus respirations are observed by abdominal movement.
- An irregular respiratory rate and short apneic spells are normal for newborns.
- Nurses can simply observe infant or young child while chest and abdomen are exposed.
- Use cardiorespiratory monitors for infants or newborns that are at risk for respiratory compromise or sustained apnea.

Gerontologic

- Aging causes ossification of costal cartilage and downward slant of ribs, resulting in more rigid rib cage, which reduces chest wall expansion. Kyphosis and scoliosis, frequent in older adults, may also restrict chest expansion.
- Depth of respirations tends to decrease with aging.
- Change in lung function with aging results in respiratory rates generally higher in older adults, with a range of 16 to 25 breaths/min.
- Some older adults depend more on accessory abdominal muscles during respiration than weakened thoracic muscles.

Home Care

- Assess for environmental factors in the home that influence patient's respiratory rate such as secondhand smoke, poor ventilation, or gas fumes.

SKILL 5-5 Assessing Arterial Blood Pressure

NSO *Vital Signs Module / Lesson 5*

Blood pressure (BP) is the force exerted by blood against the vessel walls. The peak pressure occurs when the ventricular contraction of the heart, or systole, forces blood under high pressure into the aorta. When the ventricles relax, the blood remaining in the arteries exerts a minimal or diastolic pressure. Diastolic pressure is the minimal pressure exerted against the arterial wall at all times.

The standard unit for measuring blood pressure is millimeters of mercury (mm Hg). The most common technique of measuring blood pressure is auscultation with a sphygmomanometer and stethoscope. As the sphygmomanometer cuff is deflated, the five different sounds heard over an artery are called *Korotkoff phases*.

The sound in each phase has unique characteristics (Fig. 5-9). Blood pressure is recorded with the systolic reading (first Korotkoff sound) before the diastolic (beginning of the fifth Korotkoff sound). The difference between systolic and diastolic pressure is the pulse pressure. For a blood pressure of 120/80, the pulse pressure is 40.

Hypertension

Hypertension is a major factor underlying death from heart attack and stroke in the United States and Canada. The Joint National Committee on Prevention, Detection, Evaluation, and Treatment of High Blood Pressure (NHBPEP, 2003) has set criteria for determining categories of hypertension (Table 5-2). Prehypertension is a designation for patients at high risk for developing hypertension.

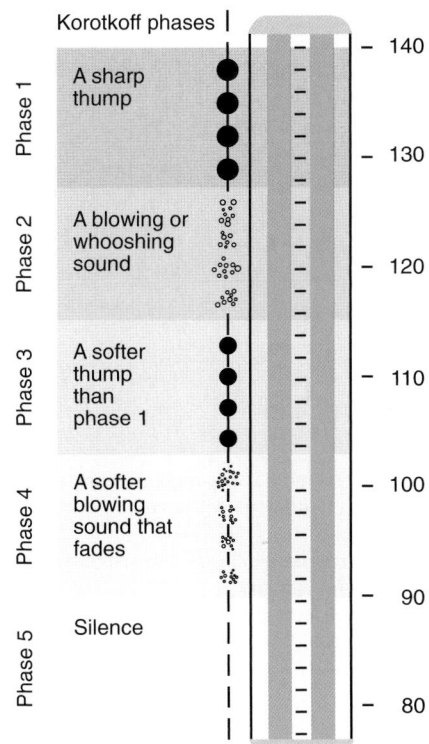

Korotkoff phases

Phase 1 — A sharp thump

Phase 2 — A blowing or whooshing sound

Phase 3 — A softer thump than phase 1

Phase 4 — A softer blowing sound that fades

Phase 5 — Silence

140
130
120
110
100
90
80

FIG 5-9 The sounds auscultated during blood pressure measurement can be differentiated into five Korotkoff phases. In this example the blood pressure is 140/90 mm Hg.

In these patients early intervention by adoption of healthy lifestyles reduces the risk of or prevents hypertension. Hypertension is defined as systolic blood pressure (SBP) of 140 mm Hg or greater, diastolic blood pressure (DBP) of 90 mm Hg or greater, or taking antihypertensive medication (NHBPEP, 2003). The diagnosis of hypertension in adults requires the average of two or more readings taken at each of two or more visits after an initial screening.

One blood pressure recording revealing a high systolic or diastolic blood pressure does not qualify as a diagnosis of hypertension. However, if you assess a high reading (e.g., 150/90 mm Hg), encourage the patient to return for another checkup within 2 months (Table 5-3).

Hypotension

Hypotension occurs when the systolic blood pressure falls to 90 mm Hg or below. Although some adults normally have a low blood pressure, for most people a low blood pressure is an abnormal finding associated with illness (e.g., hemorrhage or myocardial infarction). Orthostatic hypotension, also referred to as *postural hypotension*, occurs when a normotensive person develops symptoms (e.g., light-headedness or dizziness) and low blood pressure when rising to an upright position. In severe cases loss of consciousness may occur. Orthostatic changes in vital signs are effective indicators of blood volume depletion. Some medications cause orthostatic hypotension, especially in young patients and older adults.

Blood Pressure Equipment

You measure arterial blood pressure either directly (invasively) or indirectly (noninvasively). The direct method requires electronic monitoring equipment and the insertion of a thin catheter into an artery. The risks of invasive blood pressure monitoring require use in an intensive care setting.

TABLE 5-2	Classification of Blood Pressure for Adults Ages 18 Years and Older*		
Category	**Systolic (mm Hg)**		**Diastolic (mm Hg)**
Normal	<120	and	<80
Prehypertension	120-139	or	80-89
Stage 1	140-159	or	90-99
Stage 2	≥160	or	≥100

From National High Blood Pressure Education Program; National Heart, Lung, and Blood Institute; National Institutes of Health: The seventh report of the Joint National Committee on Prevention, Detection, Evaluation and Treatment of High Blood Pressure, *JAMA* 289(19):2560, 2003.
*Based on the average of two or more readings taken at each of two or more visits after an initial screening. Patient is not taking antihypertensive drugs and not acutely ill. When systolic and diastolic blood pressures fall into different categories, the higher category should be selected to classify the individual's blood pressure status. For example, 160/92 mm Hg should be classified as stage 2 hypertension.

TABLE 5-3	Recommendations for Blood Pressure Follow-up
Initial Blood Pressure	**Follow-up Recommended***
Normal	Recheck in 2 years.
Prehypertension	Recheck in 1 year.†
Stage 1 hypertension	Confirm within 2 months.†
Stage 2 hypertension	Evaluate or refer to source of care within 1 month. For those with higher pressure (e.g., >180/110 mm Hg), evaluate and treat immediately or within 1 week, depending on clinical situation and complications.

*Modify follow-up scheduling according to reliable information about past blood pressure measurements, other cardiovascular risk factors, or target organ damage.
†Provide advice about lifestyle modifications.

The more common noninvasive method requires use of the sphygmomanometer and stethoscope. A sphygmomanometer includes a pressure manometer, an occlusive cloth or disposable vinyl cuff that encloses an inflatable rubber bladder, and a pressure bulb with a release valve that inflates the bladder. The aneroid pressure manometer has a glass-enclosed circular gauge containing a needle that registers millimeter calibrations. Before using the aneroid manometer, make sure that the needle is pointing to zero. The release valve of the sphygmomanometer that holds the pressure constant must be clean and freely movable in either direction.

Cloth or disposable vinyl compression cuffs contain an inflatable bladder and come in several different sizes. The size selected is proportional to the circumference of the limb that you are assessing. Ideally the width of the cuff should be 40% of the circumference (or 20% wider than the diameter) of the midpoint of the limb on which the cuff is to be used (Fig. 5-10). The bladder enclosed within the cuff should encircle at least 80% of the upper arm (NHBPEP, 2003). Many adults require a large adult cuff. A regular-size cuff holds a bladder in the width of 12 to 13 cm (4.8 to 5.2 inches) and the length of 22 to 23 cm (8.5 to 9 inches). An improperly fitting cuff produces inaccurate blood pressure measurements (Box 5-6).

Electronic or automatic blood pressure machines consist of an electronic sensor positioned inside a blood pressure cuff attached

BOX 5-6 | Common Mistakes in Blood Pressure Assessment

Error	Effect
Bladder or cuff too wide	False low reading
Bladder or cuff too narrow or too short	False-high reading
Cuff wrapped too loosely or unevenly	False-high reading
Deflating cuff too slowly	False-high diastolic reading
Deflating cuff too quickly	False-low systolic and false-high diastolic reading
Arm below heart level	False-high reading
Arm above heart level	False-low reading
Arm not supported	False-high reading
Stethoscope that fits poorly or impairment of examiner's hearing, causing sounds to be muffled	False-low systolic and false-high diastolic reading
Stethoscope applied too firmly against antecubital fossa	False-low diastolic reading
Inflating too slowly	False-high diastolic reading
Repeating assessments too quickly	False-high systolic reading
Inaccurate inflation level	False-low systolic reading
Multiple examiners using different Korotkoff sounds for diastolic readings	False-high systolic and false-low diastolic reading

BOX 5-7 | Advantages and Limitations of Assessing Blood Pressure Electronically

Advantages
- Ease of use
- Efficient when frequent repeated measurements are indicated
- Stethoscope not required
- Allows blood pressure to be recorded more frequently, as often as every 15 seconds with accuracy

Limitations
- Expensive
- Requires source of electricity
- Requires space to position machine
- Sensitive to outside motion interference and cannot be used in patients with seizures, tremors, or shivers or patients unable to cooperate
- Not accurate for patients with irregular heart rate or hypotension or in conditions with reduced blood flow (e.g., hypothermia)
- Accuracy standards for electronic blood pressure machine manufacturers are voluntary
- Vulnerable to error among older adults and obese patients (Heinemann et al., 2008).

to an electronic processor (see Procedural Guideline 5-2). Electronic devices have limitations but are useful when frequent measurements are necessary (Box 5-7).

Delegation and Collaboration
The skill of blood pressure measurement can be delegated to nursing assistive personnel (NAP) unless the patient is considered unstable (i.e., hypotensive). The nurse instructs the NAP by:
- Explaining the appropriate limb for measurement, blood pressure cuff size, and equipment (manual or electronic) to be used.
- Communicating the frequency of measurement and factors related to the patient's history such as risk for orthostatic hypotension.
- Reviewing the patient's usual blood pressure values and significant changes or abnormalities to report to the nurse.

Equipment
- Aneroid sphygmomanometer
- Cloth or disposable vinyl pressure cuff of appropriate size for patient's extremity
- Stethoscope
- Alcohol swab
- Pen and vital sign flow sheet or electronic health record (EHR)

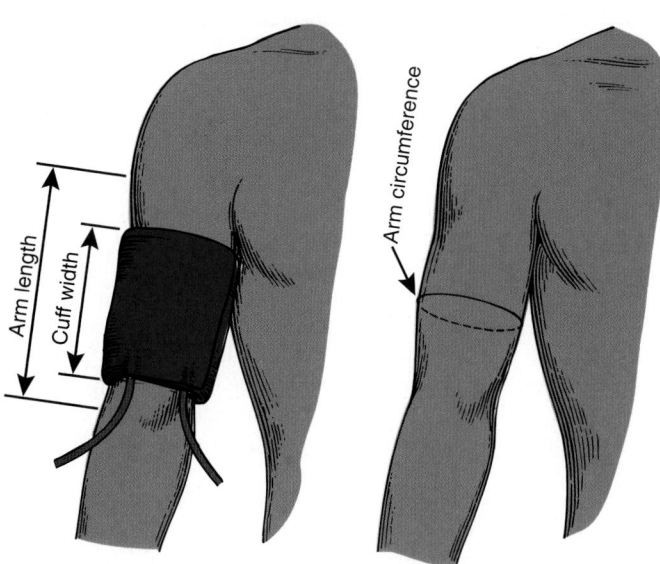

FIG 5-10 Guidelines for proper blood pressure cuff size. Cuff width equals 20% more than upper arm diameter or 40% of circumference around upper arm and two thirds of upper arm length.

STEP	RATIONALE

ASSESSMENT

1 Determine need to assess patient's blood pressure:

  a Assess risk factors for blood pressure alterations:

Certain conditions place patients at risk for blood pressure alteration.

- History of cardiovascular disease
- Renal disease
- Diabetes mellitus
- Circulatory shock (hypovolemic, septic, cardiogenic, or neurogenic)
- Acute or chronic pain
- Rapid intravenous (IV) infusion of fluids or blood products
- Increased intracranial pressure
- Postoperative status
- Toxemia of pregnancy

  b Assess for signs and symptoms of blood pressure alterations. In patients at risk for high blood pressure (HBP), assess for headache (usually occipital), flushing of face, nosebleed, and fatigue in older adults. Hypotension is associated with dizziness; mental confusion; restlessness; pale, dusky, or cyanotic skin and mucous membranes; cool, mottled skin over extremities.

Physical signs and symptoms indicate alterations in blood pressure. Hypertension is often asymptomatic until pressure is very high.

  c Assess for factors that influence blood pressure:

Allows you to anticipate factors that influence respirations, ensuring a more accurate interpretation.

- Age

Acceptable values for blood pressure vary throughout life (see Pediatric and Gerontologic Considerations).

- Gender

During and after menopause women often have higher blood pressures than men of same age.

- Daily (diurnal) variation

Blood pressure varies throughout day; pressure is highest during the day between 10:00 AM and 6:00 PM and lowest in early morning.

- Position

Blood pressure falls as person moves from lying to sitting or standing position; normally postural variations are minimal.

- Exercise

Increases in oxygen demand by the body for activity increase blood pressure.

- Weight

Obesity is an independent predictor of hypertension.

- Sympathetic stimulation

Pain, anxiety, or fear stimulates the sympathetic nervous system, causing blood pressure to rise.

- Medications

Antihypertensives, diuretics, beta-adrenergic blockers, vasodilators, calcium channel blockers, angiotensin-converting enzyme (ACE) inhibitors, angiotensin receptor blockers (ARBs), and antidysrhythmics lower blood pressure; opioids and general anesthetics also cause a drop in blood pressure.

- Smoking

Smoking results in vasoconstriction, a narrowing of blood vessels. Blood pressure rises acutely and returns to baseline approximately 15 minutes after stopping smoking (NHBPEP, 2003).

- Ethnicity

Incidence of hypertension is higher in African Americans than in European Americans. African Americans tend to develop more severe hypertension at an earlier age and have twice the risk for the complications of hypertension (i.e., stroke and heart attack). Hypertension-related deaths are also higher among African Americans.

2 Determine best site for blood pressure assessment. Avoid applying cuff to extremity when IV fluids are infusing, an arteriovenous shunt or fistula is present, or breast or axillary surgery has been performed on that side. In addition, avoid applying cuff to extremity that has been traumatized or diseased or requires a cast or bulky bandage. Use lower extremities when brachial arteries are inaccessible.

Inappropriate site selection may result in poor amplification of sounds, causing inaccurate readings. Application of pressure from inflated bladder temporarily impairs blood flow and can further compromise circulation in extremity that already has impaired blood flow.

STEP	RATIONALE
3 Determine previous baseline blood pressure and site (if available) from patient's record. Determine any report of latex allergy.	Assesses for change in condition. Provides comparison with future blood pressure measurements. If patient has latex allergy, verify that stethoscope and blood pressure cuff are latex free.
4 Assess patient's knowledge of procedure.	Encourages cooperation, minimizes risks and anxiety. Identifies teaching needs.

NURSING DIAGNOSES

- Decreased cardiac output
- Deficient fluid volume
- Excess fluid volume
- Ineffective tissue perfusion

Related factors are individualized based on patient's condition or needs.

PLANNING

1 Expected outcome following completion of procedure: • Blood pressure is within acceptable range for patient's age.	Cardiovascular status is stable.
2 Explain to patient that you will assess blood pressure. Have him or her rest at least 5 minutes before measuring lying or sitting blood pressure and 1 minute before measuring standing. Ask patient not to speak while you are measuring blood pressure.	Reduces anxiety that falsely elevates readings. Exercise causes false elevations in blood pressure. Talking to a patient during blood pressure assessment increases readings 10% to 40% (NHBPEP, 2003).
3 Be sure that patient has not exercised, ingested caffeine, or smoked for 30 minutes before assessment of blood pressure.	Smoking increases blood pressure immediately and lasts up to 15 minutes. The effects of coffee or caffeine increase blood pressure up to 3 hours (NHBPEP, 2003).
4 Have patient assume sitting or lying position. Be sure that room is warm, quiet, and relaxing.	Maintains patient's comfort during measurement. Patient's perceptions that the physical or interpersonal environment is stressful affect blood pressure.
5 Select appropriate cuff size (see Fig. 5-10) and ensure that other equipment is in the patient's room.	Use of improper-size cuff causes false-low or false-high reading (see Box 5-6).
6 Perform hand hygiene.	Reduces transmission of microorganisms.

IMPLEMENTATION

1 Assess blood pressure by auscultation: **a** Upper extremity: With patient sitting or lying, position his or her forearm at heart level with palm turned up (see illustration). If sitting, instruct patient to keep feet flat on floor without legs crossed. If supine, patient should not have legs crossed. Lower extremity: With patient prone, position patient so knee is slightly flexed.	If arm is extended and not supported, patient will perform isometric exercise that can increase diastolic pressure. Placement of arm above level of heart causes false-low reading, 2 mm Hg for each inch above heart level. Leg crossing can falsely increase blood pressure.

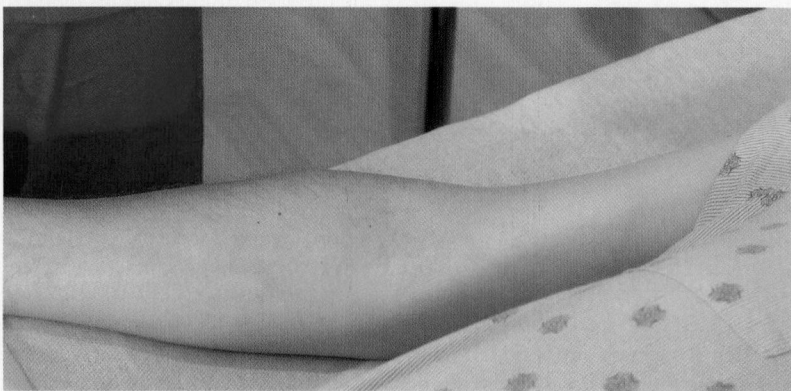

STEP 1a   Patient's forearm supported on bed.

STEP	RATIONALE
b Expose extremity (arm or leg) fully by removing constricting clothing.	Ensures proper cuff application. Do not place blood pressure cuff over clothing.
c Palpate brachial artery (arm, see illustration A) or popliteal artery (leg, see illustration B). With cuff fully deflated, apply bladder of cuff above artery by centering arrows marked on cuff over artery (see illustration C). If cuff does not have any center arrows, estimate center of bladder and place this center over artery. Position cuff 2.5 cm (1 inch) above site of pulsation (antecubital or popliteal space). With cuff fully deflated. wrap it evenly and snugly around upper arm (see illustration D).	Popliteal artery is just below patient's thigh, behind knee. Placing bladder directly over artery ensures that you apply proper pressure during inflation. Loose-fitting cuff causes false-high readings.
d Position manometer gauge vertically at eye level. You should be no farther than 1 meter (approximately 1 yard) away.	Looking up or down at scale can result in distorted readings.
e Measure blood pressure.	

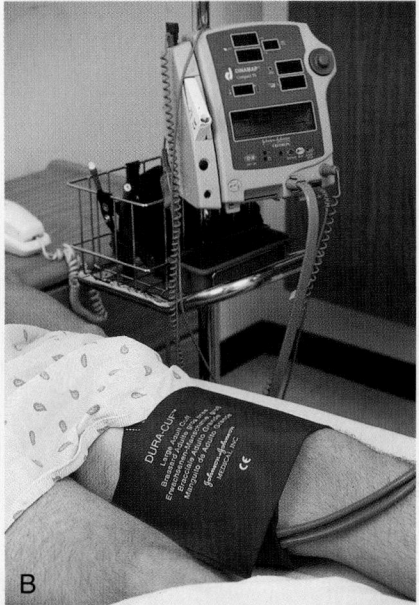

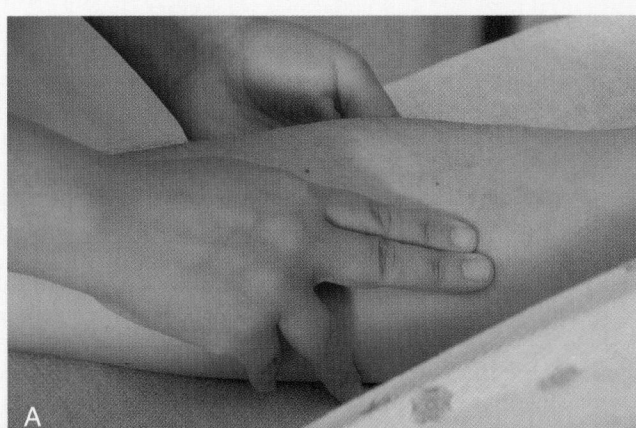

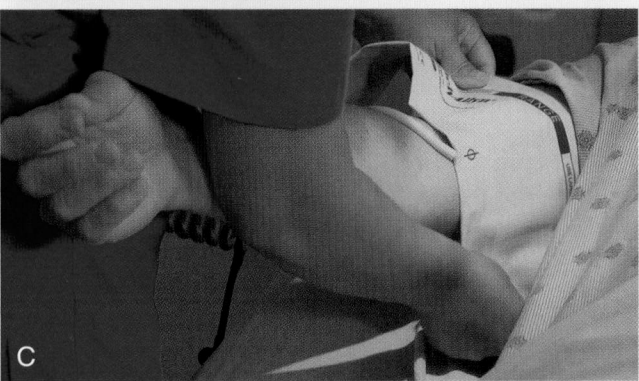

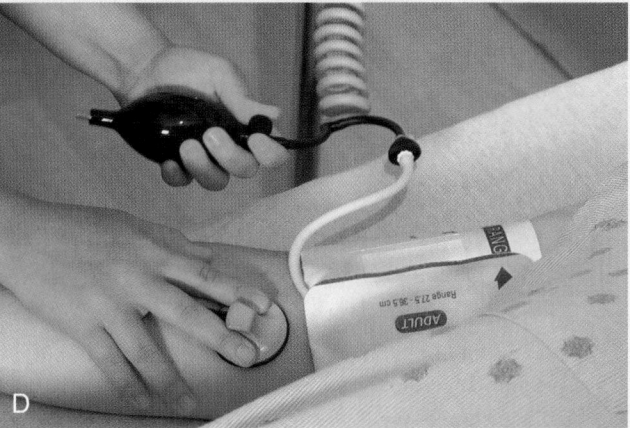

STEP 1c **A,** Palpating brachial artery. **B,** Blood pressure cuff applied around thigh. **C,** Aligning blood pressure cuff arrow with brachial artery. **D,** Blood pressure cuff wrapped around upper arm.

STEP	RATIONALE
(1) Two-step method:	
(a) Relocate brachial pulse. Palpate artery distal to cuff with fingertips of nondominant hand while inflating cuff rapidly to a pressure 30 mm Hg above point at which pulse disappears. Slowly deflate cuff and note point when pulse reappears. Deflate cuff fully and wait 30 seconds.	Estimating prevents false-low readings. Determine maximal inflation point for accurate reading by palpation. If unable to palpate artery because of weakened pulse, use an ultrasonic stethoscope (see Chapter 6). Completely deflating cuff prevents venous congestion and false-high readings.
(b) Place stethoscope earpieces in ears and be sure that sounds are clear, not muffled.	Ensure that each earpiece follows angle of ear canal to facilitate hearing.
(c) Relocate brachial artery and place bell or diaphragm chest piece of stethoscope over it. Do not allow chest piece to touch cuff or clothing.	Proper stethoscope placement ensures best sound reception. Stethoscope improperly positioned causes muffled sounds that often result in false-low systolic and false-high diastolic readings. The bell provides better sound reproduction, whereas the diaphragm is easier to secure with fingers and covers a larger area.
(d) Close valve of pressure bulb clockwise until tight. Quickly inflate cuff to 30 mm Hg above patient's estimated systolic pressure.	Tightening valve prevents air leak during inflation. Rapid inflation ensures accurate measurement of systolic pressure.
(e) Slowly release pressure bulb valve and allow manometer needle to fall at rate of 2 to 3 mm Hg/second.	Too-rapid or too-slow a decline causes inaccurate readings.
(f) Note point on manometer when you hear first clear sound. The sound will slowly increase in intensity.	First Korotkoff sound reflects systolic blood pressure.
(g) Continue to deflate cuff gradually, noting point at which sound disappears in adults. Note pressure to nearest 2 mm Hg. Listen for 20 to 30 mm Hg after last sound and allow remaining air to escape quickly.	Beginning of fifth Korotkoff sound is indication of diastolic pressure in adults (NHBPEP, 2003). Fourth Korotkoff sound involves distinct muffling of sounds and is indication of diastolic pressure in children.
(2) One-step method:	
(a) Place stethoscope earpieces in ears and be sure that sounds are clear, not muffled.	Earpieces should follow angle of ear canal to facilitate hearing.
(b) Relocate brachial artery and place bell or diaphragm chest piece of stethoscope over it. Do not allow chest piece to touch cuff or clothing.	Proper stethoscope placement ensures optimal sound reception. Stethoscope improperly positioned causes muffled sounds that often result in false-low systolic and false-high diastolic readings. Bell provides better sound reproduction, whereas diaphragm is easier to secure with fingers and covers larger area.
(c) Close valve of pressure bulb clockwise until tight. Quickly inflate cuff to 30 mm Hg above patient's usual systolic pressure.	Tightening valve prevents air leak during inflation. Inflation above systolic level ensures accurate measurement of systolic pressure.
(d) Slowly release pressure bulb valve and allow manometer needle to fall at rate of 2 to 3 mm Hg/second. Note point on manometer when you hear first clear sound. Sound will slowly increase in intensity.	Too-rapid or too-slow a decline in mercury level causes inaccurate readings. First Korotkoff sound reflects systolic pressure.
(e) Continue to deflate cuff gradually, noting point at which sound disappears in adults. Note pressure to nearest 2 mm Hg. Listen for 10 to 20 mm Hg after last sound and allow remaining air to escape quickly.	Beginning of fifth Korotkoff sound is indication of diastolic pressure in adults (NHBPEP, 2003). Fourth Korotkoff sound involves distinct muffling of sounds and is indication of diastolic pressure in children (NHBPEP, 2003).
(f) The Joint National Committee (NHBPEP, 2003) recommends the average of two sets of blood pressure measurements 2 minutes apart. Use second set of blood pressure measurements as patient's baseline.	Two sets of blood pressure measurements help to prevent false-positive readings based on patient's sympathetic response (alert reaction). Averaging minimizes effect of anxiety, which often causes first reading to be higher than subsequent measures (NHBPEP, 2003).
(g) Remove cuff from patient's arm unless you need to repeat measurement.	Continuous cuff inflation causes arterial occlusion, resulting in numbness and tingling of patient's arm.
(h) If this is first assessment of patient, repeat procedure on other arm.	Comparison of blood pressure in both arms detects circulatory problems. (Normal difference of 5 to 10 mm Hg exists between arms.)
(i) Help patient return to comfortable position and cover upper arm if previously clothed.	Restores comfort and provides sense of well-being.
(j) Discuss findings with patient as needed.	Promotes participation in care and understanding of health status. Makes patient accountable for follow-up assessment. Systolic blood pressure in leg is 10 to 40 mm Hg higher than arm but diastolic blood pressure is same.

STEP	RATIONALE
(k) Perform hand hygiene. Clean earpieces and diaphragm of stethoscope with alcohol swab as needed.	Reduces transmission of microorganisms. Controls transmission of microorganisms when nurses share stethoscope.
2 Assess systolic blood pressure by palpation:	
a Follow Steps 1a through 1d of auscultation method.	
b Locate and then continually palpate brachial, radial, or popliteal artery with fingertips of one hand. Inflate cuff to a pressure 30 mm Hg above point at which you can no longer palpate pulse.	Ensures accurate detection of true systolic pressure once pressure valve is released.

Clinical Decision Point *If unable to palpate artery because of weakened pulse, use a Doppler ultrasonic stethoscope (Fig. 5-11).*

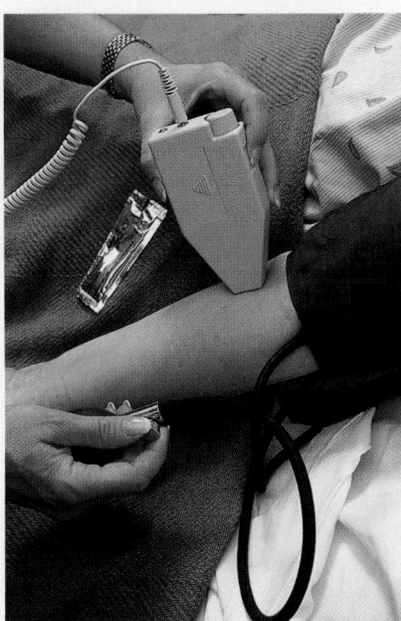

FIG 5-11   Doppler ultrasonic stethoscope over brachial artery to measure blood pressure.

c Slowly release valve and deflate cuff, allowing manometer needle to fall at rate of 2 mm Hg/second. Note point on manometer when pulse is again palpable.	Too-rapid or too-slow a decline results in inaccurate readings. Palpation helps identify systolic pressure only.
d Deflate cuff rapidly and completely. Remove cuff from patient's extremity unless you need to repeat measurement.	Continuous cuff inflation causes arterial occlusion, resulting in numbness and tingling of extremity.
e Help patient return to comfortable position and cover extremity if previously clothed.	Restores comfort and promotes sense of well-being.
f Discuss findings with patient as needed.	Promotes participation in care and understanding of health status.
g Perform hand hygiene.	Reduces transmission of microorganisms.

EVALUATION

1 If assessing blood pressure for the first time, establish baseline blood pressure if it is within acceptable range.	Used to compare future blood pressure measurements.
2 Compare blood pressure reading with patient's previous baseline and usual blood pressure for patient's age.	Allows nurse to assess for change in condition. Provides comparison with future blood pressure measurements.

Unexpected Outcomes	Related Interventions
1 Patient's blood pressure is above acceptable range.	• Repeat measurement in other extremity and compare findings. • Verify correct selection and placement of blood pressure cuff. • Have another nurse repeat measurement in 1 to 2 minutes. • Observe for related symptoms that are not apparent unless blood pressure is extremely high, including headache, facial flushing, nosebleed, and fatigue in older patient. • Report blood pressure to nurse in charge or health care provider to initiate appropriate evaluation and treatment. • Administer antihypertensive medications as ordered.
2 Patient's blood pressure is not sufficient for adequate perfusion and oxygenation of tissues.	• Compare blood pressure value to baseline. • Position patient in supine position to enhance circulation and restrict activity that decreases blood pressure further. • Repeat measurement with sphygmomanometer. Electronic blood pressure devices are less accurate in low-flow conditions. • Assess for signs and symptoms associated with hypotension, including tachycardia; weak, thready pulse; weakness; dizziness; confusion; and cool, pale, dusky, or cyanotic skin. • Assess for factors that contribute to a low blood pressure, including hemorrhage, dilation of blood vessels resulting from hyperthermia, anesthesia, or medication side effects. • Report blood pressure to nurse in charge or health care provider to initiate appropriate evaluation and treatment. • Increase rate of IV infusion or administer vasoconstriction drugs if ordered.
3 Unable to obtain blood pressure reading.	• Determine that no immediate crisis is present by obtaining pulse and respiratory rate. • Assess for signs and symptoms of decreased cardiac output; if present, notify nurse in charge or health care provider immediately. • Use alternative sites or procedures to obtain blood pressure; use Doppler ultrasonic instrument (see Chapter 6); palpate systolic blood pressure.
4 Patient experiences orthostatic hypotension.	• Maintain patient safety. • Return patient to safe position in bed or chair.

Recording and Reporting

• Record blood pressure and site assessed on vital sign flow sheet, nurses' notes, and EHR.
• Document measurement of blood pressure after administration of specific therapies in nurses' notes and EHR.
• Record any signs or symptoms of blood pressure alterations in nurses' notes and EHR.
• Report abnormal findings to nurse in charge or health care provider.

Special Considerations
Teaching

• Educate patient about risks for hypertension. Persons with family history of hypertension, premature heart disease, lipidemia, or renal disease are at significant risk. Obesity, cigarette smoking, heavy alcohol consumption, high blood cholesterol and triglyceride levels, and continued exposure to stress from psychosocial and environmental conditions are factors linked to hypertension (NHBPEP, 2003).
• Primary prevention of hypertension includes lifestyle modifications (e.g., lose weight, exercise daily, reduce sodium and saturated fat intake, and maintain adequate intake of dietary potassium and calcium). Cigarette smoking is a significant risk factor; thus encourage patients to avoid tobacco in any form (NHBPEP, 2003).
• Instruct primary caregiver to take blood pressure at same time each day and after patient has had a brief rest. Take blood pressure sitting or lying down; use same position and arm each time you take pressure.
• Instruct primary caregiver that, if the blood pressure is difficult to hear, it is probably caused by one of the following: cuff too loose, not large enough, or too narrow; stethoscope not over arterial pulse; cuff deflated too quickly or too slowly; or cuff not pumped high enough for systolic readings.

Pediatric

• Blood pressure measurement is not a routine part of assessment in children younger than 3 years.
• Blood pressure measurement can frighten children. Prepare child for squeezing feeling of inflated blood pressure cuff by comparing sensation to elastic band on finger or a tight hug on the arm.
• Obtain blood pressure in child before performing anxiety-producing tests or procedures.

- Korotkoff sounds are difficult to hear in children because of low frequency and amplitude. Using the bell of a pediatric stethoscope is often helpful.

Gerontologic
- Older adults, especially frail older adults, have lost upper-arm mass, requiring special attention to selection of blood pressure cuff size.
- Skin of older adults is more fragile and susceptible to cuff pressure when measurements are frequent. More frequent assessment of skin under cuff or rotation of measurement sites is recommended.
- Older adults have an increase in systolic pressure related to decreased vessel elasticity.
- Older adults often experience a fall in blood pressure after eating.

- Instruct older adults to change position slowly and wait after each change to avoid postural hypotension and prevent injuries.

Home Care
- Assess home noise level to determine the room that provides the quietest environment for assessing blood pressure.
- Instruct patient in the importance of an appropriate-size blood pressure cuff for home use.
- Assess family's financial ability to afford a sphygmomanometer for performing blood pressure evaluations on a regular basis. Recommend electronic devices or aneroid sphygmomanometers that have proven to be accurate according to standard testing and appropriate-size cuffs. Finger blood pressure monitors are inaccurate (NHBPEP, 2003).

PROCEDURAL GUIDELINE 5-2 Assessing Blood Pressure Electronically

NSO *Vital Signs Module / Lesson 5*

Many different styles of electronic blood pressure machines are available to determine blood pressure automatically (Fig. 5-12). Electronic machines rely on an electronic sensor to detect the vibrations caused by the rush of blood through an artery. Although electronic blood pressure machines are fast, you must consider their advantages and limitations. The devices are used when frequent assessment is required such as in critically ill or potentially unstable patients, during or after invasive procedures, or when therapies require frequent monitoring. Verify an assessment of an abnormal blood pressure by an electronic machine with a sphygmomanometer and stethoscope.

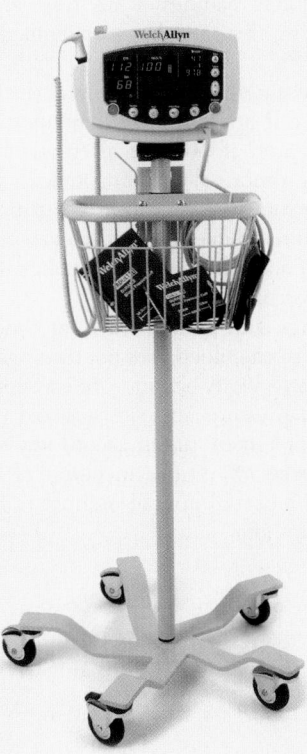

FIG 5-12 Noninvasive electronic blood pressure machine. (*Photo courtesy Welch Allyn.*)

Delegation and Collaboration

The skill of blood pressure measurement using an electronic blood pressure machine can be delegated to nursing assistive personnel (NAP) unless the patient is considered unstable (i.e., hypotensive). The nurse instructs the NAP by:
- Communicating the frequency and extremity for measurement.
- Reviewing how to select appropriate-size blood pressure cuff for designated extremity and appropriate cuff for the machine.
- Reviewing patient's usual blood pressure and report significant changes or abnormalities to the nurse.

Equipment
- ❏ Electronic blood pressure machine
- ❏ Source of electricity
- ❏ Blood pressure cuff of appropriate size as recommended by manufacturer
- ❏ Pen and vital sign flow sheet or electronic health record (EHR).

Procedural Steps

1 Determine appropriateness of using electronic blood pressure measurement. Patients with irregular heart rate, peripheral vascular disease, seizures, tremors, and shivering are not candidates for this device.

2 Determine best site for cuff placement.

3 Collect and bring appropriate equipment to patient's bedside.

4 Perform hand hygiene. Assist patient to comfortable position, either lying or sitting. Plug in and place device near patient, ensuring that connector hose between cuff and machine reaches.

5 Locate on/off switch and turn on machine to enable device to self-test computer systems.

6 Select appropriate cuff size for patient extremity (Table 5-4) and appropriate cuff for machine. Electronic blood pressure cuff and machine must be matched by manufacturer and are not interchangeable.

7 Expose extremity by removing constricting clothing to ensure proper cuff application. Do not place blood pressure cuff over clothing.

8 Prepare blood pressure cuff by manually squeezing all the air out of the cuff and connecting it to connector hose.

Continued

PROCEDURAL GUIDELINE 5-2   Assessing Blood Pressure Electronically—cont'd

TABLE 5-4	Proper Blood Pressure Cuff Size for Electronic Monitor*	
Cuff Size	**Limb Circumference (cm)**	
Small adult	17-25	
Adult	23-33	
Large adult	31-40	
Thigh	38-50	

*A 12- to 24-foot cord is required for adult blood pressure monitoring.

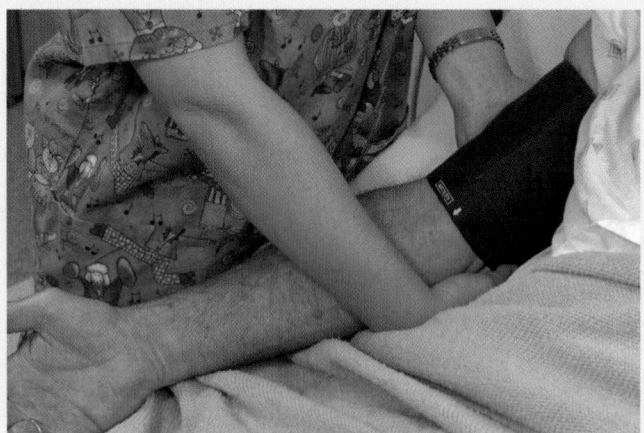

STEP 9   Aligning blood pressure cuff arrow with brachial artery.

9 Wrap flattened cuff snugly around extremity, verifying that only one finger can fit between cuff and patient's skin. Make sure that "artery" arrow marked on outside of cuff is placed correctly (see illustration).

10 Verify that connector hose between cuff and machine is not kinked. Kinking prevents proper inflation and deflation of cuff.

11 Following manufacturer directions, set frequency control for automatic or manual and press the start button. The first blood pressure measurement pumps cuff to a peak pressure of about 180 mm Hg. After this pressure is reached, the machine begins a deflation sequence that determines the blood pressure. The first reading determines peak pressure inflation for additional measurements.

12 When deflation is complete, digital display provides most recent values and flash time in minutes that has elapsed since the measurement occurred (see illustration).

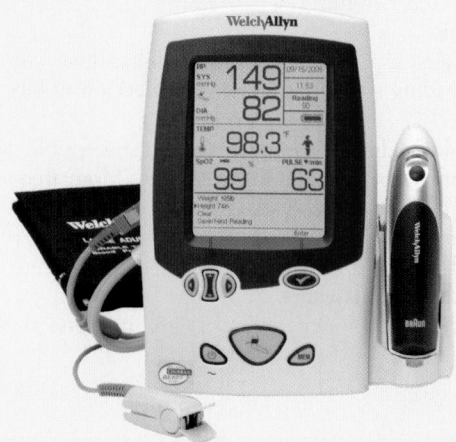

STEP 12   Digital electronic blood pressure display. (*Image courtesy Welch Allyn.*)

Clinical Decision Point *If unable to obtain blood pressure with electronic device, verify machine connections (e.g., plugged into working electrical outlet, hose-cuff connections tight, machine on, correct cuff). Repeat electronic blood pressure; if unable to obtain, use auscultatory technique (see Skill 5-5).*

13 Set frequency of measurements and upper and lower alarm limits for systolic, diastolic, and mean blood pressure readings. Intervals between measurements can be set from 1 to 90 minutes. The nurse determines frequency and alarm limits based on patient's acceptable range of blood pressure, nursing judgment, and health care provider order.

14 Obtain additional readings at any time by pressing the start button. Pressing the cancel button immediately deflates the cuff.

15 If frequent measurements are required, the cuff may be left in place. Remove it at least every 2 hours to assess underlying skin integrity and if possible alternate measurement sites. Patients with abnormal bleeding tendencies are at risk for microvascular rupture from repeated inflations. When patient no longer requires frequent blood pressure monitoring, remove and clean cuff according to agency policy to reduce transmission of microorganisms.

16 Discuss findings with patient. Perform hand hygiene.

17 Compare electronic blood pressure readings with auscultatory measurements to verify accuracy of electronic device.

18 Record blood pressure and site assessed on vital sign flow sheet, EHR, or nurses' notes; record any signs or symptoms of blood pressure alterations in narrative form in EHR and nurses' notes; report abnormal findings to nurse in charge or health care provider.

PROCEDURAL GUIDELINE 5-3 Measuring Oxygen Saturation (Pulse Oximetry)

NSO *Airway Management Module / Lesson 2*

 Video Clip

Pulse oximetry is the noninvasive measurement of arterial blood oxygen saturation, the percent to which hemoglobin is filled with oxygen. A pulse oximeter is a probe with a light-emitting diode (LED) connected by cable to an oximeter. The LED emits light wavelengths that are absorbed differently by the oxygenated and deoxygenated hemoglobin molecules. The more hemoglobin saturated by oxygen, the higher the oxygen saturation. Normally SpO_2 is greater than 95%.

The measurement of oxygen saturation is simple, painless, and has few of the risks associated with more invasive measurements of oxygen saturation such as arterial blood gas sampling. A vascular, pulsatile area is needed to detect the change in the transmitted light when making measurements with a digit or earlobe probe. Conditions that decrease arterial blood flow such as peripheral vascular disease, hypothermia, pharmacologic vasoconstrictors, hypotension, or peripheral edema affect accurate determination of oxygen saturation in these areas. For patients with decreased peripheral perfusion, you can apply a forehead sensor. Factors that affect light transmission such as outside light sources or patient motion also affect the measurement of oxygen saturation. Carbon monoxide in the blood, jaundice, and intravascular dyes can influence the light reflected from hemoglobin molecules.

In adults you can apply reusable and disposable oximeter probes to the earlobe, finger, toe, bridge of the nose, or forehead (Box 5-8). Pulse oximetry is indicated in patients who have an unstable oxygen status or are at risk for impaired gas exchange.

Delegation and Collaboration

The skill of oxygen saturation measurement can be delegated to nursing assistive personnel (NAP). The nurse instructs the NAP by:

- Communicating specific factors related to the patient that can falsely lower oxygen saturation.
- Informing NAP about appropriate sensor site and probe.
- Notifying frequency of oxygen saturation measurements for specific patient.
- Instructing to notify nurse immediately of any reading lower than SpO_2 of 95% or value for specific patient.
- Instructing to refrain from using pulse oximetry to obtain heart rate because oximeter will not detect an irregular pulse.

Equipment

☐ Oximeter
☐ Oximeter probe appropriate for patient and recommended by oximeter manufacturer
☐ Acetone or nail polish remover if needed
☐ Pen and vital sign flow sheet or electronic health record (EHR)

Procedural Steps

1 Determine need to measure patient's oxygen saturation. Assess risk factors for decreased oxygen saturation (e.g., acute or chronic compromised respiratory problems, change in oxygen therapy, chest wall injury, recovery from anesthesia).

| BOX 5-8 | Characteristics of Pulse Oximeter Sensor Probes and Sites |

Digit Probe
- Easy to apply, conforms to various sizes

Earlobe Probe
- Clip-on smaller and lighter, although more positional than digit probe
- Yields strong correlation with oxygen saturation
- Greater accuracy at lower saturations suggested in research
- Good when uncontrollable or rhythmic movements (e.g., hand tremors during exercise) are present
- Vascular bed least affected by decreased blood flow

Forehead Sensor
- Greater accuracy during decreased perfusion suggested in research
- Reliable for patients on vasoactive medications
- Detects desaturation quicker than other sites
- Does not require a pulsatile vascular bed
- Good when uncontrollable or rhythmic movements (e.g., hand tremors) are present
- Requires headband to secure sensor

Disposable Sensor Pad
- Can be applied to a variety of sites: earlobe of adult, nose bridge, palm or sole of infant
- Less restrictive for continuous oxygen saturation monitoring
- Expensive
- Contains latex
- Possible that skin under adhesive becomes moist and harbors pathogens
- Available in variety of sizes; pad can be matched to infant weight

---

2 Assess for signs and symptoms of alterations in oxygen saturation (e.g., altered respiratory rate, depth, or rhythm; adventitious breath sounds [see Chapter 6]; cyanotic nails, lips, mucous membranes, or skin; restlessness; difficulty breathing).

3 Assess for factors that influence measurement of SpO_2 (e.g., oxygen therapy; respiratory therapy such as postural drainage and percussion; hemoglobin level; hypotension; temperature; nail polish [Cicek et al., 2010], and medications such as bronchodilators).

4 Review patient's medical record for health care provider's order or consult agency procedure manual for standard of care for measurement of SpO_2.

5 Determine previous baseline SpO_2 (if available) from patient's record.

6 Determine most appropriate patient-specific site (e.g., finger, earlobe, bridge of nose, forehead) for sensor probe placement by measuring capillary refill (see Chapter 6). If capillary refill is less than 2 seconds, select alternative site.

   a Site must have adequate local circulation and be free of moisture.

Continued

PROCEDURAL GUIDELINE 5-3 Measuring Oxygen Saturation (Pulse Oximetry)—cont'd

b A finger free of polish or acrylic nail is preferred (Cicek et al., 2011).

c If patient has tremors or is likely to move, use earlobe or forehead.

d If the patient finger is too large for the clip on probe, as may be the case with obesity or edema, the clip-on probe may not fit properly (Mininni, 2009); obtain a disposable (tape-on) probe.

7 Bring equipment to the bedside and perform hand hygiene.

8 Position patient comfortably. Instruct him or her to breathe normally.

9 Attach sensor to monitoring site (see illustration). If using finger, remove fingernail polish from digit with acetone or polish remover. Instruct patient that clip-on probe will feel like a clothespin on the finger but will not hurt.

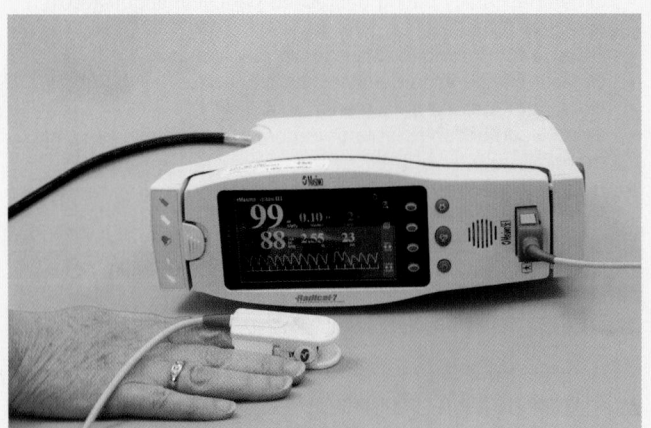

STEP 9 Oximeter sensor attached to finger.

Clinical Decision Point *Do not attach probe to finger, ear, or bridge of nose if area is edematous or skin integrity is compromised. Do not use earlobe and bridge of nose sensors for infants and toddlers because of skin fragility. Do not attach sensor to fingers that are hypothermic. Select ear or bridge of nose if adult patient has a history of peripheral vascular disease. Do not use disposable adhesive sensors if patient has a latex allergy. Do not place sensor on same extremity as electronic blood pressure cuff because blood flow to finger will be temporarily interrupted when cuff inflates and cause inaccurate reading that can trigger alarms (Skirton et al., 2011).*

10 Once sensor is in place, turn on oximeter by activating power. Observe pulse waveform/intensity display and audible beep. Correlate oximeter pulse rate with patient's radial pulse.

11 Leave sensor in place 10 to 30 seconds or until oximeter readout reaches constant value and pulse display reaches full strength during each cardiac cycle. Inform patient that oximeter alarm will sound if sensor falls off or patient moves it. Read SpO$_2$ on digital display.

12 If you plan to monitor oxygen saturation continuously, verify SpO$_2$ alarm limits preset by manufacturer at a low of 85% and a high of 100%. Determine limits for SpO$_2$ and pulse rate as indicated by patient's condition. Verify that alarms are on. Assess skin integrity under sensor probe every 2 hours; relocate sensor at least every 4 hours and more frequently if skin integrity is altered or tissue perfusion compromised.

13 If you plan intermittent or spot-checking of SpO$_2$, remove probe and turn oximeter power off. Cleanse sensor and store sensor in appropriate location.

14 Discuss findings with patient. Perform hand hygiene.

15 Compare SpO$_2$ with patient's previous baseline and acceptable SpO$_2$.

16 Record SpO$_2$ on vital sign flow sheet, EHR, or nurses' notes; indicate type and amount of oxygen therapy used by patient during assessment; record any signs or symptoms of alterations in oxygen saturation in narrative form in nurses' notes and EHR; report abnormal findings to nurse in charge or health care provider.

❓ Critical Thinking Exercises

You are assigned to Mr. Augsten, a 56-year-old university professor. He is admitted from the trauma unit following a motorcycle-automobile accident. Mr. Augsten has a fractured left humerus and pelvis. Although he was wearing a helmet, he suffered a concussion. When doing your admissions assessment you note a cast on his left arm and an intravenous (IV) line in his right antecubital fossa. He received IV narcotics in the emergency department and is very sleepy. He awakens only to touch.

1 Which admission vital signs can you assign to the nursing assistive personnel (NAP)? Which directions do you provide the NAP regarding obtaining routine vital signs for this patient?

2 The NAP reports that the blood pressure for Mr. Augsten is 94/60 mm Hg. You note that the emergency department nurse recorded a blood pressure of 140/86 mm Hg. Which interventions should you consider at this time? What might explain the differences in blood pressure values?

3 The nurse directed the NAP to report a respiratory rate of 16 or less. The NAP documents a respiratory rate of 12 in the vital sign flow sheet but does not report the rate to you until you inquire. She states

that Mr. Augsten was speaking with her so it was not important to bother the nurse. What is your response to the NAP? Explain the significance of the respiratory rate.

4 You direct the NAP to repeat Mr. Augsten's blood pressure and respiratory rate in 30 minutes. In a half hour the NAP reports a blood pressure in the right arm of 160/100 and a respiratory rate of 20. She also notes that Mr. Augsten was sleeping quietly. What is your response?

✔ REVIEW QUESTIONS

1 The nurse is assessing the axillary temperature of a confused patient with a fever. Which actions by the nurse will best help provide an accurate measurement? (Select all that apply.)

1 Drying the axilla before placing the thermometer probe

2 Holding the thermometer probe in place

3 Placing the patient in a supine position

4 Checking that the patient has not had anything to eat or drink recently

2 After checking the tympanic temperature two consecutive times in an 82-year-old patient, the nurse finds the reading to be several degrees lower than expected. What is the most appropriate nursing action at this time?
1 Obtain a different thermometer
2 Observe for the presence of cerumen
3 Document the temperature assessed
4 Record the average between the two readings

3 A patient with abdominal ascites is having his respiratory rate assessed. Which is the best action to obtain the respiratory assessment for this patient?
1 The patient is assessed while flat, supine, and quiet.
2 The patient's head is elevated based on his desire.
3 The nurse tells the patient when to begin breathing for the assessment.
4 The nurse holds the patient's wrist while counting respirations.

4 The nurse is preparing to assess a patient's blood pressure. Which statement by the nurse will help promote an accurate reading?
1 "Just relax while I put the cuff on your arm."
2 "This is painless and will take just a minute."
3 "The cuff can go over your thin silk sleeve."
4 "Please uncross your legs while I do this."

5 Place in correct order the following sequencing steps for two-step blood pressure measurement using the brachial artery.
a Relocate brachial artery and inflate blood pressure cuff.
b Palpate brachial artery.
c Obtain proper sized cuff.
d Apply deflated cuff above brachial artery.
e Apply bell of stethoscope over artery.
f Release pressure in cuff.
g Record first and last sounds.
1 c, d, b, e, a, f, g,
2 c, b, a, d, e, g, f,
3 c, b, d, a, e, f, g,
4 b, c, d, a, e, g, f

6 Electronic blood pressure monitoring cannot be used on certain patients. Which of these patients can have an electronic blood pressure monitor?
1 The patient with constant extremity tremors
2 The patient with diabetes mellitus
3 The feverish patient who is shivering
4 The patient with an irregular heart rate

7 Mr. Marquis is 87 years old and is admitted to your medical unit for pneumonia of 4 days' duration. His temperature is 37.2° C (99° F). The NAP questions why his temperature is so low for a person with an active infection. Your best response is:
1 His body has compensated for the infection by increasing heart rate.
2 He probably had an antipyretic in the assisted-living facility where he lived.
3 He took a cool shower before he was admitted.
4 The baseline temperature of older adults is lower because of loss of subcutaneous fat.

8 You are checking the vital signs of a 75-year-old patient. The radial pulse is irregular, and about every fourth beat is different. The patient offers no complaints. What is your next action?
1 Report the findings to the health care provider immediately.
2 Obtain a blood pressure.
3 Obtain an apical heart rate.
4 Notify the nurse in charge.

9 Which of the following nursing interventions is/are correct when determining a pulse deficit? (Select all that apply.)
1 Counting for 30 seconds and multiplying by 2
2 Starting to count after the peripheral first beat is heard
3 Using a peripheral artery and apical pulse
4 Counting simultaneously with another health care provider

10 Which of the following blood pressures would classify as prehypertension? (Select all that apply.)
1 118/78
2 126/82
3 130/80
4 132/94

REFERENCES

Cicek HS, et al: Effect of nail polish and henna on oxygen saturation determined by pulse oximetry in healthy young adult females, *Emerg Med J* 28(9):783, 2011.

Davie A, Amoore J: Best practices in the measurement of body temperature, *Nurs Stand* 24(42):42, 2010.

Ebersole P, et al: *Toward healthy aging: human needs and nursing response*, ed 7, St Louis, 2008, Mosby.

Giger JN: *Transcultural nursing: assessment and intervention*, ed 6, St Louis, 2013, Mosby.

Heinemann M, et al: Automated versus manual blood pressure measurement: a randomized crossover trial, *Int J Nurs Pract* 14:296, 2008.

Hockenberry MJ, Wilson D: *Wong's nursing care of infants and children*, ed 9, St Louis, 2011, Mosby.

Lim CH, et al: Human thermoregulation and measurement of body temperature in exercise and clinical settings, *Ann Acad Med Singapore* 37:347, 2008.

Lu S, et al: The effects of measurement site and ambient temperature on body temperature values in healthy older adults: a cross-sectional comparative study, *Int J Nurs Stud* 46(11):1415, 2009.

Mininni NC, et al: Pulse oximetry: an essential tool for the busy med-surg nurse, *Am Nurs Today* 4(9):31, 2009.

National High Blood Pressure Education Program (NHBPEP); National Heart, Lung, and Blood Institute; National Institutes of Health: The seventh report of the Joint National Committee on Detection, Evaluation, and Treatment of High Blood Pressure (JNC 7), *JAMA* 289(19):2560, 2003.

Nelson D, et al: Accuracy of automated blood pressure monitors, *J Dent Hyg* 82(4):1, 2008.

Skirton H, et al: A systematic review of variability and reliability of manual and automated blood pressure readings, *J Clin Nurs* 20:614, 2011.

Thompson HJ, Kagan SH: Clinical management of fever by nurses: doing what works, *J Adv Nurs* 67 (2):359, 2010.

Valdez-Lowe C, et al: Pulse oximetry in adults, *Am J Nurs* 109(6):52, 2009.

Health Assessment

MEDIA RESOURCES

- **evolve** learning system http://evolve.elsevier.com/Perry/skills
  - Review Questions
  - ▶ Video Clips
  - Audio Glossary

- Mosby's Nursing Video Skills, 4th edition

KEY TERMS

Atrophy	Costovertebral angle (CVA) tenderness	Erythema	Orthostatic hypotension
Auscultation		Friction rub	Pallor
Bruit	Crackles	Inspection	Palpation
Cardiomegaly	Cyanosis	Intercostal space	Percussion
Cerumen	Dorsum	Nares	
Conjunctiva	Edema	Olfaction	

OBJECTIVES

Mastery of content in this chapter will enable the nurse to:
- Discuss the purposes of physical assessment.
- Describe the techniques used with each assessment skill.
- Describe proper positioning for a patient during each phase of the examination.
- Describe how to conduct a physical examination on patients from diverse cultures.
- List techniques to promote a patient's physical and psychological comfort during an examination.
- Make environmental preparations before an assessment.
- Identify data to collect from the nursing history before an examination.

- Discuss normal physical findings for patients across the life span.
- Discuss ways to incorporate health promotion and health teaching into an assessment.
- Identify self-screening assessments commonly performed by patients.
- Use physical assessment techniques and skills during routine nursing care.
- Document assessment findings on appropriate forms.
- Communicate abnormal findings to appropriate personnel.

Nurses perform systematic physical assessments on a regular basis in nearly every health care setting. In acute care settings you will perform more comprehensive assessments when patients are admitted to agencies and brief physical assessments at the beginning of each shift to identify changes in a patient's status for comparison with the previous assessment. A routine physical assessment takes 10 to 15 minutes and reveals information that supplements a patient's database. In nursing homes and home care settings, you will complete similar assessments weekly, monthly, or more frequently when a patient's health status changes. Ongoing, objective, and comprehensive assessments promote continuity in health care.

Nurses are often the first to detect changes in patients' conditions. For this reason the ability to think critically and interpret patient behaviors and physiologic changes are essential. The skills of physical assessment are powerful tools for detecting both subtle and obvious changes in a patient's health.

EVIDENCE-BASED PRACTICE

The American Cancer Society estimates that 68,130 cases of melanoma were diagnosed in 2010. The highly malignant cancer occurs slightly more often in men than women (ACS, 2011a). There are several risk factors for melanoma, including fair skin that freckles or burns easily, red or blond hair, blue or green eyes, long term treatment with ultraviolet light, and a first-degree relative having melanoma.

The ACS (2011a) recommends that people engage in regular skin self-examination (SSE). Women who have positive body image and older women are more likely to perform skin SSE (Chait et al., 2009). According to the U.S. Preventive Services Task Force, evidence showing that there is a benefit to whole body screening as a way to effectively reduce morbidity and mortality from melanoma is lacking (Wolff, 2009). The National Guideline Clearinghouse suggests that full-body screening may benefit people who have a high risk (Marret et al., 2007). Further study is needed to know whether the accuracy and cost of skin cancer screening warrant recommending it for the general public.

- Instruct patients to conduct a complete monthly SSE, noting moles, blemishes, and birthmarks. Instruct to inspect all skin surfaces.
- Perform the examination after a bath or shower, including a head to toe check.
- Use a well-lit room and mirrors for the exam. Have a partner help, increasing the chance that the self-examination is thorough.
- Instruct patient to report to their health care provider any change in size or color of moles, or skin lesions or a sore that does not heal, start to bleed, ooze, or feel different (swollen, hard, lumpy, itchy, or tender to the touch).
- Use supportive communication (Glantz et al., 2010, Mujumdar et al., 2009) to inform patients of ways to prevent skin cancer by avoiding overexposure to the sun.
- Use sunscreen and lip balms (needed most between the hours of 10 AM and 4 PM).
- Use sun protection of 30 SPF or higher and use on hazy days. Use at least one ounce to cover the average adult. Reapply every 2 hours.
- Wear a hat with a 2- to 3-inch brim. Avoid straw hats that do not offer much protection.
- Wear a shirt. Dark fabric protects more effectively than light fabric, and tightly woven fabric is preferred.
- Dry clothes protect more than wet clothes.
- Use wraparound sunglasses. These should have labels that indicate at least 99% UV protection.
- Do not use tanning beds and sunlamps.
- Seek shade, especially in the middle of the day. Test the strength of the sun. If your shadow is shorter than you, the rays of the sun are the strongest.

PATIENT-CENTERED CARE

An admission assessment involves a detailed review of a patient's condition and includes a nursing history and behavioral and physical examination. The health history comprises an interview with patients to gather subjective data about their current state of health and any presenting conditions. Conduct a patient-centered

TABLE 6-1	Development of Individualized Nursing Diagnoses		
Assessment Method	Findings	Patterns	Nursing Diagnosis
Inspection of skin	Skin along sacral area is intact. There is a 3-cm area of redness around coccyx; skin blanches on palpation. No skin lesions are observed.	There is pressure area around coccyx.	Risk for impaired skin integrity
Palpation of skin	Skin is moist from diaphoresis. There is tenderness to palpation at sacral area. Skin turgor is elastic.	Skin moisture promotes maceration.	
Historical data	Patient suffered fractured left leg. Patient is immobilized because of left leg traction.	Continued pressure is exerted over sacrum.	

interview to learn about problems from the patient's perspective. Have patients explain their symptoms by allowing them to offer details. Use open-ended questions and be sure the patients have exhausted their descriptions. For example, as a patient is describing a symptom, you can say "go on" to encourage more information sharing.

A physical assessment includes a head-to-toe review of each body system, which offers objective information about a patient. A patient's condition and response affect the extent of an examination. After gathering data, you group significant findings into patterns of data (clusters) that reveal actual or potential nursing diagnoses (Table 6-1). Each abnormal finding directs you to gather additional data. Initial assessment and examination provide a baseline for a patient's functional status and serve as a comparison for future assessment findings. In addition, the information is useful in selecting the best nursing measures to manage a patient's health problems.

The physical assessment is an ideal time to offer individualized patient teaching and to encourage promotion of health practices such as breast (Box 6-1) and genital (Box 6-2) self-examination. A patient should understand any symptoms he or she presents with as well as symptoms to look for in detecting problems. For example, educate patients about the American Cancer Society (ACS) (2012a and 2012b) guidelines for early detection of breast and genital cancers. Integrate health promotion and education into physical assessment activities. There are "teachable moments" when you can share findings and educate patients about health promotion.

Respect patients' cultural diversity and beliefs when completing a physical assessment. It is important to remember that cultural differences influence a patient's behavior. Consider the patient's health beliefs, use of alternative therapies, nutritional habits, relationships with family, and comfort with your physical closeness during the history and examination. Be culturally aware and avoid stereotyping on the basis of culture, race, sexual preference, or age. There is a difference between cultural and physical characteristics.

BOX 6-1 | Breast Self-Examination

According to the American Cancer Society (ACS) (2012), screening refers to tests and exams used to find a disease, like cancer, in people who do not have any symptoms. Breast self-examination (BSE) is optional for women starting in their 20s (ACS, 2012). Women should be told about the benefits and limitations of BSE and report any breast changes to their health professional right away.

Research has shown that BSE plays a small role in finding breast cancer compared with finding a breast lump by chance or simply being aware of what is normal for each woman. Some women feel very comfortable doing BSE regularly (usually monthly after their period), which involves a systematic step-by-step approach to examining the look and feel of their breasts. Other women are more comfortable simply looking and feeling their breasts in a less systematic approach, such as while showering or getting dressed or doing an occasional thorough exam (ACS, 2012).

A regular breast self-examination (BSE) should be done monthly so a woman becomes familiar with the usual appearance and feel of her breast. Familiarity makes it easier to notice any changes in the breast from 1 month to another. Early discovery of a change from what is "normal" is the main idea behind BSE.

For women who menstruate, the best time to do BSE is 2 or 3 days after a period ends, when the breasts are least likely to be tender or swollen. For women who no longer menstruate, pick a day such as the first day of the month to remind yourself to do BSE.

Procedure

1 Stand before a mirror. Inspect both breasts for anything unusual such as skin redness; any discharge from the nipples; puckering, dimpling, or scaling of the skin.

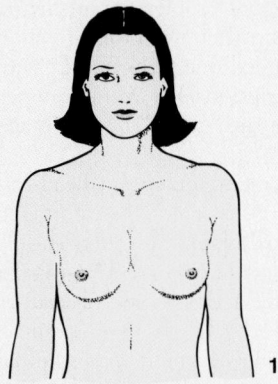

2 Watching closely in the mirror, clasp hands behind your head and bring elbows forward. Note how chest muscles tighten.

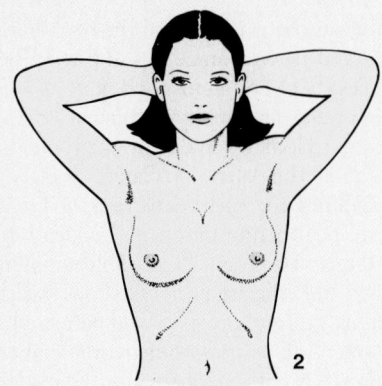

3 Next press hands firmly on hips and bow slightly toward the mirror as you pull your shoulders and elbows forward.

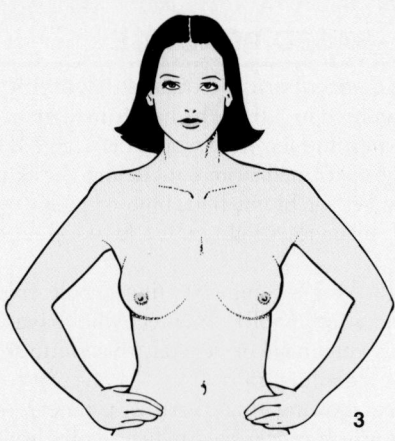

The next part of the examination may be done in the shower. Gliding fingers over soapy skin makes it easier to appreciate the texture underneath.

4 Raise your left arm. Use three or four fingers of your right hand to explore your left breast firmly, carefully, and thoroughly. Beginning at the outer edge, press the flat part of your fingers in small circles, moving the circles slowly around the breast. Gradually work toward the nipple. Be sure to cover the entire breast. Pay special attention to the area between the breast and the armpit itself. Feel for any unusual lump or mass under the skin.

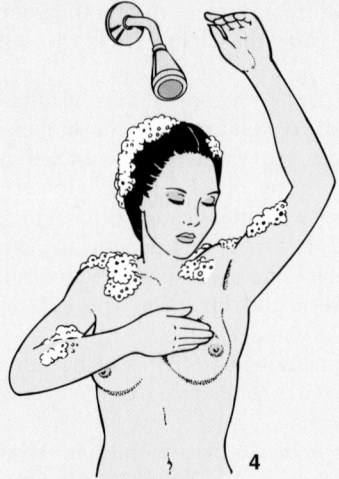

5 Gently squeeze the nipple and look for discharge. Repeat the examination on your right breast.

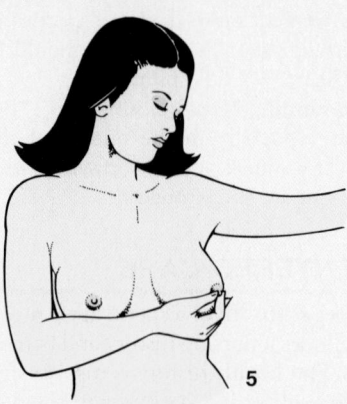

BOX 6-1	Breast Self-Examination—cont'd

6   Lie flat on your back, left arm over your head, and a pillow or folded towel under your left shoulder. This position flattens the breast and makes it easier to examine. Use the same circular motion described earlier. Repeat on your right breast.

Call your health care provider if you find a lump or other abnormality.

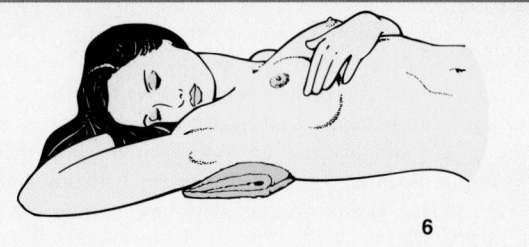

6

From American Cancer Society: Learn about cancer, American Cancer Society recommendations for early breast cancer detection, http://www.cancer.org/Cancer/BreastCancer/DetailedGuide/breast-cancer-detection, accessed May 19, 2012; Seidel HM et al: *Mosby's guide to physical examination*, ed 7, St Louis, 2011, Mosby.
BSE, Breast self-examination.

BOX 6-2	Genital Self-Examination

All men 15 years and older should perform this examination monthly. Perform the examination during or after a warm bath or shower when the scrotal sac is relaxed. Call your health care provider if you find a lump or any other abnormality.

Penile Examination
1   Stand naked in front of a mirror and hold the penis in your hand and examine the head. Pull back the foreskin if uncircumcised.
2   Inspect and palpate the entire head of the penis in a clockwise motion, looking carefully for any bumps, sores, or blisters.
3   Look for any bumpy warts.
4   Look at the opening at the end of the penis for discharge.
5   Look along the entire shaft of the penis for the same signs.
6   Separate pubic hair at the base of the penis and carefully examine the skin underneath.

Testicular Examination
1   Look for swelling or lumps in the skin of the scrotum while looking in the mirror.
2   Use both hands, placing the index and middle fingers under the testicles and the thumb on top.
3   Gently roll the testicle, feeling for hard lumps; smooth, rounded bumps; or thickening.
4   Find the epididymis (feels like a small "bump" on the upper or middle outer side of the testis).
5   Feel for small, pea-size lumps on the front and side of the testicle. The lumps are usually painless and are abnormal.

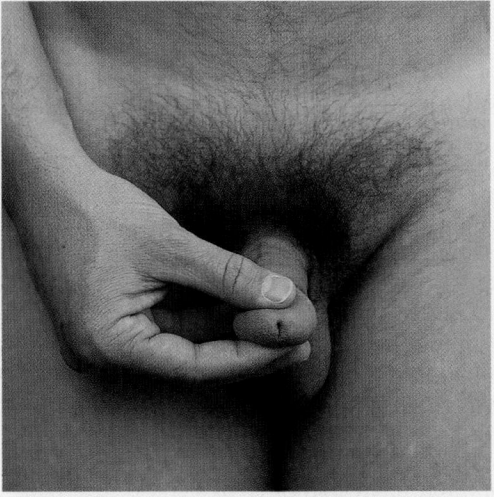

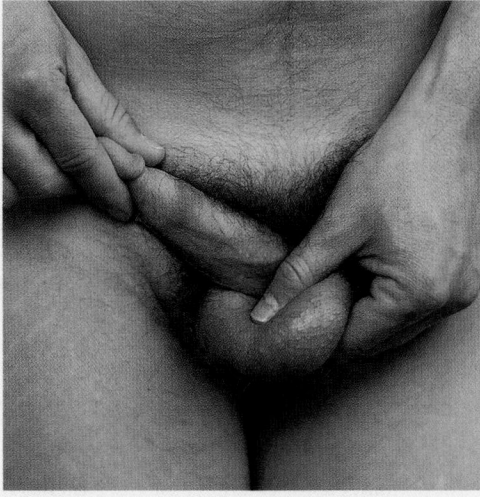

From Seidel HM et al: *Mosby's guide to physical examination*, ed 7, St Louis, 2011, Mosby.

Your recognition of cultural diversity helps to respect a patient's uniqueness and provide a higher-quality care. Improved patient outcomes can result from recognition and respect for cultural diversity (Cherry and Stuart, 2011).
  • Learn to use open-ended questions to identify sociocultural and religious values that influence health/illness beliefs and practices.

  • Communicate respect through proper use of distance, attention, eye contact, tone, and loudness of voice.
  • Use a professional interpreter familiar with a patient's culture and language.
  • Allow time for responses.
  • Observe verbal and nonverbal language and communication patterns of patients.

- Work with the established family hierarchy as identified by a patient.
- Learn words that are offensive to the culture. For example, some Southeast Asian groups do not use words such as vagina, penis, and breasts because they find them offensive.
- Obtain information about health risks common to a cultural group. Certain diseases are prevalent in some groups. For example, malaria is prevalent among Africans and Asians, and parasitic worms are prevalent among migrants from the Third World.
- Integrate knowledge of cultural differences in growth and development, physical characteristics, and norms in interpreting assessment data.
- Biologic/racial characteristics influence physical traits such as skin and mucosal color, hair texture/color, and height and weight.
- Develop awareness of healing modalities such as cupping, coining, and pinching used by some cultures, especially Asians, which may leave the skin discolored or scratched.
- It is not unusual for patients from ethnocultural groups to ask for a family member to be present during an examination to interpret for them or provide moral support.
- Use gender-congruent health care providers to perform a physical assessment.
- Ask permission before you touch a patient.
- Drape a patient thoroughly and use the bedside screen or curtains.

Safety Guidelines

1 Prioritize an assessment based on a patient's presenting signs and symptoms or health care needs. For example, when a patient develops sudden shortness of breath, first assess the lungs and thorax. If a patient is acutely ill, you may choose to assess only the involved body systems. Use judgment to ensure that an examination is relevant and inclusive.

2 Organize an examination. Compare both sides of the body for symmetry. If a patient becomes fatigued, offer rest periods. Perform painful or intrusive procedures near the end of an examination.

3 Use a head-to-toe approach following the sequence of inspection, palpation, percussion, and auscultation (except during abdominal assessment). This sequence facilitates an effective assessment.

4 Encourage a patient's active participation. Patients usually know about their physical condition. Often a patient can let you know when certain findings are normal or when there have been changes.

5 Always identify a patient using at least two identifiers other than the room number. For example, use the patient's name and date of birth, comparing them with the identification band or medical record (The Joint Commission [TJC], 2012). In long-term care settings, identification bands are not used; however, pictures are available for identification. CAUTION: Patients with sensory impairments or altered level of consciousness (LOC) may answer to a name other than their own.

6 Follow standard precautions for infection control. During an assessment you may have contact with body fluids and discharge. Always wear clean gloves when there are breaks in the skin, lesions, or wounds or when having contact with mucous membranes. In some circumstances you will need to wear a gown.

7 Consider the possibility of latex allergy. The incidence of serious allergic reaction to latex has increased dramatically (Seidel et al., 2011).

8 Record quick notes to facilitate accurate documentation. Inform a patient that you will be recording the data.

9 Record a summary of the assessment using appropriate medical terminology and in the sequence that findings are gathered. Use commonly accepted medical abbreviations to keep notes concise. Be thorough and descriptive, especially for abnormal findings.

ASSESSMENT TECHNIQUES

Use assessment techniques during each patient contact, including activities such as bathing, administering medications, other therapies, or while talking with a patient. This practice will help you learn to become more observant and better able to identify changes quickly.

Inspection, palpation, percussion, auscultation, and olfaction are the five basic assessment techniques. Each skill allows you to collect a broad range of physical data about patients. Nurses need experience to recognize normal variations among patients and ranges of normal for an individual. Remember, cultural diversity is one factor that influences both normal variations and potential alterations that you may find during an assessment. It is important to take the time needed to carefully assess each body part. Hurrying causes you to overlook significant signs and make incorrect conclusions about a patient's condition.

Inspection is the visual examination of body parts or areas. An experienced nurse learns to make multiple observations almost simultaneously while becoming very perceptive of any abnormalities. The secret is to always pay attention to patients. Watch all movements and look carefully at the body part that you are inspecting. It is important to recognize normal physical characteristics of patients of all ages before trying to distinguish abnormal findings.

Inspection requires good lighting and full exposure of body parts. Inspect each area for size, shape, color, symmetry, position, and the presence of abnormalities. If possible inspect each area compared with the same area on the opposite side of the body. When necessary, use additional light such as a penlight to inspect body cavities such as the mouth and throat. *Do not hurry. Pay attention to detail.* Verify and clarify all abnormalities with subjective patient data. In other words, ask the patient for further information about each abnormality or change such as whether the change is recent.

Palpation uses the sense of touch. Through palpation the hands make delicate and sensitive measurements of specific physical signs. Palpation detects resistance, resilience, roughness, texture, temperature, and mobility. You often use palpation with or after visual inspection. You often use different parts of the hand to detect specific characteristics. For example, the dorsum (back) of the hand is sensitive to temperature variations. The pads of the fingertips detect subtle changes in texture, shape, size, consistency, and pulsation of body parts. The palm of the hand is especially sensitive to vibration. You measure position, consistency, and turgor by lightly grasping a body part with the fingertips.

Help a patient relax and assume a comfortable position because muscle tension during palpation impairs the ability to palpate correctly. Asking a patient to take slow, deep breaths enhances muscle relaxation. Palpate tender areas last because they could cause a patient to become tense and impede the assessment. Ask a patient to point out areas that are more sensitive and note any nonverbal signs of discomfort. Patients appreciate clean, warm hands; short fingernails; and a gentle approach. Palpation is either light or deep and is controlled by the amount of pressure applied with the fingers or hand. Light palpation precedes deep palpation. Consider a patient's condition, the area being palpated, and the reason for using palpation. For example, when a patient is admitted to the emergency department after an automobile accident, consider the factors surrounding the patient's injury and inspect the chest wall carefully before performing any palpation around the area of the ribs.

For light palpation apply pressure slowly, gently, and deliberately, depressing approximately 1 cm (½ inch) (Fig. 6-1, A). Check tender areas further, using light intermittent pressure. After light palpation you may use deeper palpation to examine the condition of organs (Fig. 6-1, B). Depress the area that you are examining by approximately 2 cm (1 inch). Caution is the rule. Bimanual palpation involves one hand placed over the other while applying pressure. The upper hand exerts downward pressure as the other hand feels the subtle characteristics of underlying organs and masses. Seek the assistance of a qualified instructor before attempting deep palpation.

Percussion involves tapping the body with the fingertips to vibrate underlying tissues and organs. The vibration travels through body tissues, and the character of the resulting sound reflects the density of underlying tissue. The denser the tissue, the quieter the sound is. By knowing various densities of organs and body parts, you learn how to locate organs or masses, map their edges, and determine their size. An abnormal sound suggests a mass or substance such as air or fluid in a body cavity. The skill of percussion is used more often by advanced practice nurses (APNs) than by nurses in daily practice at the bedside.

The most commonly used percussion technique is the indirect technique. You perform the indirect technique by placing the middle finger of your nondominant hand firmly against the body surface. With palm and fingers remaining off the skin, the tip of the middle finger of the dominant hand strikes the base of the distal joint of the finger (Fig. 6-2). Use a quick, sharp stroke, keeping the forearm stationary. Relax the wrist to deliver the proper blow. Once the finger has struck, the wrist snaps back. If the blow is not sharp, if the hand is held loosely, or if the palm rests on the body surface, the sound is softened; and you will not detect the presence of underlying structures. A light, quick blow produces the clearest sounds. Table 6-2 describes the five different percussion sounds.

Auscultation is listening with a stethoscope to sounds produced by the body. To auscultate correctly, listen in a quiet environment for both the presence of sound and its characteristics. To be successful in auscultation, you must first recognize normal sounds from each body structure, including the passage of blood through an

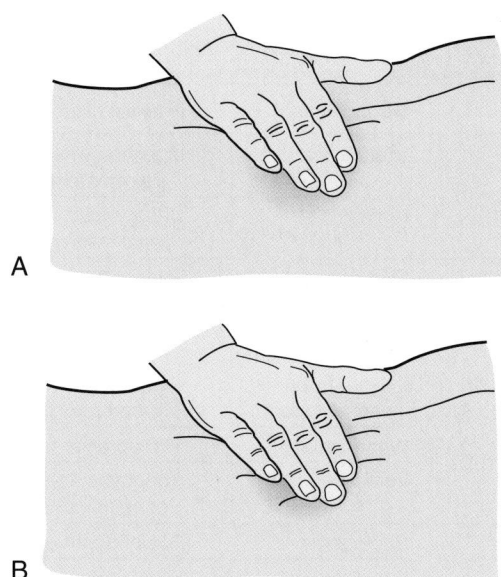

A

B

FIG 6-1 **A,** During light palpation gentle pressure against underlying skin and tissues can be used to detect areas of irregularity and tenderness. **B,** During deep palpation depress tissue to assess condition of underlying organs.

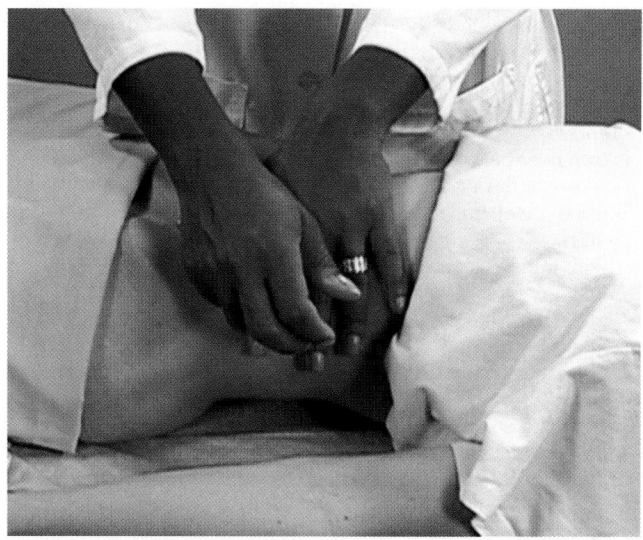

FIG 6-2 Percussion of abdomen. (*From Seidel HM et al: Mosby's guide to physical examination, ed 6, St Louis, 2006, Mosby.*)

TABLE 6-2	Sounds Produced by Percussion				
Sound	**Intensity**	**Pitch**	**Duration**	**Quality**	**Common Location**
Tympany	Loud	High	Moderate	Drumlike	Gastric air bubble, puffed-out cheek
Resonant	Loud	Low	Long	Hollow	Healthy lung
Hyperresonant	Very loud	Low	Longer than resonance	Booming	Emphysematous lung
Dull	Soft to moderate	Moderate to High	Moderate	Thudlike	Over liver
Flat	Soft	High	Short	Very dull	Over muscle

artery, heart sounds, and movement of air through the lungs. These sounds vary according to the location in which they can be most easily heard. Likewise you become familiar with areas that normally do not emit sounds. Practice listening to many normal sounds so you can recognize abnormal sounds when they arise.

To auscultate you need good hearing acuity, a good stethoscope, and knowledge of how to use the stethoscope properly (Box 6-3).

Nurses with hearing disorders may purchase stethoscopes with greater sound amplification and may need to ask colleagues to verify some findings through auscultation. It is essential to place the stethoscope directly on a patient's skin because clothing obscures and changes sound. Through auscultation the nurse notes that there are four characteristics of sound:

- *Frequency*: Number of sound wave cycles generated per second by a vibrating object. The higher the frequency, the higher the pitch of a sound and vice versa.
- *Loudness*: Amplitude of a sound wave. Auscultated sounds are described as loud or soft.
- *Quality*: Sounds of similar frequency and loudness from different sources. Terms such as *blowing* or *gurgling* describe quality of sound.
- *Duration*: Length of time that sound vibrations last. Duration of sound is short, medium, or long. Layers of soft tissue dampen the duration of sounds from deep internal organs.

A nurse cannot be successful at auscultation without knowing how to use a stethoscope properly. Chapter 5 describes the parts of the acoustic stethoscope and use of the bell and diaphragm.

Olfaction uses the sense of smell to detect abnormalities that go unrecognized by any other means. Some alterations in body function and certain bacteria create characteristic odors (Table 6-3).

BOX 6-3 | Using a Stethoscope

1 Place earpieces in both ears with tips of earpieces turned toward the face. *Lightly* blow against the diaphragm (flat side of chest piece). Now place the earpieces in both ears with the tips turned toward the back of the head and again blow against the diaphragm. Compare comfort in the ears and amplification of sounds with earpieces in both directions. Earpieces pointing toward the face should fit snugly and comfortably.

2 If the stethoscope has both a diaphragm (flat side) and a bell (bowl shaped with a rubber ring), put earpieces in ears and lightly blow against the diaphragm. The chest piece can be turned to allow sound to be carried through either side (bell or diaphragm) of the chest piece. If sound is faint, lightly blow into the bell. Then turn the chest piece and blow again against both the diaphragm and the bell. The diaphragm is used for higher-pitched heart sounds, bowel sounds, and lung sounds. The bell is used for lower-pitched heart sounds and vascular sounds.

3 With earpieces in place and using the diaphragm, move the diaphragm lightly over the hair on your arm. The bristling sound mimics a sound heard in the lungs. When listening for significant sounds, hold the diaphragm still and firmly make a tight seal against the skin to eliminate extraneous sounds.

4 Place the diaphragm over the front of your chest directly on your skin and listen to your own breathing, comparing the bell and the diaphragm. Repeat the process while listening to your own heartbeat. Ask someone to speak in a conversational tone and note how the speech detracts from hearing clearly. When using a stethoscope, both you and the patient should remain quiet.

5 With the earpieces in your ears, gently tap the tubing. Note that it generates extraneous sounds. When listening to a patient, maintain a position that allows the tubing to extend straight and hang free. Movement may allow it to rub or bump objects, creating extraneous sounds. Kinked tubing muffles sounds.

6 Care of a stethoscope: Remove earpieces regularly and clean or remove cerumen (earwax). Keep the bell and diaphragm free of dust, lint, and body oils. Keep the tubing away from your body oils. Avoid draping the stethoscope around the neck next to the skin. To clean, wipe the entire stethoscope (e.g., diaphragm, tubing) with alcohol or soapy water. Be sure to dry all parts thoroughly. Follow manufacturer recommendations.

7 Infection control: Harmful bacteria, even antibiotic-resistant microorganisms, can be transferred from patient to patient when using portable equipment such as stethoscopes (Uneke et al., 2010). Follow agency infection control guidelines, especially contact precautions, to decrease this risk. Clean a stethoscope (diaphragm/bell) with a disinfectant before reuse on another patient. Using a disinfectant such as isopropyl alcohol (with or without chlorhexidine), benzalkonium, and sodium hypochlorite is effective in reducing the number of bacterial colonies. Earpieces of stethoscopes are also sources of transferable bacteria when you inadvertently touch your ears and then care for a patient. Potential pathogens could contaminate earpieces. Using hand hygiene before and after patient contact decreases the risk of transmitting microorganisms from your ear to your patient (Uneke et al., 2010).

TABLE 6-3 | Assessment of Characteristic Odors

Odor	Site or Source	Potential Causes
Alcohol	Oral cavity	Ingestion of alcohol; diabetes mellitus
Ammonia	Urine	Urinary tract infection, renal failure
Body odor	Skin, particularly in areas where body parts rub together (e.g., under arms, beneath breasts, perineal area)	Poor hygiene, excess perspiration (hyperhidrosis), foul-smelling perspiration (bromhidrosis)
	Wound site	Wound abscess; infection
	Vomitus	Abdominal irritation, contaminated food
Feces	Rectal area	Bowel obstruction
	Vomitus/oral cavity (fecal odor)	Fecal incontinence; fistula
Fetid, sweet odor	Tracheostomy or mucus secretions	Infection of bronchial tree (*Pseudomonas* bacteria)
Foul-smelling stools in infants	Stool	Malabsorption syndrome
Halitosis	Oral cavity	Poor dental or oral hygiene, gum disease; sinus infection
Musty odor	Casted body part	Infection inside cast
Stale urine	Skin	Uremic acidosis
Sweet, fruity ketones	Oral cavity	Diabetic acidosis
Sweet, heavy, thick odor	Draining wound	*Pseudomonas* (bacterial) infection

PREPARATION FOR ASSESSMENT

Preparation of the environment, equipment, and patient facilitates a smooth assessment. Provide patients privacy to promote their comfort and the efficiency of an examination. In a health care agency, close the door and pull privacy curtains. In the home examine the patient in the bedroom. A comfortable environment includes a warm, comfortable temperature; a loose-fitting gown or pajamas for a patient; adequate direct lighting; control of outside noises; and precautions to prevent interruptions by visitors or other health care personnel. If possible, place the bed or examination table at waist level so you can assess a patient easily. During an examination you must protect a patient from falls and injury and return the bed to a safe height at the completion of the assessment (TJC, 2012).

Preparing the Patient

Prepare patients both physically and psychologically for accurate assessments. A tense, anxious patient may have difficulty understanding, following directions, or cooperating with your instructions. To prepare a patient:

1 Provide comfort by allowing the opportunity to empty the bowel or bladder (a good time to collect needed specimens).
2 Provide privacy.
3 Minimize a patient's anxiety and fear by conveying an open, receptive, and professional approach. Using simple terms, thoroughly explain what will be done, what the patient should expect to feel, and how he or she can cooperate. Even if a patient appears unresponsive, it is still important to explain your actions.
4 Provide access to body parts while draping areas that are not being examined.
5 Reduce distractions. Turn down volume or turn off radio or television.
6 Eliminate drafts, control room temperature, and provide warm blankets.
7 Help patients assume positions during assessments so body parts are accessible and patients stay comfortable (Table 6-4). A patient's ability to assume positions depends on physical strength and limitations. Some positions are uncomfortable or embarrassing; keep a patient in position no longer than is necessary.
8 Pace assessment according to an individual's physical and emotional tolerance.
9 Use a relaxed tone of voice and facial expressions to put a patient at ease.
10 Encourage a patient to ask questions and report discomfort felt during the examination.
11 Have a third person of patient's gender in the room during assessment of genitalia. This prevents a patient from accusing you of behaving in an unethical manner.
12 At conclusion of an assessment, ask the patient if there are any concerns or questions.

| TABLE 6-4 | Positions for Physical Assessment |

Position	Areas Assessed	Rationale	Limitations
Sitting	Head and neck, back, posterior thorax and lungs, anterior thorax and lungs, breasts, axillae, heart, vital signs, upper extremities	Sitting upright provides full expansion of lungs and better visualization of symmetry of upper body parts.	Physically weakened or developmentally disabled patient is sometimes unable to sit. Use supine position with head of bed elevated instead.
Supine	Head and neck, anterior thorax and lungs, breasts, axillae, heart, abdomen, extremities, pulses	This is most normally relaxed position. It provides easy access to pulse sites.	If patient becomes short of breath easily, raise head of bed.
Dorsal recumbent	Head and neck, anterior thorax and lungs, breasts, axillae, heart, abdomen	Position is for abdominal assessment because it promotes relaxation of abdominal muscles.	Patients with painful disorders are more comfortable with knees flexed.
Lithotomy	Female genitalia and genital tract	This position provides maximal exposure of genitalia and facilitates insertion of vaginal speculum.	Lithotomy position is embarrassing and uncomfortable; thus examiner minimizes time that patient spends in it. Keep patient well draped. Patients with arthritis or other joint deformities may be unable to tolerate the position.

Continued

TABLE 6-4 | Positions for Physical Assessment—cont'd

Position	Areas Assessed	Rationale	Limitations
Sims'	Rectum and vagina	Flexion of hip and knee improves exposure of rectal and genitourinary areas.	Joint deformities hinder patient's ability to bend hip and knee.
Prone	Musculoskeletal system	This position is for assessing extension of hip joint, skin, and buttocks.	Patients with respiratory difficulties do not tolerate this position well.
Lateral recumbent	Heart	This position aids in detecting murmurs.	Patients with respiratory difficulties do not tolerate this position well.
Knee-chest	Rectum	This position provides maximal exposure of rectal area.	This position is embarrassing and uncomfortable. Patients with arthritis or other joint deformities may be unable to assume it.

PHYSICAL ASSESSMENT OF VARIOUS AGE-GROUPS

Children and Adolescents

1 Routine assessments of children focus on health promotion and illness prevention, particularly for care of well children with competent parenting and no serious health problems (Hockenberry and Wilson, 2011). Focus on growth and development, sensory screening, dental examination, and behavioral assessment.
2 Children who are chronically ill, disabled, in foster care, or foreign-born adopted may require additional assessments because of unique health needs.
3 When obtaining histories of infants and children, gather all or part of the information from parents or guardians.
4 Children who are chronically ill, disabled, in foster care, or adopted from a foreign country may require additional assessment because of their unique health risks.
5 Parents may think that the examiner is testing or judging them. Offer support during examination and do not pass judgment.
6 Call children by their preferred name and address parents as "Mr. and Mrs. Brown" rather than by first names.
7 Open-ended questions often allow parents to share more information and describe more of the child's problems.
8 Older children and adolescents respond best when treated as adults and individuals and often can provide details about their health history and severity of symptoms.

9 An adolescent has a right to confidentiality. After talking with parents about historical information, arrange to be alone with the adolescent to speak privately and perform the examination.

Older Adults

1 Do not assume that aging is always accompanied by illness or disability. Older adults are able to adapt to change and maintain functional independence (Touhy and Jett, 2010).
2 A thorough assessment of an older adult provides critical information that can be used to maximize independence (Cress, 2012).
3 Provide adequate space for an examination, particularly if a patient uses a mobility aid.
4 Plan the history and examination, taking into account an older adult's energy level, physical limitations, pace, and adaptability. You may need more than one session to complete the assessment (Touhy and Jett, 2010).
5 Measure performance under the most favorable conditions. Take advantage of natural opportunities for assessment (e.g., during bathing, grooming, mealtime) (Touhy and Jett, 2010).
6 Sequence an examination to keep position changes to a minimum. Be efficient throughout the examination to limit patient movement.
7 Be sure that an examination of an older adult includes review of mental status.

SKILL 6-1   General Survey

The general survey begins a review of a patient's primary health problems, and it includes assessment of vital signs, height and weight, general behavior, and appearance. It provides information about characteristics of an illness, a patient's hygiene, skin condition and body image, emotional state, recent changes in weight, and developmental status. The survey reveals important information about a patient's behavior that influences how you communicate instructions and continue an assessment.

Delegation and Collaboration

The skill of completing the general survey cannot be delegated to nursing assistive personnel (NAP). The nurse directs the NAP to:

- Measure the patient's height and weight.
- Obtain vital signs (not the initial set, but subsequent measurements if patient is stable).
- Monitor oral intake and urinary output.
- Report a patient's subjective signs and symptoms to the nurse.

Equipment

- ❑ Stethoscope
- ❑ Sphygmomanometer and cuff
- ❑ Thermometer
- ❑ Digital watch or wristwatch with second hand
- ❑ Tape measure
- ❑ Clean gloves (use nonlatex if necessary)
- ❑ Tongue blade
- ❑ Appropriate electronic record or documentation form

STEP	RATIONALE

ASSESSMENT

	STEP	RATIONALE
1	Note if patient has had any acute distress: difficulty breathing, pain, anxiety. If such signs are present, defer general survey until later and focus immediately on affected body system.	Signs establish priorities regarding which part of the examination to conduct first.
2	Review graphic sheet for previous vital signs and consider factors or conditions that may alter values (see Chapter 5).	Provides baseline and historical data about patient's vital signs.
3	Determine patient's primary language. If you identify a need for an interpreter, determine the availability of a professional interpreter. It is best to have an interpreter of the same gender who is older and mature. Have the interpreter translate verbatim if possible.	Facilitates patient understanding and promotes accuracy of information provided by patient.
4	After reviewing history, confirm primary reason patient has sought health care.	Keeps assessment focused on patient to ensure that his or her expectations are addressed.
5	Identify patient's normal height, weight, and body mass index. If a sudden gain or loss in weight has occurred, determine amount of weight change and period of time in which it occurred. Assess if patient has recently been dieting or following an exercise program. Use growth chart for children under 18 years of age.	Generally a body mass index of 25 to 29.9 for men and women is overweight, whereas 30 and over is obese (Seidel et al., 2011). Fluid retention is one factor that must be ruled out. A person's weight can fluctuate daily because of fluid loss or retention (1 L of water weighs 1 kg [2.2 pounds]).
6	Review patient's past fluid intake and output (I&O) records.	Fluid and electrolyte balance affects health and function in all body systems. Intake includes all liquids taken orally, by feeding tube, and parenterally. Liquid output includes urine, diarrhea stool, vomitus, drainage from fistulas and gastric suction, and drainage from postsurgical tubes such as chest tubes or Jackson-Pratt drains.
7	Identify patient's general perceptions about personal health.	Assessment of patient's general appearance coupled with patient's own perceptions may reveal specific problem areas.
8	Assess for evidence of latex allergy, which may include contact dermatitis or systemic reactions. Ask if patient has risk factors such as food allergies (papaya, avocado, banana, peach, kiwi, or tomato); has high latex exposure (housekeepers, food handlers, health care worker); or must avoid products containing latex (rubber bands, adhesive tape, certain paints or carpets).	Gloves are worn during certain aspects of the assessment. Repeated exposure to latex may result in more serious reactions, including asthma, itching, and anaphylaxis (Ball and Bindler, 2010; Seidel et al., 2011).

NURSING DIAGNOSES

- Anxiety
- Bathing self-care deficit
- Deficient fluid volume
- Excess fluid volume
- Fear
- Imbalanced nutrition: less than body requirements or more than body requirements
- Impaired physical mobility
- Impaired skin integrity
- Ineffective breathing pattern
- Ineffective peripheral tissue perfusion
- Latex allergy response
- Pain (acute, chronic)

Related factors are individualized based on patient's condition or needs.

PLANNING

	STEP	RATIONALE
1	Expected outcomes following completion of procedure:	
	• Patient demonstrates alert, cooperative behavior without evidence of physical or emotional distress during assessment.	You use a calm and confident approach during assessment. Patient has no abnormal findings.
	• Patient provides appropriate subjective data related to physical condition.	Patient is able to cooperate with assessment.

STEP	RATIONALE
2 *Prepare patient*: Tell patient that you will be doing a routine process to check for areas of concern. Ask patient to tell you if any area that you examine hurts when touched.	Understanding promotes patient's cooperation. Pain is an important finding during assessment.
3 Perform hand hygiene. Assemble necessary equipment. Position patient initially, either sitting or lying supine with head of bed elevated.	Prevents transmission of microorganisms. Promotes efficiency of exam.

IMPLEMENTATION

1 Throughout assessment note patient's verbal and nonverbal behaviors. Determine patient's level of consciousness (LOC) and orientation by observing and talking to him or her (Box 6-4).	Behaviors may reflect specific physical abnormalities. Dementia and LOC influence ability to cooperate.
2 Obtain temperature, pulse, respirations, and blood pressure unless taken within last 3 hours or if a serious potential change is noted (e.g., change in LOC or difficulty breathing) (see Chapter 5). Inform patient of vital signs.	Vital signs provide important information regarding physiologic changes in relation to oxygenation and circulation.
3 Note the patient's gender and race, and ask their age. Note patient's external physical features.	Gender influences type of examination performed and manner in which you make assessments. Different physical characteristics and predisposition to illnesses are related to gender and race.
4 If uncertain whether patient understands a question, rephrase or ask a similar question.	Inappropriate response from a patient may be caused by language barriers or deterioration of mental status, preoccupation with illness, or decreased hearing acuity.
5 If patient's responses are inappropriate, ask short, to-the-point questions regarding information patient should know, for example: "Tell me your name." "What is the name of this place?" "Tell me where you live." "What day is this?" "What month is this?" or "What season of the year is this?"	Measures patient's orientation to person, place, and time. You may note this in documentation as "Oriented × 3." If disoriented in any way, include subjective and/or objective data rather than just documenting "disoriented."
6 If patient is unable to respond to questions of orientation, offer simple commands, for example, "Squeeze my fingers" or "Move your toes."	LOC exists along a continuum, ranging from full responsiveness, to inability to consciously initiate meaningful behaviors, to unresponsiveness to stimuli.
7 Assess affect and mood: Note if verbal expressions match nonverbal behavior and if appropriate to situation.	Reflects patient's mental and emotional status, consciousness, and feelings.
8 Watch patient interact with spouse or partner, older-adult child, or caregiver. Be alert for indications of fear, hesitancy to report health status, or willingness to let caregiver control assessment interview. Does partner or caregiver have a history of violence, alcoholism, or drug abuse? Is the person unemployed, ill, or frustrated with caring for a patient? Note if patient has any obvious physical injuries.	Suspect abuse in patients who have suffered obvious physical injury or neglect, show signs of malnutrition, or have ecchymoses (bruises) on the extremities or trunk. Health care providers are often the first to identify evidence of abuse because patients may not be able to tell family or friends. Partners or caregivers may have history of abusive or addictive behaviors.

BOX 6-4 | **Characteristics of Dementia**

Cognition
- Memory impaired: trouble recalling recent conversations, events, and appointments
- Frequently misplaces objects

Speech/Language
- Struggles to find words
- Conversation possibly incoherent

Activity
- Unchanged from usual behavior
- Difficulty performing tasks that require many steps

Mood and Affect
- Depressed
- Apathetic
- Uninterested

Delusions/Hallucinations
- Can be some delusions
- No hallucinations

Modified from Seidel et al: *Mosby's guide to physical examination*, ed 7, St Louis, 2011, Mosby.

STEP	RATIONALE

Clinical Decision Point *Be discreet in how you conduct the interview. Ask direct questions about abuse in private. It is often necessary to delay assessment to a later time when the partner or caregiver is not present. Asking a partner or caregiver to leave during an assessment creates an awkward situation, but inquiring about possible abuse in front of an abuser puts a patient at risk for further abuse. Patients are more likely to reveal any problems when the suspected abuser is absent from the room.*

9 Observe for signs of abuse:

   a *Child*: Blood on underclothing, pain in genital area, difficulty sitting or walking, pain on urination, vaginal or penile discharge, itching or unusual color in genital area, physical injury inconsistent with parent's or caregiver's account of how injury occurred.

     Indicates child sexual abuse (Hockenberry and Wilson, 2011; Seidel et al., 2011). Suggests child physical abuse.

   b *Female patient*: Injury or trauma inconsistent with reported cause or obvious injuries to head, face, neck, breasts, abdomen, and genitalia (e.g., black eyes, abrasions, bruises/ welts, broken nose, lacerations, broken teeth, strangulation marks, burns, human bites, orbital fractures, fractured skull).

     Suggests domestic abuse (Hegarty et al., 2008; Seidel et al., 2011). These signs also apply to male patient being abused by female partner.

   c *Older adult*: Injury or trauma inconsistent with reported cause, injuries in unusual locations (e.g., neck or genitalia), pattern injuries (left when an object with which a person is struck leaves an imprint), parallel injuries (e.g., bilateral ecchymosis on the upper arms suggesting that patient was held and shaken), burns (shaped like a cigarette, iron, rope), fractures, poor hygiene, and poor nutrition.

     Indicates elder abuse/neglect (Seidel et al., 2011; Touhy and Jett, 2010). Prolonged interval between injury and time patient sought medical care also indicates older adult abuse or neglect.

Clinical Decision Point *A pattern of findings indicating abuse usually mandates a report to a social service center (refer to state guidelines). Obtain immediate consultation with health care provider, social worker, and other support staff to facilitate placement in a safer environment.*

10 Assess posture and position, noting alignment of shoulders and hips while patient stands and/or sits. Observe whether patient is slumped, erect, or has a bent posture (see illustration).

     Reveals musculoskeletal problem, mood, or presence of pain.

   Assess body movements. Are they purposeful? Are there tremors of the extremities? Are any body parts immobile? Are movements coordinated or uncoordinated?

     May indicate neurologic or muscular problem or emotional stress (see Skill 6-7).

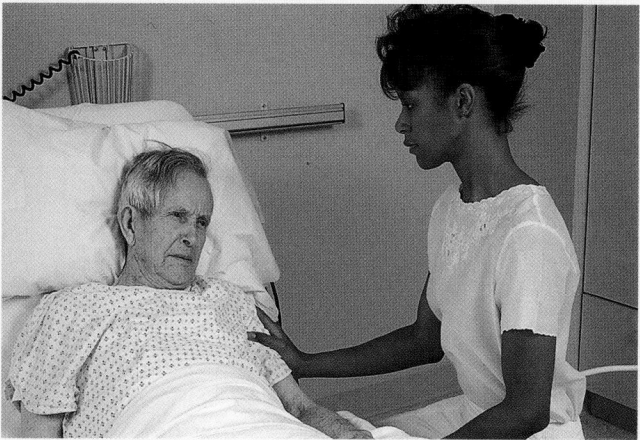

STEP 10 Observe patient's position and posture.

11 Assess speech. Is it understandable and moderately paced? Is there an association with patient's thoughts?

     Alterations reflect neurologic impairment, injury or impairment of mouth, improperly fitting dentures, differences in dialect or language, and some mental illnesses.

12 Observe hygiene and grooming for presence or absence of makeup, type of clothes (hospital or personal), and cleanliness. Hair, teeth, and nails are good places to assess for hygiene status.

     Grooming may reflect activity level before examination, resources available to purchase grooming supplies, patient's mood, and self-care practices. It may also reflect culture, lifestyle, economic status, and personal preferences.

   a Observe color, distribution, quantity, thickness, texture, and lubrication of hair.

     Changes in hair may reflect hormonal changes, changes from aging, poor nutrition, or use of certain hair-care products.

STEP	RATIONALE
b Inspect condition of nails (hands and feet). Note color, length, symmetry, cleanliness, and shape. Nails are normally transparent, smooth, and well rounded, with smooth, intact cuticle.	Changes indicate inadequate nutrition or grooming practices, nervous habits, or systemic diseases.
c Assess presence or absence of body odor.	Body odor may result from physical exercise, deficient hygiene, or physical or mental abnormalities. Inadequate oral hygiene or unhealthy teeth cause bad breath.
13 Inspect exposed areas of skin and ask if patient has noted any changes, including:	Determines presence of abnormalities and cancerous lesions. Melanoma is an aggressive form of skin cancer; detection and prompt treatment are critical (Box 6-5).
a Pruritus, oozing, bleeding	Itching could result from dry skin. Oozing could indicate infection, and bleeding may indicate a blood disorder.
b Appearance of a mole (nevus), bump, or nodule; change in sensation; itchiness, tenderness, or pain	These are key indicators that a lesion may be cancerous.
c Petechiae (pinpoint-size red or purple spots on skin caused by small hemorrhages in the skin layers)	Petechiae may indicate serious blood clotting disorder, drug reaction, or liver disease.
14 Inspect skin surfaces. Compare color of symmetric body parts, including areas unexposed to sun. Look for any patches or areas of skin color variation.	Changes in color can indicate pathologic alterations (Table 6-5).

BOX 6-5 | Malignant Melanoma Mnemonics

The ABCDE Rule of Melanoma
Here is a simple way to remember the characteristics that should alert you to the possibility of malignant melanoma.

A *Asymmetry* of lesion: One side different than the other
B *Borders:* Irregular (uneven, lumpy edges)
C *Color:* Blue/black or variegated; pigmentation not uniform; variations/multiple colors (tan, black) with areas of pink, white, gray, blue, or red
D *Diameter* greater than 6 mm
E *Evolving:* Change in size, shape, color; itching or bleeding

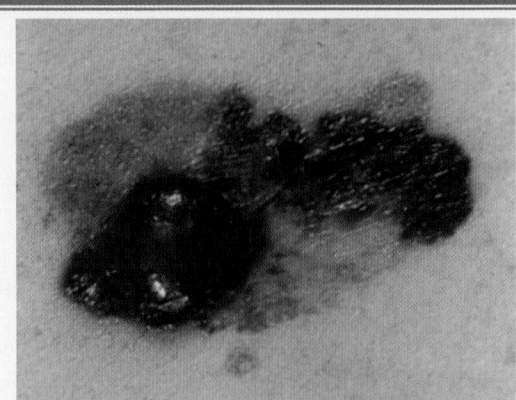

Malignant melanoma. (From Zitelli B, Davis H: *Atlas of pediatric physical diagnosis,* ed 5, St Louis, 2007, Mosby.)

From American Academy of Dermatology (AAD): *How to examine your skin,* Washington, DC, 2011, AAD; and American Cancer Society (ACS): *Can melanoma be prevented,* Atlanta, 2011a, The Society.

TABLE 6-5 | Skin Color Variations

Color	Condition	Cause	Assessment Location
Bluish (cyanosis)	Related to hypoxia (late sign of decreased oxygen levels)	Heart or lung disease, cold environment	Nail beds, lips, base of tongue, skin (severe cases)
Pallor (decrease in color)	Reduced amount of oxyhemoglobin	Anemia Shock	Face, conjunctivae, nail beds, palms of hands
	Reduced visibility of oxyhemoglobin resulting from decreased blood flow		Skin, nail beds, conjunctivae, lips
Loss of pigmentation	Vitiligo	Congenital autoimmune condition causing lack of pigment	Patchy areas on skin over face, hands, arms
Yellow-orange (jaundice)	Increased deposit of bilirubin in tissues	Liver disease, destruction of red blood cells	Sclerae, mucous membranes, skin
Red (erythema)	Increased visibility of oxyhemoglobin caused by dilation or increased blood flow	Fever, direct trauma, blushing, alcohol intake	Face, area of trauma, and areas at risk for pressure such as sacrum, shoulders, elbows, and heels
Tan-brown	Increased amount of melanin	Suntan, pregnancy	Areas exposed to sun: face, arms; areolae, nipples

STEP	RATIONALE

Clinical Decision Point *Be alert for basal cell carcinomas such as an open sore that does not heal, a shiny nodule, a pink or reddish growth, or scarlike area. These are often seen in sun-exposed areas and frequently occur in sun-damaged skin.*

15 Carefully inspect color of face, oral mucosa, lips, conjunctiva, sclera, palms of hands, and nail beds.

Abnormalities are easier to identify in areas of body where melanin production is lowest.

Clinical Decision Point *When assessing the skin of a patient with bandages, cast, restraints, or other restrictive devices, note report of pain or tingling and areas of pallor, decreased temperature, decreased movement, and impaired sensation, which may indicate impaired circulation. Immediate release of pressure from the restrictive device may be necessary.*

16 Use ungloved fingertips to palpate skin surfaces to feel texture and moisture of intact skin.

Changes in texture may be the first indication of skin rashes in dark-skinned patients. Hydration, body temperature, and environment may affect the skin. Older adults are prone to xerosis, presenting as dry, scaly skin (Touhy and Jett, 2010).

   a Stroke skin surfaces lightly with fingertips to detect texture of surface of skin. Note whether skin is smooth or rough, thick or thin, or tight or supple and if localized areas of hardness or lesions are present.

Localized texture changes result from trauma, surgical wounds, or lesions.

   b Palpate any areas that appear irregular in texture.

Allows detection of localized areas of hardness and/or tenderness within subcutaneous skin layers.

   c Using dorsum (back) of hand, palpate for temperature of skin surfaces. Compare symmetric body parts. Compare upper and lower body parts. Note distinct temperature difference and localized areas of warmth.

Skin on dorsum of hand is thin, which allows detection of subtle temperature changes. Cool skin temperature often indicates decreased blood flow. A stage I pressure ulcer may cause warmth and erythema (redness) of an area. Environmental temperature and anxiety may also affect skin temperature.

Clinical Decision Point *In patients who receive routine injections (e.g., insulin, heparin), localized areas of hardness may be palpated over injection sites. Develop a plan to rotate injection sites systematically. Site rotation prevents local skin changes from repeated injections (Lewis et al., 2011).*

17 Apply clean gloves. Inspect character of any secretions; note color, odor, amount, and consistency (e.g., thin and watery, thick and oily). Remove gloves.

Description of secretions helps to indicate type of lesion, presence of infection, or wound healing.

18 Assess skin turgor by grasping fold of skin on sternum, forearm, or abdomen with fingertips. Release skinfold and note ease and speed with which skin returns to place (see illustration).

With reduced turgor skin remains suspended or "tented" for a few seconds before slowly returning to place, indicating decreased elasticity and possible dehydration. With altered turgor, provide measures for prevention of pressure ulcers (see Chapter 18).

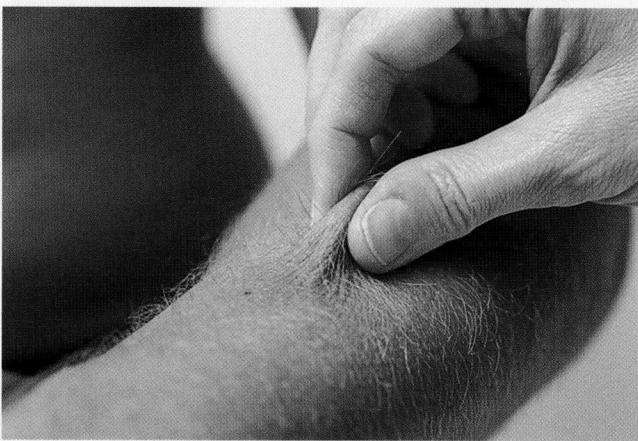

STEP 18 Checking skin turgor.

19 Assess condition of skin for pressure areas, paying particular attention to regions at risk for pressure (e.g., sacrum, greater trochanter, heels, occipital area, clavicles). If you see areas of redness, place fingertip over area, apply gentle pressure, and release. Look at skin color.

Normal reactive hyperemia (redness) is a visible effect of localized vasodilation, the normal response of the body to lack of blood flow to underlying tissue. Affected area of skin normally blanches with fingertip pressure. If area does not blanch, suspect tissue injury.

STEP	RATIONALE

Clinical Decision Point *With evidence of normal reactive hyperemia, reposition patient and develop a turning schedule if he or she is dependent (see Chapter 18).*

20 When you detect a lesion, use adequate lighting to inspect color, location, texture, size, shape, and type (Box 6-6). Also note grouping (e.g., clustered or linear) and distribution (e.g., localized or generalized).

Observation of skin lesions allows for accurate description and identification.

   a Use gloves if lesion is moist or draining. Gently palpate any lesion to determine mobility, contour (e.g., flat, raised, or depressed), and consistency (e.g., soft or hard).

Gentle palpation prevents rupture of underlying cysts. Gloves reduce transmission of microorganisms.

   b Note if patient reports tenderness with or without palpation.

   c Measure size of lesion (height, width, depth) with a centimeter ruler.

Tenderness may indicate inflammation or pressure on body part. Provides for a baseline to assess changes in lesion over time.

21 Remove gloves. Discard used supplies and gloves in proper receptacle. Assist patient to comfortable position. Perform hand hygiene.

Prevents transmission of infections.

BOX 6-6 | Types of Skin Lesions

Macule: Flat, nonpalpable change in skin color; smaller than 1 cm (0.4 inch) (e.g., freckle, petechia)

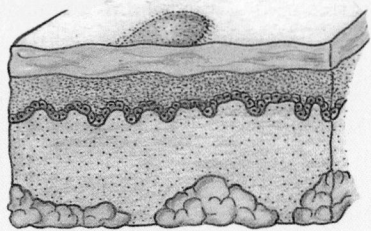

Vesicle: Circumscribed elevation of skin filled with serous fluid; smaller than 0.5 cm (0.2 inch) (e.g., herpes simplex, chickenpox)

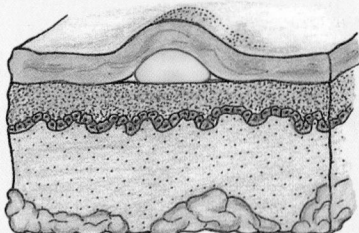

Papule: Palpable, circumscribed, solid elevation in skin; smaller than 0.5 cm (0.2 inch) (e.g., elevated nevus)

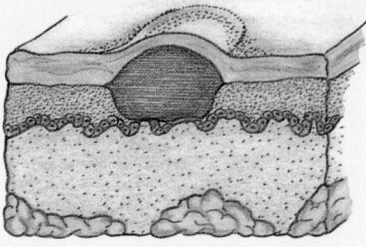

Ulcer: Deep loss of skin surface that may extend to dermis and frequently bleeds and scars; varies in size (e.g., venous stasis ulcer)

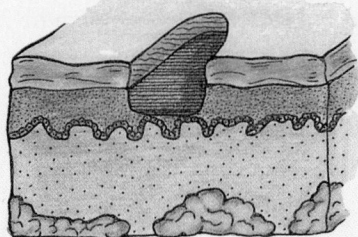

Tumor: Solid mass that may extend deep through subcutaneous tissue; larger than 1 to 2 cm (0.4 to 0.8 inch) (e.g., epithelioma)

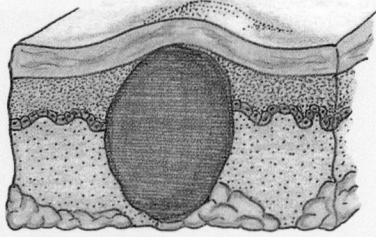

Atrophy: Thinning of skin with loss of normal skin furrow with skin appearing shiny and translucent; varies in size (e.g., arterial insufficiency)

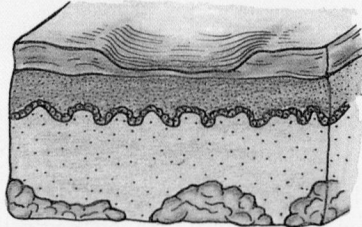

STEP	RATIONALE

BOX 6-6 | Types of Skin Lesions—cont'd

Pustule: Circumscribed elevation of skin similar to vesicle but filled with pus; varies in size (e.g., acne, staphylococcal infection)

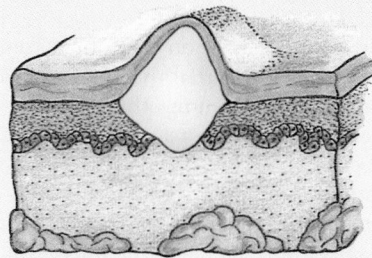

Nodule: Elevated solid mass, deeper and firmer than papul; 0.5 to 2 cm (0.2 to 0.8 inch) (e.g., wart)

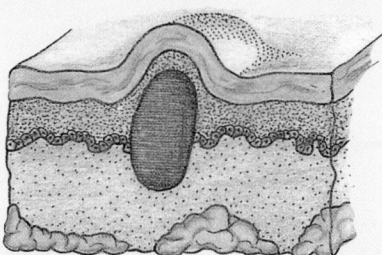

Wheal: Irregularly shaped, elevated area or superficial localized edema; varies in size (e.g., hive, mosquito bite)

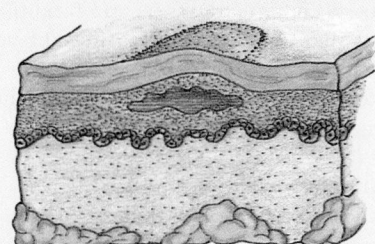

EVALUATION

1 Observe throughout assessment for evidence of physical or emotional distress, which may alter assessment data.

Interaction during assessment reveals emotional problems. Maneuvers used during physical examination reveal presence of physical problems.

2 Compare assessment findings with previous observations.

Determines if change has occurred.

3 Ask patient if there is information about physical condition that you have not discussed.

Some patients think that they are bothering you by asking questions unless the opportunity for questions is provided.

Unexpected Outcomes

1 Patient demonstrates acute distress (e.g., shortness of breath, acute pain, severe anxiety).

2 Patient has abnormal skin condition (e.g., dry texture, reduced turgor, lesions, or erythema).

3 Patient is unwilling or unable to provide adequate information relating to identified concerns.

Related Interventions

- Respond immediately to identified need (e.g., repositioning, oxygen, or medication as appropriate).
- Obtain vital signs.
- Notify health care provider.

- Identify contributing factors and prevent continued irritation or damage as appropriate (see Chapter 18).

- Seek information from family members if present.
- Review patient's record for baseline data.

Recording and Reporting

- Record patient's vital signs on vital sign flow sheet.
- Record description of alterations in patient's general appearance.
- Describe patient's behaviors using objective terminology. Include patient's self-report of signs and symptoms.
- Report abnormalities and acute symptoms to nurse in charge or health care provider.

Special Considerations
Teaching

- During general survey inform patient about normal range of vital signs for age and physical condition and normal weight for height and body frame.
- If patient is on established diet, discuss any problems that he or she has preparing a diet or selecting food. The best form of weight reduction is to achieve gradual weight loss by increasing

exercise and decreasing caloric intake. Refer to clinical dietitian for specific information.

Pediatric

- Measurement of physical growth is a key element in evaluation of a child's health status. These physical growth parameters include height, length, weight, skinfold thickness, and arm and head circumference (Hockenberry and Wilson, 2011). Use growth charts specific to child's age and condition.
- Weigh infants nude. Weigh children in light underclothes or gown.
- A child's interactions with parents provide valuable information regarding the child's behavior.

Gerontologic

- An older adult's presenting signs and symptoms are sometimes deceiving. An older adult has a diminished physiologic reserve that sometimes masks the usual, or "classic," signs and symptoms of a disease. In older adults signs and symptoms are often blunted or atypical (Touhy and Jett, 2010).
- Common skin changes with aging include dryness, thinning, decreased elasticity, and prominent small blood vessels. Common lesions include seborrheic keratosis (pigmented raised, warty lesion); cherry angioma (bright, ruby-red round papules);

cutaneous tags (soft pinkish-tan to light-brown pedunculated lesions); and solar lentigines (gray-brown, irregular macular lesions on sun-exposed areas) (Seidel et al., 2011).

- Inspection of the feet is critically important in the presence of impaired circulation, impaired vision, and diabetes mellitus. Common foot conditions include ulceration, fungal infection, corns, calluses, bunions, plantar warts, and hammer toe.

Home Care

- In the home the focus may be on the patient's ability to perform basic self-care tasks. Be sure that the home assessment builds on all health concerns identified in other settings.
- The home health nurse takes a small portable scale to monitor weight changes.

Long-Term Care

- The minimum data set (MDS) is a tool that includes a comprehensive assessment of residents in the long-term care setting. It provides an ongoing comprehensive assessment of each resident, emphasizing functional ability and both a physical and a psychosocial profile. Only a registered nurse (RN) can function as the assessment coordinator (Cress, 2012). All members of the interdisciplinary team make contributions.

SKILL 6-2   Head and Neck Assessment

Examination of the head and neck includes assessment of the head, eyes, ears, nose, mouth, and sinuses. Assessment of the head and neck uses inspection, palpation, and auscultation, with inspection and palpation often used simultaneously.

Delegation and Collaboration

The skill of assessing the head and neck cannot be delegated to nursing assistive personnel (NAP). The nurse directs the NAP to:

- Observe for nasal discharge and nasal bleeding.
- Report any findings found during routine care (e.g., oral care, bathing) to the nurse for further assessment.

Equipment

- ❏ Stethoscope
- ❏ Clean gloves (use nonlatex if necessary)
- ❏ Tongue blade
- ❏ Pen light

STEP	RATIONALE
ASSESSMENT	
1 Assess for history of headache, dizziness, pain, or stiffness.	Headaches and dizziness are signs of stress, a symptom of another underlying problem such as high blood pressure, or a result of injury.
2 Determine if the patient has a history of eye disease, diabetes mellitus, or hypertension.	Common conditions predispose patients to visual alterations requiring health care provider referral.
3 Ask if patient has experienced blurred vision, flashing lights, halos around lights or a reduced visual field.	These common symptoms indicate visual problems.
4 Ask if patient has experienced ear pain, itching, discharge, vertigo, tinnitus (ringing in the ears), or change in hearing.	These signs and symptoms indicate infection or hearing loss.
5 Review patient's occupational history.	Patient's occupation can create a risk of injury, potential for eye fatigue, or prolonged noise exposure.
6 Ask if patient has a history of allergies, nasal discharge, epistaxis (nosebleeds), or postnasal drip.	History is useful in determining source of nasal and sinus drainage.
7 Determine if patient smokes or chews tobacco.	Tobacco users have greater risk for mouth and throat cancer (ACS, 2012b.)

NURSING DIAGNOSES

- Deficient knowledge
- Impaired oral mucous membranes
- Ineffective health maintenance
- Risk for injury

Related factors are individualized based on patient's condition or needs.

STEP	RATIONALE

PLANNING

1 Expected outcomes following completion of procedure: No abnormalities identified.
- Patient recognizes warning signs and symptoms of eye, ear, sinus, and mouth disease. / Awareness of warning signs improves adherence with reporting problems to healthcare provider.
- Patient takes appropriate safety precautions for occupational injury related to the head and neck. / Awareness of safety precautions improves adherence to healthful behaviors.
- Patient exhibits good visual acuity, normal hearing, moist and intact oral mucosa, and head and neck without masses or lesions. / Patient has no abnormal findings.

2 Prepare patient. Tell him or her that you will be completing a routine examination of the head and neck to check for areas of concerns. / Understanding promotes patient's cooperation.

3 Anticipate teaching topics so that during the exam, you can instruct patient on common symptoms of eye, ear, sinus, and mouth problems, and occupational health safety. / Enables you to incorporate teaching during examination.

4 Perform hand hygiene. Assemble necessary equipment. / Prevents transmission of microorganisms. Promotes efficiency of exam.

IMPLEMENTATION

1 Position patient sitting upright if possible. / Provides for more thorough examination of head and neck structures.

2 Inspect the head.
Note head position and facial features. Look for symmetry. / Head tilting to one side may indicate hearing or visual loss. Neurologic disorders such as paralysis often affect facial symmetry.

3 Assess the eyes:
  a Inspect position of eyes, color, condition of conjunctiva, and movement. / Asymmetric positioning may reflect trauma or tumor growth. Differences in color are sometimes congenital; changes in color of conjunctiva may be the result of local infection or symptomatic of another abnormality (e.g., pale conjunctiva is associated with anemia).

  b Assess patient's near vision (ability to read newspaper or magazines) and far vision (ability to follow movement, read clock, watch television, or read signs at a distance). / A patient with visual acuity or visual field loss indicates need for supporting self-care measures (e.g., feeding, bathing, hygiene, dressing) and teaching.

  c Inspect pupils for size, shape, and equality (see illustration). / Normal pupils are round, regular, and equal in size and shape.

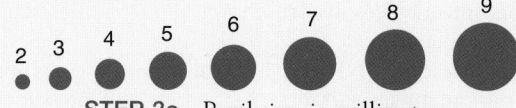

STEP 3c   Pupil sizes in millimeters.

  d Test pupillary reflexes. To test reaction to light, dim room lights. If you cannot dim lights, cup hand over eye to temporarily shield the light. As patient looks straight ahead, move penlight from side of patient's face and direct light on pupil. Observe pupillary response of both eyes, noting briskness and equality of reflex (see illustrations A and B). / Darkened room normally ensures brisk response of pupils to light. Pupil that is illuminated constricts. Pupil in other eye should constrict equally (consensual light reflex).

STEP	RATIONALE

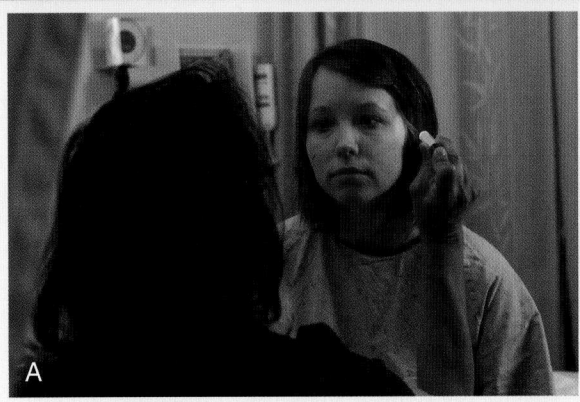 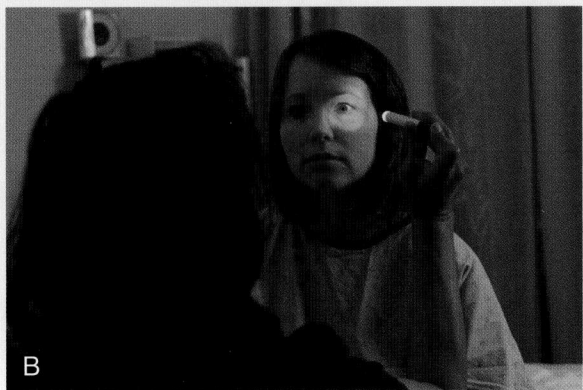

STEP 3d   A, Holding penlight to side of patient's face. **B,** Illumination of pupil causes pupillary constriction.

(1)   Test for accommodation by asking patient to focus on a distant object, which dilates the pupil. Then have the patient shift to a near object about 7 to 8 cm (3 inches) from the nose and observe for pupil constriction and convergence of the eyes. NOTE: You can also ask patient to follow an object (e.g., finger, pen) with eyes from far to near point.

Absence of constriction, convergence or an asymmetric response requires further ophthalmologic assessment (Seidel et al., 2011).

4   Assess hearing. Note patient's response to questions and presence/use of a hearing aid. If you suspect a patient has hearing loss, ask him or her to repeat random words that you state. Use one- or two-syllable words. Repeat, gradually increasing voice intensity until patient correctly repeats the words.

Patients normally hear 3 to 6 sounds clearly when whispered (Seidel et al., 2011). For patient with obvious hearing impairment, speak clearly and concisely, stand so patient can see your face, stand toward patient's good ear, use a low pitch, and avoid yelling.

Clinical Decision Point *If hearing deficit is present, have a qualified nurse inspect patient's ears because impaired hearing may be the result of impacted cerumen, external otitis, or swelling in ear canal because of allergic reactions to materials in hearing aids.*

5   Inspect nose externally for shape, skin color, alignment, drainage, and presence of deformity or inflammation. Note color of mucosa and any lesions, discharge, swelling, or presence of bleeding. If drainage appears infectious, consult with health care provider about obtaining a specimen.

Character of discharge and inflammation indicates allergy or infection. Perforation and erosion of septum and puffiness and/ or increased vascularity of mucosa indicate habitual drug use.

6   In patients with a nasogastric (NG), nasointestinal (NI), or nasotracheal tube, inspect nares for excoriation, inflammation, or discharge. Using a penlight, look up into each naris. Stabilize tube as needed.

Swallowing or coughing reflex causes movement of tubes against nares, and pressure against tissues and mucosa can result in tissue erosion.

7   Inspect sinuses by palpating gently over frontal and maxillary areas. Use thumbs to apply pressure up and under the eyebrows to assess frontal sinuses. Use thumbs to apply pressure over maxillary sinuses, about 1 inch below eyes.

Infection, allergy, or drug use sometimes causes tenderness.

8   Assess the mouth:

   a Apply clean gloves. Inspect the lips for color, texture, hydration, and lesions. Have females remove their lipstick.

Normal lips are pink, moist, symmetrical, and smooth.

   b Inspect the teeth, and note position and alignment. Note the color of teeth and presence of dental caries, tartar, and extraction sites.

Reveals quality of hygiene and discoloring effects of cola, coffee, and tobacco, Teeth are normally smooth, white, and shiny.

   c Inspect the mucosa and gums. Determine if patient wears dentures or retainers and if they are comfortable. Remove dentures to visualize and palpate gums. Use a tongue blade to lightly depress the tongue and inspect the oral cavity with a penlight (see illustration). Inspect the oral mucosa, tongue, teeth, and gums for color, hydration, texture, and obvious lesions.

Dentures and retainers can cause chronic irritation. Normal mucosa is glistening, pink, smooth and moist. Precancerous lesions can go unnoticed and progress rapidly.

   d If oral lesions are present, palpate gently with a gloved hand for tenderness, size, and consistency.

Cancerous lesions tend to be hard and non-tender.

STEP	RATIONALE

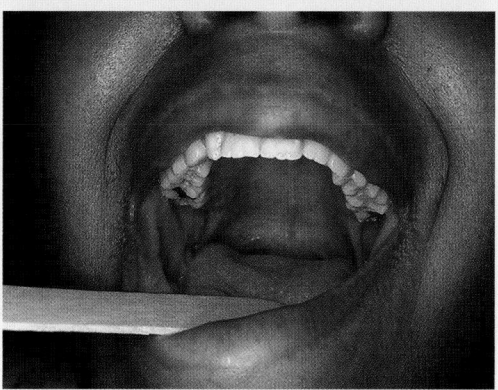

STEP 8c   Inspect mouth.

9 Inspect and palpate the neck.

  a Ask patient if there is a history of neck pain or difficulty moving the neck.

  b Neck muscles: Inspect neck for bilateral symmetry of muscles. Ask patient to flex and hyperextend neck and turn head side to side.

  c Lymph nodes.
   (1) With patient's chin raised and head tilted slightly, inspect area where lymph nodes are distributed and compare both sides (see illustration).

Assesses function of all neck structures, including neck muscles; lymph nodes; thyroid glands; and trachea.

May indicate muscle strain, head injury, local nerve injury, or swollen lymph nodes.

Detects muscle weakness, strain, and range of motion (ROM).

Lymph nodes are sometimes enlarged from infection or various diseases such as cancer.

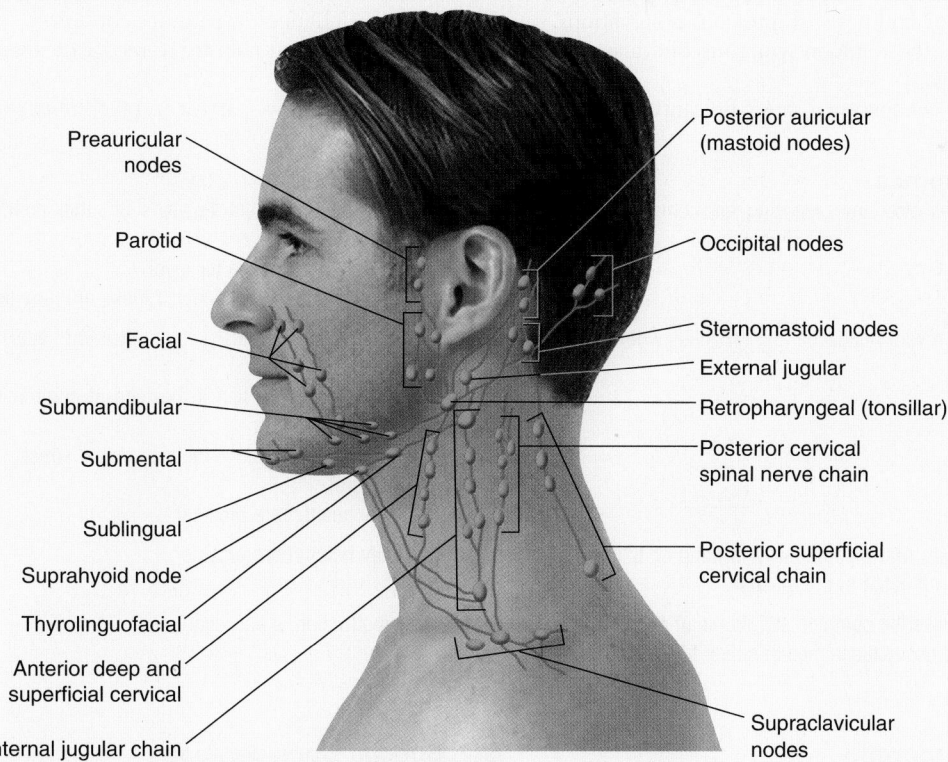

STEP 9c(1)   Palpable lymph nodes of head and neck. (*From Seidel HM et al:* Mosby's guide to physical examination, *ed 7, St Louis, 2011, Mosby.*)

   (2) To examine lymph nodes, have patient relax with neck flexed slightly forward. To palpate, face or stand to side of patient and use pads of middle three fingers of hand (see illustration). Palpate gently in a rotary motion for superficial lymph nodes.

This position relaxes tissues and muscles.

STEP	RATIONALE

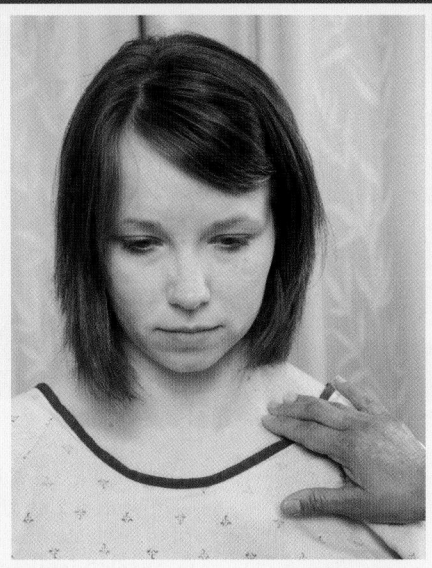

STEP 9c(2) Palpation of cervical lymph nodes.

(3) Note if lymph nodes are large, fixed, inflamed, or tender.	Large, fixed, inflamed, or tender lymph nodes indicate local infection, systemic disease, or neoplasm.
10 Remove gloves. Discard used supplies and gloves in proper receptacle. Assist patient to comfortable position. Perform hand hygiene.	Reduces transmission of infection.

EVALUATION

1 Compare assessment findings with previous observations.	Identifies changes in patient's condition.
2 Ask patient to describe common symptoms of eye, ear, sinus, or mouth disease.	Measures patient's ability to recognize abnormalities.
3 Ask patient to list occupational safety precautions.	Knowledge allows patient to take safety precautions.

Unexpected Outcomes

1 Patient has yellow nasal discharge, sneezing, and complaint of sinus pain.

2 Patient complains of severe headache and dizziness when standing.

3 Patient has mouth sore that bleeds easily, a lump or thickening in the cheek, or a white or red patch in the mucosa.

4 Patient is unable to describe common symptoms of eye, ear, sinus, and mouth problems, and occupational health safety factors.

Related Interventions

- Reposition into semi-Fowler's or other comfortable position to relieve sinus pain.
- Monitor temperature for fever.
- Notify health care provider if these are new findings.
- Respond immediately by obtaining vital signs, especially blood pressure.
- Return patient to bed in position of comfort to minimize dizziness and relieve headache.
- Identify contributing factors (e.g., stress, pain, or elevated blood pressure).
- Notify health care provider.
- Notify health care provider.
- Reinstruction is necessary.

Recording and Reporting

- Record all findings, including any abnormal findings such as hearing or visual loss, pain and its location, current infection, and character of drainage in nurses' notes, electronic health record (EHR), or flow sheet.
- Report any unexpected findings or changes to charge nurse or health care provider.

Special Considerations
Teaching

- Explain the common visual changes associated with aging, including reduced acuity (presbyopia), loss of or a reduction in peripheral vision, reduced tearing, and sensitivity to glare or bright lights. Inform patients when to seek help from an eye-care professional.

- Teach the visually impaired patient and family how to adjust room arrangements at home to promote safer ambulation. Self-help aids are available to assist patient with functioning independently with daily activities.

Pediatric

- Some infants resist eye examination by closing eyes. Using distraction encourages eye opening (Hockenberry and Wilson, 2011).
- Headaches in children are usually caused by loss of sleep, poor nutrition, eye fatigue, and allergies. Children as young as 3 years of age can develop severe migraine headaches, but the symptoms are vague and difficult to diagnose (Hockenberry and Wilson, 2011).

Gerontologic

- Older adults commonly have loss of peripheral vision caused by changes in the lens.
- Instruct patients older than age 65 to have regular hearing checks.
- Measuring visual acuity helps determine level of assistance that patient requires with daily living activities and ability of patient to safely ambulate and function independently within home.

SKILL 6-3 Thorax and Lung Assessment

Assessment of the thorax and lungs requires review of the ventilatory and respiratory functions of the lungs. It is a critical part of assessment because alterations can be life-threatening. Changes in respiration can occur quickly as a result of immobility, infection, and fluid overload. Use data from all body systems to determine the nature of pulmonary alterations. You will use inspection, palpation, and auscultation during the examination.

Before assessing the thorax and lungs, know the landmarks of the chest (Fig. 6-3, A-C). These landmarks help you identify findings and use assessment skills correctly. A patient's nipples, angle of Louis at the sternum, suprasternal notch, costal angle, clavicles, and vertebrae are key landmarks. Keep a mental image of the location of the lobes of the lung and the position of each rib (Fig. 6-4, A-C).

Locating the position of each rib is critical to visualizing the lobe of the lung being assessed. To begin, locate the angle of Louis by palpating the "speed bump" at the manubriosternal junction, where the second rib connects with the sternum. The angle is often visible and palpable. Count the ribs and intercostal spaces (between the ribs) from this point. The number of each intercostal space corresponds with that of the rib just above it. The spinous process of the third thoracic vertebra and the fourth, fifth, and sixth ribs help to locate the lung lobes laterally. The lower lobes project laterally and anteriorly (Fig. 6-4, B). Posteriorly the tip or inferior margin of the scapula lies approximately at the level of the seventh rib (Fig. 6-4, C).

During the examination, you will use auscultation to listen to breath sounds using a stethoscope. You can hear these sounds best when the person breathes deeply through the mouth. Adventitious sounds (abnormal sounds) result from air passing through fluid, mucus, or narrowed airways or from an inflammation between the pleural linings. The four types of adventitious sounds include crackles, rhonchi, wheezes, and pleural friction rubs (Table 6-6). Note the location and characteristics of the sounds, diminished breath sounds, or the absence of breath sounds. Determine where in the respiratory cycle the abnormal sounds are heard.

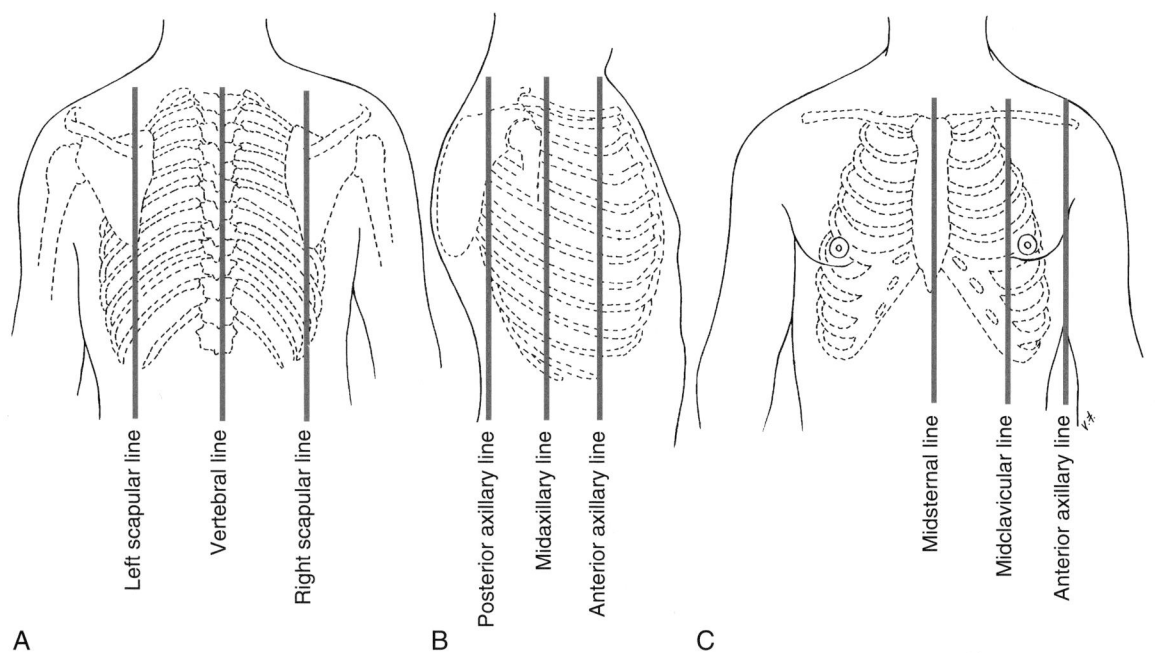

FIG 6-3 Anatomic landmarks and order of progression for examination of thorax. **A,** Posterior thorax. **B,** Anterior thorax. **C,** Lateral thorax.

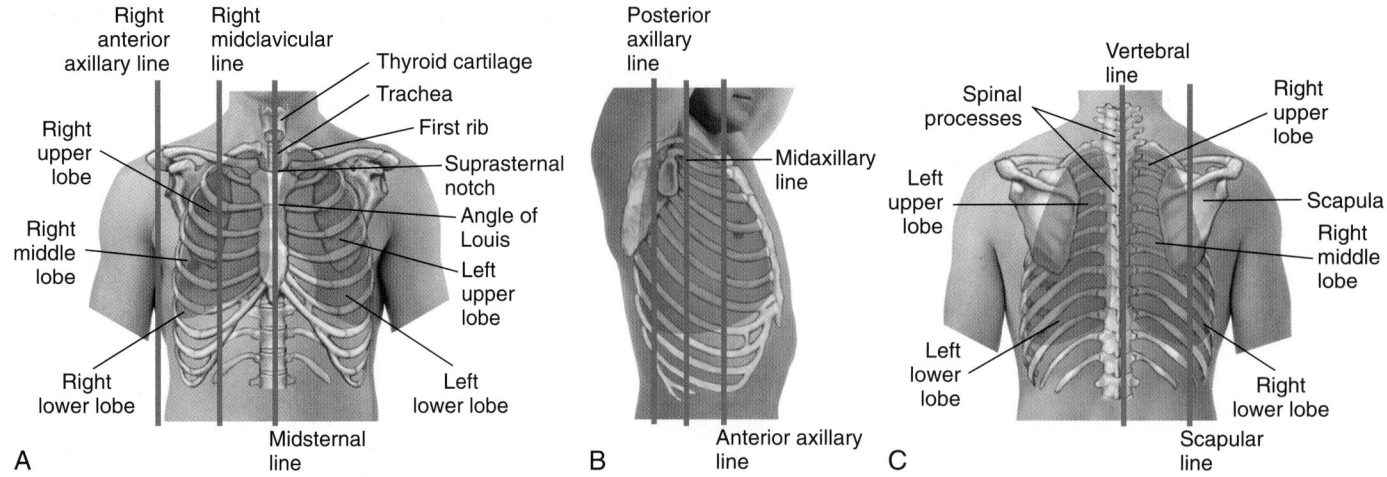

FIG 6-4 Position of lung lobes in relation to anatomical landmarks. **A,** Anterior position. **B,** Lateral position. **C,** Posterior position. (*From Seidel HM, et al: Mosby's guide to physical examination, ed 7, St Louis, 2007, Mosby.*)

TABLE 6-6	Adventitious Breath Sounds		
Sound	**Site Auscultated**	**Cause**	**Character**
Crackles (formerly called rales)	Most common in dependent lobes: right and left lung bases	Random, sudden reinflation of groups of alveoli; also related to increase in fluid in small airways	Fine, short, interrupted crackling sounds heard during end of inspiration, expiration, or both; may or may not change with coughing; sound like crushing cellophane Medium crackles: lower, moister sounds heard during middle of inspiration; not cleared with coughing Coarse crackles: loud bubbly sounds heard during inspiration; not cleared with coughing
Rhonchi (sonorous wheeze)	Heard primarily over trachea and bronchi; if loud enough, can be heard over most lung fields	Fluid or mucus in larger airways causing turbulence; muscular spasm	Loud, low-pitched, continuous sounds heard more during expiration; sometimes cleared by coughing Sound like blowing air through fluid with a straw
Wheezes (sibilant wheeze)	Heard over all lung fields but more distinct over posterior lung fields	High-velocity airflow through severely narrowed or obstructed bronchus	High-pitched, musical sounds such as a squeak heard continuously during inspiration or expiration; usually louder on expiration Do not clear with coughing
Pleural friction rub	Heard over anterior lateral lung field (if patient is sitting upright)	Inflamed pleura, parietal pleura rubbing against visceral pleura	Has grating quality heard best during inspiration; does not clear with coughing; heard loudest over lower lateral anterior surface

Data from Seidel HM et al: *Mosby's guide to physical examination*, ed 7, St Louis, 2011, Mosby.

Delegation and Collaboration

The skill of assessing the lungs and thorax cannot be delegated to nursing assistive personnel (NAP). The nurse directs the NAP to:

- Measure the patient's respirations after vital signs confirm patient is stable.
- Report respiratory distress, difficulty breathing, and changes in rate and depth.
- Keep head of bed elevated for a patient who has respiratory difficulties.

Equipment

❑ Stethoscope

STEP	RATIONALE

ASSESSMENT

1 Assess history of tobacco or marijuana use, including type of tobacco, duration (number of years), and amount in pack-years. Pack-years equal number of years smoking times the number of packs per day (e.g., 4 years × ½ pack per day equals 2 pack-years). If patient has quit, determine the length of time since smoking stopped.

Smoking is a major cause of lung cancer, heart disease, and chronic lung disease (emphysema and chronic bronchitis). Risk factors for lung cancer include history of smoking for over 20 years, exposure to environmental pollution, and secondhand smoke (ACS, 2012b).

2 Ask if patient experiences any of the following: *persistent cough* (productive or nonproductive), sputum production, *blood-streaked sputum*, *chest pain*, shortness of breath, orthopnea, dyspnea during exertion, activity intolerance, or *recurrent attacks of pneumonia or bronchitis*.

Symptoms of respiratory alterations help to localize objective physical findings. (Warning signals for lung cancer are in italics.)

3 Determine if patient works in environment containing pollutants (e.g., asbestos, arsenic, coal dust, or chemical irritants) or requiring exposure to radiation. Does patient have exposure to secondhand cigarette smoke?

Patients with chronic respiratory disease, particularly asthma, have symptoms aggravated by change in temperature and humidity, irritating fumes or smoke, emotional stress, and physical exertion.

4 Review history for known or suspected human immunodeficiency virus (HIV) infection, substance abuse, low income, residence or employment in nursing home or shelter, homelessness, recent imprisonment, being a family member of patient with tuberculosis (TB), and immigration to the United States from a country where TB is prevalent (Furlow, 2010).

These are known risk factors for exposure to and/or development of TB.

5 Ask if patient has history of persistent cough, hemoptysis (bloody sputum), unexplained weight loss, fatigue, night sweats, and/or fever.

These are signs and symptoms for both TB and HIV infection.

6 Does patient have history of chronic hoarseness?

Hoarseness indicates laryngeal disorder or abuse of cocaine or opioids (sniffing).

7 Assess for history of allergies to pollen, dust, or other airborne irritants and to any foods, drugs, or chemical substances.

Allergic response is associated with wheezing on auscultation, dyspnea, cyanosis, and diaphoresis.

8 Review family history for cancer, TB, allergies, or chronic obstructive pulmonary disease (COPD).

Familial history places patient at risk for lung disease.

NURSING DIAGNOSES

- Fatigue
- Impaired gas exchange
- Ineffective airway clearance
- Ineffective breathing pattern
- Pain (acute, chronic)
- Risk for infection

Related factors are individualized based on patient's condition or needs.

PLANNING

1 Expected outcomes following completion of procedure:

a Respirations are passive, diaphragmatic or costal, and regular (12 to 20/min in adult) with symmetric expansion.

Characteristics of normal respirations.

b Breath sounds are clear to auscultation and equal bilaterally.

Air flows without interference or obstruction. Corresponding sides should sound the same.

c Patient is able to describe factors that predispose to lung disease.

Awareness of risks can improve patient adherence to healthy behavior.

d Patient assumes appropriate posture for best breathing.

Patient can learn about benefits of good posture as examination maneuvers are performed.

2 Anticipate teaching topics so that during the exam, you can instruct patient on predisposing factors for lung disease.

Allows you to incorporate teaching during assessment process.

3 Perform hand hygiene. Assemble necessary equipment.

Prevents transmission of microorganisms. Promotes efficiency of exam.

STEP	RATIONALE

IMPLEMENTATION

1 Position and prepare patient for examination:

  a Position patient sitting upright. For bedridden patient elevate head of bed 45 to 90 degrees. If unable to tolerate sitting, use the supine and side-lying positions.

Promotes full lung expansion during examination. Patients with chronic respiratory disease may need to sit up throughout the examination because of shortness of breath. May require assistance of another caregiver to position unresponsive patients.

  b Remove gown or drape first from posterior chest, keeping front of chest and legs covered. As examination progresses, remove gown from area being examined.

Avoids unnecessary exposure and provides full visibility of thorax. Allows direct placement of diaphragm or bell on patient's skin, which enhances clarity of sounds.

  c Explain all steps of procedure, encouraging patient to relax and breathe normally through the mouth.

Anxiety alters respiratory function. Breathing through the mouth decreases extraneous sounds from air passing through the nose.

2 Posterior thorax:

  a If possible, stand behind patient. Inspect thorax for shape and symmetry. Note any deformities, position of spine, slope of ribs, or symmetric expansion during inspiration. Note the anteroposterior diameter.

Allows for identification of impairment in chest expansion and any symptoms of respiratory distress. Normal chest contour is symmetrical. In a child, the shape of chest is almost circular, with anteroposterior (AP) diameter in 1:1 ratio. In an adult the AP is one third to one half of the side-to-side diameter. Chronic lung disease causes ribs to be more horizontal and increases AP diameter, resulting in a "barrel chest." Patients with breathing problems assume postures that improve ventilation.

Clinical Decision Point *When a patient holds the chest wall during breathing, this indicates localized chest pain. Assess the nature of pain, including onset, severity, precipitating factors, quality, region, and radiation.*

  b Determine the rate and rhythm of breathing (see Chapter 5). Examine the thorax as a whole. Have patient relax.

This is a good time to count respirations, with patient relaxed and unaware of inspection. Awareness could alter respirations.

  c Systematically palpate the thoracic muscles and skeleton for lumps, masses, pulsations, and unusual movement (see illustration). If the patient voices pain or tenderness, avoid deep palpation. If there is a suspicious mass, palpate lightly for shape, size, and qualities of a lesion (see Skill 6-1). Do not palpate painful areas deeply.

Palpation assesses further characteristics and confirms or supplements findings from inspection. Localized swelling or tenderness indicates trauma to ribs or underlying cartilage. A fractured rib fragment could be displaced.

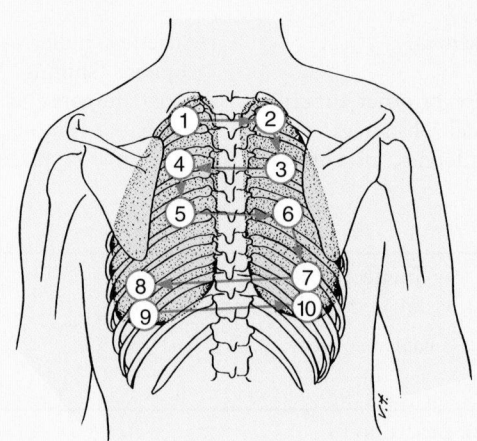

STEP 2c   Pattern for assessment of posterior thorax.

STEP	RATIONALE

d Assess chest excursion by standing behind patient and placing thumbs along spinal processes at tenth rib, with palms lightly contacting posterolateral surfaces (see illustration A). Keep thumbs about 5 cm (2 inches) apart, with thumbs pointing toward spine and fingers pointing laterally. Press hands toward patient's spine to form small skinfold between thumbs. After exhalation patient takes deep breath. Note movement of thumbs (see illustration B) and symmetry of chest wall movement. Normally symmetric separation of thumbs occurs during chest excursion 3 to 5 cm (1½ to 2 inches).

Palpation of chest excursion assesses depth of patient's breathing. This technique is good measure to evaluate patient's ability to perform deep-breathing exercises (see Chapter 36). Limited movement on one side indicates that patient is voluntarily splinting during ventilation because of pain. Avoid allowing hands to slide over the skin, which gives a false measure of excursion.

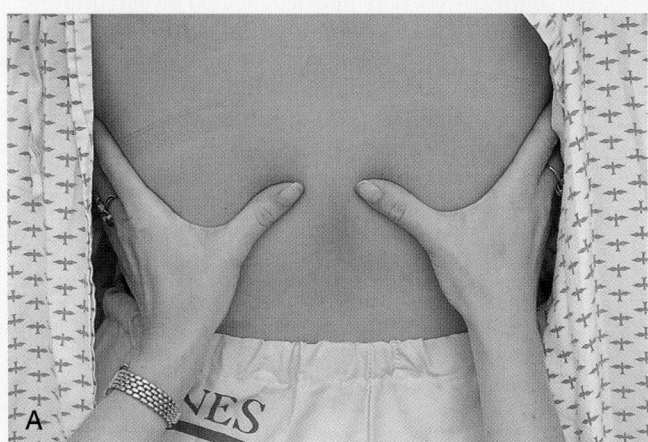
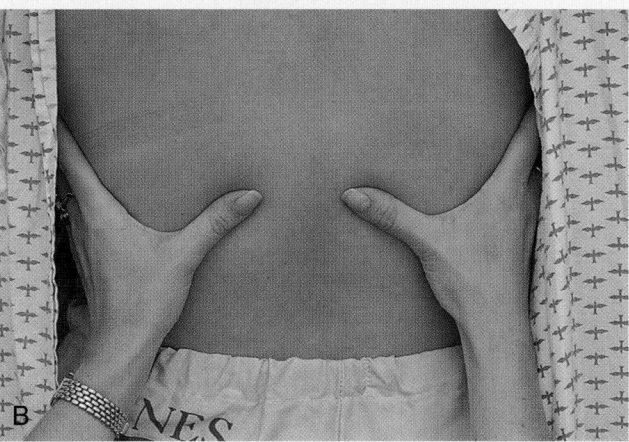

STEP 2d **A,** Position of hands for palpation of posterior thorax excursion. **B,** As patient inhales, movement of chest excursion separates nurse's thumbs.

e Auscultate breath sounds. Instruct patient to take slow, deep breaths with mouth slightly open. Place diaphragm of stethoscope firmly on skin, over the posterior chest wall and the intercostal spaces (see illustration). Have the patient fold arms in front of the chest and keep the head bent forward. Listen to an entire inspiration and expiration at each stethoscope position (see pattern in Step 2c.) If sounds are faint, as in obese patients, ask the person to breathe harder and faster temporarily. Systematically compare breath sounds over right and left sides, listening for normal and adventitious sounds.

Assesses movement of air through tracheobronchial tree (Table 6-7). Recognition of normal airflow sounds allows detection of sounds caused by mucus or airway obstruction. Characterize sounds by length of inspiratory and expiratory phases.

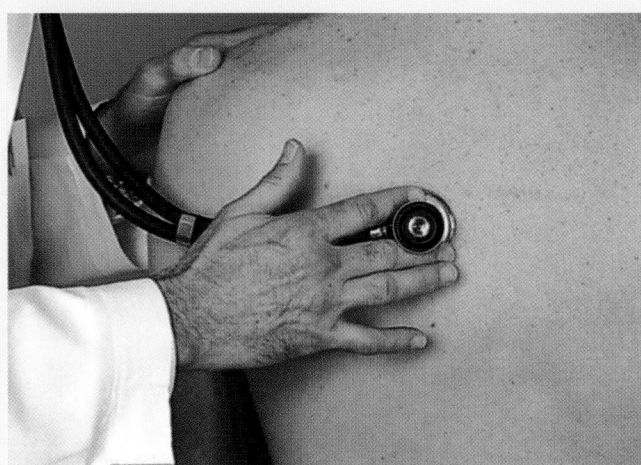

STEP 2e Use of diaphragm of stethoscope to auscultate breath sounds. (*From Seidel HM et al: Mosby's guide to physical examination, ed 6, St Louis, 2006, Mosby.*)

STEP	RATIONALE
f If you auscultate adventitious sounds, have patient cough. Listen again with stethoscope to determine if sound has cleared with coughing. See Table 6-7 for a description of adventitious breath sounds.	Coughing may clear adventitious sounds. Rhonchi often are eliminated or altered by coughing. Crackles and wheezes are not.
3 Lateral thorax:	
a Instruct patient to raise arms and inspect chest wall for same characteristics as reviewed for posterior chest.	Improves access to lateral thoracic structures.
b Extend palpation and auscultation of posterior thorax to lateral sides of chest, except for excursion measurement (see illustration).	Locates abnormalities in lateral lung fields.
4 Anterior thorax:	
a Inspect accessory muscles of breathing: sternocleidomastoid, trapezius, and abdominal muscles, noting effort to breathe.	Extent to which accessory muscles are used reveals degree of effort to breathe. The accessory muscles move little with normal passive breathing. Patients who require great effort and rely on these muscles may produce a grunting sound.
b Inspect width or spread of costal angle made by costal margins and tip of sternum. Angle is usually larger than 90 degrees between margins.	Indicates congenital, acquired, or traumatic alterations that may influence patient's chest expansion.
c Observe patient's breathing pattern, observing symmetry and degree of chest wall and abdominal movement. Respiratory rate and rhythm are more often assessed on anterior chest wall.	Assesses patient's effort to breathe: symmetric, passive movement indicates no respiratory distress. Male patient's breathing is diaphragmatic, while female's is more costal.
d Palpate anterior thoracic muscles and ribs for lumps, masses, tenderness, or unusual movement, following a systematic pattern across and down (see illustration).	Localized swelling or tenderness indicates trauma to underlying ribs or cartilage.

TABLE 6-7	**Normal Breath Sounds**		
Type	**Description**	**Location**	**Origin**
Bronchial	Loud and high-pitched sounds with hollow quality Expiration lasts longer than inspiration (3:2 ratio).	Best heard over trachea	Created by air moving through trachea close to chest wall
Bronchovesicular	Medium-pitched and blowing sounds of medium intensity Inspiratory phase equal to expiratory phase	Best heard posteriorly between scapulae and anteriorly over bronchioles lateral to sternum at first and second intercostal spaces	Created by air moving through large airways
Vesicular	Soft, breezy, and low-pitched sounds Inspiratory phase 3 times longer than expiratory phase	Best heard over periphery of lung (except over scapula)	Created by air moving through smaller airways

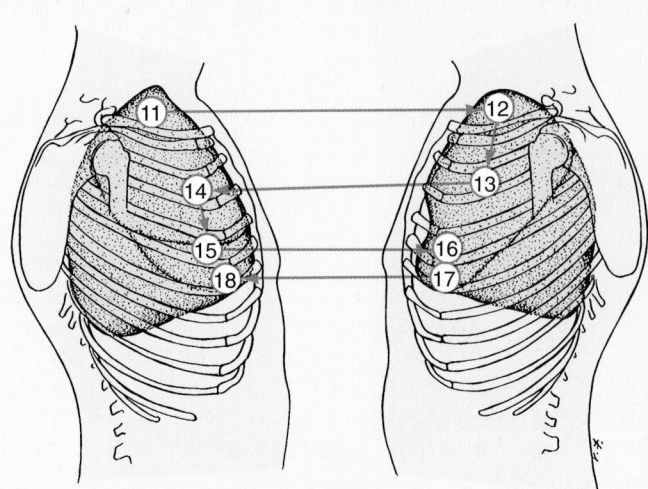

STEP 3b   Pattern for assessment of lateral thorax.

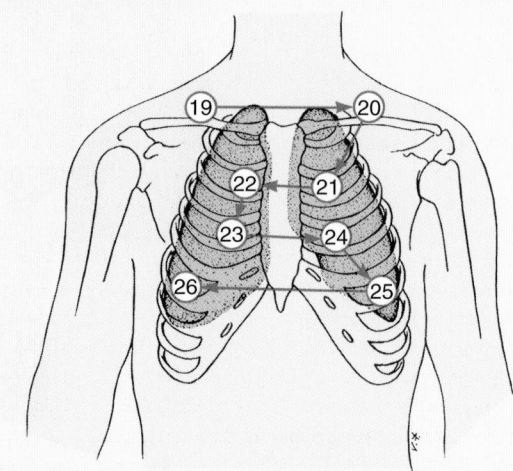

STEP 4d   Pattern for assessment of anterior chest.

STEP	RATIONALE
e Palpate anterior chest excursion. Place hands over each lateral rib cage, with thumbs approximately 5 cm (2 inches) apart and angled along each costal margin. As patient inhales deeply, thumbs should symmetrically move apart 3 to 5 cm (1½ to 2 inches), with each side expanding equally.	Assesses depth of patient's breathing and ability to perform deep-breathing exercises. Certain abnormalities are evident if expansion is not symmetric.
f With patient sitting, auscultate anterior thorax. Begin above clavicles; move across and then down as during palpation. Compare right and left sides. Give special attention to lower lobes, where mucus commonly gathers.	A systematic pattern of assessment comparing sides helps to identify abnormal sounds.
5 Clean and store stethoscope. Perform hand hygiene.	Reduces transmission of infection.

EVALUATION

1 Compare respiratory findings with assessment characteristics for thorax and lungs.	Determines presence of abnormalities.
2 Have patient identify factors leading to lung disease.	Demonstrates learning.

Unexpected Outcomes	Related Interventions
1 Patient has copious mucus production; audible inspiratory wheezing; or congested cough with thick mucus.	• Help patient cough by splinting chest; teach to inhale slowly through nose, exhale, and cough; encourage expectoration of mucus. • Auscultate breath sounds before and after cough to evaluate cough effectiveness. • Auscultate lungs for adventitious sounds. • Encourage increased oral intake (if permitted). • If unable to clear airway by coughing, suctioning may be indicated (see Chapter 25). • Monitor vital signs. • Notify health care provider.
2 Respirations are rapid or slow and irregular (see Chapter 5), and bulging of intercostal spaces is present.	• Position patient more upright if appropriate. • Auscultate lungs for adventitious sounds. • Notify health care provider.
3 Chest excursion is reduced. Depth of breathing is reduced by pain, postural deformity, or fatigue.	• Reposition patient more comfortably. • Administer analgesic if appropriate.
4 Patient is unfamiliar with risks for lung disease.	• Education is necessary.

Recording and Reporting

- Record patient's respiratory rate and character; breath sounds, including type, location, and presence on inspiration, expiration, or both; changes noted after coughing; and other physical assessment findings in nurses' notes, EHR, or flow sheet.
- Report abnormalities immediately to nurse in charge or health care provider.

Special Considerations
Teaching

- Educate patients about risks of cigarette smoking. Smoking accounts for at least 30% of all cancer deaths and 80% of lung cancer deaths (ACS, 2012b) Individuals who stop smoking have the potential to live longer than those who continue to smoke. The probability of these individuals dying from lung cancer or other related causes continues to decline with further abstinence.
- Explain to patients that exposure to radiation, arsenic, and asbestos from occupational, medical, and environmental sources; air pollution; history of TB, and secondhand smoke contribute significantly to lung cancer (ACS, 2012b).
- Discuss with patients the warning signs of lung cancer such as a persistent cough, sputum streaked with blood, chest pains, and recurrent attacks of pneumonia or bronchitis.

Pediatric

- In children observe for use of accessory muscles, which indicate respiratory distress. Retractions may involve intercostal, suprasternal, supraclavicular, or sternal muscles (Hockenberry and Wilson, 2011).
- Use the bell of the stethoscope to auscultate lung sounds in children. Breath sounds are louder in children because of their thin chest walls.
- Children younger than 7 years of age normally exhibit noticeable abdominal or diaphragmatic movement. Older children and adults exhibit more costal or thoracic movement.
- Head bobbing and nasal flaring in infants are signs of significant respiratory distress (Hockenberry and Wilson, 2011).

Gerontologic

- Older adults have a costal angle (anteriorly) of slightly less than 90 degrees. The AP diameter sometimes increases from kyphosis.
- In older adults chest expansion is reduced because of calcification of rib cartilage and partial contraction of inspiratory muscles.
- Individuals with chronic or immunosuppressing conditions, including asthma, should receive the pneumococcal vaccine before age 64. Individuals who received the vaccine before age 65 should receive another dose at age 65 or 5 years after the previous dose. Those who receive the vaccine at or after age 65 should receive only a singe dose. There is no indication to revaccinate (CDC, 2010).

SKILL 6-4 Cardiovascular Assessment

A patient who presents with signs or symptoms of heart (cardiac) problems such as chest pain may be suffering a life-threatening condition requiring immediate attention. In this situation you act quickly and perform the portions of the examination that are absolutely necessary. Conduct a more thorough assessment when the patient is more stable. This will reveal baseline heart function and any risks for heart disease. Patients tend to seek information about heart disease because it remains a leading cause of death in the United States. The heart, neck vessels, and peripheral circulation are assessed together because the systems work in unison.

Your assessment can determine the integrity of the circulatory system. Inadequate tissue perfusion results in an inadequate delivery of oxygen and nutrients to cells, a condition called *ischemia*. This is caused by constriction of vessels or occlusion (blockage) from clot formation. The effects of ischemia depend on the duration of the problem and the metabolic needs of the tissues. Ischemia results in pain. If lack of oxygen to tissues is unrelieved, tissue necrosis (death) occurs. An embolus is a blood clot that breaks loose and travels through the circulation. If the clot obstructs circulation to the lungs or brain, it can be life threatening.

You begin assessment of the heart after examining the lungs because the patient is already in a suitable position with the chest exposed. Assessment then proceeds to the neck vessels and ends with evaluating peripheral circulation. The skills of inspection, palpation, auscultation, and percussion are used during the examination.

Delegation and Collaboration
The skill of completing a comprehensive cardiovascular assessment cannot be delegated to nursing assistive personnel (NAP). The nurse directs the NAP to:
- Count peripheral pulses after vital signs confirm patient is stable.
- Recognize skin temperature and color changes of affected extremities and report any changes to the nurse.
- Recognize changes in peripheral pulses and report any changes to the nurse.

Equipment
- ❑ Stethoscope
- ❑ Doppler stethoscope (optional)
- ❑ Conducting gel (if a Doppler stethoscope is used)
- ❑ Gloves

STEP	RATIONALE

ASSESSMENT

1 Assess patient for history of smoking, alcohol intake, caffeine intake (e.g., coffee, tea, soft drinks, energy drinks, and chocolate), and use of "recreational" drugs. Determine exercise habits and dietary patterns and intake.

These contribute to risk factors for cardiovascular disease. In addition, caffeine and alcohol cause tachycardia. Insufficient exercise and intake of fatty and salty foods increase risk for cardiovascular disease.

2 Determine if patient is taking medications for cardiovascular function (e.g., antiarrhythmics, antihypertensives, beta-blockers, antianginals) and if patient knows their purpose, dosage, and side effects.

Allows you to assess patient's adherence to and understanding of drug therapies. Medications for cardiovascular function cannot be taken intermittently.

3 Ask if patient has experienced dyspnea, chest pain or discomfort, palpitations, excess fatigue, cough, leg pain or cramps, edema of the feet, cyanosis, fainting, and orthopnea. Ask if symptoms occur at rest or during exercise.

These are the cardinal symptoms of heart disease. Cardiovascular function is sometimes adequate during rest but not during exercise.

4 If patient reports chest pain, determine onset (sudden or gradual), precipitating factors, quality, region, severity, and if it radiates. Anginal pain is usually a deep pressure or ache that is substernal and diffuse, radiating to one or both arms, neck, or jaw.

Symptoms reveal acute coronary syndrome (ACS) or coronary artery disease (CAD).

5 Assess family history for heart disease, diabetes mellitus, high cholesterol and/or lipid levels, hypertension, stroke, or rheumatic heart disease.

Family history of these conditions increases risk for heart and vascular disease.

6 Ask patient about a history of any preexisting heart conditions (e.g., heart failure, congenital heart disease, CAD, dysrhythmias, or murmurs), heart surgery, or vascular disease (e.g., hypertension, phlebitis, varicose veins).

Knowledge reveals patient's level of understanding of condition. A preexisting condition influences which examination techniques to use and the expected findings.

7 Determine if patient experiences leg cramps; numbness or tingling in extremities; sensation of cold hands or feet; pain in legs; or swelling or cyanosis of feet, ankles, or hand.

These are signs and symptoms of vascular disease.

8 If patient experiences leg pain or cramping in lower extremities, ask if it is relieved by walking or standing for long periods or if it occurs during sleep.

Relationship of symptoms to exercise clarifies if problem is vascular or musculoskeletal. Pain caused by vascular condition tends to increase with activity. Musculoskeletal pain is usually not relieved when exercise ends.

9 Ask women if they wear tight-fitting underwear or hosiery and sit or lie in bed with legs crossed.

Tight hosiery around lower extremities and crossing legs can impair venous return, promoting clot formation.

STEP	RATIONALE

NURSING DIAGNOSES

- Activity intolerance
- Decreased cardiac output
- Deficient knowledge

- Ineffective peripheral tissue perfusion
- Pain (acute, chronic)

- Risk for peripheral neurovascular dysfunction

Related factors are individualized based on patient's condition or needs.

PLANNING

1 Expected outcomes following completion of procedure:

- Heart rate is 60 to 100 beats/min (adolescent through adult), without extra sounds or murmurs.

  Indicates normal rate and sinus rhythm.

- Point of maximal impulse (PMI) is palpable at fifth intercostal space at left midclavicular line in children older than 7 years of age and adults.

  Indicates normal heart position.

- Patient describes changes in own behavior that could improve cardiovascular function.

  Information may improve patient's health behavior habits.

- Patient describes schedule, dosage, purpose, and benefits of medications being taken for cardiovascular function.

  Information related to health benefits may improve adherence to therapy.

- Blood pressure is within normal limits for patient (see Chapter 5).

  This is one indicator of normal cardiovascular function.

- Carotid pulse is localized, strong, elastic, and equal bilaterally. No change occurs during inspiration or expiration; without carotid bruit.

  This indicates a patent vessel.

- Jugular veins distend when patient lies supine and flatten when patient is in sitting position.

  Venous pressure is normal.

- Peripheral pulses are equal and strong (2+); extremities are warm and pink, with capillary refill less than 2 seconds. There is no dependent edema. Peripheral hair growth is symmetric and evenly distributed, and the skin is free of lesions.

  Peripheral circulation is intact.

2 Anticipate teaching topics so that during the exam, you can instruct patient on risks for heart and vascular disease.

   Allows you to incorporate teaching during examination.

3 Perform hand hygiene. Prepare necessary supplies.

   Reduces transmission of infection. Promotes efficient examination.

IMPLEMENTATION

1 Help patient be as relaxed and comfortable as possible.

   An anxious or uncomfortable patient can have mild tachycardia, which alters findings.

2 Have patient assume semi-Fowler's or supine position.

   Provides adequate visibility and access to left thorax and mediastinum. Patient with heart disease often experiences shortness of breath while lying flat.

3 Explain procedure. Avoid facial gestures reflecting concern.

   Patients with previously normal cardiac history may become anxious if you show concern.

4 Be sure that room is quiet.

   Subtle, low-pitched heart sounds are difficult to hear.

5 Assess the heart:

   a Form a mental image of the exact location of the heart (see illustration). The base of the heart is the upper portion, and the apex is the bottom tip. The surface of the right ventricle constitutes most of the anterior surface of the heart.

   Visualization improves ability to assess findings accurately and determines possible source of abnormalities.

   b Find the angle of Louis, felt as a ridge in the sternum approximately 5 cm (2 inches) below the suprasternal notch (between the sternal body and the manubrium). Slip fingers down each side of angle to feel adjacent ribs. The intercostal spaces are just below each rib.

   Provides you with landmarks to locate and assess heart sounds.

   c Find the following anatomic landmarks (see illustration):

   Familiarity with landmarks allows you to describe findings more clearly and ultimately may improve assessment.

STEP	RATIONALE

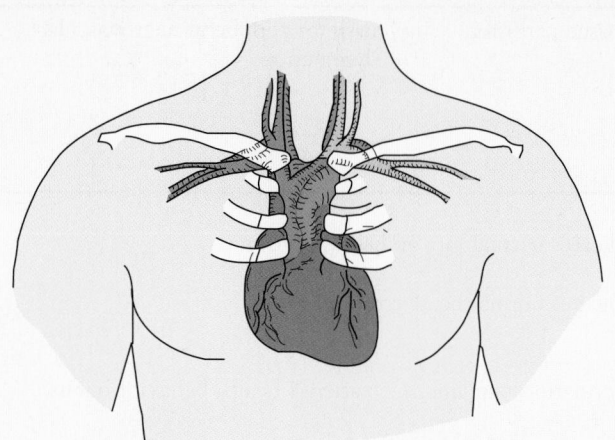

STEP 5a   Anatomic position of heart.

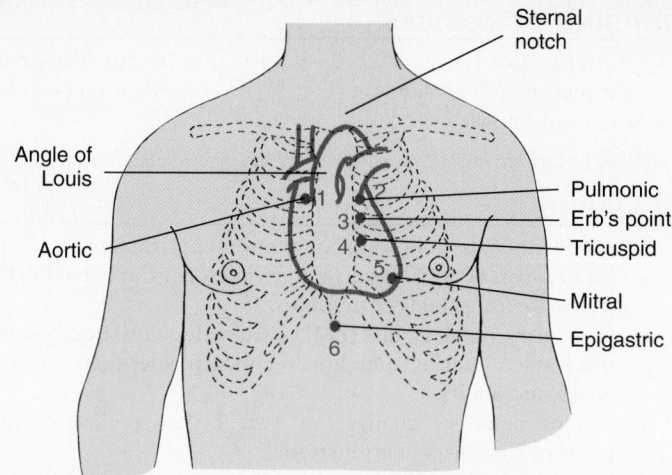

STEP 5c   Anatomic sites for assessment of cardiac function.

(1)   The aortic area is at the second intercostal space, right of patient's sternum, close to the sternal border *(1)*.

(2)   The pulmonic area is at the second intercostal space, left of patient's sternum, close to the sternal border *(2)*.

(3)   The second pulmonic area is found by moving down the left side of the sternum to the third intercostal space, close to the sternal border *(3)*, also referred to as *Erb's point.*

(4)   The tricuspid area *(4)* is located at the fourth left intercostal space along the sternum, close to the sternal border.

(5)   The mitral area is found by moving fingers laterally to patient's left to locate fifth intercostal space at left midclavicular line *(5)*.

(6)   The epigastric area *(6)* is at the inferior tip of the sternum.

Listening to the heart sounds from too far away from the sternal border decreases the ability to hear them clearly.

d   Stand to patient's right to inspect and palpate the precordium with patient supine. Note any visible pulsations and more exaggerated lifts. Closely inspect the area of the apex. Palpate for pulsations (placing proximal half of four fingers together and then alternating with ball of hand at all anatomic landmarks).

Reveals size and symmetry of the heart. The apical impulse may be visible at the midclavicular line in the fifth intercostal space. The apical impulse (PMI) may become visible only when the patient sits up, bringing the heart closer to the anterior wall. Obesity obscures the ability to visualize the PMI. There should be no pulsations or vibrations. A thrill is a continuous palpable sensation, such as the purring of a cat. A thrust is the upward lift felt when palpating the chest wall.

STEP	RATIONALE

e Locate the PMI by palpating with fingertips along the fifth intercostal space in midclavicular line (see illustration). Note a light, brief pulsation in an area 1 to 2 cm (½ to 1 inch) in diameter at the apex.

In the presence of serious heart disease, the PMI is located to the left of the midclavicular line related to the enlarged left ventricle. In chronic lung disease the PMI may be to the right of the midclavicular line as a result of right ventricular enlargement.

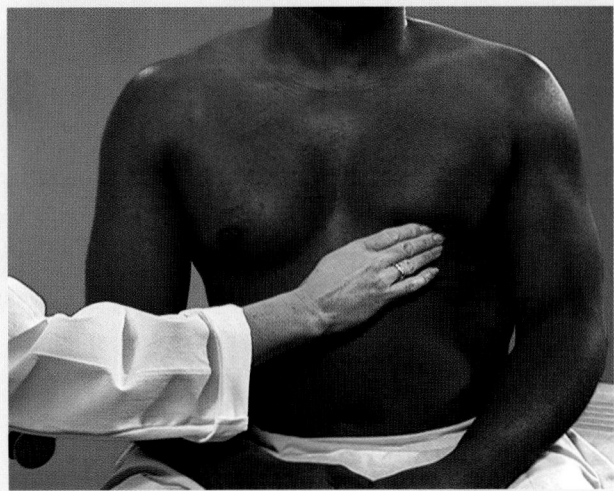

STEP 5e Palpation of point of maximal impulse. (*From Seidel HM et al: Mosby's guide to physical examination, ed 7, St Louis, 2011, Mosby.*)

Clinical Decision Point *Presence of a palpable thrill is not normal and indicates a disruption of blood flow caused by a defect in closure of a heart valve or atrial septal defect. Report to health care provider.*

Clinical Decision Point *A stronger than expected impulse is a heave or lift, which indicates increased cardiac output or left ventricular hypertrophy. Report to health care provider.*

f If palpating PMI is difficult, turn patient onto left side.

Maneuver moves the heart closer to the chest wall.

g Inspect epigastric area and palpate abdominal aorta. Note you should feel a localized strong beat.

Rules out reduced blood flow or diffuse pulse, which indicates an abnormality.

h Auscultate heart sounds.

Different positions help to clarify type of sounds heard. Sitting position is best to hear high-pitched murmurs (if present). Supine is a common position to hear all sounds. Left lateral recumbent is the best position to hear low-pitched sounds.

  (1) Have patient sit up and lean slightly forward; then have him or her lie supine; and end the examination with patient in a left lateral recumbent position (see illustration A to C). In a female patient it may be necessary to lift the left breast to hear heart sounds more effectively.

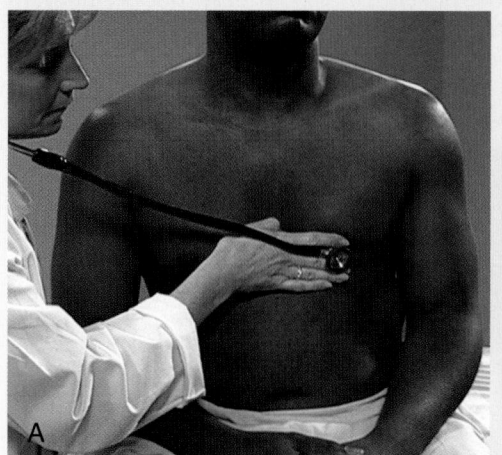
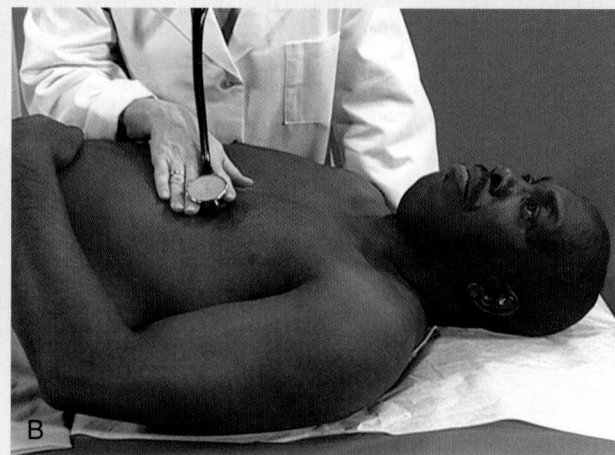
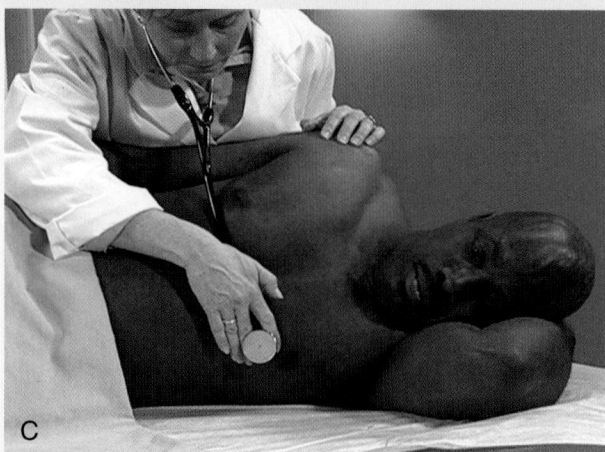

STEP 5h(1) Patient positions for auscultation of heart sounds. **A,** Sitting. **B,** Supine. **C,** Left lateral. *(From Seidel HM et al: Mosby's guide to physical examination, ed 7, St Louis, 2011, Mosby.)*

(2) While auscultating sounds at each anatomic landmark, ask patient not to speak but to breathe comfortably. Begin with the diaphragm of the stethoscope; alternate with the bell. Use very light pressure for the bell. Inch the stethoscope along; avoid jumping from one area to another. Do not try to hear all heart sounds at once.

Auscultation requires you to isolate each heart sound at all auscultation sites, especially in patients with soft heart sounds.

(3) Begin at the apex or PMI; move systematically to the aortic area, pulmonic area, Erb's point, tricuspid area, and mitral area (see illustration in Step 5c). (NOTE: Some examiners use reverse sequence.) S_1 is loudest at the apex and is simultaneous with the carotid pulse. NOTE: a helpful mnemonic for remembering heart sound locations: **A P**ig **E**ats **T**oo **M**uch (Aortic, Pulmonic, Erb's point, Tricuspid, Mitral).

At normal slow rates S_1 is high pitched and dull in quality and sounds like a "lub." This sound precedes the systolic phase of heart contraction.

(4) Listen for S_2 at each site. This sound is loudest at the aortic area. Heart sounds vary by pitch, loudness, and duration, depending on the auscultatory site (Table 6-8).

Normal sounds S_1 and S_2 are high pitched and best heard with the diaphragm. S_2 precedes the diastolic phase and sounds like "dub."

(5) After both sounds are heard clearly as "lub-dub," count each combination of S_1 and S_2 as one heartbeat. Count the number of beats for 1 minute.

Determines apical pulse rate.

STEP	RATIONALE

(6) Assess heart rhythm by noting the time between S_1 and S_2 (systole) and then the time between S_2 and the next S_1 (diastole). Listen to the full cycle at each auscultation area. Note regular intervals between each sequence of beats. There should be a distinct pause between S_1 and S_2.

Failure of heart to beat at regular intervals is a dysrhythmia, which interferes with the ability of the heart to pump effectively.

(7) When the heart rate is irregular, compare apical and radial pulses (Table 6-9). Auscultate the apical pulse and then immediately palpate the radial pulse. A colleague can assess the radial pulse while assess the apical pulse.

Determines if a pulse deficit (radial pulse is slower than apical) exists. Deficit indicates that ineffective contractions of the heart fail to send pulse waves to the periphery.

i Auscultate for extra heart sounds at each site. Note pitch, loudness, duration, timing, location on chest wall, and where it is heard in cardiac cycle.

Abnormal sounds include murmurs. Characteristics of murmurs help to identify contributing factors.

(1) Use the stethoscope bell and listen for low-pitched extra heart sounds such as S_3 and S_4 gallops, clicks, and rubs. S_3, or a ventricular gallop, occurs just after S_2 at the end of ventricular diastole. It sounds like "lub-dub-ee" or "Ken-tuc-ky." S_4, or an atrial gallop, occurs just before S_1 or ventricular systole. It sounds like "dee-lub-dub" or "Ten-nes-see."

Premature rush of blood into a ventricle that is stiff or dilated or an atrial contraction pushing against a ventricle that is not accepting blood causes gallops.

(2) With patient leaning forward or lying on the left side, listen for friction rubs as "squeaky" or rubbing sounds.

Rubs result from lungs or inflamed visceral and parietal layers of the pericardium of the heart rubbing against one another.

TABLE 6-8 | Heart Sounds According to Auscultatory Area

	Aortic	Pulmonic	Second Pulmonic	Mitral	Tricuspid
Pitch	$S_1 < S_2$	$S_1 < S_2$	$S_1 < S_2$	$S_1 > S_2$	$S_1 = S_2$
Loudness	$S_1 < S_2$	$S_1 < S_2$	$S_1 < S_2$*	$S_1 > S_2$†	$S_1 > S_2$
Duration	$S_1 > S_2$	$S_1 > S_2$	$S_1 > S_2$	$S_1 > S_2$	$S_1 > S_2$

Modified from Seidel HM et al: *Mosby's guide to physical examination*, ed 7, St Louis, 2011, Mosby.
*S_1 is relatively louder in second pulmonic area than in aortic area.
†S_1 may be louder in mitral area than in tricuspid area.

TABLE 6-9 | Abnormalities in Rates and Rhythms

Type	Findings	Description
Atrial fibrillation	Rapid, random contractions of atria cause irregular ventricular beats >100 beats/min and atrial beats at 200-350 beats/min	Atria discharge very rapidly, with some impulses not reaching ventricles. This condition occurs in rheumatic heart disease and mitral stenosis. It causes reduced cardiac output.
Sinus arrhythmia	Pulse rate changes during respiration, increasing at peak of inspiration and decreasing during expiration.	Blood is momentarily trapped in lungs during inspiration, causing a fall in stroke volume of heart.
Sinus bradycardia	Pulse rhythm is regular, but rate is <60 beats/min.	Sinoatrial node fires less frequently. This is common in well-conditioned athletes and with use of antiarrhythmic medications.
Sinus tachycardia	Pulse rhythm is regular, but rate is accelerated to >100 beats/min.	Exercise, emotional stress, and caffeine or alcohol ingestion are common factors that cause increased firing of sinoatrial node.
Premature ventricular contraction	Premature beat occurs before regularly expected heart contraction. Underlying rhythm can be any rate.	Ventricle contracts prematurely because of electrical impulse bypassing normal conduction pathway. It may occur so early that it is difficult to detect as second beat. It may be followed by a pause.

STEP	RATIONALE
j Auscultate for heart murmurs over each of the auscultation sites.	Murmurs are sustained swishing or blowing sounds heard at the beginning, middle, or end of systole or diastole. Increased blood flow through a normal valve, forward flow through a stenotic valve or into a dilated vessel or chamber, or backward flow through a valve that fails to close causes murmurs.
(1) When you detect a murmur, listen carefully to note where you hear it best. Note the intensity of the murmur.	Intensity is related to rate of blood flow through the heart or the amount of blood regurgitated.
(2) Note if the murmur is low, medium, or high in pitch, using the bell for low-pitched sounds.	Pitch depends on velocity of blood flow through the valves.
6 Assess neck vessels:	
a To assess carotid arteries: have patient remain in sitting position.	Allows easier mobility of neck to expose artery for inspection and palpation.
b Inspect neck on both sides for obvious arterial pulsations. Sometimes a pulse wave can be seen.	Carotids are the only sites to assess quality of pulse wave (see illustration). Experience is required to evaluate wave in relation to events of cardiac cycle.
c Palpate each carotid artery separately with index and middle fingers around medial edge of sternocleidomastoid muscle. Ask patient to raise chin slightly, keeping the head straight (see illustration) or slightly away from artery. Note rate and rhythm, strength, and elasticity of artery. Also note if pulse changes as patient inhales and exhales.	If both arteries were occluded simultaneously, patient could lose consciousness from reduced circulation to the brain. Turning the head improves access to artery. A change indicates a sinus arrhythmia.

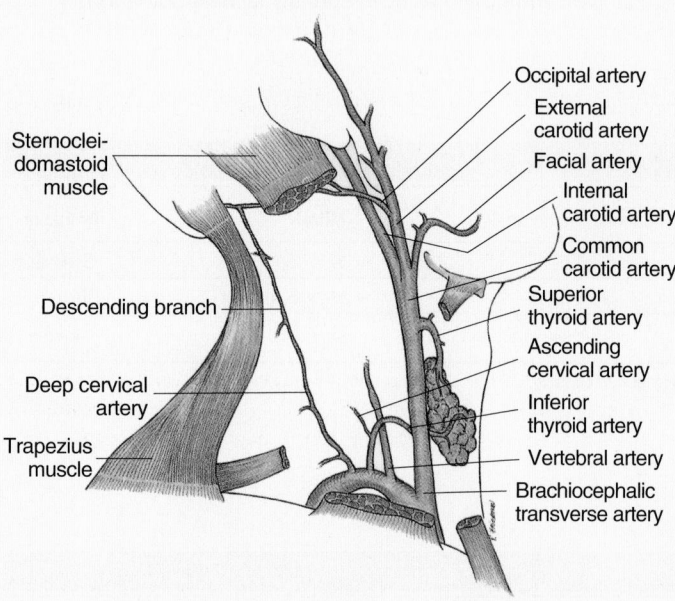

STEP 6b   Anatomic position of carotid artery.

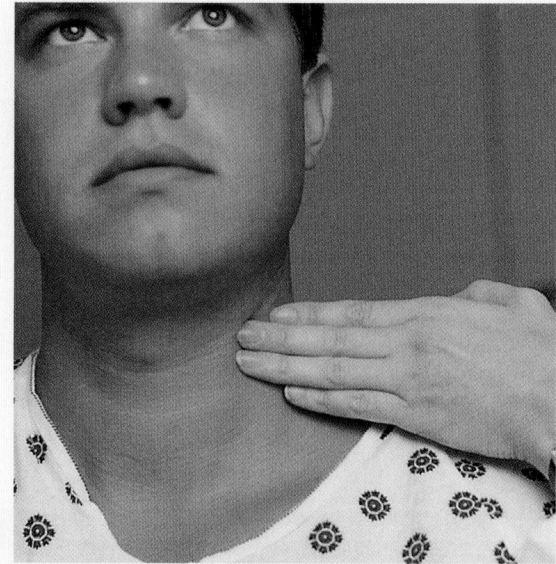

STEP 6c   Palpate each carotid artery separately.

Clinical Decision Point *Do not palpate or massage the carotid artery vigorously. Stimulation of carotid sinus causes a reflex drop in heart rate and blood pressure.*

d Place bell of stethoscope over each carotid artery, auscultating for blowing sound (bruit) (see illustration). Ask patient to hold a breath for a few heartbeats so respiratory sounds do not interfere with auscultation (Seidel et al., 2011).	Narrowing of the lumen of the carotid artery by arteriosclerotic plaques causes disturbance in blood flow. Blood passing through narrowed section creates turbulence and emits blowing or swishing sound. Normally you do not hear a bruit.

STEP	RATIONALE

e To assess jugular venous pressure (JVP), have patient assume a supine position. Raise the head of the bed 45 degrees, avoiding neck hyperextension or flexion. Locate the highest point along the internal jugular vein where a pulsation can be seen (good lighting helps). Locate the sternal angle with a centimeter ruler and measure the vertical distance between the sternal angle and the meniscus of the internal jugular vein (see illustration).

Normal veins are flat when patient is sitting, and pulsations become evident as you lower patient's head. A height of pulsation greater than 2.5 cm (1 inch) indicates fluid overload or right-sided heart failure.

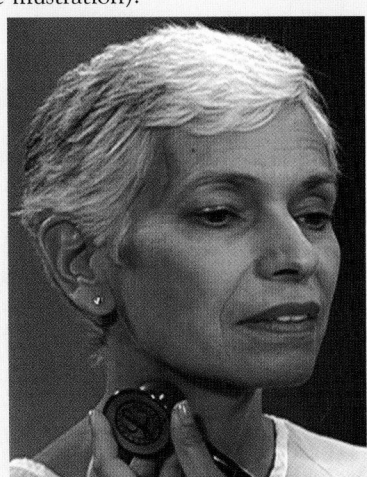

STEP 6d Auscultation for carotid artery bruit. (*From Seidel HM et al: Mosby's guide to physical examination, ed 7, St Louis, 2011, Mosby.*)

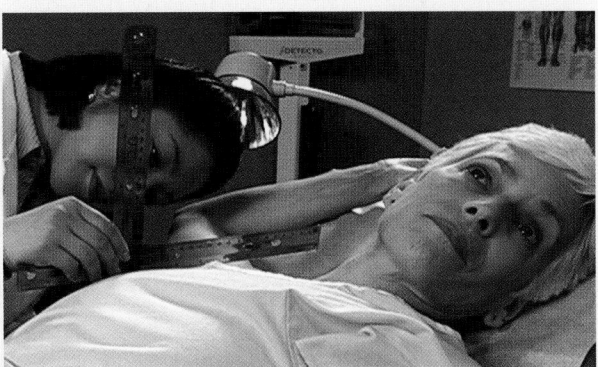

STEP 6e Position for assessment of jugular vein distention. (*From Seidel HM et al: Mosby's guide to physical examination, ed 7, St Louis, 2011, Mosby.*)

7 Peripheral vascular assessment:

   a Inspect lower extremities for changes in color and condition of skin (Table 6-10). Note skin and nail texture, hair distribution, venous patterns, edema, and scars or ulcers. Compare skin color with patient lying and standing.

Changes may reflect impaired peripheral circulation.

   b Palpate edematous areas, noting mobility, consistency, and tenderness.

Assists in determining extent of edema.

   c Assess for pitting edema by pressing area firmly with one finger for 5 seconds and releasing. Depth of indentation determines severity (see illustration).

      2 mm: 1+ edema
      4 mm: 2+ edema
      6 mm: 3+ edema
      8 mm: 4+ edema

   Use a tape measure to measure the circumference of the extremity.

Unilateral edema of affected leg is the most common physical finding of deep vein thrombosis (DVT), although symptoms are similar to other conditions, making diagnosis difficult (Carter, 2010).

Measuring circumference establishes a baseline for future comparison.

TABLE 6-10 | Signs of Venous and Arterial Insufficiency

Assessment Criterion	Venous	Arterial
Pain	Aching; increases in evening and with dependent position	Burning, throbbing, cramping; increases with exercise
Paresthesia	None	Numbness, tingling, decreased sensation
Temperature	Normal to touch	Cool to touch
Color	Normal or cyanotic	Pale; worsened by elevation of extremity; dusky red when extremity is lowered
Capillary refill	Not applicable	>2 seconds
Pulse	Present	Decreased or absent
Skin changes	Brown pigmentation around ankles	Thin, shiny skin; decreased hair growth; thickened nails
Ulcerations	Shallow ulcers around ankles (chronic venous stasis); edema apparent	Deep, well defined at site of trauma or tips of toes

STEP	RATIONALE

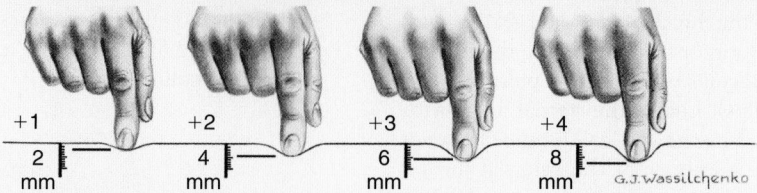

STEP 7c Assessing for pitting edema. *(From Seidel HM et al: Mosby's guide to physical examination, ed 7, St Louis, 2011, Mosby.)*

d Check capillary refill by grasping patient's fingernail or toenail and noting color of nail bed. Apply gentle, firm pressure to nail bed. Release quickly, watching for color change. Circulation is restored and normally returns to pink color in less than 2 seconds.

Capillary refill is measured in seconds; less than 2 seconds is brisk, whereas greater than 4 seconds is sluggish.
Cold environmental temperature with vasoconstriction and vascular disease can delay refill. Local pressure from a cast or bandage also slows refill.

e Ask if patient experiences pain or tenderness and gently palpate for heat, firmness, or localized swelling of the calf muscle, which are signs of phlebitis or DVT.

Patients who have been immobilized for at least 3 days and who have bone or joint disease, lengthy surgery, surgical correction of joint or bone, heart failure, shock, varicose veins, or pain are at risk for impaired tissue perfusion (Carter, 2010).

Clinical Decision Point *Homans' sign (pain in calf on dorsiflexion of foot) is no longer considered a reliable indicator for the presence or absence of DVT (Carter, 2010; Seidel et al., 2011) and should not be considered a reliable test. Trauma to a vein or muscle, reduced mobility, and increased blood clotting are reliable risk factors. If calf is swollen, tender, or red, notify patient's health care provider for further assessment and evaluation. If there is a strong suspicion of DVT, testing for Homans' sign is contraindicated. If a clot is present, it may become dislodged from its original site during this test. This could result in a pulmonary embolism.*

f Palpate peripheral arteries.
   (1) Start at the most distal part of each extremity. Palpate each peripheral artery for equality, comparing side to side; elasticity of vessel wall (depress and release artery, noting ease with which it springs back to shape); and strength of pulse (force of blood against arterial wall) using the following rating scale (Seidel et al., 2011):
   0 Absent, not palpable
   1+ Diminished, pulse barely palpable, weak and thready, and easy to obliterate
   2+ Normal pulse, easy to palpate
   3+ Full, easy to palpate, increases
   4+ Strong, bounding against fingertips, and cannot be obliterated

Comparison of both arteries allows you to determine any localized obstruction or disturbance in blood flow. Pulses should be symmetric side to side. If asymmetry is noted, look for other factors related to impaired circulation.

   (2) Palpate radial pulse by lightly placing tips of first and second fingers in groove formed along radial side of forearm, lateral to flexor tendon of wrist (see illustration).

Pulse is relatively superficial and should not require deep palpation.

   (3) Palpate ulnar pulse by placing fingertips along ulnar side of forearm (see illustration).

Palpated when arterial insufficiency to hand is expected or when you assess for radial occlusion (e.g., during arterial blood gas sampling) which may affect circulation to hand (see Chapter 43).

   (4) Palpate brachial pulse by locating groove between biceps and triceps muscles above elbow at antecubital fossa (see illustration). Place tips of first two fingers in muscle groove.

Artery runs along medial side of extended arm, requiring moderate palpation. If difficult to palpate, hyperextend arm to bring pulse site closer to the surface.

   (5) Have patient lie supine with feet relaxed and palpate dorsalis pedis pulse. Gently place fingertips between great and first toe; slowly move fingers along groove between extensor tendons of great and first toe until pulse is palpable (see illustration).

Artery lies superficially and does not require deep palpation. Pulse may be congenitally absent.

   (6) Palpate posterior tibial pulse by having patient relax and extend feet slightly. Place fingertips behind and below medial malleolus (ankle bone) (see illustration).

Artery is easily palpable with foot relaxed.

STEP	RATIONALE
(7) Palpate popliteal pulse by having patient slightly flex knee with foot resting on table or bed. Instruct patient to keep leg muscles relaxed. Palpate deeply into popliteal fossa with fingers of both hands placed just lateral to midline. Patient may also lie prone to achieve exposure of artery (see illustration).	Flexion of knee and muscle relaxation improve accessibility of artery. Popliteal pulse is one of the more difficult pulses to palpate.

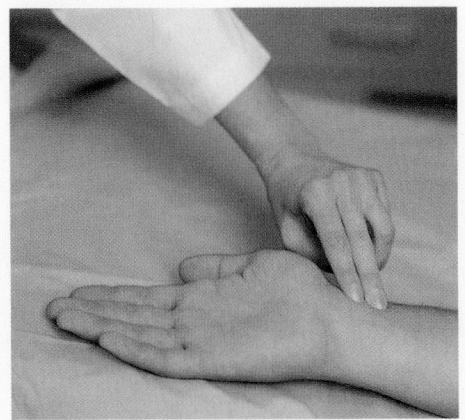

STEP 7f(2)   Palpation of radial pulse.

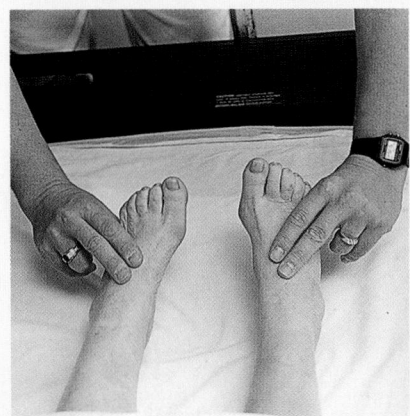

STEP 7f(5)   Palpation of dorsalis pedis pulses.

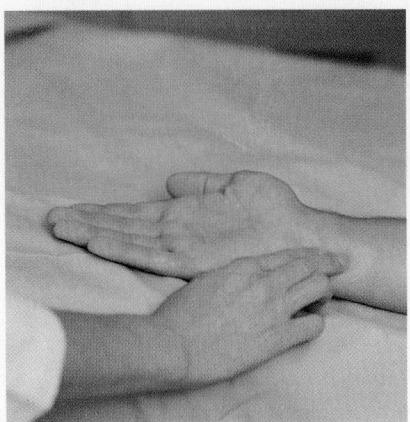

STEP 7f(3)   Palpation of ulnar pulse.

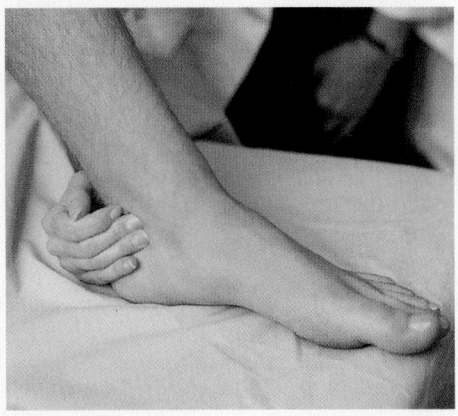

STEP 7f(6)   Palpation of posterior tibial pulse.

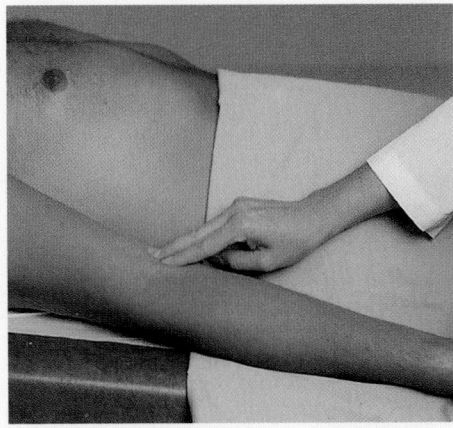

STEP 7f(4)   Palpation of brachial pulse.

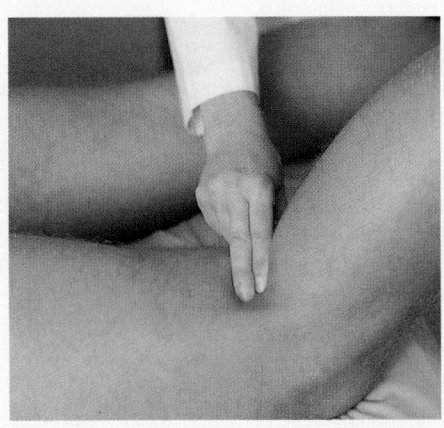

STEP 7f(7)   Palpation of popliteal pulse with patient prone.

STEP	RATIONALE
(8) Apply clean gloves. With patient supine, palpate femoral pulse by placing first two fingers over inguinal area below inguinal ligament, midway between pubic symphysis and anterosuperior iliac spine (see illustration).	Supine position prevents flexion in groin area, which interferes with artery access.
g If pulses are difficult to palpate or are not palpable, use a Doppler instrument over the pulse site:	Doppler amplifies sounds, allowing you to hear low-velocity blood flow through peripheral arteries.
(1) Apply conducting gel to patient's skin over pulse site or onto transducer tip of probe. Turn Doppler on.	
(2) Gently apply ultrasound probe to skin, changing Doppler angle until pulsation is audible. Adjust volume as needed (see illustration). Wipe off gel from patient and Doppler.	
8 Remove gloves and discard used supplies and gloves in proper receptacle. Assist patient to comfortable position. Perform hand hygiene.	Reduces transmission of infection.

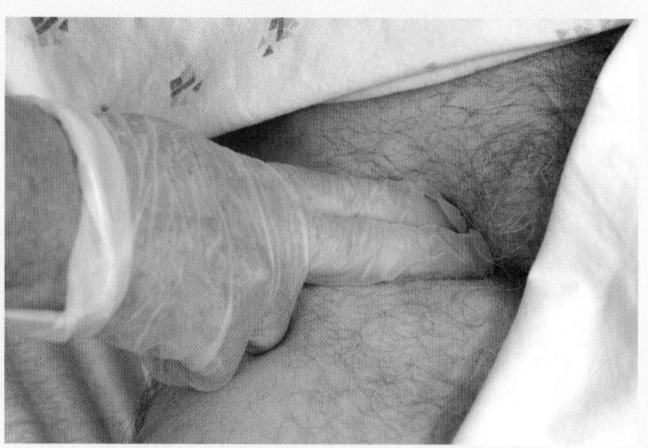
STEP 7f(8) Palpation of femoral pulse.

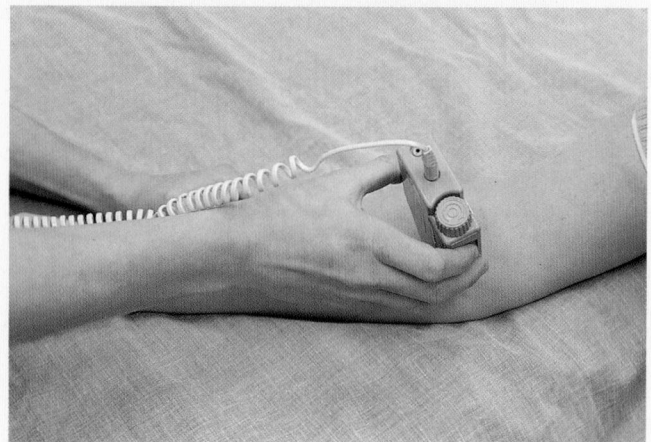
STEP 7g(2) Use of Doppler to assess brachial pulse.

EVALUATION

1 Compare findings with normal assessment characteristics of heart and vascular system.	Determines presence of abnormalities.
2 If heart sounds are not audible or pulses are not palpable, ask another nurse to confirm assessment.	Validates abnormal assessment findings.
3 Ask patient to describe behaviors that increase risk for heart and vascular disease.	Demonstrates learning.
4 Compare pulses and capillary refill bilaterally with previous assessment.	Demonstrates change from baseline measures.

Unexpected Outcomes

1 Abnormal findings that differ from previous assessments require you to **notify the health care provider**. These include:
- Pulsations, vibrations, or both are palpable. These are the result of valvular problem, murmur, or both.
- PMI is to the left of midclavicular line, which is the result of cardiomegaly.
- Extra heart sounds S_3 or S_4 are auscultated. Extra sounds indicate atrial or ventricular gallop.
- Murmur is auscultated. Impaired blood flow through heart indicates need for immediate medical attention. Some murmurs are benign.
- JVP is elevated. This is a sign of right-sided heart failure or fluid overload.

Related Interventions

- Prepare to obtain or assist with electrocardiogram (ECG).

Unexpected Outcomes

2 Heart rate is irregular, with rate less than 60 beats/min or more than 100 beats/min.

3 Pulse deficit is noted. There is risk for inadequate cardiac output.

4 Patient is unable to explain risks for heart or vascular disease.

5 Previously palpable dorsalis pedis pulses are diminished or absent, indicating circulatory compromise.

6 Patient's lower extremities have pale, cool, thin, and shiny skin, with reduced hair growth and thickened nails, indicating chronic arterial insufficiency.

Related Interventions

- Check blood pressure. If low, dysrhythmia is contributing to inadequate cardiac output.
- Observe for sensations or reports of dizziness or feeling "faint."
- Prepare to obtain ECG.

- Obtain vital signs.
- Additional education is needed.
- Elevate extremity.

- Instruct patient in proper foot care.
- Refer to podiatrist for nail trimming.
- Inspect feet for signs of impaired skin integrity.

Recording and Reporting

- Document quality (clear or muffled), intensity (weak or pounding), rate, and rhythm (regular, regularly irregular, or irregularly irregular) of heart sounds and peripheral pulses on nurses' notes, EHR, or flow sheet.
- Document additional cardiac findings, jugular venous pressure, and condition of extremities in nurses' notes, EHR, or flow sheet.
- Document activity level and subjective data related to fatigue, shortness of breath, and chest pain.
- Report immediately to health care provider any irregularities in heart function and indications of impaired arterial blood flow.
- Report to health care provider changes in peripheral circulation, which may indicate circulatory compromise, which may result in permanent nerve damage or tissue death if untreated.

Special Considerations

Teaching

- Explain risk factors for heart disease: high dietary intake of saturated fat or cholesterol, lack of regular aerobic exercise, smoking, excess weight, stressful lifestyle, hypertension, and family history of heart disease.
- Refer patient (if appropriate) to resources available for controlling or reducing risks (e.g., nutrition counseling, exercise class, and stress-reduction programs).
- Encourage patient to discuss with health care provider the need for periodic C-reactive protein (CRP) testing. CRP levels assess a patient's cardiovascular disease risk.

- Help patient to find resources to assist in quitting smoking because this lowers the risk for coronary heart disease and coronary vascular disease (ACS, 2011b). Nicotine in cigarette smoke causes vasoconstriction.
- Patients who are at risk benefit from taking a daily low dose of aspirin. Consult health care provider before starting therapy.

Pediatric

- PMI is at fourth intercostal space at left midclavicular line in children younger than 7 years of age (Hockenberry and Wilson, 2011).
- Capillary refill in infants is usually less than 1 second.
- It is not uncommon for children to have third heart sounds (S_3). Sinus arrhythmia occurs normally in many infants and children (Hockenberry and Wilson, 2011).
- Children have louder, higher-pitched heart sounds because of their thin chest walls.

Gerontologic

- PMI may be difficult to find in an older adult because anteroposterior diameter of the chest deepens.
- Accidental massage of the carotid sinus during palpation of the carotid artery is a particular problem for older adults, causing a sudden drop in heart rate from vagal nerve stimulation.
- Older adults with hypertension benefit from regular monitoring of blood pressure (daily, weekly, or monthly). Home monitoring kits are available. Teach patient how to use them correctly.

SKILL 6-5 Abdominal Assessment

Abdominal assessment is complex because of the multiple organs located within and near the abdominal cavity. This area of the body is associated with many health complaints; and many people are embarrassed by bowel or bladder dysfunction, reproductive problems, or urinary elimination problems. Abdominal pain is one of the most common symptoms that patients report when seeking medical care. It can be caused by alterations in organs such as the stomach, gallbladder, or intestines; or the pain may be the result of spinal or muscular injury. An accurate assessment requires matching the patient's history with a careful assessment of the location of physical symptoms (Table 6-11).

To perform an effective abdominal assessment you need to know the location and function of the underlying structures involved, including the lower pelvis, kidneys, rectum, genitalia, liver, gallbladder, stomach, spleen, appendix, pancreas, intestines, and reproductive organs (Fig. 6-5). An abdominal assessment is routine after abdominal surgery, for any patient who has undergone invasive diagnostic tests of the gastrointestinal (GI) tract, and for patients with abnormalities affecting GI function (see Chapter 44). The order of an abdominal assessment differs from that of other assessments. You begin with inspection and follow with auscultation. It is important to auscultate before palpation and percussion because these maneuvers alter the frequency and character of bowel sounds.

Delegation and Collaboration

The skill of abdominal assessment cannot be delegated to nursing assistive personnel (NAP). The nurse directs the NAP to:

- Report the development of abdominal pain and changes in the patient's bowel habits or dietary intake to the nurse.

Equipment

- ❑ Stethoscope
- ❑ Tape measure
- ❑ Examination light
- ❑ Water-based marking pen
- ❑ Drapes

TABLE 6-11	Common Causes of Abdominal Pain	
Condition	**Physical Alteration**	**Physical Signs and Symptoms**
Appendicitis	Obstruction of appendix associated with inflammation, perforation, and peritonitis Patient often lies on back or side with knees flexed to decrease pain	Sharp pain directly over the irritated peritoneum 2-12 hours after onset. Often pain localizes in right lower quadrant (McBurney's point) between anterior iliac crest and umbilicus. Associated with rebound tenderness. Accompanied by anorexia, nausea, and vomiting.
Celiac disease	Damage to small intestine mucosa from ingestion of barley, rye, oats, and wheat	Foul-smelling diarrhea, abdominal distention, and symptoms of malnutrition may be present.
Cholecystitis	Obstruction of cystic duct causing inflammation or distention of the gallbladder	*Murphy's sign*: Apply gentle pressure below right subcostal arch and liver margin. Sharp pain and increased respiratory rate occur when patient takes a deep breath (Seidel et al, 2011).
Constipation	Disruption in normal bowel pattern, which may occur with opioid use or inadequate fiber and fluid intake	Generalized discomfort accompanied by distention and palpation of a hard mass in the left lower quadrant. Nausea and vomiting may begin after several days.
Crohn's disease	Chronic inflammatory lesion of the ileum	Steady colicky pain in the right lower quadrant, with cramping, tenderness, flatulence, nausea, fever, and diarrhea. Often associated with bloody stools, weight loss, weakness, and fatigue. A tender mass of thickened intestine may be palpated in right lower quadrant.
Gastroenteritis	Inflammation of the stomach and intestinal tract	Generalized abdominal discomfort accompanied by anorexia, nausea, vomiting, diarrhea, abdominal cramping.
Pancreatitis	Inflammation of the pancreas associated with alcoholism, drug reaction, and gallbladder disease	Steady severe epigastric pain close to umbilicus radiates to back. Associated with abdominal rigidity and vomiting. Pain is unrelieved by vomiting, worsens by lying supine.
Paralytic ileus	Obstruction of the small bowel that occurs after abdominal surgery, from abdominal radiation, or from use of anticholinergic medications	Generalized severe abdominal distention, nausea, and vomiting. Decreased/absent bowel sounds.
Peptic ulcers (gastric and duodenal)	Damage of gastrointestinal (GI) mucosa at any area of the GI tract. May be caused by bacterial infection (*Helicobacter pylori*) or nonsteroidal antiinflammatory drugs (NSAIDs) Thought to be unrelated to stress Aggravated by smoking and excessive alcohol use	*Gastric ulcer*: Dull epigastric pain, localized midline. Early satiety; not usually relieved by food or antacids. *Duodenal ulcer*: Pain is episodic, lasting 30 minutes to 2 hours. It is located midline in epigastric region, may radiate around costal border to back; described as aching, burning, or gnawing. Typically occurs 1-3 hours after meals and at night (12 midnight to 3 AM). Often relieved by food/antacid. *Both (dyspepsia syndrome)*: Complaints of fullness, epigastric discomfort, vague feeling of nausea, abdominal distention, and bloating; anorexia; weight loss.

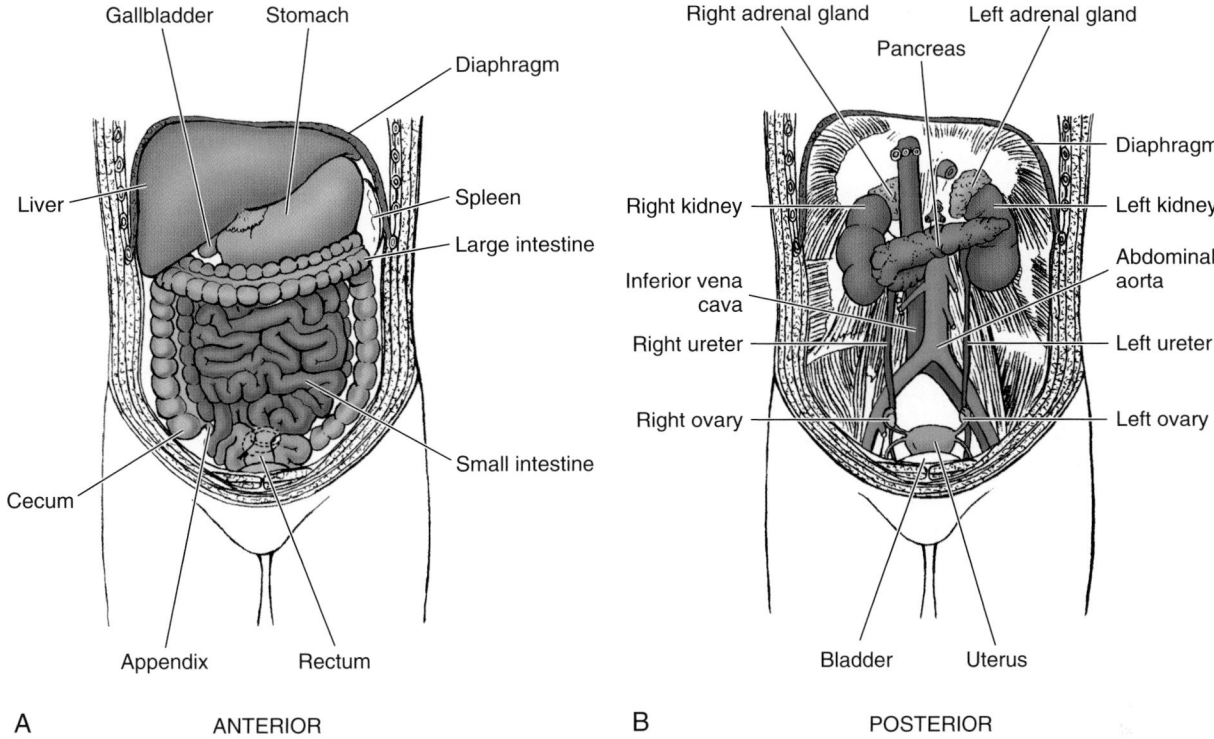

Gallbladder Stomach

Diaphragm

Liver

Spleen

Large intestine

Cecum

Small intestine

Appendix Rectum

A ANTERIOR

Right adrenal gland Left adrenal gland

Pancreas

Diaphragm

Right kidney

Left kidney

Abdominal aorta

Inferior vena cava

Right ureter

Left ureter

Right ovary

Left ovary

Bladder Uterus

B POSTERIOR

FIG 6-5 Location of organs in abdomen. **A,** Anterior. **B,** Posterior. (*Modified from* Mosby's expert 10 minute physical examinations, *ed 2, St Louis, 2005, Mosby.*)

STEP	RATIONALE

ASSESSMENT

1 If patient has abdominal or low back pain, assess the character of pain in detail (location, onset, frequency, precipitating factors, aggravating factors, type of pain, severity, course).

Knowing pattern of characteristics of pain helps determine its source.

2 Carefully observe patient's movement and position such as lying still with knees drawn up, moving restlessly to find a comfortable position, or lying on one side or sitting with knees drawn up to chest.

Positions assumed by patient reveal nature and source of pain (e.g., peritonitis, kidney stone, appendicitis). Patients with peritonitis lie still because movement aggravates the pain. The supine position worsens acute pancreatitis pain; a flexed knee, curved-back position brings relief. Patients with appendicitis lie on side or back with knees flexed in an attempt to decrease muscle strain on the abdominal wall.

3 Assess patient's normal bowel habits: frequency of stools; character of stools; recent changes in character of stools; measures used to promote elimination such as laxatives, enemas, and dietary intake; and eating and drinking habits.

Data compared with information from physical assessment may help identify cause and nature of elimination problems.

4 Determine if patient has had abdominal surgery, trauma, or diagnostic tests of the GI tract.

Surgery or trauma to the abdomen may result in altered position of underlying organs. Diagnostic tests may change character of stool.

5 Assess if patient has had recent weight changes or intolerance to diet (nausea, vomiting, cramping, especially in past 24 hours).

Changes may indicate alterations in upper GI tract (e.g., stomach or gallbladder) or lower colon.

6 Assess for difficulty in swallowing, belching, flatulence, bloody emesis (hematemesis), black or tarry stools (melena), heartburn, diarrhea, or constipation.

Indicative of GI alterations.

7 Determine if patient takes antiinflammatory medications (e.g., aspirin, steroids, and nonsteroidal antiinflammatory drugs [NSAIDs]), or antibiotics.

These medications may cause GI upset or bleeding.

8 Review family history of cancer, kidney disease, alcoholism, hypertension, or heart disease.

Information may reveal risk for significant abdominal alterations. Chronic alcohol ingestion causes GI and liver problems.

STEP	RATIONALE
9 Review patient's history for health care occupation, hemodialysis, intravenous drug use, household or sexual contact with hepatitis B virus (HBV) carrier, sexually active heterosexual person (more than one sex partner in previous 6 months), sexually active homosexual or bisexual man, international traveler in area of high HBV prevalence.	These are risk factors for HBV exposure. Abdominal findings for hepatitis include jaundice, hepatomegaly, anorexia, abdominal and gastric discomfort, tea-colored urine, and clay-colored stools (Lewis et al., 2011).

NURSING DIAGNOSES

- Constipation
- Deficient knowledge
- Diarrhea

- Imbalanced nutrition: less than body requirements
- Nausea

- Imbalanced nutrition: more than body requirements
- Ineffective health maintenance
- Pain (acute, chronic)

Related factors are individualized based on patient's condition or needs.

PLANNING

1 Expected outcomes following completion of procedure:	
• Abdomen is soft and symmetric, with smooth and even contour. No mass, distention, or tenderness is palpable. There are no forceful visible pulsations.	These are normal abdominal assessment findings.
• Bowel sounds are active and audible in all four quadrants.	Indicates normal peristaltic activity.
• No costovertebral angle (CVA) tenderness is present.	Indicates no inflammation of kidney.
• Patient denies discomfort or worsening of existing discomfort following examination.	Proper examination procedures have been implemented.
• Patient is able to list warning signs of colorectal cancer.	Demonstrates learning.
2 Anticipate teaching topics so that during the exam, you can instruct patient about warning signs of colorectal cancer.	Allows you to incorporate instruction during physical assessment.
3 Perform hand hygiene. Prepare necessary supplies.	Reduces risk of transmission of infection. Ensures efficiency during examination.

IMPLEMENTATION

1 Prepare patient for abdominal assessment:	
a Ask if patient needs to empty bladder or defecate.	Palpation of full bladder causes discomfort and feeling of urgency and makes it difficult for patient to relax.
b Keep upper chest and legs draped.	Maintains patient's comfort during examination, promoting relaxation.
c Be sure that room is warm.	Promotes patient's comfort. Reduces risk of patient tensing abdominal muscles.
d Have patient lie supine or in a dorsal recumbent position with arms down at sides and knees slightly bent. Place a small pillow under patient's knees.	Placing arms under the head or keeping knees fully extended causes abdominal muscles to tighten. Tightening of muscles prevents adequate palpation.
e Move sheet or blanket to expose area from just above xiphoid process down to symphysis pubis.	Provides full visualization of abdomen.
f Maintain conversation during assessment except during auscultation. Explain steps calmly and slowly.	Patient's ability to relax during assessment improves accuracy of findings. Talking interferes with hearing bowel sounds.
g Ask patient to point to tender areas.	Assess painful areas last. Manipulation of body part increases patient's pain and anxiety and makes remainder of assessment difficult to complete.
2 Abdominal assessment:	
a Identify landmarks that divide abdominal region into quadrants. Boundary begins at tip of xiphoid process to symphysis pubis with line crossing and intersecting umbilicus, dividing abdomen into four equal sections (see illustration).	Location of findings by common reference point helps successive examiners confirm findings and locate abnormalities.

STEP	RATIONALE

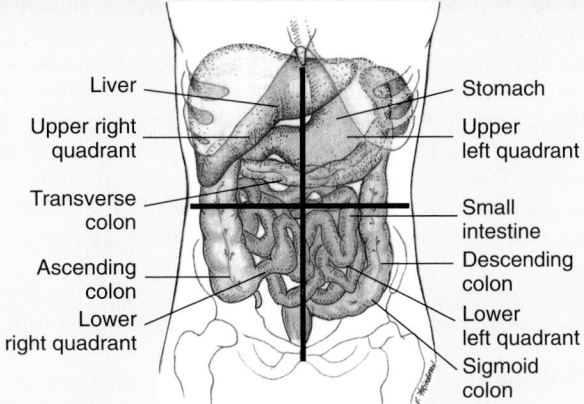

STEP 2a   Division of abdomen into quadrants.

b Inspect skin of surface of abdomen for color, scars, venous patterns, rashes, lesions, silvery white striae (stretch marks), and artificial openings (stomas). Observe skin lesions for characteristics described in Skill 6-1.

Scars reveal evidence that patient has had past trauma or surgery. Striae indicate stretching of tissue from growth, obesity, pregnancy, ascites, or edema. Venous patterns reflect liver disease (portal hypertension). Artificial openings indicate bowel or urinary diversion (see Chapter 35).

c If you note bruising, ask if patient self-administers injections (e.g., heparin or insulin).

Frequent injections may cause bruising and hardening of underlying tissues. Bruising also indicates physical abuse, accidental injury, or bleeding disorders.

d Inspect contour, symmetry, and surface motion of abdomen. Note any masses, bulging, or distention. (Flat abdomen forms a horizontal plane from xiphoid process to symphysis pubis. Round abdomen protrudes in convex sphere from horizontal plane. Concave abdomen sinks into muscular wall. All are normal.)

Changes in symmetry or contour reveal underlying masses, fluid collection, or gaseous distention. An everted umbilicus (protruding outward) indicates distention. A hernia also causes the umbilicus to protrude upward.

e If abdomen appears distended, note if distention is generalized. Look at the flanks on each side.

Distention may be caused by the nine F's (*fat, flatus, feces, fluids, fibroid, full bladder, false pregnancy, fatal tumor, and fetus*) (Seidel et al., 2011). If gas causes distention, flanks do not bulge. If fluid causes distention, flanks bulge. A tumor may cause a more unilateral bulging or distention. Pregnancy causes symmetric bulge in lower abdomen.

f If you suspect distention, measure size of abdominal girth by placing tape measure under patient and around abdomen at level of umbilicus (see illustration). Use marking pen to indicate where tape measure was applied.

Consecutive measurements show any increase or decrease in abdominal distention. Make all subsequent measurements at same level of umbilicus to provide objective means to evaluate changes. Use a water-based pen to make a mark on abdomen for subsequent measurements.

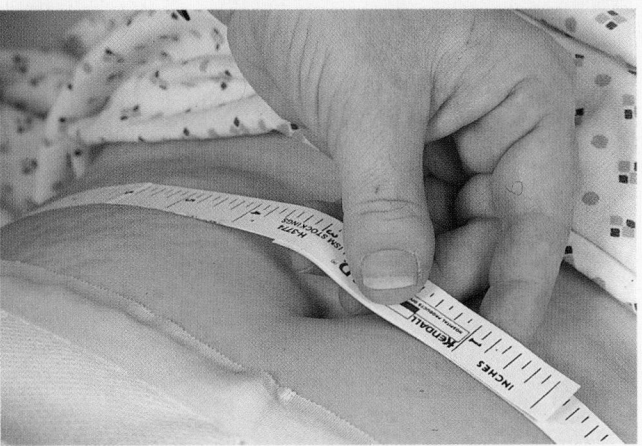

STEP 2f   Measuring abdominal girth at level of umbilicus.

STEP	RATIONALE

g If patient has a nasogastric (NG) or nasointestinal (NI) tube connected to suction, turn off momentarily.

Sound of suction obscures bowel sounds.

h To auscultate bowel sounds, place the diaphragm of the stethoscope lightly over each of the four abdominal quadrants. Ask patient not to talk. Listen until you hear repeated gurgling or bubbling sounds in each quadrant (minimum of once in 5 to 20 seconds). Describe sounds as normal, hyperactive, hypoactive, or absent. Listen 5 minutes over each quadrant before deciding that bowel sounds are absent.

Normal bowel sounds occur irregularly every 5 to 15 seconds. Absence of sounds indicates cessation of gastric motility. Hyperactive bowel sounds not related to hunger or a recent meal may indicate diarrhea or early intestinal obstruction. Hypoactive or absent bowel sounds indicate paralytic ileus or peritonitis. It is common for bowel sounds to be hypoactive after surgery for 24 hours or more, especially following abdominal surgery.

Clinical Decision Point *Nausea and vomiting, increasing distention, and inability to pass flatus may accompany severe paralytic ileus.*

i Place the bell of the stethoscope over the epigastric region of the abdomen and each quadrant. Auscultate for vascular (whooshing) sounds.

Determines presence of turbulent blood flow (bruit) through thoracic or abdominal aorta, which may indicate an aneurysm.

Clinical Decision Point *If aortic bruit is auscultated, suggesting presence of an aneurysm, stop assessment and notify health care provider immediately. Percussion or palpation over abdominal bruit could cause rupture of an already weakened vessel wall in the presence of an abdominal aneurysm.*

j With patient supine, gently percuss each of the four abdominal quadrants systematically. Note areas of tympany and dullness.

Reveals presence of air or fluid in stomach and intestines. Normal percussion is tympanic because of swallowed air in GI tract. Presence of fluid or underlying masses is revealed by dull percussion.

k To determine if fluid or air is causing distention, percuss for a fluid wave. Ask a colleague to assist by pressing gently and firmly at midline of abdomen (see illustration).
Place your fingertips along both sides of lower abdomen in lumbar region. Thrust quickly into patient's side with your dominant hand, keeping nondominant hand in place. If fluid is present, you will palpate a fluid wave with the nondominant hand.

If you do not feel a fluid wave, air is causing the distention. Presence of a fluid wave indicates ascites, found in cirrhosis, peritonitis, metastatic carcinoma, ovarian carcinoma, and pancreatitis. Jaundice, pruritus, dependent edema, and enlarged superficial abdominal veins often accompany ascites from liver congestion (Lewis et al., 2011).

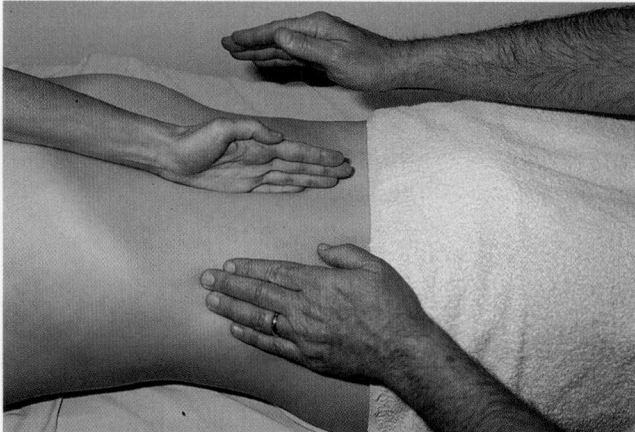

STEP 2k Testing for fluid wave. (*From Seidel HM et al: Mosby's guide to physical examination, ed 6, St Louis, 2006, Mosby.*)

l Ask patient if abdomen feels unusually tight and determine if this is a recent development.

Continued sensation of fullness helps to detect distention. A feeling of fullness after a heavy meal causes only temporary distention. Tightness is not felt with obesity.

STEP	RATIONALE

m With patient sitting, gently but firmly percuss over each CVA along scapular lines (see illustration A). Use ulnar surface of fist indirectly by placing nondominant hand flat against CVA and percussing with dominant hand or percuss directly against patient's skin (see illustration B). Note if patient experiences pain.

Determines presence of kidney inflammation.

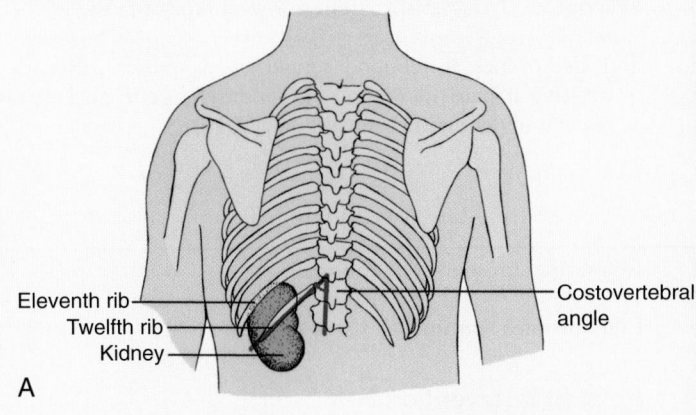

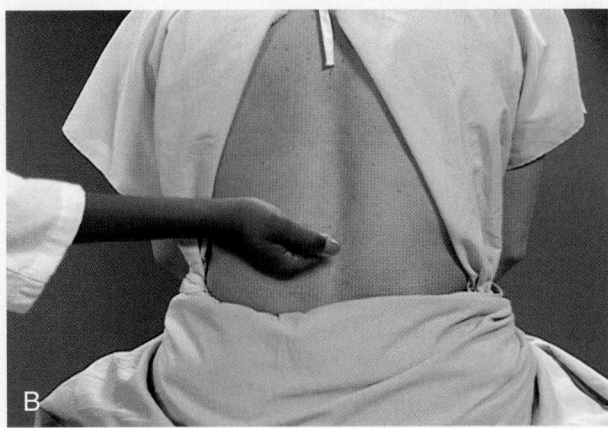

Eleventh rib
Twelfth rib
Kidney
Costovertebral angle

A

B

STEP 2m **A,** Position of kidney in relation to costovertebral angle. **B,** Direct percussion of kidney for costovertebral angle tenderness. *(From Seidel HM et al: Mosby's guide to physical examination, ed 6, St Louis, 2006, Mosby.)*

n Lightly palpate over each abdominal quadrant, laying palm of hand with fingers extended and approximated lightly on abdomen. Keep palm and forearm horizontal. The pads of the fingertips depress the skin no more than 1 cm (½ inch) in a gentle dipping motion (see illustration). Palpate painful areas last.

Detects areas of localized tenderness, degree of tenderness, and presence and character of underlying masses or fluid. Palpation of sensitive area causes guarding (voluntary tightening of underlying abdominal muscles).

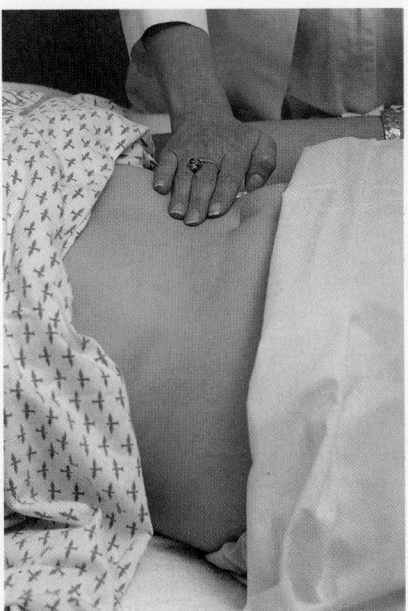

STEP 2n Light palpation of abdomen.

(1) Note muscular resistance, distention, tenderness, and superficial masses or organs while observing patient's face for signs of discomfort.

Patient's verbal and nonverbal cues may indicate discomfort from tenderness. Firm abdomen indicates active obstruction with buildup of fluid or gas.

(2) Note if abdomen is firm or soft to touch.

Soft abdomen is normal or reveals that obstruction is resolving.

STEP	RATIONALE
o Just below umbilicus and above symphysis pubis, palpate for a smooth, rounded mass. While applying light pressure, ask if patient has sensation of need to void.	Detects presence of dome of distended bladder.

Clinical Decision Point *Routinely check for distended bladder if patient has been unable to void, patient has been incontinent, or an indwelling Foley catheter is not draining well or has been removed recently.*

STEP	RATIONALE
p If masses are palpated, note size, location, shape, consistency, tenderness, mobility, and texture.	Descriptive characteristics help to reveal type of mass.
q When tenderness is present, press one hand slowly and deeply into the involved area and let go quickly. Note if pain is aggravated.	Test determines if rebound tenderness is present. Results are positive if pain increases. This indicates peritoneal irritation such as appendicitis (Seidel et al., 2011).

EVALUATION

1 Compare assessment findings with previous assessment characteristics to identify changes.	Determines presence of abnormalities.
2 Ask patient to describe signs and symptoms of colorectal cancer.	Demonstrates learning.

Unexpected Outcomes

1 Abdomen is asymmetric, with palpable mass, and dull to percussion, suggesting a tumor.

2 Abdomen protrudes symmetrically with skin taut; patient complains of tightness, and/or bowel sounds are absent. GI motility has ceased. Patient is vomiting. Signs suggest an obstruction.

3 Hyperactive bowel sounds are evident with GI motility. Commonly they result from anxiety, diarrhea, overuse of laxatives, inflammation of the bowel, or reaction of the intestines to certain foods.

4 Rebound abdominal tenderness is noted.

5 Bladder is palpable over symphysis pubis and distended.

6 Patient is unable to describe signs and symptoms of colorectal cancer.

Related Interventions

- Report to health care provider.

- Keep patient on nothing by mouth (NPO) status and encourage ambulation.
- Notify health care provider.
- Gastric decompression following insertion of NG tube sometimes may be necessary.

- Patient may need to be NPO.
- Contact health care provider if patient needs antidiarrheal medication.

- Avoid palpating area.
- Notify health care provider if this is a new finding.
- Place patient on NPO status.

- Facilitate voiding by placing patient in sitting position or encouraging him or her to bear down (if not contraindicated); run water within hearing distance or have patient place hand in basin of warm water.
- Use bladder scan to determine extent of bladder fullness.
- If unable to void, urinary catheterization is necessary (see Chapter 33).

- Additional education is necessary.

Recording and Reporting

- Document appearance of abdomen, quality of bowel sounds, presence of distention, abdominal circumference, and presence and location of tenderness in nurses' notes, EHR, or flow sheet.
- Record patient's ability to void and defecate, including description of output.
- Record content of any patient instruction.
- Report serious abnormalities such as absent bowel sounds, presence of a mass, or acute pain to nurse in charge and health care provider.

Special Considerations

Teaching

- Explain that factors such as diet, regular exercise, limited use of over-the-counter drugs causing constipation, establishment of regular elimination schedule, and adequate fluid intake promote normal bowel elimination.

- If patient is a health care worker or has contact with blood or body fluids of affected people, encourage him or her to receive series of three HBV vaccine doses.

Pediatric

- Most common palpable abdominal mass in child is feces, usually palpated in right lower quadrant (Hockenberry and Wilson, 2011).
- Have a child stand erect and then lie supine during inspection of abdominal surface. Normal abdomen of infants and young children is cylindric in erect position and flat in supine position. School-age children may have a rounded abdomen until 13 years of age when standing.
- In infants and children skin of abdomen is usually taut and without wrinkles or creases.
- Infants and children until the age of 7 years are abdominal breathers.

- Some children perceive superficial palpation as tickling. Drawing attention to their laughter only causes it to increase. Have the children help by placing their hand on top of yours or have them place their hand on their abdomen with their fingers separated and then palpate between their fingers.

Gerontologic

- Older adults often lack abdominal tone; underlying organs are more easily palpable.

- Constipation along with nausea, flatulence, and heartburn is common.
- Stress to older adults importance of adequate fluid intake, regular exercise, and a diet with at least four servings daily of fresh fruit, vegetables, and high-fiber food to promote normal defecation.

SKILL 6-6 Genitalia and Rectum Assessment

The best time to examine a patient's external genitalia is while performing routine hygiene measures or preparing to insert or care for a urinary catheter. An examination of female and male external genitalia is part of preventive health screenings. You examine adolescent and young adults because of the growing incidence of sexually transmitted infections (STIs). The average age of menarche among girls has declined, and most male and female teenagers are sexually active by age 19 (Hockenberry and Wilson, 2011). You can easily combine rectal and anal assessments with this examination because the patient assumes a lithotomy or dorsal recumbent position.

Delegation and Collaboration

The skill of assessing the genitalia and rectum cannot be delegated to nursing assistive personnel (NAP). The nurse directs the NAP to:

- Report changes in patient's genitourinary function and presence of drainage in the perineal area.

Equipment

❏ Examination light
❏ Clean gloves (use nonlatex if necessary)
❏ Drapes

STEP	RATIONALE

ASSESSMENT

1 Assessment: female patients:

a Determine if patient has signs and symptoms of vaginal discharge, painful or swollen perianal tissues, or genital lesions.

b Determine if patient has symptoms or history of genitourinary problems, including burning during urination (dysuria), frequency, urgency, nocturia, hematuria, or incontinence.

c Ask if the patient has had signs of bleeding outside of normal menstrual cycle or after menopause or has had unusual vaginal discharge.

d Determine if patient has received human papillomavirus (HPV) vaccine.

e Determine if patient has history of HPV (condyloma acuminatum, herpes simplex, or cervical dysplasia); had first pregnancy before age of 17; smokes cigarettes; is obese; eats diet low in fruits and vegetables; has had multiple full-term pregnancies.

f Determine if patient is older than 63; is obese; has history of ovarian dysfunction, breast or endometrial cancer, or endometriosis; has family history of reproductive cancer; has history of infertility or nulliparity; or uses estrogen (alone) as hormone replacement therapy.

These signs and symptoms are consistent with an STI or other pathologic condition.

Urinary problems are associated with gynecologic disorders, including STIs.

These are warning signs for cervical and endometrial cancer or a vaginal infection.

The CDC (2011) recommends that all 11 or 12 year old girls get the 3 doses of HPV vaccine (Gardasil or Cervarix) to protect against cervical cancer. Gardasil also protects against most genital warts and some cancers of the vulva, vagina, and anus. Girls and young women ages 13 through 26 should get HPV vaccine if they have not received any or all doses when they were younger. CDC also recommends Gardasil for all boys aged 11 or 12 years, and for males aged 13 through 21 years who did not get any or all of the three recommended doses when they were younger. All men should confer with their doctor about vaccination.

These are risk factors for cervical cancer (ACS, 2011c).

These are risk factors for ovarian cancer (ACS, 2011d).

STEP	RATIONALE
g Determine if patient is postmenopausal, obese, or infertile; had early menarche or late menopause; has history of hypertension, diabetes mellitus, gallbladder disease, or polycystic ovary disease; has family history of endometrial, breast, or colon cancer; or has a history of estrogen-related exposure (estrogen replacement therapy, tamoxifen use).	These are risk factors for endometrial cancer (ACS, 2011e).
h Determine patient's knowledge of the risk factors and signs of cervical and other gynecologic cancers.	Provides baseline for patient education.
2 Assessment of male patients:	
a Review normal elimination pattern, including frequency of voiding; history of nocturia; character and volume of urine; daily fluid intake; symptoms of burning, urgency, and frequency; difficulty starting stream; and hematuria.	Urinary problems are directly associated with genitourinary problems because of anatomic structure of men's reproductive and urinary systems.
b Ask if patient has noted penile pain or swelling, genital lesions, or urethral discharge.	These are signs and symptoms of STIs.
c Determine if patient has noted heaviness or painless enlargement or irregular lumps of testis.	These signs and symptoms are early warning signs for testicular cancer.
d Determine if patient reports any enlargement in inguinal area and assess if intermittent or constant, associated with straining or lifting, and painful. Assess whether coughing, lifting, or straining at stool causes pain.	Signs and symptoms indicate potential inguinal hernia.
e Ask if patient has experienced weak or interrupted urine flow, inability to urinate, difficulty in starting or stopping urine flow, polyuria, nocturia, hematuria, or dysuria. Determine if patient has continuing pain in lower back, pelvis, or upper thighs.	These are warning signs of prostatic cancer (ACS, 2011f). Symptoms also may indicate infection or prostate enlargement.
f Assess patient's knowledge of risk factors and signs of prostate and testicular cancer.	Provides baseline for patient education.
3 Assessment of all patients:	
a Determine whether patient has rectal bleeding, black or tarry stools (melena), rectal pain, or change in bowel habits (constipation or diarrhea).	These are warning signs of colorectal cancer (ACS, 2011g) or other GI alterations.
b Determine whether patient has personal or strong family history of colorectal cancer, polyps, or chronic inflammatory bowel disease. Ask if patient is over age 50.	These are risk factors for colorectal cancer (ACS, 2011g).
c Inquire about dietary habits, including high fat intake, diet high in processed or red meats, diet high in meats cooked at high temperatures (frying, broiling, grilling), or deficient fiber content (inadequate fruits and vegetables).	Colon cancer is often linked to dietary intake of fat, red meat, high cooking temperatures, or insufficient fiber intake (ACS, 2011g).
d Determine if patient is obese, physically inactive, smokes, has type 2 diabetes, or consumes alcohol.	These are risk factors for colorectal cancer (ACS, 2011g).
e Assess medication history for use of laxatives or cathartic medications.	Repeated use causes diarrhea and eventual loss of intestinal muscle tone.
f Assess for use of codeine or iron preparations.	Codeine causes constipation. Iron turns stool black and tarry.
g Assess patient's knowledge of risks and signs of colorectal cancer.	Provides baseline for patient education.

NURSING DIAGNOSES

- Deficient knowledge
- Ineffective health maintenance
- Pain (acute, chronic)
- Readiness for enhanced immunization status

Related factors are individualized based on patient's condition or needs.

PLANNING

1 Expected outcomes following completion of procedure:	
• Patient denies discomfort or worsening of existing discomfort following examination.	Proper examination procedures have been implemented.
• Patient is able to list warning signs of colorectal cancer: female patient: cervical, endometrial, and ovarian cancer; male patient: testicular and prostate cancer.	Demonstrates learning.
• Patient is able to discuss guidelines for HPV immunization.	Demonstrates learning.

STEP	RATIONALE
2 Anticipate teaching topics so that during the exam, you can instruct patient about warning signs of colorectal cancer.	Prepares you for incorporating teaching into assessment activities.
3 Perform hand hygiene. Prepare necessary supplies.	Reduces transmission of infection.

IMPLEMENTATION

STEP	RATIONALE
1 Prepare patient for assessment:	
a Ask if patient needs to empty bladder or defecate.	Palpation of full bladder causes discomfort and feeling of urgency and makes it difficult for patient to relax.
b Keep upper chest and legs draped and keep room warm.	Maintains patient's comfort during examination, promoting relaxation.
c Position patient: Female should lie in a dorsal recumbent position with arms down at sides and knees slightly bent. Place a small pillow under her knees. Male should lie supine with chest, abdomen, and lower legs draped; or have him stand during examination.	Placing the arms under the head or keeping knees fully extended causes tightening of the abdominal muscles.
d Apply clean gloves.	
2 Female genitalia examination.	
a Expose perineal area, repositioning sheet.	
b Inspect surface characteristics of perineum and retract labia majora; observe for inflammation, edema, lesions, or lacerations. Note if there is any vaginal discharge. Presence of discharge may indicate need for a culture.	Skin of perineum is smooth, clean, and slightly darker than other skin. Mucous membranes are dark pink and moist. Labia majora are symmetric; may be dry or moist. Normally there is no vaginal discharge.
3 Male genitalia examination.	
a Expose perineal area. Observe genitalia for rashes, excoriations, or lesions.	Normally skin is clear without lesions.
b Inspect and palpate penile surfaces.	
(1) Inspect corona, prepuce (foreskin), glans, urethral meatus, and shaft. Retract foreskin in uncircumcised males. Observe for discharge, lesions, edema, and inflammation. Return foreskin to normal position.	Glans should be smooth and pink along all surfaces. Urethral meatus is slitlike and normally positioned at tip of glans. Foreskin should retract easily. Area between foreskin and glans is a common site for venereal lesions.
c Inspect and palpate testicular surfaces.	
(1) Inspect size, color, shape, and symmetry; also gently palpate for lesions and edema.	Left testicle is normally lower than right. Scrotal skin is usually loose, surface is coarse, and skin color is more deeply pigmented than body skin.
d Palpate testes.	
(1) Note size, shape, and consistency of tissue.	Testes are normally ovoid and approximately 2 to 4 cm (0.8 to 1.6 inches) in size; feel smooth and rubbery, and are free from nodules. Most common symptom of testicular cancer is an irregular, nontender fixed mass.
(2) Ask if patient experiences tenderness with palpation.	Testes are normally sensitive but not tender.
5 Assess rectum.	
a Female patient remains in dorsal recumbent position or assumes side-lying (Sims') position.	These positions allow for optimum visualization of the rectum.
b Male patient stands and bends forward with hips flexed and upper body resting across examination table; examine nonambulatory patient in Sims' position.	
c View perianal and sacrococcygeal areas by gently retracting buttocks using your nondominant hand.	Perianal skin is smooth, more pigmented, and coarser than skin covering buttocks.
d Inspect anal tissue for skin characteristics, lesions, external hemorrhoids (dilated veins that appear as reddened skin protrusion), ulcers, inflammation, rashes, and excoriation.	Anal tissues are moist and hairless; voluntary sphincter holds anus closed.
6 Remove and discard gloves. Discard disposable supplies. Assist patient to comfortable position. Perform hand hygiene.	Prevents transmission of infection.

EVALUATION

STEP	RATIONALE
1 Compare assessment findings with previous assessment characteristics to identify changes.	Determines presence of abnormalities.
2 Ask patient to list warning signs of colorectal cancer: female patient: cervical, endometrial, and ovarian cancer; male patient: testicular and prostate cancer.	Demonstrates learning.
3 Ask patient to identify guidelines for HPV vaccination.	Demonstrates learning.

Unexpected Outcomes	Related Interventions
1 Patient has vaginal/penile drainage and burning sensation during voiding. Women may have vaginal bleeding between menstrual periods. Symptoms may suggest STI.	• Notify health care provider. • Prepare to collect a culture of discharge.
2 Patient is unable to list warning signs of colorectal cancer: female patient: cervical, endometrial, and ovarian cancer; male patient: testicular and prostate cancer.	• Provide additional education.

Recording and Reporting

- Record results of assessment in nurses' notes, EHR, or flow sheet.
- Record patient's ability to void, including description of output.
- Record content of any patient instruction.
- Report any abnormalities such as presence of a mass or acute pain to nurse in charge and health care provider.

Special Considerations

Teaching

- Discuss the guidelines of the ACS (2011g) for early detection of colorectal cancer for both men and women. The ACS (2011g) recommends the following examination schedules beginning at age 50:
  1. Tests that detect polyps and cancer; one of the following: (1) flexible sigmoidoscopy (every 5 years), (2) colonoscopy (every 10 years), (3) double-contrast barium enema (every 5 years), (4) computed tomographic colonoscopy (every 5 years).
  2. Tests that primarily detect cancer: (1) guaiac-based fecal occult blood test (gfobt), or fecal immunochemical test (FIT) with high sensitivity for cancer (every year), (2) stool deoxyribonucleic acid (DNA) (interval unclear).
- Discuss warning signs of colorectal cancer, including long-term progressive weight loss, change in bowel habits, and blood in stools.
- Discuss dietary planning and healthy lifestyle choice to maintain or improve colon health.

Female Health Teaching

- Instruct patient about purpose and recommended frequency of Papanicolaou (Pap) smears and GYN examinations.

- Explain warning signs of STIs: pain or burning on urination, pain during sex, pain in pelvic area, bleeding between menstruation, itchy rash around vagina, and abnormal vaginal discharge.
- Teach measures to prevent STIs (e.g., male partner's use of condoms, restricting number of sexual partners, avoiding sex with persons who have several other partners, and perineal hygiene measures).
- Reinforce the importance of performing perineal hygiene (as appropriate).

Male Health Teaching

- Explain warning signs of STIs: pain on urination and during sex, abnormal penile discharge, swollen lymph nodes, or rash or ulcer on skin or genitalia.
- Teach measures to prevent STIs: use of condoms, avoiding sex with infected partner, avoiding sex with persons who have multiple partners, and using regular perineal hygiene. Tell patients with an STI to inform their sexual partners of the need to have an examination. Instruct patient to seek treatment as soon as possible if partner becomes infected with an STI.
- Instruct patient in how to perform genital self-examination (see Box 6-2).

Pediatric

- When examining the testes in a male infant, avoid stimulating the cremasteric reflex, which causes the testes to pull higher into the pelvic cavity.

SKILL 6-7 Musculoskeletal and Neurologic Assessment

You use the skills of inspection and palpation during the musculoskeletal and neurologic assessment. During the general survey you inspect gait, posture, and body position. A more thorough assessment of major bone, joint, and muscle groups and sensory, motor, and cranial nerve (CN) function is indicated in the presence of abnormalities. The assessment can be performed as you examine other body systems. For example, while assessing head and neck structures assess neck range of motion (ROM) and examine select CNs. Integrate assessment into routine activities of care (e.g., while bathing or positioning the patient). Assessment of these systems is important when a patient reports pain, loss of sensation, or impairment of muscle function. Prolonged illness or immobility may result in muscle weakness and atrophy. Neurologic assessment is often conducted simultaneously because muscles may be weakened as a result of nerve involvement.

Delegation and Collaboration

The skill of assessing musculoskeletal and neurologic function cannot be delegated to nursing assistive personnel (NAP). The nurse directs the NAP to:

- Report patients' problems with gait, ROM, and muscle strength.
- Be informed of patients at risk for falls (unsteady gait, foot dragging, weakness of lower extremities).
- Assist patients with muscular weakness with transfer and ambulation.

Equipment

- ❑ Cotton balls or cotton-tipped applicators
- ❑ Penlight
- ❑ Opposite tip of cotton swab or tongue blade broken in half
- ❑ Tape measure
- ❑ Tongue blade
- ❑ Tuning fork
- ❑ Reflex hammer

STEP	RATIONALE

ASSESSMENT

1 Review patient history for use of alcohol intake of more than 2 drinks/day; inadequate intake of protein, vitamin D, or calcium; thin and light body frame; family history of osteoporosis; white or Asian ancestry; sedentary lifestyle; long-term use of certain medications (e.g., corticosteroids, phenytoin [Dilantin], or heparin); and certain medical conditions (e.g., anorexia nervosa, hyperthyroidism) (Jaffe et al., 2011).

These factors increase the risk for osteoporosis.

2 Determine if patient has been screened for osteoporosis.

Women age 65 and older need routine screening for osteoporosis. There is insufficient evidence that men require screening for osteoporosis (Jaffe et al., 2011).

3 Ask patient to describe history of alteration in bone, muscle, or joint function (e.g., recent fall, trauma, lifting heavy objects, bone or joint disease with sudden or gradual onset) and location of alteration.

History assists in assessing nature of musculoskeletal problem. It is estimated that 25 million Americans have osteoporosis and an additional 34 million have osteopenia (USPSTF, 2011).

4 Assess nature and extent of patient's musculoskeletal pain: location, duration, severity, predisposing and aggravating factors, relieving factors, and type of pain. If patient reports pain or cramping in lower extremities, ask if walking relieves or aggravates it. Assess distance walked and characteristics of pain before, during, and after activity.

Pain frequently accompanies alterations in bone, joints, or muscle. Pain has implications for comfort and also ability to perform activities of daily living. Pain caused by certain vascular conditions tends to increase with activity.

5 Assess height and weight (see Skill 6-1). Note if there is a decrease in women older than 50 by subtracting current height from recall of maximum adult height.

Body mass index less than 22 is a risk factor, and loss of height more than 7.5 cm (3 inches) is one of the first clinical signs of osteoporosis (Touhy and Jett, 2010).

6 Determine if patient uses analgesics, antipsychotics, antidepressants, nervous system stimulants, or recreational drugs.

These medications alter level of consciousness (LOC) or cause behavioral changes. Abuse sometimes causes tremors, ataxia, and changes in peripheral nerve function.

7 Determine if patient has recent history of seizures/convulsions: clarify sequence of events (aura, loss of muscle tone, falling, motor activity, loss of consciousness); character of any symptoms; and relationship to time of day, fatigue, or emotional stress.

Seizure activity often originates from central nervous system (CNS) alteration. Characteristics of seizure help determine its origin.

8 Screen patient for headache, tremors, dizziness, vertigo, numbness or tingling of body part; visual changes; weakness; pain; or changes in speech.

These symptoms commonly result from CNS dysfunction. Identifying patterns aids in diagnosis.

9 Discuss with spouse, family member, or friends any recent changes in patient's behavior (e.g., increased irritability, mood swings, memory loss, change in energy level).

Behavioral changes may result from intracranial pathology.

10 Assess patient for history of change in vision, hearing, smell, taste, or touch.

Major sensory nerves originate from brainstem. These symptoms help to localize nature of problem.

11 If patient displays sudden acute confusion (delirium), review history for drug toxicity (e.g., anticholinergics, digoxin, antihistamines, antipsychotics, benzodiazepines, opioid analgesics, sedative/hypnotics, steroids); serious infections, metabolic disturbances (e.g., diabetes mellitus); heart failure; and severe anemia.

Delirium is one of the most common mental disorders in older persons (Touhy and Jett, 2010), but it also occurs in children.

12 Review history for head or spinal cord injury, meningitis, congenital anomalies, neurologic disease, or psychiatric counseling.

These neurologic symptoms or behavioral changes help to focus assessment on possible cause.

NURSING DIAGNOSES

- Activity intolerance
- Impaired physical mobility
- Impaired walking
- Ineffective peripheral tissue perfusion
- Pain (acute, chronic)
- Risk for injury
- Risk for peripheral neurovascular dysfunction
- Risk for trauma
- Self-care deficit (bathing/hygiene, dressing/grooming, feeding, or toileting)

Related factors are individualized based on patient's condition or needs.

PLANNING

1 Expected outcomes following completion of procedure:
- Patient demonstrates erect posture; strong grasp; steady gait, with arms swinging freely at side.

Indicates normal alignment, gait, and neuromuscular muscle strength.

STEP	RATIONALE
• There is bilateral symmetry of extremities in length, circumference, alignment, position, and skinfolds.	
• Full active ROM is present in all joints with good muscle tone and absence of contractures, spasticity, or muscular weakness.	Indicates normal ROM of joints.
• Patient is alert and oriented to person, place, and time. Behavior and appearance appropriate for condition/situation.	Indicates normal cerebral function.
• Patient demonstrates normal pupil reaction to light and accommodation (see Skill 6-2); external ocular muscles (EOMs) intact; facial sensation intact; symmetric facial expressions; soft palate and uvula midline and rise on phonation; gag reflex intact; speech clear without hoarseness; no difficulty swallowing.	Indicates normal functioning of CNs III, IV, V, VI, VII, IX, and X.
• Patient distinguishes between sharp and dull sensations and light touch on symmetric areas of extremities. Position sense intact to lower extremities.	Indicates normal function of sensory nerves.
• Gait coordinated, steady with appropriate stance and swing phases. Romberg test negative.	Indicates normal cerebellar and motor system functioning.
2 Perform hand hygiene. Prepare necessary supplies.	Reduces transmission of infection.

IMPLEMENTATION

1 Prepare patient: **a** Integrate musculoskeletal and neurologic assessments during other portions of physical assessment or during nursing care (e.g., when patient moves in bed, rises from chair, or walks).	You can conduct the assessment as a patient performs activities or goes through movements required during complete physical examination. Integration with care conserves patient's energy and allows observation of patient performing more naturally.
b Plan time for short rest periods during assessment.	Movement of body parts and various maneuvers may tire patient. Always plan rest periods with older adult and very ill patients.
2 Assess musculoskeletal system. **a** Observe ability to use arms and hands for grasping objects (e.g., pen, utensils) (see illustration).	Assesses coordination and muscle strength.
b Assess muscle strength of upper extremities by applying gradual increase in pressure to muscle group.	Upper and lower extremity on patient's dominant side normally is stronger than that on nondominant side. Pain rather than weakness may cause reduced muscle strength; however, long-term pain can lead to muscle weakening.
c To assess hand grasp strength, cross your hands and have patient grasp index and middle fingers of both of your hands and squeeze them as hard as possible (see illustration).	It is common for the patient's dominant hand to be slightly stronger than nondominant hand. By crossing your hands, patient's right hand grasps your right hand. This helps with recall of which is patient's right/left hand.

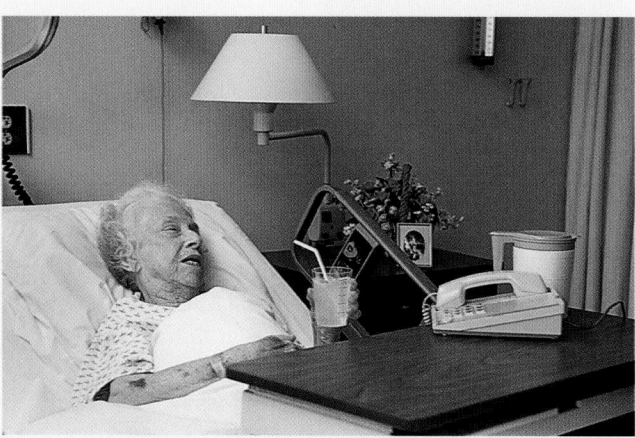

STEP 2a   Observe use of arms and hands.

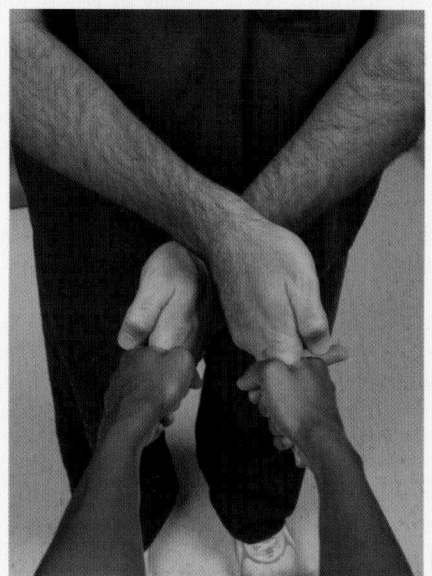

STEP 2c   Assessing strength of hand grasps, comparing sides.

STEP	RATIONALE
d Place hand on lower arm or leg and have patient move major joint (e.g., elbow, knee) against resistance (e.g., flex elbow). Have patient maintain pressure until told to stop. Compare symmetric muscle groups. Note weakness and compare right with left.	Compares strength of symmetric muscle groups. Rate muscle strength on scale of 0 to 5 as follows: 0 No voluntary contraction 1 Slight contractility, no movement 2 Full ROM, passive 3 Full ROM, active 4 Full ROM against gravity, some resistance 5 Full ROM against gravity, full resistance
e Observe body alignment for sitting, supine, prone, or standing positions. Muscles and joints should be exposed and free to move to allow for accurate measurement.	Each joint or muscle group requires different position for measurement.
f Inspect gait as patient walks. Have patient use his or her assistive device (e.g., cane, walker) if appropriate. Observe for foot dragging, shuffling or limping, balance, presence of obvious deformity in lower extremities, and position of trunk in relation to legs.	Gait is more natural if patient is unaware of your observation. Assesses for a neuromusculoskeletal disorder.
g Perform Get Up and Go Test: From a sitting position have patient stand without using arms for support. Observe gait and ability to stand.	The Get Up and Go Test is an assessment that should be conducted as part of a routine evaluation of older adults. The test detects risk for falls.
h Stand behind patient and observe postural alignment (position of hips relative to shoulders). Look sideways at cervical, thoracic, and lumbar curves (see illustration).	Abnormal curves of posture include lordosis (swayback, increased lumbar curvature), kyphosis (hunchback, exaggerated posterior curvature of thoracic spine), and scoliosis (lateral spinal curvature). Postural changes indicate muscular, bone, or joint deformity; pain; or muscular fatigue. Head should be held erect.

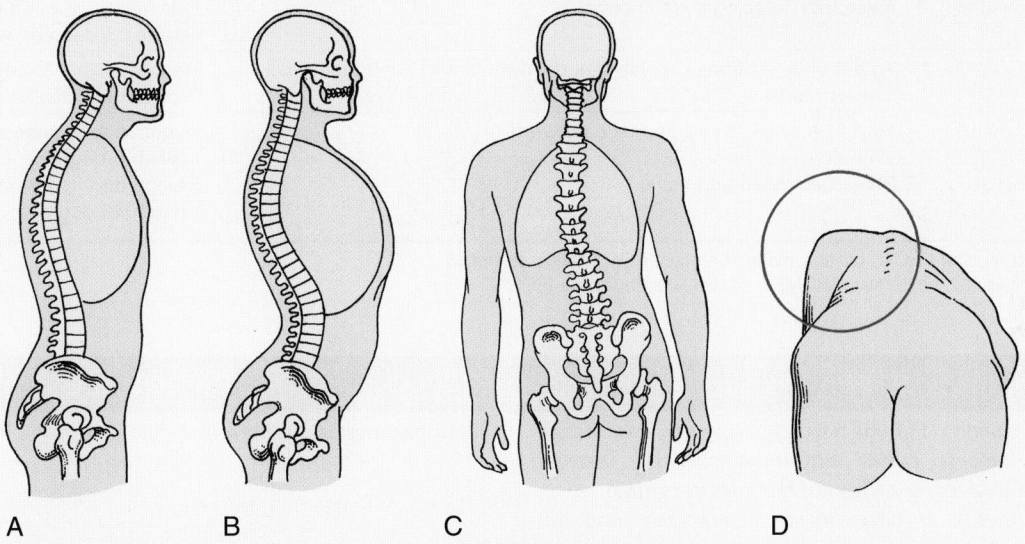

STEP 2h Observe spinal deformities. **A,** Kyphosis. **B,** Lordosis. **C,** Scoliosis. **D,** Scoliosis with patient bending forward.

STEP	RATIONALE
i Make a general observation of extremities. Look at overall size, gross deformity, bony enlargement, alignment, and symmetry.	General review pinpoints areas requiring in-depth assessment.
j Gently palpate bones, joints, and surrounding tissue in involved areas. Note any heat, tenderness, edema, or resistance to pressure.	Reveals changes resulting from trauma or chronic disease. Do not attempt to move joint when fracture is suspected or joint is apparently "frozen" by lack of movement over a long period of time.
k Ask patient to put major joint through its full ROM (Table 6-12). Patients with deformities, reduced mobility, joint fixation, or weakness will require passive ROM assessment. Observe equality of motion in same body parts:	Assessment of patient's normal ROM provides baseline for assessing later changes after surgery or inactivity.

TABLE 6-12 | Assessing Range of Motion*

Body Part	Assessment Procedure	ROM
Upper Extremities		
Neck	Bend head forward and then backward. Bend neck side to side. Turn head to look over each shoulder.	Flexion, hyperextension, lateral flexion, rotation
Shoulders	Raise both arms to vertical position level at sides of head. Bring arm across upper chest to touch opposite shoulder. Place both hands behind neck, with elbows out to sides. Place both hands behind small of back. Have patient make small circles with hands, with arms extended at shoulder level.	Flexion Adduction External rotation and abduction Internal rotation Circumduction
Elbows	Bend and straighten elbows. Place hands at waist with elbows flexed.	Flexion and extension Internal rotation
Wrists	Flex and extend wrist (bend and straighten). Bend wrist to radial and then ulnar side. Turn palm upward and then downward.	Flexion and extension Radial and ulnar deviation Supination and pronation
Hands	Make a fist with both hands; open hand. Extend and spread fingers and thumb outward; bring back together.	Flexion and extension Adduction and abduction
Lower Extremities		
Hips (with patient supine)	With knees extended, raise one leg upward. Cross leg over other leg. Swing legs laterally. With knee flexed, hold ankle and rotate leg inward and outward.	Flexion: Expect 90 degrees Abduction: Expect 45 degrees Adduction: Expect 30 degrees Internal and external rotation: Expect 40-45 degrees
Knees (with patient sitting)	Raise foot, keeping knee in place.	Extension: Expect full extension and up to 15 degrees hyperextension
Ankles	With foot held off floor, point toes downward and bring them back toward knee.	Plantar flexion: Expect 45 degrees Dorsiflexion: Expect 20 degrees
Toes	Turn foot (sole) inward and sole outward. Bend toes down and back.	Inversion and eversion: Expect to reach 5 degrees Flexion and hyperextension: Expect to reach 40 degrees

AROM, Active range of motion; *PROM,* passive range of motion; *ROM ,* range of motion.
*This may be done actively by the patient (AROM) or passively by the nurse (PROM).

STEP	RATIONALE
(1) *Active motion:* (Patient needs no support or assistance and is able to move joint independently.) Instruct patient in moving each joint through its normal range. Sometimes it is necessary to demonstrate and ask patient to mimic your movements.	Identifies muscle strength and detects limited ROM.
(2) *Passive motion:* (Joint has full ROM, but patient does not have strength to move it independently.) Have patient relax and move same joints passively until end of range is felt. Support extremity at joint. Do not force joint if there is pain or muscle spasm.	Determines ability to perform joint motion in presence of muscle weakness. Forcing joint causes injury and pain.
l Palpate joint for swelling, stiffness, tenderness, and heat; note any redness.	Indicates acute or chronic inflammation. ROM causes pain or injury.
m Assess muscle tone in major muscle groups. Normal tone causes mild, even resistance to movement through entire ROM.	If muscle has increased tone (hypertonicity), any sudden movement of joint is met with considerable resistance. Hypotonic muscle moves without resistance. Muscle feels flabby.
3 Neurologic assessment	
a Assess LOC and orientation by asking patient to identify name, location, day of week, and year; note behavior and appearance. This can be completed during the general survey.	A fully conscious patient responds to questions spontaneously. As consciousness declines patient may show irritability, shortened attention span, or unwillingness to cooperate. As consciousness continues to deteriorate patient becomes disoriented to name, time, and place. Behavior and appearance reveal information about patient's mental status.

STEP	RATIONALE
b Assess cranial nerves (CNs):	
(1) For CNs III (oculomotor), IV (trochlear), and VI (abducens), assess extraocular movement (EOM). Ask patient to follow movement of your finger through the six cardinal positions of gaze; measure pupillary reaction to light reflex and accommodation (see Skill 6-2) using penlight.	These CNs are those most likely to be affected by increasing intracranial pressure (ICP), which causes change in response or size of pupil; pupils may change shape (more oval) or react sluggishly. ICP impairs movements of EOMs. Accommodation is ability of the eye to adjust vision from near to far.
(2) For CN V (trigeminal), apply light sensation with a cotton ball to symmetric areas of face.	Sensations should be symmetric; unilateral decrease or loss of sensation may be caused by CN V lesion.
(3) For CN VII (facial) note facial symmetry. Have patient frown, smile, puff out cheeks, and raise eyebrows.	Expressions should be symmetric; Bell's palsy causes drooping of upper and lower face; CVA causes asymmetry.
(4) For CNs IX (glossopharyngeal) and X (vagus), have patient speak and swallow. Ask him or her to say "ah" while using tongue blade and penlight. Check for midline uvula and symmetric rise of uvula and soft palate. Use tongue blade and place on posterior tongue to elicit gag reflex.	Damage to CN IX causes impaired swallowing; damage to CN X causes loss of gag reflex, hoarseness, nasal voice. When palate fails to rise and uvula pulls toward normal side, this indicates a unilateral paralysis.
c Assess extremities for sensation. Perform all sensory testing with patient's eyes closed so patient is unable to see when or where a stimulus strikes the skin.	
(1) *Pain:* Ask patient to indicate when sharp or dull sensation is felt as you alternately apply sharp and blunt ends of tongue blade to skin surface. Apply in symmetric areas of extremities.	Patient should be able to distinguish sharp or dull sensations. Impaired sensations indicate disorders of spinal cord or peripheral nerve roots.
(2) *Light touch:* Apply light wisp of cotton to different points along surface of skin in symmetric areas of extremities.	Patient should be able to distinguish when touched.
(3) *Position:* Grasp finger or toe, holding it by its sides with your thumb and index finger. Alternate moving finger or toe up and down. Ask patient to state when finger is up or down. Repeat with toes.	Patient should be able to distinguish movements of a few millimeters. Decreased/absent position sense may occur in spinal anesthesia, paralysis, or other neurologic disorders.
d Assess motor and cerebellar function:	
(1) *Gait:* Have patient walk across room, turn, and come back. Similarly note use of assistive devices. This is a good time to instruct on proper use of assistive devices.	Neurologic and musculoskeletal disorders impair gait and balance.
(2) *Romberg's test:* Have patient stand with feet together, arms at sides, both with eyes open and eyes closed (for 20 to 30 seconds). Protect patient's safety by standing at side; observe for swaying.	Romberg's test should be negative; slight swaying is considered normal.
e Assess deep tendon reflexes (DTRs):	
(1) In patients with back pain or surgery, CVA, or spinal cord compression, it is appropriate to monitor DTRs (Seidel et al., 2011). This requires an advanced level of skill. In most settings this is not part of routine physical assessment.	Muscle spasticity and hyperactive reflexes may result from disorders such as stroke and paralysis. Diminished DTRs and muscle weakness may suggest electrolyte abnormalities or lower motor neuron disorders (e.g., amyotrophic lateral sclerosis [ALS] or Guillain-Barré syndrome).
(2) For each reflex tested, compare sides and assign a grade on the following scale: 0 No response 1+ Sluggish or diminished response 2+ Normal, active or expected response 3+ More brisk than expected; slightly hyperactive 4+ Very brisk; hyperactive, with clonus.	Grade indicates extent of neuron dysfunction. Clonus is described as repeated spasms of muscular contraction and relaxation.
(3) *Knee reflex:* Palpate patellar tendon just below patella. Tap pointed end of reflex hammer briskly on tendon (see illustration).	Knee reflex is the most common DTR assessment performed. The normal response is knee extension.
(4) *Plantar response (Babinski's reflex):* Using handle end of reflex hammer, stroke lateral aspect of sole from heel to ball of foot.	Toes should flex inward and downward (see illustration).

STEP	RATIONALE

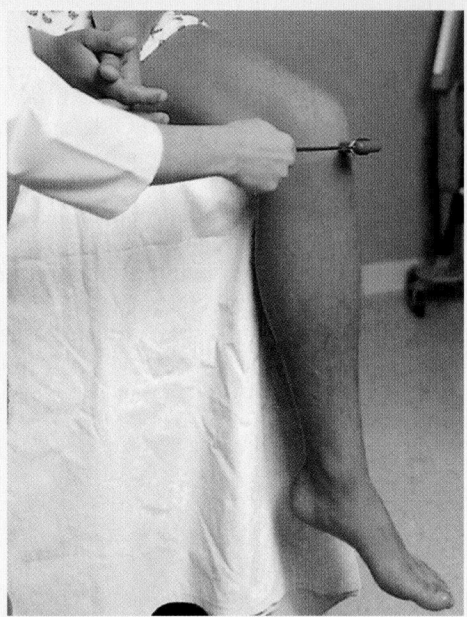

STEP 3e(3) Assessing knee reflex. Knee should extend.

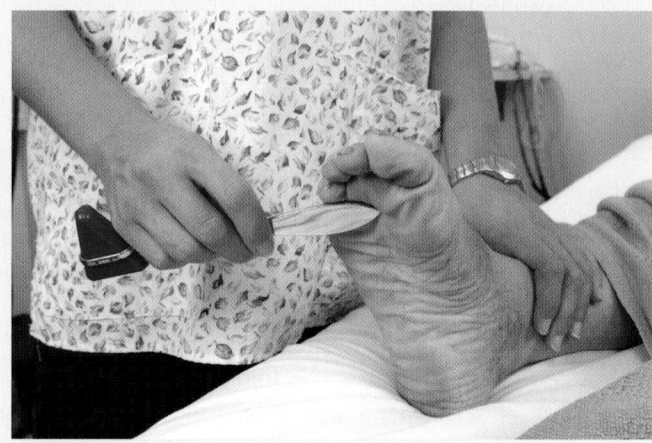

STEP 3e(4) Assessing plantar response. Toes should flex inward and downward.

(5) After stroking soles of feet, if Babinski's reflex is present, great toe dorsiflexes, accompanied by fanning of the other toes.

4 Dispose of supplies. Perform hand hygiene.

Indicates CNS dysfunction. Dorsiflexion of great toe and fanning of the others are normal in a child younger than age 2 (Hockenberry and Wilson, 2011).

Reduces transmission of infection.

EVALUATION

1 Compare muscle strength and ROM with previous physical assessment.

Determines presence of abnormalities.

2 Compare neurologic status with previous physical assessment.

Determines presence of abnormalities.

3 Evaluate level of patient's discomfort following procedure, using appropriate pain scale.

Determines if manipulation of musculoskeletal structures intensifies patient's discomfort.

Unexpected Outcomes	Related Interventions
1 Joints are prominent, swollen, and tender with nodules or overgrowth of bone in distal joints, indicating signs of arthritis.	• Instruct patient in proper ROM. • Determine patient's knowledge regarding use of antiinflammatory medications and nonpharmacologic measures (see Chapter 15).
2 ROM is reduced in one or more major joints: shoulder, elbow, wrist, fingers, knee, hip.	• Assess further for pain during movement with joint unstable, stiff, painful, or swollen or with obvious deformity. • Notify health care provider. • Reduce mobility in extremity until cause of abnormal joint motion is determined.
3 Patient demonstrates weakness in one or more major muscle groups or has difficulty with gait or ability to walk and sit during Get Up and Go Test, indicating a fall risk.	• Place patient on fall precautions. • Provide patient safety when ambulating (see Chapter 10). • Notify health care provider.
4 Patient has changes in mental status and pupillary response or other neurological deficits.	• Notify health care provider immediately. • Continue to assess patient's vital signs and LOC closely. • Place on fall precautions.

Recording and Reporting

- Record posture, gait, muscle strength, and ROM in nurses' notes, EHR, or appropriate assessment flow sheet.
- Record LOC, orientation, pupillary response, sensation, and reflex responses in nurses' notes, EHR, or appropriate assessment flow sheet.
- Report to nurse in charge or health care provider acute pain or sudden muscle weakness, change in LOC, or change in size or pupillary reaction, which require immediate treatment.

Special Considerations
Teaching

- Instruct patient about correct postural alignment. Consult with physical therapist to provide patient with exercises for improving posture.
- To reduce bone demineralization, instruct older-adult patient in a proper weight-bearing exercise program (e.g., walking, low-impact aerobics) to be followed three or more times a week.
- Encourage intake of calcium to meet the recommended daily allowance. Increased vitamin D aids calcium absorption (400 to 800 international units daily). Recommendation for daily calcium supplements for adults over age 50: 1200 mg/day. Instruct patient to take no more than 500 mg of calcium supplements at one time (Touhy and Jett, 2010).
- Explain to patients with low back pain that they can benefit from modification of work-related risk factors (e.g., lifting heavy weights, use of protective equipment), regular aerobic exercise, exercises that strengthen the back and increase trunk flexibility, and learning how to lift properly.
- Explain measures to ensure safety (e.g., use of ambulation aids or safety bars in bathrooms or stairways) for patients with sensory or motor impairments.

Pediatric

- Examine infants carefully for musculoskeletal anomalies resulting from genetic or fetal insults. An examination includes review of posture, generalized movement, symmetry and skin creases of the extremities, muscle strength, and hip alignment.
- Normally the back of a newborn is rounded or C shaped from the thoracic and pelvic curves.
- Scoliosis, lateral curvature of the spine, is an important childhood problem, especially in females, usually identified at puberty. (For closer examination have child stand erect wearing only underclothes. Observe from behind, looking for asymmetry of shoulders and hips. Then observe from the back as child bends forward.) Uneven dress hems or trouser hems or uneven fit of clothing at the waist is an indication of scoliosis.
- Watching a child during play reveals information about musculoskeletal function.
- Children age 13 to 19 years need 1300 mg of calcium daily with 400 international units of vitamin D (Hockenberry and Wilson, 2011).

Gerontologic

- Instruct older adults about fall prevention. Make modifications in the home environment to reduce the risk of falls (see Chapter 42).
- Instruct older adults and those with osteoporosis in proper body mechanics, ROM exercises, and moderate weight-bearing exercises (e.g., swimming, walking) to minimize trauma.
- Functional assessment is a measurement of older person's ability to perform basic self-care tasks (Cress, 2012). When patient is unable to perform self-care easily, determine need for assistive devices (e.g., zippers on clothing instead of buttons, elevation of chairs to minimize bending of knees and hips).
- Older adults tend to assume a stooped, forward-bent posture with hips and knees somewhat flexed, arms bent at the elbows, and level of arms raised.

PROCEDURAL GUIDELINE 6-1 Monitoring Intake and Output

 Video Clip

Measuring and recording intake and output (I&O) during a 24-hour period is part of the assessment database for fluid and electrolyte balance (Table 6-13). You are responsible for accurate recording of all intake (liquids taken orally, by enteral feedings, and parenterally) and all output (urine, diarrhea, vomitus, gastric suction, and drainage from surgical tubes). Monitoring a patient on I&O requires cooperation and assistance from the patient and family. Accuracy is critical as physicians will use findings in prescription of medications and IV fluids.

Monitor I&O for patients with a fever or edema, receiving intravenous (IV) or diuretic therapy, or on restricted fluids. It is also important when a patient has electrolyte losses associated with vomiting, diarrhea, gastrointestinal drainage, or extensive open wounds such as burns. Total and evaluate I&O at the end

---

TABLE 6-13	Adult Average Fluid Gains and Losses			
Fluid Intake and Output	**Volume (mL)**	**Fluid Intake and Output**	**Volume (mL)**
Fluid Intake		**Fluid Output**	
Oral fluids	1300	Kidneys	1500
Solid foods	1000	Skin	600
Oxidative metabolism	300	Lungs	300
		Gastrointestinal	200
Total gains	**2600**	**Total losses**	**2600**

From Metheny N: *Fluid and electrolyte balance: Nursing considerations,* ed 5, Sudbury, Mass, 2012, Jones and Bartlett.

Continued

PROCEDURAL GUIDELINE 6-1   Monitoring Intake and Output—cont'd

of each shift or at specified times such as every 8 hours. Significant alterations are apparent by comparing 24-hour totals over several days. Because fluid imbalance occurs at any time, be aware of I&O for all patients, even when documentation is not required.

Delegation and Collaboration

The skill of assessing I&O totals at the end of each shift; comparing 24-hour totals over several days; and monitoring and recording intravenous (IV) therapy, wound or chest tube drainage, and tube feedings cannot be delegated to nursing assistive personnel (NAP). The nurse emphasizes maintaining standard precautions related to body fluids, accurately measuring and recording I&O, and using the metric system with standard containers. The nurse directs the NAP to:

- Measure and record oral intake, urinary output, liquid diarrheal stools, vomitus, and wound drainage device output.
- Report changes in patient's condition such as alteration in intake or changes in color, amount, or odor of output.

Equipment

❑ Sign to alert personnel of I&O measurement
❑ Daily I&O record form or computer graphic
❑ Graduated measuring container
❑ Bedpan, urinal, bedside commode, or urine "hat" (a receptacle that fits under the toilet seat)
❑ Clean gloves
❑ Mask, eye protection, and gown (optional)

Procedural Steps

1 Identify patients with conditions that increase fluid loss (e.g., fever, diarrhea, vomiting, surgical wound drainage, chest tube drainage, gastric suction, major burns, or severe trauma).
2 Identify patients with impaired swallowing, unconscious patients, and patients with impaired mobility.
3 Identify patients on medications that influence fluid balance (e.g., diuretics and steroids).
4 Assess signs and symptoms of dehydration and fluid overload (e.g., bradycardia versus tachycardia, hypotension versus hypertension, and reduced skin turgor versus edema).
5 Weigh patients daily using the same scale, the same time of day, and with comparable clothing.
6 Monitor laboratory reports:
   a Urine specific gravity (normal is 1.010 to 1.030)
   b Hematocrit (Hct) (normal range is 38% to 47% for females and 40% to 54% for males).
7 Assess patient's and family's knowledge of purpose and process of I&O measurement.
8 Explain to patient and family the reasons that I&O are important.
9 Perform hand hygiene.
10 Measure and record all fluid intake:
   a Liquids with meals, gelatin, custards, ice cream, popsicles, sherbets, ice chips (recorded as 50% of measured volume [e.g., 100 mL of ice chips equals 50 mL of water]). Convert household measures to the metric system: 1 ounce equals 30 mL; therefore 12 ounces (soda can) equals 360 mL.
   b Count liquid medicines such as antacids and fluids with medications as fluid intake.
   c Calculate fluid intake from tube feedings (see Chapter 31).

d Calculate fluid intake from parenteral fluids, blood components, and total parenteral nutrition solutions (see Chapters 28 and 29).

> **Clinical Decision Point** *Record intake as soon as you measure it to maintain accuracy. If more than one patient is in the same room, each must have urine receptacles labeled with name and bed location.*

11 Instruct patient and family to call you or the NAP to empty contents of urinal, urine hat, or commode each time patient uses it. Have patient and family monitor incontinence, vomiting, and excessive perspiration and report it to the nurse.
12 Inform patient and family that Foley catheter drainage bag and wound, gastric, or chest tube drainage are closely monitored, measured, and recorded and who is responsible for this. Each patient must have a graduated container clearly marked with name and bed location and used only for the patient indicated.
13 Apply clean gloves. Measure drainage at the end of the shift or as indicated, using appropriate containers and noting color and characteristics. If splashing is anticipated, wear mask, eye protection, and/or gown.
   a Measure urine drainage using a "hat" into which patient voids or a graduated container (see illustration).
   b Observe color and characteristics of urine in Foley tubing and drainage bag. Sometimes a measuring device is part of the drainage bag (see illustration). Otherwise measure using a graduated container.
   c Measure chest tube drainage by marking and recording the time on the collection chamber at specified intervals (see illustration) (see Chapter 26). Chest tube collection devices are changed when they become full.
   d Measure Jackson-Pratt/Hemovac drainage using a medicine cup (see illustration) (see Chapter 38).
   e Measure gastric drainage or larger drainage pouches by opening clamp and pouring into graduated cup with a 240-mL capacity (see illustration).

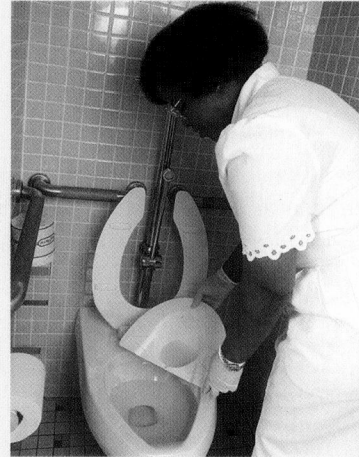

STEP 13a   Measuring and emptying the urine "hat."

PROCEDURAL GUIDELINE 6-1 Monitoring Intake and Output—cont'd

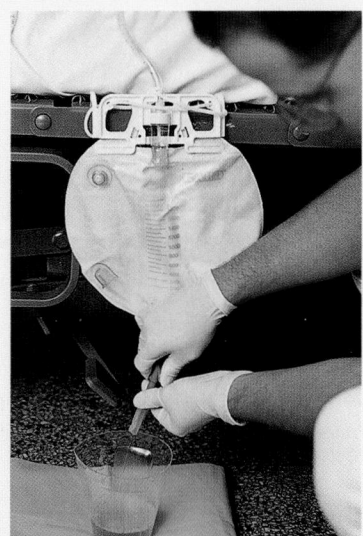

STEP 13b Device for monitoring hourly urine output.

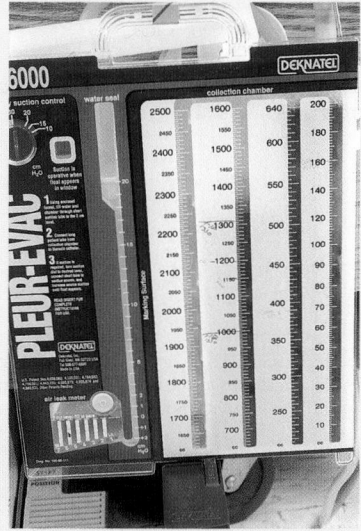

STEP 13c Collection chamber for measuring chest tube drainage.

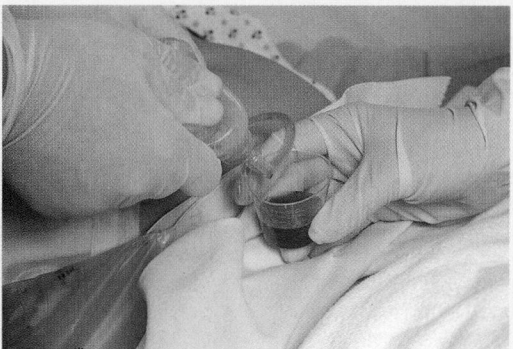

STEP 13d Measuring wound drainage through Jackson-Pratt drain.

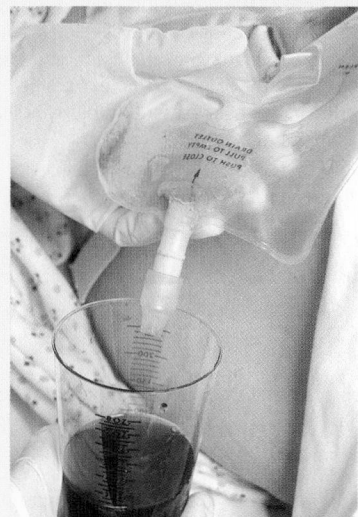

STEP 13e Measuring drainage from large drainage pouch.

14 Remove gloves and dispose of them in appropriate receptacle. Perform hand hygiene.

15 Note I&O balance or imbalance and report to health care provider any urine output less than 30 mL/hr or significant changes in daily weight.

16 Document on I&O forms or electronic record.

[?] Critical Thinking Exercises

You are caring for Mrs. Williams, a 73-year-old retired schoolteacher who underwent a right hip arthroplasty. This is her first postoperative day on your clinical unit. The night nurse reported that patient had an "uneventful" night. She has an intravenous infusion in her right hand, a right hip dressing, Foley catheter to gravity, and a Jackson-Pratt surgical drain in place.

1 Which body systems would you assess for this patient? Describe key elements in these assessments.
2 On auscultation of her posterior lung field bases, you hear a crackling noise on inspiration. You also assess and note that her breathing is shallow. What is this sound, and what does it indicate? Which nursing diagnosis is a priority to consider at this time?
3 You next assess her cardiac status: she has a heart rate of 86 beats/min, rhythm regular. What does this assessment indicate?
4 Mrs. Williams complains of right hip pain and requests pain medication. After you administer the medication, you inspect and then auscultate her abdomen. After listening for 60 seconds at a site below and to the right of the umbilicus, you are unable to hear bowel sounds. What is the best assessment of this situation?
5 While assisting Mrs. Williams with the bath, you assess the peripheral neurovascular status of her lower extremities. Which key elements are included in this assessment? Which findings indicate deep vein thrombosis?

[✓] REVIEW QUESTIONS

1 A nurse in orientation is performing an abdominal assessment. Which action would indicate that further practice and study are indicated?
   1 The bowel is auscultated before being palpated.
   2 The nurse determines any tenderness before touching the patient.
   3 Inspection is done before percussion.
   4 The abdomen is palpated before auscultation is done.
2 A nurse is performing a neurologic assessment. Which approach is most effective in obtaining accurate data when testing sensory pathways?
   1 Perform each test quickly.
   2 Have the patient as relaxed as possible.
   3 Compare symmetric areas.
   4 Use a predictable order of assessment.
3 An older-adult female patient presents with a history of vomiting and diarrhea. Assessment findings reveal lethargy, decreased skin turgor, a weight loss of 5 pounds (2.27 kg) in 3 days, and a hematocrit of 51%. Which other assessment data would the nurse expect to find?
   1 Hypoactive bowel sounds and an elevated urine specific gravity of 1.026
   2 Concentrated urine and hyperactive bowel sounds
   3 Moist mucous membranes and a low urine specific gravity of 1.008
   4 Increased capillary refill time and brisk reactive pupils
4 During the respiratory assessment the nurse thinks that he hears some crackles in his older-adult patient. What should the nurse do to ensure that the assessment is correct?
   1 Ask patient if he has ever had crackles in his lungs
   2 Ask patient to breathe in through his nose
   3 Have patient breathe in deeper when bases are auscultated
   4 Check patient's medical record to determine if they were previously heard on auscultation
5 Calculate patient's intake in milliliters based on the following amounts: 3 ounces of orange juice, half carton of milk (240 mL per carton), 3-ounce popsicle, 12 ounces of cola, and an 8-ounce cup of ice.

6 In conducting a general survey of a patient, the nurse knows that the survey should include which of the following? (Select all that apply.)
   1 Appearance
   2 Obtaining peripheral pulses
   3 Measuring chest excursion
   4 Conducting a detailed history
   5 Behavior
   6 Pupillary response
   7 Posture
7 In teaching a patient about skin lesions, the nurse knows that teaching has been successful when the patient identifies which lesion as abnormal?
   1 A symmetric lesion
   2 A lesion with regular edges and borders
   3 One that is blue/black or varied in color
   4 One that is less than 7 mm in diameter
8 On respiratory assessment the nurse notes high-pitched, musical sounds on auscultation. The nurse interprets these sounds as:
   1 Normal; vesicular.
   2 Rhonchi.
   3 Crackles.
   4 Wheezes.
9 The nurse determines that the patient has an audible S_2 on auscultation during cardiovascular assessment. After documenting the finding, the nurse should:
   1 Reposition the patient for comfort.
   2 Report the finding to the health care provider.
   3 Initiate fluid restriction.
   4 Do nothing because this is a normal finding.
10 Place the following components of the abdominal assessment in the correct order:
   1 Palpation
   2 Inspection
   3 Auscultation
   4 Percussion

REFERENCES

American Cancer Society (ACS): Learn about cancer, American Cancer Society recommendations for early breast cancer detection, 2012a, http://www.cancer.org/Cancer/BreastCancer/DetailedGuide/breast-cancer-detection, accessed May 19, 2012.

American Cancer Society (ACS): *Cancer facts and figures 2012*, Atlanta, 2012b, The Society.)

American Cancer Society (ACS): *Can melanoma be prevented*, Atlanta, 2011a, The Society.

American Cancer Society (ACS): *Human papilloma virus (HPV), cancer, and HPV vaccines 2011*, Atlanta, 2011b, The Society.

American Cancer Society (ACS): *Cervical cancer: causes, risk factors, and prevention topics 2011*, Atlanta, 2011c, The Society.

American Cancer Society (ACS): *Ovarian cancer: causes, risk factors, and prevention topics 2011*, Atlanta, 2011d, The Society.

American Cancer Society (ACS): *Endometrial (uterine) cancer: causes, risk factors, and prevention topics 2011*, Atlanta, 2011e, The Society.

American Cancer Society (ACS): *Prostate cancer: causes, risk factors, and prevention topics 2011*, Atlanta, 2011f, The Society.

American Cancer Society (ACS): *Colorectal cancer early detection 2011*, Atlanta, 2011g, The Society.

Ball JW, Bindler RC: *Child health nursing: partnering with children and families*, Upper Saddle River, NJ, 2010, Pearson Prentice Hall.

Carter K: Identifying and managing deep vein thrombosis, *Primary Health Care* 20(1):30, 2010.

Centers for Disease Control and Prevention: Updated recommendations for prevention of invasive pneumococcal disease among adults using the 23-valent pneumococcal polysaccharide vaccine (PPSV23). *MMWR* 59(34):1102, 2010.

Centers for Disease Control and Prevention: Vaccines and preventable diseases – HPV vaccine questions and answers, 2011, http://www.cdc.gov/vaccines/vpd-vac/hpv/vac-faqs.htm, accessed May 24, 2012.

Chait SR, et al: Relationship of body image to breast and skin self-examination intentions and behaviors, *Body Image* 6:60, 2009.

Cherry C, Stuart J: *Pocket guide to culturally sensitive health care*, Philadelphia, 2011, Davis.

Cress C: *Handbook of geriatric care management*, ed 3, Sudbury, 2012, Jones and Bartlett.

Furlow B: Tuberculosis: a review and update, *Radiol Technol* 82(1):33, 2010.

Glanz K, Schoenfeld ER, Steffen A: Randomized trial of tailored skin cancer prevention messages for adults: Project SCAPE, *Amer J Public Health* 100(4):735–741, 2010.

Hegarty K, et al: Violence between intimate partners: working with the whole family, *Br Med J* 337:346, 2008.

Hockenberry MJ, Wilson D: *Wong's nursing care of infants and children*, ed 9, St Louis, 2011, Mosby.

Jaffe S, et al: Osteoporosis prevention, *CINAHL Inf Sys* 3:2p, 2011.

Lewis S, et al: *Medical-surgical nursing: assessment and management of clinical problems*, ed 8, St Louis, 2011, Mosby.

Marret L, et al: *Screening for skin cancer: a clinical practice guideline, evidence-based series no. 15-11*, Toronto, 2007, Cancer Care Ontario.

Mujumdar UJ, et al: Sun protection and skin self-examination in melanoma survivors, *Psychooncology* 18(10):1106–1115, 2009.

Seidel HM, et al: *Mosby's guide to physical examination*, ed 7, St Louis, 2011, Mosby.

The Joint Commission (TJC): *2012 Comprehensive accreditation manual for hospitals: the official handbook*, Oakbrook Terrace, Ill, 2012, The Commission.

Touhy T, Jett K: *Ebersole and Hess' gerontological nursing & healthy aging*, ed 3, St Louis, 2010, Mosby.

Uneke C, et al: Bacterial contamination of stethoscopes used by health workers: public health implications, *J Infect Dev Ctries* 4(7):436, 2010.

US Preventive Services Task Force (USPSTF): Screening for osteoporosis. U.S. Preventive Services Task Force recommendation sheet, *Ann Intern Med* 154(5):356, 2011.

Wolff T, et al: Screening for skin cancer: an update of the evidence for the US Preventive Services Task Force, *Ann Intern Med* 150(3):194, 2009.

Medical Asepsis

SKILLS AND PROCEDURES

MEDIA RESOURCES

- evolve http://evolve.elsevier.com/Perry/skills
  learning system
  - Review Questions
  - Video Clips
  - Audio Glossary

- Mosby's Nursing Video Skills, 4th edition
- NSO Nursing Skills Online

KEY TERMS

Asepsis	Infection	Health care–associated	Surgical asepsis
Aseptic technique	Invasive procedure	infection	Transmission-based
Colonized	Isolation	Pathogen	precautions
Contamination	Medical asepsis	Rhinorrhea	
Immunocompromised	Microorganism	Standard precautions	

OBJECTIVES

Mastery of content in this chapter will enable the nurse to:

- Discuss how to apply critical thinking in the prevention of the transmission of infection.
- Explain the difference between medical and surgical asepsis.
- Identify nursing care measures intended to break the chain of infection.

- Explain how each element of the infection chain contributes to infection.
- Describe the factors that influence nursing staff compliance with hand hygiene.
- Perform proper procedures for hand hygiene.
- Perform correct isolation techniques.

Infection prevention and control practices that reduce or eliminate sources and transmission of infection help to protect patients and health care providers from disease. Patients in all health care settings are at risk of becoming colonized or infected as a result of an impaired immune response, exposure to an increased number of pathogenic organisms, and performance of invasive procedures (Fardo, 2011). Health care-associated infections (HAIs) result from delivery of health services in a health care setting and were not present at the time of admission. A hospital is one of the most likely settings for acquiring an HAI because staff, patients, and environmental factors support a high population of pathogens that are resistant to antibiotics. Health care workers transmit many HAIs by direct contact during the delivery of care. Although protecting patients from HAIs is an obvious priority, nurses are also at risk because of contact with infectious materials or exposure to a communicable disease.

The presence of a pathogen does not mean that an infection will occur. Infection occurs in a cycle, often referred to as the *chain of infection*, which depends on the presence of all of the following elements:

1. An infectious agent or pathogen
2. A reservoir or source for pathogen growth
3. A portal of exit from the reservoir
4. A mode of transmission
5. A portal of entry to the host
6. A susceptible host

An infection develops if this chain remains intact (Fig. 7-1). In patient care it is important to use infection control practices to break an element of the chain so as not to transmit infection (Table 7-1). Steps taken to minimize the onset and spread of infection are based on asepsis and the principles of aseptic technique. Asepsis is the absence of pathogenic (disease-producing) microorganisms (Iwamoto, 2011). The two types of aseptic technique that nurses practice are medical and surgical asepsis.

Medical asepsis, or clean technique, includes procedures used for reducing the number of organisms and preventing

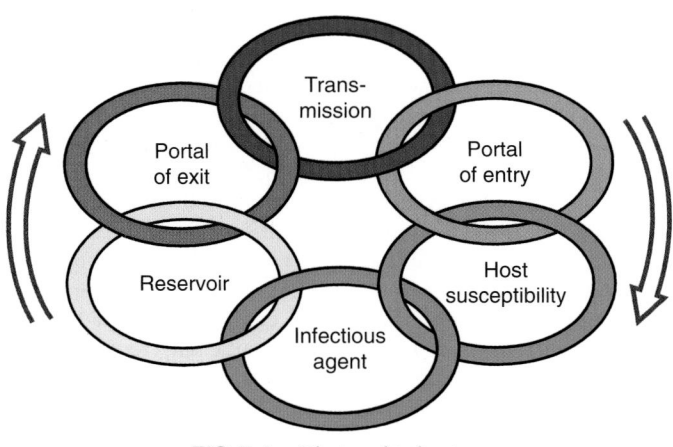

FIG 7-1 Chain of infection.

their transfer. Hand hygiene, barrier techniques, and routine environmental cleaning are examples of medical asepsis. Principles of medical asepsis are common in the home, as in the case of washing hands before preparing food.

Surgical asepsis, or sterile technique, includes procedures used to eliminate all microorganisms from an area. Sterilization destroys all microorganisms and their spores (Rutala and Weber, 2011). Nurses in the operating room, labor and delivery area, and procedural areas practice sterile technique when using sterile instruments and supplies.

Use sterile technique on nursing units when performing certain invasive procedures (e.g., insertion of a central line or an indwelling urinary catheter). The techniques for maintaining surgical asepsis is more rigid than those performed under medical asepsis (see Chapter 8).

TABLE 7-1	**Breaking the Chain of Infection**
Element of Infection Chain	**Medical Asepsis Practices**
Infectious agent (pathogenic organism capable of causing disease)	Clean contaminated objects. Clean, disinfect, and sterilize.
Reservoir (site or source of microorganism growth)	Control sources of body fluids and drainage. Perform hand hygiene. Bathe patient with soap and water or disposable bath. Change soiled dressings. Dispose of soiled tissues, dressings, or linen in moisture-resistant bags. Place syringes, uncapped hypodermic needles, and intravenous needles in designated puncture-proof containers. Keep table surfaces clean and dry. Do not leave bottled solutions open for prolonged periods. Keep solutions tightly capped. Keep surgical wound drainage tubes and collection bags patent. Empty and dispose of drainage suction bottles according to agency policy.
Portal of exit (means by which microorganisms leave a site)	Respiratory • Avoid talking, sneezing, or coughing directly over wound or sterile dressing field. • Cover nose and mouth when sneezing or coughing. • Wear mask if suffering respiratory tract infection. Urine, feces, emesis, and blood • Wear clean gloves when handling blood and body fluids. • Wear gowns and eyewear if there is a chance of splashing fluids. • Handle all laboratory specimens as if infectious.
Transmission (means of spread)	Reduce microorganism spread. • Perform hand hygiene. • Use personal set of care items for each patient. • Avoid shaking bed linen or clothes; dust with damp cloth. • Avoid contact of soiled item with uniform. • Discard any item that touches the floor. • Follow standard precautions or select transmission-based isolation precautions.
Portal of entry (site through which microorganism enters a host)	Skin and mucosa • Maintain skin and mucous membrane integrity, lubricate skin, offer frequent hygiene, turn and position. • Cover wounds as needed. • Clean wound sites thoroughly. • Dispose of used needles in puncture-proof container. Urinary • Keep all drainage systems closed and intact, maintaining downward flow.
Host (patient)	Reduce susceptibility to infection. Provide adequate nutrition. Ensure adequate rest. Promote body defenses against infection. Provide immunization.

EVIDENCE-BASED PRACTICE

For generations handwashing with soap and water was considered the best method to prevent transmission of infection from health care workers to patients. However, recent research shows that handwashing with plain soap sometimes results in paradoxical increases in bacterial counts on the skin (WHO, 2009). Alcohol-based products are more effective for standard handwashing or hand antisepsis than soap or antiseptic soaps (WHO, 2009). Alcohol-based hand sanitizers reduced infections in a variety of settings from intensive care units to long-term care facilities (Herud, 2009). Moreover, brisk alcohol-based rinses or gels containing emollients cause substantially less skin irritation and dryness than plain or antimicrobial soaps (Haas, 2011). Soap and water are still necessary for hand hygiene if hands are visibly soiled or when caring for patients infected with *Clostridium difficile* or multidrug-resistant organisms (MDROs) such as methicillin-resistant *Staphylococcus aureus* (MRSA) or vancomycin-resistant enterococcus (VRE). Studies show that health care workers with chipped nail polish or long or artificial nails have high numbers of bacteria on their fingertips.

- Health care workers should not wear artificial nails and extenders (Longtin et al., 2011)
- No rings or bracelets should be worn during patient care (Fagernes and Lingaas, 2009; Longtin et al., 2011).
- Fingernails should not be longer than 0.625 cm (¼ inch) in length and nail polish should not be chipped. There are no recommendations regarding nail polish color (Cook, 2011).
- Whenever possible, use alcohol-based products that contain emollients (Longtin et al., 2011).

PATIENT-CENTERED CARE

As a nurse you are responsible for educating patients about infection prevention. Patient and family teaching needs to include information concerning signs and symptoms of infection, modes of transmission, and methods of prevention. Knowledge of the infectious process, disease transmission, and critical thinking skills associated with use of aseptic techniques and barrier protection is essential. The Joint Commission (TJC) National Patient Safety Goals (2012) support patients' rights to question health care workers about infection control and prevention practices, including hand hygiene. For example, it is believed that, if patients ask health care providers if they have washed their hands, health care providers' compliance will increase. Through education you play a vital role in the prevention of infection.

When a patient requires isolation in a private room, remember that loneliness can easily develop. Isolation disrupts normal social relationships with visitors and caregivers. Some patients who suffer from an infectious disease also experience self-concept or body image changes. Other cultures rely on alternative health care practices (e.g., the use of Chinese herbs to treat illness and optimize health) (University of Minnesota, 2011). When a patient from another culture requires isolation, use caution to be sure that the patient and family understand the therapeutic purpose of isolation. For example, the isolation of a loved one is considered disrespectful and uncaring behavior in collectivistic cultures (Hispanics, Africans, and Asians). Unless you act to minimize feelings of psychological and physical isolation, the patient's emotional state could interfere with recovery.

Safety Guidelines

1. Hand hygiene with an appropriate alcohol-based hand antiseptic or soap and water is an essential part of patient care and infection prevention.
2. Always know a patient's susceptibility to infection. Age, nutritional status, stress, disease processes, and forms of medical therapy can place patients at risk.
3. Recognize the elements of the chain of infection and initiate measures to prevent its onset and spread.
4. Consistently incorporate the basic principles of asepsis into patient care.
5. Ensure that patients cover their mouth and nose when coughing or sneezing, use tissues to contain respiratory secretions, and dispose of tissues in the waste receptacle.
6. Use clean gloves when you anticipate contact with body fluids, nonintact skin, or mucous membranes when there is a risk of drainage.
7. Use gown, mask, and eye protection when there is a splash risk.
8. Protect fellow health care workers from exposure to infectious agents through proper use and disposal of equipment.
9. Be aware of body sites where HAIs are most likely to develop (e.g., urinary or respiratory tract). This enables you to direct preventive measures.

SKILL 7-1 Hand Hygiene

NSO *Infection Control Module / Lessons 1 and 2*

 Video Clip

The most important and basic technique in preventing and controlling transmission of infection is hand hygiene. Hand hygiene is a general term that applies to handwashing, antiseptic hand wash, antiseptic hand rub, or surgical hand antisepsis. Handwashing refers to washing hands with plain soap and water. An antiseptic hand wash is defined as washing hands with water and soap or other detergents containing an antiseptic agent. An antiseptic hand rub means applying an antiseptic hand rub product to all surfaces of the hands to reduce the number of microorganisms present. Surgical hand antisepsis is the use of an antiseptic hand wash or antiseptic hand rub before surgery by surgical personnel to eliminate transient and reduce resident hand flora. Antiseptic detergent preparations often have persistent antimicrobial activity (WHO, 2009).

The decision to perform hand hygiene depends on four factors: (1) the intensity or degree of contact with patients or contaminated objects, (2) the amount of contamination that may occur with the contact, (3) the patient or health care worker's susceptibility to infection, and (4) the procedure or activity to be performed (Haas, 2011). Longtin et al. (2011) found that hand-hygiene compliance among health care workers found an overall compliance rate below 40%. *Hand hygiene is not optional.* It is a critical responsibility for all health care workers. Follow these guidelines for hand hygiene (CDC, 2002; WHO, 2009):

1 Wash hands with either plain soap and water or an antibacterial soap and water when hands are visibly dirty, soiled with blood or other body fluids, before eating, and after using the toilet.

2 Wash hands if exposed to spore-forming organisms such as *Clostridium difficile* or *Bacillus anthracis*.

3 If hands are not visibly soiled, use an alcohol-based hand rub for routinely decontaminating hands in the following clinical situations:

   a Before and after having direct contact with patients.

   b Before applying sterile gloves and inserting an invasive device such as indwelling urinary catheters and peripheral vascular catheters

   c After contact with body fluids or excretions, mucous membranes, and nonintact skin

   d After contact with wound dressings (if hands are not visibly soiled)

   e When moving from a contaminated body site to a clean body site during patient care

   f After contact with inanimate objects (e.g., medical equipment) in the immediate vicinity of a patient

   g After removing gloves

Delegation and Collaboration

The skill of hand hygiene is performed by all caregivers. Hand hygiene is not optional.

Equipment

❑ Antiseptic hand rub
❑ Alcohol-based waterless antiseptic containing emollients
❑ Handwashing
   • Easy-to-reach sink with warm running water
   • Antimicrobial or regular soap
   • Paper towels or air dryer
   • Disposable nail cleaner (optional)

STEP	RATIONALE

ASSESSMENT

1 Inspect surface of hands for breaks or cuts in skin or cuticles. Cover any skin lesions with a dressing before providing care. If lesions are too large to cover, you may be restricted from direct patient care.	Open cuts or wounds can harbor high concentrations of microorganisms. Agency policy may prevent nurses from caring for high-risk patients if open lesions are present on hands (WHO, 2009).
2 Inspect hands for visible soiling.	Visible soiling requires handwashing with soap and water.
3 Inspect condition of nails. Natural tips should be no longer than 0.625 cm (¼ inch) long. Be sure that fingernails are short, filed, and smooth.	Subungual areas of hand harbor high concentrations of bacteria. Long nails and chipped or old polish increase the number of bacteria residing on hands. Artificial applications increase microbial load on hands (Boyce and Pittet, 2008, CDC, 2002).

NURSING DIAGNOSES

This skill is required for patients with a variety of nursing diagnoses
Related factors are individualized based on patient's condition or needs.

PLANNING

1 Expected outcomes following completion of procedure: • Hands and areas under fingernails are clean and free of debris.	Transient bacteria have been removed.

IMPLEMENTATION

1 Push wristwatch and long uniform sleeves above wrists. Avoid wearing rings. If worn, remove during hand hygiene.	Provides complete access to fingers, hands, and wrists. Wearing rings increases number of microorganisms on hands (Longtin et al., 2011).
2 *Antiseptic hand rub* a Dispense ample amount of product into palm of one hand (see illustration).	Many microorganisms on hands come from the subungual region (beneath fingernails). Use enough product to thoroughly cover hands.

STEP	RATIONALE

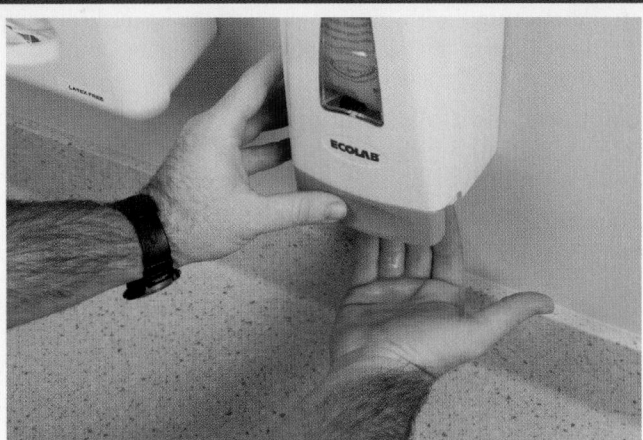

STEP 2a   Apply waterless antiseptic to hands.

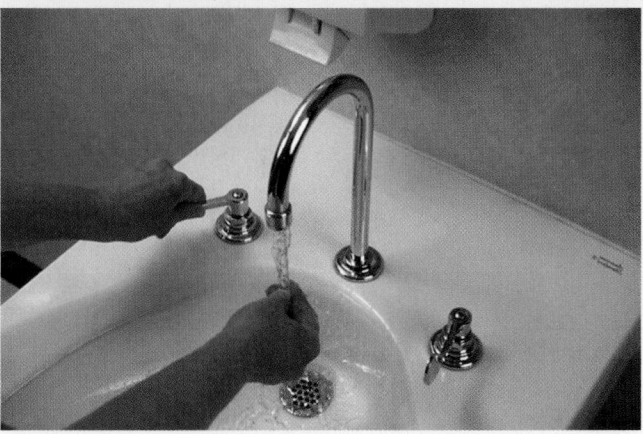

STEP 3b   Turn on water.

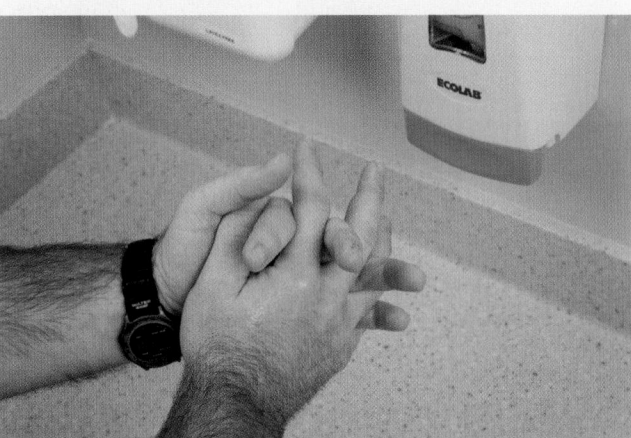

STEP 2b   Rub hands thoroughly.

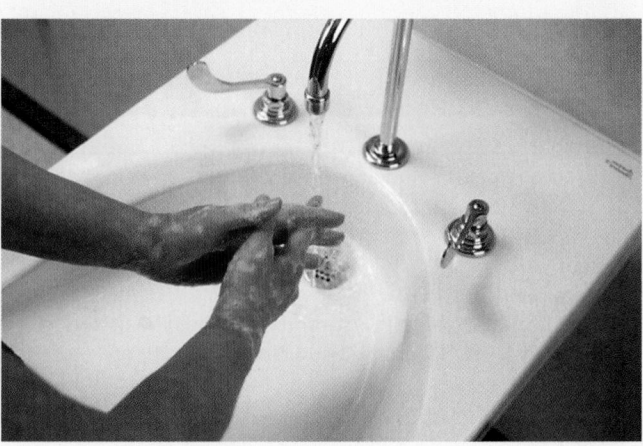

STEP 3f   Lather hands thoroughly.

b Rub hands together, covering all surfaces of hands and fingers with antiseptic (see illustration).	Provides enough time for product to work.
c Rub hands together until the alcohol is dry. Allow hands to completely dry before applying gloves.	Ensures complete antimicrobial action.
3 *Handwashing using regular or antimicrobial soap*	
a Stand in front of sink, keeping hands and uniform away from sink surface. (If hands touch sink during handwashing, repeat sequence.)	Inside of sink is a contaminated area. Reaching over sink increases risk of touching edge, which is contaminated.
b Turn on water. Turn faucet on (see illustration) or push knee pedals laterally or press pedals with foot to regulate flow and temperature.	Knee pads within the operating room and treatment areas are preferred to prevent hand contact with faucet. Faucet handles are likely to be contaminated with organic debris and microorganisms (AORN, 2011).
c Avoid splashing water against uniform.	Microorganisms travel and grow in moisture.
d Regulate flow of water so temperature is warm.	Warm water removes less of protective oils on hands than hot water.
e Wet hands and wrists thoroughly under running water. Keep hands and forearms lower than elbows during washing.	Hands are most contaminated parts to wash. Water flows from least to most contaminated area, rinsing microorganisms into sink.
f Apply 3 to 5 mL of antiseptic soap and rub hands together (see illustration).	Ensure that all surfaces of hands and fingers are cleaned.

STEP	RATIONALE
g Perform hand hygiene using plenty of lather and friction for at least 15 to 20 seconds. Interlace fingers and rub palms and back of hands with circular motion at least 5 times each. Keep fingertips down to facilitate removal of microorganisms.	Soap cleans by emulsifying fat and oil and lowering surface tension. Friction and rubbing mechanically loosen and remove dirt and transient bacteria. Interlacing fingers and thumbs ensures that all surfaces are cleaned. Adequate time is needed to expose skin surfaces to antimicrobial agent.
h Areas underlying fingernails are often soiled. Clean them with fingernails of other hand and additional soap or with disposable nail cleaner.	Area under nails can be highly contaminated, which increases risk for transmission of infection from nurse to patient.

Clinical Decision Point *Do not tear or cut skin under or around nail.*

STEP	RATIONALE
i Rinse hands and wrists thoroughly, keeping hands down and elbows up (see illustration).	Rinsing mechanically washes away dirt and microorganisms.
j Dry hands thoroughly from fingers to wrists with paper towel, single-use cloth, or warm air dryer.	Drying from cleanest (fingertips) to least clean (wrist) avoids contamination. Drying hands prevents chapping and roughened skin.
k If used, discard paper towel in proper receptacle.	Prevents transfer of microorganisms.
l To turn off hand faucet, use clean, dry paper towel; avoid touching handles with hands (see illustration). Turn off water with foot or knee pedals (if applicable).	Wet towel and hands allow transfer of pathogens from faucet by capillary action.

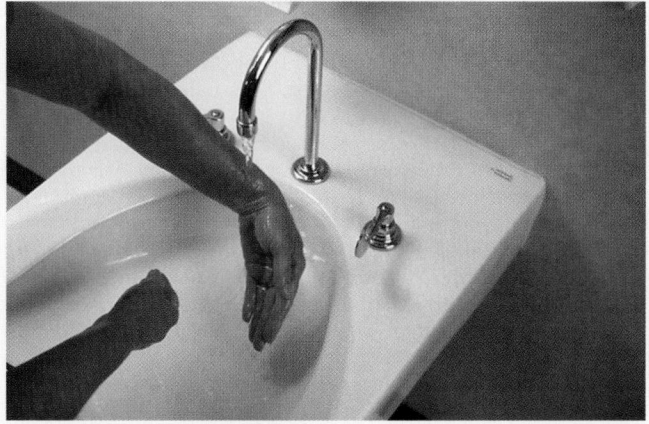

STEP 3i   Rinse hands.

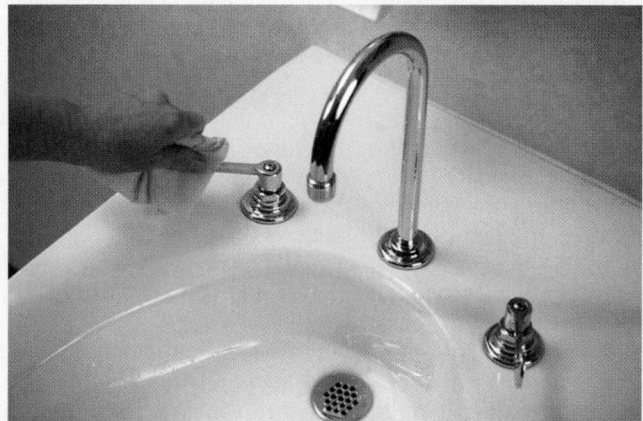

STEP 3l   Turn off faucet.

STEP	RATIONALE
m If hands are dry or chapped, use a small amount of lotion or barrier cream dispensed from an individual use container.	Helps to minimize skin dryness. There is risk of organism growth in lotion, so only apply after patient care activities are complete.

EVALUATION

1 Inspect surface of hands for obvious signs of dirt or other contaminants.	Determines if hand hygiene is adequate.

Unexpected Outcomes

1 Hands or areas under fingernails remain soiled.

2 Repeated use of soaps or antiseptics causes dermatitis or cracked skin.

Related Interventions

- Repeat handwashing with soap and water.

- Rinse and dry hands thoroughly after using soap and water; avoid excessive amounts of soap or antiseptic; try various products.

- Use approved hand lotions or barrier creams. Small individual-use containers are preferred because large containers have been found to harbor pathogens.

Special Considerations
Teaching Considerations
- Instruct patient and family caregiver in proper techniques and situations for hand hygiene.
- When patients are educated about the risks for infections, they play an important role in improving hand hygiene compliance in health care settings by reminding visitors and health care workers to perform hand hygiene.

Gerontologic Considerations
- The impact of infections is greater in older adults. Hand hygiene by staff attending older adults is of utmost importance and should be an ongoing continuing-education requirement.

Home Care
- Evaluate patient and primary caregiver to determine their understanding of the transmission of microorganisms and their ability and motivation to perform hand hygiene correctly.
- Evaluate the hand hygiene facilities in the home to determine the possibility of contamination, proximity of the facilities to the patient, and the ability to maintain supplies and equipment.

SKILL 7-2   Caring for Patients Under Isolation Precautions

 Video Clip

When a patient has a known or suspected source of colonization or infection, health care workers follow specific infection prevention and control practices to reduce the risk of cross-contamination to other patients. Certain procedures performed at a patient's bedside require the application of personal protective equipment (PPE) such as a mask, cap, eyewear, gown, or gloves. Standard precautions require you to wear clean gloves before coming in contact with mucous membranes, nonintact skin, blood, body fluids, or other infectious material. You wear gloves routinely when performing a variety of procedures (e.g., nasogastric tube insertion). Masks are worn when there is the risk of splash during a procedure or when certain sterile procedures such as changing a central line dressing are performed. Protective eyewear and masks become important when there is a risk for splash of blood or other body fluids to the eyes or mouth.

The majority of organisms causing health care–associated infections are in the colonized body substances of patients, regardless of whether or not a culture has confirmed infection and a diagnosis has been made (Saint et al., 2008). Body substances such as feces, emesis, urine, mucus, and wound drainage contain potentially infectious organisms. Assess the need for PPE for each task you plan and for all patients, regardless of their diagnoses. Because of increased attention to the prevention of bloodborne pathogens and tuberculosis (TB) (Box 7-1), the Centers for Disease Control and Prevention (CDC) (2007a, 2007b) and the Occupational Safety and Health Administration (OSHA) (2010) have stressed the importance of barrier protection.

In 2007 the Hospital Infection Control Practices Advisory Committee (HICPAC) of the CDC published revised guidelines for isolation precautions. These recommendations were based on current epidemiologic information regarding disease transmission in health care settings. Although primarily intended for care of patients in acute care, you can apply the recommendations to patients in subacute care or long-term care facilities. HICPAC recommends that hospitals modify the recommendations according to their needs and as dictated by federal, state, or local regulations (CDC, 2007b).

The guidelines contain recommendations for respiratory hygiene/cough etiquette as part of standard precautions. Standard precautions, or tier one precautions, are for the care of all patients, regardless of risk or presumed infection status (Box 7-2). Standard precautions are the primary strategies for prevention of infection transmission and apply to contact with blood, body fluids, nonintact skin, and mucous membranes and with equipment or surfaces

BOX 7-1 | Special Tuberculosis Precautions

In 1994 the Centers for Disease Control and Prevention (CDC) published guidelines for preventing tuberculosis (TB) transmission in health care agencies in response to a resurgence of TB in the United States associated with the increasing incidence of human immunodeficiency virus (HIV) infection, TB infection transmission in health care settings, and increasing immigration from countries with a high incidence of TB (CDC, 2011a). The current CDC guidelines for preventing and controlling TB focus on early detection of infection, preventing close contact with patients with active TB disease, and applying effective infection control measures in health care settings. Suspect TB in any patient with respiratory symptoms lasting longer than 3 weeks accompanied by other suspicious symptoms such as unexplained weight loss, night sweats, fever, and a productive cough often streaked with blood. Also consider the potential for infectious pulmonary or laryngeal TB from documented positive acid-fast bacilli (AFB) smear or culture, cavitation on chest x-ray film, or history of recent TB exposure. Isolation for patients with suspected or confirmed TB includes placing the patient on airborne precautions in a single-patient negative-pressure room.

Occupational Safety and Health Administration (OSHA) and CDC guidelines require health care workers who care for patients with suspected or confirmed TB to wear special respirators (e.g., N95 or P100) (CDC, 2010). These respirators are high-efficiency particulate masks that have the ability to filter particles at a 95% or better efficiency. Health care workers who use these respirators must be fit tested in a reliable way to obtain a face-seal leakage of 10% or less (Roberge, 2008). OSHA also requires employers to provide training concerning transmission of TB, especially in areas where the risk of exposure is high. In addition, the CDC now recommends the use of the QuantiFERON-TB Gold test (QFT-GIT) or the T-SPOT (CDC, 2011b), a blood test, in place of the traditional TB skin test. The advantages of the QFT-GIT test are that it does not boost responses measured by subsequent tests and the results are not subject to reader bias.

---

contaminated with these potentially infectious materials. The strategy of respiratory hygiene/cough etiquette applies to any person with signs of respiratory infection, including cough, congestion, rhinorrhea, or increased production of respiratory secretions when entering a health care site. Educating health care staff, patients, and visitors to cover the mouth and nose with a tissue when coughing, dispose properly of used tissues, and perform hand hygiene is among the elements of respiratory hygiene.

The second tier (see Box 7-2) includes precautions designed for care of patients who are known or suspected to be infected, or colonized, with microorganisms transmitted by the contact, droplet, or

| BOX 7-2 | Centers for Disease Control and Prevention Isolation Guidelines |

Standard Precautions (Tier One) for Use with All Patients

- Standard precautions apply to blood, blood products, all body fluids, secretions, excretions (except sweat), nonintact skin, and mucous membranes.
- Perform hand hygiene before, after, and between direct contact with patients. (e.g., between contact: cleaning hands after a patient care activity, moving to a nonpatient care activity, and cleaning hands again before returning to perform patient contact).
- Perform hand hygiene after contact with blood, body fluids, secretions, and excretions; after contact with surfaces or articles in a patient room; and immediately after gloves are removed.
- When hands are visibly soiled or contaminated with blood or body fluids, wash them with either a nonantimicrobial soap or an antimicrobial soap and water.
- When hands are not visibly soiled or contaminated with blood or body fluids, use an alcohol-based hand rub to perform hand hygiene.
- Wash hands with nonantimicrobial soap and water if contact with spores (e.g., *Clostridium difficile*) is likely to have occurred.
- Do not wear artificial fingernails or extenders if duties include direct contact with patients at high risk for infection and associated adverse outcomes.

- Wear gloves when touching blood, body fluids, secretions, excretions, nonintact skin, mucous membranes, or contaminated items or surfaces is likely. Remove gloves and perform hand hygiene between patient care encounters and when going from a contaminated to a clean body site.
- Wear personal protective equipment when the anticipated patient interaction indicates that contact with blood or body fluids may occur.
- A private room is unnecessary unless the patient's hygiene is unacceptable (e.g., uncontained secretions, excretions, or wound drainage).
- Discard all contaminated sharp instruments and needles in a puncture-resistant container. Health care agencies must make available needleless devices. Any needles should be disposed of uncapped; or a mechanical safety device is activated for recapping.
- Respiratory hygiene/cough etiquette—Have patients:
  - Cover the nose/mouth when coughing or sneezing.
  - Use tissues to contain respiratory secretions and dispose in nearest waste container.
  - Perform hand hygiene after contacting respiratory secretions and contaminated objects/materials.
  - Contain respiratory secretions with procedure or surgical mask.
  - Sit at least 91.4 cm (3 feet) away from others if coughing.

Transmission-Based Precautions (Tier Two) for Use With Specific Types of Patients

Category	Infection/Condition	Barrier Protection
Airborne precautions (droplet nuclei smaller than 5 microns)	Measles, chickenpox (varicella), disseminated varicella zoster, pulmonary or laryngeal tuberculosis	Private room, negative-pressure airflow of at least 6 to 12 exchanges per hour via HEPA filtration; mask or respiratory protection device, N95 respirator required (depending on condition)
Droplet precautions (droplets larger than 5 microns; being within 3 feet of patient)	Diphtheria (pharyngeal), rubella, streptococcal pharyngitis, pneumonia or scarlet fever in infants and young children, pertussis, mumps, *Mycoplasma* pneumonia, meningococcal pneumonia or sepsis, pneumonic plague	Private room or cohort patients; mask or respirator required (depending on condition) (refer to agency policy)
Contact precautions (direct patient or environmental contact)	Colonization or infection with multidrug-resistant organisms such as VRE and MRSA, *Clostridium difficile*, *Shigella*, and other enteric pathogens; major wound infections; herpes simplex; scabies; varicella zoster (disseminated); respiratory syncytial virus in infants, young children, or immunocompromised adults	Private room or cohort patients (see agency policy), gloves, gowns
Protective environment	Allogeneic hematopoietic stem cell transplants	Private room; positive airflow with 12 or more air exchanges per hour; HEPA filtration for incoming air; mask to be worn by patient when out of room during times of construction in area

Modified from Centers for Disease Control and Prevention (CDC), Hospital Infection Control Practice Advisory Committee: Guidelines for isolation precautions in hospitals, *MMWR Morb Mortal Wkly Rep* 57/RR-16:39, 2007.
HEPA, High-efficiency particulate air; *MRSA,* methicillin-resistant *Staphylococcus aureus*; *VRE,* vancomycin-resistant enterococcus.

airborne route (CDC, 2007a; Brisko, 2011) or by contact with contaminated surfaces. The three types of transmission-based precautions—airborne, droplet, and contact—may be combined for diseases that have multiple routes of transmission (e.g., chickenpox). When used either singly or in combination, you use them in addition to standard precautions. Box 7-2 summarizes the types of patients who are cared for under transmission-based precautions.

One important aspect of care for a patient in isolation is compliance with hand hygiene and the changing of gloves between exposures to body sites and patient equipment. Inadequate glove changes and hand hygiene can lead to contamination of previously uncolonized sites (Haas, 2011). Noncompliance with glove changing and hand hygiene increases the risk of HAIs.

Delegation and Collaboration

The skill of caring for patients on isolation precautions can be delegated to nursing assistive personnel (NAP). However, the nurse must assess the patient's status and isolation indications. The nurse instructs the NAP to:

- Take special precautions regarding individual patient needs such as transportation to diagnostic tests.
- Take precautions about bringing equipment into the patient's room.
- Be aware of high-risk factors for infection transmission that pertain to the assigned patient.

Equipment

❑ Barrier protection determined by type of isolation required; clean gloves, mask, eyewear or goggles, face shield, and gown (gowns may be disposable or reusable, depending on agency policy)
❑ Other patient care equipment (as appropriate) (e.g., hygiene items, medications, dressing supplies, sharps container, disposable blood pressure cuff)
❑ Soiled linen bag and trash receptacle
❑ Sign for door indicating type of isolation and/or for visitors to come to the nurses' station before entering room

STEP	RATIONALE

ASSESSMENT

1 Assess patient's medical history for possible indications for isolation (e.g., risk factors for TB, major draining wound, or purulent productive cough). Review precautions for the specific isolation system, including appropriate barriers to apply (see Box 7-2).	Mode of transmission for infectious microorganism determines type and degree of precautions followed. Ensures adequate protection.
2 Review laboratory test results (e.g., wound culture, acid-fast bacillus [AFB] smears, changes in WBC count).	Reveals type of microorganism for which patient is being isolated, body fluid in which it was identified, and whether patient is immunosuppressed.
3 Consider types of care measures that you will perform while in patient's room (e.g., medication administration or dressing change).	Allows you to organize care items for procedures and time spent in patient's room.
4 Review nursing care plan notes or confer with colleagues regarding patient's emotional state and reaction/adjustment to isolation. Also assess patient's understanding of purpose of isolation.	Determines patient's need for emotional support and teaching.

NURSING DIAGNOSES

- Deficient knowledge regarding purpose of isolation
- Impaired social interaction
- Ineffective protection
- Risk for infection

Related factors are individualized based on patient's condition or needs.

PLANNING

1 Expected outcomes following completion of procedure:	
• Patient asks for information about disease transmission.	Active interaction reveals patient's willingness and/or ability to communicate and be taught and understand information.
• Patient explains purpose of isolation.	Instruction about precautions improves patient's ability to cooperate in care.

IMPLEMENTATION

1 Perform hand hygiene (see Skill 7-1).	Reduces transmission of microorganisms.
2 Prepare all equipment needed in patient's room. In many cases, dedicated equipment such as stethoscopes should remain in the room until patient is discharged.	Prevents you from making more than one trip into room. The CDC recommends use of dedicated noncritical patient care equipment (CDC, 2007a).
3 Prepare for entrance into isolation room. Prior to applying PPE, step into patient's room and stay by door. Introduce yourself and explain the care that you are providing.	Proper preparation ensures protection from microorganism exposure. Allows patient to see you without PPE and without exposing yourself to risk of infection transmission.
a Apply gown, being sure that it covers all outer garments. Pull sleeves down to wrist. Tie securely at neck and waist (see illustration).	Prevents transmission of infection; protects you when patient has excessive drainage, discharges.

STEP	RATIONALE

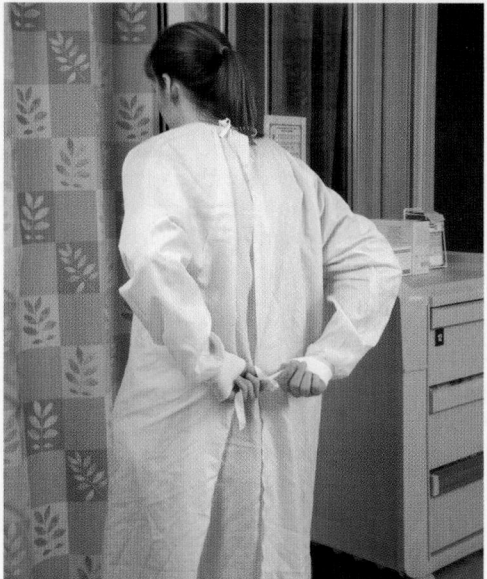

STEP 3a Tie isolation gown.

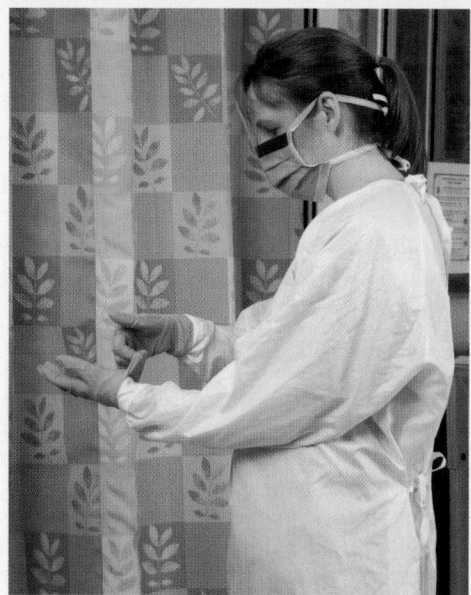

STEP 3d Bring glove cuffs over edge of gown sleeves.

b Apply either surgical mask or fitted respirator around mouth and nose (type and fit-testing depend on type of isolation and agency policy). You must have a medical evaluation and be fit-tested before using a respirator.

Prevents exposure to airborne microorganisms or microorganisms from splashing of fluids.

c If needed apply eyewear or goggles snugly around face and eyes. If you wear prescription glasses, side shields may be used.

Protects you from exposure to microorganisms that may occur during splashing of fluids.

d Apply clean gloves. (NOTE: Wear unpowdered gloves latex-free gloves if you, the patient, or another health care worker has a latex allergy.) Bring glove cuffs over edge of gown sleeves (see illustration).

Reduces transmission of microorganisms.

4 Enter patient's room. Arrange supplies and equipment. (NOTE: if equipment will be reused, place on a clean paper towel).

Prevents extra trips entering and leaving room. Minimizes contamination of care items.

5 Explain purpose of isolation and precautions for patient and family to take. Offer opportunity to ask questions.

Improves patient's and family's ability to participate in care and minimizes anxiety. Identifies opportunity for planning social interaction and diversional activities.

6 Assess vital signs (see Chapter 5).

a Reusable equipment brought into room must be thoroughly disinfected when removed from room.

Decreases the risk of infection being transmitted to another patient.

b If stethoscope is to be reused, clean earpieces and diaphragm or bell with 70% alcohol or agency-approved germicide. Set aside on clean surface.

Systematic disinfection of stethoscopes with 70% alcohol or approved germicide minimizes chance of spreading infectious agents between patients (CDC, 2007b).

c Use individual or disposable thermometers and blood pressure cuffs when available.

Prevents cross-contamination.

Clinical Decision Point *If patient is infected or colonized with a resistant organism (e.g., vancomycin-resistant enterococcus [VRE], methicillin-resistant Staphylococcus aureus [MRSA]), equipment remains in room whenever possible (CDC, 2011c). This includes stethoscope and blood pressure cuff.*

Clinical Decision Point *If disposable thermometer indicates a fever, assess for other signs/symptoms of infection. Confirm fever using an alternative thermometer. Do not use electronic thermometer if patient is suspected or confirmed to have Clostridium difficile (Cohen et al., 2010).*

7 Administer medications (see Chapters 20, 21, and 22).

a Give oral medication in wrapper or cup.

b Dispose of wrapper or cup in plastic-lined receptacle.

Handle and discard supplies to minimize transfer of microorganisms.

c Wear gloves when administering an injection.

Reduces risk of exposure to blood.

d Discard disposable syringe and uncapped or sheathed needle into designated sharps container.

Reduces risk of needlestick injury.

STEP	RATIONALE
e Place reusable plastic syringe (e.g., Carpuject) on clean towel for eventual removal and disinfection.	Prevents added contamination of syringe.
f If you are not wearing gloves and hands contact a contaminated article or body fluids, perform hand hygiene as soon as possible.	Reduces transmission of microorganisms.
8 Administer hygiene, encouraging patient to ask any questions or express concerns about isolation. Provide informal teaching at this time.	Hygiene practices further minimize transfer of microorganisms. Quality time should be spent with patient when in room.
a Avoid allowing isolation gown to become wet; carry washbasin outward away from gown; avoid leaning against wet tabletop.	Moisture allows organisms to travel through gown to uniform.

Clinical Decision Point *When there is a risk for excess soiling, wear a gown impervious to moisture.*

STEP	RATIONALE
b Help patient remove own gown; discard in leak-proof linen bag.	Reduces transfer of microorganisms.
c Remove linen from bed; avoid contact with isolation gown. Place in leak-proof linen bag.	Handle linen soiled by patient's body fluids to prevent contact with clean items.
d Provide clean bed linen and set of towels.	
e Change gloves and perform hand hygiene if gloves become excessively soiled and further care is necessary. Reglove.	
9 Collect specimens (see Chapter 43).	
a Place specimen containers on clean paper towel in patient's bathroom.	Container will be taken out of patient's room; prevents contamination of outer surface.
b Follow agency procedure for collecting specimen of body fluids (see Chapter 43).	
c Transfer specimen to container without soiling outside of container. Place container in plastic bag and place label on outside of bag or per agency policy. Label specimen in front of patient (TJC, 2012). Perform hand hygiene and reglove if additional procedures are needed.	Specimens of blood and body fluids are placed in well-constructed containers with secure lids to prevent leaks during transport. Proper labeling prevents diagnostic error.
d Check label on specimen for accuracy. Send to laboratory (warning labels are often used, depending on agency policy). Label containers of blood or body fluids with a biohazard sticker (see illustration).	Ensures that health care providers who transport or handle containers are aware of infectious contents.
10 Dispose of linen, trash, and disposable items.	
a Use single bags that are impervious to moisture and sturdy to contain soiled articles. Use double bag if necessary for heavily soiled linen or heavy wet trash.	Linen or refuse should be totally contained to prevent exposure of personnel to infectious material.
b Tie bags securely at top in knot (see illustration).	
11 Remove all reusable pieces of equipment. Clean any contaminated surfaces with hospital-approved disinfectant (CDC, 2007b) (see agency policy).	All items must be properly cleaned, disinfected, or sterilized for reuse.

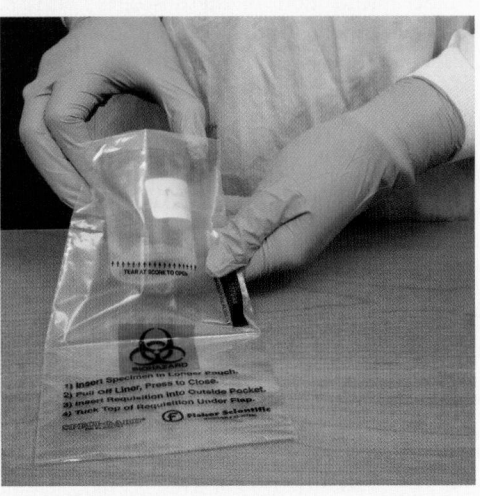

STEP 9d   Place specimen container in biohazard bag.

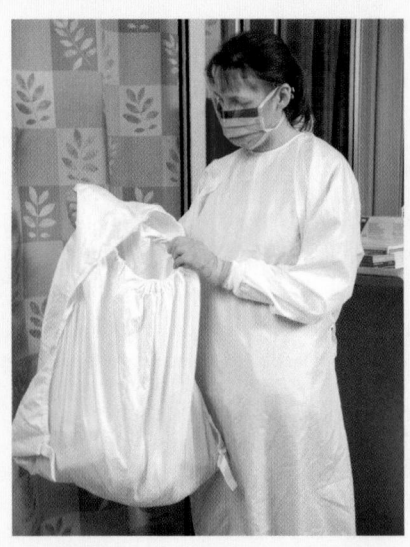

STEP 10b   Tie bag securely.

STEP	RATIONALE
12 Resupply room as needed. Have staff colleague hand new supplies to you.	Limiting trips of personnel into and out of room reduces your and patient's exposure to microorganisms.
13 Leave isolation room. Order of removal of PPE depends on what you wear in room. This sequence describes steps to take if all barriers are worn.	Order of removal minimizes exposure to any infectious material on barriers.
a Remove gloves. Remove one glove by grasping cuff and pulling glove inside out over hand. Hold removed glove in gloved hand (see illustration). Slide fingers of ungloved hand under remaining glove at wrist. Peel glove off over first glove. Discard gloves in proper container.	Technique prevents contact with outer surface contaminated of glove.
b Remove eyewear, face shield, or goggles. Handle by headband or earpieces. Discard in proper container.	Outside of goggles is contaminated. Hands have not been soiled.
c Untie neck strings and then untie back strings of gown. Allow gown to fall from shoulders (see illustration); touch inside of gown only. Remove hands from sleeves without touching outside of gown. Hold gown inside at shoulder seams and fold inside out into a bundle; discard in laundry bag.	Hands do not come in contact with soiled front of gown.
d Remove mask. If mask secures over ears, remove elastic from ears and pull mask away from face. For a tie-on mask, untie *bottom* mask string and then top strings, pull mask away from face (see illustration), and drop into trash receptacle. (Do not touch outer surface of mask.)	Ungloved hands will not be contaminated by touching only elastic or mask strings. Prevents top part of mask from falling down over uniform.
e Perform hand hygiene.	Reduces transmission of microorganisms.
f Retrieve wristwatch and stethoscope (unless items must remain in room) and record vital sign values on note paper.	Clean hands can contact clean items.
g Explain to patient when you plan to return to room. Ask whether patient requires any personal care items. Offer books, magazines, audiotapes.	Diversions can help to minimize boredom and feeling of social isolation.
h Dispose of all contaminated supplies and equipment in manner that prevents spread of microorganisms to other persons (see agency policy). Perform hand hygiene.	

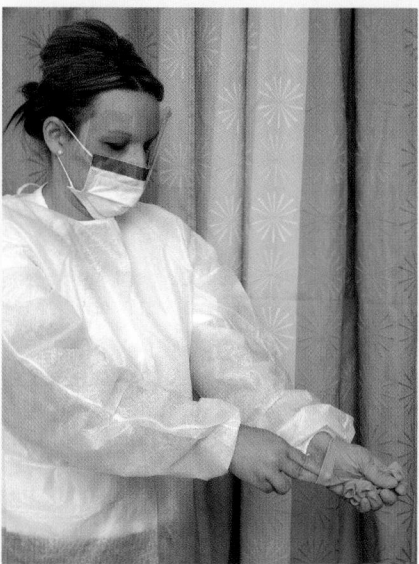

STEP 13a   Hold removed glove in gloved hand and pull remaining glove.

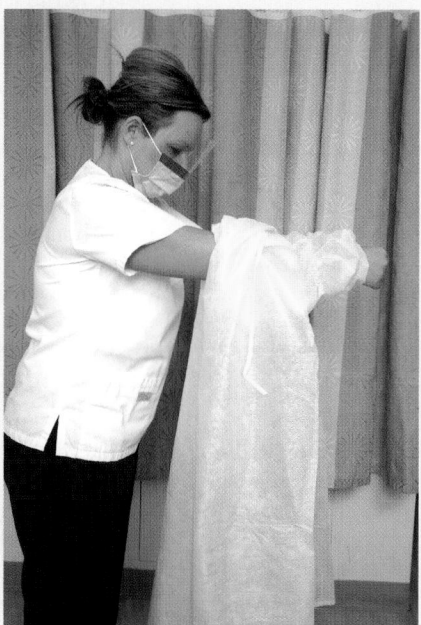

STEP 13c   Remove gown by allowing it to fall from shoulders.

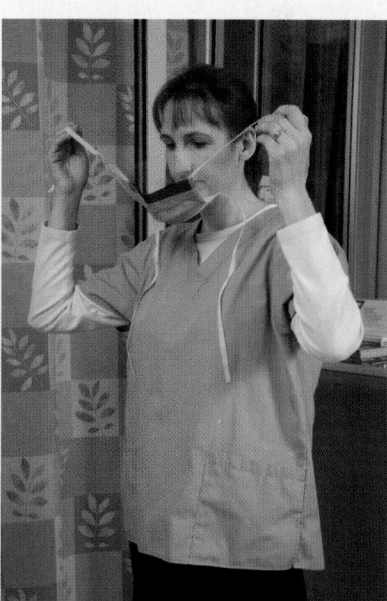

STEP 13d   Pull mask away from face.

STEP	RATIONALE
i Leave room and close door if necessary. Close door if patient is on airborne precautions or in negative airflow room.	Maintains negative airflow environment and reduces transmission of microorganisms.

EVALUATION

1 While in room, ask if patient has had sufficient chance to discuss health problems, course of treatment, or other topics important to him or her.	Measures patient's perception of adequacy of discussions with caregivers.
2 Ask patient to describe purpose of isolation and offer chance to ask questions.	Feedback demonstrates learning.

Unexpected Outcomes
1 Patient avoids social and therapeutic discussions.

2 Patient or health care worker may have an allergy to latex gloves.

Related Interventions
- Confer with family and/or significant other and determine best approach to reduce patient's sense of loneliness and depression.
- Notify physician/employee health and treat sensitivity or allergic reaction appropriately.
- Use latex-free gloves for future care activities.

Recording and Reporting
- Document procedures performed and patient's response to social isolation. Also document any patient education performed and reinforced.
- Document type of isolation in use and the microorganisms (if known).

Special Considerations
Teaching Considerations
- Teach visitors and family members how to follow the recommended isolation precautions when visiting a patient.

Pediatric Considerations
- Isolation creates a sense of separation from family and loss of control. Strange environment adds to the confusion that a child feels during isolation. Preschoolers are unable to understand cause-effect relationship for isolation. Older children may be able to understand cause but still fantasize.
- Children require simple explanations (e.g., "You need to be in this room to help you get better.") Show all barriers to a child.

Actively involve parents in any explanations. Nurses let child see their faces before applying masks so child does not become frightened.

Gerontologic Considerations
- Isolation can be a particular concern for older adults, especially those who have signs and symptoms of confusion or depression. Many times patients become more confused when they are confronted with a nurse using barrier precautions or when they are left in a room with the door closed. Nurses must assess need for closing door (negative-airflow room) along with safety of patient and additional safety measures that may need to be taken.
- Assess older adults for signs of depression such as loss of appetite or decrease in verbal communications. If necessary, report to the health care team for appropriate interventions.

Home Care Considerations
- Although isolation precautions followed in the hospital are not directly applicable to home care, caregivers should be aware of potential sources of contamination in the home (see Box 7-2).

PROCEDURAL GUIDELINE 7-1 Caring for Patients with Multidrug-Resistant Organisms (MDRO) and *Clostridium difficile*

Multidrug-resistant organisms (MDROs) such as methicillin-resistant *Staphylococcus aureus* (MRSA) and vancomycin-resistant enterococcus (VRE) have become increasingly common as a cause of colonization and health care–associated infections (HAIs). MRSA is a frequently identified pathogen associated with increased mortality. In recent reports MRSA caused upward of 19% of health care-associated bloodstream infections (Becker and Kahl, 2011). VRE, another MDRO, poses a greater risk to immune-compromised and debilitated patients (Archibald, 2011). *Clostridium difficile* infection is one of the most common and costly HAIs (Gerding, 2011). In most instances patient susceptibility to *C. difficile* infection requires prior treatment with antibiotics.

Unlike MRSA and VRE, *C. difficile* is more difficult to eliminate from the environment because it is a spore-forming organism, meaning that it can remain on surfaces in its dormant state for long periods of time. No matter which MDRO is involved, the most common means of transmission is by way of a health care worker's hands. To reduce the risk of cross-contamination among patients, use contact precautions in addition to standard precautions when caring for these patients.

Delegation and Collaboration
Assessment of a patient's status and type of care required cannot be delegated to nursing assistive personnel (NAP). Basic care

PROCEDURAL GUIDELINE 7-1   Caring for Patients with Multidrug-Resistant Organisms (MDRO) and *Clostridium difficile*–cont'd

procedures performed using contact precautions can be delegated to NAP. The nurse instructs the NAP to:

- Clarify personal precautions used under contact precautions.
- Explain the type of clinical changes to report.

Equipment

☐ Clean gloves, gown, protective eyewear, surgical mask (based on patient's clinical condition)

☐ Basic care items (e.g., medication equipment, hygiene items)

Procedural Steps

1 Perform hand hygiene.
2 Prepare all equipment needed in patient's room.
3 Before entering room apply gown, being sure that it covers all outer garments. Pull sleeves down to wrists. Tie securely at neck and waist.

4 Apply clean gloves.
5 Explain purpose of contact precautions to patient and family.
6 Provide personal care and treatments.
7 Leave room after telling patient when you will return and asking if he or she has questions concerning his or her care.
8 Remove gloves and discard per agency policy.
9 Untie neck and waist ties on gown. Remove gown, allowing it to fall from shoulders. Discard in appropriate receptacle per agency policy.
10 Perform hand hygiene. If patient is being treated for *C. difficile* infection, clean hands with soap and water. Alcohol-based hand rubs are not effective against the spores of *C. difficile*.

Critical Thinking Exercises

Joe is assigned to care for Mr. Nesbitt, a 78-year-old nursing home resident. After greeting Mr. Nesbitt, Joe begins to conduct a physical assessment.

1 As Joe turns Mr. Nesbitt to check the condition of his skin, he notices moisture on his own hand. Joe looks more closely and realizes that the moisture is from an open, oozing lesion on Mr. Nesbitt's sacral area. What should Joe do next?

2 A few hours later Joe prepares to enter Mr. Nesbitt's room. Wearing gloves, he assesses the wound and quickly checks the position and function of Mr. Nesbitt's indwelling urinary catheter. He performs hand hygiene before leaving Mr. Nesbitt's room. Critique Joe's approach. Did he use correct aseptic technique?

3 After Joe places Mr. Nesbitt on contact precautions, he observes a student nurse preparing to go into the patient's room with a mask. Is the student nurse's use of a mask appropriate?

REVIEW QUESTIONS

1 A health care worker has visible dirt on his hands. Which method of hand hygiene is most appropriate?
1 Using an alcohol-based disinfectant
2 Washing with water and then an alcohol-based hand rub
3 Using an alcohol gel containing an emollient
4 Washing with soap and water
2 Which aspect of handwashing is most effective to loosen dirt and transient bacteria?
1 Using hot water instead of warm water
2 Using plenty of lather with friction
3 Drying the hands vigorously from wrists to fingers
4 Applying lotion to the hands

3 When a patient is to be placed on isolation precautions, there are many factors to consider regarding his or her care. (Select all that apply.)
1 The need for social interaction
2 The type of isolation required
3 The patient's cultural background
4 Education of family and friends regarding the isolation
5 Organization of care to minimize trips in and out of the isolation room
6 How the patient contracted an infection
4 The use of a mask when the nurse is closer than 3 feet to a patient involves which type of precautions?
1 Airborne
2 Droplet
3 Contact
4 Standard
5 A nurse goes in and out of a patient's room and only needs a gown when coming into contact with the patient. What should the nurse do on leaving the room? (Select all that apply.)
1 Leave the used gown hanging on a hook inside the room for the next time it is needed
2 Leave the used gown hanging on a hook outside the room for the next time it is needed
3 Discard the gown after using it
4 Perform hand hygiene
6 A nurse enters the room of a patient who has been diagnosed with pneumonia. The nurse instructs the patient to cover the mouth when coughing. This reduces transmission of infection by:
1 Contact.
2 Small droplets.
3 Vector.
4 Splashing.

7 A nurse applies clean gloves when collecting a urine specimen. How does this technique break the chain of infection? (Select all that apply.)
   1 Blocks the portal of entry for microorganisms
   2 Blocks the portal of exit
   3 Reduces susceptibility of the host
   4 Controls a reservoir source of organisms

8 *C. difficile* organisms can be passed easily from patient to patient. An infection prevention practice used to reduce possible transmission includes:
   1 Wearing a surgical mask when entering the patient's room.
   2 Using soap and water when performing hand hygiene.
   3 Instructing the patient on the source of the organism.
   4 Maintaining droplet precautions.

9 The most likely means of transmitting infection between patients is:
   1 Exposure to another's cough.
   2 Sharing equipment among patients.
   3 Discarding soiled linen in a shared laundry bag.
   4 Contact with health care workers' hands.

10 A patient is isolated for pulmonary tuberculosis. The nurse notes that the patient seems angry but knows that this is a normal response to isolation. The best intervention is to:
   1 Provide a dark, quiet room to calm the patient.
   2 Reduce the level of precautions to relax the patient.
   3 Explain the reason for isolation and answer the patient's questions.
   4 Limit family and caregiver visits to reduce the risk of spreading the infection.

REFERENCES

Archibald L: Enterococci. In Carrico R, et al, editors: *APIC text of infection control and epidemiology*, ed 3, Washington, DC, 2011, Association for Professionals in Infection Control and Epidemiology (APIC).

Association of Operating Room Nurses (AORN): *Standards, recommended practices, and guidelines*, Denver, 2011, The Association.

Becker K, Kahl B: Staphylococci. In Carrico R, et al, editors: *APIC text of infection control and epidemiology*, ed 3, Washington, DC, 2011, Association for Professionals in Infection Control and Epidemiology (APIC).

Boyce JM, Pittet D: *HICPAC/SHEA/APIC/IIDA Hand Hygiene Task Force and the CDC Healthcare Control Practices Advisory Committee guidelines for hand hygiene in healthcare settings*, Atlanta, 2008, WHO Press.

Brisko V: Isolation precautions. In Carrico R, et al, editors: *APIC text of infection control and epidemiology*, ed 3, Washington, DC, 2011, Association for Professionals in Infection Control and Epidemiology (APIC).

Centers for Disease Control and Prevention (CDC), Hospital Infection Control Practice Advisory Committee and the HICPAC/SHEA/APIC/IDSA Hand Hygiene Task Force: Guideline for hand hygiene in healthcare settings, *MMWR Recomm Rep* 51(No. RR-16), 2002.

Centers for Disease Control and Prevention (CDC): Guideline for isolation precautions: preventing transmission of infectious agents in healthcare settings, 2007a, available at http://www.cdc.gov/hicpac/2007IP/2007isolationPrecautions.html, accessed February 17, 2012.

Centers for Disease Control and Prevention (CDC), Hospital Infection Control Practices Advisory Committee: Guidelines for isolation precautions in hospitals, *MMWR Morb Mortal Wkly Rep* 57(RR-16), 2007b.

Centers for Disease Control and Prevention (CDC): Respiratory protection in health care settings, 2010, available at http://www.cdc.gov/tb/publications/factsheets/prevention/rphcs.pdf, accessed May 17, 2012.

Centers for Disease Control and Prevention (CDC): Basic TB facts, 2011a, available at http://www.cdc.gov/tb/topic/basics/default.htm, accessed May 17, 2012.

Centers for Disease Control and Prevention (CDC): Treatment for latent TB, 2011b, available at http://www.cdc.gov/tb/topic/treatment/default.htm, accessed May 17, 2012.

Centers for Disease Control and Prevention (CDC): Precautions to prevent the spread of MRSA in healthcare settings, 2011c, available at http://www.cdc.gov/mrsa/prevent/healthcare.html, latest update August 2011, accessed February 17, 2012.

Cohen SH, et al: Clinical Practice Guidelines for *Clostridium difficile* infection in adults: update by the Society for Healthcare Epidemiology of America (SHEA) and the Infectious Diseases Society of America (IDSA), *Infect Control Hosp Epidemiol* 31(5):341, 2010.

Cook K: The hands have it! Hand hygiene in the OR, *OR Nurse* 5(6):14-16, 2011.

Fagernes M, Lingaas E: Impact of finger rings on transmission of bacteria during hand contact, *Infect Control Hosp Epidemiol* 30(5):427, 2009.

Fardo R: Geriatrics. In Carrico R, et al, editors: *APIC text of infection control and epidemiology*, ed 3, Washington, DC, 2011, Association for Professionals in Infection Control and Epidemiology (APIC).

Gerding D: *Clostridium difficile* infection and pseudomembranous colitis. In Carrico R, et al, editors: *APIC text of infection control and epidemiology*, ed 3, Washington, DC, 2011, Association for Professionals in Infection Control and Epidemiology (APIC).

Haas J: Hand hygiene. In Carrico R, et al, editors: *APIC text of infection control and epidemiology*, ed 3, Washington, DC, 2011, Association for Professionals in Infection Control and Epidemiology (APIC).

Herud T: Association between use of hand hygiene products and rates of healthcare-associated infections in a large university hospital in Norway, *Am J Infect Control* 35(4):311, 2009.

Iwamoto P: Aseptic technique. In Carrico R, et al, editors: *APIC text of infection control and epidemiology*, ed 3, Washington, DC, 2011, Association for Professionals in Infection Control and Epidemiology (APIC).

Longtin Y, et al: Hand hygiene, *N Engl J Med* 364(13):e24, 2011.

Occupational Safety and Health Administration (OSHA): Infectious disease: final rule, 29 CFR Part 1910, *Fed Reg* 75:87, 2010.

Roberge R: Evaluation of the rationale for concurrent use of N95 filtering face piece respirators with loose-fitting powered air-purifying respirators during aerosol generating medical procedures, *J Infect Control* 36(2):135, 2008.

Rutala W, Weber D: Disinfection and sterilization of patient-care items. In Carrico R, et al, editors: *APIC text of infection control and epidemiology*, ed 3, Washington, DC, 2011, Association for Professionals in Infection Control and Epidemiology (APIC).

Saint S, et al: Preventing hospital-acquired urinary tract infection in the United States: a national study, *Clin Infect Dis* 46:243, 2008.

The Joint Commission (TJC): *National Patient Safety Goals*, Oakbrook Terrace, Ill, 2012, The Commission, available at http://www.jointcommission.org/standards_information/npsgs.aspx.

University of Minnesota: How does culture affect healthcare? Taking charge of your health, 2011, available at www.takingcharge.csh.umn.edu, accessed February 12, 2012.

WHO guidelines on hand hygiene care, Geneva, Switzerland, 2009, World Health Organization (WHO) Press.

Sterile Technique

MEDIA RESOURCES

- evolve http://evolve.elsevier.com/Perry/skills
  - Review Questions
  - ▶ Video Clips
  - Audio Glossary

- Nursing Skills Online
- NSO Mosby's Nursing Video Skills, 4th edition

KEY TERMS

Asepsis	Pathogenic microorganisms	Sterile field	Transmission-based
Latex allergy reaction	Standard precautions	Strike through	precautions
Microorganisms	Sterile	Surgical asepsis	

OBJECTIVES

Mastery of content in this chapter will enable the nurse to:
- Discuss settings where surgical aseptic techniques are used.
- Describe conditions when surgical asepsis is used.
- Identify the principles of surgical asepsis.
- Explain the importance of organization and caution when using surgical aseptic techniques.

- Apply and remove a cap, mask, and protective eyewear correctly.
- Identify individuals at risk for a latex allergy.
- Perform the following skills: Applying sterile gloves using open-glove method, preparing a sterile field, and applying a sterile drape correctly.

Surgical asepsis or aseptic techniques and practices are designed to make and maintain objects and areas free from pathogenic microorganisms (Iwamoto, 2009). Sterilization destroys all microorganisms and their spores. The most common means of sterilizing objects used in the operating room (OR) is by steam sterilization. As in medical asepsis, hand hygiene with an appropriate cleaner or antiseptic is essential before the initiation of an aseptic procedure. Although nurses commonly practice surgical asepsis in ORs, labor and delivery areas, and major diagnostic or special procedure areas, they also use surgical aseptic techniques at a patient's bedside (Box 8-1) in three primary situations:

- During procedures that require intentional perforation of a patient's skin (e.g., insertion of central intravenous [IV] catheters [see Chapter 28])
- When the integrity of the skin is broken because of a surgical incision or burns (see Chapters 38 and 39)
- During procedures that involve insertion of devices or surgical instruments into normally sterile body cavities (e.g., insertion of a urinary catheter [see Chapter 33])

A nurse in an OR follows a series of steps to maintain sterile technique, including applying a mask, protective eyewear, and a cap; performing a surgical hand scrub; applying a sterile gown; and applying sterile gloves. In contrast, a nurse performing a sterile dressing change at a patient's bedside or in the home setting may only wash his or her hands and apply sterile gloves. In 2007 the Centers for Medicare and Medicaid Services (CMS) identified a list of conditions viewed to be reasonably preventable by applying evidence-based guidelines. Among these conditions are hospital-acquired vascular and urinary catheter–associated infections. Since October 1, 2008, hospitals receive no additional funds for treating these conditions. As of January 2012, CMS has identified 10 hospital-acquired conditions that are preventable based on evidence-based guidelines (CMS, 2012). In many instances this has led agencies to encourage staff to speak up if they see a break in sterile technique by a co-worker. Regardless of the procedures followed or the setting, all individuals involved in surgical asepsis have a responsibility to provide and maintain a safe environment by following aseptic principles (AORN, 2011; Iwamoto, 2009).

BOX 8-1 | Principles of Surgical Asepsis

1 All items used within a sterile field must be sterile.
2 A sterile barrier that has been permeated by punctures, tears, or moisture must be considered contaminated.
3 Once a sterile package is opened, a 2.5-cm (1-inch) border around the edges is considered unsterile.
4 Tables draped as part of a sterile field are considered sterile only at table level.
5 If there is any question or doubt about the sterility of an item, the item is considered to be unsterile.
6 Sterile persons or items contact only sterile areas; unsterile persons or items contact only unsterile areas.
7 Movement around and in the sterile field must not compromise or contaminate the sterile field.
8 A sterile object or field out of the range of vision or an object held below a person's waist is contaminated.
9 A sterile object or field becomes contaminated by prolonged exposure to air; stay organized and complete any procedure as soon as possible.

In treatment areas and at the bedside it is important to have a patient's full cooperation to minimize contamination of a work area. Be sure to prepare a patient before any procedure. Certain patients may fear moving or touching objects during a sterile procedure, whereas others even try to assist. Explain how you will perform a procedure and what a patient can do to avoid contaminating sterile items, including avoiding sudden body movement, refraining from touching sterile supplies, and avoiding coughing or talking over a sterile area.

The Centers for Disease Control and Prevention (CDC) (2007) established standard precautions as the minimum standard for infection control (see Chapter 7). Use standard precautions for potential contact with blood and all body fluids. The use of standard precautions calls for wearing masks in combination with eye protection devices such as goggles or glasses with solid side shields whenever splashes, sprays, splatter, or droplets of blood or other potentially infectious fluids may occur. These barriers are not sterile but are designed to keep the eyes, nose, and mouth free from exposure. Similarly, you wear gowns when there is risk of being splattered with blood or other infectious materials. All health care agencies need to provide personal protective equipment (PPE) and instructions for their use to all employees at risk for exposure (OSHA, 1994).

EVIDENCE-BASED PRACTICE

In 1860 Joseph Lister promoted the use of carbolic acid as a surgical hand scrub. Since then using an antiseptic on the hands of surgical team members has been an accepted practice. Bacteria on the hands of health care workers can lead to wound infections when introduced into surgical wounds. Studies found that surgical staff may transmit pathogens from contact with patients or with contaminated items such as tourniquets, linens, or surfaces (e.g., doorknobs, countertops) (Cook, 2011). Studies show that antiseptics containing 60% to 90% alcohol alone or 50% to 95% alcohol when combined with other selected antiseptics (e.g., chlorhexidine) lower bacterial counts on the skin more effectively then do other antiseptics without alcohol (Cook, 2011). In addition, bacteria appear to reproduce slowly on the hands after a surgical scrub with alcohol. For this reason an alcohol-based hand rub may be

used as a preoperative hand scrub after an initial 15-second prewash with plain soap and water (AORN, 2011).

The subungual area (under a fingernail) of the hand is a source of high concentrations of bacteria, most frequently coagulase-negative staphylococci and gram-negative rods. Even after thorough hand hygiene, large numbers of potential pathogens exist under the subungual spaces (Cook, 2011). Health care workers who wear artificial nails or nail extenders are more likely to harbor gram-negative pathogens on their fingertips both before and after hand hygiene. Fungal growth frequently occurs under artificial nails as a result of moisture becoming trapped between the natural and artificial nail (AORN, 2011). Many health care agencies have banned artificial nails and extenders in all clinical areas, with the rationale that all patients are at risk for infection.

- Health care workers having direct contact with patients should not wear artificial nails (Church and Berjke, 2009; Cook, 2011).
- Use an additional antiseptic such as chlorhexidine to reduce bacterial count on the skin (AORN, 2011; Cook, 2011).
- Carefully clean under the fingernail during hand hygiene and before applying sterile gloves.
- Maintain fingernails no longer than $\frac{1}{4}$ inch in length, and nail polish should not be chipped (Cook, 2011).

PATIENT-CENTERED CARE

Whether performed in a hospital, ambulatory care setting, or health care provider's office, invasive procedures such as starting an IV line or inserting a urinary catheter pose a risk for infection. It is your responsibility to protect patients from infection by adhering strictly to the principles of surgical asepsis when performing such procedures and, when assisting with such a procedure, to intervene to stop it when a break in sterile technique occurs. The Joint Commission (TJC) encourages nurses to "speak up" in these instances (TJC, 2012).

Regardless of a patient's background, beliefs, or attitudes, it is important to maintain sterile asepsis for invasive procedures. In these cases patient-centered education of patients and families before any aseptic procedure reduces fears and misconceptions about any sterile asepsis attire. In addition, such education provides time for patients and families to ask any questions about their concerns. In some cases a person's cultural background requires gender-congruent care providers.

Safety Guidelines

1 Follow standard precautions with all patients.
2 Review agency policies and procedures before conducting a sterile procedure.
3 Assess a patient's potential for infection before choosing the barrier to be used such as masks or protective eyewear.
4 Use barrier techniques to decrease the transmission of microorganisms from health care personnel and the environment to a patient.
5 Remain organized while performing any sterile procedure; keep bedside surfaces clutter free.
6 Remember that hand hygiene is essential before initiating any sterile procedure.
7 Incorporate the principles of surgical asepsis when conducting any sterile procedure.

SKILL 8-1   Applying and Removing Cap, Mask, and Protective Eyewear

NSO *Nursing Skills Online Infection Control Module / Lesson 1*

Although masks and caps are usually worn in surgical procedure areas (e.g., the operating room [OR]), certain aseptic procedures performed at a patient's bedside also might require these barriers. For example, it may be agency policy for a nurse to wear a mask during the changing of a central line dressing or insertion of a peripherally inserted central catheter (PICC). Other policies might require that a nurse wear a mask and a cap to secure hair during dressing changes on a patient with extensive burns or a central line (Lynn-McHale Wiegand, 2011). When there is a risk of splattering blood or body fluid, there is also the need to apply protective eyewear (OSHA, 2012).

Assess a patient's potential for acquiring an infection before applying a mask (e.g., Does the patient have a large open wound? Do you have a respiratory infection? Is the patient immunosuppressed?). If you wear a mask, change it when it becomes moist or soiled (e.g., splattered with blood). Some nurses choose to wear a surgical cap to secure loose hair that might contaminate a sterile area (Church and Bjerke, 2009). Wear eyewear when there is a risk for body fluids splashing into your eyes.

Delegation and Collaboration

The skill of applying and removing cap, mask, and protective eyewear is required of all caregivers when working in sterile areas. However, the procedures performed at a patient's bedside that require cap and mask generally cannot be delegated to nursing assistive personnel (NAP). The nurse determines if protective barriers are necessary for the other staff. The nurse instructs the NAP about:

- The procedure to be performed and how to assist with positioning and obtaining supplies
- Performing hand hygiene after glove removal

Equipment

- ❑ Surgical mask (different types are available for people with different skin sensitivities)
- ❑ Surgical cap (NOTE: Use in OR or if agency policy requires. Use to secure hair if there is a possibility of contamination of a sterile field.)
- ❑ Hairpins, rubber bands, or both
- ❑ Protective eyewear (e.g., goggles or glasses with appropriate side shields)

STEP	RATIONALE
ASSESSMENT	
1 Review type of sterile procedure to be performed and consult agency policy for use of mask/caps/protective eyewear.	Not all sterile procedures require mask, cap, or protective eyewear. Ensures that nurse and patient are properly protected.
2 If you have symptoms of a respiratory infection, either avoid participating in procedure or apply a mask.	A greater number of pathogenic microorganisms reside within the respiratory tract when infection is present.
3 Assess patient's actual or potential risk for infection when choosing barriers for surgical asepsis (e.g., older adult, neonate, or immunocompromised patient).	Some patients are at a greater risk for acquiring an infection; thus use additional barriers.
NURSING DIAGNOSES	
• Ineffective protection	
• Risk for infection	
Related factors are individualized based on patient's condition or needs.	
PLANNING	
1 Expected outcome following completion of procedure:	
• Patient does not develop signs of localized infection (e.g., redness, tenderness, edema, drainage) or systemic infection (e.g., fever, change in white blood cell [WBC] count) 24 hours after procedure.	Indicates lack of microorganism transfer to patient and sterile field.
2 Prepare equipment and inspect packaging for integrity and exposure to sterilization.	Ensures availability of equipment and sterility of supplies before procedure begins.
IMPLEMENTATION	
1 Perform hand hygiene	Reduces transient microorganisms on skin.
2 Apply a cap.	
a If hair is long, comb back behind ears and secure.	Cap must cover all hair entirely.
b Secure hair in place with pins.	Ensures that long hair does not fall down or cause cap to slip and expose hair.
c Apply cap over head as you would apply hairnet. Be sure that all hair fits under edges of cap (see illustration).	Loose hair hanging over sterile field or falling dander contaminates objects on sterile field.

STEP	RATIONALE

3 Apply a mask.

   a Find top edge of mask, which usually has thin metal strip along edge.

   b Hold mask by top two strings or loops, keeping top edge above bridge of nose.

   c Tie two top strings at top of back of head, over cap (if worn), with strings above ears (see illustration). Alternatively place loops over ears.

   d Tie two lower ties snugly around neck with mask well under chin (see illustration).

   e Gently pinch upper metal band around bridge of nose.

4 Apply protective eyewear.

   a Apply protective glasses, goggles, or face shield comfortably over eyes and check that vision is clear (see illustration).

   b Be sure that face shield fits snugly around forehead and face.

5 Apply sterile gloves if needed (see Skill 8-3).

6 Remove protective barriers.

   a Remove gloves first if worn (see Skill 8-3).

   b Untie bottom strings of mask.

   c Untie top strings of mask and remove mask from face, holding ties securely. Discard mask in proper receptacle (see illustrations).

Pliable metal fits snugly against bridge of nose.

Prevents contact of hands with clean facial portion of mask. Mask covers all of nose.

Position of ties at top of head provides tight fit. Strings over ears may cause irritation.

Prevents escape of microorganisms through sides of mask as you talk and breathe.

Prevents microorganisms from escaping around nose and eyeglasses from steaming up.

Positioning affects clarity of vision.

Ensures that eyes are fully protected.

Prevents contamination of hair, neck, and facial area.

Prevents top part of mask from falling down over uniform. If mask falls and touches uniform, uniform will be contaminated.

Avoids contact of nurse's hands with contaminated mask.

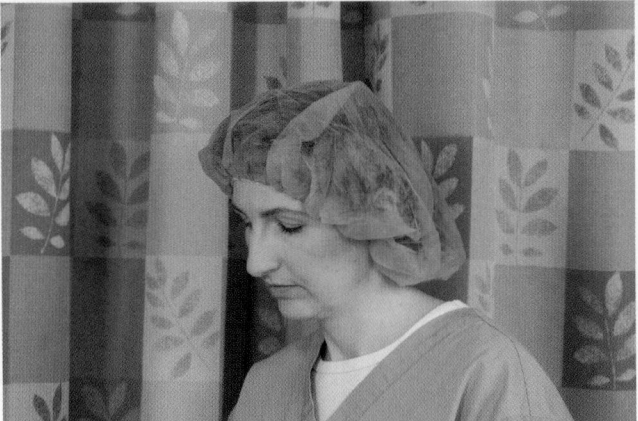

STEP 2c   Apply cap over head, covering all hair.

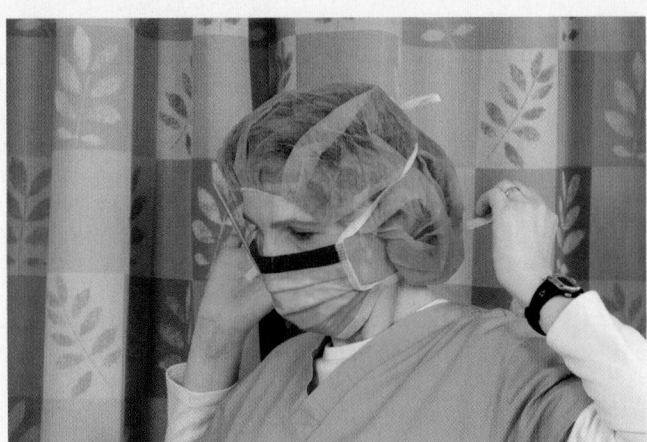

STEP 3d   Tie bottom strings of mask.

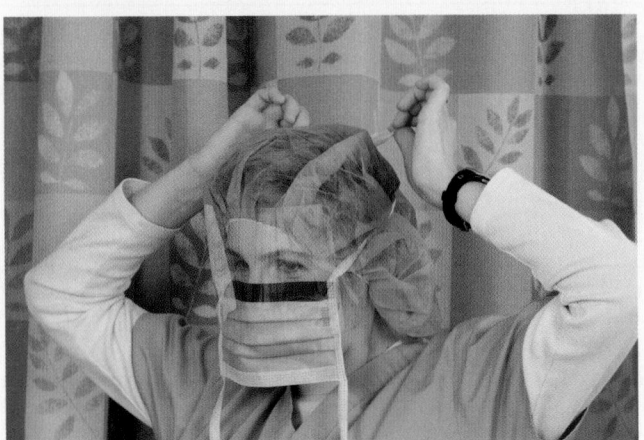

STEP 3c   Tie top strings of mask.

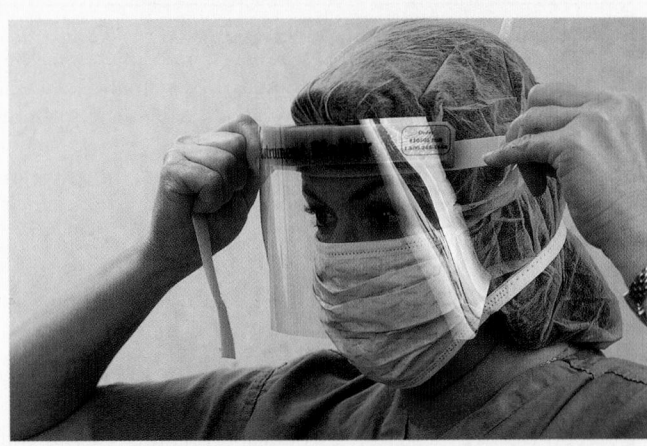

STEP 4a   Apply face shield over cap.

STEP	RATIONALE

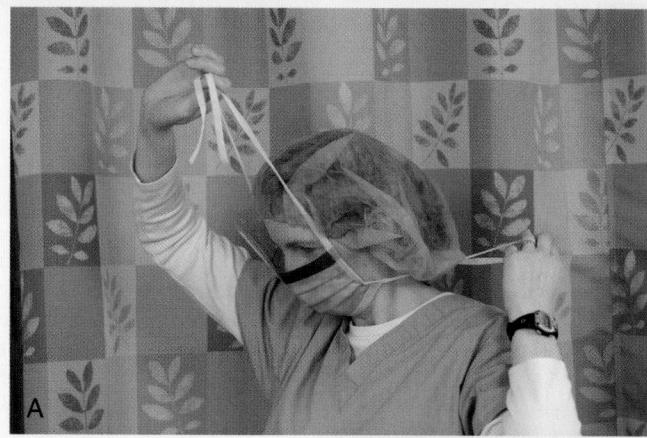 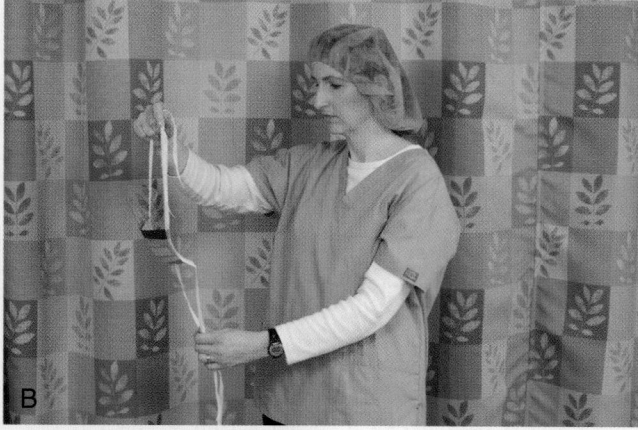

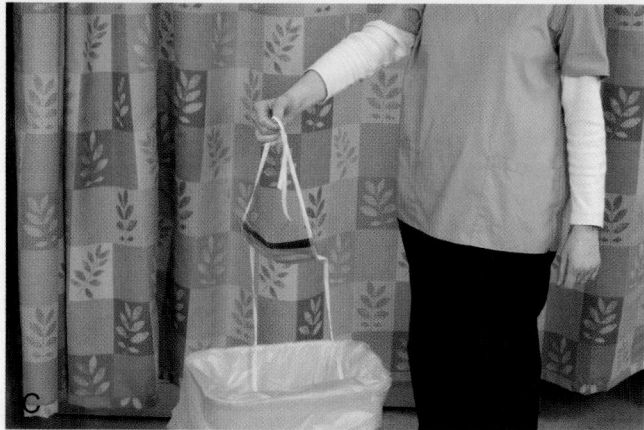

STEP 6c **A,** Untie top mask strings. **B,** Remove mask from face. **C,** Discard mask.

d Remove eyewear, avoiding placing hands over soiled lens. If wearing face shield, remove it before removal of mask. NOTE: A combination mask and eyewear is available in some agencies.	Prevents transmission of microorganisms.
e Grasp outer surface of cap and lift from hair.	Minimizes contact of hands with hair.
f Discard cap in proper receptacle and perform hand hygiene.	Reduces transmission of infection.

EVALUATION

1 Following the procedure, assess area of body treated for drainage, tenderness, edema, or change in temperature or color of skin.	Rules out presence of localized infection.

Unexpected Outcomes
1 Redness, heat, edema, pain, or purulent drainage develops at wound or treatment site, indicating possible infection.

Related Interventions
• Notify health care provider of change in condition of affected area and initiate appropriate treatments as ordered.

Recording and Reporting
• No recording or reporting is required for this set of skills. Record specific procedure performed in nurses' notes and electronic health record (EHR), and describe patient's status.

Special Considerations
Home Care
• Instruct family caregiver about specifics of when to apply cap, mask, and protective eyewear in the home.
• Determine ability of family caregiver to safely implement sterile procedure.
• Instruct patient and family caregiver about the signs and symptoms of infection.

SKILL 8-2 Preparing a Sterile Field

NSO *Nursing Skills Online Infection Control Module / Lesson 3*

 Video Clip

When performing sterile aseptic procedures, you need a sterile work area in which objects can be handled with minimal risk for contamination. A sterile field provides a sterile surface for placement of sterile equipment. It is an area considered free of microorganisms and may consist of the inside of a sterile kit or tray, a work surface draped with a sterile towel or wrapper, or a table covered with a large sterile drape (Iwamoto, 2009). Sterile drapes establish a sterile field around a treatment site such as a surgical incision, venipuncture site, or site for introduction of an indwelling urinary catheter. Drapes also provide a work surface for placing sterile supplies and manipulating items with sterile gloves. They are available in cloth, paper, and plastic. They may be wrapped in individual sterile packages or included within sterile kits or trays. These kits or trays contain external and internal sterile (chemical) indicators that indicate that the item has completed a sterilization process. After the kit is opened, the inside surface of the cover can be used as a sterile field. Most drapes are fluid resistant.

Drapes come in various styles, shapes, and sizes. For example, bladder catheterization kits and tracheal suction kits contain sterile items that can be moved within the tray and containers into which sterile solutions can be poured. Once you create a sterile field, you are responsible for performing the procedure without contaminating the field. The skill of preparing a sterile field includes opening sterile packages, preparing a sterile drape, adding sterile supplies to a field, and pouring sterile solutions.

Delegation and Collaboration

The skill of preparing a sterile field cannot be delegated to nursing assistive personnel (NAP). Surgical technicians may prepare a sterile field (see agency policy). However, NAP may assist in positioning patients and obtaining extra supplies. The nurse directs the NAP to:

- Assist with patient positioning and obtaining any necessary supplies.

Equipment

- ☐ Sterile pack (commercial or institution wrapped)
- ☐ Sterile drape or kit that is to be used as a sterile field
- ☐ Sterile gloves
- ☐ Sterile solution and equipment specific to a procedure
- ☐ Waist-high table/countertop surface
- ☐ Appropriate personal protective equipment (PPE): gown, mask, protective eyewear (see agency policy)

STEP	RATIONALE

ASSESSMENT

1 Verify that procedure requires surgical aseptic technique.

Some procedures require medical rather than surgical aseptic technique.

2 Assess patient's comfort, oxygen requirements, and elimination needs before preparing for procedure.

Certain procedures that require a sterile field may last a long time. Anticipates patient's needs so patient can relax and avoid any unnecessary movement that might disrupt procedure.

3 Instruct patient not to touch the work surface or equipment during procedure.

Prevents contamination of sterile field.

4 Assess for latex allergies.

A review may reveal latex allergies and determine use of latex-free supplies.

5 Check sterile package integrity for punctures, tears, discoloration, moisture, or any other signs of contamination. If using commercially packaged supplies or those prepared by agency, check for sterilization indicator (a marker that changes color when exposed to heat or steam).

The inspection of packaging ensures that only sterile items are presented to sterile field (AORN, 2011).

6 Anticipate number and variety of supplies needed for procedure.

Not all sterile kits contain sufficient amounts or types of supplies. Failure to have necessary supplies causes you to leave sterile field, increasing risk for contamination.

NURSING DIAGNOSES

- Ineffective protection
- Risk for infection

Related factors are individualized based on patient's condition or needs.

PLANNING

1 Expected outcomes following completion of procedure:
- The sterile field is not contaminated.
- Patient is not exposed to microorganisms.

Correct surgical aseptic practice is performed.

STEP	RATIONALE
2 Complete all other priority tasks (e.g., medication administration, suctioning patient) before beginning procedure.	Prepare sterile fields as close as possible to time of use to reduce potential for contamination (AORN, 2011).
3 Ask visitors to step out briefly during procedure. Discourage movement by staff assisting with procedure.	Traffic or movement can increase potential for contamination through spread of microorganisms by air currents.
4 Prepare equipment at bedside.	Ensures availability before procedure and prevents break in sterile technique (Torch, 2011). [NOTE: Povidone-iodine and chlorhexidine are not considered sterile solutions and require separate work surfaces for prepping.]
5 Position patient comfortably for specific procedure to be performed. If a body part is to be examined or treated, position patient so area is accessible. Have NAP assist with positioning as needed.	Patient should be able to lie still in one position comfortably during procedure. Movement can contaminate sterile items.
6 Explain to patient purpose of procedure and importance of sterile technique.	Ensures patient's ability to cooperate. Teaching before procedure eliminates need to talk during procedure, which can cause air-droplet contamination of sterile area.

IMPLEMENTATION

1 Apply PPE as needed (consult agency policy) (see Skills 8-1 and 8-3).	Controls spread of airborne microorganisms.
2 Select a clean, flat, dry work surface above waist level.	A sterile object below person's waist is considered contaminated.
3 Perform hand hygiene (see Chapter 7).	Reduces carriage of microorganisms on hands, which may be transmitted to patient. Do not allow rinse water to run down arms onto clean hands (i.e., arms are considered dirty).
4 Prepare sterile work surface.	
a **Using sterile commercial kit or pack containing sterile items.**	
(1) Place sterile kit or pack containing sterile items on clean, dry, flat work surface above waist level.	Items placed below waist level are considered contaminated.
(2) Open outside cover (see illustration) and remove package from dust cover. Place on work surface.	Inner kit remains sterile.
(3) Grasp outer surface of tip of outermost flap.	Outer surface of package is considered unsterile. There is a 2.5-cm (1-inch) border around any sterile drape or wrap that is considered contaminated.
(4) Open outermost flap away from body, keeping arm outstretched and away from sterile field (see illustration).	Reaching over sterile field contaminates it.

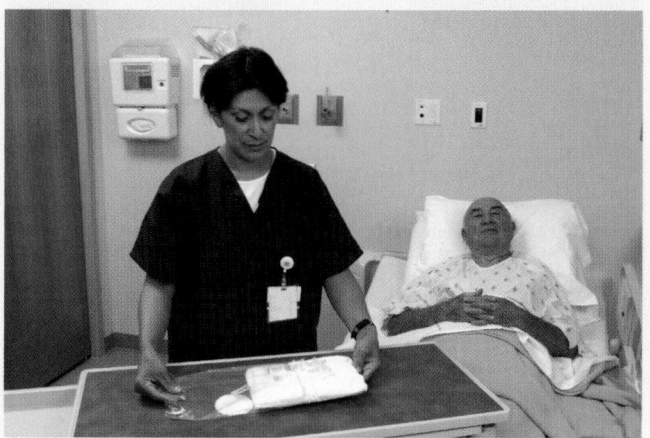

STEP 4a(2) Open outside cover of sterile kit.

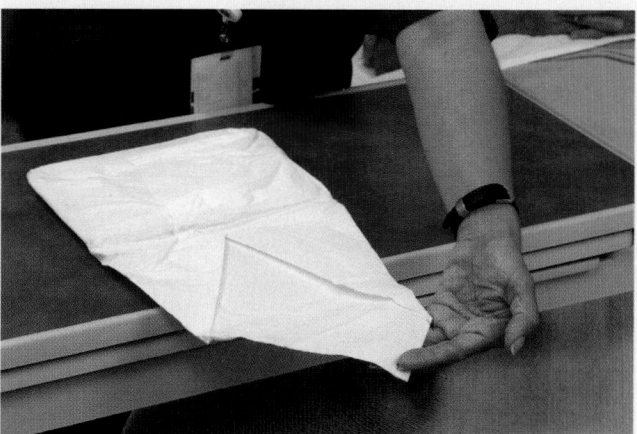

STEP 4a(4) Open outermost flap of sterile kit away from body.

STEP	RATIONALE
(5) Grasp outside surface of edge of first side flap.	Outer border is considered unsterile.
(6) Open side flap, pulling to side, allowing it to lie flat on table surface. Keep arm to side and not over sterile surface (see illustration).	Drape or wrapper should lie flat so it does not accidentally rise up and contaminate inner surface or sterile contents.
(7) Repeat Step (6) for second side flap (see illustration).	
(8) Grasp outside border of last and innermost flap (see illustration). Stand away from sterile package and pull flap back, allowing it to fall flat on table.	Outer border is considered unsterile. Never reach over a sterile field.

b Open sterile linen-wrapped package.

STEP	RATIONALE
(1) Place package on clean, dry, flat work surface above waist level.	Items placed below waist level are considered contaminated.
(2) Remove sterilization tape seal and unwrap both layers following same steps (see Steps 4a(2) through 4a(8)) as for sterile kit (see illustration).	Linen-wrapped items have two layers. The first is a dust cover. The second layer must be opened to view chemical indicator. If item is dropped on floor, it is considered contaminated.
(3) Use opened package wrapper as sterile field.	Inner surface of wrapper is considered sterile.

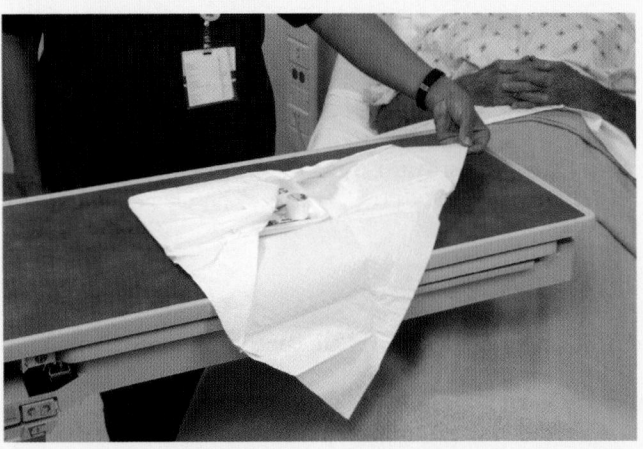

STEP 4a(6)   Open first side flap, pulling to side.

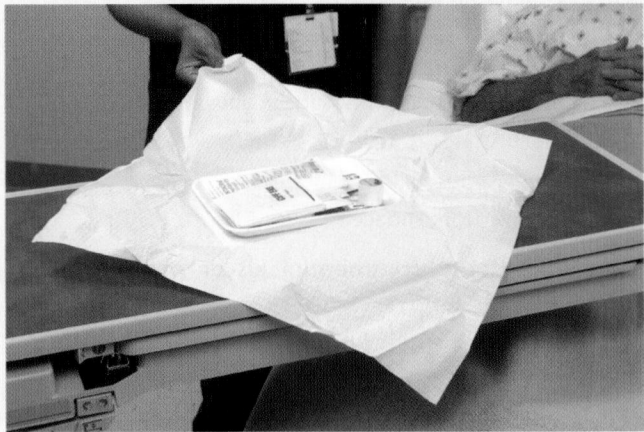

STEP 4a(8)   Open last and innermost flap.

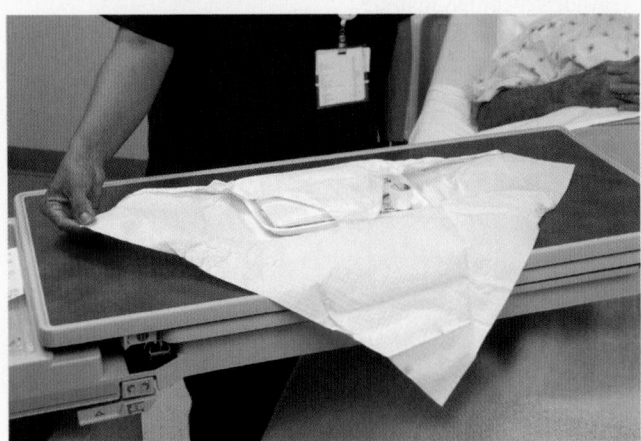

STEP 4a(7)   Open second side flap, pulling to side.

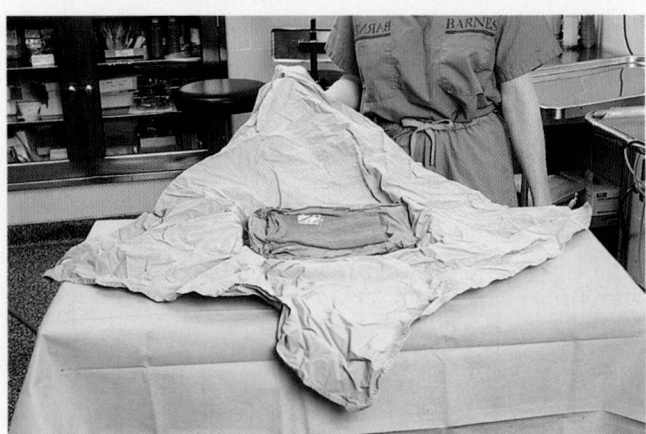

STEP 4b(2)   Open sterile linen-wrapped package.

STEP	RATIONALE
c Prepare sterile drape.	
(1) Place pack containing sterile drape on flat, dry surface and open as described (see Steps 4a(2) through 4a(8)) for sterile package.	Ensures sterility of packaged drape.
(2) Apply sterile gloves (*optional,* see agency policy). You may touch outer 2.5-cm (1-inch) border of drape without wearing gloves.	A sterile object remains sterile only when touched by another sterile object. Gloves are not necessary as long as fingers grasp the 2.5-cm (1-inch) unsterile border of the drape.
(3) Grasp folded top edge of drape with fingertips of one hand. Gently lift drape up from its wrapper without touching any object.	If sterile object touches any nonsterile object, it becomes contaminated.
(4) Allow drape to unfold, keeping it above waist and work surface and away from body. (Carefully discard wrapper with other hand.)	Object held below waist or above chest is contaminated.
(5) With other hand grasp adjacent corner of drape. Hold drape straight over work surface (see illustration).	Drape can now be placed properly with two hands.
(6) Holding drape, position bottom half over top half of intended work surface (see illustration).	Prevents nurse from reaching over sterile field.
(7) Allow top half of drape to be placed over bottom half of work surface (see illustration).	Creates flat, sterile work surface for placement of sterile supplies.

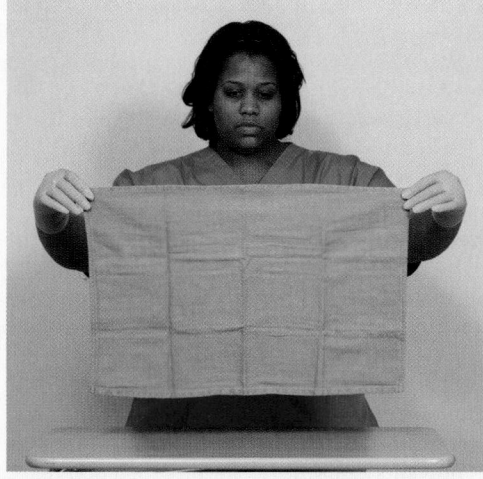

STEP 4c(5)   Hold corners of sterile drape up and away from body.

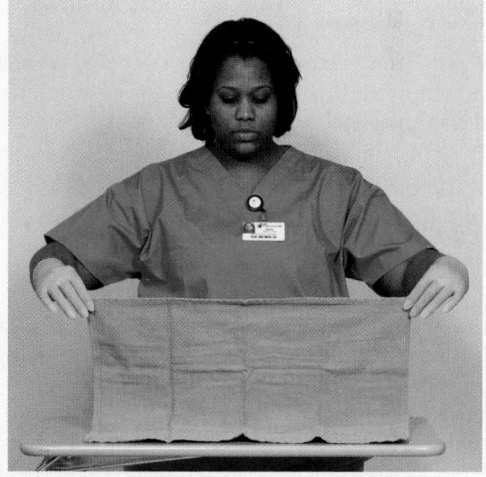

STEP 4c(6)   Position bottom half of sterile drape over top half of work surface.

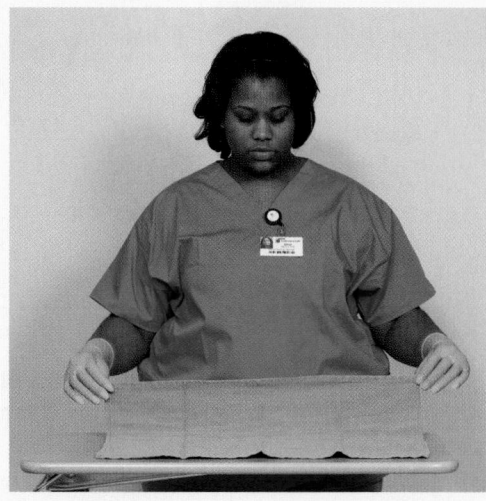

STEP 4c(7)   Allow top half of drape to be placed over bottom half of work surface.

STEP	RATIONALE

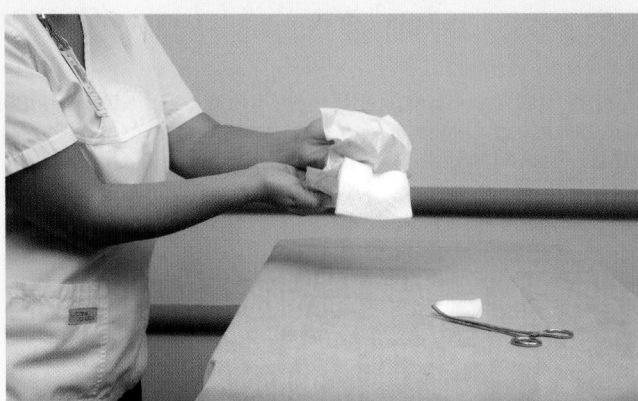

STEP 5c   Add items to sterile field.

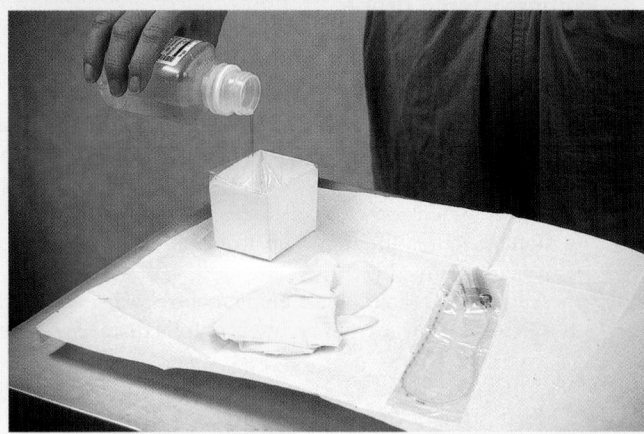

STEP 6d   Pour solution into receiving container on sterile field.

5   Add sterile items to sterile field.
   a Open sterile item (following package directions) while holding outside wrapper in nondominant hand.

Frees dominant hand for unwrapping outer wrapper.

   b Carefully peel wrapper over nondominant hand.

Item remains sterile. Inner surface of wrapper covers hand, making it sterile.

   c Being sure that wrapper does not fall down on sterile field, place item onto field at an angle (see illustration). **Do not hold arm over sterile field.**

Secured wrapper edges prevent flipping wrapper and contaminating contents of sterile field (AORN, 2011).

Clinical Decision Point *Do not flip or toss objects onto sterile field.*

   d Dispose of outer wrapper.

Prevents accidental contamination of sterile field.

6   Pour sterile solutions.
   a Verify contents and expiration date of solution.

Ensures proper solution and sterility of contents.

   b Be sure that receptacle for solution is located near table/work surface edge. Sterile kits have cups or plastic molded sections into which fluids can be poured.

Prevents reaching over sterile field during pouring of solution.

   c Remove sterile seal and cap from bottle in upward motion.

Prevents contamination of bottle lip.

   d With solution bottle held away from field and bottle lip 2.5 to 5 cm (1 to 2 inches) above inside of sterile receiving container, slowly pour needed amount of solution into container. Hold bottle with label facing palm of hand (see illustration).

Edge and outside of bottle are considered contaminated. Slow pouring prevents splashing. Sterility of contents cannot be ensured if cap is replaced.

Prevents label from becoming wet and illegible

Clinical Decision Point *When liquids permeate sterile field or barrier, it is called strike through, resulting in contamination.*

EVALUATION

1   Observe for break in sterile technique.

Break in sterile field requires you to set up new sterile field.

Unexpected Outcomes

1   Sterile field comes in contact with contaminated object or liquid splatters onto drape, causing strike through.

2   Sterile item falls off sterile field.

Related Interventions

•   Discontinue field preparation and start over with new equipment.

•   Open package containing new sterile item and add to field, unless field becomes contaminated.

Recording and Reporting

- No recording or reporting is required for this set of skills. Record sterile procedure performed in nurses' notes and EHR, and describe patient's status.

Special Considerations
Home Care

- Most care procedures in the home setting involve clean technique. In the event that a sterile environment is ordered, patient and family need to be aware of the principles that apply to the sterile environment. For example, teach family how to correctly use package wrapper as a sterile drape/barrier when applying a sterile dressing or teach family the correct procedure for removing sterile item from package.
- Assess patient's and family's understanding and ability to provide a sterile environment when needed to perform a specific procedure.

SKILL 8-3   Sterile Gloving

NSO *Nursing Skills Online Infection Control Module / Lesson 4*

 Video Clip

Sterile gloves help prevent the transmission of pathogens by direct and indirect contact. Nurses apply sterile gloves before performing sterile procedures such as inserting urinary catheters or applying sterile dressings. It is important to select the proper size glove. The gloves should not stretch so tightly over the fingers that they can easily tear, yet they need to be tight enough that objects can be picked up easily. Sterile gloves are available in various sizes (e.g., 6, 6½, 7). They are also available in a "one size fits all" style or in "small," "medium," and "large." Always remember that sterile gloves do not replace hand hygiene.

It is important to choose not only the right size of glove but also the correct material. Many patients and health care workers are allergic to latex, the natural rubber used in most gloves and other medical products (Church and Bjerke, 2009). Box 8-2 lists risk factors for a latex allergy. Latex proteins enter the body through skin or mucous membranes, intravascularly, or via inhalation. The powder that is used to make latex gloves slip on easily is a carrier of the latex proteins (AORN, 2011; Molinari and Harte, 2009). When you apply or remove gloves, the powder particles become airborne and can remain so for hours. The latex can then be inhaled or settle on clothing, skin, or mucous membranes. Reactions to latex are mild to severe (Box 8-3). For individuals at high risk or with suspected sensitivity to latex, it is important to choose latex-free or synthetic gloves. More health care agencies are implementing latex-safe environments for workers (AORN, 2011). If only sterile latex gloves are available, don a pair of synthetic gloves first because these provide a barrier between the skin and the latex gloves.

Once you apply gloves, always be conscious of the position of your hands during procedures. If a sterile glove touches a clean, contaminated, or questionably contaminated object, it becomes unsterile, and a new sterile glove must be applied. It is helpful to interlock the fingers and hold the hands together in front of the body and above waist level while waiting to handle sterile items. If a tear develops in a sterile glove, apply a new glove immediately. Once gloved, keep your hands clasped about 30 cm (12 inches) in front of your body, above waist level and below the shoulders, until you are ready to perform the procedure.

Delegation and Collaboration

Assisting with skills that include the application and removal of sterile gloves may be delegated to nursing assistive personnel (NAP). However, many procedures that require the use of sterile gloves cannot be delegated to NAP. The nurse instructs the NAP about:

- The reason for using sterile gloves for a specific procedure.

Equipment

- ❏ Package of proper-size sterile gloves, latex or synthetic nonlatex (NOTE: Hypoallergenic, low-powder, and low-protein latex gloves may still contain enough latex protein to cause an allergic reaction [Molinari and Harte, 2009].)

BOX 8-2 | Individuals at Risk for Latex Allergy

- Spina bifida
- Congenital or urogenital defects
- History of indwelling catheters or repeated catheterizations
- History of using condom catheters
- High latex exposure (e.g., health care workers, housekeepers, food handlers, tire manufacturers, workers in industries that use gloves routinely)
- History of multiple childhood surgeries
- History of food allergies

Modified from Molinari J, Harte J: Dental services. In Carrico R, editor: *APIC text of infection control and epidemiology*, Washington, DC, revised 2009, Association for Professionals in Infection Control and Epidemiology (APIC).

BOX 8-3 | Levels of Latex Reactions

The three types of common latex reactions (in order of severity) are:
1. *Irritant dermatitis*: A nonallergic response characterized by skin redness and itching.
2. *Type IV hypersensitivity*: Cell-mediated allergic reaction to chemicals used in latex processing. Reaction, including redness, itching, and hives, can be delayed up to 48 hours. Localized swelling, red and itchy or runny eyes and nose, and coughing may develop.
3. *Type I allergic reaction*: A true latex allergy that can be life-threatening. Reactions vary based on type of latex protein and degree of individual sensitivity, including local and systemic. Symptoms include hives, generalized edema, itching, rash, wheezing, bronchospasm, difficulty breathing, laryngeal edema, diarrhea, nausea, hypotension, tachycardia, and respiratory or cardiac arrest.

Cleveland Clinic: *Latex allergy*, 2012, available at http://www.clevelandclinic.org/health/health-info/docs/1900/1955.asp?index=8623, accessed February 19, 2012.

STEP	RATIONALE

ASSESSMENT

1 Consider the type of procedure to be performed and consult agency policy on use of sterile gloves.	Ensures proper use of sterile gloves when needed.
2 Consider patient's risk for infection (e.g., a preexisting condition and size or extent of area being treated).	Directs you to follow added precautions (e.g., use of additional protective barriers) if necessary.
3 Select correct size and type of gloves and then examine glove package to determine if it is dry and intact with no water stains.	Torn or wet package is considered contaminated. Signs of water stains on package indicate previous contamination by water.
4 Inspect condition of hands for cuts, hangnails, open lesions, or abrasions. In some settings you are allowed to cover any open lesion with a sterile, impervious transparent dressing (check agency policy). In some cases presence of such lesions may prevent you from participating in a procedure.	Cuts, abrasions, and hangnails tend to ooze serum, which possibly contains pathogens. Breaks in skin integrity permit microorganisms to enter and increase the risk for infection for both patient and nurse (AORN, 2011).
5 Assess patient for the following risk factors before applying latex gloves:	Determines level of patient's risk for latex allergy.
a Previous reaction to the following items within hours of exposure: adhesive tape, dental or face mask, golf club grip, ostomy bag, rubber band, balloon, bandage, elastic underwear, intravenous (IV) tubing, rubber gloves, condom	Items known to lead to latex allergy.
b Personal history of asthma, contact dermatitis, eczema, urticaria, rhinitis	
c History of food allergies, especially avocado, banana, peach, chestnut, raw potato, kiwi, tomato, papaya	
d Previous history of adverse reactions during surgery or dental procedure	Suggests allergic response.
e Previous reaction to latex product	Suggests allergic response.

NURSING DIAGNOSES

• Ineffective protection	• Risk for infection	• Risk for injury

Related factors are individualized based on patient's condition or needs.

PLANNING

1 Expected outcomes following completion of procedure:	
• Patient does not develop signs or symptoms of infection after procedure.	Indicates that microorganisms are not introduced into sterile body cavities or sites (such as skin or urinary tract).
• Patient does not develop latex sensitivity or latex allergy reaction.	Patient at risk for latex allergy is not exposed to latex proteins.

Clinical Decision Point *Synthetic nonlatex gloves are necessary for patients at risk or if nurse has sensitivity or allergy to latex.*

IMPLEMENTATION

1 Apply sterile gloves.	
a Perform thorough hand hygiene. Place glove package near work area.	Reduces number of bacteria on skin surfaces and transmission of infection. Ensures availability before procedure.
b Remove outer glove package wrapper by carefully separating and peeling apart sides (see illustration).	Prevents inner glove package from accidentally opening and touching contaminated objects.
c Grasp inner package and lay on clean, dry, flat surface at waist level. Open package, keeping gloves on inside surface of wrapper (see illustration).	Sterile object held below waist is contaminated. Inner surface of glove package is sterile.

STEP	RATIONALE
d Identify right and left glove. Each glove has a cuff approximately 5 cm (2 inches) wide. Glove dominant hand first.	Proper identification of gloves prevents contamination by improper fit. Gloving of dominant hand first improves dexterity.
e With thumb and first two fingers of nondominant hand, grasp glove for dominant hand by touching only inside surface.	Inner edge of cuff will lie against skin and thus is not sterile.
f Carefully pull glove over dominant hand, leaving a cuff and being sure that cuff does not roll up wrist. Be sure that thumb and fingers are in proper spaces (see illustration).	If outer surface of glove touches hand or wrist, it is contaminated.
g With gloved dominant hand, slip fingers underneath cuff of second glove (see illustration).	Cuff protects gloved fingers. Sterile touching prevents glove contamination.
h Carefully pull second glove over nondominant hand (see illustration).	Contact of gloved hand with exposed hand results in contamination.

Clinical Decision Point *Do not allow fingers and thumb of gloved dominant hand to touch any part of exposed nondominant hand. Keep thumb of dominant hand abducted back.*

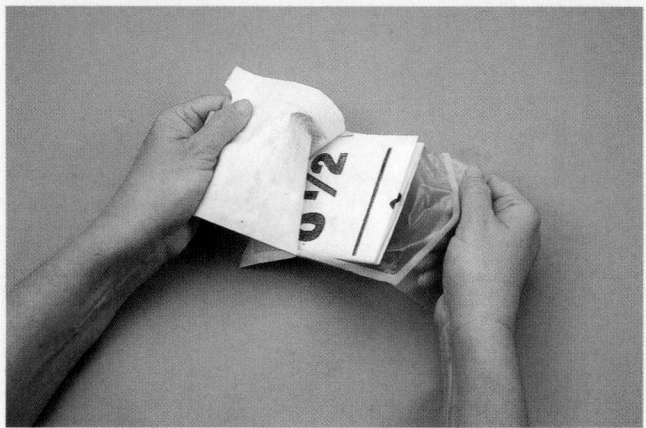

STEP 1b Open outer glove package wrapper.

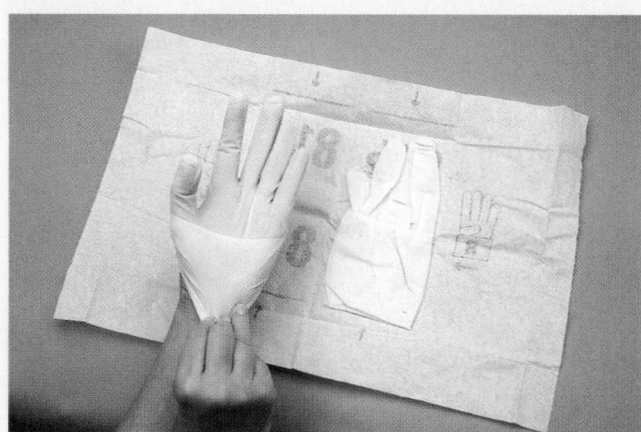

STEP 1f Pick up glove at cuff for dominant hand and insert fingers; pull glove completely over dominant hand (example is for left-handed person).

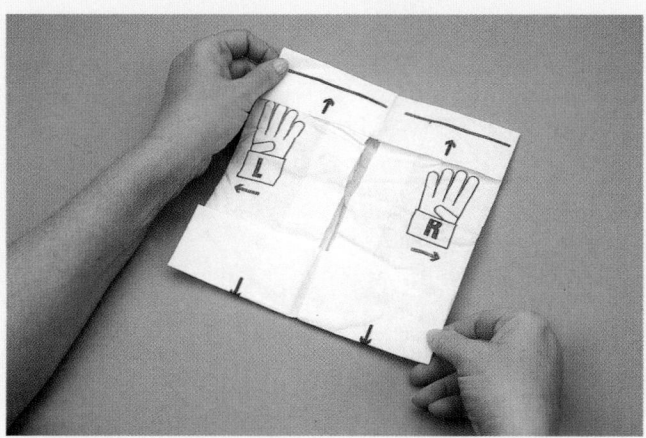

STEP 1c Open inner glove package on work surface.

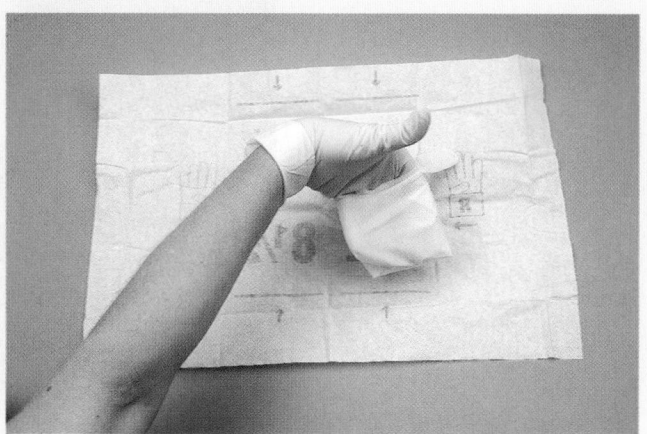

STEP 1g Pick up glove for nondominant hand.

STEP	RATIONALE

i After second glove is on, interlock hands together above waist level. The cuffs usually fall down after application. Be sure to touch only sterile sides (see illustration).

Ensures smooth fit over fingers.

2 Remove gloves.

   a Grasp outside of one cuff with other gloved hand; avoid touching wrist.

Minimizes contamination of underlying skin.

   b Pull glove off, turning it inside out, and place it in gloved hand.

Outside of glove does not touch skin surface.

   c Take fingers of bare hand and tuck inside remaining glove cuff (see illustration). Peel glove off inside out and over previously removed glove. Discard both gloves in receptacle

Fingers do not touch contaminated glove surface.

   d Perform thorough hand hygiene.

Protects health care worker from contamination resulting from any unseen tears or pinholes in gloves; also removes powder from hands to prevent skin irritation.

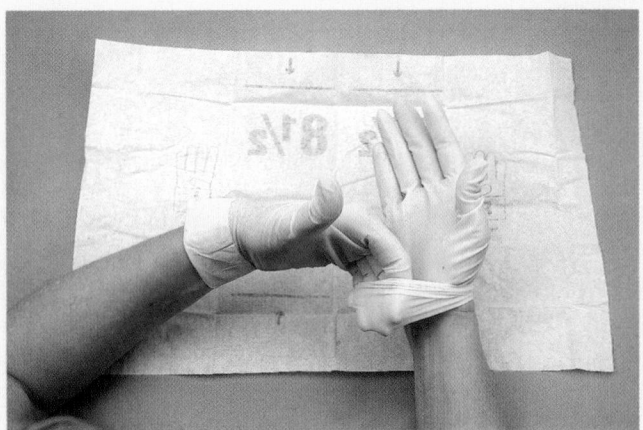

STEP 1h   Pull second glove over nondominant hand.

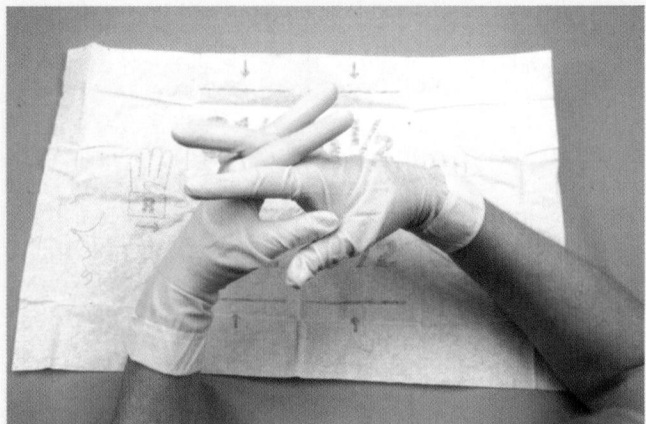

STEP 1i   Interlock gloved hands.

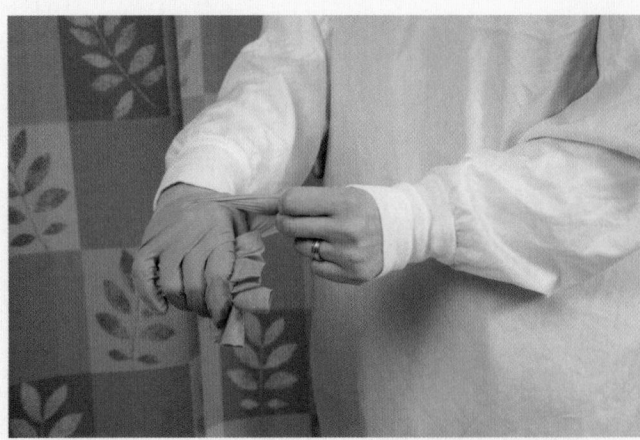

STEP 2c   Remove second glove by turning it inside out.

STEP	RATIONALE

EVALUATION

1 Assess patient for signs of infection, focusing on area treated.

2 Evaluate patient for signs of latex allergy.

Improper technique contributes to development of an infection.

Establishes baseline for patient's reaction to latex.

Unexpected Outcomes

1 Patient develops localized signs of infection (e.g., urine becomes cloudy or odorous; wound becomes painful, edematous, or reddened with purulent drainage).

2 Patient develops systemic signs of infection (e.g., fever, malaise, increased white blood cell count).

3 Patient develops allergic reaction to latex (see Box 8-3).

Related Interventions

- Contact health care provider and implement appropriate treatments as ordered.

- Contact health care provider and implement appropriate treatments as ordered.
- Immediately remove source of latex.
- Bring emergency equipment to bedside. Have epinephrine injection ready for administration, and be prepared to initiate IV fluids and oxygen.

Recording and Reporting

- It is not necessary to record application of gloves. Record specific procedure performed and patient's response and status.
- In the event of a latex allergy reaction, record patient's response in nurses' notes, EHR, and vital sign flow sheet. Note type of response and patient's reaction to emergency treatment.

Special Considerations
Teaching

- Nurse or patient with a known latex allergy should wear a medical alert bracelet or tag and carry a wallet card stating "latex allergy."
- Individuals with known latex allergies should carry a quick-acting oral antihistamine and an epinephrine autoinjector at all times.

[?] Critical Thinking Exercises

You are assigned to Mrs. Lorenzo, a 78-year-old grandmother who is blind and is being admitted for a cholecystectomy. You enter her room to begin a series of procedures: inserting an indwelling urinary catheter, irrigating a nasogastric tube, suctioning the oral cavity, and measuring the patient's blood pressure.

1 Which procedure requires use of sterile gloves?

2 Mrs. Lorenzo tells you that she has allergic reactions when she eats bananas or tomatoes. Based on this information, what would you ask Mrs. Lorenzo and which actions would you take?

3 Mrs. Lorenzo's physician is planning to insert a central venous line. You obtained the necessary equipment, prepared a sterile drape, and opened the sterile pack. You removed the outer wrapper and placed the item on the sterile field. While doing this, you noticed that the item touched the drape 5 cm (2 inches) from the border of the drape. What would you do next?

☑ REVIEW QUESTIONS

1 A nurse with a latex allergy needs to perform a sterile procedure and finds that the only sterile gloves available are latex. Which action by the nurse would be most effective in solving the problem?
   1 Rubbing petroleum jelly on the hands to provide a barrier between the hands and the gloves
   2 Putting a pair of synthetic gloves on before donning the latex sterile gloves
   3 Using a larger pair of sterile gloves so they're not as tight
   4 Rinsing the hands with cold water before putting on the sterile gloves

2 When opening a sterile pack, which action compromises the sterility of the contents?
   1 Keeping the contents of the pack away from the table edge
   2 Holding or moving the object below the waist
   3 Opening the pack just before the procedure
   4 Allowing movement around the sterile field that does not touch near the sterile field

3 A nurse is preparing to change a dressing using sterile gloves. It is most important to remember which concept when putting them on?
   1 Grab only the inside of the glove with the ungloved hand.
   2 Grab only the cuffs of the gloves with the bare hand.
   3 Wear a glove that is as tight as possible.
   4 Keep the glove fingertips parallel to the body.

4 A teenager with spina bifida is to have a urinary catheter inserted. Which action is most important before performing this procedure?
   1 Washing the insertion area with soap and water before insertion of the catheter
   2 Positioning the patient as comfortably as possible
   3 Asking the patient if he or she is allergic to eggs
   4 Obtaining a nonlatex catheter for the procedure

5 A nurse is supervising a nursing student setting up for a sterile dressing change. Which action by the nursing student would require intervention from the nurse?
   1 The first flap of the sterile package is opened away from the student's body.
   2 The glove for the dominant hand is pulled on first.
   3 When pouring a solution on to the sterile field, the label of the solution bottle is facing the floor.
   4 The bottle of solution is kept above the student's waist.

6 Sterilization of surgical instruments and surgical dressings is accomplished by using:
1 An autoclave.
2 Soap and water.
3 Ethylene oxide gas.
4 Chemicals such as alcohol.

7 A nurse has a cold and needs to change a dressing on a patient who is immunocompromised. Which action by the nurse would be most appropriate?
1 Asking another nurse to change the dressing
2 Wearing a gown and mask when changing the dressing
3 Performing hand hygiene for a longer time before putting on sterile gloves
4 Asking the patient if it's all right with him if he changes the dressing

8 In setting up a sterile field, which of the listed actions would require intervention?
1 The bottle of solution is poured with the label facing up.
2 The sterile drape is allowed to unfold above the waist.
3 The first flap of the sterile package is opened toward the nurse.
4 The glove for the dominant hand is pulled on first.

9 When performing a sterile procedure at the bedside, the NAP can help by assisting the nurse to _____ the patient.

10 Place an S next to the procedures requiring sterile (aseptic) technique. (Select all that apply.)
1 Urinary catheterization
2 Insertion of a feeding tube
3 Tracheal suctioning
4 Lumbar puncture
5 Insertion of a rectal suppository
6 Sitz bath

REFERENCES

Association of periOperative Registered Nurses (AORN): *Standards, recommended practices, and guidelines,* Denver, 2011, The Association.

Centers for Disease Control and Prevention, Hospital Infection Control Practice Advisory Committee: Guidelines for isolation precautions in healthcare settings 2007, available at http://www.cdc.gov/ncidod/dhap/pdf/guidelines/Isolation2007.

Centers for Medicare and Medicaid Services (CMS): Evidence-based guidelines for selected and previously considered hospital-acquired infections 2012, available at https://www.cms.gov/Medicare/Medicare-Fee-for-Service-Payment/HospitalAcqCond/Downloads/Evidence-Based-Guidelines.pdf, accessed June 26, 2012.

Church N, Bjerke N: Surgical services. In Carrico R, editor: *APIC text of infection control and epidemiology,* Washington, DC, revised 2009, Association for Professionals in Infection Control and Epidemiology (APIC).

Cook K: The hands have it! Hand hygiene in the OR, *OR Nurse* 5(6):14-16, 2011.

Iwamoto P: Aseptic technique. In *APIC text of infection control and epidemiology,* Washington, DC, revised 2009, Association for Professionals in Infection Control and Epidemiology (APIC).

Lynn-McHale Wiegand D: *AACN procedure manual for critical care,* ed 6, Philadelphia, 2011, Saunders.

Molinari J, Harte J: Dental services. In *APIC text of infection control and epidemiology,* Washington, DC, revised 2009, Association for Professionals in Infection Control and Epidemiology (APIC).

Occupational Safety and Health Administration (OSHA): Respiratory protection: proposed rule, *Fed Reg* 59(219):58884, 1994.

Occupational Safety and Health Administration (OSHA): Blood-borne pathogens, *Fed Reg* 77:19934, 2012.

The Joint Commission (TJC): *National Patient Safety Goals,* Oakbrook Terrace, Ill, 2012, The Commission, available at http://www.jointcommission.org/standards_information/npsgs.aspx.

Torch J: Raising the Red Flag, *Prev Strategist* 4 (3):44, 2011.

Safe Patient Handling, Transfer, and Positioning

MEDIA RESOURCES

- **evolve** learning system http://evolve.elsevier.com/Perry/skills
  - Review Questions
  - ▶ Video Clips
  - Audio Glossary
- Mosby's Nursing Video Skills, 4th edition
- **NSO** Nursing Skills Online

KEY TERMS

Balance	Footdrop	Hoyer lift (mechanical/ hydraulic lift)	Paralysis
Base of support	Friction		Paresis
Body alignment	Hand rolls	Leverage	Posture
Body mechanics	Hemiparesis	Line of gravity	Proprioceptive function
Center of gravity	Hemiplegia	Logrolling	Weight
Drawsheet		Orthostatic hypotension	

OBJECTIVES

Mastery of content in this chapter will enable the nurse to:
- Describe body mechanics and its importance in caring for patients.
- Describe principles of safe patient handling, transfer, and positioning.
- Describe normal body alignment for standing, sitting, and lying down.
- Assess for alterations in body alignment.

- Describe procedures for safety and use of equipment needed for lifting patients.
- Describe positioning techniques for the supported Fowler's, supine, prone, 30-degree lateral side-lying, and Sims' positions.
- Describe the procedures for helping a patient move up in bed, helping a patient to a sitting position, logrolling a patient, and transferring a patient from a bed to a chair.

Health care agencies are required to provide employees with safety information and training to use when transferring, positioning, and lifting patients. Refer to the policies and procedures of the agency in which you work. The National Institute of Occupational Safety and Health Administration (NIOSHA) has guidelines for back safety and the prevention of musculoskeletal injuries (NIOSHA, 2009).

Before lifting or transferring patients, consider principles of safe patient transfer and positioning (Box 9-1). Before lifting, assess the weight to be lifted and what assistance, if any, you need (Nelson et al., 2009; NIOSHA, 2009). If you need help, assess if a second person is adequate or if mechanical assistance is needed. Once you assess the amount of assistance, use the following steps for proper body mechanics:

- Keep back, neck, pelvis, and feet aligned and avoid twisting. Twisting your spine can lead to serious injury.

- Tighten stomach muscles and tuck pelvis; this provides balance and protects the back.
- Bend at the knees; this helps to maintain your center of gravity and lets the strong muscles of the legs do the lifting.
- Keep the weight to be lifted as close to the body as possible; this action places the weight in the same plane as the lifter and close to the center of gravity for balance.
- Maintain the trunk erect and knees bent so multiple muscle groups work together in a synchronized manner.
- The best height for lifting vertically is approximately 2 feet off the ground and close to the lifter's center of gravity.
- The person with the heaviest load coordinates efforts of the personnel involved in lifting or transferring.

BOX 9-1	Principles of Safe Patient Transfer and Positioning

Mechanical lifts and lift teams are essential when the patient is unable to assist. When a patient is able to assist, remember these principles:

- The lower the center of gravity, the greater the stability of the nurse.
- The equilibrium of an object is maintained as long as the line of gravity passes through its base of support.
- Facing the direction of movement prevents abnormal twisting of the spine.
- Dividing balanced activity between arms and legs reduces the risk for back injury.
- Leverage, rolling, turning, or pivoting requires less work than lifting.
- When friction is reduced between the object to be moved and the surface on which it is moved, less force is required to move it.

Body mechanics is the coordinated effort of the musculoskeletal and nervous systems to maintain balance, posture, and body alignment during lifting, bending, moving, and performing activities of daily living (ADLs). Body mechanics also facilitates body movement so a person can carry out a physical activity without using excessive muscle energy.

Many patients have conditions resulting in immobility or require limitations in activity imposed by their treatment plan. It is an important nursing role to safely position and move patients effectively to reduce the risks related to immobilization. Positioning patients to maintain correct body alignment is essential in preventing complications. These complications include pressure ulcers (see Chapter 18), which can develop in less than 24 hours and require months to heal (Institute for Healthcare Improvement, 2008); and contractures, which can occur within a few days when muscles, tendons, and joints become less flexible because of lack of mobility and incorrect alignment. Pillows placed under the knees or an elevated knee Gatch can produce knee and hip contractures and increase pressure on the sacrum, thus creating risk for pressure ulcers.

Some patients are at high risk for complications from improper positioning and have increased risk for injury during transfer. Examples include patients with poor nutrition, poor circulation, loss of sensation, alterations in bone formation or joint mobility, and impaired muscle development. The application of proper body mechanics, alignment, and the use of safe patient transfer and positioning techniques help patients achieve an optimal level of independence without resultant injury to health care providers.

EVIDENCE-BASED PRACTICE

Musculoskeletal disorders are the most prevalent and debilitating occupational health hazard among nurses. There has been little improvement in the incidence of musculoskeletal injuries in health care workers. The total recordable injury incidence rate for hospitals is 5.2 per 100 full-time employees (Bureau of Labor Statistics, 2011). Back injuries among health care workers are estimated to cost $10,689 per case; thus back injuries alone prove to be an economic burden and a major health concern (CDC, 2009; NIOSHA, 2009).

- Complete an ergonomics hazard assessment based on patient population, patient handling tasks, and physical environment.
- Train staff on devices, equipment, and handling policies.

- Organizations can develop a "no lift" policy that discourages manual lifting and requires the use of equipment and devices as needed (ANA, 2011).
- Use lift devices to reduce on-the-job injuries (Kutash et al., 2009; Sedlak et al., 2009; Zadvinskis and Salsbury, 2010).
- Knowledge about safe, efficient lifting techniques and proper use of assistive equipment and devices promotes safe patient transfer without injury to a patient or health care worker (ANA, 2011).

PATIENT-CENTERED CARE

Ultimately it is a patient's choice to increase his or her mobility and activity level. Consider a patient's knowledge, cultural beliefs, and circumstances surrounding the loss of independent activity when developing a plan of care. Take some time to assess a patient's knowledge and provide information about the complications of immobility. This may be all that is needed to elicit a patient's cooperation in ambulating after surgery. It is also important to consider a patient's cultural and ethnic beliefs. Assessing these beliefs guides you to incorporate appropriate interventions that match them. For example, some patients have a fear of becoming addicted to a narcotic after one dose, but pain is preventing them from increasing their mobility. With this knowledge you can individualize the patient's plan of care and explain the safe and proper use of narcotics for pain control. In addition, taking into consideration the circumstances surrounding the loss of independent activity and mobility is crucial in developing a plan of care that is realistic and attainable. For example, a patient with pulmonary disease who has recently undergone surgery may be expected to ambulate a prescribed number of feet on the second postoperative day. This information prompts the nurse to alter the patient's plan of care based on his or her activity limitation to achieve a reasonable level of mobility and activity.

Safety Guidelines

1 Know how physiologic influences on body alignment and mobility affect patients throughout the life span. Inactive older adults are at risk for muscle atrophy, loss of bony mass, contractures of joints, and pressure ulcers (Touhy et al., 2010).

2 Know the pathologic conditions that affect a patient's body alignment and mobility. Postural abnormalities affect body mechanics. For example, a patient with severe kyphosis cannot lie supine or lift an object safely because the center of gravity is not in alignment.

3 Know the history of underlying chronic conditions (e.g., diabetes, chronic obstructive pulmonary disease) or malnutrition. Patients with chronic conditions are at risk for skin breakdown and other hazards of immobility and as a result require more frequent position changes.

4 Control factors that indirectly affect body mechanics by altering the safety of the environment. Cluttered hallways and bedside areas increase a patient's risk of falling (see Chapters 13 and 41).

5 Know a patient's fluid balance status. Dehydration or edema may require more frequent position changes because patients are prone to skin breakdown. Dehydration also predisposes patients to orthostatic hypotension. Identify patients with incontinence or profuse sweating. Moisture from incontinence or sweating can alter the resiliency of skin to external forces (Stechmiller et al., 2008).

6 Know a patient's range of motion. Contractures or spasticity limit joint and muscle mobility; take care not to position a patient's limb in an unnatural position. This could result in injury or dysfunction of the affected limb (see Chapter 10).

7 Determine a patient's level of sensory perception. Loss of sensation increases vulnerability to the hazards of immobility because of the inability to sense pain or need for repositioning. Patients with decreased sensation must have their positions evaluated and changed frequently to avoid damage to the integumentary and musculoskeletal systems.

SKILL 9-1   Using Safe and Effective Transfer Techniques

NSO *Nursing Skills Online: Safety Module / Lesson 3*

 Video Clip

Transferring is a nursing skill to help a dependent patient or a patient with restricted mobility attain positions to regain optimal independence as quickly and safely as possible. Physical activity maintains and improves joint motion, increases strength, promotes circulation, relieves pressure on skin, and improves urinary and respiratory functions. It also benefits a patient psychologically by increasing social activity and mental stimulation and providing a change in environment (Janelli et al., 2009; Schneider et al., 2008).

One of the major concerns during transfer is the safety of the patient and the nurse. The nurse prevents self-injury by using correct posture, minimal muscle strength, effective body mechanics and lifting techniques, and appropriate lift devices. Consider individual patient problems during transfer. For example, a patient who has been immobile for several days or longer may be weak or dizzy or may develop orthostatic hypotension (a drop in blood pressure) when transferred. If there is any doubt about safe transfer, use a transfer belt and obtain assistance when transferring patients.

Delegation and Collaboration

The skill of effective transfer techniques can be delegated to nursing assistive personnel (NAP). The nurse directs the NAP by:

- Assisting and supervising when moving patients who are transferred for the first time after prolonged bed rest, extensive surgery, critical illness, or spinal cord trauma.
- Explaining the patient's mobility restrictions, changes in blood pressure, or sensory alterations that may affect safe transfer.
- Explaining what to observe and report back to the nurse, such as dizziness or the patient's ability to assist.

Equipment

- ☐ Transfer belt, sling, or lap board (as needed)
- ☐ Nonskid shoes, bath blankets, pillows
- ☐ Slide board (friction-reducing board)
- ☐ Bedside chair with arms or wheelchair: Position chair at 45-degree angle to bed, lock brakes, remove footrests, lock bed brakes
- ☐ Stretcher: Position next to bed, lock brakes on stretcher, lock brakes on bed
- ☐ Optional: Mechanical/hydraulic lift: Use frame, canvas strips or chains, and hammock or canvas strips; stand-assist lift device
- ☐ Sphygmomanometer and stethoscope

STEP	RATIONALE

ASSESSMENT

1 Assess physiologic capacity of a patient to transfer and the need for special adaptive techniques (see Chapter 6). Assess the following:	Determines patient's ability to tolerate and assist with transfer and whether special adaptive techniques are necessary.
a Muscle strength (legs and upper arms)	Immobile patients have decreased muscle strength, tone, and mass. Affects ability to bear weight or raise body.
b Joint mobility and contracture formation	Immobility or inflammatory processes (e.g., arthritis) may lead to contracture formation and impaired joint mobility.
c Paralysis or paresis (spastic or flaccid)	Patient with central nervous system (CNS) damage may have bilateral paralysis (requiring transfer by swivel bar, sliding bar, mechanical lift) or unilateral paralysis, which requires belt transfer to strong side. Weakness (paresis) requires stabilization of knee while transferring. Flaccid arm must be supported with sling during transfer.
d Bone continuity (trauma, amputation), or calcium loss from long bones	Patients with trauma to one leg or hip may be non–weight bearing when transferred. Amputees may use sliding board to transfer. Osteoporosis increases risk for injury.
2 Assess presence of weakness, dizziness, or postural hypotension.	Determines risk for fainting or falling during transfer. The move from supine to vertical position redistributes about 500 mL of blood; immobile patients may have decreased autonomic nervous system response to equalize blood supply, resulting in orthostatic hypotension (Lewis et al., 2011).

STEP	RATIONALE
3 Assess level of endurance:	
a Assess level of fatigue during activity.	Ability to transfer may be limited by fatigue. Estimates ability to participate in transfer. Assess endurance by patient's participation in activities of daily living (ADLs). Planned rest periods before transfer may enhance function.
b Assess vital signs.	Vital sign changes such as increased pulse and respiration may indicate activity intolerance (see Chapter 5). Patient with low blood pressure may not tolerate sudden position change and is at risk for orthostatic hypotension.
4 Assess patient's proprioceptive function (awareness of posture and changes in equilibrium):	Determines stability of patient's balance for transfer.
a Ability to maintain balance while sitting in bed or on side of bed	Determines risk for fainting or falling during transfer.
b Tendency to sway or position self to one side	Patients with brain dysfunction may have proprioceptive losses. This may cause them to lean to one side or lose balance during transfer.
5 Assess patient's sensory status, including adequacy of central and peripheral vision, adequacy of hearing, and presence of peripheral sensation loss.	Determines influence of sensory loss on ability to make transfer. Visual field loss decreases patient's ability to see in direction of transfer. Peripheral sensation loss decreases proprioception. Patients with visual and hearing losses need transfer techniques adapted to deficits. Patients with cerebrovascular accident (CVA) may lose area of visual field, which profoundly affects vision and perception.

Clinical Decision Point *Patients with hemiplegia may "neglect" one side of the body (inattention to or unawareness of one side of body or environment), which distorts perceptions of the visual field.*

STEP	RATIONALE
6 Assess patient for pain (e.g., joint discomfort, muscle spasm) and measure level of pain using scale of 0 to 10. Offer prescribed analgesic 30 minutes before transfer.	Pain reduces patient's motivation and ability to be mobile. Pain relief before transfer enhances patient participation (Quinlan-Colwell, 2009).
7 Assess patient's cognitive status:	Determines patient's ability to follow directions and learn transfer techniques.
a Ability to follow verbal instructions	May indicate patient is at risk for injury.
b Short-term memory	Patient with short-term memory deficit may have difficulty with transfer, initial learning, or consistent performance.
c Recognition of physical deficits and limitations to movement	Patient's knowledge of deficits can help you plan a safe transfer.
8 Assess patient's level of motivation, such as his or her eagerness versus unwillingness to be mobile.	Altered psychological states often reduce patient's desire to engage in activity.
9 Assess previous mode of transfer (if applicable).	Determines mode of transfer and assistance required to provide continuity. Transfer (gait) belts should be used with patients who need assistance (Nelson et al., 2009; OSHA, 2011).
10 Determine if a lift device is needed and the number of people needed to assist with transfer. Do not start procedure until all required caregivers are available.	Ensures safe patient transfer.

NURSING DIAGNOSES

- Activity intolerance
- Acute or chronic pain
- Acute confusion
- Risk for falls
- Impaired physical mobility
- Impaired skin integrity
- Risk for injury

Related factors are individualized based on patient's condition or needs.

STEP	RATIONALE

PLANNING

1 Expected outcomes following completion of procedure:

- Patient dangles legs or sits without dizziness, weakness, or orthostatic hypotension.
- Patient tolerates increased activity.

- Patient can bear more weight.

- Patient transfers without injury.
- Patient is more motivated to be mobile.
- Patient transfers with minimal discomfort.

2 Explain procedure to patient. Repeat instructions simply and with continuity to patient with cognitive dysfunction.

Precautions during transferring prevent vascular compromise.

Gradual increase in number of transfers and period of time out of bed increases tolerance and endurance.
Repeated transfers usually result in improved endurance and greater independence of patient.
Proper techniques avoid injury.

Transfer procedures performed correctly.
Promotes understanding and cooperation, reducing anxiety.

IMPLEMENTATION

1 Perform hand hygiene.

Reduces transfer of microorganisms.

2 Assist patient to sitting position (bed at waist level):

Clinical Decision Point *If patient is in hospital bed, use electrical controls to raise him or her to a sitting position in bed.*

a Place patient in supine position.

b Face head of the bed at 45-degree angle and remove pillows.

c Place feet in wide base of support with foot closer to head of bed in front of other foot.
d Place hand nearer head of bed under patient's shoulders, supporting patient's head and cervical vertebrae.
e Place other hand on bed surface.
f Raise patient to sitting position by shifting weight from front to back leg.
g Push against bed using arm that is placed on bed surface.

Enables you to assess patient's body alignment continually and administer additional care such as suctioning or hygiene needs.
Proper positioning reduces twisting of your body when moving patient. Pillows may cause interference when patient is sitting up in bed.
Improves balance and allows transfer of body weight while moving patient to sitting position.
Maintains alignment of head and cervical vertebrae and allows for even lifting of patient's upper trunk.
Provides support and balance.
Improves balance, overcomes inertia, and transfers your weight in direction in which patient is moved.
Divides activity between your arms and legs and protects back from strain. By bracing one hand against mattress and pushing against it as patient is lifted, part of weight that would be lifted by your back muscles is transferred through your arms onto mattress.

3 Assist patient to sitting position on side of bed with bed in low position, using electrical bed:

a With patient in supine position, raise head of bed 30 degrees.

b Turn patient onto side, facing you on side of bed on which patient will be sitting (see illustration).
c Stand opposite patient's hips. Turn diagonally so you face patient and far corner of foot of bed.
d Place feet apart in wide base of support with foot closer to head of bed in front of other foot (see illustration).
e Place arm nearer head of bed under patient's shoulders, supporting head and neck.
f Place other arm over patient's thighs (see illustration).

g Move patient's lower legs and feet over side of bed. Pivot toward rear leg, allowing patient's upper legs to swing downward.

h At same time shift weight to rear leg and elevate patient (see illustration).

Decreases amount of work needed by patient and nurse to raise patient to sitting position.
Prepares patient to move to side of bed and protects from falling.

Places your center of gravity nearer patient. Reduces twisting of body because you are facing direction of movement.
Increases balance and allows you to transfer weight as patient is brought to sitting position on side of bed.
Maintains alignment of head and neck as you bring patient to sitting position.
Supports hip and prevents patient from falling backward during procedure.
Decreases friction and resistance. Weight of patient's legs when off bed allows gravity to lower legs, and weight of legs assists in pulling upper body into sitting position.
Allows you to transfer weight in direction of motion.

STEP	RATIONALE

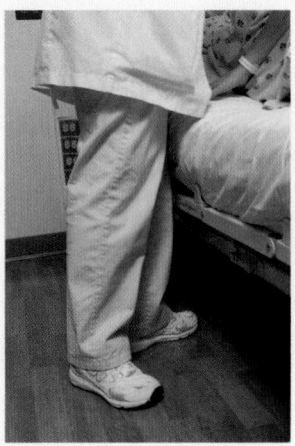

STEP 3b   Side-lying position.

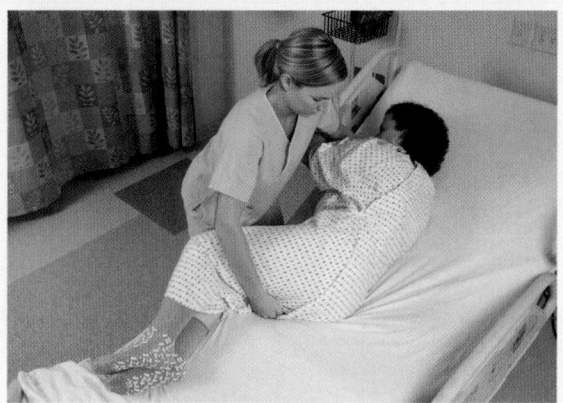

STEP 3f   Nurse places arm over patient's thighs.

STEP 3d   Proper foot placement.

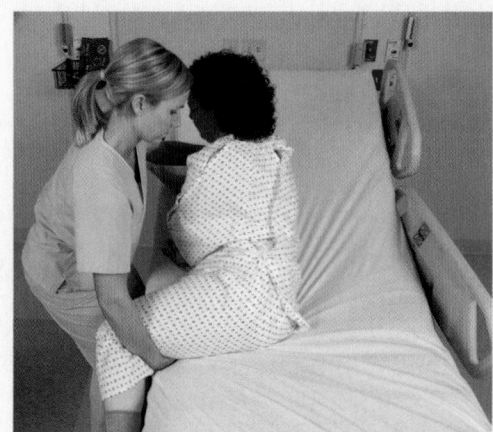

STEP 3h   Nurse shifts weight to rear leg and elevates patient.

Clinical Decision Point *Remain in front until patient regains balance and continue to provide physical support to weak or cognitively impaired patient.*

4   **Transfer patient from bed to chair with bed in the low position:**

  a If patient has partial weight bearing with upper body strength, use bariatric transfer aid with minimum of two or three caregivers (see illustration).

The use of mechanical lift devices is strongly recommended to transfer a patient to reduce risk for musculoskeletal injury (Baptiste et al., 2008; Nelson et al., 2009).

STEP	RATIONALE

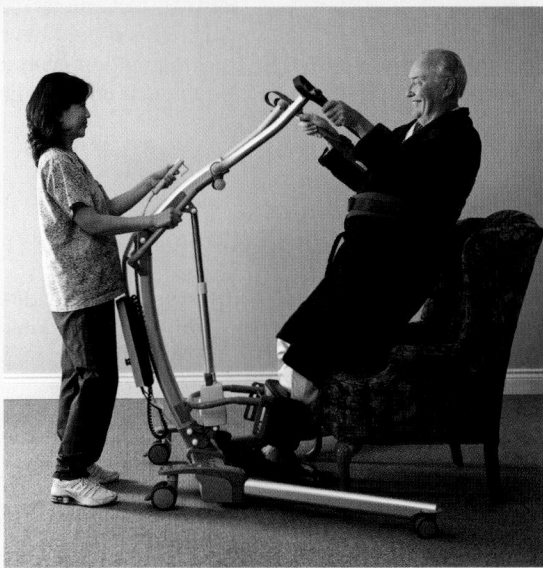

STEP 4a   Stand-assist lift device. *(Courtesy Waverly Glen Systems, a Prism Medical Co.)*

Clinical Decision Point *If patient demonstrates weakness or paralysis of one side of the body, place chair on patient's strong side.*

b If patient has normal weight bearing and upper body strength, first assist him or her to sitting position on side of bed (see Steps 3a to h). Have chair in position at 45-degree angle to bed. If using wheelchair, make sure that wheels are locked. Allow patient to sit on side of bed (dangling) for a few minutes before transferring to chair. Ask if he or she feels dizzy. Do not leave patient unattended during dangling.

Positions chair within easy access for transfer. Dangling or allowing a patient to sit on side of bed before transfer helps equilibrate blood pressure by preventing a sudden change in position, reducing risk for dizziness or fainting when standing (Thompson et al., 2011).

c Apply transfer belt (see illustration) or use transfer board. Place board across bed to chair so patient can slide across it. Patient's arm should be in sling if flaccid paralysis is present.

Transfer belt allows you to maintain stability of patient during transfer and reduces risk for falling (OSHA, 2011). Transfer board makes sliding over to chair easy with less physical effort. Transfer belt is contraindicated after abdominal surgery.

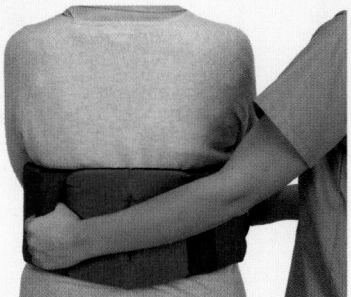

STEP 4c   Transfer belt with handles. *(Courtesy The Posey Company, Arcadia, Calif.)*

d Help patient apply stable, nonskid shoes. Place patient's weight-bearing, or strong, leg forward, with weak foot back.

Nonskid soles decrease risk for slipping during transfer. Always have patient wear shoes during transfer; bare feet increase risk for falls. Patient will stand on stronger, or weight-bearing, leg.

e Spread your feet apart.

Ensures balance with wide base of support.

f Flex hips and knees, aligning knees with patient's knees (see illustration).

Flexing knees and hips lowers your center of gravity to object to be raised; aligning knees with patient's allows for stabilization of knees when patient stands.

STEP	RATIONALE
g Grasp transfer belt along patient's sides.	Transfer belt allows you to move patient at center of gravity. Patients should never be lifted by or under arms.
h Rock patient up to standing position on count of three while straightening hips and legs and keeping knees slightly flexed (see illustration). While rocking patient in back-and-forth motion, make sure that your body weight is moving in the same direction as patient's to ensure that you and patient are moving in same direction simultaneously. Unless contraindicated, patient may be instructed to use hands to push up if applicable.	Rocking motion gives patient's body momentum and requires less muscular effort to lift him or her.
i Maintain stability of patient's weak or paralyzed leg with your knee.	Ability to stand can often be maintained in paralyzed or weak limb with support of knee to stabilize.
j Pivot on foot farther from chair.	Maintains support of patient while allowing adequate space for patient to move.
k Instruct patient to use armrests on chair for support and ease into chair (see illustration).	Increases patient stability.
l Flex hips and knees while lowering patient into chair (see illustration).	Prevents injury from poor body mechanics.

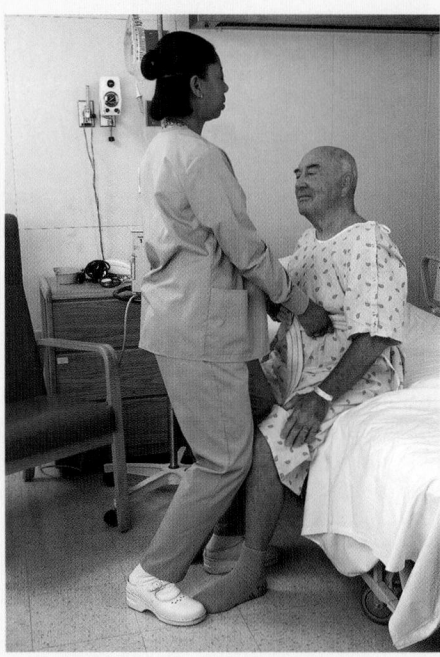

STEP 4f   Nurse flexes hips and knees, aligns knees with patient's knee, and grasps transfer belt.

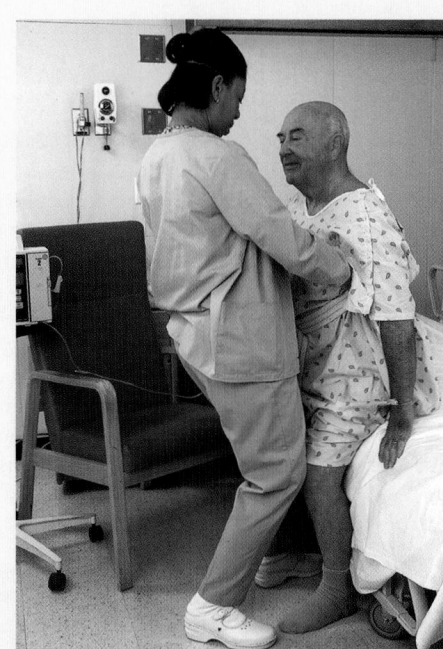

STEP 4h   Nurse rocks patient to standing position.

STEP	RATIONALE

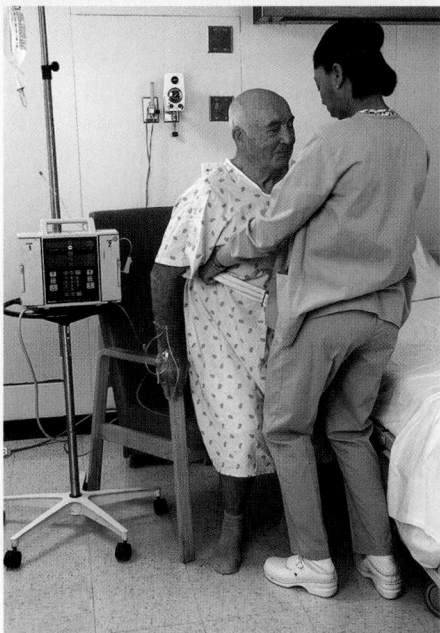

STEP 4k   Patient uses armrests for support.

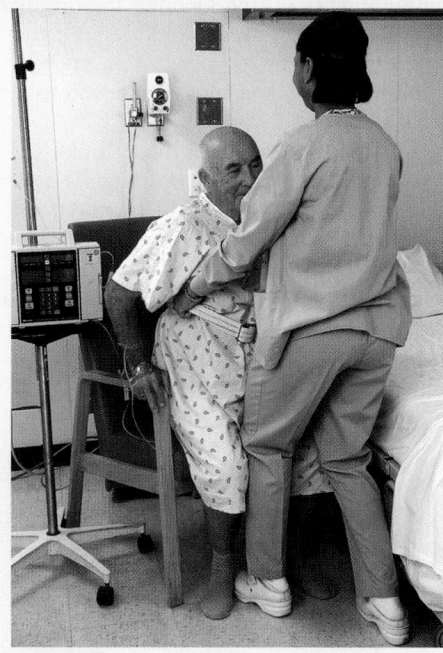

STEP 4l   Nurse eases patient into chair.

m Assess patient for proper alignment in sitting position. Provide support for paralyzed extremities. Lap board or sling supports flaccid arm. Stabilize leg with bath blanket or pillow.

Prevents injury to patient from poor body alignment.

n Proper alignment for sitting position: head is erect, and vertebrae are in straight alignment. Body weight is evenly distributed on buttocks and thighs. Thighs are parallel and in horizontal plane. Both feet are supported on floor, and ankles are comfortably flexed. A 2.5- to 5-cm (1- to 2-inch) space is maintained between edge of seat and popliteal space on posterior surface of knee.

Prevents stress on intravertebral joints. Prevents increased pressure over bony prominences and reduces damage to underlying musculoskeletal system.

o Praise patient's progress, effort, and performance.

Continued support and encouragement provide incentive for patient perseverance.

5 Perform horizontal transfer from bed to stretcher using slide board or friction-reducing board (see illustration):

The three-person lift for horizontal transfer from bed to stretcher is no longer recommended and in fact is discouraged (NIOSHA, 2009; Waters et al., 2011). Physical stress can be decreased significantly by using slide board or friction-reducing board positioned under drawsheet beneath patient. In addition, patient is more comfortable using this method.

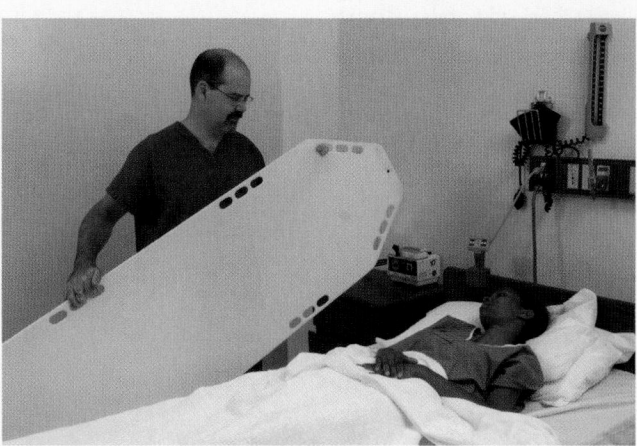

STEP 5   Slide board.

STEP	RATIONALE
a Determine number of staff required to horizontally transfer patient safely (three nurses recommended).	During any patient transferring task, if any caregiver is required to lift more than 15.9 kg (35 lbs) of a patient's weight, the patient is considered fully dependent, and an assist device is used.
b Lower head of bed as much as patient can tolerate. Be sure to lock bed brakes.	Maintains alignment of spinal column. Ensures that bed does not move inadvertently.
c Cross patient's arms on chest.	Prevents injury to arms during transfer.
d Lower side rails. To place slide board under patient, position two nurses on side of bed to which patient will be turned. Position third nurse on other side of bed.	Distributes weight equally between nurses.
e Fanfold drawsheet on both sides.	Provides strong handles to grip drawsheet without slipping.
f On count of three turn patient onto side toward the two nurses. Turn patient as one unit with a smooth, continuous motion.	Maintains body in alignment, preventing stress on any part.
g Place slide board under drawsheet (see illustration).	Prevents friction from contact of skin with board.

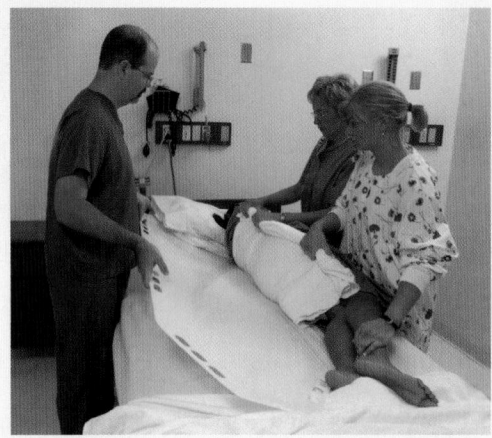

STEP 5g   Placing slide board under drawsheet.

STEP	RATIONALE
h Gently roll patient back onto slide board.	
i Line up stretcher with bed. Lock brakes on stretcher.	Ensures that stretcher does not move inadvertently during transfer.
j Two nurses position themselves on side of stretcher while the third nurse positions self on side of bed without stretcher.	

Clinical Decision Point *A nurse may also be positioned at the head of patient's bed to protect and support his or her head and neck if patient is weak or unable to assist.*

STEP	RATIONALE
k Fanfold drawsheet; using count of three, the two nurses pull drawsheet with patient onto stretcher while the third nurse holds slide board in place (see illustration).	Slide board remains stationary and provides slippery surface to reduce friction and allows patient to transfer easily to stretcher.
l Position patient in center of stretcher. Raise head of stretcher if not contraindicated. Raise stretcher side rails. Cover patient with blanket.	Provides for patient comfort.

STEP	RATIONALE
6 Use mechanical/hydraulic lift to transfer patient from bed to chair:	Research supports use of mechanical lifts to prevent musculoskeletal injuries (ANA, 2011; Nelson et al., 2009). Use of ceiling-mounted lifts is becoming more popular choice because of availability of lift in each patient's room (see illustration).

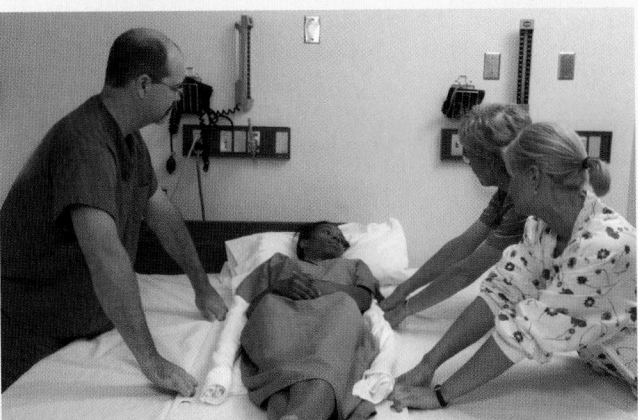

STEP 5k Transfer of patient to stretcher using slide board.

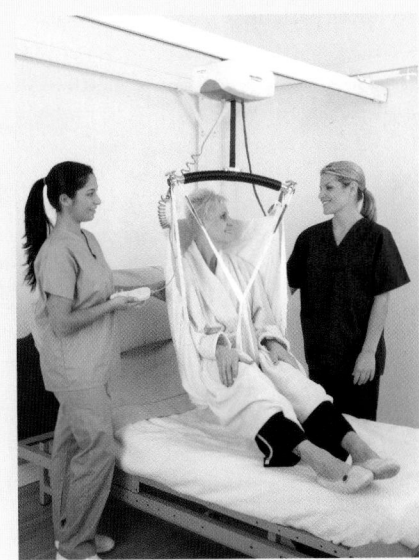

STEP 6 Ceiling lift. (*Courtesy Waverly Glen Systems, a Prism Medical Co.*)

STEP	RATIONALE
a Bring lift to bedside or lower ceiling lift and position properly.	Ensures safe elevation of patient off bed.
b Position chair near bed and allow adequate space to maneuver lift.	Prepares environment for safe use of lift and subsequent transfer.
c Raise bed to high position with mattress flat. Lower side rail on side near chair.	Allows you to use proper body mechanics.
d Raise opposite side rail unless a second nurse is assisting.	Maintains patient safety.
e Roll patient on side away from you.	Positions patient for placement of lift sling.
f Place hammock or canvas strips under patient to form sling. With two canvas pieces, lower edge fits under patient's knees (wide piece), and upper edge fits under patient's shoulders (narrow piece).	Two types of seats are supplied with mechanical/hydraulic lift: hammock style is better for patients who are flaccid, weak, and need support; canvas strips can be used for patients with normal muscle tone. Hooks should face away from patient's skin. Place sling under patient's center of gravity and greatest portion of body weight.
g Raise bed rail.	Maintains patient safety.
h Go to opposite side of bed and lower side rail.	
i Roll patient to opposite side and pull hammock (strips) through and smooth over bed surface.	Completes positioning of patient on mechanical/hydraulic sling.
j Roll patient supine onto canvas hammock.	Sling should extend from shoulders to knees (hammock) to support patient's body weight equally.
k Remove patient's glasses if appropriate.	Swivel bar is close to patient's head and could break eyeglasses.
l Place horseshoe bar of lift under side of bed (on side with chair).	Positions lift efficiently and promotes smooth transfer.
m Lower horizontal bar to sling level by following manufacturer directions. Lock valve if required.	Positions hydraulic lift close to patient. Locking valve prevents injury to patient.
n Attach hooks on strap (chain) to holes in sling. Short chains or straps hook to top holes of sling; longer chains hook to bottom of sling.	Secures hydraulic lift to sling.
o Elevate head of bed.	Positions patient in sitting position.
p Fold patient's arms over chest.	Prevents injury to patient's arms.
q Pump hydraulic handle using long, slow, even strokes until patient is raised off bed (see illustration). For ceiling lift turn on control device to move lift.	Ensures safe support of patient during elevation.

STEP	RATIONALE
r Use steering handle to pull lift from bed and maneuver patient to chair.	Moves patient from bed to chair.
s Roll base around chair.	
t Release check valve slowly (turn to left) and lower patient into chair (see illustration). For ceiling lift again use control device to lower patient.	Positions lift in front of chair into which patient is to be transferred. Safely guides patient into back of chair as seat descends.

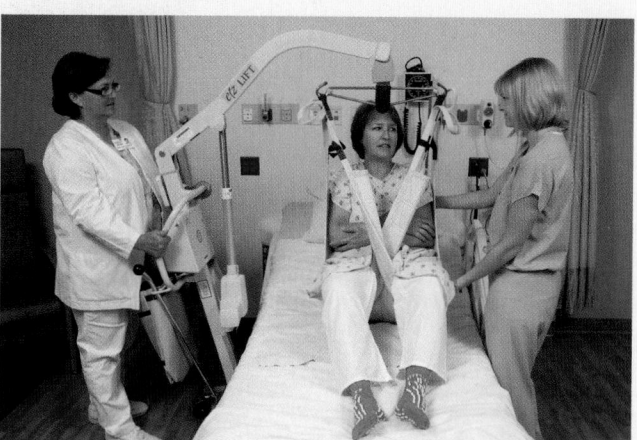

STEP 6q   Sling under patient and attached to lift.

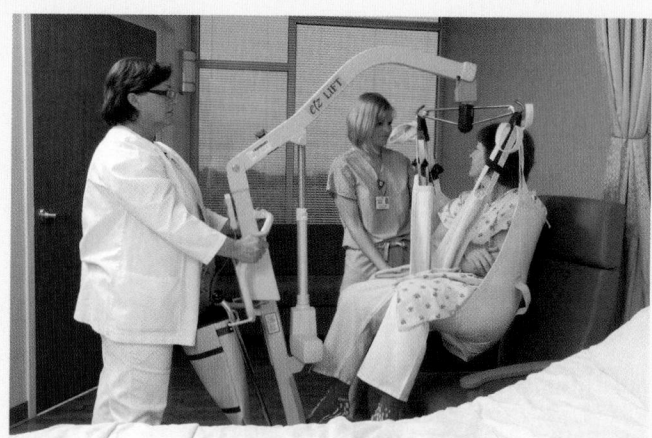

STEP 6t   Use of hydraulic lift to lower patient into chair.

u Close check valve or turn off control device as soon as patient is down and straps can be released.	If valve is left open or device left on, boom may continue to lower and injure patient.
v Remove straps and mechanical/hydraulic lift.	Prevents damage to skin and underlying tissues from canvas or hooks.
w Check patient's sitting alignment, and correct if necessary (see Step 4n).	Prevents injury from poor posture.
7 Perform hand hygiene.	Reduces transmission of microorganisms

EVALUATION

1 Monitor vital signs. Ask if patient feels dizzy or fatigued.	Evaluates patient's response to postural changes and activity.
2 Note patient's behavioral response to transfer.	Reveals level of motivation and self-care potential.
3 Ask if patient experienced pain during transfer.	Determines need for additional pain control or alteration in technique of transferring (e.g., additional assistance).
4 Have patient who transfers to chair attempt to bear weight with nurse at side.	Determines tolerance to weight bearing.

Unexpected Outcomes

1 Patient is unable to comprehend and follow directions for transfer.

Related Interventions

- Reassess continuity and simplicity of instruction.
- Transfers may be difficult when patient is fatigued or in pain; assess before transfer (allow for a rest period before transferring or medicate for pain if indicated).

2 Patient sustains injury on transfer.

- Evaluate incident that caused injury (e.g., inadequate assessment, change in patient status, improper use of equipment).
- Complete incident report according to agency policy.

3 Patient's level of weakness does not permit active transfer.

- Increase bed activity and exercise to heighten tolerance.

4 Patient is unable to stand for time required to transfer.

- Provide for additional nurses to provide adequate assistance during transfer.

Recording and Reporting

- Record procedure, including pertinent observations: weakness, ability to follow directions, weight-bearing ability, balance, ability to pivot, number of personnel needed to assist, and amount of assistance (muscle strength) required.
- Report transfer ability and assistance needed to next shift or other caregivers. Report progress or remission to rehabilitation staff (physical therapist, occupational therapist).

Special Considerations

Teaching

- Teach family and patient transfer skills, including principles of body mechanics and hazards of immobility. Incorporate return demonstration in discharge planning.

Pediatric

- Whenever possible, transporting child by stretcher, stroller, or wheelchair outside confines of room increases environmental stimuli and provides social contact with others (Hockenberry et al., 2011).
- Children confined to bed for any length of time such as those in traction need to have dependent skin surfaces assessed at least three times in a 24-hour period.

Gerontologic

- A major health concern that threatens the function of an older adult is the risk for falls (Touhy et al., 2010). Concern increases when an older adult enters a hospital. Assess the patient for the risk for falls on admission and implement a protocol to prevent falls (Lewis et al., 2011) (see Chapter 13).
- Use a drawsheet to avoid shearing force during repositioning in bed. This protects an older adult patient who has fragile skin.

Home Care

- Have family or caregiver practice transfer in hospital to achieve success before taking patient home. Alternatively have patient (if living alone) practice transfer skills in bed that will be used at home. Teach patient to transfer to chair with arms for ease of rising and sitting.
- Home should be free of hazards (e.g., throw rugs, electric cords, slippery floors). If wheelchair is used, access must be possible through all doors, and space for transfer must be available in bedroom and bathroom (see Chapter 41).
- Aids that enhance transfer ability are shower stools, commode elevators, handrails on tub, and nonskid shower surface. Many self-care devices are available for wheelchair-bound patients or patients with weak or poor muscle function. Medical supply stores provide excellent information and catalogs of such supplies.

PROCEDURAL GUIDELINE 9-1   Wheelchair Transfer Techniques

Transferring a patient from a bed to a wheelchair encompasses many of the same principles discussed in Skill 9-1. The following procedural guideline focuses on the safety precautions that need to be considered when using a wheelchair. Several additional steps must be taken to maintain safety of a patient and nurse to prevent injury when transferring from or to a wheelchair (Pierson and Fairchild, 2008). Check wheelchair locks and footplates for proper functioning before use.

Delegation and Collaboration

The skill of transferring a patient to or from a wheelchair can be delegated to nursing assistive personnel (NAP). The nurse directs NAP by:

- Assisting and supervising when moving patients who are transferring for the first time after prolonged bed rest, extensive surgery, critical illness, or spinal cord trauma.
- Explaining the patient's mobility restrictions, changes in blood pressure, or sensory alterations that may affect safe transfer.
- Reminding NAP to back a wheelchair into or out of an elevator to avoid tipping forward.

Equipment

❑ Transfer belt, nonskid shoes, wheelchair

1 **Transferring patient from a wheelchair to bed (patient is cooperative and weight bearing)**
   a Adjust the height of the bed to the level of the seat of the wheelchair.
   b Position wheelchair at a 45-degree angle next to the bed.
   c Face the wheelchair toward the foot of the bed midway between the head and foot of the bed.
   d Lock the wheelchair. Locks are located above the rims of the wheels. Push handle forward to lock.

e Raise the footplates.
f Place transfer belt on patient.
g Assist patient to move to the front of the wheelchair.
h Position yourself slightly in front of patient to guard and protect him or her throughout the transfer. If patient has sufficient upper body strength, use a slide board during transfer (see illustration).

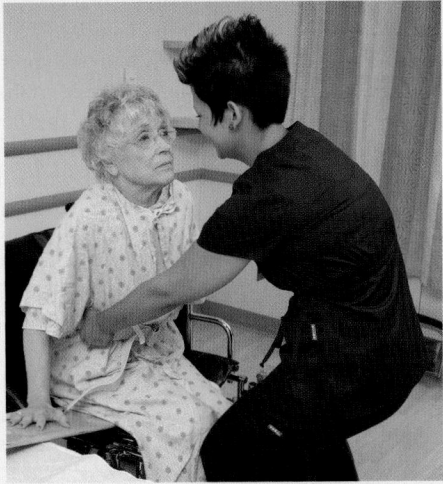

STEP 1h   Transfer from wheelchair to bed using a slide board.

i Coordinate transfer to bed by having patient stand and then pivot to the side of the bed. Then have patient sit on the side of the mattress.
j With patient sitting on the side of the bed, place your arm nearest the head of the bed under his or her shoulder while supporting the head and neck. Place your other arm under patient's knees. Bend your knees and keep your back straight.

Continued

PROCEDURAL GUIDELINE 9-1 Wheelchair Transfer Techniques—cont'd

k Tell patient to help lift the legs when you begin to move. On a count of three, standing with a wide base of support, raise patient's legs as you pivot his or her body and lower the shoulders onto the bed. Remember to keep your back straight.

2 **Transferring a patient from a bed to a wheelchair**
a Adjust the height of the bed to the level of the seat of the wheelchair.
b Position the wheelchair at a 45-degree angle next to the same side of the bed as patient's strong side.
c Face the wheelchair toward the foot of the bed midway between the head and foot of the bed.
d Lock the wheelchair. Locks are located above the rims of the wheels. Push handle forward to lock.
e Raise the footplates.

f Sit patient on the side of the bed (see Skill 9-1).
g Place transfer belt on patient.
h Assist patient to move to the edge of the mattress.
i Position yourself slightly in front of patient to guard and protect him or her throughout the transfer.
j Coordinate transfer to chair with patient by counting to three (see Skill 9-1).
k Lower the footplates after transfer and place patient's feet on them.
l Unlock the wheelchair. Pull lock toward you to release.
m Ensure that patient is positioned well back in the seat.
3 Monitor vital signs as needed. Ask if patient feels dizzy or fatigued.
4 Note patient's behavioral response to transfer.

SKILL 9-2 Moving and Positioning Patients in Bed

NSO *Nursing Skills Online: Safety Module / Lesson 4*

 Video Clip

Correctly positioning patients is crucial for maintaining body alignment and comfort; preventing injury to the musculoskeletal and integumentary systems; and providing sensory, motor, and cognitive stimulation. A patient with impaired mobility, decreased sensation, impaired circulation, or lack of voluntary muscle control can develop damage to the musculoskeletal and integumentary systems while lying down. You must minimize this risk by maintaining unrestricted circulation and correct body alignment while moving, turning, or positioning a patient. The term *body alignment* refers to the condition of the joints, tendons, ligaments, and muscles in various body positions. When the body is aligned, whether standing, sitting, or lying, no excessive strain is placed on these structures. Body alignment means that the body is in line with the pull of gravity and contributes to body balance. Without this balance the center of gravity is displaced, which increases the force of gravity and predisposes a person to falls and injuries. Body balance is achieved when a wide base of support exists, the center of gravity falls within the base of support, and a vertical line can be drawn from the center of gravity through the base of support (Fig. 9-1).

Delegation and Collaboration
The skills of moving and positioning patients in bed and maintaining correct body alignment can be delegated to nursing assistive personnel (NAP). The nurse directs the NAP by:
- Explaining about any moving and positioning restrictions (e.g., avoid prone position, patient has one-sided weakness).
- Designating specific times throughout the shift that NAP must reposition the patient.
- Providing information regarding patient's individual needs for body alignment (i.e., patient with spinal cord injury).

Equipment
- ❏ Pillows, drawsheet
- ❏ Friction-reducing device
- ❏ Therapeutic boots/splints (optional)
- ❏ Trochanter roll
- ❏ Sandbag
- ❏ Hand rolls

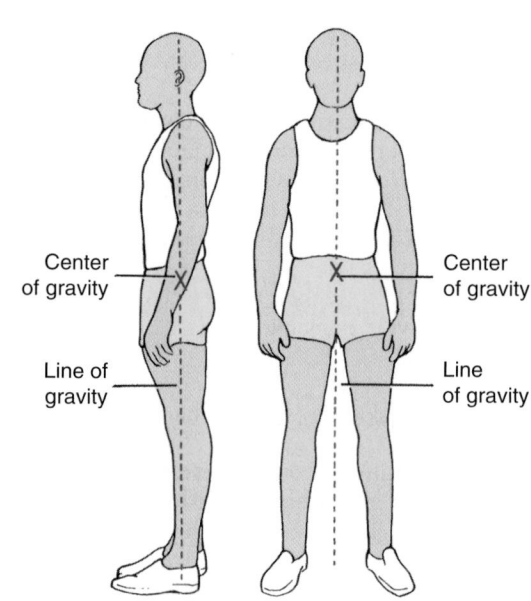
FIG 9-1 Body alignment when standing.

STEP	RATIONALE

ASSESSMENT

1 Assess patient's range of motion (ROM) (see Chapter 10), body alignment, and comfort level while patient is lying down.

Provides baseline data for later comparisons. Determines ways to improve position and alignment.

2 Assess for risk factors that contribute to complications of immobility:

Increased risk factors require patient to be repositioned more frequently.

   a *Sensation:* Decreased from cerebrovascular accident (CVA), paralysis, neuropathy.

Paralysis impairs movement; muscle tone changes; sensation is affected. Because of difficulty in moving and poor awareness of involved body part, patient is unable to position body part and protect it from pressure.

   b *Impaired mobility:* Traction, arthritis, hip fracture, joint surgery, or other contributing disease processes

Traction, bone fractures, surgery, or arthritic changes of affected extremity result in decreased ROM.

   c *Impaired circulation:* Arterial insufficiency

Decreased circulation predisposes patient to pressure ulcers.

   d *Age:* Very young, older adult

Premature and young infants require frequent turning because their skin is fragile. Normal physiologic changes associated with aging predispose older adults to greater risks for developing complications of immobility.

3 Assess patient's level of consciousness.

Determines need for special aids or devices. Patients with altered levels of consciousness may not understand instructions and may be unable to help.

4 Assess condition of patient's skin, especially over bony prominences.

Provides baseline to determine effects of positioning.

5 Assess patient's physical ability to help with moving and positioning, which may be affected by age, level of consciousness, disease process, strength, ROM, and coordination.

Enables you to use patient's mobility, strength, and coordination. Determines need for additional help. Ensures patient and nurse safety.

6 Assess for presence of incisions, drainage tubes, and equipment (e.g., traction). Empty drainage bags before positioning.

Alters positioning procedure and type of positions to use. Determines approach needed for instruction. Eliminates barrier to moving patient.

7 Assess motivation of patient and ability of family caregivers to participate in moving and positioning.

Indicates whether instruction is necessary before discharge.

8 Check health care provider's orders before positioning patient.

Some positions may be contraindicated in certain situations (e.g., spinal cord injury; hip fracture; respiratory difficulties; certain neurologic conditions; presence of incisions, drains, or tubing).

NURSING DIAGNOSES

- Activity intolerance
- Acute confusion
- Impaired physical mobility
- Impaired skin integrity
- Risk for impaired skin integrity

Related factors are individualized based on patient's condition or needs.

PLANNING

1 Expected outcomes following completion of procedure:
   - Patient retains ROM.

Correct positioning allows patient to achieve optimal joint mobility and alignment.

   - Patient's skin shows no evidence of breakdown.

Frequent position changes decrease risk for skin breakdown.

   - Patient's comfort level increases.

Proper positioning reduces stress on joints.

   - Patient's level of independence in completing activities of daily living (ADLs) increases.

Maintaining good body alignment and joint mobility increases patient's overall mobility. Patient with inadequate joint mobility may need assistance to carry out ADLs.

2 Raise level of bed to comfortable working height.

Raises level of work toward nurse's center of gravity and reduces risk for back injuries.

3 Remove all pillows and devices used in previous position.

Reduces interference from bedding during positioning procedure.

4 Get extra help as needed.

Provides for patient and nurse safety.

5 Explain procedure to patient.

Helps to decrease anxiety and increase cooperation.

STEP	RATIONALE

IMPLEMENTATION

1 Perform hand hygiene.

2 Close door to room or bedside curtains.

3 **Help patient move up in bed:**

a Can patient assist?

    (1) Fully able to assist, nurse assistance is not needed; nurse stands by to assist.

    (2) Partially able to assist; patient can assist using positioning cues or aides (e.g., drawsheet or friction-reducing device).

4 **Help patient move up in bed using a drawsheet (two to three nurses assist):**

a Place patient supine with head of bed flat. Place height of bed appropriate for all staff. A nurse stands on each side of bed.

b Remove pillow from under head and shoulders and place it at head of bed.

c Turn patient side to side to place drawsheet under him or her, extending from shoulders to thighs.

d Return patient to supine position.

e Fanfold drawsheet on both sides, with each nurse grasping firmly near patient.

f Place feet apart with forward-backward stance. Flex knees and hips. On count of three, shift weight from front to back leg and move patient and drawsheet to desired position in bed (see illustrations).

Reduces transmission of infection.

Provides for patient privacy.

This is not a one-person task unless patient can fully assist (NIOSHA, 2009).

Determines degree of risk in repositioning patient and technique required to safely assist patient.

Enables you to assess body alignment. Reduces pull of gravity on patient's upper body.

Prevents striking patient's head against head of bed.

Supports patient's body weight and reduces friction during movement.

Even distribution of weight makes lifting easier.

Provides strong handles to grip drawsheet without slipping.

Facing direction of movement ensures proper balance. Shifting weight reduces force needed to move patient. Flexing knees lowers nurses' center of gravity and uses thighs instead of back muscles.

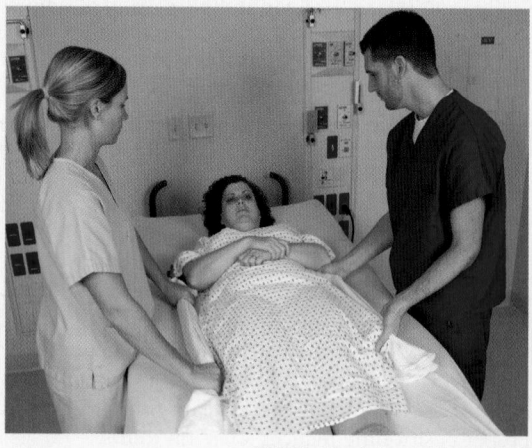 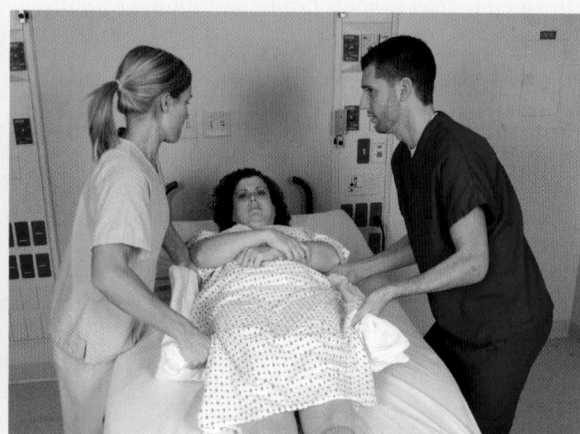

STEP 4f   Moving immobile patient up in bed with drawsheet.

5 **Help patient move up in bed using a friction-reducing device (two or three nurses assist):**

a Position patient as in Steps 4a-c.

b Place friction-reducing device under drawsheet by having patient turn side to side.

A minimum of three or four caregivers is recommended if the patient's weight is greater than 71.4 kg (157 lbs) (Waters et al., 2011).

Supine position on drawsheet prepares patient for placement of friction-reducing device.

Prevents friction from contact of skin with board.

STEP	RATIONALE

c Move patient up in bed by having two nurses grasp drawsheet, and one nurse holds onto friction-reducing device. Follow Steps 4e and f, moving patient up in bed.

Slide board remains stationary, provides a slippery surface to reduce friction, and allows patient to move up in bed easily.

Clinical Decision Point *Protect patient's heels from shearing force by having another caregiver lift heels while moving patient up in bed.*

6 Position patient in one of the following positions using correct body alignment. Protect pressure areas. Begin with patient lying supine and move up in bed following either Step 4 or 5.

Prevents injury to musculoskeletal system.

a Position patient in supported semi-Fowler's (see illustration) or Fowler's position:

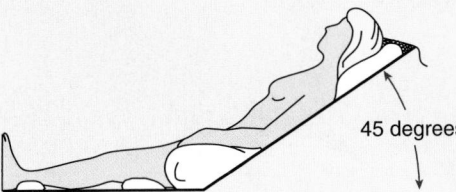

STEP 6a   Supported semi-Fowler's position.

(1) With patient lying supine, elevate head of bed 45 to 60 degrees if not contraindicated.

Increases comfort, improves ventilation, and increases patient's opportunity to socialize or relax.

(2) Rest head against mattress or on small pillow.

Prevents flexion contractures of cervical vertebrae.

(3) Use pillows to support arms and hands if patient does not have voluntary control or use of hands and arms.

Prevents shoulder dislocation from effect of downward pull of unsupported arms, promotes circulation by preventing venous pooling, and prevents flexion contractures of arms and wrists.

(4) Position small pillow at lower back.

Supports lumbar vertebrae and decreases flexion of vertebrae.

(5) Place small pillow or roll under thigh.

Prevents hyperextension of knee and occlusion of popliteal artery from pressure from body weight.

(6) Support calves with pillows.

Heels should not be in contact with bed to prevent prolonged pressure of mattress on heels. This is sometimes referred to as *floating* heels.

b Position hemiplegic patient in supported semi-Fowler's or Fowler's position:

(1) Position patient in supine position. Elevate head of bed 45 to 60 degrees.

Increases comfort, improves ventilation, and increases patient's opportunity to relax. Adjust head of bed according to patient's condition. For example, those with increased risk for pressure ulcers remain at 30-degree angle (see Chapter 18).

(2) Position patient in Fowler's position as straight as possible.

Counteracts tendency to slump toward affected side. Improves ventilation and cardiac output; decreases intracranial pressure. Improves patient's ability to swallow and helps prevent aspiration of food, liquids, and gastric secretions.

(3) Position head on small pillow with chin slightly forward. If patient is totally unable to control head movement, avoid hyperextension of neck.

Prevents hyperextension of neck. Too many pillows under head may cause or worsen neck flexion contracture.

(4) Provide support for involved arm and hand by placing arm away from patient's side and supporting elbow with pillow.

Paralyzed muscles do not automatically resist pull of gravity as they do normally. As a result, shoulder subluxation, pain, and edema may occur.

(5) Place rolled blanket (trochanter roll) firmly alongside patient's legs.

Ensures proper alignment. Prevents external rotation of hips, which contributes to contractures.

(6) Support feet in dorsiflexion with therapeutic boots or splints.

Prevents plantar flexion contractures or footdrop by positioning patient's ankle in neutral dorsiflexion. Position foot so heel is aligned in opening of splint to prevent pressure. Other therapeutic boots or splints are manufactured with thick padding to cushion heel and prevent pressure ulcers.

c Position patient in supported supine position:

(1) Place patient supine with head of bed flat.

Necessary for properly aligning patient.

(2) Place small rolled towel under lumbar area of back.

Provides support for lumbar spine.

(3) Place pillow under upper shoulders, neck, and head.

Maintains correct alignment and prevents flexion contractures of cervical vertebrae.

STEP	RATIONALE
(4) Place trochanter rolls or sandbags parallel to lateral surface of patient's thighs.	Reduces external rotation of hip.
(5) Place patient's feet in therapeutic boots or splints.	Maintains feet in dorsiflexion. Prevents plantar flexion contractures or footdrop.
(6) Place pillows under pronated forearms, keeping upper arms parallel to patient's body (see illustration).	Reduces internal rotation of shoulder and prevents extension of elbows. Maintains correct body alignment.

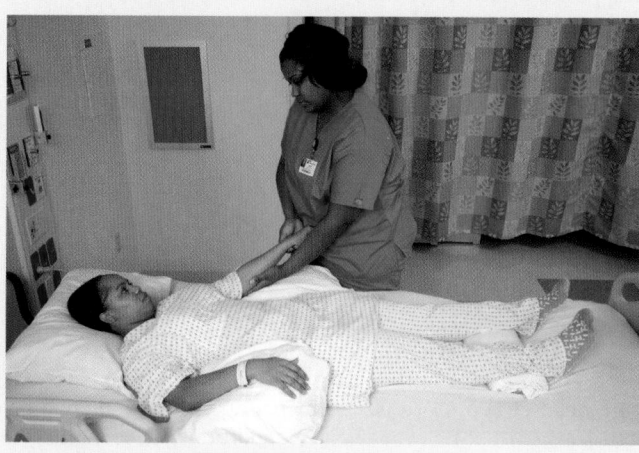

STEP 6c(6) Supine position with pillows in place.

STEP	RATIONALE
(7) Place hand rolls in patient's hands. Consider physical therapy referral for use of hand splints.	Reduces extension of fingers and abduction of thumb. Maintains thumb slightly adducted and in opposition to fingers.
d Position hemiplegic patient in supine position:	
(1) Place head of bed flat.	Necessary for positioning in supine position.
(2) Place folded towel or small pillow under shoulder or affected side.	Decreases possibility of pain, joint contracture, and subluxation. Maintains mobility in muscles around shoulder to permit normal movement patterns.
(3) Keep affected arm away from body with elbow extended and palm up. Position the affected hand in one of recommended positions for flaccid or spastic hand. (Alternative is to place arm out to side, with elbow bent and hand toward head of bed.)	Maintains mobility in arm, joints, and shoulder to permit normal movement patterns. (Alternative position counteracts limitation of ability of arm to rotate outward at shoulder [external rotation]. External rotation must be present to raise arm over head without pain.)
(4) Place folded towel under hip of involved side.	Diminishes effect of spasticity in entire leg by controlling hip position.
(5) Flex affected knee 30 degrees by supporting it on pillow or folded blanket.	Slight flexion breaks up abnormal extension pattern of leg. Extensor spasticity is most severe when patient is supine.
(6) Support feet with soft pillows at right angle to leg.	Maintains foot in dorsiflexion and prevents footdrop. Pillows prevent stimulation to ball of foot by hard surface, which has tendency to increase muscle tone in patient with extensor spasticity of lower extremity.
e Position patient in prone position, using two nurses:	In certain patients with pulmonary conditions such as acute respiratory distress syndrome use of prone position can help improve oxygenation.
(1) With head of bed flat and one nurse standing on each side of bed, roll patient to one side while placing arm on side to be turned alongside of body. For patients with hemiplegia, move toward unaffected side.	Prepares patient for positioning.
(2) Roll patient over arm positioned close to body, with elbow straight and hand under hip. Position on abdomen in center of bed.	Positions patient correctly so alignment can be maintained.
(3) Turn patient's head to one side and support head with small pillow.	Reduces flexion or hyperextension of cervical vertebrae.
(4) Place small pillow under patient's abdomen below level of diaphragm.	Reduces pressure on breasts of some female patients and decreases hyperextension of lumbar vertebrae and strain on lower back. Improves breathing by reducing mattress pressure on diaphragm.

STEP	RATIONALE
(5) Support arms in flexed position level at shoulders.	Maintains proper body alignment. Support reduces risk for joint dislocation.
(6) Support lower legs with pillow to elevate toes (see illustration).	Prevents footdrop. Reduces external rotation of legs. Reduces mattress pressure on toes.

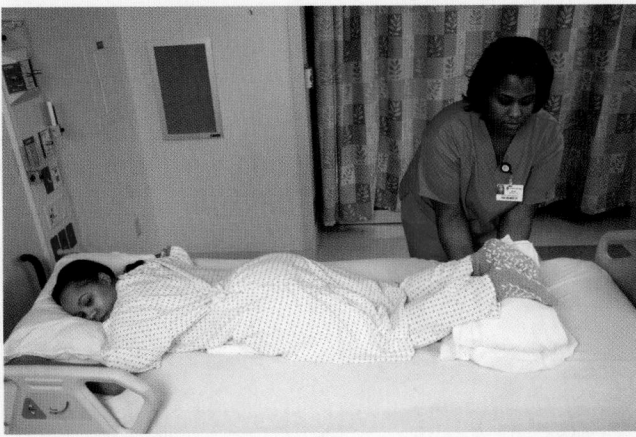

STEP 6e(6)   Prone position with pillows supporting lower legs.

f Position hemiplegic patient in prone position using two nurses:

(1) Move patient toward unaffected side.	Ensures proper alignment in center of bed when patient is rolled onto abdomen.
(2) While rolling patient onto side, place pillow on patient's abdomen.	Prevents sagging of abdomen when patient is rolled over; decreases hyperextension of lumbar vertebrae and strain on lower back.
(3) With one nurse standing on each side of bed, roll patient onto abdomen by positioning involved arm close to patient's body, with elbow straight and hand under hip. Roll patient carefully over arm.	Prevents injury to affected side.
(4) Turn head toward involved side.	Promotes development of neck and trunk extension, which is necessary for standing and walking.
(5) Position involved arm out to side with elbow bent, hand toward head of bed, and fingers extended (if possible).	Counteracts limitation of ability of arm to rotate outward at shoulder (external rotation). External rotation must be present to raise arm over head without pain.
(6) Flex knees slightly by placing pillow under legs from knees to ankles.	Flexion prevents prolonged hyperextension, which could impair joint mobility.
(7) Keep feet at right angle to legs by using pillow high enough to keep toes off mattress.	Maintains feet in dorsiflexion.

g Position patient in 30-degree lateral (side-lying) position (one nurse):

(1) Lower head of bed completely or as low as patient can tolerate.	Provides position of comfort for patient and removes pressure from bony prominences on back.
(2) Lower side rail and position patient on side of bed opposite direction toward which patient is to be turned. Move upper trunk, supporting shoulders first; then move lower trunk, supporting hips.	Provides room for patient to turn to side.
(3) Raise side rail and go to opposite side of bed.	
(4) Flex patient's knee that will not be next to mattress. Keep foot on mattress. Place one hand on patient's upper bent leg near hip, and place other hand on patient's shoulder.	Use of leverage makes turning to side easy.
(5) Roll patient onto side toward you.	Rolling decreases trauma to tissues. In addition, patient is positioned so leverage on hip makes turning easy.
(6) Place pillow under patient's head and neck.	Maintains alignment. Reduces lateral neck flexion. Decreases strain on sternocleidomastoid muscle.
(7) Place hands under patient's dependent shoulder and bring shoulder blade forward.	Prevents patient's weight from resting directly on shoulder joint.

STEP	RATIONALE
(8) Position both arms in slightly flexed position. Support upper arm with pillow level with shoulder; other arm, by mattress.	Decreases internal rotation and adduction of shoulder. Supporting both arms in slightly flexed position protects joint. Ventilation improves because chest is able to expand more easily.
(9) Place hands under dependent hip and bring hip slightly forward so angle from hip to mattress is approximately 30 degrees.	The 30-degree lateral position reduces pressure on trochanter; designed to prevent pressure ulcer.
(10) Place small tuck-back pillow behind patient's back. (Make by folding pillow lengthwise. Smooth area is slightly tucked under patient's back.)	Provides support to maintain patient on side.
(11) Place pillow under semiflexed upper leg level at hip from groin to foot (see illustration).	Flexion prevents hyperextension of leg. Maintains leg in correct alignment. Prevents pressure on bony prominences.

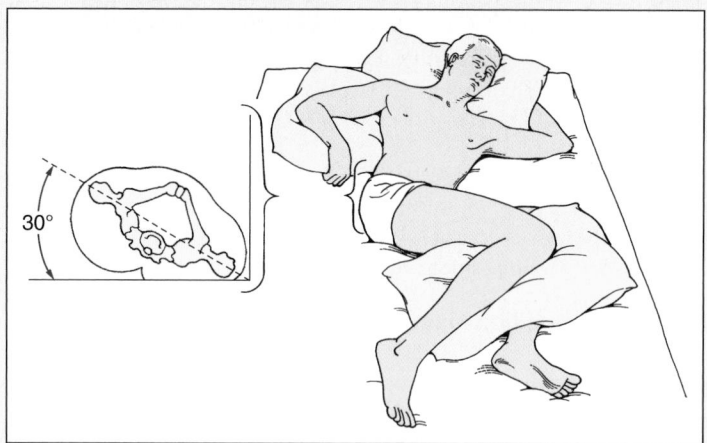

STEP 6g(11)   Thirty-degree lateral position with pillows in place.

(12) Place sandbags parallel to plantar surface of dependent foot. May use ankle-foot orthotic on feet if available.	Maintains dorsiflexion of foot.
h Position patient in Sims' (semiprone) position (one nurse):	
(1) Lower head of bed completely.	Provides for proper body alignment while patient is lying down.
(2) Place patient in supine position and position him or her on side of bed opposite direction toward which he or she is to be turned. Move upper trunk, supporting shoulders first, followed by moving lower trunk, supporting hips.	Prepares patient for position.
(3) Move to other side of bed and turn patient on side. Position in lateral position, lying partially on abdomen, with dependent shoulder lifted out and arm placed at patient's side.	
(4) Place small pillow under patient's head.	Maintains proper alignment and prevents lateral neck flexion.
(5) Place pillow under flexed upper arm, supporting arm level with shoulder.	Prevents internal rotation of shoulder. Maintains alignment.
(6) Place pillow under flexed upper legs, supporting leg level with hip.	Prevents internal rotation of hip and adduction of leg. Flexion prevents hyperextension of leg. Reduces mattress pressure on knees and ankles.
(7) Place sandbags parallel to plantar surface of foot (see illustration).	Maintains foot in dorsiflexion. Prevents plantar flexion contractures or footdrop.

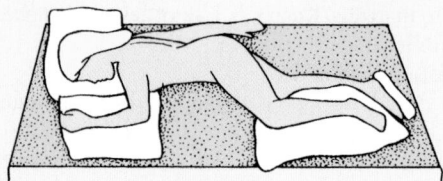

STEP 6h(7)   Sandbag supporting right foot in dorsiflexion.

STEP	RATIONALE

i Logroll patient (three nurses):

Clinical Decision Point *A nurse should supervise and aid NAP when there is a health care provider's order to logroll a patient. Patients with a spinal cord injury or who are recovering from neck, back, or spinal surgery often need to keep the spinal column in straight alignment to prevent further injury.*

STEP	RATIONALE
(1) Place small pillow between patient's knees.	Prevents tension on spinal column and adduction of hip.
(2) Cross patient's arms on chest.	Prevents injury to arms.
(3) Position two nurses on side toward which patient is to be turned and one nurse on side where pillows are to be placed (see illustration).	Distributes weight equally between nurses during turning.
(4) Fanfold drawsheet alongside of patient that will be turning.	Provides strong handles to grip drawsheet without slipping.
(5) With one nurse grasping drawsheet at lower hips and thighs and the other nurse grasping drawsheet at patient's shoulders and lower back, roll patient as one unit in a smooth, continuous motion on count of three (see illustration).	Maintains proper alignment by moving all body parts at the same time, preventing tension or twisting of spinal column.
(6) Nurse on opposite side of bed places pillows along length of patient for support (see illustration).	Maintains patient in side-lying position.
(7) Gently lean patient as a unit back toward pillows for support.	Ensures continued straight alignment of spinal column, preventing injury.
7 Perform hand hygiene.	Reduces transmission of microorganisms.

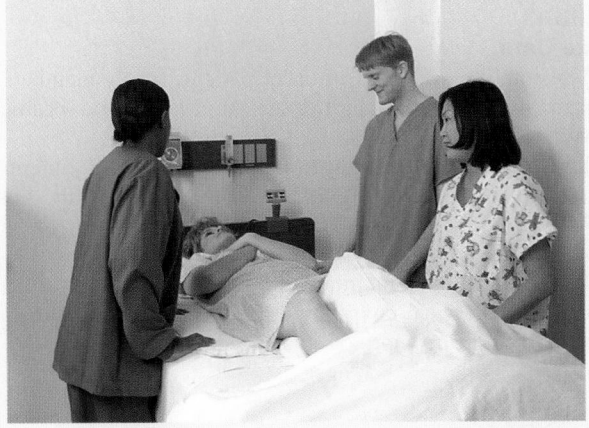

STEP 6i(3) Preparing patient for logrolling.

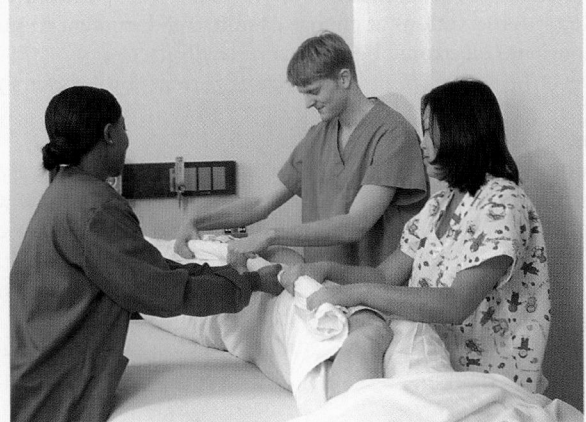

STEP 6i(5) Logrolling patient.

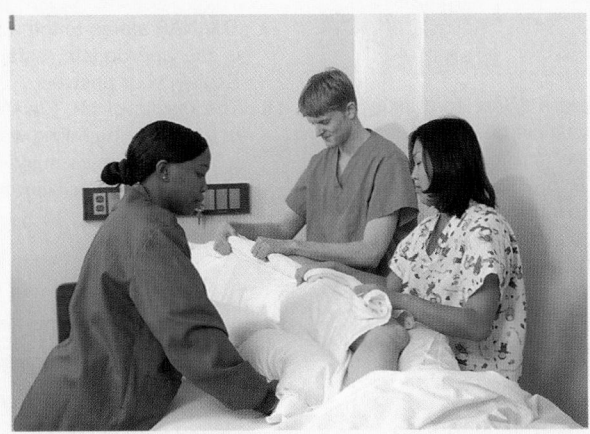

STEP 6i(6) Place pillows along patient's back for support.

STEP	RATIONALE

EVALUATION

1 Assess patient's body alignment, position, and level of comfort. Patient's body should be supported by adequate mattress, and vertebral column should be without observable curves.

2 Measure ROM.

3 Observe for areas of erythema or breakdown involving skin.

Determines effectiveness of positioning. Additional supports (e.g., pillows, bath blankets) may be added or removed to promote comfort and correct body alignment.

Determines if joint contracture is developing.

Provides ongoing observation regarding patient's skin and musculoskeletal systems. Indicates complications of immobility or improper positioning of body part.

Unexpected Outcomes

1 Joint contractures develop or worsen.

2 Skin shows localized areas of erythema and breakdown.

3 Patient avoids moving.

Related Interventions

- Increase frequency of ROM exercises to affected and immobilized areas (see Chapter 10).

- Increase frequency of repositioning.
- Place turning schedule above patient's bed.

- Medicate with analgesia as ordered by health care provider to ensure patient's comfort before moving.
- Allow pain medication to take effect before proceeding.

Recording and Reporting

- Record procedure and observations (e.g., condition of skin, joint movement, patient's ability to assist with positioning).
- Report observations at change of shift and document in nurses' notes and electronic health record (EHR).
- Record time and position change of patient throughout shift.

Special Considerations

Teaching

- Teach family members how to position patient, especially when caring for infant, young child, or confused or unconscious patient.
- Teach patient ways to help with positioning and provide opportunity for return demonstration.
- Teach patient and family signs and symptoms of pressure ulcers and contractures.

Pediatric

- Children who are unable to move require passive exercise and movement (see Chapter 10).

Gerontologic

- Reposition older adult patients at least every 1 to 2 hours and maintain a regular program of ROM exercises (Touhy et al., 2010).

Home Care

- Assess ability and motivation of patient, family members, and primary caregiver to participate in moving and positioning patient in bed.
- Assess home to determine compatibility of environment with assistive devices (e.g., over-bed trapeze, Hoyer lift, hospital bed).

Long-Term Care

- Patients who have maintained bed rest for a long period may revert back to a favorite position. Frequently assess these patients and turn more often as needed.

❓ Critical Thinking Exercises

Mr. Clark is a 37-year-old man who suffered a spinal cord injury in a motor vehicle accident. He has sustained multiple deep lacerations on his face and trunk and facial fractures of the maxillary and zygomatic bones. He rates his pain at 9 on a scale of 0 to 10. He weighs approximately 88 kg (193.6 lbs). You are preparing to transfer him to a stretcher.

1 The emergency department nurse was extremely busy and was unable to provide a complete report. Which other information would you obtain about this patient before transferring him to a stretcher?

2 Mr. Clark is scheduled immediately for a computed tomography (CT) scan of the head and spine. He refuses to allow you to move him onto the stretcher. Which interventions would you select to elicit his cooperation? (Select all that apply.)

  1 Administer pain medication as ordered by the physician.

  2 Explain the purpose and importance of the CT scan.

  3 Describe the method by which you will move him onto the stretcher.

  4 Tell him that it is the health care provider's order and must be carried out.

  Explain your choice(s).

3 The NAP states to the nurse that he or she will turn Mr. Clark. What is the appropriate, safe action in response to turning Mr. Clark? Explain your answer.

4 The results of Mr. Clark's CT scan showed no injuries to his spine or neck and log rolling was no longer needed. Considering his weight and other injuries sustained from the accident, what is the safest method to transfer him from the stretcher to the bed? Explain your answer.

✓ REVIEW QUESTIONS

1 A 65-year-old patient who weighs 998 kg (260 lbs) is to be transferred from his bed to a stretcher. The patient is unable to bear full weight on one leg. His upper body strength is good. Which technique is the *least* appropriate technique for transfer?

  1 Use of a transfer board

  2 Use of a bariatric transfer device

  3 Use of a three-person carry

  4 Use of a ceiling lift

2 A patient who has suffered a stroke will be taken care of by his daughter at home. Which statement by the daughter regarding body mechanics indicates that learning has occurred?
   1 "I'm glad I have a strong back."
   2 "As I twist to place my father in his chair, I'll make sure that he doesn't fall."
   3 "I'll keep my knees bent and trunk erect so my muscles work together."
   4 "I'll tighten my back muscles and push my pelvis forward to provide balance when lifting my father."

3 The nurse is transferring a patient from the bed to the chair for the first time after abdominal surgery. Which initial step in the transfer is most appropriate for the nurse and the patient?
   1 Apply a transfer belt around the patient's waist.
   2 Use the under-axilla support technique to prevent pulling on the abdominal area.
   3 Have the patient sit on the side of the bed and dangle for a few minutes.
   4 Observe this patient's response while she transfers to increase his or her independence.

4 A patient has arrived on the unit after undergoing extensive abdominal surgery. He is awake and alert but refuses to be repositioned in bed. What should the nurse assess first to determine the reason for his refusal to move?
   1 Oxygen saturation level
   2 Pain level
   3 Level of consciousness
   4 The amount of equipment present

5 A young adult is admitted with an unstable spinal cord injury. What is the most appropriate method of moving this patient from her side to her back?
   1 Use a slide board to move her from side to side.
   2 Logroll the patient using three people.
   3 Allow the patient to move herself to promote independence.
   4 Use a step-by-step method: move the trunk, then the hips, and finally the leg.

6 A patient has been on bed rest for several days. When he attempted to stand from a sitting position, he became dizzy and nauseated. These symptoms indicate which of the following conditions?
   1 Rebound hypertension
   2 Orthostatic hypotension
   3 Dysfunctional proprioception
   4 Central nervous system rebound hypotension

7 A patient who weighs145.5 kg (320 lbs) is being transferred from his bed to a chair. The patient is on partial weight bearing as a result of bilateral reconstructive knee surgery. Which of the following is the best technique for transfer?
   1 Transfer board
   2 Stand-assist device
   3 Three-person carry
   4 Ceiling lift

8 An adolescent has been admitted with an unstable spinal cord injury sustained from a motor vehicle accident. The patient needs to be taken to the operating room. What is the most appropriate method to move this patient to a stretcher for transport?
   1 Use a step-by-step method: move the trunk, then the hips, and finally the legs.
   2 Logroll the patient; place a slide board; and slide the patient to the stretcher as one unit, maintaining body alignment.
   3 Allow the patient to stand and transfer to the stretcher.
   4 Use a mechanical lift device to transfer to the stretcher.

9 To increase stability during patient transfer, you increase the base of support by performing which action?
   1 Leaning slightly backward
   2 Tensing and tightening the back muscles
   3 Keeping the knees in a locked position
   4 Spacing your feet farther apart

10 Two NAPs ask for the nurse's assistance to transfer a 56.8 kg (125 lbs) patient from the bed to the stretcher. The patient is unable to assist. What is the best response?
   1 "As long as we use proper body mechanics, no one will get hurt."
   2 "The patient only weighs 125 pounds. You don't need my assistance."
   3 "The three-man lift technique is recommended to ensure your safety and that of the patient."
   4 "Use the slide board; it is more comfortable for the patient and will lessen the chance of injury to us."

REFERENCES

American Nurses Association (ANA): Safe patient handling tip sheet, 2011, available at http://nursingworld.org/MainMenuCategories/WorkplaceSafety/SafePatient/TipSheet.html, accessed June 5, 2012.

Baptiste A, et al: Proper sling selection and application while using patient lifts, *Rehabil Nurs* 33:22, 2008.

Bureau of Labor Statistics: Occupational industries and illnesses: industry data, 2011, available at http://stats.bls.gov/bls/occupation.htm, accessed June 5, 2012.

Centers for Disease Control and Prevention (CDC) and National Institute of Occupational Health and Safety: State of the Sector/Healthcare and Social Assistance, 2009, available at http://www.cdc.gov/niosh/docs/2009-139/pdfs/2009-139.pdf, accessed June 5, 2012.

Hockenberry MJ, et al: *Wong's nursing care of infants and children*, ed 9, St Louis, 2011, Mosby.

Institute for Healthcare Improvement: *5 Million lives campaign. Getting started kit: Prevent pressure ulcers how-to guide*, Cambridge, MA, 2008, Institute for Healthcare Improvement, available at http://www.ihi.org/IHI/Programs/Campaign/Pressureulcers.htm, accessed June 5, 2012.

Janelli L, et al: Can an exercise program enhance mood among Hispanic elders? *Medsurg Nurs* 18:356, 2009.

Kutash M, et al: The lift team's importance to a successful safe patient handling program, *J Nurs Admin* 39(4):170, 2009.

Lewis S, et al: *Medical-surgical nursing: assessment and management of clinical problems*, ed 8, St Louis, 2011, Mosby.

National Institute of Occupational Health and Safety Administration: Ergonomics for the Prevention of Musculoskeletal Disorders: Guidelines for Nursing Homes, NIOSH 318; revised 2009, available at http://www.NIOSH.gov/ergonomics/guidelines/nursinghome/final_nh_guidelines.html, accessed June 5, 2012.

Nelson A, et al: *Safe patient handling and movement*, New York, 2009, Springer.

Occupational Safety and Health Administration (OSHA): Activity 6—Everyone benefits from an ergonomic program, 2011, available at http://www.osha.gov/SLTC/healthcarefacilities/training/activity_6.html, accessed June 5, 2012.

Pierson M, Fairchild S: *Principles & Techniques of Patient Care*, ed 4, St Louis, 2008, Saunders.

Quinlan-Colwell A: Understanding the paradox of patient pain and patient satisfaction, *J Holist Nurs* 27:177, 2009.

Sedlack C, et al: Development of the National Association of Orthopaedic Nurses guidance statement on safe patient handling and movement in the orthopaedic setting, *Orthop Nurs* 28(2S):S2, 2009.

Schneider J, et al: Cognitive-behavioral therapy, exercise, and older adults' quality of life, *West J Nurs Res* 30:704, 2008.

Stechmiller J, et al: Guidelines for the prevention of pressure ulcers, *Wound Repair Regeneration* 16:151, 2008.

Thompson P, et al: Non-pharmacological treatments for orthostatic hypotension, *Age Aging* 40(3):292, 2011.

Touhy T, et al: *Ebersole and Hess's Gerontological nursing and healthy aging*, ed 3, St Louis, 2010, Mosby.

Waters T, et al: AORN ergonomic tool 1: lateral transfer of a patient from a stretcher to an OR bed, *AORN J* 93(3):223, 2011.

Zadvinskis I, Salsbury SL: Effects of a multifaceted minimal-lift environment for nursing staff: pilot results, *West J Nurs Res* 32:47, 2010.

10

Exercise and Ambulation

SKILLS AND PROCEDURES

MEDIA RESOURCES

- **evolve** *learning system* http://evolve.elsevier.com/Perry/skills
  - Review Questions
  - ▶ Video Clips
  - Audio Glossary

- Mosby's Nursing Video Skills, 4th edition

KEY TERMS

Abduction
Active range-of-motion exercises
Active-assisted range-of-motion exercises
Activity tolerance
Adduction
Atrophy
Bed rest
Circumduction
Contractures

Crutch gait
Crutch palsy
Deep vein thrombosis (DVT)
Dorsal
Dorsiflexion
Eversion
Exercise
Extension
External rotation
Flexion

Foot pump
Gait
Gait belt
Hyperextension
Immobility
Internal rotation
Inversion
Isometric contraction
Isometric exercise
Lateral flexion
Mobility

Opposition
Orthostatic hypotension
Osteoblastic
Osteoclastic
Passive range-of-motion exercises
Plantar flexion
Pronation
Rotation
Supination
Thrombus

OBJECTIVES

Mastery of content in this chapter will enable the nurse to:

- Discuss indications for assisting with ambulation or using devices to assist with ambulation.
- Discuss indications for performing range-of-motion and isometric exercises.
- Identify complications that may develop in a patient wearing either elastic stockings or a sequential compression device.
- Identify significant assessment data to be noted before and during the use of a continuous passive motion machine.
- Identify significant assessment data to be noted before assisting with ambulation and range-of-motion and isometric exercises.

- Demonstrate the following skills on selected patients: assisting with ambulation, assisting with ambulation with the use of an ambulation aid, assisting with range-of-motion exercises, assisting with isometric exercises, applying a continuous passive motion machine, and applying elastic stockings and sequential compression device.
- Develop teaching plans for selected patients for safety precautions to use at home while using an ambulation aid, applying and monitoring effects of elastic stockings and sequential compression devices, using the continuous passive motion machine, and performing range-of-motion and isometric exercises.

Mobility refers to an ability to move about freely, whereas immobility refers to a person's inability to move about freely. Mobility and immobility are best understood as the end points on a continuum, with many degrees of partial mobility in between. Some patients move back and forth on the mobility-immobility continuum as a result of disease or injury. Other patients experience immobility for an indefinite period.

The level of mobility has a significant impact on an individual's physiological, psychosocial, and developmental well-being (Janelli et al., 2009). When mobility is altered, many body systems are at risk for impairment. Impaired mobility can result in altered cardiovascular functioning, disruption of normal metabolic functioning, increased risk for pulmonary complications, the development of pressure ulcers, and urinary elimination alterations (Huether and McCance 2008; Lewis et al., 2011).

The severity of mobility impairment depends on a patient's age, overall health status, nutritional status, and degree of immobility experienced. For example, pronounced effects of immobility develop more quickly in older adults with chronic illness than in younger patients (Touhy et al., 2010). Older adults are at greater risk for developing orthostatic hypotension, syncope, confusion, increased risk for fractures, and functional incontinence as a result of decreased mobility from bed rest (Craig et al., 2010; Johnson et al., 2009). Increase in activity and exercise may reduce length of stay and cost for hospitalized older adults.

Alterations in mobility may have profound psychosocial and developmental effects. Immobilization often leads to emotional, intellectual, sensory, and sociocultural alterations. For young and older adults, immobility may alter employment, family role functions, and social interactions. Such changes can lead to altered self-concept, lowered self-esteem, and depression. Children also are affected by immobility. Activity for them is a way of releasing energy and expressing themselves. When deprived of physical activity, children become restless and may even show signs of anger and aggression (Hockenberry and Wilson, 2011).

Changes in a patient's mobility result from a variety of health problems. For example, musculoskeletal conditions such as fractured extremities or muscle sprains, neurologic conditions such as spinal cord trauma, degenerative neurologic conditions such as myasthenia gravis, and head injuries. Some patients are immobilized for therapeutic reasons (e.g., prescribed bed rest or reduced activity). Nursing measures attempt to maintain and/or restore optimal mobility and decrease the hazards associated with immobility. Frequent repositioning, deep-breathing and coughing exercises, muscle and joint exercises, increased fluid intake, and dietary intake of foods containing fiber are examples of measures that help to reduce the hazards of immobility.

EVIDENCE-BASED PRACTICE

Older adults have a decline in physical activity and some changes in joints that may predispose them to problems with mobility. In a recent study, time spent in active physical activities, even ½ hour per day, resulted in significantly lower (15% to 35%) mortality risks compared with no time in active activities (Paganini-Hill et al., 2011). There is strong evidence that exercise and physical activity help older adults maintain an active lifestyle, improve quality of life, and prevent injury (see Procedural Guideline 10-1).

- Implement and provide resources for planned exercise programs. Weight-bearing and resistance exercises slow further bone loss and prevent fractures in the older adult with osteoporosis (De Kam et al., 2009; Touhy et al., 2010).
- Recommend resistance- and agility-training programs. These forms of exercise reduce fear of falling and increase sense of well-being in older adults (De Kam et al., 2009; Sherrington et al., 2008).
- Consult a health care provider before beginning an exercise program, particularly in the presence of heart or lung disease and other chronic illnesses (Chodzko-Zajko et al., 2009).
- When developing an exercise program for any older adult, consider not only the person's current activity level, range of motion, muscle strength and tone, and response to physical activity, but also their interests, capacities, and limitations.

PATIENT-CENTERED CARE

Assess each patient's expectations concerning activity and exercise and determine his or her perception of what is normal or acceptable is of utmost importance. For example, one of the factors affecting physical activity is freedom from pain. If exercising is painful or tiresome to a patient, commitment to the desired interventions may be lacking. It is important to consider that some patients are content with their present physical activity and fitness and do not perceive a need for improvement.

When assisting with range-of-motion exercises or ambulation, keep in mind that these activities may place patients in positions that can be embarrassing. Provide a garment that protects a patient's privacy. Many cultures emphasize modesty, and patients from these cultures may not participate in treatment measures for fear of being exposed. For example, Muslim females need to be fully covered when in public because of the emphasis on *hijab*, or female modesty (Simpson et al., 2008).

Safety Guidelines

1 Obtain and become familiar with any type of assistive device to be used. Knowledge of proper preparation and use of devices is needed to teach patients to use them safely and correctly.
2 Prepare patients. Make sure that they are rested and not fatigued. Obtain extra personnel to assist; use safety devices and flat, nonskid shoes for a patient.
3 Address a patient's fear of falling if present.
4 Determine the type and frequency of intervention. Activity that is appropriate for 1 day or one shift can change, resulting in an increased or decreased need for assistance with ambulation or a change in the type of intervention.
5 Know a patient's home care plan. A patient may need to continue the exercise regimen or use an assistive device at home.

PROCEDURAL GUIDELINE 10-1 Performing Range-of-Motion Exercises

Range-of-motion (ROM) exercises may be active, passive, or active assisted. They are active if a patient is able to perform the exercise independently and passive if the exercises are performed for a patient by the caregiver. In every aspect of activities of daily living (ADLs), encourage patients to be as independent as possible. Encourage and supervise patients to perform active and passive ROM exercises. Incorporate active ROM exercises in a patient's ADLs (Table 10-1). Incorporate passive ROM into bathing and feeding activities. Collaborate with a patient to develop a schedule for ROM activities.

Delegation and Collaboration

The skill of performing ROM exercises can be delegated to nursing assistive personnel (NAP). Patients with spinal cord or orthopedic trauma usually require ROM exercises by professional nurses or physical therapists. The nurse directs the NAP to:

- Perform exercises slowly and provide adequate support to each joint being exercised.
- Not exercise joints beyond the point of resistance or to the point of fatigue or pain.
- Discuss a patient's individual limitations or preexisting conditions such as arthritis, which may affect ROM.

Equipment

❑ No mechanical or physical equipment needed
❑ Clean gloves (optional)

Procedural Steps

1 Review patient's chart for physical assessment findings, health care provider's orders, medical diagnosis, medical history, and progress.
2 Obtain data on patient's baseline joint function. Observe for limitations in joint mobility, redness, or warmth over joints; joint tenderness; deformities; or crepitus produced by joint motion.
3 Determine patient's or family caregiver's readiness to learn. Explain all rationales for the ROM exercises and describe and demonstrate exercises to be performed.
4 Assess patient's level of comfort (on a scale of 0 to 10 with 10 being the worst pain) before exercises. Determine if patient would benefit from pain medication before beginning ROM exercises.
5 Perform hand hygiene and apply clean gloves if wound drainage or skin lesions are present.
6 Help the patient to a comfortable position, preferably sitting or lying down.
7 When performing active-assisted or passive ROM exercises (Table 10-2), support joint by holding distal portion of extremity or using cupped hand to support joint (see illustration).

TABLE 10-1	Incorporating Active Range-of-Motion Exercises into Activities of Daily Living

Joint Exercised	Activity of Daily Living	Movement
Neck	Nodding head yes	Flexion
	Shaking head no	Rotation
	Moving right ear to right shoulder	Lateral flexion
	Moving left ear to left shoulder	Lateral flexion
Shoulder	Reaching to turn on overhead light	Flexion, extension
	Reaching to bedside stand for book	Hyperextension
	Rotating shoulders toward chest	Abduction
	Rotating shoulders toward back	Adduction
Elbow	Eating, bathing, shaving, grooming	Flexion, extension
Wrist	Eating, bathing, shaving, grooming	Flexion, extension, ulnar/radial deviation
Fingers and thumb	All activities requiring fine-motor coordination (e.g., writing, eating, painting)	Flexion, extension, abduction, adduction, opposition
Hip	Walking	Flexion, extension, hyperextension
	Moving to side-lying position	Flexion, extension, abduction
	Moving from side-lying position	Extension, adduction
	Rolling feet inward	Internal rotation
	Rolling feet outward	External rotation
Knee	Walking	Flexion, extension
	Moving to and from side-lying position	Flexion, extension
Ankle	Walking	Dorsiflexion, plantar flexion
	Moving toe toward head of bed	Dorsiflexion
	Moving toe toward foot of bed	Plantar flexion
Toes	Walking	Extension, hyperextension
	Wiggling toes	Abduction, adduction

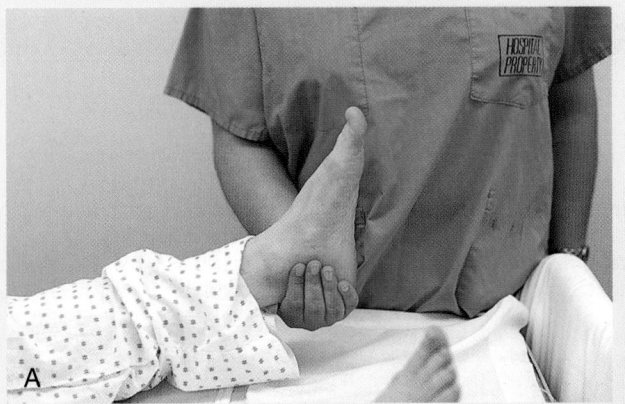
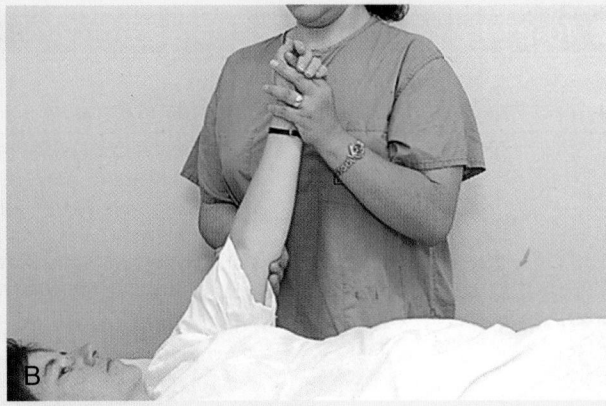
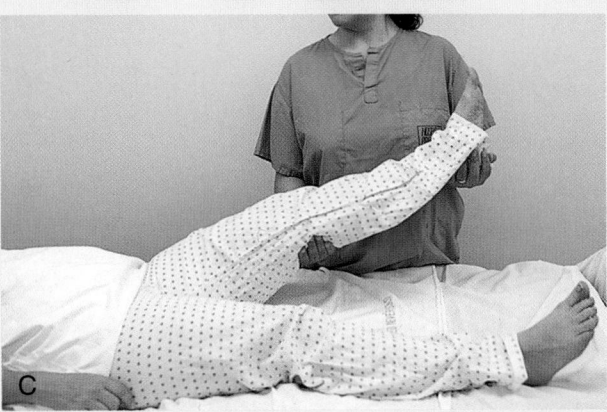

STEP 7 **A,** Support joint by holding distal and proximal areas adjacent to joint. **B,** Support joint by cradling distal portion of extremity. **C,** Use cupped hand to support joint.

8 Complete exercises in head-to-toe sequence. Repeat each movement 5 times during exercise period. Inform patient how these exercises can be incorporated into ADLs (see Table 10-1). If worn, remove gloves. Perform hand hygiene.

9 Observe patient performing ROM activities.
10 Measure joint motion as needed.
11 Monitor pain throughout ROM exercise period.

Clinical Decision Point *When resistance is noted within a joint, do not force joint motion. Consult with health care provider or physical therapist.*

| **TABLE 10-2** | Range-of-Motion Exercises |

Body Part	Type of Joint	Type of Movement	Range (Degrees)	Primary Muscles
Neck, cervical spine	Pivotal	Flexion: Bring chin to rest on chest.	45	Sternocleidomastoid
		Extension: Return head to erect position.	45	Trapezius
		Hyperextension: Bend head back as far as possible.	10	Trapezius
		Lateral flexion: Tilt head as far as possible toward each shoulder.	40-45	Sternocleidomastoid
		Rotation: Turn head as far as possible in circular movement.	180	Sternocleidomastoid, trapezius

TABLE 10-2 | Range-of-Motion Exercises—cont'd

Body Part	Type of Joint	Type of Movement	Range (Degrees)	Primary Muscles
Shoulder	Ball and socket	Flexion: Raise arm from side position forward to position above head.	45-60	Coracobrachialis, deltoid, pectoralis major
		Extension: Return arm to position at side of body.	180	Latissimus dorsi, teres major, triceps brachii
		Hyperextension: Move arm behind body, keeping elbow straight.	45-60	Latissimus dorsi, teres major, deltoid
		Abduction: Raise arm to side to position above head with palm away from head.	180	Deltoid, supraspinatus
		Adduction: Lower arm sideways and across body as far as possible.	320	Pectoralis major
		Internal rotation: With elbow flexed, rotate shoulder by moving arm until thumb is turned inward and toward back.	90	Pectoralis major, latissimus dorsi, teres major, subscapularis
		External rotation: With elbow flexed, move arm until thumb is upward and lateral to head.	90	Infraspinatus, teres major, deltoid
		Circumduction: Move arm in full circle, (circumduction is combination of all movements of ball-and-socket joint).	360	Deltoid, coracobrachialis, latissimus dorsi, teres major
Elbow	Hinge	Flexion: Bend elbow so lower arm moves toward its shoulder joint and hand is level with shoulder.	150	Biceps brachii, brachialis, brachioradialis
		Extension: Straighten elbow by lowering hand.	150	Triceps brachii

TABLE 10-2 | Range-of-Motion Exercises—cont'd

Body Part	Type of Joint	Type of Movement	Range (Degrees)	Primary Muscles
Forearm	Pivotal	Supination: Turn lower arm and hand so palm is up.	70-90	Supinator, biceps brachii
		Pronation: Turn lower arm so palm is down.	70-90	Pronator teres, pronator quadratus
Wrist	Condyloid	Flexion, move palm toward inner aspect of forearm.	80-90	Flexor carpi ulnaris, flexor carpi radialis
		Extension: Move fingers and hand posterior to midline.	80-90	Extensor carpi radialis brevis, extensor carpi radialis longus, extensor carpi ulnaris
		Hyperextension: Bring dorsal surface of hand back as far as possible.	80-90	Extensor carpi radialis brevis, extensor carpi radialis longus, extensor carpi ulnaris
		Radial deviation: Bend wrist medially toward thumb.	Up to 30	Flexor carpi radialis brevis, extensor carpi radialis brevis, extensor carpi radialis longus
		Ulnar deviation: Bend wrist laterally toward fifth finger.	30-50	Flexor carpi ulnaris, extensor carpi ulnaris
Fingers	Condyloid hinge	Flexion: Make fist.	90	Lumbricales, interosseus volaris, interosseus dorsalis
		Extension: Straighten fingers.	90	Extensor digiti quinti proprius, extensor digitorum communis, extensor indicis proprius
		Hyperextension: Bend fingers back as far as possible.	30-60	Extensor digitorum
		Abduction: Spread fingers apart.	30	Interosseus dorsalis
		Adduction: Bring fingers together.	30	Interosseus volaris
Thumb:	Saddle	Flexion: Move thumb across palmar surface of hand.	90	Flexor pollicis brevis
		Extension: Move thumb straight away from hand.	90	Extensor pollicis longus, extensor pollicis brevis
		Abduction: Extend thumb laterally (usually done when placing fingers in abduction and adduction).	30	Abductor pollicis brevis and longus
		Adduction: Move thumb back toward hand.	30	Adductor pollicis obliquus, adductor pollicis transversus
		Opposition: Touch thumb to each finger of same hand.		Opponens pollicis, opponens digiti minimi

Continued

TABLE 10-2 | Range-of-Motion Exercises—cont'd

Body Part	Type of Joint	Type of Movement	Range (Degrees)	Primary Muscles
Hip	Ball and socket	Flexion: Move leg forward and up.	90-120	Psoas major, iliacus, sartorius
		Extension: Move leg back beside other leg.	90-120	Gluteus maximus, semitendinosus, semimembranosus
		Hyperextension: Move leg behind body as far as possible.	30-50	Gluteus maximus, semitendinosus, semimembranosus
		Abduction: Move leg laterally away from body.	30-50	Gluteus medius, gluteus minimus
		Adduction: Move leg back toward medial position and beyond if possible.	30-50	Adductor longus, adductor brevis, adductor magnus
		Internal rotation: Turn foot and leg toward other leg.	90	Gluteus medius, gluteus minimus, tensor fasciae latae
		External rotation: Turn foot and leg away from other leg.	90	Obturatorius internus, obturatorius externus, quadratus femoris, piriformis, gemellus superior and inferior, gluteus maximus
		Circumduction: Move leg in circle.	120-130	Psoas major, gluteus maximum, gluteus medius, adductor magnus

TABLE 10-2 | Range-of-Motion Exercises—cont'd

Body Part	Type of Joint	Type of Movement	Range (Degrees)	Primary Muscles
Knee	Hinge	Flexion: Bring heel back toward back of thigh.	120-130	Biceps femoris, semitendinosus, semimembranosus, sartorius
		Extension: Return leg to floor.	120-130	Rectus femoris, vastus lateralis, vastus medialis, vastus intermedius
Ankle	Hinge	Dorsal flexion: Move foot so toes are pointed upward.	20-30	Tibialis anterior
		Plantar flexion: Move foot so toes are pointed downward.	45-50	Gastrocnemius, soleus
Foot	Gliding	Inversion: Turn sole of foot medially.	10 or less	Tibialis anterior, tibialis posterior
		Eversion: Turn sole of foot laterally.	10 or less	Peroneus longus, peroneus brevis
Toes	Condyloid	Flexion: Curl toes downward.	30-60	Flexor digitorum, lumbricalis pedis, flexor hallucis brevis
		Extension: Straighten toes.	30-60	Extensor digitorum longus, extensor digitorum brevis, extensor hallucis longus
		Abduction: Spread toes apart.	15 or less	Abductor hallucis, interosseus dorsalis
		Adduction: Bring toes together.	15 or less	Adductor hallucis, interosseus plantaris

SKILL 10-1 Performing Isometric Exercises

In addition to range-of-motion (ROM) exercises, some immobilized patients are able to perform muscle-strengthening exercises. Isotonic muscle contractions cause a change in muscle length. Examples of exercises that cause isotonic muscle contractions are walking, performing aerobics, and moving arms and legs against light resistance. Performing these types of exercises regularly positively affects heart and lung function, improves muscle tone, and has beneficial effects on the entire body if performed properly (Burtin et al., 2009; Chrysant, 2010; Granacher et al., 2011). Some individuals are unable to tolerate such increases in activity. For these individuals isometric exercises are more appropriate and are easily accomplished when patients are in bed. Isometric or static exercises involve tightening or tensing of muscles without moving body parts (isometric contractions). They increase muscle tension but do not change the length of muscle fibers.

Isometric exercises involve the contraction of a muscle while pushing against a stationary object or resisting the movement of an object. Examples are performing push-ups and hip lifting. In hip lifting the individual, who is in a sitting position, pushes with the hands against a sitting surface such as a chair to raise the hips. Isometric exercises help to promote muscular strength and provide the necessary stress for bone maintenance and growth. Without sufficient stress against bone, osteoclastic activity (activity by cells responsible for bone tissue absorption) increases over osteoblastic activity (activity by bone-forming cells) (Huether and McCance, 2008). The result is demineralization of the bone and eventual osteoporosis.

Delegation and Collaboration

The skill of performing isometric exercises can be delegated to nursing assistive personnel (NAP). However, patients with cardiovascular disease or musculoskeletal disorders require assessment by a nurse when initially performing these exercises. The nurse directs the NAP by:

- Discussing the amount of time and frequency of the prescribed isometric exercises.
- Reminding NAP to perform exercises slowly at a patient's pace.
- Discussing a patient's individual limitations or preexisting conditions such as arthritis, which may affect ROM needed for isometric exercises.

STEP	RATIONALE

ASSESSMENT

1 Review patient's chart for contraindications to isometric exercises such as cardiovascular disease.

Isometric exercises may raise blood pressure and pulse. The presence of a preexisting medical condition such as a history of cardiac problems may be a contraindication.

2 Assess patient's baseline vital signs.

Isometric exercises may raise blood pressure. Baseline vital signs offer a measure for determining whether exercises cause deterioration in vital signs (Huether and McCance, 2008).

3 Assess patient's baseline muscle strength:

Allows you to compare muscle strength before and after exercise.

a Ask patient to perform task against resistance (e.g., push one foot against palm of hand).

b Assess grasp strength by having patient grasp your hands. Note whether hand grasps are equal.

c Have patient grasp two fingers of your right hand with patient's left hand and two fingers of your left hand with patient's right hand.

d Observe patient's ability to do daily activities (e.g., whether patient has adequate strength to bathe self, pull self up in bed, move from bed to chair).

e Obtain patient's subjective statements related to muscle strength. Does he or she feel weaker?

4 Assess patient's nutritional status.

Proper nutrition is essential if patient is to be able to perform exercises. Promotion of protein anabolism involves conservation and replenishment of energy stores (Touhy, 2010).

5 Assess level of comfort: pain severity (using a scale of 0 to 10). *Option:* Administer ordered analgesic 30 to 60 minutes before exercise.

Pain may reduce patient's motivation to perform isometric exercises. Pain relief before attempting exercises may enhance patient's participation.

6 Assess patient's or family caregiver's understanding of isometric exercises to be used.

Allows patient to verbalize concerns and identifies educational needs of patient or caregiver.

NURSING DIAGNOSES

- Activity intolerance
- Deficient knowledge regarding exercises
- Fatigue
- Impaired physical mobility
- Pain (acute, chronic)

Related factors are individualized based on patient's condition or needs.

PLANNING

1 Expected outcomes following completion of procedure:
- Patient increases number of exercise repetitions.

Patient gradually becomes stronger and is able to increase number of repetitions.

- Vital signs remain stable.

Documents patient's activity tolerance.

2 Explain procedure and demonstrate exercises.

Relieves anxiety and encourages patient cooperation.

3 Help patient to comfortable position.

Reduces stress and promotes patient participation.

IMPLEMENTATION

1 Provide privacy.

Prevents patient embarrassment.

2 Instruct patient to perform the following isometric exercises usually prescribed by a physical therapist. Each exercise prescription is individualized according to patient's needs and limitations. Exercises are as follows:

Gradual build-up of exercise repetitions improves both muscle strength and endurance (Peterson et al., 2011).

Clinical Decision Point *Teach patients to exhale while exerting effort during isometric exercises. Many persons hold their breath (Valsalva maneuver), which increases intrathoracic pressure, causing a decrease in venous return to heart.*

a Quadriceps isometric exercises:

Quadriceps muscles enable person to ambulate and get out of chair; large muscles of thigh (quadriceps) must be strong enough for patient to extend knees and stabilize them.

STEP	RATIONALE
(1) Assist patient to supine recumbent position.	
(2) Instruct patient to press back of knee against mattress while trying to lift heel from bed (see illustration).	
(3) Hold muscles tightly contracted for 5 to 15 seconds and then relax completely for several seconds.	Nurse can assist patient in learning this exercise by placing hand between back of patient's knee and mattress and asking patient to press hand against mattress with back of knee.
(4) Repeat exercise five times.	
b Gluteal muscle isometric exercises:	Improves patient's balance when sitting.
(1) Help patient to supine position.	
(2) Instruct patient to pinch buttocks muscles together and hold for 5 to 15 seconds and then relax completely for several seconds (see illustration).	
(3) Repeat exercise five times.	
c Abdominal muscle isometric exercises:	Improves trunk stability.
(1) Have patient pull abdominal muscles in as tightly as possible (see illustration)	
(2) Hold for 5 to 15 seconds. Release muscles gradually.	
(3) Repeat exercise five times.	
d Foot muscle isometric exercises:	Increases muscle activity in leg and thereby promotes venous return to heart.
(1) Instruct patient to flex foot toward and away from knee, holding muscles tightly in each position for 5 to 15 seconds.	
(2) Repeat exercise five times.	
e Hand muscle isometric exercises:	Strengthens grip to hold onto crutch or walker more effectively.
(1) Obtain sponge rubber ball. (Size of ball depends on size of patient's hand.)	
(2) Have patient grip ball with entire hand 5 to 10 times.	
(3) Dig each fingertip, one at a time, into ball 5 to 10 times each.	
(4) Gradually increase frequency of exercise until patient can grip ball. Exercise once or twice a day.	
f Biceps isometric exercises:	Strengthens biceps and thereby helps with ambulation if ambulatory assistive device is used.
(1) Have patient raise arms to shoulder height and interlock fingertips of both hands.	
(2) Use arm muscles to try to pull hands apart.	
(3) Hold for 5 to 15 seconds.	
(4) Relax muscles.	
(5) Repeat exercise five times.	

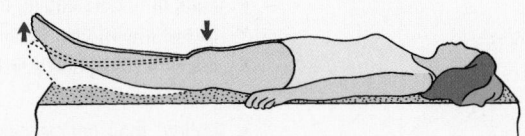

STEP 2a(2) Lift heels while pressing back of knees against mattress.

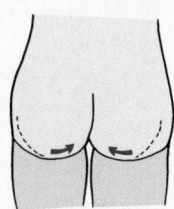
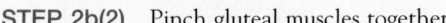

STEP 2b(2) Pinch gluteal muscles together.

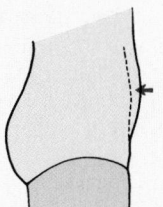

STEP 2c(1) Pull abdominal muscles in tightly.

STEP	RATIONALE
g Triceps muscle isometric exercises:	Strengthens triceps to assist with transfer techniques and use of crutches or walker. Patient must have enough strength to extend and stabilize elbows when lifting or shifting body weight.

(1) Arm exercises (see illustration)
    (a) Have patient raise arms to shoulder height.
    (b) Make fist with one hand and place against palm of other hand.
    (c) Push hands together as hard as possible and hold for 5 to 15 seconds.
    (d) Relax and repeat exercise five times.
  (2) Sitting exercises (see illustration)
    (a) Help patient to sitting position on edge of bed or in chair. If mattress is soft, place blocks or books on bed under patient's hands.
    (b) Instruct patient to try to lift buttocks off bed or seat of chair by pressing down on mattress or chair seat with hands.
    (c) Hold muscles tight for 5 to 15 seconds and then relax.
    (d) Repeat exercise as tolerated.
	To use crutches or walker effectively, patient must have enough strength in triceps to extend and stabilize elbows while lifting or shifting body weight.

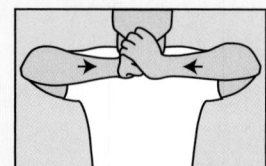

STEP 2g(1) Triceps muscle isometric exercises.

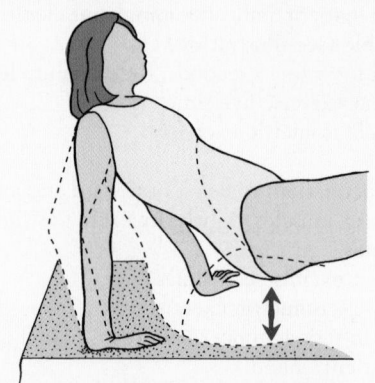

STEP 2g(2) Triceps muscle resistive isometric exercises.

EVALUATION

1 Observe patient's ability to perform exercises.	Demonstrates patient's learning.
2 Evaluate patient's level of energy, muscular strength, and comfort following exercises.	Determines whether patient is performing exercises accurately and whether exercises are increasing muscle strength.
3 Obtain vital signs after one or two repetitions.	Determines patient's tolerance to activity.
4 Ask patient to rate pain level on a scale of 0-10.	Determines patient's pain status post isometric exercises and if pre exercise analgesia was effective.

Unexpected Outcomes	Related Interventions
1 Patient is unable to perform exercises. Patient may be too weak.	• Continue ROM exercises and reposition patient to try to increase strength. • Make sure that nutrition and rest are adequate.
2 Patient is unwilling to perform exercises.	• Lack of understanding of significance of exercises may be the problem. • Stress importance of exercises. • Be sure that patient is not experiencing distracting symptoms such as nausea or pain.
3 Muscular strength is not increasing.	• Patient may not be performing exercises as described or as often as instructed. • Stress importance of following routine.
4 Patient's blood pressure and heart rate increase significantly during exercises.	• Patient may not be able to tolerate procedure. • Discontinue exercises and consult health care provider.

Recording and Reporting
- Record in the nurses' notes and electronic health record (EHR) the type of isometric exercises used; length of time contractions held; number of repetitions of each exercise; assessment of patient's muscular strength and comfort after exercises, vital signs, subjective statements regarding muscular strength, and ability to perform exercises.

Special Considerations
Teaching
- Instruct patient to perform exercises before regular activities such as breakfast or work. Building exercises into routine activities increases likelihood of adherence to exercise program.
- Instruct patient to gradually increase exercise activity each day.

Pediatric
- Incorporate exercises into a child's activity plan.
- Children are more likely to exercise as part of a game or in groups as opposed to exercising alone (Hockenberry and Wilson, 2011).

Gerontologic
- Physical exercise is important for older adults to maintain health, preserve functional status, and improve general quality of life (Peterson et al., 2011; Touhy, 2010).
- For the older adult who has not previously participated in exercise, it is important to start with only 5 minutes of exercise and gradually work up to a 20- to 30-minute daily routine (Peterson et al., 2011).

SKILL 10-2   Continuous Passive Motion Machine

The continuous passive motion (CPM) machine is designed to exercise various joints such as the hip, ankle, knee, shoulder, and wrist. The CPM machine is most commonly used after knee surgery. It is usually prescribed on the day of surgery or the first postoperative day, depending on the surgeon's preference and patient's condition (Lewis et al., 2011). An initial setting is typically 20 to 30 degrees of flexion and full extension at two cycles per minute. However, this setting varies according to a patient's condition and health care provider's preference (Ignatavicius and Workman, 2009). The purpose of the CPM machine is to mobilize the joint to prevent contractures, muscle atrophy, venous stasis, and thromboembolism (Long, 2008). It helps to alleviate pain, edema, stiffness, and dislocation and potentially can shorten a patient's hospital stay.

The electronically controlled CPM machine flexes and extends a joint to a prescribed degree and at a set speed as ordered by the health care provider. Velcro straps secure the extremity. When the device is turned on, the frame slides slowly back and forth, gently moving the joint through a preset range of motion (ROM). The CPM machine can weigh up to 25 pounds. Using two hospital personnel to lift the machine reduces the risk for caregiver back strain and prevents risk of damage to a patient's extremity.

Delegation and Collaboration
The skill of using the CPM machine cannot be delegated to nursing assistive personnel (NAP). The nurse directs the NAP by:
- Instructing them to immediately report increase in patient's pain, skin breakdown, or joint inflammation.

Equipment
- ❑ CPM machine
- ❑ Clean gloves

STEP	RATIONALE
ASSESSMENT	
1 Assess CPM machine for electrical safety. If you suspect a problem, notify the electrical safety department.	All electrical equipment in health care settings is checked routinely for safety. Routine observation of electrical cord and functioning of equipment each time it is used further monitors safety.
2 Assess setup of machine before placing on bed: check stability of frame, flexion/extension controls, padding of exposed metal parts or hard surfaces, and on/off switch.	Ensures that all pieces of equipment are operational and prevents damage to patient's joint. Ensures that metal parts are padded to prevent skin breakdown or chafing of skin rubbing against metal or hard surfaces.
3 Assess patient's pain on a scale of 0 to 10 (10 being the worst pain) before and during use.	Establishes comfort baseline. Determines how patient tolerates CPM machine and need for analgesia.
4 Assess patient's vital signs.	Provides baseline to measure exercise tolerance.
5 Assess patient's knowledge about CPM and ability and willingness to learn about CPM machine.	Determines readiness to learn, reduces anxiety, and promotes patient participation.
6 Assess nature of patient's condition and ROM limits prescribed by health care provider.	Procedure must be ordered by health care provider.

NURSING DIAGNOSES
- Activity intolerance
- Acute pain
- Deficient knowledge regarding CPM machine
- Fatigue
- Impaired physical mobility

Related factors are individualized based on patient's condition or needs.

STEP	RATIONALE

PLANNING

1 Expected outcomes following completion of the procedure:
- Patient increases length of time and flexion of joint as prescribed.
- Patient's vital signs remain stable.
- Patient denies increased discomfort during or after CPM exercise.

2 Explain procedure and demonstrate CPM machine.

3 Assist patient to comfortable supine position.

CPM machine facilitates joint range of motion and prevents formation of adhesions, edema, stiffness, deformity.
Patient tolerates activity.
Analgesia is effective in promoting exercise tolerance.

Relieves anxiety and encourages patient cooperation.
Reduces stress and promotes patient participation.

IMPLEMENTATION

1 Perform hand hygiene.

2 Identify patient using two identifiers (i.e., name and birthday or name and account number, according to agency policy). Compare identifiers with information on patient's identification bracelet.

3 Provide analgesia 20 to 30 minutes before CPM machine is needed.

4 Apply clean gloves if wound drainage is present.

5 Place elastic stockings on patient if ordered (Procedural Guideline 10-2).

6 Place CPM machine on bed.

7 Set limits of flexion and extension as prescribed by health care provider and set speed control to slow or moderate range.

8 Put machine through one full cycle.

9 Stop CPM machine when in extension. Place sheepskin on CPM machine.

10 Support patient's joints while placing extremity in CPM machine (see illustration).

Reduces transmission of microorganisms.
Ensures correct patient. Complies with The Joint Commission standards and improves patient safety (TJC, 2012).

Pain control assists patient in tolerating exercise (see Chapter 15).
Reduces nurse's risk for exposure to bloodborne viruses or bacteria.
Elastic stockings promote venous return from lower extremities.

Prevents injury by setting machine at safe limits.

Ensures that CPM machine is working properly.
Ensures that all exposed hard surfaces are padded to prevent rubbing and chafing patient's skin.

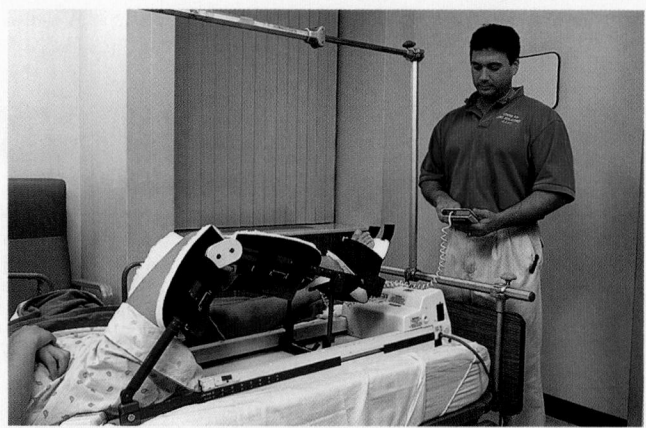

STEP 10 Leg positioned in CPM machine cradle.

11 Adjust CPM machine to patient's extremity. Lengthen and shorten appropriate sections of frame.

12 Center patient's extremity on frame.

13 Align patient's joint with mechanical joint of CPM.

14 Secure patient's extremity on CPM machine with Velcro straps (see illustration). Apply loosely.

Avoids pressure areas on extremity.

STEP	RATIONALE

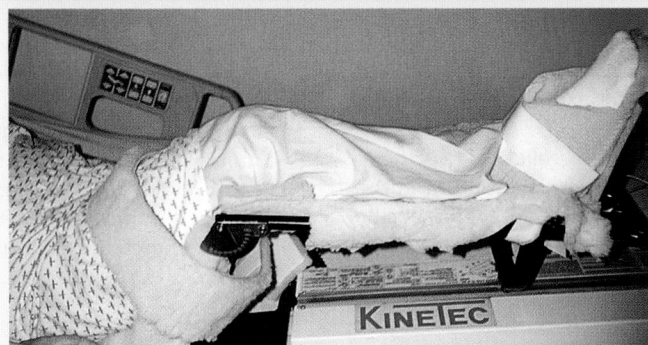

STEP 14   Patient's extremity properly placed and secured on CPM machine.

15 Start machine. When it reaches flexed position, stop it and check degree of flexion.	Prevents possible complications and ensures correct settings.
16 Start CPM machine and observe for two full cycles.	Ensures that CPM machine is fully operational at preset extension and flexion modes.
17 Make sure that patient is comfortable.	
18 Instruct patient to turn CPM machine off if malfunctioning or if he or she is experiencing pain. Instruct him or her to notify nurse immediately.	Prevents excessive stress on joint.
19 Provide patient with on/off switch.	Allows patient to turn CPM machine on and off if it malfunctions or discomfort develops.
20 Discard gloves and perform hand hygiene.	Prevents transmission of microorganisms.

EVALUATION

1 Inspect bony prominences and areas of skin in contact with machine at least every 2 hours.	Identifies potential skin breakdown.
2 Ask patient to rate pain on scale of 0 to 10.	Determines if analgesia is effective.
3 Check patient's alignment and positioning at least every 2 hours.	Promotes comfort and ensures proper extension and flexion of joint.
4 Observe patient and CPM machine with each increase in flexion and extension.	Prevents complications and ensures that CPM machine is functioning properly.

Unexpected Outcomes

1 Patient does not tolerate increase in flexion or extension.

2 Patient experiences increased pain when using CPM machine.

3 Patient develops reddened areas on bony prominences or extremity.

Related Interventions

- Consult with health care provider and physical therapist to plan additional therapies to increase flexion and extension of joint.
- Provide rest periods throughout day to rest the joint.
- Consider modification of current analgesia plan before using CPM machine.
- Determine efficacy of current analgesia and obtain new orders to change dosage or medication.
- Determine cause of increased pain.
- Determine if hard surfaces on CPM machine are well padded.
- Monitor patient's alignment and positioning at least every 2 hours.
- Provide skin care at least every 2 hours.

Recording and Reporting

- Record in the nurses' notes and EHR the patient's tolerance for CPM machine, rate of cycles per minute, degree of flexion and extension used, condition of extremity and skin, condition of operative site if present, length of time CPM machine in use.
- Report immediately to nurse in charge or health care provider any resistance to range of motion; increased pain; swelling, heat, or redness in joint.

Special Considerations
Teaching

- Instruct patient in the use and importance of the CPM machine, including length of time that CPM is used and any adverse conditions such as increased pain, swelling, or redness in joint. Instruct a patient to call the health care provider if any of these conditions is present.

Pediatric

- During therapy arrange for social or creative activities that are developmentally appropriate for the child's age (Hockenberry and Wilson, 2011).
- Relieve a child's anxiety by demonstrating use of the CPM machine, using a large doll or stuffed animal, before applying it.

Gerontologic

- Older adults have increased risk for skin breakdown because of decreased elasticity and fragility of the skin. Pressure from the CPM machine increases the risk for pressure ulcers, especially on the heel (Touhy, 2010).

- Encourage older adults to move at their own speed. Relaxation exercises decrease anxiety, ease muscle tension, and assist with pain relief (Christo et al., 2011). Special attention to nonverbal cues and additional instruction in pain management are often necessary to ensure an older adult's comfort.

Home Care

- Home care physical therapist may assist patient/family in continuing CPM machine in the home.
- Patient/family must have specific instructions regarding the use of the CPM machine, length of time for each session, and expected outcomes.

PROCEDURAL GUIDELINE 10-2 Applying Elastic Stockings and Sequential Compression Device

 Video Clip

A patient may develop a deep vein thrombosis (DVT) for many reasons. Some common risk factors include injury to a vein from a fracture or surgery, immobility caused by a cast or prolonged sitting, inherited clotting disorders, obesity, smoking, and a family history (Harvard Health Publications, 2009). Three factors (known as *Virchow's triad*): hypercoagulability of the blood, venous wall damage, and blood flow stasis, contribute to DVT development (Lewis et al., 2011). If a DVT is suspected, keep the patient calm and quiet in bed, and notify the health care provider. Prevention, which can include anticoagulant medications, is the best approach for DVTs; however, movement of the extremities, wearing compression stockings, and use of foot pumps are equally important. Elastic stockings help reduce blood stasis and venous wall injury by promoting venous return and limiting venous dilation, which decreases the risk of endothelial tears. Sequential compression devices (SCDs) pump blood into deep veins, thus removing pooled blood and preventing venous stasis. Another venous plexus foot pump promotes circulation by mimicking the natural action of walking (Fig. 10-1).

Delegation and Collaboration

The skill of applying elastic stockings and SCDs may be delegated to nursing assistive personnel (NAP). The nurse initially determines the size of elastic stockings and assesses the patient's lower extremities for any signs and symptoms of DVTs or impaired circulation. The nurse directs the NAP to:

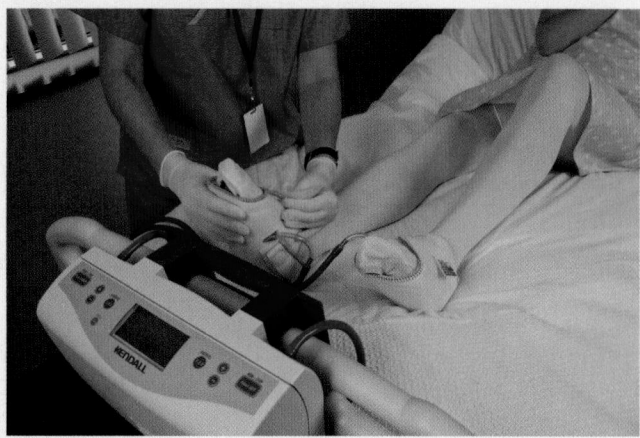

FIG 10-1 Venous plexus foot pump with bedside controls. (*Courtesy Tyco Healthcare Group LP.*)

- Remove the SCD sleeves before allowing a patient to get out of bed.
- Report to the nurse if a patient's calf appears larger than the other or is red or hot or if there are signs of allergic reactions to elastic (redness, itching, irritation).

Equipment

- ❏ Tape measure
- ❏ Powder or cornstarch (optional)
- ❏ Elastic support stockings
- ❏ SCD motor, disposable SCD sleeve(s), tubing assembly

Procedural Steps

1. Assess patient for risk factors in Virchow's triad:
   a. Hypercoagulability (e.g., clotting disorders, fever, dehydration)
   b. Venous wall abnormalities (e.g., orthopedic surgery, varicose veins, atherosclerosis)
   c. Blood stasis (e.g., immobility, obesity, pregnancy)
2. Observe for contraindications for use of elastic stockings or SCDs:
   a. Dermatitis or open skin lesions
   b. Recent skin graft to lower leg
   c. Decreased arterial circulation in lower extremities as evidenced by cyanotic, cool extremities and/or gangrenous conditions affecting the lower limb(s)
3. Assess condition of patient's skin and circulation to the legs (e.g., presence of pedal pulses, edema, discoloration of skin, temperature, lesions).
4. Obtain health care provider's order.
5. Perform hand hygiene.
6. Identify patient using at least two patient identifiers (e.g., name and birthday or name and account number, according to agency policy). Compare identifiers with information on patient's identification bracelet.
7. Explain procedure and reason for applying elastic stockings and SCDs.
8. Position patient in supine position. Elevate head of bed to comfortable level. Use tape measure to measure patient's leg to determine proper elastic stocking or SCD size.
9. *Option:* Apply a small amount of powder or cornstarch to legs provided patient does not have sensitivity.
10. Apply elastic stocking:
    a. Turn elastic stocking inside out by placing one hand into sock, holding heel of sock with other hand, and pulling. Pull until reaching the heel (see illustration).

PROCEDURAL GUIDELINE 10-2 Applying Elastic Stockings and Sequential Compression Device—cont'd

b Place patient's toes into foot of elastic stocking up to heel, making sure that sock is smooth (see illustration).

c Slide remaining portion of sock over patient's foot, making sure that toes are covered. Make sure that foot fits into toe and heel position of sock. Sock will now be right side out (see illustration).

d Slide sock up over patient's calf until sock is completely extended. Be sure that sock is smooth and that no ridges or wrinkles are present (see illustration).

e Instruct patient not to roll socks partially down.

11 Apply SCD sleeve(s):

a Remove SCD sleeves from plastic cover; unfold and flatten.

b Arrange SCD sleeve under patient's leg according to leg position indicated on inner lining of sleeve (see illustration).

c Place patient's leg on SCD sleeve. Back of ankle should line up with ankle marking on inner lining of sleeve.

d Position back of knee with popliteal opening on sleeve (see illustration).

e Wrap SCD sleeve securely around patient's leg. Check fit of SCD sleeve by placing two fingers between patient's leg and sleeve (see illustration).

12 Attach SCD sleeve connector to plug on mechanical unit. Arrows on connector line up with arrows on plug from mechanical unit (see illustration).

13 Turn mechanical unit on. Green light indicates that unit is functioning. Monitor functioning SCD through one full cycle of inflation and deflation.

14 Remove elastic stockings or SCD sleeves at least once per shift (e.g., long enough to inspect skin for irritation or breakdown).

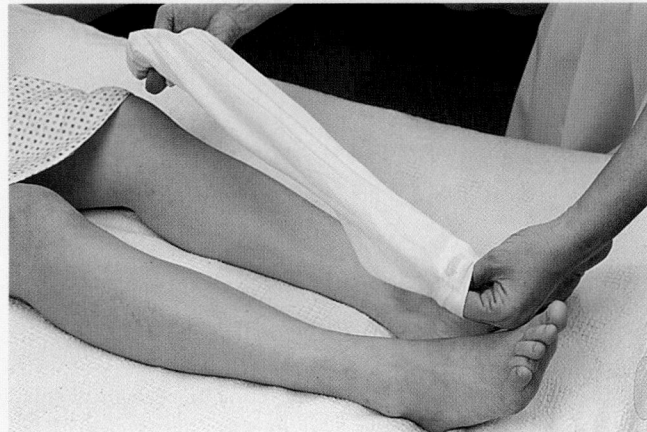

STEP 10a Turn stocking inside out; hold heel and pull through.

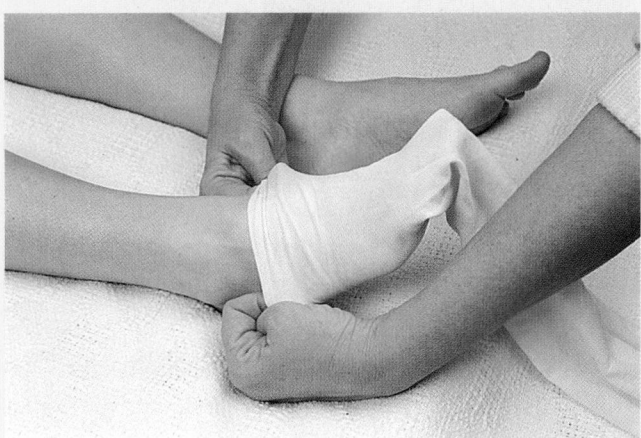

STEP 10c Slide remaining portion of sock over foot.

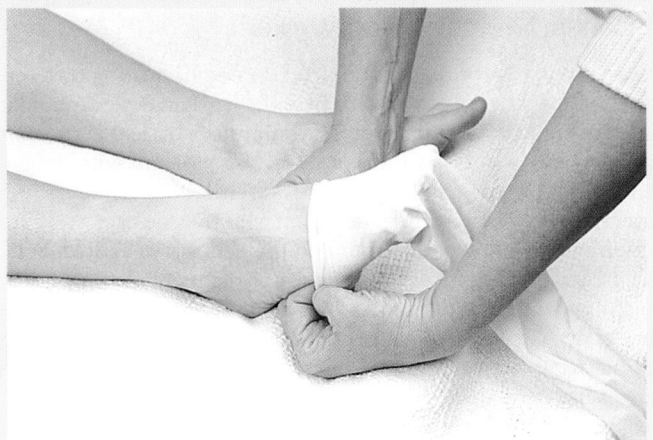

STEP 10b Place toes into foot of stocking.

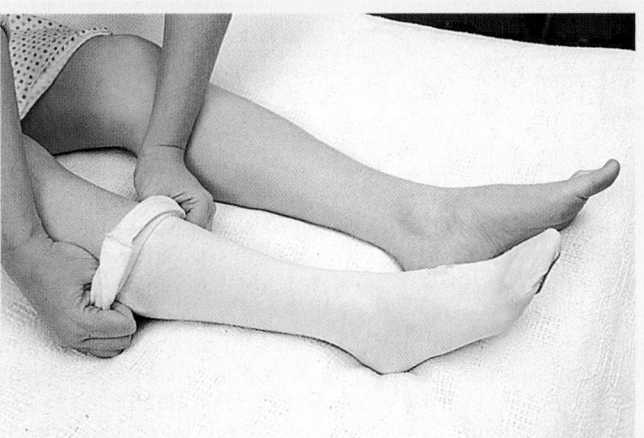

STEP 10d Slide sock up leg until completely extended.

Continued

PROCEDURAL GUIDELINE 10-2 Applying Elastic Stockings and Sequential Compression Device—cont'd

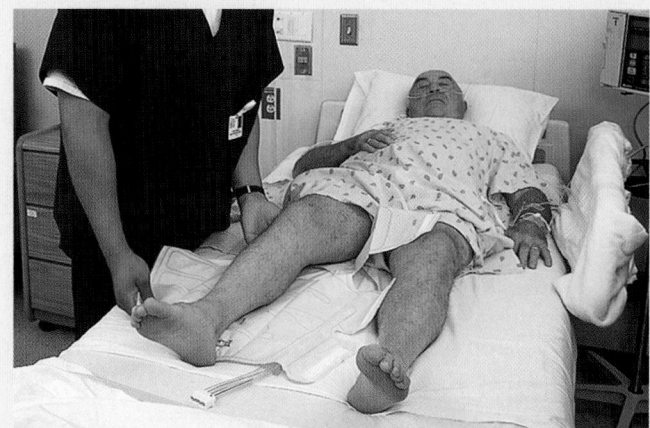

STEP 11b   Correct positioning of leg on inner lining of SCD.

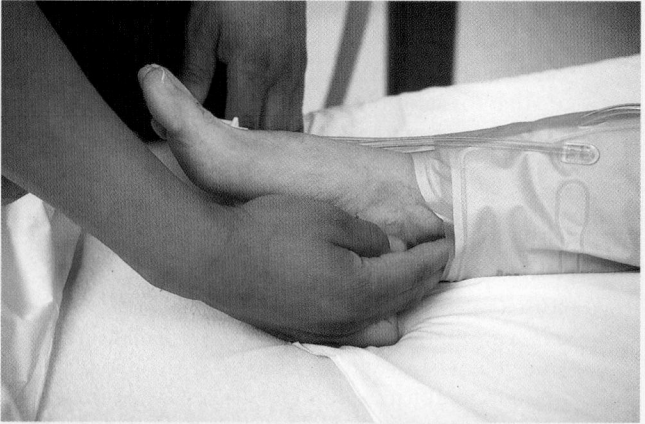

STEP 11e   Check fit of SCD sleeve.

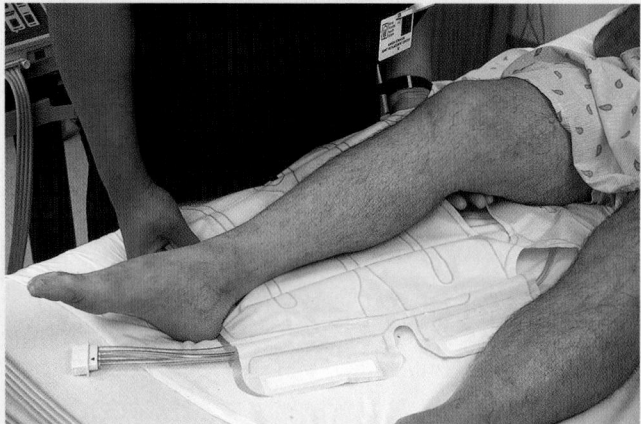

STEP 11d   Position back of patient's knee with the popliteal opening.

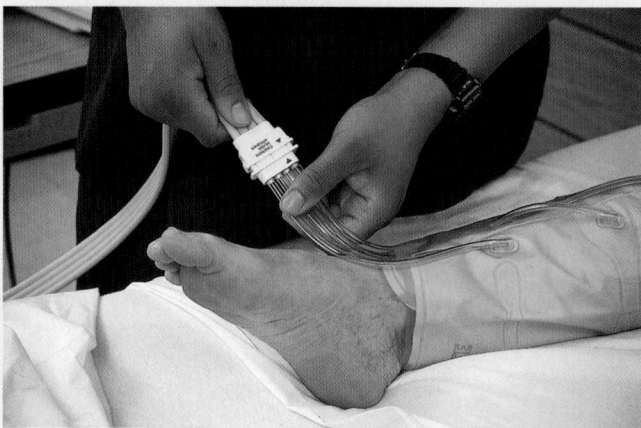

STEP 12   Align arrows when connecting to mechanical unit.

SKILL 10-3   Assisting with Ambulation and Use of Canes, Crutches, and Walker

 Video Clip

Patients who are immobile for even a short time may require assistance with ambulation. Have patients wear gait belts and stand on their stronger side. Then, if the patient begins to fall, you can pull him or her toward you on the stronger side. Whenever assisting a patient up and out of bed or a chair, there is a risk for orthostatic hypotension. Orthostatic hypotension or postural hypotension is a drop in blood pressure that occurs when a patient changes from a horizontal to a vertical position. A drop in blood pressure greater than 20 mm Hg in systolic pressure or 10 mm Hg in diastolic pressure with symptoms of dizziness, light-headedness, nausea, tachycardia, pallor, and fainting indicates orthostatic hypotension (Lewis et al., 2011; Thompson et al., 2011). Before ambulating patients use interventions to maintain muscle tone, increase venous return to the heart, and decrease stasis of blood in the lower extremities. Use safety precautions before and during ambulation to control for orthostatic hypotension and subsequent falling.

A patient may require the use of an assistive device to aid in ambulation. Use of an assistive device increases stability, supports weak extremities, or reduces the load on weight-bearing structures such as hips, knees, or ankles. These devices range from standard canes, which provide balance and minimal physical support, to crutches and walkers, which are used by patients with weight-bearing limitations on one or more of their legs. When assisting a patient to ambulate while using an assistive device, have the person wear a gait belt and stand on the person's weak side. Selection of the appropriate device depends on a patient's age, diagnosis, muscular coordination, and ease of maneuverability (Pierson and Fairchild, 2008). Use of assistive devices may be temporary (e.g., during recuperation from a fractured extremity or orthopedic surgery) or permanent (e.g., a patient with paralysis or permanent weakness of the lower extremities).

Canes are lightweight, easily movable devices that extend approximately waist high and are made of wood or metal. They help to maintain balance by widening the base of support. They are indicated for patients with hemiparesis and are used to ease the strain on weight-bearing joints. Canes are not recommended for patients with bilateral leg weakness; crutches or walkers are more appropriate for such patients (Pierson and Fairchild, 2008). There are three types of commonly used canes. The *standard crook* cane provides the least support and is used by patients requiring only minimal assistance to walk. It has a half-circle handle, which allows it to be hooked over chairs. The *tripod cane* (pyramid cane) has three legs, and the *quad cane* has four legs; the additional legs provide a wide base of support. These types of canes are useful for patients with unilateral or partial leg paralysis. They also have the advantage of standing alone, freeing the arms to help a patient rise from a chair.

A crutch is a wooden or metal staff that reaches from the ground almost to the axilla. Crutches remove weight from one or both legs. They are used by patients who must transfer more weight to their arms than is possible with canes. There are three types of crutches: *axillary*, *Lofstrand*, and *platform*. Patients of all ages often use an axillary crutch on a short-term basis. The Lofstrand crutch has a handgrip and a metal band that fits around a patient's forearm. Both the metal band and the handgrip are adjusted to fit a patient's height. This type of crutch is useful for patients with a permanent disability such as paraplegia. The metal armband stabilizes and helps to guide the crutch. It also offers other advantages. First, the encircling armband allows patients to use their hands for other activities such as opening doors without dropping the crutches. Second, the anterior opening of the band allows patients to free themselves of the crutches if a fall occurs. Patients who are unable to bear weight on their wrists use a platform crutch. It has a horizontal trough on which patients can rest their forearms and wrists and a vertical handle for patients to grip.

A walker is an extremely lightweight, movable device that stands about waist high, consisting of a metal frame with handgrips, four widely placed sturdy legs, and one open side. Because it has a wide base of support, the walker provides great stability and security. A walker can be used by a patient who is weak or has problems with balance (Pierson and Fairchild, 2008). In addition to the standard walker, several other models are available: a foldable version that is easy to transport, one with a fold-down seat, and one with wheels on the front legs. Walkers with wheels are useful for patients who have difficulty lifting the walker as they walk because of limited balance or endurance. However, the disadvantage is that the walker can roll forward when weight is applied.

Delegation and Collaboration

The skill of assisting patients with ambulation can be delegated to nursing assistive personnel (NAP). The nurse directs the NAP by:

- Instructing them to have a patient dangle following lying in bed before ambulation (see Chapter 9).
- Instructing them to immediately return a patient to the bed or chair if he or she is nauseated, dizzy, pale, or diaphoretic and to report these signs and symptoms to the nurse immediately.
- Discussing the importance of applying safe, nonskid shoes and ensuring that the environment is free of clutter and there is no moisture on the floor before ambulating patient.

Equipment

- ❏ Ambulation device (crutch, walker, cane)
- ❏ Safety device (gait belt)
- ❏ Well-fitting, flat, nonskid shoes for patient
- ❏ Robe
- ❏ Goniometer (*optional*)

STEP	RATIONALE

ASSESSMENT

1 Review patient's chart, including:

   a Patient's medical history.

   b Patient's previous activity level.

   c Current activity order

2 Assess patient's physical readiness:

   a Obtain patient's heart rate; blood pressure; and orientation to time, place, and person.

   b Assess range of motion (ROM), muscle strength, coordination, and whether there is the presence of foot deformities.

   c Assess patient for any visual, perceptual, or sensory deficits.

   d Assess environment for potential threats to patient safety.

   e Assess patient's pain on a scale of 0-10, 10 being the worst pain.

3 Determine patient's or family caregiver's understanding of technique of ambulation to be used.

4 Determine optimal time for ambulation.

5 Assess degree of assistance that patient needs.

Rationale column:

Certain medications, chronic illness, and history of falling may influence patient's ability to ambulate independently.

Identifies patient's activity tolerance. Patient may tire easily or be prone to orthostatic hypotension if bed rest has been prolonged.

Verifies if an ambulation aid is needed and specifies amount of activity permitted.

Ambulation following immobility can be fatiguing and stressful. Baseline is needed to detect orthostatic hypotension. Baseline vital signs also offer a means for comparison after exercise. The oriented patient is able to understand instructions.

Determines if patient has enough flexibility and muscle strength to ambulate safely and if he or she needs muscle-strengthening exercises. Determines presence of foot deformities affecting ambulation.

Determines if patient can use assistive device safely. Ambulation after immobility can be fatiguing and stressful.

Protects patient from potential injury.

Patient may be in pain or fear pain resulting from exercise. If necessary, administer analgesic 30 to 60 minutes before exercise.

Allows patient to verbalize concerns. Patients who have been immobile for a long time may be hesitant to ambulate. Caregiver may be hesitant to learn how to help with ambulation.

Patient's personal habits must be considered when planning activities.

For safety, another person may be needed initially to assist with patient ambulation. Allow patient as much independence as possible.

STEP	RATIONALE

NURSING DIAGNOSES

- Activity intolerance
- Decreased cardiac output
- Deficient knowledge regarding use of assistive device
- Fatigue
- Impaired physical mobility
- Ineffective peripheral tissue perfusion
- Risk for falls
- Risk for injury

Related factors are individualized based on patient's condition or needs.

PLANNING

1 Expected outcomes following completion of procedure:

- Patient ambulates without injury.

- Patient is able to ambulate without excessive fatigue or dizziness.
- Patient demonstrates correct gait.
- Patient resumes social and self-care activities.

2 Preparing patient for ambulation:

a Explain reasons for exercise and demonstrate specific gait technique to patient or family caregiver.

b Decide with patient how far to ambulate.

c Schedule ambulation around patient's other activities.

d Place bed in low position and slowly help patient to Fowler's upright position (see Chapter 9). If in chair, have patient sit upright with feet flat on floor.

e Help patient in bed to dangling position on side of bed (see illustration). Apply gait belt.

Precautions prevent orthostatic hypotension. Appropriate level of assistance on device ensures patient's safety.
Assistive device chosen requires minimal exertion.

Demonstrates learning.
Progressive ambulation increases patient's endurance and independence.

Teaching and demonstration enhance learning, reduce anxiety, and encourage cooperation.
Determines mutual goal.
Taking scheduled rest periods between activities reduces patient fatigue.
Allows a few minutes for circulation to equilibrate. Prevents orthostatic hypotension and potential injuries.

Movement of legs in dangling position promotes venous return.

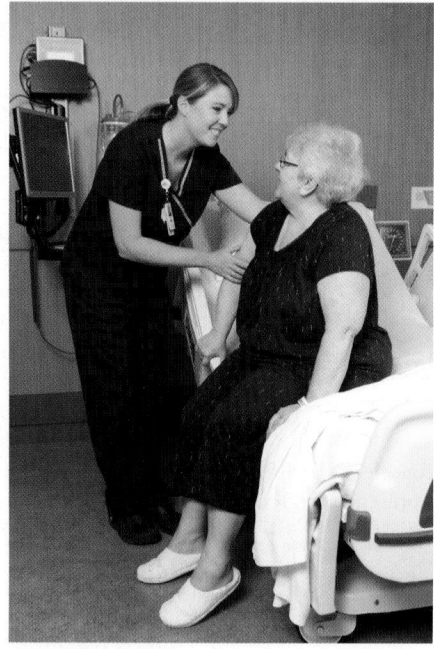

STEP 2e   Assisting patient to side of bed.

f Help sitting patient to standing position and allow to stand until balance is gained. Support by holding gait belt.

g Ask if patient feels dizzy or light-headed. If patient appears light-headed, sit him or her back down and recheck blood pressure.

h Care must be taken if patient has intravenous (IV) tubing or a Foley catheter. Obtain an IV pole with wheels that can be pushed as patient walks. Urinary catheter drainage bags must stay at or below level of bladder; a second person may be needed to assist.

Allows you to detect orthostatic hypotension before ambulation begins.

Allows patient to ambulate unencumbered.
Urine in tubing must not reenter bladder, which would increase risk of infection.

STEP	RATIONALE

Clinical Decision Point *Remove obstacles from pathways, including throw rugs, and wipe up any spills immediately. Avoid crowds. Crowds increase the risk of the crutch, cane, or walker being kicked or jarred and patient losing balance.*

3 Determining appropriate height of ambulation device, if used:

  a *Crutch measurement:* Includes three areas: Patient's height, distance between crutch pad and axilla, and angle of elbow flexion. Use one of two methods:

    (1) *Standing:* Position crutches with crutch tips at 15 cm (6 inches) to side and 15 cm in front of patient's feet (tripod position) and crutch pads 5 cm (2 inches) below axilla (Pierson and Fairchild, 2008) (see illustration).

    (2) *Supine:* Crutch pad is approximately 5 cm (2 inches) or two-to-three finger widths under axilla with crutch tips positioned 15 cm (6 inches) lateral to patient's heel (Pierson and Fairchild, 2008) (see illustration).

    (3) Instruct patient to report any tingling or numbness in upper torso.

    (4) Following correct crutch adjustment, two to three fingers must fit between top of crutch and axilla (see illustration).

Promotes optimal support and stability.

Radial nerve passes under axillary area superficially. If crutch is too long, it can cause pressure on axilla and radial nerve. Injury to radial nerve causes paralysis of elbow and wrist extensors, commonly called crutch palsy. *In addition, if crutch is too long, shoulders are forced upward, and patient cannot push body off the ground. If ambulation device is too short, patient is bent over and uncomfortable.*

May mean that crutches are being used incorrectly or that they are wrong size.

Adequate space prevents crutch palsy.

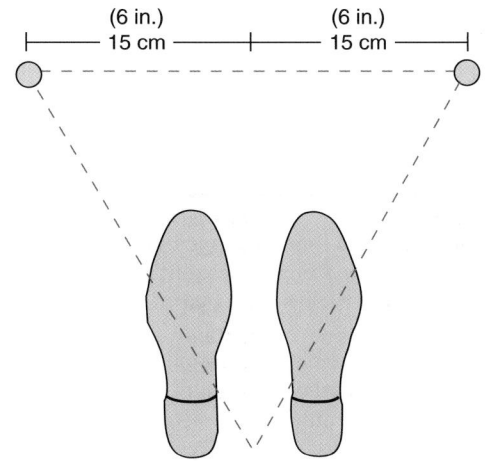

STEP 3a(1)   Tripod position.

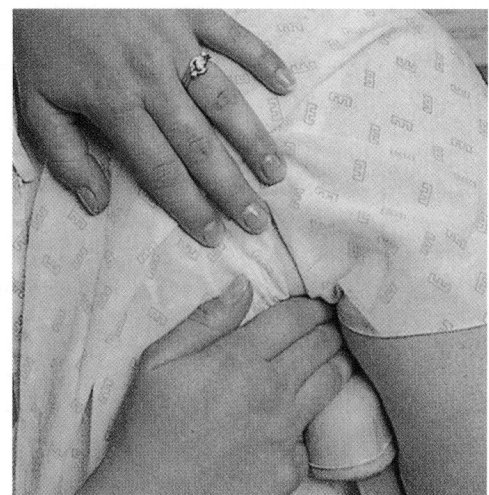

STEP 3a(4)   Top of crutch.

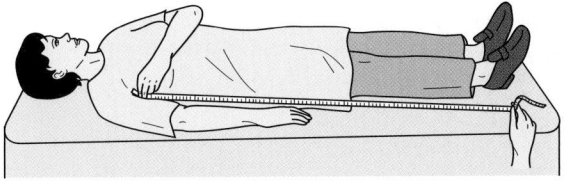

STEP 3a(2)   Supine method.

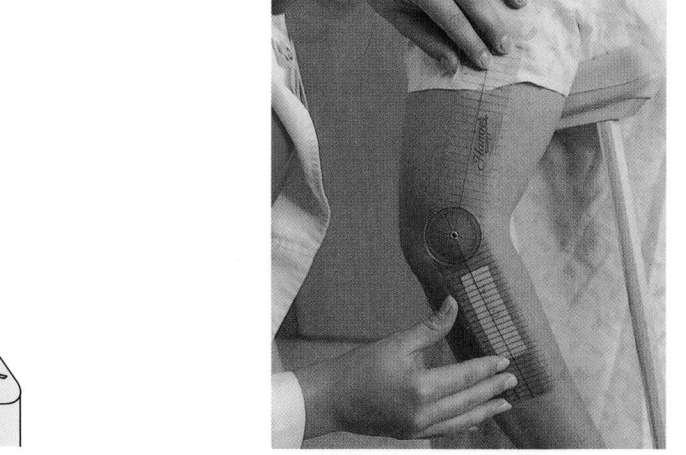

STEP 3a(5)   Elbows flexed. Verification of elbow flexion.

STEP	RATIONALE
(5) With either measurement method, elbows are flexed 15 to 30 degrees. Verify elbow flexion with goniometer (see illustration).	Angle ensures that arms can push body off ground. Obtain goniometer from physical therapy department.
(6) In addition to overall *length* of axillary crutch, *height* of handgrip is important. Both dimensions are adjustable on a well-made crutch, and ability to adjust these dimensions is an important feature for a growing child. Adjust handgrip so patient's elbow is slightly flexed.	If handgrip is too low, radial nerve damage can occur even if overall crutch length is correct because extra length between handgrip and axillary bar can force bar up into axilla as patient stretches down to reach handgrip. If handgrip is too high, patient's elbow is sharply flexed, and strength and stability of arms are decreased.
b *Cane measurement:* Patient holds cane on uninvolved side 10 to 15 cm (4 to 6 inches) to side of foot. Cane extends from greater trochanter to floor while it is held 15 cm (6 inches) from foot. Allow approximately 15 to 30 degrees of elbow flexion.	Offers most support when cane is placed on stronger side of body. Cane and weaker leg work together with each step. If cane is too short, patient has difficulty supporting weight and is bent over and uncomfortable. As weight is taken on by hand and affected leg is lifted off floor, complete extension of elbow is necessary.
c *Walker measurement:* Top of walker should match crease in wrist when patient stands up straight (American Academy of Orthopaedist Surgeons, 2011). Elbows are flexed at approximately 15 to 30 degrees when patient is standing inside walker with hands on handgrips.	Walker should be at proper height so patient does not bend forward.
4 Make sure that ambulation device has rubber tips.	Rubber tips prevent device from slipping.
5 Make sure that surface patient will walk on is clean and dry. Remove any objects that might obstruct pathway.	Prevents falls and injuries.

IMPLEMENTATION

1 Assisted ambulation with one nurse:	
a Before beginning ambulation, reconfirm that patient does not feel light-headed.	Helps patient gain balance before attempting ambulation and ensures that patient will not become faint while walking.
b Perform hand hygiene. Be sure gait belt is secure. Help patient to standing position; observe balance.	Reduces transmission of microorganisms. Prevents injury. Gait belt encircles patient's waist and has space for you to hold while patient walks. If patient appears weak or unsteady, return him or her to bed.
c Have patient take a few steps while you stand on his or her stronger side. If assistive device (e.g., cane, walker) is used, stand on patient's weak side.	If patient has hemiplegia (one-sided paralysis) or hemiparesis (one-sided weakness), stand next to patient's strong, unaffected side and support him or her by placing arm closest to him or her on gait belt.
d Stand and grasp gait belt in middle of patient's back.	If patient begins to fall, this position allows you to move him or her to stronger side and reduce injury. Provides support at waist so patient's center of gravity remains midline.
e Take a few steps forward with patient. Then assess for strength and balance.	Ensures that patient has satisfactory strength and balance to continue.
f If patient becomes weak or dizzy, return him or her to bed or chair, whichever is closer.	Allows patient to rest.
g If patient begins to fall, gently ease him or her to floor by holding firmly onto gait belt; stand with feet apart to provide broad base of support, extend leg, and let patient gently slide to floor. As patient slides, bend your knees to lower body (see illustrations).	You can cause more damage to self and patient by trying to catch patient.
2 Assisted ambulation with two nurses:	
a Follow Steps 1a and b.	
b Have a nurse stand on either side of patient.	
c Both nurses grasp gait belt in middle of patient's back.	Provides secure grip for each nurse.
d Step forward in unison with patient, keeping speed and step size same as patient's.	Ensures patient's stability.
e Gradually increase distance walked.	Strengthens muscles, increases endurance, and prevents patient from becoming too fatigued.
f If patient becomes weak or dizzy, follow Step 1f.	

STEP	RATIONALE

3 Ambulation with assistive devices:

a Help patient crutch walk by choosing appropriate crutch gait:

To use crutches, patient supports self with hands and arms; therefore strength in arm and shoulder muscles, ability to balance body in upright position, and stamina are necessary. Type of gait patient uses in crutch walking depends on amount of weight that he or she is able to support with one or both legs.

  (1) Four-point gait:

This is the most stable crutch gait because it provides at least three points of support at all times. Patient must be able to bear weight on both legs. Patient moves each leg alternately with each opposing crutch so that three points of support are on the floor all the time. Often used when patient has some form of paralysis, such as for children with spastic cerebral palsy (Hockenberry and Wilson, 2011). May also be used for arthritic patients.

   (a) Begin in tripod position. Place crutches 15 cm (6 inches) in front and 15 cm (6 inches) to side of each foot. Have patient place weight on handgrips, not under arms [see Planning Step 3a(1)].

Improves patient's balance by providing wide base of support. Patient should have a posture of erect head and neck, straight vertebrae, and extended hips and knees.

   (b) Move right crutch forward 10 to 15 cm (4 to 6 inches) (see illustration A).

Crutch and foot position is similar to arm and foot position during normal walking.

   (c) Move left foot forward to level of left crutch (see illustration B).

   (d) Move left crutch forward 10 to 15 cm (4 to 6 inches) (see illustration C).

   (e) Move right foot forward to level of right crutch (see illustration D).

   (f) Repeat above sequence.

  (2) Three-point gait:

Requires patient to bear all weight on one foot. Weight is borne on strong leg and then on both crutches. Affected leg does not touch ground during early phase of three-point gait. May be useful for patient with broken leg or sprained ankle.

   (a) Begin in tripod position (see illustration A).

Improves patient's balance by providing wide base of support.

   (b) Advance both crutches and affected leg (see illustration B).

   (c) Move stronger leg forward, stepping on floor (see illustration C).

   (d) Repeat sequence.

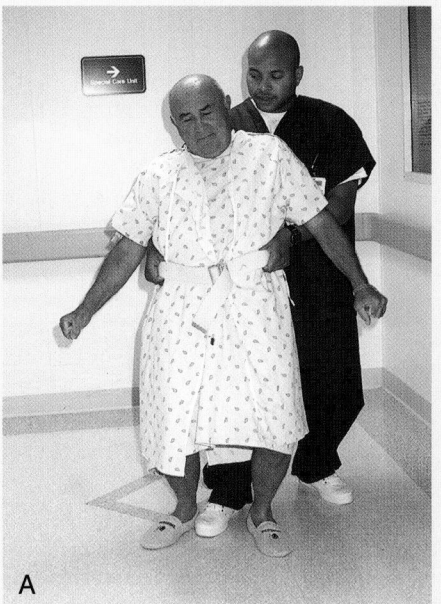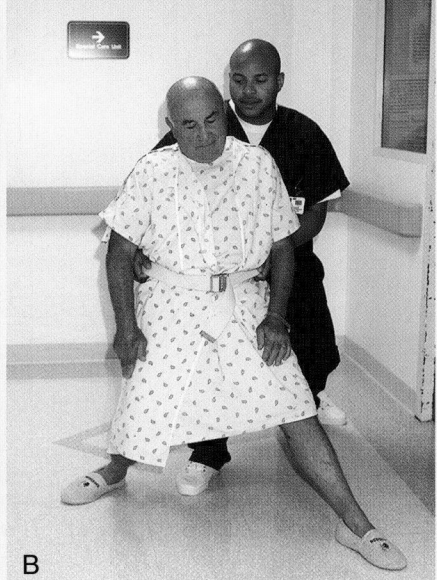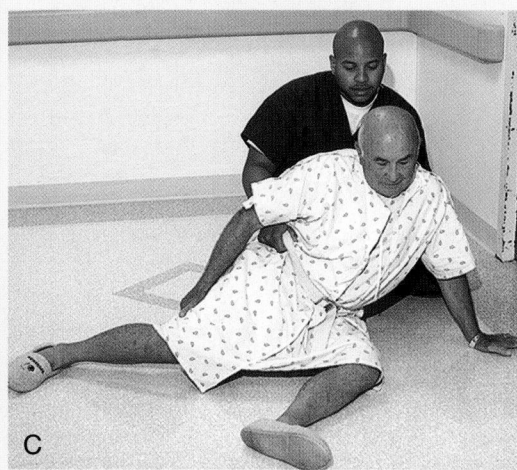

STEP 1g   **A,** Stand with feet apart to provide broad base of support. **B,** Extend one leg and let patient slide against it to the floor. **C,** Bend knees to lower body as patient slides to floor.

STEP	RATIONALE
(3) Two-point gait:	Requires at least partial weight bearing on each foot. Is faster than the four-point gait. Requires more balance because only two points support body at one time.
(a) Begin in tripod position (see illustration A).	Improves patient's balance by providing wide base of support.
(b) Move left crutch and right foot forward (see illustration B).	Crutch movements are similar to arm movement during normal walking; patient moves crutch at same time as opposing leg.
(c) Move right crutch and left foot forward (see illustration C).	
(d) Repeat sequence.	
(4) Swing-to gait:	Frequently used by patients whose lower extremities are paralyzed or who wear weight-supporting braces on their legs.
(a) Begin in tripod position.	This is the easier of two swinging gaits. It requires ability to partially bear body weight on both legs.
(b) Move both crutches forward.	
(c) Lift and swing legs to crutches, letting crutches support body weight.	
(d) Repeat two previous steps.	
(5) Swing-through gait:	Requires that patient have ability to bear partial weight on both feet.

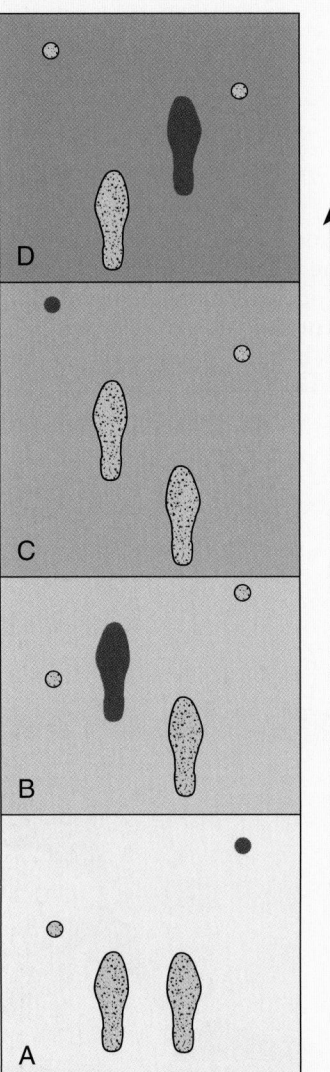

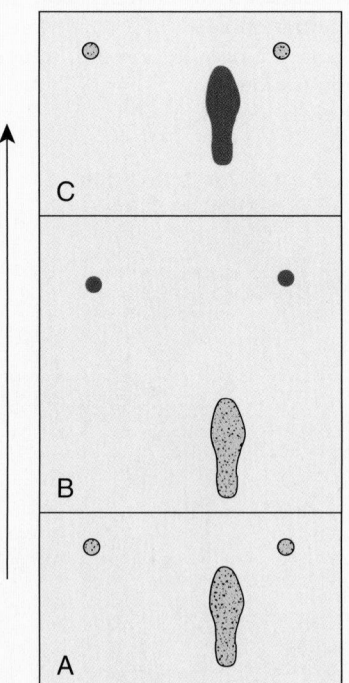

STEP 3a(1)(b-e)   Four-point gait. Solid feet and crutch tips show foot and crutch tip movement in each of four phases. (Read from bottom to top.) **A**, Right tip moves forward. **B**, Left foot moves toward left crutch. **C**, Left crutch tip moves forward. **D**, Right foot moves toward right crutch.

STEP 3a(2)(a-c)   Three-point gait with weight borne on unaffected right leg. Solid foot and crutch tips show weight bearing in each phase. (Read from bottom to top.)

STEP	RATIONALE
(a) Begin in tripod position.	Improves patient's balance by providing wide base of support.
(b) Move both crutches forward.	Initial placement of crutches is to increase patient's base of support so, when the body swings forward, patient is moving center of gravity toward additional support provided by crutches.
(c) Lift and swing legs through and beyond crutches.	
b Helping patient climb stairs with crutches:	
(1) Begin in tripod position.	Improves patient's balance by providing wide base of support.
(2) Patient transfers body weight to crutches (see illustration).	Prepares patient to transfer weight to strong leg when ascending first stair.

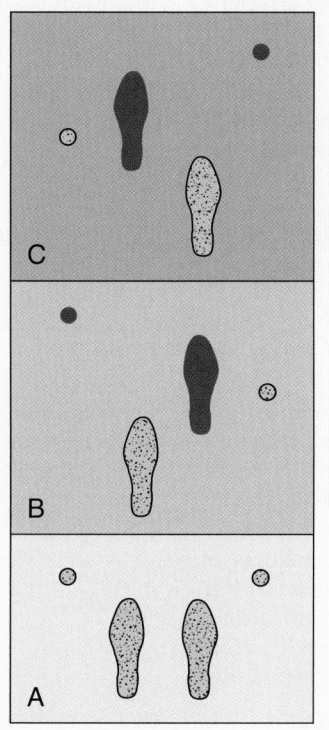

STEP 3a(3)(a-c)   Two-point gait. Solid areas indicate weight-bearing leg and crutch tips. (Read from bottom to top.)

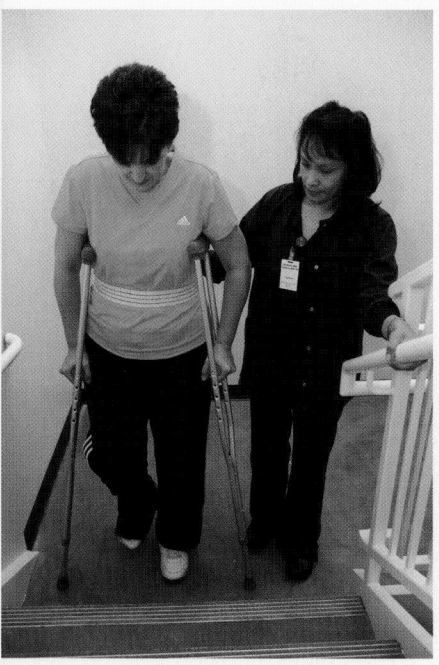

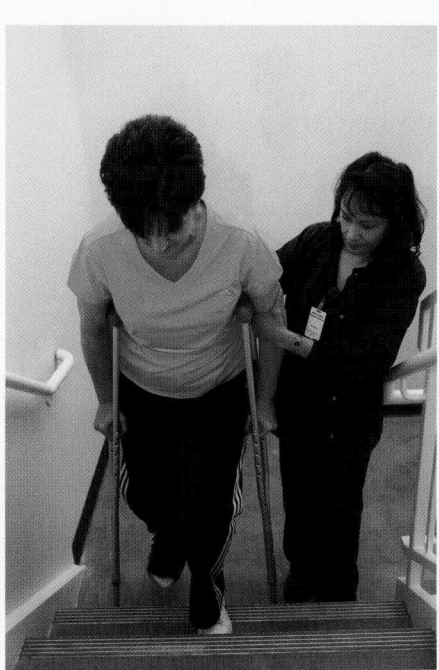

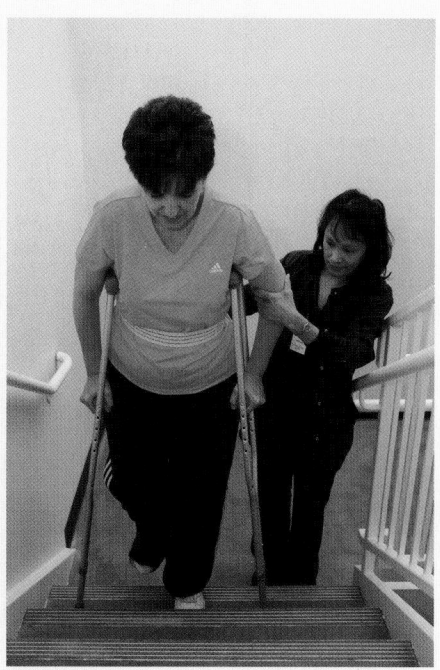

STEP 3b(2)   Transfer body weight to crutches.   **STEP 3b(3)**   Advance unaffected leg to stair.   **STEP 3b(4)**   Align crutches with unaffected leg.

STEP	RATIONALE
(3) Patient advances strong, unaffected leg to stair (see illustration).	Crutch adds support to affected leg. Patient then shifts weight from crutches to strong leg.
(4) Both crutches are aligned with strong, unaffected leg on stairs (see illustration).	Maintains balance and provides wide base of support.
(5) Repeat sequence until patient reaches top of stairs.	
c Helping patient descend stairs with crutches:	
(1) Begin in tripod position.	Improves patient's balance by providing wide base of support.
(2) Patient transfers body weight to unaffected, strong leg, and aligns with crutches (see illustration).	Prepares patient to release support of body weight maintained by crutches.
(3) With weight on unaffected, strong leg, patient positions crutches firmly on lower stair and steps down with affected leg. Weight is supported by crutches (see illustration).	Maintains balance and provides base of support.
(4) Unaffected leg is brought down to lower stair, aligned with crutches, and tripod position is resumed (see illustration).	
(5) Repeat sequence until stairs are descended.	
d Helping patient ambulate with walker (see illustration):	Patients who are able to bear partial weight use walkers. Walkers do need to be picked up, so patient needs sufficient strength to be able to pick it up. Four-wheeled models do not need to be picked up; however, they are not as stable.
(1) Have patient stand straight in the center of walker and grasp handgrips on upper bars.	Patient balances self before attempting to walk.
(2) Have patient lift walker; move it 15 to 20 cm (6 to 8 inches) forward; and then set it down, making sure that all four feet of walker stay on floor. Patient then takes a step forward with either foot and follows through with the other leg.	Provides broad base of support between walker and patient. Patient then moves center of gravity toward walker. Keeping all four feet of walker on floor is necessary to prevent tipping walker.
(3) After walker is advanced, if unilateral weakness is present, instruct patient to step forward with weaker leg, support self with arms, and follow through with strong leg. If patient is unable to bear weight on one leg, after advancing walker have patient swing into it, supporting weight on hands.	

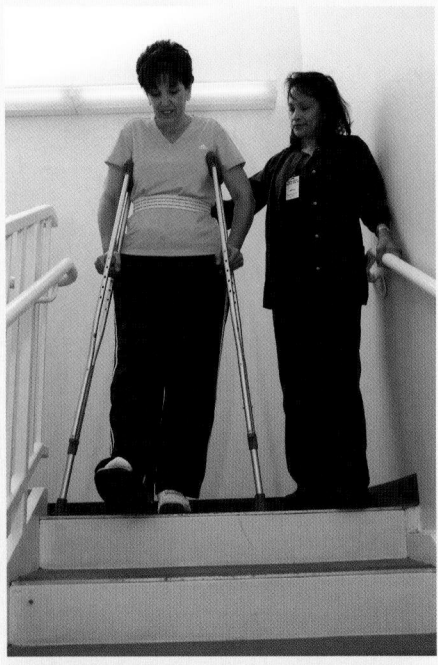

STEP 3c(2) Body weight is transferred to unaffected leg.

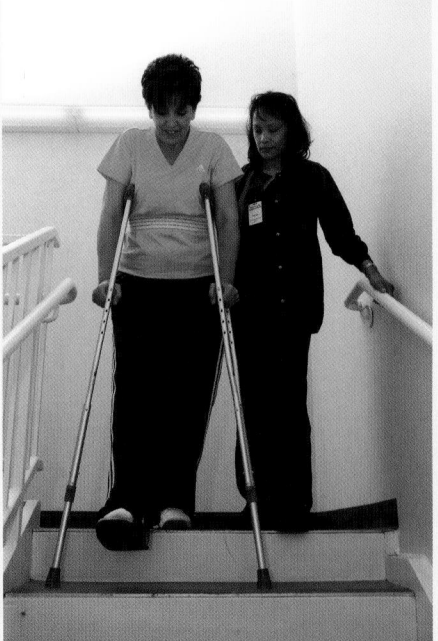

STEP 3c(3) Transfer weight to crutches.

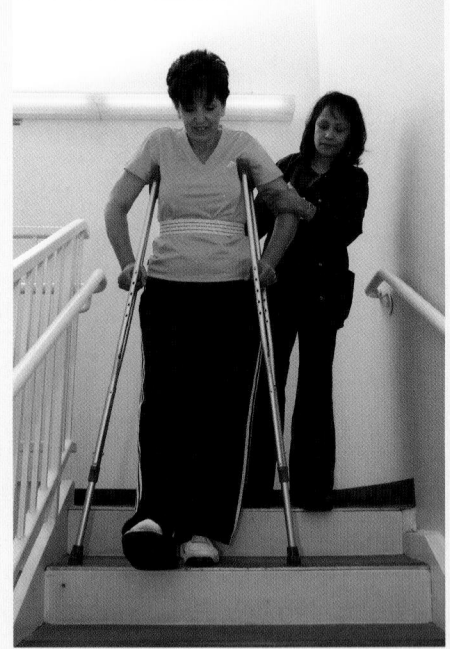

STEP 3c(4) Move unaffected leg and align crutches.

STEP	RATIONALE
e **Helping patient ambulate with cane (steps are same with standard or quad canes) (see illustrations):**	
(1) Begin by having patient place cane on side of strong leg.	Provides added support for weak or impaired side.
(2) Place cane forward 15 to 25 cm (6 to 10 inches), keeping body weight on both legs.	Distributes body weight equally.
(3) Have patient stand straight, look straight ahead, and move involved leg forward, even with cane.	Body weight is supported by cane and uninvolved leg.
(4) Advance strong leg past cane.	Body weight is supported by cane and strong leg.

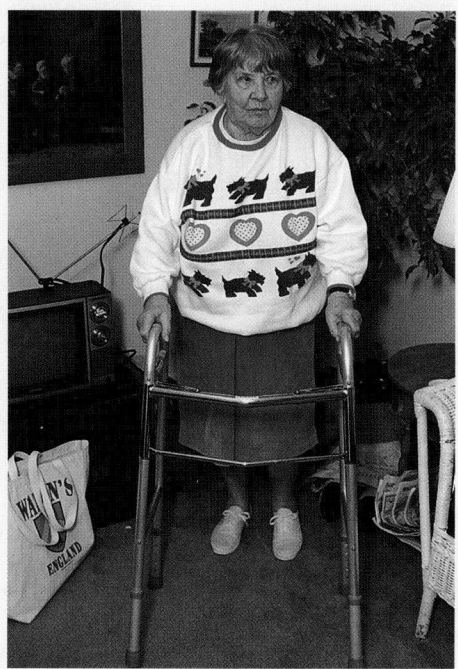

STEP 3d   Walker.

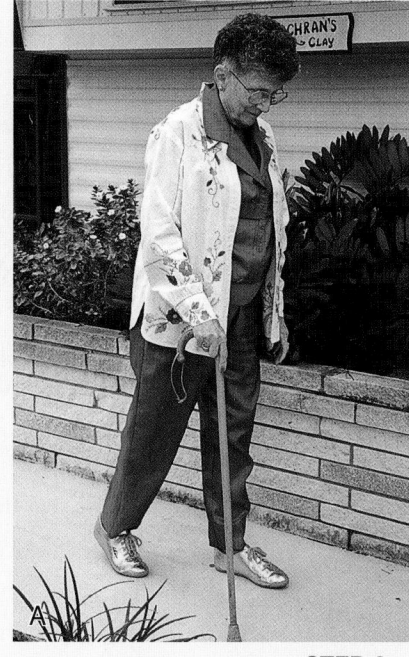

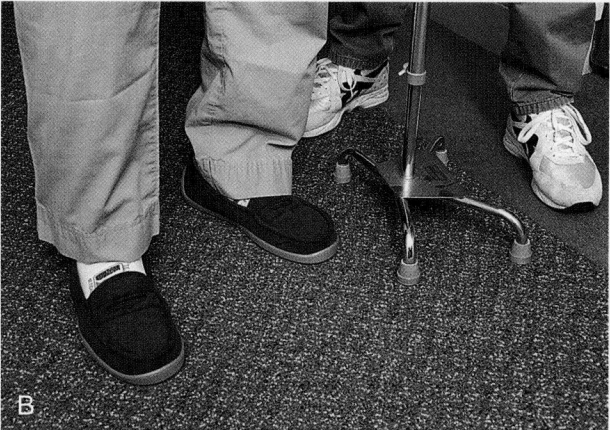

STEP 3e   **A**, Standard cane. **B**, Quad cane.

STEP	RATIONALE
(5) Move involved leg forward, even with strong leg.	Aligns patient's center of gravity. Returns patient's body weight to equal distribution.
(6) Repeat these steps.	

EVALUATION

1 After ambulation, obtain patient's vital signs, observe skin color, and ask about patient's level of comfort and energy level.

2 Evaluate patient's subjective statements regarding experience.

3 Evaluate gait of patient, observing body alignment in standing position and balance.

4 Observe patient's ability to perform self-care activities.

Evaluates how patient tolerated procedure and whether there was progress in ambulation. Assesses stage of patient's illness and degree of convalescence when evaluating the process.

Evaluates activity tolerance.

Determines if patient is using supportive aids for ambulation correctly. Keep in mind patient's previous manner of ambulating when assessing gait.

Level of ambulation progresses.

Unexpected Outcomes

1 Patient is unable to ambulate because of fear of falling, physical discomfort, upper body muscles that are too weak to use ambulation device, and lower extremities that are too weak to support body.

2 Patient sustains injury.

3 When using cane or walker, patient bends over, does not stand straight.

Related Interventions

- Initiate isometric exercise program to strengthen upper body muscles.
- Provide analgesia if needed.

- Notify health care provider. Return patient to bed if injury stable.
- Reinforce correct posture.

Recording and Reporting

- Record in the nurses' notes and EHR the type of gait patient used, assist device, amount of assistance required, distance walked, and activity tolerance.
- Immediately report any injury sustained during attempts to ambulate, alteration in vital signs, or inability to ambulate to nurse in charge or health care provider.

Special Considerations
Teaching

- Instruct patient that exercises such as squeezing a rubber ball, raising and lowering both arms in a slow and rhythmic manner while holding weights, pushups, and pull-ups help to strengthen the upper extremities.
- Teach patients using walkers to examine the frame daily. When inspecting a walker, the patient should observe for signs of bending or deformation of the frame, protruding screws that can scratch, and loose or missing screws that weaken the joints of the frame. Assess handgrips for any cracks or signs of being loose.
- Instruct patients to use the arms of a chair rather than the walker to give them leverage when getting up from a chair; the walker is likely to tip if used for this purpose.
- Blistering or soreness of the hands can result from continual pressure between the hand and the handle of a crutch. Advise patient to release pressure intermittently and wear gloves or pad the handle to reduce friction.

- Instruct patient that, if wearing shoes with varying heel sizes, the crutches need to be adjusted to maintain two-to-three fingers between the axilla and the crutch.

Pediatric

- For rehabilitation of a small child who has not yet learned to walk or who is unsteady, special crutches with three or four legs provide needed stability to allow the child to maintain an upright posture and learn to walk (Hockenberry and Wilson, 2011).
- Another option for children who are just learning to walk would be front- or rear-rolling walkers.

Gerontologic

- The older adult may require additional time in the morning before resuming activities.

Home Care

- Teach patient how to use the ambulation aid on various terrains (e.g., carpet, stairs, rough ground, inclines). Teach him or her how to maneuver around obstacles such as doors and how to use the aid when transferring to and from a chair, toilet, and tub.
- Teach family caregivers how to assist and what to observe to ensure that an assistive device is used correctly.

Long-Term Care

- Conduct safety and maintenance checks of ambulation devices on a routine basis.
- Perform periodic assessments to ensure that the patient is using the ambulation device properly.

Critical Thinking Exercises

Mr. Timber, 78 years old, is hospitalized for a right total knee replacement. He has a medical history of diabetes mellitus. He is now 1 day postoperative following right knee replacement. He rates his pain as 8 on a scale of 0 to 10. Postoperative orders include ambulating with crutches today and using the continuous passive motion (CPM) machine 4 times a day.

1 As you discuss the plan of care with Mr. Timber for the day, you include the need for ambulation with crutches. He states, "I'm not getting out of bed; I hurt and just had surgery." Discuss nursing interventions that will facilitate this patient's cooperation and participation.

2 Mr. Timber has several risk factors associated with the occurrence of orthostatic hypotension. Identify the nursing interventions needed to minimize orthostatic hypotension.

3 You are preparing to apply the CPM machine to Mr. Timber's right leg. Discuss several measures to ensure proper and safe functioning of this machine before application.

4 Mr. Timber needs crutches for approximately 4 to 6 weeks during his recovery. He is allowed no weight bearing on his right leg for the first week. What is the appropriate crutch gait for Mr. Timbers? Discuss several teaching considerations associated with the use of crutches.

REVIEW QUESTIONS

1 The nurse notes that a patient's left elbow is resistant to extension and flexion while performing range-of-motion exercises. What is the appropriate nursing action at this time?
1 Move the joint through the full range of motion.
2 Perform range of motion to the left elbow only until resistance is met.
3 Omit all the range-of-motion exercises until the health care provider is notified.
4 Tell the health care provider that the patient is uncooperative with exercising.

2 A patient has been immobile for more than 2 weeks. He notices dizziness the first time the nurse has him sit up, and he states feeling tired. He is now able to begin performing isometric exercises. Which nursing diagnosis best relates to the safety of this patient?
1 Fatigue
2 Impaired skin integrity
3 Disturbed body image
4 Risk for activity intolerance

3 The nurse suspects that a patient has a deep vein thrombosis (DVT) in the left lower leg. What is the priority nursing intervention at this time?
1 Perform test for Homans' sign immediately.
2 Massage the area gently to promote circulation.
3 Keep the patient calm and quiet in bed; notify physician.
4 Apply the ordered elastic stockings and sequential compression devices.

4 Which of the following activities may be delegated to nursing assistive personnel (NAP) related to helping patients with ambulation?
1 Checking the patient's medications to determine if they may influence the ability to ambulate independently
2 Instructing the patient about the correct use of a walker
3 Inspecting the environment for potential threats to patient safety
4 Evaluating the patient's ability to perform crutch walking

5 The nurse is preparing to ambulate a patient with left-sided weakness. Which action demonstrates appropriate care of this patient during ambulation?
1 Assign the strongest health care worker to ambulate her.
2 Stand on the left side of the patient during ambulation.
3 The patient holds her cane in her left hand while the nurse is behind her during ambulation.
4 The nurse should walk on the patient's right side.

6 A patient who is going to be using crutches asks about wearing shoes with varying size heels. What statement by the nurse is most accurate?
1 "You should wear shoes with the same size heel."
2 "Try to wear the same shoes for stability and safety."
3 "If you change heel sizes, the crutches will need adjusting."
4 "Wearing shoes with different heel sizes is fine as long as you're comfortable."

7 A patient with a left-sided weakness uses a cane. Where should the nurse stand while ambulating this patient?
1 On the patient's left side
2 On the patient's right side
3 Slightly in front on the patient's left side
4 Slightly behind the patient's right side

8 A patient is being taught how to get up from the chair to his walker. The nurse knows that teaching has been successful when the patient statement includes which of the following?
1 "Use the walker's handgrips to give myself leverage."
2 "Get toward the back of the chair."
3 "Rock myself several times to get up."
4 "Use the arms of the chair to push up to the walker."

9 A patient using a continuous passive motion (CPM) machine reports a sore area on the heel of the affected leg. Which intervention by the nurse would be done first?
1 Checking the functioning of the CPM machine
2 Performing skin care on the affected extremity
3 Notifying the health care provider
4 Assessing the skin on both lower extremities

10 The nurse is helping a patient to the side of the bed and recognizes that the patient is experiencing orthostatic hypotension. Which of the following signs and symptoms alert the nurse to this condition? (Select all that apply.)
1 Pallor
2 Bradycardia
3 Nausea
4 Dizziness
5. Irritability

REFERENCES

American Academy of Orthopaedist Surgeons: How to use crutches, canes, and walkers, available at http://orthoinfo.aaos.org/topic.cfm?topic=A00181, accessed December 2011.

Burtin C, et al: Early exercise in critically ill patients enhances short-term functional recovery, *Crit Care Med* 37(9):2499, 2009.

Chodzko-Zajko WJ, et al: Exercise and physical activity for older adults, *Med Sci Sports Exercise* 41(7):1500, 2009.

Christo P, et al: Effective treatments for pain in the older patient, *Curr Pain Headache Rep* 15:22, 2011.

Chrysant S: Current evidence on the hemodynamic and blood pressure effects of isometric exercise in normotensive and hypertensive persons, *J Clin Hypertension* 12(9):721, 2010.

Craig L, et al: Early mobilization after stroke: an example of an individual patient data meta-analysis of a complex intervention, *Stroke* 41(11):2632, 2010.

De Kam D, et al: Exercise interventions to reduce fall-related fractures and their risk factors in individuals with low bone density: a systematic review of randomized controlled trials, *Osteoporosis Int* 20(12):2111, 2009.

Granacher U, et al: An intergenerational approach in the promotion of balance and strength for fall prevention—a mini review, *Gerontology* 57:304, 2011.

Harvard Health Publications: On the alert for deep-vein blood clots, *Harvard Heart Lett* 19(9):4, 2009.

Hockenberry MJ, Wilson D: *Wong's nursing care of infants and children*, ed 9, St Louis, 2011, Mosby.

Huether S, McCance K: *Understanding pathophysiology*, ed 4, St Louis, 2008, Mosby.

Ignatavicius D, Workman L: *Medical surgical nursing: critical thinking for collaborative care*, ed 6, St Louis, 2009, Mosby.

Janelli L, et al: Can an exercise program enhance mood among Hispanic elders? *Medsurg Nurs* 18:356, 2009.

Johnson K, et al: Physiological rationale and current evidence for therapeutic positioning of critically ill patients, *AACN Adv Crit Care* 20(3):228, 2009.

Lewis S, et al: *Medical-surgical nursing: Assessment and management of clinical problems*, ed 8, St Louis, 2011, Mosby.

Long F: A healing machine, *Rehabil Manage Interdiscip J Rehabil* 21(5):34, 2008. http://www.rehabpub.com/issues/articles/2008-06_07.asp, accessed June 13, 2012.

Paganini-Hill A, et al: Activities and mortality in the elderly: the Leisure World Cohort Study, *J Gerontol* 66A(5):559, 2011.

Peterson M, et al: Resistance exercise for the aging adult: clinical implications and prescription guidelines, *Am J Med* 124(3):194, 2011.

Pierson F, Fairchild S: *Principles & techniques of patient care*, ed 4, St Louis, 2008, Saunders/Elsevier.

Schneider J, et al: Cognitive-behavioral therapy, exercise, and older adults' quality of life, *West J Nurs Res* 30:704, 2008.

Sherrington D, et al: Effective exercise for the prevention of falls: a systematic review and meta-analysis, *J Am Geriatr Soc* 56(12):2234, 2008.

Simpson J, et al: Muslim women's experience with health care providers in a rural area of the United States, *J Transcult Health Care* 19(1):16, 2008.

The Joint Commission (TJC): *National Patient Safety Goals*, Oakbrook Terrace, Ill, 2012, The Commission, available at http://www.jointcommission.org/standards_information/npsgs.aspx.

Thompson P, et al: Non-pharmacological treatments for orthostatic hypotension, *Age Aging* 40(3):292, 2011.

Touhy T, et al: *Ebersole and Hess's Gerontological nursing and healthy aging*, ed 3, St Louis, 2010, Mosby.

Orthopedic Measures

SKILLS AND PROCEDURES

MEDIA RESOURCES

- **evolve** http://evolve.elsevier.com/Perry/skills

  - Review Questions
  - Audio Glossary

KEY TERMS

Cast	External fixation	Reduction	Thomas splint
Cast saw	Pearson attachment	Spica cast	Traction
Comminuted fracture	Petaling	Spreader bar	Traction boot
Compartment syndrome	Pulleys	Stockinette	Walking cast boot
Countertraction			

OBJECTIVES

Mastery of content in this chapter will enable the nurse to:

- Discuss the purposes of different orthopedic immobilization devices.
- Describe neurovascular assessments for a patient with an orthopedic injury.
- Describe how to assist in the application of a cast.
- Describe how to care for a patient with a casted extremity.

- Explain the purposes of placing a patient into skeletal or skin traction.
- Explain turning and positioning techniques for patients with impaired mobility.
- Describe strategies to prevent complications from immobility.
- Discuss nursing considerations for the patient with an immobilization device.

Trauma or disease to the musculoskeletal system often requires immobilization, stabilization, and support to affected body parts. Traction, casts, and immobilization devices are examples of methods used to accomplish these purposes and enhance the healing process. When using any of these devices, it is essential that integumentary tissues must remain healthy and intact, both inside and outside of a device. Assessment of the skin includes the detection of pressure, inflammation, irritation, or lesions that could lead to the development of pressure ulcers or infection. Turning, positioning, and range-of-motion (ROM) exercises help to maintain the health of the integumentary tissues and the comfort of the extremity. Orthopedic devices are used to correct or improve deformities or joint contractures. They are also used to treat joint dislocation; reduce, immobilize, and align a fracture (Box 11-1); and prevent and manage muscle spasms. By controlling spasms

and fractured bones, these devices prevent further soft tissue damage. Finally preoperative and postoperative positioning and alignment, skeletal lengthening, and rest of a damaged joint are managed using one or more of these devices.

Traction involves a pulling force applied through use of weights on a part of the body while a second force called *counter traction* pulls in the opposite direction. Age, condition of a patient, and purpose of the traction determine the amount of weight on the pulling force. In straight or running traction the force pulls against the long axis of the body while a patient's body supplies the counter traction. In balanced-suspension skeletal traction (BSST) the amount of force in the traction is equal to the amount of force in the counter traction. A sling or hammock and a system of weights attached to an over-bed frame support the affected part while weight is attached to the pin or wire traversing the femoral bone.

BOX 11-1	Types of Fractures

Closed fracture: Skin intact over fracture
Open or compound fracture: Skin punctured by bone ends
Comminuted: Having three or more bone fragments
Depressed: Bone fragments pushed inward
Displaced: Two parts of fracture that have moved out of alignment
Impacted: Bone ends pushed into one another
Longitudinal: Fracture that runs parallel with bone
Oblique: Facture that slants across bone
Pathologic: Results from minor stress applied to pathologically
    weakened bone
Segmental: Segment of bone fractured and detached
Spiral: Twisting around the bone
Transverse: Across the bone

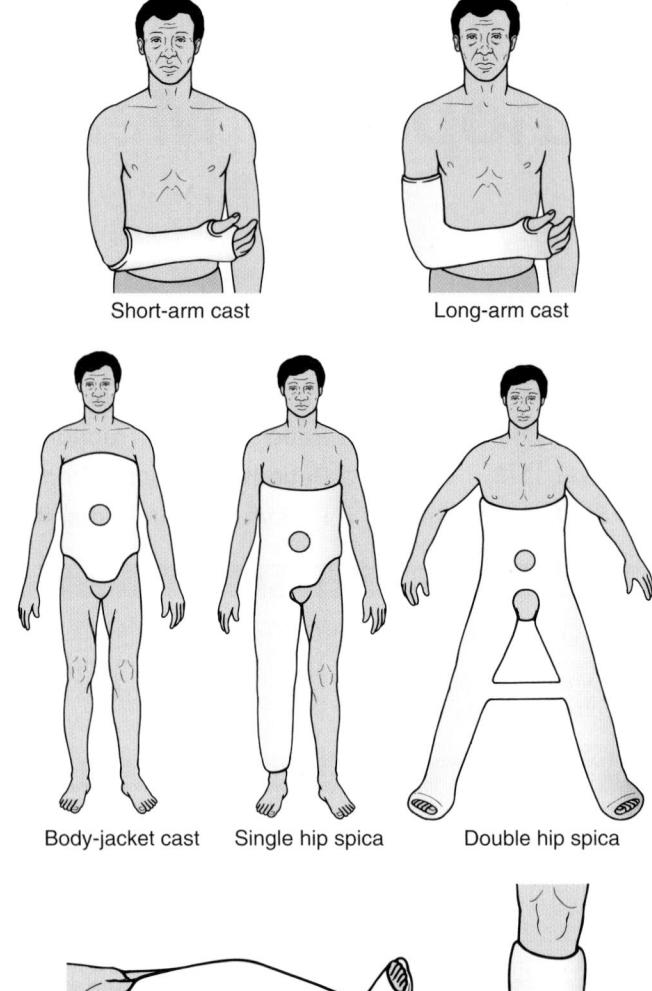

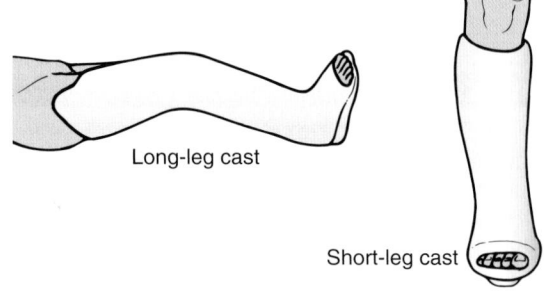

FIG 11-1 Common types of casts.

Although there are many types of traction, there are six general principles of traction care: (1) maintain the established line of pull, (2) maintain the traction equipment, (3) maintain counter traction, (4) maintain continuous traction unless otherwise ordered, (5) maintain correct body alignment, and (6) prevent friction and pressure on the skin (Whiting, 2008).

A second treatment method for immobilization involves the use of a cast (Fig. 11-1). Applied externally, a cast immobilizes injured or deformed musculoskeletal tissues in proper position to promote healing. Therefore tissue structures must be in optimal position for healing when the cast is applied. An advantage of using a cast is that it permits early ambulation and in some cases partial weight bearing on the injured extremity.

A third treatment device used with musculoskeletal injury or disorder is the orthotic device. These devices immobilize a body part, prevent deformity, protect against injury, relieve pain and muscle spasm, maintain position until healing is complete, and assist with function. Immobilization devices are applied externally to the body and are available in many varieties, ranging from arm slings to back braces and finger splints. They are made from different materials such as rubber, leather, metal, and plastic.

Walker boots manage soft tissue injury, sprains, stable toe and ankle fractures, and promote postoperative early weight bearing for internal fixation with ligament tears. They provide musculoskeletal stabilization and support through the use of pneumatics. Research has shown that there is no loss of stability when a walker boot is used (Hyer et al., 2010).

EVIDENCE-BASED PRACTICE

The treatment of complicated fractures often includes the use of pins and plates to stabilize the bones and promote healing. The use of external fixation devices allows for early mobilization of patients, increase in patient comfort and compliance, and discharge to home. One of the most common complications is pin tract infections; thus meticulous pin care is essential. To date there is insufficient evidence to be able to identify a single effective strategy of pin-site care that minimizes infection rates (Lethaby et al., 2011). The level of evidence for pin-site care is low, but guidelines outlined by Voda (2011) parallel recommendations made by the National Association of Orthopedic Nurses (Holmes & Brown, 2005):

- Perform pin-site care once a day, twice a day, or weekly, depending on the amount of drainage, the stability of the bone, and pin sites.
- Clean pin site with chlorhexidine 2 mg/mL solution on stable pins (0.9% sodium chloride solution is used in many

agencies but has not been shown to be more effective than chlorhexidine).
- Antimicrobial ointment may be ordered for pin sites.
- Cover pin sites with sterile gauze or leave open to air.

PATIENT-CENTERED CARE

When a patient has had a musculoskeletal injury, patient-centered care focuses on minimizing pain managing stabilization and immobilization devices competently and recognizing how the injury affects a patient's general well-being. Routine assessment ensures that you can identify pain early and find appropriate comfort measures.

Explanation of procedures helps to minimize a patient's anxiety and fear. With orthopedic injuries the treatment often results in some degree of immobility and restriction. Lack of ability to function in a normal role may lead to feelings of frustration and even depression.

It is also important to understand a patient's cultural beliefs and values related to issues of immobility. For example, Muslim patients do not accept instructions regarding the use of the alternative hand for hygiene after toileting since in that culture the right hand is traditionally used for clean tasks, and the left for dirty tasks.

Maintain privacy of a patient in a cast or in traction by draping him or her adequately and closing the bedside curtain. Most likely the extremity will be elevated, which may inadvertently leave the patient exposed. Female modesty is valued in many cultures (Spector, 2008).

Safety Guidelines

1 Frequently assess a patient's neurovascular status to identify early impairment of any sensory changes. It is essential to monitor the five P's (pain, pallor, pulselessness, paresthesia, and paralysis) of neurovascular status because permanent damage results if circulation is not maintained or restored.

2 Determine the permitted ROM for the extremity in a cast or traction. Although it is important to maintain the mobility of the joint, do not move the extremity beyond the limitations of the cast or traction device. Excessive movement impairs wound healing, limits new bone growth, and affects alignment of the extremity.

3 Determine a patient's prior level of functioning. Knowing what a patient was able to do assists in determining what level of assistance is now required.

4 Determine a patient's normal pattern of elimination. Immobility and analgesics can alter it.

5 Review the type of analgesic frequency ordered for the patient by the health care provider. During the first few days the patient may experience acute continuous pain as part of the inflammatory stage, with or without muscle spasms, and needs aggressive pain assessment and management (Voda, 2011).

SKILL 11-1   Assisting with Cast Application

A cast immobilizes an injured extremity to protect it from further injury, provides alignment of a fracture by holding the bone fragments in reduction and alignment during the healing process, and promotes comfort. In addition, a cast maintains a limb in alignment to prevent or correct deformity. Casts are used in many different ways. The use and type of application materials depend on the anatomic area of injury.

Casts materials are natural (plaster of Paris), synthetic acrylic, fiberglass free, latex-free polymer, or a combination of materials. Plaster of Paris is composed of several layers of open-weave cotton roll or strips covered with calcium sulfate crystals. When moistened with water, this material molds easily during application; but drying takes anywhere from 24 to 72 hours, depending on the size of the cast. During drying the cast must be exposed to air, well supported on a firm surface, handled with palms (not fingertips) to avoid indentations, and turned regularly so it dries evenly. Weight bearing is delayed until a cast is completely dry.

Synthetic casting materials are composed of open-weave fiberglass tape covered with a polyurethane resin that is activated by water. This cast sets very quickly, in approximately 15 minutes, and withstands pressure and weight bearing after 20 minutes. It forms a lightweight, sturdy cast that is radiolucent and waterproof. Different colors of this casting material are also available (e.g., pink, purple, navy), which appeal to children and help to maintain the appearance of the cast. These casts are more expensive than plaster casts.

This skill includes frequent assessments before, during, and after cast application, including peripheral neurovascular status. In addition, optimal skin care is important, including removal of dirt and debris before cast application and removal of any plaster crumbs after application.

Delegation and Collaboration

The skill of assisting with cast application may be delegated to nursing assistive personnel (NAP). The nurse instructs the NAP by:

- Instructing them in the method of positioning a specific patient with mobility restrictions.
- Explaining the patient self-reports (e.g., pain, numbness in fingers or toes) to report to a nurse as soon as possible.

Equipment (may be on cast cart) (Fig. 11-2)

❏ Plaster rolls (sizes include 2-, 3-, 4-, and 6-inch rolls) or cast materials such as fiberglass, casting tape, or plastic, depending on purpose of cast or specific patient condition
❏ Padding material (felt, stockinette, Webril, or gore lining)
❏ Plastic-lined bucket or basin filled three-fourths full with warm water
❏ Clean gloves, apron, or protective cover
❏ Cart, chair, and fracture table scissors
❏ Paper or plastic sheets
❏ Cast cutter (if old cast is to be removed)
❏ Clean cast saw blades

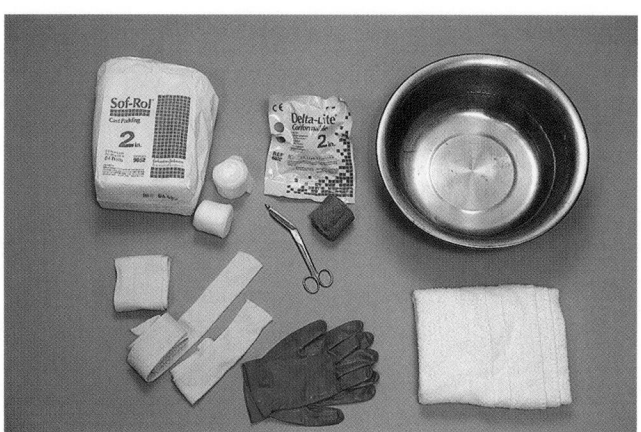

FIG 11-2   Casting materials.

STEP	RATIONALE

ASSESSMENT

1 Assess patient's ability to cooperate and level of understanding concerning the cast application process.

Sudden movement during procedure could cause injury.

2 Inspect condition of skin that will be under the cast. Specifically note any areas of skin breakdown, rashes, bruising, or incisional wound.

Determines need for additional skin care before cast application. Provides baseline for close observation after cast is applied.

Clinical Decision Point *Patients with skin breakdown or skin lesions may not be candidates for casting.*

3 Assess neurovascular status of area to be casted. Specifically note alteration of motor and sensory function and skin color, temperature, and capillary refill. Compare with opposite extremity or surrounding tissues. Pay attention to tissues distal to the cast.

Changes in neurovascular status may occur after casting; thus it is important to know baseline status.

4 Assess patient's pain status on a scale of 0 to 10.

Pain scale provides baseline to determine efficacy of nursing comfort measures.

5 Determine extent to which patient will be able to use casted extremity.

Predicts degree of assistance that is needed for self-care and/or ambulation.

6 Assess patient's understanding of the normal bone healing process.

Serves as a baseline for teaching patient how to care for casted extremity in the home.

NURSING DIAGNOSES

- Acute pain
- Bathing, dressing, and toileting self-care deficit
- Deficient knowledge

- Impaired home maintenance
- Impaired physical mobility
- Ineffective peripheral tissue perfusion
- Risk for impaired skin integrity

- Risk for injury
- Risk for peripheral neurovascular dysfunction

Related factors are individualized based on patient's condition or needs.

PLANNING

1 Expected outcomes following completion of procedure:
- Patient has edema of ≥1+, soreness, mild pain, and some limitation of range of motion (ROM), but less than 25% decrease in active ROM of affected extremity after cast application.

Cast limits normal function of affected tissues.

- Skin of tissues below cast is warm and pink, with capillary refill of less than 2 seconds. Pulses distal to cast are palpable, strong, and regular.

Neurovascular function to body part is maintained (Boyd et al., 2009).

- Patient verbalizes no abnormal or unusual sensations and is able to move fingers or toes below casted part.
- Cast remains clean, without indentations or fraying, until removal.

Skin is free of pressure and friction from cast edges.

- Patient requires minimal assistance with usual activities of daily living (ADLs) after extremity is casted.

Cast may interfere with ability to dress, feed, or bathe oneself.

- Patient verbalizes comfort after cast in place. Rates pain less than 4 on a scale of 0 to 10.

Injured tissues and bone are stabilized.

- Patient verbalizes cast care techniques.

Verbalizes cast care instructions and techniques.

2 Instruct patient, parent, and other caregivers how to facilitate application of cast by maintaining affected part in desired position.

Cast holds tissues in position in which they are held during cast application. Patient teaching reduces anxiety and increases cooperation.

IMPLEMENTATION

1 Identify patient using two identifiers (i.e., name and birthday or name and account number) according to agency policy. Compare identifiers with information on patient's identification bracelet.

Ensures correct patient. Complies with The Joint Commission standards and improves patient safety (2012).

2 Administer analgesic before cast application: oral (PO), 30 to 40 minutes before; intramuscular (IM), 20 to 30 minutes before; intravenous (IV) 2 to 5 minutes before. If patient has a patient-controlled analgesic pump (PCA), instruct him or her to administer a dose 2 to 5 minutes before the cast application.

Reduces pain during cast application. Provides optimal analgesic effect. Often muscle spasms are treated more effectively with skeletal muscle relaxants than with opioids.

STEP	RATIONALE
3 Perform hand hygiene and apply clean gloves. NOTE: Use latex-free gloves if there is a risk of an allergic reaction.	Reduces transmission of microorganisms. Synthetic cast can leave gluelike resin on hands. Prevents exposure to latex allergen.
4 Help health care provider or certified technician position patient and injured extremity as desired, depending on type of cast to be used and area to be casted.	Parts to be casted must be supported and in optimal alignment.
5 Prepare skin that will be enclosed in cast. Clean skin with mild soap and water and change dressing (if present). Skin must be completely dry before application of cast.	Reduces complications to underlying tissues after casting. Gentle manipulation prevents pain or additional injury.
6 Explain that patient may experience warmth during cast application process.	Plaster and fiberglass cast materials give off heat from a chemical reaction when drying. This warmth usually dissipates after approximately 15 to 30 minutes. Make sure there that is enough padding to decrease chance of thermal injury as cast is setting (Boyd et al., 2009).
7 Assist with application of padding material around body part to be casted (see illustration). Apply minimum of four layers of padding. Avoid wrinkles or uneven thickness.	Prevents pressure points under cast. Four layers of padding have been shown to decrease incidence of burning when cast is removed (Satryb et al., 2011).
8 Hold body part or parts to be casted or assist with preparation of cast materials.	Support of body part may also require application of slight manual traction.
a *Plaster cast:* Mark end of roll by folding one corner of material under itself. With your thumb under outer edge, submerge plaster roll under water in casting bucket or plastic basin until bubbles stop; squeeze slightly and hand roll to person applying cast.	Once dampened, the end of the casting tape may be difficult to find. Dampened plaster rolls are unrolled and molded to fit extremity or body part being casted.
b *Synthetic cast:* Submerge cast roll in lukewarm water for 10 to 15 seconds. Squeeze to remove excess water. You can use a water bottle to apply water to casting material.	The polyurethane prepolymer is activated by the application of water.
9 Continue to hold body part(s) as necessary as cast is applied (see illustration) or supply additional rolls of casting tape as needed.	Support of body part involves applying slight manual traction, if desired, to maintain optimal position. Thickness of cast determines strength.

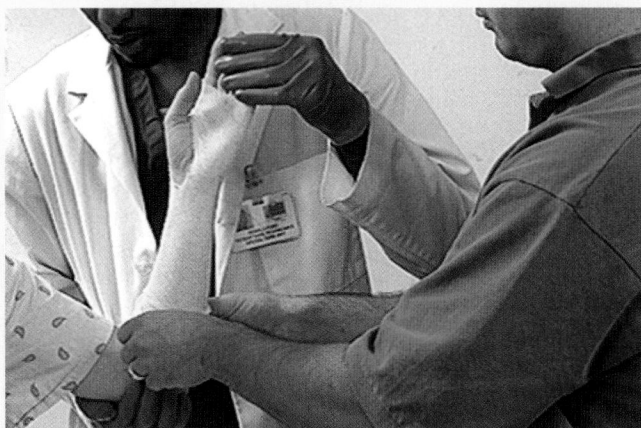

STEP 7   Padding under cast is smooth.

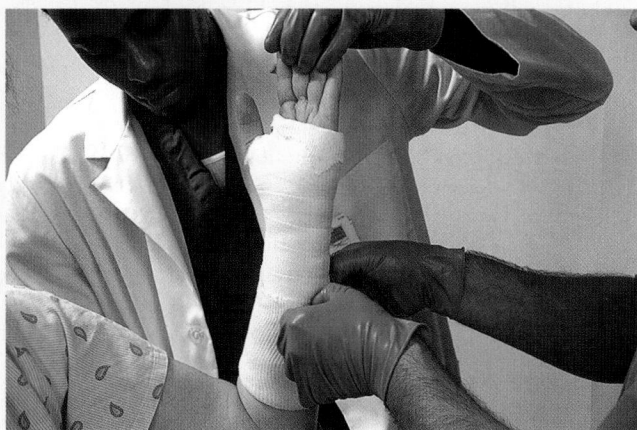

STEP 9   Supporting extremity during cast application.

STEP	RATIONALE
10 Hold body part while casting tape is applied and molded. Synthetic tape is applied with slight tension. When wrapping is complete, gently compress with hands (see illustration).	Casting tape has synthetic adhesive or glass-fiber materials that dry quickly and are lightweight. Compression promotes bonding of cast layers. Plaster cast materials are smoothed at the end to finish outside of cast and ensure that plaster has bonded to other layers as well.

STEP	RATIONALE

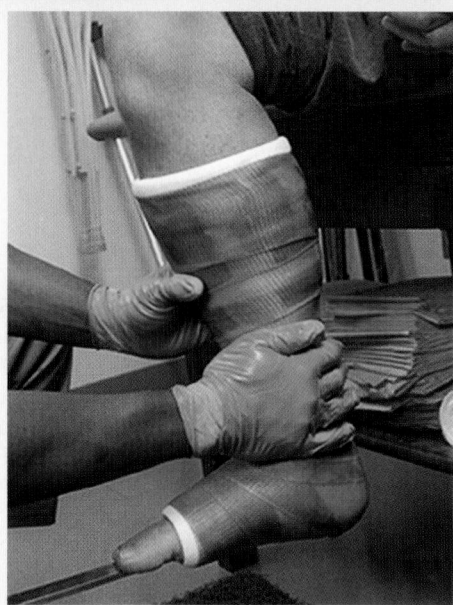

STEP 10   Applying synthetic cast roll.

11 Provide walking heel, cast brace, bar, or other cast stabilization material as requested by health care provider.

Ambulation may be permitted with partial weight bearing on affected extremity after cast has dried. Bars stabilize spica cast, or "posts" (metal poles) stabilize four-poster cast. Braces incorporated into cast assist in joint motion and mobility.

12 Assist with "finishing" cast by folding edge of stockinette over outer edge of cast to provide smooth edge. Unroll dampened plaster roll over stockinette to hold it in place. Cushion any rough edges of cast with tape or moleskin.

Smooth edges decrease chance of skin irritation or tissue injury. By finishing cast with stockinette, later petaling with tape is not required when cast is dry (Boyd et al., 2009).

13 Using scissors, trim cast around fingers, toes, or thumb as necessary.

Cast should be snug but should not constrict uninvolved joint movement or circulation.

14 Depending on tissue to be casted:

   a Elevate casted tissue to heart level on two or three cloth-covered pillows or in a sling. Avoid completely encasing cast. Air dry. If ice is ordered, place to the side of casted extremity to prevent indentations on the top.

Pillows prevent indentations, which could harden and cause underlying pressure. Elevation enhances venous return and decreases edema. Covering cast delays or impedes drying.

   b When applying a sling, ensure that sling supports but does not encase cast.

Covering (encasing) impedes air movements and delays drying.

15 Remove and dispose of gloves and other disposable equipment into appropriate receptacle. Perform hand hygiene.

Reduces transmission of microorganisms.

16 Using palms of hands to support casted areas, help patient with transfer to stretcher or wheelchair for return to nursing unit or preparation for discharge. Use additional personnel to transfer patient safely, especially in spica or other body cast.

Safety in transfer requires additional personnel, use of pillows to support cast, side rails, and in some cases restraints.

Clinical Decision Point *Synthetic casts are dry or set in 7 to 15 minutes. Soft tissues around affected area may swell from processes of "reducing" or manipulating before cast was applied.*

17 Reposition patient every 2 hours. Do not rest heel of the cast on bed or pillow.

Prevents any one area of cast from receiving continuous pressure. Avoids indentation of cast.

18 Inform patient to notify care provider of any alteration in sensation, numbness, tingling, burning, pain on passive motion, or inability to move fingers or toes in affected extremity (Voda, 2011).

Edema within casted extremity causes pressure on nerves, blood vessels, and muscle tissue. This leads to compartment syndrome, neurovascular deficit, and tissue necrosis.

STEP	RATIONALE

EVALUATION

1 Observe patient for signs of pain or anxiety: ask him or her to rate pain on a scale of 0 to 10, observe for discolored or pale fingers or nail beds, inability to move body parts distal to cast, pain on passive motion of distal body parts, hyperventilation, nausea and/or vomiting, tachycardia, and blood pressure elevation.

These are signs of compartment syndrome, cast syndrome, or severe claustrophobia (common for patients in spica or body cast) from snugness of cast. Reposition patient and reassess extremity. If unresolved, need to immediately notify health care provider.

2 Perform neurovascular assessment every 1 to 2 hours for first 24 hours. Assess for pain, pallor, pulselessness, paresthesia, and paralysis (Table 11-1). Compare findings with precasting application neurovascular assessment (see illustration).

Neurovascular status reflects vascular supply or pressure to tissues, indicating functioning and viability of tissues.

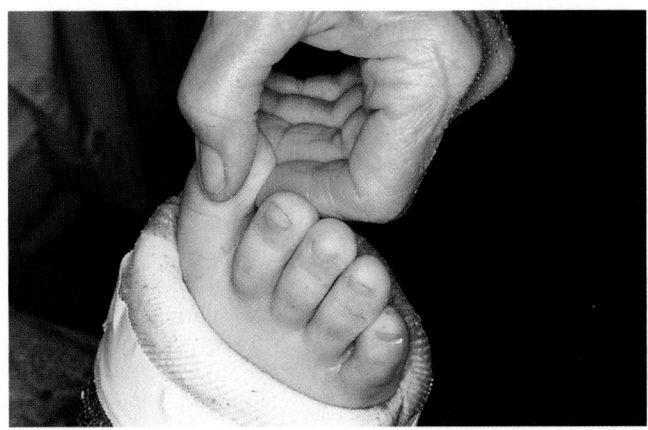

STEP 2 Assessing capillary refill.

3 Observe condition of cast and assess for edema of tissues distal to cast.

Broken edges of cast can cause skin irritation. Drainage on cast can indicate underlying infection. Edema results from trauma or venous stasis. Rarely does heat from plaster drying contribute to development of edema.

4 Palpate temperature of tissues around casted area for warmth and assess hot spots, which could indicate underlying infection.

Warmth of tissues distal to cast usually indicates adequate perfusion.

5 Ask patient to perform ADLs and ROM within limitations of cast. Compare ROM in noncasted extremity.

Determines change in ROM or ability to perform self care.

6 After cast is dry, observe patient perform and verbalize knowledge of cast care.

Return demonstration objectively measures patient's learning.

Unexpected Outcomes

1 Patient experiences impaired mobility related to cast application.

2 Patient develops pressure ulcer over bony prominence, or skin irritation occurs at cast edges.

3 Patient reports increased severity in pain after cast application.

Related Interventions

- Assist with ROM exercises every 3 to 4 hours.
- Teach isometric exercises.

- Position off bony prominence and turn frequently.
- Health care provider may split, window, bivalve, or remove cast.
- Cut small pieces (petals) of adhesive tape or moleskin 2.5 to 5 cm (1 to 2 inches) and tape smoothly over edge of cast. Pay close attention to edges where there may be more movement such as around fingers and toes.

- Elevate casted extremity on a pillow. Adjust elevation of pillows as necessary.
- Apply ice bags along sides of cast.
- Increase frequency of neurovascular checks.
- Assess tightness of cast by checking with two fingers around edges. Cast should be snug but not tight.
- If pain continues, notify health care provider before administering analgesics (analgesics do not relieve edema and could mask symptoms).

4 Patient develops compartment syndrome with severe pain unrelieved by analgesics; change in neurovascular status such as cold extremity, decreased capillary refill, swelling, pallor, diminished pulse, numbness, tingling, or altered motion of distal parts occurs.

- Notify health care provider immediately.
- Prepare to bivalve cast using cast cutter. Cut through underlying wadding and padding.

5 Patient in body or hip spica cast develops nausea, vomiting, feeling of abdominal fullness or pain, which indicate cast syndrome (superior mesenteric artery syndrome), in which the duodenum is compressed between the superior mesenteric artery and the spine.

- Change patient from supine to prone position.
- Give nothing by mouth.
- Notify health care provider and prepare to cut abdominal window, bivalve cast, and/or insert nasogastric tube.

6 Patient is unable to demonstrate cast care.

- Reinstruction is necessary. May need to incorporate teach-back method to ascertain level of understanding.

Recording and Reporting

- Document cast application, condition of the skin, status of circulation (before and after application), and motion of distal part.
- Record instructions given to patient and family.
- Report abnormal or unusual findings from neurovascular assessments and symptoms of compartment syndrome immediately.
- Record odor and drainage from cast. Report to health care provider.

Special Considerations
Teaching

- Teach patient to realign pillows to promote cast drying.
- Teach patient about effects of pressure from cast on underlying skin and tissue.
- Prepare patient for itching sensations under cast. Patient should avoid sticking objects down or in cast to scratch because these objects can cause breaks in underlying skin and subsequent infections. The patient's health care provider can order medication to control itching. May teach patient to tap onto cast, blow cold air with hair dryer at sides of cast (Musher, 2010), or try scratching on the opposite extremity.

- If patient must use crutches, instruct in crutch-walking techniques (see Chapter 10).
- Teach patient proper ROM and isometric exercises for affected extremity.
- Caution patient against drying wet cast with hair dryer; this can cause plaster to crack or skin underneath to be damaged. Using a hair dryer does not dry the cast thoroughly and leads to development of mold.

Pediatric

- Teach parents or other caregivers to protect cast from moisture or unnecessary wear. Plastic wrap placed around perineal area during urination or defecation prevents soiling. Protect cast with a plastic bag or plastic wrap when the child bathes or showers. With a spica cast, tuck the ends of a small disposable diaper around the edges of the casted area to cover and protect the perineum in babies (Hockenberry and Wilson, 2011).
- Children are particularly prone to placing objects into casts to scratch. Assess edges of cast to ensure that the child has not done this (Hockenberry and Wilson, 2011).
- Use antihistamines and a hair dryer set to *cool* for itching (Hockenberry and Wilson, 2011).

TABLE 11-1	**Five P's of Neurovascular Assessment**	
Criteria	**Assessment**	**Rationale**
Pain	Determine amount and severity of pain if present. Ask patient for descriptions; avoid coaching patient with words to describe pain.	Manipulation and reduction may produce dull, aching pain as a result of pressure on nerve endings. Patients vary in perception and tolerance of pain. Further assess pain on passive motion, unrelenting pain, or pain out of proportion because it may signify compartment syndrome. Sudden increase in pain may signify thrombus formation.
Pallor	Observe color of tissues distal to cast. Older adults may have bluish color normally; however, no other signs of circulatory compromise should be present.	Pink indicates that arterial perfusion is normal, whitish color signifies decreased arterial supply, and bluish color signifies venous stasis.
Pulselessness	When possible, palpate distal pulse of casted extremity; note presence and strength of pulse. Assess capillary refill by pressing on toenail or fingernail (if cast is on extremity), releasing, and noting "pinking" of nail; nail should "pink up" in 2 seconds or less.	Weak or absent pulse may indicate decreased circulation to casted area. Blanching on pressure with subsequent capillary refill indicates arterial perfusion. Capillary refill is too sluggish if refill takes more than 3 seconds. It takes 2 seconds to say "capillary refill" slowly and 4 seconds to repeat it once.
Paresthesia	Assess for numbness, tingling, or abnormal sensations.	Abnormal sensations may indicate nerve damage and/or development of compartment syndrome.
Paralysis	Assess for ability to move fingers, toes, or extremity.	Paralysis may indicate nerve damage and/or development of compartment syndrome.

Gerontologic
- Some older nonverbal patients do not express pain, leading you to believe that there is none. Patients may express pain through crying, agitation, or restlessness (Ebersole et al., 2008). Older adults with changes in mental status make pain assessment difficult.
- Lightweight, synthetic casts are better for older adults. Cast is less restrictive, and the light weight assists patients to maintain better balance.
- Age-related decreased muscle strength in older adults is a result of loss of skeletal muscle and may cause difficulty in ambulating with a cast.
- Some older adults have reduced sensation as a result of decreased skin receptors and are less able to detect compression.

Home Care
- Instruct patient that rest, ice, and elevation of affected extremity help to reduce swelling. Instruct him or her to place ice on either side of cast, not directly on top.

- Inform patient to inspect cast daily and petal any rough edges to reduce risk for trauma to underlying skin and need for cast changes.
- Have patient inspect cast daily for foul odor, which indicates skin excoriation or infection under cast; monitor neurovascular status, paying particular attention to blueness or paleness of nails, pain, feeling of tightness, numbness, or tingling sensation.
- Instruct patient to keep plaster of Paris cast dry. When bathing, patient must not submerge casted extremity because cast absorbs water, which can lead to its crumbling. If cast becomes wet, dry immediately. Instruct patient to inform health care provider of wet or damaged cast.
- Clean synthetic casts with warm water and mild soap.

PROCEDURAL GUIDELINE 11-1 Care of a Patient During Cast Removal

When caring for patients with casts, it is also important to understand the techniques for cast removal, which consist of removing the cast and padding, followed by skin care to the affected areas. The cast is removed with a noisy cast saw, but the procedure is painless because the saw vibrates and does not cut the skin. However, it is necessary to adequately prepare the patient for cast removal. A small child or confused patient may need gentle restraint during removal to prevent any injury. When removing a synthetic cast (with gore lining), it is important to remove gently to prevent burns from the heat generated by the vibrating saw. After cast removal the patient may experience some tenderness, soreness, muscle weakness and atrophy, and a buildup of dead skin cells.

Delegation and Collaboration
The skill of assisting with cast removal can be delegated to nursing assistive personnel (NAP) who have specific training; but the nurse is responsible for assessing the patient's condition. The nurse directs the NAP by:
- Informing them about preferred positioning methods for specific patients.
- Informing them about the proper method of treating the skin following cast removal.

Equipment
- ❏ Cast saw
- ❏ Plastic sheets or paper
- ❏ Cold water enzyme wash
- ❏ Skin lotion
- ❏ Basin, water, washcloths, and towels
- ❏ Scissors
- ❏ Clean gloves
- ❏ Eye protection for patient and health care provider

Procedural Steps
1. Assess patient's understanding of and response to upcoming cast removal.
2. Help with positioning patient.
3. Describe the physical sensations to expect during cast removal (vibration of cast saw generates heat) (see illustration).

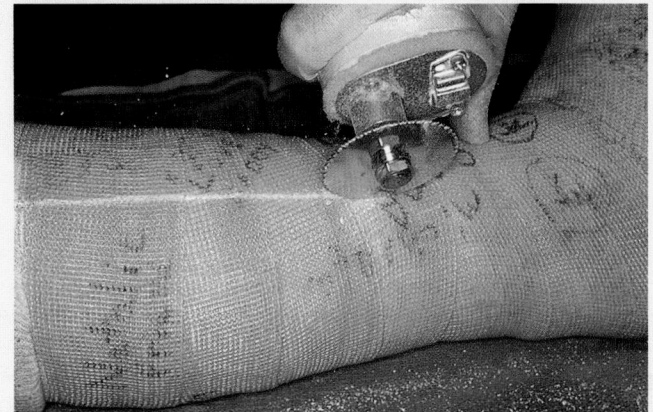

STEP 3 Vibration of cast cutter generates heat.

4. Describe the expected appearance of the extremity. Skin under cast is often scaly with dead cells that slough off. Muscle atrophy occurs from disuse.
5. Describe and demonstrate the loud noise of the cast saw.
6. Perform hand hygiene. Apply clean gloves and eye goggles or protective glasses to self and patient.
7. Stay with patient and explain progress of procedure as cast and underlying padding are removed (see illustration).

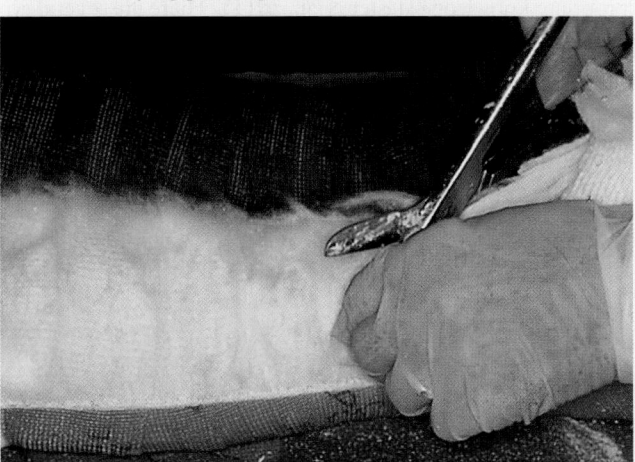

STEP 7 Cutting through wadding under cast with scissors.

Continued

PROCEDURAL GUIDELINE 11-1   Care of a Patient During Cast Removal—cont'd

8 Inspect tissues underlying cast after removal.

9 If skin is intact, apply cold-water enzyme wash (if available) to skin and leave on for 15 to 20 minutes. Use oil or mild soap and water to soften crusts. Do not scrub skin.

10 Gently wash off enzyme wash or soap and water. If possible, immerse tissues in basin or tub to assist in dead cell removal.

11 Pat extremity dry. Apply generous coat of lotion to patient's skin.

12 Dispose of used supplies and equipment. Remove and dispose of gloves. Perform hand hygiene.

13 After cast removal, explain and provide written skin care procedures for patient before discharge (Box 11-2).

14 Obtain health care provider order to perform active and passive range of motion and clarify level of activity allowed.

15 Instruct patient to observe for swelling and continue to elevate extremity no higher than the heart to manage edema (Satryb et al., 2011).

BOX 11-2 | **Care After Cast Removal**

Skin Care
- Apply enzyme wash solution such as Woolite or Delicare and leave in place for at least 20 minutes. The enzymes in the solution loosen dead cells and emulsify fatty or crusty lesions but cause no skin irritation.
- After 20 minutes, immerse the area in warm water and gently swab with a soft cloth.
- Rinse with clear warm water and pat dry.
- Apply a moisturizing skin lotion or a little oil, gently massaging it in to help maintain the integrity of the tissues.
- Repeat these steps in 24 to 48 hours, after which the area should need no special care.

Relieving Edema
- Apply cloth-covered ice bags if there is significant edema. Do not apply ice directly to the skin.
- Elevate affected extremity for 24 hours or when swelling occurs.

Managing Tenderness, Weakness, and Discomfort
- Take prescribed analgesic every 3 to 4 hours to develop a therapeutic blood level and continue the medication for 24 to 48 hours.
- Immerse the part or the entire body in warm water and gently exercise the muscles under water.
- Begin to reuse affected tissue and muscles slowly to decrease resulting pain. Explain that usually it takes twice as long as the part was in a cast to regain full function.
- Perform prescribed muscle exercises with 5 to 10 repetitions every 4 hours while awake to aid in regaining muscle strength. Take a non-narcotic analgesic and soak in warm water before exercise if muscle soreness persists. Soreness should lessen as muscle gains strength. Health care provider may prescribe a consultation with a physical therapist to prescribe appropriate exercises to increase mobility and strength.

SKILL 11-2   Care of a Patient in Skin Traction

Skin traction is the application of a pulling force directly to the skin and soft tissue that indirectly pulls on the skeletal system. It immobilizes a fracture and relieves muscle spasms and pain through the use of continuous traction. Skin traction is usually used for temporary immobilization until the fracture can be repaired surgically by open reduction and internal fixation (ORIF) or by skeletal traction (Wheeles, 2011). The health care provider issues written orders for specific traction weights, bed position, and turning regimen. Skin traction is applied by skilled practitioners with appropriate knowledge (Jester et al., 2011). There are several types of skin traction.

1 *Buck's extension*: It is the most common type of adult skin traction. It is applied to one or both legs using straps or a commercially prepared foam boot with Velcro straps (Fig. 11-3). This is then attached to a spreader bar, and a weight is attached to the end of the extremity. No more than 7 lbs of weights are used. Buck's extension provides temporary immobilization of hip fracture and reduces muscle spasms, contractures, and dislocations.

2 *Dunlop's traction*: This type of traction applies 7 to 10 lbs of weight to an upper limb for treatment of contractures or fractures of the humerus or elbow (Fig. 11-4).

3 *Russell's traction*: This type of traction uses skin traction on the lower leg; a padded sling is placed under the knee. There are two lines of pulling force: one is along the longitudinal plane of the lower leg, and one is perpendicular to the leg. The hip and knee are immobilized in a flexed position (Fig. 11-5).

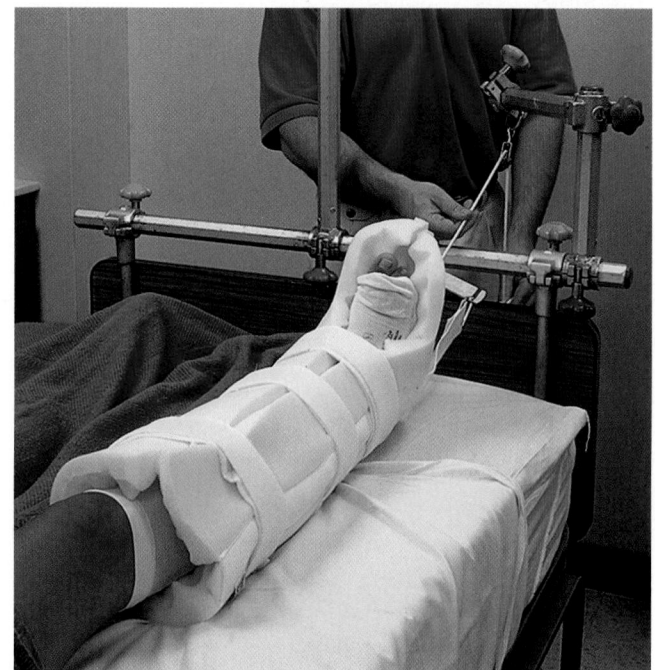

FIG 11-3   Buck's extension.

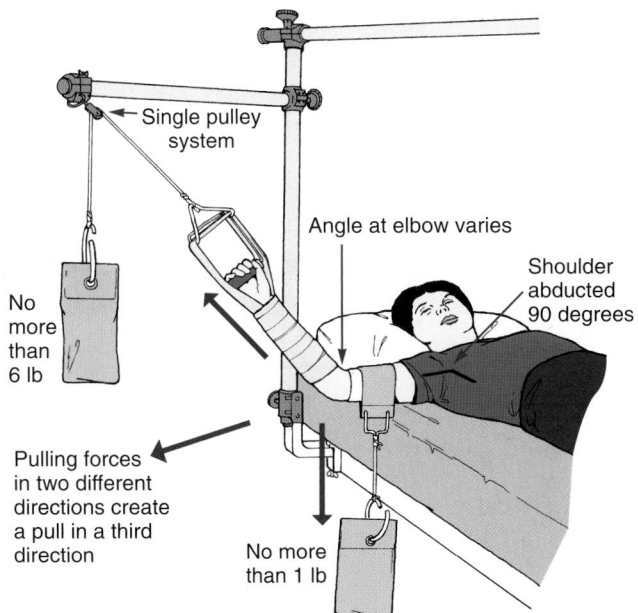

FIG 11-4   Dunlop's traction.

Single pulley system

Angle at elbow varies

Shoulder abducted 90 degrees

No more than 6 lb

Pulling forces in two different directions create a pull in a third direction

No more than 1 lb

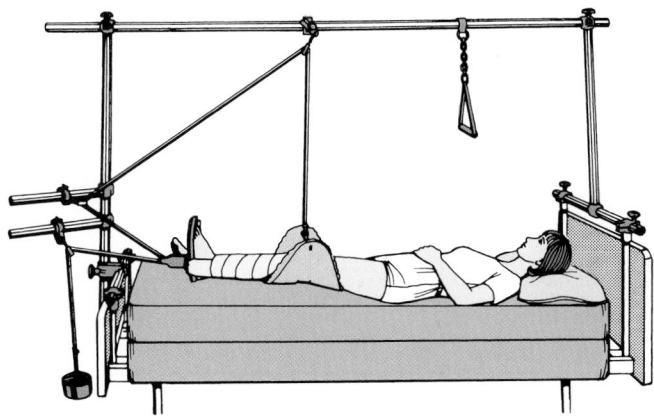

FIG 11-5   Russell's traction.

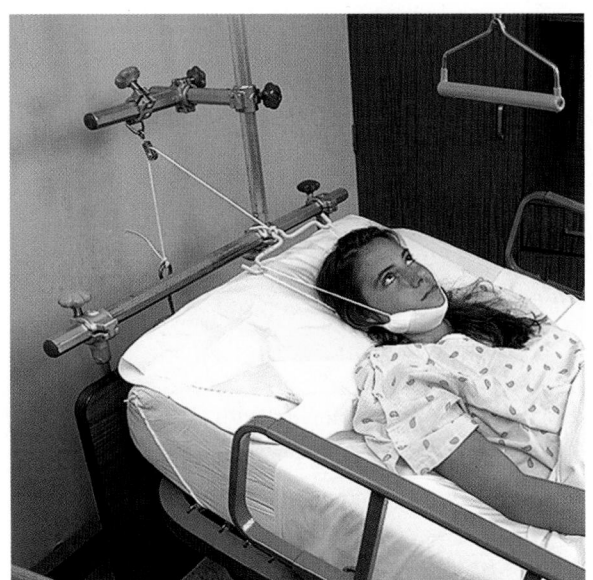

FIG 11-6   Cervical traction.

4 *Cervical traction:* Cervical traction uses a head halter with a cutout for the ears and face. The halter cradles the chin and has straps leading to a bar attached to ropes, pulleys, and weights (Fig. 11-6). Between 7 and 10 lbs of weight are applied. Cervical traction immobilizes conditions of the cervical vertebrae, not fractures. It may be removed periodically.

The more weight applied to traction, the greater the risk of skin breakdown. Contraindications to the use of skin traction include pressure ulcers, dermatitis, burns, or abrasions. Older patients and patients with tissue perfusion problems are at increased risk of skin breakdown.

When caring for patients in skin traction, regularly monitor them for correct maintenance of the traction device and proper musculoskeletal alignment. Agency policy may specify the frequency of assessment, but it should be at least every 4 hours. Traction maintenance involves monitoring the weights, the direction of pull, the ropes and pulleys, and all connections (Box 11-3).

BOX 11-3 | Traction Assessment

1 Maintain the Established Line of Pull
The direction of pull should be along the long axis of the bone. Weights hang freely, not hitting the bed or resting on the floor. Recheck the position of the weights if the level of the bed is altered. Avoid (1) bumping against the weights when walking near the bed, and (2) allowing the weights to sway. Both movements can cause pain for a patient in traction. It is preferred that the weights not hang over a patient; if this is necessary, tape the ropes so the weights will not fall on a patient.

2 Maintain Traction Equipment
Traction rope rests in the groove of the pulley and moves easily. Monitor the rope for fraying. Securely tie the knots in the traction rope and tape the rope ends. Ensure that the rope knots are not lodged against the pulley because this will interfere with the line of pull. Ensure that the pulley, spreader bar, and footplate do not rest against the foot of the bed.

3 Maintain Counter traction
To provide traction ensure that counter traction is maintained by the weight of the patient's body, the pull of the weights in the opposite direction, or elevation of the bed. For example, the feet of a patient in Buck's traction do not touch the foot of the bed; or, if a patient is in cervical traction, the head does not touch the head of the bed.

4 Maintain Continuous Traction Unless Ordered Otherwise
Maintain continuous traction unless the health care provider orders intermittent traction. To change a patient's position in bed, do not lift or adjust the weights if traction is continuous. Ensure that the correct amount of weight is used. For intermittent traction gently place and slowly remove the weights, avoiding jerking or suddenly moving the weights because these could jar a patient.

5 Maintain Correct Body Alignment
Be sure patients have correct body alignment while lying centered in the bed. Instruct patients about any restricted positions. Be sure that a patient does not angle the body or lean off the side of the bed because the line of traction pull would then be changed or interrupted.

6 Prevent Friction to the Skin
Remove skin traction and reapply daily. The usual amount of weight used for skin traction in adult patients is 5 to 8 lbs. With any traction monitor the skin for evidence of redness, bruising, or skin breakdown. Avoid friction or pressure from the equipment.

Modified from Jester R et al: *Oxford handbook of orthopaedic nursing*, New York, 2011, Oxford University Press.

Delegation and Collaboration

Neurovascular assessment of the patient's condition cannot be delegated. The skill of assisting with application of skin traction may be delegated to nursing assistive personnel (NAP) who have had specific training. The nurse instructs the NAP by:

- Instructing how to adapt the skill for specific patients.
- Instructing to inform the nurse if patient demonstrates any change in skin condition or complains of discomfort.

Equipment

- ❏ Overhead frame for attachment of traction
- ❏ Traction bar
- ❏ Cross clamp and pulley
- ❏ Buck's extension boot or moleskin and elastic bandages
- ❏ 1- to 7-lb weights
- ❏ Spreader bar

STEP	RATIONALE

ASSESSMENT

1 Assess patient's knowledge of reason for traction.

Determines concerns and need for further teaching.

2 Assess patient's overall health condition, including degree of functional mobility, current medical conditions, and ability to perform activities of daily living (ADLs).

Determines patient's ability to tolerate traction, self-care ability, and need for assistance.

3 Assess integrity and condition of skin before application of traction.

Establishes baseline for skin integrity.

4 Assess patient's position in bed: supine, perpendicular to ends of bed, with affected limb in proper body alignment.

Ensures that pull of traction is at proper angle in relation to patient's body.

5 Assess patient's severity of pain using scale of 0 to 10 and determine need for analgesics before application of traction.

Analgesics decrease patient's discomfort while traction is applied, and assessment serves as baseline for later comparison and evaluation.

6 Assess neurovascular status of extremity distal to traction, including skin color, temperature, capillary refill, presence of distal pulses, sensation, and patient's ability to move digits.

Establishes baseline for early detection of neurovascular deficits.

7 Review medical record for amount of weight to be used in traction.

Ensures appropriate weight is applied at all times.

NURSING DIAGNOSES

- Acute pain
- Bathing, dressing, and toileting self-care deficit

- Ineffective peripheral tissue perfusion
- Deficient knowledge
- Impaired physical mobility

- Risk for impaired skin integrity
- Risk for peripheral neurovascular dysfunction

Related factors are individualized based on patient's condition or needs.

PLANNING

1 Expected outcomes following completion of procedure:

- Patient participates in ADLs as much as possible within limitations.

Activities are performed safely and without injury.

- Skin under traction boot or elastic warp remains intact, without redness or breakdown.

Skin is free of pressure and/or pulling.

- Patient verbalizes increase in comfort after traction application and rates pain as 4 or lower on a scale of 0 to 10 after repositioning and administering analgesics.

Injured tissues and bone are stabilized.

- Neurovascular status remains stable. Distal skin tissue remains warm, pink, with capillary refill of 3 seconds or less. Patient verbalizes no abnormal sensations and is able to move fingers or toes distal to fracture site.

There is no evidence of increased pressure within muscle compartment and no neurovascular deficit (Parvizi, 2010).

- Patient verbalizes understanding of procedure, including traction setup and mobility restrictions.

Promotes cooperation and reduces anxiety. Having patient teach back procedure allows for assessment of understanding.

- Patient moves all extremities independently by discharge date.

No neuromuscular injury occurs.

IMPLEMENTATION

1 Identify patient using two identifiers (i.e., name and birthday or name and account number) according to agency policy. Compare identifiers with information on patient's identification bracelet.

Ensures correct patient. Complies with The Joint Commission standards and improves patient safety (TJC, 2012).

2 Prepare patient by discussing procedure.

Assists with decreasing anxiety.

3 Administer analgesic for acute pain and a muscle relaxant for spasms in advance of traction application.

Allows drugs to reach peak effect at time of traction application, thereby reducing pain and resultant muscle spasm.

STEP	RATIONALE
4 Perform hand hygiene.	Reduces transmission of microorganisms.
5 *Buck's extension:* Position patient supine and nearly flat with no more than 30 degrees of elevation, with affected leg halfway between edge and middle of bed.	Maintains pull of traction at proper angle in relation to patient's body.
6 Apply clean gloves and wash affected extremity gently and pat dry. Do not shave extremity.	Shaving might nick skin, which could become inflamed and infected under traction straps.
7 Apply foam boot, moleskin, or elastic bandages to affected extremity, proceeding from distal to proximal. For *Buck's extension:*	Applying in distal-to-proximal pattern prevents trapping of blood in distal region.
a Before placing foam boot, wrap leg in soft roll. Ensure that boot fits snugly.	Boot that is too tight applies pressure to skin, peroneal nerve, and vasculature structures.
b Seat heel properly in traction boot. Do not pad at heel.	Prevents pressure on patient's heel.

Clinical Decision Point *Skin traction that is too tight puts pressure on nerves and vascular structures, putting patient at risk for an irreversible neurovascular deficit. Skin traction that is too loose will slip.*

STEP	RATIONALE
c Do not apply traction boot over sequential pneumatic compression devices. Instead use foot pumps.	Causes pressure on tissues and does not allow compression device to function.
8 Attach weight to boot gradually and gently at end of bed. Health care provider determines exact amount of weight to be applied and position to be maintained.	Traction is applied slowly to avoid muscle spasm or pain for patient.

Clinical Decision Point *Assess for peroneal nerve damage by noting if there is decreased sensation between patient's great and second toes and an inability to dorsiflex the foot and extend the toes.*

STEP	RATIONALE

9 Inspect traction equipment, making sure that:
  • Knots are secure.
  • Ropes are in pulleys and not frayed.
  • Weights are hanging freely, not caught on bed or resting on floor.
  • Bed linens and bedclothes are not interfering with traction equipment.
  • Check the four P's of traction maintenance: pounds, pressure, pull, and pulleys.
	Observation of these checkpoints maintains the appropriate amount of traction and effective immobilization.

10 Before health care provider leaves, assess patient's position and ask about additional permissible positions for patient and bed.	Ensures patient's safety and position for effective traction.
a *Buck's extension:* Patient is primarily on back but may be allowed to turn to unaffected side for brief periods (10 to 15 minutes).	Positioning on side permits back care and relief of pressure to tissues.
b *Dunlop's traction:* Patient must lie on back. Bed may be tilted on low shock blocks toward side opposite traction. Head of bed is kept flat.	Tilting uses body for some countertraction.
c *Russell's traction:* Patient lies on back; head of bed may be elevated 30 to 45 degrees, depending on injury.	Low-Fowler's position creates most effective traction pull.
11 Release and reapply traction and provide skin care according to health care provider's order. Traction boot is removed every 4 to 8 hours.	Permits visualization of skin and opportunity to provide skin care.
12 Remove and dispose of gloves. Perform hand hygiene. Gather unused materials and return to storage areas.	Reduces transmission of microorganisms.

EVALUATION

1 Observe patient's ability to perform ADLs.	Encourages level of independence in self-care activities to give patients a sense of accomplishment.
2 Frequently assess condition of skin around traction straps or bandages for signs of pressure, color changes, edema, or tenderness.	Ensures early identification of irritation or breakdown. Patient is limited in making minor adjustments skin positioning and may need assistance.
3 Observe patient for correct alignment.	Ensures that traction is being maintained.

STEP	RATIONALE
4 Ask patient to rate discomfort on scale of 0 to 10 and to report muscle spasms.	May indicate misalignment of bones or presence of muscle spasms. Initial reaction may be slight increase in soreness or pain until patient is able to relax and allow traction to perform as designed.
5 Assess neurovascular status of extremity distal to traction every 30 minutes after application of skin traction twice, then every 2 hours for 24 hours, and every 4 hours thereafter (see agency policy). Check skin temperature, capillary refill, presence of distal pulses, sensation, and patient's ability to move digits.	Provides objective data concerning peripheral perfusion to tissues.
6 Observe patient's use of trapeze and ability to reposition self correctly.	Prevents pressure ulcers and gives early feedback regarding skin condition.

Unexpected Outcomes

1 Patient complains of increased pain, soreness, or stiffness after traction is applied.

2 Patient experiences muscle spasms from traction.

3 Patient experiences reddened areas on extremity under traction.

Related Interventions

- Administer analgesics as prescribed.
- Remove traction (if permitted by health care provider) and reapply.
- Realign body and/or extremity.
- If pain is unrelieved or occurs on passive motion, notify health care provider of possible neurovascular deficit.
- Administer skeletal muscle relaxants.
- Obtain health care provider order to remove foam boot for 1 hour to relieve pressure.
- Ensure that you can insert one finger between patient's skin and foam boot.
- Increase frequency of skin assessment.
- Apply protective barrier agent (e.g., Aloe Vista or Sween cream) to affected extremity.
- Ensure that heels do not rest on bed or pillow.

Recording and Reporting

- Record assessment of skin underneath traction apparatus, type of traction, and nursing interventions to maintain skin integrity.
- Record neurovascular assessment on flow sheet or nurses' notes and electronic health record (EHR).
- Record length of time that patient is in or out of specific traction.
- Report any neurovascular deficits to health care provider immediately.

Special Considerations

Teaching

- When traction time is decreased or discontinued, teach patient to ambulate slowly within medical guidelines, gradually increasing length of time out of bed and distance walked.
- Teach patient to alert health care provider of changes in level of pain, muscle spasms, and increased numbness.

Pediatric

- Infants and young children have difficulty remaining still and in alignment.

Gerontologic

- Some older adults may have keratoses, rashes, or other lesions that become irritated in skin traction; thus skin traction should not be used in these cases.

- Some older adults have long-standing conditions of musculoskeletal tissues such as arthritis or gout that could lead to inflamed tissues and skin breakdown.
- Older and chronically ill patients may have increased need for position changes as a result of limitations caused by osteoporosis, osteomalacia, weakened muscles, or increased risk for skin breakdown.
- Older adults' skin heals more slowly, tears more easily, loses its elasticity, and becomes thinner than that of a younger adult (Ebersole et al., 2008). Use pressure-relief devices to reduce the risk for skin breakdown.

Home Care

- Before discharge home, teach family or family caregivers how to manage traction, including positioning, level of mobility, rest, and nutritional considerations.
- Teach family caregivers how to maintain integrity of traction by inspecting at least once daily; weights are free hanging; traction ropes rest in groove of pulley and hang freely; not caught on bed or resting on floor.

SKILL 11-3 Care of a Patient in Skeletal Traction and Pin Site Care

Skeletal traction immobilizes fractures of the cervical spine, fractures of the femur below the trochanter, and some fractures of the bones of the arm or ankle. It is also used for immobilizing the femoral head when there is an acetabular fracture. Skeletal traction is being used less frequently because of newer surgical repair procedures and new trauma management (Musher, 2010). This type of traction is used for patients with multiple traumas who cannot have an immediate surgical repair.

A common form of skeletal traction is balanced-suspension skeletal traction (BSST), which is used for a fractured femur (Fig. 11-7). BSST relieves muscle spasms, realigns the fracture fragments, and promotes callus formation. Callus formation is the development of new supportive bone around the injured site. BSST temporarily stabilizes the patient's condition while waiting for surgical insertion of an internal fixation device such as a plate, screw, or nail. Balanced suspension involves a sling attached to splints around the leg and a Steinmann pin or Kirschner wire supplying the traction (Fig. 11-8, A and B). Sufficient weight to overcome the quadriceps and hamstring muscle spasms ranges between 30 to 40 lbs.

Other common forms of skeletal traction are sidearm traction (with a pin drilled through the lower humerus) and external fixation (used for comminuted fractures with soft tissue injury, skull and facial fractures, and pelvic fractures). For cervical spine fractures, Crutchfield or Garner-Wells tongs are inserted into the skull. Halo traction is frequently used for neurologically intact patients, stabilizing the spinal vertebra and preventing further injury to the spinal cord (Fig. 11-9).

External fixation is a form of skeletal traction that consists of a frame or apparatus to hold pins placed into or through bones above and below a fracture site. External fixation promotes early ambulation and use of other joints while maintaining immobilization of affected bones. A variety of external fixation devices are used for skull and facial fractures, ribs, bones of the extremities, and pelvic bones (Fig. 11-10).

Skeletal traction involves piercing the skin at the site where the pin enters and exits (Fig. 11-8, C). In the case of external fixation or halo traction, the device attaches to the bone through the skin (Sarro et al., 2010). Slow healing requires longer periods of traction (6 to 8 weeks) to promote bone repair. This prolonged immobilization influences nursing care, which is focused on activities of daily living (ADLs), maintaining traction, and preventing fat embolism and complications of immobility (e.g., skin breakdown, pulmonary emboli).

Because skeletal traction involves placement of a pin, meticulous pin-site care reduces the risk for pin-tract infections. Up to 10% of external fixation pins develop infections (Parvizi, 2010).

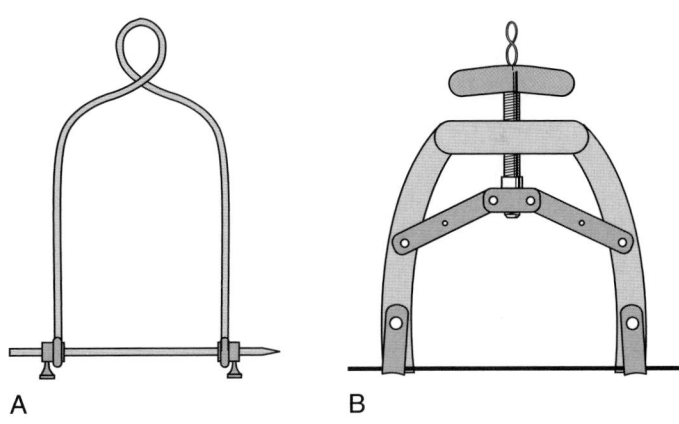

A   B

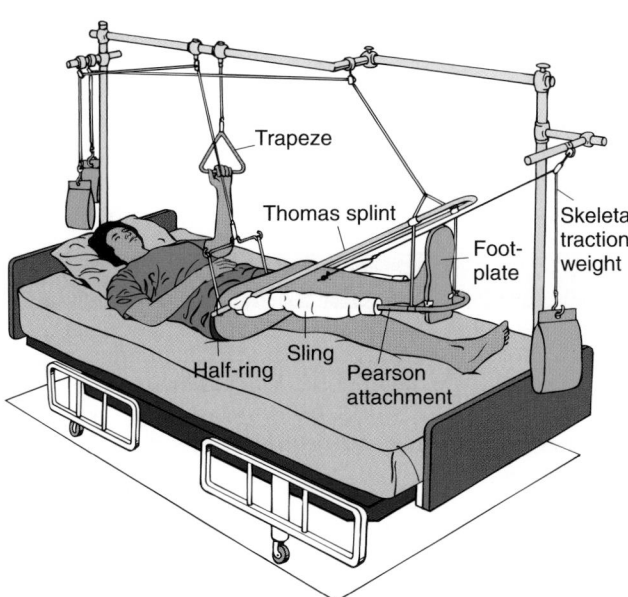

FIG 11-7 Balanced-suspension skeletal traction. Traction is applied via Kirschner wire through proximal portion of tibia. Limb is supported by Thomas splint beneath thigh and Pearson attachment beneath lower leg. Footplate attachment prevents footdrop. Weights apply countertraction to Thomas splint and suspend its lower end. Patient can shift position of hips without change in amount of traction.

Labels in Fig 11-7: Trapeze, Thomas splint, Footplate, Skeletal traction weight, Sling, Half-ring, Pearson attachment

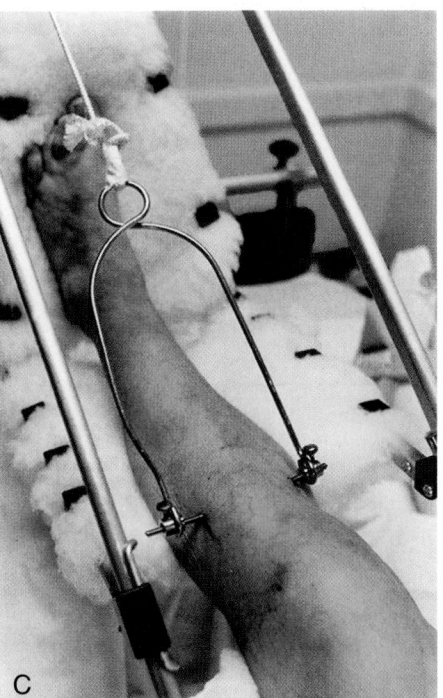

C

FIG 11-8 **A,** Steinmann pin and holder. **B,** Kirschner wire and tractor. **C,** Steinmann pin placed in tibial plateau for treatment of distal femoral fracture.

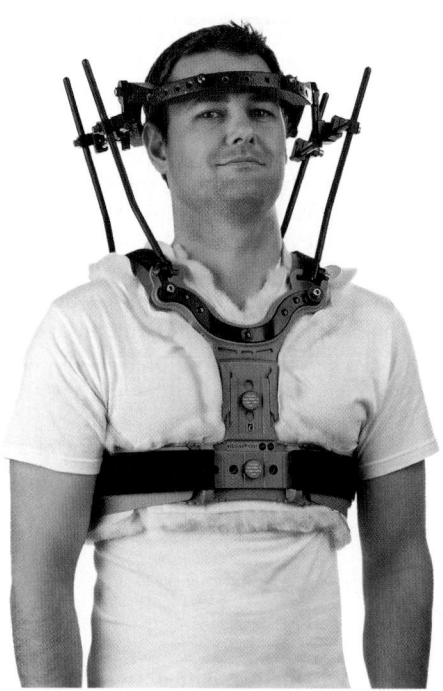

FIG 11-9 Halo traction and vest. *(Image courtesy Össur Americas. All rights reserved.)*

Pin-site care can reduce the risk of infection and must be implemented using current evidence-based practice guidelines (Rose, 2010). Some agencies have policies outlining pin-site care. Chlorhexidine 2 mg/mL solution or 0.9% sodium chloride solution is recommended for stable pins (Voda, 2011). Some agencies require health care provider orders that specify the frequency of pin care and the cleaning agent to be used.

Delegation and Collaboration
Assessment of the patient's condition and status in skeletal traction cannot be delegated. The skill of assisting with insertion of skeletal pins and pin site care may be delegated to nursing assistive personnel (NAP) once adequately trained in the principles of surgical asepsis. The nurse directs the NAP by:
• Instructing to report any signs and symptoms of inflammation or infection at the pin insertion site.

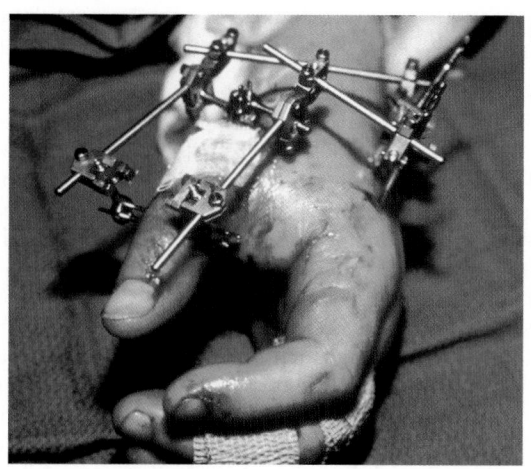

FIG 11-10 External fixator,

Equipment
Balanced-Suspension Skeletal Traction
❑ Ropes, pulleys, weights, weight holders
❑ Thomas splint
❑ Pearson attachment with sheepskin padding
❑ Footplate
❑ Trapeze bar
❑ Clean gloves
Halo Traction
❑ Halo ring with four pins
❑ Molded vest jacket
❑ Vertical metal bars connecting ring to jacket
❑ Tracheostomy tray (for emergency resuscitation)
❑ Allen wrench (allows removal of screws for resuscitation)
Pin-site Care
❑ Sterile cotton-tipped applicators
❑ Prescribed cleaning agent. Preferred agent chlorhexidine, 2 mg/mL solution, or 0.9% sodium chloride solution (check agency policy)
❑ Split 2 × 2-inch gauze barrier (*optional*)
❑ Topical antibiotic ointment (check agency policy)
❑ Clean gloves

STEP	RATIONALE

ASSESSMENT

1 Assess patient's knowledge of the reason for traction, including nonverbal behaviors and responses. | Determines anxiety and need for further teaching.
2 Inspect integrity and condition of skin over bony prominences and under devices in use. Consider need for special bed or mattress. | Determines baseline status of dependent tissues at risk for pressure ulcer formation.
3 Assess for proper alignment of extremity. | Ensures that pull of traction is at proper angle in relation to patient's body.
4 Assess patient's degree of mobility, ability to reposition and perform ADLs, and current medical condition. | Determines baseline status of patient's health status.
5 Assess patient's level of pain using scale of 0 to 10 and determine need for analgesics before procedure begins. | Decreases patient's discomfort during traction application and serves as baseline for later comparison.
6 Following application, assess traction setup: weights hanging freely, ordered amount of weight applied, ropes move freely through pulleys, all knots tight in roles and away from pulleys. | Ensures that traction functions correctly.

STEP	RATIONALE
7 Prior to application, assess neurovascular status of extremity distal to traction, including skin color, temperature, capillary refill, presence of distal pulses, sensation, and patient's ability to move digits.	Provides baseline information and detects neurovascular deficits.
8 Following pin insertion, assess pin sites for redness, edema, discharge, and odor.	Provides baseline for condition of pin insertion site.
9 Assess respiratory rate, depth, rhythm, and chest expansion.	Pulmonary embolus can occur in patients with spinal cord injury or on prolonged bed rest. Fat embolism syndrome (FES) can occur with long-bone fractures.

NURSING DIAGNOSES

- Acute pain
- Anxiety
- Bathing, dressing, and toileting self-care deficit
- Deficient knowledge
- Impaired physical mobility
- Risk for impaired skin integrity
- Risk for infection
- Risk for injury
- Risk for peripheral neurovascular dysfunction

Related factors are individualized based on patient's condition or needs.

PLANNING

1 Expected outcomes following completion of procedure:	
• Patient's skeletal deformity is reduced, alignment is maintained, and injury is healed.	Skeletal traction promotes healing of fractures.
• Patient performs ADLs independently to all unaffected areas.	Self-care activities help patient to reduce risk for complications of immobility and give him or her a sense of control.
• Patient's skin remains intact without redness, inflammation, or purulent drainage, especially over pressure points.	Indicates no development of pressure ulcers or infection.
• Patient is free of neurovascular deficits following application of skeletal traction. Patient verbalizes no abnormal sensations and is able to move fingers or toes below fracture site.	Adequate neurovascular functioning is essential to health and well-being of extremity (Parvizi, 2010).
• Patient performs range of motion in unaffected extremities.	Routine exercise prevents contractures and muscle wasting.
• Patient demonstrates correct use of trapeze.	Prevents injury, allows patient to participate in repositioning.
• Patient describes purpose of skeletal traction and follows activity restrictions.	Demonstrates learning and acceptance of restrictions. Able to repeat back purpose of traction and associated restrictions.
• Skin around pin sites remains free of redness, edema, or drainage.	No pin site infection present.

IMPLEMENTATION

1 Identify patient using two identifiers (i.e., name and birthday or name and account number) according to agency policy). Compare identifiers with information on patient's identification bracelet.	Ensures correct patient. Complies with The Joint Commission standards and improves patient safety (TJC, 2012).
2 Discuss procedure with patient.	Decreases patient anxiety.
3 Perform hand hygiene.	Reduces transmission of infection.
4 Initial traction setup:	
a Apply clean gloves and position patient per health care provider's order. Support limb at joint above and below fracture to be placed in traction. Do not move distal parts unnecessarily. Patient will likely be placed in supine position with head of bed slightly elevated.	Ensures proper alignment during and after traction application. Movement can cause severe pain or additional trauma.
b Health care provider wears sterile gloves and gown while cleaning skin over pin sites and injecting local anesthetic.	Anesthetic desensitizes pin insertion area. Patient feels pressure during drilling but should not experience pain. Procedure requires surgical asepsis.
c Assist (usually by holding spreader bar, splint, or Pearson attachment) while health care provider continues to use drill to insert number of pins needed for traction. Support area of joints not at injury site. Do not move distal portion unnecessarily.	Movement can cause severe pain or additional trauma.
d Once traction setup is applied, attach weights and gently lower until rope is taut.	Reduces spasm and discomfort.

STEP	RATIONALE
e Inspect traction setup; ensure that: • Knots are secure and footplate is in place. • Ropes and pulleys are not frayed. • Weights are hanging freely, not caught on bed or resting on floor. • Bedclothes are not interfering with traction apparatus.	Ensures that traction and immobilization are effective.

Critical Decision Point *Irreversible muscle and tissue damage can occur within 6 to 8 hours (Hockenberry and Wilson, 2011).*

STEP	RATIONALE
5 Provide pin-site care according to agency policy or health care provider's order. a Apply clean gloves and remove gauze dressings from around pins and discard in appropriate receptacle. b Inspect pin sites for redness, edema, or purulent drainage. NOTE: Clear drainage and crusting are expected findings. Remove and discard gloves and perform hand hygiene. c Prepare supplies. d Apply clean gloves and clean each pin site with prescribed cleaning solution by placing tip of moistened sterile applicator close to pin and cleaning away from insertion site. Dispose of applicator. Use new sterile applicator for each swipe. e Repeat process for each pin site. f Using sterile applicator, apply small amount of topical antibiotic ointment to pin site (see health care provider order or according to agency policy). g Cover with sterile 2×2-inch split gauze dressing or leave site open to air (see health care provider order or according to agency policy).	 These are signs and symptoms of infection. Reduces transmission of infection. Removes infectious material without contaminating pin site. May reduce development of infection. Some health care providers prefer plain soap and water for cleaning pins.
6 Provide routine traction care. a Inspect skin (bony prominences, heels, elbows, sacrum, and areas under appliances) for signs of pressure. Use pressure-relief devices as appropriate. Try to reposition any areas under pressure if possible. Do not massage areas of pressure if there is tenderness, reactive hyperemia (increase in blood flow), or areas of skin breakdown.	 Massage to compromised tissues increases risk for breakdown.
7 Provide nonpharmacologic and pharmacologic pain relief as indicated (see Chapter 15).	Pain relief will improve patient's ability to remain active within mobility limitations.
8 Encourage use of unaffected extremities for ADLs and active and passive exercises. Encourage use of trapeze bar for repositioning.	Prevents muscle atrophy and maintains muscle tone for later ambulation.
9 For elimination, provide a fracture pan if needed.	Smaller bedpan is more comfortable and easier to place under patient.
10 Raise appropriate number of side rails as needed.	Provides for patient's safety. Side rails can be considered a restraint.
11 Remove and dispose of gloves if used, gather equipment and supplies, and return to proper storage places. Perform hand hygiene.	Provides for safety and cleanliness and prevents transmission of infection.

EVALUATION

1 Inspect body part in traction for correct alignment.	Determines if traction is functioning as desired.
2 Monitor neurovascular status and peripheral tissue perfusion every 2 hours for the first 24 hours and every 4 hours thereafter (see agency policy).	Permanent neurovascular deficits can occur in as little as 6 hours. Edema in muscle compartment is most likely to develop in first 24 hours after injury. Determines peripheral perfusion to tissues and identifies any neurovascular deficits.
3 Evaluate for presence of pain and muscle spasms on scale of 0 to 10.	Determines response to traction and need for analgesics and muscle relaxants.
4 Observe for local and systemic signs of infection, including purulent drainage and inflammation of pin sites; fever; elevated white blood cell count; continuous, dull, aching pain; redness; or warmth in extremity.	May indicate signs of osteomyelitis (infection of the bone) (Miller, 2008).

STEP	RATIONALE

5 Monitor respiratory status for FES, atelectasis, and pulmonary embolism every shift.

6 Inspect skin, especially around ankle, elbow, foot, or distal tibia, for fracture blisters. Do not rupture blister. Apply hydrocolloid dressing to ruptured blister (see Chapter 39).

Restlessness, tachycardia, and petechiae of chest are early signs of FES (Miller, 2008).

Fracture blisters are associated with increased interstitial pressure from posttraumatic edema.

Unexpected Outcomes

1 Patient has severe edema; marked increase in pain; inability to actively move joints; or increased pain on passive movement, indicating compartment syndrome.

2 Patient develops signs of infection or osteomyelitis. This is especially a concern with open fractures and extensive soft tissue injury.

3 Patient experiences nerve damage:
- Peroneal nerve: Footdrop with inability to evert and dorsiflex foot.
- Radial or median nerve at wrist: Inability to approximate thumb and fingers (radial) and numbness and tingling of thumb, index, middle fingers (median) with wrist drop.

4 Patient experiences FES, which is common in pelvic and long-bone fractures. Symptoms include hypoxia, restlessness, mental changes, tachycardia, tachypnea, dyspnea, hypotension, and petechial rash over upper chest and neck.

5 Patient experiences deep vein thrombosis with possible pulmonary embolus. Symptoms include dyspnea, chest pain, tachypnea, apprehension, tachycardia, cyanosis, and circulatory collapse.

Related Interventions
- Compartment syndrome is an emergent situation. Notify health care provider immediately.

- Cultures of drainage may be ordered by health care provider.
- Notify health care provider.
- Be prepared to administer ordered intravenous (IV) antibiotics and/or irrigate site with antibiotic solution.
- Encourage fluid intake and provide comfort measures for fever.

- Notify health care provider.
- Eliminate pressure if possible according to type of traction in place.
- Maintain foot in dorsiflexion according to health care provider order (e.g., pillows or orthotic).

- This is a life-threatening emergency. Notify health care provider and initiate resuscitation efforts if indicated.

- Do not massage lower extremity.
- Elevate head of bed (if conscious), administer oxygen, and notify health care provider immediately.

Recording and Reporting
- Record in nurses' notes and EHR the type of traction, site to which traction was applied, time of application, amount of weights, and patient's initial response. It may be helpful to draw a diagram for the chart and post in the room to maintain the correct traction configuration while the patient remains in traction.
- Record in nurses' notes and EHR the site care performed and appearance of pin sites.
- Record on flow sheet specific assessments and frequency of assessments.

Special Considerations
Teaching
- Before discharge teach patient use of ambulatory aid (cane, walker, or crutches); give written instructions to patient and family caregivers.
- Supply patient with dietary instructions with emphasis on protein and calcium to aid in bone and tissue healing.
- Teach patient to notify health care provider of any increase in pain; muscle spasms; increased numbness or tingling; appearance of drainage, redness, or soreness at operative or traction pin sites; and increased temperature over 101° F (38.3° C).

Pediatric
- Blood loss from a fracture poses a greater danger because the blood volume in a child is 70% to 85% of total body weight and only about 60% in an adult (Hockenberry and Wilson, 2011).
- Parents and other caregivers must work together to prevent boredom for children in traction. Parents need to be aware of the possibility of regressive behaviors. School work can be obtained when the child is able to perform those tasks.
- Assure children that someone will always be available to help them while they are in traction.

Gerontologic
- Older adults need lower initial doses of opioids because of the physiologic changes of aging (Meiner, 2011).
- Loss of functional independence may lead to depression (Meiner, 2011).

Home Care
- Following removal of skeletal traction, teach patient to dangle before ambulation, proceed slowly with ambulation, and gradually increase the time and distance ambulated.
- Teach family and patients home safety methods to prevent further injury.

SKILL 11-4   Care of a Patient with an Immobilization Device

Immobilization devices increase stability, support an extremity, or reduce the load on weight-bearing structures such as hips, knees, or ankles. A splint immobilizes and protects a body part. Temporary splints reduce pain and prevent tissue damage from further motion immediately after an injury such as a fracture or sprain. Air splints, Thomas splints, and improvised splints from material on hand are examples of temporary splints applied in emergency situations. Upper-extremity fractures are sometimes managed with splints such as hand and digital splints or sugar-tong splints. Slings support splints, casts, or injured upper extremities (Fig. 11-11). They are available commercially or can be made for almost any body part. Velcro or buckle closures permit these devices to be adjusted to fit a body part of almost any size and shape.

The abduction splint or pillow, used after hip replacement surgery, maintains a patient's legs in an abducted position (Fig. 11-12). This permits a patient to be turned without changing the position of the healing limb and prevents dislocation of the hip prosthesis. The splint is removed easily for nursing care (e.g., skin care, dressing changes, and neurovascular assessments) and ambulation with physical therapy. A posterior splint with elastic wraps is sometimes used to support an extremity.

Cloth and foam splints, known as *immobilizers*, provide long-term immobilization (Fig. 11-13). Immobilizers treat sprains and dislocations that do not require complete and continuous immobilization in a cast or traction. Other common types of immobilizers include cervical collars (hard or soft), vinyl wrist forearm splints, belt-type shoulder immobilizers, and knee immobilizers. Molded splints made of plastic provide support to patients with chronic injuries or diseases such as arthritis. They maintain the body part in a functional position to prevent contractures and minimize muscle atrophy during periods of disuse. Splints and immobilizers can be removed quickly for assessment of the skin or a wound.

Braces support weakened structures during weight bearing. For this reason they are made of sturdy materials such as leather, metal, and molded plastic. Chest and abdominal braces such as the Boston brace immobilize the thoracic and lumbar vertebral column to treat scoliosis (curvature of the spine). The brace does not correct the curve but instead prevents progression. Lumbar braces support lumbar and sacral tissues after spinal surgery. Leg braces hold the thigh, leg, and foot in functional positions for weight bearing and ambulation. Both short- and long-leg braces support weak leg muscles, aid in the control of involuntary muscle movement, and maintain surgical correction during the postoperative healing process.

Delegation and Collaboration

The skill of caring for a patient wearing a brace, sling, splint, or other immobilization device can be delegated to nursing assistive personnel (NAP). The nurse directs the NAP by:

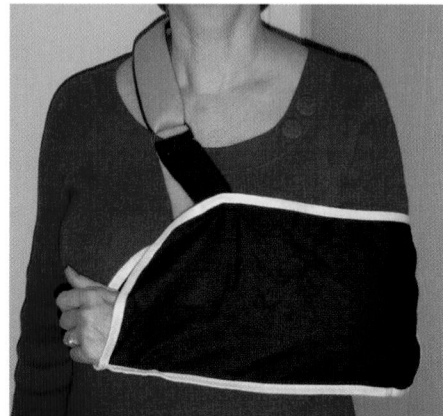

FIG 11-11   Sling for shoulder/arm immobilization. (*Courtesy Wanda Dubuisson.*)

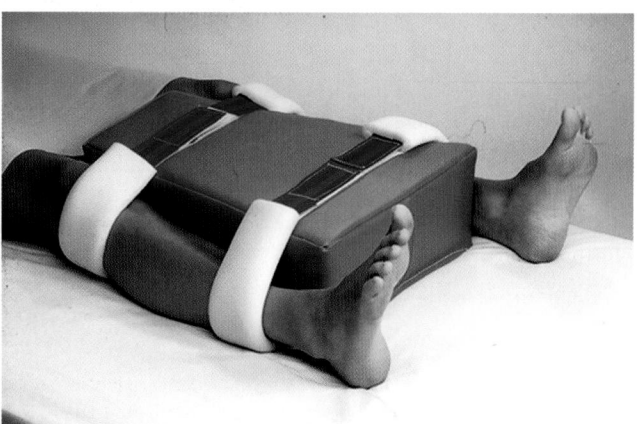

FIG 11-12   Abduction pillow.

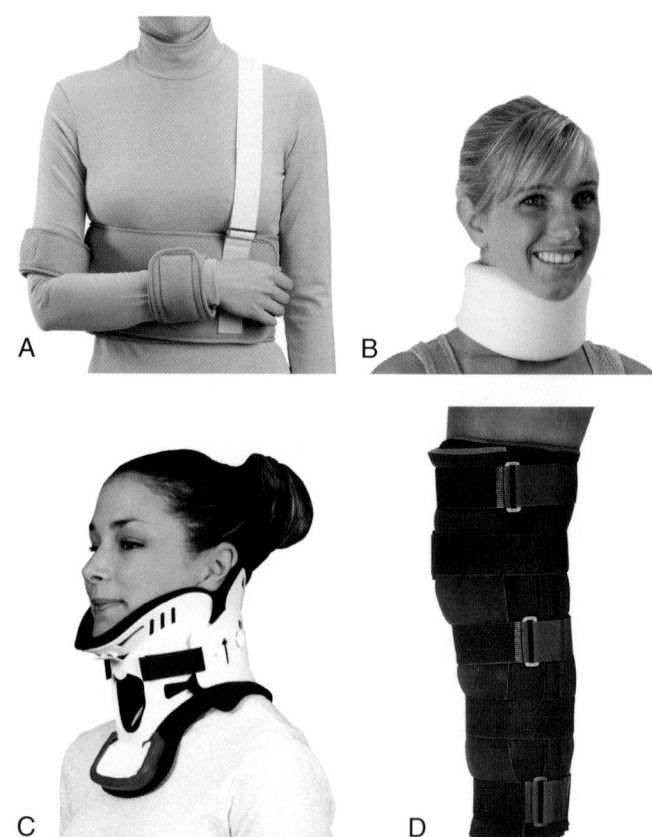

FIG 11-13   Examples of immobilizers. **A,** Shoulder immobilizer. **B,** Soft cervical collar. **C,** Hard cervical collar. **D,** Knee immobilizer.

- Reviewing correct application of the brace/splint/sling and positioning of any ties or straps.
- Reviewing prescribed schedule of wear and activities permitted while in the brace/splint/sling.
- Instructing to inform the nurse if the patient complains of any pain, rubbing, or pressure from the brace or immobilization device or if a change occurs in the patient's skin condition.

Equipment
- ❏ Brace/splint/commercially prepared sling or triangular bandage and safety pin
- ❏ Cotton shirt or gown
- ❏ Clean gloves

STEP	RATIONALE

ASSESSMENT

1 Review patient's medical history; previous and current activity level; and description of condition requiring immobilization.	Reveals patient's current and previous health status and purpose for brace/splint/sling.
2 Determine patient's previous experience with braces/splints/slings.	Provides patient's baseline knowledge and need for instruction.
3 Assess patient's level of pain using a scale of 0 to 10.	Provides baseline to determine if immobilization device affects comfort.
4 Assess patient's understanding of reason for brace/splint/sling and its care, application, and schedule of wear.	Determines level of instruction needed. Ask patient to teach back to determine level of understanding
5 Inspect areas of skin that will be in contact with support device.	Provides baseline to monitor patient for skin breakdown. Immobilized and older patients are particularly vulnerable to skin breakdown (Meiner, 2011).
6 Refer to occupational or physical therapy consultation to determine type of brace to be used, desired position, and amount of activity and movement permitted.	Ensures proper use of device.
7 Assess patient's additional need for an assistive device such as walker, cane, or crutches.	Patients may need an assistive device to provide support and promote balance during ambulation.

NURSING DIAGNOSES

- Acute pain
- Bathing and dressing self-care deficit
- Deficient knowledge
- Disturbed body image
- Impaired home maintenance
- Impaired physical mobility
- Risk for impaired skin integrity
- Risk for injury
- Risk for peripheral neurovascular dysfunction
- Risk for ineffective tissue perfusion

Related factors are individualized based on patient's condition or needs.

PLANNING

1 Expected outcomes following completion of procedure:	
• Patient and family caregiver verbalize purpose, correct application, and care of device.	Demonstrates learning and ability to manage self-care.
• Patient reports transitory increase in pain on a scale of 0 to 10 during device application.	Indicates proper fit of device and permits safer ambulation.
• Skin distal to brace/splint/sling is intact, warm to touch, without signs of pressure, and with normal sensation.	Reveals that there are no neurovascular deficits following application of device.
• Patient uses device correctly, including schedule of wear, activity limitations, and positioning.	Demonstrates correct application of principles of immobilization device.

IMPLEMENTATION

1 Identify patient using two identifiers (i.e., name and birthday or name and account number) according to agency policy. Compare identifiers with information on patient's identification bracelet.	Ensures correct patient. Complies with The Joint Commission standards and improves patient safety (TJC, 2012).
2 Explain reasons for brace/splint/sling and demonstrate how device works.	Teaching and demonstration enhance learning, reduce anxiety, and encourage cooperation.
3 Perform hand hygiene. Help patient to a comfortable position: apply upper-extremity braces/splints/slings with patient sitting upright; apply lower-extremity braces with patient lying down.	Reduces transmission of infection. Facilitates correctly aligned brace.
4 Apply clean gloves and prepare skin that will be enclosed in brace/splint/sling with soap and water, rinse, pat dry, and change any dressings (if present). If applying back brace, put thin cotton shirt or gown on patient. Ensure that there are no wrinkles to cause pressure.	This protects skin and keeps brace/splint/sling clean. Smooth cotton clothing between device and skin protects skin from irritation and absorbs moisture.

STEP	RATIONALE
5 Inspect device for wear, damage, or rough edges.	Decreases potential for skin breakdown and maintains correct alignment.
6 Apply brace/splint/sling as directed by health care provider, orthotist, physical therapist, or occupational therapist.	Proper application of brace/splint/sling is important to avoid skin breakdown, pressure ulcers, neurovascular compromise, calluses, or worsening of deformity.
a Apply even tension while wrapping a bandage from distal to proximal.	Prevents trapping of blood and fluid distal to immobilization device.
b Prevent padding from gathering or bunching.	Prevents irritation to underlying tissues.
c Support joints when placing a device.	Reduces risk of musculoskeletal injury during application.
7 Apply sling using triangular bandage:	
a Position one end of bandage over shoulder of unaffected arm (see illustrations).	Commercially available slings secure arm to chest for added support and have padding on strap for comfort.

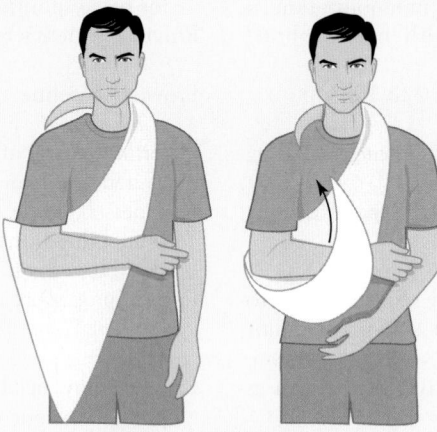

STEP 7a   Applying a sling.

STEP	RATIONALE
b Take remaining bandage and place material against chest and under and over affected arm, cradling arm.	Position supports arm.
c Position pointed end of triangle toward elbow.	
d Tie two ends of triangle at side of neck.	Avoids placing knot over cervical spine, causing pressure and discomfort.
e Fold pointed end of sling at elbow in front and secure with safety pin, closing end of sling.	
f Be sure that sling supports limb comfortably without interfering with circulation.	Prevents skin irritation and pressure to back of neck.
8 Remove and dispose of gloves. Perform hand hygiene.	Reduces transmission of infection.
9 Teach patient prescribed schedule of wear and activities while in brace/splint/sling as directed by health care provider, physical therapist, or occupational therapist.	Proper use of brace/splint/sling facilitates healing and mobility and reduces pain and stress.
10 Reinforce instruction regarding signs of skin breakdown, pressure, or rubbing to report.	Brace/splint/sling may need to be adjusted. Changes may be required because of growth or atrophy, when muscles regain or lose strength, or after reconstructive surgery.
11 Help patient ambulate with brace/splint/sling in place.	Ensures patient safety during ambulation and assesses fit of device.
12 Have patient or family caregiver apply and remove brace/splint/sling.	Promotes patient independence; demonstration confirms level of learning skill.

EVALUATION

1 Inspect areas of skin underneath brace/splint/sling for signs of pressure, including redness or breakdown.	Ensures early identification of irritation or breakdown.
2 Observe patient using brace/splint/sling.	Reinforces learning of permitted activities and related restrictions.
3 Ask patient to rate level of pain on scale of 0 to 10 after brace/splint/sling application.	Indicates proper fit of device to ensure safe ambulation.
4 Palpate temperature, pulse, and sensation of extremity distal to brace/splint/sling.	Neurovascular status reflects vascular supply or pressure on tissues.
5 Inspect alignment of limb after device application.	Ensures proper application of device to promote healing.

Unexpected Outcomes

1 Patient is unable to use brace/splint/sling correctly.

2 Patient develops areas of pressure, redness, or skin breakdown.

3 Patient reports increased severity of pain after application of device.

Related Interventions

- Reassess patient for correct fit.
- Reassess level of comfort.
- Assess muscle strength in uninvolved extremities.
- Obtain referral for physical or occupational therapy.
- Reconsult orthotist if brace not performing as designed.

- Inspect device for proper fit and positioning and for areas of damage, wear, or rough edges.
- Inform health care provider.
- Inform orthotist, physical therapist, or occupational therapist so adjustments to brace/splint can be made.

- Reposition extremity.
- Administer analgesics as ordered to maintain comfort.
- Increase frequency of neurovascular checks.
- Inform health care provider.

Recording and Reporting

- Record specific assessments related to skin integrity, neurovascular status, type of brace/splint/sling applied, schedule of wear, activity level and movement permitted, and patient's tolerance of procedure in nurses' notes and EHR.
- Document instructions given to patient and family.
- Record observations regarding patient's ability to apply, ambulate, and remove the brace/splint/sling.
- Immediately report any injury sustained by patient while using the brace/splint/sling.

Special Considerations
Teaching
- Teach patient and family caregiver how to care for brace/splint/sling:
  - When not in use, store metal braces upright in safe but easily accessible location to prevent bending or deforming.
  - Store splints of molded materials away form heat.
  - Treat leather braces or splints with a leather preservative to prevent drying and cracking.
  - Keep immobilization devices clean, dry, and in good working order. Clean plastic parts with damp cloth. Clean metal joints with pipe cleaner and oil weekly (using oil recommended by manufacturer). Remove rust with steel wool and clean metal parts with proper solvent.

- Refer to brace manufacturer or orthotist if brace is in need of maintenance or repair.
- Teach patients to avoid lotions or powders that may irritate skin.
- Teach patient appropriate range-of-motion exercises within limitation of device.
- Instruct patient and family caregiver of signs and symptoms of impaired skin integrity to report.

Pediatric
- Recognize that bracing in an adolescent affects body image and self-esteem.
- Adolescents may seek out chat rooms or social networking sites to share experiences with peers.
- Monitor children closely to ensure that they do not remove the immobilization device.

Geriatric
- Lightweight immobilization devices are less restrictive.
- Older adults may have decreased sensation (Ebersole, 2008).

Home Care
- Assess for environmental factors that interfere with safe ambulation in the home (e.g., scatter rugs).
- Remind patient to inspect and clean braces/splints/slings weekly.
- Remind patient to inspect skin daily for pressure or areas of breakdown.

? Critical Thinking Exercises

An 85-year-old woman is admitted to the orthopedic unit after falling down 12 steps. She sustained an intertrochanteric fracture of her right femur and a right Colles fracture of her right wrist. A fiberglass cast is placed on her right forearm in the emergency department, and 5 lbs of Buck's traction applied to her right leg. The plan is for an open reduction and internal fixation (ORIF) of her femur fracture in the morning.

1 Which of the following describes the correct way to position the casted arm?
  1 Carefully with palms of your hands to ensure that there are no indentations.
  2 On a plastic-covered pillow to prevent the linens from becoming damp.
  3 On several pillows, elevating the casted extremity with the hand higher than the elbow to decrease swelling.
  4 With a cradle over it to ensure air flow for proper drying.

2 The patient is using a patient-controlled analgesic (PCA) pump for pain control and receiving an opioid analgesic intravenously. She is using the pump appropriately, administering her doses of opioids; but, as the afternoon progresses, she complains of increased pain and a jumping, squeezing feeling in her right thigh. As her nurse, you would first:
  1 Massage her right thigh to relax her muscles.
  2 Medicate her with a muscle relaxant to decrease muscle spasms.
  3 Medicate her with a bolus dose of opioid analgesic for breakthrough pain.
  4 Release the Buck's traction briefly to decrease the pain.

3 It has been 12 hours, and the patient's fingers are becoming more swollen. Her cast has been further elevated to the level of her heart, and ice packs have been applied to either side of the cast. In spite of these interventions, her pain continues to increase. Which action should you take?
   1 Apply a heating pad circumferentially.
   2 Apply additional ice packs to the top and bottom of the cast.
   3 Obtain an order to change the analgesic to another one.
   4 Notify the physician, and prepare for bivalving the cast.

✔ REVIEW QUESTIONS

1 To assist in caring for a short-arm plaster cast, the nurse recommends to a family that they should do which of the following:
   1 Completely cover the cast with plastic wrap to keep it clean.
   2 Cushion any sharp edges of the cast with tape or moleskin.
   3 Scrape rough edges off the cast with a blunt knife.
   4 Blow dry the cast following a shower.

2 Place the steps of cast removal in the correct order.
   A Describe the vibration of the cast saw and the feeling of warmth the saw causes.
   B Help with positioning the patient.
   C Inspect the tissues underlying the cast.
   D Gently wash intact skin with cold-water enzyme.
      1 A, B, C, D
      2 B, A, C, D
      3 A, B, D, C
      4 B, A, D, C

3 The nurse is helping to apply a traction boot for Buck's extension; he or she should perform the following actions. (Select all that apply.)
   1 Shave the affected leg
   2 Ensure that the boot fits snugly
   3 Pad the heel of the traction boot
   4 Attach weight to the boot gradually and gently at the end of the bed
   5 Reassess neurovascular status of the extremity proximal to the traction

4 In the first 24 hours following application of skeletal traction, how often should the nurse perform neurovascular assessment distal to the traction? (Short answer)

5 After application of a cast, the patient develops severe pain and swelling of the tissues beneath it. Identify the appropriate actions the nurse should take: (Select all that apply.)
   A Assess tightness of cast.
   B Elevate casted extremity on pillows.
   C Increase frequency of neurovascular checks.
   D Lower the casted extremity.
   E Notify health care provider before administering analgesics.
   F Apply warm compresses to sides of cast.
   G Apply ice bags along sides of cast.

6 The nurse is teaching a patient how to use and care for a back brace. Which of the following directions should he or she provide the patient?
   1 Place no clothing between the brace and the skin.
   2 Inspect the brace for wear, damage, or rough edges daily.
   3 Clean the metal joints with a small steel brush and apply emollient cream to the joints weekly.
   4 Clean the plastic parts of the brace with ammonia weekly.

7 Which of the following may indicate an infection from a Steinmann pin inserted for skeletal traction?
   1 Crusting
   2 Ashen skin color
   3 Clear drainage at the pin sites
   4 Erythema at the pin sites

8 Which of the following nurses' actions are appropriate when assessing a patient's balanced-suspension skeletal traction (BSST) setup?
   1 Adding weight to the traction if it does not seem to be exerting enough force
   2 Adjusting the position of the weights if they are not hanging freely at the end of the bed
   3 Altering the line of pull of the ropes to ensure that they are at a 45-degree angle
   4 Reinserting a slipped Steinmann pin back into place

9 In developing a plan of care for a patient in skeletal traction to the leg, the nurse would take which precaution?
   1 Avoid using an overhead trapeze.
   2 Remove weights when moving the patient in bed.
   3 Maintain alignment of the injured limb with the trunk.
   4 Release the traction for 15 minutes every 8 hours.

10 Which instructions should the nurse provide to a casted patient experiencing itching under the cast?
   1 "The health care provider can provide medication for the itching."
   2 "If you can reach the area with your fingers, it is appropriate to itch that area."
   3 "You should not physically scratch under the cast; itching is part of the healing process."
   4 "You should use a tongue blade to itch instead of your fingernails."

REFERENCES

Boyd A, et al: Principles of casting and splinting, *Am Fam Physician* 79(1):16, 2009.

Ebersole P, et al: *Geriatric nursing and healthy aging*, ed 3, St Louis, 2008, Mosby.

Hockenberry MJ, Wilson D: *Wong's nursing care of infants and children*, ed 9, St Louis, 2011, Mosby.

Holmes SB, Brown SJ: Skeletal pin site care: National Association of Orthopaedic Nurses guidelines for orthopaedic nursing, *Orthop Nurs* 24(2):99, 2005.

Hyer C, et al: Early weight bearing of calcaneal fractures fixated with locked plates, *Foot Ankle Spec* 3(6):320, 2010.

Jester R, et al: *Oxford handbook of orthopaedic nursing*, New York, 2011, Oxford University Press.

Lethaby A, et al: Pin site care for preventing infections associated with external bone fixators and pins, *Cochrane Database Syst Rev* 4, 2011, CD004551. DOI: 10.1002/14651858.CD004551.pub2.

Meiner S: *Gerontologic nursing*, ed 4, St Louis, 2011, Elsevier.

Miller D: *Review of orthopaedics*, ed 5, Philadelphia, 2008, Saunders.

Musher C: *An introduction to orthopaedic nursing*, ed 4, Chicago, 2010, National Association of Orthopaedic Nurses.

Parvizi J: *High yield orthopaedics*, Philadelphia, 2010, Elsevier.

Rose RAC: Pin site care with the Ilizarov circular fixator, *Internet J Orthop Surg* 16(1): DOI: 10.5580/28c0, 2010.

Sarro A, et al: Developing a standard of care for halo vest and pin site care including patient and family education: a collaborative approach among three greater Toronto area teaching hospitals, *J Neurosci Nurs* 42(3):169, 2010.

Satryb SA, et al: Casting: all wrapped up, *Orthop Nurs* 30(1):37, 2011.

Spector R: *Cultural diversity in health and illness*, ed 7, Upper Saddle River, 2008, Prentice Hall.

The Joint Commission (TJC): *National Patient Safety Goals*, Oakbrook Terrace, Ill, 2012, The Commission, available at http://www.jointcommission.org/standards_information/npsgs.aspx.

Voda S: Bad breaks: a nurse's guide to distal radius fractures, *Nursing 2011* 41(8):37, 2011.

Wheeles C: *Wheeles' textbook of orthopaedics*, Durham, 2011, Data Trace Publishing.

Whiting N: Fractures: pathophysiology, treatment, and nursing care, *Nurs Standard* 23(2):17, 2008.

Support Surfaces and Special Beds

SKILLS AND PROCEDURES

MEDIA RESOURCES

- **evolve** http://evolve.elsevier.com/Perry/skills
  learning system

  - Review Questions
  - Audio Glossary

KEY TERMS

Air-fluidized bed	Egg-crate mattress	Kinesthetic	Rotokinetic bed
Air-suspension bed	Flotation pad	Pressure ulcers	Waffle mattress
Bariatric bed			

OBJECTIVES

Mastery of content in this chapter will enable the nurse to:
- Identify the different types of support surfaces and specialty beds used for pressure redistribution.
- Explain why preventive nursing care is still essential when using support surfaces and specialty beds.
- Describe guidelines for placing patients on support surfaces and specialty beds.
- Compare and contrast differences between mattress overlays and mattress replacements.

- Describe mechanisms by which skin breakdown can occur on an air-suspension or an air-fluidized bed, a bariatric bed, a Rotokinetic bed, or a support surface mattress or wheelchair seat cushion.
- Describe the steps for correct placement of a patient on an air-fluidized bed, an air-suspension bed, a bariatric bed, a Rotokinetic bed, or a support surface mattress.

Despite increasing technologic advances in health care, pressure ulcers remain a major problem that affects patient comfort, length of stay in a health care agency, and health care costs. Although an interdisciplinary team approach is key to reducing pressure ulcers, you are at the forefront of prevention and treatment of pressure ulcers in health care settings (WOCN, 2010). The National Pressure Ulcer Advisory Panel (NPUAP, 2009) defines pressure ulcers as localized injury to the skin and/or underlying tissue, usually over a bony prominence, as a result of pressure or pressure in combination with shear and/or friction. Pressure ulcers occur in any age-group or ethnic population, regardless of socioeconomic status. The occurrence of pressure ulcers is a serious and expensive health care problem in the United States. The National Quality Forum (NQF, 2010) considers prevention of pressure ulcers safe practices and development of pressure ulcers, especially stage III and IV ulcers, in a care setting a serious reportable event.

The pressure ulcer objective in *Healthy People 2020* is to reduce the rate of pressure ulcer–related hospitalizations among older adults to show a 10% improvement in pressure ulcer–related hospitalizations compared to baseline (USDHHS, 2011). To meet this challenge, along with the challenges of health care reform and cost reduction, it is essential to identify patients at risk for skin breakdown and pressure ulcer formation. Factors contributing to pressure ulcer formation are both extrinsic (e.g., pressure, moisture, friction, and shear) and intrinsic (e.g., malnutrition, loss of sensation, impaired mobility, aging skin, impaired mental status, infection, incontinence, and low arteriolar pressure).

The major cause of pressure ulcers is unrelieved pressure. The greater the pressure and the longer it is applied, the greater the likelihood for pressure ulcer development. To stay healthy, body tissues require an adequate supply of oxygen and nutrients and removal of carbon dioxide and other waste products of metabolism. This requires maintenance of adequate blood flow through the capillaries, which is normally 12 to 32 mm Hg. When external pressure on the tissues exceeds 32 mm Hg (the capillary closing pressure), the network of capillaries collapses. This interrupts the supply of oxygen and nutrients to the cells and the removal of metabolic waste products. As a result, there is tissue ischemia and, if unrelieved, tissue death or necrosis.

Support surfaces are one important aspect of pressure ulcer prevention. The NPUAP (2009) defines support surfaces as specialized devices for "pressure redistribution designed for management of tissue loads, micro-climate, and/or other therapeutic functions (e.g., any mattresses, integrated bed system, mattress replacement, overlay, or seat cushion or seat cushion overlay)." Several types of support surfaces can be used in beds or wheelchairs.

Thus support surfaces have differing purposes, including pressure redistribution, repositioning, and support of morbidly obese patients. They are used in acute, rehabilitative, long-term, and home care settings. Support surfaces are essential to help prevent pressure ulcers or promote wound healing by reducing capillary closing pressure. They reduce pressure by redistributing it over a larger surface area. The extent to which a support surface reduces pressure is characterized in two ways. The first is preventive, in which pressure is not consistently reduced below 32 mm Hg (e.g., foam, air, or gel overlay). The second is therapeutic, in which pressure is consistently reduced below 32 mm Hg (e.g., powered overlay air mattress or low-air-loss mattress). Preventive surfaces are for patients at risk for skin breakdown and partial-thickness ulcers. Therapeutic surfaces are for patients with stage III and IV pressure ulcers (NPUAP, 2009). Support surfaces are one intervention for redistributing pressure; they are used in conjunction with other pressure ulcer risk-reduction strategies (see Chapter 18). Although the effectiveness of certain general interventions to prevent pressure ulcers is well documented, you should tailor these interventions to individual patients based on the specific risk factors identified during assessment (Anton, 2012).

At-risk patients left sitting in chairs sometimes develop deeper and more serious pressure ulcers than patients left in their beds because a patient's body is exerting greater pressure on a smaller surface area (i.e., the buttocks). A patient lying in bed has pressure distributed over a greater surface area but is also at risk for developing pressure ulcers over bony prominences because they receive greater pressure than other parts of the body. Never place patients at high risk for pressure ulcer development on ordinary chairs or hospital mattresses. Use specialized support surfaces (e.g., foam, air, or gel mattresses, beds, and cushions) to reduce pressure. Pressure-redistribution surfaces are classified as nonpowered (formerly called *static*) support surfaces or powered (formerly called *dynamic*) support surfaces (NPUAP, 2009). Nonpowered support surfaces include mattresses or mattress overlays filled with air, water, gel, foam, or a combination of any of these. Powered support surfaces change the pressure beneath a patient, reducing the duration of any applied pressure. Many studies have reported the benefits demonstrated by pressure-redistribution surfaces in the prevention of pressure ulcers (McInnes et al., 2011).

Several support surfaces also reduce friction, shear, and moisture. Support surfaces with a slick surface help decrease friction and shear. Surfaces with porous covers allow airflow, which reduces moisture, resulting in decreased risk for skin maceration. Table 12-1 provides a comparison of support surfaces.

Frequent repositioning, which temporarily relieves pressure, is the backbone of prevention protocols. No bed or mattress totally eliminates the need for competent nursing care. It is your responsibility to use appropriate turning schedules for patients in bed or in a chair. Use lift teams and lifting devices to transfer patients from a regular bed to a special support surface (see Chapter 9). Although useful, turning devices still injure soft tissues, requiring a nurse to be especially observant for signs of pressure formation.

EVIDENCE-BASED PRACTICE

Sustained pressure on areas that support the body leads to reduced blood supply and eventually necrosis of the skin and underlying muscles. Pressure reduction and relief are major nursing interventions for the prevention of pressure ulcers (McInnes et al., 2011; WOCN, 2010). The three approaches to pressure redistribution are frequent positioning of the patient to reduce sustained pressure, use of support surfaces to distribute the body weight over a large area, and use of an alternating support surface where inflatable cells alternately inflate and deflate. Pressure-redistribution surfaces need to serve as adjuncts and not replacements for repositioning protocols (WOCN, 2010).

Systematic reviews of existing research have concluded that there is insufficient evidence to recommend one support surface over another (McInnes et al., 2011; Reddy et al., 2008).

- Encourage patients to be up as soon as medically possible in a specialty chair or wheelchair equipped with a tailored support surface for pressure relief.
- Measure seat cushions so they are properly fitted to the person's body type and chair size to prevent friction and pressure.
- Use support surfaces in the operating room for patients at high risk for pressure ulcer development.
- During the postoperative period observe the skin for signs of breakdown or injury.
- Instruct patients who had their surgeries in ambulatory care settings to observe for signs of skin injury.

PATIENT-CENTERED CARE

When making decisions about the best support surface for a patient, you must first complete thorough patient assessment, including individual needs, health care provider needs, and location of the patient. Ultimately the features of the support surface must match a patient's unique needs. Always describe to a patient and family members which interventions will be instituted and allow time for questions as needed. Some cultural groups may hesitate to question or ask for help, especially when they have limited English communication. If a patient or family members will be permitted to use any of the features of the support surface, you should provide for demonstration and return demonstration of these features.

Safety Guidelines

1 Perform complete assessment to determine patient's risk for pressure ulcers and selection of appropriate special mattresses and beds. A complete patient assessment includes use of appropriate pressure ulcer risk scales, which include factors such as presence of shear and friction and a patient's mobility and continence status (see Chapter 18).
2 Know the reason for and extent of a patient's reduced mobility. A patient who is not easy to reposition or who has pressure ulcers involving multiple surfaces benefits from pressure-redistribution support devices.
3 The use of incontinence pads increases peak pressure by 20% to 25%. Have an incontinence management plan in place (Norton et al., 2011).

TABLE 12-1	Support Surfaces		
Category and Mechanism of Action	**Indications for Use**	**Advantages**	**Disadvantages**
Support Surfaces and Overlays			
Foam Overlay (Available as an Overlay or in a Full Mattress)			
Reduces pressure; the cover (top) can reduce friction and shear. Base height of 7.5-10 cm (3-4 inches); see manufacturer guidelines regarding amount of body weight supported.	Use for moderate- to high-risk patients.	One-time charge No setup fee Cannot be punctured Available in various sizes (e.g., bed, chair, operating room table) Little maintenance Does not need electricity	Elevated body temperature Hot and may trap moisture Limited life span Plastic protective sheet needed for incontinent patients or patients with draining wounds Not indicated for those with existing stage III or IV pressure ulcers
Water Overlay (Available as an Overlay or in a Full Mattress)			
Reduces pressure and pressure points because surface provides flotation with pressure reduction by evenly redistributing patient's weight over entire support surface.	Use for high-risk patients.	Readily available Some control over motion sensations Easy to clean	Easily punctured Heavy Fluid motion may make procedures (e.g., dressing changes, CPR) difficult Maintenance needed to prevent microorganism growth Patient transfers out of bed are difficult Difficult to raise and lower head of bed
Gel Overlay			
Reduces pressure and pressure points because surface provides flotation by evenly redistributing patient's weight over entire support surface.	Use for moderate- to high-risk patients. Use for patients who are wheelchair dependent.	Low maintenance Easy to clean Multiple-patient use Impermeable to needle punctures	Heavy Expensive Lacks air flow for moisture control Variable friction control
Nonpowered Air-Filled Overlay			
Reduces pressure by lowering mean interface pressure between patient's tissue and mattress.	Use for moderate- to high-risk patients. Use for patients who can reposition themselves.	Easy to clean Multiple-patient use Low maintenance Potential repair of some air-filled products Durable	Damaged by punctures from needles and sharps Requires routine monitoring to determine adequate inflation pressure Patient transfers out of bed are difficult
Low-Air-Loss Overlay (Available as an Overlay or in a Full Mattress)			
Maintains constant and slight air movement against skin to prevent buildup of moisture and skin breakdown.	Use for moderate- to high-risk patients.	Easy to clean Maintains a constant inflation Deflates to facilitate transfer and CPR Moisture control Fabric covering overlay is air permeable, bacteria impermeable, and waterproof Reduces shear and friction Setup provided by manufacturer	Damaged by needles and sharps Noisy Requires electricity, but some are available with short backup battery In home may need to purchase backup generator in case of loss of electrical power
Specialty Beds			
Air-Fluidized Bed			
Bed frame contains silicone-coated beads and incorporates both air and fluid support. Silicone-coated beads become fluidized when air is pumped through beads.	Use for high-risk patients. Use for patients with stage III or IV pressure ulcers or burns.	Less frequent turning or repositioning Improved patient comfort Quickly becomes firm for CPR or other treatments when device is turned "off" Reduces shear, friction, and edema to site May facilitate management of copious wound drainage or incontinence Setup provided by manufacturer	Continuous circulation of warm, dry air may increase patient risk for dehydration Possible increase in room temperature Patient may experience disorientation Patient transfer difficult Heavy Expensive May not be wide enough for use with obese patients or patients with contractures Patient cannot lay prone because of risk of suffocation

Continued

TABLE 12-1 | Support Surfaces—cont'd

Category and Mechanism of Action	Indications for Use	Advantages	Disadvantages
Low-Air-Loss Bed Bed frame with series of connected air-filled pillows. Amount of pressure in each pillow is controlled and can be calibrated to patient need.	Use for patients who need pressure relief, those who cannot be repositioned frequently, or those who have skin breakdown on more than one surface. Contraindicated in patients with unstable spinal column.	Can raise and lower head and foot of bed Easy transfer in and out of bed Less frequent turning schedule Pillows can be transferred to stretcher with patient Setup provided by manufacturer	Portable motor is noisy Bed surface material is slippery; patients can easily slide down mattress or out of bed when being transferred
Kinetic Therapy Provides continuous passive motion to promote mobilization of pulmonary secretions and low air loss, which provides pressure relief.	Use primarily for patients needing spinal stabilization. Should not be used when the patient is hemodynamically unstable.	Reduces pulmonary complications associated with restricted mobility Reduces the risk for urinary stasis and urinary tract infections Reduces venous stasis	Does not reduce shear or moisture Cannot be used with cervical or skeletal traction Possible motion sickness initially Possible sensations of claustrophobia

CPR, Cardiopulmonary resuscitation.
Data from Wound, Ostomy and Continence Nurses (WOCN): *Guideline for prevention and management of pressure ulcers*, Glenview, Ill: 2010, The Association; McInnes E, et al: Support surfaces for pressure ulcer prevention, *Cochrane Database Syst Rev* 13(4):CD001735, 2011.

4 Continue to provide basic prevention care measures against the hazards of immobility (e.g., regular skin assessment, turning, correct positioning, or range-of-motion exercises).
5 Use safe patient-handling techniques and proper body mechanics when positioning or working with patients (see Chapter 9).
6 Follow all safety measures to prevent injury to patients from accidental falls or improper positioning when placing them on special beds or mattresses.
7 Encourage patients to remain as mobile as possible within the limits of their physical conditions and prescribed activity levels.
8 Educate family caregivers about the advantages/disadvantages and methods of operation of all support devices to ensure their proper use in all settings.
9 Collaborate and consult with health care professionals who have expertise in this area.

PROCEDURAL GUIDELINE 12-1   Selection of Pressure-Reducing Support Surfaces

Delegation and Collaboration

The selection of a pressure-reducing support device cannot be delegated to nursing assistive personnel (NAP).

Equipment

❑ Pressure ulcer risk assessment tool (see agency policy) (see Chapter 18)
❑ Body chart, tape measure, and/or camera to document existing areas of impaired skin integrity
❑ Documentation form or electronic health record
❑ Skin care products

Procedural Steps

1 Assess patient's risk for skin breakdown using a risk assessment tool (e.g., Braden Scale).
2 Assess patient's existing pressure ulcers, including location, stage, areas of blistering, abnormal reactive hyperemia, and abrasion.
3 Assess patient's level of comfort using a pain scale of 0 to 10.
4 Determine the need for a pressure-reduction surface from assessment data. Place "at risk" patients on a pressure-reduction surface and not an ordinary mattress (McInnes et al., 2011).

5 Identify patient factors when selecting an appropriate surface (Fig. 12-1):
   a Does patient need pressure redistribution (e.g., you cannot reposition the patient, or there is an existing pressure ulcer)?
   b Is the surface needed for short- or long-term care? A short-term surface is usually needed for an acute illness and hospitalization. A long-term surface is usually needed for extended or home care.
   c What is the potential comfort level achieved by the surface? If patient is sensitive to noise, a device with a loud motor will increase his or her discomfort.
   d Are the patient, family, and caregivers cooperative and adherent to repositioning? In addition, are they aware that a support surface should never replace repositioning? Is adequate assistance available for repositioning? In a home setting a support surface is often necessary when the family, caregiver, or patient is unable to independently reposition or assist with repositioning.
   e Does the support surface have a potential to interfere with patient's independent functioning? The height of the overlay and its soft edge may affect patient's ability to

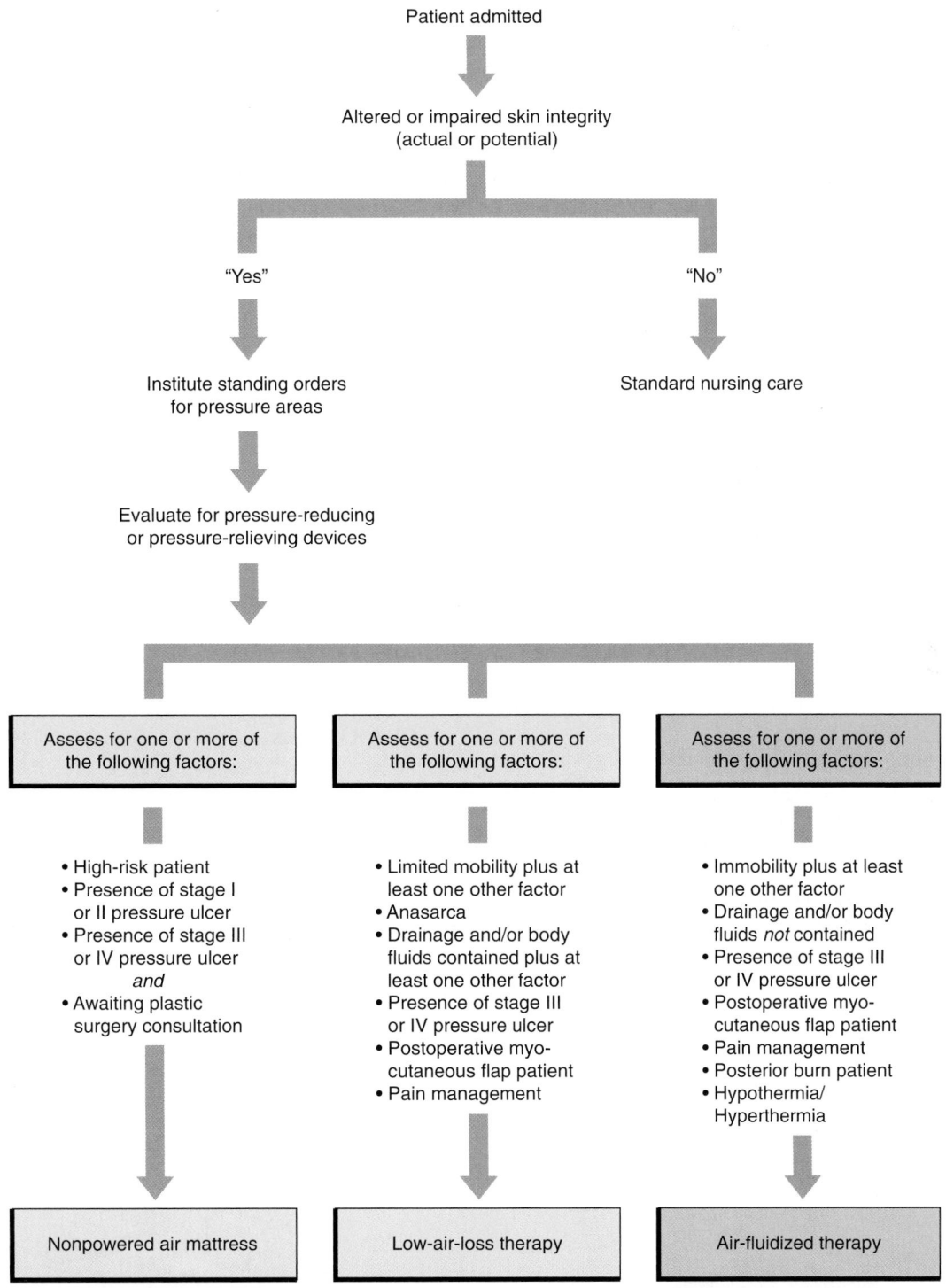

Patient admitted

Altered or impaired skin integrity
(actual or potential)

"Yes"

"No"

Institute standing orders
for pressure areas

Standard nursing care

Evaluate for pressure-reducing
or pressure-relieving devices

Assess for one or more of the following factors:	Assess for one or more of the following factors:	Assess for one or more of the following factors:
• High-risk patient • Presence of stage I or II pressure ulcer • Presence of stage III or IV pressure ulcer *and* • Awaiting plastic surgery consultation	• Limited mobility plus at least one other factor • Anasarca • Drainage and/or body fluids contained plus at least one other factor • Presence of stage III or IV pressure ulcer • Postoperative myo-cutaneous flap patient • Pain management	• Immobility plus at least one other factor • Drainage and/or body fluids *not* contained • Presence of stage III or IV pressure ulcer • Postoperative myo-cutaneous flap patient • Pain management • Posterior burn patient • Hypothermia/ Hyperthermia
Nonpowered air mattress	Low-air-loss therapy	Air-fluidized therapy

FIG 12-1   Flow diagram for ordering specialty beds.

PROCEDURAL GUIDELINE 12-1   Selection of Pressure-Reducing Support Surfaces—cont'd

transfer, and a high-air-loss bed is not appropriate for a patient who needs to get in and out of bed frequently.

f   What are patient's financial limitations?

g   If the patient is using the device in the home, what are the environmental limitations? Will the home and existing electrical service accommodate the surface selected? Can the caregivers and family in the home manage the surface?

h   How durable is the product? Is the surface easily subjected to puncture? How easily can the surface be cleaned?

i   Does patient need pressure-relief surfaces in a chair/ wheelchair? Has the family or caregiver been instructed on appropriate inflation of the device?

6   Choose the appropriate surface (see Table 12-1).

a   Pressure-redistribution devices redistribute pressure over bony prominences. Surfaces providing pressure redistribution include therapeutic mattress replacements, nonpowered and powered (i.e., moving) surfaces, low-air-loss beds and mattresses, and air-fluidized beds (WOCN, 2010).

Continued

PROCEDURAL GUIDELINE 12-1   Selection of Pressure-Reducing Support Surfaces—cont'd

Pressure-redistribution surfaces are also used in the operating room for individuals who are at high risk or for lengthy procedures (McInnes et al., 2011).

b Use a nonpowered support surface if patient can assume a variety of positions without bearing weight on a pressure ulcer without bottoming out. Bottoming out makes the support surface ineffective. To assess for bottoming out, place a hand (palm up) under the mattress or cushion below the area of risk for pressure areas (e.g., patient's pressure points when lying or sitting on surface). If there is less 2.5 cm (1 inch) of support material felt, patient has bottomed out (WOCN, 2010).

c Select a powered support surface when patient cannot assume a variety of positions without bearing weight on a pressure ulcer, if patient fully compresses the static support surface, or if the pressure ulcer does not show evidence of healing. Alternating or powered mattresses are associated with lower incidence of pressure ulcers compared with standard mattresses (Gray, 2009; WOCN, 2010).

d High-specification foam is effective in decreasing the incidence of pressure ulcers in fairly high-risk patients, including older adults and patients with fractures of the neck of the femur (McInnes et al., 2011; WOCN, 2010).

e Patients with stage III or IV pressure ulcers on multiple turning surfaces often benefit from an air-fluidized bed (WOCN, 2010).

f There is limited evidence that low-air-loss beds reduce the incidence of pressure ulcers in intensive care (WOCN, 2010).

g When excess moisture is a potential risk, a support surface that provides airflow is important in drying the skin and reducing the incidence of pressure ulcers (NPUAP, 2009).

7 Check agency policy regarding implementing a support surface.

a Obtain a health care provider's order. This is usually required for a patient to obtain third-party reimbursement.

b Consult with agency case manager or social worker to assist with patient's financial eligibility and terms and length of third-party reimbursement for the surface.

c Consult with agency home care or discharge planning if the device is anticipated for long-term use. Specific procedures and evaluations are needed for continuity of surface when patient is transferred to extended care or discharged home.

8 Perform hand hygiene. Inspect condition of skin regularly according to agency policy to evaluate changes in skin and effectiveness of therapy.

9 Inspect existing pressure ulcers for evidence of healing.

10 Observe for side effects associated with specific pressure-reducing surface (e.g., nausea, dizziness).

11 Document pressure ulcer risk assessment and skin assessment in patient's record. Document the support surface selected and patient response to the surface (see specific skills for recording and reporting details).

SKILL 12-1   Placing a Patient on a Support Surface

Numerous support surfaces reduce pressure on tissues overlying bony prominences. These devices are recommended for preventive measures for patients with reduced mobility and risk for developing pressure ulcers. Most of the devices are easy to apply and keep clean. The extent to which the devices actually reduce pressure and prevent skin breakdown is highly variable.

Support surfaces are categorized as mattress (or wheelchair) overlays (Fig. 12-2), mattress replacements, or specialty beds. An overlay rests on top of a hospital mattress and uses foam, air, water,

gel, or combinations of these products to provide pressure relief. Mattress overlays and mattress replacements are either nonpowered (e.g., foam, gels) or powered (e.g., alternating-pressure surfaces).

A flotation pad is made of a silicone or polyvinyl chloride gel enclosed in a vinyl-covered square. The pad serves as an artificial layer of fat to protect bony surfaces such as the sacrum and greater trochanters. These flotation pads are available for the bed or wheelchair (Fig. 12-3).

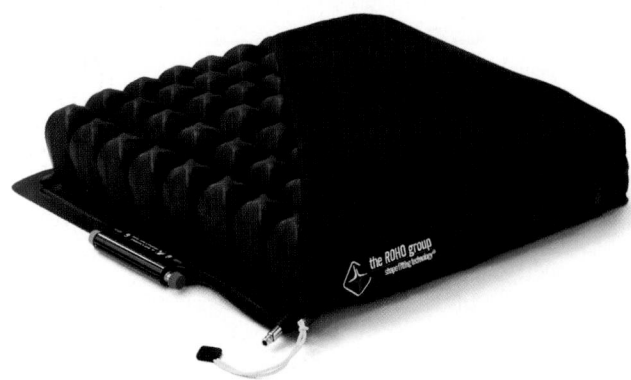

FIG 12-2 ROHO cushion for a wheelchair. (©ROHO Group. Reprinted with permission. All rights reserved.)

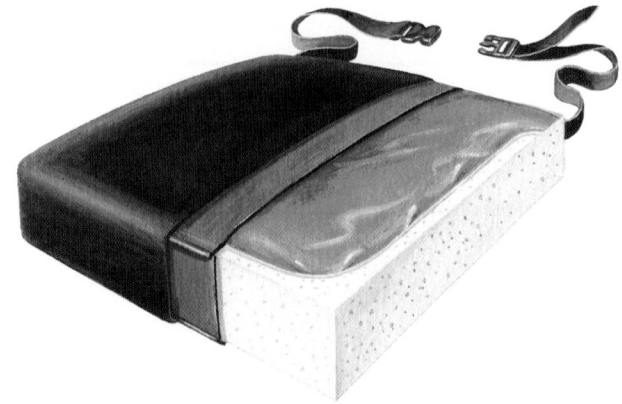

FIG 12-3 Gel cushion for wheelchair. (©Skil-Care Corp. Reprinted with permission. All rights reserved.)

There are two types of foam mattresses. One is the foam mattress overlay, which has a flat smooth surface, foam rubber peaks (egg-crate, Fig. 12-4), or a cut surface. Place one on top of a bed mattress and place a sheet over the foam mattress pad overlay to prevent soiling and provide ease of cleaning. The second type is the foam specialty mattress, which completely replaces the hospital mattress and is covered by a loose-fitting cover intended to protect the mattress and minimize friction and shear. Foam mattresses are used more for comfort than for pressure redistribution. Some of the newer foam mattresses have memory and an increased life span. The memory foam molds to the shape of the body and reduces pressure to the area in contact with the foam.

One type of air mattress is fully integrated into the hospital bed or designed to be placed in a wheelchair (Fig. 12-5). You can adjust this bed surface to a patient's comfort level by adding or removing air through buttons within the patient's reach, or you can automatically adjust pressures to a patient's position and movement when in the automatic mode. Always use a bedsheet to cover an air mattress to prevent skin from touching the plastic surface.

Air mattress overlays are either nonpowered or powered and consist of interconnected air cells or cushions inflated by the use of a motorized blower (Fig. 12-6). More complex air mattresses contain several layers of tubes or support cells. These mattresses use a pressure-cycling device to intermittently inflate and deflate or to maintain a constant inflation and slight air movement in the mattress.

A nonpowered mattress is inflated with a simple air blower after placing the mattress on a bed. An integrated air mattress connects with a pressure-cycling device that intermittently inflates and deflates sections of the mattress, creating a cycling effect that minimizes pressure on bony prominences (Fig. 12-7).

Replacement mattresses have foam, gel, air, or fluid sections that you can customize to the needs of a specific patient with moderate-to-high risk for skin breakdown. Another available option is an air-integrated replacement mattress instead of the conventional mattress. These mattresses may also be fully integrated into the bed. Air mattresses are usually for patients with moderate-to-high risk for skin breakdown. You must deflate air mattresses before initiating cardiopulmonary resuscitation (CPR). Many agencies have purchased replacement mattresses to replace their standard hospital mattresses because of improved skin and wound outcomes.

Another preventive intervention is a low-pressure seat cushion (Fig. 12-8) overlaid on a wheelchair or a dry, nonpowered flotation

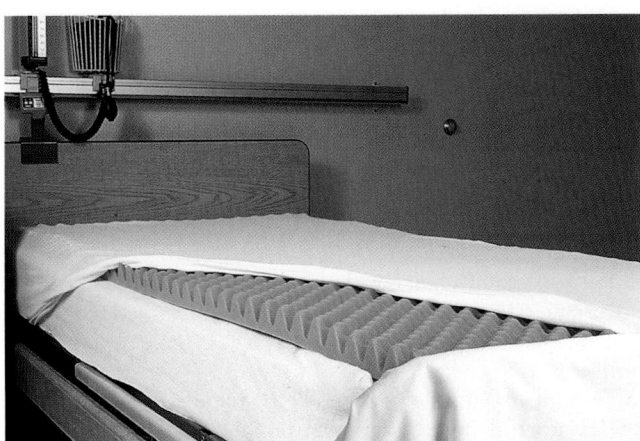

FIG 12-4 Egg-crate foam overlay is primarily for comfort.

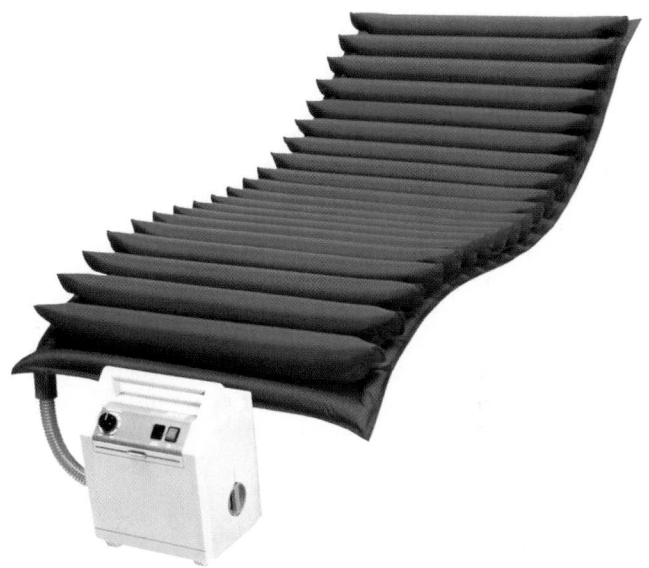

FIG 12-6 Dynamic air mattress overlay. (©2002 Hill-Rom Services. *Reprinted with permission. All rights reserved.*)

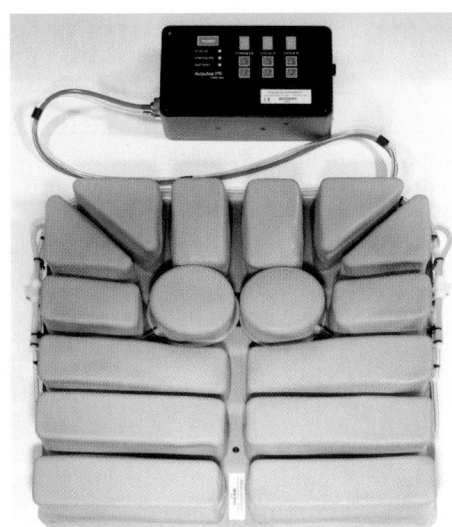

FIG 12-5 Air-filled cushion for wheelchair. (©*Aquila Corporation, Reprinted with permission. All rights reserved.*)

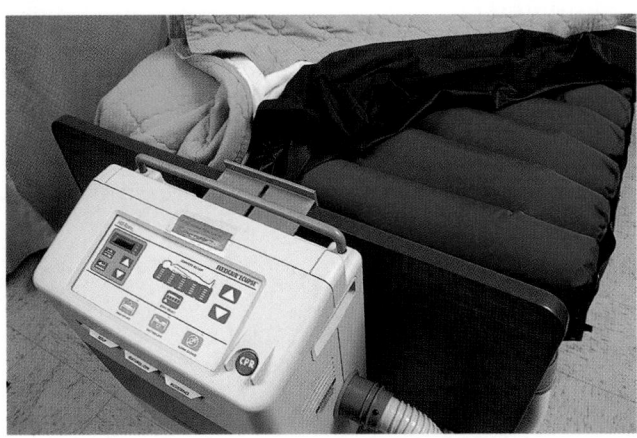

FIG 12-7 Motor for integrated air mattress.

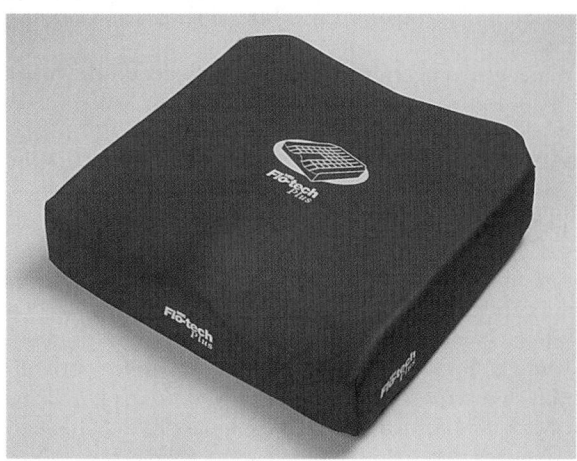

FIG 12-8   Low-pressure seat cushion. (*Reproduced with permission from Medical Support Systems Ltd.*)

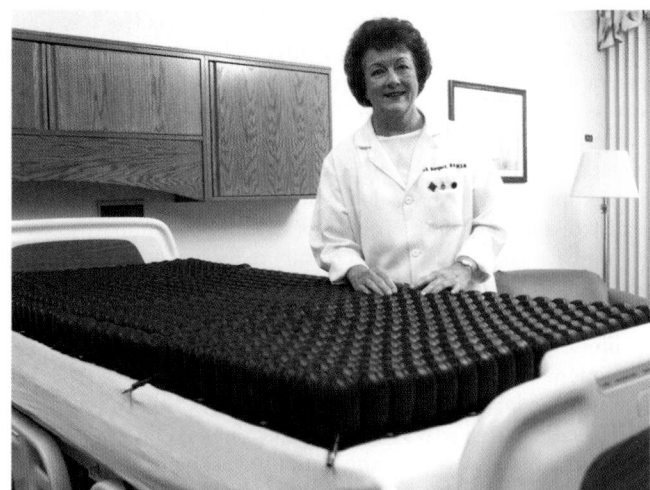

FIG 12-9   ROHO dry flotation mattress for a bed. (*©The ROHO Group. Reprinted with permission. All rights reserved.*)

mattress system (Fig. 12-9) that you overlay on a bed. Through a system of controlled dynamics, a cushion maintains low pressures by distributing pressure across a patient's body surface, reducing friction and shear.

Support surfaces aid in reducing pressure on a patient's skin but do not replace regular repositioning, meticulous skin care, or range-of-motion exercises. The decision to place a patient on a pressure-redistribution surface and the selection of this surface is a nursing responsibility (see Procedural Guideline 12-1).

Delegation and Collaboration

The skill of placing a patient on a support surface can be delegated to nursing assistive personnel (NAP). However, you must first complete the assessment, determine the need for a support surface, and select the specific surface. Some types of support surfaces require that a manufacturer's representative set up and maintain the support system. The nurse directs the NAP to:

- Notify the nurse of any changes in a patient's skin; the nurse then evaluates condition of the skin.

- Continue to regularly turn and reposition a patient and seek assistance for patient position changes as necessary in bed or wheelchair.
- Monitor the normal functioning of the support device such as inflation and deflation cycles and report to the nurse any changes in these cycles or leakage of air, water, or gel.

Equipment

- ❏ Pressure ulcer risk assessment tool (see agency policy) (see Chapter 18)
- ❏ Mattress and/or chair overlay support surface of choice: foam overlays, air mattress overlay, bed with integrated surface, air-integrated replacement mattress
- ❏ Sheet(s)
- ❏ Clean gloves (if soiled linen is being handled)
- ❏ Standard bed frame (with mattress) if overlay is to be used (*optional*)

STEP	RATIONALE

ASSESSMENT

1 Perform hand hygiene.	Reduces transmission of microorganisms.
2 Determine patient's risk for pressure ulcer formation using a valid assessment tool (e.g., Braden Scale) and assess for risk factors for pressure ulcers (e.g., nutritional deficits, shear stress, friction, alterations in mobility and sensory perception, moisture, and abnormal serum albumin and hemoglobin levels) (see Chapter 18).	Risk assessment tools provide an objective measure of risk consistent over time (WOCN, 2010).

Clinical Decision Point *Patients with unstable conditions do not always tolerate turning or positioning required for thorough assessment or the application of a support surface mattress.*

3 Perform skin assessment (see Chapter 18). Inspect condition of skin, especially over dependent sites and bony prominences (see Chapter 18).	Provides baseline to determine a change in skin integrity or in an existing pressure ulcer.
4 Assess patient's level of comfort using a pain scale of 0 to 10.	Provides baseline to determine patient's response to therapy and comfort needs.

STEP	RATIONALE

Clinical Decision Point *Some patients experiencing pain need pain medication before application of support surface of choice or transfer to another bed (NPUAP, 2009).*

5 Assess patient's understanding of purpose of support surface. | Misconceptions affect patient's cooperation in use of mattress.
6 Verify health care provider's order for type of support surface. | Health care provider's order is usually required to ensure third-party payment of support surface.

NURSING DIAGNOSES

- Deficient knowledge regarding use of support surface mattress
- Impaired physical mobility
- Impaired skin integrity
- Ineffective tissue perfusion
- Pain (acute, chronic)
- Risk for impaired skin integrity
- Risk for infection

Related factors are individualized based on patient's condition or needs.

PLANNING

1 Expected outcomes following completion of procedure:
  - Patient's skin is without erythema or mottling.

  - Existing pressure ulcer shows signs of healing.

  - Patient expresses improved level of comfort.
  - Patient is removed from therapeutic surface when risk for pressure ulcers decreases.
2 Explain purpose of mattress and method of application to patient and family caregiver.

Mottling represents hypoxia, which is an abnormal physiologic response in tissues under pressure.
Skin remains free of new pressure ulcers. Support surface does not interfere with circulation to dependent areas.
Equalized pressures have eliminated localized areas of discomfort.
Provides for efficient, cost-effective care while maintaining high-quality outcomes.
Reduces anxiety and promotes cooperation.

IMPLEMENTATION

1 Close room door or bedside curtain. | Provides patient privacy and considerate care during application of mattress to bed or transfer to alternative bed.

2 Perform hand hygiene. Apply clean gloves (if linens are soiled or wet). Obtain assistance to position patient and/or mattress as needed. | Prevents transmission of microorganisms. Assistance from other caregivers reduces risk for friction and shear in transfer to new surface.

3 Identify patient using two identifiers (i.e., name and birthday or name and account number) according to agency policy. Compare identifiers with information on patient's identification bracelet. | Ensures correct patient. Complies with The Joint Commission standards and improves patient safety (TJC, 2012).

4 Apply support surface to bed or prepare alternative bed (bed may be occupied or unoccupied). Keep sharp objects away from air mattress or air-surface bed.
  a Replacing mattress:
    (1) Apply mattress to bed frame after removing standard hospital mattress. | Hospital mattress needs to be stored. In some instances mattress replacements are standard procedure.
    (2) Apply sheet over mattress. Keep linens between surfaces to a minimum. | Sheet reduces soiling. Multiple layers decrease surface effectiveness in reducing pressure (WOCN, 2010).
  b Preparing an air mattress/overlay:
    (1) Apply deflated mattress flat over surface of bed mattress. (There may be directions on pad indicating which side to place up.) | Provides smooth, even surface.

    (2) Bring any plastic strips or flaps around corners of bed mattress. | Secures air mattress in place.

    (3) Attach connector on air mattress to inflation device. Inflate mattress to proper air pressure determined by air pump or blower. | Mattresses vary as to requiring one-time or continuous inflation cycle. Check inflation daily. Manufacturer directions indicate desired air pressure designed to distribute patient's body weight evenly. Directions are included with each mattress.

    (4) Place sheet over air mattress, being sure to eliminate all wrinkles. | Prevents soiling of mattress, reduces direct contact of skin with plastic surface. Wrinkles can cause pressure.
    (5) Check air pumps to be sure that pressure cycle alternates. | Alternating airflow mattress produces intermittent cycling, inflating only parts of mattress at any one time. Intermittent cycle continually alternates pressure against skin and soft tissue.

    (6) Help patient transfer in and out of bed. | Mattress surface is less firm and slippery. This makes it difficult for some patients to transfer from bed to chair/stretcher.

STEP	RATIONALE
c Using an air-surface bed: (1) Obtain and place linen on bed.	In some instances an air-surface bed is available in patient rooms. If not, an ordering system exists to obtain one as needed (see agency policy).
(2) Place switch in the "prevention" mode.	In the "prevention" mode, surface pressures change automatically with patient position to equalize pressure and eliminate points of pressure.

Clinical Decision Point *Most pressure-relieving beds in the hospital and home care are equipped with a CPR switch to instantly lower head section from an elevated position and deflate the mattress to provide a firm surface for chest compressions (Fig. 12-10). Note this on the Kardex.*

5 Position patient comfortably as desired over support surface. Reposition routinely.	Location of existing pressure ulcer might influence type of positioning (WOCN, 2010).
6 Remove and dispose of gloves and perform hand hygiene.	Reduces transmission of microorganisms.

EVALUATION

1 Reassess patient's risk for pressure ulcer formation at routine intervals.	Documents change in status, which is critical for evaluating continued need for therapeutic surface.
2 Inspect and compare condition of patient's skin every 8 hours or according to agency policy to determine changes in skin integrity, pressure ulcer status, and effectiveness of support surface.	Determines if pressure sores develop or if condition of existing sores changes.
3 Ask patient to rate comfort on a scale of 0 to 10.	If pressure-relief mattress is effective, patient generally experiences less discomfort.
4 Evaluate functioning of support surface periodically.	Regular inspection of mechanical components of mattress ensures proper functioning.

Unexpected Outcomes	Related Interventions
1 Patient develops localized areas of abnormal reactive hyperemia for longer than 30 minutes (WOCN, 2010), mottling, swelling, and tenderness with evidence of breakdown.	• Modify skin care regimen. • Increase frequency of skin assessment. • Increase types of pressure-relief interventions. • Check for proper inflation of support surface. • Revise turning schedule. • Consult with skin care expert. • Notify health care provider.
2 Existing pressure areas fail to heal or increase in size or depth.	• Modify skin care regimen. • Revise turning schedule. • Consult with skin care expert. • Notify health care provider.
3 Patient expresses discomfort while on support surface.	• Evaluate need for analgesia or mild sedation. • Evaluate need to modify support surface. • Reposition patient more frequently. • Unless contraindicated, provide back massage. Do not massage reddened areas or bony prominences because massage to these areas contributes to skin breakdown (WOCN, 2010).
4 Bed or mattress develops leak (air, water, gel).	• Take corrective action according to agency or manufacturer policies/directions.

Recording and Reporting

- Record type of support surface applied, extent to which patient tolerated procedure, and condition of patient's skin in nurses' notes, electronic health record (EHR), and/or skin assessment flow sheet. Record any patient teaching and validation of understanding in nurses' notes and EHR.
- Report evidence of pressure ulcer formation to nurse in charge or health care provider.

Special Considerations
Teaching

- Explain risks of immobility and pressure ulcer formation to patient and family members (see Chapter 18).
- Instruct in proper use of body mechanics, positioning, and pressure relief methods.
- Explain purpose and function of the pressure-redistribution surface. Include reminder that the surface augments care and

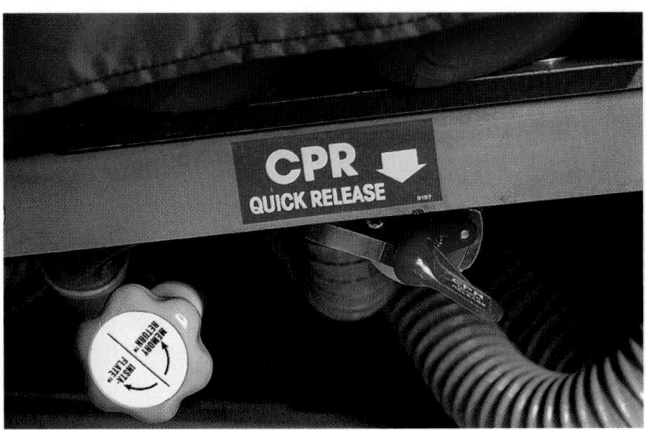

FIG 12-10 Cardiopulmonary resuscitation switch deflates low-air-loss bed to provide hard surface.

does not replace the need for turning and pressure-relief maneuvers.
• Explain precautions regarding sharp objects and fire hazard.

Pediatric
• Various pain assessment tools have been developed specifically for use in children (see Chapter 15).

• Parents can support children in being able to express their pain an treatment preferences (Hockenberry and Wilson, 2011).

Gerontologic
• Implement preventive measures because aging skin is drier, thinner, and less pressure sensitive, increasing the risk for skin breakdown.
• Adding mattress overlays changes the bed height. Use care when transferring and teaching family members to transfer a patient from bed to chair.

Home Care
• Most of the devices may be adapted for home use on a standard twin bed or hospital bed.
• Base selection on patient needs and environmental audit. For example, a patient on total bed rest who smokes is not an ideal candidate for a foam mattress because of the potential for fire; a patient with pets that sleep in the bed is not suited for an air-filled mattress because of the risk for puncture.
• Address concerns in the home setting related to need for a back-up generator or other plan to maintain the support surface during power outages.

SKILL 12-2 Placing a Patient on an Air-Suspension or Air-Fluidized Bed

Air-suspension beds are designed for patients who are immobile or confined to bed. The air-suspension bed supports a patient's weight on air-filled cushions. There are two types of systems: low-air-loss and high-air-loss. A low-air-loss system minimizes pressure and reduces shear. If a patient has large stage III or IV pressure ulcers on multiple turning surfaces of the skin, a low-air-loss bed or air-fluidized bed may be indicated (WOCN, 2010).

High-air-loss beds provide for selective drying and do not have the effect of substantially increasing insensible fluid losses. For patients requiring high air loss under a body part (e.g., under the buttocks) you can substitute high-air-loss cushions. It is also possible to adapt the air-suspension beds to individual patient needs with specialty cushions for positioning, foot support, and lateral arm supports.

Another adaptation of the air-suspension bed is the kinetic low-air-loss bed (Fig. 12-11). This bed is used in intensive care areas and has the ability to provide a pressure-relief surface while rotating approximately 30 to 35 degrees continuously. Do not use this surface with a patient who has an unstable spine or who is in traction (see Chapter 11).

An air-fluidized bed is a powered device designed to distribute a patient's weight evenly over its support surface (Fig. 12-12). The contact pressure of the patient's body against the filter sheet stays at 11 to 16 mm Hg. The bed minimizes pressure and reduces shearing force and friction through the principle of fluidization. Fluidization is created by forcing a gentle flow of temperature-controlled air upward through a mass of fine ceramic microspheres. The microspheres fluidize and take on the appearance of boiling milk and all the properties of a fluid. The patient lies directly on a polyester filter sheet that allows air to pass through but does not allow the microspheres to escape. Patients feel as though they are floating on a surface such as a warm waterbed.

Air-fluidized beds are useful in the care of patients who require minimal movement to prevent skin damage by shearing force and

for patients who experience significant pain when being turned or positioned (e.g., burn patients, those who have undergone extensive skin grafts or have existing pressure ulcers, and victims of multiple trauma). Patients tend to perspire and lose body fluids while on the bed because the surface of the filter sheet warms. As patients perspire, moisture is quickly absorbed into the circulating microspheres. Diaphoresis often goes undetected; thus insensible fluid loss is not always evident until a patient develops fluid and electrolyte imbalances. Therefore you need to monitor the patient's fluid balance status carefully.

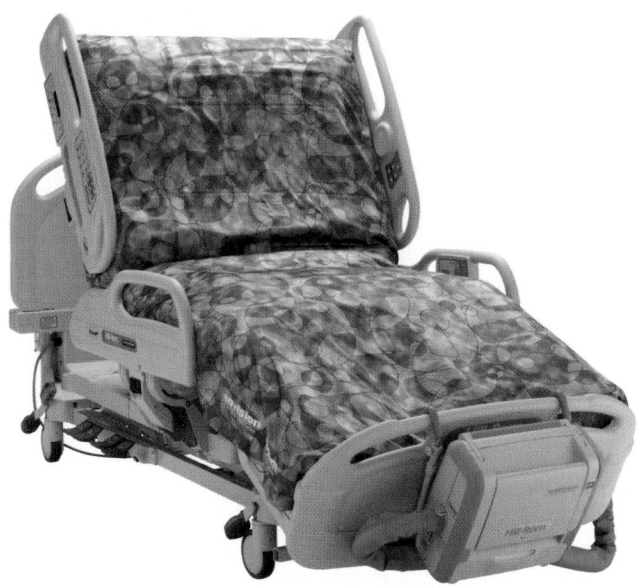

FIG 12-11 Low-air-loss bed. (©2002 Hill-Rom Services. Reprinted with permission. All rights reserved.)

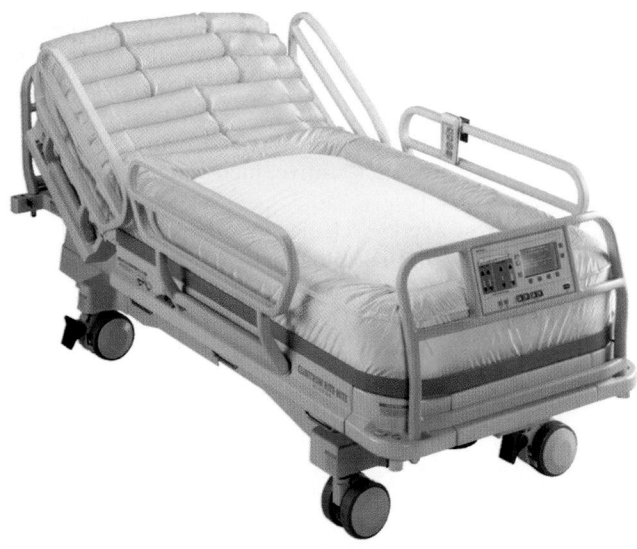

FIG 12-12 Combination air-fluidized, low-air-loss bed. (©2008 Hill-Rom Services. Reprinted with permission. All rights reserved.)

Conventional fluidized beds do not allow for head-of-bed position changes. Use foam wedges to elevate the head. Combinations of fluidized-low-air-loss beds that allow head-of-bed elevation are also available. These beds use air to lift the upper body while the lower body stays on a fluidized bed surface. The weight of the bed structure makes transport extremely difficult. A pediatric version of this bed is available.

Delegation and Collaboration

The skill of placing a patient on an air-suspension or air-fluidized bed can be delegated to nursing assistive personnel (NAP). However, first you complete the assessment, determine the need for a support surface, and select the specific surface. Some types of support surfaces require that the manufacturer representative set up and maintain the support system. The nurse directs the NAP to:

- Notify the nurse of any changes in the patient's skin.
- Continue to regularly turn and reposition the patient and seek assistance for patient position changes as necessary. This is not always necessary for patients who are placed on a lateral rotation air-suspension bed.
- Monitor the normal functioning of the air-suspension bed such as inflation and deflation cycles and report to the nurse any changes in these cycles.
- Notify the nurse if the patient becomes disoriented, restless, or complains of nausea.

Equipment

Air-suspension Bed
- ❏ Gore-Tex sheet (supplied by manufacturer)
- ❏ Disposable bed pads, if indicated
- ❏ Clean gloves (*optional*)

Air-fluidized Bed
- ❏ Foam positioning wedges if indicated
- ❏ Filter sheet (supplied by manufacturer)
- ❏ Clean gloves (*optional*)

STEP	RATIONALE

ASSESSMENT

1 Perform hand hygiene.	Reduces transmission of microorganisms.
2 Determine patient's risk for pressure ulcer formation using a valid assessment tool (e.g., Braden Scale) and assess for risk factors for pressure ulcers, including nutritional deficits, shear stress, friction, alterations in mobility and sensory perception, moisture, and abnormal serum albumin and hemoglobin levels (see Chapter 18).	Risk assessment tools as suggested by the Agency for Healthcare Research and Quality (AHRQ) and WOCN (e.g., Braden Scale) provide an objective measure of risk consistent among nurse assessors over time (WOCN, 2010).
3 Identify patients who will benefit from air-suspension therapy or air-fluidized therapy (e.g., immobilized or burn patients).	Beds effectively minimize pressure on fragile tissues and dependent body parts. Selected for patients who require pressure relief for treatment or prevention of pressure ulcers.

Clinical Decision Point *Do not use this surface with a patient who has an unstable spine or who is in traction.*

4 Inspect condition of skin, especially over dependent sites and bony prominences. Note appearance of existing ulcers and determine stage of ulcer (see Chapter 18).	Provides baseline to determine a change in skin integrity or in an existing pressure ulcer over time.
5 Assess patient's level of comfort using a pain scale of 0 to 10.	Provides baseline to determine patient's comfort needs. Nerve endings related to pressure, touch, temperature, and limb position are in the skin (WOCN, 2010). Patients usually require less analgesia while on the bed.
6 Review health care provider orders.	A health care provider's order is usually required to obtain third-party reimbursement for cost of bed.
7 Assess patient's level of orientation.	Baseline used to detect change while patient is on bed. Some patients may become confused or disoriented from the flotation sensation of the bed (WOCN, 2010).
8 Assess patient's and family members' knowledge about therapy and understanding of purpose of bed.	Blowers maintain bed inflation; they make a sound that creates anxiety for some patients.
9 Review patient's serum electrolyte levels if available.	Movement of air through the mattress increases patient's risk for dehydration (WOCN, 2010).

STEP	RATIONALE
10 Determine if patient needs frequent weights.	Scales are available in some air-suspension beds and as underbed units for patients who need to be weighed frequently or those who cannot be moved for weighing.
11 Assess risk of complications from air-fluidized beds.	
a Dehydration	Patients may become dehydrated with use of this bed because of insensible fluid loss.
b Aspiration	Inability to elevate head of bed is limited to placing foam wedges under patient's head and shoulders.
c Difficulty with patient positioning	Repositioning is limited to use of foam wedges.
d Assess level of orientation	Patients may be at risk for developing delirium from dehydration and floating sensation with air-fluidized bed.

NURSING DIAGNOSES

- Anxiety
- Deficient fluid volume
- Deficient knowledge regarding use of support surface mattress

- Impaired physical mobility
- Impaired skin integrity
- Ineffective tissue perfusion

- Pain (acute, chronic)
- Risk for impaired skin integrity

Related factors are individualized based on patient's condition or needs.

PLANNING

1 Expected outcomes following completion of procedure:	
• Patient's skin remains warm, clean, and intact or existing lesions show evidence of healing.	Skin is free from pressure effects of immobility.
• Existing pressure ulcers show evidence of healing by formulation of granulation tissue.	Low-pressure surface of bed facilitates healing of existing pressure ulcers.
• Patient expresses improved sense of comfort.	Surface of bed is soft, minimizing pain stimulation.
• Patient experiences no complications from remaining on air-fluidized bed.	Patient does not experience sensory perceptual changes or dehydration.
2 Review instructions provided by manufacturer.	Promotes safe and correct use of bed.
3 Explain procedure and purpose of bed to patient and caregiver.	Reduces anxiety and promotes patient's cooperation.
4 Obtain additional personnel needed to transfer patient to bed.	Ensures safety by having sufficient personnel for transfer.
5 For patients with moderate-to-severe pain, premedicate approximately 30 minutes before transfer to bed.	Promotes patient's comfort and ability to cooperate during transfer to bed. Decreases patient's energy expenditure (WOCN, 2010).

IMPLEMENTATION

1 Close patient's room door or bedside curtain.	Maintains patient's privacy during transfer.
2 Identify patient using two identifiers (i.e., name and birthday or name and account number) according to agency policy. Compare identifiers with information on patient's identification bracelet.	Ensures correct patient. Complies with The Joint Commission standards and improves patient safety (TJC, 2012).
3 Perform hand hygiene and apply clean gloves (if linen or surface is soiled or wet).	Reduces transmission of microorganisms.
4 Transfer patient to bed using appropriate transfer techniques (see Chapter 9). Bed surface is sometimes slippery; thus do not attempt transfers without assistance.	Appropriate safe patient-handling techniques maintain alignment and reduce risk of injury during procedure. Manufacturer representative adjusts bed to patient's height and weight.
5 Once patient has been transferred, release Instaflate, fluidize, or turn bed on by depressing switch; regulate temperature.	Releasing Instaflate or turning on bed allows pressure cushions to automatically adjust to preset levels to minimize pressure, friction, and shear.
6 Position patient and perform range-of-motion exercises as appropriate.	Promotes comfort and reduces contracture formation.
7 To turn patient, position bedpans, or perform other therapies, turn on Instaflate setting. Once you have completed the procedure, release Instaflate. With air-fluidized bed, use foam wedges to position patient as needed.	Instaflate firms bed surface to facilitate turning and handling patient. Patient does not receive pressure relief while bed is in this mode.
8 Use special features of bed as needed.	
a Scales	Facilitates ease of routine weights.
b Portable transport units to maintain inflation when primary power is interrupted	Provides for continuous pressure reduction.

STEP	RATIONALE
c Specialty cushions for positioning, providing pressure relief, reducing moisture, preventing patient from sliding down in bed, or relieving weight from orthopedic devices	Reduces pressure, friction, and shearing forces.

Clinical Decision Point *A patient should never be placed in prone position on an air-fluidized bed because of the chance of suffocation.*

d Lateral rotation (Fig. 12-13), which allows approximately 30 degrees of turning	Helps to reduce risk and prevent pulmonary and urinary complications of reduced mobility (WOCN, 2010).
9 Assess effectiveness of pressure-relief mattress or seat cushion by placing hand beneath support surface under a bony prominence.	Underinflation or improper functioning of certain overlays may result in tissue damage. Likewise, overinflation can result in too firm a surface and create pressure damage.
10 Remove and dispose of gloves. Perform hand hygiene.	Reduces transmission of microorganisms.

EVALUATION

1 Inspect condition of patient's skin periodically while patient is on bed, using the National Pressure Ulcer Advisory Panel (NPUAP) staging system.	Determines if any new pressure areas are forming.
2 Observe existing pressure ulcers for evidence of healing.	Evaluates healing progress of any existing pressure ulcers.
3 Ask patient to rate level of comfort on scale of 0 to 10.	Flotation effects of bed minimize pain stimuli.
4 Assess patient's level of orientation.	Determines onset of perceptual changes.

Unexpected Outcomes	Related Interventions
1 Existing areas of skin breakdown or pressure areas fail to heal or increase in size or depth.	• Modify skin care regimen. • Revise turning schedule. • Consult with skin care expert. • Notify health care provider.
2 Patient is restless, confused, or agitated.	• Determine need for antianxiety medication and consult with physician. • Evaluate alternative pressure-relief devices.
3 Patient becomes nauseated.	• Provide short-term antiemetic, such as Compazine. If using lateral rotation, obtain order to give Compazine around the clock. • Notify health care provider. • If using lateral rotation, decrease cycle frequency.
4 Bed malfunctions.	• Maintain patient safety. • Follow agency or manufacturer policy.

FIG 12-13 Lateral rotation bed. (*Tria Dyne*™ *Therapy System. Courtesy KCI Licensing, Inc., 2012.*)

Recording and Reporting

• Record transfer of patient to bed, amount of assistance needed for transfer, tolerance of procedure, and condition of skin in nurses' notes, EHR, and/or skin assessment flow sheet. Record any patient teaching and validation of understanding in nurses' notes and EHR.
• Report changes in condition of skin, level of orientation, and electrolyte levels to health care provider.

Special Considerations
Teaching

• Explain function and purpose of air-suspension or air-fluidized bed.
• Explain the need to continue to change position at intervals to diminish the effects of immobility.
• Explain the need for adequate fluid intake because bed surface sometimes causes dehydration.

Pediatric

• The air-suspension bed is used commonly with older children and for children with significant burns. Make sure that instructions are age appropriate and include any restrictions such as raising the head of the bed.

- Parents need to know that the child will have some dizziness or nausea when first placed on the air-fluidized bed. This is because of the flotation sensation and will disappear as the child becomes adjusted to the bed.

Gerontologic
- Some hospitalized older adults experience misperceptions of their environment that are intensified by the constant flotation of these types of beds. Proprioception abnormalities affecting older adults are the result of nervous system and muscle changes (WOCN, 2010).

Home Care
- The air-fluidized bed weighs between 1700 and 2100 pounds; therefore the company leasing the bed needs to inspect the home for accessibility and structural support.
- Consult with social worker or case manager to determine third-party reimbursement. Thorough documentation of skin condition is essential in obtaining reimbursement.

- A version of the air-fluidized bed is available for home use for rent or purchase; the bed rental company is responsible for proper cleaning.
- Instruct family in importance of maintaining patient hydration and skin care.
- Instruct family regarding steps to take in the event of a power failure. This may include purchasing a back-up generator for the home.

Long-Term Care
- Nurses and NAPs need to be instructed on proper use and inflation of the bed.
- Post signs and have protocols in place for procedures in the event of the need to perform cardiopulmonary resuscitation (CPR) (e.g., how to deflate the bed to provide a flat surface for compressions).

SKILL 12-3   Placing a Patient on a Bariatric Bed

A valuable resource in the care of a morbidly obese patient (a person who weighs more than 100 lbs above ideal weight) is the bariatric bed (Fig. 12-14). The bariatric bed is capable of allowing upright or sitting positions, patient transport, and in-bed scale use. It is equipped with hand controls that allow self-positioning and facilitate independence for an obese patient. The full-function hand controls also allow you to change the bed position and thus facilitate care while reducing risk for staff injury when moving a patient. The in-bed scale provides you with a means of obtaining accurate weights and thus improves health care and patient dignity. The bed is slightly wider than a standard hospital bed, yet it is within the guidelines for standard door width, which allows

movement into and out of a room without difficulty. Because the bariatric bed is capable of supporting weights up to 850 lbs, it provides a stable balanced surface that limits hospital liability should the standard bed frame collapse or the electric motor burn out.

A full- or double-wide bariatric bed can accommodate a patient up to 1000 lbs. However, when using this bed, you must assemble it in the patient's room and not use it for transfers because it is too large to fit through standard hospital doorways.

A limitation of this bed is the lack of pressure reduction or relief in the mattress. An at-risk obese patient needs to have some type of pressure-redistribution mattress placed on the bariatric bed. Choices for pressure redistribution include air or gel type of mattresses and low-air-loss replacement systems. These beds also have cardiopulmonary resuscitation (CPR) switches, which permit an immediate hard surface for chest compressions.

Delegation and Collaboration
The skill of placing a patient on a bariatric bed can be delegated to nursing assistive personnel (NAP). However, you must first complete the assessment, determine the need for a support surface, and select the specific surface. Some types of specialty beds require that the manufacturer's representative set up and maintain the system. The nurse directs the NAP to:
- Notify the nurse of any changes in patient's skin.
- Continue to regularly turn and reposition the patient and seek assistance for patient position changes as necessary.
- Monitor specifics on applying, cleaning, and maintaining support surface.

Equipment
- ❏ Bariatric bed
- ❏ Pressure-relief mattress overlay
- ❏ Sheets
- ❏ Overhead frame (optional)
- ❏ Heavy-duty lift
- ❏ Clean gloves

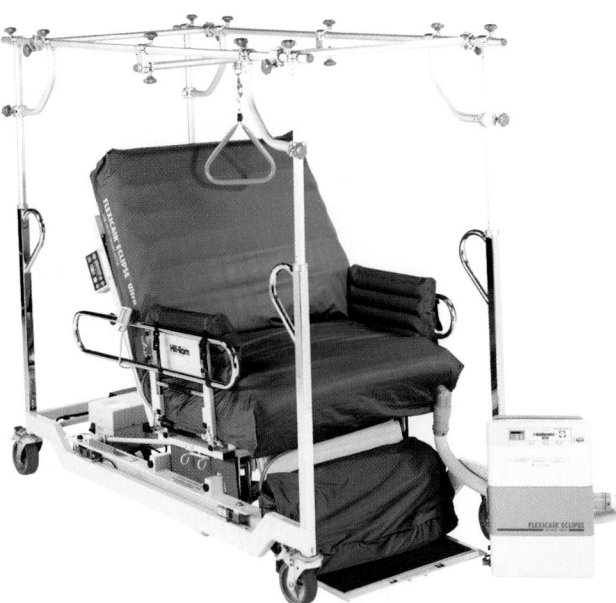

FIG 12-14   Bariatric bed with low-air-loss mattress replacement. (©2008 Hill-Rom Services. Reprinted with permission. All rights reserved.)

STEP	RATIONALE

ASSESSMENT

1 Perform hand hygiene.

Reduces transmission of microorganisms.

2 Determine patient's risk for pressure ulcer formation using a valid assessment tool (e.g., Braden Scale) and assess for risk factors for pressure ulcers, including nutritional deficits, shear stress, friction alterations in mobility and sensory perception, moisture, and abnormal serum albumin and hemoglobin levels (see Chapter 18).

Provides an objective measure of risk consistent among nurse assessors over time (WOCN, 2010).

3 Identify patients who will benefit from the bariatric bed system and assess their mobility status.

Selected for patients who are morbidly obese and have the potential to be independent in positioning with assistance of a stable surface.

4 Assess condition of patient's skin, paying particular attention to potential pressure sites and skinfolds. Assistance may be needed to turn patient to observe all skin surfaces. Determine need for patient to have pressure-redistribution mattress placed on bariatric bed.

Data provide baseline to determine any change in patient's condition while on the bed.

5 Assess patient's and family members' understanding of purpose of bed.

Improves patient and family cooperation.

6 Review health care provider's orders.

Health care provider's order is usually needed to obtain third-party reimbursement for cost of bed.

7 Assess need for patient to be weighed.

Scales are available in many bariatric beds or as underbed scales for beds without in-bed scales.

8 Determine the number of people needed to assist in safe patient transfer from regular bed to bariatric bed.

Reduced risk of injury by ensuring safe patient handling.

NURSING DIAGNOSES

- Deficient knowledge regarding use of support surface mattress
- Impaired physical mobility
- Impaired skin integrity
- Ineffective tissue perfusion
- Pain (acute, chronic)
- Risk for impaired skin integrity

Related factors are individualized based on patient's condition or needs.

PLANNING

1 Expected outcomes following completion of procedure:
   - Patient is independent for position changes.
   - Patient's skin remains intact, or existing lesions show evidence of healing.
   - Patient remains free of injury.

Bed surface is adaptable by hand-operated controls.
Skin is free from pressure effects of immobility.

Bed is stable to allow for positioning without tipping or bending.

2 Explain procedure and purpose of bed to patient and family.

Reduces anxiety and promotes patient's cooperation.

3 Review instructions supplied by bed manufacturer.

Promotes safe and correct use of bed.

Clinical Decision Point *Do not exceed weight limits indicated by the manufacturer and do not use with spinal cord–injured patients.*

4 For patients with moderate-to-severe pain, medicate approximately 30 minutes before transfer.

Promotes patient's comfort and ability to cooperate during transfer to bed. Decreases patient's energy expenditure (WOCN, 2010).

5 Obtain any additional personnel identified during assessment to transfer patient to bed.

Ensures safety of patient and staff by having sufficient personnel to assist in transferring.

IMPLEMENTATION

1 Close patient's room door or bedside curtain.

Maintains patient's privacy during transfer.

2 Identify patient using two identifiers (i.e., name and birthday or name and account number) according to agency policy. Compare identifiers with information on patient's identification bracelet.

Ensures correct patient. Complies with The Joint Commission standards and improves patient safety (TJC, 2012).

3 Perform hand hygiene and put on clean gloves (if needed) before helping patient to bed using appropriate transfer techniques (see Chapter 9). Current safe patient-handling protocols mandate the use of a mechanical lift to move or transfer obese patients.

Appropriate transfer techniques maintain alignment and reduce risk for injury to patient and health care workers during the procedure. The recommended safe limit for nurses to lift in patient care is 35 lbs (Nelson et al., 2009). One nurse can safely logroll a patient weighing up to 78 lb; two caregivers are required if the patient weighs more than 78 lb but not more than 156 lb; and three caregivers are needed if the patient weighs more than 156 lb but not more than 234 lb (Gonzalez, 2009).

STEP	RATIONALE
4 Place pull sheet, slide board, hydraulic lifts, or other assistive devices under patient and transfer safely.	Reduces trauma from friction and shear to patient's skin.
5 Cover and position patient and place hand controls within reach. Be certain that out-of-bed alarm is on if needed. Attach overhead frame if needed.	Allows for maximal patient independence. Alarm alerts caregiver that patient has left bed surface.
6 Encourage patient to initiate frequent position changes and move in bed as much as possible.	Morbidly obese patients quickly increase pressure over bony prominences. Frequent removal (e.g., every 30 to 60 minutes) of pressure from these points helps to reduce risk for pressure ulcer formation.
7 Remove gloves and perform hand hygiene.	Reduces transmission of microorganisms.

EVALUATION

1 Inspect condition of patient's skin according to agency policy while patient is on bed.	Evaluates healing of any existing pressure ulcers. Determines if any new pressure areas are forming.
2 Ask patient to rate sense of comfort using pain scale of 0 to 10.	Identifies patient comfort or need for pain medication.
3 Evaluate patient's risk for injury.	Surface is balanced and allows maximal patient independence.
4 Evaluate patient's ability to move in bed.	Evaluates effectiveness of bed and education to promote independence.

Unexpected Outcomes

1 Existing areas of skin breakdown or pressure areas fail to heal or increase in size or depth.

2 Patient is unable to operate bed for position changes independently.

Related Interventions

- Modify skin care regimen.
- Consult with skin care expert.
- Notify health care provider.

- Reassess patient's level of independence and ability to understand instructions.
- Reinstruct patient and family in how to operate bed.
- Provide for return demonstration regarding bed operation.

Recording and Reporting

- Record transfer of patient to bed, tolerance of procedure, and condition of skin in nurses' notes, EHR, and/or skin assessment flow sheet. Record patient teaching and validation of understanding in nurses' notes and EHR.
- Report changes in condition of skin to nurse in charge or health care provider.

Special Considerations
Teaching

- Explain function and purpose of bariatric bed and pressure-relief mattress overlay.
- Explain the need to continue to change position at intervals to diminish effects of immobility.

SKILL 12-4 Placing a Patient on a Rotokinetic Bed

The Rotokinetic bed helps maintain skeletal alignment while providing constant rotation (Fig. 12-15). It is used in the care of patients with spinal cord injuries or multiple traumas. The support structure of the bed outlines the body parts and maintains proper alignment when secured properly. This bed improves skeletal alignment with constant side-to-side rotation up to 90 degrees. It rotates from side to side at a 60- to 90-degree angle every 7 minutes. You may adjust turning angles to meet a patient's needs. Constant rotation reduces pressure ulcer development and stimulates body systems. It is recommended that the bed stay in the rotation mode for at least 20 hours a day. There is an emergency lever that can quickly interrupt rotation when needed. To initiate cardiopulmonary resuscitation (CPR), return the bed to the horizontal position and lock in place.

The constant motion often leads to sensory distress for a patient, especially older adults. This is associated with the constant kinetic stimulation, the limited visual field, and inner ear disequilibrium. Be aware of these complications and provide necessary emotional support.

Delegation and Collaboration
The skill of placing a patient on a Rotokinetic bed cannot be delegated to nursing assistive personnel (NAP). The nurse directs the NAP to:

- Notify the nurse of any changes in the patient's skin while warning the NAP to not stop rotation, move, or reposition patient without the RN's assistance.
- Monitor the exact rotation frequency of the bed.
- Stop the rotation only for selected aspects of care determined by the nurse (e.g., bathing, oral hygiene, enemas).
- Immediately notify the nurse if the patient experiences confusion, nausea, and pain.

Equipment
- Rotokinetic bed with support packs, bolsters, and safety straps
- Top sheet
- Pillowcases for bolsters

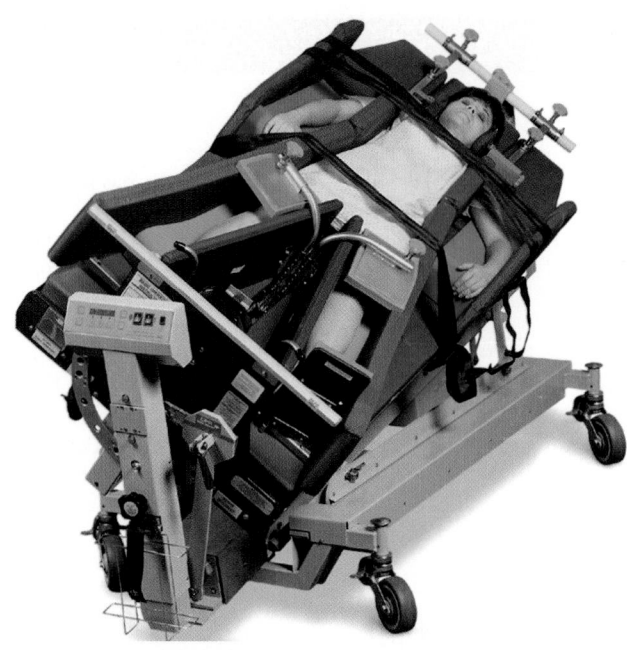

FIG 12-15   Rotokinetic bed. (*RotoRest, Courtesy Kinetic Concepts, San Antonio, Tex.*)

STEP	RATIONALE

ASSESSMENT

1 Perform hand hygiene.	Reduces transmission of microorganisms.
2 Determine patient's risk for pressure ulcer formation using a validated assessment tool (e.g., Braden Scale) and assess for risk factors for pressure ulcers, including nutritional deficits, shear stress, friction, alterations in mobility and perception, moisture, and abnormal serum albumin and hemoglobin levels (see Chapter 18).	Risk assessment tools suggested by the Agency for Health Care Policy and Research (AHCPR) and WOCN (e.g., Braden Scale) provide an objective measure of risk consistent among nurse assessors over time (WOCN, 2010).
3 Perform skin assessment. Inspect condition of skin, especially over dependent sites, under skin folds, and bony prominences (see Chapter 18).	Provides baseline to measure ongoing data to determine a change in skin integrity or in an existing pressure ulcer.
4 Review health care provider's orders.	Health care provider's order is needed to receive third-party reimbursement for cost of bed.
5 Assess patient's level of comfort using pain scale of 0 to 10.	Provides baseline to determine patient's comfort needs. Nerve endings related to pressure, touch, temperature, and limb position are located in the skin (WOCN, 2010).
6 Assess patient's level of orientation.	Baseline used to detect change while patient is on bed. Constant motion often leads to sensory distress.
7 Perform pulmonary assessment and obtain vital signs.	Provides baseline of patient's pulmonary status and vital signs. Patients with severe injuries or spinal cord injuries are at risk for accumulation of pulmonary secretions. In addition, when these patients are first placed on the bed, they are at risk for changes in pulse and blood pressure because of motion of bed.
8 Determine the number of people needed to assist in safe patient transfer from regular bed to rotokinetic bed.	Reduces risk of injury by ensuring safe patient handling.
9 Assess patients' and family members' knowledge and understanding of purpose of bed.	Appearance and movement of bed creates anxiety for patient and family members.

NURSING DIAGNOSES

- Anxiety
- Deficient knowledge regarding the use of Rotokinetic bed
- Impaired physical mobility
- Impaired skin integrity
- Ineffective tissue perfusion
- Pain (acute, chronic)
- Risk for impaired skin integrity
- Risk for infection

Related factors are individualized based on patient's condition or needs.

STEP	RATIONALE
PLANNING	
1 Expected outcomes following completion of procedure:	
• Patient's skin remains intact without evidence of abnormal reactive hyperemia or mottling.	Skin is free from pressure effects of immobility.
• Existing pressure ulcers show evidence of healing.	Patient is experiencing benefits of bed.
• Patient's musculoskeletal system is properly aligned and free of contractures.	Device provides support and alignment to trunk and extremities.
• Patient's breath sounds improve from baseline assessment or remain clear to auscultation.	Patient's pulmonary congestion is improving or absent.
• Patient remains alert, oriented, and cooperative.	Patient does not experience sensory perceptual changes from bed positions.
• Patient denies nausea or dizziness.	Motion of bed is not negatively affecting patient.
• Patient's blood pressure remains consistent with baseline vital signs.	Patient is not experiencing cardiovascular disturbances.
2 Explain procedure and purpose of bed to patient and family.	Reduces anxiety and promotes cooperation.
3 Review instructions supplied by bed manufacturer.	Promotes safe and correct use of bed.
4 Premedicate for moderate-to-severe pain approximately 30 minutes before transfer.	Promotes patient's comfort and ability to cooperate during transfer to bed. Decreases patient's energy expenditure (WOCN, 2010).
5 Obtain any additional personnel needed to transfer patient to bed.	Ensures patient's safety.
IMPLEMENTATION	
1 Close patient's room door or bedside curtain.	Maintains patient's privacy during transfer.
2 Identify patient using two identifiers (i.e., name and birthday or name and account number) according to agency policy. Compare identifiers with information on patient's identification bracelet.	Ensures correct patient. Complies with The Joint Commission standards and improves patient safety (TJC, 2012).
3 Place Rotokinetic bed in horizontal position and remove all bolsters, straps, and supports. Close posterior hatches.	
4 Unplug electrical cord. Lock gatch.	Prevents accidental rotation during transfer.
5 Perform hand hygiene and apply clean gloves.	Reduces transmission of microorganisms.
6 Maintaining proper alignment of patient and using appropriate transfer techniques (see Chapter 9), transfer patient to Rotokinetic bed.	Reduces risk for further tissue injury during transfer. Will need other health care providers to assist in transfer.
7 Secure thoracic panels, bolsters, head and knee packs, and safety straps.	Maintains proper alignment and prevents sliding during rotation.
8 Cover patient with top sheet.	Prevents unnecessary exposure.
9 Plug in bed.	
10 Have manufacturer representative set optional angle as ordered by health care provider. Gradually increase rotation.	Health care provider determines rotational angle based on patient's overall condition and tolerance to constant motion.
11 Increase degree of rotation gradually according to patient's tolerance.	Reduces or prevents nausea, dizziness, and orthostatic hypotension.
12 It is difficult to maintain eye contact when talking with patients during rotation. Provide space for caregivers and family to move around bed to facilitate communication.	Allows opportunity to meet patient's psychosocial needs.
13 Stop bed for assessment and procedures. To stop bed, permit it to rotate to desired position, turn motor off, and push knob into lock position. If necessary, you can manually reposition bed.	Allows nurse to easily access patient for any procedure.
14 Inform patient that there will be a sensation of light-headedness or falling. However, reassure patient that he or she will not fall because pads prevent this and are checked by two people to ensure proper placement.	Informing patient of what to expect decreases anxiety.
EVALUATION	
1 Inspect condition of skin (occipital region, ears, axillae, elbows, sacrum, groin, heels) and musculoskeletal alignment every 2 hours or more often if indicated by patient's condition.	Evaluates healing process of any existing pressure ulcers and determines effectiveness of Rotokinetic therapy.

STEP	RATIONALE
2 Inspect patient's pressure ulcers for evidence of healing.	Evaluates healing process.
3 Observe alignment and range of motion of all joints.	Determines if complications have developed.
4 Auscultate lung sounds every shift and compare with baseline.	Provides ongoing pulmonary assessment.
5 Determine patient's level of orientation once per shift while on bed or more often if patient's condition changes.	Evaluates if sensory overload has developed from excess kinetic stimulation.
6 Ask whether patient is experiencing nausea or dizziness.	Determines if patient is having inner ear disturbance.
7 Monitor blood pressure.	Determines if patient experiences orthostatic hypotension from position rotation.

Unexpected Outcomes

1 Existing areas of skin breakdown or pressure areas fail to heal or increase in size or depth.

2 Patient experiences hypotension.

3 Patient becomes disoriented, confused, nauseated, and anxious.

4 Patient develops abnormal lung sounds.

5 Bed fails to rotate.

Related Interventions

- Evaluate rotation schedule; bed needs to remain in rotation 20 hours per day to prevent skin breakdown.
- Modify skin care regimen.

- If severe drop in blood pressure, stop rotation, notify health care provider, remain with patient, and monitor vital signs every 5 minutes.
- For less severe blood pressure changes, decrease rotational angle. Gradually increase rotation angle as patient adjusts to rotation.

- Reorient patient to person, place, time.
- Provide audio stimulation via radio or tapes.
- Provide television adapted to Rotokinetic bed (available from manufacturer).
- Hang mirror on ceiling so patient is able to view surroundings.
- Provide symptomatic relief of motion sickness, and obtain order for anti-emetic to be given around the clock.

- Increase frequency of pulmonary hygiene measures (e.g., cough and deep breathe, suctioning).
- Have patient use incentive spirometry.

- Provide for patient safety.
- Position bed flat.
- Follow manufacturer/agency policies.

Recording and Reporting

- Record transfer of patient to bed, time of transfer, degree of rotation, tolerance of procedure, and condition of skin before placement on bed in nurses' notes, EHR, and/or skin assessment flow sheet. Record patient teaching and validation of understanding in nurses' notes and EHR. Take a photograph to document skin condition and provide a baseline for later assessments for progress in healing.
- Record and report subjective data indicating response to the constant rotation and presence/absence of dizziness or nausea or blood pressure changes.
- Use a flow sheet to document routine assessment and care, including the length of time the bed rotation stopped. The bed needs to be rotating at least 20 hours out of every 24 hours and stopped for no more than 30 minutes at a time.
- Report changes in condition of skin to nurse in charge or health care provider.

Special Considerations
Teaching
- Explain function and purpose of Rotokinetic bed to patient and family members.
- Explain that patient will feel sensation of light-headedness or falling. However, patient will not fall because pads are positioned to prevent this.

Pediatric
- Provide age-appropriate education for the child. It is important that the child understand that he or she is secure in the bed and will not fall out as the bed turns.
- Distraction such as talking books, videos, and music help the older child adjust to the bed and the restricted mobility.

Gerontologic
- Older adults are at increased risk for sensation of light-headedness or dizziness.

Critical Thinking Exercises

You are assigned to admit Mr. Sachiko Hoji, a 48-year-old male who was involved in a motor vehicle accident that resulted in quadriplegia (causing loss of sensation and movement below the neck). The patient is unable to change positions or transfer without assistance. He also has a language barrier, and communicating instructions about his care is difficult. The nurse has arranged for the services of a qualified interpreter to assist in breaching the language barrier.

1   You anticipate that this patient will need a support surface. Before selecting this surface, what assessments will you make?

2   Which category of support surface will you select? What is your rationale for this selection?

3   Following consultation with physical therapy and social service, the health care provider orders an air-suspension bed with lateral rotation because Mr. Hoji has some blistering over bony prominences, and his impaired mobility and sensation increase his risk for developing pressure ulcers. Mr. Hoji begins experiencing a small amount of nausea and restlessness when initially placed on the air-suspension bed. He tells his wife, "I'm afraid that I'll fall out of this bed when it tilts. Will I?" Which actions should you implement for Mr. Hoji's nausea and anxiety?

REVIEW QUESTIONS

1   A patient at risk for pressure areas is placed on a specialty bed. Dehydration and/or electrolyte imbalances can occur with which type of specialty bed/mattress?
    1   Egg-crate mattress
    2   Air-suspension bed
    3   Aid-fluidized bed
    4   Bariatric bed

2   A nurse is caring for a patient on a Rotokinetic type of bed when he complains of sudden dizziness. The nurse checks his blood pressure and notes that on lateral rotation he develops orthostatic hypotension. What should the nurse's initial actions be?
    1   Have the nursing assistive personnel (NAP) notify the health care provider while the nurse assesses the patient
    2   Stop the rotation of the bed for a few minutes to further assess the patient
    3   Talk to the patient and assess for other factors that can make him hypotensive
    4   Increase his oral fluids and assess the patient again after he has been hydrated

3   A nurse is caring for a patient who can change position independently on an air-filled overlay on the mattress. While conducting a skin assessment, the nurse notices skin breakdown over the coccyx and left hip, even though this patient has received meticulous skin care and routine repositioning. What is the appropriate nursing action?
    1   Maintain the present mattress
    2   Increase repositioning frequency
    3   Check functioning and filling of the mattress
    4   Consider changing to a pressure-relief device

4   A patient needs to be placed on a bariatric bed. Which factor would be least considered when determining the need for the larger bed?
    1   The patient's ability to assist with transfer to the bed
    2   Availability of personnel to reposition the patient
    3   The ability of the environment to accommodate the bed
    4   The integrity of the skin on pressure areas and in skinfold regions

5   A patient on an air-fluidized bed needs to be turned. Which nursing intervention indicates that the nurse needs additional teaching about using this type of bed?
    1   The nurse prepares to place the patient in prone position on the bed.
    2   The nurse uses foam wedges to support the patient's head for comfort.
    3   The nurse asks the patient how much she can do before turning her.
    4   The nurse assesses visible skin areas before and after turning the patient.

6   A patient with paraplegia is sitting on a Roho cushion and self-adjusting the inflation during the day when he is up in his wheelchair. The home caregiver notes that the patient has small areas of continuing redness on his ischia. Which interventions are indicated? (Select all that apply.)
    1   The caregiver should report the situation to the nurse or case manager immediately.
    2   The caregiver should instruct the patient to not change the chair cushion inflation.
    3   The caregiver should check for proper inflation of the cushion.
    4   The caregiver should reinflate the cushion appropriately while the patient is sitting on it and wait to reevaluate the skin condition later.
    5   The caregiver should increase frequency of checking the patient's skin.

7   To check the inflation of a seat cushion in the wheelchair, the nurse should:
    1   Place a set of keys under the cushion and ask the patient if he can feel them.
    2   Visually inspect that the person's buttocks are not sitting directly on the seat.
    3   Manually check with a hand under the cushion to be sure that the person's ischia are cushioned appropriately.
    4   Avoid checking after inflating the cushion exactly according to the manufacturer's instructions.

8   In determining whether or not a mechanical lift should be used to transfer a person from a regular bed to a bariatric bed, which of the following statements reflects best practice? (Select all that apply.)
    1   All morbidly obese patients should be moved with a mechanical lift to prevent caregiver injury.
    2   Only patients weighing over 180 lbs who are completely dependent require the use of a mechanical lift.
    3   The appropriate use of mechanical lifts has been shown in numerous studies to reduce injury to nurses.
    4   The recommended safe limit for one nurse to logroll a patient is 156 lb.
    5   A lift team should be called to physically lift all patients from the bed to the chair.

9   The best guideline to use when selecting a pressure-relieving support surface for a patient is to:
    1   Consider the individual's specific risk factors when selecting a device.
    2   Choose the least expensive type of device.
    3   Consider staffing patterns and staff's current knowledge.
    4   Choose the most expensive type of device to ensure quality.

10 Place the following steps for applying an air mattress overlay in the correct order:
    1   Check air pumps to be sure that pressure cycle alternates.
    2   Bring any plastic strips or flaps around corners of bed mattress.
    3   Apply deflated mattress flat over surface of bed mattress.
    4   Place sheet over air mattress, being sure to eliminate all wrinkles.
    5   Attach connector on air mattress to inflation device and inflate to proper pressure.

REFERENCES

Anton PM: Maintaining skin integrity. In Mauk KL, editor: *Rehabilitation nursing: A contemporary approach to practice*, Sudbury, Mass, 2012, Jones and Bartlett.

Gonzalez C, et al: Safe patient handling, *Orthop Nurs* 28(2):S9–S12, 2009.

Gray M: Context for WOC practices: assessment, prevention, and intervention in wound, ostomy, and continence care, *J Wound Ostomy Continence Care* 36(1):11, 2009.

Hockenberry MJ, Wilson J: *Wong's nursing care of infants and children*, ed 9, St Louis, 2011, Mosby.

McInnes E, et al: Support surfaces for pressure ulcer prevention, *Cochrane Database Syst Rev* 13(4):CD001735, 2011.

National Pressure Ulcer Advisory Panel Support Surfaces Standard Initiative (NPUAP): *Pressure ulcer treatment recommendations: clinical practice guidelines*, Washington, DC, 2009, National Pressure Ulcer Advisory Panel.

National Quality Forum (NQF): *National voluntary consensus standards for public reporting or patient safety event information consensus report*, Washington, DC, 2010, NQF.

Nelson A, et al: *The illustrated guide to safe patient handling and movement*, New York, NY, 2009, Springer Publishing.

Norton L, et al: Beds: practical pressure management for surfaces/mattresses, *Adv Skin Wound Care* 24(7):325, 2011.

Reddy M, et al: Treatment of pressure ulcers: a systematic review, *JAMA* 300(22):2647, 2008.

The Joint Commission (TJC): *National Patient Safety Goals*, Oakbrook Terrace, Ill, 2012, The Commission, available at http://www.jointcommission.org/standards_information/npsgs.aspx.

US Department of Health and Human Services (USDHHS): *Older adults*, 2011, available at http://healthypeople.gov/2020/topicsobjectives2020/pdfs/OlderAdults.pdf, accessed February 7, 2012.

Wound, Ostomy, and Continence Nurses Society (WOCN): *Guideline for prevention and management of pressure ulcers*, Glenview, Ill, 2010, The Association.

Safety and Quality Improvement

MEDIA RESOURCES

- evolve http://evolve.elsevier.com/Perry/skills
  - Review Questions
  - Video Clips
  - Audio Glossary
- NSO Nursing Skills Online
- Mosby's Nursing Video Skills, 4th edition

KEY TERMS

Aspiration	Material safety data sheet (MSDS)	Mummy restraints	Seizure
Belt restraints	Mitten restraints	Physical restraint	Seizure precautions
Extremity restraints		Polypharmacy	Sentinel event

OBJECTIVES

Mastery of content in this chapter will enable the nurse to:
- Describe how safety principles are enhanced through a patient-centered care approach.
- Discuss current evidence in the area of fall prevention.
- Discuss the importance of a nursing assessment in providing for patient safety.
- Describe nursing interventions taken in the event of a fire and electrical shock.
- Describe nursing interventions specific for reducing patients' risks for falls.
- Describe steps in the design of a restraint-free environment.
- Discuss precautions used to prevent injury in patients who are restrained.
- Describe nursing interventions for a patient who experiences generalized seizures.
- Describe methods to evaluate safety interventions.
- Describe how to conduct a root cause analysis of a sentinel event.

Safety, often defined as freedom from psychological and physical injury, is a basic human need. Health care provided in a safe manner and a safe environment is essential for a patient's survival and well-being. A safe environment reduces the risk for illness and injury and contains the costs of health care by preventing extended lengths of treatment and/or hospitalization, improving or maintaining a patient's functional status, and increasing the patient's sense of well-being. The Institute of Medicine report *"To Err Is Human: Building a Safer Health System"* (IOM, 2000) was a pivotal publication that brought patient safety to the forefront of health care in the United States. This report indicated that 44,000 to 98,000 people were dying each year as a result of preventable medical errors. Many health care organizations (e.g., The Joint Commission [TJC], The National Quality Forum [NQF], and The Centers for Medicaid and Medicare Services [CMS] now develop and monitor key health care safety initiatives and provide information to health care organizations and the public to promote patient safety. For example, the NQF (2011a) published *"Safe Practices for Better Healthcare—2011 Update,"* which includes 29 safe practices and 12 new proposed safe practices that have been demonstrated to be effective in reducing the occurrence of adverse events. Health care organizations foster a patient-centered safety culture by continually focusing on performance-improvement endeavors and risk-management findings and safety reports; providing current reliable technology; integrating evidence-based practice (EBP) into procedures; designing a safe work environment and atmosphere; and providing adequate staff educational opportunities.

As part of the health care team, a nurse is responsible to engage in activities that support a patient-centered safety culture. Patient-centered is defined by Quality and Safety Education for Nurses (QSEN) as recognizing a patient as the source of control and full partner in providing compassionate and coordinated care based on respect for patient's preferences, values, and needs (QSEN, 2011). There is an emphasis on improving the education of student nurses so they become more competent in promoting safe health care practices. The QSEN project was developed to meet the challenge of preparing future nurses who will have the knowledge, skills, and attitudes (KSAs) necessary to continuously improve the quality and safety of the health care systems within which they work (QSEN, 2011). The QSEN safety competency for nurses is defined as "Minimizes risk of harm to patients and providers through both system effectiveness and individual performance." The QSEN skills for safety competency include:

- Demonstrate effective use of technology and standardized practices that support safety and quality.
- Demonstrate effective use of strategies to reduce risk of harm to self or others.
- Use appropriate strategies to reduce reliance on memory.
- Communicate observations or concerns related to hazards and errors to patients, families, and the health care team.

As a nurse you are responsible for incorporating critical thinking skills when using the nursing process, assessing each patient and his or her environment for hazards that threaten safety, and planning and intervening appropriately to maintain a safe environment.

The Joint Commission requires hospitals to have a process for patients and their families to report concerns about safety such as asking caregivers if they have washed their hands. The Joint Commission launched a national campaign urging patients to "Know Your Rights," part of the Commission's Speak Up program (TJC, 2007). The program encourages people to take an active role in their own health care by speaking up if they have questions, paying attention to the care they receive, educating themselves about their diagnosis and treatment plan, and knowing and understanding their medications. In addition, TJC encourages patients to participate in all decisions about their treatment, making them partners in care (TJC, 2012a).

EVIDENCE-BASED PRACTICE

There continues to be significant research in the area of fall prevention, both in community and health care settings. In a review of studies designed to reduce the incidence of falls among community-living older adults, multifactorial programs were successful for older adults with a previous fall history (Costello and Edelstein, 2008). A multifactorial fall prevention program uses multiple interventions because individuals are at risk for falls for a variety of reasons. Research shows that medication and vision assessment, exercise, and home-hazard assessment with modifications may be beneficial in reducing falls in the home (Beer et al, 2011). Exercise alone is effective in reducing falls and should include a comprehensive program that combines muscle

strengthening, balance, and/or endurance training for at least 12 weeks. Tai chi shows improvements in body balance and ambulation (Bula et al., 2011). Improved balance confidence is important to avoid unnecessary, self-imposed restrictions of activity.

- Apply multifactorial interventions that match patients' risks and behaviors.
- Conduct a thorough medication assessment to identify polypharmacy (more than five medications).
- Determine potential withdrawal of certain at-risk medications such as psychotropics and sedatives.
- After a vision assessment, follow up with patients to determine their adherence in obtaining new glasses or other prescribed treatment.
- Provide educational information about fall risks and why modifications are beneficial following a home hazard assessment.
- Including an occupational therapist or physical therapist in a home-hazard assessment may have added benefit.

PATIENT-CENTERED CARE

Being hospitalized places patients at risk for injury in an unfamiliar and confusing environment. The experience is usually at least minimally frightening. Normal life cues such as a bed without side rails and the direction one usually takes to the bathroom are absent. Thought processes and coping mechanisms are affected by illness and its accompanying emotions. Thus patients are more vulnerable to injury. For patients of diverse cultural backgrounds, this vulnerability may be intensified. It is a nurse's responsibility to diligently protect all patients, regardless of their socio-economic status and cultural background. Most untoward events are related to failures of communication. Health care providers must be particularly attentive to communication during assessment. For example, nurses must use approaches that recognize a patient's cultural background so appropriate questions can be raised to clearly reveal health behaviors and risks. You enhance a patient's safety by considering him or her in light of the whole person and seeing each care situation through "the patient's eyes" and not just your perspective. Here are some specific patient-centered safety guidelines:

- When restraints are needed, clarify their meaning to the patient and the family. For example, some Asian families view the restraining of older adults as disrespectful. Similarly some survivors of war or persecution view restraints as imprisonment or punishment.
- Collaborate with family members in accommodating a patient's cultural perspectives regarding restraints. Removing the restraints when family members are present shows respect and caring for the patient.
- Be familiar with agency restraint protocol. Identify potential areas for negotiation with the patient's and family's preferences such as using a jacket versus arm restraints.
- When seizure precautions are necessary, explain and demonstrate the therapeutic regimen to the patient/family. Some cultures observe different caring practices for a person with seizures.

■ Safety Guidelines

1 Accurate patient identification is crucial to safety before any procedures (TJC, 2012b).
2 Safety begins with a patient's immediate environment. The call light/bed control system allows patients to adjust bed positions

and signal caregivers. Explain to patients and visiting family members how to operate a call system correctly.

3 Always be alert to conditions within a patient's environment that pose risks for patient injury (e.g., hazards along walking paths, liquid spilled on the floor, poorly functioning equipment).

4 Communicate clearly to other health care providers the plan of care, including procedures to be performed, procedures completed, and patient response. Communicate important test results to the right staff person in a timely manner (TJC, 2012b).

SKILL 13-1 Fall Prevention in a Health Care Agency

NSO *Safety Module / Lessons 1 and 2*

Patient falls are the most common type of inpatient accident, with approximately 1 million inpatient falls occurring in the United States each year (Oliver, Healey, and Haines, 2010). Between 1% and 3% of these falls result in fractures. A systematic review of studies examining the effectiveness of hospital fall prevention programs revealed no conclusive evidence that the programs can reduce the number of falls or fallers (Coussement et al., 2008). However, this is likely because falls are multifactorial and many studies focus on single interventions. Risk factors for falls among inpatients include a history of falling, muscle weakness, agitation and confusion, urinary incontinence or frequency, postural hypotension, and use of high-risk medications (e.g., benzodiazepine, opioids and antihistamines, and sedative hypnotics) (Chang et al., 2011; Oliver, Healey, and Haines, 2010).

Disease also plays a role in falls. For example, patients with cancer appear to have a higher fall rate compared with medicine and neurology patients and have the highest injury rate because of disease-related factors (e.g., osteoporosis, coagulation disorders) (Allan-Gibbs, 2010). Because a variety of factors create fall risks for patients, it is very important for nurses and other health care providers to perform thorough fall risk assessments and use fall prevention techniques individualized to the patients' risks and behaviors. The Centers for Medicare and Medicaid Services (CMS) have identified select serious adverse events as "Never Events" (i.e., adverse events that should never occur in a health care setting) (DHHS, 2008). One of these "Never Events" is hospital-acquired injury from external causes (e.g., fractures, head injury, crushing injury), as in the case of falls. The CMS denies hospitals higher payment for any hospital-acquired condition resulting from or complicated by the occurrence of a "Never Event."

Another area of risk includes wheelchair-related falls involving older adults and persons with disabilities. Patients are at risk for falls during transfer tasks and reaching while seated in a wheelchair. Wheelchair-related injuries from falls include fractures, concussions, dislocations, amputations, and serious head and spinal injuries (Opalek, Graymire, and Redd, 2009). An example of a wheelchair characteristic that increases risk for falls is having smaller and harder front wheels that cause a chair to tip when striking uneven terrain. Caregivers are also at risk for injury by not handling patients correctly or not asking for assistance. Injuries can occur while caregivers transfer patients who are agitated, fearful, unsteady, or too weak to transfer. Tripping over the front foot or leg rest and leaning over the back of the wheelchair to engage or disengage the wheel lock are common sources of injury.

The Joint Commission recommends that hospitals have formal fall-reduction programs, which include the evaluation of program effectiveness (TJC, 2012a). A fall-reduction program includes a fall risk assessment of every patient, which is usually conducted on admission to a hospital and then routinely (see agency policy) until the patient's discharge. Most health care agencies use fall risk assessment tools designed to identify levels of risk such as low and high. A variety of tools are available, but not all have been well tested. The Hendrich II Fall Risk Model is one example of a fall assessment tool that has been shown to successfully identify high-risk patients (Ang et al., 2011).

It is important for nurses to identify patients' fall risks and communicate these risks to patients, their visiting family members, and members of the health care team. Patient-centered care is important, with nurses making patients their partners in recognizing fall risks and taking preventive action. Fall prevention strategies must be targeted to specific patient risks. For example, if a patient has postural hypotension, a nurse might choose a low bed and the practice of dangling the patient for 5 minutes on the side of the bed before trying to ambulate. Or a patient with a history of urinary incontinence might be given a bedside commode to use. Remember that patient situations change. Preventing falls and fall-related injuries requires diligent ongoing nursing assessment and engagement of the entire health care team in the implementation of patient-specific interventions (ICSI, 2010). The Joint Commission has a Speak Up campaign created for patients to follow in the home and hospital (Zhani, 2010). It offers tips and actions for helping people reduce their risk of falling, whether at home or in a medical facility.

Nurses are responsible for making a patient's bedside safe. Fig. 13-1 shows a variety of environmental interventions for patient safety. The call light/bed control system allows patients to adjust the position of a bed and signal caregivers for assistance. A full set of raised side rails (two to a bed or four to a bed) is a physical restraint. Traditionally health care providers used side rails for patient protection; however, patients have become entrapped or entangled in them. Raising only one of two, or three of four, side rails gives patients room to exit a bed safely and move around within the bed. It is also important to keep a bed in low position with wheels locked when stationary. Finally, always check a bed for structural risks (e.g., wobbly rails, damaged rails, or soft mattresses).

Electronic bed and chair alarms warn nursing staff when patients try to leave the bed or chair on their own. One type of alarm is a pressure-sensitive strip that is placed beneath a patient and under the buttocks on a bed or chair. As a patient rises off the sensor, an alarm sounds to alert staff. Another warning device is a tab alarm that connects to a patient in a chair or bed by a wire tether. When a patient moves beyond the length of the tether, the alarm sounds. An Ambularm is a device that a patient wears on a leg. The alarm signals when the leg is in a dependent position such as over a side rail or on the floor.

Additional devices to use at a patient's bedside are a gait belt, a bedside commode, a nonskid floor mat, an overhead trapeze, and a ceiling lift (see Fig. 13-1). All of these devices help patients either move in bed or transfer out of bed more safely.

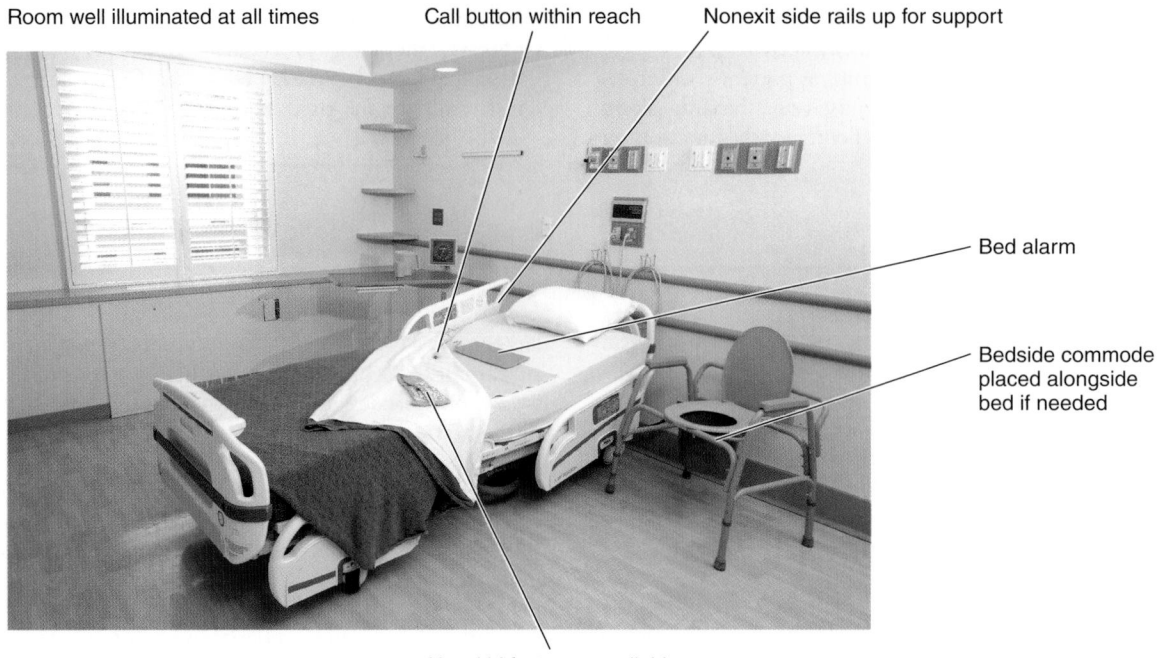

Room well illuminated at all times   Call button within reach   Nonexit side rails up for support

Bed alarm

Bedside commode placed alongside bed if needed

Nonskid footwear available

FIG 13-1   Safe patient room environment with bed in low position, bed alarm activated, nonskid floor mat and call light in place, and bedside commode positioned along bedside.

Delegation and Collaboration

The skill of assessing and communicating a patient's fall risks cannot be delegated to nursing assistive personnel (NAP). However, the skills used to prevent falls can be delegated. The nurse directs the NAP by:

- Explaining a patient's mobility limitations and specific measures needed to minimize risks.
- Teaching specific environmental safety precautions to use (e.g., bed locked in low position, nonskid footwear).
- Explaining patient behaviors (e.g., disorientation, wandering, anxiety) that are precursors to falls and that should be reported immediately.

Equipment

- ❏ Fall risk assessment tool
- ❏ Hospital bed with side rails
- ❏ Wedge cushion
- ❏ Call light
- ❏ Seat belt
- ❏ Gait belt
- ❏ Wheelchair
- ❏ Bed alarm

STEP	RATIONALE

ASSESSMENT

1. Assess patient's fall risks using an agency fall risk assessment tool. Assess patient's age (over 65), number of co-morbidities, impaired memory and cognition (ability to cooperate), incontinence or urinary frequency/urgency, decreased hearing, decreased night vision, orthostatic hypotension or dizziness/vertigo, impaired gait, weak lower extremities, fatigue, need for transfer assistance, history of stroke, and decreased peripheral sensation (Kojima et al, 2011; Viera, Freund-Heritage, and da Costa, 2011).

   Certain physiologic factors predispose patients to fall (e.g., incontinence or urgency and the attempt to rush to a bathroom or find a urinal).

2. Determine if patient has a history of recent falls (TJC, 2012a) or other injuries within the home. Assess previous falls; be specific and follow the acronym SPLATT (Meiner, 2011):
   - Symptoms at time of fall
   - Previous fall
   - Location of fall
   - Activity at time of fall
   - Time of fall
   - Trauma after fall

   Key symptoms are often helpful in identifying cause for falls. Onset, location, and activity associated with a fall provide further details on causative factors and how to prevent future falls.

STEP	RATIONALE
3 Review patient's medication history, including over-the-counter (OTC) medications and herbal products and antidepressants, anticonvulsants, antihypertensives, antihistamines, anti-Parkinson drugs, antipsychotics, anxiolytics, corticosteroids, diuretics, histamine (H_2) receptors, hypnotics (especially benzodiazepines), hypoglycemics, and muscle relaxants. Also assess for polypharmacy (use of more than five medications).	Certain medications have been associated with patient falls (Chang et al., 2011; Gribbin et al., 2010; Kojima et al., 2011; Viera, Freund-Heritage, and da Costa, 2011). Multiple use of medications (polypharmacy) is also associated with falls, especially in older adults (Beer et al, 2011).
4 Assess patient for fear of falling; consider patients who are over 75 years of age, female, lower income, or single and have poor perceived general health and history of falling in last 3 months (Boyd and Stevens, 2009).	Fear and fear of falling are interrelated problems; each is a risk factor for the other (Scheffer et al., 2008).
5 Assess risk factors in health care agency (e.g., being attached to equipment such as sequential compression hose, intravenous [IV] or oxygen tubing, improperly lighted room, obstructed walkway to bathroom, clutter of supplies and equipment).	Environmental barriers pose risk for falls.
6 Assess condition of equipment.	Equipment in poor repair (e.g., uneven legs on bedside commode) increase fall risk.
7 Perform the timed "get up and go" (TGUG) test if patient is able to ambulate: • Have patient rise from sitting position without using arms for support. • Instruct patient to walk 10 feet (3 m), turn around, and walk back to the chair. • Have patient return to chair and sit down without using arms for support. • Look for unsteadiness in patient's gait.	Examination easily incorporated into clinical encounters with patient is measure of physical performance, with low scores associated with risk for falling (Khazzani et al., 2009). Patient taking less than 20 seconds to complete test is adequate for independent mobility. Patient who takes longer than 30 seconds is dependent and at risk for fall.
8 Assess patient for: osteoporosis, anticoagulant therapy, history of previous fracture, and recent chest or abdominal surgery.	Factors increase likelihood of injury from a fall.
9 Use patient-centered approach and determine what patient knows about risks for falling and steps that he or she takes to prevent falls.	Patient's own knowledge of risks influences ability to take necessary precautions in reducing falls.
10 After assessment apply color-coded wristband (e.g., yellow) for patients at risk for falling. Some organizations institute fall risk signs on doors and special yellow labels on patient charts and assignment boards.	Color-coded bands are easily recognizable. National efforts in a majority of states have resulted in the standardization of yellow as a color for fall risk wrist bands.

NURSING DIAGNOSES

• Activity intolerance	• Impaired physical mobility	• Impaired walking
• Deficient knowledge	• Impaired transfer ability	• Risk for falls
• Impaired memory	• Impaired urinary elimination	• Risk for injury

Related factors are individualized based on patient's condition or needs.

PLANNING

1 Expected outcomes following completion of procedure:	
• Patient's environment is free of hazards.	Environmental hazards predispose patient to potential injury.
• Patient and/or family member is able to identify safety risks.	Patient awareness of risks promotes cooperation and understanding of treatment plan.
• Patient and/or family member verbalizes understanding of fall prevention interventions.	Makes patient and family partners in prevention strategies.
• Patient does not suffer a fall or injury.	Fall precautions are successful in preventing a fall.

IMPLEMENTATION

1 Introduce yourself to patient, including both name and title or role.	Reduces patient uncertainty.
2 Explain plan of care. Specifically discuss reasons that patient is at risk for falling.	Promotes patient cooperation. Younger patients are very independent and often believe they are not likely to fall.
3 Gather equipment and perform hand hygiene.	Promotes organization and reduces transmission of microorganisms.

STEP	RATIONALE

4 Provide privacy. Assign patient to bed that allows an exit toward his or her stronger side. Position and drape patient as needed.

    Maintains patient's self-esteem. Enhances patient's ability to move in bed and transfer out of bed.

5 Adjust bed to low position with wheels locked (see illustration). Place padded mats on floor at side of bed.

    Allows for proper body mechanics. Height of bed allows ambulatory patient to get in and out of bed easily and safely. Pads provide nonslippery surface on which to stand.

6 Encourage patient to wear properly fitted skid-proof footwear. *Option:* Place nonslip padded floor mat on exit side of bed.

    Prevents falls from slipping on floor.

7 Orient patient to surroundings and call light/bed control system:
  a Provide patient's hearing aid and glasses.
  b Explain and demonstrate how to turn call light/intercom system on and off at bedside and in bathroom (see illustration). Have patient perform return demonstration.

    Enables patient to remain alert to conditions in environment.
    Knowledge of location and use of call light is essential to patient safety.

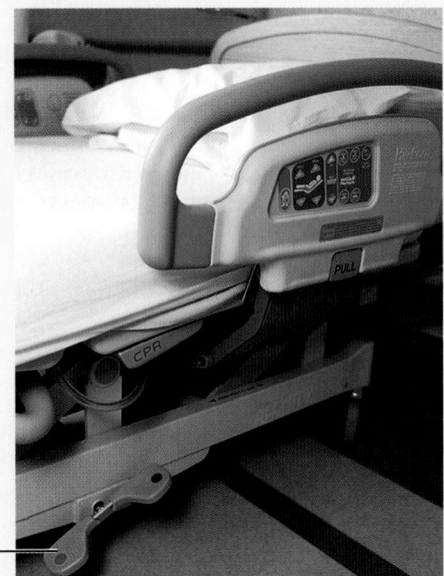

STEP 5   Hospital bed should be kept in lowest position with wheels locked and side rails up (as appropriate).

Brake lock

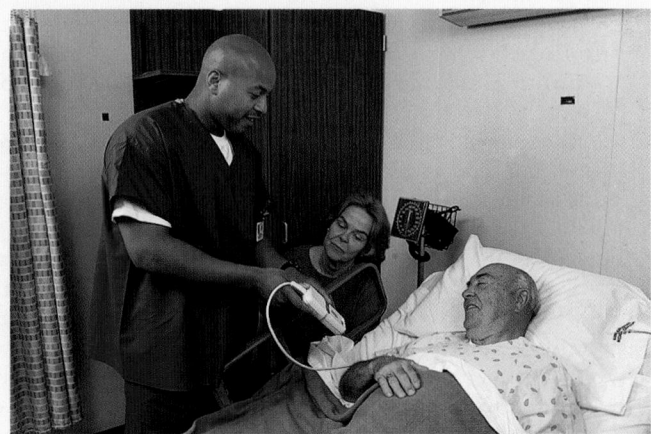

STEP 7b   Nurse demonstrates use of call light to patient.

  c Explain to patient and family when and why to use call system (e.g., report pain, get out of bed, go to bathroom).

    Increases likelihood of nurse being able to respond.

  d Consistently secure call light/bed control system to an accessible location within patient's reach.

    Ensures that patient is able to reach device immediately when needed.

8 **Use of hospital side rails (acute care):**
  a Explain to patient and family the main reason for using side rails: moving and turning self in bed.

    Promotes patient and family cooperation.

  b Check agency policies regarding side rail use.
    (1) Dependent, less mobile patients:
      In a two-side rail bed, keep both rails up. (NOTE: Rails on newer hospital beds allow for room at foot of bed for patient to safely exit bed.) In a four-side rail bed, leave two upper rails up.

    Side rails are a restraint device if they immobilize or reduce ability of patient to move his or her arms, legs, body, or head freely (CMS, 2008).

    (2) Patient able to get out of bed independently: In a four-side rail bed, leave only one upper side rail up.
      In a two-side rail bed, keep only one rail up.

    Allows for safe exit from bed.

Clinical Decision Point   *Assess for excessive gaps and openings between mattress, bedframe, and side rails.*

9 Provide environmental interventions:
  a Remove excess equipment, supplies, and furniture from rooms and halls.

    Reduces likelihood of falls from tripping.

STEP	RATIONALE
b Keep floors clutter and obstacle free, particularly path to bathroom. Coil and secure excess electrical, telephone, and other cords or tubing.	Reduces likelihood of falls from tripping.
c Clean all spills promptly. Post sign indicating wet floor. Remove sign when floor is dry.	Reduces falls from slipping on wet surface.
d Ensure adequate glare-free lighting: use night-light at night.	Reduces fall risk since glare is a problem for older adults because of normal visual changes.
e Have assistive devices (e.g., walker, cane, bedside commodes) located on exit side of bed.	Provides added support when transferring out of bed. Commode eliminates need to get up to walk to bathroom.
f Arrange necessary items (e.g., water pitcher, eyeglasses, dentures, telephone) within patient's easy reach.	Prevents patient from reaching and allows him or her to perform self-care activities safely.
g Secure locks on beds, stretchers, and wheelchairs.	Prevents accidental movement of devices during patient transfer.
10 Additional interventions for patients at high risk (based on fall risk assessment):	Level of risk defined by fall risk assessment tool.
a Prioritize call light responses to patients at high risk, using a team approach,	Ensures rapid response to calls from patients.
b Monitor and assist patients in following daily schedules.	Patients are less likely to try an activity on their own when they have a defined schedule.
c Establish elimination schedule, using bedside commode when appropriate.	Proactive toileting keeps patients from being unattended with sudden urge to use toilet.
d Stay with patient during toileting.	
e Place patients in geri chair or wheelchair with wedge cushion. Use wheelchair only for transport, not for sitting an extended time.	Designed to maintain alignment and comfort and makes it difficult to exit chair.
f Use low bed that has low height above floor and floor mats.	Reduces fall-related injuries.
g Activate bed alarm for patient.	
11 When ambulating patient, have patient wear gait belt and walk along patient's strong side (see Chapter 10).	Gait belt gives you secure hold on patient during ambulation.
12 Explain to patient that hourly rounds will be conducted to reassess for fall risks, provide toileting needs, and attend to symptom management.	Use of hourly rounds has been shown to reduce incidence of falls (Halm, 2009).
13 Explain to patient specific safety measures to prevent falls (e.g., wear well-fitting, flat footwear with nonskid soles; dangle feet for a few minutes before standing; walk slowly; ask for help if dizzy or weak).	Promotes patient understanding and cooperation. Dangling provides adjustment to orthostatic hypotension, allowing blood pressure to stabilize before ambulating (see Chapter 10).
14 Consult with physical therapist about possibility of gait training and muscle-strengthening exercises.	There is evidence that sustained exercise programs may reduce falls (Oliver, Healey, and Haines, 2010).
15 Discuss with health care provider and pharmacist possibility of adjusting patient's medications to reduce side effects and interactions.	Evidence shows that medication assessment with modification (e.g., eliminating unnecessary medications, adjusting dosages) can reduce incidence of falls in home setting (Costello and Edelstein, 2008). Drug interactions can also have effects that place patients at risk in an acute care setting.
16 Safe transport using a wheelchair:	
a During transfer position wheelchair on same side of bed as patient's strong or unaffected side (see Chapter 9).	Facilitates patient's ability to assist in transfer to chair.
b Place wedge cushion in chair (see illustration).	Wedge cushion prevents patient from slipping out of chair.

STEP	RATIONALE

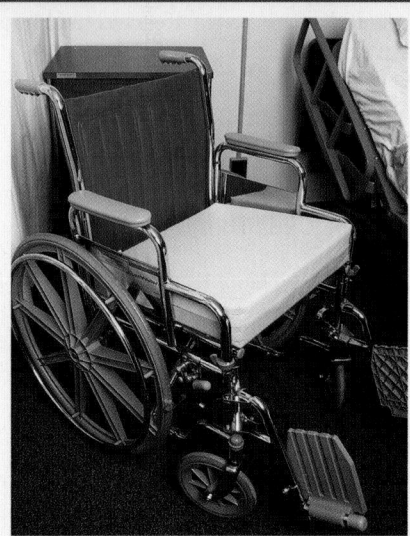

STEP 16b   Wheelchair with footplates raised and wedge cushion in place.

c Securely lock brakes on both wheels when transferring patient into or out of wheelchair.	Keeps chair steady and secure.
d Raise footplates before transfer (see illustration for Step b); lower footplates, placing patient's feet on them after he or she is seated.	Prevents tripping over footplate.
e Have patient sit with buttocks well back in seat. *Option:* Apply a quick-release seat belt.	Prevents patient from sliding out of chair.
f Back wheelchair into and out of elevator or door, leading with large rear wheels first.	Prevents smaller front wheels from catching in crack between elevator and floor, causing chair to tip.

EVALUATION

1 Conduct hourly rounds.	Monitors patient for ongoing risks of falling.
2 Observe patient's immediate environment for presence of hazards.	Ensures that there are no obstacles or barriers to patient's freedom of movement.
3 Evaluate patient's ability to use assistive devices.	Determines if instruction or clarification is needed.
4 Ask patient or family member to identify safety risks.	Determines extent of learning.
5 Evaluate motor, sensory, and cognitive status and review if any falls or injuries have occurred.	Determines how effective nursing interventions are in reducing actual or potential threats to patient's safety.

Unexpected Outcomes

1 Patient/family member is unable to identify safety risks.

2 Patient starts to fall while ambulating with a caregiver.

3 Patient found after suffering a fall.

Related Interventions

- Reinforce identified risks with patient or review needed safety measures with family.

- Put both arms around patient's waist or grasp gait belt.
- Stand with feet apart to provide broad base of support.
- Extend one leg and let patient slide against it to the floor (Fig. 13-2, *A*).
- Bend knees and lower body as patient slides to floor (Fig. 13-2, *B*).

- Call for assistance.
- Assess patient for injury and stay with him or her until assistance arrives.
- Notify primary health care provider and family members.
- Follow agency occurrence or sentinel event reporting policy.
- Note pertinent events related to fall and treatment provided in medical record.
- Evaluate patient and environment; determine whether fall could have been prevented.
- Reinforce identified risks with patient and measures recommended to prevent fall recurrence.
- Monitor patient closely after fall to assess for possible injury.

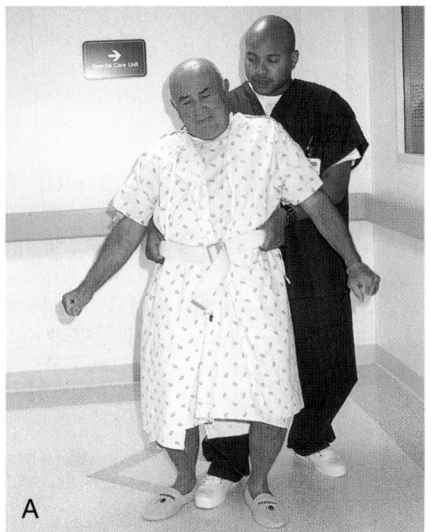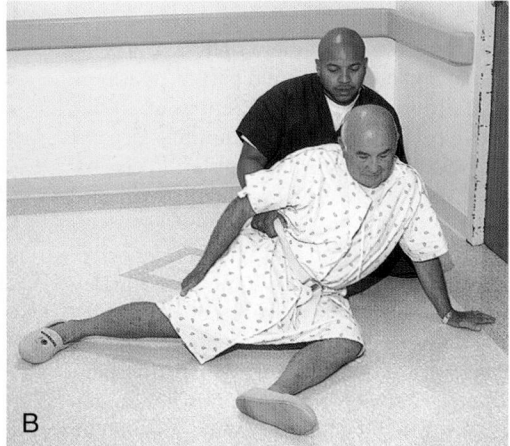

FIG 13-2 **A,** Stand with feet apart to provide broad base of support; extend one leg against which patient can slide to floor. **B,** Bend knees and lower body as patient slides to floor.

Recording and Reporting
- Record fall risk assessment findings and specific interventions, including instructions, used to prevent falls in nurses' notes, electronic health record (EHR), and/or care plan.
- Report to health care personnel specific risks to patient's safety and measures taken to minimize risks.
- If patient suffers a fall, inform primary health care provider. Document what occurred, including description of the fall as given by patient or witness. Be sure to include baseline assessment, any injuries noted, tests or treatments given, follow-up care, and additional safety precautions taken after fall.

Special Considerations
Teaching
- Make available to patients and families the website for the Centers for Disease Control and Prevention (CDC), which has resources on fall prevention at http://www.cdc.gov/HomeandRecreationalSafety/Falls/index.html.
- Encourage patients to have annual vision and hearing examinations. Adaptive devices such as a hearing aid or glasses are sometimes necessary or need modification.
- Emphasize to patients the need to always look ahead when ambulating and use good posture.
- Instruct patients on how to use assistive devices and keep them in good repair.

Pediatric
- Falls are the leading cause of nonfatal injuries for all children ages 0 to 19 (CDC, 2009). Encourage parents to follow these CDC recommendations:

- *Play safely.* Be sure that playground equipment that a child uses is properly designed and maintained and that there is a safe, soft landing surface below.
- *Make home safety improvements.* Use home safety devices such as guards on windows that are above ground level, stair gates, and guard rails.
- *Keep sports safe.* Be sure that a child wears protective gear such as wrist guards, knee and elbow pads, and a helmet for biking or skating when playing active sports.
- *Supervision is key.* Supervise young children at all times around fall hazards, whether at home or out to play.
- Children's activity levels and curiosity increase risk for falls. Eliminate places for the child to climb. Consider using a crib hood if child is hospitalized.
- Keep side rails of hospital beds down to allow toddlers and preschoolers easy exit and to decrease the need to crawl over the rails (Hockenberry and Wilson, 2011).
- When caring for infants, keep a hand on a child when you turn away from the bedside.

Gerontologic
- Interventions to improve balance confidence has shown benefits, including multicomponent behavioral group interventions and exercise (including tai chi), which increases lower body strength and dynamic balance (Bula et al., 2011).

Home Care
- See Chapter 41.

SKILL 13-2   Designing a Restraint-Free Environment

NSO *Safety Module / Lesson 1*

 Video Clip

Physical and chemical restraints restrict a patient's physical activity or normal access to the body and are not a usual part of treatment indicated by a patient's condition or symptoms. Serious and often fatal complications can develop from the use of restraints. Because of the risks associated with restraint use, current legislation emphasizes reducing their use. A restraint-free environment is the first goal of care for all patients.

Patients at risk for falls or wandering present special safety challenges when trying to create a restraint-free environment. Wandering is the meandering, aimless, or repetitive locomotion that exposes a patient to harm and is often in conflict with boundaries, limits, or obstacles (NANDA, 2012). This is a common problem in patients who are confused or disoriented. Interrupting a wandering patient can increase distress. The Department of Veterans Affairs has suggestions for managing wandering, most of which are environmental adaptations. Some of these include hobbies, social interaction, regular exercise, and circular design of a care unit (VA NCPS, 2010). Environmental modifications are effective alternatives to restraints. More frequent observation of patients, involvement of family during visitation, and frequent reorientation are also helpful measures. *There are many alternatives to the use of restraints. Use these alternatives before applying restraints.*

Delegation and Collaboration

The skills of assessing patient behaviors and orientation to the environment and determining the type of restraint-free interventions to use cannot be delegated to nursing assistive personnel (NAP). However, actions for promoting a safe environment can be delegated to NAP. The nurse instructs the NAP about:

- Using specific diversional or activity measures for making the environment safe.
- Applying appropriate alarm devices.
- Reporting patient behaviors and actions (e.g., confusion, getting out of bed unassisted, combativeness) to the nurse.

Equipment

- ❏ Visual or auditory stimuli (e.g., calendar, clock, radio, television, pictures)
- ❏ Diversional activities (e.g., puzzle, game, audio books, DVD)
- ❏ Wedge cushion
- ❏ Wrap-around belt (Fig. 13-3)
- ❏ Ambularm or pressure-sensitive bed or chair alarm
- ❏ Bed enclosure system

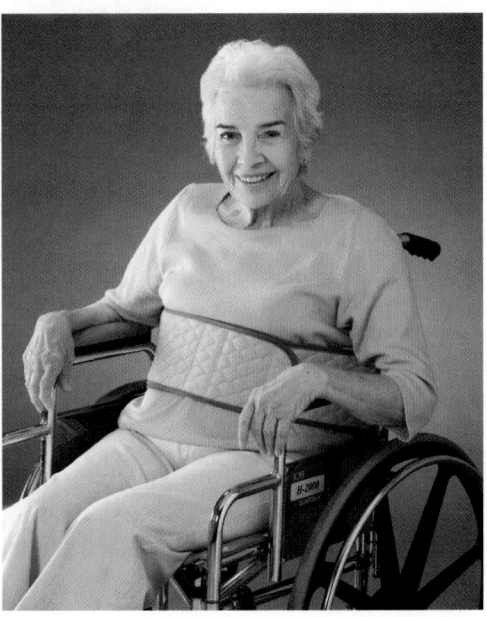

FIG 13-3   Wrap-around belt. (*Courtesy Posey Company, Arcadia, Calif.*)

STEP	RATIONALE

ASSESSMENT

1 Assess patient's medical history for dementia and depression.

2 Assess patient's behavior (e.g., orientation, level of consciousness, ability to understand and follow directions, combative behaviors, restlessness, agitation), balance, gait, vision, hearing, bowel/bladder routine, level of pain, electrolyte and blood count values, and presence of orthostatic hypotension.

3 Review over the counter (OTC) and prescribed medications (see Skill 13-1) for interactions and untoward effects.

4 Assess patient's knowledge of condition and prescribed treatments.

5 For patients who wander or have known dementia, assess for cognitive decline using the Mini-Mental State Examination (MMSE) (see Chapter 6).

6 Assess degree of wandering behavior using Revised Algase Wandering Scale (RAWS) (Nelson and Algase, 2007).

7 For patients with dementia, ask family or friends about his or her usual communication style and cues to indicate pain, fatigue, hunger, need to urinate or defecate (Evans and Cotter, 2008).

Wandering is associated with these common conditions (Futrell, Melillo, and Remington, 2008).

Accurate assessment identifies patients with safety risks and the physiologic causes for patient behaviors that prompt caregivers to use restraints. Ensures proper selection of nonrestraint interventions.

Medication interactions or side effects often contribute to falling or altered mental status.

Knowledge of treatment protocols and rationales increases patient's cooperation.

Determines cause and nature of wandering, which leads to effective intervention selection.

The RAWS provides a quantitative measure for wandering in several domains as reported by caregivers, including persistent walking, spatial disorientation, and eloping behavior (Futrell, Melillo, and Remington, 2008).

Enables you to use best method to determine patient needs, which often prompt wandering when need is unmet.

STEP	RATIONALE

NURSING DIAGNOSES

- Deficient knowledge
- Risk for falls
- Risk for injury
- Risk for trauma
- Wandering

Related factors are individualized based on patient's condition or needs.

PLANNING

1 Expected outcomes following completion of procedure:
- Patient is injury free and/or does not inflict injury on others while in a restraint-free environment.

Restraints and/or alternatives are successful in preventing injury.

IMPLEMENTATION

1 Orient patient and family to surroundings, introduce to staff, and explain all treatments and procedures. Be sure that patient is able to read your name badge.

Promotes patient understanding and cooperation.

2 Assign same staff to care for patient as often as possible. Encourage family and friends to stay with patient. In some agencies, volunteers are effective companions.

Increases familiarity with individuals in patient's environment, decreasing anxiety and restlessness. Companions are often helpful, preventing patient from being alone.

3 Place patient in room that is easily accessible to caregivers, close to nurses' station.

Allows for frequent observation to reduce falls in high-risk patients (VA NCPS, 2010).

4 Be sure that patient has glasses, hearing aid, or other sensory-aid devices on and that all are functioning.

Improves patient's level of orientation to environment.

5 Provide visual and auditory stimuli meaningful to patient (e.g., clock, calendar, radio/MP3 player [with patient's choice of music], television, and family pictures).

Orients patient to day, time, and physical surroundings. You must individualize stimuli for this to be effective.

6 Anticipate patient's basic needs (e.g., toileting, relief of pain, relief of hunger) as quickly as possible.

Basic needs provided in timely fashion decreases patient discomfort, anxiety, and restlessness.

Clinical Decision Point *Getting out of bed for toileting purposes is one of the most common events leading to a patient's fall (Tzeng, 2010), especially during evening or night hours, when rooms are often dark.*

7 Provide scheduled ambulation, chair activity, and toileting (e.g., ask patient every hour about toileting needs). Organize treatments so a patient has uninterrupted periods throughout the day.

Regular opportunity to void avoids risk of patient trying to reach bathroom alone. Provides for sleep and rest periods. Constant activity overstimulates patients.

8 Position intravenous (IV) catheters, urinary catheters, and tubes/drains out of patient view. Use camouflage by wrapping IV site with bandage or stockinette. Place undergarments on patient with urinary catheter or cover abdominal feeding tubes/drains with loose abdominal binder.

Maintains medical treatment and reduces patient access to tubes/lines.

9 Decrease wandering by eliminating stressors from environment such as cold at night, changes in daily routines, and extra visitors (Futrell, Melillo, and Remington, 2008).

Reduced stress allows patient's energy to be channeled more appropriately.

10 Use stress-reduction techniques such as back rub, massage, and guided imagery (see Chapter 15).

11 Use diversional activities such as puzzles, games, music therapy, pet therapy, activity apron, performing purposeful activity (e.g., folding towels, drawing/coloring). Be sure that it is an activity in which patient has interest. Involve a family member in the activity.

Meaningful diversional activities provide distraction, help to reduce boredom, and provide tactile stimulation. Minimize occurrences of wandering.

12 Position patient on wedge cushion and apply wraparound belt.

Cushion prevents slipping in chair and makes it difficult for patient to get out of chair without assistance. Wraparound belt allows patient to lift flap for self-release.

13 Use pressure-sensitive bed or chair pad with alarms:
  a Explain use of device to patient and family.
  b When in the bed, position device so that it is under the patient's mid-to-low back or under buttocks.
  c Test alarm by applying and releasing pressure.

Alarms alert staff to patient who is standing or rising without assistance.

Alarm activates sooner if placed under back. By the time buttocks are off the sensor, patient may be almost out of bed.

Ensures that alarm is audible through call light system.

STEP	RATIONALE
14 Use an Ambularm monitoring device.	
a Explain use of device to patient and family.	Reinforces person's risk for falling or wandering.
b Measure patient's thigh circumference just above knee to determine appropriate size: leg circumference less than 18 inches (45 cm) requires regular size; 18 inches or greater requires large size.	Band that is too loose slips off; one that is too tight irritates skin or interferes with circulation.
c Test battery and alarm by touching snaps to corresponding snaps on leg band.	
d Apply leg band just above knee and snap battery securely in place (see illustration).	
e Instruct patient that alarm will sound unless he or she keeps leg in horizontal position (see illustration).	
f Deactivate alarm to ambulate patient; unsnap device from leg band.	
15 Place patient in bed enclosure system (see illustration).	Restraint alternative that allows patient freedom of movement within a protected environment.

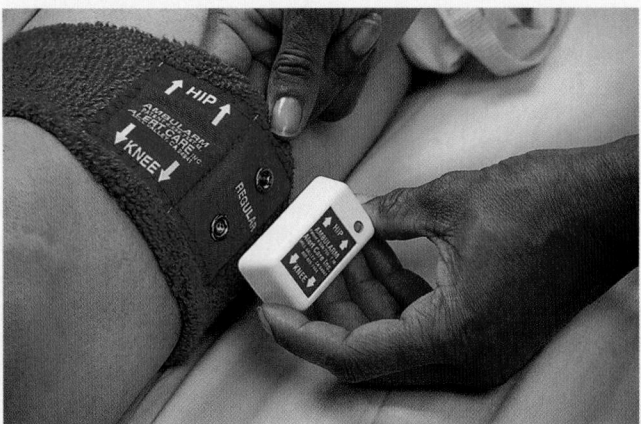

STEP 14d Snap battery in place to activate alarm. (*Courtesy Alert Care, Tiburon, Calif.*)

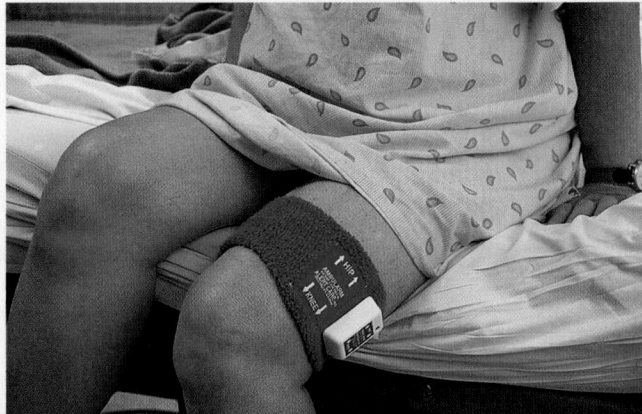

STEP 14e Audio alarm sounds when patient approaches near-vertical position when getting out of bed. (*Courtesy Alert Care, Tiburon, Calif.*)

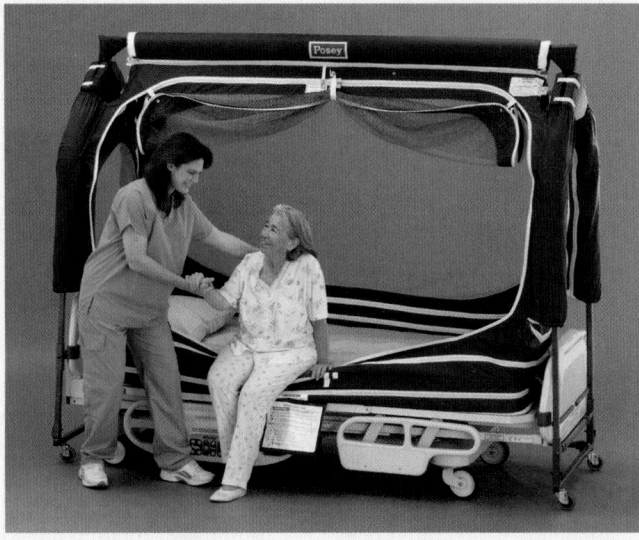

STEP 15 Bed enclosure system.

STEP	RATIONALE
16 Consult with physical, speech, and occupational therapy for activities that provide stimulation and exercise. 17 Minimize invasive treatments (e.g., tube feedings, blood sampling) as much as possible.	Involvement in meaningful and purposeful activities reduces tendency to wander. Exercise improves balance and coordination. Stimuli increase patients' restlessness.

EVALUATION

1 Observe patient for any injuries.	Patient should be injury free.
2 Observe patient's behavior toward staff, visitors, and other patients.	Ensures that patient's behavior does not cause injury to others.
3 Determine need for continuation of invasive treatments and whether you can substitute less invasive treatment.	Eliminates cause and reason for restraint.

Unexpected Outcomes

1 Patient displays behaviors that increase risk for injury to self or others.

2 Patient sustains injury or is out of control, placing others at risk for injury.

Related Interventions

- Review episodes for pattern (e.g., activity, time of day) that indicates alternatives that would eliminate behavior.
- Discuss with all caregivers and family alternative interventions.
- Notify health care provider and complete incident or occurrence report according to agency policy.
- Identify alternative measures for safety or behavioral control.
- Apply physical restraint (see Skill 13-3) only after all other interventions are unsuccessful.

Recording and Reporting

- Record restraint alternatives attempted, patient behaviors that relate to cognitive status, and interventions to mediate these behaviors in nurses' notes, EHR, and/or care plan.

Special Considerations
Teaching

- Teach family members ways to involve patient in their visits, keeping patient appropriately stimulated.
- Teach the family how to adapt the home environment (see Chapter 42) to minimize patient wandering.

Gerontologic

- Keep older adults active and ambulatory to increase endurance and function.
- Reminiscence helps older adults remain oriented.

Home Care

- Patients at risk for self-injury or violence to others need intensive supervision. Family and health care providers need to recognize this and take appropriate preventive measures.
- Have family members set up an area in the home where it is safe for an older adult to wander.

SKILL 13-3 Applying Physical Restraints

NSO *Safety Module / Lesson 2*

 Video Clip

A physical restraint is any manual method, physical or mechanical device, material, or equipment that immobilizes or reduces the ability of a patient to move his or her extremities, body, or head freely (CMS, 2008). A drug may be considered a chemical restraint when it is given to manage behavior or restrict freedom of movement and is not part of the standard treatment for a patient's condition (NAPHS, 2007). Physical or chemical restraints should be the last resort and used only when reasonable alternatives fail (see Skill 13-2).

Restraints are most commonly used in hospitals to prevent the disruption of therapy, such as pulling out intravenous (IV) tubes or removing urinary catheters. Restraint use is more common in critical care settings, where nurses are concerned that disruption of therapy can significantly injure patients (Mion, 2008). The use of physical restraints is no longer a safe strategy, yet many nurses still believe that they are needed to control behavioral symptoms

and prevent falls in older adults with dementia (Evans and Cotter, 2008). The Centers for Medicare and Medicaid Services (CMS, 2008) and The Joint Commission (TJC, 2009a) have set standards for reducing the use of restraints in health care settings and using them only with extreme caution. In 2011 the National Quality Forum (NQF) released its National Voluntary Consensus Standards for Public Reporting of Patient Safety Events (NQF, 2011b). The report provides a framework for publicly reporting patient safety information, including adverse events, about health care organizations to consumers. The NQF has endorsed a select list of serious reportable events, one of which is patient death or serious disability associated with the use of restraints or bedrails while being cared for in a health care agency.

The CMS (2008) released revisions to the Medicare conditions of participation, outlining standards for the safe use of restraints in hospitals and defining patients' rights and choices regarding restraints. It requires that a restraint be used only under the following circumstances: (1) to ensure the immediate physical safety of the patient, a staff member, or others; (2) when less restrictive interventions have been ineffective; (3) in accordance with a written modification to the patient's plan of care; (4) when it is the least restrictive intervention that will be effective to protect the patient, staff member, or others from harm; (5) in accordance with safe and appropriate restraint techniques as determined by hospital policies; and (6) it is discontinued at the earliest possible time.

Restraints are a temporary means to maintain patient safety. However, there is no evidence that they prevent falls, reduce wandering, or prevent medical devices from being pulled out (Ebersole et al., 2008). Research has shown that patients suffer fewer injuries if left unrestrained (Knox and Holloman, 2012). The use of mechanical or physical restraints requires a licensed health care provider's order and must be based on a face-to-face patient assessment. The order must be current, specifying the type of restraint and the duration and circumstances or patient behaviors under which the restraint is to be used. Orders should be renewed according to agency policy (usually every calendar day) and based on reassessment and reevaluation of the restrained patient. A patient's or family member's informed consent is necessary in the long-term care setting.

The use of restraints is associated with serious complications, including pressure ulcers, hypostatic pneumonia, constipation, incontinence, and death. The Food and Drug Administration (FDA) regulates restraints as medical devices and requires manufacturers to label them "prescription only." Most patient deaths in the past have resulted from strangulation from a vest or jacket restraint. Numerous agencies no longer use vest restraints. For these reasons this text does not describe their use.

Delegation and Collaboration

The skills of assessing a patient's behavior and level of orientation, the need for restraints, the appropriate restraint type, and the ongoing assessments required while a restraint is in place cannot be delegated to nursing assistive personnel (NAP). Applying and routinely checking a restraint can be delegated to NAP. The Joint Commission (2009a) requires training on first aid for anyone who monitors patients in restraints. The nurse directs the NAP by:

- Reviewing correct placement of the restraint and how to routinely check the patient's circulation, skin condition, and breathing.
- Reviewing when and how to change a patient's position and provide range-of-motion (ROM) exercises, toileting, and skin care.
- Instructing NAP to notify nurse immediately if there is a change in level of patient agitation, skin integrity, circulation of extremities, or patient's breathing.

Equipment

- ❏ Proper restraint (e.g., belt, wrist, mitten)
- ❏ Padding (if needed)

STEP	RATIONALE
ASSESSMENT	
1 Assess patient's behavior (e.g., confusion, disorientation, agitation, restlessness, combativeness, repeated removal of tubing or other therapeutic devices, and inability to follow directions).	If patient's behavior continues despite treatment or restraint alternatives, use of restraint is indicated.
2 Follow agency policies regarding restraints. Check health care provider's order for purpose, type, location, and time or duration of restraint. Determine if signed consent for restraint use is needed.	In acute care settings a licensed health care provider who is responsible for care of patient must order least restrictive type of restraint. Each original restraint order is limited to 4 hours for adults 18 years of age and older, 2 hours for children ages 9 through 17, and 1 hour for children under age 9 (TJC, 2009a). Original orders may be renewed up to maximum of 24 hours (CMS, 2008).

Clinical Decision Point *If a nurse or qualified health provider (see agency policy) restrains a patient in an emergency situation because of violent or aggressive behavior that presents an immediate danger, a face-to-face health care provider assessment within 1 hour is necessary (TJC, 2012a).*

3 Review manufacturer instructions for correct restraint application and determine most appropriate size of restraint.	You need to be familiar with all devices used for patient care and protection. Incorrect application of restraint device can result in patient injury or death.
4 Inspect area where restraint is to be placed. Note if there is any nearby tubing or devices. Assess condition of skin, sensation, adequacy of circulation, and ROM.	Provides baseline to monitor patient's response to restraint. Provides baseline data to monitor patient's skin integrity.

NURSING DIAGNOSES

- Anxiety
- Risk for impaired skin integrity
- Risk for impaired physical mobility.
- Risk for injury
- Risk for peripheral neurovascular dysfunction
- Risk for self-directed or other-directed violence

Related factors are individualized based on patient's condition or needs.

STEP	RATIONALE

PLANNING

1 Expected outcomes following completion of procedure:

- Patient maintains intact skin integrity, pulses, temperature, color, and sensation of restrained body part.

Restraints applied and monitored correctly.

- Patient is free from injury.

Restraints removed in timely manner.

- Patient's therapy (e.g., IV tube, catheters) is uninterrupted.

Disruption of therapy causes patient injury, pain, or discomfort and increases risk for infection.

- Patient maintains self-esteem and sense of dignity.

Physical restraints have detrimental effect on psychosocial well-being of patient.

- Restraint is discontinued as soon as possible.

Limits period of time patient is at risk for injury.

IMPLEMENTATION

1 Gather equipment and perform hand hygiene.

Promotes organization and reduces transmission of microorganisms.

2 Use calm approach and introduce yourself to patient, including both name and title or role.

Reduces patient anxiety and uncertainty.

3 Identify patient using two identifiers (i.e., name and birthday or name and account number) according to agency policy. Compare indentifiers with information on patient's identification bracelet.

Ensures correct patient. Complies with The Joint Commission standards and improves patient safety (TJC, 2012b).

4 Provide privacy. Explain to patient and family purpose of restraint. Be sure that patient is comfortable and in correct anatomic position.

May promote cooperation. Positioning prevents contractures and neurovascular impairment.

5 Adjust bed to proper height and lower side rail on side of patient contact.

Allows you to use proper body mechanics and prevent injury.

6 Pad skin and bony prominences (as necessary) that will be covered by restraint.

Reduces friction and pressure from restraint to skin and underlying tissue.

7 Apply proper-size restraint: *Follow manufacturer directions.*

   a Belt restraint:

      Have patient in sitting position. Apply belt over clothes, gown, or pajamas. Make sure to place restraint at waist, not chest or abdomen. Remove wrinkles or creases in clothing. Bring ties through slots in belt. Help patient lie down if in bed. Avoid applying belt too tightly (see illustrations).

Restrains center of gravity and prevents patient from rolling off stretcher, sitting up while on stretcher, or falling out of bed. Tight application or misplacement can interfere with ventilation. This type of restraint may be contraindicated in patient who had abdominal surgery.

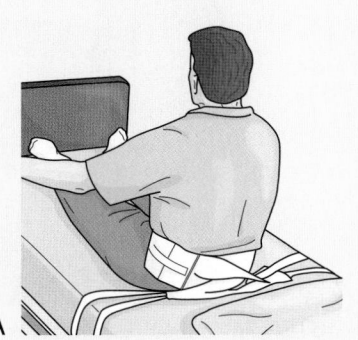 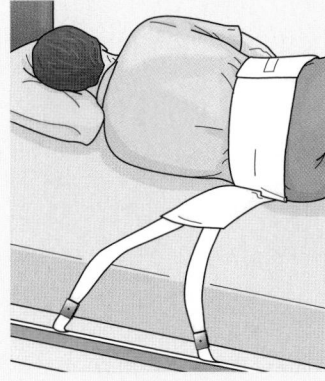

STEP 7a   A, Apply belt restraint with patient sitting. **B**, Properly applied belt restraint allows patient to turn in bed. (**A** *from Sorrentino SA:* Mosby's textbook for nursing assistants, *ed 7, St Louis, 2008, Mosby.*)

   b Extremity (ankle or wrist) restraint:

      Commercially available limb restraints are made of sheepskin with foam padding. Wrap limb restraint around wrist or ankle with soft part toward skin and secure snugly (not tightly) in place by Velcro straps. Insert two fingers under secured restraint (see illustration).

Restraint immobilizes one or all extremities to protect patient from fall or accidental removal of therapeutic device (e.g., IV tube, Foley catheter).

Tight application interferes with circulation and causes neurovascular injury.

STEP	RATIONALE

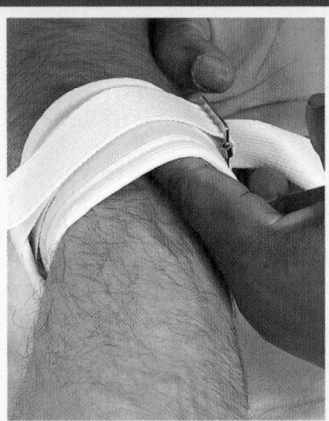

STEP 7b Securing an extremity restraint. Check restraint for constriction by inserting two fingers under restraint. *(From Sorrentino SA: Mosby's textbook for nursing assistants, ed 7, St Louis, 2008, Mosby.)*

Clinical Decision Point *Patient with extremity restraints is at risk for aspiration if placed in supine position. Place patient in lateral position or with head of bed elevated rather than supine.*

c Mitten restraint:
Thumbless mitten device restrains patient's hands. Place hand in mitten, being sure that Velcro strap(s) are around wrist and not forearm (see illustration).

Prevents patients from dislodging invasive equipment, removing dressings, or scratching; yet allows greater movement than wrist restraint.

d Elbow restraint (freedom splint):
Restraint consists of rigidly padded fabric that wraps around arm and is closed with Velcro. Upper end has a clamp that hooks to patient's gown sleeve (see illustration). Insert patient's arm so elbow joint rests against padded area, keeping joint rigid.

Commonly used with infants and children to prevent elbow flexion (e.g., when IV line placed in antecubital fossa). May also be used for adults.

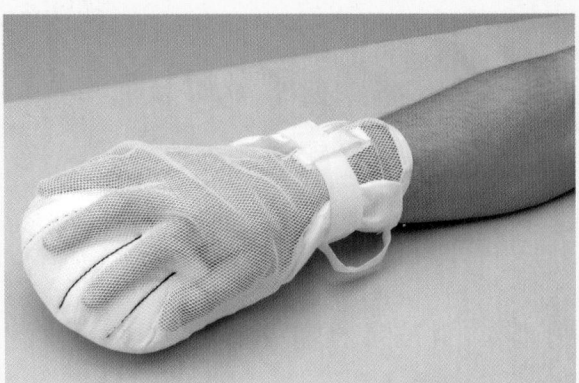

STEP 7c Mitten restraint. *(Courtesy Posey Company, Arcadia, Calif.)*

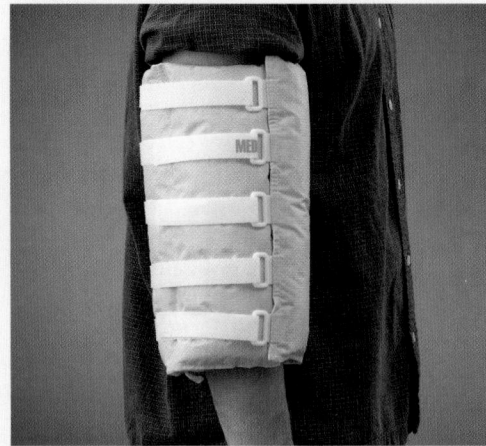

STEP 7d Elbow restraint. *(Courtesy Posey Company, Arcadia, Calif.)*

8 Attach restraint straps to portion of bedframe that moves when raising or lowering head of bed. Be sure that straps are secure. *Do not attach to side rails.* Restraints can be attached to frame of chair or wheelchair as long as ties are out of patient's reach.

Patient will be injured if restraint is secured to side rail and bed is then lowered.

9 Secure restraints with quick-release tie (see illustrations), buckle, or adjustable seat belt–like locking device. *Do not tie in a knot.*

Allows for quick release in emergency.

10 Double-check and insert two fingers under secured restraint.

Checking for constriction prevents neurovascular injury.

STEP	RATIONALE

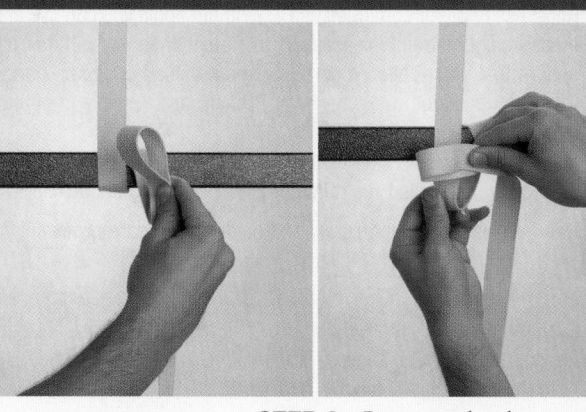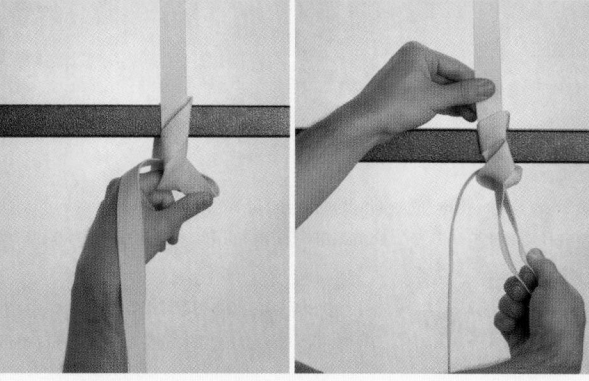

STEP 9   Posey quick-release tie. (*Courtesy Posey Company, Arcadia, Calif.*)

Clinical Decision Point *Restraint should not interfere with equipment such as an IV line or be placed over other types of access devices such as an arteriovenous shunt.*

STEP	RATIONALE
11 Assess proper placement of restraint, including skin integrity, pulses, temperature, color, and sensation of restrained body part.	Provides baseline to later evaluate if injury develops from restraint use.
12 Remove restraints at least every 2 hours (TJC, 2012a) or according to agency policy and assess patient each time. If patient is violent or noncompliant, remove one restraint at a time and/or have staff assist while removing restraints.	Removal provides opportunity to change patient's position, offer nutrients, perform full ROM, toilet and exercise patient.

Clinical Decision Point *Do not leave violent or aggressive patient unattended while restraints are off.*

STEP	RATIONALE
13 Secure call light or intercom system within reach.	Allows patient, family, or caregiver to obtain assistance quickly.
14 Leave bed or chair with wheels locked. Keep bed in lowest position.	Locked wheels prevent bed or chair from moving if patient tries to get out. Placing bed in lowest position reduces chance of injury if patient falls out of bed.
15 Perform hand hygiene.	Reduces transmission of microorganisms.

EVALUATION

1 Following application, evaluate patient's condition for signs of injury every 15 minutes (e.g., circulation, nutrition and hydration, ROM in extremities, vital signs, hygiene and elimination, physical and psychological status, and readiness for discontinuation). Visual checks can be performed if patient is too agitated to approach (TJC, 2012a).	Frequent assessments prevent injury to patient and allows for removal of restraint at earliest possible time.
2 Evaluate patient for any complications of immobility.	Limitation in movement can result in complications (e.g., pressure ulcers, ventilation impairments).
3 Observe IV catheters, urinary catheters, and drainage tubes routinely.	Determines if therapeutic devices are positioned correctly and that therapy remains uninterrupted.
4 Evaluate patient's need for restraints on an ongoing basis (see agency policy). When restraint is used for violent or self-destructive behavior, licensed health care provider must evaluate patient in person within 1 hour of initiation of restraints.	Ensures that restraint application continues to be medically appropriate. Orders may be renewed within these limits: 4 hours for adults 18 and over, 2 hours for children ages 9 through 17, and 1 hour for children under 9 years of age (TJC, 2009a). Original orders may be renewed up to a maximum of 24 hours (CMS, 2008).

Unexpected Outcomes	Related Interventions
1 Patient experiences impaired skin integrity.	• Reassess need for continued use of restraint and if you can use alternative measures. If restraint is necessary to protect patient or others from injury, ensure that you applied it correctly and provided adequate padding. • Check skin under restraint for abrasions and remove restraints more frequently. • Institute appropriate skin/wound care. • Change wet or soiled restraints to prevent skin breakdown.
2 Patient has altered neurovascular status of an extremity (e.g., cyanosis, pallor and coldness of skin) or complaints of tingling, pain, or numbness.	• Remove restraint immediately and notify health care provider.
3 Patient has increased confusion, disorientation, and agitation.	• Evaluate cause for altered behavior and attempt to eliminate cause. • Provide appropriate sensory stimulation, reorient as needed, attempt restraint alternatives, involve family.
4 Patient releases restraint and suffers a fall or other traumatic injury.	• Attend to patient's immediate physical needs, inform health care provider of fall or injury, and reassess type of restraint and its correct application.

Recording and Reporting

• Record patient's behavior before and after restraints were applied, level of orientation, and patient's or family member's statement of understanding of purpose of restraint and consent (when required).
• Record restraint alternatives tried and patient's response in nurses' notes and EHR.
• Record reason for restraint, the type and location, the time applied, the time ending the restraints, and the routine observations made every 15 minutes (e.g., skin color, pulses, sensation, vital signs, behavior) in the nurses' notes and EHR and flow sheets.

Special Considerations

Teaching

• Explain thoroughly the use of restraints. Caution family against removing, repositioning, or retying restraint.

Pediatric

• Limit the use of restraints to clinically appropriate and adequately justified situations (e.g., examination or treatment that involves the head and neck) after using all appropriate alternatives. Remain with infant while restrained and remove restraint immediately after treatment is completed.

• When a child needs to be restrained for a procedure, it is best if the person applying the restraint is not the child's parent or guardian.
• When an infant or small child requires a restraint, a papoose board with straps or a mummy wrap using a blanket or sheet effectively controls his or her movements (Hockenberry and Wilson, 2011).

Gerontologic

• Restrained older adults often respond with anger, fear, depression, humiliation, demoralization, discomfort, and resignation.
• Consider the risks associated with restraints (e.g., pressure ulcers, impaired strength and balance) for older adults (Meiner, 2011). All of the complications of immobility are amplified, leading to greater risk for functional decline.

Home Care

• A health care provider's order is needed for use of a restraint in the home. Provide clear, detailed instructions to the family caregiver, with a return demonstration of restraint application. Do not send a restraint home with family unless device is necessary to protect patient from injury. Carefully assess the family caregiver for competency and understanding of intent for using restraint.

PROCEDURAL GUIDELINE 13-1   Fire, Electrical, and Chemical Safety

Fires in health care settings are typically electrical or anesthetic related. Although smoking is not allowed in health care agencies, smoking-related fires still pose a significant risk because of unauthorized smoking in beds or bathrooms. In the home setting oxygen-related fires are a risk for patients requiring continuous oxygen therapy (see Chapter 23). Health care agencies need to routinely check and maintain all electrical devices. Every biomedical device (e.g., suction machine, infusion pump) must have a safety inspection sticker with an expiration date applied to it. Electrical equipment in good working order requires a three-prong electrical plug for proper grounding. If a patient brings an electrical device to the hospital, an engineer must inspect the device for safe wiring and function before use. Always discourage patients from bringing nonessential electrical devices (e.g., hair dryers or electric toothbrushes) into a health care agency. Many patients with disabilities use battery chargers for mobility equipment function. These devices need to be inspected by hospital engineers as well.

Prevention is the key to fire safety. Nursing measures include complying with agency smoking policies, using equipment correctly, and keeping combustible materials away from heat sources. If a fire occurs, health care personnel report the exact location of the fire, contain it, and extinguish it only if it is safe and possible. All personnel are then mobilized to evacuate patients if needed. Most agencies have fire doors that are held open by magnets and close automatically when a fire alarm sounds. Fire doors should *never* be blocked.

PROCEDURAL GUIDELINE 13-1 Fire, Electrical, and Chemical Safety—cont'd

Chemicals in many medications (e.g., chemotherapy drugs), anesthetic gases, cleaning solutions, and disinfectants are potentially toxic. They injure the body after skin or mucous membrane (e.g., eyes) contact, ingestion, or vapor inhalation. Health care agencies provide employees access to a material safety data sheet (MSDS) for each hazardous chemical in the workplace. An MSDS form contains information about the properties of the particular chemical and information for handling the substance in a safe manner (e.g., storage, disposal, protective equipment, and spill-handling procedures).

Delegation and Collaboration

The skill of protecting patients from fire, electrical, and chemical hazards can be delegated to nursing assistive personnel (NAP). When an event occurs, a nurse leads the health care team in an emergency response. In the event of fire the health care team collaborates with the local fire department. In the event of an electrical or chemical event the team collaborates with the safety officer of the agency. The nurse directs the NAP to:

- Identify patients requiring the most assistance to evacuate or protect.
- Alert the nurse to any risk for chemical exposure.

Equipment
Fire
❏ Appropriate fire extinguisher for fire: type A, B, C, or ABC
Chemical
❏ Appropriate personal protective equipment: clean gloves, mask, gown
❏ MSDS form

Procedural Steps

1 Review agency guidelines for rapid response to fire, electrical, and chemical emergency. Know your responsibilities such as initiating fire alarm and patient evacuation.
2 Know the location of fire alarms, emergency equipment (e.g., fire extinguishers), MSDS forms, emergency eyewash stations, and emergency exit routes.
3 Assess patient's mental status and ability to ambulate, transfer, or move to anticipate the procedures that will be needed to evacuate him or her.
4 Be alert to situations that increase the risk of fire (e.g., a patient on oxygen charging a cell phone while in the bed).
5 Know which patients are on oxygen. Oxygen delivery may be shut off in the event of a severe fire.
6 Inspect equipment for current maintenance sticker. Check electrical equipment for basic safety features (i.e., intact cords and plugs, intact casing). Know agency process for tagging and reporting broken or unsafe equipment.
7 Fire safety:
  a Follow the acronym RACE**.**
    (1) Rescue patient from immediate injury by removing from area or shielding from fire to avoid burns.
    (2) Activate fire alarm immediately. Follow agency policy for alerting staff to respond. (In many situations perform Steps (1) and (2) simultaneously by using call system to alert staff while you help patients at risk.)
    (3) Contain the fire by:
      (a) Closing all doors and windows.
      (b) Turning off oxygen and electrical equipment.
      (c) Placing wet towels along base of doors.

    (4) Evacuate patients:
      (a) Direct ambulatory patients to walk by themselves to a safe area. Know the fire exits and emergency evacuation route.
      (b) If patient is on life support, maintain respiratory status manually until you remove him or her from fire area.
      (c) Move bedridden patients by stretcher, bed, or wheelchair.
      (d) For patients who cannot walk or ambulate (*Options*):
        i Place on blanket and drag patient out of area of danger.
        ii *Use two-person swing*: Place patient in sitting position and have two staff members form a seat by clasping forearms together. Lift patient into "seat" and carry out of area of danger (see illustrations A and B).

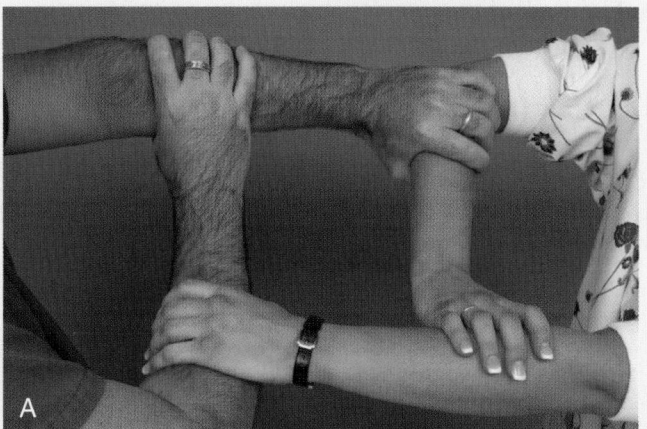

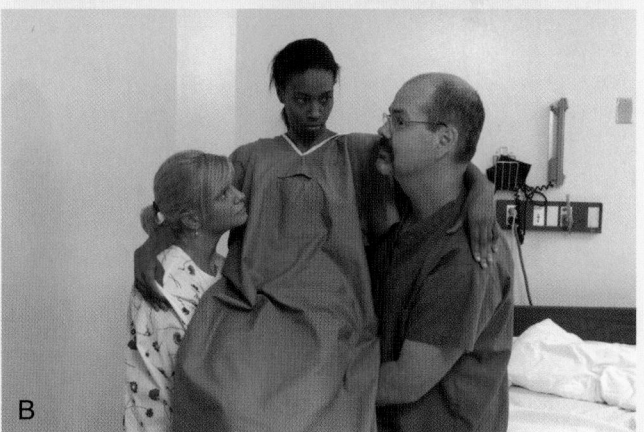

STEP 7a(4)(d)ii A, Hands positioned to form two-person evacuation swing. **B,** Patient seated firmly on swing and holding shoulders of nurses for evacuation.

        iii *Use "back-strap" method*: Stand in front of patient and place his or her arms around your neck. Grasp patient's wrists firmly against your chest. Pull patient onto your back and carry out of danger.

Continued

PROCEDURAL GUIDELINE 13-1 Fire, Electrical, and Chemical Safety—cont'd

(5) If fire department personnel are on the scene, they will help with evacuation of patients.

Clinical Decision Point *Know the weight and size of patients and their self-help ability when choosing an evacuation carry. Use safe patient-handling techniques. Use of a two-person carry versus trying to carry patient independently reduces risk for injury.*

b Extinguish fire using appropriate fire extinguisher: type A for ordinary combustibles (e.g., wood, cloth, paper, most plastics), type B for flammable liquids (e.g., gasoline, grease, paint, anesthetic gas), type C for electrical equipment, type ABC for any type of fire (most common extinguisher in use).

   (1) To use an extinguisher, follow the acronym PASS:

     (a) Pull the pin (see illustration A).

     (b) Aim nozzle at base of fire.

     (c) Squeeze extinguisher handles (see illustration B).

     (d) Sweep from side to side to coat area evenly. (See illustration C).

8 Electrical safety:

a If patient receives an electrical shock, immediately unplug the electrical source and assess for presence of a pulse. *Caution:* When disengaging electrical source, check for presence of water on floor.

Clinical Decision Point *Do not touch a person who is being shocked while he or she is still engaged with the electrical source. If unable to disconnect source, call emergency number for assistance.*

b Once the source of electricity is disconnected, provide appropriate interventions. If patient is pulseless, institute emergency resuscitation (see Chapter 27).

c Notify emergency personnel and patient's health care provider.

d If patient has a pulse and remains alert and oriented, obtain vital signs and assess the skin for signs of thermal injury.

9 Chemical safety:

a Attend to any person exposed to a chemical. Treat chemical splashes to the eyes immediately; flush eyes with water. Use clean, lukewarm tap water for 15 to 20 minutes; stand under a shower, or place head under running faucet. Remove contact lenses if flushing does not remove them (see Chapter 19).

b Notify persons in the immediate area of the spill and evacuate all nonessential personnel from area.

c Refer to MSDS; if spilled material is flammable, turn off electrical and heat sources.

d Avoid breathing vapors of spilled material; apply appropriate respirator.

e Use appropriate personal protective equipment (refer to MSDS) to clean up a spill.

f Dispose of any materials used in cleanup as hazardous waste.

10 Regularly inspect patient's room for fire or electrical hazards.

11 Follow agency policy for reporting a sentinel event (Procedural Guideline 13-2). Documentation will likely be made as a sentinel event report and not in nurses' notes or EHR.

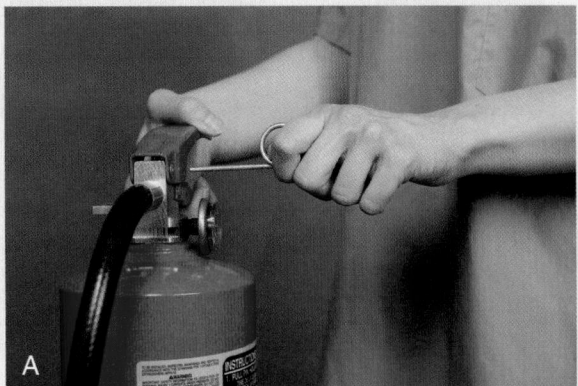
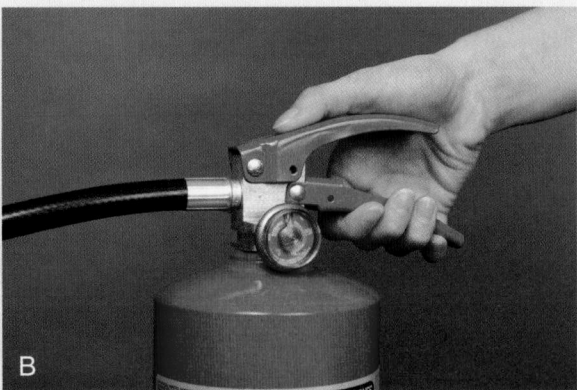
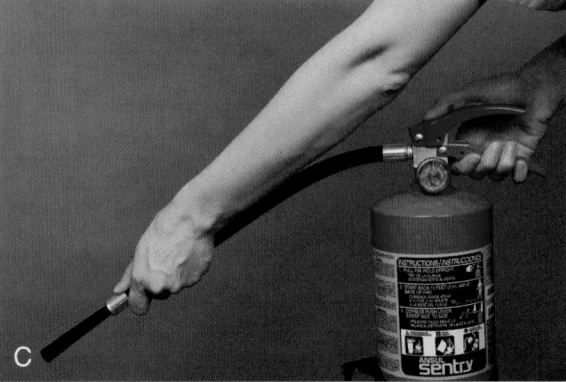

STEP 7b(1)(a-c) **A,** Pull safety pin from fire extinguisher. **B,** Aim nozzle of hose at base of fire. **C,** Squeeze handle while sweeping side to side with nozzle.

SKILL 13-4   Seizure Precautions

Seizures are sudden, abnormal, and excessive electrical discharges from the brain that change motor or autonomic function, consciousness, or sensation. Seizures are epileptic and nonepileptic. Epileptic seizures result from epilepsy, a neurologic condition in which a brain abnormality causes recurrent seizure activity. Nonepileptic seizures are a response to a stimulus outside of the central nervous system such as alcohol withdrawal, high fever, drug toxicity, and poisoning. The two basic types of seizures are partial (simple and complex) and generalized. A partial seizure starts in a specific part of the brain. In a simple seizure a patient does not lose consciousness. In a partial complex seizure a patient loses consciousness. Generalized seizures, of which there are several types, affect the whole brain and cause both nonconvulsive and convulsive seizures. Status epilepticus, characterized by prolonged seizures lasting more than 10 minutes or a series of seizures that occur in rapid succession over 30 minutes, is a medical emergency (Eliahu et al., 2008).

Your role as a nurse is to protect patients who have a seizure disorder from harm. The most immediate risks from a generalized seizure are traumatic injury and choking, requiring you to protect the patient physically and assist with airway management as needed. After that you assess cardiopulmonary effects and administer ordered antiseizure medications. Because each type of seizure has a unique combination of clinical features, it is important to assess a patient carefully if you witness a seizure. Careful observation may help to determine the type of seizure. For example, a generalized seizure lasts from 1 to 2 minutes. A cry, loss of consciousness, tonicity (muscle rigidity), clonicity (rhythmic muscle jerking), and incontinence are all characteristics. Following the seizure there is a postictal phase, which lasts for up to an hour.

During a seizure perform interventions to keep the patient's airway open. Traditionally nurses have used oral airways to maintain the patient's airway. However, forcing an object into a patient's mouth can injure the jaw, tongue, or teeth and cause stimulation of the gag reflex, causing vomiting, aspiration, and respiratory distress (NINDS, 2011). Forcing an airway or tongue blade into a patient's mouth is no longer recommended. Insert an airway only when there is clear access for insertion, possibly after the seizure resolves and there is a need for airway support.

Delegation and Collaboration

The skill of assessing a patient on seizure precautions cannot be delegated to nursing assistive personnel (NAP). However, the skills for making a patient's environment safe can be delegated. The nurse directs NAP by:

- Explaining the patient's prior seizure history and factors that may trigger a seizure.
- Instructing to inform the registered nurse immediately when seizure activity develops.
- Explaining how to protect the patient in the event of a seizure.
- Emphasizing not to try to restrain the patient or place anything in the patient's mouth during a seizure.

Equipment

- ❏ Suction machine
- ❏ Oral airway
- ❏ Oral Yankauer suction catheter
- ❏ Oxygen via nasal cannula or face mask
- ❏ Equipment for vital signs (see Chapter 5)
- ❏ Equipment for intravenous access (see Chapter 31)
- ❏ Emergency medications (e.g., IV diazepam, lorazepam, valproate [Depacon], phenytoin [Dilantin])
- ❏ Clean gloves

STEP	RATIONALE

ASSESSMENT

1 Assess patient's seizure history (e.g., new diagnosis, frequent seizures, seizure within last year) and knowledge of precipitating factors. Ask patient to describe frequency of past seizures, presence and type of aura (e.g., metallic taste, perception of breeze blowing on face, or noxious odor), and body parts affected if known. Use family as resource if necessary.

Knowledge about seizure history enables nurse to anticipate onset of seizure activity and take appropriate safety measures.

2 Assess for medical and surgical conditions, including history of head trauma, electrolyte disturbances (e.g., hypoglycemia, hyperkalemia), heart disease, excess fatigue, alcohol or caffeine consumption.

Common conditions lead to seizures or worsen existing seizure condition.

3 Assess medication history (e.g., antidepressants and antipsychotics). Assess for patient's adherence to anticonvulsants and therapeutic drug levels if test results available.

Certain medications lower seizure threshold.

If patient does not take seizure medications as prescribed and stops them suddenly, this often precipitates seizure activity.

4 Inspect patient's environment for potential safety hazards (e.g., extra furniture) if seizure occurs. Keep bed in low position, side rails up at head of bed, patient in side-lying position when possible.

Protects patient from injury sustained by striking head or body on furniture or equipment.

5 Assess patient's individual and cultural perspective about the meaning of seizures and their treatment.

Some cultures follow different caring practices for a person with seizures.

STEP	RATIONALE

NURSING DIAGNOSES

- Deficient knowledge
- Noncompliance
- Risk for aspiration
- Risk for ineffective airway clearance
- Situational low self-esteem

Related factors are individualized based on patient's condition or needs.

PLANNING

1 Expected outcomes following completion of procedure:
- Patient remains free of traumatic injury while experiencing seizure.
- Patient's airway remains patent during seizure activity.

- Patient does not experience lowered sense of self-esteem following seizure episode.

Seizure precautions prevent patients from incurring injury from a fall or generalized seizure activity.

Airway occlusion and aspiration are potential complications of seizure activity.

Loss of bowel or bladder control is common in generalized seizures, causing patient to feel embarrassment or shame.

IMPLEMENTATION

1 For patients with a history of seizures, keep bed in lowest position with side rails up (see agency policy). Pad rails if patient is at risk for head injury. Have oral suction and oxygen equipment ready for use.

2 Patient with history of seizures should be in room close to nurse's station or room with video monitor.

3 Seizure response:

a Position patient safely

(1) If standing or sitting, guide patient to floor and protect head in your lap or place pillow under head. Turn patient onto side with head tilted slightly forward. Do not lift patient from floor to bed during seizure.

(2) If patient is in bed, turn him or her onto side and raise side rails.

b Note time seizure began and call for help. Track duration of seizure. Have health care provider notified immediately. Have staff member bring emergency cart to bedside and clear surrounding area of furniture.

c Keep patient in side-lying position, supporting head and keeping it flexed slightly forward.

d If possible, provide privacy. Have staff control flow of visitors in area.

e Do not restrain patient; if patient is flailing limbs, hold them loosely. Loosen restrictive clothing/gown.

f *Never force any object into patient's mouth* such as fingers, medicine, tongue depressor, or airway when teeth are clenched.

Reduces risk of fall and injury. Equipment ensures prompt intervention directed toward maintaining a patent airway. Padded side rails are used only when patient is at risk for head injury (Clore, 2010; Lewis et al., 2011).

Improves likelihood of quick response with emergency equipment.

Position protects patient from aspiration and traumatic injury, especially head injury.

Reduces exposure to injury. Description of seizure may help in ultimate identification of type of seizure.

Position prevents tongue from blocking airway and promotes drainage of secretions, reducing risk of aspiration.

Embarrassment is common after a seizure, especially if others witnessed it.

Prevents musculoskeletal injury. Promotes free ventilatory movement of chest and abdomen.

Prevents injury to mouth and possible aspiration.

Clinical Decision Point *Injury can result from forcible insertion of a hard object into the mouth. Soft objects break and become aspirated. Insert a bite block or oral airway in advance if you recognize the possibility of a generalized seizure.*

g Maintain patient's airway; suction orally as needed. Check patient's level of consciousness and oxygen saturation. Provide oxygen by nasal cannula or mask if ordered. *Use oral airway only if you can easily access oral cavity* (see Chapter 27).

h Observe sequence and timing of seizure activity. Note type of seizure activity (tonic, clonic, staring, blinking); whether more than one type of seizure occurs; sequence of seizure progression; level of consciousness; character of breathing; presence of incontinence; presence of autonomic signs of lip smacking, mastication, or grimacing; rolling of eyes.

Prevents hypoxia during seizure activity.

Continued observation helps to document, diagnose, and treat seizure disorder.

STEP	RATIONALE

i As patient regains consciousness, assess vital signs and reorient and reassure him or her. Explain what happened and answer patient's questions. Stay with patient until fully awake.

Informing patients of type of seizure activity experienced helps them to participate knowledgeably in their care. Some patients remain confused for a period of time after the seizure or become violent.

4 Status epilepticus is a medical emergency.

   a Call health care provider and response team immediately.

Medical emergency requires rapid response.

   b Insert oral airway (see Chapter 27) when jaw is relaxed (between seizure activity).

Provides route for intravenous (IV) medication.

   c Access oxygen and suction equipment; keep airway patent.

   d Prepare for IV insertion (if one is not in place) and administration of IV antiseizure medications.

5 After seizure assist patient to side-lying position in bed with padded side rails (if needed) up and bed in lowest position (see illustration). Place call light or intercom system within reach and provide quiet, nonstimulating environment. Instruct patient not to get out of bed without assistance.

Provides for continued safety. Patients are often confused and lethargic following a seizure (postictal).

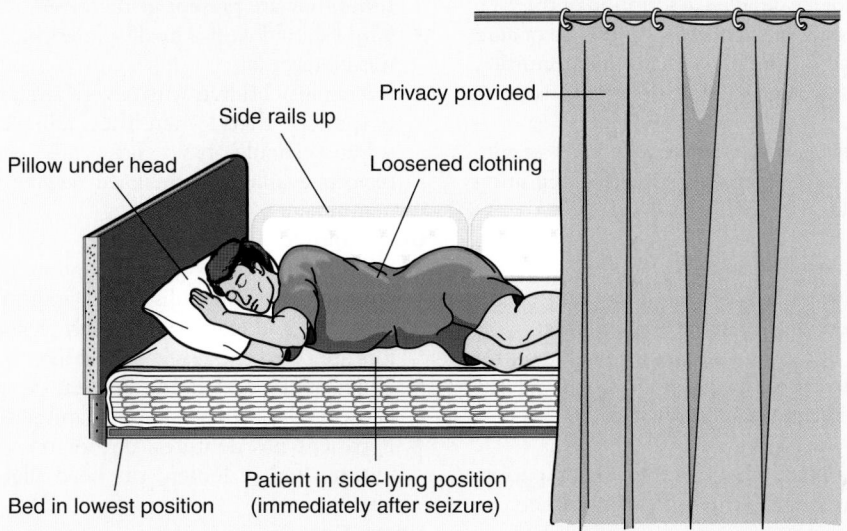

STEP 5 Position of patient following seizure and when on seizure precautions.

6 As patient regains consciousness, reorient and reassure. Explain what happened and provide time for him or her to express feelings and concerns.

Patients may be confused postictal. Patients who understand disease are better prepared to manage their seizure activity and have higher self-esteem.

7 Perform hand hygiene.

Reduces transmission of microorganisms.

EVALUATION

1 Check vital signs and oxygen saturation every 15 minutes during postictal phase and maintain patent airway.

Determines patient's cardiopulmonary status and response to seizure episode.

2 Examine patient for injury, including oral cavity (broken teeth, laceration of tongue or mucosa) and extremities.

Determines presence of any traumatic injuries resulting from seizure activity.

Clinical Decision Point *If onset of seizure was not witnessed and you suspect that patient fell and struck head, treat as a closed head injury or spinal injury. Place a cervical collar on patient before attempting to turn or reposition.*

3 Evaluate patient's mental status after seizure (level of consciousness, confusion, hallucinations). Encourage him or her to verbalize feelings.

Temporary mental status changes are common following a seizure. Therapeutic interaction enables patient to recognize feelings associated with having a seizure disorder.

STEP	RATIONALE
Unexpected Outcomes 1 Patient suffers traumatic injury.	**Related Interventions** • Attend to patient's immediate physical needs. • Administer prescribed treatments. • Inform health care provider • Reassess patient's environment to ensure that environment is free of safety hazards.
2 Patient aspirates.	• Turn onto side, insert oral airway (if possible; see Chapter 27), and apply suction to remove material in oral pharynx and maintain patent airway. • Administer oxygen as needed.

Recording and Reporting

• Record in nurses' notes and EHR what you observed before, during, and after seizure. Provide detailed description of the type of seizure activity and sequence of events (e.g., presence of aura [if any], level of consciousness, color, movement of extremities, incontinence, patient's status immediately following seizure, and time frame of events).

• Alert primary health care provider immediately as seizure begins. Status epilepticus is an emergency situation requiring immediate medical therapy.

Special Considerations
Teaching

• Instruct patient to avoid seizure triggers such as caffeine.
• Patients need to know that antiseizure medications help control epilepsy. Warn them to take prescribed medications regularly. They should never stop medications suddenly because this precipitates seizures.
• Advise patient to avoid alcohol, which is often incompatible with anticonvulsive medications and intensifies central nervous system depression.
• Proper oral hygiene and frequent dental care are necessary when patient takes phenytoin (Dilantin) long term, since gingival hyperplasia is a side effect.
• Encourage patient to wear a medical alert bracelet or carry identification card noting presence of seizure disorder and listing medications taken.
• Fatigue, stress, and illness can potentiate seizures. Teach patients to eat a balanced diet at regular intervals, get adequate sleep, and consult their health care provider promptly when ill.
• A seizure disorder usually imposes driving limitations. It is recommended that a waiting period of 1 seizure-free year elapse before patient attempts to drive or operate dangerous equipment (see state law).

Pediatric

• Teach parents for what to observe in seizures because many times they are present at the onset.
• Child should wear a medical alert bracelet noting presence of a seizure disorder.
• Encourage children with severe atonic seizures to wear helmets to protect them when they fall. A child with generalized seizures should have side rails padded and suction and oxygen available to manage respiratory secretions for airway maintenance.

Gerontologic

• Older adults often have symptoms that make it difficult to recognize a seizure disorder. Confusion lasting several days, receptive and expressive speech problems, and unusual behaviors are often the result of a seizure.
• Older adults metabolize antiseizure medications more slowly, allowing drugs to accumulate and possibly result in toxicity.
• If patient has dentures, do not try to remove them during a seizure. If they loosen, tilt head slightly forward and remove after seizure.

Home Care

• Instruct family members about steps to take when patient experiences a seizure.
• Assess patient's home for environmental hazards that could increase the risk of injury in the event of a fall.
• Until a seizure condition is well controlled (usually for at least 1 year), make sure that patient does not take a tub bath or engage in activities such as swimming unless a knowledgeable family member is present.
• Refer patient to the Epilepsy Foundation or a similar community resource for support groups.

PROCEDURAL GUIDELINE 13-2 Conducting a Root Cause Analysis

Root cause analysis (RCA) is a process of responding to sentinel events with the purpose of discovering the causes of the event and developing an effective plan for preventing future events (e.g., falls, injuries, and medication errors). The Joint Commission requires an RCA of sentinel events with a resultant action plan (TJC, 2009b). An RCA needs to be relevant and thorough. It is not about placing blame or relieving accountability; it is about looking at all the details that may have contributed to an error. Most health care agencies have a safety department that includes a specially trained team to lead all RCAs. The people closest to an error and the people close to any system processes that may have contributed to the error must participate in the RCA. The process is valuable for genuine practice improvement and the prevention of similar events in the future.

Delegation
The skill of conducting an RCA is the responsibility of a multidisciplinary team.

Procedural Steps
1 In response to a sentinel event (e.g., injury from a restraint, patient fall) ensure that immediate needs of patient/family are met. Report the event according to agency policy.
2 The designated safety team reviews the event, identifies the professionals involved, and ensures that all professional groups are represented in the analysis.
3 The team analyzes factors leading to and associated with the sentinel event by asking these questions:
   a What happened? Describe details of event, when it occurred, and area within agency affected.
   b Why did it happen? Describe process or activity in which the event occurred. Use a flow chart to show steps in the process.
   c What factors contributed to the event? Describe steps contributing to the event, the people involved, equipment performance, environmental factors, and factors beyond organization control.

4 For each question the team decides if any element was a root cause and if action is needed.
5 Further analysis asks why the event happened in more detail and the proximate factors contributing to it. Examples are:
   a Human Resource issues—Staffing, competence, staff performance
   b Educational issues—Can orientation and training improve?
   c Information management issues—To what degree was all necessary information available, accurate, and complete?
   d Leadership issues—Does the work unit culture support risk identification and reduction? What barriers exist for communicating need to prevent adverse events?
6 Here are examples of approaches for analyzing data in an RCA:
   a Six Sigma (Smith and Erwin, 2011)
      (1) Define problem.
      (2) Map process.
      (3) Gather data.
      (4) Conduct cause/effect analysis seeking root cause.
      (5) Verify root cause with data.
      (6) Identify solutions and prevention steps.
      (7) Create pilot of implementation (with evaluation).
      (8) Implement.
      (9) Control/monitor plan.
      (10) Lessons learned
   b Fish Diagram (see illustration) (Gano, 2007)
      (1) Arrange a list of causal factors in a fish diagram. Depending on the model used, there are predetermined categories (e.g., People, Equipment, Environment) into which causes for events should be able to be identified.
7 Develop an action plan for risk reduction—For each factor in the analysis that needs an action, develop a plan.
8 Implement the plan—Consider if pilot testing the planned improvement is needed.
9 Evaluate results.

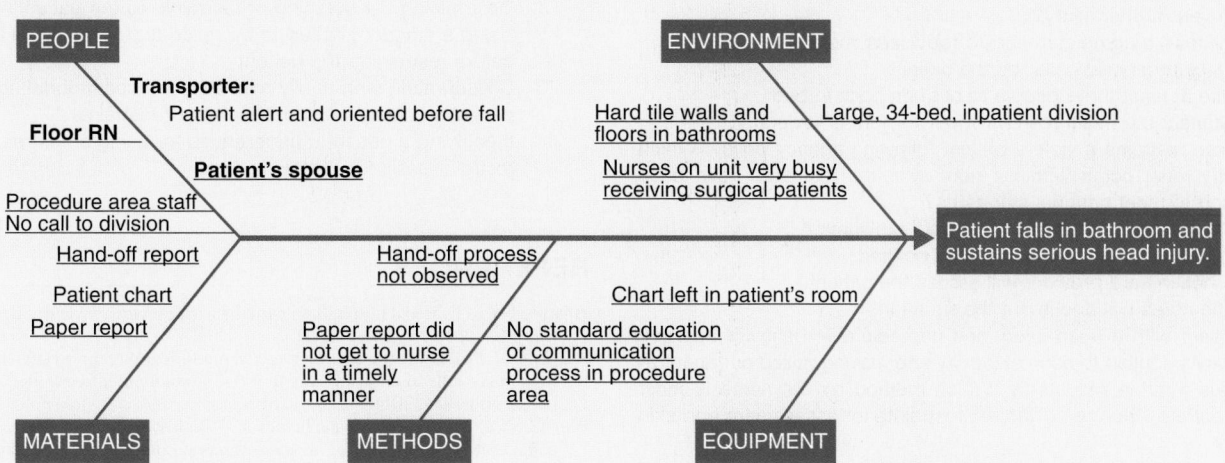

STEP 6b Root cause analysis for patient fall. (*Adapted from the Institute for Healthcare Improvement, IHI, 2004.*)

Critical Thinking Exercises

Daniel Werneck is a 78-year-old patient who entered the hospital for lower gastrointestinal bleeding. During the morning nurses administered a series of enemas to Mr. Werneck before diagnostic tests of the colon. He has a history of high blood pressure, which is well controlled on medications. He has some weakness in his left leg as a result of an old back injury. As the evening nurse you assess Mr. Werneck and find that he is having diarrhea and abdominal cramping. His wife stays with him until visiting hours conclude. He is alert and tells you, "I'm fine. I just feel a bit worn out from the testing today."

1 Which factors in Mr. Werneck's case place him at risk for falling?
2 Which interventions can you implement for fall prevention?
3 At 11 PM you enter Mr. Werneck's room and find him lying on the floor. What are your first two actions?

REVIEW QUESTIONS

1 A nurse is providing information to nursing assistive personnel (NAP) regarding a patient who is having frequent seizures. Which instructions are most important for the nurse to include?
1 If a seizure occurs, turn the patient on his side and insert an oral airway.
2 Hold the patient firmly during the seizure so he does not bump his head.
3 If a seizure occurs, be sure to lower the bed side rails.
4 If a seizure occurs, stay with him while watching his ability to breathe.

2 An elderly patient with a seizure disorder wears dentures. If the patient has a seizure, when should the nurse remove the dentures?
1 When the patient experiences an aura, right before the seizure begins
2 During the most active part of the seizure so the airway stays open
3 As soon as the seizure is over
4 During the postictal period if the dentures are loose

3 A patient is found unconscious on the floor and may have sustained a head injury. Which immediate action should the nurse implement to prevent further injury?
1 Perform a complete head-to-toe assessment
2 Place a cervical collar on the patient
3 Use at least three people to put him back in bed
4 Contact the health care provider for further orders

4 A nurse restrains a violent patient following agency policy. Which activity must occur within 1 hour after the restraints have been applied to meet national standards?
1 The patient will receive a detailed explanation.
2 The patient's next-of-kin will be notified.
3 A health care provider will assess the patient.
4 The nurse will document the situation.

5 A patient with a head injury and unpredictable behavior has soft restraints applied to each extremity after having pulled out an intravenous (IV) line repeatedly. Which method by the nurse is most appropriate when removing the restraints for assessment and skin care?
1 Remove one hand and one leg restraint at the same time.
2 Remove the upper-extremity restraints at the same time and then the lower ones.
3 Remove one restraint at a time with another staff member present.
4 Remove all of the restraints at the same time with another staff member present.

6 How would you demonstrate Quality and Safety Education for Nurses (QSEN) skills for safety competency in which of the following behaviors? (Select all that apply.)
1 During rounds on three different patients you use your memory to recall which patient needs to get an analgesic in the next 30 minutes.
2 You place a patient on a new bed alarm system without having attended an in-service on the system.
3 You follow evidence guidelines in your assessment of a patient's fall risk.
4 During a change of shift report you include a fall occurrence involving a patient for whom you cared.

7 A nurse working in a home health agency is collaborating with other nurses to develop a fall prevention program for patients in the community. Using evidence from the literature on fall prevention, the nurses would likely include which of the following strategies?
1 Developing a recommended set of diversional activities for patients to use in the home
2 Conducting a standard vision assessment when visiting patients the first time
3 Developing guidelines for using restraints for persons with dementia
4 Instituting the use of the Revised Algase Wandering Scale (RAWS)

8 A fire is discovered in a trash can in a patient's room. Which action by the nurse should be questioned?
1 Turning off the oxygen sources
2 Getting the patient out of the room
3 Asking the patient to place her blanket over the trash can
4 Calling for help

9 A nurse enters a patient's room, finds the patient asleep, and notices sparks and fire coming from an electrical outlet. The patient is in traction for fractures to the legs. Place the following steps for the nurse's response to the fire in their correct order.
_____ 1 Contain the fire by turning off all oxygen in the room.
_____ 2 Rescue the patient by moving the bed away from the outlet.
_____ 3 Alert a staff member to activate the fire alarm.
_____ 4 Evacuate the patient from the room.

10 A nurse uses a patient-centered approach for any safety interventions to minimize a patient's vulnerability and diligently protect the patient from injury. Which of the following approaches are patient-centered when applying a restraint? (Select all that apply.)
1 Determining the meaning of restraints to the patient's family
2 Using a standard assessment guide that is evidence based before restraining the patient
3 Collaborating with family members in accommodating a patient's cultural perspectives about restraints
4 Identifying a patient's preferences for using an extremity restraint or mitten restraint

REFERENCES

Allan-Gibbs R: Falls and hospitalized patients with cancer: a review of the literature, *Clin J Oncol Nurs* 14(6):784, 2010.

Ang E, et al: Evaluating the use of a targeted multiple intervention strategy in reducing patient falls in an acute care hospital: a randomized controlled trial, *J Adv Nurs* 67(9):1984, 2011.

Beer C, et al: Quality use of medicines and health outcomes among a cohort of community dwelling older men: an observational study, *Br J Clin Pharmacol* 71(4):592, 2011.

Boyd R, Stevens JA: Falls and fear of falling: burden, beliefs and behaviours, *Age Ageing* 38(4):423, 2009.

Bula CJ, et al: Interventions aiming at balance confidence improvement in older adults: an updated review, *Gerontology* 57(3):276, 2011.

Centers for Medicare and Medicaid Services (CMS): *Revisions to Medicare conditions of participation,* 37, Bethesda, Md, 2008, US Department of Health and Human Services.

Centers for Disease Control and Prevention (CDC): *Protect the ones you love: child injuries are preventable*, 2009, available at http://www.cdc.gov/SafeChild/Falls/, accessed May, 2011.

Chang CM, et al: Medical conditions and medications as risk factors of falls in inpatient older people: a case-control study, *Int J Geriatr Psychiatry* 26(6):602, 2011.

Clore E: Seizure precautions for pediatric bedside nurses, *Pediatr Nurs* 36(4):191, 2010.

Costello E, Edelstein JE: Update on falls prevention for community-dwelling older adults: review of single and multifactorial intervention programs, *J Rehabil Res Dev* 45(8):1135, 2008.

Coussement J, et al: Interventions for preventing falls in acute- and chronic-care hospitals: a systematic review and meta-analysis, *J Am Geriatr Soc* 56(1):29, 2008.

Department of Health and Human Services (DHHS) Office of Inspector General: *Adverse events in hospitals: overview of key issues*, OEI-06-07-00470, Washington, DC, 2008, DHHS.

Ebersole P, et al: *Toward healthy aging: human needs and nursing process*, ed 7, St Louis, 2008, Mosby.

Eliahu SF, et al: I. Status epilepticus, *South Med J* 101(4):400, 2008.

Evans LK, Cotter VT: Avoiding restraints in patients with dementia: understanding, prevention, and management are keys, *Am J Nurs* 108(3):40, 2008.

Futrell M, Melillo KD, Remington R: *Wandering*, Iowa City, Ia, 2008, University of Iowa Gerontological Nursing Interventions Research Center, Research Translation Dissemination Core.

Gano DL: *Apollo root cause analysis-a new way of thinking: comparison of common root cause analysis tools and methods*, 2007, http://www.apollorca.com/_public/site/files/ARCA_Appendix.pdf. Accessed June 15 2012.

Gribbin J, et al: Risk of falls associated with antihypertensive medication: population-based case-control study, *Age Ageing* 39(5):592, 2010.

Halm MA: Hourly Rounds: what does the evidence indicate? *Am J Crit Care* 18:581, 2009.

Hockenberry MJ, Wilson D: *Wong's nursing care of infants and children*, ed 9, St Louis, 2011, Mosby.

Institute for Clinical Systems Improvement (ICSI): *Prevention of falls (acute care)*, revised 2010, available at http://www.guideline.gov/summary/summary.aspx?ss=15&doc_id=13697&nbr=007031&string=patient+AND+falls#s23, accessed through National Guidelines Clearinghouse (NGC) May 2011.

Institute of Medicine (IOM) Committee on Quality of Health Care in America: *To err is human: building a safer health system*, Washington, DC, 2000, National Academies Press.

Khazzani H, et al: The relationship between physical performance measures, bone mineral density, falls, and the risk of peripheral fracture: a cross-sectional analysis, *BMC Public Health* 9:297, 2009.

Knox D, Holloman G: Use and avoidance of seclusion and restraint: consensus statement of the American Association for Emergency Psychiatry Project BETA Seclusion and Restraint Workgroup. *West J Emerg Med* 13(1):36, 2012.

Kojima T, et al: Association of polypharmacy with fall risk among geriatric outpatients, *Geriatr Gerontol Int* 11(4):438, 2011.

Lewis SL, et al: *Medical-surgical nursing: assessment and management of clinical problems*, ed 8, St Louis, 2011, Mosby.

Meiner SE: *Gerontologic nursing*, ed 4, St Louis, 2011, Mosby.

Mion LC: Physical restraint in critical care settings: will they go away? *Geriatric Nurs* 29(6):421, 2008.

NANDA International: *NANDA International: nursing diagnoses, definitions and classification, 2012-2014*, Philadelphia, 2012, NANDA International.

National Association of Psychiatric Health Systems (NAPHS): Restraint and seclusion: implementing the CMS hospital patients' rights conditions of participation final rule, 2007, available at http://www.naphs.org/documents/patientrightsfinalrule_000.ppt, accessed 6/4/2011.

National Institute of Neurological Disorders and Stroke (NINDS): *Seizures and epilepsy: hope through research*, Bethesda, Md, updated 2011, National Institutes of Health, available at http://www.ninds.nih.gov/disorders/epilepsy/detail_epilepsy.htm#188543109, accessed November 22, 2011.

National Quality Forum (NQF): *National Quality Forum Safe Practices for Better Healthcare—2011 Update*, Washington, DC, 2011a, NQF, available at http://www.qualityforum.org/Publications/2011/04/Safe_Practices_for_Better_Healthcare_-_2011_Update.aspx, accessed August 17, 2012.

National Quality Forum (NQF): *National voluntary consensus standards for public reporting of patient safety events*, 2011b, available at http://www.qualityforum.org/Publications/2011/02/National_Voluntary_Consensus_Standards_for_Public_Reporting_of_Patient_Safety_Event_Information.aspx, accessed May 2011.

Nelson AL, Algase DL: *Evidence-based protocols for managing wandering behavior*, New York, 2007, Springer Publishing.

Oliver D, Healey F, Haines TP: Preventing falls and fall-related injuries in hospitals, *Clin Geriatr Med* 26(4):645, 2010.

Opalek JM, Graymire VL, Redd D: Wheelchair falls: 5 years of data from a level I trauma center, *J Trauma Nurs* 16(2):98, 2009.

Quality and Safety Education for Nurses, 2011, available at http://www.qsen.org, accessed November 12, 2011.

Scheffer AC, et al: Fear of falling: measurement strategy, prevalence, risk factors, and consequences among older persons, *Age Aging* 37:19, 2008.

Smith ML, Erwin JA: Final solution via root cause analysis, Six Sigma, available at http://www.isixsigma.com/index.php, accessed November 24, 2011.

The Joint Commission (TJC): The Joint Commission's New Speak Up™ program urges patients to "know your rights," *The Joint Commission News Release* 2007.

The Joint Commission: *Provision of care, treatment, and services: restraint/seclusion for hospitals that use TJC for deemed status purposes*, Chicago, 2009a, TJC.

The Joint Commission (TJC): *A framework for a root cause analysis and action plan in response to a sentinel event*, Sentinel Event Forms and Tools, 2009b, TJC. available at http://www.jointcommission.org/Framework_for_Conducting_a_Root_Cause_Analysis_and_Action_Plan/, accessed November 22, 2011.

The Joint Commission (TJC): *2012 Comprehensive accreditation manual for hospitals: the official handbook*, Oakbrook Terrace, Ill, 2012a, The Commission.

The Joint Commission (TJC): *National Patient Safety Goals*, Oakbrook Terrace, Ill, 2012b, The Commission, available at http://www.jointcommission.org/standards_information/npsgs.aspx.

Tzeng HM: Understanding the prevalence of inpatient falls associated with toileting in adult acute care settings, *J Nurs Care Qual* 25(1):22, 2010.

VA National Center for Patient Safety (VA NCPS): *VHA NCPS escape and elopement management*, 2010, available at http://www4.va.gov/ncps/CogAids/EscapeElope/index.html#page=page-13, accessed May 2011.

Viera ER, Freund-Heritage R, da Costa BR: Risk factors for geriatric patient falls in rehabilitation hospital settings: a systematic review, *Clin Rehabil* 25(9):788, 2011.

Zhani EE: The Joint Commission: Joint Commission Urges Americans to 'Speak Up' to Prevent Falls. *The Joint Commission News Release* 2010.

14

Disaster Preparedness

MEDIA RESOURCES

- **e**volve *learning system* http://evolve.elsevier.com/Perry/skills

  - Review Questions
  - Audio Glossary

KEY TERMS

Biologic agent

Biologic disaster

Bioterrorism/bioterrorist attack

Chemical warfare agent

Decontamination

Department of Homeland Security (DHS)

Detection and surveillance

Disaster response

Epidemic

Field triage tag

First responders

Hazard/hazard identification

Incident Command System (ICS)

International Nursing Coalition for Mass Casualty Education (INCMCE)

Manmade disaster

Mutual aid agreement

Natural disaster

Nuclear event

Pandemic

Shelter-in-place

Strategic national stockpile (SNS)

Triage

Weapons of mass destruction (WMD)

OBJECTIVES

Mastery of content in this chapter will enable the nurse to:

- Describe elements of the Centers for Disease Control and Prevention strategic plan for disasters.
- Discuss the characteristics of different types of disasters.
- Identify actions to take in the event of biologic, chemical, and radiation exposure.
- Discuss guidelines for patient care in the event of a mass casualty incident.
- Describe psychosocial effects of disasters on patients.

Although disaster preparedness and the possibility of terrorist attacks has been a subject of discussion and research for over 20 years, the attacks on the World Trade Center and Pentagon on September 11, 2001, forever changed the reality and sense of security felt by citizens of the United States. They demonstrated the vulnerabilities, including the lack of preparedness of the health care community, in the event of a mass casualty incident (MCI). The attacks increased public awareness of not only probable future terrorist attacks but also the more common natural or environmental disasters affecting individuals on a more regular basis. National preparedness has progressed considerably during the last decade. Hospitals have plans and disaster drills for internal and external disasters (Veenema, 2011). Medical and public health professionals have joined the disaster preparedness community; the U.S. Federal government increased investment in preparedness; and community partners and participants are involved in disaster preparedness (Inglesby, 2011). In addition, The Institute of Medicine (IOM) issued a report, *Guidance for Establishing Crises Standards of Care for Use in Disaster Situations*, designed to assist schools, hospitals, health care and emergency systems, and community agencies in developing policies and protocols for standards of care in disasters, where resources are scarce (IOM, 2009).

Throughout history nurses have played a role in the multidisciplinary approach in preparing for and responding to disasters. Information gathered from post-disaster evaluations have provided a considerable body of knowledge and experience to improve the response of an entire health care team and the many agencies/individuals involved (e.g., police, firefighters, administrators, and paramedics) in a disaster response. The Department of Homeland Security has identified preparedness and education of the nation as an essential component to national security against domestic and foreign threats (DHS, 2008).

DISASTER DEFINED

A disaster is any unexpected event the effect of which leads to significant destruction and/or adverse consequences. More specifically, a disaster is any event in which needs exceed available resources. Box 14-1 provides common disaster terminology definitions. Although these definitions standardize the events of an MCI, it is important to understand that each disaster is unique in the way it affects individuals, families, and communities.

When most Americans hear the term *disaster*, they immediately think terrorist attack. In reality the most common forms of disaster are natural or manmade (e.g., major fires, hurricanes, tornadoes, and floods). If the public is not adequately protected, the spread of natural-borne disease can create a natural disaster.

An **epidemic** is an infectious disease or condition that attacks many people at the same time in the same geographic area. A **pandemic** is an epidemic that occurs in many parts of the world. History tells us that there are approximately three influenza pandemics every 100 years that result in the death of millions of people. Experts believe that the world is due for another pandemic influenza virus to which virtually no one is immune. A pandemic flu is highly contagious from person to person (CDC, 2011a). Surveillance by the World Health Organization continues for such infections as severe acute respiratory syndrome (SARS) and avian influenza (bird flu) for indications of mutations and increased transmission (Boxes 14-2 and 14-3). If a pandemic flu occurs, it will take months for a vaccine to be developed and, once manufactured, doses would first be rationed to persons with a compromised immune system, older adults, and health care workers (CDC, 2011b; WHO 2011a). To be adequately prepared, citizens need education on preventing the spread of influenza (see Chapter 7).

HOMELAND SECURITY

The National Strategy for Homeland Security and the Homeland Security Act (HSA) of 2002 were enacted to secure the homeland from terrorist attack. Since the development of the HSA, the Department of Homeland Security (DHS) has evolved and strengthened their mission, vision, and core values to provide a unifying core as the basis for efforts to prevent and discourage terrorist attacks. This governmental agency coordinates the efforts of multiple organizations to secure and maintain the safety of the United States.

BOX 14-1 | Disaster Definitions and Types

- **Disaster:** A catastrophic and/or destructive event that disrupts normal functioning; it may include any anticipated or unexpected event, the effects of which lead to significant destruction and/or adverse consequences
- **Mass casualty incident or event (MCI):** Any event or situation that results in multiple casualties and/or deaths; an MCI exists when health care needs exceed health care resources
- **All-hazards event:** Multiple manmade or natural events with destructive capacity to cause multiple casualties
- **All-hazards preparedness:** The comprehensive preparedness necessary to manage casualties resulting from a disaster, regardless of etiology
- **Casualty:** Any individual who is ill, injured, missing, or killed as a result of an MCI
- **Medical disasters:** Catastrophic events that result in human casualties that overwhelm the available health care resources
- **Natural/environmental disasters:** Catastrophic events that result from an ecologic event that exceeds the capacity of the community (e.g., the impact of hurricanes or tornados on a community)
- **Manmade disasters:** Catastrophic events the principal direct cause of which is attributable to human action
- **Technologic disasters:** Catastrophic events in which people, property, community infrastructure, and economic welfare are adversely affected by the disruption of technology (e.g., industrial accidents, unplanned release of nuclear waste)

BOX 14-2 | Severe Acute Respiratory Syndrome (SARS)

- A viral respiratory illness caused by a coronavirus (SARS-CoV).
- Spread by close person-to-person contact through respiratory droplets. Strict adherence to contact and droplet precautions, along with eye protection, seems to prevent SARS-CoV transmission in most instances.
- In 2003 8098 people worldwide became sick with SARS; of these 774 died.
- Onset of a high fever; other symptoms include headache and body aches.
- About 10% to 20% have diarrhea. After 2 to 7 days SARS patients may develop a dry cough.
- Most SARS patients develop pneumonia.
- Treatment may consist of various therapies, including antibiotics, antivirals, corticosteroids, alternative medicine (i.e., glycyrrhizin), and assisted ventilation.
- Research for vaccine development is ongoing.

Data from Centers for Disease Control and Prevention: *Severe, acute respiratory syndrome (SARS)*, 2011, available at http://www.cdc.gov/sars/index.html, accessed February 12, 2012.

BOX 14-3 | Avian Influenza ("Bird Flu")

- It is an infectious disease of birds that is highly contagious among poultry; it has also been documented in pigs, tigers, leopards, ferrets, domestic cats, and the stone marten (a weasel-like animal).
- More than 200 cases among humans have been reported worldwide; approximately half of the people reported as infected have died.
- It is believed to be transmitted primarily through close contact with live or dead diseased birds or contaminated surfaces; person-to-person transmission is rare. No evidence of disease is spread through poorly cooked food.
- Incubation period is 2 to 8 days, possibly as long as 17 days.
- Initial symptoms include a high fever and flulike symptoms (i.e., fever, cough, sore throat, and muscle aches). Watery diarrhea and vomiting have also been reported as early symptoms. Eye infection (conjunctivitis) and pneumonia may occur. Clinical deterioration is rapid, with respiratory distress and multi-organ dysfunction.
- Antiviral drugs (e.g., oseltamivir phosphate [Tamiflu]) can improve survival when administered within 48 hours of symptom onset.
- On April 17, 2007 the U.S. Food and Drug Administration announced approval of a vaccine against one strain of the avian flu H5N1 virus. The vaccine has been purchased by the federal government and is being held in the strategic national stockpile. Research continues for vaccines against other strains of the H5N1 virus.
- Concern is that the virus could start a pandemic; however, currently the virus does not spread easily from person to person and is not sustainable among humans.

Data from World Health Organization (WHO): *Avian influenza fact sheet*, 2011, available at http://www.who.int/mediacentre/factsheets/avian_influenza/en/, February 12, 2012.

Terrorism Preparedness

In addition to the activities of the DHS, the Centers for Disease Control and Prevention (CDC) is a leading federal agency designed to protect the health and safety of people at home and abroad. The mission of the CDC Coordinating Office for Terrorism Preparedness and Emergency Response (COTPER) is to protect the health and life of all people related to community emergency preparedness and response (CDC, 2009). The CDC strategic plan in the event of a disaster first focuses on preparedness, which is key to the impact that any disaster has on the individuals or communities involved. Preparedness requires that nurses have a basic understanding of the science of a disaster and an understanding of the key components of any plan to deal with an MCI (CDC, 2010a,b).

In the event of a biologic, chemical, or radiation attack, the CDC strategic plan includes the following:

- *Preparedness and prevention*: The comprehensive preparedness required to manage self, family, and/or the community when an event occurs that is likely to result from a catastrophic and or destructive event that disrupts normal functioning
- *Detection and surveillance*: Awareness of the environment, recognizing what is unusual or different and knowing what these differences possibly mean for purpose of mitigation or prevention (DHS, 2011a)
- *Diagnosis and characterization of biologic, chemical, and radiologic agents*: The ability of an individual to recognize or identify clusters of data indicating that a biologic, chemical, or radiologic MCI event has occurred
- *Response*: The systematic, coordinated, and effective delivery of services when disaster strikes
- *Communication*: The establishment of protocols and standing orders in the event of a disaster to successfully manage health care and use the media for communicating information to the public (e.g., directions to treatment facilities, evacuation routes) (Traditional modes of communication will likely be interrupted in the event of an MCI; therefore part of disaster preparedness involves backup plans for maintaining public and intraagency/interagency communication [e.g., use of two-way radios and satellite phones].)

Although the CDC plan is for mass casualty disaster events or community-wide incidents, the plan clearly applies to any disaster event. The CDC and the American Red Cross advocate preparedness and coordination of prompt, effective emergency efforts. This preparedness coordination includes outreach to other agencies or groups through mutual aid agreements. These agreements might include the willingness of one agency to provide shelter (e.g., a church, school, or recreation center) and other agencies to provide clothing (e.g., department stores, the Salvation Army, or Goodwill). Some agreements might include identifying and caring for the deceased (e.g., funeral homes); still other agencies agree to provide vehicular support in the time of a disaster. Disaster planning is not only a multidisciplinary task but also a multiagency task. Although the average citizen, government agency, and other health care workers play a vital role in disaster preparedness, nurses will always have unique responsibilities within this multidisciplinary and multiagency coalition.

Disaster Preparedness

To further support the need for health care providers to increase their preparedness, some states are enacting new laws that require disaster training as part of the continuing education requirement for licensure. However, only disaster planning, education, training, and drills on a local, national, and global level will effectively prepare health care providers, volunteers, and other individuals needed in the event of an MCI. Nurses need to influence, develop, and practice policies that will improve the safety and quality of health care at the time of an MCI (USDHHS, 2010).

It is essential that, in addition to the preparation of government officials and first responders for disasters, the public must also be aware of and prepared for them. To facilitate public awareness of disasters the DHS established The National Terrorism Advisory System (NTAS) to provide government officials, first responders, and public citizens with information regarding the nature and degree of terrorist threat (Fig. 14-1) (DHS, 2011b).

The D-I-S-A-S-T-E-R Paradigm

A series of National Disaster Life Support (NDLS) courses provide coordinated training with an all-hazards approach to MCIs (AMA, 2011). The D-I-S-A-S-T-E-R model put forth in the training program standardizes methods for recognizing a disaster, managing the scene, and providing care to disaster victims.

Detection

Detection is the first goal in an MCI and includes (a) determining the presence of an MCI or public health emergency (PHE), (b) recognizing the cause of the incident, and (c) becoming aware of the environment or more specifically changes in the environment (e.g., an unusual pattern of patient presentation, unusual smells, or suspicious individuals). Although many events have a clear cause,

Alert Is Issued	
Elevated Threat Alert Warns of a credible terrorist threat against the United States	**Imminent Threat Alert** Warns of a credible, specific, and impending terrorist threat against the United States

Information Included in Alert		
Summary	Details, including affected areas	Duration of alert
How you can help	Steps to stay prepared	How to stay informed

Sunset Provision
An individual threat alert is issued for a specific time period and then automatically expires. It may be extended if new information becomes available or the threat evolves.

FIG 14-1 National Terrorism Advisory System overview. (*Department of Homeland Security—Adapted from data available at http://www.dhs.gov/xlibrary/assets/ntas/ntas-public-guide.pdf.*)

others have an insidious onset. For example, if a large number of otherwise healthy young adults start showing up in an emergency department (ED) with similar but unexplained symptoms, nurses and other health care providers should suspect that something is not right. Detection is sometimes simply the awareness of an unusual health care situation.

Remember, to be able to provide care, you first need to ensure personal safety. It is essential that rescue and health care workers avoid becoming victims, which may go against your initial instinct to help others. When the scene of a disaster is in a clearly designated area outside the health care agency, you need to determine the security of the scene. Always consider external scenes of disasters such as sites of explosions or severe storm damage unsafe until trained professionals arrive and determine that the scene is safe.

The use of biologic agents is a considerable terrorist threat because they are easy to disperse and affect large numbers of people at a relatively low cost (Box 14-4). Incubation periods and common initial clinical symptoms make detection of a biologic attack difficult.

Another form of MCI is the dissemination, or spreading, of a toxic chemical agent. There are a number of methods for spreading toxic chemical agents (e.g., fire or explosion). Health care providers are often at risk for becoming secondary victims when chemical agents create an MCI. Chemical agents are categorized based on their mechanism of injury (CDC, 2006a). These include pulmonary agents, blistering agents, blood agents, and nerve agents.

The thought of nuclear and radiologic incidents creates considerable fear for many individuals. Most often the cause for disseminating radioactive material is generally known. A fire or an explosion is often associated with nuclear attacks; however, devices designed to disseminate radioactive material are not always obvious (e.g., a "dirty bomb"). The effects of nuclear and radiologic events depend on the amount of radiation exposure. Most victims will have delayed onset of symptoms (including nausea, vomiting, and diarrhea), but some will have obvious burns. Generally the sooner symptoms appear, the greater the exposure to radioactive material.

Incident Command

Incident command is the need for the emergency system to be activated when a threat or hazard is suspected. For most individuals this means activating the 9-1-1 system so emergency responders can be brought in to assume command. Emergency responders initially remain outside the possible contaminated area. Therefore the impact of the disaster on roads, traffic, and availability of resources can delay or prevent their arrival. An Incident Command System (ICS), also referred to as an incident management system (IMS), provides a standard approach to managing emergencies when multiple agencies are involved. ICSs are used by all forms of government and the private sector during an emergency situation and help guide five major functions: (1) command, (2) operations, (3) planning, (4) logistics, and (5) finance/administration (DHS, 2011c). Fig. 14-2 offers an example of a general chain of command in an MCI.

Scene Security and Safety

Nurses are not responsible for determining the security and safety of a disaster scene. This task is the responsibility of trained emergency personnel (e.g., firefighters and police). When a health care agency is the scene of the disaster or a secondary site for a disaster, trained personnel determine scene security and safety. A health care agency becomes a secondary disaster site when contaminated by the agent from the original disaster scene. For example, a patient has been exposed to mustard gas, an oily chemical that is difficult to remove from a patient's body. If not properly decontaminated, the victim contaminated by the mustard gas will inadvertently contaminate health care providers and others (CDC, 2010a). The same is true for many biologic agents. The first priority at any disaster scene is to protect yourself and other team members. The second priority is to protect the public, patients, and the environment (Box 14-5).

Knowing which personal protective equipment (PPE) to use minimizes the risk for contact with contaminated materials or individuals. Proper use of many advanced forms of PPE requires training, fitting, and an understanding that not all PPE protects against all potential hazards. When used inappropriately, PPE becomes a hazard (e.g., dehydration, decreased vision, mobility,

---

BOX 14-4	Potential Organisms for Bioterrorism by CDC Category

Category A—Greatest Threat
- Can be easily disseminated or transmitted person to person
- Cause high mortality with a potential for major public health impact, including:
  Anthrax (*Bacillus anthracis*)
  Botulism (*Clostridium botulinum* toxin)
  Plague (*Yersinia pestis*)
  Smallpox (variola major)
  Viral hemorrhagic fevers (Ebola, Marburg, Lassa, Machupo)

Category B—High Risk
- Moderately easy to disseminate
- Cause moderate morbidity and low mortality, including:
  - Brucellosis (*Brucella* species)
  - Epsilon toxin of *Clostridium perfringens*
  - Food safety threats (e.g., *Salmonella, Escherichia coli, Shigella*)
  - Ricin toxin from *Ricinus communis* (castor beans)
  - Staphylococcal enterotoxin B
  - Water safety threats (e.g., *Vibrio cholerae, Cryptosporidium parvum*)

Category C—Emerging Biologic Weapons for Terrorist Use
- Pathogens that could be engineered for mass dissemination, including:
  Nipah virus
  Hantavirus

BOX 14-5	The Do's and Don'ts of Scene Safety and Security

DO	DON'T
• Stay out of a disaster scene unless well trained and invited. • Call 9-1-1.	• Don't enter the scene unless invited. • Don't needlessly disturb the scene; important evidence could be lost or contaminated by an eager but untrained helper. • Don't interfere with the services of other emergency personnel when uninvited or untrained. • Don't open suspicious packages.

HOSPITAL EMERGENCY INCIDENT COMMAND SYSTEM

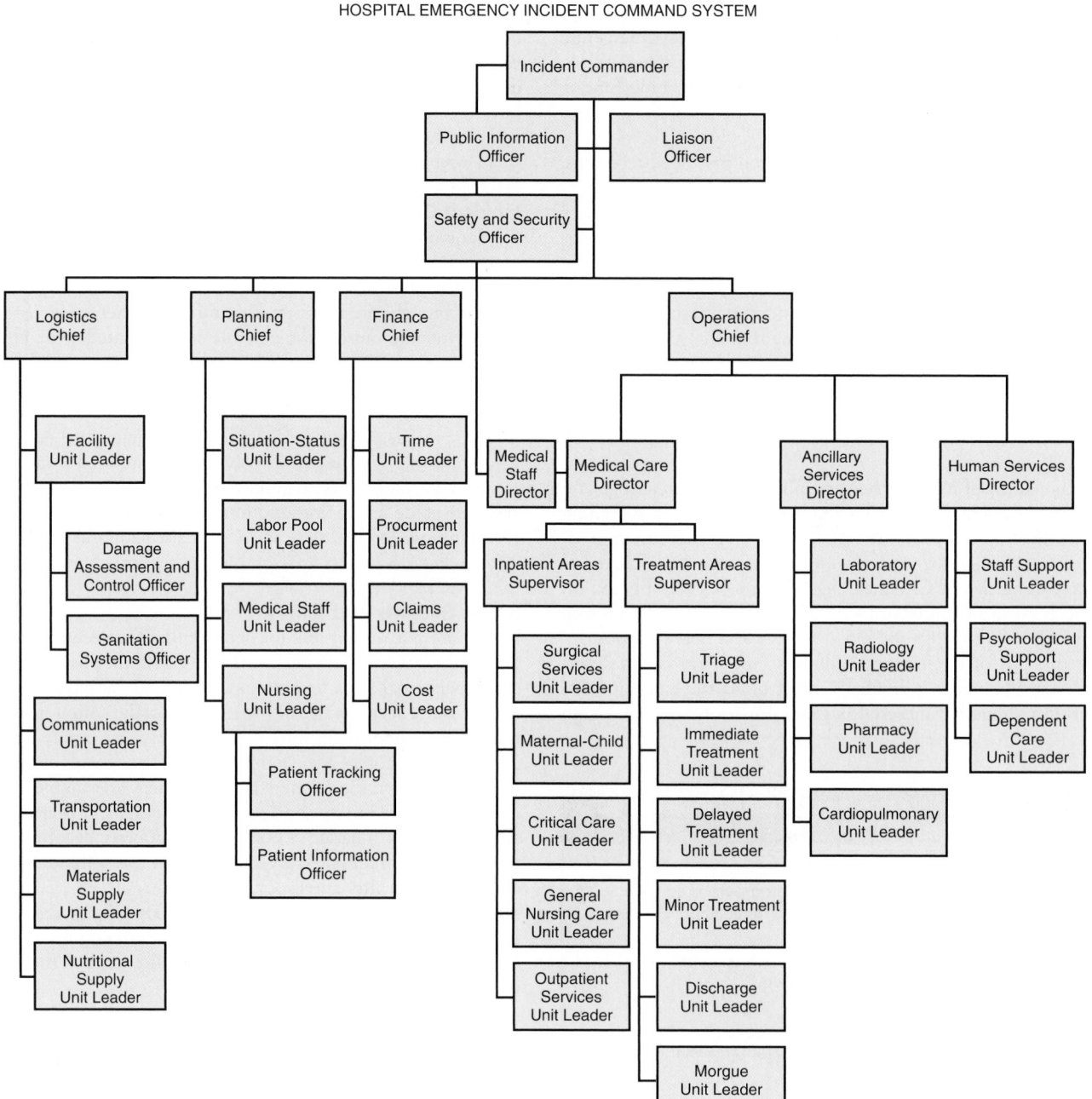

FIG 14-2 The Hospital Emergency Incident Command System prepares all response teams to work smoothly in a disaster situation.

and ability to communicate). Some of these hazards result because, while using advanced forms of PPE, the user is unable to eat, drink, or go to the bathroom.

PPEs are categorized by levels A to D for the level of safety provided. Level A is selected when the greatest level of skin, respiratory, and eye protection is required. It provides maximum protection because it offers a self-contained breathing apparatus, total encapsulating chemical-protective suit, coveralls, undergarments, chemical-resistant boots and gloves, hard hat, and disposable protective suit worn over the encapsulating suit (Fig. 14-3). Highly trained personnel use level A protection in heavily contaminated areas. If you are not wearing this type of protection and you are near an area where level A PPE is being used, the general rule is to get out or do not enter. Level B provides the highest level of

respiratory protection but less skin protection. Used by trained responders, this PPE includes a self-contained breathing apparatus; hooded chemical-resistant suit; and face, boot, and glove protection. Level B protection also requires training and fitting. First responders (emergency personnel first on the scene) and hospital personnel are trained and fitted to use level C protection, which involves knowing the concentration and type of airborne substance(s) and the criteria for using air-purifying respirators. Level C constitutes the use of full-face or half-mask, air-purifying respirators (National Institute for Occupational Safety and Health [NIOSH] approved), hooded chemical resistant clothing, and protective gloves and boots. Because of the garment protection worn with levels A, B and C, the user is at risk for dehydration and hyperthermia.

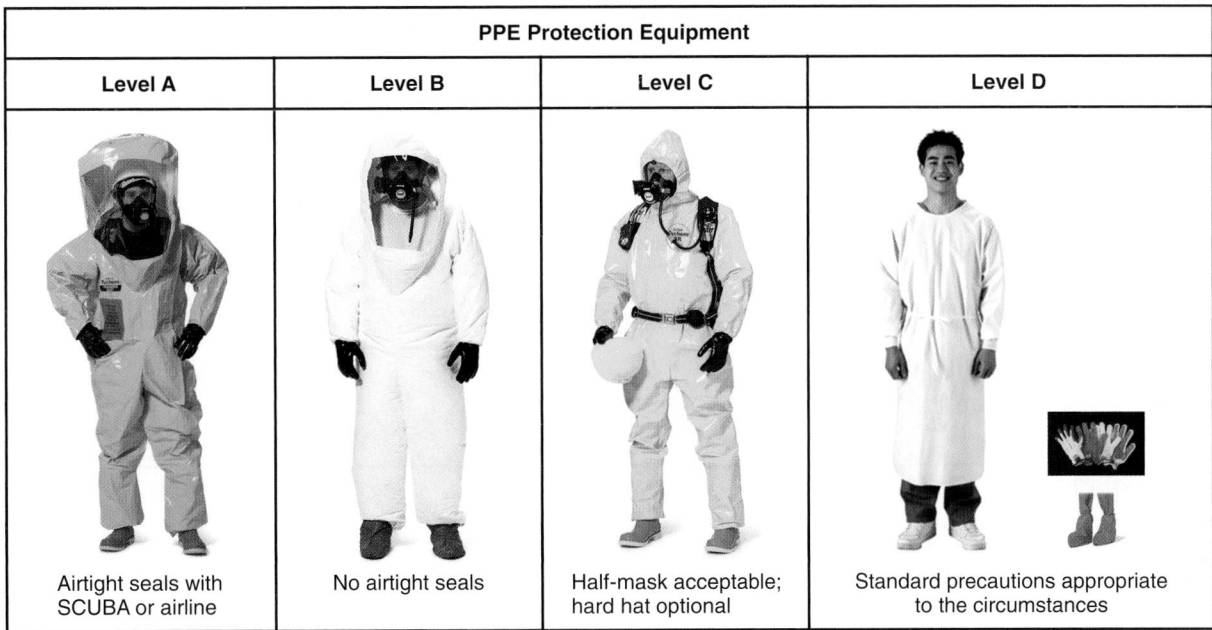

PPE Protection Equipment			
Level A	Level B	Level C	Level D
Airtight seals with SCUBA or airline	No airtight seals	Half-mask acceptable; hard hat optional	Standard precautions appropriate to the circumstances

FIG 14-3 The Occupational Safety and Health Administration (OSHA) defines personal protective equipment for the four levels of hazardous exposure. *PPE*, Personal protective equipment; *SCUBA*, self-contained underwater breathing apparatus.

For level D protection standard work uniform or work clothes are appropriate and used for nuisance contamination only. The users must wear coveralls and chemical resistant shoes; and, depending on the contaminant, gloves, goggles, mask, face shield, and hard hats may also be worn. There is no respiratory protection. It is important to take standard precautions when using level D protection. Depending on the circumstances, some health care providers also choose to use a fluid-impermeable gown, cap, eye protection, mask, gloves, and shoe covers (OSHA, 2011).

The most recently labeled level of protection is BioPPE. BioPPE requires the use of standard work clothes along with contact and respiratory protection. Double gloving and an N95 mask (see Chapter 7) or better respirator are recommended. Hand hygiene that includes washing with soap and water followed by use of an alcohol gel is important not only at this level but also at all other levels. BioPPE protection is not adequate when caring for patients exposed to toxic chemicals; however, it provides adequate protection against radiologic and biologic agents.

Assessment

Assessing hazards is more important than knowing the exact cause of a disaster. By allowing trained individuals to assess a disaster scene, you will avoid becoming a victim. Health care providers and volunteers need to learn to shift thinking and realize that the MCI can result in secondary hazards that come in many forms (Box 14-6).

Support

In terms of a disaster, *support* means, "Give me what I need to get the job done." The earlier you ask for support, the better. Support varies with the situation and task at hand. Support resources necessary during a disaster include human resources, agencies, facilities, supplies, and vehicles. For example, although there are not enough hospitals to accommodate all victims, a school or recreation center could easily be turned into a makeshift hospital if there has been preparation for unforeseen disasters.

BOX 14-6 | Potential Hazards at the Scene of a Disaster

- Downed power lines
- Smoke/toxic gases
- Debris that can result in trauma
- Fractured/leaking gas lines
- Fire resulting in burns
- Structural collapse
- Blood and other body fluids
- Inclement weather
- Hazardous materials
- Nuclear, biologic, or chemical exposure
- Flooding and the threat of drowning
- Radiation exposure
- Explosion, particularly secondary explosions
- Snipers
- Darkness
- Infection
- High-velocity projectiles and the pressure wave after an explosion
- Becoming incapacitated and unable to protect yourself or your patient

---

The CDC has developed a strategic national stockpile (SNS) that contains large amounts of medical equipment in the event of a disaster (CDC, 2011c). Most local communities will be prepared to provide essential resources for up to 72 hours (via hospitals, pharmacies) to support local needs. Once local and federal authorities confirm the need for the SNS and on request of the governor's office of the affected state, the 12-hour push package is flown or transported within 12 hours to any state in the United States. The 12-hour push package contains approximately 100 steel containers that hold pharmaceuticals (prepackaged 10-day supplies of antibiotics, antidotes, narcotics, epinephrine, albuterol, prednisone, and other medications), intravenous (IV) fluids and IV supplies,

BOX 14-7	ID-ME—Assess, Treat, and Send			
IMMEDIATE (RED)	**DELAYED (YELLOW)**	**MINIMAL (GREEN)**	**EXPECTANT (BLACK)**
• Unconscious or unresponsive • Altered mental status • Experiencing hypoxia or near-hypoxia • Chest pain • Chest wounds • Full-thickness burns over 20% to 60% of the body • Uncontrollable bleeding • Amputations above elbow or knee • Rapid or weak pulse • Open abdominal wounds	• Deep lacerations • Open fractures with controlled bleeding and strong pulses • Multiple fractures • Finger amputations • Abdominal injuries with stable vital signs • Closed head injuries without altered level of consciousness	• Abrasions • Contusions • Sprains • Minor lacerations • No apparent injuries • Other injuries of similar severity	• Victims still alive but so severely injured as to have little chance of survival • Victims who have died

ID-ME, Immediate, delayed, minimal, expectant.

ventilators, suction equipment, airway supplies, tablet-counting machines, and other emergency provisions (CDC, 2011c).

Chaos is common in every disaster. It is manageable, but it is difficult to control. In the event of a disaster many "worried well" (injured individuals who are able to transport themselves to a health care agency or even frightened individuals who fear contamination) will leave a disaster scene. Within 30 minutes these individuals will overrun the hospital nearest the disaster scene, leaving the most highly injured individuals at the site of the disaster. Adding to the chaos at the health care agency is the responsibility to care for sick and injured individuals already admitted to the hospital or ED.

First responders must quickly distinguish between actual victims with exposure to the weapon of mass destruction (chemical, biologic, or nuclear) that led to the MCI and the worried well. Regardless of the lethality of any biologic, nuclear, or chemical terrorist attack, the "shock" to the community and society often serves the intended purpose of the terrorist. You need to recognize the worried well as victims because they are obviously suffering fear and anxiety. However, do not let them distract you from the job of rescuing as many potential survivors as possible. Quickly differentiating worried well from actual injured patients prevents wasting valuable time.

Also consider the security of a health care agency in disaster planning. Health care providers offer a valuable resource and cannot spend time maintaining the security of the health care agency. The local police in collaboration with agency administration and security personnel are responsible to maximize the protection of lives and assets of the health care agency. Keep security officers informed about the incident history, current status, and potential problems. As part of this protection, roadblocks, checkpoints, and agency lockdown procedures are often put in place.

Triage, Treat, and Evacuate

Triage is the sorting of individuals by the seriousness of their condition and the likelihood of their survival (Box 14-7). There are many different modern triage systems to classify, tag, and treat victims of MCI. These systems use a variety of symbols, colors, and other devices to classify individuals as to the need for treatment. Mass casualty triage is an initial sorting of victims into groups. The disaster triage model described in this section is the SALT (Sort-Assess-Lifesaving Interventions-Triage/Treatment) triage system.

The SALT triage system was developed by a workgroup of emergency medical services (EMS) physicians who were funded by the CDC and tasked with reviewing current triage systems and making recommendations for a national standard (Lerner et al, 2011). The group could not find a model that had enough research evidence or all the elements of a system that they deemed necessary to recommend as a national standard. They developed the SALT triage system instead, using the best features of several widely accepted models. All victims are first sorted into groups based on mobility. They are then individually assessed, sorted into categories, and evacuated for treatment as needed (Fig. 14-4). The ultimate goal is to sort, assess, and perform lifesaving measures as quickly as possible to large numbers of victims.

At a disaster, Step One in the SALT triage model is to "sort" individuals into one of three categories before they are assessed individually. Category one consists of persons who are not moving and have obvious life-threatening injuries. Category two consists of persons who can wave or have purposeful movements. Category three consists of persons who can walk. Step Two of the SALT triage system involves individual assessment and further sorting of patients into categories. These categories include (1) those minimally injured, (2) people who will survive even with delayed treatment, (3) those who need immediate intervention, and (4) people expected to die. Lifesaving interventions will be administered according to which category the person is labeled. Step Three involves treatment and/or transport of victims. As with any emergency, reassessment is always necessary. During reassessment rescue workers need to consider patient conditions, resources, and scene safety.

EVIDENCE-BASED PRACTICE

When disaster strikes, unexpected problems may occur. Because there are many types of disasters, the American Nurses Association recommends that nurses need to know their disasters because the type of disaster has a direct impact on nursing actions (ANA, 2010). When the first plane hit the World Trade Center in 2001, calls overwhelmed hospital telephone systems. After the Madrid, Spain terrorist bombing in 2004, the CDC developed a disaster plan for nursing care. Working with the assumption that aid will not come for at least 72 hours, the plan was designed to treat 300 injured patients for up to 72 hours (CDC, 2010b). This plan includes the following recommended actions:

- Be able to rapidly increase nursing staff.
- Maintain a list of employees with their proximity to the hospital.

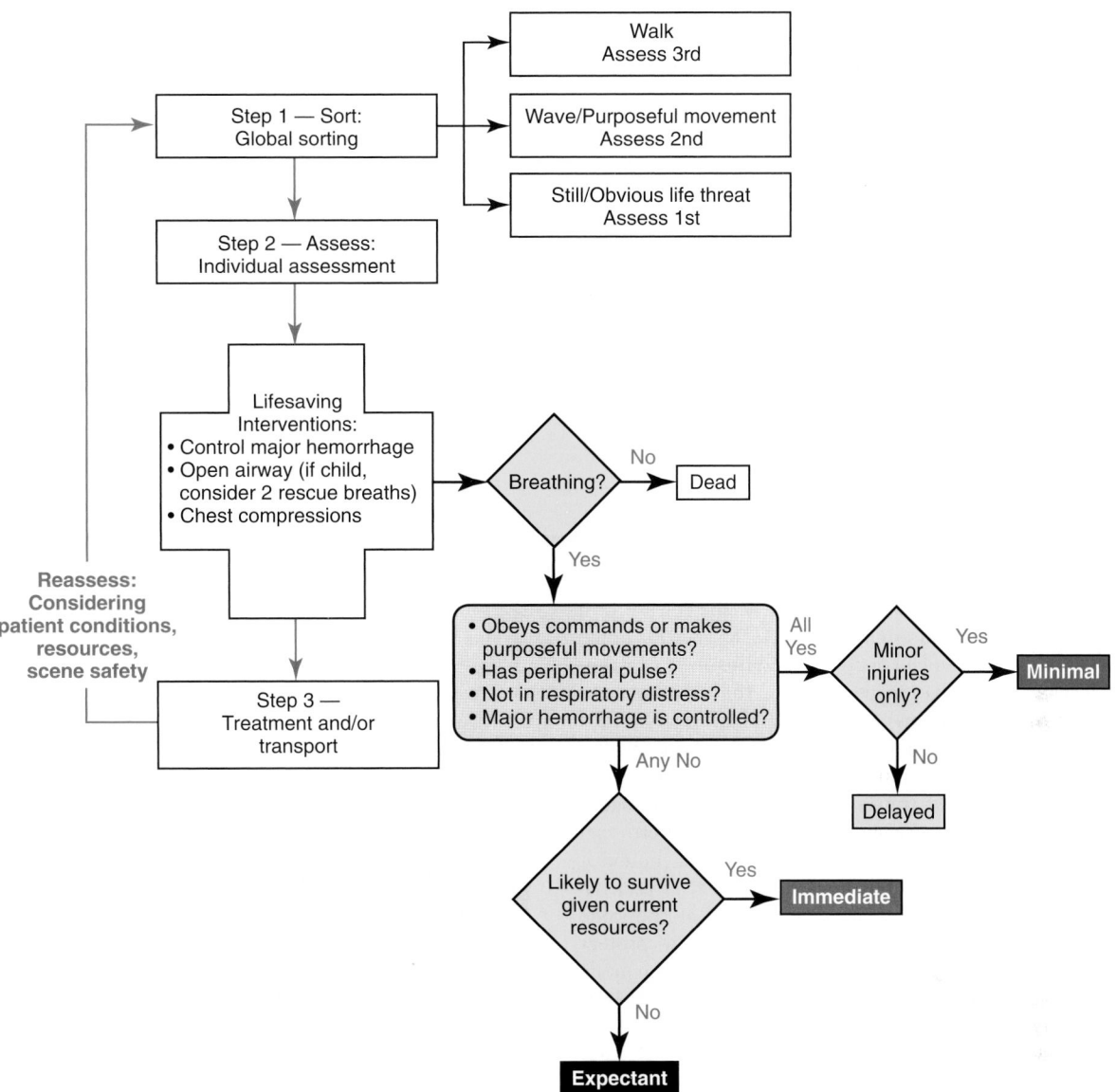

FIG 14-4   SALT Mass casualty triage algorithm (Sort, Assess, Lifesaving interventions, Treatment/ transport). (*US Department of Health and Human Services: Adapted from Lerner EB et al: Mass casualty triage: an evaluation of the science and refinement of a national guideline,* Disaster Med Public Health Prep 5(2):129, 2011.)

- Consider using a rapid response model for accessing nursing staff.
- Have protocols in place for tiered staffing.
- Have just-in-time nursing training about bomb blast injuries and treating pediatric bomb injuries available. Have a plan to deploy pediatric nurses quickly.
- Provide nurse training for the rapid influx and treatment of patients (Tillman, 2011).
- Implement rapid discharge procedures.
- Maintain a centralized database with staff competencies (Strangeland, 2010).
- Have a plan for hospitals to implement a drill with EMS at least once a year to prepare for an MCI.
- Quickly critique and share the information with participants.

Many lessons have been learned from previous disasters, and failure of communication systems is identified as a major issue. Communication is essential, and preparing for interruptions during disasters is recommended by both the Federal Emergency Management Agency (FEMA) and the Federal Communications Commission (FCC, 2011). Other lessons learned include the following:

- When it becomes necessary to evacuate patients, the Agency for Healthcare Research and Quality (AHRQ) recommends that a discharge summary go with the patient. The discharge summary should include current medications, allergies, current orders, and a brief history (USDHHS, 2010).
- Some staff had difficulty passing through roadblocks in previous disasters; thus it is now recommended that all staff keep their hospital identification with them.
- The need for diversional activities to reduce stress deserves important consideration. Staff could share items such as musical instruments or a DVD player and movies.

PATIENT-CENTERED CARE

To provide the highest standard of care while in a disaster situation it is essential to acknowledge the cultural diversity of all individuals involved. A lack of cultural considerations of victims leads to the impression of insensitivity and biases toward patients who are different racially, sexually, or ethnically. Regardless of cultural differences and perhaps language difficulties, it is important to convey compassion and work closely with people within the community for disaster recovery. As noted with bereavement counseling, existing support networks are often more effective. Emergency responders need to support rather than further disrupt these networks (Mendez, 2010). Some disaster events result in a changed culture for individuals, families, and communities.

Safety Guidelines

When considering all forms of disaster, there are basic safety guidelines for a nurse or other health care provider to follow:
1 Rapid response is crucial. Know your agency policies for disaster response and the specific role that each member must perform.
2 Health care providers are responsible for ensuring that the contaminated, the injured, and those concerned about potential exposure to a hazardous agent are medically treated in an efficient manner.
3 The potential for public alarm and major disruption of everyday life is enormous because of widespread fear of the unknown. Know crisis intervention and stress-management techniques.
4 A health care agency such as a hospital is part of a community. Hospitals and other agencies need to work with their communities in developing and instituting plans for notification and communication.
5 In an MCI the majority of people, whether contaminated, exposed, or not, will self-triage and go directly to a local hospital, bypassing triage and treatment. Plans are needed to transfer patients to other medical facilities.

SKILL 14-1   Care of a Patient After Biologic Exposure

Bioterrorism or a biologic attack is the result of the release of a biologic agent into a specified environment (CDC, 2007). Some biologic attacks are unannounced or covert, and the onset of symptoms is delayed by an incubation period (i.e., the time between exposure and onset of symptoms). Differing biologic agents have incubation periods from 1 or 2 days to several weeks, during which some of these agents may be transmitted as an infected patient exposes others. The mode of transmission of the biologic agent determines the severity of the disaster. Recognition of bioterrorism is a challenge because early signs and symptoms mimic the flu or produce a rash mistaken for a viral illness (Fig. 14-5, A and B). Sometimes several biologic agents are disseminated at the same time, further confusing the issue. To understand how to protect yourself from becoming a victim, you need to understand the mode of transmission and precautions to take for biosafety (Table 14-1).

Delegation and Collaboration

The skill of assessment of a patient exposed to a biologic agent cannot be delegated to nursing assistive personnel (NAP). The nurse directs the NAP to:
- Use appropriate personal equipment (PPE) to prevent exposure during care activities.
- Use proper techniques for handling a body after death to prevent contamination.

Equipment

Choice of equipment depends on the route of transmission of the infecting agent. The following is a general list of supplies needed in the event of release of the most contagious biologic agents. Not all equipment is needed in all situations.
- ❏ Biohazard bags with label
- ❏ Soap and water
- ❏ 0.5% diluted bleach or Environmental Protection Agency (EPA)–approved germicidal agent
- ❏ Negative-pressure room (high-efficiency particulate air [HEPA] filtration may be required) with anteroom
- ❏ Clean gloves
- ❏ Gown
- ❏ Shoe covers
- ❏ Head covers
- ❏ Mask
- ❏ Standard face mask
- ❏ N95 mask
- ❏ Face shield
- ❏ Equipment for physical examination
- ❏ Oxygen therapy
- ❏ Airway maintenance supplies
- ❏ Intravenous therapy supplies

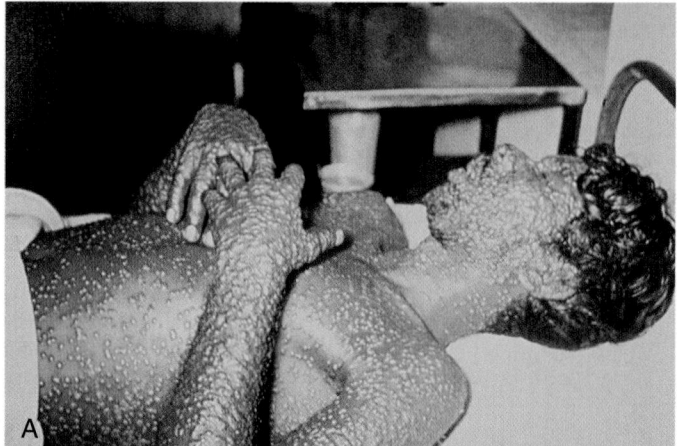
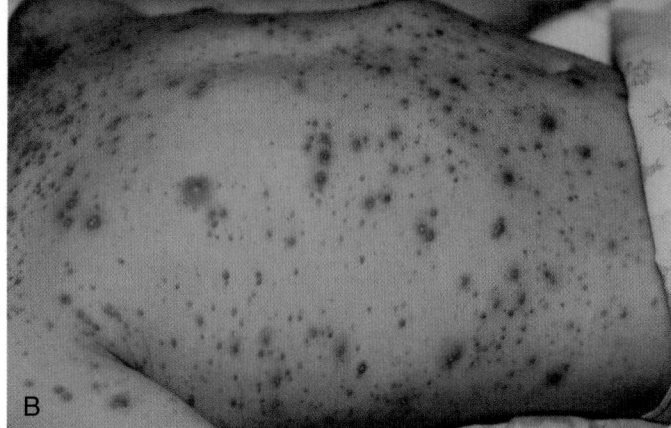

FIG 14-5   Differences in distribution of smallpox versus chickenpox. **A,** Man with smallpox. *Courtesy CDC/NIP/Barbara Rice.* **B,** Chickenpox covering patient torso. *Courtesy David Effron, MD.*

| TABLE 14-1 | Summary of Selected Class A Biologic Warfare Agents |

Disease/Infectious Agent	Form and Incubation/Onset of Symptoms	Untreated Course of Disease		Probable Route of Contamination for Use as a Biologic Warfare Agent	Treatment of Mass Casualties	Prophylaxis/Vaccine
		Early-Onset Symptoms	Late-Onset Symptoms			
Bacterial Biologic Agents						
Anthrax *Bacillus anthracis*, a gram-positive bacillus that can remain stable in spore form	Inhalation or pulmonary (usually within 48 hours but may incubate for up to 60 days)	Febrile flulike symptoms (malaise, low-grade fever, dry cough, and headache)	Severe respiratory distress, hemodynamic failure, and death	Aerosol; no person-to-person transmission	Ciprofloxacin or doxycycline	Ciprofloxacin (Cipro) or, if susceptible, doxycycline; vaccine available but in short supply
	Cutaneous (1-12 days)	Local urticaria; painless papular lesions usually located on head, forearms, or hands	Papular lesions become vesicular, later developing black eschar and edema	Person-to-person transmission with direct contact with skin lesions		
	Gastrointestinal (1-7 days)	Abdominal pain, nausea, vomiting, and diarrhea	Gastrointestinal bleeding, fever; usually followed by toxic sepsis and death	Contaminated food and/or water		
Plague Acute, severe bacterial infection secondary to a gram-negative bacillus, *Yersinia pestis*	Bubonic Onset of symptoms dependent on route of transmission (1-6 days)	Swollen, tender lymph nodes (most notable femoral and inguinal), high fever, rapid pulse	Hypotension, extreme exhaustion, death	Aerosol and then human-to-human by droplet inhalation	Ciprofloxacin or doxycycline	Ciprofloxacin or doxycycline; no vaccine available at the present time
	Pneumonic (1-6 days)	High fever, chills, tachycardia, headache	Fulminate pneumonia (foamy hemoptysis, tachypnea, and dyspnea), sepsis, and death			
Botulism Anaerobic gram-positive bacillus that produces a potent muscle-paralyzing neurotoxin	Foodborne (12-36 hours)	Nausea, vomiting, diarrhea	Symmetric cranial nerve paralysis, descending flaccid paralysis (progressive paralysis of arms, respiratory muscles, and legs), and death	Contaminated food	Passive immunization (antitoxin); supportive care	Passive immunization (antitoxin); antitoxin available in short supply
	Inhalational (2 hours–8 days)	No fever, no changes in mental status	Symmetric cranial nerve paralysis, descending flaccid paralysis (progressive paralysis of arms, respiratory muscles, and legs), and death	Inhalation of aerosolized toxin		

Continued

TABLE 14-1	Summary of Selected Class A Biologic Warfare Agents—cont'd

Disease/Infectious Agent	Form and Incubation/Onset of Symptoms	Untreated Course of Disease		Probable Route of Contamination for Use as a Biologic Warfare Agent	Treatment of Mass Casualties	Prophylaxis/Vaccine
		Early-Onset Symptoms	Late-Onset Symptoms			
Typhoidal tularemia *Francisella tularensis*, an extremely infectious bacteria	Contaminated water or food or via aerosol distribution (1-14 days)	Flulike symptoms (headache, cough, fever and chills, malaise)	Pharyngeal ulcers, pleuritic chest pain, pneumonia, pericarditis, respiratory failure, sepsis, and death	Inhalation of aerosolized bacteria	Ciprofloxacin or doxycycline	Ciprofloxacin or doxycycline; vaccine available, only limited supply; vaccine offers incomplete protection
Major Viral Biological Agent of Concern—Smallpox						
Smallpox variola virus	Distribution via airborne droplets, aerosols, and fomites (7-17 days; weaponized smallpox when delivered aerosolized has an incubation period of only 3-5 days)	Acute viral symptoms (high fever, myalgia, headache, and backache)	Continued viral symptoms, high fever, prostration, synchronous onset of rash progressing from macules to papules to vesicles, and eschar formation Vesicles more abundant on extremities and face, and all develop at the same time; pustules appear on palms of hands and soles of feet (unlike chickenpox)	Transmitted person to person by large droplets; therefore spread may be by inhalation of aerosolized virus, oral secretions, infected human vector exposure, or exposure to contaminated objects	Supportive therapy only (ventilator)	None; vaccine available in short supply

STEP	RATIONALE

ASSESSMENT

1 Perform hand hygiene. Don proper personal protective equipment (PPE).

Proper PPE provides safety to personnel and helps prevent spread of infectious agent to health care provider.

2 Conduct a focused health history and physical examination (e.g., pulmonary assessment—oxygen saturation, lung sounds, sputum character; cardiac—heart sounds; neurologic—Glasgow Coma Scale, reflexes). Review history of patient's presenting symptoms and determine if pattern exists.

Symptom identification and clustering of data assist in accurately determining exposure to type of biologic agent and patient's response.

3 Measure patient's vital signs and include assessment of pain on a scale of 0 to 10.

Provides baseline to later evaluate patient's response to therapy.

4 Review results of diagnostic tests and consult with health care provider.

Initial signs and symptoms of exposure to biologic agent suggest common disorders (e.g., flu). Further review of diagnostic findings helps to rule out other common disorders.

5 Assess patient for health risks (e.g., history of heart disease, pulmonary disease, cancer) that complicate effects of exposure to biologic agent.

Patients with preexisting medical conditions often require additional treatment or are at greater risk for death.

STEP	RATIONALE
6 Stay calm and assess patient's immediate psychological response after exposure. Some patients present with dissociative symptoms (e.g., feeling as though "not there" or sensing that everything is outside of the person): disorientation, depression, anxiety, psychosis, and an inability to care for self. Even without direct exposure to a biologic agent, many individuals, spurred by feelings of fear and doom, will present for emergency services.	Aids in providing appropriate crisis intervention and stress management. Remaining calm and projecting confidence while assessing individuals for clinical symptoms help to reduce anxiety of the ill and worried well as they experience the general sense of panic associated with a biologic event.
7 Identify all patient contacts (names, addresses, and phone numbers) in the emergency department (ED) waiting room.	All patient contacts need to be identified for proper follow-up by the public health department. Often patients will self-triage and transport to the ED.
8 Identify resources available (e.g., critical incident stress debriefing teams, counselors, psychiatric/mental health nurse practitioners).	Expert resources help to assess extent of psychological impact of disaster.

Clinical Decision Point *You should consider a biologic event when large numbers of ill persons present who have unexplained yet similar symptoms; when there are unexplained deaths, particularly among young and healthy populations; when there is an unusual pattern associated with the symptoms (e.g., geographic, seasonal, patient population); when a patient fails to respond to traditional therapy; when a single patient presents with symptoms suggestive of an uncommon agent (e.g., anthrax or smallpox). Once you suspect a biologic event, notify incident command immediately.*

NURSING DIAGNOSES

- Acute confusion
- Acute pain
- Anxiety/fear
- Decreased cardiac output
- Impaired gas exchange
- Impaired oral mucous membrane

- Impaired skin integrity
- Impaired swallowing
- Ineffective airway clearance
- Nausea
- Post-trauma syndrome

- Risk for imbalanced body temperature
- Risk for imbalanced fluid volume
- Risk for peripheral neurovascular dysfunction

Related factors are individualized based on patient's condition or needs.

PLANNING

1 Expected outcomes following completion of procedure:	
• Patient is comforted.	In some cases care is only palliative, with comfort as the focus. Do not underestimate the value of *comfort* as *care*.
• Patient's vital signs return to baseline.	When there are no underlying medical conditions and *if* the patient's disease process is responsive to treatment (when available), vital signs will return to normal, taking days or weeks.
• Patient's work of breathing decreases.	Indicates improved gas exchange and cardiac output.
• Patient's skin integrity returns to baseline.	Antibiotic and antitoxin therapy will aid in resolution/healing of lesions over time.
• Patient's level of consciousness (LOC) returns to baseline.	Treatment measures restore neurologic function and oxygenation status.
• Patient's mental health status returns to a pre-trauma level of functioning.	Crisis intervention is successful in reducing patient's anxiety, fear, and dissociative symptoms.
2 Dispense timely and accurate information, including an accurate description of agent to which patient is exposed and implications to patient and family.	Information helps to relieve anxiety and fear.

IMPLEMENTATION

1 Perform hand hygiene.	Reduces transmission of microorganisms.
2 Institute transmission-based isolation precautions (see Chapter 7). (See Table 14-1 for mode of transmission of category A biologic agents.) Use strict isolation with smallpox because of its communicability from person to person. Use airborne precautions, contact precautions, and a negative pressure room for patients suspected of having smallpox.	Reduces transmission of microorganisms and the likelihood of additional secondary sites of contamination.

STEP	RATIONALE
3 Decontaminate as instructed by health care provider. If you suspect anthrax, have patient remove clothing and place in labeled plastic biohazard bag. CAUTION: *Do not pull over patient's head; instead cut garments off.* Instruct patient to shower thoroughly using soap and water.	Handle clothing minimally to avoid agitation. Showering with soap and water aids in decontaminating and reducing exposure (CDC, 2006 a,b).
4 Administer appropriate antibiotics and/or antitoxins.	Various biologic agents are commonly treated with ciprofloxacin (Cipro) and/or doxycycline (e.g., anthrax, plague, typhoidal tularemia). Botulism requires supportive care and use of an antitoxin. For some viral pathogens treatment is only supportive.
5 Administer immunizations (e.g., smallpox).	In the event that smallpox is the biologic weapon, the best treatment is prevention by immunization with vaccine before the onset of symptoms. Vaccination within 3 days of exposure completely prevents the disease or significantly reduces its effect. Vaccination 4 to 7 days after exposure offers some protection from disease or decreases its severity (CDC, 2011c).
6 Administer fluid and nutrition therapy.	Biologic agents commonly cause gastrointestinal (GI) disturbances that sometimes result in dehydration.
7 Administer oxygen therapy.	Various biologic agents (e.g., pulmonary anthrax) commonly cause respiratory symptoms that will result in an altered gas exchange.
8 Provide supportive care (e.g., comfort measures, including pain management).	Some victims of a biologic attack will not survive; palliative care is essential (see Chapter 16).
9 Counsel patient and family on acute and potential long-term psychological effects of exposure. Offer access to trained counselors. Support survivors of a disaster by identifying resources available.	Reaction of patients will include shock, fear, and immobilization. Long-term psychological effects can arise without proper counseling. Social support networks foster coping in the days following a disaster event.

Clinical Decision Point *Collaborate with the health care provider and other rescue workers for an ongoing plan for managing patients exposed to a biologic agent. You will need to do this while caring for other patients who are already present in the health care agency seeking care for illness unrelated to the current MCI.*

EVALUATION

1 Observe for improved airway maintenance, breathing, circulation, LOC, and neurologic functioning.	Evaluates patient's response to available treatment and/or supportive care.
2 Evaluate vital signs and level of pain.	Evaluates patient's response to treatment.
3 Inspect condition of patient's skin; note character of remaining lesions.	Evaluates patient's response to antibiotic therapy.
4 Query patient, "Tell me how you feel right now." Check level of orientation and ability to conduct conversation.	Evaluates patient for changes that suggest either improvement or deterioration of psychological status.

Unexpected Outcomes

Related Interventions

1 Patient's physical symptoms progress despite appropriate treatment.
- Notify health care provider.
- Continue to provide comfort care.

2 Patient becomes more anxious or delusional or develops suicidal ideations.
- Notify mental health treatment team.
- Remain calm, offer reassurance, and protect self and others from physical harm.
- Continue to provide comfort measures.

3 Patient death occurs.
- When handling bodies, take into account continued risk for contamination; make sure that everyone is fully informed regarding proper procedure.

4 Secondary contamination of rescue workers.
- Rescue workers immediately report symptoms to a health care provider or nursing supervisor.

Recording and Reporting

- Report suspected cases of a biologic incident to health care provider or ED officer. In the event of an ED exposure to a communicable disease, the department will be locked down immediately. Public health officials (e.g., the emergency officer) will determine if the hospital should be locked down.
- Create checklists that can be used quickly and use them in a disaster event to record specific data regarding patient status, treatment administered, and response to treatment and/or comfort measures.
- Report any unexpected outcome to health care provider in charge.

Special Considerations
Teaching

- Preparation for an MCI goes a long way toward preventing casualties and chaos. Public education of the likelihood of a mass casualty biologic event is necessary and includes information about types of biologic agents, mode of transmission, symptoms, treatment, and locations of shelters and disaster treatment sites.

- Encourage families to prepare for the unexpected (see Home Care Considerations).

Pediatric

- Children are one of the most vulnerable populations, and many facets influence the impact of disaster on children. These facets often include age, sex, family dynamics, and the level of and direct exposure to disaster (Hockenberry and Wilson, 2011).
- Children often have both physical and emotional needs during disasters. They often show fear and may have temporary changes in behavior after the disaster. These changes are usually related to stress (Hockenberry and Wilson, 2011).
- Many disasters result in the need to relocate, which creates stress and unique challenges in children. Stress may be increased by changes in children's cultural, psychological, and social environment. Reactions of their parents and other family members contribute to how well the child will cope with relocation and whether or not he or she will be able to stay connected with friends and familiar activities (Hockenberry and Wilson, 2011).
- Children are particularly vulnerable to the adverse effects of environmental chemicals and toxins because (1) pound for pound children take in larger doses of toxins through food, water, and air; (2) their organ systems are less mature and unable to remove some of the toxins; and (3) their life expectancy is longer, and long-term effects of exposure to toxins is unknown (Hockenberry and Wilson, 2011).
- Disasters disrupt infrastructure and may cause large-scale displacement, leading to unsafe water, lack of access to health care, and decreases in vector control and infectious agents (WHO, 2011b). Outbreaks of communicable diseases have been reported after natural disasters, and children are more likely to develop infections secondary to immature immune systems (Hockenberry and Wilson, 2011).
- It is important to keep the family together after a disaster. Family togetherness provides reassurance to a child and alleviates fears of being abandoned and unprotected (Hockenberry and Wilson, 2011).
- Media has an enormous influence over children and may impact development and behavior. Encourage parents to limit their children's exposure to media reports of the disaster and to watch television with them whenever possible to clarify information and answer questions (Hockenberry and Wilson, 2011).
- The death of a child, regardless of the situation, is always traumatic; parents may have a compelling need to be present during pediatric resuscitation and at the time of death; ideally you should allow it. It is important for a nurse to be present to explain to the parent what is happening and facilitate the grieving process (Hockenberry and Wilson, 2011).

Gerontologic

- Under disaster conditions triage older adults according to injuries, not age.
- Because the older adult often has several concurrent illnesses, possible exposure to a biologic agent often worsens these conditions and results in the need for more immediate care than an initial triage may suggest.

Home Care

- Assemble a disaster kit before disaster strikes. FEMA and the American Red Cross offer free literature on establishing home care preparedness (Boxes 14-8 and 14-9).

BOX 14-8 | Basic Disaster Supply Kit

- Water: 1 gallon of water per person per day (minimum of 3-day supply)
- Food: minimum of 3-day supply for evacuation/2-week supply for home
- Manual can opener
- Plastic resealable bags
- Utility knife
- Disposable cups, plates, and utensils
- Several flashlights
- Battery-powered radio or television
- Fresh batteries
- Matches in waterproof container
- First-aid kit
- Medications (7-day supply)
- One complete change of clothing and footwear for each person
- Blankets
- Sanitation and hygiene items (e.g., hand sanitizer, toilet paper)
- Small fire extinguisher
- Shut-off valve wrench

Additional Considerations

- Items for infants, seniors, or disabled persons
- Pet-care items
- Entertainment items for small children
- Extra set of keys and identification
- Copies of medical prescriptions in plastic sealable bags

Additional Supplies for Sheltering-in-Place (in the Event of a Chemical or Radiologic Hazard)

- Roll of duct tape and scissors
- Plastic sheeting precut to fit shelter-in-place room openings (10 square feet per person will provide sufficient air to prevent carbon dioxide buildup for up to 5 hours)
- Additional supplies in preparation for a pandemic flu (Have a 2-week supply of basic items so you can survive without outside help or going out in public.)
- Thermometer, nonaspirin pain reliever, prescription medication
- Household-cleaning supplies (e.g., disinfectant sprays, bleach)
- Extra bath and hand soap

Data from American Red Cross (ARC) and Centers for Disease Control and Prevention (CDC): Emergency preparedness and response, 2011, available at http://www.emergency.cdc.gov/preparedness/kit/disasters/, accessed August 19, 2012.

BOX 14-9 | Suggested Foods for a Disaster Supply Kit

- Ready-to-eat canned meats, fruits, and vegetables
- Protein or fruit bars
- Peanut butter
- Dry cereal or granola
- Nuts
- Dried fruit
- Canned juices
- Nonperishable pasteurized milk
- Comfort/stress foods

Data from American Red Cross (ARC) and Centers for Disease Control and Prevention (CDC): Emergency preparedness and response, 2011, available at http://www.emergency.cdc.gov/preparedness/kit/disasters/, accessed August 19, 2012.

- Individuals with special needs (e.g., hearing impairment, impaired mobility, individuals without vehicles, and individuals with special diets) require additional planning to be prepared in the event of a disaster.
- In case of a disaster many schools and employers have disaster plans; individuals need to familiarize themselves with these plans along with their own home disaster plan.
- Post emergency telephone numbers by the telephone and teach children how and when to call 9-1-1.
- Family members need to have a mechanism in place to ensure that they are able to stay in contact in case they are separated (e.g., a designated meeting place, a friend to call to notify when separated from the family).
- An individual of the family needs to know how to turn off water, gas, and electricity in case of a disaster because emergency management personnel often make this request of civilians in the event of a disaster.
- Install a high-efficiency particulate air (HEPA) filter in the return duct of the furnace. These filters will filter out most biologic agents but not chemical agents.
- Have as many members of the family as possible take a first aid class to reduce the risk of complications from a biologic infectious agent during a disaster. Individuals need to maintain a first-aid kit in an accessible location in the home and know which type of PPE will protect the family from secondary exposure.

- Listen to the radio or television for instructions when a biologic disaster becomes a reality. However, limit media exposure to reduce reliving the event and further traumatization. Children and older adults are prone to the emotional stressors of such continuous reporting, which leads to a sense of helplessness.
- Remain isolated and advise friends and relatives not to visit if family members are symptomatic.
- Use the appropriate PPE needed to protect the family; this can include sheltering-in-place.
- Maintain strict hand hygiene for both well and symptomatic family members after using the bathroom, before eating and drinking, and after contact with pets.
- Have family caregivers wear gloves (vinyl or latex) when in contact with a sick individual's blood or body fluids.
- When a sick individual's symptoms worsen, transport to the nearest designated hospital.
- Change the sick person's clothing and bed linens frequently; wash them separately from those of other family members, using any commercial detergent.
- Disinfect any surfaces with which the symptomatic person comes in contact, using an appropriate disinfectant (e.g., Lysol), especially when soiled by blood or other body fluids.
- Family caregiver's highest priority is to avoid becoming a victim. This individual needs to get plenty of rest, drink fluids frequently, and eat a healthy diet. If the caregiver develops symptoms, obtain appropriate medical care immediately.

SKILL 14-2   Care of a Patient After Chemical Exposure

A chemical disaster is the dispersal of a toxic chemical agent into the environment. The mechanism of dispersal is not always known. In fact, the dispersal mechanism such as an explosion or fire can be a secondary terrorist attack designed to create greater fatalities. Explosions spread a toxic chemical in uncontrolled directions, creating more victims. Symptoms from chemical exposure are usually apparent within minutes, but some are delayed up to 24 hours. Early recognition of a chemical event is a priority because you will need to administer many chemical antidotes quickly. Toxic chemical incidents such as biologic events are often unannounced or overt. Terrorists often intend for chemical agents to cause mass casualties and induce fear and/or mass hysteria.

Chemical events are generally confined to small areas, although larger dispersal of these agents may occur (e.g., via a crop duster). The nature and scale of contamination depends on the state of the agent used (e.g., gas versus liquid), characteristics of the chemical used (e.g., heavy or lighter than air), and where the event occurs (e.g., indoors, where ventilation systems affect dispersal, or outdoors, where wind and velocity affect speed and direction of dispersal). For safety reasons, rescue workers should be upwind and uphill from a toxic chemical disaster scene to avoid exposure. The exception is when cyanide gas has been released. Cyanide is lighter than air and thus will travel uphill. It has the unique smell of bitter almonds. If you detect the smell, evacuate the area immediately, although exposure may have already occurred (CDC, 2008).

Because symptoms are almost immediate, it is important to evacuate victims as quickly as possible from the contaminated zone to a decontamination zone. Special respiratory and skin personal protective equipment (PPE) prevent contamination of rescue workers. Before decontamination victims are a potential source of contamination for rescue workers. It is imperative that a nurse protect against toxic chemical contamination when in contact with a contaminated patient. Secondary contamination is high

with toxic chemical incidents. Table 14-2 summarizes common chemical warfare agents, presenting symptoms, and untreated course of exposure.

The rapid chemical decontamination of victims of a toxic chemical incident is more important than determining the exact

TABLE 14-2	Summary of Selected Chemical Warfare Agents	
Chemical Agent	**Onset of Symptoms**	**Untreated Course of Chemical Exposure**
"Lethal" agents —nerve agents (tabun, sarin, soman, and VX)	Symptoms are generally immediate.	Pinpoint pupils and shortly thereafter salivation, runny nose, dyspnea, chest tightness, nausea, muscle twitching, coma, seizures, and death
"Blood" agents —hydrogen cyanide	Rapid onset of symptoms though cyanide poisoning is often associated with the smell of bitter almonds	Death caused by asphyxiation
"Blister" agents —mustard and lewisite	Symptoms may be immediate or delayed.	Skin irritation and blistering
"Choking" agents— phosgene and chlorine	Symptoms can be immediate or delayed up to 24 hours.	Coughing, choking, and disruption in pulmonary function that can lead to death

toxic chemical. When decontamination is necessary, trained personnel are required. Decontamination is either gross or technical, which generally occurs at the scene. The hospital also provides decontamination when a contaminated individual presents for treatment. A nurse and all other health care personnel need to use appropriate precautions to avoid becoming victims.

Delegation and Collaboration

The skill of assessing a patient exposed to a chemical agent cannot be delegated to nursing assistive personnel (NAP). The nurse directs the NAP to:

- Use appropriate PPE to prevent chemical exposure.
- Use techniques for handling a body after death to prevent contamination.

Equipment

The following is a general list of supplies needed in the event of release of the most toxic chemical agents:

- ❏ Decontamination room or area (adult decontamination rooms may not meet the needs of children requiring decontamination; decontamination areas for ambulatory victims will not meet the needs of those who are not ambulatory)
- ❏ Scissors or a tool to cut off clothing
- ❏ Biohazard bags with labels
- ❏ Large volumes of water, decontamination shower (Fig. 14-6)
- ❏ Appropriate PPE
- ❏ Equipment for physical examination

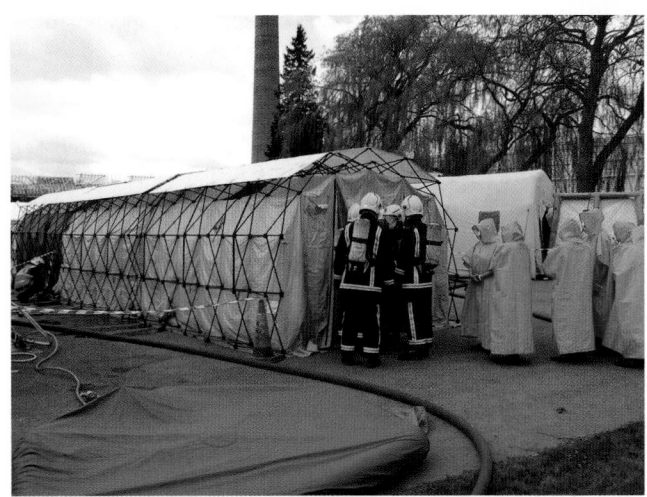

FIG 14-6   Inflatable decontamination shower for ambulatory victims. (*Courtesy Professional Protection Systems, Ltd.*)

STEP	RATIONALE

ASSESSMENT

	STEP	RATIONALE
1	Perform hand hygiene. Don proper personal protective equipment (PPE).	Proper PPE provides safety to personnel and helps prevent spread of infectious agent to health care provider.
2	Assess patient's symptoms and level of pain (on a scale of 0 to 10). Perform appropriate focused physical examination (see Skill 14-1).	Symptom identification and clustering of data accurately identify patient's problem and response.
3	Observe for presence of liquid on patient's skin or clothing and odor (e.g., chlorine). Note condition of skin.	Common conditions present when chemical exposure has occurred.
4	Assess patient for preexisting medical conditions that will complicate the effects of the toxic chemical exposure.	Patients with preexisting medical conditions will likely require additional treatment and sometimes are at greater risk for death.

Clinical Decision Point *Consider a toxic chemical event when large numbers of ill persons present who have unexplained yet similar symptoms. The primary objective for initial care is decontamination, the process used to remove harmful contaminants from the surface of the skin. You achieve this by removing clothing; scrubbing the skin; and hydrolysis, a process of chemical dilution using large volumes of water.*

	STEP	RATIONALE
5	Calmly assess patient's immediate psychological response following exposure. Some patients present with dissociative symptoms, disorientation, depression, anxiety, psychosis, and inability to care for self. Even without direct exposure to a chemical agent, many individuals, spurred by feelings of fear and doom, will present for emergency services and quickly overwhelm available emergency services.	Aids in being able to provide appropriate crisis intervention and stress management. Remaining calm and projecting confidence reduces the anxiety of the ill and worried well as they experience the general sense of panic associated with chemical exposure.
6	Identify resources available (e.g., critical incident stress debriefing teams, counselors, psychiatric/mental health nurse practitioners).	Expert resources assess extent of psychological impact of disorders.

STEP	RATIONALE

NURSING DIAGNOSES

- Acute confusion
- Acute pain
- Anxiety/fear
- Decreased cardiac output
- Impaired gas exchange

- Impaired oral mucous membrane
- Impaired skin integrity
- Impaired swallowing
- Impaired verbal communication
- Ineffective airway clearance

- Nausea
- Post-trauma syndrome
- Risk for imbalanced fluid volume
- Risk for peripheral neurovascular dysfunction

Related factors are individualized based on patient's condition or needs.

PLANNING

STEP	RATIONALE
1 Expected outcomes following completion of procedure:	
• Patient is comforted.	Because of the fatal nature of many chemical agents, the only care available is palliative.
• Patient's vital signs return to baseline.	When there are no underlying medical conditions and *if* the patient's condition is responsive to treatment (when available), vital signs will return to normal within days or weeks.
• Patient's work of breathing decreases.	Indicates improved gas exchange and cardiac output.
• Patient's skin integrity returns to baseline.	Minimizing exposure of skin to chemical agent reduces severity and extent of skin lesions.
• Patient's level of consciousness (LOC) returns to baseline.	Neurologic stability is achieved by minimizing exposure to chemical and giving antitoxin quickly.
• Patient's mental health status returns to a pre-trauma level of functioning.	Crisis intervention is successful in reducing patient's anxiety, fear, and dissociative symptoms.
2 Explain care to patient and family, including decontamination and treatment. Explain your role, orient to location and activities to perform, explain what patient has experienced, and ask, "How are you feeling right now?" Assure them that a medical professional will see them shortly.	Information helps to calm anxiety and fear.

IMPLEMENTATION

STEP	RATIONALE
1 Perform hand hygiene.	Reduces transmission of and injury from toxic chemicals.
2 Prepare for decontamination. Only trained personnel using required PPE may decontaminate patients with toxic chemical contamination.	Reduces likelihood of secondary toxic chemical contamination to untrained personnel attempting decontamination.

Clinical Decision Point *Hold victim outside decontamination area until preparations are completed for decontamination procedure. If patient is grossly contaminated, consider decontamination before entry into building.*

STEP	RATIONALE
3 Provide for patient privacy by closing room curtains or door.	Prevents discomfort and embarrassment when clothing is removed.
4 Decontaminate patient:	
a Act quickly; avoid touching contaminated parts of clothing as much as possible.	
b Remove all of patient's clothing. CAUTION: *Do not pull over patient's head; instead cut garments off.*	Cutting off clothing prevents contamination of head and hair.
c Use large amounts of soap and water to wash patient thoroughly.	Will lead to chemical dilution and in some cases will prevent patient death.
d If eyes are burning or vision is blurred, rinse eyes with plain water for 10 to 15 minutes. If patient wears contacts, remove and place with contaminated clothing; do not reinsert in eyes. Wash eyeglasses with soap and water; reapply when completed.	Flushes toxins from the eye.
5 Dispose of patient's contaminated clothing in an appropriate biohazard bag and seal. Place bag in another plastic bag and seal (see agency policy).	Reduces likelihood of secondary chemical contamination.
6 Initiate treatment for chemical agent using appropriate chemical agent protocol.	Appropriate chemical agent protocol varies with patient exposure (e.g., linesterase, nerve agent, chlorine, and lewisite) (Box 14-10).
7 Establish airway if needed; administer oxygen therapy.	Various chemical agents commonly cause respiratory problems that will result in altered gas exchange.

STEP	RATIONALE
8 Control bleeding.	Various chemical agents cause extensive bleeding.
9 Administer fluid and nutrition therapy.	Various chemical agents commonly cause gastrointestinal disturbances that can result in dehydration.
10 Provide supportive care (e.g., comfort measures, including pain management).	Some victims will not survive; it is essential for a nurse to provide palliative symptom control.
11 Counsel patient and family on both acute and potential long-term psychological effects of exposure. Offer access to trained counselors.	Reaction of patients to exposure includes shock, immobilization, and fear. Long-term psychological effects can arise without proper counseling.

Clinical Decision Point *Collaborate with the health care provider and other rescue workers for an ongoing plan to manage patients exposed to a toxic chemical agent. You will need to do this while also caring for other patients who are already present in the health care agency seeking care for illness unrelated to the current MCI.*

EVALUATION

1 Observe status of airway maintenance, breathing, circulation, LOC, and neurologic functioning. Assess vital signs.	Evaluates patient's physical response to available treatment and/or supportive care.
2 Ask patient to rate pain level on a 0-to-10 scale.	Determines if comfort measures are effective.
3 Inspect condition of skin; note extent of blistering.	Determines extent of healing.
4 Evaluate patient's level of orientation, ability to problem solve, and perception of condition.	Evaluates patient's psychological status and ability to make decisions.

Unexpected Outcomes / Related Interventions

Unexpected Outcomes	Related Interventions
1 Secondary contamination of rescue workers occurs.	• Rescue workers immediately remove their clothing, scrub their bodies, and use copious amounts of soap and water. • Contain clothes in appropriate biohazard bags. • Provide clean clothes.
2 Patient's physical symptoms progress despite appropriate treatment.	• Notify health care provider in charge. • Continue to provide comfort care.
3 Patient's psychological symptoms progress despite appropriate treatment. Patient exhibits anxiety, disorientation, and suicidal ideation.	• Notify mental health treatment team. • Remain calm, offer reassurance, and protect self and others from physical harm. • Continue to provide comfort measures.
4 Patient death occurs.	• When handling bodies, take into account continued risk for contamination; make sure that everyone is fully informed regarding proper procedures. When delegating preparation of the deceased, always take into account the level of training of those managing the body.

BOX 14-10 | Examples of Chemical Exposure Protocols

CHLORINE PROTOCOL

1 Dyspnea?
  • Try bronchodilators
  • Admit to hospital
  • Oxygen by mask
  • Chest x-ray examination
2 Treat other problems and reevaluate (consider phosgene)
3 Respiratory system OK?
  • Yes—Go to 5
4 Is phosgene poisoning possible?
  • Yes—Go to Phosgene Protocol on the CDC website
5 Give supportive therapy: treat other problems or discharge

MUSTARD PROTOCOL

1 Airway obstruction?
  • Yes—Tracheostomy
2 If there are large burns:
  • Establish IV line—Do not push fluids as for thermal burns
  • Drain vesicles—Unroof large blisters and irrigate area with topical antibiotics
3 Treat other symptoms appropriately:
  • Antibiotic eye ointment
  • Sterile precautions prn
  • Morphine prn

CDC, Centers for Disease Control and Prevention; *IV,* intravenous; *prn,* as needed.
Modified from Centers for Disease Control and Prevention: *Emergency room procedures in chemical hazard emergencies: a job aid,* 2010, available at http://www.cdc.gov/nceh/demil/articles/initialtreat.htm, accessed February 12, 2012.

Recording and Reporting

- Report suspected cases of a toxic chemical event to health care provider or emergency officer.
- Record in nurses' notes and electronic health record (EHR) patient's status, decontamination and treatment procedures, and response to treatment and/or comfort measures.
- Report any unexpected outcome to health care provider in charge.

Special Considerations

Teaching

- Preparation for an MCI goes a long way toward preventing casualties and chaos. Public education about the likelihood of a mass casualty chemical event is necessary. This education needs to include information regarding types of chemical agents, mode of dissemination, symptoms, and treatment.
- Education of the public needs to include locations of shelters and disaster treatment sites.
- See Skill 14-1 for family disaster plan and preparation.

Pediatric

- To avoid becoming a secondary victim, emergency responders need to consider potential contamination of children before picking them up and holding them. Often decontamination consists of providing fresh air and a large volume of low-pressure warm water. Observe children for potential hypothermia because they are more susceptible.
- Adult decontamination facilities are not always appropriate to meet the needs of children. The special protective equipment worn by rescue workers may frighten young children. The cleaning process and possible separation from uncontaminated parents will likely cause considerable stress and anxiety. Additional health care workers are often necessary to ensure that adequate decontamination has taken place. Verbal encouragement and praise will be effective in facilitating the process.
- See Skill 14-1 for further pediatric considerations.

Gerontologic

- See Skill 14-1 for gerontologic considerations.

Home Care

- Keep upwind and uphill from the release of the toxic chemical unless it is cyanide.
- Use appropriate PPE needed to protect the family; this includes sheltering-in-place.
- See Skill 14-1 for further home care considerations.

SKILL 14-3   Care of a Patient After Radiation Exposure

Radiologic events differ from nuclear events. A radiologic event is the dispersal of radioactive material via a "dirty bomb," by deliberate contamination of food or water supplies, or over the terrain. A nuclear event involves a device that releases nuclear energy in an explosive manner as a result of a nuclear chain reaction. Early symptoms of radiation exposure are similar to those experienced by anxious individuals. Thus, once radiation release becomes publicly recognized, an enormous number of worried well will compromise incident management, scene security, and triage (CDC, 2011b).

Radiation comes in a variety of forms. Alpha particles are the least dangerous, traveling only a few centimeters. They do not penetrate materials easily and are harmful only if ingested. An individual's clothing block alpha particles from reaching the skin. Beta particles penetrate a short distance into the skin. Protective clothing is necessary for protection. Gamma rays pose the greatest health risk because the waves penetrate deeply, causing severe burns and internal injury. Lead shielding protects against gamma rays. Blasts caused by a nuclear explosion cause not only injury from radiation exposure but also traumatic injuries and burns. Some victims will present with many combined forms of injury requiring treatment. The sooner symptoms begin to appear, the greater the patient's exposure to the radiation. Early symptoms, within a few hours, suggest that the individual has received a lethal dose of radiation. They include nausea, vomiting, diarrhea, and a possible burn. For some, hair begins to fall out, and the victim quickly becomes immunocompromised.

Nuclear incidents usually result in wide destruction requiring specialized equipment and resources at the scene to assess structural damage and levels of radioactivity. Radiologic events usually cover much smaller areas, but they are often difficult to define. Table 14-3 presents characteristic differences between a nuclear event and a radiologic event. Specialized equipment and training are required to assess the source of radioactivity, determine the scope of contamination, and perform decontamination. Decontamination is important with radiation exposure; however, it needs to occur in an area where there is not continued radiologic release (CDC, 2011d,e). The principles to follow to protect individuals from exposure involve distance, time, and shielding.

Delegation and Collaboration

The skill of assessment of a patient exposed to a radiologic agent cannot be delegated to nursing assistive personnel (NAP). The nurse directs the NAP to:

- Use appropriate personal protective equipment (PPE) to prevent exposure.
- Use techniques for handling a body after death to prevent contamination.

Equipment

The following is a general list of supplies needed in the event of release of the most radiologic exposure:

- ❏ Decontamination room or area (adult decontamination rooms do not always meet the needs of children requiring

TABLE 14-3	Characteristics of a Nuclear Event and a Radiologic Event	
Characteristics	**Nuclear Event**	**Radiologic Event**
Event recognition	Obvious	Not obvious
Thermonuclear explosion	Yes	No
Casualties	Large	Small
Amount of radiation release and contamination	Large	Small
Likelihood of terrorism	No	Yes

From American Medical Association: *Core Disaster Life Support: provider manual*, version 1.01, Chicago, 2002, The Association. Used with permission of the American Medical Association.

decontamination; decontamination of ambulatory victims will not meet the needs of those who are not ambulatory)
❏ Scissors or some other tool to cut off clothing
❏ Clothing containers; type depends on the kind of radiologic exposure
❏ Appropriate personal protective equipment (PPE) for use by personnel in area of radiation release

❏ Appropriate PPE for health care workers in hospital setting (i.e., surgical masks, N95 masks, recommended if available)
❏ Radiation meter available to survey hands and clothing at frequent intervals (CDC, 2011d)
❏ Equipment for select specimen collection
❏ Equipment for physical examination

STEP	RATIONALE

ASSESSMENT

1 Assess patient's symptoms by performing a focused physical examination (see Skill 14-1).

Symptom identification and clustering of data are the first steps to determining patient's condition and response.

Clinical Decision Point *Before assessment, a specially trained technician conducts a radiation survey of the patient, initially conducting a scan of the face, hands, and feet with a radiation survey instrument. If meter results are positive, a thorough survey (5 to 8 minutes per person) is conducted.*

2 Assess patient for secondary traumatic wounds: location, drainage, size, appearance.

Radioactive fragments are sometimes embedded in a wound. Very high localized levels of internal contamination indicate radioactive fragments.

Clinical Decision Point *Do not touch the wound if you suspect that radioactive fragments are present.*

3 Assess patient for preexisting medical conditions that will complicate effects of the radiologic exposure.

4 Determine patient's allergies, specifically allergy for iodine sensitivity.

5 Assess individual psychological response to radiologic event. Some patients present with dissociative symptoms (e.g., feeling as though "not there," sensing that experiences are outside the person), disorientation, depression, anxiety, psychosis, and an inability to care for self. Ask patient, "How do you feel now?" Determine level of orientation, ability to follow conversation.

6 Identify resources available (e.g., critical incident stress debriefing teams, counselors, psychiatric/mental health nurse practitioners).

Patients with preexisting medical conditions can require additional treatment or are at greater risk for death.

Patients with iodine sensitivity need to avoid taking potassium iodide, the treatment of choice for radioactive iodine exposure.

Aids a nurse in being able to provide appropriate crisis intervention and stress management. Remaining calm and projecting confidence while assessing individuals for clinical symptoms versus feelings of panic goes a long way toward reducing the anxiety of the ill and worried well as they experience the general sense of panic associated with a radiologic event.

Expert resources assess extent of psychological impact of disaster.

Clinical Decision Point *A radiologic event is the event most feared by most individuals. Many are uneducated regarding the dangers of and differences among radiation materials. Health care agencies will likely have many anxious, frightened individuals who can potentially create a danger to the environment.*

NURSING DIAGNOSES

- Acute pain
- Anxiety
- Deficient fluid volume

- Diarrhea
- Fear
- Impaired tissue integrity

- Nausea
- Post-trauma syndrome
- Risk for infection

Related factors are individualized based on patient's condition or needs.

PLANNING

1 Expected outcomes following completion of procedure:
- Patient is comforted.
- Patient is successfully decontaminated.

- Patient's vital signs return to baseline.

- Patient is free of nausea and diarrhea.

- Patient's skin integrity returns to baseline.

In some cases the only care that is available is palliative.
Decontamination procedures remove radioactive materials from patient's skin.
When there are no underlying medical conditions and *if* the patient's disease process is responsive to treatment (when available), vital signs will return to normal within days or weeks.
Gastrointestinal alterations following radiation exposure typically respond to antidiarrheal and antiemetic medications.
Radiologic burns are minimized through successful decontamination procedures.

STEP	RATIONALE
• Patient's immune system (e.g., complete blood count [CBC]) returns to baseline.	Exposure to radiation is successfully minimized.
• Patient's work of breathing decreases.	Indicates improved gas exchange and cardiac output.
2 Explain care to patient and family. Explain your role, orient to location and activities to perform, explain what patient has experienced, and ask, "How are you feeling right now?" Assure them that medical personnel will see them shortly.	Crisis intervention reestablishes patient's orientation and sense of reality.

IMPLEMENTATION

STEP	RATIONALE
1 Perform hand hygiene.	Reduces transmission of microorganisms.
2 Only trained personnel use required PPE to decontaminate patients with radiologic contamination.	Reduces likelihood of secondary radiologic contamination to untrained personnel attempting decontamination.
3 Provide for patient privacy by closing room curtains or door.	Prevents anxiety or embarrassment when clothes are removed.
4 Decontaminate patient:	
a Remove patient's clothing.	Normally eliminates up to 90% of contamination.
b Wash patient's skin thoroughly with water and soap, taking care not to abrade or irritate the skin. Do not allow radioactive material to be incorporated into any wounds.	Use of large amounts of water is critical in decontamination.
c Have radiation technician resurvey patient after washing. Rewash as necessary.	Determines if radiation residual is present.
d Isolate and cover any area of the skin that is still positive for radiation by using a plastic bag or wrap.	The area is washed until no further reduction in contamination is achieved (verified by survey instrumentation) and then covered to reduce exposure of health care workers.
5 Bag and tag patient's contaminated clothing for further evaluation and place in appropriate biohazard container.	Reduces likelihood of secondary contamination when you use containers designed to contain the radiologic particle.

Clinical Decision Point *Collaborate with the health care provider and other rescue workers for an ongoing plan to manage patients exposed to radiologic materials. You will need to do this while also caring for other patients who are already present in the health care agency seeking care for illness unrelated to the current nuclear or radiologic event.*

STEP	RATIONALE
6 Prepare for possibly obtaining a CBC, urinalysis, fecal specimen, and swabs of body orifices (see Chapter 43).	CBC establishes baseline to determine patient's immunologic status over time. A health care provider who suspects internal contamination will order collection of urine, feces, and body orifice swabs to analyze for radionuclides.
7 Treat symptoms according to ordinary treatment practices: provide intravenous fluid support, antidiarrheal therapies, antiemetic medications, and potassium iodide tablets (CDC, 2011d,e).	Patient exposed to radiation is at risk for gastrointestinal (GI) alterations and fluid imbalance. Potassium iodide reduces risk for thyroid cancer from radioactive iodine exposure.

EVALUATION

STEP	RATIONALE
1 Observe skin integrity, fluid balance, respiratory and GI status, level of consciousness, and neurologic functioning. Look for improvement of other radiologic agent–specific symptoms. Evaluate vital signs.	Evaluates patient's physical response to available treatment and/or supportive care.
2 Monitor CBC and other laboratory tests.	Determines patient's immune response.
3 Evaluate patient's level of consciousness, orientation, and ability to relate events. Ask if patient remembers what has occurred; observe affect.	Determines if psychological status has improved.

Unexpected Outcomes	Related Interventions
1 Secondary contamination of rescue workers occurs.	• Institute appropriate decontamination of worker.
2 Patient's symptoms progress despite appropriate treatment.	• Notify health care provider in charge.
	• Continue to provide comfort care.
3 Patient's psychological state deteriorates with development of disorientation, suicidal ideation, violence toward others.	• Notify mental health treatment team.
	• Remain calm, offer reassurance, and protect self and others from physical harm.
	• Continue to provide comfort care.
4 Patient death occurs.	• When handling bodies, take into account continued risk for contamination; make sure that everyone is fully informed about proper procedure. When delegating preparation of the deceased, take into account the level of training of those managing the body.

Recording and Reporting

- Record in nurses' notes and EHR patient's status and response to treatment and/or comfort measures.
- Report presence of open wound and any suspected radioactive fragment to health care provider in charge.
- Report any unexpected outcomes to health care provider.

Special Considerations

Teaching
- See Skill 14-1.

Pediatric
- Children are vulnerable to radiation because (1) their organ systems are more sensitive than those of adults, and (2) they have more years of life expectancy over which to develop complications from the radiologic exposure.
- See Skills 14-1 and 14-2 for further pediatric considerations.

Gerontologic
- Because some older adults have many concurrent illnesses, it is possible that radiologic agents will worsen these conditions and result in the older adult needing more immediate care than an initial triage had indicated.
- See Skill 14-1 for further gerontologic considerations.

Home Care
- When a radiologic or nuclear event becomes reality, listen to the radio or television for special instructions, including appropriate means for maintaining a safe shelter.
- Keep upwind and uphill from the release of the radioactive materials.
- See Skill 14-1 for further home care considerations.

? Critical Thinking Exercises

Victims of an explosion involving a chemical are arriving in the emergency department (ED). Authorities state that the substance is unknown at this time, but there were reports by people in the area of a "funny smell" earlier in the day.

1 What are some safety measures that a rescue worker should take to avoid exposure?
2 Victims on the scene are triaged. How would the following patients be color coded, and which would receive the highest priority? A 22-year-old with cyanosis, a respiratory rate of 35, and confusion; a 14-year-old with a diffuse red rash on the extremities; a 56-year-old with controlled bleeding of deep lacerations received from falling debris; a 41-year-old with burns on 50% of the body.
3 What should the nurse working in the ED expect the initial care to be, and how is it achieved?
4 Yvette is an 18-year-old patient who arrived in the ED for treatment. Her clothing appears to be saturated with the unknown chemical. How should Yvette's clothing be handled?
5 Among the victims to be treated is a 3-year-old. What special considerations need to be taken when decontaminating children?

✓ REVIEW QUESTIONS

1 A hospital committee formed to work on an emergency response plan is meeting initially to discuss how to proceed with the process. Why is a clearly defined, executable, and practiced emergency response plan the best indicator that an agency will be successful in a disaster situation?
  1 Practice makes staff more familiar with disaster protocols in the event of a true disaster.
  2 Practice of protocols helps to meet all of the regulatory agency guidelines.
  3 Practice prevents the likelihood of acute traumatic stress disorder in the staff.
  4 Practice is cost-effective in the long term because fewer staff will be required to handle the disaster as a result of the preparation of the staff members.
2 A major traffic accident involving multiple vehicles and an explosion has sent numerous patients to the local ED. Which experienced nurse has the most difficult assignment and a greater chance for demonstrating signs and symptoms of acute traumatic stress disorder?
  1 A nurse who has been delegated to care for the community patients currently admitted to the ED
  2 A nurse assigned to triage disaster victims transported to the ED but able to walk in to the triage area
  3 A nurse who is assigned to care for patients on an as-needed basis
  4 A nurse who must inform a mother that her three children did not survive
3 Four victims from a disaster arrive at the ED at the same time. Which victim should receive the highest level of priority for care?
  1 A disaster victim who arrives at the ED without a pulse
  2 A disaster victim who arrives at the ED with labored respirations, cool skin, a pulse of 120 beats/min, and a blood pressure of 90/60 mm Hg
  3 A disaster victim who is a noted politician with an open fracture of his left arm
  4 A disaster victim who is under the age of 6 years, regardless of the extent of his injuries
4 A patient arrives at the ED with suspected cutaneous anthrax. Which type of precautions should be used with this patient?
  1 Standard
  2 Contact
  3 Respiratory
  4 Airborne
5 A practice emergency drill is being held in the ED. The drill would be considered successful if which group of people were initially protected at the disaster scene?
  1 The health care workers
  2 The patient(s)
  3 The news crews reporting the event
  4 The family members of the victim(s)
6 In the case of a biologic exposure, delegation and collaboration are important. Which of the following tasks may be delegated to the nursing assistive personnel (NAP)?
  1 Conducting a focused health history
  2 Assessing the patient for health risk
  3 Reviewing diagnostic test results
  4 Gathering appropriate personal protective equipment (PPE)
7 A patient exposed to toxic chemical agents arrives at the ED. When caring for the patient, which action is most important?
  1 Determining what the toxic chemical agent is
  2 Decontaminating the patient
  3 Assessing the patient's immediate psychological response to exposure
  4 Assessing the patient for preexisting medical conditions

8 Understanding the levels of personal protective equipment is important to both rescue workers and health care providers. Most hospital personnel are trained and fitted to use which level of protection?
   1 Level A
   2 Level B
   3 Level C
   4 Level D

9 During a radiologic event the treatment of choice is:
   1 Potassium iodide.
   2 Potassium chloride.
   3 Potassium hypochlorite.
   4 Potassium carbonate.

10 In the event that smallpox is the biologic weapon, which is the best treatment to reduce the effects of exposure?
   1 Administering antibiotics
   2 Decontaminating the person
   3 Providing supportive care
   4 Immunizing with vaccine

REFERENCES

American Medical Association (AMA): National Disaster Life Support Program. 2011, available at http://www.ama-assn.org/go/ndls. accessed February 12, 2012.

American Nurses Association (ANA): *Who will be there? Ethics, the law, and a nurse's duty to respond in a disaster*, Washington, DC, 2010, The Association.

Centers for Disease Control and Prevention (CDC): Chemical agents: facts about personal cleaning and disposal of contaminated clothing. 2006a, available at http://www.bt.cdc.gov/planning/personalcleaningfacts.asp. accessed February 12, 2012.

Centers for Disease Control and Prevention (CDC): Chemical agents: facts about sheltering in place. 2006b, available at http://www.bt.cdc.gov/planning/shelteringfacts.asp. accessed February 12, 2012.

Centers for Disease Control and Prevention (CDC): Bioterrorism: frequently asked questions about smallpox vaccine. 2007, available at http://www.bt.cdc.gov/agent/smallpox/vaccination/faq.asp#vaccine. accessed February 12, 2012.

Centers for Disease Control and Prevention (CDC): Potassium cyanide. 2008, available at http://www.cdc.gov/NIOSH/ershdb/EmergencyResponseCard_29750037.html, accessed August 28, 2012.

Centers for Disease Control and Prevention (CDC): About CDC organization COTPER. 2009, available at http://www.cdc.gov/healthywater/at_cdc/ophpr.html. accessed February 12, 2012.

Centers for Disease Control and Prevention (CDC): Emergency room procedures in chemical hazard emergencies: a job aid. 2010a, available at http://www.cdc.gov/nceh/demil/articles/initialtreat.htm. accessed February 12, 2012.

Centers for Disease Control and Prevention (CDC): Updated in a moment's notice: surge capacity for terrorist bombings—challenges and proposed solutions. 2010b, available at http://www.bt.cdc.gov/masscasualties/pdf/CDC_Surge-508.pdf. accessed February 12, 2012.

Centers for Disease Control and Prevention (CDC): Influenza (flu) vaccine. 2011a, available at http://www.cdc.gov/flu/about/qa/research.htm. accessed February 12, 2012.

Centers for Disease Control and Prevention (CDC): Severe, acute respiratory syndrome (SARS). 2011b, http://www.cdc.gov/sars/index.html. accessed February 12, 2012.

Centers for Disease Control and Prevention (CDC): Strategic national stockpile. 2011c, available at http://www.cdc.gov/phpr/stockpile/stockpile.htm. accessed February 12, 2012.

Centers for Disease Control and Prevention (CDC): Public health and radiation emergency preparedness. 2011d, available at http://www.cdcradiationconference.com/index.html. accessed February 12, 2012.

Centers for Disease Control and Prevention (CDC): Shelter in place in a radiation emergency. 2011e, available at http://www.bt.cdc.gov/radiation/shelter.asp. accessed February 12, 2012.

Department of Homeland Security (DHS): Strategic plan—one team one mission—securing our homeland. 2008, available at http://www.hsdl.org/?view&did=235371, accessed August 29, 2012.

Department of Homeland Security (DHS): If you see something say something campaign. 2011a, available at http://www.dhs.gov/files/reportincidents/see-something-say-something.shtm. accessed February 12, 2012.

Department of Homeland Security (DHS): National terrorism advisory system. 2011b, available at http://www.dhs.gov/national-terrorism-advisory-system, accessed August 30, 2012.

Department of Homeland Security (DHS): Incident command system overview. 2011c, available at http://www.fema.gov/emergency/nims/IncidentCommandSystem.shtm#item1. accessed February 12, 2012.

Federal Communications Commission (FCC): FEMA and FCC unveil tips on communicating during disaster. 2011, available at http://www.fcc.gov/document/fema-and-fcc-unveil-tips-communicating-during-disasters. accessed February 12, 2012.

Hockenberry M, Wilson D: *Wong's Nursing care of infants and children*, ed 9, St Louis, 2011, Mosby.

Inglesby TV: Progress in disaster planning and preparedness since 2011, JAMA 306(12):1372, 2011.

Institute of Medicine: *Guidance for establishing crisis standards of care for use in disaster situations: A letter report*, Washington, DC, 2009, National Academies Press.

Lerner EB, et al: Mass casualty triage: an evaluation of the science and refinement of a national guideline, *Disaster Med Public Health Prep* 5(2):129, 2011.

Mendez T: Disaster planning for vulnerable populations: mental health, *Crit Care Clin North Am* 22(4):493, 2010.

Occupational Safety and Health Administration (OSHA): OSHA Fact Sheet: Personal protective equipment (PPE) reduces exposure to bloodborne pathogens, 2011, available at www.osha.gov/OshDoc/data_BloodborneFacts/bbfact03.pdf, accessed August 19, 2012.

Stangeland P: 2010 Disaster nursing: a retrospective review, *Crit Care Nurs Clin North Am* 22(4):421, 2010.

Tillman P: Disaster preparedness for nurses: a teaching guide, *J Contin Educ Nurs* 42(9):404, 2011.

US Department of Health and Human Services (USDHHS), Agency for Healthcare Research and Quality: Public health emergency preparedness. 2010, available at http://www.ahrq.gov/about/cp3/cp3syscap.htm. accessed February 12, 2012.

Veenema TG: Disaster preparedness 10 years after 911, *Am J Nurs* 111(9):7, 2011.

World Health Organization (WHO): Avian influenza fact sheet. 2011a, available at http://www.who.int/mediacentre/factsheets/avian_influenza/en/. accessed February 12, 2012.

World Health Organization (WHO): Disaster risk management for health: communicable diseases. 2011b, available at http://www.who.int/hac/events/drm_fact_sheet_communicable_diseases.pdf. accessed February 12, 2012.

Pain Assessment and Basic Comfort Measures

MEDIA RESOURCES

- **evolve** *learning system* http://evolve.elsevier.com/Perry/skills

  - Review Questions
  - Video Clips
  - Audio Glossary

KEY TERMS

Acute pain	Effleurage	Opioid Naïve	Physical dependence
Addiction	Epidural analgesia	Oversedation	Preemptive analgesia
Analgesia	Guided imagery	Pain intensity	Pseudoaddiction
Anaphylaxis	Massage	Pain rating scales	Rational polypharmacy
Chronic pain/persistent pain	Multimodal analgesia	Patient-controlled analgesia	Sedation scale
Cutaneous stimulation	Nonopioids	(PCA)	Sleep apnea
Drug tolerance	Opioids	Pétrissage	Splinting

OBJECTIVES

Mastery of content in this chapter will enable the nurse to:
- Assess a patient's level of comfort.
- Assess a patient's level of pain.
- Assess a patient's level of sedation.
- Identify skills appropriate for relieving a patient's reported pain.
- Plan care based on a patient's history, including pain history and physical assessment.
- Describe delivery of medication through a patient-controlled analgesia (PCA) device.
- Teach a patient to use a PCA device.

- Monitor and manage a patient receiving epidural analgesia.
- Monitor and manage a patient receiving a local anesthetic infusion pump.
- Identify and discuss various nonpharmacologic pain-relief measures.
- Monitor and manage a patient receiving nonpharmacologic measures to relieve pain.
- Evaluate the effectiveness of pain-management techniques.

Pain is a complex problem that is physical and/or mental in nature while being subjective and highly individualized. It is tiring and demands a person's physical, emotional, and mental energy. It interferes with personal relationships and even influences the meaning of life. Although certain types of pain create predictable signs and symptoms, you primarily assess it by relying on a patient's self-report. The patient is the only one who knows whether pain is present and what the experience is like. The International Association for the Study of Pain (IASP) defines pain as an unpleasant subjective sensory and emotional experience associated with actual or potential disuse damage or described in terms of such damage (IASP, 2010).

The Joint Commission requires that a patient's reports of pain are to be addressed and appropriately treated (Box 15-1). Optimal pain management is considered the right of every patient. Many people receive inadequate pain relief for conditions that could be treated or managed (IOM, 2011; Pasero and McCaffery, 2011). When you care for a patient with cognitive impairments, pain management represents a special challenge. It is important that you carefully observe a patient's behavior and nonverbal responses to pain when he or she is unable to self-report (Box 15-2) (Herr et al., 2011).

Pain is difficult to categorize, but the literature commonly identifies three types: acute, chronic/persistent, and cancer

BOX 15-1	The Joint Commission Pain Standards

The Joint Commission calls on health care organizations to do the following:
- Recognize the right of patients to appropriate assessment and management of pain
- Assess pain in all patients
- Record the assessment in a way that facilitates regular reassessment and follow-up
- Educate providers/patients and families
- Establish policies that support appropriate prescription or ordering of pain medicines
- Include patient needs for symptom control in discharge planning
- Collect data to monitor effectiveness and appropriateness of pain management

From The Joint Commission: *Comprehensive accreditation manual for hospitals: the official handbook*, Oak Brook Terrace, Ill, 2012, The Joint Commission.

BOX 15-2	Pain Assessment in a Nonverbal Patient

Recommended Assessment Approaches
- Attempt a self-report of pain using simple yes/no responses or vocalizations or a numeric rating scale.
- Explain why a self-report cannot be used.
- Search for the potential cause of pain by using physical examination techniques (e.g., palpation).
- Assume that pain is present after ruling out other causes (infection or constipation).
- Identify pathologic conditions or procedures that may cause pain.
- Observe patient behaviors (e.g., confusion, pacing, facial expressions, vocalizations, body movements such as guarding) that indicate pain. These vary based on patient's developmental level.
- Ask family members, parents, and caregivers for a proxy report of patient's pain.
- Attempt an analgesic trial if pathologic conditions or procedures that may induce pain are present.

Using a Behavioral Pain Assessment Tool
- Use reliable and valid tools to ensure that appropriate criteria are used in assessment (e.g., the NOPPAIN for older adults).
- Select an appropriate scale for each patient (e.g., visual analog scale or FACES scale); no one scale is required for all specific groups of patients.
- Vital signs are not sensitive indicators for the presence of pain.

NOPPAIN: *Noncommunicative Patient's Pain Assessment Instrument.*
Modified from Bell L: Pain assessment in the adult nonverbal or sedated patients, *Am J Crit Care*19:356, 2010; Herr K et al: *Pain in the nonverbal patient: position statement with clinical practice recommendations*, The American Society for Pain Management Nursing, 2011, ASPMN.

BOX 15-3	Pain Categories

Acute/Transient Pain
- Protective and has an identifiable cause
- Has a rapid onset
- Varies in intensity
- Is of short duration
- Generally disappears with healing (Mackey, 2011)

Chronic/Persistent Pain
- Extends beyond the period of healing, eventually becoming a disease in its own right, not a symptom
- Often lacks identified pathology
- Rarely has autonomic signs; vital signs no longer indicate pain (Drew and St. Marie, 2011)
- Does not provide a protective function
- Disrupts sleep and other activities of daily living (ADLs)
- Degrades health and function of the individual

Cancer Pain
- May be acute, chronic, or intermittent (More cancer patients are living longer with chronic pain.) (APS, 2009)
- Usually related to tumor recurrences or treatments

BOX 15-4	Terminology Related to the Use of Opioids in Pain Treatment

Physical Dependence
A state of adaptation that is manifested by a drug class–specific withdrawal syndrome produced by abrupt cessation, rapid dose reduction, decreasing blood level of an opioid, and/or administration of a drug that can act as an antagonist.

Addiction
A primary, chronic, neurobiologic disease, with genetic, psychosocial, and environmental factors influencing its development and manifestations. Addictive behaviors include one or more of the following: impaired control over drug use, compulsive use, continued use despite harm, and craving.

Drug Tolerance
A state of adaptation in which exposure to a drug induces changes that result in a diminution of one or more of the effects of the drug over time.

Approved by the Boards of Directors of the American Academy of Pain Medicine, The American Pain Society and American Society of Addiction Medicine, February 2011, American Pain Society, 2011.

pain (APS, 2009). Because cancer pain differs from chronic non-cancer pain in significant ways (time frame, pathology, treatment strategies), currently it is in a different category (Box 15-3).

The most effective pain management combines pharmacologic and nonpharmacologic strategies with the administration of pharmacologic agents. There are three types of analgesics: (1) nonopioids, including acetaminophen (Tylenol) and nonsteroidal antiinflammatory drugs (NSAIDs); (2) opioids (traditionally called *narcotics*); and (3) adjuvants or coanalgesics (e.g., antidepressants and muscle relaxants) that enhance analgesics or have analgesic properties. Timely administration before a patient's pain becomes severe is crucial for optimal relief. Pain is easier to prevent than to treat. In most situations administration of pharmacologic agents "around-the-clock" rather than on an "as-needed" (prn) basis is preferable. This approach alleviates pain before it becomes severe and facilitates an earlier recovery. Although nonpharmacologic strategies are sometimes omitted in the acute care setting because of time constraints, you should make every effort to include complementary/integrative methods, which generally do not require a health care provider's order (check agency policy). Complementary strategies for pain relief provide an opportunity for a patient to assume an active role in achieving a higher level of comfort and in some instances freedom from pain (NIH, 2011).

Knowing and understanding the terms related to opioid use (Box 15-4), teaching your patient and his or her family about pain treatment, and having an attitude of dignity and caring will allow you to individualize a patient's pain control plan. Using an integrated approach that considers both pharmacologic and nonpharmacologic therapies in managing pain is recommended (Baird et al., 2010).

EVIDENCE-BASED PRACTICE

Pain is considered a co-morbid medical condition and not simply a symptom of a pathologic state. The current trend in health care is to prevent it. Preemptive analgesia is a method of preventing pain while reducing overall opioid use. Understanding the influence of genes (Young and Plenge, 2010) and gender and age (deTovar et al., 2010; Herr, 2011) on pain management is essential. In addition, nonpharmacologic interventions to pain management help to control acute and chronic pain (Allred et al., 2010; Baird et al., 2010). The goal is to develop an individualized pain-management plan to provide optimum pain relief with minimal adverse effects.

- Assess for causes of pain or conditions that intensify or moderate it.
- When possible, talk with family caregivers to identify behavioral changes associated with pain in patients who are unable to effectively report their level of pain (e.g., young children, critically ill patients, patients with cognitive impairments) (Herr et al., 2011).
- Post any behavioral changes in a patient's care plan to alert other caregivers.
- Premedicate with analgesia when therapy or a painful procedure is to be performed (e.g., dressing change, diagnostic testing).
- Cautiously use nonopioids, which may have more dangerous side effects than opioids, especially for the elderly. For example, acetaminophen and NSAIDS have some very serious side effects (e.g., liver damage, gastrointestinal bleeding), even when given in recommended dosages (Rahme and Bernatsky, 2010; USFDA, 2009).
- Your primary goal should be pain relief and whatever measures it takes accomplish the goal. Some patients may need opioids the rest of their lives, just as some patients need insulin the remainder of their lives (APS and AAPM, 2009; Gloth, 2011).
- Individualize patient care and avoid misconceptions regarding pain control (Table 15-1). All health care professionals need to consider common misconceptions about pain when planning patient care.
- A method of using smaller doses of more medications is a new practice called *rational polypharmacy* or *multimodal dosing*. When these are combined, there are fewer side effects and greater analgesia (Pasero and McCaffery, 2011).

PATIENT-CENTERED CARE

Pain is unique to each individual, and it is important to recognize all factors influencing a patient's pain and integrate them into an individualized plan for pain management. To effectively design this plan, carefully assess a patient's coping style, physical status, past experiences with pain, culture and ethnicity, expectations for pain relief, and emotional health. A timely, factual, and accurate pain assessment requires you to work closely with patients and their families. You need to learn and understand what pain means in the eyes of the patient. Be objective, listen carefully, and explore any symptoms that a patient expresses. Effective communication and caring are keys to gathering all the information needed to

TABLE 15-1	Misconceptions: Barriers to the Assessment and Treatment of Pain
Misconception	**Correction**
• The best judge of the existence and severity of a patient's pain is the health care provider or nurse caring for the patient.	• The patient's self-report is the most reliable indicator of the existence and intensity of pain.
• Clinicians should use their personal opinions and beliefs about the truthfulness of a patient to determine a patient's true pain status.	• Allowing each clinician to act on personal beliefs presents the potential for different pain assessments by different clinicians, leading to different interventions from each clinician. This results in inconsistent and often inadequate pain management. It is essential to establish a patient's self-report of pain as the standard for pain assessment.
• Visible signs, either physiologic or behavioral, always accompany pain and can be used to verify its existence and severity.	• Even with severe pain, periods of physiologic and behavioral adaptation occur, leading to periods of minimal or no observable signs of pain. Lack of pain expression does not necessarily mean lack of pain.
• The pain rating scale preferred for use in daily clinical practice is the visual analog scale (VAS).	• The preferred pain rating scale depends on a patient's cognitive and physical ability, culture, developmental level, and availability.
• Cognitively impaired older adults are unable to use pain rating scales.	• When an appropriate pain rating scale is used and a patient is given sufficient time to process information and respond, many cognitively impaired older adults can use a pain rating scale.
• If patients hurt enough, they will tell you.	• Patients are often hesitant to report pain for fear of being labeled as complainers, hypochondriacs, or addicts.
• Psychosocial interventions alone will reduce or alleviate pain.	• Nonpharmacologic interventions are synergistic with medications but are not a substitute for pharmacologic management of pain.

Modified from Pasero C, McCaffery M: *Pain: assessment and pharmacological management*, St Louis, 2011, Mosby.

accurately determine a patient's pain and its impact. Knowing these factors will help you intervene effectively to manage your patient's pain.

Pain assessment tools, along with explanations of how to use them, are now available in many different languages (Pasero and McCaffery, 2011). Cultures vary in recognition of pain, expression of pain, when to seek treatment, and what treatments are desirable. For example, some cultures tend to be stoic, whereas others tend to be more expressive (Finley et al., 2009; Giordano et al., 2010).

Be sure to assess for cultural, ethnic, and genetic variations in tolerance and metabolism of analgesics and other medications (Manougian, 2010; Tennant, 2010). Be aware of cultural variables that may influence the operation of equipment such as PCA pumps. For example, Orthodox Jews may not use electrical equipment during the Sabbath and Holy Days; thus alternative methods of pain relief are needed during these times (Spector, 2008).

Explore a patient's beliefs about pain/discomfort. For example, cultures with a holistic worldview of health and illness mix religious/spiritual, natural (hot and cold), and the supernatural in their belief systems. When necessary use an interpreter to explain the pain tools and help a patient report the pain.

Safety Guidelines

1 Know a patient's medical history, type of therapies used, and medications, including over-the-counter (OTC) products. Many patients do not mention using these for fear of being criticized or because they do not want them taken away.

2 Patients currently receiving opioids for chronic pain often require higher doses of analgesics to alleviate new or increased pain; this is tolerance, not an early sign of addiction (see Box 15-4). Be aware of individualized dosages and ensure that all caregivers are aware of this individualization.

3 Drug-drug interactions, including enhanced or reduced effects or side effects, often occur with the multiple drug use required by people with chronic pain. This practice is termed *rational polypharmacy* or *multimodal analgesia* (Manougian, 2010; Pasero and McCaffery, 2011).

4 While 0 is an ideal goal for a pain level, in some chronic/persistent pain situations it is not realistic. Many patients are able to do most of the things they desire at a pain intensity of 1 or 2, even 3. If a patient's goal is above 3, reassess understanding of the pain scale.

BOX 15-5 | **Sedation Scale***

S = Sleep, easy to arouse
1 = Awake and alert
2 = Slightly drowsy, easily aroused
3 = Frequently drowsy, arousable, drifts off to sleep during conversation
4 = Somnolent, minimal-or-no response to physical stimulation

Remember—sedation precedes respiratory depression.
*Many institutional sedation scales include nursing actions to be taken for each level of sedation.
From Pasero C, McCaffery M: *Pain assessment and pharmacologic management,* St Louis, 2011, Mosby.

---

5 Communicate to the health care provider any significant changes in a patient's comfort level and need for changes in the pain-management regimen.

6 Know your agency policy for frequency of pain assessment and timing for follow-up assessments. The first 24 hours on opioids requires frequent assessment, at least every 4 hours.

7 Determine the safety of the equipment used for pain management. Correct programming of the PCA pump and correct functioning of any pump is vital for patient safety.

8 When using a PCA pump, the patient is the only person who should press the button to administer pain medication.

9 Respiratory depression can be a side effect of opioids, whether oral, intravenous, or epidural, and especially with opioid-naïve patients. Using a standard sedation scale can prevent respiratory depression by observing for and intervening for oversedation (Box 15-5).

SKILL 15-1   Providing Pain Relief

The assessment of pain aims to find the cause of a person's pain, identify his or her perception of pain, and determine the effect of pain on the individual. Accurate and factual pain assessment is necessary for determining a patient's response, arriving at a proper nursing diagnoses, and selecting appropriate therapies. A comprehensive pain assessment helps you understand the impact of pain on a patient's life (Hadjistavropoulos et al., 2009). Effectively managing a patient's pain does not necessarily mean eliminating it, but it does mean getting it to an acceptable level for him or her. Pain management requires you to work with a patient and family to prevent pain whenever possible and identify an acceptable intensity of pain and level of other factors, especially sleep, that allows maximum patient function.

The nursing process offers a systematic method for pain management that results in improved pain relief for most patients. This process recognizes distinct and unique differences in patient perceptions and responses to pain. The nursing process guides you in learning to know a patient and develop an individualized plan of care. The American Society for Pain Management Nursing (ASPMN) developed clinical practice guidelines for pain assessment and associated treatment principles (Herr et al., 2011).

Delegation and Collaboration

Assessment of a patient's pain cannot be delegated to nursing assistive personnel (NAP). The NAP may screen patients for pain and

provide selected nonpharmacologic strategies (e.g., back rubs, heat, cold, elevation) as instructed by the nurse. The nurse directs the NAP to:

- Eliminate environmental conditions that aggravate pain (e.g., an excessively warm, noisy room).
- Provide maximum rest periods; a written schedule for all to follow is ideal.
- Turn and place patients in a position of comfort at least every 2 hours or remind patients to turn themselves. Encourages patient to use a pillow for splinting if needed.
- Observe for behavioral signs of pain for a patient who is unable to self-report (see Box 15-2).
- Ask patient to report pain using the pain-intensity scale chosen by patient and nurse.
- Report in a timely manner any patient reports of pain intensity above predetermined goal and nonverbal behaviors suggestive of pain.
- Screen for pain during patient transfer or other activity that might provoke pain.

Equipment
❏ Pain rating scale (check agency policy)

STEP	RATIONALE

ASSESSMENT

1 Assess patient's risk for pain (e.g., those undergoing invasive procedures, anxious patients, those unable to communicate).

Allows you to anticipate patient's needs and intervene in a timely manner, possibly preventing pain.

2 Ask patients if they are in pain.

There is no objective test to measure pain.

Older adults and patients from various cultures may not admit to having pain. Try using other terms such as *hurt* or *discomfort*.

Accept patient's self-report of pain (APS, 2009; Pasero and McCaffery, 2011). Observe for nonverbal indicators of pain; ask significant others if they believe patient is in pain (Herr et al., 2011).

3 Assess patient's response to previous pharmacologic interventions, especially ability to function (e.g., sleeping, eating, and other activities of daily living [ADLs]).

Determines extent to which therapies have or have not been successful in the past (Gloth, 2011).

Determine if any analgesic side effects are likely based on medication and patient's previous responses (e.g., itching or nausea).

Some side effects, especially the itching that can occur with morphine, are often poorly tolerated by the patient and indicate a need to identify another analgesic.

4 Examine site of patient's pain or discomfort when possible. Inspect (discoloration, swelling, drainage), palpate (change in temperature, area of altered sensation, painful area, areas that trigger pain), and assess range of motion of involved joints. Percussion and auscultation can help to identify abnormalities (e.g., underlying mass or lung crackles) and determine cause of pain (Chapter 6). When assessing abdomen, always auscultate first and then inspect and palpate.

Reveals the nature of the pain and directs you toward appropriate interventions.

5 Assess physical, behavioral, and emotional signs and symptoms of pain:

Signs and symptoms may reveal source and nature of pain. Nonverbal responses to pain are useful in assessing pain in patients who are cognitively impaired or nonverbal.

  a Moaning, crying, whimpering, groaning, vocalizations

  b Decreased activity

  c Facial expressions (e.g., grimace, clenched teeth)

  d Change in usual behavior (e.g., less active, irritable)

  e Abnormal gait (e.g., shuffling) and posture (e.g., bent, leaning)

  f Guarding a body part

  g Diaphoresis

  h Increased blood glucose level reflecting stress of unrelieved pain

The stress of unrelieved pain causes the endocrine system to release excessive amounts of hormones (especially cortisol) and decreased levels of insulin (Pasero and McCaffery, 2011).

  i Decreased gastrointestinal (GI) motility, constipation, nausea, and vomiting

Signs and symptoms of pain originate from involvement of visceral organs with stimulation of the parasympathetic nervous system, which decreases GI tract activity (Drew and St. Marie, 2011).

  j Insomnia, anorexia, and fatigue

  k Depression, hopelessness, anger, fear, social withdrawal

Depression frequently occurs in patients with chronic pain and increases perception and intensity of pain (Drew and St. Marie, 2011).

  l Concomitant symptoms: Symptoms that often occur with pain (e.g., headache, constipation). Note: constipation can also develop from opioids.

Multiple symptoms increase complexity in care of patient.

> **Clinical Decision Point** *Physiologic responses (e.g., tachycardia, hypertension) to acute pain are of short duration and return to normal within minutes. Be aware that with persistent pain a patient does not usually exhibit physical signs and symptoms. Never use physiologic responses alone to determine pain therapy selected, even with acute pain (Pasero and McCaffery, 2011).*

6 Assess characteristics of pain. Follow agency policy regarding frequency of assessment. Use the PQRSTU pain assessment.

Guides clinician in collecting complete information about patient's pain experience.

  a Provocative/Palliative factors (e.g., "What makes your pain better or worse?"): Consider patient's experience with over-the-counter (OTC) drugs (including herbals and topicals) that have helped to reduce pain in the past.

Identifies the nature and source of pain and what patient uses to reduce discomfort. A combination of interventions is often the most effective approach to pain relief (APS, 2009).

  b Quality: Use open-ended questions such as "Tell me what your pain feels like."

Assists in determining underlying pain mechanism (e.g., somatic versus neuropathic pain).

STEP	RATIONALE
c Region/Radiation (e.g., "Show me everywhere your pain is."). Have patient use finger (if possible) to point out areas of pain.	Identify location of pain and possible causative factors for acute/transient pain.
d Severity: Use a valid pain rating scale appropriate to patient's age, developmental level, and comprehension (see illustrations). Ask patient to rate pain before any intervention. Also assess patient's pain when he or she is moving, not just lying in bed or sitting in a chair.	An appropriate pain rating scale is reliable, easily understood, and reflects changes in pain intensity (Herr, 2011).
e Timing: Ask patient if pain is constant, intermittent, continuous, or a combination. Does pain increase during specific times of the day, with particular activities, or in specific locations?	Environmental stimuli such as loud noises, bright lights, strong odors, or temperature extremes sometimes alter patient's response to pain.
f How is pain affecting *U* (patient) regarding ADLs, work, relationships, and enjoyment of life?	Provides important baseline information to later gauge effectiveness of interventions.

NURSING DIAGNOSES

- Activity intolerance
- Anxiety
- Deficient knowledge
- Disturbed sleep pattern
- Fatigue

- Fear
- Ineffective coping
- Chronic pain
- Impaired physical mobility

- Acute pain
- Powerlessness
- Readiness for enhanced comfort
- Risk for constipation

Related factors are individualized based on patient's condition or needs.

PLANNING

1 Expected outcomes following completion of procedure:

• Patient verbalizes full or partial relief from pain.	Patient's self-report of pain is single most reliable indicator of pain (Pasero and McCaffery, 2011).
• Patient displays nonverbal behaviors such as relaxed face and absence of squinting.	Nonverbal behaviors can be valid and reliable indicators of pain and pain relief in the cognitively impaired (Herr et al., 2011).
• Patient's sleep, nutrition, physical activity, and personal relationships improve.	Adequate pain relief usually permits patient to participate in usual ADLs.

IMPLEMENTATION

1 Perform hand hygiene and apply clean gloves if indicated.	Reduces transmission of microorganisms.
2 Identify patient using two identifiers (i.e., name and birthday or name and account number) according to agency policy. Compare identifiers in MAR/medical record with information on patient's identification bracelet and/or ask patient to state name.	Ensures correct patient. Complies with The Joint Commission standards and improves patient safety (TJC, 2012).
3 Prepare patient's environment. • Temperature suited to patient • Lighting • Sound • Eliminate unnecessary interruptions and coordinate care activities; allow for rest.	Temperature and sound extremes can enhance patient's perception of pain. Bright or very dim lighting can aggravate pain sensation. Fatigue increases pain perception.
4 Teach patient how to use pain rating scale. Explain range of intensity scores and how they relate to measure pain.	Accurate reporting by patient or family improves pain assessment and treatment.
5 Set pain-intensity goal with patient (when able).	Pain is unique to each individual. Patient sets individual goal for tolerable pain severity.
6 Prepare and administer pain-relieving medications per health care provider's order (see Chapter 20).	Analgesics are the cornerstone of pain management but should not be the only intervention.
7 Remove or reduce painful stimuli.	Reduction of pain stimuli and pressure receptors maximizes responses to pain-relieving interventions.
a Help patient turn and reposition to a comfortable position in good body alignment.	
b Smooth wrinkles in bed linens.	Reduces pressure and irritation to skin.
c Loosen any constrictive bandage (if appropriate to purpose of bandage) or loosen or remove device (e.g., blood pressure cuff, elastic hose, intravenous [IV] dressings, and identification band).	Bandage or device encircling extremity can restrict circulation and cause pain (see Chapter 39).
d Reposition underlying tubes or equipment.	

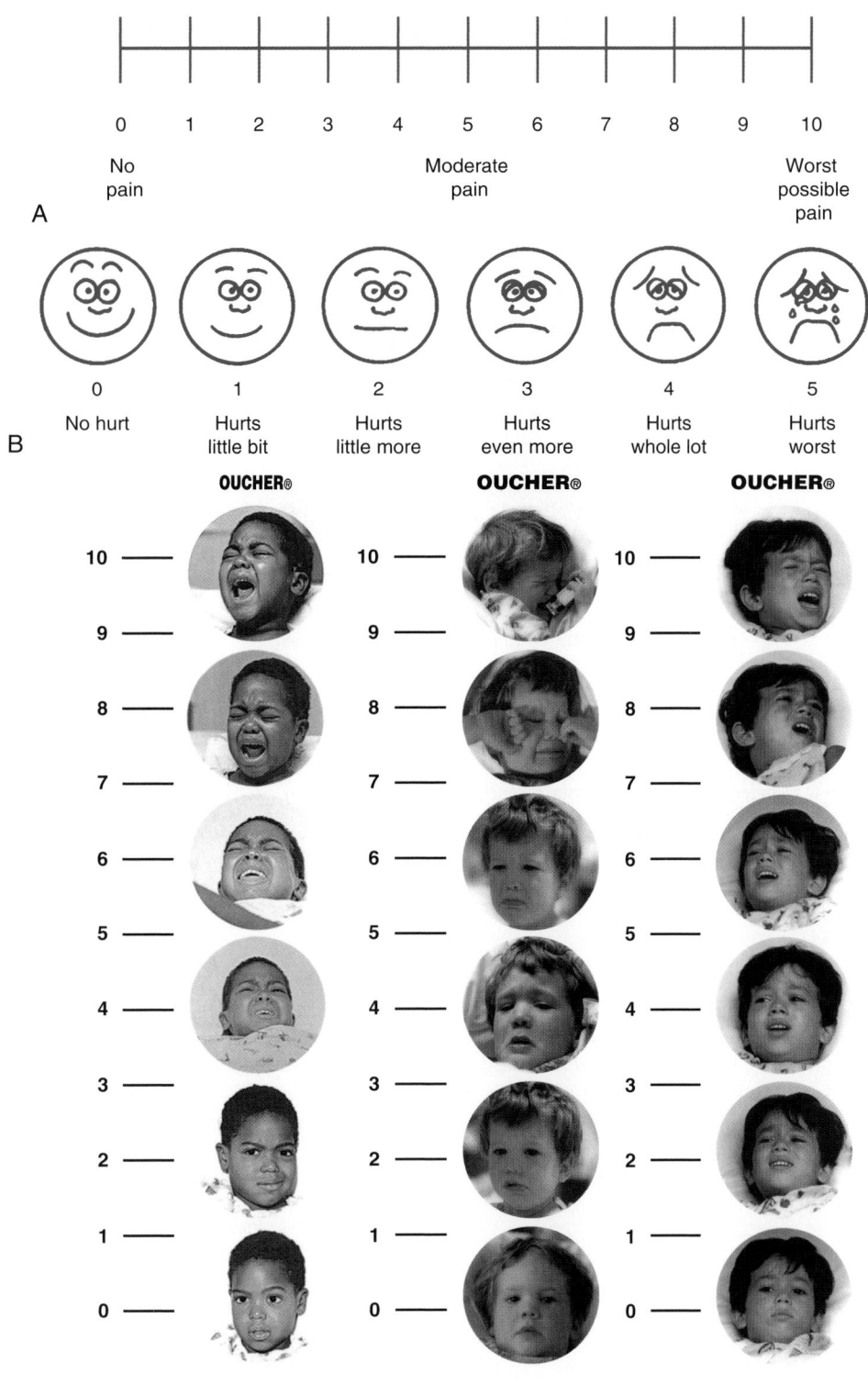

STEP 6d A, Pain rating scale. *From McCaffery M, Pasero C: Pain: clinical manual, ed 2, St Louis, 1999, Mosby.* **B,** Wong-Baker FACES pain rating scale. *From Wong DL et al.: Whaley and Wong's nursing care of infants and children, ed 7, St Louis, 2003, Mosby.* **C(1),** African-American version of Oucher pain scale. *Developed and copyrighted in 1990 by Mary J. Denyes, PhD, RN, Wayne State University and Antonia M. Villarruel, PhD, RN, University of Michigan. Cornelia P. Porter, PhD, RN, and Charlotta Marshall, RN, MSN, contributed to the development.* **C(2),** Caucasian version of Oucher pain scale. *Developed and copyrighted in 1983 by Judith E. Beyer, PhD, RN, University of Missouri-Kansas City School of Nursing, Kansas City, Mo.* **C(3),** Hispanic version of Oucher pain scale. *Developed and copyrighted in 1990 by Antonia M. Villarruel, PhD, University of Michigan, and Mary J. Denyes, PhD, RN, Wayne State University.*

STEP	RATIONALE
8 Teach patient how to splint over the site of pain using either a pillow or hand.	Splinting reduces pain by minimizing muscle movement.
a Explain purpose of splinting.	Promotes patient's cooperation.
b Place pillow or blanket over site of discomfort and help patient place hands firmly over area of discomfort (see illustration).	Splinting immobilizes painful area.

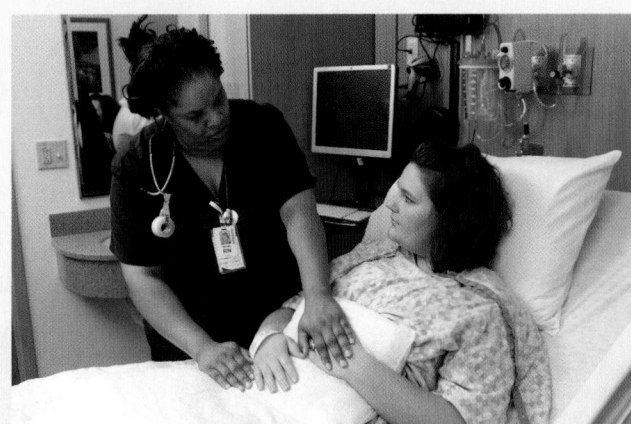

STEP 8b   Patient splinting painful area.

STEP	RATIONALE
c Have patient hold area firmly while coughing, deep breathing, and turning.	Splinting decreases movement and subsequent pain during activity.
9 Reduce or eliminate emotional factors that increase pain experiences.	Helps patients relax. Thoughts influence feelings, which change perception and behaviors, including a perception of pain relief (Baird et al., 2010).
a Offer information that reduces anxiety (e.g., explaining the cause of pain if known).	
b Offer patient opportunity to pray (if appropriate).	
c Spend time to allow patient to talk about pain.	
10 If used, remove and dispose of gloves. Perform hand hygiene.	Reduces transmission of microorganisms.

EVALUATION

1 Within 1 hour of an intervention (e.g., when the drug used is at its peak effect), ask patient to describe level of relief using a scale of 0 to 10.	Evaluates effectiveness of pain-relieving interventions in a timely manner (Pasero and McCaffery, 2011).
2 Compare patient's current pain with personally set pain-intensity goal.	Assists in determining appropriate changes to the pain-management plan.
3 Compare patient's ability to function and perform ADLs before and after pain interventions.	Contributes to determining effectiveness of pain-relieving interventions, especially in nonverbal patients (APS, 2009; Gloth, 2011; Herr et al., 2011).
4 Observe patient's nonverbal behaviors.	Determines effectiveness of pain-relieving interventions (Herr et al., 2011).
5 Evaluate for analgesic side effects.	Side effects of analgesics may be controlled by reducing the dose, increasing time intervals, or administering other medications (D'Arcy, 2008).

Unexpected Outcomes

1 Patient verbalizes continued pain that exceeds pain-intensity goal or displays nonverbal behavior reflecting worsening pain.

2 Patient experiences unexpected or adverse reaction to medication.

Related Interventions

- Perform a complete pain assessment.
- Implement nonpharmacologic pain relief measures.
- Ask family members what might be helpful.
- Notify health care provider.

- Assess unexpected effects on patient.
- Notify health care provider immediately.
- Be prepared to administer antidote if indicated (e.g., antiemetic, antihistamine, opioid-reversing agent such as naloxone [Narcan]).
- Monitor for effectiveness of antidote; antidote may have a shorter half-life than the opioid; a repeat dose of antidote may be needed.
- Complete adverse reaction documentation according to agency policy.

Recording and Reporting

- Record and report character of pain before intervention, therapies used, and patient response to interventions in nurses' notes and electronic health record (EHR).
- Record inadequate pain relief (not reaching goal), a reduction in patient function, adverse effects from pain interventions (pharmacologic and nonpharmacologic), and any patient or family education given.
- Report continued inadequate pain relief to health care provider.

Special Considerations
Teaching
- Review patient's and family's understanding of the pain rating scale used and how to use it when providing pain therapies.
- Explain to patient and family about behavioral changes that may result from pain (Elhoaris and Resnik, 2010).
- Ask patient and family about fear of addiction, a common primary concern, or other misconceptions that could undermine the patient's pain relief (see Table 15-1).

Pediatric
- Although validity and reliability scores of pain rating scales generally increase with age, you can use some rating scales with a child as young as 3 years of age (deTovar et al., 2010; Finley et al., 2009).
- Some children are reluctant to report pain because they have misconceptions about the cause of their pain or they fear the consequences (e.g., another painful procedure or an injection).
- Infants and children experience pain but respond to it differently than adults. For example, they cry and thrash about, have sleep disturbances, have a shortened attention span, suck or rock, refuse to eat or play, or are quiet and withdrawn. Variations in pain response are related to the child's personality, developmental level, and previous pain experiences (Hockenberry and Wilson, 2011).
- Parents are a helpful source of information when assessing a child's pain and planning pain-relief therapies. Most parents know how their child exhibits pain and which pain relief interventions have been successful (Riddell and Racine, 2009).
- Children with verbal skills can rate their level of pain on the Wong-Baker FACES pain rating scale or the Oucher pain scale (deTovar et al., 2010).

Gerontologic
- Many geriatric patients understand a categorical pain scale such as none, mild, moderate, severe more than they do a numeric scale (Deane and Smith, 2008; Pasero and McCaffery, 2011).
- Some older adults may require more time for you to explain the pain assessment scale that you select.
- Pain is not a natural occurrence of aging, although older adults are at risk for experiencing more pain-producing conditions.
- Nonverbal older adults experiencing pain typically receive fewer analgesics than similar patients who are able to report their pain (Hadjistavropoulos et al., 2009; Herr et al., 2011). Thus be sure your assessment is thorough and evaluate a patient's response critically.

Home Care
- Consider home conditions such as type of bed, stairs, and environmental stimuli. A supportive bed and quiet environment enhance sleep and promote pain management.
- Assess the pain-management attitudes of the primary home care provider (significant other) and provide necessary education to achieve successful pain control (Viclop et al., 2009).

SKILL 15-2 Patient-Controlled Analgesia

 Video Clip

Patient-controlled analgesia (PCA) is an interactive method of pain management that permits a patient control over pain through self-administration of analgesics (D'Arcy, 2008; Wells et al., 2008). It is a safe method of analgesic administration for acute and chronic pain, including conditions such as postoperative pain, cancer, and end-of-life pain. Commonly prescribed medications delivered via PCA include morphine sulfate, hydromorphone (Dilaudid), and fentanyl. PCA devices are individually programmed to automatically deliver a specific health care provider–prescribed continuous infusion (basal rate) of medication, a bolus dose (patient initiated), or both. PCA prevents overdosing by having a preprogrammed delay time or "lockout" (usually 6 to 16 minutes) between patient-initiated doses. In addition, the health care provider may limit the total amount of opioid that a patient receives in 1 to 4 hours. A patient depresses the button on a PCA device to deliver a regulated dose of analgesic. It is crucial that candidates for PCA be able to understand how, why, and when to self-administer the medication (APS and AAPM, 2009). Available routes of PCA administration include subcutaneous, intravenous (IV) (the most common), and epidural. Monitoring levels of sedation are essential with the use of PCA. This is especially true for patients who are "opioid naïve" (i.e., those who have never taken any opioids for any reason or who have not taken opioids in the past 5 weeks) (Pasero and McCaffery, 2011). In addition, oversedation is a risk in patients with sleep apnea (brief cessation of respirations during sleep) or obese patients with short, thick, necks who commonly have undiagnosed sleep apnea (see Box 15-5).

PCA has several advantages. It allows more constant serum levels of an opioid and avoids peaks and troughs of a large bolus. Patients receive better pain relief and fewer side effects from opioids because blood levels are maintained at a level of minimum effective analgesia concentration. Increased patient control and independence are other advantages for patients. Because PCA provides medication on demand, the total amount of opioid use can be reduced.

Concerns involving PCA use are patient related, pump failure, or health care provider errors. Patients may misunderstand how PCA therapy works, mistake the PCA button for a nurse call button, or have family members operate the demand button (Wells et al., 2008). A pump may fail to deliver a drug on demand, have a faulty alarm or low battery, or lack free-flow protection. Health care providers may incorrectly program a dose, concentration, or rate. Incorrect programming is the most common type of error. Other errors include failing to clamp or unclamp tubing, improperly loading syringe or cartridge, failing to monitor for side effects/overdose, and not responding to alarms (D'Arcy, 2008). PCA requires careful monitoring; never try to operate it without fully understanding the particular model in use.

Delegation and Collaboration
The skill of administration of PCA cannot be delegated to nursing assistive personnel (NAP). The nurse directs the NAP to:

- Immediately report any new symptom or change in patient status, including unrelieved pain or oversedation, to the nurse.
- Never administer a PCA dose for the patient.

Equipment
- ❏ PCA system and tubing
- ❏ Identification label and time tape (may come attached and completed by pharmacy)
- ❏ Needleless connector
- ❏ Alcohol swab
- ❏ Adhesive tape
- ❏ Clean gloves (when applicable)
- ❏ Equipment for vital signs and pulse oximeter, capnography (CO_2) monitoring equipment

STEP	RATIONALE

ASSESSMENT

1 Check accuracy and completeness of each MAR or computer printout with the health care provider's order for name of medication, dosage, frequency of medication (continuous or demand or both), and lockout settings. Verify that patient is not allergic to medication.	Requires health care provider's order required for opioid medication. Ensures that patient receives right medication. *This is the first check for accuracy.*

Clinical Decision Point *Nausea is not an allergic reaction and can be treated. Itching alone is not an allergic reaction but is a common side effect of opioids. Itching is also treatable and should not preclude use of PCA.*

2 Assess patient's cognitive and physical ability to press device button.	Determines if patient is able to use PCA for pain management.
3 Assess character of patient's pain, including physical, behavioral, and emotional signs and symptoms (see Skill 15-1).	Establishes baseline to determine patient's response to analgesia.
4 Obtain pulse oximetry or capnography reading.	Provides baseline of patient's oxygenation status for later determination of patient's response to analgesic.
5 Assess environment for factors that could contribute to pain (e.g., noise, temperature of room).	Elimination of irritating stimuli may be effective in reducing pain perception.
6 If patient has had surgery, apply clean gloves and inspect incision. Gently palpate around the area for tenderness. Use sterile gloves if placing hand directly on the incision.	Reveals evidence of tissue trauma or damage, which stimulates peripheral pain receptors to transmit impulses to cortex to create conscious awareness of pain (Drew and St. Marie, 2011).
7 When giving an IV, assess existing IV infusion line (peripheral or central) and surrounding tissue for patency and condition of site for infiltration or inflammation (see Chapter 28).	IV line must be patent with fluid infusing for medication to reach venous circulation safely and effectively. Never attach PCA to an IV line with blood running or to IV lines with incompatible drugs infusing. If necessary, start another IV site.
8 Assess patient's knowledge and effectiveness of previous pain-management strategies, especially previous PCA use.	Response to pain-control strategies helps to identify learning needs and affects patient's willingness to try therapy.

NURSING DIAGNOSES

• Activity intolerance	• Chronic pain	• Fear
• Acute pain	• Deficient knowledge regarding use of	• Ineffective coping
• Anxiety	PCA	• Impaired physical mobility

Related factors are individualized based on patient's condition or needs.

PLANNING

1 Expected outcomes following completion of procedure:	Drug is given safely and is effective in providing pain control.
• Patient verbalizes pain relief	Supports successful pain relief.
• Patient exhibits a relaxed facial expression and body position.	Nonverbal cues of pain relief
• Patient remains alert and oriented.	Indicates freedom from overly sedating effects of opioids. Sleepiness is usually from fatigue and not necessarily a sign of oversedation.
• Patient increasingly participates in self-care activities.	Suggests successful pain relief.
• Patient correctly operates PCA device.	Demonstrates safe and appropriate use of PCA device.
2 Explain purpose and demonstrate function of PCA to patient and family:	Effective explanations allow patient participation in care and independence in pain control (Pasero and McCaffery, 2011).

STEP	RATIONALE

IMPLEMENTATION

1 Perform hand hygiene.

2 Prepare analgesic while following the "six rights" for administration of medication (see Chapter 20). NOTE: Pharmacy prepares medication cartridge.

3 Identify patient using two identifiers (i.e., name and birthday or name and account number) according to agency policy. Compare identifiers in MAR/medical record with information on patient's identification bracelet and/or ask patient to state name.

4 At the bedside compare the MAR or computer printout with the name of medication on the drug cartridge. Have a second registered nurse (RN) confirm the health care provider's order and the correct setup of the PCA. The second RN should check the health care provider's order and the device independently and not just look at the existing setup.

5 Before initiating analgesia, explain purpose of PCA and demonstrate its function to patient and family, as follows:

  a Explain type of medication in PCA device.

  b Explain that the device safely administers self-initiated small but frequent amounts of medication prn to provide comfort and minimize side effects from analgesia. Tell patient that self-dosing before repositioning, walking, or coughing and deep breathing will help in performing activities.

  c Explain that device is programmed to deliver ordered type and dose of pain medication, lockout interval, and 1- to 4-hour dosage limits. Explain how lockout time prevents overdose.

  d Demonstrate to patient how to push medication demand button on PCA device.

  e Instruct patient to notify a nurse for possible side effects, problems in attaining pain relief, changes in severity or location of pain, alarms sounding, or questions.

6 Check infuser and patient-control module for accurate labeling or evidence of leaking.

7 Program computerized PCA pump as ordered to deliver prescribed medication dose and lockout interval.

8 Insert drug cartridge into infusion device (see illustration) and prime tubing.

9 Apply clean gloves. Attach needleless adapter to tubing adapter of PCA module.

10 Wipe injection port of main IV line with alcohol.

Reduces transmission of microorganisms and possible infection.

Ensures safe and appropriate medication administration. *This is the second check for accuracy.*

Ensures correct patient. Complies with The Joint Commission standards and improves patient safety (TJC, 2012).

Ensures that the correct patient receives the right medication. *This is the third check for accuracy.*

Thorough explanation allows patient participation in care and independence in pain control. Preoperative education about PCA improves postoperative pain relief (D'Arcy, 2011).

Helps patient understand how to control pain effectively. Small, frequent dosing with PCA produces a constant serum drug level with minimal fluctuation (Lehne, 2011).

Confirms with patient the safety of the PCA device.

Gives patient control of pain.

Ensures that you respond to problems that arise.

Avoids medication error and injury to patient.

Ensures safe, therapeutic drug administration.

Locks system and prevents air from infusing into IV tubing.

Prevents transmission of microorganisms. Connects device with IV line.

Alcohol is a topical antiseptic that minimizes entry of surface microorganisms during needle insertion.

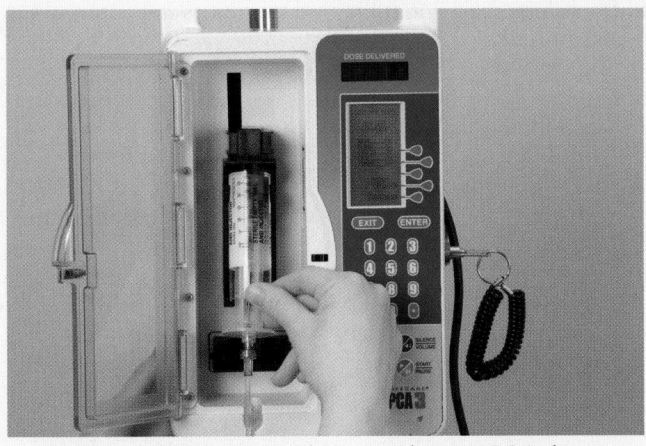

STEP 8 Nurse inserting drug cartridge into PCA device.

STEP	RATIONALE
11 Insert needleless adapter into injection port nearest patient.	Establishes route for medication to enter main IV line.
12 Secure connection with tape and anchor PCA tubing. Label PCA tubing and remove gloves.	Prevents dislodging needleless adapter from port. Label prevents errors from connecting tubing from different device to PCA (TJC, 2012).
13 Administer loading dose of analgesia if prescribed.	A one-time dose (bolus) may be given manually by you or programmed into PCA pump.
14 If patient is experiencing pain currently, have him or her demonstrate use of PCA system (see illustration); if not, have patient verbally repeat instructions given earlier.	Repeating instructions reinforces learning. Return demonstration reveals patient's understanding and ability to manipulate device.

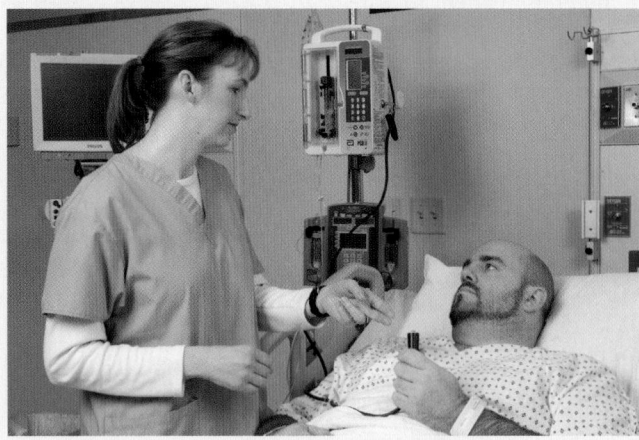

STEP 14   Patient learns to press PCA device button.

15 To discontinue PCA: **a** Obtain necessary PCA information from pump for documentation, including amount infused and amount to discard.	Two RNs must witness wastage of opioids (narcotics) and sign the record to meet requirements of the Federal Controlled Substances Act for scheduled drugs.
b Perform hand hygiene. Apply clean gloves. Turn pump off. Disconnect PCA tubing from IV maintenance line but maintain IV access.	Ensures continued IV therapy.
c Dispose of empty cartridge according to agency policy. Remove gloves and discard. Perform hand hygiene.	Controlling and dispensing opioids are regulated by the Federal Controlled Substances Act.

EVALUATION

1 Have patient use pain rating scale to evaluate pain intensity following treatments, procedures, and according to agency policy.	Determines response to PCA dosing.
2 Monitor patient's level of sedation, vital signs, and pulse oximetry or capnography every 1 to 2 hours for the first 12 hours (APS and AAPM, 2009).	Oversedation precedes respiratory depression.
3 Observe patient for adverse reactions, especially excessive sedation.	Serious problems require immediate action; oversedation can lead to life-threatening respiratory depression and must be treated.
4 Have patient demonstrate dose delivery.	Evaluates skill in use of PCA.
5 Evaluate number of attempts (number of times patient pushed button); delivery of demand doses (number of times drug actually given); and basal dose, if ordered, according to agency policy (usually every 4 to 8 hours).	Assists in evaluating effectiveness of PCA dose and frequency in relieving pain. Maintains compliance with Federal Controlled Substances Act.

Unexpected Outcomes	Related Interventions
1 Patient verbalizes continued or worsening discomfort or displays nonverbal behaviors indicative of pain.	• Perform complete pain reassessment. • Assess for possible complications other than pain. • Inspect IV site for possible catheter occlusion or infiltration. • Evaluate number of attempts and deliveries initiated by patient. • Check that maintenance IV fluid is running continuously. • Evaluate pump for operational problems. • Consult with health care provider.
2 Patient is sedated and not easily aroused.	• Stop PCA. • Notify health care provider. • Elevate head of bed 30 degrees unless contraindicated. • Instruct patient to take deep breaths. • Apply oxygen at 2 L/min per nasal cannula (if ordered). • Assess vital signs. • Evaluate amount of opioid delivered within past 4 to 8 hours. • Ask family members if they pressed the button without patient's knowledge. • Review MAR for other possible sedating drugs. • Prepare to administer an opioid-reversing agent. • Observe patient frequently (APS, 2009).
3 Patient unable to manipulate PCA device to maintain pain control.	• Consult with health care provider regarding alternative medication route or possibly a basal (continuous dose). • If agency allows, assess patient support system for significant other who can responsibly manipulate PCA device (Pasero and McCaffery, 2011).

Recording and Reporting

• Record drug, concentration, dose (basal and/or demand), time started, lockout time, and amount of IV solution infused and remaining solution. Many agencies have special PCA documentation forms.
• Record regular assessment of patient response to analgesia on PCA medication form, in nurses' notes and EHR, on pain assessment flow sheet, or on other documentation according to agency policy. This includes vital signs, oximetry or capnography, sedation status, pain rating, status of vascular access site.

Teaching Considerations

• Give instructions during pain-free or pain-reduced states and before initiating therapy. Instruct surgical patients before surgery.
• Encourage patients to push button on timing unit at the earliest indication of pain. Teach preemptive pain management.
• Explain regimen to family so they can support and help patient (but not push button for patient).
• Inform patient of nonpharmacologic pain-management strategies that supplement or enhance pharmacologic intervention (see Skill 15-5).
• Inform patient and family that patient will not overdose with PCA if only the patient pushes the button.

Pediatric Considerations

• PCA is an effective means of pain control in children who can understand the concept. When selecting children for PCA use, consider a patient's developmental level, cognitive level, and motor skills. Ordinarily PCA use is safe and effective for patients as young as 5 years old (deTovar et al., 2010). From a developmental perspective, use of PCA is particularly effective with adolescents because it leads to feelings of control.
• Some agencies have provided specific guidelines and training to allow parents to push the button for children too young or unable to use the device on their own.
• Pharmacologic pain support is safe and effective in pediatric patients when dose is calibrated according to child's weight (Klieber et al., 2011).
• There are no reports of addiction secondary to the use of PCA in pediatric patients (APS and AAPM, 2009). Untreated pain in children may also become chronic.

Gerontologic Considerations

• Older patients sometimes appear more sensitive to analgesics and experience more opioid side effects (D'Arcy, 2009; Deane and Smith, 2008; Gloth, 2011). Older adults' reduced renal and liver function slows opioid metabolism and excretion. This causes a faster peak effect and a longer duration of action of the opioid. Dosages should be started low and titrated upward slowly until pain relief is achieved (Drew and St. Marie, 2011; Gloth, 2011).
• If patient confusion occurs while using PCA, call to get orders to lower the dose, lengthen the lockout, or add a nonopioid analgesic to reduce the opioid dose; nurse-activated around-the-clock dosing is another alternative; refusing to medicate is not the answer; confusion may be caused by pain, not the medications (D'Arcy, 2009; Pasero & McCaffery, 2011).

SKILL 15-3   Epidural Analgesia

Administration of analgesics into the epidural space is an efficient intervention to manage acute pain during labor; following surgery; and for chronic pain, especially for patients with cancer (D'Arcy, 2011). Epidural analgesia is effective during labor and does not result in any adverse effects or increased frequency of cesarean delivery (Gerli et al., 2011; James, 2011). Patient-controlled epidural analgesia (PCEA) has been shown to provide excellent postoperative pain control when compared with intravenous (IV) patient-controlled analgesia (PCA) (Ferguson et al., 2009). Use of PCEA is safe and efficient, and complications from this technique are rare. Epidural opioids reduce the total amount of opioid medication required to control pain and thus produce fewer opioid-related side effects (D'Arcy, 2011).

The epidural space is a potential space that contains a network of vessels, nerves, and fat located between the vertebral column and the dura mater, the outermost meninges covering the spinal cord (Fig. 15-1). Analgesics delivered into this space distribute by (1) diffusion through the dura mater into the cerebrospinal fluid (CSF), where they act directly on the receptors in the dorsal horn of the spinal cord; (2) blood vessels in the epidural space and deliver systemically; and/or (3) absorption by fat in the epidural space, creating a depot where the analgesia is slowly released systemically. An analgesic acts by binding to opiate receptors in the dorsal horn of the spinal column, thus blocking pain impulse transmission to the cerebral cortex.

Opioids and local anesthetics, separately or in combination, are often used in epidural analgesia. Opioids are delivered close to their site of action (central nervous system) and thus require much smaller doses to achieve the same pain relief (D'Arcy, 2009; D'Arcy, 2011). Common opioids administered epidurally include morphine, hydromorphone (Dilaudid), fentanyl, and sufentanil. These opioids differ by their lipophilic "fat-loving" and hydrophilic "water-loving" properties, which affect absorption rate and duration of action. Fentanyl and sufentanil are fat-loving, causing them to have a quicker onset and shorter duration of action (2 hours). Morphine and hydromorphone are water-loving, resulting in longer onset and duration of action (24 hours).

A patient should be placed in the lateral side-lying or sitting position with the shoulders and hips in alignment and the hips and head flexed during insertion of an epidural catheter. An anesthesia provider places a catheter into the epidural space below the second lumbar vertebra, where the spinal cord ends (Fig. 15-2). However, epidurals may also be placed at the thoracic level of the spinal cord. Catheters intended for temporary or short-term use are not sutured in place and exit from the insertion site on the back. A catheter intended for permanent or long-term use is "tunneled" subcutaneously and exits on the side of the body (Fig. 15-3) or on the abdomen. Tunneling reduces infection and catheter dislodgement. A sterile occlusive dressing covers the catheter exit site and is secured to the patient. An x-ray film is the only way to confirm epidural catheter placement.

A health care provider administers epidural medication intermittently via a bolus or a patient can inject intermittently on demand (PCEA) through a pump. An epidural infusion can also be given continuously via a controlled delivery system such as an implanted infusion pump (Fig. 15-4) (D'Arcy, 2011). The use of epidural opioids requires astute nursing observation and care. The catheter poses a threat to patient safety because of its anatomic location, its potential for migration through the dura, and its proximity to spinal nerves and vessels (Pasero and McCaffery, 2011). Catheter migration into the subarachnoid space can produce dangerously high medication levels. Monitor a patient's motor and sensory function, including any onset of urinary retention. You should not administer other supplemental opioids or sedatives when patients are on an epidural because the combined effect may cause respiratory depression. In many health care agencies anesthesiologists and nurse anesthetists are the only health care providers who may initiate epidural opioid infusions or administer a medication bolus.

Delegation and Collaboration

The skill of epidural analgesia administration cannot be delegated to nursing assistive personnel (NAP). The nurse directs the NAP to:

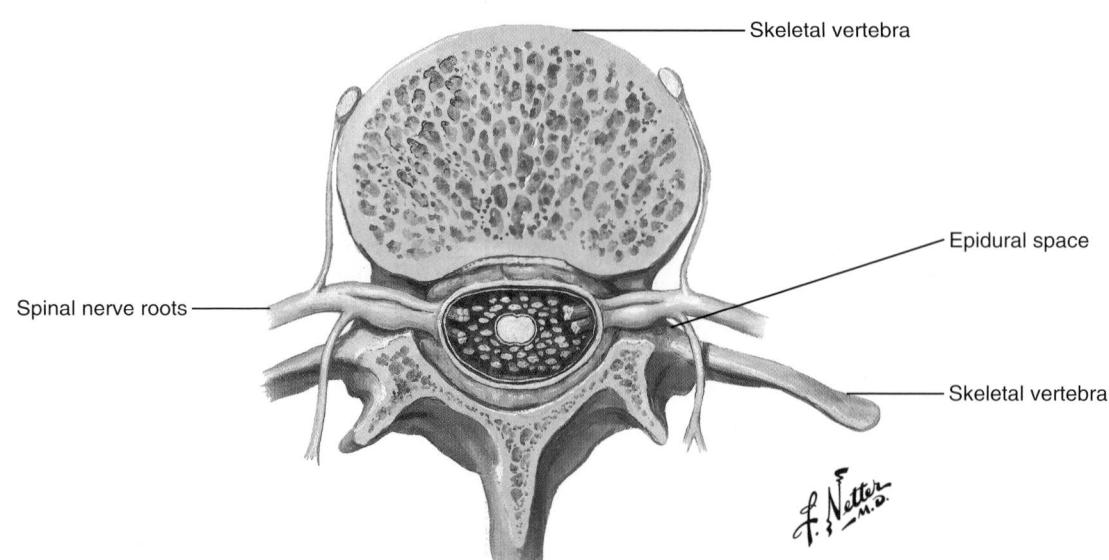

FIG 15-1   Anatomic drawing of epidural space. (*Reprinted from www.netterimages.com © Elsevier, Inc. All rights reserved.*)

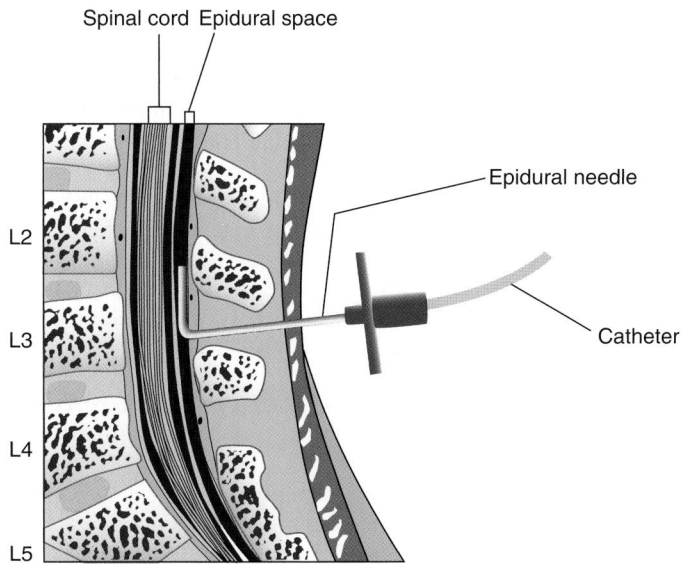

FIG 15-2 Placement of epidural catheter.

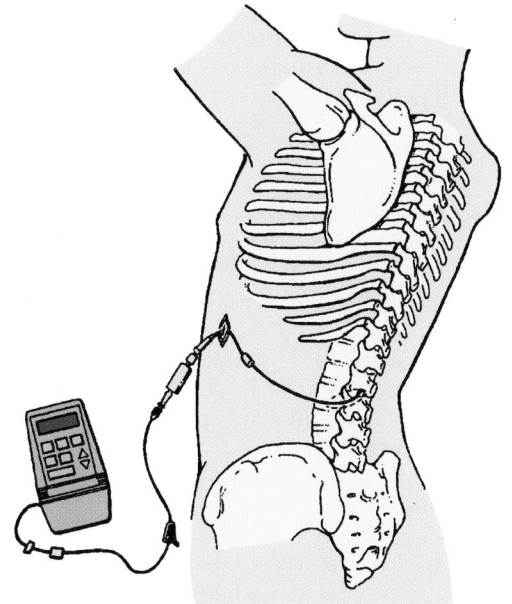

FIG 15-3 Epidural catheter attached to ambulatory infusion pump. (*Image courtesy Astra Zeneca Pharmaceuticals, Wilmington, Del. All rights reserved.*)

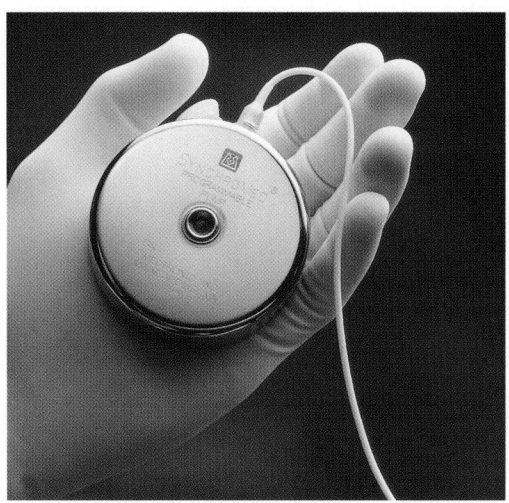

FIG 15-4 SynchroMed implantable pump. (*Courtesy Medtronic, Inc., Columbia Heights, Minn. All rights reserved.*)

- Pay particular attention to the insertion site when repositioning or ambulating patients to prevent catheter disruption.
- Avoid pulling patient up in bed while he or she is lying flat on the back, which can dislodge the epidural catheter.
- Immediately report to the nurse any change in level of consciousness.
- Report any catheter disconnection immediately.
- Immediately report to the nurse any change in patient status or comfort level.

Equipment
- ❏ Clean gloves
- ❏ Sterile gloves (if removing epidural dressing)
- ❏ Prediluted preservative-free opioid as prescribed by health care provider for use in IV infusion pump (usually prepared by pharmacy)
- ❏ Infusion pump and compatible tubing (Do not use Y-ports for infusion; some infusion pumps have color-coded tubing for intraspinal use)
- ❏ Anti-bacterial filter
- ❏ Tape
- ❏ Label (for injection port)
- ❏ Equipment for vital signs and pulse oximetry, or capnography (see agency policy)

STEP	RATIONALE

ASSESSMENT

1 Assess if patient has completed informed consent and is aware of risk/benefits of epidural analgesia (See agency policy).

Epidural analgesia is a significant procedure with specific and potentially serious complications, requiring informed consent.

2 Assess level of patient's comfort and character of patient's pain (see Skill 15-1).

Establishes baseline pain level.

3 Assess presenting medical/surgical condition and appropriateness for epidural analgesia (e.g., major abdominal or thoracic surgery, women in labor, advanced cancer, and patients predisposed to cardiopulmonary complications from preexisting medical conditions or surgery). Consult with health care provider on findings.

Certain conditions make epidural analgesia the treatment of choice.

STEP	RATIONALE
4 For cognitively impaired or non-English–speaking patients, assess nonverbal pain responses.	Cognitively impaired patients or patients for whom English is a second language may have difficulty understanding the therapy, especially if PCEA is used. Nonverbal responses provide baseline pain assessment.
5 Check to see if patient recently received anticoagulants.	Recent anticoagulation may contraindicate the placement of epidural catheter because of risk for epidural site hematoma (Pasero and McCaffery, 2011).
6 Assess if patient routinely takes herbal medications; document the complete list.	Some herbal medications interfere with the clotting mechanism (e.g., ginkgo biloba, ginseng, ginger). Currently there is no contraindication to their use (NIH, 2011).

Clinical Decision Point *Contraindications to epidural analgesia include coagulopathies, abnormal clotting test results, history of multiple abscesses, and sepsis. Additional contraindications include skeletal or spinal abnormalities (Pasero and McCaffery, 2011).*

STEP	RATIONALE
7 Assess for history of drug allergies.	Avoids placing patient at risk for allergic reaction.
8 Assess patient's sedation level by assessing level of wakefulness or alertness, ability to follow commands, and drowsiness (see Box 15-5).	Establishes a baseline before first dose. Sedation always precedes respiratory depression from opioids.
9 Assess rate, pattern, and depth of respirations; pulse oximetry; and blood pressure (see Chapter 5).	Establishes baseline. Vasodilation can occur, causing hypotension, including orthostatic hypotension. Respiratory depression may also occur.
10 Assess initial motor and sensory function of lower extremities (see Chapter 6). Test sensation in lower extremities. Have patient flex both feet and knees and raise each leg off the bed. Pay special attention to patients with preexisting sensory or motor abnormalities.	Establishes a baseline. Monitoring of motor and sensory function ensures that neural blockage does not affect motor function (D'Arcy, 2011).

Clinical Decision Point *For all patients on PECA assess for muscle impairment (e.g., sensation or strength) before ambulation or transfer (D'Arcy, 2011).*

STEP	RATIONALE
11 Verify that catheter is secured to patient's skin from the back, side, or front.	Prevents catheter dislodgement or migration.
12 Assess catheter insertion site for redness, warmth, tenderness, swelling, and drainage. Apply sterile gloves when removing occlusive dressing.	Catheter sites are at risk for local infections. Purulent drainage is a sign of infection. Clear drainage may indicate CSF leaking from punctured dura. Bloody drainage may indicate that catheter entered blood vessel.
13 Verify health care provider's order against MAR for name of medication, dosage, route, infusion method (bolus, continuous, or demand), and lockout settings.	Ensures that right drug is administered to patient. *This is the first check for accuracy.*
14 Check patency of IV tubing and check infusion pump for proper calibration and operation. Keep IV line patent for 24 hours after epidural analgesia has ended.	Kinked or clamped tubing will interrupt analgesic infusion; may cause clotting at end of IV catheter and require replacement. Patent IV line allows IV access in case medications are needed to counteract adverse reactions.

NURSING DIAGNOSES

- Activity intolerance
- Anxiety
- Deficient knowledge regarding epidural analgesia
- Acute pain
- Chronic pain
- Impaired physical mobility
- Risk for infection
- Risk for injury

Related factors are individualized based on patient's condition or needs.

PLANNING

1 Expected outcomes following completion of procedure: • Patient verbalizes pain relief within 30 to 60 minutes of initiating epidural infusion.	Indicates that drug and dose are effective in relieving pain, catheter is intact, and equipment is functioning properly in compliance with health care provider's order.
• Patient has no headache during epidural infusion or after discontinuation.	Indicates that catheter is in epidural space. No CSF leakage.
• Patient remains normotensive, and heart rate remains at or above baseline.	Indicates absence of some of the side effects of epidural opioids.

STEP	RATIONALE
• Patient is alert, oriented, and easily aroused.	Indicates absence of excessive sedation/oversedation (see Box 15-5).
• Patient's respirations are regular, of adequate depth, and equal to or greater than 8 breaths/min. Pulse oximetry is within normal range.	Indicates adequate ventilation and reduced risk for respiratory depression from opioids (Maddox et al., 2008).
• Patient voids without difficulty; averages a minimum of 30 mL/hr.	Indicates absence of urinary retention (a potential side effect of opioid medications).
• Patient has no or minimal pruritus and no paresthesias of lower extremities.	Indicates absence of potential side effect of epidural medications.
• Epidural system remains intact and functioning.	Infusion system is patent; no interruption in medication delivery to epidural space.
2 Explain purpose and function of epidural analgesia and expectations of patient during procedure (e.g., ask patient to call for assistance before getting out of bed).	Proper explanation enhances patient cooperation and assists with effective results (Elhoaris and Resnik, 2010).

IMPLEMENTATION	RATIONALE
1 Place patients receiving epidural analgesia close to the nurses' station.	Ensures close supervision during infusion (Rowbotham et al., 2010).
2 Prepare analgesic, following "six rights" for administration of medications (see Chapter 21). Note: Pharmacy prepares medication for pump. In the case of a bolus injection, draw up prediluted, preservative-free opioid solution through filter needle into syringe.	Ensures safe and appropriate medication administration. *This is the second check for accuracy.*
3 Identify patient using two identifiers (i.e., name and birthday or name and account number, according to facility policy). Compare identifiers with information on patient's medication administration record (MAR) or medical record.	Ensures correct patient. Complies with The Joint Commission standards and improves patient safety (TJC, 2013).
4 Explain purpose and function of epidural analgesia and expectations of patient during procedure (e.g., having patient call for assistance to get out of bed). Demonstrate to patient how to use pump on demand.	Proper explanation of therapy enhances patient cooperation.
5 Attach an "epidural line" label to the epidural infusion tubing. Be sure that there are no Y ports on the tubing. Epidural infusions should be labeled 'For Epidural Use Only".	Labeling helps to ensure that analgesic is administered into correct line and the epidural space. Labeling of high-risk catheters prevents connection with an inappropriate tube or catheter (TJC, 2006). The epidural infusion system between pump and patient should be considered as closed, with no injection or Y ports (Rowbotham, 2010).
6 At the bedside compare the MAR or computer printout with the name of medication on the drug container.	*This is the third check for accuracy* and ensures that the right patient receives right medication.
7 Perform hand hygiene and apply clean gloves.	
8 Administer epidural analgesic.	
a Administer continuous infusion.	
(1) Attach container of diluted preservative-free medication to infusion pump tubing and prime the tubing (see Chapter 22).	Tubing filled with solution and free of air bubbles avoids an air embolus.
(2) Insert tubing into infusion pump (see Chapter 23) and attach distal end of tubing to antibacterial filter, and then connect to epidural catheter (Rowbotham et al., 2010).	Pump propels fluid through tubing. Filter reduces entrance of microorganisms into infusion line.
(3) Check infusion pump for proper calibration, setting and operation. Many agencies have two nurses check settings.	Ensures that patient is receiving proper dosing.
(4) Tape all connections. Start infusion (see Chapter 22).	Taping maintains a secure closed system to prevent infection.
b Administer bolus dose of analgesic via infusion pump.	
(1) Perform steps 8a (1)-(4). Adjust infusion pump setting for pre-set limit for maximum bolus size. Initiate pump to deliver ordered bolus.	Prevents accidental infusion of an over dose.

STEP	RATIONALE
c Administer dose on demand. Refer to Skill 13.3 for preparation of patient to be able to initiate intermittent dose from pump. Perform steps 8a(1)-(4). Set pump for lock out time (as ordered). (1) Have patient initiate demand dose as needed	Gives patient control over administration of analgesic.
9 Explain that nurses will monitor patient's response to epidural analgesic routinely. Also instruct patient on signs or problems to report to nurse.	Builds trust to encourage patient to be a partner in care.
10 Remove and dispose of gloves. Perform hand hygiene.	Reduces transmission of microorganisms.
11 Before removal of epidural catheter, check for presence of therapeutic anticoagulation. Check agency policy for removal while patient is receiving anticoagulation therapy.	Removal of epidural catheter while patient is anticoagulated increases risk for spinal hematoma because of anticoagulation and inability to compress vessels.

EVALUATION

1 Evaluate patient's comfort level using a pain rating scale of 0 to 10.	Evaluates effectiveness of epidural infusion.
2 Evaluate sedation level: respiratory rate, rhythm, depth, and pattern; and pulse oximetry or capnography based on patient's clinical condition. Generally measured more frequently in the first 12 hours of infusions (e.g. hourly) (see agency policy), after bolus infusions or changes of infusion rate, and in periods of cardiovascular or respiratory instability (Rowbotham et al., 2010).	Oversedation occurs before respiratory depression and should be closely monitored to prevent respiratory depression (Maddox et al., 2008; Pasero and McCaffery, 2011).
3 Monitor blood pressure and pulse. Assist patient when changing positions to avoid postural hypotension.	Postural hypotension, vasodilation, and heart rate changes may occur from pain or medication side effects (Pasero and McCaffery, 2011).
4 Monitor intake and output. Assess for bladder distention. Observe for frequency or urgency of urination.	Urinary retention may occur as a result of effects of medication on spinal nerves innervating the bladder.
5 Observe for pruritus, especially of face, head, neck, and torso. Inform patient that this is a side effect but is often not an allergic response.	Pruritus *alone* is rarely an allergy to opioids (Pasero and McCaffery, 2011).
6 Observe for nausea and vomiting and presence of headache.	Nausea from epidural analgesia worsens by movement. Headache and CSF fluid leakage may occur from a dural puncture.
7 Evaluate catheter insertion site every 2 to 4 hours for redness, warmth, tenderness, swelling, or drainage. Note character of drainage (e.g., bloody, clear, or purulent).	Bloody drainage may occur if catheter has migrated into a vessel. Report immediately and treat as an emergency (Pasero and McCaffery, 2011).
8 Evaluate for motor weakness or numbness and tingling of lower extremities (paresthesias).	Reducing epidural dose may help eliminate unwanted motor and sensory deficits (Pasero and McCaffery, 2011).
9 Inspect site for disruption or displacement of catheter.	

Unexpected Outcomes	Related Interventions
1 Patient states that pain is still present or has increased. Primary causes are insufficient drug dose or catheter blockage, breakage, or improper position.	• Check all tubing, connections, medication doses, and pump settings. • Report to health care provider adequacy of medication dose.
2 Patient is sedated or not easily aroused.	• Stop epidural infusion and elevate patient's head of bed 30 degrees (unless contraindicated). • Prepare to administer opioid-reversing agent per health care provider's order. • Monitor all vital signs, pulse oximetry, and sedation level continuously until patient is easily aroused.
3 Patient experiences periods of apnea; or respirations are less than 8 breaths/min, shallow, or irregular.	• Instruct patient to take deep breaths. • Notify health care provider. • Prepare to administer opioid-reversing agent such as naloxone (Narcan) per health care provider's order (agency procedure manual may have protocol). • Monitor at least every 30 minutes until respirations are at least 8 or more per minute and of adequate depth for 2 hours.

4 Patient reports sudden headache. Clear drainage is present on epidural dressing, or more than 1 mL of fluid is aspirated from catheter. Possible indication that catheter has migrated into the subarachnoid space.	• Stop infusion. • Notify health care provider.
5 Blood is present on epidural dressing or aspirated from the catheter. Probable indication that catheter has punctured a blood vessel.	• Stop infusion. • Notify health care provider.
6 Redness, warmth, tenderness, swelling, exudate is noted at catheter insertion site. Patient is febrile. These are signs and symptoms of infection.	• Notify health care provider.
7 Patient experiences minimal urinary output, urinary frequency or urgency, bladder distention, pruritus, or nausea and vomiting.	• Consult with health care provider about reducing the dose of opioid and discuss treatment for side effects.

Reporting and Recording

- Record drug, dose, method (bolus, demand, or continuous), and time given (if injection) or time begun and ended (if demand or continuous) on appropriate medication record. Specify concentration and diluent.
- With continuous or demand infusion, obtain and record pump readout hourly for first 24 hours after infusion begins and then every 4 hours. Review pump settings and usage together with staff coming on the next shift.
- Record regular periodic assessments of patient's status in nurses' notes, in EHR, and/or on appropriate flow sheet, including vital signs, pulse oximetry, intake and output (I&O), sedation level, pain severity score, neurologic status, appearance of epidural site, presence or absence of adverse reactions to medication, and presence or absence of complications resulting from placement and maintenance of epidural catheter (Pasero and McCaffery, 2011).
- Report any adverse reactions or complications to health care provider immediately.

Teaching Considerations

- Describe catheter placement and use to patient as appropriate. Drawing or showing pictures often helps.
- Teach patient and family members the purpose, action, and signs and symptoms of adverse reactions to opioid or local anesthetic. Teach when and which signs and symptoms to report to a nurse.
- Teach patient to report pain level with acceptable (to patient) pain scale.
- Inform patient of other pain-management strategies that supplement or enhance pharmacologic intervention (e.g., imagery, distraction, relaxation) (Allred et al., 2010; NIH, 2011).
- Some patients may attempt to ambulate without assistance or overdo other activities. Caution them to begin slowly to avoid injury and to always call for nurse to assist with any activity.

Explain that the first attempt to ambulate may feel strange secondary to decreased sensation, but motor (leg) function should be unaffected.

Pediatric Considerations

- Apply EMLA cream to the epidural site a minimum of 60 minutes before catheter insertion.
- Epidural analgesia can be used in selected situations (Hockenberry and Wilson, 2011).

Gerontologic Considerations

- Older adults are at the same risk for complications and medication adverse effects as other adult patients (Deane and Smith, 2008).

Home Care Considerations

- Patients needing long-term therapy are discharged with a tunneled catheter. Before considering catheter placement and care in the home, assess patient's fine-motor skills, cognitive ability, stage of disease and prognosis, and degree of involvement of family caregiver.
- Teach patient and caregiver proper dosage and administration of medication. Evaluating patient's technique for catheter care, administering medication, and reinforcing instructions are priorities.
- Teach patient and caregiver aseptic technique for medication administration as needed and for all catheter care procedures, including dressing changes. Instruct patient to change dressing every week (policy varies with home care agency). Teach signs and symptoms of infection and instruct patient to report to nurse or health care provider immediately should signs and symptoms appear.
- Teach patient and caregiver about signs and symptoms of adverse reactions to medication being used and interventions to alleviate mild side effects in the home.
- Give patient and family phone numbers of health care providers to contact in emergency and resources in the community.

SKILL 15-4 Local Anesthetic Infusion Pump for Analgesia

During surgery for joint replacement some surgeons insert a one-way catheter into the surgical site and attach it to an infusion pump (Fig. 15-5). The pump delivers a local anesthetic (e.g., bupivacaine [Marcaine], lidocaine, ropivacaine [Naropin], or mepivacaine [Carbocaine]) directly into the wound bed to provide pain relief to the surgical site. Patients may still require oral analgesics, but the total dosage is often reduced (ISMP, 2011). The pump has a demand (4 to 6 mL/bolus) and a continuous (basal) rate (2 to 4 mL/hr) feature. Continuous flow reservoirs hold 100 mL, whereas patient-controlled units have a 60-mL reservoir. The device is one-time use only and usually remains in place for about 48 hours.

Rarely is the pump removed during hospitalization. Patients learn how to remove the catheter at home. Nursing care focuses on assessment of catheter site and connections, evaluation of local anesthetic side effects, and patient teaching.

Delegation and Collaboration

The skill of managing local anesthetic infusion pump analgesia cannot be delegated to nursing assistive personnel (NAP). The nurse directs the NAP to:

- Pay close attention to the insertion site when providing care to avoid dislocation.

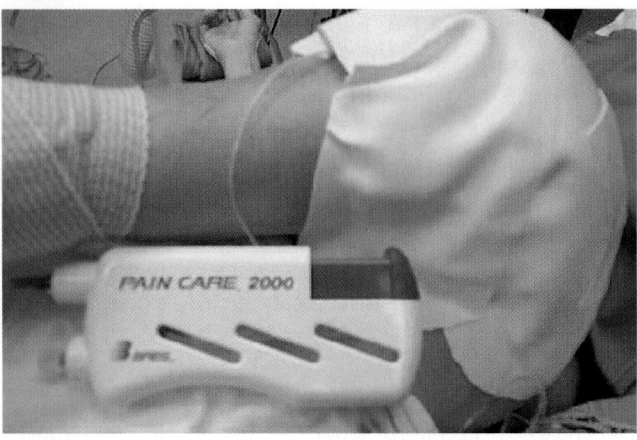

FIG 15-5 Local anesthetic infusion pump in use after shoulder surgery. *Image courtesy Breg, Inc, Vista, Calif. All rights reserved.*

- Report if the dressing becomes moist; report any catheter disconnection immediately.
- Notify nurse immediately of a change in patient's status or level of comfort.

Equipment
❑ Pump in place from surgery
Home Catheter Removal
❑ Clean gloves
❑ Sterile 4 × 4–inch gauze pads
❑ Tape
❑ Plastic bag

STEP	RATIONALE

ASSESSMENT

1 Perform hand hygiene, apply clean gloves, and assess surgical dressing and site of catheter insertion. Dressing should be dry and intact. | Determines if catheter is placed properly.

2 Assess catheter connections. If connections become detached, do *not* reattach; instead notify surgeon immediately. | Reattachment could lead to infection. Misconnections could lead to infusion of inappropriate agents into joint site.

3 Perform a complete pain assessment (see Skill 15-1). | Provides baseline to determine efficacy of analgesia.

4 Review surgeon's operative report for position of catheter. | Confirms catheter location.

5 Read label on device and compare to MAR or health care provider's order. | Provides information regarding type of anesthetic, concentration, volume, flow rate, date and time prepared.

6 Assess for presence of blood backing up in tubing. If blood is present, stop infusion and notify health care provider. | Indicates possible displacement of catheter into blood vessel.

7 Determine the level of extremity activity that patient can perform per health care provider's orders. | Excessive activity can cause catheter displacement.

8 Assess for signs of local anesthetic toxicity: hypotension, dizziness, tremor, severe itching, swelling of the skin or throat, irregular heartbeat, palpitations, confusion, ringing in the ears, muscle twitching, numbness around the mouth, metallic taste, seizures. | Early identification of toxicity prevents or lessens the possibility of complications.
Local anesthetics can have serious systemic effects (ISMP, 2011).

9 Assess patient's and family caregiver's knowledge of infusion pump. | Assesses level of teaching and support required.

NURSING DIAGNOSES

- Acute pain
- Anxiety
- Risk for infection
- Deficient knowledge regarding purpose of infusion pump
- Impaired physical mobility

Related factors are individualized based on patient's condition or needs.

PLANNING

1 Expected outcomes following completion of procedure:
- Patient verbalizes full or partial relief from pain. | Patient's self-report of pain is the single most reliable indicator of pain.
- Patient achieves reduction of nonverbal behaviors indicative of pain such as grimacing, clenching teeth, rocking. | Nonverbal behaviors are valid and reliable indicators of pain in the absence of self-report (Herr et al., 2011).
- Patient is free of adverse drug reactions.
- Patient moves about in bed, sleeps and eats better, is more active, and communicates easily with family and friends. | Adequate pain relief allows patient to participate in activities of daily living (ADLs).
- Catheter is removed correctly without injury to patient. | Patient and family caregiver are able to follow instructions for catheter removal.

STEP	RATIONALE

IMPLEMENTATION

1 Identify patient using two identifiers (i.e., name and birthday or name and account number) according to agency policy. Compare identifiers in MAR/medical record with information on the patient's identification bracelet and/or ask patient to state name.

Ensures correct patient. Complies with The Joint Commission standards and improves patient safety (TJC, 2012).

2 When repositioning or ambulating patient, use caution to avoid catheter dislodgement.

3 Teach patient or family caregiver how to remove catheter (may also be done by home health nurse).

  a Teach patient or family caregiver how to perform hand hygiene and apply clean gloves.

Decreases transmission of microorganisms.

  b Have patient assume a relaxed position in bed or chair with lower extremity in normal alignment.

Relaxes joint muscles, reducing traction from muscle tension, and provides distraction.

  c Gently remove surgical dressing.

Provides access to infusion catheter.

  d Explain to patient what he or she will feel when removing the catheter.

Helps patient anticipate procedure and reduces anxiety.

  e Place a 4 × 4–inch gauze over site. Grasp catheter firmly and pull outward from skin with steady motion. If resistance occurs, stop pulling. Reposition extremity and try again. If tubing continues to stretch and demonstrates resistance, stop pulling, cover area with sterile dressing, and notify surgeon.

Approach designed to minimize tissue trauma.

  f Observe for mark on end of catheter tip.

Indicates complete removal of catheter; retaining a part of catheter could lead to inflammation, infection, and/or an embolus (Pasero and McCaffery, 2011).

  g After catheter is removed, place a new sterile dressing over the area and apply pressure for at least 2 minutes.

Prevents hematoma formation.

  h Place catheter in bag using standard precautions. Remove gloves and perform hand hygiene.

Patient is to bring catheter to surgeon's office on first visit. Reduces transmission of microorganisms and helps prevent infection.

4 Remind patient or family caregiver of follow-up appointment with surgeon.

Increases patient adherence.

EVALUATION

1 Ask patient to rate pain intensity using appropriate scale at both rest and with activity.

Determines patient response to local infusion of medication.

2 Observe for signs of adverse drug reaction and report any signs immediately.

Local analgesics can result in systemic adverse effects if absorbed by veins (Pasero and McCaffery, 2011).

3 Observe patient's position, mobility, relaxation, participation in activities of daily living, and any nonverbal behaviors.

Indicates successful pain management.

4 Inspect condition of surgical dressing.

A wet dressing indicates possible catheter migration out of wound, especially if drainage is clear.

5 During follow-up visit inspect catheter exit site.

Determines if area has healed without infection.

Unexpected Outcomes

1 Patient verbalizes pain intensity greater than previously determined goal or demonstrates nonverbal behaviors indicative of pain. Catheter may be displaced or clogged, or surgical site may be developing complications.

2 Patient reports symptoms of local anesthetic adverse reaction. Possible hypersensitivity to local anesthetic, displacement of catheter into vein, or pump failure (releasing too much drug into site).

Related Interventions

• Check reservoir for presence of medication.
• Check patency of tubing.
• Notify health care provider.

• Stop infusion (ISMP, 2011).
• Notify health care provider.

Reporting and Recording

• Record drug, concentration, date inserted, and type of demand feature (continuous or demand) in medication record.
• Record location of catheter, patient's pain rating, response to anesthetic, and additional comfort measures given in nurses' notes and EHR.

• Record additional analgesics necessary to control pain.
• Record any adverse reactions to local anesthetic (ISMP, 2011).
• Report damp dressing and/or displaced catheter to surgeon.

Teaching Considerations

• Provide preoperative teaching because device is placed in operating room.

- If device is on demand (not continuous), instruct patient to depress button every 6 hours.
- Instruct patient to inform nurse if pain exceeds pain-intensity goal because additional oral and/or intravenous analgesics are available for breakthrough pain.

Pediatric Considerations

- Local continuous infusion pumps have been used for children undergoing orthopedic surgery. Instruct parents and the child as described under Home Care Considerations. Explain special precautions not to dislodge the catheter.

Gerontologic Considerations

- Continuous dosing is sometimes administered, but demand doses require a mentally competent adult (Herr et al., 2011). In addition, take special precautions to protect the catheter.

Home Care Considerations

- Instruct patient to notify health care provider if excessive fluid or bleeding on the dressing occurs.
- Provide written instructions regarding any possible adverse reactions and reporting them to the health care provider immediately.
- Provide verbal and written instructions regarding how and when to discontinue device when at home. Remind patient to place catheter in a plastic bag and bring it to first follow-up visit with health care provider.
- Provide instructions regarding extremity movement.
- Home-health nurse may be ordered to remove pump via surgeon's order.

SKILL 15-5 Nonpharmacologic Pain Management

 Video Clip

Effective pain management does not always mean the elimination of pain. A variety of nonpharmacologic interventions are available to lessen a patient's pain in any health care setting. Some of these interventions are also classified as complimentary or alternative therapies, and there is evidence to support pain relief (NIH, 2011). Use these interventions in combination with pharmacologic interventions, not in place of them. Nonpharmacologic techniques diminish the physical effects of pain, alter a patient's perception of pain, and provide a patient with a greater sense of control. Distraction, relaxation, guided imagery, and cutaneous stimulation such as massage and acupressure are a few examples of effective nonpharmacologic measures.

Many nonpharmacologic techniques trigger a relaxation response by stimulating the parasympathetic nervous system (PNS). Because pain often causes muscle tension and anxiety, PNS stimulation relieves these disturbing responses (Baird et al., 2010; Drew and St. Marie, 2011). Nonpharmacologic interventions are appropriate for patients who find such interventions appealing, express anxiety or fear, may benefit from avoiding or reducing drug therapy, and have incomplete pain relief with pharmacologic interventions alone. You will have an excellent opportunity to help patients control their pain by teaching them to add a variety of nonpharmacologic techniques (Box 15-6). Patients and families today are more aware of complementary techniques and should be encouraged to continue whatever has worked for them. Because everyone responds differently, finding new methods that work for a patient may take more time than finding pharmacologic techniques.

CUTANEOUS STIMULATION

Massage

A gentle massage, a form of cutaneous stimulation, is the application of touch and movement to muscles, tendons, and ligaments without manipulation of the joints. A proper massage not only blocks perception of pain impulses but also helps relax muscle tension and spasm that otherwise might increase pain. Massage hastens the elimination of wastes stored in muscles, improves oxygenation of tissues, and stimulates the relaxation response in the nervous system. A superficial massage of the back, shoulders, and lower part of the neck is sometimes referred to as a backrub. Offering a backrub after a bath or before a patient prepares for sleep promotes relaxation and comfort. An effective backrub takes 3 to 6 minutes and is an important intervention for decreasing pain and improving sense of well-being. Massage also involves the feet and hands (Asadizker et al., 2011). Do not perform massage over bruised, swollen, or inflamed areas or bones of spine.

BOX 15-6	Nonpharmacologic Strategies for Pain Management*

Relaxation and Power of the Mind
- Self-comfort
- Progressive muscle relaxation
- Autogenics training
- Breathing exercises
- Music relaxation
- Visual imagery
- Yoga

Put Your Body to Work
- Exercise
- Pacing
- Energy conservation
- Body mechanics

Spirituality and Reflection
- Engaging in religious practices
- Humor
- Setting aside time to focus on what *is*
- Sharing your stress with others
- Journaling
- Praying

What To Do When Pain Flares
- Cold and hot therapies
- Ball therapy
- Contrast baths
- Hand massage
- Herbals†

*Should be used along with analgesia medications.
†Contact health care provider before using herbals, which could interact with prescribed analgesics.

Heat and Cold

Heat and cold applications relieve pain and promote healing. The selection of heat versus cold varies with a patient's preference and condition. The application of heat or cold in a health care agency or home health environment requires a health care provider's order. Although the physiologic responses to heat and cold differ, superficial heat or cold applications provide comfort in similar conditions such as muscle spasms, strains, and localized joint pain (see Chapter 40 for a review of warm and cold therapy).

Relaxation

Relaxation is a cognitive and/or physical strategy that provides pain relief or reduces pain to an acceptable level, usually in conjunction with pharmacologic methods when pain is severe. A patient's full participation and cooperation are necessary for relaxation techniques to be effective. The techniques are particularly useful for chronic pain, labor pain, and relief of procedure-related pain. Relaxation interventions involve progressive muscle relaxation, massage, quiet breathing, deep breathing, guided imagery, or a combination (Chen and Francis, 2009; Gloth, 2011; NIH, 2011).

Guided Imagery

Guided imagery is a creative sensory experience that effectively reduces pain perception and minimizes reaction to pain. It draws on internal experience of memories, dreams, fantasies, and visions; explores the inner world of experience; protects the privacy of a patient; and fosters the imagination. The goal of imagery is to have a patient use one or several of the senses to create an image of a desired result. This image creates a positive psychophysiologic response. Focus of the imagination helps patients change their perceptions about their disease, treatment, and healing ability, which helps relieve pain, tension, or stress. Choosing images that patients find pleasant requires a careful assessment. Otherwise you may mistakenly describe images of objects or things that a patient fears or dislikes. For example, a scene of rolling waves at the seashore is restful to one patient but may be frightening to another (Baird et al., 2010).

Distraction

Distraction is a technique that diverts an individual's attention away from mild or even moderate pain sensation. By introducing meaningful stimuli, you help a patient refocus attention. Some believe that a person can consciously attend to only one stimulus, thus diverting the attention away from pain. Distraction strategies you can offer a patient include changing activity, listening to music (Allred et al., 2010; Leibovici et al., 2009), reading, focusing on another person, walking, napping, writing, concentrating on a mental and physical activity simultaneously (playing a musical instrument), learning something new (completing a crossword puzzle), and listening to or watching a comedy program (NIH, 2011). Therapeutic communication with a nurse is another example of distraction. When the distraction is removed, a patient may have a heightened awareness of pain.

Delegation and Collaboration

Assessment of a patient's pain cannot be delegated to nursing assistive personnel (NAP). The skill of nonpharmacologic pain management strategies can be delegated to NAP. The nurse directs the NAP to:
- Identify and explain which nonpharmacologic measures work best for the patient.
- Explain the importance of eliminating environmental conditions that enhance pain.
- Identify the need to adapt strategies to patient restrictions (e.g., massage in side-lying versus prone position).

Equipment

- ❏ Pain rating scale
- ❏ *Massage:* Lotion or oil (consider aroma therapy lotion), folded sheet, bath towel
- ❏ *Relaxation:* Patient's music preference, radio or CD player, relaxation tape and tape player
- ❏ *Distraction:* Based on patient preference (e.g., reading material, puzzles, video games)

STEP	RATIONALE
ASSESSMENT	
1 Using pain rating scale, have patient identify pain intensity or discomfort.	Pain score establishes baseline to determine effects of intervention.
2 Assess physiologic, behavioral, and emotional signs and symptoms of pain, including patient self-report (see Skill 15-1).	Responses serve as means to evaluate effectiveness of pain-relief measures. Overt signs and symptoms are usually not present with chronic pain. Physical signs and symptoms indicate change in comfort level.
3 Assess characteristics of pain and possible underlying cause (see Skill 15-1).	Establishes baseline to determine if nonpharmacologic approaches are appropriate.

Clinical Decision Point *It helps to administer an analgesic before implementing a nonpharmacologic strategy so a patient is able to gain a level of comfort needed to practice these approaches.*

STEP	RATIONALE
4 Examine the site of patient's pain or discomfort. Include inspection (discoloration, swelling, drainage), palpation (change in temperature, area of altered sensation, painful area, areas that trigger pain), and range of motion of involved joints (if applicable).	Clinical observations may clarify information from patient. Site of discomfort may direct you to specific types of pain-relief measures.
5 Review health care provider's orders for pain relief.	In some acute care settings a medical order is necessary to perform nonpharmacologic therapies.

STEP	RATIONALE
6 Assess patient's understanding of pain and willingness to receive nonpharmacologic pain-relief measures.	Participation increases effectiveness of pain-relief measure. If patient is reluctant to try activity, provide information about suggested therapy.
7 Assess preferred patient activities (e.g., puzzles, crocheting or knitting, board games, music, imagery, and relaxation tapes).	Doing these activities in health care setting increases patient participation.
8 Assess patient's language level and identify descriptive terms to use when providing nonpharmacologic pain-relieving strategies.	Provides clarification of information.

NURSING DIAGNOSES

- Activity intolerance
- Acute pain
- Anxiety
- Chronic pain

- Deficient knowledge regarding nonpharmacologic methods of pain control

- Ineffective coping
- Powerlessness

Related factors are individualized based on patient's condition or needs.

PLANNING

1 Expected outcomes following completion of procedures:	
• Patient demonstrates and describes pain-relief measures.	Demonstrates patient understanding and learning.
• Patient is relaxed and comfortable after technique as evidenced by slow, deep respirations; calm facial expressions; calm tone of voice; relaxed muscles; relaxed posture.	Nonpharmacologic strategies help patient relax and experience less discomfort. Physiologic response to relaxation procedures and massage is deep relaxation.
• Patient verbalizes pain relief.	Patient's subjective expression is the most reliable indicator of the presence of pain.
2 Explain purpose of technique and what you expect of patient during activity.	Proper explanation of activity enhances patient participation.
3 Plan time to perform technique when patient is able to concentrate (e.g., after voiding, awakening from a nap).	Increases opportunity for success.
4 Administer an analgesic 30 minutes before implementing a nonpharmacologic strategy.	Patient is able to gain a level of comfort needed to perform these approaches.

IMPLEMENTATION

1 Prepare patient's environment.	
• Temperature suited to patient	Temperature and sound extremes can enhance patient's perception of pain. Bright or very dim lighting can aggravate pain sensation.
• Lighting	
• Sound	
• Eliminate unnecessary interruptions and coordinate care activities; allow for rest.	
2 Massage	

Clinical Decision Point *Massage is contraindicated in cases of muscle, bone, or joint injury.*

a Perform hand hygiene.	Reduces transmission of microorganisms.
b Place patient in comfortable position such as prone or side-lying. Have patients with difficulty breathing lie on side of bed with head of bed elevated.	Enhances relaxation and exposes areas to be massaged.
c Adjust bed to comfortable position for you; lower upper side rail on side where you are standing.	Ensures proper body mechanics and prevents strain on back.
d Turn on music to patient's preference.	Promotes relaxation.
e Ensure that patient is not allergic to lotion; warm lotion in hands or in basin of warm water. NOTE: If you massage the head and scalp, delay use of lotion until completed.	Warm lotion is soothing, and warmth helps to produce local muscle relaxation.
f Choose stroke technique based on desired effect or body part.	Ensures fuller relaxation of body part.
(1) Effleurage: Massaging upward and outward from vertebral column and back again (see illustration).	A light, gliding stroke used without manipulating deep muscles smoothes and extends muscles, increases nutrient absorption, and improves lymphatic and venous circulation.

STEP	RATIONALE
(2) Pétrissage (see illustration).	Kneading tense muscle groups promotes relaxation and stimulates local circulation.
(3) Friction	Strong circular strokes bring blood to surface of skin, increasing local circulation and loosening tight muscle groups.
g Encourage patient to breathe deeply and relax during massage.	Potentiates effects of massage.
h Standing behind patient, stimulate scalp and temples.	
i Supporting patient's head, use friction to rub muscles at base of head.	Strong circular strokes (friction) stimulate local circulation and relaxation.
j With patient in supine position, massage hands and arms as appropriate:	Releases tension in hands and arms. Studies indicate that anxious behaviors may be significantly reduced with hand massage (Asadizker et al., 2011).
(1) Support hand and apply friction to palm using both thumbs.	
(2) Support base of finger and work each finger in corkscrew-like motion.	
(3) Complete hand massage using effleurage strokes from fingertips to wrist.	
(4) Knead muscles of forearm and upper arm between thumb and forefinger.	Encourages relaxation; enhances circulation and venous return.
k After determining that patient has no neck injury or condition that contraindicates neck manipulation, massage neck as appropriate:	
(1) Place patient prone unless contraindicated.	Provides access to neck muscles.
(2) Knead each neck muscle between thumb and forefinger.	Reduces tension that often localizes in neck muscles.
(3) Gently stretch neck by placing one hand on top of shoulders and other at base of head. Gently move hands away from one another.	Helps relax muscle body.
l Massage back as appropriate:	Patient with back injury, surgery, or epidural infusion should not receive back massage.
(1) Keep patient in prone position unless contraindicated; side-lying position is an option.	Provides access to muscle groups in back.
(2) Do not allow hands to leave patient's skin.	Continuous contact with surface of skin is soothing and stimulates circulation to tissues. Breaking contact with skin can startle patient.
(3) Apply hands first to sacral area; massage in circular motion. Stroke upward from buttocks to shoulders. Massage over scapulas with smooth, firm stroke. Continue in one smooth stroke to upper arms and laterally along sides of back down to iliac crest (see illustration). Continue massage pattern for 3 minutes.	General, firm pressure applied to all muscle groups promotes relaxation.

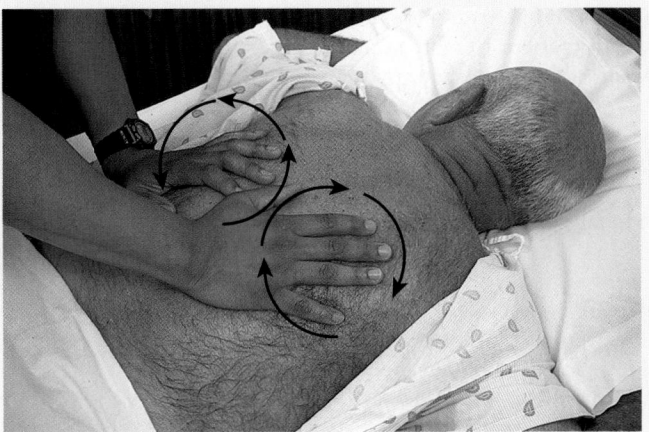

STEP 2f(1) Effleurage.

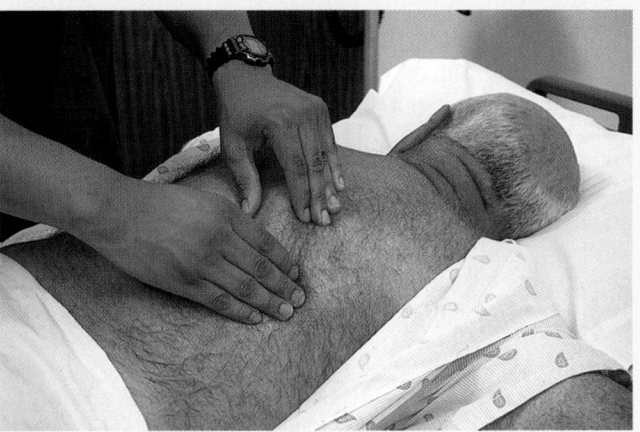

STEP 2f(2) Pétrissage.

STEP	RATIONALE

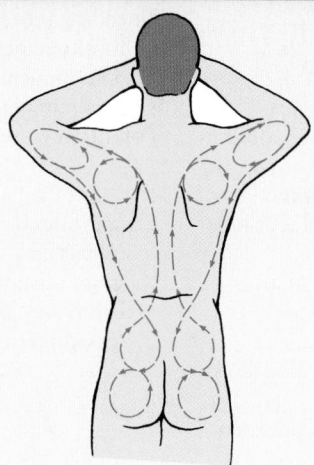

STEP 2I(3) Circular massage.

(4) Use effleurage along muscles of spine in upward and outward motion.	Massage follows distribution of major muscle groups.
(5) Use pétrissage on muscles of each shoulder toward front of patient.	Area often tightens because of tension.
(6) Use palms in upward and outward circular motion from lower buttocks to neck.	Brings blood to surface of skin.
(7) Knead muscles of upper back and shoulder between thumb and forefinger.	These muscles are thick and can be massaged vigorously.
(8) Use both hands to knead muscles up one side of back and then the other.	
(9) End massage with long, stroking effleurage movements.	Most soothing of massage movements.
m Massage feet as appropriate:	
(1) Place patient in supine position.	Returns patient to comfortable anatomic position.
(2) Hold foot firmly. Support ankle with one hand or support sides of foot with each hand while performing massage.	Maintains joint stability during massage (Asadizker et al., 2011).
(3) Make circular motions with thumb and fingers around bones of ankle and top of foot.	All massage strokes help to relax muscles.
(4) Trace space between tendons with firm finger pressure, moving from toe to ankle.	
(5) Massage sides and top of each toe.	
(6) Use top of fist to make circular motions on bottom of foot.	
(7) Knead sides of foot between index finger and thumb.	
(8) Conclude with firm, sweeping motions over top and bottom of foot.	Too light strokes may tickle.
n Tell patient that you are ending massage.	Informs and prepares patient for inhalation and exhalation.
o When procedure is complete, instruct patient to inhale deeply and exhale. Caution him or her to move slowly after resting a few minutes.	Returns patient to more awake and alert state. When deeply relaxed, patient may experience dizziness on arising too rapidly, need time for vessels to redistribute blood supply.
p Wipe excess lotion or oil from patient's body with bath towel.	Excess lotion or oil can irritate skin and lead to breakdown.
q Return bed to low position and raise side rails as appropriate when massage is finished. Perform hand hygiene.	Side rails cannot be used as a restraint.
3 Progressive relaxation	
a Instruct patient to take several slow, deep, diaphragmatic breaths.	Increased oxygen lessens anxiety and prevents shortness of breath with relaxation breathing technique. Avoids hyperventilation.
b Have patient close eyes if desired.	Helps patient maintain focus.
c Have patient alternate tightening for 3 to 4 seconds and then relaxing all muscle groups for 6 to 7 seconds, beginning at feet and working upward toward head.	Alternating tension and relaxation in muscle groups allows patient to feel the difference.

STEP	RATIONALE
(1) Instruct patient to tighten muscles during inhalation and relax muscles during exhalation.	Relaxation is an integrated response associated with diminished sympathetic nervous system arousal; decreased muscle tension is desired outcome. Relaxation decreases pulse and respiration rates, and blood pressure and helps reduce anxiety (Baird et al., 2010).
(2) As each muscle group relaxes, ask patient to enjoy relaxed feeling and allow mind to drift and think how nice it is to be relaxed. Have patient breathe deeply.	Distracts patient from perceiving pain. Enhances relaxation response. Breathing deeply prevents the Valsalva maneuver, which increases intrathoracic pressure and compromises cardiac function.
d Calmly explain that patient will feel sensations of tingling, heaviness, floating, or warmth as relaxation occurs.	Prevents anxiety if sensation occurs without warning.
e Ask patient to continue slow, deep breaths.	Allows opportunity to enjoy feelings of relaxation.
f When exercise is complete, instruct patient to inhale deeply, exhale, and then initially move about slowly after resting a few minutes.	Returns patient to more awake and alert state. Rising too rapidly can cause dizziness.
4 Deep breathing	
a Instruct patient to sit comfortably with feet uncrossed. If patient is unable to sit, move to supine position with small pillow under head.	Encourages relaxation.
b Have patient place one hand on chest and the other on abdomen.	Allows patient to focus on chest and then abdomen.
c Coach patient to inhale deeply through the nose, allowing the abdomen to rise and the hand to move outward.	Provides steady timing of inhalation and focuses the patient on stretching abdominal muscles.
d When the abdomen is partially expanded, tell patient to continue to breathe and allow chest to expand, moving the upper hand outward.	Affords maximal inhalation.
e Pause for a few seconds. Then have the patient exhale slowly through pursed lips to ensure slow, controlled release of air. Repeat for 4 to 6 minutes.	Permits optimal exchange of oxygen and carbon dioxide.
5 Guided imagery	
a Direct patient through guided imagery exercise.	
(1) Instruct patient to imagine that inhaled air is ball of healing energy.	Developing specific images helps to remove pain perception.
(2) Imagine that inhaled air travels to area of pain.	Patient's ability to concentrate decreases pain perception.
b Alternatively you may direct imagery.	
(1) Ask patient to imagine a pleasant place such as beach or mountains. Choose an image peaceful for the patient.	Directs imagery after selection of restful place.
(2) Direct patient to experience all sensory aspects of restful place (e.g., for beach: warm breeze, warm sand between toes, warmth of sunshine, rhythmic sound of waves, smell of salt air, gulls gliding and swooping in air).	Helps patient concentrate and relax through stimulation of numerous senses (Baird et al., 2010). Make sure that it is something in their experience, not just yours.
(3) Direct patient to continue deep, slow, rhythmic breathing.	Promotes relaxation through muscle relaxation.
(4) Direct patient to count to three, inhale, and open eyes. Suggest that patient move about slowly initially.	
c Provide patient time to practice exercise without interruption.	Guided imagery requires an intense level of concentration that takes time to achieve. Practice relaxation tapes are available almost everywhere; libraries are an excellent source.
6 Distraction	
a Direct patient's attention away from pain with distraction techniques.	Redirection of attention can alter emotional or cognitive aspects of pain (Allred et al., 2010).
b Ask patient to close eyes or to focus on single object in room.	Directs attention inward and protects patient from external distraction.
c Instruct patient to concentrate on slow, rhythmic breathing. Guide breathing or instruct patient to control and concentrate on breathing by thinking: "in, one, two; out, one, two."	Promotes relaxation by concentrating on kinesthetic action, thus reducing ability to concentrate on pain (Leibovici et al., 2009).
d Continue distraction using patient preferred technique.	
(1) Use music of patient's choosing. Emphasize listening to rhythm and adjust volume as pain increases or decreases.	Focusing on an activity helps divert attention from painful sensation.

STEP	RATIONALE
(2) Direct patient to give detailed account of an event or story.	Stress details of event to enhance distraction from painful stimulus.
(3) Engage patient in conversation; encourage participation of family members and visitors.	Visitors can help direct attention away from mild-to-moderate pain. Rarely is someone in severe pain able to use distraction. 

EVALUATION

1 Observe character of respirations, body position, facial expression, tone of voice, mood, mannerisms, verbalization of discomfort.	Determines effectiveness of procedure, level of relaxation, degree of pain relief achieved, and which procedures were the most effective.
2 Ask patient to use a pain rating scale to rate comfort level.	Measures change in pain intensity.
3 Observe patient perform pain-control measures.	Confirms learning.

Unexpected Outcomes
1 Patient is not able to concentrate on technique because pain intensity is unchanged or escalating or demonstrates nonverbal behaviors indicative of pain.

Related Interventions
- Reassess character of pain and determine if further analgesia is necessary.
- Ensure that environment is conducive to learning and using technique.
- Consult with health care provider on an increase in dose or alternate medication.
- Consider a different technique or a combination of complementary strategies.

Recording and Reporting
- Record in nurses' notes and EHR patient's assessment findings, procedure and technique(s) used, preparation given to patient, patient's response to procedure or technique, change in overall condition, and further comfort needs related to event. Incorporate pain-relief technique into nursing care plan.
- Report patient's response to nonpharmacologic interventions to the staff at change of shift or in a care plan meeting.
- Report any unusual responses to techniques (e.g., uncontrolled or aggravated pain, or muscle spasms) to nurse in charge or health care provider.

Teaching Considerations
- Provide patient information about each nonpharmacologic therapy, including purpose, rationale for how pain is relieved, how patient can maximize benefits. If NAP performs massage, you still need to provide patient education.
- Some techniques require more practice before patients achieve results. Pharmacologic intervention is sometimes required to lessen pain so patient can relax.
- Teach patient to rest between periods of activity at home and hospital because fatigue increases pain perception.
- Teach family member how to perform massage (if not contraindicated) as part of home care.

Pediatric Considerations
- You can use nonpharmacologic pain-management therapies successfully with children. Adapt distraction and relaxation strategies to the developmental level of the child (e.g., use a pacifier for an infant, offer reading or playing a recording of a favorite story for a preschooler, encourage a teenager to listen to music on a CD player with headphones) (Allred et al., 2010; Finley et al., 2009; Hockenberry and Wilson, 2011). Play therapists are usually available at large pediatric hospitals and are good resources for appropriate distraction techniques.
- Because children usually have an active imagination, relaxation is often a powerful adjuvant in pain control.
- Parents are very helpful in providing pain relief. For example, they provide comfort by their presence, conversation, and holding and cuddling their child.

Gerontologic Considerations
- Visual, hearing, cognitive, and motor impairments make it difficult for older adults to be able to effectively use procedures such as distraction, relaxation, or guided imagery. Make certain that glasses, hearing aids, and other assistive devices are in place. Do not assume that complementary techniques will not work on the elderly (NIH, 2011).

Home Care Considerations
- Family members need to collaborate on planning time to reduce noise and other stimuli in the home to promote patient's relaxation.

[?] Critical Thinking Exercises

Mrs. Silver is an 85-year-old newly admitted widow. She has a history of stroke, pulmonary emboli (blood clots in the lungs), a myocardial infarction (heart attack), heart failure, and a broken right hip over the past 8 years. In the past 3 years she was declared legally blind as a result of macular degeneration in both eyes. She is confined to a wheelchair, unable to stand or walk, and is very depressed because she can no longer read, her favorite pastime.

When you do a pain assessment on Mrs. Silver, you discover that she has difficulty using the numeric rating scale of 0 to10 and becomes frustrated when people ask her to use it. She asks you to decide the number for her because she "just doesn't understand." She describes her pain to you as deep, aching pain in her right leg, hip, and shoulder that keeps her awake at night and makes it very difficult to turn on her right side.

Mrs. Silver has an order for morphine 10 mg by mouth every 3 hours as needed; she had been taking this at home for several months. She tells you that, when she requested the pain pill at 4 AM this morning, the night nurse told her that she has to be very careful because she could become a drug addict if she takes morphine. She says that she is in pain right now but is afraid to take anything. Her vital signs are BP 98/70, P76, R16, and T97. Her bowel sounds are slightly hypoactive. She reports she has not had a bowel movement for 3 days.

1 How often will you assess this patient's pain, and which pain assessment tool will you use?
2 Which nonpharmacologic pain control approaches are appropriate for Mrs. Silver? Provide rationale.
3 The patient says to her nurse, "do you think my pain medicine is causing my constipation"? What should be the nurse's answer?

[✓] REVIEW QUESTIONS

1 What should you do if a postoperative patient activates (pushes the button) the patient-controlled analgesia (PCA) three times as frequently as the medication is ordered?
   1 Realize that this is normal and there is no need for any nursing action
   2 Explain that pain is to be expected after surgery
   3 Thoroughly reassess patient's pain and call the health care provider who prescribed the PCA to request orders to increase the dose or change or add a medication
   4 Tell the patient that he is only allowed to push the button three times an hour
2 Which patient is the BEST candidate for use of a PCA pump?
   1 A very confused older adult having minor surgery
   2 An obese adult with sleep apnea
   3 An older teenager having an appendectomy
   4 A middle-age adult having major surgery who requires an interpreter
3 Which patient is the *worst* candidate for use of a PCA pump?
   1 A very confused older adult having minor surgery
   2 An obese adult with sleep apnea
   3 An older teenager having an appendectomy
   4 A middle-age adult having major surgery who requires an interpreter
4 What is the most common health care provider error associated with PCA therapy?
   1 Giving the wrong medication
   2 Using a wrong concentration of a medication (e.g., Dilaudid 1 mg/mL is ordered; Dilaudid 2 mg/mL is placed in the machine)
   3 Presence of a faulty alarm
   4 Programming the PCA machine incorrectly

5 Which nursing measure is key to preventing oversedation with opioids?
   1 Awakening a patient at least once a shift
   2 Frequently monitoring a patient using a standard sedation scale
   3 Assessing the quality of respirations once a shift
   4 Medicating as ordered, even if a patient is extremely sleepy
6 On a patient's medical record you discover that a prior pain assessment was made using a behavioral pain scale for nonverbal patients. According to the nurse the patient was unable to use a numeric scale for pain intensity. Prioritize the nursing actions by marking 1 next to the highest priority; 2 next to the second priority; 3 next to the third priority, and 4 next to the lowest priority.
   _____ Look at the chart for any indication that the patient was nonverbal at one time and see when it (the behavioral scale) was last used.
   _____ Administer the appropriate pain medication based on your patient's self-report.
   _____ Educate the patient on the 0-to-10 scale and assess his or her pain intensity using it. Document the number of the pain intensity and the reason for the change in assessment tool.
   _____ Assist the patient in repositioning, turn room lights low, and administer a backrub.
7 Vital signs are always reliable indicators of the intensity of a patient's pain.
   1 True
   2 False
8 Older patients should not be given opioids for pain because they are too potent, even at low doses.
   1 True
   2 False
9 The best approach for giving analgesics for postoperative pain involves:
   1 Around-the-clock (ATC) on a fixed schedule
   2 Only when a patient requests it
   3 Only when the nurse decides that a patient has moderate-or-greater pain intensity
   4 Every hour while awake unless a patient refuses it
10 Why would a patient request an increased dose of pain medication?
   1 The patient is experiencing increased anxiety.
   2 The patient is requiring more staff and/or family attention.
   3 The patient is experiencing increased pain.
   4 The patient is experiencing beginning symptoms of addiction.

REFERENCES

Allred K, et al: The effect of music on postoperative pain and anxiety, *Pain Manage Nurs* 11(1):15, 2010.

American Pain Society (APS) and American Association of Pain Medicine (AAPM): Opioids guideline panel-Part 1, *J Pain* 10(2):113 e22, 2009.

American Pain Society (APS): *Principles of analgesic use in the treatment of acute pain and cancer pain*, ed 6, Glenview, Ill, 2009, American Pain Society.

Asadizker M, et al: The effect of foot and hand massage on postoperative cardiac surgery pain, *Int J Nurs Midwifery* 3(10):165, 2011.

Baird C, et al: Efficacy of guided imagery with relaxation for osteoarthritis symptoms and medication intake, *Pain Manage Nurs* 11(1):56, 2010.

Chen Y, Francis A: Relaxation imagery for chronic, nonmalignant pain: effects on pain symptoms, quality of life and mental health, *Pain Manage Nurs* 11(3):159, 2009.

D'Arcy Y: Keep your patient safe during PCA, *Nursing 2008* 38(1):50, 2008.

D'Arcy Y: Avoid the dangers of opioid therapy, *Am Nurse Today* 4(5):18, 2009.

D'Arcy Y: New thinking about postoperative pain management, *OR Nurse* 5(6):29, 2011.

Deane G, Smith H: Overview of pain management in older persons, *Clin Geriatr Med* 24:185, 2008.

deTovar C, et al: Postoperative self-report of pain in children: interscale agreement, response to analgesic, and preference for a FACES scale and a visual analog scale, *Pain Res Manage* 15(3):163, 2010.

Drew DJ, St Marie BJ: Pain in critically ill patients with substance abuse disorder or long-term opioid use for chronic pain, *AACN Adv Crit Care* 22 (3):238, 2011.

Elhoaris H, Resnik C: An educational strategy for treating chronic and noncancer pain (CNCP) with opioids: a pilot test, *J Pain* 11(12):1368, 2010.

Ferguson S, et al: A prospective randomized trial comparing patient-controlled epidural analgesia to patient-controlled intravenous analgesia on postoperative pain control and recovery after major open gynecologic cancer surgery, *Gynecol Oncol* 114(1):111, 2009.

Finley G, et al: Cultural influences on assessment of children's pain, *Pain Res Manage* 14(1):33, 2009.

Gerli S, et al: Effect of epidural analgesia on labor and delivery: a retrospective study, *J Matern Fetal Neonatal Med* 24 (3):458, 2011.

Giordano J, et al: Pain, neurotechnology and the treatment-enhancement debate, *Practical Pain Manage* 10(4):1, 2010.

Gloth M: Pharmacological management of persistent pain in older persons: focus on opioids and nonopioids, *J Pain* 12(3 suppl):S14, 2011.

Hadjistavropoulos T, et al: Does routine pain assessment result in better care? *Pain Res Manage* 14(3):211, 2009.

Herr K: Pain assessment strategies in older patients, *J Pain* 12(3 suppl):S3, 2011.

Herr K, et al: Pain assessment in the patient unable to self-report: position statement with clinical practice guidelines, *Pain Manag Nurs* 12(4):230, 2011.

Hockenberry M, Wilson D: *Wong's nursing care of infants and children*, ed 9, St Louis, 2011, Mosby.

Institute of Medicine (IOM): *Relieving pain in America: a blueprint for transforming prevention, care, education and research*, Washington, DC, 2011, National Academic Press, available at http://www.iom.edu/Reports/2011/Relieving-Pain-in-America-A-Blueprint-for-Transforming-Prevention-Care-Education-Research.aspx, accessed March 16, 2012.

Institute for Safe Medication Practices (ISMP): *Medication safety alert: process for handling elasomere pain relief balls (On-Q Painbuster and others) requires safety improvements*, ISMP Acute Care Quarterly Action Agenda, 2011, available at http://www.ismp.org/Newsletters/acutecare/articles/20090716.asp, accessed March 16, 2012.

International Association of the Study of Pain (IASP): Pain items, 2010, available at http://www.iasp-pain.org/Content/NavigationMenu/GeneralResourceLinks/PainDefinitions/default.htm#Pain, accessed March 20, 2012.

James DC: Routine obstetrical interventions, *J Perinat Neonat Nurs* 25(2):148, 2011.

Klieber C, et al: Evidence-based pediatric pain management in emergency departments of a rural state, *J Pain* 12(8):900, 2011.

Lehne R: *Pharmacology for nursing care*, ed 7, St Louis, 2011, Mosby.

Leibovici V, et al: Effects of virtual reality immersion and audiovisual distraction techniques for patients with pruritus, *Pain Res Manage* 14(4):283, 2009.

Mackey S: Why acute postoperative pain becomes chronic and can it be prevented? *Practical Pain Manage* 11(5):1, 2011.

Maddox R, et al: Continuous respiratory monitoring and a "smart" infusion system improve safety of patient-controlled analgesia in the postoperative period, *Advances in Patient Safety: New Directions and Alternative Approaches* 4:1, 2008.

Manougian E: Why some patients require high dose opioid therapy, *Practical Pain Manage* 10(6):1, 2010.

National Institutes of Health (NIH), National Center for Complementary and Alternative Medicine (NCCAM): Selected results of NCCAM funded research on CAM research, 2011, available at http://nccam.nih.gov/research, accessed March 16, 2012.

Pasero C, McCaffery M: *Pain assessment and pharmacologic management*, St Louis, 2011, Mosby.

Rahme E, Bernatsky S: NSAIDs and risk of lower GI bleeding, *Lancet* 576(9736):146, 2010.

Riddell R, Racine N: Assessing pain in infancy: the caregiver context, *Pain Res Manage* 14(1):27, 2009.

Rowbotham D, et al: *Best practice in the management of epidural analgesia in the hospital setting*, Faculty of Pain Medicine of The Royal College of Anaesthetists, Nov 2010, London.

Spector R: *Cultural diversity in health and illness*, ed 7, Upper Saddle River, NJ, 2008, Pearson Prentice Hall.

Tennant F: Making practical sense of cytochrome p450, *Practical Pain Manage* 10(4):12, 2010.

The Joint Commission (TJC): *National Patient Safety Goals*, Oakbrook Terrace, Ill, 2012, The Commission, available at http://www.jointcommission.org/standards_information/npsgs.aspx.

US Food and Drug Administration (USFDA): FDA Drug Safety Communication: prescription acetaminophen products to be limited to 325 mg. per dosage unit, a boxed warning will highlight, 2009, available at http://www.nccam.nih.gov/research/results/spotlight. Accessed March 16, 2012.

Viclop T, et al: Opioid prescribing practices in chronic pain management: guidelines do not sufficiently influence clinical practice, *J Pain* 10(10):1051, 2009.

Wells N, et al: Improving the quality of care through pain assessment and management. In Hughes RG, editor: *Patient safety and quality: an evidence-based handbook for nurses*, Rockville, MD, 2008, Agency for Healthcare Research and Quality (AHRQ).

Young J, Plenge R: Genomic technology applied to pharmacological traits, *JAMA* 306(6):652, 2010.

Palliative Care

MEDIA RESOURCES

- **evolve** http://evolve.elsevier.com/Perry/skills
  learning system
  - Review Questions
  - Audio Glossary

KEY TERMS

Advance directives	Brain death	Hospice	Palliative care
Autopsy	Grief	Organ/tissue donation	Postmortem care

OBJECTIVES

Mastery of content in this chapter will enable the nurse to:
- Identify a nurse's role in assisting patients and families in grief and at the end of life.
- Discuss principles of palliative care.
- Describe hospice care.
- Describe approaches to symptom management at the end of life.

- Discuss a nurse's role in facilitating autopsy and organ and tissue donation requests.
- Describe physiologic changes in impending death.
- Describe elements of postmortem care.

Nurses have historically played a vital role in the care of patients and families facing serious, life-limiting illness and death. They continue to expand their knowledge, leading the way in the development of compassionate, evidence-based palliative care (Ferrell and Coyle, 2010). The World Health Organization (2011) defines palliative care as an "approach that improves the quality of life of individuals and their families facing life-threatening illness, through the prevention and relief of suffering by means of early identification and impeccable assessment and treatment of pain and other problems, physical, psychological and spiritual." When patients receive relief from the symptoms caused by disease or treatment, they have a higher quality of life and are better able to participate in making health care decisions. Although this chapter focuses on end-of-life care, patients of all ages with any diagnosis receive palliative care, even as they seek treatment and cure for their illness.

At the end of life palliative care interventions help patients experience a "good death," often through hospice care. Hospice, an interdisciplinary, patient- and family-centered program of total palliative care, helps people live as well as possible through the dying process. Patients are eligible for hospice care as a Medicare or Medicaid benefit during the final phase of a terminal illness, usually the last 6 to 12 months of life. Because hospice is a philosophy of care, not necessarily a place, the services can be provided at home; in freestanding hospice facilities; or in nursing home, extended care, or acute care settings.

To receive hospice care at home, a family caregiver must be available to provide care when a patient is no longer able to function alone. Hospice team members offer 24-hour accessibility and coordinate care between the home and inpatient settings. As the time of a patient's death comes closer, the hospice team provides intensive support to the patient and family. Hospice benefits include respite for family caregivers, limited hospitalization for acute symptom management, and bereavement care after death (Hospice Foundation of America, 2010). Unfortunately many patients enter hospice care only a few days or weeks before death, limiting the amount of time they have to benefit from the nurses, physicians, social workers, volunteers, and spiritual care providers who make up the interdisciplinary team. Be familiar with the scope of hospice services qualifying criteria and educate patients and family members about this option for end-of-life care.

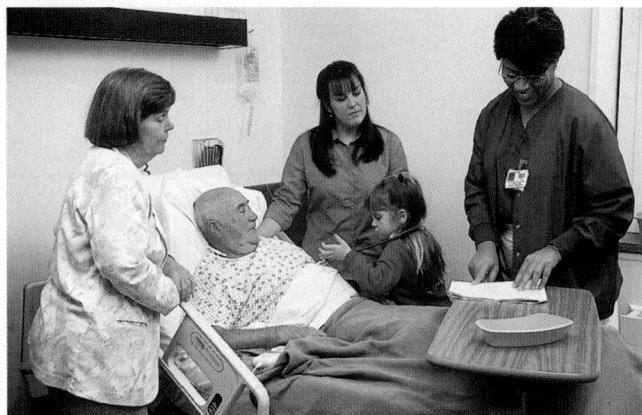

FIG 16-1 The nurse collaborates to develop an effective approach to symptom management.

Grief experiences in situations of serious illness and at the end of life have profound physical, psychological, social, and spiritual effects on dying persons, family members, friends, and caregivers. The grief associated with serious illness or death arises from many sources: fear of the unknown, pain, sadness about leaving loved ones behind, loss of control, or unresolved guilt. A nurse listens carefully to understand the significance of the loss to the patient or family members, identifies concerns, and assesses their ability to sustain hope and move forward in life.

Many symptoms that patients and families experience are caused by grief, illness, or medical treatments at the end of life. Examples of a patient's physical symptoms include pain, alterations in bowel and bladder elimination, nausea, loss of appetite, fatigue, shortness of breath, and mental status changes. Patients or family members also experience psychological symptoms such as anxiety, depression, or uncertainty because of lack of understanding of the disease, prognosis, or treatment plan. Spiritual distress often heightens a patient's perceptions of discomfort. Assess a patient's or family member's needs and strengths and initiate a plan of care for symptom management (Fig. 16-1).

At the time of death nurses provide compassionate care to patients and family members by offering information, guidance, and support and facilitating communication. As described in Skill 16-3, nurses provide postmortem care (i.e., care of the body after death) in a dignified manner, consistent with a patient's religious and cultural beliefs.

EVIDENCE-BASED PRACTICE

An extensive body of research supports the development of evidence-based palliative care. Research continues on the type and prevalence of symptoms, symptom management, pharmacologic interventions, use of advance directives, caregiver and nurse coping, and family decision making (Aoun et al., 2011; Benzein and Saveman, 2008; Daaleman et al., 2008; Johnstone and Kanitsaki, 2009).

Above all, nurses strive for positive patient-centered outcomes at the end of life. Researchers are studying what patients and family members perceive as important at the end of life, helping caregivers focus on behaviors that bring about the highest degree of patient and family satisfaction.

A systematic review of research literature focused on caregiver interventions that patients and family members described as satisfying care. The dominant themes of satisfaction that surfaced in the research studies include accessibility, coordination of care, competence, communication and relationships, education, emotional support, personalization of care, and support for patient decision making (Dy et al., 2008). Research supports the use of the following strategies for expert palliative care nursing:

- Patients and family members are most satisfied when they receive attentive, compassionate care. Novice nurses who are grounded in authentic, openhearted, holistic nursing care practices are capable of providing valuable care to patients at the end of life.
- Personalize your plan of care. Discuss priorities and preferences for care with patients and family members regularly as changes in a patient's condition may shift care preferences and needs.
- Develop competence in providing symptom management, comfort care, emotional support, and caring personal interactions.
- Give as much time as needed to discuss a sensitive topic, maintain contact, and respond to requests promptly.
- Use teamwork and interdisciplinary communication to ensure coordination of care.
- Support patients' decision making and provide assistance with advance care planning to help them maintain a sense of control.

PATIENT-CENTERED CARE

Nurses caring for patients receiving palliative and hospice care maintain a patient-centered focus by developing a plan of care that gives highest priority to patient's values, quality of life, and care preferences. Because patients near the end of life depend on family caregivers to maintain a high quality of life and death, a nurse's care extends to family members and the patient. Patients and family caregivers know their needs and preferences and should be encouraged to share their care priorities and be given as many options as possible in making decisions (Wasserman, 2008).

Patients with life-limiting chronic illness often want to determine their own approaches to living with illness and symptom management and participate in self-care activities as long as possible (Johnston, 2010). Patient-centered care focuses on encouraging patients to set realistic goals and helps them identify ways to achieve them so they can maintain their usual routines and a sense of normalcy.

When patients with advanced illness are no longer able to participate in making decisions, they can communicate their values and preferences in an advance directive. Advance directives specify medical interventions such as mechanical ventilation that a patient does not want in certain situations and are also used to communicate the care a patient wants (e.g., pain relief) to the fullest extent possible (Mahon, 2010).

Patients describe their life values orally or in writing, indicating which types of treatments are acceptable or unacceptable to them should they lose their capacity to make health care decisions. There are many forms available to help guide patients and their family caregivers through the advance directive process (Five Wishes, 2011). Patients may also designate a person, a durable power of attorney (DPOA) for health care decisions who knows a patient's values well enough to make decisions when they are no longer able to do so. The Patient Self-Determination Act of 1991 requires that all health care agencies serving Medicaid and Medicare patients provide patients with information regarding advance directives.

Nurses facilitate the optimal use of advance directives. As helpful as advance directives are, many people do not have one or need help understanding their usefulness and how to prepare one

(Johnstone and Kanitsaki, 2009). Discussions about advance directives and goals of care involve the patient, DPOA, family members, and the interdisciplinary health care team. Communicate to the health care team a patient's desire to complete an advance directive and help the patient access the appropriate resources. If a patient has an advance directive, make sure to place a copy in the medical record and instruct him or her to give copies to their health care provider and family members. Be familiar with agency policies and state laws because they often differ from place to place.

Cardiopulmonary resuscitation (CPR), an emergency procedure providing artificial ventilation and manual external cardiac massage, is used in cases of cardiac and/or pulmonary arrest. CPR is performed on a patient who has a cardiopulmonary arrest unless the patient's health care provider has written and signed a "do not resuscitate" (DNR) or "no CPR" order. Adults in consultation with the health care team may consent to a DNR status verbally or in writing. Assure patients who choose not to be resuscitated that they will continue to receive full palliative care and symptom relief. Patients who are receiving hospice care in an agency must also specifically designate their DNR status to agency personnel.

Patient-centered care respects patients' cultural heritage. Human responses to illness, death, and grief are transmitted from generation to generation through family and culture. Cultural norms influence family, gender, and community roles at the time of death. Culture also affects the meaning of pain and suffering, how one expresses grief and emotion, and ideas about an afterlife. Given the wide range of cultural beliefs, first engage in self-reflection on your own cultural and personal beliefs regarding loss and death. Gather knowledge on common end-of-life cultural or religious practices and then validate through nurse-patient discussions the relevance of those practices for a particular patient of that culture or religion (Giger, 2013).

Cultural differences influence communication at the end of life. For some people discussing death is taboo. Some people believe in the authority of the healer or the power of words. They fear that informing a patient that he or she has a serious disease brings about a poor outcome. Contrast this belief with Western cultural practices of full disclosure, honesty, informed consent, and the belief that "talking through" things helps with emotional adjustment (Erichsen et al., 2010). Caregivers who rely on biomedical interventions in the face of serious illness or impending death feel conflict with patients and families who rely mainly on spiritual interventions or afterlife considerations.

Cultural differences also influence processes such as obtaining informed consent or making life-support decisions. Research shows that ethnicity and culture are strongly related to attitudes toward life-sustaining treatments during terminal illness and the use of hospice services (Washington et al., 2008). Religious and cultural practices also govern how to care for a body near or after death (Pattison, 2008). An overview of selected religious and cultural considerations in the care of the body near or after death can be found in Box 16-1.

Safety Guidelines

1 Patients receiving palliative or hospice care are particularly vulnerable and need nurse advocates.

BOX 16-1 Religious and Cultural Considerations in Care of the Body Near and After Death

Buddhism—People prefer a quiet place for death. A Buddhist monk may chant to promote a peaceful, accepting mind in the dying person. Incense may be used. When the person has died, the body should be covered with a cotton sheet. Others should not touch the body, and the deceased's mouth and eyes are left open. Maintain strict silence after death. Autopsy and organ donation are permitted.

Christianity—Christianity has many denominations with varying practices, as do other world religions. Bible texts may be read near or at the time of death. Protestant Christians receive the sacraments of Holy Communion or sometimes baptism. Christians in the Roman Catholic tradition often request sacraments of Penance, Anointing of the Sick, and Holy Communion at the end of life. Many Christian groups offer prayers and anointing and view death as "going home" to Jesus. There are no prescribed rituals for body preparation, and autopsy and organ donation are usually permissible.

Hinduism—Persons prefer to die at home or in a quiet setting. Because of a belief in reincarnation, efforts are made to resolve relationships before death. The head of a person nearing death should face the east with a lamp placed near the head. If the dying person is unable to chant his mantra, a family member can chant it into the right ear. Passages from the Bhagavad Gita are recited. Family members prefer to wash the body after death and are present to chant, pray, and use incense. Hindus prefer cremation of the body.

Islam—A Muslim reader recites verses from the Qur'an when the person is near death. Family members prepare the body, and non-Muslims should not touch it. After death the person's eyes should be closed, and arms and legs straightened. Autopsy or organ donation is generally not permissible, except as required by law.

Judaism—Deathbed confessional, blessings, and readings from the Torah are traditional in Orthodox Judaism. A family member remains with the body until burial, which takes place within 24 hours, not on the Sabbath. A family member closes the deceased's eyes on death. Synagogue burial societies may prepare the body, which is wrapped in white linen. Organ donation prohibitions may exist in Orthodox Judaism, but not for all Jews. Autopsies may be considered if organs are not removed.

---

2 Patients at the end of life frequently receive potent medications for symptom management, are often weak or frail, and have limited reserves. Medication errors can cause an earlier-than-anticipated death or may postpone the time of death or cause prolonged suffering (Dietz et al., 2010).

3 Patients at the end of life or with cognitive deficits lose their capacity to report side effects, evaluate treatments, or participate in decision making. Caregivers must make frequent assessments and carefully observe patient behaviors and responses.

4 Proper patient identification, especially in communicating the patients' DNR or CPR status, ensures that caregivers will not initiate unwanted and unhelpful medical interventions. Know your agency's methods for designating a patient's resuscitation status.

SKILL 16-1 Supporting Patients and Families in Grief

People suffer losses and experience grief throughout life. Losses are described in several ways: necessary, actual, perceived, maturational, and situational. Necessary losses such as leaving friends after high school graduation are a natural part of life. Such losses are usually replaced by something different or better. Some necessary losses such as the death of a loved one are more difficult and never seem acceptable. A person experiences an actual loss when an object or person can no longer be felt, heard, or experienced. Examples include the loss of a person or a destroyed home. Perceived losses are uniquely interpreted by an individual and are often not obvious to others. For example, one person perceives a failure to get into a specific college as a lost opportunity, whereas for another person that event is a relief. Maturational losses occur as a part of normal life development. For instance, a parent feels loss when a child moves away from home. Situational losses include loss from sudden, unpredictable external events such as natural disasters. All types of loss can cause grief and a need for adjustment.

Hospitalization, chronic illness, and disability involve multiple losses. Hospitalized patients lose privacy and control over normal routines. With chronic illness a person's body no longer functions as it once did, leading to a loss of self-esteem and social roles. Disability creates financial insecurity and often threatens interpersonal relationships. Death separates people from the physical presence of a person in their lives.

Grief

Grief is the emotional response to a loss, manifested in ways unique to an individual and based on personal experiences, cultural expectations, and spiritual beliefs (Walter and McCoyd, 2009). Coping with grief involves a period of mourning (i.e., the outward, social expressions of grief and the behavior associated with loss). Mourning behaviors and rituals help grieving individuals adapt to loss, receive social support, adjust expectations, and go forward in life. Most mourning rituals are culturally influenced, learned behaviors. Bereavement includes grief and mourning (i.e., the inner emotional responses and outward behaviors in response to loss) (ELNEC, 2008). A person's psychological makeup, personal experiences, family, cultural expectations, and spiritual beliefs influence how he or she grieves (Hooyman and Kramer, 2008). The depth and duration of grief (i.e., one's inner emotional response to loss) depends on the type of loss and the person's perception of the loss.

As a nurse help patients by understanding types of grief. Normal or uncomplicated grief is evidenced by feelings, behaviors, and reactions associated with loss such as sadness, anger, crying, resentment, and loneliness. Families may feel the presence of the lost person and yearn for his or her return. They may find it difficult to resume life as it was before their loss. An uncomplicated grief experience often helps a person mature and develop life perspective. Anticipatory grief occurs before an actual loss or death and involves gradual disengagement from what is being lost. For example, if the dying process extends over a long period of time, the patient and family prepare for death before it occurs and sometimes, but not always, display fewer common grief responses at the time of death (Simon, 2008). Complicated grief occurs when a person has difficulty moving through the grief experience (Field and Filanosky, 2010). Grief may be chronic (lasting over long periods of time), delayed (suppressed until a much later and unexpected time), exaggerated (overwhelming grief that is expressed in self-destructive behaviors), or masked (unaware that disruptions in normal functions are a result of the loss).

Remember that people do not experience grief in the same way. Some people do not report feeling distressed or depressed, and others feel distressed for a lifetime without negative consequences. Not all people want to process the emotional experience of grief and focus instead on resilience, growth, or positive outcomes after a loss (Holman et al., 2010).

Use basic knowledge of grief responses to support patients and their families and to address other common psychosocial and spiritual symptoms at the end of life such as fear and loneliness. Personality type and culture influence the extent to which individuals share emotions or find it helpful to talk about their grief. Some patients talk openly about their approaching death, and others choose not to acknowledge it. Health care providers, depending on their own personal and cultural understandings of grief and death, often avoid initiating conversations on these difficult topics. Provide opportunities for discussion, paying close attention to a patient's response and indications of a desire to talk further (Wittenberg-Lyles, 2010).

Delegation and Collaboration

The skills of assessing patient's or family member's grief reactions and designing appropriate interventions cannot be delegated to nursing assistive personnel (NAP). The nurse directs the NAP to:

- Inform the nurse when a patient or family member exhibits behavior commonly associated with grief (e.g., crying, anger, withdrawal).
- Form supportive relationships with patients and families and inform the nurse when patients or family members have questions or concerns.
- Alert the nurse to the arrival of family members so the nurse can discuss the plan of care and offer support.

STEP	RATIONALE

ASSESSMENT

1 Sit near patient in a quiet, private location. Center yourself and establish a quiet presence. Establish eye contact. Be aware that use of eye contact in some cultures conveys disrespect or discomfort.	Presence expresses caring and creates healing moments (Gauthier, 2008; Newman, 2008). Privacy protects confidentiality and promotes a sense of safety for patient when expressing thoughts and emotions.
2 Consider the influence of patient's age, gender, race, language, religion, culture, and socioeconomic status on communication.	Individual differences influence patient's grief response and communication style (Hooyman and Kramer, 2008).
3 Listen carefully, observing patient responses. Use open communication to develop a genuine, caring nurse-patient relationship.	A nurse establishes trust in a caring relationship, listens to the patient, and demonstrates a desire for communication (Galvin and Todres, 2009; Lowey, 2008).

STEP	RATIONALE
4 Determine meaning of the loss to patient and its type, suddenness, and when it occurred. Use open-ended questions such as: • "Tell me about your family." • "What concerns do you have about how your illness will affect your family?"	The type, meaning, suddenness, and time elapsed since the loss influence the grief experience and coping methods.
5 Combine knowledge of grief theory with observation of patient behaviors. Validate observations by sharing them with patient; paraphrase, clarify, or summarize, as in the following examples: • "You've mentioned several times that you feel hopeless." • "It seems that this is hard for you to talk about." • "You look sad. Is there something in particular that brought on your tears?"	Use information about type and stage of grief to guide discussion, not to judge patient's responses. Confirms accuracy of your observations and validates patient's feelings. Prompts patient to continue.
6 Encourage patient to describe the loss and its impact on daily life (e.g., "You said your diagnosis changed your life forever. Tell me more.").	Listening to patient's description helps to minimize assumptions.
7 Ask patient to describe the coping strategies that he or she uses most often in difficult times (e.g., "What or who helps you in times of crisis?").	Familiar, effective coping strategies are often helpful in the current crisis, loss, or grief experience.
8 Assess family caregivers' unique needs and resources. Note if patient receives care at home and who gives the care.	Illness significantly affects family relationships. Although family members experience similar issues, their needs may differ.
9 Assess patient's spiritual needs and resources, focusing on aspects likely to be involved (e.g., trust, life purpose, faith/belief, and hope).	Situations of loss and grief often challenge or strengthen spiritual concepts such as meaning, hope, community, and a sense of God's presence (Daaleman, 2008; Penman et al., 2009).

NURSING DIAGNOSES

- Caregiver role strain
- Complicated grieving
- Compromised family coping
- Death anxiety
- Fear

- Grieving
- Ineffective coping
- Ineffective denial
- Readiness for enhanced family coping
- Readiness for enhanced hope

- Readiness for enhanced spiritual well-being
- Risk for caregiver role strain
- Risk for complicated grieving
- Risk for spiritual distress

Related factors are individualized based on patient's condition or needs.

PLANNING

1 Expected outcomes following completion of procedures: • Patient maintains relationships with significant people. • Patient expresses grief in keeping with his or her cultural and religious practices. • Patient uses effective coping strategies. • Patient maintains normal life routines.	Patient in grief or loss retains connections with social network. Patient receives support necessary to retain cherished values and ways of being. Patient identifies a sense of relief. Patient adjusts to life-changing circumstances and maintains a sense of control.

IMPLEMENTATION

1 Show an empathic understanding of patient's strengths and needs.	Promotes nurse-patient trust, caring, and reciprocity (Betcher, 2010; Wright et al., 2009).
2 Offer information about patient's illness and clarify misunderstandings or misinformation.	Misunderstanding adds to patient's uncertainty, anxiety, and suffering.
3 Encourage patient to sustain relationships with others to help maintain independence and receive necessary help. Include patient-identified support persons in discussions.	Affiliation with others offers support and helps patient stay engaged in life.
4 Help patient achieve short-term goals (e.g., symptom relief, completion of tasks, resolution of relational problems).	Helping patients identify and meet their personal goals contributes to their quality of life.
5 Provide frequent opportunities for patient and family members to express their fears and concerns. Be attentive to expressions of intense emotions.	Emotions change quickly and frequently at stressful times and complicate communication for nurses and patients (Hultman et al., 2008).
6 Help patients and family caregivers identify and solve problems. Encourage use of available resources (e.g., hospice, respite care, palliative care team, and support groups).	Facilitates family grief resolution and reduces caregiving stress. Solving caregiving problems results in better patient care (Spichiger, 2008).

STEP	RATIONALE
7 Instruct patient in relaxation strategies, guided imagery, meditation, hand massage, healing touch, or acupressure.	Complementary therapies effectively reduce stress and provide useful coping strategies (Mariano, 2010; Osaka et al., 2009).
8 Encourage visits with loved ones, life review with stories or photographs, or projects such as organizing photo albums or journal writing.	Patient sees that life still has meaning and dignity and creates a legacy (Butler, 2009; McSherry, 2011).
9 Address patient's spiritual needs by facilitating religious/spiritual practices and connections with religious community, prayer, music, and providing a listening presence. Make a referral to a spiritual care provider.	Spiritual interventions help patients maintain hope and connect with the things at the core of their identity. Caregivers who connect meaningfully with patient need to initiate interventions (Benzein and Saveman, 2008; Daaleman, 2008).

EVALUATION

1 Note patient descriptions of relationships and activities with others.	Provides information on the extent to which patient retains relational ties.
2 Observe patient's behaviors during ongoing interactions.	Demonstrates patient's ability to express grief and coping.
3 Elicit patient perceptions of benefit gained from use of coping interventions.	Evaluates efficacy of interventions.
4 Discuss progress toward performing routine activities at home.	Evaluates patient's achievement of desired goals or need for goal revision.

Unexpected Outcomes

1 Patient does not acknowledge loss and shows signs of extreme sorrow, anger, withdrawal, or denial.

2 Family and patient relationships do not give patient needed support.

Related Interventions

• Consider referral to a grief specialist professional (e.g., nurse practitioner, psychologist, spiritual care provider).

• Share and validate observations of family strain or patient concern over family interactions.

• Consider a family-patient discussion with health care team.

Recording and Reporting

• Record interventions used to support patient coping and note patient's verbal and nonverbal responses in nurses' notes and electronic health record (EHR).

• Report patient's grief reactions to members of the interdisciplinary team, noting behaviors that affect health outcomes such as treatment refusals or prolonged inactivity.

Special Considerations
Teaching

• Give family caregivers basic information about common grief responses and how to offer support. Coach them on ways to provide emotional and spiritual support to patient and one another (e.g., listening attentively, avoiding false reassurances, allowing for the expression of difficult emotions, talking about normal family activities).

Pediatric

• Children's understanding of death, influenced by age and developmental level, differs from that of adults. Respect parents' wishes about when and what to tell children about illness or death. When discussing sensitive topics with children, encourage parents to offer caring explanations at a level a child is able to understand.

• Play therapy or drawing helps children express thoughts, emotions, or fears about illness or death.

• Be alert to all family members' grief reactions because they may feel guilt, resentment, or helplessness with the illness or death of a sibling, child, or grandchild. Facilitate communication with family members who must be separated from the child.

• Surrogate decision makers, usually the parents, need to make health care decisions for infants and young children. Some decisions are difficult because outcomes in children are often unpredictable.

Gerontologic

• Many older adults have coexisting medical conditions that add to their symptom burden. They have also lived long enough to have experienced cumulative losses, including members of their family and support group, which complicates their grief experience (Derby et al., 2010).

SKILL 16-2 Symptom Management at the End of Life

Quality palliative care centers on vigilant symptom management. Patients living with life-limiting illness often experience multiple, complex physical, emotional, and spiritual symptoms (Aoun et al., 2011). Managing patients' symptoms at the end of life begins by understanding the impact that these symptoms have on patients' lives from their point of view (Fig. 16-2). Assess all symptoms thoroughly because a patient's fear of not being heard or believed compounds the magnitude of symptoms. Patients identify pain as their most common and severe symptom (see Chapter 15). In addition to the psychological and spiritual interventions discussed in Skill 16-1, nurses manage physiologic symptoms at the end of life.

Delegation and Collaboration

The skill of symptom management can be delegated to nursing assistive personnel (NAP). The nurse must conduct the initial

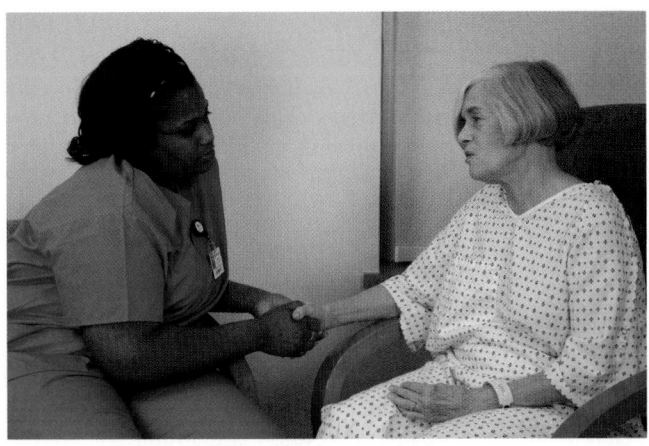

FIG 16-2 Nurses use their presence and therapeutic communication to assess how symptoms affect a patient's life.

assessments of symptoms, but the NAP can assist with supportive care. The nurse directs the NAP to:

- Notify the nurse if patient reports new symptoms or if existing symptoms worsen or change.
- Provide basic comfort care such as positioning, room temperature control, hygiene, and mouth care.
- Report possible adverse effects of drug therapy as instructed by the nurse.
- Speak to unconscious or dying patients because hearing is the last sense to diminish.

STEP	RATIONALE

ASSESSMENT

1 Ask patients to describe symptoms in their own words. Use open-ended prompts such as "Describe your leg pain to me," or "Tell me about how you are sleeping since you started taking this medication."

Allows patients to describe their personal perceptions and experiences of symptoms.

2 Allow sufficient time for patients to describe their symptoms and encourage them to say more:
- "Is there anything else bothering you?"
- "You've told me about your ____ pain. Do you have pain anywhere else?"

Ensures a more complete assessment. Prevents you from making assumptions about patient's symptoms, prematurely stopping the assessment process.

3 Assess patient's pain severity on a scale of 0 to 10 and assess other characteristics of pain routinely with all new reports (see Chapter 15).

Consistent use of a standard pain scale helps assess changes in patient pain levels and evaluate effectiveness of pain interventions (Paice, 2010).

4 Perform hand hygiene.

Reduces transmission of microorganisms.

5 Assess respiratory rate, breathing patterns, and lung sounds. Ask if patient feels that he or she is getting enough air. Assess for presence of airway secretions.

Dyspnea, air hunger, or shortness of breath results from metabolic or respiratory changes. Near the end of life, Cheyne-Stokes respirations are common and are characterized by alternating periods of apnea and hyperpnea.

6 Observe condition of skin, especially back, heels, and buttocks (see Chapter 6).

Decreased peripheral circulation and activity level contribute to skin breakdown.

7 Inspect patient's oral cavity, including mucosa, tongue, and teeth (see Chapter 6).

Dehydration, difficulty swallowing, and inflammation of the mouth are common. Bacterial colonization of the mouth increases with age, reduced salivary flow, medications, and immunosuppression (Rohr et al., 2010).

8 Assess bowel function (see Chapter 34):
a Determine usual bowel elimination pattern (frequency, character, usual time of day) and effectiveness of usual bowel-management routines.

Patients experience constipation because of decreased intestinal motility, fluid intake, and activity and increased anal sphincter tone from pain medications, especially opioids (Kyle, 2010).
Diarrhea results from infections, diseases, or medications (e.g., antibiotics or chemotherapy).

b If patient is passing liquid stool, assess for presence of a fecal impaction (see agency policy).

Watery stool leaking around blockage indicates fecal impaction.

c Review medication regimens, prescription and over-the-counter drugs known to cause constipation (e.g., opioids, antacids).

Medications can alter bowel elimination patterns.

d Identify typical food and fluid intake over 1 week and activity levels.

Bowel elimination patterns are influenced by oral intake and activity levels.

9 Assess urinary elimination (see Chapter 33) and ability to control urination. If incontinent, assess for potential complications (e.g., skin breakdown or patient discomfort).

Urinary incontinence results from progressive disease (e.g., spinal cord involvement and reduced level of consciousness) (Kyle, 2010).

STEP	RATIONALE
10 Assess patient's appetite and for presence of nausea or vomiting.	Medications, pain, depression, disease progression, or decreased blood flow to digestive organs near death often contribute to nausea, vomiting, and decreased appetite.
11 Assess daily food and fluid intake in relation to patient's condition and preferences.	Intake affects fluid balance.
12 Assess fatigue using a general scale in patients near the end of life (none, moderate, severe). Ask if fatigue limits patient's ability to perform desired activities (see Chapter 10).	Metabolic demands of a disease and treatments cause weakness and fatigue.
13 Assess for excessive restlessness in patient near death.	Terminal restlessness (delirium) causes significant patient and caregiver stress (Heidrick and English, 2010).
a Assess for pain, nausea, dyspnea, full bladder or bowel, poor sleep patterns, anxiety, or joint pain from immobility.	Determines presence of common physical problems that need to be treated or ruled out as causative factors.
b Review medical record for hypercalcemia, hypoglycemia, hyponatremia, or dehydration.	Metabolic imbalances cause restlessness or delirium.
c Review patient's medications.	Unintended responses to medications result in changed activity states.
d Determine if patient has unresolved emotional or spiritual issues.	Spiritual distress contributes to restlessness or increased pain.

NURSING DIAGNOSES

• Acute pain	• Diarrhea	• Ineffective breathing pattern
• Anxiety	• Fatigue	• Ineffective tissue perfusion
• Chronic pain	• Nausea	• Risk for constipation
• Constipation	• Impaired oral mucous membrane	• Total urinary incontinence
• Deficient fluid volume	• Impaired swallowing	

Related factors are individualized based on patient's condition or needs.

PLANNING

1 Expected outcomes following completion of procedure:	
• Patient reports acceptable level of pain.	Indicates pain control.
• Patient reports feeling warm and comfortable.	Warming interventions help reverse effects of reduced peripheral circulation.
• Patient reports comfortable eating and drinking patterns.	Optimal food and fluid intake are based on patient preferences and comfort.
• Patient has soft, formed bowel movements.	Indicates adequate bowel function and peristaltic activity.
• Skin remains free of irritation or breakdown.	Interventions to protect the skin from bowel or urinary incontinence are effective.
• Patient is not restless.	Therapies have a calming effect.
• Patient reports less distress from fatigue.	Energy conservation methods are effective; patient adjusts to changes in activity level.
• Patient experiences less respiratory distress.	Patient is less apprehensive and breathes easily.

IMPLEMENTATION

1 Perform hand hygiene.	Reduces transmission of microorganisms.
2 Administer medications and initiate nonpharmacologic pain management interventions (see Chapter 15):	Well-timed interventions keep pain from escalating. Pain decreases patient's sense of well-being and activity.
a Provide patient education on causes and patterns of pain and explain interventions.	Patient's knowledge of pain and interventions allows him or her to maintain some control (Paice, 2010).
3 Provide general comfort measures:	
a Provide bath and skin care based on patient's preferences and hygiene needs (see Chapters 17 and 18).	Daily baths are not always desired or necessary at end of life if they cause discomfort, fatigue, or increased pain.
b Provide eye care and use artificial tears in patients with decreased consciousness (see Chapter 19).	Eye irritation causes pain. Blink reflex diminishes near death, causing drying of cornea.
c Reposition frequently; do not position on tubes or other objects.	Prolonged, even slight pressure from weight of patient's body or objects causes skin injury.

STEP	RATIONALE
4 Provide oral hygiene after meals and at bedtime while awake and more frequently in mouth-breathing or unconscious patients (see Chapter 17).	Mouth rinses are effective in removing oral debris and cleaning the mouth. Dehydration develops as patient experiences metabolic changes and fluid intake declines.
a Use antifungal oral rinses as prescribed or sodium bicarbonate or normal saline rinses.	Patients near death breathe through the mouth, drying oral mucosa.
b Moisten lips with nonpetroleum balm.	
5 Initiate bowel-management regimen to reduce risk for constipation:	Interventions improve peristalsis and soften fecal mass (Enck, 2009).
a Increase fluid intake if medically tolerated and preferred by patient.	
b Encourage physical activity (e.g., walking) if tolerated.	
c Administer daily stool softener or laxative, especially in patients using opioids for pain management; give enemas as needed.	
6 Provide low-residue diet for diarrhea; treat infections or discontinue medications if possible. Administer antidiarrheal medications.	Patients with chronic diarrhea require rigorous skin care to promote comfort. They are also at risk for dehydration and thirst (Kyle, 2010).
7 Address urinary incontinence with intervention appropriate for patient's conditions (e.g., condom catheter, indwelling urinary catheter, adult incontinence pads [see Chapter 33]).	Urinary output declines near death, making it possible to manage incontinence without an indwelling catheter. Consider an indwelling catheter if skin integrity, patient preference, or fatigue from bed changes becomes an issue.
8 Offer patient favorite foods in amount and at time patient desires. Do not overly encourage patients to eat.	Near-death patients have little desire for food and water as body functions slow. Little evidence exists that anorexia or dehydration causes patient discomfort (Acreman, 2009).
a Treat nausea by administering antiemetics rectally as prescribed. As nausea subsides, offer clear liquids and ice chips. Avoid caffeinated liquids, milk, and fruit juices.	Gastrointestinal (GI) mucosa tolerates clear liquids more readily. Certain liquids increase stomach acidity.
b Consider presence of nausea in patients receiving enteral feedings.	Patients who have decreased consciousness are unable to report nausea.
9 Manage fatigue.	
a Balance activity and rest periods according to patient's priorities, energy level, and preferred time of day. Eliminate extra steps in activities.	Strategies to conserve energy and reduce fatigue allow for completion of desired activities. Conserve patient energy by modifying environment (Kehl, 2008).
b Explain care activities before performing and include patient in setting daily schedule.	Minimizes anxiety and maintains patient's autonomy and involvement
c Assist ambulatory patients with physical activity.	Fatigued patients may need assistance and monitoring to ensure patient safety.
d Incorporate safe exercise (e.g., walking, yoga) in activity plan for patients with advanced stage cancer.	Research has shown that, even for people with advanced stage cancer, exercise decreases anxiety, stress, and fatigue (Albrecht and Taylor, 2012).
10 Support patient's ventilatory efforts.	
a Position for comfort in semi-Fowler's or Fowler's position.	Promotes maximal ventilation, lung expansion, and drainage of secretions.
b Position patient near death on side to decrease noisy respirations. Elevate head to facilitate postural drainage. Turn from side to side to mobilize and drain secretions. Suction only if necessary.	Deep airway suctioning causes discomfort and is not effective in reducing airway noise or secretion clearance (Hipp and Letizia, 2009).
c Provide ordered anticholinergic medications.	Medications reduce saliva and excessive secretions.
d Stay with patients experiencing dyspnea or air hunger. Use interventions that patients perceive as relieving their shortness of breath (choice of oxygen delivery modes, fan near face, body position). Administer opioids or anxiolytics as prescribed. Keep room cool with low humidity.	Sharing control with patients reduces anxiety that contributes to feelings of air hunger. Morphine relieves perception of dyspnea and dries secretions. Air movement stimulates trigeminal nerve in cheek, which decreases dyspneic sensation. Use of oxygen has little benefit unless patient feels better using it (Balkstra, 2010).
11 Manage restlessness.	
a Keep patient's room quiet with soft lighting and at comfortable temperature. Offer family members opportunities to maintain close contact. Encourage use of soft music, prayer, or reading from patient's favorite book.	Reduces unnecessary external stimulation and provides a comforting space. Privacy allows family members chance to provide verbal assurances and touch. The presence of a family member to hold a hand provides a calming effect (Pasacreta et al., 2010).

STEP	RATIONALE
b Use least-sedating pharmacologic means possible to control restlessness. Consult with interdisciplinary team for titration of medication (haloperidol or lorazepam). Discontinue all nonessential medication. Use subcutaneous, transdermal, sublingual, or rectal medication delivery routes.	Reduce delirium without making patient unconscious. Control of restlessness relieves family's concern that patient is in pain or distress. Discontinuation of unnecessary medications makes drug interactions less likely. Use least-invasive route for patient comfort (Balkstra, 2010).

EVALUATION

1 Ask patient to rate pain on scale of 0 to 10 (see Chapter 15) and evaluate pain characteristics. Assess behavior in nonverbal patients.	Determines extent of pain relief.
2 Ask patient to describe mouth comfort and inspect oral cavity.	Evaluates condition of oral cavity and ability to chew or swallow.
3 After patient defecates inspect feces.	Determines character of stool.
4 Observe skin condition.	Determine if skin tears or areas of pressure are present.
5 Ask patient to rate fatigue (scale of 0 to 10). Observe for fatigue or shortness of breath when patient performs activities.	Determines if patient is less distressed with activity.
6 Observe patient's respiratory patterns and ask him or her if breathing is easy and comfortable.	Determines if respiratory distress is relieved.
7 Observe patient's behavior or ask family to report on it. Note level of restlessness.	Determines level of comfort and extent of restlessness.

Unexpected Outcomes	**Related Interventions**
1 One or several symptoms remain unresolved, with patient reporting little or no relief.	• Increase frequency of or change an intervention. Try combination therapies.
2 Patient becomes anxious, fearful, or exhausted as a result of continued symptoms.	• Give patients therapy choices and try different interventions. Explain goals of therapies and possible reasons for symptoms. • Answer call lights quickly and explain plan of care throughout the day.

Recording and Reporting

- Record detailed description of patient symptoms in nurses' notes, EHR, and/or appropriate flow sheets. Use consistent descriptors for comparison over time.
- Record type of interventions used and patient's response in nurses' notes and EHR. Note successful interventions in the care plan.
- Report unexpected new symptoms or uncontrolled existing symptoms to health care provider.

Special Considerations
Teaching

- Involve family members in the patient's care (Fig. 16-3). With proper instruction they can perform most symptom

FIG 16-3 Involve family in patient's care.

management interventions, deliver personal care (e.g., bathing, oral hygiene), and administer medications in the home setting.

Pediatric

- Allow young children to visit a dying parent or grandparent if desired. Encourage parents to express their concerns about how to talk about death and loss with their child.
- Teach parents how to recognize and assess pain in a nonverbal child.
- Encourage involvement of siblings of a child who is dying, based on their needs and readiness.

Gerontologic

- Include older adults in conversations and accommodate communication limits (e.g., hearing deficits).
- Older adults need companionship and maintenance of self-esteem. Detached caregiver behaviors such as being slow to respond to physical discomforts, failing to keep room odor free, and speaking in hushed tones of voice are often perceived by the person as abandonment. Encourage a family member, friend, sitter, or hospice volunteer to stay with the patient during the night. Some older adults who have developed a lifestyle around aloneness prefer solitude. Be sensitive to patient's preferences (Ebersole et al., 2008).
- Assessing and addressing pain in an older adult who is cognitively impaired or nonverbal is sometimes difficult and involves proactive symptom management.

Home Care

- Recommend that family members monitor their own energy levels and request respite care when they need relief. Suggest resources for help with meals, shopping, or staying with the patient while family goes out.

SKILL 16-3 Care of a Body After Death

Nurses provide postmortem care in home and institutional settings, caring for a deceased person's body with sensitivity and in a manner consistent with a patient's religious or cultural beliefs. Maintaining the integrity of rituals and mourning practices gives families a sense of some familiarity and control in the face of death. Individual variations exist within cultural and religious groups (see Box 16-1).

Two legal considerations arise at the time of death. First, the 1986 Omnibus Budget Reconciliation Act (OBRA) legally requires that a patient's survivors be made aware of the option of organ and tissue donation. In most states citizens can sign the back of their driver's license if they wish to be an organ or tissue donor. However, a family member still usually gives consent for donation at the time of death. Patients may indicate their wish to donate organs and tissue in an advance directive.

In the case of vital organ donation (e.g., heart, lungs, liver, pancreas, or kidneys), a patient must remain on life support until the organs are surgically removed. A nurse's role in organ procurement includes helping to identify potential organ donors, providing care for the donor's body, and caring for the family throughout the donation process (Matzo and Hill, 2010). Family members often need help understanding what "brain death" (i.e., the irreversible absence of all brain function, including the brainstem) means for a person who has died. Patients appear to still be alive because life support keeps the deceased's organs functioning until they can be retrieved. Tissues such as eyes, bone, and skin are retrieved from deceased patients not on life support. Because of the sensitive nature of making requests for organ donation, professionals educated in organ procurement often assume that responsibility. They inform family members of their options for donation, provide information about costs (no cost to the family), and inform them that donation does not delay funeral arrangements.

Nurses also play a role in the donation request process. Facilitate the conversation by providing a private place and helping to identify the surrogate to be involved in the request. Sometimes you notify the local donor registry to determine if a patient qualifies for organ donation because certain medical conditions prohibit donation. Reinforce explanations of the procedure and inform the family about how you will care for the deceased's body. Above all, honor the family's cultural and religious practices concerning organ and tissue donation and support their final decision. Donor families often report that donating organs helped them in their grief and that they felt positive about the experience.

The second procedure of legal and medical significance often performed after a death is an autopsy, or postmortem examination. An autopsy, the surgical dissection of a body after death, helps determine the exact cause and circumstances of a death, discover the pathway of a disease, or provide data for research purposes. It is not performed in every death. State laws determine when autopsies are required, but they are usually performed in circumstances of unusual death (e.g., violent trauma; unattended, unexpected death in the home) and when death occurs within 24 hours of hospital admission (Matzo and Hill, 2010). Be available to answer questions and support the family's choices. Autopsies normally do not delay burial or change the appearance of the deceased, but there may be a cost to families. The patient's legal representative and the health care provider or designated requester must sign a consent form. If appropriate, explain the value that autopsies have for advancing medical knowledge.

After death the body undergoes many physical changes, including loss of skin elasticity and change in body temperature (algor mortis), purple discoloration of the skin (livor mortis), and a stiffening of the body (rigor mortis). Provide postmortem care as soon as possible to prevent tissue damage or disfigurement. To prevent livor mortis of the face, elevate the head of the bed 30 degrees immediately after death and before beginning other activities.

Delegation and Collaboration

The skill of care of a body after death can be delegated to nursing assistive personnel (NAP). However, it is often best for the nurse and NAP to work together in providing postmortem care. The nurse directs the NAP to:

- Follow agency policy in cases of autopsy or organ and tissue donation.
- Honor family cultural or religious rituals when performing postmortem care.
- Handle the body with dignity and respect for privacy.

Equipment

- ❑ Clean gloves and isolation gown
- ❑ Plastic bag for hazardous waste disposal
- ❑ Washbasin, washcloth, warm water, and bath towel
- ❑ Clean gown or disposable gown for body as indicated by agency policy
- ❑ Shroud kit with name tags
- ❑ Syringes for removing urinary catheter
- ❑ Scissors
- ❑ Small pillow or towel
- ❑ Paper tape, gauze dressings
- ❑ Paper bag, plastic bag, or other suitable receptacle for patient's belongings to be returned to family members
- ❑ Valuables envelope

STEP	RATIONALE

ASSESSMENT

1 Ask health care provider to establish time of death and determine if he or she has requested an autopsy. If an autopsy is planned or a possible crime is involved, use special precautions to preserve evidence (see agency policy).	Certifies patient's death. Autopsy requested to determine cause of death and learn more about a disease.
2 Determine if family members or significant others are present and if they have been informed of the death. Identify patient's surrogate (next of kin or durable power of attorney [DPOA]).	Verifies that family has been notified of patient's death to avoid inappropriate communication of this sensitive information.

STEP	RATIONALE
3 Determine if patient's surrogate has been asked about organ and tissue donation and validate that donation request form has been signed. Notify organ request team per policy.	Federal guidelines require documentation that request has been made.
4 Provide family members and friends a private place to gather. Allow them time to ask questions or discuss grief.	Creates safe environment for grieving family. Questions provide information about how they are coping with loss and their needs.
5 Ask family members if they have requests for preparation or viewing of the body (e.g., position of body, special clothing, shaving). Determine if they wish to be present or assist with care of the body.	Respects individuality of patient and family and supports their right to having cultural or religious values and beliefs upheld. Provides closure for those who wish to help with body preparation.
6 Contact a support person (spiritual care provider or staff member) to stay with family members not helping to prepare the body.	Provides family support during an emotional time.
7 Consult health care providers' orders for special care directives or specimens that are to be collected.	Specimens may be used in determining cause of death.
8 Perform hand hygiene; apply clean gloves, gown, or protective barriers.	Reduces transmission of microorganisms.
9 Assess general condition of the body and note presence of dressings, tubes, and medical equipment. (If leaving room at this time, remove personal protective equipment and perform hand hygiene.)	Validates if tissue damage was present before postmortem care.

NURSING DIAGNOSES

For patients:	For family members and significant others:
• Risk for impaired skin integrity	• Compromised family coping • Ineffective coping • Deficient knowledge regarding organ donation • Grieving • Powerlessness

Related factors are individualized based on the patient's, family's, and significant others' needs.

PLANNING

1 Expected outcomes following completion of procedure: • Body is free of new skin damage.	Careful handling of body prevents lacerations, bruises, or abrasions during postmortem care.
• Significant others express grief.	Significant others feel supported through their loss.

Clinical Decision Point *Immediately after death and before proceeding with other activities, place body in supine position and elevate head of bed 30 degrees to decrease livor mortis.*

2 Place body in a private room if possible. If patient has a roommate, explain and move roommate to another location temporarily.	Provides staff with larger area for postmortem care and for family members to gather in a private setting.
3 Direct NAP to gather needed equipment and arrange at bedside.	Because this is often an emotional time for family members, organized care is important.

IMPLEMENTATION

1 Help family members notify others of the death. Promptly notify the mortuary, as chosen by the family, and discuss plans for postmortem care.	Following a death, grieving persons have difficulty focusing on details and often need guidance. Being informed increases a sense of control.
2 If patient has made tissue donation, consult agency policy for care of the body guidelines.	Retrieval of tissues (e.g., eyes, bone, skin) may require special procedures.
3 Perform hand hygiene; apply clean gloves, gown, or protective barriers.	Reduces transmission of microorganisms.

Clinical Decision Point *If family caregivers are assisting in postmortem care, have them wear a gown and gloves to protect them from body fluids.*

4 Identify patient using two identifiers (i.e., name and birthday or name and account number) according to agency policy. Compare identifiers with information on patient's identification bracelet. Tag the body and leave on the body as directed by agency policy.	Ensures correct patient. Complies with The Joint Commission standards and improves patient safety (TJC, 2012).

STEP	RATIONALE
5 Remove indwelling devices (e.g., urinary catheter, endotracheal tube). Disconnect and cap off (no need to remove) intravenous lines. Do not remove indwelling devices in cases of autopsy (follow agency policy).	Creates a normal appearance for family viewing of the body. Removing intravenous catheters allows fluids to leak out. Removal of tubes and lines is contraindicated if an autopsy is planned.
6 Place dentures in mouth for viewing. If they do not stay securely in mouth, place in denture cup and transport with body to mortuary. If culturally appropriate, close mouth with rolled-up towel under chin.	Gives face a more natural appearance. Jaw muscles relax after death, making it difficult to keep dentures in place. Mortuary personnel remove dentures to clean and seal mouth.
7 Place small pillow under head or position according to cultural preferences. Do not tie hands together on top of body. Check agency policy regarding need to secure hands and feet. Use only circular gauze bandaging on body.	Patient appears natural. Weight of limp arms causes skin damage and discoloration if hands are tied. Some agencies require securing appendages to prevent tissue damage when body is being moved.
8 Close eyes by gently pulling eyelids over them. Some cultures prefer that eyes remain open.	Closed eyes convey to some people a more peaceful and natural appearance.
9 Shave male facial hair unless prohibited by cultural practices or if patient wore a beard.	Presents patient in his normal appearance. Honors cultural or religious preferences.
10 Wash soiled body parts. Some cultural practices require that family members clean the body.	Prepares body for viewing and reduces odors. Mortuary personnel provide complete bath.
11 Remove soiled dressings and replace with clean dressings, using paper tape or circular gauze bandaging.	Changing dressings controls odors and creates more acceptable appearance. Paper tape minimizes skin damage when tape is removed.

Clinical Decision Point *Turning a recently dead body to the side sometimes causes the flow of exhaled air. This is a normal event and not a sign of life.*

STEP	RATIONALE
12 Place absorbent pad under buttocks.	Relaxation of sphincter muscles at time of death causes release of urine or feces.
13 Place clean gown on the body. Some agencies require gown removal before placing body in the shroud.	Provides privacy and prepares body for viewing.
14 Brush and comb hair. Remove any clips, hairpins, or rubber bands.	The deceased appears cared for. Hard objects damage or discolor face and scalp.
15 Identify personal belongings that stay with the body and those to be given to the family.	Prevents loss of valuable or meaningful property.
16 If family requests viewing, place clean sheet over body up to chin with arms outside covers. Remove medical equipment from the room. Provide soft lighting and chairs.	Maintains respect for patient and those viewing the body. Prevents exposure of body parts. Removing medical equipment provides more peaceful, natural setting.
17 Allow family time alone with the body and encourage them to say goodbye with religious rituals and in a culturally appropriate manner. Some cultural practices include maintaining silence at the time of death. Persons in other cultures express grief with intense emotional displays, loud wailing, or "falling out." Do not rush any grieving process.	Compassionate care provides family members with a meaningful experience during the early phase of grief. Ensure privacy and a safe environment. Provide chair at bedside for family member who might collapse.
18 After viewing, remove linens and gown per agency policy. Place body in shroud provided by the agency (see illustration).	Shroud protects injury to skin, avoids exposure of body, and provides barrier against potentially contaminated body fluids.

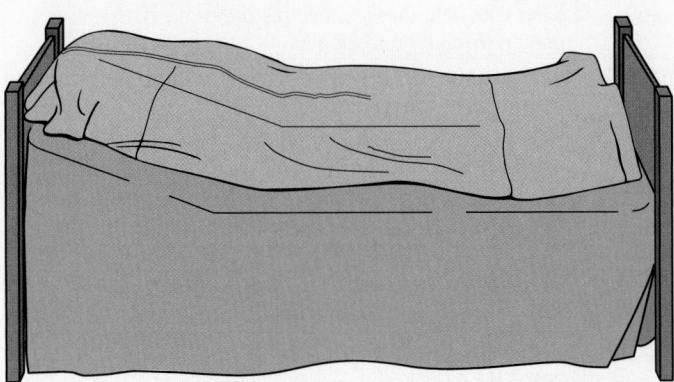 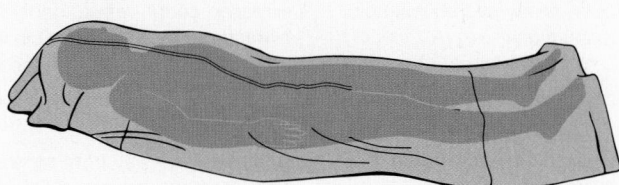

STEP 18 Body in shroud.

STEP	RATIONALE
19 Place identification label on outside of shroud if required by agency policy. Follow agency policy for marking a body that poses an infectious risk to others. Remove and dispose of personal protective equipment and perform hygiene.	Ensures proper identification of the body. Reduces exposure of morgue and mortuary staff to contamination.
20 Arrange prompt transportation of the body to the mortuary. If you anticipate a delay, transport body to the morgue.	Mortuary personnel get the best results if embalming occurs before full rigor mortis (i.e., stiffening of the body after death) occurs.

EVALUATION

1 Observe family members', friends', and significant others' response to the loss.	The need for referral or assistance is based on evaluation of person's unique response to loss.
2 Note appearance and condition of patient's skin during preparation of the body.	Provides information for postmortem care documentation.

Unexpected Outcomes

1 A family member becomes immobilized by grief and has difficulty functioning.

2 A grieving person becomes very agitated and threatens or strikes out against others.

3 Lacerations, bruises, or abrasions are noted on the body. Positioning or preparation of the body results in skin injury.

Related Interventions

- Enlist the help of a trusted friend or family member to provide direction and support.
- Call for assistance from a psychiatric nurse practitioner, spiritual care provider, or social worker who has a relationship with the family.
- Enlist help of security staff or crisis intervention professional if safety is a concern.
- Document according to policy.

Recording and Reporting

- Record time of death in the nurses' notes and EHR and other appropriate forms, describe any resuscitative measures taken (if applicable), and note the name of the professional certifying the death.
- Record any special preparation of the body for autopsy or organ/tissue donation. Note whom you called and who made the request for organ/tissue donation.
- Record names of mortuary and names of family members consulted at the time of death and their relationship to the deceased.

- Record on appropriate form personal articles left on the body (e.g., teeth or glasses), jewelry taped to skin, or tubes and lines left in place. Note how valuables and personal belongings were handled and who received them. Secure signatures as required by agency policy.
- Record time the body was transported and its destination. Note the location of body identification tags.

Pediatric Considerations

- Arrange for family members, especially parents, to be with the child throughout the dying process and at the time of death if they wish.

TABLE 16-1 | Physical Signs and Symptoms in the Final Stages of Dying

Physical Signs and Symptoms	Rationale	Intervention
Coolness, color, and temperature change in hands, arms, feet, and legs; mottling of legs; perspiration	Peripheral circulation diminished as blood shunts to vital organs. Patient may feel cool to touch, but core temperature normal	Place socks on feet. Cover with light blanket. Do not use electric blanket because person is unable to report excess heat.
Increased sleeping	Decreased energy, psychological withdrawal, medications	Spend time with person; hold his or her hand. Speak to person, even if no response.
Disorientation, confusion of time, place, person	Metabolic changes, medications, changing sleep/wake cycles, decreased oxygenation	Identify self by name; reorient person to time and place. Decrease environmental stimuli.
Incontinence of urine and/or bowel	Decreased muscle tone and consciousness	Change bedding as appropriate. Use bed pads; try not to use indwelling catheters.
Upper airway secretions; noisy respirations	Decreased cough reflex, inability to expectorate secretions or clear throat, relaxation of glottis, decreased muscle tone	Elevate head with pillow or raise head of bed; turn head to side to drain secretions. Suction minimally.
Restlessness	Metabolic changes and decrease in oxygen to brain	Calm patient by speech and action; reduce light, rub back, stroke arms, or read aloud. Do not use restraints.
Decreased intake of food and fluids, nausea	Blood shunted away from gastrointestinal (GI) tract, causing decreased GI motility and anorexia; ketosis	Do not force patient to eat or drink; give ice chips or popsicles if desired. Provide mouth care.

Modified from Ebersole P et al: *Toward healthy aging*, ed 7, St Louis, 2008, Mosby.

- Parents frequently want to hold their child's body after death. Parents of deceased newborns often want a memento of their baby (e.g., picture, article of clothing, footprint, or lock of hair). Make every effort to honor parent requests.

Gerontologic Considerations

- Some older adults have very small families and surviving circles of friends. Nurses and other care providers are sometimes the only human presence during death. Arrange for someone to be with the person when death is imminent.

Home Care Considerations

- Educate family members caring for a patient dying at home about what to expect at the time of death (Table 16-1).

Encourage family members to talk with patient and say their goodbyes because research suggests that hearing remains intact near death.

- Consider the type of support that family members will need at the time of death and make arrangements.
- After death in the home, follow agency guidelines for body preparation and transfer and for disposal of durable medical equipment (e.g., tubing, needles, syringes), soiled dressings or linens, and medications. Instruct family members in safe and proper handling and disposal of medical waste.

? Critical Thinking Exercises

You are caring for Mr. Corbin, a 79-year-old man hospitalized for abdominal pain, anorexia, weight loss, and weakness. He was treated 10 years earlier for prostate cancer. Test results now confirm that he has a large tumor in his abdomen and the cancer has spread to the lymph nodes. No medical interventions are available to cure his disease. When you enter the room, Mr. Corbin tells you in an angry voice that he wants to transfer to a different hospital where people will help him fight his cancer.

1   What should you do first in response to Mr. Corbin's statement?
2   The next day Mr. Corbin reports mild abdominal pain and mentions that he has not had a bowel movement for 3 days. His wife reports to you that he has not had anything to eat or drink for 24 hours. Which action will you take first on the basis of this information?
   1   Assure the patient that it is not abnormal to have infrequent bowel movements with decreased intake.
   2   Further assess Mr. Corbin's pain and bowel patterns.
   3   Ask Mr. Corbin's wife to describe what his pain was like when he first came to the hospital.
   4   Encourage Mr. Corbin to increase his fluid intake and activity to improve peristalsis.
3   Four weeks later you take care of Mr. Corbin again. His symptoms include weight loss, anorexia, abdominal pain, depression, and anxiety. His wife tells you that the nurse practitioner told them about home hospice care. His wife says to you, "I'm still not sure if hospice would be best for us." Which key points would you include in a discussion with Mr. Corbin and his wife about hospice care?

✓ REVIEW QUESTIONS

1   A patient with cancer is admitted into hospice care. Which question by a nurse demonstrates an understanding of a primary goal of palliative care?
   1   "What arrangements have been made for your funeral and burial?"
   2   "Are you sure that you no longer want treatment for your disease?"
   3   "What are the most important things we can do to help during this time?"
   4   "Is pain your primary problem at the current time?"
2   A mother who recently lost her only son in a motorcycle accident does not feel like going back to work after the funeral and often believes that she hears her son's motorcycle outside. Which type of grief would the nurse suspect that the mother is experiencing?

   1   Disenfranchised
   2   Anticipatory
   3   Normal
   4   Overwhelming
3   A woman experiences the loss of a very early–term pregnancy. Her friends do not mention the loss, and someone suggests to her that she can "always try again." The woman feels confusion over her sadness and stops talking about it with others. Which type of grief response might she be experiencing?
   1   Delayed
   2   Anticipated
   3   Exaggerated
   4   Disenfranchised
4   A home care nurse is asked by a family member what he should do if the patient's serious chronic illness worsens even with increased medical interventions. How would the nurse best begin a conversation about the goals of care at the end of life?
   1   Initiate a discussion about advance directives with the patient, family, and health care team
   2   Avoid the discussion about advance directives because that has to do with medical, not nursing, diagnoses
   3   Encourage the family to think more positively about the patient's new therapy
   4   Begin the discussion by asking the family member what he believes the goals should be
5   Mrs. Worth asks you for advice on how she might get her husband to eat more. She believes that if he ate more he would get stronger and enjoy life more. She feels sad that he refuses the meals she prepares. How would you best begin your conversation with her?
   1   "You might let him plan the menu so he can select what he wants."
   2   "Several nutritional supplements are available that might help him gain weight."
   3   "His appetite is decreased because he is not getting enough activity. If you encourage him to walk more, he might feel hungry at mealtimes."
   4   "It must be distressing to see him lose his interest in eating. Loss of appetite is common and normal in people with serious illness."
6   A family member of a recently deceased patient talks casually with a nurse at the time of the patient's death and expresses relief that she will not have to visit at the hospital anymore. Which type of grief may apply to this family member?
   1   Complicated
   2   Anticipatory
   3   Dysfunctional
   4   Disenfranchised
7   A nurse suggests that a patient receive a palliative care consultation for symptom management related to anxiety and increasing pain. A family member asks the nurse if this means that the patient is dying and is now "in hospice." What should the nurse tell the patient and family about the care that she is receiving?

1 Hospice (end-of-life care) and palliative care are the same thing.
2 Palliative care is for any patient, any time, any disease, in any setting.
3 Palliative care strategies are primarily designed to treat the patient's illness.
4 Palliative care interventions relieve the symptoms of illness and treatment.
5 1 and 3
6 2 and 4

8 Which of the following nursing actions best reflects sensitivity to cultural differences related to end-of-life care?
1 Practice honesty with everyone, telling patients about their illness, even if the news is not good.
2 Ask family members if they would like to assist with the care of the body after death.
3 Provide postmortem care at the time of death to relieve family members of this difficult job.
4 Value patient self-determination, understanding that each person makes his or her own decisions.
5 1, 2, and 4
6 2 and 4

9 Regarding the request for organ and tissue donation at the time of death, a nurse should be aware that:
1 Specially educated personnel make the donation request.
2 Requests are usually made by the nurse caring for the patient at the time of death.
3 Only patients who have given prior instruction regarding donation can become donors.
4 Professionals should be very selective in whom they ask for organ and tissue donation.

10 A nurse has the responsibility of managing a deceased patient's postmortem care. Arrange the steps for postmortem care in the proper order.
1 Bathe the deceased's body.
2 Collect any needed specimens.
3 Remove all drains and indwelling tubes.
4 Position the body for family visit/viewing.
5 Speak to the family members about their possible participation.
6 Confirm that request for organ/tissue donation and/or autopsy has been made.
7 Notify a support person (e.g., spiritual care provider, bereavement specialist) for the family.
8 Accurately tag the body, indicating deceased's identity and safety issues regarding infection control.
9 Elevate the head of the bed.

REFERENCES

Acreman S: Nutrition in palliative care, Br J Commun Nurs 14(10):127, 2009.

Albrecht TA, Taylor AG: Physical activity in patients with advanced stage cancer: a systematic review, Clin J Oncol Nurs 16(3):293, 2012.

Aoun S, et al: Measuring symptom distress in palliative care: psychometric properties of the symptom assessment scale, Palliat Med 14(3):315, 2011.

Balkstra C: Dyspnea. In Matzo M, Sherman D, editors: Palliative care nursing: quality care at the end of life, ed 3, New York, 2010, Springer.

Benzein G, Saveman B: Health-promoting conversations about hope and suffering with couples in palliative care, Int J Palliat Nurs 14(9):439, 2008.

Betcher D: Elephant in the room project: improving caring efficacy through effective and compassionate communication with palliative care patients, Medsurg Nurs 19(2):101, 2010.

Butler F: Telling life stories, J Psychosocial Nurs 47(11):21, 2009.

Daaleman T, et al: An exploratory study of spiritual care at the end of life, Annals Fam Med 6(5):406, 2008.

Dietz I, et al: Medical errors and patient safety in palliative care: a review of current literature, J Palliat Med 13(12):1469, 2010.

Derby S, et al: Elderly patients. In Ferrell B, Coyle N, editors: Textbook of palliative nursing, New York, 2010, Oxford University Press.

Dy S, et al: A systematic review of satisfaction with care at the end of life, J Am Geriatr Soc 56(1):124, 2008.

Ebersole P, et al: Toward healthy aging, ed 7, St Louis, 2008, Mosby.

Enck R: An overview of constipation and newer therapies, Am J Hospice Palliat Med 26(3):157, 2009.

End-of-Life Nursing Education Consortium (ELNEC), American Association of Colleges of Nursing (AACN) and City of Hope National Medical Center, 2008. Washington, DC, http://www.aacn.nche.edu/elnec/about/fact-sheet. Accessed June 19 2012.

Erichsen E, et al: A phenomenological study of nurses' understanding of honesty in palliative care, Nurs Ethics 17(1):39, 2010.

Ferrell B, Coyle N: Textbook of palliative nursing, ed 3, New York, 2010, Oxford University Press.

Field N, Filanosky C: Continuing bonds, risk factors for complicated grief and adjustment to bereavement, Death Studies 34:1, 2010.

Five wishes: available at http://www.agingwithdignity.org/forms/5wishes.pdf, accessed September 10, 2011.

Galvin K, Todres L: Embodying nursing openheartedness, J Holistic Nurs 27(2):141, 2009.

Gauthier D: Challenges and opportunities: communication near the end of life, Medsurg Nurs 17(5):291, 2008.

Giger J: Transcultural nursing: assessment and intervention, ed 6, St Louis, 2013, Mosby.

Heidrick D, English N: Delirium, confusion, agitation, and restlessness. In Ferrell B, Coyle N, editors: Textbook of palliative nursing, New York, 2010, Oxford University Press.

Hipp B, Letizia M: Understanding and responding to the death rattle in dying patients, Medsurg Nurs 18(1):17, 2009.

Holman, EA, et al: The myths of coping with loss in undergraduate psychiatric nursing books, Res Nurs Health 33:486, 2010.

Hooyman N, Kramer B: Living through loss: interventions across the lifespan, New York, 2008, Columbia University Press.

Hospice Foundation of America. Available at http://www.hospicefoundation.org/. Accessed June 19, 2012.

Hultman T, et al: Improving psychological and psychiatric aspects of palliative care: the national consensus project and the national quality forum preferred practices for palliative and hospice care, Omega 57(4):323, 2008.

Johnston B: Can self-care become an integrated part of end of life care? Implications for palliative nursing, Int J Palliat Nurs 16(5):212, 2010.

Johnstone L, Kanitsaki O: Ethics and advance care planning in a culturally diverse society, J Transcult Nurs 20(4):405, 2009.

Kehl K: Caring for the patient and the family in the last hours of life, Home Health Care Manage Pract 20(5):408, 2008.

Kyle B: Bowel and bladder care at the end of life, Br J Nurs 19(7):408, 2010.

Lowey S: Communication between the nurse and family caregiver in end of life care: a review of the literature, J Hosp Palliat Nurs 10(1):35, 2008.

Mahon M: Advanced care decision making: asking the right people the right questions, J Psychosocial Nurs 48(7):13, 2010.

Mariano C: Holistic integrative therapies in palliative care. In Matzo M, Sherman D, editors: Palliative care nursing: quality care to the end of life, New York, 2010, Springer.

Matzo M, Hill J: Peri-death nursing care. In Matzo M, Sherman D, editors: Palliative care nursing: quality care at the end of life, New York, 2010, Springer.

McSherry C: The inner life at end of life, J Hospice Palliat Nurs 13(2):112, 2011.

Newman M: Transforming presence, Philadelphia, 2008, Davis.

Osaka I, et al: Endocrinological evaluations of brief hand massage in palliative care, J Altern Comp Med 15(9):981, 2009.

Paice J: Pain at the end of life. In Ferrell B, Coyle N, editors: Textbook of palliative nursing, New York, 2010, Oxford University Press.

Pasacreta JV, et al: Anxiety and depression. In Ferrell B, Coyle N, editors: Textbook of palliative nursing, ed 3, New York, 2010, Oxford University Press.

Pattison N: Care of patients who have died, Nurs Stand 22(28):42, 2008.

Penman J, et al: Spirituality and spiritual engagement as perceived by palliative care clients and caregivers, Aust J Adv Nurs 26(4):29, 2009.

Rohr Y, et al: Oral discomfort in palliative care: results of an exploratory study of the experiences of terminally ill patients, Int J Palliat Nurs 16(9):439, 2010.

Simon J: Anticipatory grief: recognition and coping, J Palliat Med 11(9):1280, 2008.

Spichiger E: Living with terminal illness: patient and family experiences of hospital end of life care, Int J Palliat Nurs 14(5):220, 2008.

The Joint Commission (TJC): National Patient Safety Goals, Oakbrook Terrace, Ill, 2012, The Commission, available at http://www.jointcommission.org/standards_information/npsgs.aspx.

Walter C, McCoyd J: Grief and loss across the lifespan: a biopsychosocial perspective, New York, 2009, Springer.

Washington K, et al: Barriers to hospice use among African Americans: a systematic review, Health Soc Work 14(4):267, 2008.

Wasserman L: Respectful death: a model for end-of-life care, Clin J Oncol Nurs 12(4):621, 2008.

Wittenberg-Lyles E: The COMFORT initiative: palliative nursing and the centrality of communication, J Hosp Palliat Nurs 12(5):282, 2010.

World Health Organization: WHO Definition of Palliative Care, 2011, available at http://www.who.int/cancer/palliative/definition/en/, accessed September 9, 2011.

Wright D, et al: Human relationships at the end of life, J Hosp Palliat Nurs 11(4):219, 2009.

Personal Hygiene and Bed Making

SKILLS AND PROCEDURES

MEDIA RESOURCES

- **evolve** learning system http://evolve.elsevier.com/Perry/skills
  - Review Questions
  - ▶ Video Clips
  - Audio glossary

KEY TERMS

Alopecia	Gag reflex	Mastication	Podiatrist
Aspiration	Gingivae	Mucositis	Pruritus
Buccal	Gingivitis	Necrotic	Sebaceous gland
Cheilosis	Halitosis	Neuropathy	Sebum
Cuticle	Hygiene	NPO	Slough
Dental caries	Incontinence-Associated	Periodontal	Stomatitis
Dermatitis	Dermatitis	Periodontitis	Tepid
Eschar	Maceration	Plaque	Xerostomia
Flossing			

OBJECTIVES

Mastery of content in this chapter will enable the nurse to:
- Discuss guidelines used to provide personal hygiene to patients.
- Identify principles of aseptic technique applied while administering a bed bath.
- Administer a complete bed bath.

- Explain precautions to take when assisting patients with a tub bath or shower.
- Discuss precautions used to minimize transmission of infection during perineal care.
- Identify guidelines to follow when administering oral hygiene.

- Explain differences in providing oral hygiene to dependent versus unconscious patients.
- Discuss precautions used to prevent breakage of dentures.
- Identify guidelines for administering hair, nail, and foot care.
- Comb, brush, and shampoo the hair of a bed-bound patient.
- Shave a male or female patient.
- Identify risk factors for foot and nail problems.
- Safely administer nail care.
- Change the linen on an unoccupied and occupied bed.

Many patients who are totally dependent on someone else require assistance with personal hygiene or must learn or adapt new hygiene techniques. Hygiene is important for promoting and preserving health. Maintenance of personal hygiene is necessary for an individual's health, comfort, safety, and sense of well being. When performing hygiene, you have the opportunity to interact with patients to discuss emotional, social, and health-related concerns. Always convey sensitivity and respect for a patient's personal beliefs and habits and ensure a patient has as much privacy as possible. In addition, performing hygiene is an excellent time to conduct a physical assessment (see Chapter 6).

THE SKIN

Skin, the largest human body organ, protects the body from heat, light, injury and infection and serves to (1) help regulate body temperature; (2) store water, vitamin D, and fat; (3) help sense pain and other stimuli; and (4) prevent the entry of bacteria. Three primary layers make up the skin: the epidermis, dermis, and subcutaneous tissue. The skin covers the entire surface of the body and is continuous with mucous membranes of the mouth, eyes, ears, nose, vagina, and rectum. Thorough hygiene is essential for the integrity and function of each skin layer.

The epidermis, or outer skin layer, is the first line of defense against external injury and infection. It contains several thin layers of cells undergoing different stages of maturation. Sebum, secreted from hair follicles from sebaceous glands, provides an acidic coating. This acidic coating protects the epidermis against penetration by chemicals and microorganisms. It also minimizes loss of water and plasma proteins.

Two types of sweat glands, the eccrine and apocrine glands, are distributed over the surface of the skin. Eccrine glands secrete a watery fluid (sweat) that assists in temperature control through evaporation. The apocrine glands secrete sweat in the axillary and genital areas. Bacterial decomposition of sweat from the apocrine glands causes body odor.

The subcutaneous tissue layer contains blood vessels, nerves, lymph tissue, and loose connective tissue filled with fat cells. Fatty tissue insulates the body. Subcutaneous tissue also provides support for upper skin layers.

Bacteria reside on the outer surface of the skin. The resident bacteria are normal flora that do not cause disease but prevent disease-causing microorganisms from reproducing. Because a portion of the skin is usually exposed to environmental irritants and is an active organ sensitive to physiologic changes within the body, some skin problems commonly occur (Table 17-1). Assess for skin conditions while providing hygiene and suggest measures to alleviate these conditions. Skin problems cause changes that affect a patient's appearance and body image. Be sensitive to his or her feelings while attempting to care for a skin problem.

THE MOUTH

The oral cavity, which is lined with a normally moist and intact light pink mucous membrane, contains the teeth and gums. The membranous lining protects underlying organs; secretes mucus to keep the oral cavity lubricated; and absorbs water, salts, and other solutes. Saliva, a clear viscous fluid secreted by the mucous and salivary glands of the mouth, helps to prevent dental caries and plaque formation and lubricates the oral cavity. Lubrication of the oral cavity aids in chewing and swallowing. In addition, saliva provides a means for removing cellular and bacterial debris that can cause infection, particularly fungal infection (Sjögren's Syndrome Foundation, 2011). Hyposalivation results in dry mouth, or xerostomia, and compromises taste, swallowing, digestion, nutrition, and denture fit (Yasny and Silvay, 2010).

The teeth are organs of chewing, or mastication. Dentin, a hard, ivorylike substance that surrounds the pulp cavity, forms the major part of a tooth (Fig. 17-1). A layer of enamel, visible in the oral cavity, covers the upper portion of the tooth, or crown. The periodontal membrane, just below the gum margins, surrounds the tooth root and holds it firmly in place. A tooth receives its blood, lymph, and nerve supply from the base of the tooth socket within the jaw. Healthy teeth are smooth, shiny, and properly aligned.

The gums, or gingivae, are mucous membranes with underlying supportive fibrous tissue. They encircle the necks of erupted teeth to hold them firmly in place. The gums are normally pink, moist, firm, and relatively inelastic. Regular oral hygiene is necessary to maintain the integrity of teeth surfaces and prevent gingivitis, or gum inflammation.

THE HAIR

Hair grows from follicles located within the dermis of the skin (Fig. 17-2). Tiny blood vessels supply each follicle with nourishment necessary for normal hair growth. Each hair has a shaft extending from the follicle. Sebaceous glands secrete the oily substance (i.e., sebum) into each follicle, which lubricates the hair and scalp. The hair shaft is normally shiny and pliant and is not excessively oily, dry, or brittle.

The primary function of hair is protection. For example, hair protects the scalp from injury. Eyebrows and eyelashes protect the eyes from foreign particles. Special hair-care practices focus primarily on care for scalp, axilla, and pubic areas. Hair growth, distribution, and pattern are indicators of a person's health status. Hormonal changes, emotional and physical stress, aging, intake of toxins (e.g., arsenic, cocaine), gender, race, nutrition, infection, and certain diseases affect hair characteristics. A person's appearance and sense of well-being often depend on the way the hair looks and feels. Illness or disability sometimes prevents patients from maintaining daily hair care. An immobilized patient's hair soon becomes tangled if not brushed or combed regularly. Dressings may leave sticky

TABLE 17-1 | Common Skin Problems

Problem	Characteristics	Implications	Interventions
Dry skin	Flaky, rough texture resulting from lack of moisture in outer stratum corneum, resulting in less pliable epidermis; most common on anterior surfaces of lower legs, knees, elbows, and backs of hands	Skin may crack, bleed, and become inflamed. As a result, redness, pruritus, and discomfort may develop.	Effective treatment of dry skin does not include limiting frequency of bathing but lies in bathing with warm, not hot, water and use of moisturizers. Use super-fatted soap (e.g., Dove) for cleaning. Rinse body of all soap well because residue left can cause irritation and breakdown. Add moisture to air through use of humidifier. Increase fluid intake when skin is dry.
Acne (From James WD, et al: *Andrew's diseases of the skin: Clinical dermatology,* ed 10, Philadelphia, 2007, Saunders.)	Inflammatory, papulopustular skin eruption, usually involving bacterial breakdown of sebum; appears on face, neck, shoulders, and back	Infected material within pustule can spread if area is squeezed or picked. Permanent scarring can result.	Wash hair and skin each day with warm water and soap to remove oil. Use cosmetics sparingly because oily cosmetics or creams accumulate in pores and tend to make condition worse. Implement necessary dietary restrictions by eliminating foods found to aggravate condition. Use prescribed topical antibiotics for severe acne.
Hirsutism (From Goyal D, et al: Coffin-Siris syndrome with Mayer-Rokitanksy-Küster-Hauser syndrome: A case report, *J Med Case Report* 4:354, 2010; DOI: 10.1186/1752-1947-4-354.)	Excessive growth of body and facial hair, especially in women	Hirsutism may cause negative body image by giving female a male appearance.	Shaving is safest method to remove hair. Electrolysis and laser permanently remove hair. Tweezing and bleaching are temporary.
Skin rashes	Skin eruption that results from overexposure to sun or moisture or from allergic reaction; may be flat or raised, localized or systemic, pruritic or nonpruritic	If skin is continually scratched, inflammation and infection may occur. Rashes also cause discomfort.	Wash area thoroughly and apply antiseptic spray or lotion to prevent further itching and aid healing process. Warm or cold soaks may relieve inflammation.
Contact dermatitis (From Lewis SL, et al: *Medical-surgical nursing: Assessment and management of clinical problems,* ed 8, St Louis, 2011, Mosby.)	Acute or chronic eczematous rash characterized by abrupt onset with well-defined geometric margins of erythema, pruritus, pain, and appearance of scaly, oozing lesions; appears on head, neck, scalp, hands, legs, dorsum of feet, and trunk	Dermatitis is often difficult to eliminate because person is usually in continual contact with substance causing skin reaction. Substance may be hard to identify.	Identify and avoid contributing agents (e.g., cleaners, poison ivy or oak, cosmetics, latex, shoes/rubber). Treatment consists of removing contributing agent, if identified, and applying over-the-counter topical steroids or calamine lotion. In some cases prescription steroids may be ordered. Patients may also find comfort with tepid baths.
Abrasion (From Cottran SR et al: From the teaching collection of the Department of Dermatology, University of Texas, Southwestern Medical School, Dallas.)	Scraping or rubbing away of epidermis may result in localized bleeding and later weeping of serous fluid	Infection occurs easily as result of loss of protective skin layer.	Nurses should always be careful not to scratch patients with their jewelry or fingernails. Wash abrasions with mild soap and water. Dressing or bandage could increase risk for infection because of retained moisture.

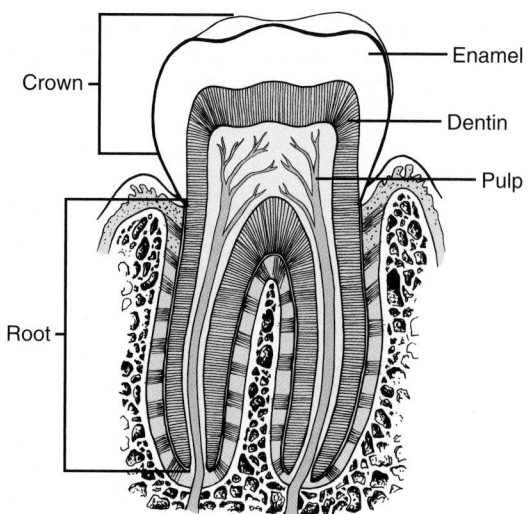

FIG 17-1   Normal tooth.

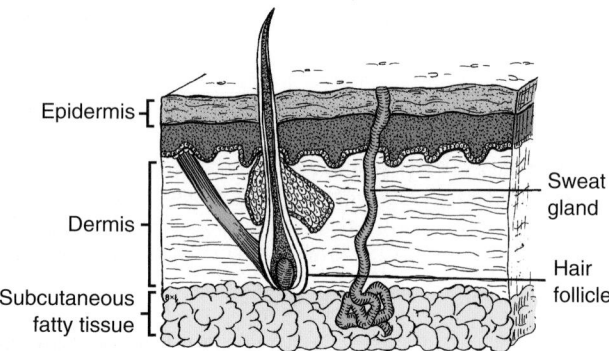

FIG 17-2   Cross section of hair follicle and supporting structures.

adhesive, blood, or antiseptic solutions on the hair. Diaphoresis leaves hair oily and unmanageable. Proper hair care is important to a person's body image.

THE NAILS

The nails are epithelial tissues that grow from the root of the nail bed, located in the skin at the nail groove. A normal, healthy nail is transparent, smooth, and convex, with a pink nail bed and translucent white tip. A normal color indicates adequate oxygenation to peripheral tissues. Pigment deposits or bands are common in nail beds of patients with dark skin. The nail is surrounded by a cuticle, which slowly grows over the nail and must be regularly pushed back with a soft nail brush.

The feet and nails require special care to prevent infection, odor, and injury. Problems typically result from abuse or poor care. Foot pain can often change a walking gait, causing strain on different muscle groups.

EVIDENCE-BASED PRACTICE

Evidence-based protocols for bathing and oral hygiene decrease hospital-acquired complications such as infection and skin ulceration (Eigsti, 2011). Concern with the number of patients with methicillin-resistant *Staphylococcus aureus* (MRSA), vancomycin-resistant enterococci (VRE), and *Clostridium difficile* infection (CDI) is related to cross-contamination and whether health care providers use antimicrobial soaps (Jury et al., 2011).

- A disposable bath is an all-in-one bathing package, which can decrease the spread of infection through decreased cross-contamination and washcloth-associated dermatitis (Johnson et al., 2009).
- Cost-effectiveness and a decrease in the time taken to administer a bath are also associated with disposable all-in-one bath products (Eigsti, 2011).
- Use of chlorhexidine gluconate–impregnated bathing cloths is well tolerated by the skin and is an effective broad antiseptic product (Eigsti, 2011).
- Moisturizer and skin protectant should be applied with each cleansing.

Adequate oral hygiene is important in preventing systemic illnesses (Wiech and Bayer, 2012; Stein and Henry, 2009). Critically ill patients in intensive care settings are especially prone to infection when oral hygiene is not performed. Approximately one fourth to one half of critically ill patients require mechanical ventilation (Grap, 2009), putting them at risk for ventilator-associated pneumonia (VAP). VAP results from the colonization of bacteria in the oral pharynx and is associated with increased morbidity and mortality (Munro et al., 2009; Wiech and Bayer, 2012). Current recommendations to reduce the risk of VAP include (Wiech and Bayer, 2012):

- Toothbrushing every 12 hours before the application of chlorhexidine
- Chlorhexidine 0.12% applied orally every 12 hours
- Head of bed elevated 30 degrees or more unless contraindicated

PATIENT-CENTERED CARE

Each culture is unique in how the provision and customs of personal hygiene are performed. Take patient's preferences and customs into consideration when providing hygiene. Having an understanding of transcultural nursing concepts and translating them into practice is key in providing culturally sensitive health care (Buschemi, 2011). Hygiene is a personal matter, and it is important to encourage patients to participate in their hygienic care. Consider patients' normal oral and bathing hygiene routines, including type of products used and the time of day when hygiene is routinely performed. Individualize your care based on patients' preferences. The nature of nursing is to provide compassionate care to patients and their families, which embodies the original focus of patient-centered care (Epstein and Street, 2011). Depending on the cultural considerations and the ability of the patient, it may be beneficial to involve a family member or significant other in the hygienic care of the patient so complete culturally sensitive patient-centered care is provided. For example, in some cultures it is not appropriate to expose the lower torso and arms, and the left hand is used for cleansing the perineal area. In other cultures, health care providers must be gender congruent whenever possible.

 Safety Guidelines

1   Always assess the environment for safety before administering hygiene care to a patient. Check floors for spills and make sure that equipment is working properly.
2   When not performing procedures, patient's bed should be in the locked and low position with at least two, but not more than three side rails raised.
3   Keep all personal care items within a patient's reach. When the head of the bed is raised, the bedside stand is usually not within

easy reach and must be moved forward. If a patient must leave the bed to go to the bathroom, be sure that there is a clear pathway.

4 Observe standard precautions when providing care, which includes wearing clean gloves. Additional precautions requiring other personal protective equipment (PPE) may be necessary, depending on the patient's condition (see Chapter 7).

5 Be sure that the call light is easily accessible to a patient at all times. Often a patient has multiple intravenous (IV) lines

and drainage tubes connected to portable poles and suction machines, which make it difficult for him or her to get to out-of-reach items. This puts the patient at risk for falling or for an injury from a dislodged tube or IV catheter.

6 Monitor laboratory findings, such as coagulation studies before administering oral care to prevent bleeding.

7 Monitor patients who have a decrease in sensory perception such as peripheral neuropathy.

SKILL 17-1 Bathing a Patient

 Video Clip

Bathing removes sweat, oil, dirt, and microorganisms from the skin. It also stimulates circulation and provides a refreshed and relaxed feeling. For some patients a bath is a time for socialization and pleasure, especially for those who are bedridden or seriously disabled.

The National Pressure Ulcer Advisory Panel and The European Pressure Ulcer Advisory Panel revised the stages of pressure ulcers and redefined important points for skin care (NPUAP and EPUAP, 2010). Although these were intended for pressure ulcer prevention, they provide sound principles for good bathing techniques.

- Clean the skin at the time of soiling and at routine intervals. Individualize frequency of cleaning according to patient need and preference. Problems such as incontinence, wound drainage, or excessive diaphoresis often require bathing several times a day.
- Avoid hot or excessively cold water and use a mild cleansing agent that minimizes irritation.
- Avoid use of force and friction when bathing a patient. Avoid massaging reddened areas, especially over bony prominences.
- Minimize environmental factors that lead to skin drying such as low humidity (less than 40%) and exposure to cold. Depending on the patient's age and physical condition, maintain room temperature between 20° and 23°C (68° and 74°F). Infants, older adults, and acutely ill patients may need a warmer temperature. However, certain critically ill patients require cooler room temperatures to lower the metabolic demands of the body. Controlling drafts and eliminating lingering odors from draining wounds, vomitus, bedpans, or urinals also improve a patient's comfort.
- Protect patients from injury by assessing and controlling bath water temperature. This is important for older adults and others with reduced sensation such as patients with diabetes or peripheral neuropathy or spinal cord–injury patients. It is also important for patients who are unable to communicate.
- Use bathing as a time to interact with and assess a patient. When giving a complete bath, perform a physical assessment of all body systems and discuss issues of concern for a patient.
- During bathing assist patients through normal joint range-of-motion (ROM) exercises to promote circulation and joint integrity.
- For patients who tire easily, consider giving a partial versus complete bed bath.

There are two categories of baths: cleansing and therapeutic. Cleansing baths include the bed bath, tub bath, sponge bath at the

sink, shower, and prepackaged disposable bed bath (Box 17-1). The type of cleansing bath to use depends on the assessment of a patient's physical capabilities and the degree of hygiene required. When a person is unable to perform personal care because of illness or disability, you are responsible for helping with bathing. This includes time for cleaning and grooming hair, shaving, and cleaning of nails. You can perform many of these procedures during or immediately after a bath.

Health care providers generally order therapeutic baths for a specific effect such as soothing the skin or for promoting the healing process. Types of therapeutic baths include:

- *Sitz bath:* Cleans and reduces pain and inflammation of perineal and anal areas. They are used for a patient who has undergone rectal or perineal surgery or childbirth or has local irritation from hemorrhoids or fissures. The patient sits in a special tub or basin (see Chapter 40).
- *Medicated bath (addition of over-the-counter, herbal, or health care provider–ordered ingredient to bath):* Relieves skin irritation and creates an antibacterial and drying effect.

Perineal care (see Procedural Guideline 17-1) involves thorough cleaning of a patient's external genitalia and surrounding skin. A patient routinely receives perineal care during a bath. However,

---

BOX 17-1 | Types of Baths

- **Complete bed bath**: Bath administered to totally dependent patient in bed.
- **Partial bed bath**: Bed bath that consists of bathing only body parts that would cause discomfort if left unbathed such as the hands, face, axilla, and perineal area. Partial bath also includes washing back and providing back rub. Dependent patients in need of partial hygiene or self-sufficient bedridden patients who are unable to reach all body parts receive a partial bed bath.
- **Sponge bath at the sink**: Involves bathing from a bath basin or sink with patient sitting in a chair. Patient is able to perform a portion of the bath independently. Nurse helps with hard-to-reach areas.
- **Tub bath**: Involves immersion in a tub of water that allows more thorough washing and rinsing than a bed bath. Patients may require nurse's assistance. Some institutions have tubs equipped with lifting devices that facilitate positioning dependent patients in the tub.
- **Shower**: Patient sits or stands under a continuous stream of water. The shower provides more thorough cleaning than a bed bath but can be tiring.
- **Disposable bed bath/travel bath**: The bag bath contains several soft, nonwoven cotton cloths that are premoistened in a solution of no-rinse surfactant cleaner and emollient. The bag bath offers an alternative because of the ease of use, reduced time bathing, and patient comfort (Barrick et al., 2008; Meiner, 2010).

patients at risk for acquiring an infection need more frequent perineal care. These include patients who have incontinence-associated dermatitis (IAD), an indwelling Foley catheter, are postpartum, or are recovering from rectal or genital surgery.

Delegation and Collaboration

Assessment of the patient's skin, pain level, and ROM cannot be delegated to nursing assistive personnel (NAP). The skill of bathing can be delegated to nursing assistive personnel (NAP). The nurse instructs the NAP about:

- Not massaging reddened skin areas during bathing.
- Contraindications to soaking a patient's feet or trimming toenails.
- Reporting any signs of impaired skin integrity to the nurse.
- Proper ways to position male and female patients with musculoskeletal limitations or an indwelling Foley catheter or other equipment (e.g., intravenous [IV] tubing).

Equipment

- ❏ Washcloths and bath towels
- ❏ Bath blanket
- ❏ Cleansing product for bath
- ❏ Toiletry items (deodorant, lotion)
- ❏ Disposable wipes
- ❏ Warm water
- ❏ Clean hospital gown or patient's own pajamas or gown
- ❏ Laundry bag
- ❏ Clean gloves
- ❏ Washbasin
- ❏ Disposable all-in-one package bath product (if basin and water baths are not performed)
- ❏ Eye patch/shield and nonallergenic tape (for unconscious patient)

STEP	RATIONALE

ASSESSMENT

1 Assess environment for safety (e.g., check room for spills, make sure that equipment is working properly and that bed is in locked, low position).

Identifies safety hazards in patient environment that could cause or potentially lead to harm (QSEN Quality/Safety Competencies, 2012).

2 Assess patient's fall risk status (if partial bathing out of bed or self-bath is to be performed), tolerance for bathing and activity, comfort level, cognitive ability, musculoskeletal function, and presence of shortness of breath.

Determines patient's ability to perform bathing and what type of bath to administer (e.g., complete bath, partial bed bath).

3 Assess patient's visual status, ability to sit without support, hand grasp, ROM of extremities (see Chapter 6).

Determines degree of assistance needed for bathing.

4 Assess for presence and position of external medical device/equipment (e.g., IV line or oxygen tubing).

Affects how you will plan bathing activities.

5 Assess patient's bathing preferences, including frequency, time of day, and type of hygiene products used.

Allows patient to participate in plan of care. Promotes patient's comfort and willingness to cooperate.

6 Ask if patient has noticed any problems related to condition of skin and genitalia.

Provides information to direct physical assessment of skin and genitalia during bathing. Also influences selection of skin-care products.

7 Before or during bath, assess condition of patient's skin. Note the presence of dryness, indicated by flaking, redness, scaling, and cracking or excessive moisture, inflammation, or pressure ulcers (see Chapter 18).

Provides baseline for comparison of skin integrity over time.

8 Identify risks for skin impairment. *Option:* Use a pressure ulcer assessment tool (e.g., Braden Scale; see Chapter 18).

Risk factors increase the likelihood of injury to the skin because of pressure, impaired tissue synthesis, softening of or friction on tissues, and impaired circulation.

a Immobilization (e.g., patients with paralysis, immobilized extremities, traction; weakened or disabled patients)

Risk for pressure on dependent body parts.

b Reduced sensation (e.g., paresthesias, circulatory insufficiency, neuropathies)

Requires caution in regulating temperature of bath water to prevent risk of injury or burns to the skin.

c Nutritional and hydration alterations

Affects condition of skin with decreases in skin turgor, thickness, and elasticity. Skin integrity is easily susceptible to infections or breaks in skin.

d Excessive moisture on skin, particularly on skin surfaces that rub against one another (e.g., under breasts, perineal area)

Skinfolds trap moisture and cause friction between surfaces, which can lead to breaks in skin integrity and result in infection.

e Vascular insufficiencies

Result in poor circulation to skin.

f External devices applied to or around skin (e.g., casts, braces, restraints, dressings, catheters, tubes)

Improperly placed medical devices or movable devices that can cause pressure or friction can result in skin breakdown.

g Older-adults

Older adults with decreased appetites may have deficits in nutrients and fluids that increase risk of impaired skin integrity. Physical changes with age and decreased skin elasticity also contribute to higher incidence of impaired skin integrity.

STEP	RATIONALE

h Shear or friction (sliding down in bed)
Causes damage to skin and underlying tissues.

i Incontinence (bowel or bladder)
Requires more frequent bathing to prevent skin maceration and infection.

9 Assess patient's comfort on a 0 to 10 pain scale.
Bath can soothe and comfort patient.

10 Assess patient's knowledge of skin hygiene in terms of its importance, preventive measures to take, and common problems encountered (see Table 17-1).
Determines patient's learning needs.

11 Review orders for specific precautions concerning patient's movement or positioning.
Prevents accidental injury to patient during bathing activities. Determines level of assistance required by patient.

NURSING DIAGNOSES

- Activity intolerance
- Bathing/self-care deficit
- Deficient knowledge regarding skin care
- Impaired physical mobility
- Impaired skin integrity
- Risk for impaired skin integrity
- Risk for infection

Related factors are individualized based on patient's condition or needs.

PLANNING

1 Expected outcomes following completion of procedure:
- Skin is free of excretions, drainage, or odor. — Skin is clean.
- Skin shows decreased redness, cracking, flaking, and scaling. — Indicates reduction in skin dryness.
- Joint ROM remains same or improves from previous measurement. — Repeated ROM exercise during bathing helps prevent contractures and promotes joint movement.
- Patient expresses sense of comfort and relaxation. — Bath relaxes patient and removes sources of discomfort.
- Patient tolerates bath without fatigue or chilling. — Fatigue during bathing indicates worsening of chronic cardiopulmonary conditions.
- Patient describes benefits and techniques of proper hygiene and skin care. — Demonstrates learning with ability to repeat back to demonstrate understanding.

2 Gather equipment and supplies.
Avoids interrupting procedure or leaving patient unattended to retrieve missing equipment.

3 Adjust room temperature and ventilation.
Warm room that is free of drafts prevents rapid loss of body heat during bathing.

4 Explain procedure and ask patient for suggestions on how to prepare supplies. If partial bath, ask how much of bath patient wishes to complete.
Promotes patient's cooperation and participation and promotion of self-care as appropriate.

5 If it is necessary to leave the room, be sure that call light is within reach of patient.
Provides for patient's safety.

Clinical Decision Point *Never leave the bedside without ensuring that at least two but not more than three side rails are raised and the bed is in the locked, low position. The number of side rails depends on the patient's fall risk assessment; however, having all side rails raised is considered a restraint. Check agency policy.*

IMPLEMENTATION

1 Close room doors and windows and draw room divider curtain.
Privacy ensures patient's mental and physical comfort.

2 Offer patient bedpan or urinal. Provide towel and moist washcloth.
Patient will feel more comfortable after voiding. Prevents interruption of bath.

3 Perform hand hygiene. Apply clean gloves.
Reduces transmission of microorganisms.

4 Place supplies on bedside table, including a washbasin two-thirds full with warm water. Check water temperature and have patient place fingers in water to test temperature tolerance. Place plastic container of bath lotion in bath water to warm if desired.
Warm water promotes comfort, relaxes muscles, and prevents unnecessary chilling. Testing temperature prevents accidental burns. Bath water warms lotion for application to patient's skin.

5 Raise bed to comfortable working height. Lower side rail closest to you and help patient assume comfortable supine position, maintaining body alignment. Bring patient toward side closest to you.
Aids access to patient. Maintains patient's comfort throughout procedure. Uses proper body mechanics, thus minimizing strain on back muscles.

6 Place bath blanket over patient. Have patient hold top of bath blanket and remove top sheet from under bath blanket without exposing patient. Place soiled linen in laundry bag.
Blanket provides warmth and privacy. Take care to avoid linen contacting uniform.

7 Remove patient's gown or pajamas.
Provides full exposure of body parts during bathing.

STEP	RATIONALE

a Whether or not patient has an IV line, simply unsnap sleeves and remove gown.

b If an extremity is *injured* or has reduced mobility, begin removal from *unaffected* side first.

c If patient has an IV line and gown with no snaps, remove gown from arm *without* IV line first. Then remove gown from arm with IV line (see illustration). Pause IV fluid infusion by pressing appropriate sensor on IV pump. Remove IV tubing from pump, then use regulator to slow IV infusion. Remove IV container from pole (see illustration) and slide IV container and tubing through arm of patient's gown (see illustration). Rehang IV container (see illustration), reconnect tubing to pump, open regulator clamp, and restart IV fluid infusion by pressing appropriate sensor on IV pump. If IV fluids are infusing by gravity, check IV flow rate and regulate if necessary. *Do not disconnect IV tubing to remove gown.*

Undressing unaffected side first allows easier manipulation of gown over body part with reduced ROM.

Manipulation of IV tubing and container can disrupt flow rate.

8 Remove pillow if allowed. Raise head of bed 30 to 45 degrees. Place bath towel under patient's head. Place second bath towel over patient's chest.

Removal of pillow makes it easier to wash patient's ears and neck. Placement of towels prevents soiling of bed linen and bath blanket.

9 Wash face.

   a Inquire if patient is wearing contact lenses.

Prevents accidental injury to eyes.

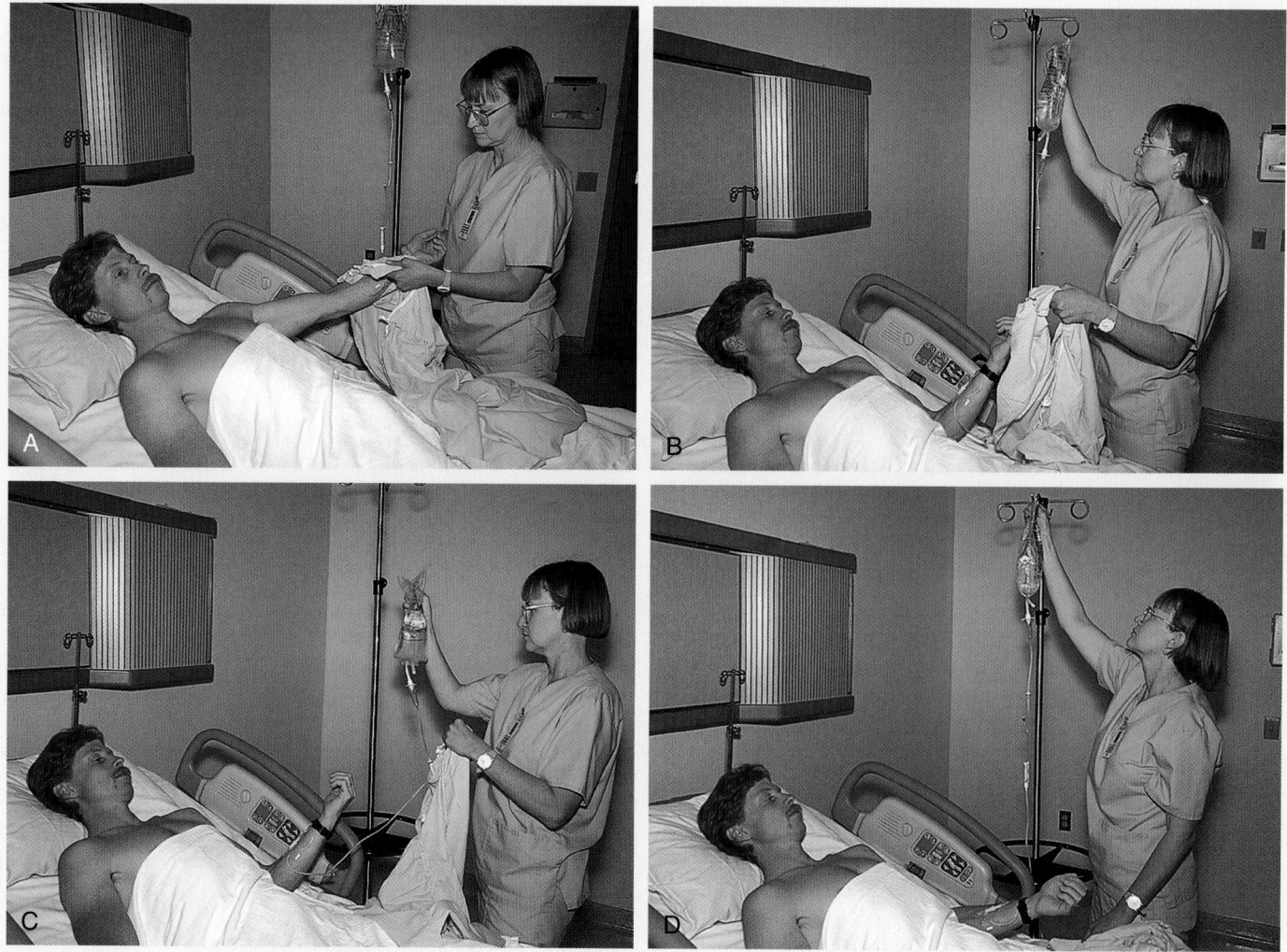

STEP 7c   **A,** Remove patient's gown. **B,** Remove IV bag from pole. **C,** Slide IV tubing and bag through arm of patient's gown. **D,** Rehang IV bag.

STEP	RATIONALE
b Form a mitt with washcloth (see illustration). Immerse in water and wring thoroughly.	Mitt retains water and heat better than loosely held washcloth; keeps cold edges from brushing against patient and prevents splashing.
c Wash patient's eyes with plain warm water, using a clean area of cloth for each eye and bathing from inner to outer canthus (see illustration). Soak any crusts on eyelid for 2 to 3 minutes with a warm, damp cloth before attempting removal. Dry around eyes gently and thoroughly.	Soap irritates eyes. Use of separate sections of mitt reduces infection transmission. Bathing eye gently from inner to outer canthus prevents secretions from entering nasolacrimal duct. Pressure causes internal injury.
d Ask if patient prefers to use soap on face. Wash, rinse, and dry forehead, cheeks, nose, neck, and ears without using soap. Ask men if they want to be shaved (see Skill 17-4).	Soap tends to dry face, which is exposed to air more than other body parts.
e Provide eye care for unconscious patient.	Patients who are unconscious have lost the normal protective corneal reflex of blinking, increasing the risk for corneal drying, abrasions, and eye infection.
(1) Instill eye drops or ointment per health care provider's order (see Chapter 21).	
(2) In the absence of blink reflex, keep eyelids closed. Close eye gently, using back of your fingertip, before placing eye patch or shield. Place tape over patch or shield. Do not tape eyelid.	When blink reflex is absent, patient loses a protective mechanism. Keeping eyelids closed maintains eye moisture and prevents injury.
10 Wash upper extremities and trunk.	
a Remove bath blanket from patient's arm that is closest to you. Place bath towel lengthwise under arm. Bathe with water and minimal soap using long, firm strokes from distal to proximal (fingers to axilla).	Long, firm strokes promote venous return.
b Raise and support arm above head (if possible) to wash axilla, rinse, and dry thoroughly (see illustration). Apply deodorant to underarms as needed or desired.	Movement of arm exposes axilla and exercises normal ROM of joint. Deodorant controls body odor.

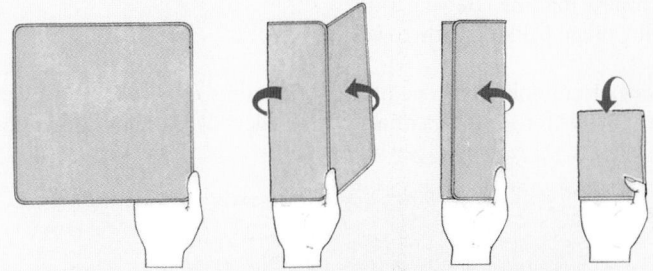

STEP 9b Steps for folding washcloth to form a mitt.

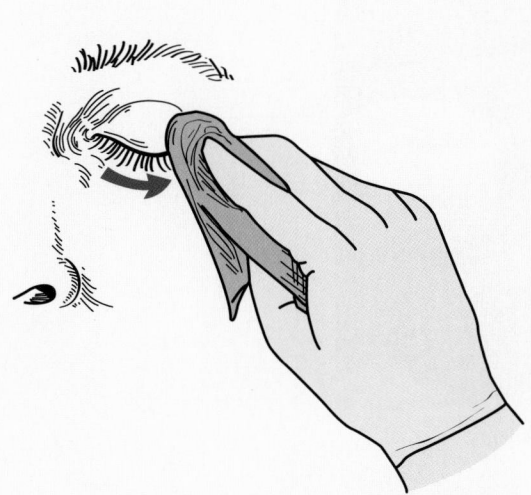

STEP 9c Wash eye from inner to outer canthus.

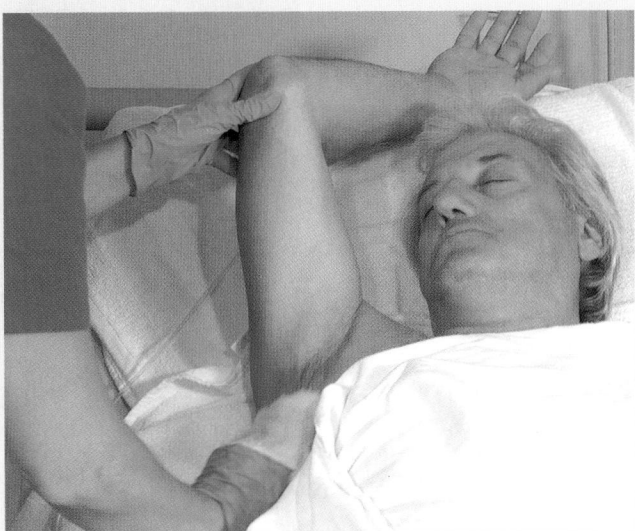

STEP 10b Positioning arm to wash axilla.

STEP	RATIONALE

c Move to other side of bed and repeat steps with other arm.

d Cover patient's chest with bath towel and fold bath blanket down to umbilicus. Bathe chest using long, firm strokes. Take special care with skin under female patient's breasts, lifting breast upward, if necessary with back of hand. Rinse and dry well.

Draping prevents unnecessary exposure of body parts. Towel maintains warmth and privacy. Secretions and dirt collect easily in areas of tight skinfolds. Skin under breasts is vulnerable to excoriation if not kept clean and dry.

11 Wash hands and nails.

a Fold bath towel in half and lay it on bed beside patient. Place basin on towel. Immerse patient's hand in water. Allow hand to soak for 3 to 5 minutes (if necessary) before cleaning fingernails (see Skill 17-5). Remove basin and dry hand well. Repeat for other hand.

Soaking softens cuticles and calluses of hand, loosens debris beneath nails, and enhances feeling of cleanliness. Thorough drying removes moisture from between fingers.

12 Check temperature of bath water and change water if necessary; otherwise continue.

Warm water maintains patient's comfort.

13 Wash abdomen.

a Place bath towel lengthwise over chest and abdomen. (You may need two towels.) Fold bath blanket down to just above pubic region. Bathe, rinse, and dry abdomen with special attention to umbilicus and skinfolds of abdomen and groin. Keep abdomen covered between washing and rinsing. Dry well.

Keeping skinfolds clean and dry helps prevent odor and skin irritation. Moisture and sediment that collects in skinfolds predispose skin to maceration.

b Apply clean gown or pajama top by dressing affected side first. *Option:* You may omit this step until completion of bath.

Maintains patient's warmth and comfort. Allows easier manipulation of gown over body part with reduced ROM.

Clinical Decision Point *If one extremity is injured or immobilized, always dress affected side first.*

14 Wash lower extremities.

a Cover chest and abdomen with top of bath blanket. Expose near leg by folding blanket toward midline. Be sure that other leg and perineum remain draped. Place bath towel under leg.

Prevents overexposure.

b Wash leg using long, firm strokes from ankle to knee and knee to thigh (see illustration). Assess for signs of redness, swelling, or pain along leg.

Promotes circulation and venous return. Assessment is a key to identifying signs and symptoms of venous thrombosis.

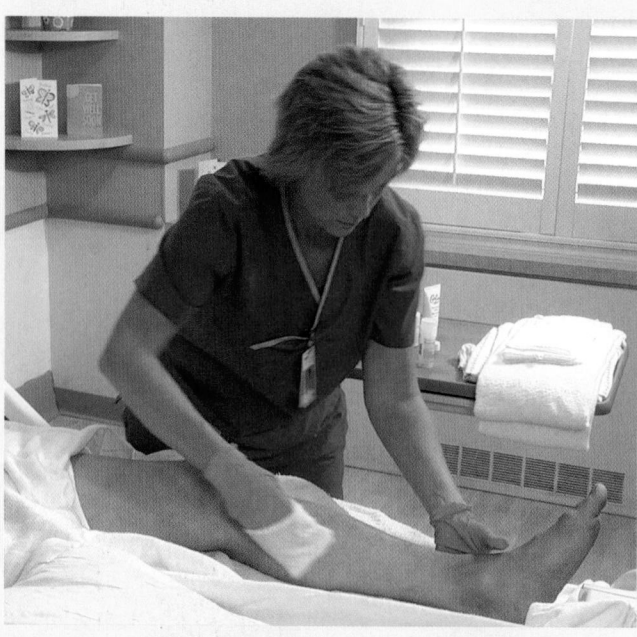

STEP 14b Washing patient's leg.

STEP	RATIONALE

Clinical Decision Point *During the bath assess for signs of warmth, redness, swelling, tenderness, and pain in the lower extremities because these might be early signs of deep vein thrombosis (DVT) (Emanuele, 2008).*

STEP	RATIONALE
c Clean foot, making sure to bathe between toes. Clean and file nails as needed (check agency policy) (see Skill 17-5). Dry toes and feet completely. Soaking feet in warm water for 10 minutes can help maintain cleanliness of the nails and feet; however, *do not soak feet of patients with diabetes mellitus.*	Secretions and moisture are often present between toes, predisposing patient to maceration and skin breakdown. Can impair wound healing and cause maceration of tissue.
d Raise side rail; remove towel; move to opposite side of bed, lower side rail, place dry towel under second leg, and repeat Steps 14b and c for other leg and foot. Apply light layer of moisturizing lotion to both feet. When finished, remove used towel.	Moisturizers are effective in reducing dry skin; however, in excess they can cause maceration.
e Cover patient with bath blanket, raise side rail, and change bath water.	Decreased bath water temperature causes chilling. Clean water reduces microorganism transmission.
15 While patient is supine, provide perineal care (see Procedural Guideline 17-1).	
16 Wash back.	
a Apply clean gloves. Lower side rail. Help patient assume prone or side-lying position (as applicable). Place towel lengthwise along patient's side.	Exposes back and buttocks for bathing.
b If fecal material is present, enclose in fold of underpad or toilet tissue and remove with disposable wipes.	Skinfolds near buttocks and anus may contain fecal secretions and microorganisms. Maintains warmth and prevents unnecessary exposure.
c Keep patient draped by sliding bath blanket over shoulders and thighs during bathing. Wash, rinse, and dry back from neck to buttocks using long, firm strokes. Pay special attention to folds of buttocks and anus.	
d Clean buttocks and anus, washing front to back (see illustration). Clean, rinse, and dry area thoroughly. If needed, place clean absorbent pad under patient's buttocks.	Cleaning buttocks after back prevents contamination of water.

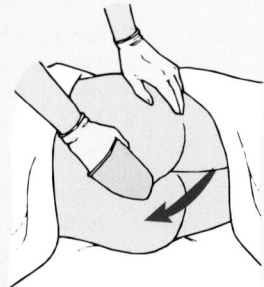

STEP 16d Clean from perineum to rectum (front to back).

STEP	RATIONALE
17 Remove gloves and massage back if patient desires (see Chapter 15).	Promotes patient relaxation.
18 Apply body lotion to skin and topical moisturizing agents to dry, flaky, reddened, or scaling areas.	Dry skin results in reduced pliability and cracking. Moisturizers help to prevent skin breakdown.

Clinical Decision Point *Massage is contraindicated in the presence of acute inflammation and where there is the possibility of damaged blood vessels or fragile skin (NPUAP and EPUAP, 2010). Massage of the legs is also contraindicated because of the possible presence of a blood clot, which could become dislodged.*

STEP	RATIONALE
19 Place clean gown on patient and adjust any external lines and equipment.	Ensures patient privacy and comfort.
20 Assist patient with grooming, oral hygiene, shaving, hair care, and application of makeup (if desired).	Promotes patient's body image.
21 Make patient's bed (see Procedural Guidelines 17-5 and 17-6).	Provides clean environment.
22 Check function and position of external devices (e.g., indwelling catheters, nasogastric tubes, IV tubes, braces).	Ensures that bathing activities did not disrupt systems.

STEP	RATIONALE
23 Remove soiled linen and place in dirty laundry bag. Do not allow linen to contact uniform. Clean and replace bathing equipment. Replace call light and personal possessions. Place bed in low, locked position with at least two but no more than three side rails raised. Make sure that patient is as comfortable as possible.	Prevents transmission of infection. Clean environment promotes patient's comfort. Keeping call light and articles of care within reach promotes patient's safety.
24 Perform hand hygiene and leave room.	Reduces transmission of microorganisms.

EVALUATION

1 Observe skin; pay particular attention to areas that were previously soiled, reddened, flaking, scaling, or cracking or that showed early signs of breakdown. Inspect areas normally exposed to pressure.	Bathing should leave skin clean and clear. If there are signs of skin irritation (e.g., redness, blistering), take steps to reduce pressure.
2 Observe ROM during bathing.	Measures joint mobility.
3 Ask patient to rate level of comfort (on a scale of 0 to 10).	Determines changes in level of comfort during bathing.
4 Ask if patient feels tired.	Determines patient's tolerance of bathing activities.

Unexpected Outcomes

1 Areas of excessive dryness, rashes, irritation, or pressure ulcer appear on skin.

2 Patient becomes excessively tired and unable to cooperate or participate in bathing.

3 Patient seems unusually restless or complains of discomfort.

Related Interventions

- Review agency skin-care policy regarding special cleansing and moisturizing products.
- Limit frequency of complete baths.
- Complete pressure ulcer assessment (see Chapter 18).
- Institute turning and positioning measures to keep patient off pressure ulcer.
- Obtain special bed surface if patient is at risk for skin breakdown.
- Notify health care provider and/or obtain wound consultation.
- Reschedule bathing to a time when patient is more rested.
- Patients with cardiopulmonary conditions and breathing difficulties require pillow or elevated head of bed during bathing.
- Notify health care provider about changes in patient's fatigue level.
- Perform hygiene measures in stages between scheduled rest periods.
- Use a less stressful method of bathing such as a disposable bath-in-a-bag product (see Procedural Guideline 17-2).
- Consider analgesia before bathing.
- Schedule rest periods before bathing.

Recording and Reporting

- Record procedure, including the amount of patient participation and how the patient tolerated procedure.
- Record condition of skin and any significant findings (e.g., reddened areas, bruises, nevi, joint or muscle pain) in nurses' notes and electronic health record (EHR).
- Report evidence of alterations in skin integrity, break in suture line, or increased wound secretions to nurse in charge or health care provider.

Special Considerations

Teaching

- Teach patients how to inspect surfaces between skinfolds for signs of irritation or breakdown.

Pediatric

- Some adolescents require and/or prefer more frequent bathing as a result of more active sebaceous glands.

- Young adolescent girls should learn basic perineal hygiene measures and know why they are predisposed to urinary tract infections.

Gerontologic

- When caring for cognitively impaired older adults, approach bathing in a calm manner and use the same bathing method and when possible the same caregiver.
- It is best to use the least distressing method first such as soaking in a bathtub or using a disposable bag bath. These approaches must be modified for each patient (i.e., soaking the feet rather than the whole body) (Barrick et al., 2008; Meiner, 2010).
- Older adults with incontinence need meticulous skin care to reduce incontinence-associated dermatitis and the risk of infection.

Home Care
- Type of bath chosen depends on assessment of the home, availability of running water, and condition of bathing facilities.
- In the home setting set up equipment according to established routines. Patient is the best resource for what works in terms of convenience and saving time.
- Patients at risk for falls may benefit from the following:

- Installation of grab bars in shower
- Adhesive strips applied to shower or tub floor
- Addition of a shower chair or placement of a chair or stool

Long-Term Care
- Tubs in long-term care settings frequently come equipped with electronic thermometers to measure water temperature. The tubs also have hydraulic lifts to help residents into the tub.

PROCEDURAL GUIDELINE 17-1 Perineal Care

Perineal care involves thorough cleansing of the patient's external genitalia and surrounding skin. A patient routinely receives perineal care during a complete bed bath. However, patients who have fecal or urinary incontinence, an indwelling Foley catheter, or rectal or genital surgery may need more frequent perineal care. Wear gloves during perineal care because of the risk of contacting infectious organisms present in fecal, urinary, or vaginal secretions. To avoid embarrassment, always act in a professional and sensitive manner and provide privacy at all times.

Delegation and Collaboration
The skill of perineal care can be delegated to nursing assistive personnel (NAP). The nurse instructs the NAP to:
- Avoid any physical restriction that affects proper positioning of patient.
- Properly position a patient with an indwelling Foley catheter.
- Inform the nurse of any perineal drainage, excoriation, or rash observed.

Equipment
- Washcloths, bath towels, and bath blanket
- Cleansing product, disposable wipes
- Warm water
- Laundry bag
- Wash basin, waterproof pad or bedpan
- Clean gloves
- Additional supplies when perineal care is provided other than during a bath (cotton balls or swabs, solution bottle or container filled with warm water or prescribed rinsing solution, waterproof bag).

Procedural Steps
1 Assess environment for safety (e.g., check the room for spills, make sure that equipment is working properly and that bed is in locked, low position).
2 Provide privacy and explain procedure and importance in preventing infection.
3 Perform hand hygiene. Apply clean gloves.

4 **Perineal care for a female.**
a If patient is able to maneuver and handle washcloth, allow to clean perineum on own.
b Help patient assume dorsal recumbent position. Note restrictions or a limitation in patient's positioning. Position waterproof pad under patient's buttocks.
c Drape patient with bath blanket placed in shape of a diamond. Lift lower edge of bath blanket to expose perineum.
d Fold lower corner of bath blanket up between patient's legs onto abdomen and under hip (see illustration). Wash and dry patient's upper thighs.
e Wash labia majora. Use nondominant hand to gently retract labia from thigh. Use dominant hand to wash carefully in skinfolds. Wipe in direction from perineum to rectum (front to back). Repeat on opposite side using separate section of washcloth. Rinse and dry area thoroughly.
f Gently separate labia with nondominant hand to expose urethral meatus and vaginal orifice. With dominant hand wash downward from pubic area toward rectum in one smooth stroke (see illustration). Use separate section of cloth for each stroke. Clean thoroughly over labia minora, clitoris, and vaginal orifice. Avoid tension on indwelling catheter if present and clean area around it thoroughly.
g Rinse and dry area thoroughly, using front-to-back method.
h If patient uses bedpan, pour warm water over perineal area and dry thoroughly.
i Fold lower corner of bath blanket back between patient's legs and over perineum. Ask patient to lower legs and assume comfortable position.

5 **Perineal care for a male.**
a If patient is able to maneuver and handle washcloth, allow him to clean perineum on his own.
b Help patient to supine position. Note restriction in mobility.
c Fold lower half of bath blanket up to expose upper thighs. Wash and dry thighs.
d Cover thighs with bath towels. Raise bath blanket to expose genitalia. Gently raise penis and place bath towel

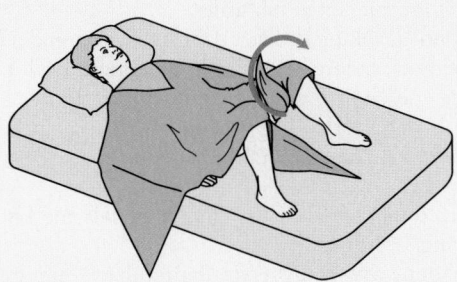
STEP 4d Drape patient for perineal care.

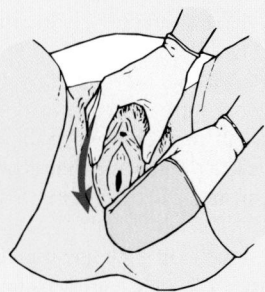
STEP 4f Clean from perineum to rectum (front to back)

Continued

PROCEDURAL GUIDELINE 17-1   Perineal Care—cont'd

underneath. Gently grasp shaft of penis. If patient is uncircumcised, retract foreskin. If patient has an erection, defer procedure until later.

e Wash tip of penis at urethral meatus first. Using circular motion, clean from meatus outward (see illustration). Discard washcloth and repeat with clean cloth until penis is clean. Rinse and dry gently and thoroughly.

f Return foreskin to its natural position.

Clinical Decision Point *After administering male perineal care for uncircumcised males, make sure that foreskin is in its natural position. This is extremely important in patients with decreased sensation in their lower extremities. Tightening foreskin around shaft of penis causes local edema; discomfort; and, if not corrected, permanent urethral damage.*

g Gently clean shaft of penis and scrotum by having patient abduct legs. Pay special attention to underlying surface of penis. Lift scrotum carefully and wash underlying skinfolds. Rinse and dry thoroughly.

h Fold bath blanket back over patient's perineum and help him to comfortable position.

6 Observe perineal area for any irritation, redness, or drainage that persists after perineal hygiene.

7 Dispose of gloves in receptacle and perform hand hygiene.

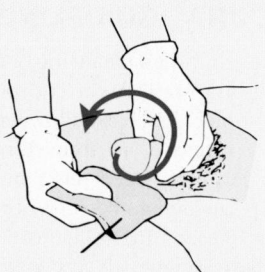

STEP 5e Use circular motion to clean tip of penis.

PROCEDURAL GUIDELINE 17-2   Use of Disposable Bed Bath, Tub, or Shower

Delegation and Collaboration

The skill of bathing in a tub or shower or using a disposable bed bath can be delegated to nursing assistive personnel (NAP). The nurse instructs the NAP to:

- Not massage reddened skin areas during bathing.
- Properly position male and female patients with musculoskeletal limitations or an indwelling Foley catheter or other equipment (e.g., intravenous tubing).
- Report changes in skin or perineal area or signs of impaired skin integrity to the nurse.

Equipment

❑ Washcloths and bath towels (for tub or shower); bath blanket, cleansing product, toiletry items (deodorant, lotion), disposable wipes, clean hospital gown or patient's own pajamas or gown, laundry bag

❑ Prepackaged, disposable bathing system (alternative to soap and water)

❑ Clean gloves

Procedural Steps

1 Assess environment for safety (e.g., check room for spills, make sure that equipment is working properly and bed is in locked, low position) and provide privacy.

2 Perform hand hygiene and apply clean gloves if there is a risk of exposure to body fluids.

3 **Disposable bed bath.**

a Position patient supine or in a position of comfort. Warm package in a microwave, following package directions. Do not use a microwave that is used for food preparation. The cleansing pack contains 8 to 10 premoistened towels.

b Use a single towel for each general body part cleansed. Follow the same order of cleaning as for total or partial bed bath (see Skill 17-1).

c Allow skin to air dry for 30 seconds. It is permissible to lightly cover patient with bath towel to prevent chilling.

d NOTE: If there is excessive soiling (e.g., in perineal region), use an extra cleansing pack or conventional washcloths, soap and water, and towels.

4 **Tub bath or shower.**

a Assess patient's fall risk status, consider patient's condition, and review orders for precautions concerning his or her movement or positioning. A health care provider's order usually is needed for tub bath or shower.

b Schedule use of shower or tub.

c Check tub or shower for cleanliness. Use cleaning techniques outlined in agency policy. Place rubber mat on tub or shower bottom. Place skid-proof disposable bath mat or towel on floor in front of tub or shower.

d Collect all hygienic aids, toiletry items, and linens requested by patient. Place within easy reach of tub or shower.

e Help patient to bathroom if necessary. Have him or her wear robe and skid-proof slippers to bathroom.

f Demonstrate how to use call signal for assistance. Place "occupied" sign on bathroom door.

g Fill bathtub halfway with warm water. Check temperature of bath water, have patient test it, and adjust it if it is too warm or too cold. Explain which faucet controls hot water. *Do not use bath oil in tub water.*

h If patient is taking shower, turn shower on and adjust water temperature before he or she enters shower stall. Use shower seat or tub chair if available (see illustration).

i Instruct patient that you will not allow him or her to remain in tub longer than 20 minutes.

j Check on patient every 5 minutes.

k Return to bathroom when patient signals and knock before entering.

l For patient who is unsteady, drain tub of water before he or she attempts to get out. Place bath towel over patient's

---

PROCEDURAL GUIDELINE 17-2   Use of Disposable Bed Bath, Tub, or Shower—cont'd

shoulders. Help him or her get out of tub as needed and help with drying. If possible have a shower chair available for patient to sit.

m Help patient as needed to don clean gown or pajamas, slippers, and robe. (In home, extended care, or rehabilitation setting, encourage patient to wear regular clothing.)

n Help patient to room and to comfortable position in bed or chair.

o Evaluate patient's tolerance and fatigue level.

p Clean tub or shower according to agency policy. Remove soiled linen and place in dirty laundry bag. Discard disposable equipment in proper receptacle. Place "unoccupied" sign on bathroom door. Return supplies to storage area.

q Perform hand hygiene.

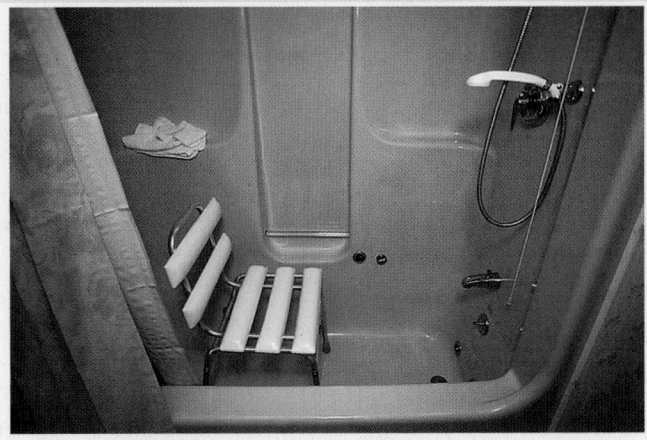

STEP 4h   Shower seat for patient safety.

SKILL 17-2   Oral Hygiene

Maintenance of daily oral hygiene, including brushing, flossing, and rinsing, is essential for the prevention and control of plaque-associated oral diseases. In addition to preventing inflammation and infection, oral hygiene promotes comfort, nutrition, and verbal communication. Brushing cleans the teeth of food particles, plaque (the cause of dental caries), and bacteria; massages the gums; and relieves discomfort from unpleasant odors and tastes. Flossing removes tartar that collects at the gum line. Rinsing removes dislodged food particles and excess toothpaste.

When a patient becomes ill, many factors influence the need for oral hygiene. Offer oral hygiene assistance as required, from preparing needed supplies to actually brushing a patient's teeth. It is also your responsibility to determine the frequency that patients require oral hygiene. Plan the frequency of care based on the condition of the oral cavity and the patient's level of comfort.

In addition to recommendations for the general population, oral-care regimens have been developed to help relieve and facilitate healing of chemotherapy- and radiation therapy–related mucositis, stomatitis, and xerostomia. These lesions are very painful and interfere with a patient's nutrition. Specific regimens are discussed later in this chapter.

Delegation and Collaboration

The skill of oral hygiene (including toothbrushing, flossing, and rinsing) can be delegated to nursing assistive personnel (NAP). However, the nurse is responsible for assessing the patient's gag reflex to determine if the patient is at risk for aspiration. The nurse instructs the NAP to:

• Note types of changes in oral mucosa (e.g., presence of lesions or open areas) for which to observe and report to the nurse.

• Report patient's complaints of pain or occurrence of bleeding during oral care.

• Be aware of special precautions such as aspiration precautions, including:

a Keeping head of bed (HOB) raised to no lower than 30 degrees.

b Explaining need to report excessive coughing or choking during procedure.

Equipment

❑ Soft-bristled toothbrush (hard toothbrush damages enamel and gums) or toothette sponges for patients for whom a toothbrush is contraindicated

❑ Nonabrasive fluoride toothpaste or dentifrice

❑ Dental floss

❑ Tongue depressor

❑ Penlight

❑ Water glass with cool water, straw

❑ Alcohol-free antiseptic mouth rinse (*optional*)

❑ Emesis basin

❑ Bath towels to place over patient's chest

❑ Clean gloves

STEP	RATIONALE

ASSESSMENT

1 Assess environment for safety (e.g., check room for spills, make sure that equipment is working properly and that bed is in locked, low position.

2 Perform hand hygiene and apply clean gloves.

3 Instruct patient not to bite down. Using a penlight and tongue depressor, inspect integrity of lips, teeth, buccal mucosa, gums, palate, and tongue (see Chapter 6).

4 Identify presence of common oral problems.

   a *Dental caries:* Chalky-white discoloration of tooth or presence of brown or black discoloration

   b *Gingivitis:* Inflammation of gums.

   c *Periodontitis:* Receding gum lines, inflammation, gaps between teeth

   d *Halitosis:* Bad breath

   e *Cheilosis:* Cracking lips

   f *Stomatitis:* Inflammation of mouth tissues or structures

   g *Mucositis:* Inflammation of oral mucous membrane

   h Dry, cracked, coated tongue

5 Remove gloves and perform hand hygiene.

6 Review medical record and assess risk for oral hygiene problems:

   a Dehydration: Inability to take fluids or food by mouth, health care provider's order prohibiting food or fluids by mouth (NPO) for a procedure or because of patient's condition

   b Presence of nasogastric or oxygen tubes; mouth breathers

   c Chemotherapeutic drugs

   d Radiation therapy to head and neck

   e Presence of artificial airway (e.g., endotracheal tube)

   f Blood-clotting disorders (e.g., leukemia, aplastic anemia)

   g Oral surgery, trauma to mouth

   h Aging

   i Chemical injury

   j Diabetes mellitus

7 Determine patient's oral hygiene practices.

   a Frequency of toothbrushing and flossing

   b Type of toothpaste, dentifrice, and mouth rinse used

   c Last dental visit

   d Frequency of dental visits

8 Assess patient's ability to grasp and manipulate toothbrush.

RATIONALE:

Identifies safety hazards in patient environment that could cause or potentially lead to harm. (QSEN Quality/Safety Competencies, 2012).

Reduces transmission of microorganisms in blood or saliva.

Determines status of patient's oral cavity and extent of need for oral hygiene.

Helps determine type of hygiene patient requires and information patient requires for self-care.

Periodontal disease.
Periodontal disease.

Periodontal disease.

Prevents spread of microorganisms.

Certain conditions increase likelihood of impaired oral cavity integrity and need for preventive care.

Causes excess drying and fragility of mucous membranes and lips; increases accumulation of secretions on tongue and gums.

Causes drying of mucosa.

Drugs kill rapidly multiplying cells, including sloughing of normal cells lining oral cavity. Mucositis with ulcers and inflammation can develop.

Reduces salivary flow and lowers pH of saliva; leads to stomatitis and tooth decay (Sjögren's Syndrome Foundation, 2011).

Increases irritation to gums and mucosa. Excess secretions accumulate on teeth and tongue.

Predisposes to inflammation and bleeding of gums.

Break in mucosa increases risk for infection. Vigorous brushing can disrupt suture lines.

With advancing age mucosa becomes thin and less elastic.

Results from irritants such as alcohol, tobacco, acidic foods or side effects of medications (e.g., antibiotics, steroids, antidepressants).

Prone to dryness of mouth, gingivitis, periodontal disease, and loss of teeth.

Identifies errors in patient's technique, deficiencies in preventive oral hygiene, patient's level of knowledge regarding dental care.

American Dental Association (ADA) (2011) recommends brushing teeth at least twice a day with ADA-accepted fluoride toothpaste and once-a-day flossing.

Antimicrobial mouth rinses and toothpastes decrease bacteria and stop bacterial growth in dental plaque, which can cause an early, reversible form of gum disease called *gingivitis* (ADA, 2011).

Regular dental visits (e.g., every 6 months) are recommended by the ADA; however, frequency of visits can vary for each patient and should be determined by his or her dentist (ADA, 2011).

Assessment determines level of assistance required from nurse. Some older patients or persons with musculoskeletal or nervous system alterations are unable to hold toothbrush with firm grip or manipulate brush. Large-handled toothbrushes or a toothbrush handle pushed through a small rubber ball may be of assistance.

STEP	RATIONALE

NURSING DIAGNOSES

- Bathing/self-care deficit
- Deficient knowledge regarding oral hygiene care
- Impaired oral mucous membrane
- Risk for infection

Related factors are individualized based on patient's condition or needs.

PLANNING

1 Expected outcomes following completion of procedure:
- Patient expresses feeling of mouth cleanliness.
- Oral cavity structures have normal characteristics:
  - Oral mucosa is moist, intact, and of normal color.
  - Gums are pink, firm, and adherent to neck of teeth.
  - Teeth are clean, smooth, and shiny.
  - Tongue is pink and without secretions or coating.
- Patient describes correct oral hygiene techniques and necessary frequency.
- Patient makes choices regarding hygiene procedure and helps by flossing and brushing.

2 Gather equipment and supplies.

3 Explain procedure to patient and discuss preferences regarding use of hygiene aids.

Hygiene measures remove secretions and thickened mucosa. Maintains integrity of teeth and healthy oral mucosa.

Demonstrates understanding of instruction.

Patient is able to manage self-care.

Avoids interrupting procedure or leaving patient unattended to retrieve missing equipment.

Some patients feel uncomfortable about having nurse care for their basic needs. Patient involvement with procedure minimizes anxiety.

IMPLEMENTATION

1 Close room doors and windows and draw room divider curtain.

2 Prepare and have supplies ready at bedside arranged within easy reach.

3 Raise bed to comfortable working height. Raise HOB to at least semi-Fowler's position (unless contraindicated) and lower side rail. Move patient or help patient move close to side from which you choose to work. A side-lying position can be used.

4 Place towel over patient's chest.

5 Perform hand hygiene. Apply clean gloves.

6 Apply toothpaste to brush bristles. Hold brush over emesis basin. Pour small amount of water over toothpaste.

7 Patient may help by brushing. Hold toothbrush bristles at 45-degree angle to gum line (see illustration). Be sure that tips of bristles rest against and penetrate under gum line. Brush inner and outer surfaces of upper and lower teeth by brushing from gum to crown of each tooth. Clean biting surfaces of teeth by holding top of bristles parallel with teeth and brushing gently back and forth (see illustration). Brush sides of teeth by moving bristles back and forth (see illustration).

Privacy ensures patient's mental and physical comfort.
Creates organized workspace.

Raising bed and positioning patient promotes good body mechanics and prevents nurse from muscle strain. Semi-Fowler's position helps prevent patient from choking or aspirating.

Prevents soiling of patient's gown.
Prevents transmission of microorganisms in body fluids.
Moisture aids in distribution of toothpaste over tooth surfaces.

Angle allows brush to reach all tooth surfaces and to clean under gum line where plaque and tartar accumulate. Back-and-forth motion loosens food particles caught between teeth and along chewing surfaces.

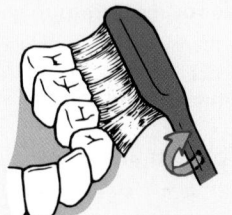 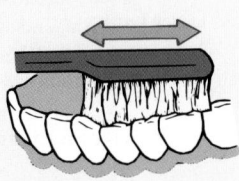 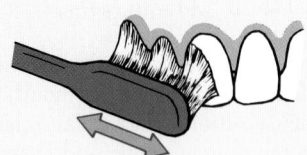

STEP 7 Directions of brush for toothbrushing.

8 Have patient hold brush at 45-degree angle and lightly brush over surface and sides of tongue (see illustration). Avoid initiating gag reflex.

Microorganisms collect and grow on surface of tongue and contribute to bad breath. Gagging may cause aspiration of toothpaste.

STEP	RATIONALE

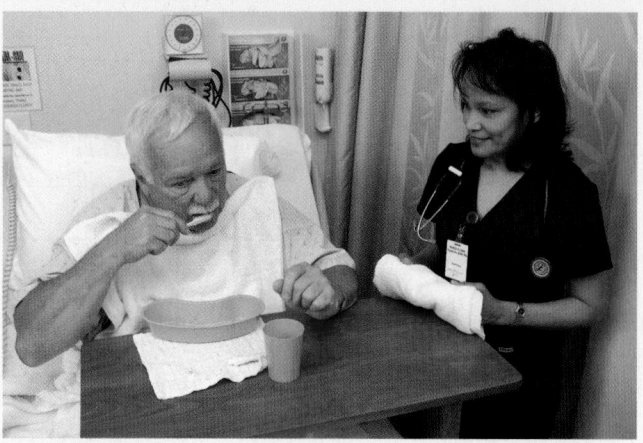

STEP 8 Nurse observes patient's toothbrushing technique.

9 Allow patient to rinse mouth thoroughly with water by taking several sips of water (may use straw), swishing water across all tooth surfaces, and spitting into emesis basin. Use this time to observe patient's brushing technique and teach importance of brushing teeth twice a day.	Rinsing removes food particles.
10 Have patient rinse teeth with alcohol-free antiseptic mouthwash for 30 seconds. Then have him or her spit rinse into emesis basin.	The ADA (2011) recommends that an antiseptic mouthwash is as effective as flossing for reducing plaque and gingivitis between teeth; effect on dental caries prevention has not been determined. Avoid using commercial brands of mouthwash that contain alcohol, which is drying to oral mucosa.
11 Help to wipe patient's mouth.	Promotes sense of comfort.
12 Allow patient to floss. Floss between all teeth. Hold floss against tooth while moving it up and down sides of teeth. Instruct patient in importance of daily flossing (see illustrations). Check to be sure that flossing is not contraindicated.	Flossing once daily removes plaque and decay-causing bacteria between teeth and under gum line, preventing gum disease. Immunocompromised patients are sometimes on precautions that prohibit use of floss or water-piks because of dislodging of bacteria and possible bleeding of gums.

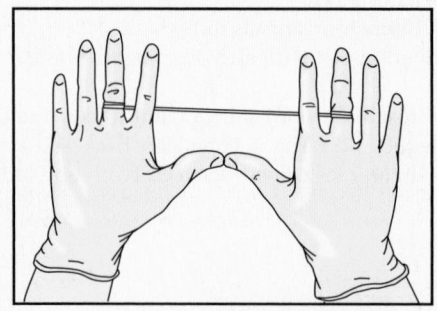 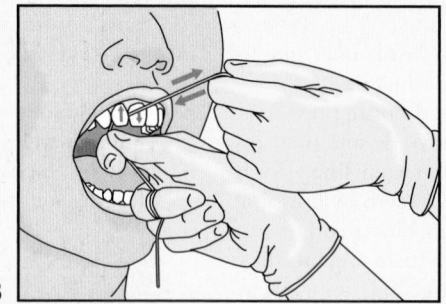 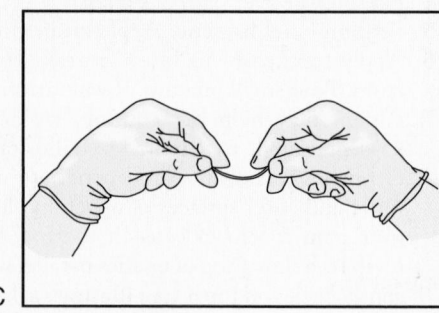

A B C

STEP 12 Flossing. **A,** Dental floss is held between middle fingers to floss upper teeth. **B,** Floss is moved in up-and-down motions between teeth. Floss is moved up and down from crown to gum line. **C,** Floss is held with index fingers to floss lower teeth.

13 Allow patient to rinse mouth thoroughly with cool water and spit into emesis basin. Help to wipe his or her mouth.	Rinsing removes plaque and tartar from oral cavity.
14 Help patient to comfortable position, remove emesis basin and over-bed table, raise side rail if appropriate, and lower bed to original position.	Provides for patient comfort and safety.
15 Wipe off over-bed table, discard soiled linen in dirty laundry bag, remove soiled gloves, and return equipment to proper place.	Proper disposal of soiled equipment prevents spread of infection.
16 Perform hand hygiene.	Reduces transmission of microorganisms.

STEP	RATIONALE

EVALUATION

1 Ask patient if any area of oral cavity feels uncomfortable or irritated.

Pain indicates need for further inspection for possible breaks in oral mucosa or identification of stomatitis or infection.

2 Apply clean gloves and inspect condition of oral cavity.

Determines effectiveness of hygiene and rinsing.

3 Ask patient to describe proper hygiene techniques and recommended frequency.

Evaluates patient's learning. Establish regular oral hygiene routine that is easy for patient to follow at home. The ADA (2011) currently recommends brushing at least twice per day and flossing daily.

4 Observe patient brushing and flossing.

Evaluates patient's ability to demonstrate correct technique.

Unexpected Outcomes

1 Mucosa is dry and inflamed. Tongue has thick coating.

2 Cheilosis—Dry, cracked lips

3 Gum margins are retracted from teeth, with localized areas of inflammation. Bleeding occurs around gum margins.

4 Mucosa becomes inflamed from repeated chemotherapy administration, and a lesion from sloughing of tissue develops. These conditions can also be caused by radiation therapy used to treat head and neck cancers.

Related Interventions

- Increase patient's hydration.
- Increase frequency of tongue brushing.
- Apply moisturizing lubricant to patient's lips.
- Report findings because patient may have an underlying bleeding tendency.
- Switch to softer-bristled toothbrush.
- Avoid vigorous brushing and flossing.
- Determine best-practice oral regimen for chemotherapy- and radiation therapy–related mucositis and stomatitis. Common regimens used to promote healing and comfort include:
  - Use a fluoride toothpaste.
  - Use one of the following rinses made with salt and/or baking soda (National Cancer Institute, 2011):
    - 1 teaspoon salt in 4 cups of water
    - 1 teaspoon baking soda in 1 cup (8 ounces) of water
    - $\frac{1}{2}$ teaspoon salt and 2 tablespoons baking soda in 4 cups of water
    - An antibacterial rinse 2 to 4 times a day for gum disease; rinse for 1 to 2 minutes
- If dry mouth (xerostomia) and hyposalivation occur such as with radiation therapy of the head and neck, additional rinses to increase moisture may be used. Brushing and gentle flossing should be continued as well.

Recording and Reporting

- Record procedure and note condition of oral cavity in nurses' notes and EHR.
- Report bleeding, pain, or presence of lesions to nurse in charge or health care provider.

Special Considerations
Teaching

- Use a variety of teaching formats (e.g., brochures, videos, DVDs) that are consistent with patient's health literacy level.
- Educate patients about methods to prevent tooth decay (e.g., reduce intake of carbohydrates, especially sweet sticky snacks between meals; brush within 30 minutes of eating sweets; rinse mouth thoroughly with water or alcohol-free antiseptic mouth rinse; use fluoride toothpaste).
- Educate patients to visit a dentist regularly (every 6 months) for professional cleaning and oral examination; however, frequency of visits can vary for each patient and should be determined by his or her dentist (ADA, 2011).
- When teaching special oral-care regimens, include family caregivers.
- Avoid mints if there are conditions of the mouth that are associated with ulcerations of the oral mucosa.

Pediatric

The following are recommended by the ADA (2011):

- Clean baby's gums with warm water and gauze after every feeding, even before teeth are formed. A dentist should be consulted before using fluoride toothpaste. The use of fluoride toothpaste usually begins at 2 years of age.
- Teach parents that infants should not be put to bed with a bottle; this causes tooth decay and ear infections.
- Limit snacks to three to four per day. Avoid sugary snacks and drinks and sticky candy.
- Notify dentist if family uses bottled or well water. A prescription for fluoride may be ordered.
- Dentist will evaluate for need of sealants for molars.
- Flossing requires parental supervision until at least 10 years of age.
- The first dental examination should be within 6 months after the first tooth comes in and no later than the first birthday, followed by dental examinations every 6 months.

Gerontologic

- A number of normal age-related changes occur in the oral cavity. Thinning of the oral mucosa and decreased vascularity of the gingivae predispose older adults to injury and periodontal disease. Loss of tissue elasticity and decreased mass and strength of the muscles make chewing more difficult. Loss of the alveolar bone can loosen natural teeth.

- The number of taste buds declines with advancing age. In an attempt to enhance the taste of food, some older adults choose salty and sugary foods, which erode tooth enamel and expose dentin (Lau, 2008).
- Plaque retention is a problem in older adults, worsened by existing teeth restorations, missing teeth, gingival recession, and wearing of removable prosthesis. Some older adults may also

experience difficulty with maintaining good oral hygiene with flossing and brushing because of decreased dexterity and decreasing eyesight.

Home Care

- During the initial admission visit document the condition of the patient's mouth, teeth, and gums, thus providing a baseline for assessing the patient's ability to comply with special diets and fluid intake and carry out oral hygiene practices.

PROCEDURAL GUIDELINE 17-3   Care of Dentures

 Video Clip

Oral bacteria from multiple strains and *Candida* species are found on acrylic dentures (Busscher et al., 2010). Encourage patients who wear dentures to continue to care for them and provide this care as frequently as with natural teeth. Loose dentures can cause discomfort and make it difficult for patients to chew food and speak clearly. Routine denture care reduces the risk for gingival infection. Some patients are unable to care for their dentures, and nurses become responsible for providing denture and oral care. Dentures are a patient's personal property; thus be sure to handle them with care because they are easy to break. Store them in an enclosed, labeled cup and soak them when not worn (e.g., at night, during surgery). Reinsert them as soon as possible.

Delegation and Collaboration
The skill of denture care can be delegated to nursing assistive personnel (NAP). The nurse instructs the NAP to:
- Not use hot or excessively cold water when caring for dentures.
- Inform the nurse if there are cracks in dentures.
- Inform the nurse if the patient has any oral discomfort.

Equipment
- ❑ Soft-bristled toothbrush or denture toothbrush
- ❑ Denture dentifrice or toothpaste, denture adhesive (*optional*)
- ❑ Glass of water
- ❑ Emesis basin or sink
- ❑ 4 × 4–inch gauze
- ❑ Washcloth
- ❑ Denture cup (for storage)
- ❑ Clean gloves

Procedural Steps
1 Assess environment for safety (e.g., check room for spills, make sure that equipment is working properly and that bed is in locked, low position).
2 Ask patient if dentures fit and if there is any gum or mucous membrane tenderness or irritation. Ask patient about denture care and product preferences.
3 Determine if patient can clean dentures independently or requires assistance. Dentures need cleaning as often as natural teeth.
4 Fill emesis basin with tepid water. (If using sink, place washcloth in bottom of sink and fill sink with approximately 2.5 cm [1 inch] of water.)
5 Perform hand hygiene. Apply clean gloves.
6 Ask patient to remove dentures. If patient is unable to do this independently, grasp upper plate at front with thumb and

index finger wrapped in gauze and pull downward. Gently lift lower denture from jaw and rotate one side downward to remove from patient's mouth. Place dentures in emesis basin or sink lined with washcloth and 2.5 cm (1 inch) of water.
7 Apply cleaning agent to brush and brush surfaces of dentures (see illustration). Hold dentures close to water. Hold brush horizontally and use back-and-forth motion to clean biting surfaces. Use short strokes from top of denture to biting surfaces to clean outer teeth surfaces. Hold brush vertically and use short strokes to clean inner teeth surfaces. Hold brush horizontally and use back-and-forth motion to clean undersurface of dentures (see Skill 17-2).

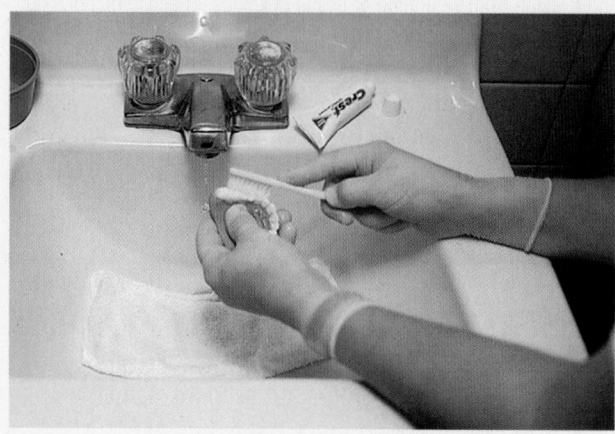

STEP 7   Brushing surface of dentures.

8 Rinse thoroughly in tepid water. If water is too cold, dentures can crack. If it is too hot, dentures can become warped and no longer fit.
9 Some patients use an adhesive to seal dentures in place. Apply a thin layer to undersurface before inserting.
10 If patient needs help with inserting dentures, moisten upper denture and press firmly to seal it in place. Insert moistened lower denture (if applicable). Ask if denture(s) feel comfortable.
11 Some patients prefer to store their dentures to give gums a rest and reduce risk for infection. Store in tepid water in denture cup. Keep denture cup in a secure place labeled with patient's name to prevent loss.
12 Dispose of supplies. Remove and discard gloves and perform hand hygiene.

SKILL 17-3 Performing Mouth Care for an Unconscious or Debilitated Patient

Unconscious or debilitated patients pose challenges because of their risk for alterations of the oral cavity from drying of the mucous membrane, thickened secretions, and the inability to eat or drink. They are susceptible to infection because of the change in the normal flora of the oral cavity and at risk for infection because of increased plaque formation from the dryness of the mouth and decreased salivation. Dryness of the oral mucosa is also caused by mouth breathing and oxygen therapy. Respiratory secretions often are thick and place patients at risk for ineffective airway clearance, requiring suction. They are also at risk for aspiration. Although saliva production is decreased, saliva is present and can pool in the back of the oral cavity, which is another contributing factor to placing the patient at risk of aspiration. The secretions in the oral cavity change very rapidly to gram-negative pneumonia-producing bacteria if aspiration occurs.

The critically ill patient faces the same risk factors for oral problems as other patients such as dehydration, dryness of the oral mucosa, chemical injury to the mucosa, and oral trauma. Once intubated, an endotracheal tube causes a bypass of normal defenses, which also causes a rapid change in the normal oral flora (Browne et al., 2011). Some patients require mouth care as often as every 1 to 2 hours until the mucosa returns to normal. Optimal oral care should focus on plaque removal and stimulation of salivary flow (Munro et al., 2009). Chlorhexidine rinse or gel is an antibacterial solution used in critically ill patients and has been shown to prevent ventilator-associated pneumonia (VAP) (Labeau et al., 2011). Currently more research is underway in establishing oral-care regimens for all critically ill patients.

Many patients have no gag reflex as a result of change in consciousness or a neurologic injury. While providing oral care to an unconscious patient, protect him or her from choking and aspiration. The safest technique is to have two nurses provide care. You provide oral care while another nurse or nursing assistive personnel (NAP) suctions oral secretions as necessary with a Yankauer suction tip. You can also delegate oral care to two NAPs with instructions. Place the unconscious or unresponsive patient in a Sim's or side-lying position with the head in a dependent position. Raise the head of bed (HOB) to at least 30 degrees, with patient's head turned to the side and toward the mattress in a dependent position. Proper oral hygiene requires keeping the oral mucosa moist and removing secretions that lead to infection. Use a moisturizing emollient for the lips as well.

Evaluate the level and frequency of oral care on a daily basis during assessment of the oral cavity. Routine suctioning of the mouth and pharynx is required to manage oral secretions to reduce the risk for aspiration. Chlorhexidine 2% gel or mouth rinse every 12 hours has been shown to effectively prevent VAP (Labeau et al., 2011). Research also suggests that toothbrushing provides additional benefit in reducing colonization of dental plaque (Berry et al., 2011). For patients who are not on ventilated-assisted breathing, toothbrushing and chlorhexidine are also effective.

Delegation and Collaboration

The skill of providing oral hygiene to an unconscious or debilitated patient can be delegated to nursing assistive personnel (NAP). The nurse must first assess the patient for a gag reflex. The nurse instructs the NAP to:

- Properly position patient for mouth care.
- Be aware of special precautions such as aspiration precautions.
- Use an oral suction catheter for clearing oral secretions (see Skill 25-1).
- Report signs of impaired integrity of oral mucosa to the nurse.
- Report any bleeding of mucosa or gums, excessive coughing or choking to the nurse.

Equipment

- ❏ Small pediatric, soft-bristled toothbrush or toothette sponges for patients for whom brushing is contraindicated.
- ❏ Antibacterial solution per organization protocol (e.g., chlorhexidine)
- ❏ Fluoride toothpaste
- ❏ Water-based mouth moisturizer
- ❏ Tongue blade
- ❏ Penlight
- ❏ Oral suction equipment
- ❏ Oral airway (uncooperative patient or patient who shows bite reflex)
- ❏ Water-soluble lip lubricant
- ❏ Water glass with cool water
- ❏ Face and bath towel
- ❏ Emesis basin
- ❏ Clean gloves

STEP	RATIONALE
ASSESSMENT	
1 Assess environment for safety (e.g., check the room for spills, make sure that equipment is working properly and that bed is in locked, low position).	Identifies safety hazards in patient environment that could cause or potentially lead to harm (QSEN Quality/Safety Competencies, 2012).
2 Perform hand hygiene, and apply clean gloves.	Reduces transmission of microorganisms in blood or saliva.
3 Test for presence of gag reflex by placing tongue blade on back half of tongue.	Helps in determining aspiration risk.

Clinical Decision Point *Patients with impaired gag reflex require oral care but are at risk for aspiration. Keep suction equipment available when caring for patients who are at risk for aspiration.*

STEP	RATIONALE
4 Inspect condition of oral cavity (see Chapter 6).	Determines condition of oral cavity and need for hygiene.
5 Remove gloves. Perform hand hygiene.	Prevents spread of infection.
6 Assess patient's risk for oral hygiene problems (see Skill 17-2).	Certain conditions increase likelihood of alterations in integrity of oral cavity mucosa and structures, necessitating more frequent care.
7 Assess patient's respirations on a regular schedule.	Ensures early recognition of aspiration.

NURSING DIAGNOSES

- Impaired oral mucous membrane
- Risk for aspiration

Related factors are individualized based on patient's condition or needs.

PLANNING

1 Expected outcomes following completion of procedure:	
• Buccal mucosa and tongue are pink, moist, and intact. Gums are moist and intact. Teeth are clean, smooth, and shiny. Tongue is pink and without coating. Lips are moist, smooth, and without cracks.	Degree of improvement in condition of oral cavity structures depends on extent of secretions or changes that existed before care.
• Debilitated patient expresses feeling of mouth cleanliness.	Comfort achieved.
• Oropharynx remains clear of secretions.	Secretions removed, thus avoiding aspiration.
2 Gather equipment and supplies.	Avoids interrupting procedure or leaving patient unattended to retrieve missing equipment.
3 Explain procedure.	

IMPLEMENTATION

1 Pull curtain around bed or close room door.	Provides privacy.
2 Perform hand hygiene and apply clean gloves.	Reduces transfer of microorganisms.
3 Place towel on over-bed table and arrange equipment. If needed turn on suction machine and connect tubing to suction catheter.	Prevents soiling of tabletop. Equipment prepared in advance ensures smooth, safe procedure. Supplies within reach create organized workspace.
4 Raise bed to appropriate working height; lower side rail. Unless contraindicated (e.g., head injury, neck trauma), lower side rail and position patient in Sims' or side-lying position. Turn patient's head toward mattress in dependent position with HOB elevated at least 30 degrees.	Use of good body mechanics with bed in high position prevents injury. Allows secretions to drain from mouth instead of collecting in back of pharynx. Prevents aspiration.
5 Place towel under patient's head and emesis basin under chin.	Prevents soiling of bed linen.
6 Remove dentures or partial plates if present.	Allows for thorough cleaning of prosthetics later (see Procedural Guideline 17-3). Provides clearer access to oral cavity.
7 If patient is uncooperative or having difficulty keeping mouth open, insert an oral airway. Insert upside down and turn airway sideways and over tongue to keep teeth apart. Insert when patient is relaxed if possible. Do not use force (see illustration).	Prevents patient from biting down on nurse's fingers and provides access to oral cavity.

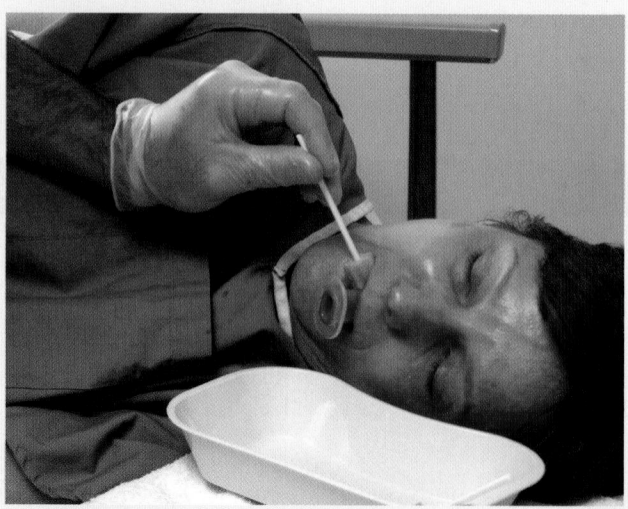

STEP 7   Cleaning around oral airway with toothette.

STEP	RATIONALE

Clinical Decision Point *Never place fingers into the mouth of an unconscious or debilitated patient. The normal response is to bite down.*

8 Clean mouth using brush moistened in water. Apply toothpaste or use antibacterial solution first to loosen crusts. Clean tooth surfaces using an up-and-down gentle motion. A toothette sponge can be used for patients for whom toothbrushing is contraindicated. Suction any accumulated secretions. Clean chewing and inner tooth surfaces first. Clean outer tooth surfaces (see Skill 17-2). Moisten brush with chlorhexidine solution to rinse. Use brush or toothette to clean roof of mouth, gums, and inside cheeks. Gently brush tongue but avoid stimulating gag reflex (if present). Repeat rinsing several times and use suction to remove secretions.

Brushing action removes food particles between teeth, along chewing surfaces and crusts for mucosa. Do not use commercial swabs because they do not clean teeth. Repeated rinsing removes all debris and aids in moistening mucosa.

Suction removes secretions and fluids that collect in posterior pharynx. Reduces risk for aspiration.

9 Use brush or toothette sponge to apply thin layer of water-soluble moisturizer to lips (see illustration).

Lubricates lips to prevent drying and cracking.

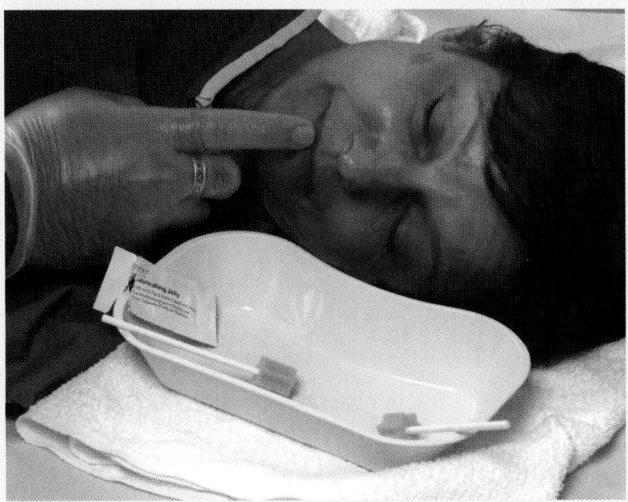

STEP 9   Application of water-soluble moisturizer to lips.

10 Inform patient that procedure is completed. Return him or her to comfortable and safe position.

Provides meaningful stimulation to unconscious or less-responsive patient.

11 Raise side rails as appropriate and return bed to locked, low position.

Reduces risk of falls from bed.

12 Clean equipment and return to its proper place. Place soiled linen in dirty laundry bag.

Proper disposal of soiled equipment prevents spread of infection.

13 Remove and dispose of gloves in proper receptacle and perform hand hygiene.

Reduces transmission of microorganisms.

EVALUATION

1 Apply clean gloves and inspect oral cavity.

Determines efficacy of cleaning. Once thick secretions are removed, underlying inflammation or lesions may be revealed.

2 Ask debilitated patient if mouth feels clean.

Evaluates level of comfort.

Unexpected Outcomes	Related Interventions
1 Secretions or crusts remain on mucosa, tongue, or gums.	• Provide more frequent oral hygiene.
	• Provide more frequent oral hygiene with toothette sponges.
	• Apply a water-based mouth moisturizer to provide moisture and maintain integrity of oral mucosa.
	• Chemotherapy and radiation can cause mucositis (inflammation of mucous membranes in mouth) because of sloughing of epithelial tissue. Room temperature saline rinses, bicarbonate and sterile water rinses, and oral care with a soft-bristled toothbrush decrease severity and duration of mucositis.
3 Lips are cracked or inflamed.	• Apply moisturizing gel or water-soluble lubricant to lips.
4 Patient aspirates secretions.	• Suction oral airway as secretions accumulate to maintain airway patency (see Chapter 25).
	• Elevate patient's HOB to facilitate breathing.
	• If aspiration is suspected, notify health care provider. Prepare patient for chest x-ray examination.

Recording and Reporting

• Record procedure on medical record. Include patient's ability to cooperate and whether suction is necessary for oral care.
• Document and report any pertinent observations (e.g., presence of gag reflex, presence of bleeding gums, dry mucosa, ulcerations, and crusts on tongue).
• Report any unusual findings to nurse in charge or health care provider.

Special Considerations
Teaching

• Family members may care for debilitated patient in the home. Instruction in mouth care is necessary so family understands how to protect patient from aspirating while thoroughly cleaning oral cavity. Observe family caregiver perform mouth care procedure.

Home Care

• Irrigate oral cavity with bulb syringe; if unavailable, substitute gravy baster or large syringe. Caution family caregiver against instilling a large amount of water or rinsing agent in the oral cavity because of the risk of aspiration.
• Encourage family caregiver to clean patient's mouth at least twice a day. If patient breathes through mouth, a soft-bristled toothbrush moistened and used every 1 to 2 hours will keep mouth moist and fresh.

SKILL 17-4 Hair Care–Combing and Shaving

A person's appearance and sense of well-being are influenced by how the hair looks and feels. Brushing, combing, and shampooing are basic measures for all patients unable to provide self-care. Having the hair groomed makes a person feel more comfortable. Most long-term care facilities have beauty shops where patients can go for professional hair care.

Fever, malnutrition, emotional stress, and depression affect the condition of the hair. Diaphoresis leaves the hair oily and unmanageable. Excessively dry or oily hair may be associated with hormone changes. Dry, brittle hair occurs with aging and excessive use of shampoo.

Certain chemotherapy agents and radiation therapy cause loss of hair (alopecia). Many patients choose to wear a wig; however, some choose to wear hair scarves or turbans. Table 17-2 describes common hair and scalp conditions and nursing interventions.

Dependent patients with beards or mustaches need assistance keeping the facial hair clean, especially after eating. Food particles easily collect in the hair. Shaving facial hair is a task most men prefer to do for themselves daily. Because some religions and cultures forbid cutting or shaving any body hair, be certain to obtain consent from these patients.

Delegation and Collaboration

The skills of combing and shaving can be delegated to nursing assistive personnel (NAP). The nurse instructs the NAP to:

• Properly position a patient with head or neck mobility restrictions.
• Report how the patient tolerated the procedure and any concerns (e.g., neck pain).
• Use an electric razor for any patient at risk for bleeding tendencies.

Equipment
Hair Care
❑ Wide-tooth comb and hairbrush
Shaving with Razor
❑ New disposable or electric razor
❑ Clean gloves
❑ Bath towel(s), mirror, washcloth, washbasin
❑ Shaving cream or soap, aftershave lotion (if patient desires and not contraindicated)
Mustache Care
❑ Scissors, brush or comb
❑ Bath towel
❑ Gooseneck lamp or overhead light

TABLE 17-2 | Hair and Scalp Problems

Characteristics	Implications	Interventions
Dandruff—Scaling of scalp accompanied by itching; in severe cases dandruff on eyebrows	Dandruff causes embarrassment; if it enters eyes, conjunctivitis may develop.	Shampoo regularly with medicated shampoo; in severe cases obtain health care provider's advice.
Ticks—Small gray-brown parasites that burrow into skin and suck blood	Ticks transmit several diseases, including Rocky Mountain spotted fever, Lyme disease, and tularemia.	Do not pull ticks from skin because sucking apparatus remains and may become infected; placing drop of oil on tick or covering it with petrolatum eases removal; oil suffocates tick.
Pediculosis capitis (head lice)—Tiny gray brown–white parasitic insects that attach to hair strands; about size of a sesame seed; nits or eggs look like oval particles attached at an angle to hair shaft; bites or pustules may be observed behind ears and at hairline	Head lice are difficult to remove and, if not treated, may spread to furniture and other people.	Check entire scalp. Use medicated shampoo for eliminating lice or permethrin (Nix), available as a crème rinse. *Caution against use of products containing lindane because the ingredient is toxic and known to cause adverse reactions* (National Pediculosis Association, 2009). Remove patient's clothing before treatment and apply new clothing following treatment. Repeat treatment according to product directions. Check hair for nits and comb with nit comb for 2 to 3 days until sure all lice and nits have been removed. Manual removal of lice is best option when treatment has failed. Vacuum infested areas of home. Wash linens in hot water and dry for at least 30 minutes.
Pediculosis corporis (body lice)—Tend to cling to clothing; thus may not be easily seen; suck blood and lay eggs on clothing and furniture	Patient itches constantly; scratches on skin may become infected; hemorrhagic spots may appear on skin where lice are sucking blood. It may spread to other people.	Patient should bathe or shower thoroughly; after skin is dried, apply lotion for eliminating lice; after 12 to 24 hours another bath or shower should be taken; bag infested clothing or linen until laundered. Vacuum items that cannot be washed.
Pediculosis pubis (crab lice)—Found in pubic hair; gray-white with red legs	Lice may spread through bed linen, clothing, furniture, or sexual contact.	Shave hair of affected area; clean as for body lice; if lice were sexually transmitted, partner must be notified.
Hair loss (alopecia)—Balding patches in periphery of hairline; hair becomes brittle and broken; caused by diseases, medication side effects, and improper use of hair-care products and hair-styling devices	Patches of uneven hair growth and loss alter patient's appearance.	Offer patients access to scarves, hairpieces, or wigs. Stop hair-care practices that damage hair.

STEP	RATIONALE

ASSESSMENT

1 Inspect condition of hair and scalp. Inspect for presence of any infestation (e.g., pediculosis). NOTE: Apply clean gloves and gown if infestation is suspected. — Indicates need for medicated applications or shampoo.

2 Assess patient's hair-care and shaving product preferences (e.g., shampoo, aftershave lotion, skin conditioner). — Influences approach to grooming. Promotes patient's independence by participating in decision making.

3 Before shaving, assess if patient has bleeding tendency. Review medical history, medications, and laboratory values (e.g., platelet count, anticoagulation studies). — Determines need to use electric razor for patient's safety because of potential for bleeding.

4 Assess patient's ability to manipulate razor. — Determines level of assistance required.

NURSING DIAGNOSES

- Bathing/self-care deficit
- Dressing/self-care deficit
- Impaired physical mobility
- Risk for injury

Related factors are individualized based on patient's condition or needs.

STEP	RATIONALE

PLANNING

1 Expected outcomes following completion of procedure:

- Patient expresses sense of comfort with hair and scalp grooming.

  Scalp stimulated and areas of matted or tangled hair removed.

- Patient expresses sense of comfort, with sensation of face feeling clean and refreshed.

  Hair and soap lather are removed.

- Skin surface is smooth, well hydrated, and free of cuts.

  Patient is free from injury.

- Patient helps with procedure as tolerated.

  Participation provides sense of independence.

2 Gather equipment and supplies.

Avoids interrupting procedure or leaving patient unattended to retrieve missing equipment.

3 Explain procedure.

Promotes patient's cooperation, participation, and self-care as appropriate.

4 Ask patient to explain during procedure steps that he or she uses to comb hair and/or shave. Ask patient to indicate if he or she becomes uncomfortable.

Patient involvement lessens anxiety.

5 Position patient sitting in chair or in bed with head elevated 45 to 90 degrees (as tolerated).

Elevation of head of bed makes it easier to access all sides of head and face.

IMPLEMENTATION

1 Provide privacy; close door or pull curtain.

Improves patient comfort.

2 Arrange supplies at bedside table and adjust lighting.

Creates organized workspace.

Lighting provides clear view of patient's face.

3 Perform hand hygiene and apply clean gloves if necessary.

Reduces transmission of infection.

4 **Combing and brushing hair.**

  a Part hair into two sections and then separate hair into two more sections (see illustrations).

  Brushing and combing are more effective when small areas of hair are groomed at any one time.

  b Brush or comb from scalp toward hair ends.

  Minimizes pulling.

  c Moisten hair lightly with water, conditioner, or alcohol-free detangle product before combing.

  Makes hair easier to comb.

  d Move fingers through hair to loosen any larger tangles.

  Lessens pulling.

  e Using a wide-tooth comb, start on either side of head and insert comb with teeth upward to hair near scalp. Comb through hair in circular motion by turning wrist while lifting up and out. Continue until all hair is combed through and then comb into place to shape and style.

  Moves comb evenly through hair without pulling.

5 **Shaving with disposable razor.**

  a Place bath towel over patient's chest and shoulders.

  Prevents shaving cream or water from soiling gown.

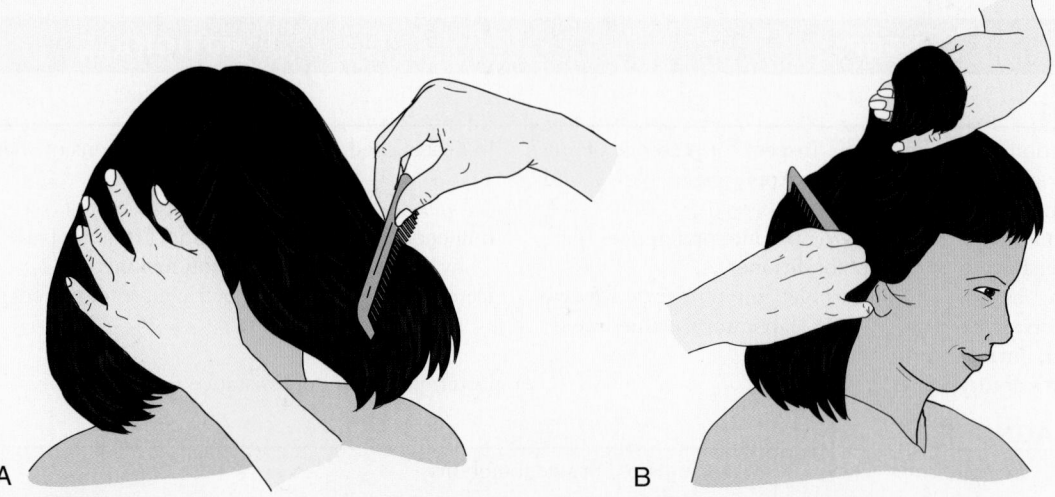

STEP 4a Parting hair. **A,** Part hair down the middle and divide it into two main sections. **B,** Part main section into two smaller sections.

STEP	RATIONALE
b Run warm water in washbasin. Check water temperature.	Warm water softens beard. Proper temperature prevents accidental burns.
c Place washcloth in basin and wring out thoroughly. Apply cloth over patient's entire face for several seconds.	Warm cloth helps soften skin and beard. Sensation of warmth can be relaxing.
d Apply approximately ¼ inch shaving cream or soap to patient's face. Smooth cream evenly over sides of face, chin, and under nose.	Cream creates additional softening effect and lubricates skin for application of razor.
e Hold razor in dominant hand at 45-degree angle to patient's skin. Begin by shaving across one side of patient's face using short, firm strokes in direction that hair grows (see illustration). Use nondominant hand to gently pull skin taut while shaving. Ask patient if he feels comfortable.	Technique facilitates shaving of facial hair. Short downward strokes work best over upper lip. Holding skin taut prevents razor cuts and discomfort during shaving. Patient is best resource to confirm if shaving technique causes discomfort.
f Dip razor blade in water because shaving cream accumulates on edge of blade.	Keeps cutting surface of razor blade clean.

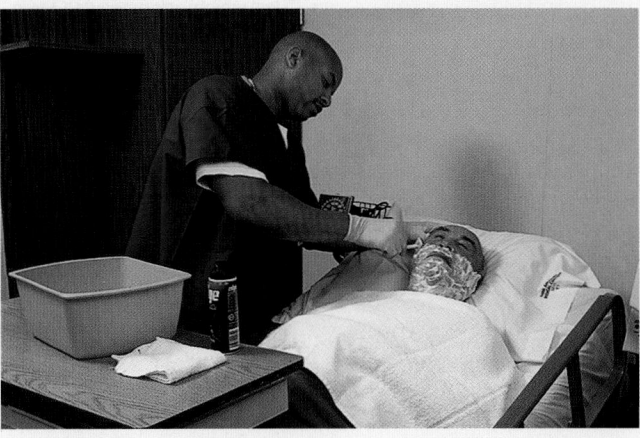

STEP 2e   Shaving patient using short, firm strokes.

STEP	RATIONALE
g After all facial hair is shaved, rinse face thoroughly with warm, moistened washcloth.	Prevents accumulation of shaving cream, which causes drying of skin.
h Dry face thoroughly and apply aftershave lotion if desired.	Retained moisture chaps skin.
6 Shaving with electric razor.	
a Place bath towel over patient's chest and shoulders.	
b Apply skin conditioner or preshave preparation.	Softens skin and beard to reduce friction from razor head.
c Turn razor on and begin by shaving across side of face. Gently hold skin taut while shaving over surface of skin. Use gentle downward stroke of razor in direction of hair growth.	Prevents pulling of beard and skin.
d After completing shave, apply aftershave lotion as desired unless contraindicated.	Stimulates and lubricates skin.
7 Mustache and beard care.	
a Place bath towel over patient's chest and shoulders.	
b If necessary gently comb mustache or beard.	Straightens hair that requires trimming.
c Allow patient to use mirror and direct areas to trim with scissors.	Allows patient to make decisions about care; maintains sense of independence.
8 Help patient to comfortable position.	
9 Return equipment to proper place. Discard soiled linen in dirty laundry bag. Perform hand hygiene.	Maintains cleanliness of patient's environment and reduces transmission of infection.

STEP	RATIONALE

EVALUATION

1 Ask patient how hair and scalp feel.	Evaluates patient's satisfaction with grooming.
2 Inspect condition of shaved area and skin underneath beard or mustache.	Reveals areas of localized bleeding from cuts and areas of dryness.
3 Ask patient if face feels clean and comfortable.	Evaluates level of patient's comfort.
4 Ask if patient is satisfied with degree of participation.	Patient maintains sense of independence.

Unexpected Outcomes

1 Patient senses tangles or discomfort in scalp.

2 Small isolated nicks or cuts appear on skin.

3 Skin surface appears dry.

Related Interventions

- Inspect scalp area. Repeat brushing/combing as needed.

- Obtain new disposable razor or change blade. If razor is reusable, be sure to clean according to agency policy.
- Change technique to glide razor over patient's skin.

- Use moisturizing shaving foam.
- Apply moisturizing lotion to patient's skin after completing shave.

Recording and Reporting

- Record shaving procedure on the clinical flow sheet or activities of daily living checklist. If there is no area indicated for shaving, make a nurse's note in the medical record. In addition, make note of how the patient tolerated procedure and any complications such as bleeding, pain, or problem skin areas.

Special Considerations

Teaching

- Shaving is a simple procedure that you can teach to a family caregiver. Teach safety precautions for shaving, especially if patient is receiving anticoagulant therapy.
- Instruct family caregiver in technique to follow in the event that patient is accidentally cut.

Pediatric

- Usually the facial hair of adolescents does not grow quickly; thus shaving daily is not necessary.
- Adolescents who shave should be asked about the frequency and allowed to perform activity as desired. Family caregivers

may wish to be involved in shaving their adolescent child if the child is unable to perform the activity on his own.

- Young girls with long hair may not tolerate brushing tangles out of hair. Tangling occurs easily in children restricted to bed. Once tangles are removed, it may be helpful to braid the hair.
- Children with lice should use a pediculocidal shampoo, followed with a visual examination for nits and removal if observed (see Table 17-2).

Gerontologic

- Usually the facial hair of older patients does not grow quickly; thus shaving daily is not necessary.
- The skin of older adults is thinner and at greater risk for injury when shaving.

Home Care

- Provide adequate towels around patient's neck to avoid spilling shaving cream or water on chest or bed.
- Perform procedure in comfortable setting with adequate lighting such as a bathroom or bedroom.

PROCEDURAL GUIDELINE 17-4   Hair Care–Shampooing

The frequency of shampooing depends on the condition of the hair and the person's daily routines and cultural preferences. Dry hair, which commonly results from aging and protein deficiency, requires less frequent shampooing than oily hair or the hair of people who actively exercise and perspire. In some health care agencies you need a health care provider's order to shampoo a patient who is dependent or has limited mobility because it is challenging to find ways to shampoo the hair without causing injury.

Remind hospitalized patients that more frequent shampooing is necessary when they remain in bed for extended periods of time, have excessive perspiration, or undergo treatments that leave blood or solutions in the hair. Two types of shampooing are available for patients: (1) traditional shampoo and water, or (2) a disposable dry shampoo cap. You can shampoo patients who are allowed to sit in a chair in front of a sink. Make sure that a patient's condition does not contraindicate neck hyperextension. Caution is needed with patients who have suffered neck injuries

because flexion and hyperextension of the neck could cause further injury. In addition, patients with positional vertigo are not able to tolerate neck hyperextension if it increases their dizziness. A folded towel placed under the neck on the edge of the sink provides added comfort. If a patient cannot sit in a chair or be transferred to a stretcher, you will need to shampoo the patient in bed, using traditional shampoo and water or a disposable shampoo product.

Delegation and Collaboration

The skill of shampooing the hair of bed-bound patients and the use of disposable shampoo product can be delegated to nursing assistive personnel (NAP). The nurse instructs the NAP about:

- Proper way to position a patient with a head or neck mobility restriction.
- Knowledge of care for lice, stressing steps to take to prevent transmission to other patients.

PROCEDURAL GUIDELINE 17-4   Hair Care–Shampooing—cont'd

Equipment

Regular Shampoo
- ❏ Clean gloves
- ❏ Bath towels (two or more), washcloth
- ❏ Shampoo, hair conditioner (*optional*), hydrogen peroxide (*optional*)
- ❏ Water pitcher with warm water
- ❏ Plastic shampoo board, wash basin
- ❏ Bath blanket, waterproof pad
- ❏ Clean comb and brush, hair dryer (*optional*)
- ❏ Saline (*optional*)

Disposable Shampoo
- ❏ Clean gloves
- ❏ Disposable shampoo cap product
- ❏ Clean comb and brush
- ❏ Bath towel

Procedural Steps

1 Assess environment for safety (e.g., check room for spills, make sure that equipment is working properly and that bed is in locked, low position).

2 Explain procedure and provide privacy.

3 Before washing patient's hair, determine that there are no contraindications to procedure. Check agency policy for health care provider order as needed. Certain medical conditions such as head and neck injuries, spinal cord injuries, and arthritis place patient at risk for injury during shampooing because of positioning and manipulation of patient's head and neck.

4 Perform hand hygiene.

5 Inspect hair and scalp before beginning shampoo. This determines if special shampoos or treatments are necessary (e.g., dandruff, lice, removal of blood). If draining head wounds are suspected, apply clean gloves. If lice are present, wear disposable gown in addition to gloves (National Pediculosis Association, 2009).

6 **Shampooing bed-bound patient with shampoo board.**

   a Apply clean gloves. Place waterproof pad under patient's shoulders, neck, and head. Position patient supine, with head and shoulders at top edge of bed. Place shampoo board under patient's head and washbasin under end of trough spout (see illustration). Be sure that trough spout extends beyond edge of mattress.

   b Place rolled towel under patient's neck and bath towel over patient's shoulders.

   c Brush and comb patient's hair.

   d Obtain pitcher with warm water.

   e Ask patient to hold towel or washcloth over eyes.

   f Slowly pour water from pitcher over hair until it is completely wet (see illustration). If hair contains matted blood, apply hydrogen peroxide to dissolve clots and rinse with saline. Apply small amount of shampoo.

   g Work up lather with both hands. Start at hairline and work toward back of neck. Lift head slightly with one hand to wash back of head. Shampoo sides of head. Massage scalp by applying pressure with fingertips.

   h Rinse hair with water. Make sure that water drains into basin. Repeat rinsing until hair is free of soap.

   i Apply conditioner or crème rinse if requested and rinse hair thoroughly.

   j Wrap patient's head in bath towel. Dry face with cloth used to protect eyes. Dry off any moisture along neck or shoulders.

   k Dry patient's hair and scalp. Use second towel if first one becomes saturated.

   l Comb hair to remove tangles and dry with dryer if desired.

   m Apply oil preparation or conditioning product to hair if desired by patient.

   n Variation for patients with coarse, curly hair: Condition hair after washing. To untangle hair, use wide teeth of comb. Beginning at nape of neck, comb small subsections of hair starting at hair ends. Continue to work through small sections until hair is free of tangles.

   o Help patient to comfortable position and complete styling of hair.

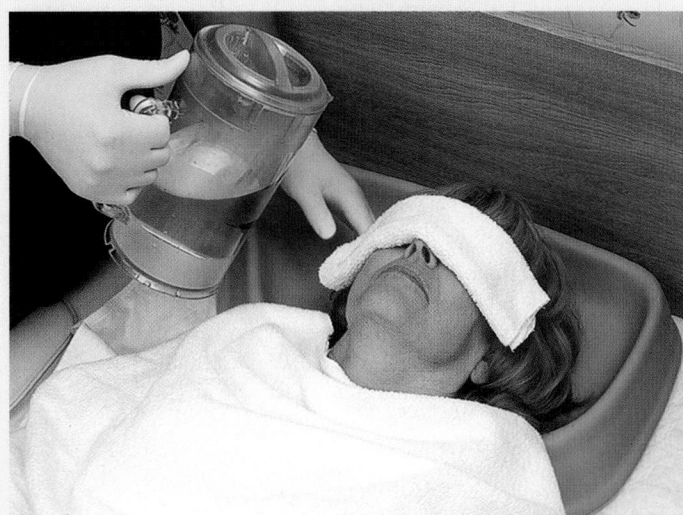

STEP 6a   Patient positioned over shampoo board. (*From Sorrentino SA: Mosby's textbook for nursing assistants, ed 8, St Louis, 2012, Mosby.*)

Continued

PROCEDURAL GUIDELINE 17-4 Hair Care–Shampooing—cont'd

p Dispose and store supplies. Remove gloves and perform hand hygiene.

7 Shampooing using disposable shampoo product.

a Patient can be sitting on chair or in bed. Apply clean gloves.

b Comb hair to remove any tangles or debris.

c Open package, apply cap, and secure all hair beneath cap (see illustration).

d Massage head through cap. Check fitting around head to maintain correct fit.

e Massage 2 to 4 minutes according to directions on package; additional time may be required for longer hair or hair matted with blood. (If blood is present, wear gloves.)

f Discard cap in trash; do not dispose of in toilet because it may clog plumbing.

g If patient desires, towel dry hair.

h Brush or comb patient's hair.

i Remove gloves. Perform hand hygiene.

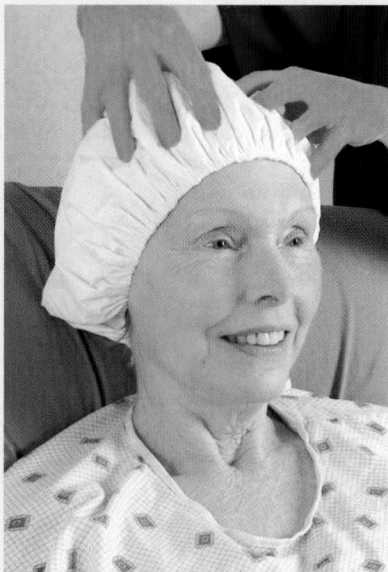

STEP 7c Patient wearing disposable shampoo cap.

SKILL 17-5 Performing Nail and Foot Care

Include nail and foot care in a patient's daily hygiene; the best time is during the bath. Many agencies require a health care provider's order before you can trim nails. Feet and nails often require special care to prevent infection, odors, pain, and injury to soft tissues. Often people are unaware of foot or nail problems until discomfort or pain occurs. Common foot and nail problems are presented in Table 17-3. For proper foot and nail care, instruct patients to protect the feet from injury, keep them clean and dry, and wear appropriate footwear. Instruct patients in the proper way to inspect the feet for lesions, dryness, or signs of infection. To maintain and promote foot and nail health, patients should visit a podiatrist when necessary. This is especially important for patients with peripheral vascular diseases (PVDs) or diabetes mellitus, older adults, and patients who are immunocompromised.

Patients most at risk for developing serious foot problems are those with peripheral neuropathy and peripheral vascular disease. These two disorders, commonly found in patients with diabetes mellitus, cause a reduction in blood flow to the extremities and a loss of sensory, motor, and autonomic nerve function. As a result, a patient is unable to feel heat and cold, pain, pressure, and positioning of the foot or feet. The reduction in blood flow impairs healing and promotes risk for infection. The development of diabetic foot ulcers has three contributing factors: (1) peripheral neuropathy (changes in the function and efficiency of the nerves), (2) ischemia (decrease in the blood flow related to plaque formation in arteries), and (3) a pivotal event (trauma caused by banging the toe or stepping on a foreign object). If foot ulcers do not heal, they can quickly become infected and lead to gangrene and subsequent amputation.

Delegation and Collaboration

The skill of nail and foot care of patients *without diabetes* or *circulatory compromise* can be delegated to nursing assistive personnel (NAP). The nurse instructs the NAP about:

- Not trimming patient's nails.
- Special considerations for patient positioning.
- Reporting any breaks in skin, redness, numbness, swelling, or pain.

Equipment

- ❑ Washbasin
- ❑ Emesis basin
- ❑ Washcloth and towel
- ❑ Nail clippers (check agency policy)
- ❑ Soft nail or cuticle brush
- ❑ Plastic applicator stick
- ❑ Emery board or nail file
- ❑ Body lotion
- ❑ Disposable bath mat
- ❑ Clean gloves

TABLE 17-3	Common Foot and Nail Problems			

Condition	Characteristics	Implications	Interventions
Callus	Thickened portion of epidermis, consisting of mass of horny, keratotic cells; usually flat, painless, and found on undersurface of foot or on palm of hand; caused by local friction or pressure	Foot calluses may cause discomfort when wearing tight-fitting shoes.	Refer patient to podiatrist and do not self-treat. Use of orthotic devices cushions and redistributes weight and pressure off calluses.
Corns	Keratosis caused by friction and pressure from shoes; mainly on toes, over bony prominence; usually cone-shaped, round, and raised; calluses with painful core	Conical shape compresses underlying dermis, making it thin and tender. Pain is aggravated by tight-fitting shoes. Patients may suffer alteration in gait because of pain.	Refer patient to podiatrist. Avoid use of oval corn pads, which increase pressure on toes. Use wider, softer shoes.
Plantar warts	Fungating lesions on sole of foot caused by papillomavirus	Warts may be contagious, are painful, and make walking difficult.	Refer patient to podiatrist.
Athlete's foot (tinea pedis)	Fungal infection of foot; scaliness and cracking of skin between toes and on soles of feet; small blisters containing fluid may appear, apparently induced by constricting footwear	Athlete's foot can spread to other body parts, especially hands. It is contagious and frequently recurs.	Feet should be well ventilated. Drying feet well after bathing and applying powder help prevent infection. Wearing clean socks or stockings reduces incidence. Health care provider orders application of griseofulvin, miconazole nitrate, or tolnaftate.
Ingrown nails	Toenail or fingernail growing inward into soft tissue around nail; results from improper nail trimming, poor shoe fit, or heredity	Ingrown nails can cause localized pain when pressure is applied.	Treatment is frequent warm soaks (exception: patient with diabetes) in antiseptic solution and removal of portion of nail that has grown into skin. Instruct patient in proper nail-trimming techniques. Refer to podiatrist.
Paronychia	Inflammation of tissue surrounding nail after hangnail or other injury; occurs in people who frequently have their hands in water; common in patients with diabetes	Area can become infected.	Treatment is warm compresses or soaks (exception: patient with diabetes) and local application of antibiotic ointments. Paronychia can be prevented by careful manicuring.
Foot odors	Result of excess perspiration promoting microorganism growth and possibly faulty foot hygiene or improper footwear	Excess perspiration causes discomfort.	Frequent washing, use of foot deodorants and powders, and clean footwear prevent or reduce this problem.

STEP	RATIONALE

ASSESSMENT

1 Assess environment for safety (e.g., check room for spills, make sure that equipment is working properly and that bed is in locked, low position).

Identifies safety hazards in patient environment that could cause or potentially lead to harm (QSEN Quality/Safety Competencies, 2012).

2 Inspect all surfaces of fingers, toes, feet, and nails. This can be done during the bath. Pay particular attention to areas of dryness, inflammation, or cracking. Also inspect areas between toes, heels, and soles of feet. Inspect socks for stains.

Integrity of feet and nails determines frequency and level of hygiene required. Heels, soles, and sides of feet are prone to irritation from ill-fitting shoes. Socks may become stained from bleeding or draining ulcer.

3 Assess color and temperature of toes, feet, and fingers. Assess capillary refill of nails. Palpate radial and ulnar pulse of each hand and dorsalis pedis pulse of foot; note character and symmetry of pulses (see Chapter 6).

Assess circulation to extremities. Peripheral artery disease (PAD) occurs when blood vessels in legs are narrowed or blocked by fatty deposits and blood flow to feet and legs decreases (American Diabetes Association, 2011).

4 Observe patient's walking gait (when appropriate). Have him or her walk down hall or walk straight line while wearing comfortable shoes or slippers (if able).

Alterations in bony structures of feet may cause pain, imbalance, and unsteady gait.

5 Ask if patient has history of leg pain on walking that is relieved with rest.

Claudicating pain is related to ischemia with diabetic and neuropathic disorders.

6 Ask patients about whether they use nail polish and polish remover frequently.

Chemicals in these products cause excessive dryness.

7 Assess type of footwear patient wears: Does patient wear socks? Are shoes tight or ill fitting? Are garters or knee-high nylons worn? Is footwear clean?

Some types of shoes and footwear predispose patient to foot and nail problems (e.g., infection, areas of friction, ulcerations).

8 Identify patient's risk for foot or nail problems.

Certain conditions increase likelihood of foot or nail problems.

   a Older adult

Poor vision, lack of coordination, or inability to bend over contributes to difficulty in performing foot and nail care. Normal physiologic changes of aging can result in brittle nails. Discolored, extremely thickened, and deformed nails can indicate infection, fungus, or disease (Malkin and Berridge, 2009).

   b Diabetes mellitus

Vascular changes associated with diabetes reduce blood flow to peripheral tissues. Break in skin integrity places patient with diabetes at high risk for skin infection.

   c Heart failure, renal disease

Both conditions increase tissue edema, particularly in dependent areas (e.g., feet). Edema reduces blood flow to neighboring tissues.

   d Cerebrovascular accident (stroke)

Presence of residual foot or leg weakness or paralysis results in altered walking patterns. Altered gait pattern causes increased friction and pressure on feet.

9 Assess for use of home remedies.

Certain preparations or applications cause more injury to soft tissue than the actual foot problem.

   a Over-the-counter (OTC) liquid preparations to remove corns or warts

Patients with diabetes or circulatory insufficiency should seek professional treatment and avoid self-treating.

   b Cutting corns or calluses with razor blade or scissors

Carries risk for cutting skin, which can lead to infection.

   c Use of oval corn pads

May exert pressure on toes, thereby decreasing circulation to surrounding tissues. Seek professional treatment.

   d Application of adhesive tape

Skin of older adult is thin and delicate and prone to tearing when adhesive tape is removed.

10 Assess patient's ability to care for nails or feet: visual alterations, fatigue, and musculoskeletal weakness.

Extent of patient's ability to perform self-care determines degree of assistance required from nurse.

11 Assess patient's knowledge of proper foot and nail care practices.

Health literacy level determines extent of teaching needed. Family caregivers should be involved in teaching process.

NURSING DIAGNOSES

- Bathing/self-care deficit
- Deficient knowledge regarding foot and nail care
- Impaired physical mobility
- Impaired skin integrity
- Ineffective tissue perfusion
- Risk for infection

Related factors are individualized based on patient's condition or needs.

STEP	RATIONALE

PLANNING

1 Expected outcomes following completion of procedure:
- Nails are smooth. Cuticles and tissues surrounding nail are clear and of normal color. Surfaces of feet are smooth.

Excess skin layers are removed. Nail integrity and cleanliness are maintained.

- Patient walks freely, without pain or unusual gait.

Patient understands importance of proper fitting footwear.

- Patient explains or demonstrates nail care correctly.

Patient learns skill.

2 Gather equipment and supplies.

Avoids interrupting procedure or leaving patient unattended to retrieve missing equipment.

3 Explain procedure to patient, including fact that proper soaking of nails on hands requires several minutes in warm water.

Patient must be willing to place fingers in basin up to 10 minutes. Patient may become anxious or fatigued.

4 Obtain health care provider's order for cutting nails (required by most clinical facilities). Obtaining order for podiatry consult should be initiated if patient has diabetes, PAD, or PVD.

Patient's skin may be cut accidentally. Certain patients are more at risk for infection, depending on their medical condition.

A podiatrist should assess and develop a regular schedule for nail care for patients with vascular insufficiency or peripheral neuropathy.

IMPLEMENTATION

1 Perform hand hygiene and apply clean gloves. Arrange equipment on over-bed table.

Reduces transmission of infection.
Easy access to equipment prevents delays.

2 Pull curtain around bed or close room door to provide privacy.

Maintaining patient's privacy reduces anxiety.

3 Help ambulatory patient sit in chair. Help bedfast patient to supine position with head of bed elevated 45 degrees. Place disposable bath mat on floor under patient's feet or place waterproof pad on mattress.

Sitting in chair facilitates immersing feet in basin. Bath mat protects feet from exposure to soil or debris.

4 Fill washbasin with warm water. Test water temperature. Place basin on floor or pad on mattress. Have patient immerse feet.

Prevents accidental burns to patient's skin.

> **Clinical Decision Point** *Patients who have diabetes mellitus, peripheral neuropathy, or PVD should not soak their hands and feet because of the increased risk of trauma, inability to sense temperature, and increased risk for infection (American Diabetes Association, 2011; Malkin and Berridge, 2009).*

5 Adjust over-bed table to low position and place it over patient's lap.

Easy access prevents accidental spills.

6 Fill emesis basin with warm water and place basin on towel on over-bed table. Test water temperature.

Warm water softens nails and thickened epidermal cells. Prevents accidental burns to patient's skin.

7 Instruct patient to place fingers in emesis basin and arms in comfortable position.

Prolonged positioning causes discomfort unless normal anatomic alignment is maintained.

8 Unless patient has diabetes mellitus, peripheral neuropathy, or PVD, allow feet and fingernails to soak 10 minutes.

Goal is to soften debris beneath nails so it can be removed easily.

9 Clean gently under fingernails with end of plastic applicator stick while fingers are immersed.

Removes debris under nails that harbors microorganisms.

10 Use soft cuticle brush or nailbrush to clean around cuticles to decrease overgrowth.

Nailbrush helps to prevent inflammation and injury to cuticles.

11 Remove emesis basin and dry fingers thoroughly.

Thorough drying impedes fungal growth and prevents maceration of tissues.

> **Clinical Decision Point** *Check agency policy for appropriate process for cleaning beneath nails. Do not use an orange stick or end of cotton swab; these splinter and can cause injury.*

12 *Check agency policy on nail care regarding filing and trimming.* Trim nails straight across at level of finger or follow curve of finger, ensuring that you do not cut down into nail grooves (see Illustration). Use disposable emery board and file nail to ensure that there are no sharp corners.

Trimming straight across avoids skin overgrowth at nail edges, which can lead to ingrown nails or infection.
Filing nail straight across to eliminate sharp nail edges minimizes nail from injuring the adjacent finger (Malkin and Berridge, 2009).

STEP	RATIONALE

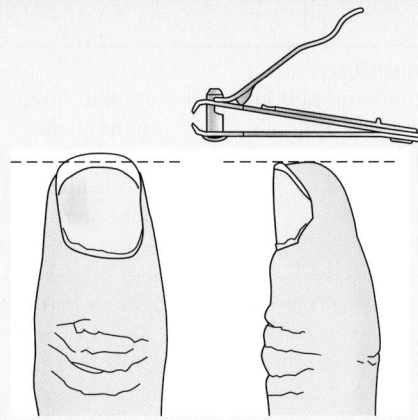

STEP 12   Trim nails straight across when using nail clipper.

13 Move over-bed table away from patient. Scrub callused areas of feet with washcloth.	Provides easier access to feet. Friction removes dead skin layers.
14 Clean between toes with washcloth.	
15 Dry feet thoroughly and trim or cut nails following Step 12.	Moisture can cause skin maceration.
16 Apply lotion to feet and hands. Rub in thoroughly. Help patient back to bed and into comfortable, safe position.	Lotion lubricates dry skin by helping to retain moisture.
17 Clean clippers with soap and water. If soiled with blood or body fluids, clean according to organizational policy and return equipment to proper place. Emery boards should be disposable. Dispose of soiled linen in dirty laundry bag. Remove gloves and perform hand hygiene.	Reduces transmission of infection.

EVALUATION

1 Inspect nails, areas between fingers and toes, and surrounding skin surfaces.	Inspection enables you to evaluate condition of skin and nails and allows you to note any remaining rough nail edges.
2 Ask patient to explain or demonstrate nail care.	Evaluates patient's level of learning techniques.
3 Observe patient's walk after foot and nail care.	Evaluate level of comfort and mobility achieved.

Unexpected Outcomes	Related Interventions
1 Cuticles and surrounding tissues are inflamed and tender to touch.	• Repeat nail care.
	• Evaluate need for antifungal cream.
2 Localized areas of tenderness occur on feet with calluses or corns at point of friction.	• Change in footwear or corrective foot surgery may be needed for permanent improvement in calluses or corns.
	• Refer patient to podiatrist.
3 Ulcerations involving toes or feet may remain.	• Institute wound care policies (see Chapters 18 and 38).
	• Consult with wound care specialist and/or podiatrist.
	• Increase frequency of assessment and hygiene.

Recording and Reporting

- Record procedure and observations in medical record (e.g., breaks in skin, inflammation, ulcerations).
- Report any breaks in skin or ulcerations to nurse in charge or health care provider.

Special Considerations
Teaching

- Use a variety of teaching formats regarding foot and nail care (e.g., brochures, videos, DVDs) that are consistent with patient's health literacy level.
- Instruct patient not to walk barefoot or use corn or callus products.

- Instruct a patient with diabetes, peripheral neuropathy, or peripheral vascular disease to do the following:
  - Inspect and bathe feet daily.
  - Inspect all surfaces of each foot.
  - Use a mirror to view bottom of each foot.
  - Clean around nails with a soft brush.
  - Dry the feet and pay special attention to drying between the toes.
  - Use lambswool between the toes if the skin stays moist or becomes macerated.
  - Wear socks made of natural fiber such as cotton that absorb perspiration and "breathe."

- Wear nonconstricting shoes with soft leather and an adequate toe box.
- See a podiatrist to develop a regular schedule for nail care.

Pediatric

- Children's nails should be assessed and trimmed to prevent injury from scratching themselves.
- Use appropriate-size clippers when clipping the nails of infants and small children (check agency policy).
- Do not use scissors.

Gerontologic

- Changes in aging skin include thinning of epidermis and subcutaneous fat and dryness because of decreased activity of oil and sweat glands. These changes are often evident in the feet. In addition, nails become discolored, thickened, deformed, and brittle.

- PVD, peripheral neuropathy, and long periods of limited exercise or bed rest impact balance, stability, and sensory impairment, resulting in impaired mobility.

Home Care

- Assess the home for any areas where a person could accidentally injure the feet such as rugs, objects that block pathways, or uneven walks or flooring.
- Avoid going barefoot or wearing open-toed shoes.
- *Alternative therapy*: Apply moleskin to friction areas of the foot or feet or wrap small pieces of lambswool around toes to reduce irritation from corns or bunions.
- Include family caregiver in foot and nail care education.
- Place contact information of podiatrist, health care provider, and home care nurse close by for easy access.

SKILL 17-6 Care of a Patient's Environment

When caring for patients who need to remain in or near their bed for an extended period, it is important to make that environment as comfortable as possible. A calm, comfortable restorative room is well ventilated; safe; and large enough to allow patients, visitors, and care providers to move about freely.

Although there are variations across health care settings, a typical room contains the following basic pieces of furniture: over-bed table, bedside stand, chairs, lamp, and bed. Long-term care and rehabilitation facilities often have similar equipment. The over-bed table rolls on wheels and can be adjusted to various heights over the bed or chair. The table provides ideal working space for nurses to perform procedures. It also provides a surface on which to place meal trays, toiletry items, and frequently used objects. Do not place the bedpan and urinal on an over-bed table. The bedside stand is for storing a patient's personal possessions and hygiene equipment. The telephone, water pitcher, and drinking cup are usually on top of the bedside stand.

Most hospital rooms contain an armless straight-backed chair or an upholstered lounge chair with arms. Straight-backed chairs are convenient when temporarily transferring a patient from the bed such as during bed making. Lounge chairs tend to be more comfortable when a patient is willing and able to sit for an extended period.

Proper lighting is necessary for everyone's safety and comfort. A brightly lit room is usually stimulating, but a darkened room is best for rest and sleep. Adjust room lighting by closing or opening drapes, regulating over-bed and floor lights, and closing or opening room doors. Position movable lights that extend over the bed from the wall for easy reach but move them aside when not in use.

Other equipment usually found in a patient's room includes a call light, a television set, a wall-mounted blood pressure gauge, oxygen and vacuum wall outlets, and personal care items. Special mattresses and bed boards are designed for comfort or positioning. Whenever using comfort and positioning equipment, check agency policy and manufacturer directions before application.

Beds

Because the bed is the piece of equipment that a patient uses most, it should be comfortable, safe, and adaptable to various positions. The typical hospital bed consists of a firm mattress on a metal frame that you can raise or lower horizontally. The frame is divided into three sections so the operator can raise and lower the head and foot of the bed separately and incline the entire bed with the head up or down. Each bed sits on four rollers, or casters, that allow you to move it easily. Table 17-4 lists common bed positions.

The position of a bed is usually changed by electric controls built into the side of the bed, at the foot of the bed, or on a bedside cable. Patients can raise or lower sections of the bed without expending much energy. It is important for you to instruct patients in the proper use of the controls and caution them against positions that will cause harm.

Often patients who are critically ill or are immobilized in traction are transported to different locations, such as the radiology department, in bed. There are beds in which scales are incorporated to facilitate routine weighing of a patient.

Beds contain a number of safety features. Use locks located on the wheels, casters, or at the center of the bed frame (Fig. 17-3) whenever a bed is stationary to prevent accidental movement during performance of a procedure (e.g., transferring a patient from bed to a stretcher). Side rails (i.e., adjustable metal frames [either four or two, depending on bed design] that you can raise or lower by pushing or pulling a knob) located on both sides of a bed help patients position themselves and provide upper-extremity support as a patient gets out of bed. Use caution when raising side rails. Research suggests that the risk for patient falls is greater when side rails on both sides of the bed are raised because patients try to climb over the rails to exit the bed. Raising only one rail (when there are only two) or three (when there are four rails) gives patients an exit route if they are able to move independently. The use of all

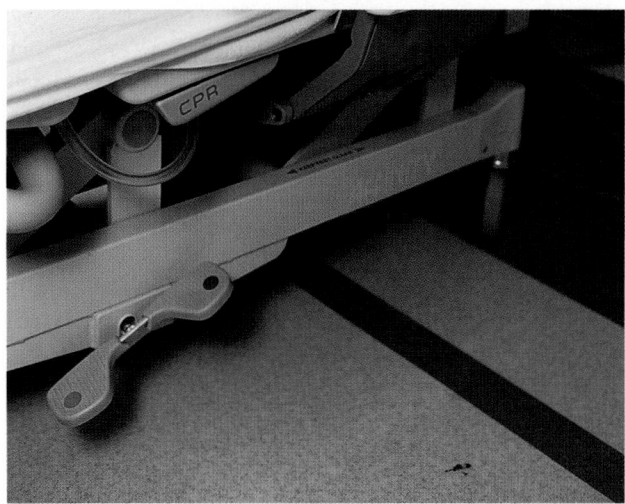

FIG 17-3 Lock on bed wheels.

side rails is considered a physical restraint (see Chapter 13). When you lower a side rail, do not leave the bedside with a patient still in bed. Most hospital beds are equipped with a bed alarm that alerts a nurse when a patient has gotten up without assistance. Each bed has a special headboard that is removable. This feature is important in emergency situations when the medical team must have easy access to a hard, flat surface to place under a patient during cardiopulmonary resuscitation (see Chapter 27).

Mattresses

Most standard mattresses are a water-repellent covered foam or pressure-reducing material that reduces pressure on bony prominences. These mattresses aid in the prevention of pressure ulcer development. In some specialized areas such as an intensive care unit (ICU) setting, foam or air therapy mattresses are used for all patients. Firm, water-repellent mattresses are still used in some areas.

TABLE 17-4	Common Bed Positions		
Position		**Description**	**Uses**
Fowler's	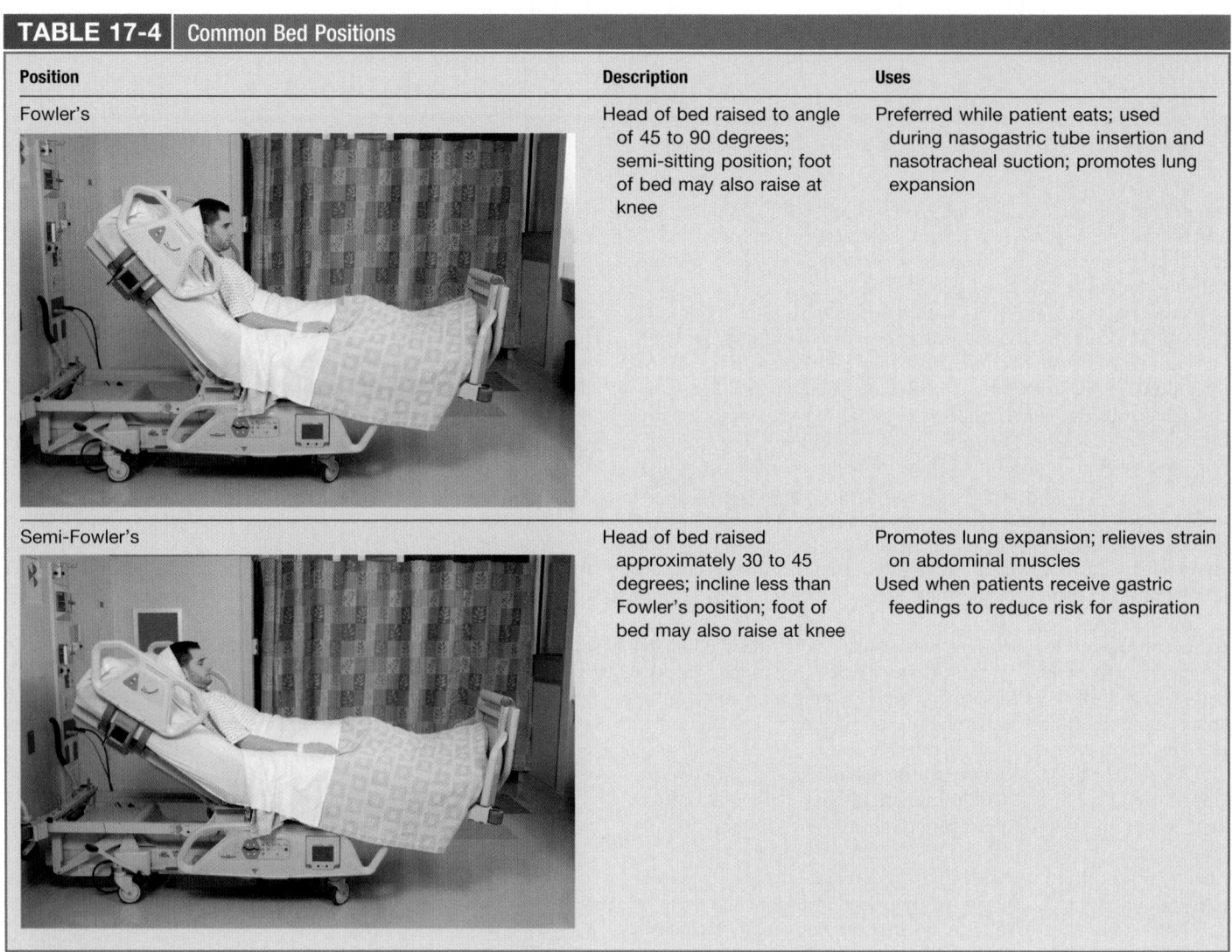	Head of bed raised to angle of 45 to 90 degrees; semi-sitting position; foot of bed may also raise at knee	Preferred while patient eats; used during nasogastric tube insertion and nasotracheal suction; promotes lung expansion
Semi-Fowler's		Head of bed raised approximately 30 to 45 degrees; incline less than Fowler's position; foot of bed may also raise at knee	Promotes lung expansion; relieves strain on abdominal muscles. Used when patients receive gastric feedings to reduce risk for aspiration

TABLE 17-4 | Common Bed Positions—cont'd

Position		Description	Uses
Trendelenburg's	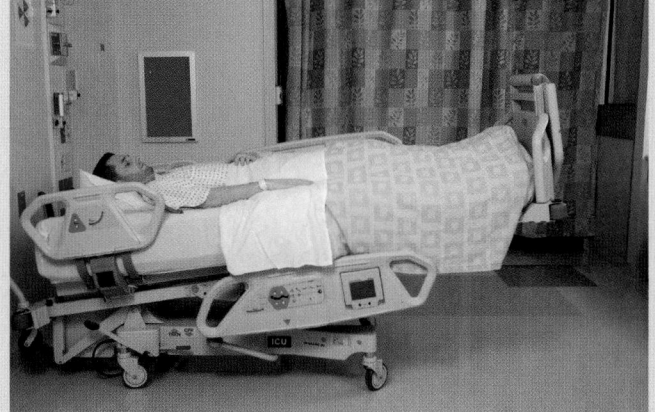	Entire bed frame tilted with head of bed down	For postural drainage; facilitates venous return in patients with poor peripheral perfusion
Reverse Trendelenburg's	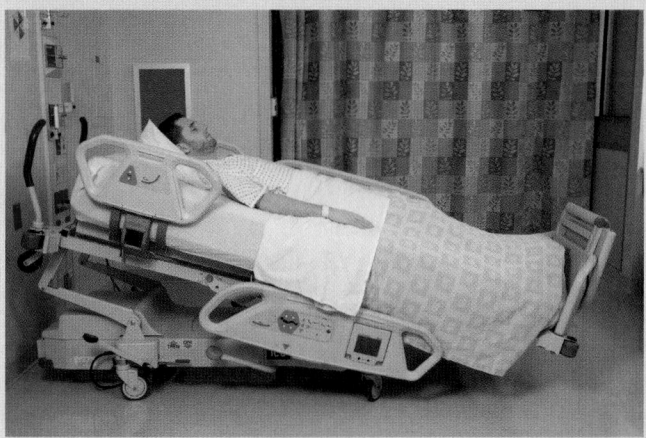	Entire bed frame tilted with foot of bed down	Used infrequently; promotes gastric emptying and prevents esophageal reflux
Supine or flat	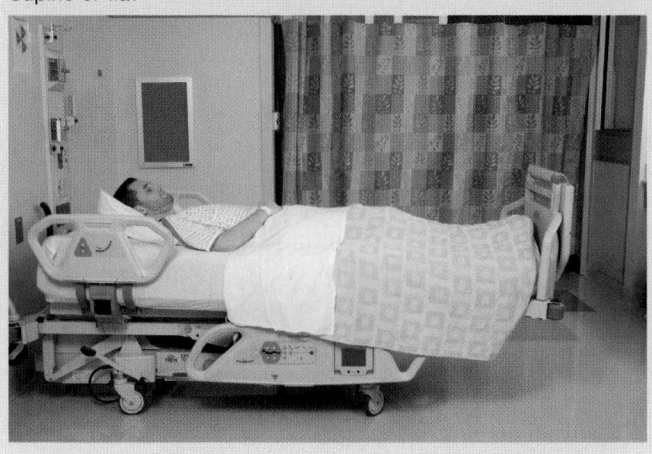	Entire bed frame horizontally parallel with floor	For patients with vertebral injuries and in cervical traction; position used for patients who are hypotensive and generally preferred by patients for sleeping

PROCEDURAL GUIDELINE 17-5   Making an Occupied Bed

At times it is necessary to make a bed that is occupied by a patient. If a patient is confined to bed, you should make the bed in a way that conserves time and the patient's energy. In addition, you need to know how to position the patient safely while the bed linens are changed. It is easier to make an occupied bed with two people. Try to keep the patient as comfortable as possible. In cases in which a patient experiences severe pain, an analgesic administered 30 to 60 minutes before a procedure helps to control pain and maintain comfort.

Even though a patient is unable to get out of bed, encourage self-help as much as possible. For example, a patient can turn, help in moving up in bed, or hold top sheets while you apply linen. These activities help maintain patient's strength and mobility and allow participation in hygiene care.

Delegation Considerations

The skill of making an occupied bed can be delegated to nursing assistive personnel (NAP). The nurse instructs the NAP about:

- Any position or activity restrictions that apply.
- Looking for wound drainage, drainage tubes, or intravenous (IV) tubing that is found in the linens.
- Obtaining help with positioning patient during linen change, observe good body mechanics, and support alignment of patient if needed.
- Using special precautions such as aspiration precautions, including:
  a Keeping head of bed (HOB) raised to no lower than 30 degrees.
  b Explaining need to report excessive coughing or choking during procedure.

Equipment

- ❏ Linen bags
- ❏ Mattress pad (change only when soiled)
- ❏ Bottom sheet (flat or fitted)
- ❏ Drawsheet (*optional*), top sheet, bedspread
- ❏ Waterproof pads (*optional*), pillowcases
- ❏ Clean gloves
- ❏ Antiseptic cleanser
- ❏ Washcloth

Procedural Steps

1 Assess environment for safety (e.g., check room for spills, make sure that equipment is working properly and that bed is in locked, low position. Pull room divider curtain or close door to provide privacy.
2 Determine if patient has been incontinent or if excess drainage is on linen.
3 Assess restrictions in mobility/positioning of patient. Explain procedure to patient, noting that patient will be asked to turn over layers of linen.
4 Perform hand hygiene and apply clean gloves if linen is soiled or there is risk of contact with blood or body fluids.
5 Assemble all equipment on bedside table.
6 Raise bed to a comfortable working height; lower HOB as tolerated, keeping patient comfortable. Remove call light. If patient is on aspiration precautions, keep HOB no lower than 30 degrees. Lower side rail from side where you are standing.
7 Loosen top linen at foot of bed.

8 Remove bedspread and blanket separately. If soiled, place in linen dirty laundry bag. If to be reused, fold into square and place over back of chair.
9 Cover patient with bath blanket, placing over top sheet. Have patient hold top edge of bath blanket or tuck blanket under shoulders. Reach beneath blanket and remove top sheet. Discard in dirty laundry bag.
10 Help patient to side-lying position facing away from you. Encourage him or her to use side rail to turn. Adjust pillow under patient's head.
11 Assess to make sure that there is no tension on any external medical devices.
12 Stand on side of bed. Loosen bottom linens, moving from head to foot. Fanfold or roll bottom sheet, drawsheet, and any cloth pads toward and under patient. Tuck edges of old bottom linen alongside patient's buttocks, back, and shoulders (see illustration).
13 Clean, disinfect, and dry mattress surface if needed.
14 Apply clean linens to exposed half of bed in separate layers. Start with mattress pad by placing lengthwise with center crease in middle of bed. Fanfold layer to center of bed alongside patient. Repeat process with bottom sheet and drawsheet (see Illustration).

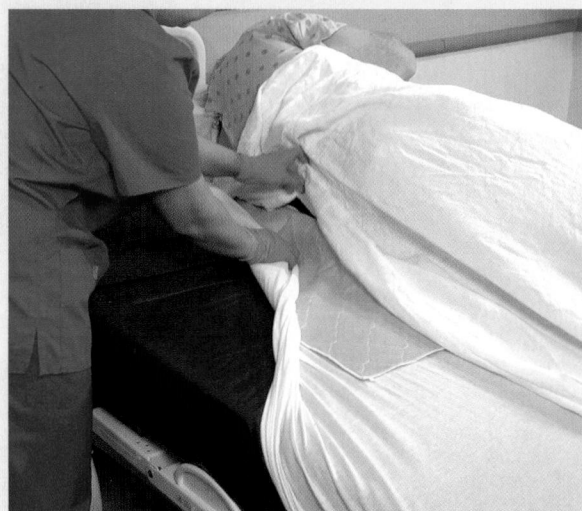

STEP 12   Soiled linen tucked alongside patient.

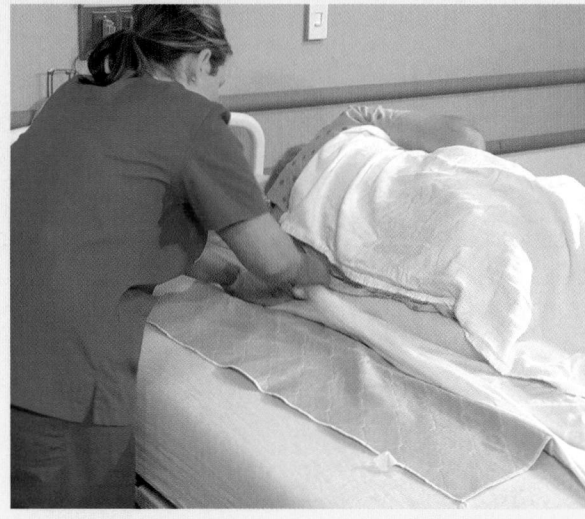

STEP 14   Apply clean linen to bed and fanfold alongside patient.

PROCEDURAL GUIDELINE 17-5 Making an Occupied Bed—cont'd

15 Pull fitted sheet smoothly over mattress corner at top and bottom of bed. If using a flat sheet, allow edge of sheet to hang about 25 cm (10 inches) over mattress edge. Be sure that lower hem of bottom sheet lies seam down and even with bottom edge of mattress.

16 If bottom sheet is flat, miter top corner at HOB. Face HOB diagonally. Place hand away from HOB under top corner of mattress, lift, and with other hand tuck edge of bottom sheet smoothly under mattress so side edges of sheet above and below mattress meet when brought together.

17 To miter a corner, pick up top of sheet at about 45 cm (18 inches) from top of mattress (see illustration A). Lift sheet and lay it on top of mattress to form a triangular fold with lower base of triangle even with mattress side edges (see illustration B).

18 Tuck lower edge of sheet, which is hanging free under mattress. Hold portion of sheet covering side of mattress in place with one hand (see illustration). With the other hand pick up triangular linen fold and bring it down over side of mattress. Tuck with palms down, without pulling triangular fold. Tuck this portion under mattress (see illustrations).

19 Tuck remaining portion of sheet under mattress, moving toward foot of bed. Keep linen smooth.

20 Place open drawsheet along middle of bed lengthwise and tuck remainder under patient's buttocks and torso. Drawsheet should be fanfolded or rolled on top of the bottom sheet. Keep linen under patient as flat as possible because patient will need to roll over new layers of linen when you are ready to make other side of bed. You may also place waterproof pad under drawsheet.

21 Raise side rail and ask patient to turn toward you; help as needed. Tell patient that he or she will be rolling over layers of linen. Make sure that patient turns slowly to keep his or her body in correct alignment (see illustration).

22 Move to opposite side of bed; lower side rail. Help patient position on other side over folds of linen.

23 Loosen edges of soiled linen from under mattress. Remove soiled linen by folding into a bundle or square.

24 Hold linen away from your body and place it in laundry bag.

25 Clean, disinfect, and dry other half of mattress as needed.

26 Pull clean, fanfolded or rolled linen, mattress pad, and optional drawsheet over edge of mattress from HOB to foot of bed. If bottom sheet is fitted, pull corners over mattress edges. If flat sheet used, unfold and pull toward you. Miter top corner of bottom flat sheet (see Steps 15 to 17).

27 Facing side of bed, grasp remaining edge of bottom flat sheet. Lean back, keep back straight, and pull while tucking excess linen under mattress from HOB to foot of bed.

28 Make sure that sheets and pad are smooth and wrinkle free.

29 Help patient roll back into supine position.

30 Place top sheet over patient with vertical centerfold lengthwise down middle of bed. Open sheet out from head to foot and unfold over patient. Be sure that top edge of sheet is even with top edge of mattress.

31 Place clean or reused bed blanket on bed over patient. Make sure that top edge is parallel with top edge of sheet and 15 to 20 cm (6 to 8 inches) from edge of top sheet. Raise side rail.

32 Go to other side of bed. Lower side rail. Spread sheet and blanket out evenly.

33 Have patient hold onto sheet and blanket while you remove bath blanket.

34 Make cuff by turning edge of top sheet down over top edge of blanket.

35 Make horizontal toe pleat; stand at foot of bed and fanfold in sheet and blanket 5 to 10 cm (2 to 4 inches) across bed. Pull

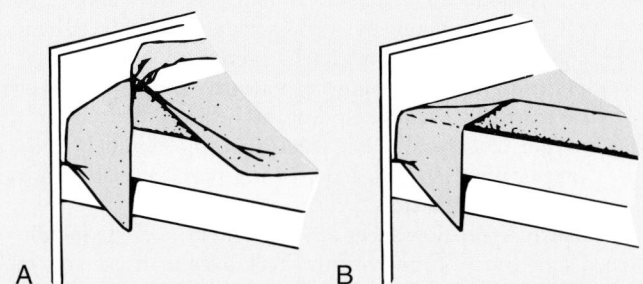

STEP 17 **A,** Top edge of sheet picked up. **B,** Sheet on top of mattress in triangular fold.

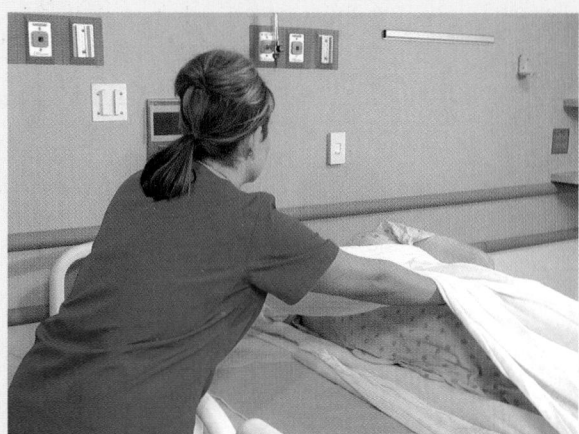

STEP 21 Patient rolling over layers of linen.

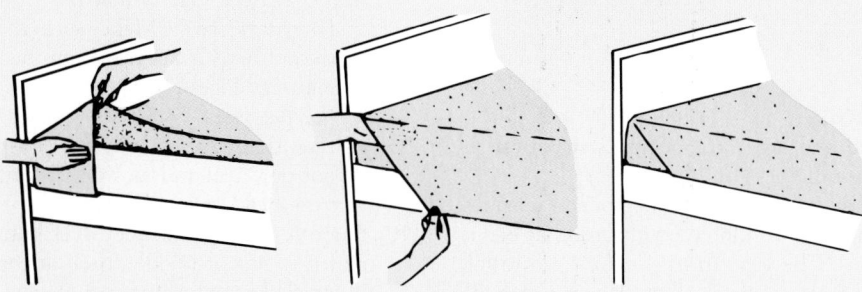

STEP 18 Triangular fold placed over side of mattress; linen tucked under mattress.

Continued

PROCEDURAL GUIDELINE 17-5 Making an Occupied Bed—cont'd

sheet and blanket up from bottom to make fold approximately 15 cm (6 inches) from bottom edge of mattress.

36 Standing at side of bed, tuck in remaining portion of sheet and blanket under foot of mattress. Tuck top sheet and blanket together. Be sure that toe pleats are not pulled out.

37 Make modified mitered corner with top sheet and blanket. After making triangular fold, do not tuck tip of triangle (see illustration).

38 Go to other side of bed. Repeat Steps 36 and 37.

39 Apply clean pillowcase.

40 Place call light within patient's reach on bedrail or pillow, return bed to locked, low position, and raise side rail (as needed).

41 Place linen in dirty laundry bag. Remove and dispose of gloves.

42 Arrange and organize patient's room and perform hand hygiene.

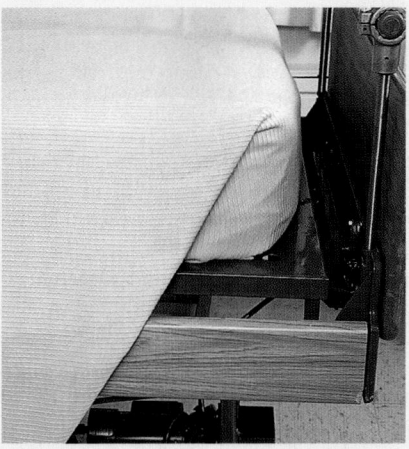

STEP 37 Modified mitered corner.

PROCEDURAL GUIDELINE 17-6 Making an Unoccupied Bed

Bedmaking may be done with the patient out of the bed (unoccupied) or in the bed (occupied). In some settings bed linen is not changed every day; however, you always need to change any wet or soiled linen promptly. An unoccupied bed is one left open with the top sheets fanfolded down. A postoperative surgical bed is prepared for patients returning from the operating room (OR) or procedural area. The bed is left with the top sheets fanfolded lengthwise and not tucked in to facilitate a patient's transfer from a stretcher. A closed bed, which is made with the top sheets pulled up to the head of the bed, is used after a patient is discharged and housekeeping cleans the unit.

Delegation and Collaboration

The skill of making an unoccupied bed can be delegated to nursing assistive personnel (NAP). The nurse instructs the NAP about:

- Position or activity restrictions that apply to patient's ability to get out of bed.
- Use of special linen instructions if patient is on an airflow mattress.

Equipment

- ❑ Linen bags
- ❑ Mattress pad (change only when soiled)
- ❑ Bottom sheet (flat or fitted)
- ❑ Drawsheet (*optional*), top sheet, bedspread
- ❑ Waterproof pads (*optional*), pillowcases
- ❑ Clean gloves
- ❑ Antiseptic cleanser
- ❑ Washcloth

Procedural Steps

1 Perform hand hygiene and apply clean gloves if patient is incontinent or excess drainage is on linen.

2 Assess environment for safety (e.g., check room for spills, make sure that equipment is working properly and that bed is in locked, low position). Check position of chair for transfer. Pull room divider curtain or close room door to provide privacy.

3 Assess activity orders or restrictions in mobility in planning if patient can get out of bed for procedure. Help patient to bedside chair or recliner.

4 Lower side rails on both sides of bed and raise bed to comfortable working position.

5 Remove soiled linen, hold away from uniform, and place in dirty laundry bag. Avoid shaking or fanning linen.

6 Reposition mattress and wipe off any moisture with a washcloth moistened in antiseptic solution (consult agency housekeeping guidelines). Dry thoroughly.

7 Apply all bottom linen on one side of bed before moving to opposite side.

   a *For fitted sheet:* Make sure that fitted sheet is placed smoothly over mattress and top and bottom mattress edge. Fit corners on one end and then the other.

   b *For flat sheet:* Place sheet over mattress. Allow about 25 cm (10 inches) to hang over side mattress edge. Lower hem of sheet should lie seam down, even with bottom edge of mattress. Pull remaining top portion of sheet over top edge of mattress. While standing at head of bed, miter top corner of bottom sheet (see Procedural Guideline 17-5, Steps 16 to 19). Tuck remaining portion of flat bottom sheet under mattress.

8 *Optional:* Apply drawsheet, laying centerfold along middle of bed lengthwise. Smooth drawsheet over mattress and tuck excess edge under mattress, keeping palms down.

9 Move to opposite side of bed and spread bottom sheet smoothly over edge of mattress from head to foot of bed.

   a *For fitted sheet:* Make sure that fitted sheet is placed smoothly over mattress from head to foot of bed and over mattress edges.

   b *For flat sheet:* Miter top corner of bottom sheet, making sure that corner is taut. Grasp remaining edge of flat bottom sheet and tuck tightly under mattress while moving from head to foot of bed.

10 Smooth folded drawsheet over bottom sheet and tuck under mattress, first at middle, then at top, and then at bottom.

11 If needed, apply waterproof pad over bottom sheet or drawsheet.

PROCEDURAL GUIDELINE 17-6 Making an Unoccupied Bed—cont'd

12 Place top sheet over bed with vertical centerfold lengthwise down middle of bed. Open sheet out from head to foot, being sure that top edge of sheet is even with top edge of mattress.

13 Tuck in remaining portion of sheet under foot of mattress. Then place blanket over bed with top edge parallel to top edge of sheet and 15 to 20 cm (6 to 8 inches) down from edge of sheet. (*Optional:* Apply additional spread over bed.)

14 Make cuff by turning edge of top sheet down over top edge of blanket and spread.

15 Standing on one side at foot of bed, lift mattress corner slightly with one hand and with other hand tuck top sheet, blanket, and spread under mattress. Be sure that toe pleats are not pulled out.

16 Make modified mitered corner with top sheet, blanket, and spread. After making triangular fold, do not tuck tip of triangle (see illustration).

17 Go to other side of bed. Spread sheet, blanket, and spread out evenly. Make cuff with top sheet and blanket (closed bed). Make modified corner at foot of bed. Alternatively fanfold sheet, blanket, and spread at foot of bed, with top layer ready to be pulled up (this leaves an open bed).

Optional: Make horizontal toe pleat; stand at foot of bed and fanfold in sheet 5 to 10 cm (2 to 4 inches) across bed. Pull sheet up from bottom to make fold approximately 15 cm (6 inches) from bottom edge of mattress.

18 Apply clean pillowcase.

19 Place call light within patient's reach on bedrail or pillow and return bed to lowest position, allowing for patient transfer. Help patient to bed.

20 Place linen bag in dirty laundry bag. Remove and dispose of gloves.

21 Arrange and organize patient's room and perform hand hygiene.

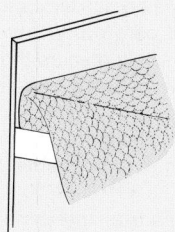

STEP 16 Modified mitered corner.

Critical Thinking Exercises

Mr. Bank is a 78-year-old male with a 3-year history of type 1 diabetes mellitus and hypertension. He was just discharged after 5 days of hospitalization with diagnoses of healing right-heel ulcer and controlled hypertension. His discharge summary notes that he requires assistance with daily dressing changes for the ulcer. Mr. Bank lives alone and is able to perform all routine activities of daily living (ADLs). During the initial home visit you assess that, although he understands the need for the daily dressing changes, he is not able to state which precautions are needed to prevent any recurrence.

1 Which three actions should Mr. Bank do to maintain good foot care?
  1 Wear properly fitting shoes
  2 Wear clean nylon socks
  3 Inspect feet daily, both top and bottom
  4 Have nails trimmed by professional
  5 Soak feet daily in warm water for 15 minutes

2 Identify a proactive foot-care intervention that Mr. Bank should perform.
  1 Self-treat corns and callus with over-the-counter products
  2 Seek a professional evaluation by a podiatrist and establish a foot-and-nail care schedule at least annually
  3 Cut toenails in a curved shape to the pink part of the nail
  4 Wear shoes without socks

REVIEW QUESTIONS

1 Provide bathing at regular intervals to:
  1 Restore normal pH of the skin from acidic to alkaline.
  2 Remove resident bacteria that normally cause disease.
  3 Clean the outer layer of skin and remove dead skin cells.
  4 Promote the maturation of new skin cells.

2 Some patients require special positioning precautions when the hair is shampooed. Special positioning precautions are most appropriate for which patient?
  1 A patient with diabetes who has hypertension
  2 A patient with a hearing deficit
  3 A patient who has an endotracheal tube
  4 A patient with arthritis in her cervical spine

3 An 88-year-old patient diagnosed with dementia frequently becomes very agitated and aggressive with caregivers. Which approach for bathing this patient would be most appropriate?
  1 Help the patient with a shower
  2 Provide a complete bed bath
  3 Avoid bathing until the patient becomes more relaxed
  4 Provide a disposable bed bath in bed

4 A Muslim woman needs to have a bed bath. Which adjustment does the female nurse need to make when performing perineal care?
  1 She needs to use gloves when performing perineal care.
  2 She needs to have another nurse in attendance while doing perineal care.
  3 She needs to use her left hand when doing perineal care.
  4 She needs to use her dominant hand when doing perineal care.

5 A patient in the intensive care unit after a head injury has been unresponsive at times and can be aroused only after painful stimuli. Which assessment by the nurse is most crucial in determining whether it is safe to perform oral hygiene?
  1 Check the patient's pupillary response
  2 Evaluate the patient using the Glasgow Coma Scale
  3 Assess the condition of the oral cavity
  4 Determine the presence of a gag reflex

6 Cleaning baths include which of the following? (Select all that apply.)
  1 Bed bath
  2 Herbal bath
  3 Tub bath
  4 Shower

7 A nurse is caring for a critically ill cardiac surgery patient who is on a ventilator. Which of the following solutions has been shown to decrease the incidence of ventilator-assisted pneumonia (VAP) in intubated patients?
1 Peroxide
2 Normal saline
3 Chlorhexidine
4 Tap water

8 While giving a complete bed bath to an unconscious patient, care is taken to:
1 Tape the eyelids shut to preserve moisture.
2 Close the eyelids with the back of the fingertip and place an eye patch or shield in place with tape.
3 Place moistened cotton balls on the eyelids to moisten the eye.
4 Allow the eyelids to stay open to help the nurse identify when the patient has regained consciousness.

9 A patient requires oral care every 2 hours. Indicate which order should be followed to safely prepare the patient for oral care.
1 Assess environment for safety and provide privacy.
2 Lower side rail.
3 Raise bed to working height.
4 Arrange supplies on over-bed table.
5 Position patient.

10 Inflammation of the mucous membrane of the mouth is called _____.

REFERENCES

American Dental Association: *Oral health topics, brushing your teeth cleaning your teeth and gums*, 2011, available at http://www.ada.org/5624.aspx?currentTab=1, accessed February 21, 2012.

American Diabetes Association: *Foot complications*, 2011, available at http://www.diabetes.org/living-with-diabetes/complications/foot-complications/, accessed February 21, 2012.

Barrick AL, et al: *Bathing without a battle: person-directed care of individuals with dementia*, ed 2, New York, 2008, Springer.

Berry AM, et al: Effects of three approaches to standardized oral hygiene to reduce bacterial colonization and ventilator pneumonia in mechanically ventilated patients: a randomized control trial, *Int J Nurs Stud* 48(6):681, 2011.

Browne J, et al: Pursuing excellence: development of an oral hygiene protocol for mechanically ventilated patients, *Crit Care Nurs Q* 34(1):25, 2011.

Buschemi C: Acculturation: state of science in nursing, *J Cultural Diversity* 18(2):39, 2011.

Busscher HJ, et al: Biofilm formation on dental restorative and implant materials, *J Dental Res* 89(7):657, 2010.

Eigsti J: Innovative solutions: beds, baths, and bottoms: a quality improvement initiative to standardize use of beds, bathing techniques, and skin care in a general critical-care unit, *Dimens Crit Care Nurs* 30(3):169, 2011.

Emanuele P: Deep vein thrombosis, *Am Assn Occup Health Nurses* 56(9):389, 2008.

Epstein RM, Street RL: The values and value of patient-centered care, *Ann Fam Med* 9:100, 2011.

Grap MJ: Not-so-trivial pursuit: mechanical ventilation risk reduction, *Am J Crit Care* 18(4):299, 2009.

Johnson D, et al: Patients' bath basins as potential sources of infection: a multicenter sampling study, *Am J Crit Care* 18(1):31, 2009.

Jury L, et al: Effectiveness of routine patient bathing to decrease the burden of spores on the skin of patients with *Clostridium difficile* infection, *Infect Control Hosp Epidemiol* 32(2):181, 2011.

Labeau SO, et al: Prevention of ventilator-associated pneumonia with oral antiseptics: a systematic review and meta-analysis, *Lancet Infect Dis* 11(11):845, 2011, Epub July 26, 2011.

Lau D: Role of food perceptions in food selection of the elderly, *J Nutr Elderly* 27(3/4):221, 2008.

Malkin B, Berridge P: Guidance on maintaining personal hygiene in nail care, *Nurs Stand* 23(41):35, 2009.

Meiner S: *Gerontologic nursing*, ed 4, St Louis, 2010, Mosby.

Munro C, et al: Chlorhexidine, toothbrushing, and preventing ventilator-associated pneumonia in critically ill adults, *Am J Crit Care* 18(5):428, 2009.

National Cancer Institute (NCI): *Oral complications of chemotherapy and head/neck radiation (PDQ)*, 2011, available at http://www.cancer.gov/cancertopics/pdq/supportivecare/oralcomplications/Patient, accessed February 21, 2012.

National Pediculosis Association: *Treatments*, 2009, available at http://www.headlice.org, accessed February 21, 2012.

National Pressure Ulcer Advisory Panel (NPUAP) and The European Pressure Ulcer Advisory Panel (EPUAP): *Pressure ulcer prevention quick reference guide*, 2010, available at kewww.npuap.org/Final_Quick_Prevention_for_web_2010.pdf accessed February 21, 2012.

Quality and Safety Education for Nurses (QSEN): *Quality/safety competencies & patient-centered care*, 2012, available at http://www.qsen.org, accessed February 21, 2012.

Sjögren's Syndrome Foundation: 2011, available at http://sjogrens.org, accessed February 21, 2012.

Stein P, Henry R: Poor oral hygiene in long-term care, *Am J Nurs* 109(6):44, 2009.

Wiech E, Bayer D: Simple interventions for ventilator-associated pneumonia, *Nursing2012 Crit Care* 7(3):19, 2012.

Yasny J, Silvay G: Geriatric patients: oral health and the operating room, *J Am Geriatr Soc* 58(7):1382, 2010.

Pressure Ulcer Care

MEDIA RESOURCES

- **evolve** *learning system* http://evolve.elsevier.com/Perry/skills
  - Review Questions
  - ▶ Video Clips
  - Audio Glossary

- **NSO** Nursing Skills Online

KEY TERMS

Debridement	Exudate	Pressure ulcer	Slough
Deep tissue injury	Ischemia	Reactive hyperemia	Topical agents
Erythema	Maceration	Shear	Undermining
Eschar	Necrosis		

OBJECTIVES

Mastery of content in this chapter will enable the nurse to:
- Describe guidelines for prevention of pressure ulcers.
- Identify risk factors for development of pressure ulcers.
- Identify outcome criteria for patients at risk for pressure ulcers or impaired skin integrity.
- Discuss the use of risk assessment tools commonly used in assessment of pressure ulcers.

- Describe patient and pressure ulcer characteristics to include in an assessment.
- Discuss indications for the use of topical agents in the treatment of pressure ulcers.
- Use topical agents correctly in the management of a pressure ulcer.
- Discuss teaching needs of patient and family regarding pressure ulcers.

A pressure ulcer is a localized area of injury to the skin and/or underlying tissue, usually over a bony prominence as a result of pressure or pressure in combination with shear and/or friction. A number of contributing factors are associated with pressure ulcers (e.g., moisture, blood flow); the significance of these factors is yet to be clarified in research (EPUAP and NPUAP, 2009). Pressure ulcers are inaccurately called *decubitus ulcers, pressure sores,* or *bedsores.* Many used to believe that only bed-bound persons developed these ulcers; however, we now know that pressure ulcers occur from unrelieved, prolonged soft tissue compression. Compression of soft tissue interferes with the blood flow to the tissue; if this compression continues for a prolonged period of time, the tissue dies from lack of blood flow, or ischemia. Ischemia develops when pressure on the skin is greater than pressure inside the vessels, causing the vessels to collapse and preventing the blood from reaching the tissue. The tissue dies from ischemic injury. Initially ischemia is often evident by skin discoloration such as redness and warmth in patients with light skin or purple and warmth in patients with darkly pigmented skin. If pressure is unrelieved or repeated, tissue will continue to break down relative to a patient's general health and tolerance for pressure. If not relieved, this pressure can cause irreversible tissue damage in as little as 90 minutes (Kosiak, 1959).

The most common sites for pressure ulcers include the sacrum, coccyx, ischial tuberosities, greater trochanters, heels, scapulas, iliac crests, and lateral and medial malleoli (Pieper, 2012). Fig. 18-1 shows pressure points over bony prominences where pressure ulcers can develop in sitting or lying positions. Pressure injury occurs on any area of skin subjected to pressure. Nonbony locations in which pressure injuries occur include the nares, usually related to pressure caused from nasogastric (NG) tubes or oxygen cannulas; the ears, resulting from oxygen tubing; or the genitalia, with ulcers resulting from Foley catheter tension. Unlike pressure ulcers, nonbony pressure injuries cannot be staged.

Factors such as incontinence, friction and shear, immobility, loss of sensory perception, level of activity, and poor nutrition all contribute to pressure ulcer formation. Chronic moisture from fecal and urinary incontinence compromises the protective barrier of the skin and may overhydrate it,

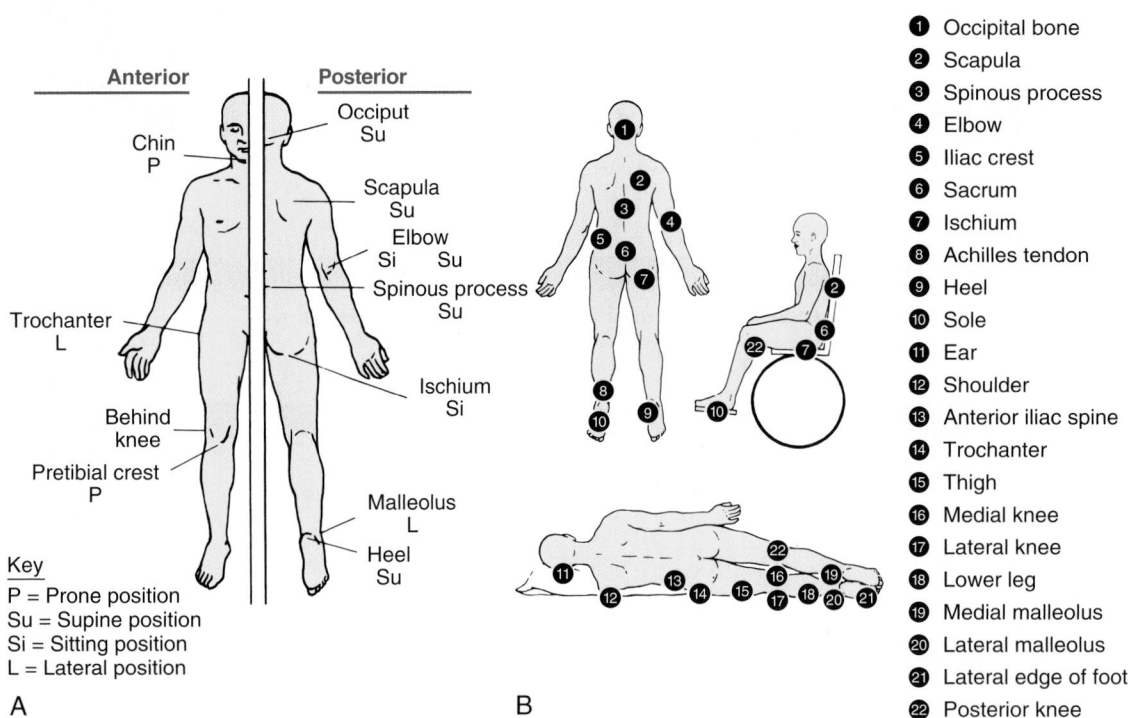

FIG 18-1 **A,** Bony prominences most frequently underlying pressure ulcers. **B,** Pressure ulcer sites. *From Trelease CC: Developing standards for wound care,* Ostomy Wound Manage 26:50, 1988.

making it more susceptible to breakdown (Black et al., 2011). Friction, the mechanical force of two surfaces moving over each other, causes surface damage such as blisters. Shear damage is caused when the skin layers adhere to the linens while the deeper tissue layers move downward (Hanson et al., 2010). This force causes reduced blood flow to the tissues.

Immobility often restricts a patient's ability to change and control body position, thus increasing the pressure over bony prominences. Loss of sensory perception decreases the individual's ability to respond to increased, prolonged pressure in an area of the body and change positions accordingly. Level of activity refers to the person's normal physical movement. A person who is bed bound is at greater risk for skin breakdown than a person who is fully or partially mobile. Research indicates that malnutrition contributes to the development of pressure ulcers (WOCN, 2010). Pressure ulcers pose serious risks to a patient's health. A break in the skin, seen in stages II to IV pressure ulcers (Box 18-1), eliminates the first line of defense of the body against infection.

Reports vary as to the number of patients who are at risk for and develop pressure ulcers, but the number of patients who develop them is significant. Patients are now older and sicker, are hospitalized for shorter periods of time, and are discharged to home or intermediate or long-term care facilities at a more acute stage of illness (Pieper, 2012). These changes contribute to an increased number of patients at risk for developing pressure ulcers. Thus it is critical to respond with an aggressive preventive approach. As a nurse you must identify the factors that place your patients at risk for the development of pressure ulcers. Once you identify these factors, begin interventions to reduce or relieve the negative effects of each factor. When a pressure ulcer develops, explore the factors that contributed to skin breakdown, vigorously attempt to minimize the effects of these variables, and use current wound-healing principles in the management of ulcers (see Chapters 38 and 39).

EVIDENCE-BASED PRACTICE

When patients enter health care settings, perform risk assessments and repeat them regularly and as frequently as required by patients' conditions (EPUAP and NPUAP, 2009):

- Educate health care professionals about how to complete an accurate and reliable risk assessment.
- Consider patients who are bedfast and/or chair fast to be at risk of pressure ulcer development (EPUAP and NPUAP, 2009).
- Document all risk assessments (WOCN, 2010).
- Use risk scores to plan care by looking at the individual risk factors, and develop a care plan to decrease or eliminate the identified risk factors.
- The risk assessment findings indicate interventions to reduce the risk associated with pressure ulcer development. For example, a patient who is incontinent of stool and urine requires a plan that includes the use of a perineal cleanser and a skin barrier. When patients are at risk for skin breakdown related to immobility, the plan of care usually includes the use of a pressure-redistribution surface, a turning schedule, and regular skin assessments (WOCN, 2010).
- Perform pressure ulcer risk assessment systematically (WOCN, 2010).

Ensure that a complete skin assessment is part of the risk assessment screening policy in place in all health care settings (EPUAP and NPUAP, 2009; WOCN, 2010). Ongoing skin assessment is necessary to detect early signs of pressure damage:

- Skin inspection should include assessment for localized heat, edema, or induration, especially in patients with darkly pigmented skin.
- Observe the skin for pressure damage caused by medical devices.

BOX 18-1	Staging of Pressure Ulcers

Staging Definition

Suspected Deep Tissue Injury

Purple or maroon localized area of discolored intact skin or blood-filled blister caused by damage of underlying soft tissue from pressure and/or shear. The area may be preceded by tissue that is painful, firm, mushy, boggy, warmer, or cooler compared with adjacent tissue.

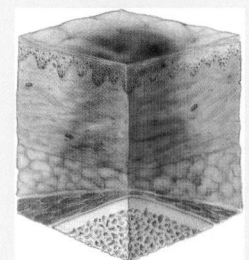 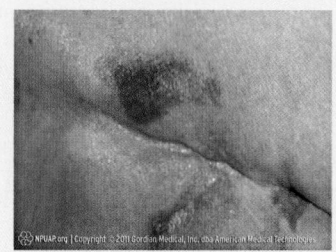

Stage I

Skin is intact with nonblanchable redness of a localized area, usually over a bony prominence. Darkly pigmented skin may not have visible blanching; its color may differ from the surrounding area.

Further description: The area may be painful, firm, soft, warmer, or cooler compared to adjacent tissue. Stage I may be difficult to detect in individuals with dark skin tones. May indicate "at-risk" person (a heralding risk).

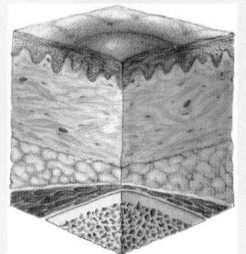 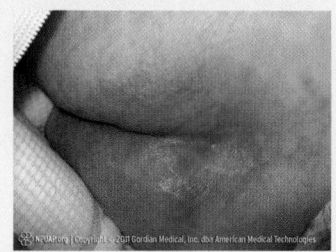

Stage II

Partial-thickness loss of dermis presents as a shallow open ulcer with a red-pink wound bed without slough. This stage may also present as an intact or open/ruptured serum-filled blister.

Further description: This stage presents as a shiny or dry shallow ulcer without slough or bruising.* This stage should not be used to describe skin tears, tape burns, perineal dermatitis, maceration, or denudement.

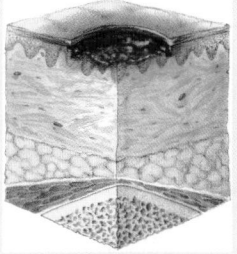 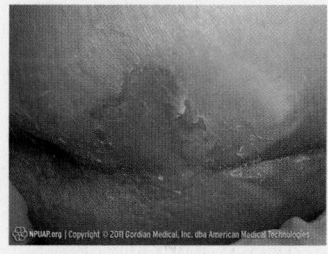

Stage III

Full-thickness tissue loss. Subcutaneous fat may be visible; but bone, tendon, or muscle is *not* exposed. Slough may be present but does not obscure the depth of tissue loss. It *may* include undermining and tunneling.

Further description: The depth of a stage III pressure ulcer varies by anatomic location. The bridge of the nose, ear, occiput, and malleolus do not have (adipose) subcutaneous tissue; and stage III ulcers can be shallow. In contrast, areas of significant adipose tissue can develop extremely deep stage III pressure ulcers. Bone or tendon is not visible or directly palpable.

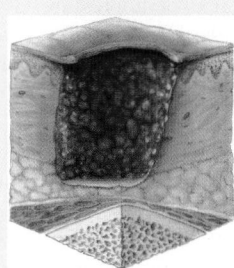 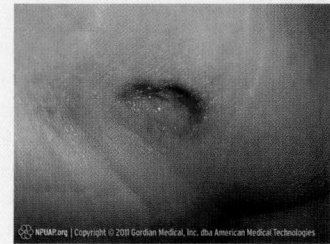

Continued

BOX 18-1 | **Staging of Pressure Ulcers—cont'd**

Stage IV

Full-thickness tissue loss with exposed bone, tendon, or muscle.
Slough or eschar may be present on some parts of the wound
bed. *Often* includes undermining and tunneling.

Further description: The depth of a stage IV pressure ulcer varies
by anatomic location. The bridge of the nose, ear, occiput, and
malleolus do not have (adipose) subcutaneous tissue; and these
ulcers can be shallow. Stage IV ulcers can extend into muscle
and/or supporting structures (e.g., fascia, tendon, or joint capsule),
making osteomyelitis possible. Exposed bone/tendon is visible or
directly palpable.

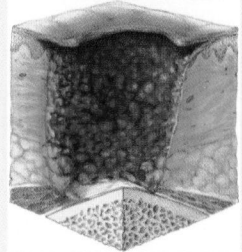 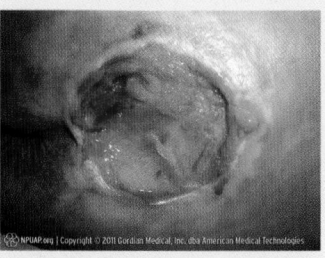

Unstageable

Full-thickness tissue loss in which the base of the ulcer is
completely obscured by slough (yellow, tan, gray, green, or brown)
and/or eschar (tan, brown, black) in the wound bed.

Further description: Until enough slough and/or eschar are removed
to expose the base of the wound, the true depth, and therefore
stage, cannot be determined. Stable (dry, adherent, intact without
erythema or fluctuance) eschar on the heels serves as "the natural
(biologic) cover of the body" and should not be removed.

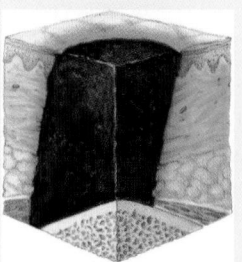 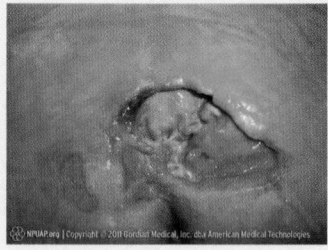

Data from European Pressure Ulcer Advisory Panel and National Pressure Ulcer Advisory Panel: *Treatment of pressure ulcers: quick reference guide,* Washington, DC, 2009, NPUAP.
Images used with permission of the National Pressure Ulcer Advisory Panel, 2012 © NPUAP.
*Bruising indicates suspected deep tissue injury.

- Document all skin assessments, noting details of any pain possibly related to pressure damage.

PATIENT-CENTERED CARE

Pressure ulcers and the associated treatments affect patients' lives emotionally, mentally, physically, and socially (Galhardo et al., 2010). Patients are aware of the amount and quality of care they receive, including levels of comfort during dressing changes and the timing of interventions. The presence of a pressure ulcer increases hospital stays and results in ongoing treatments. Given that it affects a patient's quality of life, providing culturally appropriate information about treatment and wound-healing expectations is an important aspect of care.

When planning care for a patient, consider issues such as skin tones, the issues related to patient and caregiver education, and the social effects of a pressure ulcer. Skin assessment depends on skin color, and detection becomes a challenge in dark-skinned patients (Nix, 2012). For example, redness in a dark-skinned patient is difficult to determine without the use of palpation and a comparison to other, nonaffected body parts (Box 18-2). When providing pressure ulcer care, remember that in some cultures hair has significance and should not be shaved. When shaving is absolutely necessary to prevent pain or trauma from taping hair around an ulcer, you may need the assistance of a patient's family or cultural elder.

When you educate patients and family caregivers, consider their primary language and reading ability when using printed materials. Frequently the initial use of pictures with labels can help determine if reading skills are adequate for printed educational materials. Part of the overall assessment of a patient includes how the presence of a pressure ulcer will affect the social situation (e.g., if a wound

BOX 18-2 | **Patient-Centered Care for Skin Assessment of Pressure Ulcers: Patients with Darkly Pigmented Skin**

Patients with darkly pigmented skin cannot be assessed for pressure ulcer risk by examining only skin color. Teaching points and unique considerations include the following:

1 Assess localized skin color changes. Any of the following may appear:
   - Color remains unchanged when pressure is applied.
   - Color changes that differ from patient's usual skin color occur at site of pressure ulcer.
   - If patient previously had a pressure ulcer, that area of skin may be lighter than original color.
   - Localized area of skin may be purple/blue or violet instead of red.
2 Importance of lighting for skin assessment:
   - Use natural or halogen light.
   - If possible, avoid fluorescent lamps, which can give the skin a bluish tone.
   - Avoid wearing tinted lenses when assessing skin color.
3 Tissue consistency:
   - Edema may occur with induration of more than 15 mm in diameter and may appear taut and shiny.
   - Assess for edema, swelling, and a firm or boggy feel.
4 Skin temperature:
   - Localized heat can be detected by making comparisons with the surrounding skin. An area of coolness may be a sign of tissue devitalization.

Adapted from Nix DP: Skin and wound inspection and assessment. In Bryant RA, Nix DP, editors: *Acute and chronic wounds: current management concepts,* ed 4, St Louis, 2012, Mosby.

would prevent a patient from socializing in the community). The presence of a pressure ulcer can also cause pain and resultant disability, which affect family dynamics.

Safety Guidelines

1 Routinely assess patients for individual risks for development of pressure ulcers. Select and use a risk assessment tool; the Braden Scale is one of the most widely used and researched scales (Bryant and Nix, 2012). Perform pressure ulcer risk assessment on all patients who have one or more risk factors when admitted to an acute care facility, home care, hospice, or extended care facility.

2 Assess and inspect skin at least daily. Note all pressure points; document results.

3 Redistribute the amount and duration of pressure to prevent ischemic tissue injury. The National Quality Forum (NQF) considers prevention of pressure ulcers safe practices and the development of pressure ulcers—especially stage III, stage IV, and any unstageable ulcers—in a care setting a serious reportable event (NQF, 2011). These events are called "never" events; and the Centers for Medicare and Medicaid Services (CMS) will not financially reimburse acute care hospitals if a patient acquires one of these ulcers during hospitalization (CMS, 2012).

4 Turn and reposition a patient often to redistribute pressure from the superficial capillaries and allow tissues to compensate for temporary ischemia. Use safe patient handling measures to turn and reposition patients every 1 to 2 hours as their condition

allows. Proper positioning helps minimize formation of pressure ulcers (see Chapter 9).

5 Specialized beds, overlays, and mattresses (see Chapter 12) redistribute pressure over the entire body to prevent excess pressure over bony prominences. By distributing pressure evenly over a patient's body surface, less pressure is applied at the skin level. Place patients at high risk for pressure ulcer formation on these devices as soon as possible. Consider the use of a chair cushion to redistribute pressure when a patient is seated.

6 Clean patients who are incontinent of stool or urine as soon as possible. Prolonged skin moisture and wetness from urinary and fecal incontinence is a risk factor for skin breakdown (Gray et al., 2011). Protect areas subjected to repeated episodes of incontinence with a barrier ointment or barrier paste. Containment devices are available.

7 Use approaches to minimize friction and shear. Use lift sheets when repositioning patients to reduce rubbing skin against sheets. Raise the head of the bed no more than 30 degrees (unless medically contraindicated) to prevent sliding and shear injury (WOCN, 2010).

8 Adequate nutrition helps to prevent and treat pressure ulcers (WOCN, 2010). A diet high in protein with enough calories, vitamins, and minerals helps maintain normal tissue status and promotes healing. With tissue injury the body needs more calories for healing; nutrient deficiencies may result in impaired or delayed healing. Make sure that monitoring the nutritional status is part of your total assessment (WOCN, 2010).

SKILL 18-1 Risk Assessment, Skin Assessment, and Prevention Strategies

NSO *Wound Care Module / Lessons 1 and 4*

The goal in preventing the development of pressure ulcers is early identification of an at-risk patient and the implementation of prevention strategies. In 2010 the Wound, Ostomy and Continence Nurses (WOCN) Society updated the *Guideline for Prevention and Management of Pressure Ulcers*. A panel of experts completed an extensive literature review on the prevention and management of pressure ulcers (WOCN, 2010). The panel then established a level of evidence rating that cites the best available evidence in the prevention and management of pressure ulcers. The overall management goals suggested by WOCN (2010) include the following:

1 Identify individuals at risk for developing pressure ulcers and initiate an early prevention program.

2 Implement appropriate strategies/plans to:
   a Attain/maintain intact skin.
   b Prevent complications.
   c Promptly identify or manage complications.
   d Involve patient and caregiver in self-management.

3 Implement cost-effective strategies/plans that prevent and treat pressure ulcers.

The WOCN 2010 panel recommends performing a risk assessment on entry to a health care setting and repeating this on a regularly scheduled basis or when there is a significant change in an individual's condition. For example, if a patient who was ambulatory becomes bed bound because of a surgical procedure; this person is potentially at higher risk for skin breakdown than when first admitted when ambulatory. Use risk assessment tools such as the

Braden Scale or the Norton Scale (WOCN, 2010). The Braden Scale (Table 18-1) has six parameters: sensory perception (ability to respond meaningfully to pressure-related discomfort), moisture (degree to which skin is exposed to moisture), activity (degree of physical activity), mobility (ability to change and control body position), nutrition (usual food intake pattern), and friction and shear (Ayello and Braden, 2002; Braden and Bergstrom, 1989, 1994). Risk cutoff scores vary for specific patient populations (Table 18-2). The Norton Scale, developed in 1962, includes five risk factors: physical condition, mental state, activity, mobility, and incontinence (Norton et al., 1975). It is important to understand how to interpret the meaning of a patient's total score on whichever scale you use.

Inspect patient's skin and bony prominences at least daily. Remove devices, shoes, socks, antiembolic stockings, and heel and elbow protectors for the skin inspection. Inspect all bony prominences, including back of head, shoulders, rib cage, elbows, hips, ischium, sacrum, coccyx, knees, ankles, and heels (see Fig. 18-1). Palpate any reddened or discolored areas with a gloved finger to determine if the erythema (redness of the skin caused by dilation and congestion of the capillaries) blanches (lightens in color). Blanching is normal. If you palpate an area that does not blanch (abnormal reactive hyperemia), this area is a site for potential skin breakdown.

Delegation and Collaboration

The skill of pressure ulcer risk assessment cannot be delegated to nursing assistive personnel (NAP). The nurse instructs the NAP to:

TABLE 18-1 | Braden Scale for Predicting Pressure Ulcer Risk*

Sensory Perception

Ability to respond meaningfully to pressure-related discomfort

1. *Completely limited*: Unresponsive (does not moan, flinch, or grasp) to painful stimuli because of diminished level of consciousness or sedation	2. *Very limited*: Responds only to painful stimuli Cannot communicate discomfort except by moaning or restlessness	3. *Slightly limited*: Responds to verbal commands but cannot always communicate discomfort or need to be turned	4. *No impairment*: Responds to verbal commands Has no sensory deficit that would limit ability to feel or voice pain or discomfort
or	*or*	*or*	
Limited ability to feel pain over most of body	Has a sensory impairment that limits the ability to feel pain or discomfort over half of body	Has some sensory impairment, which limits ability to feel pain or discomfort in one or two extremities	

Moisture

Degree to which skin is exposed to moisture

1. *Constantly moist*: Skin kept moist almost constantly by perspiration, urine, etc. Dampness detected every time patient is moved or turned	2. *Very moist*: Skin often but not always moist Linen must be changed at least once a shift	3. *Occasionally moist*: Skin occasionally moist, requiring extra linen change approximately once a day	4. *Rarely moist*: Skin usually dry; linen requires changing only at routine intervals

Activity

Degree of physical activity

1. *Bedfast*: Confined to bed	2. *Chair fast*: Ability to walk severely limited or nonexistent Cannot bear own weight and/or must be assisted into chair or wheelchair	3. *Walks occasionally*: Walks occasionally during day but for very short distances with or without assistance Spends most of each shift in bed or chair	4. *Walks frequently*: Walks outside room at least twice a day and inside room at least once every 2 hours during waking hours

Mobility

Ability to change and control body position

1. *Completely immobile*: Does not make even slight changes in body or extremity position without assistance	2. *Very limited*: Makes occasional slight changes in body or extremity position but unable to make frequent or significant changes independently	3. *Slightly limited*: Makes frequent though slight changes in body or extremity position independently	4. *No limitations*: Makes major and frequent changes in position without assistance

Nutrition

Usual food intake pattern

1. *Very poor*: Never eats a complete meal Rarely eats more than one third of any food offered Eats two servings or less of protein (meat or dairy products) per day Takes fluids poorly; does not take a liquid dietary supplement	2. *Probably inadequate*: Rarely eats a complete meal and generally eats only about half of any food offered Protein intake includes only three servings of meat or dairy products per day Occasionally takes a dietary supplement	3. *Adequate*: Eats over half of most meals Eats a total of four servings of protein (meat, dairy products) each day Occasionally refuses a meal but usually takes a supplement when offered	4. *Excellent*: Eats most of every meal Never refuses a meal Usually eats a total of four or more servings of meat and dairy products Occasionally eats between meals Does not require supplementation
or	*or*	*or*	
Is NPO and/or maintained on clear liquids or IV infusions for more than 5 days	Receives less than optimal amount of liquid diet or tube feeding	Is on a tube-feeding or TPN regimen that probably meets most of nutritional needs	

TABLE 18-1	Braden Scale for Predicting Pressure Ulcer Risk*—cont'd

Friction and Shear

| 1. *Problem*: Requires moderate-to-maximum assistance in moving Complete lifting without sliding against sheets impossible Frequently slides down in bed or chair; repositioning with maximal assistance Spasticity, contractions, or agitation leads to almost constant friction | 2. *Potential problem*: Moves feebly or requires minimal assistance During a move skin probably slides to some extent against sheets, chair, restraints, or other devices Maintains relatively good position in chair or bed most of the time but occasionally slides down | 3. *No apparent problem*: Moves in bed and chair independently and has sufficient muscle strength to sit up completely during move Maintains good position in bed or chair |

Adapted from Barbara Braden, PhD, RN, Creighton University School of Nursing, Omaha, Neb.
IV, Intravenous; *NPO*, nothing by mouth; *TPN*, total parenteral nutrition.
*Score patient in each of the six subscales. Maximum score is 23, indicating little or no risk. A score of ≤16 indicates "at risk"; ≤9 indicates very high risk.

TABLE 18-2	Pressure Ulcer Braden Risk Scores by Patient Population

Patient Population	High Level of Risk for Pressure Ulcer Development If Below These Scores
General population	≤16
Intensive care unit patients	≤15
Older adults	≤18
Black and Latino patients	≤18

Data from Ayello E: Predicting pressure ulcer risk, *Best Pract Nurs Care Older Adult* 5:1. 2012; Braden BJ, Bergstrom N: Clinical utility of the Braden Scale for predicting pressure sore risk, *Decubitus* 2(3):44, 1989; Bergstrom N, Braden BJ: Predictive validity of the Braden Scale among black and white subjects, *Nurs Res* 51(6):398, 2002.

- Report any redness or break in the patient's skin.
- Report any abrasion from assistive devices.

Equipment
❑ Risk assessment tool
❑ Documentation record
❑ Pressure-redistribution mattress, bed, and/or chair cushion
❑ Positioning aids
❑ Clean gloves

STEP	**RATIONALE**

ASSESSMENT

1 Assess patient's risk for pressure ulcer formation: — Determines need to administer preventive care and identifies specific factors that place patient at risk (EPUAP and NPUAP, 2009).

a Paralysis or immobilization caused by restrictive devices — Patient is unable to turn or reposition independently to relieve pressure.

b Sensory loss (e.g., hemiplegia, spinal cord injury) — Patient is unable to feel discomfort from pressure and does not independently change position.

c Circulatory disorders (e.g., peripheral vascular diseases, vascular changes from diabetes mellitus, neuropathy) — Reduce perfusion of tissue layers of skin.

d Fever — Increases metabolic demands of tissues. Accompanying diaphoresis leaves skin moist.

e Anemia — Decreased hemoglobin level reduces oxygen-carrying capacity of blood and amount of oxygen available to tissues.

f Malnutrition — Inadequate nutrition leads to weight loss, muscle atrophy, and reduced tissue mass. Nutrient deficiencies result in impaired or delayed healing (Stotts, 2012).

g Fecal or urinary incontinence — Skin becomes exposed to moist environment that contains bacteria. Excessive moisture macerates skin (Gray et al., 2011).

h Heavy sedation and anesthesia — Patient is not mentally alert and does not turn or change position independently. Sedation alters sensory perception.

STEP	RATIONALE
i Age	Neonates and very young children are at high risk, with the head being most common site of pressure ulcer occurrence (WOCN, 2010).
	There is a loss of dermal thickness in older adults, impairing ability to distribute pressure (Pieper, 2012).
j Dehydration	Results in decreased skin elasticity and turgor.
k Edema	Edematous tissues are less tolerant of pressure, friction, and shear.
l Existing pressure ulcers	Limit surfaces available for position changes, placing available tissues at increased risk.
m History of pressure ulcer	Tensile strength of skin from previously healed pressure ulcer is 80% or less; therefore this area cannot tolerate pressure as much as undamaged skin (Doughty and Sparks-Defriese, 2012).
2 Select an agency-approved risk assessment tool such as the Braden Scale or Norton Scale. Perform risk assessment when patient enters health care setting and repeat on regularly scheduled basis or when there is a significant change in patient's condition (WOCN, 2010).	Valid and reliable risk assessment tools evaluate patient's risk for developing a pressure ulcer. Identifying risk factors that contribute to the potential for skin breakdown allows you to target specific interventions for decreasing risk for skin breakdown.
3 Obtain risk score (see Tables 18-1, 18-2, and 18-3) and evaluate its meaning based on patient's unique characteristics.	Risk cutoff score depends on instrument used. The score involves identifying risk factors that contributed to it and minimizing those specific deficits.
4 Assess condition of patient's skin over regions of pressure (see Fig. 18-1).	Body weight against bony prominences places underlying skin at risk for breakdown.
a Inspect for skin discoloration (redness in light-tone skin; purplish or bluish in darkly pigmented skin) and tissue consistency (firm or boggy feel) and/or palpate for abnormal sensations (Nix, 2012).	Indicates that tissue was under pressure; hyperemia is a normal physiologic response to hypoxemia in tissues.
b Palpate discolored area, release your fingertip, and look for blanching.	If on palpation an area of redness blanches (lightens in color), this indicates normal reactive hyperemia; the tissue is not at risk for skin breakdown. Tissue that does not blanch when palpated indicates abnormal reactive hyperemia; an indication of possible ischemic injury.
c Inspect for pallor and mottling.	Persistent hypoxia in tissues that were under pressure; an abnormal physiologic response.
d Inspect for absence of superficial skin layers.	Represents early pressure ulcer formation, usually a partial-thickness wound that may have resulted from friction and/or shear.
e Inspect for localized heat, edema, or induration, especially in individuals with darkly pigmented skin (EPUAP and NPUAP, 2009).	Localized heat, edema, and induration have been identified as warning signs for pressure ulcer development. Since it is not always possible to see signs of redness on darkly pigmented skin, these additional signs should be considered in assessment (EPUAP and NPUAP, 2009).
5 Assess patient for additional areas of potential pressure injury:	Patients at high risk have multiple sites for pressure necrosis (tissue death) in addition to bony prominences.
a Nares: Nasogastric (NG) tube, oxygen cannula	
b Tongue and lips: oral airway, endotracheal (ET) tube	
c Ears: oxygen cannula, pillow	
d Drainage or other tubing	Stress against tissue at exit site or if tubing is caught under any part of the body.
e Wound drainage	Wound drainage increases risk for skin breakdown because it is caustic to skin and underlying tissues.
f Indwelling urethral (Foley) catheter	For female patients the catheter can put pressure on the labia, especially when edematous. For male patients pressure from a catheter not properly anchored can put pressure on the tip of the penis and urethra.
g Orthopedic and positioning devices	Improperly fitted or applied devices have the potential to cause pressure on adjacent skin and underlying tissue.

Clinical Decision Point *Inspect skin around and beneath orthopedic devices (e.g., cervical collar, braces, or cast). Note any abrasions or warmth in areas where devices can rub against the skin.*

TABLE 18-3	Guidelines for Pressure Ulcer Risk Assessment	
Level of Care	**Initial**	**Reassessment**
Acute care	On admission (Ayello, 2012; EPUAP and NPUAP, 2009)	• On a defined schedule (e.g., every 24 to 48 hours) • Whenever major change in patient's condition occurs
Critical care	On admission	• Every 24 hours (Ayello, 2012)
Long-term care	On admission	• Weekly for first 4 weeks after admission • Routinely on quarterly basis • Whenever patient's condition changes or deteriorates
Home care	On admission	• Every registered nurse visit

STEP	RATIONALE
6 Observe patient for preferred positions when in bed or chair.	Preferred positions result in weight of body being placed on certain bony prominences. Presence of contractures may result in pressure exerted in unexpected places.
7 Observe ability of patient to initiate and help with position changes.	Potential for friction and shear increases when patient is completely dependent on others for position changes.
8 Assess patient and caregiver understanding of risks for development of pressure ulcers.	Determines baseline knowledge for pressure ulcer risk and identifies areas for patient teaching.

NURSING DIAGNOSES

- Deficient knowledge related to pressure ulcer prevention
- Imbalanced nutrition: less than body requirements
- Impaired physical mobility
- Impaired skin integrity
- Ineffective peripheral tissue perfusion
- Risk for impaired skin integrity

Related factors are individualized based on patient's condition or needs.

PLANNING

1 Expected outcomes following completion of procedure:
  • Risk factors are identified.
  • Patient experiences no change from baseline skin assessment.
 	
  • Skin is intact with no evidence of erythema or no signs of breakdown.
	Established baseline for future assessment.
	Prevention guidelines prevent occurrence or worsening of pressure ulcer.
	Prevention strategies reduce risk factors.

2 Explain procedure(s) and purpose to patient and caregiver.	Relieves anxiety and provides opportunity for education.

IMPLEMENTATION	RATIONALE
1 Implement prevention guidelines adapted from WOCN Society *Guideline for Prevention and Management of Pressure Ulcers* (2010).	Reduces patient's risk for developing a pressure ulcer.
2 Close room door or bedside curtain and perform hand hygiene.	Maintains patient privacy.
3 If patient has open, draining wounds, apply clean gloves.	Use of standard precautions prevents accidental exposure to body fluids.

4 Inspect skin at least once a day.
  a Observe patient's skin; pay particular attention to bony prominences. If you find a reddened area, gently press the area with a gloved finger to check for blanching. If the area does not blanch, suspect tissue injury and recheck in 1 hour. Any discoloration may vary from pink to a deep red.
  b If patient has darkly pigmented skin, look for color changes that differ from his or her normal skin color, such as red, blue, or purple tones.
	Routine skin inspection is fundamental to risk assessment and in designing interventions to reduce risk (WOCN, 2010). Persistent redness when lightly pigmented skin is pressed can indicate tissue injury. If an area of redness blanches (lightens in color), this indicates that skin is not at risk for breakdown.
	Darkly pigmented skin may not blanch. Although the skin may not show direct changes in color, the color may differ from the surrounding area (EPUAP and NPUAP, 2009) (see Box 18-2).

5 Check all treatment and assistive devices (catheters, feeding tubes, casts, braces) for potential pressure points. Remove gloves.	Pressure from these devices increases the risk on bony prominences and other areas.
6 Review patient's pressure ulcer score.	Risk scores aid in identifying interventions to lessen or eliminate the present risk factors.

Clinical Decision Point *Do not massage reddened areas, because doing so may cause additional tissue trauma. Reddened areas indicate blood vessel damage, and massaging can further damage the vessel.*

7 If immobility, inactivity, or poor sensory perception is a risk factor(s) for patient, consider one of the following interventions:	Immobility and inactivity reduce patient's ability or desire to independently change position. Poor sensory perception decreases patient's ability to feel the sensation of pressure or discomfort.
a Reposition patient at least every 2 hours; use a written schedule (WOCN, 2010).	Reduces the duration and intensity of pressure. Some patients may require more frequent repositioning.
b When patient is in the side-lying position in bed, use the 30-degree lateral position (see illustration).	Reduces direct contact of the trochanter with the support surface.
c When needed use pillow bridging (see illustration).	Use of pillows prevents direct contact between bony prominences.
d Place patient (when lying in bed) on a pressure redistribution surface.	Reduces amount of pressure exerted on tissues.
e Place patient (when in a chair) on a pressure redistribution device and shift the points under pressure at least every hour (WOCN, 2010).	Reduces the amount of pressure on the sacral and ischial areas.
8 If friction and shear are identified as risk factors, consider the following interventions:	Friction and shear damage underlying skin.
a Use two nurses and a pull sheet to reposition patient. Use a slide board (see Chapter 9) to transfer patient from bed to stretcher.	Proper repositioning of patient prevents dragging along the sheets. Slide board provides slippery surface to reduce friction.

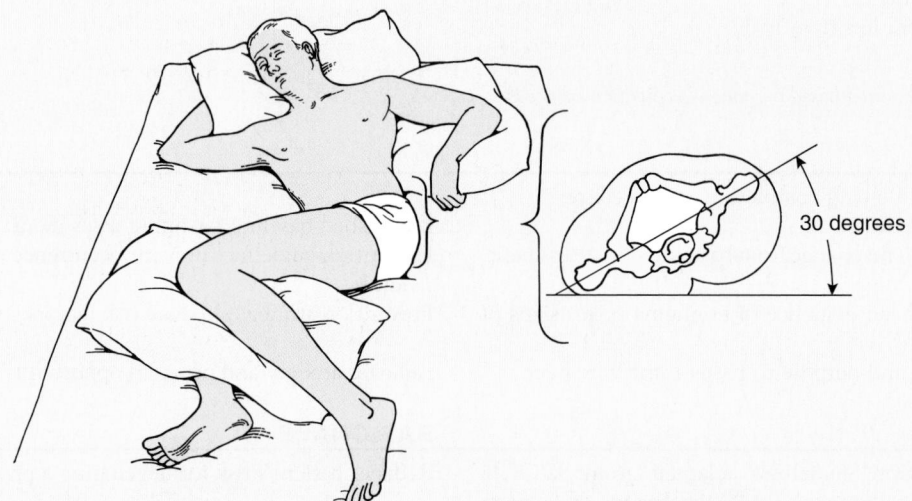

STEP 7b   Thirty-degree lateral position with pillow placement.

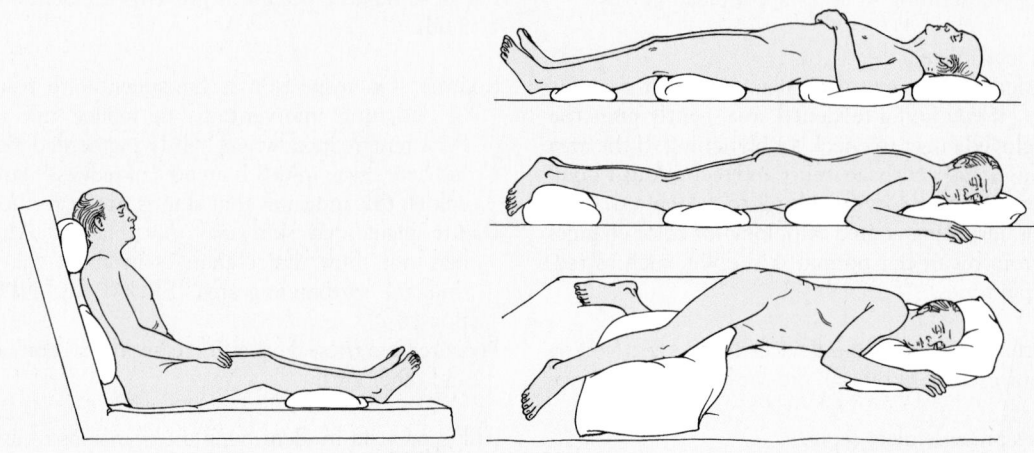

STEP 7c   Pillow bridging.

STEP	RATIONALE
b Ensure that heels are free from the surface of the bed by using a pillow under the calves to elevate the heels.	"Floating" the heels from the bed surface eliminates shear and friction.
c Maintain the head of the bed at 30 degrees.	Decreases potential for patient to slide toward foot of bed and incur a shear injury.
9 If patient receives a low score on a moisture subscale, consider one of the following interventions:	Continual exposure of body fluids on the patient's skin increases the risk for skin breakdown and pressure ulcer development.
a Apply clean gloves. Apply a moisture barrier ointment to perineum and surrounding skin after each incontinent episode.	Protects the skin from fecal or urinary incontinence.
b If skin is denuded, use a protective barrier paste after each incontinent episode.	Provides a barrier between the skin and the stool/urine, allowing for healing.
c If moisture source is from wound drainage, consider frequent dressing changes, skin protection with protective barriers, or collection devices.	Removes the frequent exposure of wound drainage from the skin.
10 Educate patient and family caregiver regarding pressure ulcer risk and prevention (WOCN, 2010).	Assists in adhering to interventions to reduce pressure ulcer risk.
11 Remove gloves and discard in appropriate receptacle. Perform hand hygiene.	Reduces transmission of microorganisms.

EVALUATION

1 Observe patient's skin for areas at risk for tissue damage, noting change in color, appearance, or texture.	Enables you to evaluate success of prevention techniques.
2 Observe tolerance of patient for position change by measuring level of comfort on a pain scale.	Position changes sometimes interfere with patient's sleep and rest pattern.
3 Compare subsequent risk assessment scores and skin assessments.	Provides ongoing comparison of patient's risk level to facilitate appropriateness of plan of care.

Unexpected Outcomes	Related Interventions
1 Skin becomes mottled, reddened, purplish, or bluish.	• Refer patient to wound, ostomy, and continence (WOC) nurse; dietitian; clinical nurse specialist (CNS); and/or physical therapist as necessary. Reevaluate position changes and bed surface.
2 Areas under pressure develop persistent discoloration, induration, or temperature changes.	• Refer patient to WOC nurse; dietitian; CNS; and/or physical therapist as necessary. • Modify patient's positioning and turning schedule.

Recording and Reporting

- Record any skin changes, patient's risk score, and skin assessment. Describe positions, turning intervals, pressure-redistribution devices, and other prevention measures. Note patient's response to the interventions.
- Report need for additional consultations for the high-risk patient to health care provider.

Special Considerations
Teaching

- Help patient and family caregiver understand multiple factors involved in preventing and treating pressure ulcers.
- Explain and demonstrate positioning options to achieve pressure redistribution.
- Explain the purpose and maintenance of pressure-redistribution devices (see Chapter 12).
- When teaching patients to change position for pressure redistribution, suggest using television programming and commercial intervals or a watch with an alarm as reminders.

Pediatric

- Infants and young children in diapers are at risk for skin breakdown.

Gerontologic

- Reevaluate sitting posture and position because body weight and muscle tone change with age.
- In older adults the dermis is not as thick. Skin over the legs and forearms is especially thin. There is less subcutaneous tissue, leading to less padding protection over bony prominences; and the time for epidermal regeneration is diminished, leading to slower healing (Wysocki, 2012).

Home Care

- Identify community resources such as neighbors and relatives to provide assistance if patient needs help with position changes.
- Closely monitor home care patients for pressure ulcer development if they have any of the following risk factors: wheelchair or bed dependence, incontinence, anemia, fracture, and or skin drainage.
- Remind patient and family caregiver that position changes need to occur while a patient is sitting in a chair. Consider shifts every 15 minutes. Small shifts such as moving or repositioning the legs redistributes pressure over bony prominences (WOCN, 2010).

SKILL 18-2   Treatment of Pressure Ulcers

 Video Clip

Treatment of patients with pressure ulcers requires a holistic approach using a thorough assessment of patients and their ability to heal. Have a good understanding of the identified goal for a patient's overall care before implementing topical pressure ulcer treatment. The principles of managing patients with pressure ulcers includes systematic support of patients, reduction or elimination of the cause of skin breakdown, and management that provides an environment conducive to healing. Once you find the cause of the pressure ulcer, take steps to control or eliminate it. For example, if the ulcer is related to unrelieved pressure, choose the appropriate pressure-redistribution surface, develop a turning schedule, or choose the appropriate chair pad. Next assess the patient's wound-healing abilities: cardiovascular and pulmonary function, nutritional status, and conditions that interfere with wound healing such as diabetes, steroid administration, and immunosuppression (Doughty and Sparks-Defriese, 2012). Wound assessment tools such as the Bates-Jensen Wound Assessment Tool (BWAT) (Nix, 2012) and the PUSH tool can assist in determining the individual treatment goals for different pressure ulcers.

The principle that guides the selection and use of topical dressings is to provide a wound environment that supports healing (Rolstad, Bryant, and Nix, 2012). The best environment for wound healing is moist and free of necrotic tissue and infection. Choose interventions and dressings designed to support a clean, moist wound bed. Perform a thorough assessment of the wound and the periwound skin before initiating wound therapy. Data obtained will help to plan the appropriate care for a patient with a pressure ulcer.

No specific studies demonstrate the benefit of using one cleanser over another for pressure ulcers. In most cases water or saline is sufficient for cleaning a clean wound (WOCN, 2010). Hydrogen peroxide was once widely used but is now known to cause tissue damage. When a wound is contaminated with debris, necrotic tissue, or heavy drainage, use a cleanser that is noncytotoxic to healthy tissue. If the tissue in the wound is devitalized, consult with a patient's health care provider to consider debridement, which is the removal of devitalized tissue. Debridement is accomplished by the choice of dressing and the use of enzyme preparations or surgical or laser techniques. The choice of the type of debridement depends on a patient's overall condition, the condition of the wound, and the type of devitalized tissue.

Choose wound dressings to meet the characteristics of the wound bed (Rolstad, Bryant, and Nix, 2012). The choice of a wound dressing depends on the type of wound tissue in the base of the wound, the amount of wound drainage, the presence or absence of infection, the location of the wound, the size of the wound, the ease of use, cost-effectiveness, and patient comfort. Categories of wound dressings include transparent films, hydrocolloids, hydrogels, foams, calcium alginates, gauze, and antimicrobial dressings (see Chapter 39). The type of dressings to use will change as the pressure ulcer characteristics change; frequent wound assessment is key.

Advanced wound care therapies used in select cases include growth factors, electrical stimulation, hyperbaric therapy, negative-pressure wound therapy, and tissue-engineered skin. Growth factors occur naturally in wound fluid and stimulate both granulation and epithelialization when applied topically. Pulsed electrical stimulation is a procedure usually performed by physical therapists with the goal of increased wound healing. Hyperbaric oxygen therapy uses increased amounts of pressurized oxygen delivered to patients in a variety of specialized methods. Negative-pressure wound therapy (NPWT) applies suction to facilitate healing and collect wound fluid (Netsch, 2012). NPWT works via a suction system and a wound filler (dressing such as foam or gauze) placed into the wound and covered with a semiocclusive dressing. This therapy applies negative pressure to a wound through suction to facilitate healing and collect wound fluid (Netsch, 2012) (see Chapter 39). Tissue-engineered skin develops living cells that you place over a clean wound bed to facilitate wound closure. Advanced wound therapies may play an important role in pressure ulcer healing, but use only after consultation with a wound care expert.

Delegation and Collaboration

The skill of treatment of pressure ulcers and dressing changes cannot be delegated to the nursing assistive personnel (NAP). The nurse instructs the NAP to:

- Report any wound drainage that might be on linens or intact skin, indicating the need to change the dressing or use an alternative dressing.
- Report any new areas of redness, blistering, or skin irritation.

Equipment

- ☐ Protective equipment: clean gloves, goggles, cover gown (if splash is a risk)
- ☐ Sterile gloves (optional)
- ☐ Plastic bag for dressing disposal
- ☐ Measuring device
- ☐ Sterile cotton-tipped applicators (check agency policy for use of sterile applicators)
- ☐ Topical agent (as ordered)
- ☐ Cleansing agent (as ordered)
- ☐ Sterile solution container
- ☐ Dressing of choice based on patient wound characteristics
- ☐ Hypoallergenic tape (if needed)
- ☐ Documentation records

STEP	RATIONALE

ASSESSMENT

1 Assess patient's level of comfort on a pain scale of 0 to 10. If patient is in pain, determine if a prn pain medication has been ordered and administer.	Dressing change should not be a traumatic event for patient; evaluate wound pain before, during, and after wound care management (Hopf et al., 2012).
2 Determine if patient has allergies to topical agents.	Topical agents could contain elements that cause localized skin reactions.
3 Review the order for topical agent(s) and/or dressings.	Ensures administration of proper medication and treatment.

STEP	RATIONALE

Clinical Decision Point *Determine if the order is consistent with established wound care guidelines and outcomes for a patient. If the order is not consistent with guidelines or varies from the identified outcome for a patient, review it with the health care team.*

4 Close room door or bedside curtains. Perform hand hygiene and apply clean gloves.

Provides privacy. Reduces transmission of microorganisms and prevents accidental exposure to body fluids.

5 Position patient to allow dressing removal and position plastic bag for dressing disposal.

Provides an accessible area for dressing change. Proper disposal of old dressing promotes proper handling of contaminated waste.

6 Assess patient's wounds using wound parameters, and continue ongoing wound assessment per agency policy. NOTE: This may be done during procedure after dressing removal.

Determines effectiveness of wound care and guides the treatment plan of care (WOCN, 2010).

  a *Wound location:* Describe the body site where the wound is located.

  b *Stage of wound:* Describe the extent of tissue destruction (see Box 18-1).

Staging is a way of assessing a pressure ulcer based on depth of tissue destruction. Wounds are documented as unstageable if the wound base is not visible (EPUAP and NPUAP, 2009).

  c *Wound size:* Length, width, and depth of the wound are measured per agency protocol. Use a disposable measuring guide for length and width. Use a cotton-tipped applicator to assess depth (see illustration).

Ulcer size changes as healing progresses; therefore the longest and widest areas of the wound change over time. Measuring the width and length by measuring consistent areas provides a consistent measurement (Nix, 2012).

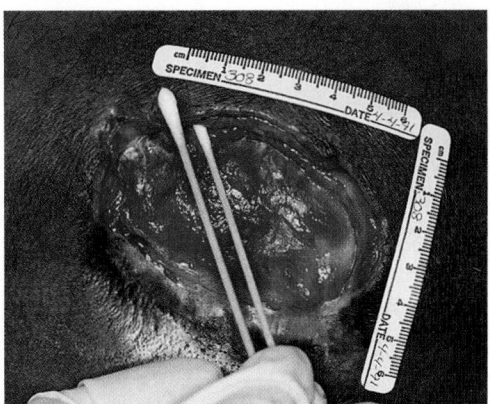

STEP 6c   Measuring wound width, length, and undermining of skin.

  d *Presence of undermining, sinus tracts, or tunnels:* Use a sterile cotton-tipped applicator to measure depth and, if needed, a gloved finger to examine the wound edges.

Wound depth determines amount of tissue loss.

  e *Condition of wound bed:* Describe the type and percentage of tissue in the wound bed.

The approximate percentage of each type of tissue in the wound provides critical information on the progress of wound healing and the choice of dressing. A wound with a high percentage of black tissue requires debridement, yellow tissue or slough tissue may indicate the presence of an infection or colonization, and granulation tissue indicates that a wound is moving toward healing.

  f *Volume of exudate:* Describe the amount, characteristics, odor, and color.

Amount and type of exudate may indicate type and frequency of dressing changes.

  g *Condition of periwound skin:* Examine the skin for breaks, dryness, and the presence of a rash, swelling, redness, or warmth. Modify assessment based on patient's skin color (see Box 18-2).

Impaired skin condition at the edge of an ulcer indicates progressive tissue damage. Maceration on periwound skin shows a need to alter the choice of wound dressing.

  h *Wound edges:* Gives information regarding epithelialization, chronicity, and etiology.

7 Remove gloves, discard appropriately, and perform hand hygiene.

Reduces transmission of microorganisms.
Repeated hand hygiene is needed as you assess other pressure areas. Different organisms contaminate different wounds.

8 Assess for factors affecting wound healing: poor perfusion, immunosuppression, or preexisting infection.

Factors will affect treatment and wound healing.

STEP	RATIONALE

9 Assess patient's nutritional status (see Chapter 30). Clinically significant malnutrition is present if (1) serum albumin level is less than 3.5 g/dL, (2) lymphocyte count is less than 1800/mm³, or (3) body weight decreases more than 15% (see illustration) (WOCN, 2010).

Delayed wound healing occurs in poorly nourished patients.

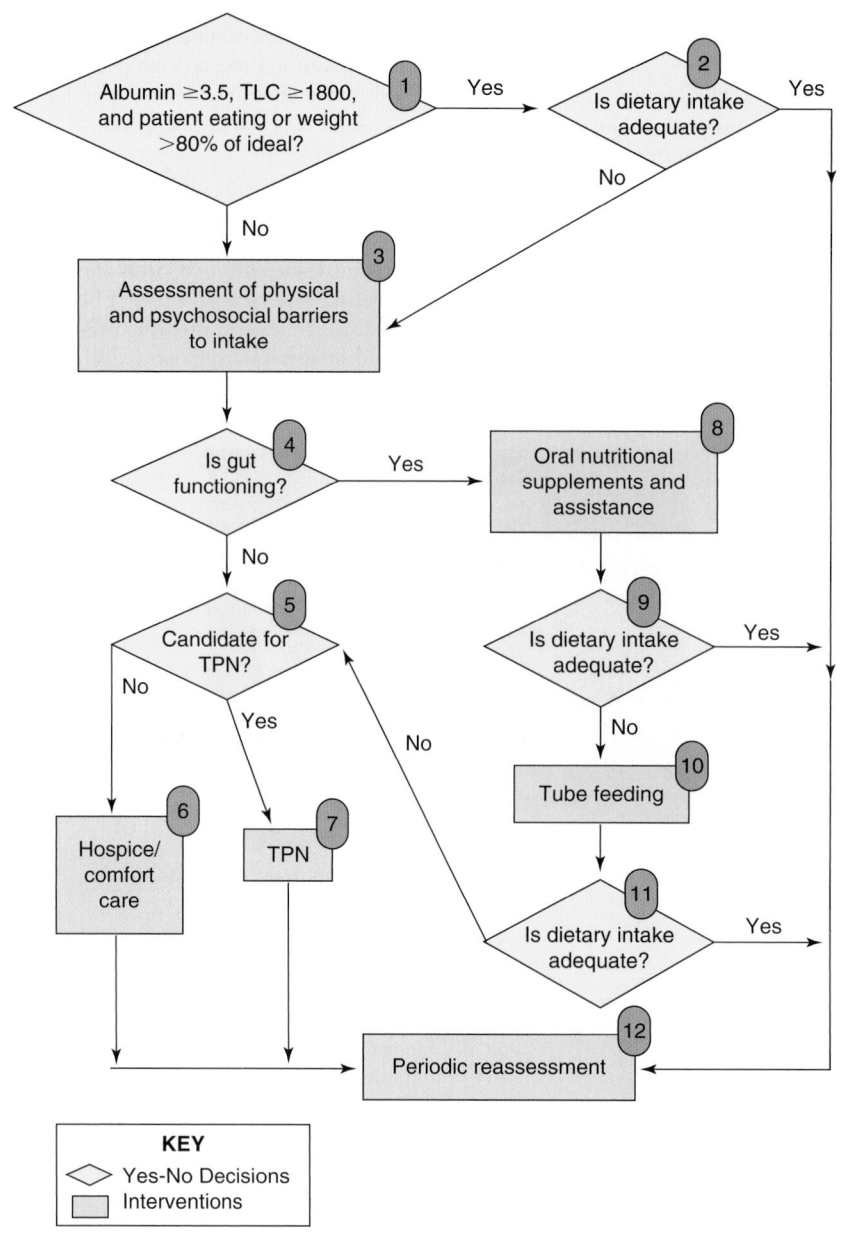

STEP 9 Nutritional assessment and support. *TLC,* Total lymphocyte count; *TPN,* total parenteral nutrition. *From Bergstrom N et al: Treatment of pressure ulcers, AHCPR Pub No. 95-0652, Rockville, Md, 1994, Agency for Health Care Policy and Research, Public Health Service, U.S. Department of Health and Human Services.*

Clinical Decision Point *When you suspect malnutrition, consider a nutritional consultation to modify patient's diet to promote wound healing.*

10 Assess patient's and caregiver's understanding of prevention, treatment, and factors contributing to recurrence of pressure ulcers (WOCN, 2010).

Patient and caregiver need to partner with health care providers to prevent further skin breakdown.

STEP	RATIONALE

NURSING DIAGNOSES

- Deficient knowledge regarding pressure ulcer treatment plan
- Imbalanced nutrition: less than body requirements
- Impaired physical mobility
- Impaired skin integrity
- Ineffective tissue perfusion
- Pain (acute, chronic)

Related factors are individualized based on patient's condition or needs.

PLANNING

STEP	RATIONALE
1 Expected outcomes following completion of procedure:	
• Ulcer drainage decreases.	Reflects decrease in inflammatory process and progress toward healing.
• Granulation tissue is present in wound base.	Evidence that wound is moving toward healing.
• Skin surrounding ulcer remains healthy and intact.	No additional damage is evident; dressing is appropriate to contain wound drainage.
• Nutritional intake meets caloric and nutrient targets.	Nutritional therapy provides adequate protein to support wound healing.
• Patient's overall skin remains intact and without further breakdown.	Patient remains at risk for further breakdown while existing ulcer heals.
2 Explain procedure to patient and family caregiver. Individualize teaching plan for older adults, taking into account normal aging changes that affect learning.	Preparatory explanations relieve anxiety, correct any misconceptions about the ulcer and its treatment, and offer an opportunity for patient and family education.
3 Prepare the following necessary equipment and supplies:	
a Normal saline or other wound-cleansing agent in sterile solution container	Clean ulcer surface before applying topical agents and new dressing.

Clinical Decision Point *Use only noncytotoxic agents to clean ulcers.*

STEP	RATIONALE
b Prescribed topical agent:	
(1) Enzyme debriding agents (Follow specific manufacturer directions for frequency of application) *or*	Enzymes debride dead tissue to clean ulcer surface. Enzymes are not applied to healthy tissue.
(2) Topical antibiotics	Topical antibiotics decrease bioburden of wound and should be considered for use if no healing is noted after 2 to 4 weeks of optimal care (WOCN, 2010).

Clinical Decision Point *If using an enzymatic debriding agent, do not use wound-cleansing agents with metals.*

STEP	RATIONALE
c Select an appropriate dressing based on pressure ulcer characteristics, principles of wound management, and patient care setting. Dressing options include (Table 18-4) (see Chapter 39):	Dressing should maintain moist environment for wound while keeping surrounding skin dry (Rolstad, Bryant, and Nix, 2012).
(1) Gauze. Apply as a moist dressing, a dry cover dressing when using enzymes or topical antibiotics, or as a means to deliver solution to a wound (see Chapter 39).	Gauze delivers moisture to a wound and is absorptive.

Clinical Decision Point *Make sure that absorbency of dressing is adequate for the amount of wound drainage. Check that wound does not dry out or surrounding skin does not become macerated.*

STEP	RATIONALE
(2) Transparent film dressing. Apply over superficial ulcers with minimal or no exudate and skin subjected to friction.	Maintains a moist environment and offers intact skin protection.

Clinical Decision Point *Use transparent dressings for autolytic debridement of noninfected superficial pressure ulcers.*

STEP	RATIONALE
(3) Hydrocolloid dressing	Maintains moist environment to facilitate wound healing while protecting wound base.

Clinical Decision Point *Use a hydrocolloid to protect skin from friction. Some brands have custom shapes available for specific anatomic parts such as heel, elbows, and sacrum.*

STEP	RATIONALE
(4) Hydrogel–Available in a sheet or in tube	Maintains moist environment to facilitate wound healing.
(5) Calcium alginate	Highly absorbent of wound exudate in heavily draining wounds.
(6) Foam dressings	Protective and prevents wound dehydration; also absorbs moderate-to-large amounts of drainage.
(7) Silver impregnated dressings/gels	Controls bacterial burden in wound.
(8) Wound fillers	Fills shallow wounds, hydrates, and absorbs
d Obtain hypoallergenic tape or adhesive dressing sheet	Used to secure nonadherent dressing. Prevents skin irritation and tearing.

TABLE 18-4 Dressings by Pressure Ulcer Stage

Pressure Ulcer Stage	Pressure Ulcer Status	Dressing	Comments*	Expected Change	Adjuvants
I	Intact	None	Allows visual assessment.	Resolves slowly without epidermal loss over 7 to 14 days	Turning schedule. Support hydration. Nutritional support. Pressure-redistribution bed or use of chair cushion.
		Transparent dressing	Protects from shear. Do not use in presence of excessive moisture.		
		Hydrocolloid	Does not allow visual assessment.		
II	Clean	Composite film	Limits shear.	Heals through reepithelialization	See previous stage. Manage incontinence.
		Hydrocolloid	Change when seal of dressing breaks, maximal wear time 7 days.		
		Hydrogel	Provides moist environment.		
III	Clean	Hydrocolloid	Change when seal of dressing breaks, maximum wear time 7 days. Apply over wound to protect and absorb moisture.	Heals through granulation and reepithelialization	See previous stages. Evaluate pressure-redistribution needs.
		Hydrogel covered with foam dressing			
		Calcium alginate	Use when there is significant exudate. Cover with secondary dressing.		
		Gauze	Use with normal saline or other prescribed solution. Wring out excess solution; unfold to make contact with wound.		
		Growth factors	Use with gauze per manufacturer instructions.		
IV	Clean	Hydrogel covered with foam dressing	See stage III clean.	Heals through granulation, scar tissue development, and reepithelialization.	Surgical consultation may be necessary for closure. See stages I, II, and III.
		Calcium alginate	Used with significant exudate; must cover with secondary dressing		
		Gauze	See stage III clean.		
Unstageable	Wound covered with eschar	Adherent film	Facilitates softening of eschar.	Eschar lifts at edges as healing progresses	See previous stages. Surgical consultation may be considered for debridement. May be considered for slow debridement.
		Gauze plus ordered solution	Delivers solution and wicks wound drainage.		
		Enzymes	Breaks down eschar, providing debridement.	Eschar loosens over time.	
		None	Rarely, if eschar is dry and intact, no dressing is used, allowing eschar to act as physiologic cover.		

*As with *all* occlusive dressings, wounds should not be clinically infected.

STEP	RATIONALE
IMPLEMENTATION	**RATIONALE**

	STEP	RATIONALE
1	Identify patient using two identifiers (i.e., name and birthday or name and account number) according to agency policy. Compare identifiers with information on patient's identification bracelet.	Ensures patient identity. Complies with The Joint Commission standards and improves patient safety (TJC, 2012).
2	Assemble supplies at beside. Close room door or bedside curtains.	Maintains patient privacy.
3	Perform hand hygiene and apply clean gloves. Open sterile packages and topical solution containers. Keep dressings sterile. Wear goggles, mask, and moisture-proof cover gown if potential for contamination from spray exists when cleaning wound.	Reduces transmission of microorganisms.
4	Remove bed linen and arrange patient's gown to expose ulcer and surrounding skin. Keep remaining body parts draped.	Prevents unnecessary exposure of body parts.
5	Remove old dressing and discard in appropriate receptacle. Assess condition of wound and amount and color of wound drainage if present. Remove gloves and discard.	With each dressing change note progress of wound healing.
6	Perform hand hygiene and change gloves.	Maintains aseptic technique during cleaning, measuring, and applying dressings. Refer to agency policy regarding use of clean or sterile gloves.
7	Clean wound thoroughly with normal saline or prescribed wound-cleansing agent (see Chapter 39) from least contaminated to most contaminated area.	Cleansing wound removes wound exudate and/or dressing residue and reduces surface bacteria.
8	Apply topical agents to wound using cotton-tipped applicators or gauze as ordered:	
	a Enzymes	Follow manufacturer directions for method and frequency of application. Be aware of which solutions inactivate enzymes and avoid their use in wound cleaning.
	(1) Apply small amount of enzyme debridement ointment directly to necrotic areas in pressure ulcer. *Do not apply enzyme to surrounding skin.*	Proper distribution of ointment ensures effective action.
	(2) Place moist gauze dressing directly over ulcer and tape in place. Follow specific manufacturer recommendation for type of dressing material to use to cover a pressure ulcer when using enzymes.	Protects wound and prevents removal of ointment during turning or repositioning.
	b Antibacterials Examples include bacitracin, metronidazole, and silver sulfadiazine.	Reduces bacterial growth.
9	Apply prescribed wound dressing:	
	a Hydrogel	
	(1) Cover surface of ulcer with a thick layer of the amorphous hydrogel, or cut a sheet to fit wound base.	Provides moist environment to facilitate wound healing.
	(2) Apply secondary dressing such as dry gauze; tape in place.	Holds hydrogel against wound surface because amorphous hydrogel (in tube) or sheet form does not adhere to wound and requires a secondary dressing to hold it in place.
	(3) If using impregnated gauze, pack loosely into wound; cover with secondary gauze dressing and tape.	A loosely packed dressing delivers the gel to the wound base and allows any wound debris to be trapped in the gauze.
	b Calcium alginate	Use in heavily draining wounds.
	(1) Lightly pack wound with alginate using sterile cotton-tipped applicator or gloved finger.	The dressing swells and increases in size; tight packing can compromise blood flow to the tissues.
	(2) Apply a secondary dressing and tape in place.	
	c Transparent film dressing; hydrocolloid; and foam dressings (see Chapter 39)	
10	Reposition patient comfortably off pressure ulcer.	Prevents pressure to ulcer.
11	Remove gloves and dispose of soiled supplies. Perform hand hygiene.	Reduces transmission of microorganisms.

STEP	RATIONALE
EVALUATION	
1 Observe skin surrounding ulcer for inflammation, edema, and tenderness.	Determines progress of wound healing.
2 Inspect dressings and exposed ulcers, observing for drainage, foul odor, and tissue necrosis. Monitor patient for signs and symptoms of infection: fever and elevated white blood cell (WBC) count.	Ulcers can become infected.
3 Compare subsequent ulcer measurements, using one of the scales designed to measure wound healing such as the PUSH Tool or the BWAT Assessment.	Allows comparison of serial measurements to evaluate wound healing. Provides standard method of data collection that demonstrates wound progress or lack thereof.

Unexpected Outcomes	Related Interventions
1 Skin surrounding ulcer becomes macerated.	• Reduce exposure of surrounding skin to topical agents and moisture. • Select a dressing that has increased moisture-absorbing capacity.
2 Ulcer becomes deeper with increased drainage and/or development of necrotic tissue.	• Review current wound care management. • Consult with multidisciplinary team regarding changes in wound care regimen. • Obtain wound cultures (see Chapter 43).
3 Pressure ulcer extends beyond original margins.	• Monitor for systemic signs and symptoms of poor wound healing such as abnormal laboratory results (WBC count, levels of hemoglobin/hematocrit, serum albumin, serum prealbumin, total proteins), weight loss, and fluid imbalances. • Assess and revise current turning schedule. • Consider further pressure-redistribution devices.

Recording and Reporting

- Record type of wound tissue present in ulcer, ulcer measurements, periwound skin condition, character of drainage or exudate, type of topical agent used, dressing applied, and patient's response.
- Report any deterioration in ulcer appearance to nurse in charge or health care provider.

Special Considerations

Teaching

- Discuss treatment and identify individual(s) who will help with care at home.
- Discuss process of wound healing and expected wound appearance. For example, discuss patient's perception about appearance of the pressure ulcer. Sometimes eschar looks like a scab to a patient, and he or she needs to understand the difference. A scab is caused by exudate, and an eschar is dead tissue that the patient should not remove.
- Discuss with patient and family caregivers perceptions about size of pressure ulcer. Some wounds, especially after debridement, may appear larger and are very troublesome to patients and support persons.
- Discuss with patient and support persons perceptions about treatment. Some patients and family caregivers believe that it is cruel for staff to keep turning and positioning a patient on a frequent basis.
- Review prevention guidelines to prevent further breakdown.
- Discuss options for maintaining good nutrition.

Gerontologic

- Wound healing is often slower in older adults (Doughty and Sparks-Defriese, 2012).

- The normal reduction in the Langerhans cells in the older adult's epidermis causes a decrease in T-cell function and immunity.
- Because older skin has a slower and less intense inflammatory reaction, monitor older patients more closely for altered responses to skin irritants.

Home Care

- Consider family caregiver time when selecting a dressing. In the home care setting caregivers may sometimes choose more expensive dressing materials to reduce the frequency of dressing changes.
- Some patients have more time than financial resources. They may choose a less expensive treatment option (e.g., dressing material), especially if there is no third-party reimbursement. Another example is to teach the family caregiver to make a normal saline solution rather than buying it ready-made.
- Identify clean storage area for dressing supplies. Determine availability of required supplies. Discuss need for home care nurse.
- Discuss need for home pressure-redistribution surface or bed. Identify adaptive equipment needed to care for patient at home.
- Medicare regulations limit reimbursement of some types of support surfaces in the treatment of pressure ulcers.

Long-Term Care

- Rehabilitation units often use a variety of support surfaces and beds.
- Some patients may be discharged to long-term care facilities that specialize in pressure ulcer and wound care.

Critical Thinking Exercises

Ms. Willet is a 72-year-old white woman who recently underwent a total hip replacement, left side. Her significant medical history includes rheumatoid arthritis and coronary artery disease. This is her first postoperative day, and she is resting in bed with an immobilizer (a foam wedge that is placed between her thighs to keep her hip in position) in place. She weighs 200 lbs and is approximately 5 feet 6 inches tall. A physical therapist is scheduled to see her today to help her get out of bed for the first time since surgery. When the physical therapist is not available, Ms. Willet is on bed rest. Skin assessment reveals a 2.5-cm (1 inch), round, black right heel ulcer and a 2-cm red warm spot located over the sacrum.

1 The Braden risk assessment tool was used to determine the risk factors that place Ms. Willet at risk for skin breakdown. Which factors in the above scenario may contribute to the potential for skin breakdown?

2 The black tissue on Ms. Willet's heel is best described as and would be staged as:
1 Granulation, stage II.
2 Eschar, nonstageable.
3 Slough, stage III.
4 Induration, stage I.

3 The red warm spot noted over her sacrum is described as:
1 Erythema.
2 Sheet burn.
3 Blistering.
4 Bruising.
Explain your choice.

4 Identify the likely cause of the red warm area over Ms. Willett's sacrum and name one approach to determine if there is skin breakdown. Explain your choice.

✓ **REVIEW QUESTIONS**

1 Which of the following patients has factors that negatively affect wound healing? (Select all that apply.)
1 A patient whose surgical wound is producing yellowish drainage and whose white blood cell count is elevated
2 A cancer patient receiving the antiinflammatory drug cortisol
3 An older adult who has been advised to add more sources of vitamin C to her diet
4 A trauma patient with an open wound that is being treated with a moist dressing

2 A nurse on a surgical unit is providing care to patients who have recently undergone major abdominal procedures. How often should a pressure ulcer risk assessment be performed for these patients?
1 At least every day of their hospital stay
2 On admission to the unit, on a regularly scheduled basis, and as their condition changes
3 Every other day until the fifth postoperative day
4 If indicated by the presence of a history of pressure ulcers

3 A patient who is completely immobile and who does not make even slight changes in body or extremity position without assistance is being assessed for risk for developing a pressure ulcer using the Braden Scale. Which intervention would be appropriate to prevent pressure ulcers in this patient?
1 Use a moisture barrier ointment at least 3 times per day.
2 Consult with the wound clinical nurse specialist about the most appropriate bed surface to reduce pressure.
3 Order a nutrition consultation to be sure that the patient has adequate vitamin and mineral intake.
4 Consult with the physical therapy staff to determine exercises to increase muscle strength.

4 A patient is recovering from abdominal surgery and has a nasogastric tube inserted for stomach decompression. An intravenous (IV) line of normal saline is infusing into the left arm at 100 drops/min. The patient uses an incentive spirometer to perform deep-breathing exercises and has a drain exiting the wound and draining fluid into a small enclosed container. The patient is at risk for a pressure injury in which area? (Select all that apply.)
1 Lips
2 Nares
3 Left arm
4 Skin

5 An order for a hydrocolloid dressing is written for a patient with a pressure ulcer. What is the rationale for using a hydrocolloid dressing?
1 It provides an antibiotic solution to decrease surface bacteria, which helps healing.
2 It protects the wound base and provides a moist environment.
3 It can be changed several times per day without damaging the wound bed.
4 It contains a debriding agent to clean a wound environment.

6 The pediatric nursing team is orienting new nurses on preventing pressure ulcers in neonates and young children. Where should the nurses check frequently for the occurrence of these ulcerations in these children?
1 Shoulders
2 Head
3 Sacrum
4 Heels

7 When using gauze moistened in normal saline for a wound dressing, why is the gauze pad wrung out before application?
1 To prevent excessive delivery of the solution to the wound
2 To keep the healing wound moist and wick any excessive drainage
3 To prevent moistening the secondary dressing and causing maceration
4 To allow the wound to become slightly dry to facilitate healing

8 What is the primary mechanism of action of a hydrocolloid dressing?
1 It covers the wound, preventing staff from viewing the affected area.
2 It forms a gel over the wound to facilitate moist healing.
3 It forms a temporary membrane over the wound, allowing oxygen transport directly to the wound.
4 It delivers epithelial growth factors to the wound base.

9 Which of the following patients is most at risk for developing a pressure ulcer?
1 An 80-year-old adult with Alzheimer's who has poor oral intake
2 A 45-year-old male who is confined to a wheelchair as a result of paraplegia
3 A 50-year-old male with type I diabetes who underwent major heart surgery 24 hours ago and has diaphoresis
4 A 60-year-old female who underwent bladder surgery and now has urinary incontinence

10 The dressing ordered for a patient's sacral pressure ulcer is a hydrocolloid dressing. Place the following steps in the correct order for the dressing application.
1 Clean wound with ordered solution.
2 Remove paper backing from dressing.
3 Explain to patient the purpose of the dressing change.
4 Position patient to gain access to the pressure ulcer.
5 Measure wound to determine correct size of dressing.
6 Place dressing over wound; apply light pressure for 30 to 60 seconds.
1 1,3,5,6,2,4
2 3,4,1,5,2,6
3 3,4,1,5,2,6
4 5,1,3,4,2,6

REFERENCES

Ayello E: Predicting pressure ulcer risk, *Best Pract Nurs Care Older Adult* 5:1, 2012.

Ayello EA, Braden B: How and why do pressure ulcer risk assessment, *Adv Wound Care* 15(3):125, 2002.

Black JM, et al: MASD Part 2: Incontinence-associated dermatitis and intertriginous dermatitis, *J Wound Ostomy Continence Nurs* 38(4):359, 2011.

Braden BJ, Bergstrom N: Clinical utility of the Braden scale for predicting pressure sore risk, *Decubitus* 2(3):44, 1989.

Braden BJ, Bergstrom N: Predictive utility of the Braden scale for predicting pressure sore risk, *Res Nurs Health* 17:459, 1994.

Bryant RA, Nix DP: Developing and maintaining a pressure ulcer prevention program. In Bryant RA, Nix DP, editors: *Acute and chronic wounds: current management concepts*, ed 4, St Louis, 2012, Mosby.

Centers for Medicare and Medicaid Services (CMS): Evidence-based guidelines for selected and previously considered hospital-acquired infections. 2012, available at https://www.cms.gov/Medicare/Medicare-Fee-for-Service-Payment/HospitalAcqCond/Downloads/Evidence-Based-Guidelines.pdf, accessed June 26, 2012.

Doughty DB, Sparks-Defriese B: Wound-healing physiology. In Bryant RA, Nix DP, editors: *Acute and chronic wounds: current management concepts*, ed 4, St Louis, 2012, Mosby.

European Pressure Ulcer Advisory Panel (EPUAP) and National Pressure Ulcer Advisory Panel (NPUAP): *Treatment of pressure ulcers: quick reference guide*, Washington, DC, 2009, NPUAP.

Galhardo V, et al: Health-relate quality of life and depression in older patients with pressure ulcers, *Wounds* 22:20, 2010.

Gray M, et al: Moisture-associated skin damage: overview and pathophysiology, *J Wound Ostomy Continence Nurs* 38(3):233, 2011.

Hanson D, et al: Friction and shear considerations in pressure ulcer development, *Adv Skin Wound Care* 23:21, 2010.

Hopf H, et al: Managing wound pain. In Bryant RA, Nix DP, editors: *Acute and chronic wounds: current management concepts*, ed 4, St Louis, 2012, Mosby.

Kosiak M: Etiology and pathology of decubitus ulcers, *Arch Phys Med Rehabil* 40:62, 1959.

National Quality Forum (NQF): *National voluntary consensus standards for public reporting or patient safety event information consensus report*. Washington, DC, 2011, NQF, available at http://www.qualityforum.org/Publicatins/2011/National_Voluntary_Consensus_Standards_for_Public_Reporting_of_Patient_Safety_Event_information.aspx, accessed June, 2012.

Netsch D: Negative pressure wound therapy. In Bryant RA, Nix DP, editors: *Acute and chronic wounds: current management concepts*, ed 4, St Louis, 2012, Mosby.

Nix DP: Skin and wound inspection and assessment. In Bryant RA, Nix DP, editors: *Acute and chronic wounds: current management concepts*, ed 4, St Louis, 2012, Mosby.

Norton D, et al: *An investigation of geriatric nursing problems in hospital*. Edinburgh, 1962, reissue 1975, Churchill Livingstone.

Pieper B: Pressure ulcers: impact, etiology, and classification. In Bryant RA, Nix DP, editors: *Acute and chronic wounds: current management concepts*, ed 4, St Louis, 2012, Mosby.

Rolstad BS, Bryant RA, Nix DP: Topical management. In Bryant RA, Nix DP, editors: *Acute and chronic wounds: current management concepts*, ed 4, St Louis, 2012, Mosby.

Stotts N: Nutritional assessment and support. In Bryant RA, Nix DP, editors: *Acute and chronic wounds: current management concepts*, ed 4, St Louis, 2012, Mosby.

The Joint Commission (TJC): *National Patient Safety Goals*, Oakbrook Terrace, Ill, 2012, The Commission, available at http://www.jointcommission.org/standards_information/npsgs.aspx.

Wound Ostomy and Continence Nurses (WOCN) Society: *Guideline for prevention and management of pressure ulcers*, WOCN clinical practice guidelines series. Mount Laurel, NJ, 2010, WOCN Society.

Wysocki A: Anatomy and physiology of skin and soft tissue. In Bryant R, Nix D, editors: *Acute and chronic wounds: current management concepts*, ed 4, St. Louis, 2012, Mosby.

Care of the Eye and Ear

MEDIA RESOURCES

- ⊖volve http://evolve.elsevier.com/Perry/skills
  - Review Questions
  - Audio Glossary

KEY TERMS

Audiologist	Prosthesis
Cerumen	Refractive error
Enucleation	

OBJECTIVES

Mastery of content in this chapter will enable the nurse to:

- Explain safety guidelines used in the proper care of eye and ear prostheses.
- Identify patient-centered care guidelines used in caring for eye and ear prostheses.
- Correctly remove, store, clean, and insert a contact lens.
- Explain the rationale for maintaining aseptic technique during care of an artificial eye.
- Correctly perform eye and ear irrigations.
- Describe techniques that determine whether a hearing aid functions properly.
- Correctly remove, clean, and reinsert a hearing aid.

Artificial sensory devices help to replace or restore sensory function. Eyeglasses and contact lenses help to restore visual loss, and hearing aids improve sound reception. A patient may also depend on a prosthetic device such as an artificial eye to maintain an attractive appearance. Artificial eyes in particular help patients maintain a normal appearance when an eye is lost as a result of injury or disease (Goiato et al., 2010).

Artificial sensory devices must fit and work properly if patients are to function optimally within their environment. Breakage or loss is expensive and may result in serious impairment that can put a patient at risk for injury and interfere with communication, isolate a patient socially, and increase patient dependence and thereby threaten self-esteem. Understandably patients are especially sensitive about care of contact lenses, hearing aids, or artificial eyes.

An artificial eye or hearing aid requires regular cleaning to ensure proper function and prevent injury. Most patients have an established routine for cleaning their devices. When patients are unable to care for their device, you must understand the correct method to clean, handle, and store contact lenses, hearing aids, and artificial eyes. Careful handling is vital to avoiding damage to these devices or to a patient's eyes or ears.

EVIDENCE-BASED PRACTICE

Often vision and hearing change as people age. However, some of these changes are beyond the normal expectation of aging. Dual sensory impairment (DSI), the concurrent losses in vision and hearing, has the potential to cause cognitive function decline or contribute to acute confusion or depression (Saunders and Echt, 2011). Furthermore, DSI in rehabilitation or long-term care settings affect a patient's success in using assistive devices and rehabilitation services and progressing to a higher level of independent function (McDonnall, 2009). Although the evidence is not conclusive, some literature suggests that DSI is more debilitating than a single sensory impairment, whereas other literature suggests that the vision impairment component of DSI has the main impact on individuals (Smith et al., 2008).

Age-related hearing loss is gradual, progressive, and often bilateral. Older adults may not actually perceive their hearing loss because initially it is mild; however, as it progresses, they usually avoid or delay hearing evaluation (Chou et al., 2011). Hearing loss is the third leading chronic condition affecting adults over 75 years of age (Cacchione, 2010). There is a high prevalence of hearing loss in nursing facility residents (Adams-Wendling, 2008).

Vision impairment is the functional limitation of the eyes (e.g., reduced visual acuity, visual field loss, contrast sensitivity reduction, glare disability) that cannot be corrected with standard glasses or contact lenses (Smith et al., 2008). There are multiple definitions and classifications of levels of vision impairment and blindness, which adds to the complexity in understanding DSI. In addition, the psychosocial and functional impacts of DSI are not well understood when compared with those of a single sensory impairment (Smith et al., 2008). A person with DSI is likely to be at greater risk for disability, but evidence is mixed.

In community settings sensory impairments negatively impact the use of community support services and health-related quality of life (McDonnall, 2009). DSI decreases independence, socialization, and quality of life of individuals and, in many cases, their families (Swann, 2008).

- Common screening tests for hearing loss can help identify patients at higher risk for hearing loss. The whispered voice test at 2 feet and a single question regarding perceived hearing loss are comparable with more detailed screening questionnaires and audiometric devices for identifying at least mild hearing loss (Chou et al., 2011).
- Identify patients at risk for hearing impairments: Male over age 65, male or female over age 75, resident in nursing facility, existing visual impairment, chronic ear infection, prolonged exposure to loud noises, and use of ototoxic medication (Cacchione, 2010; Adams-Wendling et al., 2008).
- Involving patients with DSI in volunteer work has been shown to result in fewer depressive symptoms compared to persons without sensory loss who volunteer (McDonnall, 2011).
- Patients with DSI will have unique communication needs that require a thorough assessment.
- Evaluate nursing facility residents for hearing impairment on admission and routinely thereafter (Adams-Wendling, 2008).
- Verify that patients are able to see, hear, and understand instructions about their therapy.

PATIENT-CENTERED CARE

Any intervention, device, or prosthesis needed to improve sensory perception must fit and work properly if patients are to function optimally within their environment. It is important to know a patient's preferences and have a discussion with your patients about

how to use and care for a device or prosthesis. Breakage or loss of a patient's hearing aid or eye prosthesis often results in costly repair and replacement. When a patient is without visual or hearing aids, it interferes with communication, isolates a patient socially, and increases patient dependence. In addition, especially in the case of an eye prosthesis, the loss of the device threatens a patient's self-esteem.

Hospitals, rehabilitation centers, and skilled nursing facilities are environments that make hearing difficult. The hard flooring surfaces, medical equipment, televisions, and constant need to speak with other health care professionals all produce noise. For the hearing impaired this increased background noise makes hearing even more difficult (Wallhagen and Pettengill, 2008). When a patient has visual impairments, the increased background noise in an unfamiliar environment often makes a patient more anxious and decreases his or her ability to adjust to new surroundings.

Communication is vital to people from all cultures. When vision and/or hearing is threatened or impaired, that change must be understood in terms of a patient's culture. In cultures such as the Navajo Indian and in some Asian and Middle Eastern cultures, limited eye contact is the norm and is a nonverbal form of respect (Galanti, 2008). Changes in the ability to move the eyes, as with a prosthesis, present a social difficulty because a patient is unable to lower the eyes. The Navajo Indians are comfortable with the soft-spoken word and silence (Galanti, 2008).

Hearing impairments may force a patient's family and friends to speak loudly, which is not effective. In addition, because of the comfort with silence, one can easily mistake a patient's silence for a measure of comfort and never correctly assess what he or she is able to hear or if the information is heard correctly. At times you will use touch to get the attention of a patient with decreased hearing. In some cultures such as Muslim, same-sex caregivers are required before touch can be used. Remember this before using touch to gain a patient's attention.

The following list includes interventions for patients with sensory loss. As always it is important to carefully communicate with a patient about the course of action and verify that a patient saw, heard, and understood these interventions.

- Understand the cause of a person's sensory loss and then determine the patient's own perception of the reason for the loss.
- Identify patient's usual practices in using sensory assistive devices and the preferred maintenance.
- Provide large-print educational materials for patients with visual impairments.
- Design nursing interventions based on the type of sensory loss, patient safety, and patient preference.

Safety Guidelines

1 Whenever you care for patients with sensory alterations, safety is a priority. Anticipate how the sensory alteration places a patient at risk for injury (e.g., ability to maneuver through home, climb stairs, respond to alarms).

2 Orient patient to any new environment or changes within an existing environment to minimize safety hazards. In addition, educate family and friends about the best way to help patient adapt to sensory loss.

3 When patients have visual impairments, they may have difficulty with tasks requiring visual detail (e.g., reading

prescriptions or syringes). This increases the risk of improper administration of medications in the home setting. In addition, certain eye conditions such as cataracts and macular degeneration cause a patient difficulty when adjusting to changes in contrast and brightness.

4 Provide additional time for patients with hearing loss to ask repeated questions about their care or upcoming procedure.
5 If a patient must sign a consent form for a procedure or surgery, be sure to have a method to verify that patient read, heard, and understood the procedure.

PROCEDURAL GUIDELINE 19-1 Eye Care for Comatose Patients

Comatose patients do not have natural protective mechanisms, including blinking and lubrication of the eye, to protect the cornea (Rosenberg and Eisen, 2008). The blinking reflex flushes debris out of the eye. When patients are heavily sedated or in a coma, tear production is reduced; as a result the normal lubrication of the eye surface is decreased (So et al., 2008). Tears maintain a moist environment, lubricate the eyes, wash away foreign material and cell debris, prevent organisms from adhering to the ocular surface, and transport oxygen to the outer eye surface (Marshall et al., 2008). When a patient's normal protective eye mechanisms are not effective, a nurse is responsible for providing this care. Left unprotected, damage to the cornea can occur. This damage ranges from corneal scarring to premature cataract formation or vision changes. Simple nursing measures such as protecting the eyes or administering sterile lubricant decrease the risk for or prevent damage to the cornea (Oh et al., 2008).

Delegation and Collaboration
The skill of eye care for a comatose patient can be delegated to nursing assistive personnel (NAP). However, it is the nurse's responsibility to assess a patient's eyes and administer the sterile lubricant. The nurse directs the NAP to:
- Adapt the skill for specific patients (e.g., using skin-sensitive tape to affix eye pads for patients with sensitive skin).
- Immediately report any eye drainage or irritation to the nurse for further assessment.

Equipment
- ❏ Clean gloves
- ❏ Water or normal saline solution
- ❏ Clean washcloth
- ❏ Cotton balls
- ❏ Eye pads or patches
- ❏ Paper tape
- ❏ Eyedropper bulb syringe
- ❏ Sterile lubricant or eye preparations as ordered

NOTE: A moisture chamber (e.g., polyethylene covers or swimming goggles) to completely seal off the eye from the environment may also be used; verify with agency policy.

Procedural Steps
1 Perform hand hygiene.
2 Observe patient's eyes for drainage, irritation, redness, and lesions. Apply clean gloves if drainage is present.
3 Continually explain each step of the procedure. It is unknown how much a comatose patient can hear; thus it is important to continually orient a patient to any procedure.
4 Assess for blink reflex.
5 Perform pupillary examination: Determine if pupils are equal, round, and react to light (PERRL) (see Chapter 6).
6 Observe patient's eye movements, noting symmetry of eye movement.
7 Explain procedure to patient and family members.
8 Position patient in supine position.
9 Use clean washcloth or cotton balls moistened with water or saline and gently wipe each eye from inner to outer canthus. Use a separate, clean cotton ball or corner of the washcloth for each eye.
10 Use an eyedropper to instill the prescribed lubricant (e.g., saline, methylcellulose, liquid tears) as ordered, wiping away any excess lubricant.
11 If the blink reflex is absent, gently close patient's eyes and apply eye patches, pads, or a moisture chamber. Secure patch, being careful not to tape a patient's eyes.
12 Dispose of excess material, remove gloves, and perform hand hygiene.
13 Remove eye pads or patches every 4 hours or as ordered and observe condition of patient's eyes for drainage, irritation, redness, and lesions.
14 Document eye exam findings and administration of lubricant.
15 Notify health care provider if signs of irritation or infection are present.

PROCEDURAL GUIDELINE 19-2 Taking Care of Contact Lenses

A contact lens is a thin, concave disk that fits directly over the cornea of the eye. It is transparent over at least the pupil and may be colorless or tinted. Contact lenses correct refractive errors of the eye or abnormalities in the shape of the cornea that distort vision. They are relatively easy to apply and remove.

All modern contact lenses are gas (oxygen) permeable and adhere to the cornea by surface tension. There are two basic types of contact lenses in use today: rigid gas permeable (RGP) and soft. They differ primarily in size, flexibility, and durability. Rigid contact lenses are made of firm, durable plastic and are smaller than the cornea. Soft contact lenses are made of a flexible hydrogel plastic and cover the entire cornea and a small rim of the sclera. There are many different kinds of both RGP and soft lenses to accommodate patient needs for comfort, vision correction, and convenience. Contact lenses have specific prescribed wear and replacement schedules.

It is important to remember that all lenses must be removed periodically to prevent infection and corneal damage and that proper cleaning is necessary before reinserting a lens. As contact lenses are worn, secretions and foreign matter adhere to the lens

Continued

PROCEDURAL GUIDELINE 19-2   Taking Care of Contact Lenses—cont'd

surface (American Optometric Association, 2011). It is extremely important to determine whether patients wear contact lenses, particularly when they are admitted to hospitals or agencies in unresponsive or confused states. If a seriously ill patient is wearing contact lenses and this fact goes undetected, severe corneal injury can result.

Delegation and Collaboration

The skill of taking care of contact lenses can be delegated to the nursing assistive personnel (NAP). The nurse directs the NAP to:

- Know a patient's specific type of contact lens, including cleaning solutions and routine, wear schedule, storage, and replacement schedule.
- Report immediately to the nurse any eye pain or discomfort, redness, swelling, tearing, or drainage.
- Carefully handle the lens to prevent damage and injury.

Equipment

- ❑ Bath towels or waterproof pads
- ❑ Sterile saline solution
- ❑ Sterile lens care solution(s) for cleaning, disinfecting, and rinsing
- ❑ Sterile wetting or conditioning solution (depends on care regimen)
- ❑ Sterile enzyme solution (depends on care regimen)
- ❑ Flashlight or penlight
- ❑ Clean lens storage container
- ❑ Suction cup (optional)
- ❑ Powder-free, clean gloves

Procedural Steps

1 Inspect patient's eyes or ask patient if contact lens is in place.

Clinical Decision Point *If a patient is unconscious or confused, you must assess for presence of contact lenses, which are often difficult to detect if they are colorless (untinted).*

2 Determine if patient is able to manipulate and hold contact lenses and if glasses are available for periods when contacts are not in use. Determine patient's usual routine for wearing, cleaning, and storing lenses.
3 Assess patient for any unusual visual signs/symptoms (e.g., change in visual acuity, blurred vision, halos, photophobia).
4 Review types of medication prescribed for patient: sedatives, hypnotics, muscle relaxants, antihistamines, or another medication that decreases blink reflex and subsequent lubrication of cornea.
5 Explain procedure to patient.
6 Perform hand hygiene.
7 Verify expiration date of all solutions and assemble equipment at bedside.
8 Be sure that your fingernails are short and smooth.
9 Position patient in supine or high-Fowler's position in bed.
10 Identify patient using two identifiers (i.e., name and birthday or name and account number) according to agency policy. Compare identifiers with information on patient's identification bracelet.
11 Apply clean gloves. Place towel just below patient's face.
12 **Removing lenses:**
  a Removal of soft lens: Follow Steps (1) through (6) for each eye.

(1) If you are unable to visualize the lens, shine a penlight or flashlight sideways onto the eye to locate the position of the lens.
(2) Add 2 to 3 drops of sterile saline solution to patient's eye.
(3) If possible ask patient to look straight ahead. Retract lower eyelid and expose lower edge of lens.
(4) Use pad of index finger to slide lens off cornea down onto lower sclera (white of the eye).
(5) Pull upper eyelid down gently with thumb of other hand and compress lens slightly between thumb and index finger.
(6) Gently pinch lens and lift out without allowing edges to stick together. Place lens in storage case.

Clinical Decision Point *If lens edges stick together, place lens in palm and soak thoroughly with sterile saline solution. Gently roll lens with index finger in back-and-forth motion. If necessary, soak lens in storage solution, which may return lens to normal shape.*

  b Removal of hard lenses: Follow Steps (1) through (6) for each eye.
(1) Inspect the eye to be sure that lens is positioned directly over the cornea. If you are unable to visualize the lens, shine a penlight or flashlight sideways onto the eye to locate the position of the lens.

Clinical Decision Point *If lens is not positioned directly over the cornea, have patient close eyelid, place index and middle fingers of one hand on eyelid just beside the lens and beneath, and gently attempt to massage lens back into place. If lens cannot be repositioned, an immediate referral to an ophthalmologist is needed.*

(2) Place index finger on outer corner of patient's eye and draw skin gently back toward ear.
(3) Ask patient to blink. Do not release pressure until blink is completed.

Clinical Decision Point *For patients unable to open eye or blink on command, a lens suction cup can be used to remove lens from eye. Gently apply suction cup to lens surface and lift out.*

(4) If lens does not dislodge, gently retract eyelid beyond edge of lens. Press lower eyelid gently against lower edge of lens to dislodge lens.
(5) Allow both eyelids to close slightly and grasp lens as it rises from the eye. Cup lens in hand.
(6) Inspect lens to be sure that it is intact. Place it in storage container.
  c After lenses are removed, inspect eye for redness, pain, swelling of eyelids or conjunctiva, discharge, or excess tearing.
13 **Cleaning and storage:**
Typical cleaning and disinfecting of contact lenses (verify specific method for lenses):
  a Apply 1 or 2 drops of cleaning solution to lens in palm of hand. Using index finger (soft lenses) or little finger (rigid lenses), rub lens gently but thoroughly on both sides for 20 to 30 seconds.
  b Holding lens over emesis basin, rinse thoroughly with recommended rinsing solution.

PROCEDURAL GUIDELINE 19-2 Taking Care of Contact Lenses—cont'd

Clinical Decision Point *Do not use tap water for cleaning, rinsing, or storage. Tap water contains microbes and may be absorbed into the lens, making them uncomfortable to wear. Periodic cleaning with enzymatic cleaner and/or heat disinfecting may be part of the prescribed regimen. Follow prescriber's instructions and schedules.*

    c Place lens in proper storage case compartment: "R" for right lens and "L" for left. Rigid lenses are placed inside up.

    d Fill with recommended disinfectant or storage solution.

    e Secure cover(s) over storage case. Label case with patient's name, identification number, and room number.

14 Inserting lenses:

    a Inserting a soft lens: Follow Steps (1) through (5) for each eye.

      (1) Remove right lens from storage case and rinse with recommended rinsing solution; inspect lens for foreign materials, tears, and other damage.

      (2) Hold lens on tip of index finger of dominant hand with concave side up.

      (3) Inspect lens from side at eye level to ensure that it is not inverted (see illustration).

      (4) Using middle or index finger of opposite hand, retract upper lid until iris is exposed (see illustration). Using middle finger of hand holding the lens, pull down lower lid.

      (5) Instruct patient to look straight ahead and focus on an object in the distance. Gently place lens directly on cornea and release lids slowly, starting with lower lid.

    b Inserting a rigid lens: Follow Steps (1) through (6) for each eye.

      (1) Remove right lens from storage case; attempt to lift lens straight up.

      (2) Hold lens on tip of index finger of dominant hand with concave side up.

      (3) Inspect the lens to ensure that it is moist, clean, clear, and free of chips or cracks.

      (4) Wet lens surfaces using a few drops of prescribed wetting solution.

      (5) Using middle finger of hand holding lens, pull down lower lid (see illustration).

      (6) Instruct patient to look straight ahead and focus on an object in the distance (see illustration). Gently place lens directly on cornea and release lids slowly, starting with lower lid.

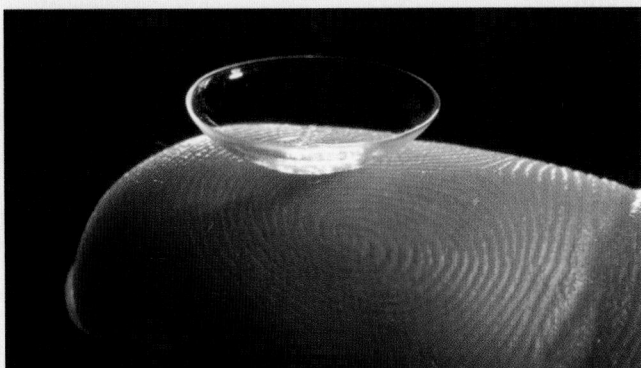

STEP 14a(3)   Correct position of soft lens before insertion.

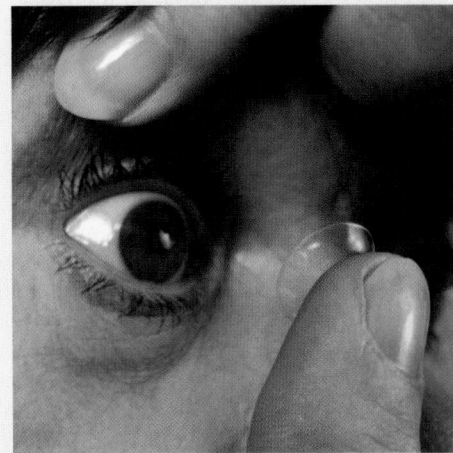

STEP 14a(4)   Correct position of hands for soft lens insertion.

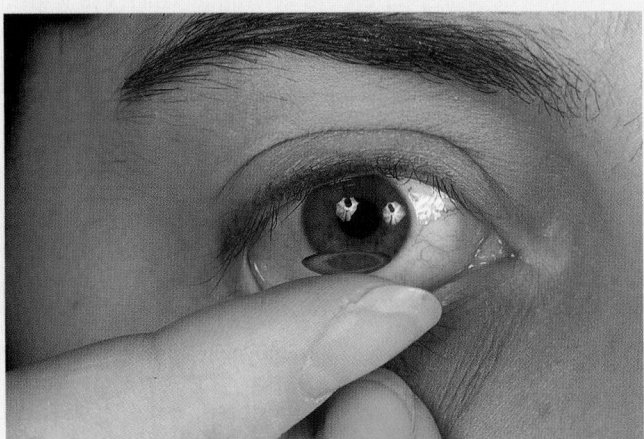

STEP 14b(5)   Hand position for rigid lens insertion.

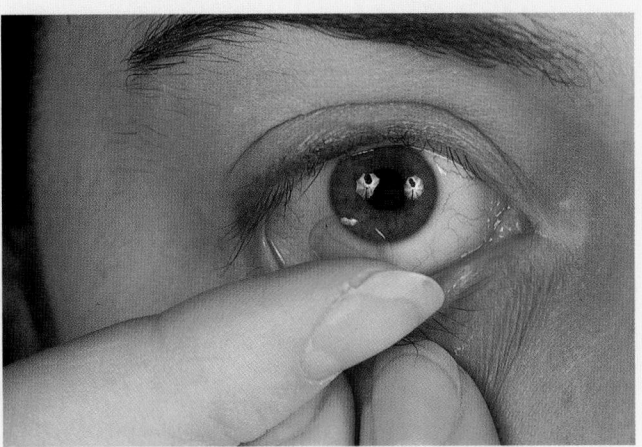

STEP 14b(6)   Instruct patient to look straight ahead and focus on an object in the distance.

Continued

PROCEDURAL GUIDELINE 19-2   Taking Care of Contact Lenses—cont'd

(a) Ask patient to close eyes briefly and avoid blinking.

15 Inspect eye to ensure that lens is on cornea.

Clinical Decision Point *If lens is on sclera rather than cornea, ask patient to slowly close eye and look toward the lens. Gentle pressure on the eyelid may help to center the lens on the cornea. Ask patient to blink a few times.*

16 Ask patient to cover other eye with hand and report if vision is clear and lens is comfortable.

17 Repeat procedure to insert lens in other eye.

18 Discard solution from storage case and rinse case thoroughly with sterile lens storage solution. Sterilize or replace case as recommended by manufacturer. Allow case to air dry. Dispose of towel, remove gloves, and perform hand hygiene.

19 Ask patient if lens feels comfortable after removal and reinsertion of lenses.

20 Observe for unexpected outcomes (e.g., blurred vision, burning, pain, foreign body sensation).

PROCEDURAL GUIDELINE 19-3   Taking Care of an Artificial Eye

As a result of tumor, infection, congenital blindness, or severe trauma to the eye, patients may undergo *enucleation,* the complete surgical removal of the eyeball. During this surgical procedure a spherical implant is placed in the orbit to maintain the natural eye structure and provide support for a cosmetic prosthesis (Goiato et al., 2010). The muscles and other tissues of the eye are sewn around the implant, holding it in place. Therefore the implant is not visible (Fig. 19-1). Modern implants are made of glass or plastic and are porous so the tissues of the eye grow into the sphere (Center for Ocular Prosthetics, 2011). Like a healthy eye, this integrated implant moves as the companion eye moves.

A concave cosmetic prosthesis is placed over the implant, resulting in a nearly normal appearance. Some implants are fitted with a peg that secures and optimally transfers implant movement to the prosthesis. The prosthesis (i.e., the artificial eye) is glass or plastic and colored to match the companion eye.

Prostheses are relatively easy to remove and insert and are usually worn day and night. Cleaning with sterile saline or soap and water is done at intervals of up to a year based on ocularist recommendations and patient's preference (Kolberg Ocular Prosthetics, 2011). Too much handling of the prosthesis causes socket irritation and increases secretions (Erickson Laboratories, n.d.). Patients are instructed to have the artificial eye checked and polished at least twice a year to avoid unnecessary discomfort as a result of protein deposits or scratches on the surface.

An artificial eye is usually replaced every 5 years (Erickson Laboratories, n.d.).

Delegation and Collaboration

The skill of taking care of an artificial eye can be delegated to nursing assistive personnel (NAP). The nurse directs the NAP to:
- Report eye pain or discomfort, inflammation, drainage, or odor.
- Understand the importance of careful handling of the prosthesis to prevent damage or injury.

Equipment

- ❏ Bath towels or waterproof pads (2)
- ❏ Sterile saline for washing prosthesis
- ❏ Irrigation bulb or large syringe (without needle)
- ❏ Sterile saline: 30 to 180 mL at 32° to 38° F (about 90° to 100° C)
- ❏ Emesis basin
- ❏ 4 × 4–inch gauze pads
- ❏ Clean gloves
- ❏ Facial tissues *(optional)*
- ❏ Washbasin with warm water and mild soap *(optional)*
- ❏ Suction device (or medicine dropper bulb) *(optional)*
- ❏ Covered plastic storage case *(optional)*

Procedural Steps

1 Perform hand hygiene
2 Ask patient or inspect eyes to determine which eye is artificial. Some implants allow movement of the prosthesis and can make distinguishing it from the natural eye difficult. An artificial eye pupil does not react to changes in light or accommodation (see Chapter 6).
3 Assess for patient's frequency and method of cleaning and length of time since last cleaning.

Clinical Decision Point *Unless a patient's eye-care practitioner advises otherwise, the prosthesis is usually not removed unless a patient experiences discomfort because excessive handling may cause irritation and increased secretions (Kolberg Ocular Prosthetics, 2011).*

4 Assess patient's ability to remove, clean, and reinsert prosthesis.
5 Before and after removal of prosthesis, assess eyelids and socket for inflammation, tenderness, swelling, drainage, or odor. Pay particular attention to the implant peg if present. Assess patient's pain or other symptoms.

FIG 19-1   Side view of orbital implant, artificial eye removed.

PROCEDURAL GUIDELINE 19-3 Taking Care of an Artificial Eye—cont'd

Clinical Decision Point *Signs/symptoms such as pain or discharge may indicate infection or injury. Infection can spread easily to neighboring eye, underlying sinuses, or brain tissue. The implant peg is a common site of infection.*

6 Discuss procedure with patient.
7 Assemble supplies at bedside. Place one towel over work area.
8 **Removing prosthesis:**
  a Position patient in sitting or supine position with head elevated. Provide privacy.
  b Perform hand hygiene. Apply clean gloves.
  c Place towel just below patient's face.
  d With thumb or forefinger of dominant hand gently retract lower eyelid against lower orbital ridge (see illustration).
  e Exert slight pressure below eyelid and slide prosthesis out (see illustration).

Clinical Decision Point *If prosthesis does not slide out, use moistened suction device to apply direct suction to it (Kolberg Ocular Prosthetics, 2011).*

  f Note presence and orientation of colored dot at margin of prosthesis.
  g Place prosthesis in palm of hand.
  h Clean prosthesis by washing with mild soap and warm water or plain saline solution by rubbing well between

thumb and index finger (see manufacturer instructions). NOTE: Never use alcohol or other products because they are harmful to the prosthesis (Erickson Laboratories, n.d.).
  i Inspect prosthesis for rough edges or surfaces. Set aside on towel.
9 If prosthesis will not be reinserted immediately, store in sterile saline in a labeled case in a documented location (see manufacturer instructions).
10 **Clean eyelid margins and socket:**
  a Wash and rinse eyelid margins with mild soap and water. Wipe from inner to outer canthus using a clean section of cloth with each wipe.
  b Retract upper and lower eyelid margins with thumb and index finger.
  c Gently irrigate socket with sterile saline solution. Note presence of discharge or odor.
  d Remove excess moisture with gauze pads by wiping from inner to outer canthus.
11 **Insert prosthesis:**
  a Moisten prosthesis in water or sterile saline.
  b Retract patient's upper eyelid with index finger or thumb of nondominant hand.
  c With dominant hand hold prosthesis so iris faces outward and colored dot is properly oriented (see illustration).
  d Gently slide prosthesis up under upper eyelid and push down lower lid to allow prosthesis to slip into place.
  e Ask patient if prosthesis fits comfortably and without pain.
12 Inspect eyelids and socket for signs of infection such as excessive, purulent, or foul drainage; excessive tearing or clear discharge; excessive itching; or lashes turned toward prosthesis.
13 Observe patient removing, cleaning, and reinserting prosthesis.
14 Teach patient and family how to inspect eye socket for redness, drainage, or excessive dryness.
15 Teach patient and family how to inspect artificial eye for damage, scratches, or areas of roughness. Alert patient to report any odor noted on eye or prosthesis to the health care provider.

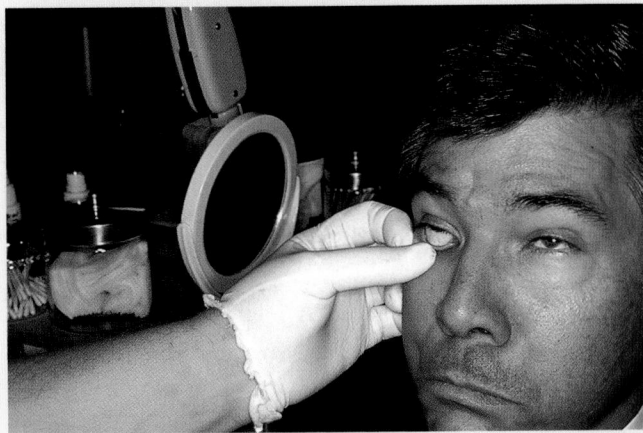

STEP 8d Retraction of lower lid to aid removal of eye prosthesis.

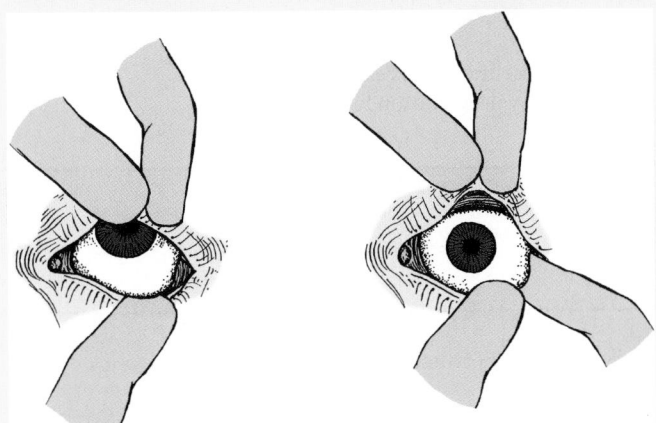

STEP 8e Exertion of pressure below eyelid and removal of prosthesis.

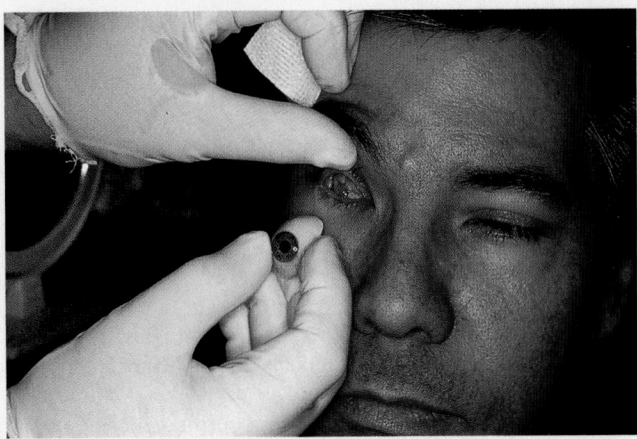

STEP 11c Prosthesis must be oriented for correct insertion.

SKILL 19-1   Eye Irrigation

Eye irrigations effectively flush out exudates, irritating solutions, or foreign bodies from the eye. The procedure is typically used in emergency situations when a foreign object or some other substance has entered the eye. When a chemical or irritating substance contaminates the eyes, irrigate immediately with copious amounts of cool water for at least 15 minutes to minimize corneal damage (U.S. National Library of Medicine, 2011b). Users of contact lenses or artificial eyes may need eye irrigation to flush out particles of dust or fibers from the eye socket. Patients with artificial eyes are also at risk for socket irritation secondary to the composite material of the artificial eye itself, and irrigation assists in relieving the irritation (Cao et al., 2009).

A chemical injury to the eye is considered an emergency and requires flushing the eye with copious amounts of irrigation fluid (Rodrigues, 2009). Often cool tap water is recommended for emergency eye flushing because it is effective, immediately available for first aid, and initially helps to dilute the concentration of the chemical. The goal in treating ocular chemical injury is to prevent or reduce visual loss caused by the burn (Rodrigues, 2009).

Chemical injuries to the eye can be from alkaline or acid solutions. In treatment settings the best type of solutions are normal saline or lactated Ringers because they are more effective in restoring pH after a chemical injury to the eye. Continue to irrigate the eye because the irrigating solution helps to dilute and flush out the chemical. Once the acute phase is over, an irrigation solution that buffers alkali or acid chemical is then selected (Babineau and Sanchez, 2008).

Delegation and Collaboration

The skill of eye irrigation cannot be delegated to nursing assistive personnel (NAP). The nurse directs the NAP to:

- Report any patient complaint of discomfort or excess tearing following irrigation.

Equipment

- ❏ Prescribed irrigating solution: volume usually 30 to 180 mL at 32° to 38° C (90° to 100° F) (For chemical flushing, use normal saline or lactated Ringers fluid in large volume to provide continuous irrigation over 15 minutes.)
- ❏ Sterile basin or bag of solution
- ❏ Curved emesis basin
- ❏ Waterproof pad or towel
- ❏ 4 × 4–inch gauze pads
- ❏ Soft bulb syringe, eyedropper, or intravenous (IV) tubing
- ❏ Clean gloves
- ❏ Penlight
- ❏ Medication administration record (MAR)

STEP	RATIONALE
ASSESSMENT	
1 Review health care provider's medication order, including solution to be instilled and affected eye(s) (right, left, or both) to receive irrigation.	Ensures safe and correct administration of irrigant.
2 Obtain history of the injury to assess reason for eye irrigation.	Determines amount and type of solution and immediacy of need for treatment.
3 Determine patient's ability to open affected eye.	Spasm of the eyelid or pain makes opening the eye difficult. Local anesthetics such as proparacaine or tetracaine cause topical numbness and are used before eye examination procedures.
4 If time permits, do a complete eye examination, including determining if pupils are equal, round, and react to light and accommodation (PERRLA) (see Chapter 6).	Provides baseline information.
5 Assess eye for redness, excessive tearing, discharge, and swelling. Ask patient about symptoms of itching, burning, pain, blurred vision, or photophobia.	Establishes baseline signs and symptoms.
6 Ask patient to rate level of pain. Use scale of 0 to 10.	Establishes baseline for level of pain.
7 Assess patient's ability to cooperate.	Determines level of assistance needed.

NURSING DIAGNOSES

• Acute pain	• Risk for infection	• Risk for injury

Related factors are individualized based on patient's condition or needs.

PLANNING

1 Expected outcomes following completion of procedure:	
• Patient demonstrates minimal anxiety during and after irrigation.	Potential for anxiety and pain is high during emergency.
• Patient verbalizes reduced pain, burning, or itching and improved visual acuity after irrigation.	Reflects effectiveness of procedure in removing irritant.
• Patient maintains normal pupillary reaction and eye movement after irrigation.	Reflects effectiveness of procedure in minimizing exposure to irritant and preventing eye damage.

STEP	RATIONALE
2 Discuss procedure with patient.	Decreases patient anxiety.
3 Check accuracy and completeness of each MAR with health care provider's written medication or procedure order. Check patient's name, irrigation solution name and concentration, route of administration, and time for administration. Compare MAR with label of eye irrigation solution.	The order sheet is the most reliable source and only legal record of drugs or procedure that patient is to receive. Ensures that patient receives correct medication.
4 Assemble supplies at bedside.	Provides easy access to supplies.
5 Help patient to side-lying position on side of affected eye. Turn head toward affected eye. If both eyes are affected, place patient supine for simultaneous irrigation of both eyes.	Position facilitates flow of solution from inner to outer canthus, preventing contamination of unaffected eye and nasolacrimal duct.

IMPLEMENTATION	RATIONALE
1 Identify patient using two identifiers (i.e., name and birthday or name and account number) according to agency policy. Compare identifiers in MAR/medical record with information on patient's identification bracelet and/or ask patient to state name.	Ensures correct patient. Complies with The Joint Commission standards and improves patient safety (TJC, 2012).
2 Perform hand hygiene. Apply clean gloves.	Reduces transmission of microorganisms. Protects hands from chemical irritants.
3 Remove any contact lens if possible (see Procedural Guideline 19-2). Remove gloves after contact lens is removed. Reapply new gloves.	Prompt removal of lenses is needed to safely and completely irrigate foreign substances from patient's eyes. Removal of gloves following contact lens removal prevents reintroduction of chemical transferred from lens to glove.

Clinical Decision Point *In an emergency such as first aid for a chemical burn, do not delay by removing patient's contact lens before irrigation. Do not remove lens unless rapid swelling is occurring. Flush eye from the inner to outer canthus with cool tap water immediately (U.S. National Library of Medicine, 2011b). Advise patient to consult health care provider before using contact lens.*

STEP	RATIONALE
4 Explain to patient that eye can be closed periodically and that no object will touch it.	Informing patients what to expect decreases anxiety and reassures them.
5 Place towel or waterproof pad under patient's face and curved emesis basin just below patient's cheek on side of affected eye.	Catches irrigation fluid.
6 Using gauze moistened with prescriber's solution (or normal saline), gently clean visible secretions or foreign material from eyelid margins and eyelashes, wiping from inner to outer canthus.	Minimizes transfer of material into eye during irrigation. Prevents secretions from entering nasolacrimal duct.
7 Explain next steps to patient and encourage relaxation: a With gloved finger gently retract upper and lower eyelids to expose conjunctival sacs. b To hold lids open, apply gentle pressure to lower bony orbit and bony prominence beneath eyebrow. Do not apply pressure over eye.	Retraction minimizes blinking and allows irrigation of conjunctiva.
8 Hold irrigating syringe, dropper, or IV tubing approximately 2.5 cm (1 inch) from inner canthus.	Direct contact with irrigation equipment may injure the eye.
9 Ask patient to look toward brow. Gently irrigate with steady stream toward lower conjunctival sac, moving from inner to outer canthus (see illustration).	Minimizes force of stream on patient's cornea. Flushes irritant out and away from the other eye and nasolacrimal duct.

STEP	RATIONALE

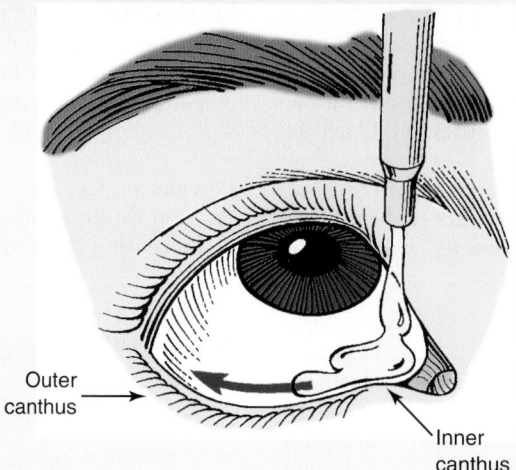

STEP 9   Irrigation of eye from inner to outer canthus.

STEP	RATIONALE
10 Reinforce importance of procedure and encourage patient by using calm, confident, soft voice.	Reduces anxiety.
11 Allow patient to blink periodically.	Lid closure moves secretions from upper conjunctival sac.
12 Continue irrigation with prescribed solution volume or time or until secretions are cleared. (NOTE: An irrigation of 15 minutes or more is needed to flush chemicals.)	Assessment of eye secretion pH may be necessary if eye was exposed to an acidic or basic solution during injury (U.S. National Library of Medicine, 2011b).
13 Blot excess moisture from eyelids and face with gauze or towel.	
14 Dispose of soiled supplies, remove gloves, and perform hand hygiene.	Reduces transmission of microorganisms.

EVALUATION

1 Observe for verbal and nonverbal signs of anxiety during irrigation.	Verifies that patient is adequately comforted.
2 Assess patient's comfort level after irrigation.	Verifies effective removal of irritant.
3 Inspect eye for movement and to determine if pupils are equal, round, react to light and accommodation (PERRLA).	Impaired reaction to light, accommodation, or movement may indicate injury.
4 Ask patient about improved visual acuity.	Corneal damage from irritant can result in altered visual acuity (e.g., blurred vision, cloudiness).

Unexpected Outcomes

1 Anxiety

2 Patient complains of pain or foreign body sensation in eye following irrigation, excessive tearing, or photophobia.

Related Interventions

- Reinforce rationale for irrigation.
- Allow patient to close eye periodically during irrigation.
- Instruct patient to take slow, deep breaths.
- Advise patient to close eye and avoid eye movement.
- Immediately notify health care provider or eye care practitioner.

Recording and Reporting

- Record in nurses' notes and electronic health record (EHR) condition of eye and patient's report of pain and visual symptoms. Record amount and type of irrigation on patient's MAR.
- Report continuing symptoms of pain or blurred vision.

Special Considerations
Teaching

- Help patient identify potential hazards at home and work and take steps to prevent accidents such as use of safety goggles while working with dust or chemicals.

- Review first-aid procedures for eye emergencies with patient and/or caregiver.
- Instruct patient to not press or rub an injured eye.

Pediatric

- A child with a foreign body or chemical in the eye may panic. It may be necessary to restrain the child to safely and quickly irrigate the eye.

SKILL 19-2 Ear Irrigation

The common indications for irrigation of the external ear are presence of foreign bodies, local inflammation, and buildup of cerumen in the ear canal. The procedure is not without potential hazards. Usually irrigations are performed with liquid warmed to body temperature to avoid vertigo or nausea in patients. The greatest danger during ear irrigation is rupture of the tympanic membrane by forcing irrigant into the canal under pressure. Damage to the external auditory meatus may occur by scratching the lining of the canal if a patient suddenly moves or if there is inadequate control of the irrigating syringe (Kraszewski, 2008; U.S. National Library of Medicine, 2011a). Improperly drying the ear may lead to acute otitis externa (infection of the outer ear).

Ear emergencies can include the presence of foreign bodies, insect bites, or percussion injuries. In addition, a patient can also have damage from inside the ear, which includes blood and drainage. Sometimes the cause of bloody drainage may be the result of a head or neck injury. If a head or neck injury is suspected, do not move patient. Cover the outside of the ear with a sterile dressing (if available), get medical help immediately, and do not irrigate the ear (U.S. National Library of Medicine, 2011a). In addition, do not irrigate the ear if vegetable matter or an insect is present in the canal; the tympanic membrane is ruptured; or a patient has otitis externa, myringotomy tubes, or a mastoid cavity (Hockenberry and Wilson, 2011).

Delegation and Collaboration
The skill of administering ear irrigation cannot be delegated to nursing assistive personnel (NAP). The nurse directs the NAP to:
- Immediately report any potential side effects of ear irrigation (e.g., pain, drainage, dizziness).
- Help a patient when ambulating because some lightheadedness may be present, which increases a patient's risk for falling.

Equipment
- Clean gloves
- Irrigation syringe
- Basin for irrigating solution (Use sterile basin if sterile irrigating solution is used.)
- Emesis basin for drainage or irrigating solution exiting the ear
- Towel
- Cotton balls or 4 × 4–inch gauze
- Prescribed irrigating solution warmed to body temperature or mineral oil, over-the-counter softener
- Medication administration record (MAR)
- Otoscope (optional)

STEP	RATIONALE
ASSESSMENT	
1 Review health care provider's medication order, including solution to be instilled and affected ear(s) (right, left, or both) to receive irrigation.	Ensures safe and correct administration of medication.
2 Review medical record for history of ruptured tympanic membrane, placement of myringotomy tubes, or surgery of the auditory canal.	These conditions contradict irrigation.
3 Inspect pinna and external auditory meatus for redness, swelling, drainage, abrasions, and presence of cerumen or foreign objects.	Findings provide baseline to monitor effects of medication or solution.
a Always attempt to remove foreign objects in ear by first simply straightening ear canal.	This may cause object to fall out.

Clinical Decision Point If vegetable matter (such as a dried bean or pea) is occluded in the canal, do not perform irrigation. The material can swell on contact with water and cause further damage to the canal.

STEP	RATIONALE
4 Use otoscope to inspect deeper portions of auditory canal and tympanic membrane.	Verifies if tympanic membrane is intact.
5 Ask if patient is experiencing discomfort, using a scale of 0 to 10. Note patient's ability to hear clearly.	Pain is symptomatic of external ear infection or inflammation. Occlusion of auditory canal by cerumen or foreign object can impair hearing.
6 Review patient's knowledge of purpose for irrigation and normal care of ears.	May indicate need for instruction regarding hygiene.

NURSING DIAGNOSES
- Deficient knowledge (regarding purpose for irrigation)
- Pain (acute or chronic)
- Risk for injury

Related factors are individualized based on patient's condition or needs.

STEP	RATIONALE

PLANNING

1 Expected outcomes following completion of procedure:	
• Patient denies pain during instillation.	Fluid is properly instilled.
• Patient demonstrates hearing conversation more clearly in affected ear.	Obstruction in ear canal is resolved.
• Patient is able to discuss purpose of irrigation and describe correct ear-care techniques.	Feedback reflects patient's learning.
• Patient's canal is clear of cerumen, foreign material, and discharge.	Inflammation, irritation, and occlusion of canal are relieved.
2 Check accuracy and completeness of each MAR with health care provider's written medication or procedure order. Check patient's name, drug name and dosage, route of administration, and time for administration. Compare MAR with label of ear irrigation solution.	The order sheet is the most reliable source and only legal record of drugs or procedure that patient is to receive. Ensures that patient receives correct medication.
3 If patient is found to have impacted cerumen, instill 1 to 2 drops of mineral oil or over-the-counter softener into ear twice a day for 2 to 3 days before irrigation.	Loosens cerumen and ensures easier removal during irrigation.
4 Explain procedure. Warn that irrigation may cause sensation of dizziness, ear fullness, and warmth.	Prepares patient to anticipate effects of irrigation and promotes cooperation.

IMPLEMENTATION

1 Identify patient using two identifiers (i.e., name and birthday or name and account number) according to agency policy. Compare identifiers in MAR/medical record with information on patient's identification bracelet and/or ask patient to state name.	Ensures correct patient. Complies with The Joint Commission standards and improves patient safety (TJC, 2012).
2 Perform hand hygiene and arrange supplies at bedside.	Reduces transfer of microorganisms; helps nurse perform procedure smoothly.
3 Close curtain or room door.	Maintains privacy.
4 Help patient to sitting or lying position with head turned toward affected ear. Place towel under patient's head and shoulder and have patient, if able, hold emesis basin under affected ear.	Position minimizes leakage of fluids around neck and facial area. Solution will flow from ear canal to basin.
5 Pour prescribed irrigating solution into basin. Check temperature of solution by pouring small drop on your inner forearm. NOTE: If sterile irrigating solution is used, sterile basin is required.	
6 Apply clean gloves. Gently clean auricle and outer ear canal with gauze or cotton balls. Do *not* force drainage or cerumen into ear canal.	Prevents infected material from reentering ear canal. Forceful instillation of solution into occluded canal can cause injury to eardrum.
7 Fill irrigating syringe with solution (approximately 50 mL).	Enough fluid is needed to provide a steady irrigating stream.
8 For adults and children over 3 years old, gently pull pinna up and back. In children 3 years or younger, pinna should be pulled down and back (Hockenberry and Wilson, 2011). Adults can lie supine. Place tip of irrigating device just inside the external meatus. Leave space around irrigating tip and canal.	Pulling pinna straightens external ear canal. Prevents obstruction of canal with device, which can lead to increased pressure on tympanic membrane.
9 Slowly instill irrigating solution by holding tip of syringe 1 cm (½ inch) above opening to ear canal. Direct fluid toward superior aspect of ear canal. Allow it to drain out into basin during instillation. Continue until canal is cleaned or solution is used (see illustration).	Slow instillation prevents buildup of pressure in ear canal and ensures contact of solution with all canal surfaces.

STEP	RATIONALE

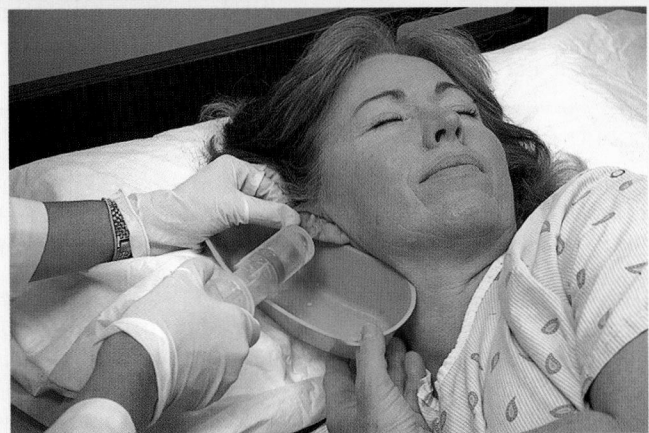

STEP 9 Tip of syringe does not occlude ear canal during irrigation.

10 Maintain flow of irrigation in steady stream until pieces of cerumen flow from canal.	Constant flow of fluid loosens cerumen.
11 Periodically ask if patient is experiencing pain, nausea, or vertigo.	Symptoms indicate that irrigating solution is too hot or too cold or instilled with too much pressure.
12 Drain excessive fluid from ear by having patient tilt head toward affected side.	Excess fluid may promote microorganism growth.
13 Dry outer ear canal gently with cotton ball. Leave cotton ball in place for 5 to 10 minutes.	Drying prevents buildup of moisture that can lead to otitis externa.
14 Help patient to a sitting position.	Maintains comfort.
15 Remove gloves, dispose of supplies, and perform hand hygiene.	Reduces transmission of infection.

EVALUATION

1 Ask patient if discomfort is noted during instillation of solution.	Fluid instilled improperly under pressure causes discomfort.
2 Ask patient about sensations of light-headedness or dizziness.	Instillation of fluid into ear can cause some light-headedness or dizziness, which can put patient at risk for falling.
3 Reinspect condition of meatus and canal.	Determines if solution relieves symptoms and removes foreign materials.
4 Measure patient's hearing acuity.	Determines if conduction deafness is relieved.
5 Ask patient to describe purpose of irrigation and proper techniques for ear care.	Reflects patient's understanding of procedure and proper hygiene.

Unexpected Outcomes	Related Interventions
1 Patient complains of increased ear pain during irrigation.	• Rupture of eardrum may have occurred. Stop irrigations immediately and notify health care provider immediately.
2 Ear canal remains occluded with cerumen.	• Repeat irrigation.
3 Foreign body remains in ear canal.	• Refer patient to otolaryngologist if foreign object remains after irrigation.
4 Patient is unable to explain ear-care practices.	• Repeat instruction and have patient explain and/or demonstrate procedure. • Include family members or caregivers if possible.

Recording and Reporting

- Record in nurses' notes, EHR, and/or MAR the procedure, amount of solution instilled, time of administration, and ear receiving irrigation.
- Record appearance of external ear and patient's hearing acuity in nurses' notes and EHR.
- Report adverse effects/patient response and/or withheld drugs to nurse in charge or health care provider.

Special Considerations
Teaching

- Instruct patient that cerumen has an antibacterial effect that maintains an acid pH in the auditory canal.
- Instruct patients to clean ears daily with a washcloth, soap, and warm water.
- Warn patients against placing objects (including cotton swabs) in ears.

Pediatric

- When cleaning the ear of a small child, be certain that child's head is immobilized to prevent puncturing eardrum. It may be necessary to have child's parent or staff participate.

Home Care

- Instruct patient to use a clean bulb syringe for irrigation. Mineral oil drops or over-the-counter otic preparations can help with removal of cerumen.

SKILL 19-3   Care of Hearing Aids

Hearing is vital for normal communication and orientation to sounds in the environment. Hearing loss is the most common sensory deficit in older adults (Adams-Wendling et al., 2008). When hearing loss occurs, it is difficult to hear doorbells, car horns, sirens, and alarms. According to the National Institute on Deafness and other Communication Disorders (2010), hearing loss affects 36 million people. In addition, 50% of residents in assisted-living and residential facilities are hearing impaired (Cacchione, 2010; Wallhagen and Pettengill, 2008). Only one out of five people who actually need a hearing aid wear one. Those who do not wear a hearing aid often say that it is because of the quality of sound that the aid produces.

Any hearing loss has social implications, and the person may not engage in social activities. There are also many safety considerations. Not only do people with hearing loss have difficulty hearing car horns and emergency sirens; they also have difficulty understanding patient education and, as a result, may not safely manage their symptoms or therapies.

For people with hearing loss, a proper hearing aid improves the ability to hear and understand spoken words. Hearing aids amplify sound so it is heard at a more effective level. All hearing aids have four basic components:

1 A microphone, which receives and converts sound into electrical signals
2 An amplifier, which increases the strength of the electrical signal
3 A receiver, which converts the strengthened signal back into sound
4 A power source (batteries)

In addition, programmable hearing aids are now available. The programmable hearing aids are in analog and digital formats. Digital technology uses a tiny processor to convert the sound before it is amplified (Kuk et al., 2010). This allows the signal to be analyzed to remove background nose and automatically adjust the volume. Patients seeking these aids need to be evaluated by a licensed audiologist to determine the type of aid and which frequencies are needed for an individual patient. These aids are adjusted to accommodate the range of a patient's residual hearing. Programmable aids independently amplify high-frequency (soft-spoken consonants) from low-frequency (loudly spoken vowels) sounds; this process occurs rapidly and continuously (Ebersole et al., 2008). Several styles of hearing aids are available to patients today (Table 19-1).

It is a challenge to adjust one's communication style to accommodate a patient with a hearing impairment. Use patient as a resource for communication techniques that are generally helpful. Be sure that a patient can see your face; speak slowly in a normal tone; and rephrase rather than repeat if he or she cannot understand you. Also remember that a patient is unable to hear alerts such as fire alarms or overhead announcements.

Hearing aids are usually worn only while a patient is awake and are cleaned as needed after removal. Remember that a hearing aid is delicate and must be protected from moisture, heat, and breakage.

Delegation and Collaboration

This skill of caring for a hearing aid can be delegated to nursing assistive personnel (NAP). The nurse directs the NAP to:

- Report ear pain, inflammation, drainage, odor, or changes in hearing.
- Identify alternative ways to communicate with a patient while the aid is not in use.
- Learn how to carefully handle the aid to prevent damage or injury.

Equipment

- ❏ Soft towel and washcloth
- ❏ Facial tissues
- ❏ Brush or wax loop
- ❏ Storage case
- ❏ Warm water and soap
- ❏ Spare battery, size depends on aid (*optional*)
- ❏ Clean gloves (if drainage present)

STEP	RATIONALE

ASSESSMENT

STEP	RATIONALE
1 Determine whether patient can hear clearly with hearing aid by talking slowly and clearly in normal tone of voice.	Inability to hear may indicate a problem with the hearing aid or battery or that that particular model is no longer effective for patient.
2 Ask if patient is able to manipulate and hold hearing aid or observe patient insert aid independently.	Determines level of assistance required in care.
3 Assess if hearing aid is working by removing from patient's ear. Close battery case and turn volume slowly to high. Cup hand over hearing aid. If you hear a squealing sound (feedback), it is working. If no sound is heard, replace batteries and test again.	May indicate malfunctioning of hearing aid.
4 Determine patient's usual hearing aid–care practices.	Provides information as to how patient cares for device and identifies patient preferences.

TABLE 19-1 | Types of Hearing Aids

Type	Advantages	Disadvantages	Cautions
In-the-ear (ITE) hearing aids fit completely in the outer ear and are used for mild-to-severe hearing loss.	Design of the aid can improve sound transmission through telephone calls.	ITE aids are damaged by earwax and ear drainage, and their small size can cause adjustment problems and feedback.	Not usually worn by children because the casings need to be replaced as the ear grows
Behind-the-ear (BTE) hearing aids are worn behind the ear and are connected to a plastic earmold that fits inside the outer ear.	Sound travels through the earmold into the ear. People of all ages wear BTE aids for mild-to-profound hearing loss.	Poorly fitting BTE earmolds can cause feedback, a whistling sound caused by the fit of the hearing aid.	May not be appropriate for children or adults who are active in sports because of potential for damage of the device
Completely-in-canal (CIC) aids are customized to fit the size and shape of the ear canal.	Used for mild to moderately severe hearing loss and are largely concealed in the ear canal.	Because of their small size, canal aids may be difficult for the user to adjust and remove and may not be able to hold additional devices such as a telecoil.	Expensive and not recommended for children Can also be damaged by earwax and ear drainage
Digital hearing aids	Digital aids analyze sounds to remove background noise; Program for low- and high-frequency sounds.	Need to be programmed and adjusted by a licensed audiologist.	Digital aids can also be damaged by earwax and ear drainage.

(Used with permission of GN Resound. All rights reserved.)

STEP	RATIONALE
5 Assess patient for any unusual physical or auditory signs/symptoms (pain, itching, redness, discharge, odor, tinnitus, decreased acuity).	May indicate injury, infection, or cerumen accumulation.
6 Inspect earmold for cracked or rough edges.	Poorly fitting hearing aids cause irritation and/or discomfort to external ear canal.
7 Inspect for accumulation of cerumen around aid and plugging of opening in aid.	Cerumen can block sound reception (U.S. National Library of Medicine, 2011c).
8 Assess patient's knowledge of and routines for cleaning and caring for hearing aid.	Determines compliance with and knowledge of self-care.

STEP	RATIONALE

NURSING DIAGNOSES

- Risk for situational low self-esteem
- Deficient knowledge regarding hearing aid care
- Impaired verbal communication
- Risk for injury

Related factors are individualized based on patient's condition or needs.

PLANNING

STEP	RATIONALE
1 Expected outcomes following completion of procedure: • Patient verbalizes comfort after removal and reinsertion of hearing aid. • Patient responds appropriately to normal conversation and environmental sounds. • Patient demonstrates proper care of hearing aid.	Hearing aid is removed or inserted properly and positioned correctly. Hearing aid and batteries are operational. Aid is secure and unobstructed. Learning is achieved.
2 Discuss procedure with patient. Explain all steps before removing aid.	Patient can assist in planning by explaining additional tips for care. Patient may be confused or anxious if verbal instructions are given after removal of hearing aid.
3 Assemble supplies at bedside. Place towel over work area.	Provides easy access to supplies. Towel catches aid if accidentally dropped and avoids breakage.
4 Have patient assume supine, side-lying, or sitting position in bed or chair.	Provides easy access for nurse. Promotes patient comfort.

IMPLEMENTATION

STEP	RATIONALE
1 Removing and cleaning hearing aid (perform Steps a through g for both ears if bilateral aids are present: **a** Perform hand hygiene. Apply clean gloves if drainage is present.	Reduces transmission of microorganisms.
b Turn hearing aid volume off, usually by turning volume control to left or toward patient's nose. Grasp aid securely and gently remove device following natural ear contour.	Prevents feedback (whistling) during removal. Prevents dropping hearing aid. Prevents injury to ear.

Clinical Decision Point *Some ITC and CIC devices have no volume control but are turned off by opening the battery door. Ask patient if this is necessary. CIC devices have a clear plastic, fiber handle for removal. Firmly grasp handle and gently pull straight out.*

STEP	RATIONALE
c Hold aid over towel and wipe exterior with tissue to remove cerumen.	Prevents breakage if dropped. Cerumen may irritate canal and interfere with fit.
d Inspect all openings in aid for accumulated cerumen. Carefully remove cerumen with wax loop or other device supplied with hearing aid.	Cerumen may block sound from receiver. Cerumen may block pressure equalization channel and create feeling of ear pressure. Makeshift tools may damage hearing aid.

Clinical Decision Point *The pressure equalization channel is a tiny hole through the entire length of the earmold and should be clear for the entire length. The receiver points into the ear through another opening. It is easily damaged. NEVER insert anything into the receiver port!*

STEP	RATIONALE
e Inspect earmold for rough edges or any frays in cords.	May irritate ear canal.
f Open battery door, place hearing aid in labeled storage container, and allow it to air dry.	Allows drying of internal components. Protects against breakage and loss.
g Assess ear for redness, tenderness, discharge, or odor.	Signs may indicate injury or infection.
h Place towel beneath patient's ear(s). Wash ear canal(s) with washcloth moistened in soap and water. Rinse and dry.	Absorbs excess water. Removes cerumen from ear canal. Removes soap residue and water that may harbor microbes or damage aid.
i Dispose of towels, remove gloves, and perform hand hygiene.	Reduces transmission of microorganisms.
j If storing hearing aid, place it in dry storage case with desiccant material. Label case with patient's name and room number. If more than one aid, note right or left. Indicate in patient's medical record where aid is stored.	Protects hearing aid against damage, moisture, and breakage. Documents how and where hearing aid is stored.
2 Inserting hearing aid (perform Steps a through g if bilateral aids are present): **a** Perform hand hygiene and apply clean gloves if patient has ear drainage.	Reduces transmission of microorganisms.

STEP	RATIONALE
b Remove hearing aid from storage case, and check battery (see assessment). Check that volume is off.	
c Identify hearing aid as either right (marked "R" or red color coded) or left (marked "L" or blue color coded).	Proper orientation prevents damage and injury.
d When possible, allow patient to insert aid. Otherwise hold hearing aid with thumb and index finger of dominant hand so canal (long portion with holes) is at bottom. Insert pointed end of earmold into ear canal. Follow natural ear contours to guide aid into place.	Prevents dropping. Proper positioning prevents injury. Pulling on ear may distort canal and make insertion more difficult.
e Anchor any separate pieces, as in case of BTE aid or body aid.	Prevents pieces from falling and breaking.
f Adjust or have patient adjust volume gradually to comfortable level for talking to patient in regular voice 3 to 4 feet away. Rotate volume control toward nose to increase volume and away from nose to decrease volume.	Gradual adjustment prevents discomfort and injury to ear.
g Close and store case. Perform hand hygiene.	Preserves desiccant. Prevents loss. Reduces transmission of microorganisms.

EVALUATION

1 Ask patient to rate level of comfort after removal or insertion.	Verifies proper technique and positioning.
2 Observe patient during normal conversation and in response to environmental sounds.	Verifies that aid is operational, correctly positioned, unobstructed, and effective.
3 Observe patient removing, cleaning, and reinserting hearing aid.	Assesses patient's understanding of and ability to perform techniques.

Unexpected Outcomes

1 Patient is unable to hear conversations or environmental sounds. Patient's verbal responses are inappropriate.

2 Patient experiences discomfort or pain, inflammation, drainage, or odor from affected ear.

3 Patient lacks knowledge and/or skills to perform hearing aid care properly.

Related Interventions

- Check function, type, and placement of battery and replace it if indicated.
- Increase volume if adjustable.
- Inspect aid and ear canal for cerumen blockage.
- Refer to audiologist for reassessment.
- Remove aid and inspect for sharp or rough edges. Refer to provider for repair.
- Assess ear for signs of injury or infection.
- Confirm R or L. Reposition hearing aid (pain).
- Teach patient and home care provider hearing aid–care skills.
- Provide written instructions and brochures with needed information.

Recording and Reporting

- Record removal of hearing aid, storage location if not reinserted after cleaning, and patient's preferred communication techniques. If family takes aid home, be sure that this information is in the patient's medical record.
- Report any signs or symptoms of infection or injury or sudden decrease in hearing acuity.

Special Considerations
Teaching

- Batteries are toxic if swallowed; keep them away from pets and children.
- Patients should insert the aid after their hair is dried and any hair spray applied. Heat from the hair dryer or perfumes and hair spray can damage the aid.
- Dogs in particular and cats are attracted to the smell of used hearing aids. Advise patient to protect the hearing aids and their pets by properly storing the aids out of reach.
- Encourage patients to identify helpful communication tips and teach them to others. Many patients find facial cues informative. Speakers must:

1 Face patient, stay within 3 to 4 feet away, and keep hands away from mouth.
2 Get patient's attention before speaking.
3 Rephrase rather than repeat when a patient cannot understand.
4 Reduce background noise or move to a quiet area.

Pediatric

- Children are more often fitted with BTE hearing aids because the ear canal is still growing.
- The aid is made less conspicuous with hair styling or becomes a statement of fashion and personality with a brightly colored or transparent case.
- Children need help to prevent acoustic feedback (whistling), which they are unable to hear. This is usually eliminated by removing and reinserting the device and making sure that no hair is caught between the earmold and canal or lowering the volume of the device (Hockenberry and Wilson, 2011).

Gerontologic

- Advise patient to protect the hearing aid from water, alcohol, hair spray or cologne, perspiration, rain, and snow and to avoid exposing the hearing aid to extremes of temperature.

- Encourage patient to store hearing aids and batteries with desiccant or in an electronic dryer to prolong life, minimize repairs, and preserve batteries.
- The small size of some hearing aids may make them difficult to manipulate, particularly for individuals with decreased dexterity or visual acuity. Consult an audiologist to identify an aid that accommodates a patient's particular need.

Home Care
- Determine presence and willingness of caregiver to perform necessary care of hearing aid.
- Assess patient's home and determine need for special precautions given patient's limited hearing.

Critical Thinking Exercises

Mr. Kupec is married and enjoys a socially active life. He and his wife have two grown children who are married with children. He has worn bilateral-in-the-ear (ITE) hearing aids for the last 10 years. He knows how to care for his aids. He is comfortable with them and is satisfied with the assistance they provide. He notes that, when the aids are working well, he hears his family and coworkers clearly, has minimal distortion in large gatherings, and is able to distinguish emergency sirens and car horns when he is driving.

1 Mr. Kupec now complains of diminished hearing in the left ear and senses drainage from the ear. The nurse decides to check the functioning of the hearing aid. Place the following steps in appropriate order for cleaning the hearing aid.
   a Wash ear canal.
   b Place hearing aid in storage case.
   c Apply clean gloves.
   d Grasp aid securely and remove from ear following natural ear contour.
   e Use brush to clean holes in the aid.
   f Have patient turn hearing aid volume off.
      1 f, d, c, a, b, e
      2 c, f, d, e, a, b
      3 c, f, d, a, e, b
      4 f, d, c, e, a, b
2 Mr. Kupec's preschool grandchildren visit frequently and are curious about the hearing aids. Which safety concerns for preschool children should the nurse teach him? (Select all that apply.)
   1 Batteries are toxic if swallowed.
   2 Tell the children to face grandpa.
   3 Keep batteries and aids out of children's reach.
   4 Show the children how the aid fits in the ear.
3 What would you teach Mr. Kupec and his wife about these aids?

REVIEW QUESTIONS

1 A patient who wears contact lenses in both eyes is scheduled for hand surgery and will have her hand in a cast for 6 weeks. What is the priority nursing diagnosis for this patient?
   1 Anxiety
   2 Self–health management
   3 Imbalanced nutrition: less than body requirements
   4 Disturbed personal identity
2 A patient is being discharged following care for severe conjunctivitis related to noncompliance with the prescribed lens care regimen. Which patient statement indicates a need for further teaching?
   1 "I should discard my open lens care solutions when I get home."
   2 "Cloudy solutions should be discarded even if they haven't expired."
   3 "Plain soap is the best thing for washing my hands before I touch my contacts."
   4 "I'm switching to disposable contacts so I won't have to worry about getting another infection."

3 A nurse who wears contact lenses splashes rubbing alcohol into his right eye. What is the priority action to take?
   1 Carefully remove the contact lens from the affected eye
   2 Gently cover the eye with a comfortable patch
   3 Test the pH of the secretions with litmus paper
   4 Irrigate the eye with water or prescribed solution
4 A patient is being discharged home after having an enucleation and an artificial eye placed. Which statement by a patient indicates a need for further teaching?
   1 "I'll clean the eye at least once a week."
   2 "I should use sterile saline for cleaning the eyes."
   3 "The colored dot is there to show me which way to put it in."
   4 "Rubbing alcohol and fingernail polish remover are bad for the eye."
5 The nurse is caring for a patient who is hearing impaired. Which approach(es) by the nurse is/are most appropriate to best facilitate communication? (Select all that apply.)
   1 Speaking slightly more loudly than usual
   2 Speaking slightly more slowly using a normal tone
   3 Standing so patient can see the nurse's face
   4 Using hand gestures to help explain what is being said.
6 The nurse is performing a neurologic assessment on a patient with an artificial eye. How would the nurse confirm identification of the natural eye?
   1 Only the natural eye would produce tears and lubrication.
   2 The artificial eye would have more natural movement.
   3 The artificial eye would respond slightly to a light stimulus.
   4 Accommodation would only be present in the natural eye.
7 A patient has just received a new hearing aid and instruction about its care. Which statement by a patient indicates a need for further teaching?
   1 "I need to store my hearing aid batteries away from my children and dogs."
   2 "I need to keep hair spray and cologne away from the hearing aid."
   3 "I can blow dry my hair while wearing my hearing aid."
   4 "I need to store my hearing aid and batteries with a desiccant."
8 A patient with bilateral hearing aids is experiencing some discomfort in his right ear. What should the nurse do for this patient initially?
   1 Ask if he understands how to care for his hearing aids
   2 Check his ears for any signs of irritation
   3 Teach him how to reposition his hearing aids if they are uncomfortable
   4 Reduce the volume of the hearing aid in his left ear
9 The nurse is caring for a comatose patient. What is the most important nursing responsibility pertaining to the patient's eye care?
   1 Performing frequent eye irrigations to remove secretions
   2 Gently securing his eyelids with paper tape
   3 Checking for the pupillary response
   4 Preventing injury to the patient's corneas
10 A patient calls the nurse at the health care provider's office about increasing pain in her left ear. What should be the nurse's initial response?
   1 "Clean your ears daily with soap and water."
   2 "Try to get as much earwax out of your ear as possible."
   3 "Put a drop or two of mineral oil in your left ear."
   4 "Tell me more about the ear pain you're having."

REFERENCES

Adams-Wendling L, et al: Evidence-Based Guideline—Nursing management of hearing impairment in nursing facility residents—The University of Iowa College of Nursing Gerontological Nursing Interventions Research Center, *J Gerontol Nurs* 34(11):9, 2008.

American Optometric Association: *What you need to know about contact lens hygiene and compliance*, available at http://www.aoa.org/documents/AOA-Contact-lens-hygiene.pdf, 2011, accessed May 2011.

Babineau MR, Sanchez LD: Ophthalmologic procedures in the emergence department, *Emerg Clin North Am* 26:17, 2008.

Cacchione PZ: Sensory changes and aging, *Insight* 35(2):24, 2010.

Cao LK, et al: Hand/face/neck localized pattern: sticky problem: resins, *Dermatol Clin* 27:227, 2009.

Center for Ocular Prosthetics: *Custom made artificial plastic eyes*, available at www.artificialeyesplastic.com/new-eye-care.htm, accessed December 2011.

Chou R, et al: *Screening for hearing loss in adults ages 50 years and older: A review of the evidence for the U.S. preventive Services Task Force*, Rockville, MD, 2011, Agency for Health Care Research and Quality.

Ebersole P, et al: *Toward healthy aging*, ed 7, St Louis, 2008, Mosby.

Erickson Laboratories: *Prosthetic care*, available at www.ericksonlaboratories.com/care.html, accessed December 2011.

Galanti GA: *Caring for patients from different cultures*, ed 4, Philadelphia, 2008, University of Pennsylvania Press.

Goiato MC, et al: Mobility, aesthetic, implants, and satisfaction of the ocular prostheses wearers, *J Craniofacial Surg* 21(1):160, 2010.

Hockenberry MJ, Wilson D: *Wong's nursing care of infants and children*, ed 9, St Louis, 2011, Mosby.

Kraszewski S: Safe and effective ear irrigation, *Nurs Stand* 22(43):45, 2008.

Kolberg Ocular Prosthetics: *Artificial eye information and patient support page*, 2011, available at http://www.artificialeye.net, accessed December 2011.

Kuk F, et al: *Digital wireless hearing aids. Part 1. A primer*, 2010, available at http://www.hearingreview.com/issues/articles/2010-03_09.asp, accessed July 2012.

Marshall AP, et al: Eye care in the critically ill: clinical practice guideline, *Aust Crit Care* 21:97, 2008.

McDonnall MC: Risk factors for depression among older adults with dual sensory loss, *Aging Mental Health* (13):569, 2009.

McDonnall MC: The effect of productive activities on depressive symptoms among older adults with dual sensory loss, *Res Aging* 33(3):234–255, 2011.

National Institute on Deafness and Other Communication Disorders: *Quick statistics*, 2010, available at http://www.nidcd.nih.gov/health/statistics/Pages/quick.aspx, accessed December 2011.

Oh EG, et al: Factors related to incidence of eye disorders in Korean patients at intensive care units, *J Clin Nurs* 18:29, 2008.

Rodrigues Z: Irrigation of the eye after alkaline and acid burns, *Emerg Nurse* 17(8):26, 2009.

Rosenberg JB, Eisen LA: Eye care in the intensive care unit: narrative review and meta-analysis, *Crit Care Med* 36(12):3151, 2008.

Saunders G; Echt, K: Dual sensory impairment in an aging population, *The ASHA Leader* 2011.

So HM, et al: Comparing the effectiveness of polyethylene covers (Glad® wrap) with lanolin (Duratears) eye ointment to prevent corneal abrasions in critically ill, *Int J Nurs Studies* 45:1565, 2008.

Smith SL, et al: Prevalence and characteristics of dual sensory impairment (hearing and vision) in a veteran population, *J Rehab Res Devel* 45(4):597–610, 2008.

Swann J: Understanding visual and hearing loss, *Nurs Residential Care* 10(4):195, 2008.

The Joint Commission (TJC): *National Patient Safety Goals*, Oakbrook Terrace, Ill, 2012, The Commission, available at http://www.jointcommission.org/standards_information/npsgs.aspx.

US National Library of Medicine: Medline Plus: Ear Emergencies, 2011a, available at http://www.nlm.nih.gov/medlineplus/ency/article/000052.htm, updated December 14, 2011, accessed December 2011.

US National Library of Medicine: Medline Plus: *Eye emergencies*, 2011b, available at http://www.nlm.nih.gov/medlineplus/ency/article/000054.htm, updated December 14, 2011, accessed December 2011.

US National Library of Medicine: Medline Plus: *Wax blockage*, 2011c, updated December 14, 2011, available at http://www.nlm.nih.gov/medlineplus/ency/article/000979.htm, accessed December 2011.

Wallhagen MI, Pettengill E: Hearing Impairment—significant but under assessed in primary care settings, *J Gerontol Nurs* 34(2):36, 2008.

Safe Medication Preparation

MEDIA RESOURCES

- evolve http://evolve.elsevier.com/Perry/skills
  learning system
  - Review Questions
  - Audio Glossary

- NSO Nursing Skills Online

KEY TERMS

Adverse drug events (ADEs)	Medication tolerance	Peak concentration	Summation
Anaphylaxis	NPO	Pharmacokinetics	Synergistic effect
Duration of action	Onset of medication action	Plateau	Therapeutic effect
Idiosyncratic reaction	Over-the-counter (OTC)	Polypharmacy	Toxic effects
Medication administration	medication	prn	Trough concentration
record (MAR)	Parenteral	Serum half-life	Unit-dose system
Medication dependence	Peak action	Side effect	Verbal order
Medication reconciliation			

OBJECTIVES

Mastery of content in this chapter will enable the nurse to:
- Discuss National Patient Safety Goals for medication administration.
- Discuss factors that contribute to medication errors.
- Discuss the types of medication actions.
- List and discuss the six rights of medication administration.

- Identify the system of measurement for a given prescribed medication.
- Accurately calculate medication doses.
- Describe the safety features of medication delivery systems.
- Identify guidelines for safe administration of medications.
- Identify steps to take in reporting medication errors.

Safe and accurate medication administration is a challenging and important nursing responsibility. A nurse is responsible for having a full understanding of medication administration and the related nursing implications. The Institute of Medicine (IOM) (2000) published the book *To*

Err Is Human: Building a Safer Health System, which created a national awareness of problems within the health care system. It is estimated that approximately 1.5 million preventable adverse drug events (ADEs) occur annually, costing more than $3.5 billion (Macdonald, 2010). The IOM has a national agenda for reducing medical errors and improving patient safety. One essential IOM recommendation is to develop standards for patient safety to establish minimum levels of performance and set expectations for health professionals. The Institute for Safe Medicine Practices (ISMP) also developed strategies to prevent harm from "high-alert medications" such as anticoagulants, sedatives, narcotics, and insulin (ISMP, 2011a). In addition, the National Quality Forum (NQF) includes a recommendation for safe medication practice that all health care organizations develop, reconcile, and communicate accurate patient medication information throughout the continuum of care (NQF, 2010).

Many factors contribute to medication errors, especially at patient care-transition points such as during hospital admission, transfer from one unit to another, and discharge to home or another agency (LaMantia et al., 2010). Almost 37% of total medication errors are related to errors of administration (Anderson and Townsend, 2010). In a recent study nurses identified factors contributing to medication errors such as being unfamiliar with the drug, the need for advanced drug preparation, and failure to recheck a medication before administration. Other factors included workload, miscommunication around verbal orders, clinician miscommunication, and not being alert while checking medications (Kim et al., 2011). In many cases drug errors occur as a result of failure of nurses to follow policy (Shane, 2009). Nurses need to make clinical judgments when administering medications and not simply give drugs automatically. This includes thorough patient assessment and an understanding of pharmacokinetics, growth and development, nutrition, and mathematics.

The Joint Commission (TJC) defines a medication error as any preventable event that may cause inappropriate medication use or jeopardize patient safety (TJC, 2012a). Medication errors include inaccurate prescribing; administering the wrong medication, route, and time interval; and administering extra doses or failing to administer a medication. Medication safety is always one of the National Patient Safety Goals (TJC, 2012b) (Box 20-1).

All professional nurses need to understand the implications involved in medication administration. Safe medication administration requires good judgment and clinical decision-making skills. Registered nurses (RNs) and licensed practical nurses (LPNs) are able to administer medications under the direction of a licensed physician and according to State Practice Acts. Advanced practice nurses (APNs) have some prescriptive authority in almost every state, but the degree of required physician involvement varies.

NSO *Safe Medication Administration Module / Lesson 1*

PATIENT-CENTERED CARE

A nurse's responsibility when administering medications safely must include effective communication with staff, pharmacy, patients, and family caregivers. Patients are an important resource for understanding the knowledge they have about their medications, their perceptions about the effects of medications, and their expectations for treatment. Consider factors that influence patient's abilities to communicate effectively such as anxiety, pain, hearing, or their cultural background. Therapeutic communication is essential to nursing practice.

A new scientific field, pharmacogenetics, involves the study of the genetic influence on drug response that occurs from inherited metabolic defects or deficiencies. As a nurse you cannot detect a genetic abnormality. However, you can learn to become aware of cultural differences in drug responses to better monitor drug therapy.

| BOX 20-1 | The Joint Commission 2012 Hospital National Patient Safety Goals: Implications for Medication Administration |

- Identify patients correctly.
- Use at least two patient identifiers (neither can be patient's room number) when providing care, treatment (e.g., medications), or services.
- Improve the effectiveness of communication among caregivers.
- Verbal or telephone orders require a verification "read-back" of the complete order or test result by the person receiving the order/test result.
- Standardize a list of abbreviations, acronyms, symbols, and dose designations that are *not* to be used throughout an organization.
- Improve the safety of using medications.
- Identify and at a minimum annually review a list of look-alike/sound-alike drugs used by the organization.
- Before a procedure, label all medications and medication containers (e.g., syringes, medicine cups) that are not labeled. Do this in areas where medicines and supplies are set up, such as on and off the sterile field in perioperative and other procedural settings. Labels include drug name, strength, amount, expiration date when not used within 24 hours, and expiration time when expiration occurs in less than 24 hours.
- Take extra care with patients who take anticoagulants. Use only oral unit-dose products and premixed infusions. When heparin is administered intravenously and continuously, use programmable infusion pumps.
- Maintain and communicate accurate patient medication information.
- Accurately and completely reconcile medications across the continuum of care.
- There is a process for comparing the patient's current medications with those ordered for the patient while under the care of the health care organization.
- Communicate a complete list of the patient's medications to the next provider of service when a patient is referred or transferred to another setting, service, or level of care. Also provide the complete list to the patient on discharge from the agency.
- Encourage patients' active involvement in their own care as a patient safety strategy.

Modified from The Joint Commission: *2012 National Patient Safety Goals*, Oakbrook Terrace, IL, 2012, The Commission, available at http://www.jointcommission.org/standards_information/npsgs.aspx.

Culturally a patient's values and beliefs affect medication response. A patient's level of education, prior experience with medication therapy, and the family's influence on actions significantly influence medication adherence. For example, in some cultures it is not acceptable to complain about gastrointestinal problems; thus it is common for patients not to report nausea, vomiting, and bowel changes related to medication use. Use of herbal and homeopathic remedies in some cultures alters response to a medication. Ethnicity needs to be considered when medications are prescribed and administered.

PHARMACOLOGIC CONCEPTS

Medication Names

Some medications have as many as three different names. The chemical name describes the drug composition and molecular structure, such as N-acetyl-para-aminophenol, commonly known as Tylenol. The chemical name provides an exact description of its composition and molecular structure. It is rarely used in clinical practice. A manufacturer who first develops a medication provides the generic name (e.g., acetaminophen is the generic name for Tylenol). The generic name is the official name that is listed in official publications such as the *United States Pharmacopeia* (USP). A medication trade name or brand name is used to market the medication. The trade name has the symbol™ at the upper right of the name, indicating a manufacturer trademark of the name (e.g., Panadol™, Tempra™, Tylenol™).

Many companies choose brand and generic names that are easy to remember and can be very similar, which contributes to medication errors. The USP identifies several problematic medications with similar names and spelling such as Lamictal for epilepsy and Lamisil for fungal infections; Levoxine for hypothyroidism and Lanoxin for heart failure; Zebeta for hypertension and Diabeta for type 2 diabetes. The ISMP (2010a) and TJC (2012a) both publish a list of medications that are frequently confused with one another. Another measure to help address the confusion around drugs having similar names includes the use of tall-man lettering (ISMP, 2011b). This measure uses capital letters in specific parts of a word and helps distinguish dissimilarities in drug names; for example, TEGretol (for seizures) can be confused with ([TRENtal), which is prescribed for intermittent claudication; but the tall-man letters emphasize the difference in the drug name).

The physical appearances of some drugs with similar color, size, and shape have led to medication errors. For example, St. Joseph's aspirin and Crestor, a lipid-lowering agent, have a similar peach color, size, and circular shape. Generic drugs are often prescribed as a more cost-efficient substitution for brand-name medications. However, there may be dramatic differences in appearance of generic drugs, depending on the manufacturer (Greene et al., 2011). Patients may be confused as to why their medication has a different color or shape when the prescription is refilled. Hospital and clinic pharmacies try to consistently dispense medications with the same trade names so nurses will become familiar with them. However, nurses find medications under a variety of different names and must be careful to obtain the exact name and spelling before administering a medication. TJC (2012a) publishes on its website (http://www.jointcommision.org) a look-alike/sound-alike drug list and recommendations for nurses, prescribers, and health care organizations to prevent mixing up look-alike/sound-alike medications.

Classification

Medications with similar characteristics are categorized by their class. Medication classification indicates the effect of a medication on a body system, the symptoms the medication relieves, or the desired effect of the medication. For example, patients with type 2 diabetes often take oral hypoglycemic medications to control their blood glucose levels. The sulfonylureas are one classification of 11 medications used to treat hyperglycemia. Many adults with type 2 diabetes are treated with more than one class of diabetic medication (Bennett et al., 2011). Some medications are part of more than one class. For example, aspirin is an analgesic, antipyretic, and antiinflammatory medication.

Medication Forms

Medications are available in a variety of forms or preparations. The form of the medication determines its route of administration. The composition of a medication influences its absorption and metabolism. Many medications are made in several forms such as tablets, caplets, or suppositories. When administering a medication, be certain to use the proper form (Table 20-1).

Pharmacokinetics

A medication must enter a patient's body; be absorbed and distributed to cells, tissues, or a specific organ; and then alter physiologic function to be therapeutic. Pharmacokinetics is the study of how medications enter the body, reach their site of action, are metabolized, and exit the body. Understanding pharmacokinetics allows you to properly time medication administration, select an administration route, and judge a patient's response to medications. Absorption is the passage of medication molecules into the blood from the site of administration. Factors that influence the rate of absorption include the administration route, ability of a medication to dissolve, blood flow to the administration site, body surface area, and lipid solubility of a medication (Table 20-2). After a medication is absorbed, it is distributed to tissues and organs and finally to the site of drug action. The rate and extent of distribution depends on circulation, cell membrane permeability, and protein binding. Poor perfusion (e.g., heart failure) alters medication distribution. A medication must pass through biologic membranes to reach certain organs. Some membranes are barriers to the passage of medications. For example, the blood-brain barrier allows only fat-soluble medications to pass into the brain and cerebrospinal fluid. The degree to which medications bind to serum proteins such as albumin affects distribution. Most medications bind to albumin to some extent. When this happens, they are unable to exert pharmacologic activity. Only the unbound, or "free," medication is active. Older adults and patients with liver disease or malnutrition have reduced albumin, which increases their risk for medication toxicity.

After a medication reaches its site of action, it becomes metabolized into a less active or inactive form. Biotransformation occurs under the influence of enzymes that detoxify, degrade (break down), and remove biologically active chemicals. Most biotransformation occurs in the liver, although the lungs, kidneys, blood, and intestines also play a role. Patients (e.g., older adults and those with chronic disease) are at risk for medication toxicity if their organs cannot metabolize medications effectively.

The final aspect of pharmacokinetics is excretion, the process by which medications exit the body through the lungs, exocrine glands, bowel, kidneys, and liver. The chemical makeup of a medication determines the organ of excretion. For example, gaseous and volatile compounds such as alcohol and nitrous oxide exit through the lungs. The site of excretion poses implications for nursing care. For example, when medications exit through sweat glands, you provide skin care to reduce irritation. You must know if a drug is excreted through the intestines because the administration of laxatives or enemas increases peristalsis, accelerates excretion, and thus lessens the time for drug effects. When patients have reduced renal function, they are at risk for medication toxicity since kidneys are the main organs for medication excretion.

TYPES OF MEDICATION ACTION

Medications vary in the way they act and their types of action. Patients do not always respond in the same way to each successive dose of a medication. Sometimes the same medication causes very different responses in different patients. Therefore it is essential to understand all the effects that medications have on patients.

Therapeutic Effects

Each medication has a therapeutic effect, the intended or desired physiologic response of a medication. For example, you administer morphine sulfate, an analgesic, to relieve a patient's pain. Sometimes a single medication has many therapeutic effects. For

TABLE 20-1	Forms of Medication
Form	**Description**
Medication Forms Commonly Prepared for Administration by Oral Route	
Solid Forms	
Caplet	Shaped like a capsule and coated for ease of swallowing
Capsule	Medication encased in a gelatin shell
Tablet	Powdered medication compressed into a hard disk or cylinder; in addition to primary medication, contains binders (adhesive to allow powder to stick together), disintegrators (to promote table dissolution), lubricants (for ease of manufacturing), and fillers (for convenient tablet size)
Enteric coated	Coated tablet that does not dissolve in stomach; coating dissolves in intestine, where medication is absorbed
Liquid Forms	
Elixir	Clear fluid containing water and alcohol; often sweetened
Extract	Syrup or dried form of pharmacologically active medication, usually made by evaporating solution
Aqueous solution	Substance dissolved in water and syrups
Suspension	Finely dissolved drug particles in liquid medium must be shaken When left standing, particles settle to bottom of container
Syrup	Medication dissolved in concentrated sugar solution
Tincture	Alcohol extract from plant or vegetable
Other Oral Forms and Terms Associated With Oral Preparations	
Troche (lozenge)	Flat, round tablet that dissolves in mouth to release medication; not meant for ingestion
Aerosol	Aqueous medication sprayed and absorbed in mouth and upper airway; not meant for ingestion
Sustained release	Tablet or capsule that contains small particles of a medication coated with material that requires a varying amount of time to dissolve
Medication Forms Commonly Prepared for Administration by Topical Route	
Ointment (salve or cream)	Semisolid, externally applied preparation, usually containing one or more medications
Liniment	Usually contains alcohol, oil, or soapy emollient applied to skin
Lotion	Liquid suspension that usually protects, cools, or cleans skin.
Paste	Medication preparation that is thicker than ointment; absorbed through skin more slowly than ointment; often used for skin protection
Transdermal patch or disk	Disk or patch embedded with medication that is applied to skin Drug absorbed through the skin over a designated period of time
Medication Forms Commonly Prepared for Administration by Parenteral Route	
Solution	Sterile preparation that contains water/normal saline with one or more dissolved compounds
Powder	Sterile particles of medication that are dissolved in a sterile liquid (e.g., water, normal saline) before administration
Medication Forms Commonly Prepared for Instillation Into Body Cavities	
Suppository	Solid dosage form mixed with gelatin and shaped in form of a pellet for insertion into body cavity (rectum or vagina) (Suppository melts when it reaches body temperature and is then absorbed.)
Intraocular disk	Small, flexible oval (similar to a contact lens) consisting of two soft outer layers and a middle layer containing medication; slowly releases medication when moistened by ocular fluid.

example, aspirin relieves pain and reduces fever and tissue inflammation. Knowing the desired therapeutic effect for each medication allows you to provide patient education and accurately evaluate its desired effect.

Side Effects/Adverse Effects

Every medication has the potential to harm a patient. No medication is totally safe and absolutely free of nontherapeutic effects. Side effects are predictable and often unavoidable secondary effects produced at a usual therapeutic drug dose. They are either harmless or cause injury. The intensity of side effects is often dose

dependent. If the side effects are serious enough to outweigh the benefits of the therapeutic action of a medication, the prescriber will likely discontinue the medication. Patients commonly stop taking medications because of side effects such as anorexia, nausea, vomiting, dizziness, drowsiness, dry mouth, constipation, and diarrhea. Report any side effect to the prescriber to ensure that it is not incorrectly interpreted as a more serious adverse medication reaction.

Adverse drug events or effects (ADEs) are unintended, undesirable, and often unpredictable. Unfortunately, although they sometimes are apparent immediately, they often take weeks or months

TABLE 20-2	Medication Absorption
Absorption Factor	**Physiologic Effects**
Route of administration	Topical applications on skin absorb slowly. Medications applied to mucous membranes and respiratory airways absorb quickly. Oral medications pass through the gastrointestinal tract and absorb slowly. The intravenous route absorbs most rapidly.
Ability to dissolve	Solutions and liquid suspensions absorb more readily than tablets or capsules. Acidic medications absorb rapidly, whereas basic medications (pH >7.0) do not absorb before reaching the small intestine.
Blood flow	When the administration site contains a rich blood supply, medications absorb rapidly.
Body surface area	A medication in contact with a large surface area (e.g., small intestine) absorbs faster than one in contact with smaller surface area (e.g., stomach).
Lipid solubility	Medications that are highly lipid soluble absorb more readily.

TABLE 20-3	Mild Allergic Reactions
Symptom	**Description**
Urticaria (hives)	Raised, irregularly shaped skin eruptions with varying sizes and shapes; reddened margins and pale centers
Eczema (rash)	Small, raised vesicles that are usually reddened; often distributed over the entire body
Pruritus	Itching of the skin; accompanies most rashes
Rhinitis	Inflammation of mucous membranes lining the nose, causing swelling and a clear watery discharge

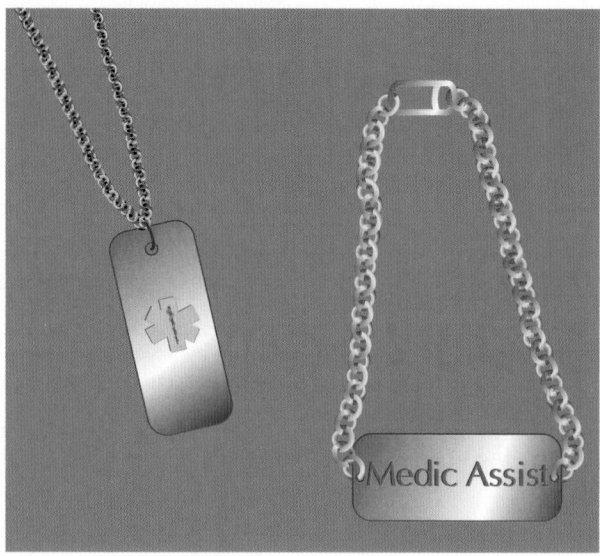

FIG 20-1 Identification bracelet and medal.

to develop. Early clinical recognition of ADEs is the important first step in identification. ADEs range from mild (e.g., rashes or photosensitivity to light) to potentially fatal (anaphylaxis). Prompt recognition and reporting of ADEs prevents serious injury to patients. Always assess patients who may be at high risk for an ADE such as pregnant women and patients with chronic disorders (e.g., hypertension, epilepsy, heart disease, psychoses) (Lehne, 2010). Health care providers report adverse events to the Food and Drug Administration (FDA) using the MedWatch program (USFDA, 2010).

Toxic Effects

Toxic effects develop after prolonged intake of a medication or when a medication accumulates in the blood because of impaired metabolism or excretion. Excess amounts of a medication within the body sometimes have lethal effects, depending on the action of the medication. For example, toxic levels of morphine, an opioid, cause severe respiratory depression and death. Antidotes are available to treat specific types of medication toxicity. For example, naloxone (Narcan), an opioid antagonist, reverses the effects of opioid toxicity.

Idiosyncratic Reactions

Medications sometimes cause unpredictable effects such as an idiosyncratic reaction, in which a patient overreacts or underreacts to a medication or has a reaction different from normal. Predicting which patients will have an idiosyncratic response is impossible. For example, lorazepam (Ativan) is an antianxiety medication that may cause agitation and delirium when given to an older adult.

Allergic Reactions

Allergic reactions also are unpredictable responses to a medication. Exposure to an initial dose of a medication causes a patient to become sensitized immunologically. The medication acts as an antigen, which causes antibodies to be produced. With repeated administration a patient develops an allergic response to the drug, its chemical preservatives, or a metabolite. An allergic reaction ranges from mild to severe, depending on the patient and the

medication (Table 20-3). Among the different classes of medications, antibiotics cause a high incidence of allergic reactions. Severe or anaphylactic reactions, which are life threatening, are characterized by sudden constriction of bronchiolar muscles, edema of the pharynx and larynx, severe wheezing, and shortness of breath. Some patients become severely hypotensive, necessitating emergency resuscitation measures.

It is common practice for hospitalized patients with known drug allergies to have their allergy information recorded in a clearly identifiable place. This allows all caregivers to be aware of each patient's allergies. In many agencies this information is recorded on the front of a patient's medical record, in the medication administration record (MAR), or on a specially designed label that is applied to the front of a patient's chart. Patients also receive color-coded allergy identification bands to wear around the wrist. *Always record a patient's allergies in the MAR.* Patients who are cared for in other settings (e.g., home or community clinics) and have a known history of an allergy to a medication or substance should wear an identification bracelet or medal, which alerts all health care providers to the allergies in case a patient is found unconscious or is unable to communicate (Fig. 20-1).

Medication Tolerance and Dependence

Medication tolerance occurs over time. It is usually noted clinically when patients receive the same medication for long periods and require higher doses to produce the desired therapeutic effect.

Medications known to produce tolerance include opium alkaloids (e.g., morphine), nitrates, and ethyl alcohol. Patients hospitalized for acute episodes of illness usually do not develop tolerance. It may take a month or longer for tolerance to occur.

Medication tolerance is not the same as medication dependence. Two types of medication dependence exist: physical or psychological (or addiction). In psychological dependence the patient desires the medication for benefit other than the intended effect. Physical dependence is a physiologic adaptation to a medication that manifests itself by intense physical disturbance when the medication is withdrawn. When patients receive medications for a short term such as for postoperative pain, dependence is rare. If a patient is dependent on alcohol, a higher-than-usual medication dose is necessary for the desired effect of the medication.

Medication Interactions

When one medication modifies the action of another medication, a medication interaction occurs. Medication interactions are common in individuals taking many medications. Some medications increase or diminish the action of other medications and alter the way in which another medication is absorbed, metabolized, or eliminated from the body. When two medications have a synergistic effect, their combined effect is greater than the effect of one drug given separately. For example, alcohol is a central nervous system depressant that has a synergistic effect with antihistamines, antidepressants, and narcotic analgesics. Sometimes a medication interaction is the desired effect. Prescribers often combine medications to create an interaction that has a therapeutic effect. For example, a patient with hypertension may receive several medications such as diuretics and vasodilators, which act together to control the blood pressure when one medication alone is not effective.

Medication Dose Responses

After administration a medication undergoes absorption, distribution, metabolism, and excretion. Except when administered intravenously, medications take time to enter the bloodstream. When a medication is prescribed, the goal is a constant blood level within a safe therapeutic range. The minimum effective concentration (MEC) is the plasma level of the medication below which the effect of the medication does not occur. The toxic concentration is the level at which toxic effects occur. The safe therapeutic range is between the MEC and the toxic concentration (Fig. 20-2). When a medication is administered repeatedly, its serum level fluctuates between doses. The highest level is called the *peak concentration*, and the lowest level is called the *trough concentration*. After peaking the serum concentration falls progressively. With intravenous (IV) infusions, the peak concentration occurs quickly, but the serum level also begins to fall immediately. Some medication doses (e.g., vancomycin or gentamicin [Garamycin]) are based on peak and trough serum levels. A patient's trough level is drawn as a blood sample 30 minutes before administering the drug, and the peak level is drawn whenever the drug is expected to reach its peak concentration. The results of the blood test reveal if the drug is reaching its therapeutic blood level.

All medications have a biologic half-life, which is the time it takes for excretion processes to lower the serum medication concentration by half. To maintain a therapeutic plateau, a patient needs to receive regular fixed doses. For example, current evidence shows that pain medications are most effective when they are given around-the-clock (ATC) rather than when the patient intermittently complains of pain because the body maintains an almost constant level of pain medication. After an initial medication dose,

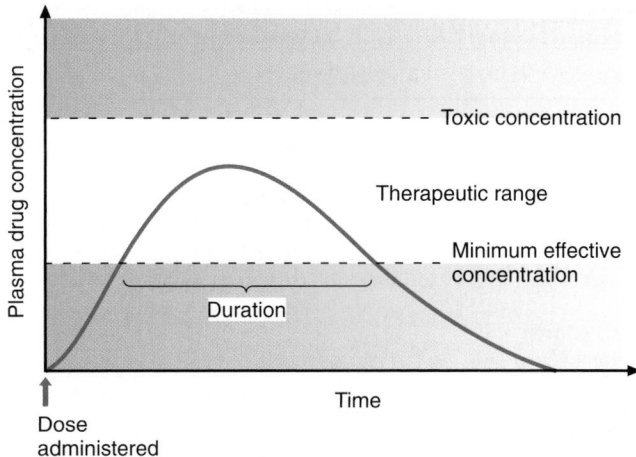

FIG 20-2 The therapeutic range of medication occurs between the minimum effective concentration and the toxic concentration. (*From Lehne R:* Pharmacology for nursing care, *ed 7, St Louis, 2010, Saunders.*)

the patient receives each successive dose when the previous dose reaches its half-life. The patient and nurse need to follow regular dosage schedules and administer prescribed doses at correct intervals. Know the following time intervals of medication action to anticipate the effect of a medication:

1 *Onset of medication action:* Period of time it takes after you administer a medication for it to produce a therapeutic effect
2 *Peak action:* Time it takes for a medication to reach its highest effective peak concentration
3 *Trough:* Minimum blood serum concentration of medication reached just before the next scheduled dose
4 *Duration of action:* Length of time during which a medication is present in a concentration great enough to produce a therapeutic effect
5 *Plateau:* Blood serum concentration reached and maintained after repeated, fixed doses

ROUTES OF ADMINISTRATION

The route prescribed for administering a medication (Table 20-4) depends on its properties and desired effect and on a patient's physical and mental condition. Because of what you know about your patients, you need to collaborate with a prescriber in determining the best route for a patient's medical condition. Table 20-5 summarizes the factors that influence the choice of administration routes.

MEDICATION DISTRIBUTION

Health care providers write medication orders, pharmacists dispense medications, and nurses deliver medications to patients. A number of technologies for medication distribution have the potential for reducing medication errors and ADEs. The technologies include computerized provider order entry (CPOE), automated medication dispensing system (AMDS), and bar coding (Agrawal, 2009; Poon et al., 2010). The use of the AMDS may reduce the chance of medication errors (Agrawal, 2009).

Computerized Provider Order Entry

CPOE is a system that allows prescribers to electronically enter orders for medications, eliminating the need for written orders.

TABLE 20-4	Routes of Medication Administration
Route	**Description**
Nonparenteral	
Oral, buccal	By mouth
Sublingual	Under the tongue
Topical	On the skin (as a cream or patch) and eyedrops/eardrops
Suppository	Into the rectum or vagina
Parenteral	
Intramuscular (IM)	Into a muscle
Subcutaneous	Into the subcutaneous tissue of the skin
Intradermal (ID)	Into the dermis of the skin
Epidural	Into the epidural space
Intravenous (IV)	Into a vein

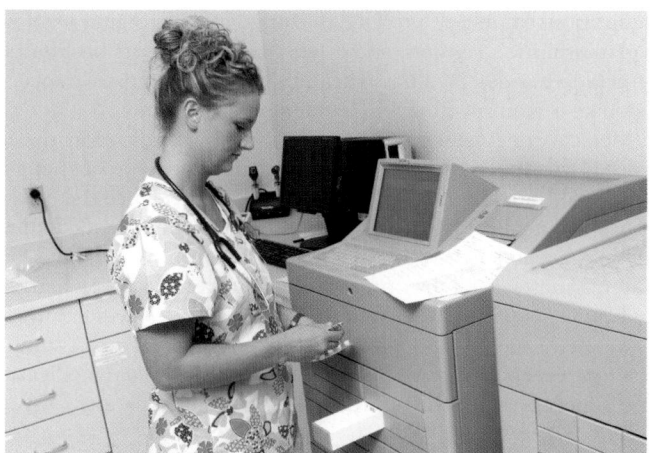

FIG 20-3   Automated medication dispensing system.

With use of CPOE, there is increased accuracy and legibility of medication orders; integration of clinical decision support into the order-entry process; and optimization of prescriber, nurse, and pharmacist time (Agrawal, 2009). Decision support software integrated into a CPOE system allows for automatic drug allergy checks, dosage indications, baseline laboratory result checks, and identification of potential drug interactions. When a prescriber enters an order through CPOE, the information about the order immediately transmits to the pharmacy and ultimately to the nurses' MAR without the need for written transcription. Use of CPOE systems may significantly reduce medication errors as much as 55% to 83% (Agrawal, 2009).

Distribution Systems

Systems for storing and distributing medications vary. Agencies providing nursing care have special areas for stocking and dispensing medications. Special medication rooms, portable locked carts, computerized medication cabinets, and individual storage units next to patients' rooms are examples of storage areas used. Medication storage areas must be locked when unattended.

Unit Dose

The standard for medication distribution is the unit-dose system. The system uses an AMDS or carts containing a drawer with a 24-hour supply of medications for each patient. Each drawer has a label with the name of the patient in the designated room. The unit dose is the ordered dose of medication that the patient receives at one time. Each medication form is wrapped in a foil or paper container separately. Liquid doses come in prepackaged foil or plastic cups. The cart also contains limited amounts of prn and stock medication for special situations. At a designated time each day the pharmacist or a pharmacy technician refills the drawers in the cart with a fresh supply. Controlled substances are not in the individual patient drawer; they are in a larger locked drawer to keep them secure. A unit-dose system is designed to reduce the number of medication errors and saves steps in dispensing medications.

Automated Medication Dispensing System

AMDSs are variations of unit-dose and floor stock systems (Fig. 20-3). The systems within the health care agency are networked with one another and with other computer systems in the agency (e.g., computerized medical record). AMDSs control the dispensing of all medications, including narcotics. Each nurse has a security code, which allows access to the system. If your agency uses a system that requires bioidentification, you have to place your finger on a screen to access the computer. Once logged onto the AMDS, you select a patient's name and medication profile. Then you select the medication, dosage, and route from a list displayed on the computer screen. The system opens the medication drawer or dispenses the medication to the nurse, records the event, and charges it to the patient. If the system is connected to the patient's medical record, information about the medication (e.g., name, dose, time) and the name of the nurse who retrieved it from the AMDS is recorded in the patient's medical record. There is evidence of an increase in reported medication errors with use of the system and a reduction in dispensing errors through the use of alerts that are embedded within the clinical decision support system (Agrawal, 2009). The use of AMDS has been shown to reduce the chance of medication errors (Agrawal, 2009).

Bar Coding

Bar-code labels are required on all medications, vaccines, and over-the-counter (OTC) drugs used in health care agencies (Poon et al., 2010). Electronic health record (EHR) technology is used to improve patient care quality and coordination and increase patient access to information in a secure format. The use of electronic bar codes on medication labels and packaging has the potential to improve patient safety in a number of ways. Bar codes electronically link with a hospital computer system. A patient's MAR entered into the computer database and encoded in the patient's wristband is accessible to a nurse through a handheld device. The device scans the patient's wristband and then displays the MAR. When administering a medication, the nurse scans the bar code on the drug and the patient's medical record number on the wristband. The computer processes the scanned information, charts it, and updates the patient's MAR record appropriately (Poon et al., 2010). The use of bar codes improves accuracy of patient identification, correct medication use, and improves medical record keeping (Poon et al., 2010).

SYSTEMS OF MEDICATION MEASUREMENT

NSO *Safe Medication Administration Module / Lesson 3*

The proper administration of medication depends on your ability to compute medication doses accurately and measure medications

TABLE 20-5	Factors Influencing Choice of Administration Routes

Advantages	Disadvantages/Contraindications
Oral, Buccal, Sublingual Routes	
Routes are easy and comfortable to administer, convenient, economical; may produce local or systemic effects; and rarely cause anxiety for patient.	Routes are avoided when patient has alterations in GI function (e.g., nausea and vomiting), with reduced GI motility (after general anesthesia or bowel inflammation), and with surgical resection of portion of GI tract.
	Gastric secretions destroy some medications. Oral administration is contraindicated in patients who are NPO and unable to swallow (e.g., patients with neuromuscular disorders, esophageal strictures, and mouth lesions).
	Do not give oral medications when patient has gastric suction or before certain diagnostic tests or surgery.
	An unconscious or confused patient is unable or unwilling to swallow or hold sublingual medication under tongue or buccal medication in cheek.
	Oral medications sometimes irritate lining of GI tract, discolor teeth, or have an unpleasant taste.
Subcutaneous, Intramuscular, Intravenous, Intradermal, Epidural Routes	
Routes provide means of administration when oral medications are contraindicated. More rapid absorption occurs than with topical or oral routes.	There are risks for introducing infection, and medications are expensive. Some patients experience pain from repeated needlesticks. Avoid Subcutaneous, IM, and ID routes in patients with bleeding tendencies.
	There is risk for tissue damage with subcutaneous injections.
IV infusion provides medication delivery when patient is critically ill or long-term therapy is necessary. If peripheral perfusion is poor, IV route is preferred over injections.	IV and IM routes have higher absorption rates, thus placing patients at higher risk for reactions.
Epidural provides excellent pain control.	It limits mobility during administration, and there is risk for infection.
Skin	
Topical	
Topical skin applications provide primarily local effect. Route is usually painless. Limited side effects occur.	Extensive applications often require dressings that are bulky for a patient when maneuvering.
	Do not apply to skin if abrasions are present, unless that is the reason for order.
	Medications can be absorbed by person applying them if gloves are not worn.
Transdermal	
Transdermal applications provide prolonged systemic effects with limited side effects.	Application leaves oily or pasty substance on skin and may soil clothing. Some patients have sensitivity to adhesive.
Mucous Membranes (Includes Eyes, Ears, Nose, Vaginal, Rectal, Buccal, and Sublingual Routes)	
Therapeutic effects are provided by local application to involved sites. Aqueous solutions are readily absorbed and capable of causing systemic effects.	Mucous membranes are highly sensitive to some medication concentrations.
	Insertion of rectal and vaginal medications often causes embarrassment.
Mucous membranes provide route of administration when oral medications are contraindicated.	Rectal suppositories are contraindicated if patients have had rectal surgery or if active rectal bleeding is present.
	If eardrum is ruptured, otic medications are usually contraindicated.
Inhalation	
Inhalation provides rapid relief for local respiratory problems. An inhaled form of insulin is also available. Route provides easy access for introduction of general anesthetic gases.	Some local agents cause serious systemic effects.
	If patients are unable to administer inhaler correctly, medication is ineffective.
	Inhalation is difficult to learn for older adults and children.
Intraocular Disk	
Route is advantageous in that it does not require frequent administration (e.g., as for eyedrops). Patient can also wear disk when sleeping or swimming. Dry eyes do not affect medication delivery.	Local reactions such as tearing, itching, or redness of the eyes occur.
	Patient needs to know how to insert disk into and remove from eye.
	Medication is often expensive.
	Medication is contraindicated in patients with eye infections.

GI, Gastrointestinal; *ID*, intradermal; *IM*, intramuscular; *IV*, intravenous; *NPO*, nothing by mouth.

correctly. A careless mistake in placing a decimal point or adding a zero to a dosage can lead to fatal errors. The prescriber and patient depend on you to check doses before administering medications. Medication therapy uses metric, apothecary, and household systems of measurement. The apothecary system is used infrequently today. The most common medication measurement system is the metric system.

Metric System

As a decimal system the metric system is the most logically organized of the measurement systems. Metric units are easy to convert and compute through simple multiplication and division. Each basic unit of measure is organized into units of 10. Multiplying or dividing by 10 forms secondary units. In multiplication the decimal point moves to the right; in division the decimal moves to the left. For example:

$$10 \text{ mg} \times 10 = 100 \text{ mg}$$

$$10 \text{ mg} \div 10 = 1 \text{ mg}$$

The basic units of measure in the metric system are the meter (length), the liter (volume), and the gram (weight). For drug calculations you will primarily use volume and weight units. In the metric system lowercase or capital letters designate the basic units:

$$\text{Gram} = g \text{ or } Gm$$

$$\text{Liter} = l \text{ or } L$$

Use only lowercase letters for abbreviations for subdivisions of major units:

$$\text{Milligram} = mg$$

$$\text{Milliliter} = mL$$

When writing medication dosages in metric units, prescribers and nurses use either fractions or multiples of a unit. Convert fractions to decimals:

$$500 \text{ mg or } 0.5 \text{ g, not } \frac{1}{2} \text{ g}$$

$$10 \text{ mL or } 0.01 \text{ L, not } \frac{1}{100} \text{ L}$$

Many actual or potential medication errors happen with the use of fractions or decimal points. Use practice standards when medications are ordered in fractions to prevent errors. For example, never use a trailing zero (e.g., 1.0 mg) and always include a zero before a decimal point (e.g., 0.1 mL) (ISMP, 2010b; TJC, 2012a).

Household Measurement

Household measures are familiar to most people, but these are not recommended for medication administration because of the variability in the size of household utensils. Household measures include drops, teaspoons, tablespoons, and cups for volume and ounces and pounds for weight. When the accuracy of a medication dose is not critical (e.g., OTC medications), it is safe to use household measures. To calculate medications accurately, you need to know common equivalents of metric and household units (Table 20-6).

TABLE 20-6	Equivalents of Measurement	
Metric	**Apothecary**	**Household**
1 mL	15-16 minims (m)*	15 drops (gtt)
5 mL	1 dram*	1 teaspoon (tsp)
15 mL	4 drams*	1 tablespoon (tbsp)
30 mL	1 fluid ounce	2 tablespoon (tbsp)
240 mL	8 fluid ounces	1 cup (c)
480 mL (approximately 500 mL)	1 pint (pt)	1 pint (pt)
960 mL (approximately 1 L)	1 quart (qt)	1 quart (qt)
3840 mL (approximately 4 L)	1 gallon (gal)	1 gallon (gal)

*Minims and drams are no longer acceptable units of measure for medication administration, although some medication cups and syringes still have them listed. Use mL for safe medication administration.

Solutions

Solutions of various concentrations are used for injections, irrigations, and infusions. A solution is a given mass of solid substance dissolved in a known volume of fluid or a given volume of liquid dissolved in a known volume of another fluid. Solutions are available in units of mass per units of volume (e.g., g/mL or g/L). You can also express the concentration of a solution as a percentage. A 10% solution is 10 g of solid dissolved in 100 mL of solution. A proportion also expresses concentrations. A 1/1000 solution represents a solution containing 1 g of solid in 1000 mL of liquid or 1 mL of liquid mixed with 1000 mL of another liquid.

SAFE MEDICATION ADMINISTRATION

Standards are actions that help ensure safe nursing practice. Standards for medication administration are set by health care agencies and the nursing profession. Most agencies have procedure manuals that contain policies about which medications nurses can and cannot deliver. The types and dosages that nurses may administer often vary from unit to unit within an agency. Professional standards such as *Nursing: Scope and Standards of Practice* (ANA, 2010) apply to the activity of safe medication administration. To prevent medication errors follow the six rights of medication administration consistently every time you administer medications. Many medication errors are linked in some way to an inconsistency in adhering to the six rights:

1 The right medication
2 The right dose
3 The right patient
4 The right route
5 The right time
6 The right documentation

Right Medication

A medication order is required for every medication that you administer to a patient. Some prescribers write orders by hand in a patient's chart. However, many agencies use CPOE, eliminating the need for handwritten orders and enhancing patient safety (Sowan et al., 2010). Regardless of how an order is received, you compare the prescriber's orders with the MAR or electronic MAR (eMAR) when the medication is ordered initially. Nurses verify medication information whenever new MARs are written or distributed or when patients transfer from one nursing unit or health care setting to another (TJC, 2012a).

The ISMP (2010a) and TJC published a list of error-prone and prohibited abbreviations that have been found to increase the incidence of errors in medication administration (Table 20-7). You are responsible for using correct abbreviations and verifying that the order was transcribed accurately.

Medication Orders

You must have a medication order before administering medications to a patient. Verbal and telephone orders are optional forms of orders when written or electronic communication between the prescriber and nurse is not possible. When you receive a verbal or telephone order, you write or enter the order on the prescriber's order sheet. The name of the prescriber and your signature are included. The prescriber will countersign the order at a later time, usually within 24 hours after making it (see agency policy). Box 20-2 provides guidelines for safely taking verbal or telephone orders for medications.

Five common types of orders based on frequency and/or urgency of medication administration orders are: standing; prn orders; and single (one-time) orders, which include stat orders and now orders. Each order needs to include the patient's name, the drug ordered, dosage, route of administration, and time(s) of administration.

You carry out a *standing order* until the health care provider cancels it by another order or until a prescribed number of days elapse. A standing order sometimes indicates a final day or number of doses. Many agencies have a policy for automatically discontinuing standing orders.

A medication can be ordered to be given only when a patient requires or requests it. This is a prn order. You must assess a patient thoroughly to determine whether he or she needs the medication. A prn order usually has a minimum interval set for the time of administration.

Single (one-time) orders are common for preoperative medications or medications given before diagnostic procedures. The medication is ordered to be given only once at a specified time. A stat order means that you give a single dose of medication immediately and only once. Stat orders are used for emergencies when a patient's condition changes suddenly. A now order is more specific and is used when a patient needs a medication quickly but not as soon as a stat order. TJC (2012a) discourages the use of range orders for prn medications. An example of a range order is morphine sulfate 2 to 6 mg IV push every 2 to 4 hours prn for pain. Range orders are often unclear and a source of medication errors.

Once you determine that information on the patient's MAR is accurate, use the MAR to prepare and administer medications. When preparing medications from bottles or containers, *compare the label of the medication container with the MAR 3 times:* (1) before removing the container from the supply drawer or shelf, (2) as the amount of medication ordered is removed from the container, and (3) at the patient's bedside before administering the medication to the patient. Never prepare medications from unmarked containers or containers with illegible labels (TJC, 2012b). With unit-dose prepackaged medications, check the label with the MAR when taking medications out of the medication dispensing system. Finally, verify all medications at the patient's bedside with the patient's MAR and use at least two identifiers before giving the patient any medications (TJC, 2012a).

If a patient questions a medication, stop and recheck to be certain there is no mistake. An alert patient or family caregiver will know whether a medication is different from those received before. In most cases the medication order has been changed or the drug is manufactured by a different company than the patient has been using at home. However, attention to a patient's question is how errors are identified and prevented.

Right Dose

The unit-dose system is designed to minimize errors. When a medication is prepared from a larger volume or strength than needed or when the prescriber orders a system of measurement different from that which the pharmacist supplies, the chance of error increases. After calculating the doses of high-risk medications such as insulin or warfarin (Coumadin) compare the calculation with one done independently by a second nurse. This is especially important if it is an unusual calculation or involves a potentially toxic drug.

After calculating doses, prepare the medication using standard measurement devices. Use graduated cups, syringes, and scaled droppers to measure medications accurately. At home teach patients to use kitchen measuring spoons rather than teaspoons and tablespoons, which vary in volume. Key principles to observe when using measuring receptacles include:

1 Pour liquid medication into a medication cup with the cup on a flat surface at eye level so you can see the desired amount accurately. The amount of poured liquid must be even with the base of the meniscus (Fig. 20-4, A and B)
2 Pour liquid medications away from a label to ensure that liquid will not run down it, making it difficult to read
3 Draw liquid medication into a syringe (without a needle) slowly to prevent air bubbles from entering the syringe. Air displaces medications and leads to inaccurate measurement of doses

Medication errors occur when pills need to be split. To promote patient safety in inpatient settings, pharmacists split medications, label and package them, and return them to the nurse for administration. Because pill splitting can be problematic in the home, determine if a patient has the manual dexterity or visual acuity to split tablets. If possible, determine if his or her pharmacy can split the pill or encourage the health care provider to order medications that do not require splitting.

Tablets are sometimes crushed and mixed with food. Be sure to clean the crushing device completely before crushing the tablet. Remnants of previously crushed medications increase concentration of the medication or result in a patient receiving a portion of an unprescribed medication. Mix crushed medications with very small amounts of food or liquid. Do not use a patient's favorite foods or liquids because medications alter their taste and decrease

---

BOX 20-2 | **Guidelines for Verbal and Telephone Orders**

- Clearly identify patient's name, room number, and diagnosis. "Read back" all orders from the health care provider (TJC, 2012a).
- Use clarification questions to avoid misunderstandings.
- Write "TO" (telephone order) or VO (verbal order), including date and time, name of patient, and complete order; sign the name of the health care provider and nurse.
- Follow agency policies; some agencies require documentation of the "read back" or two nurses to review and sign telephone or verbal orders.
- Physician or licensed health care provider co-sign the order within the time frame required by the agency (usually 24 hours; verify agency policy).

TABLE 20-7 | Institute for Safe Medication Practice List of Error-Prone Abbreviations

These abbreviations, symbols, and dose designations were reported to the Institute for Safe Medication (ISMP) though the USP-ISMP Medication Error Reporting Program for being frequently misinterpreted and involved in harmful medication errors. They should NEVER be used when communicating medical information. This includes internal communications, telephone/verbal prescriptions, computer-generated labels, labels for drug storage bins, medication administration records, and pharmacy and prescriber computer order entry screens. The Joint Commission (TJC) has established a National Patient Safety Goal that specifies that certain abbreviations must appear on the do-not-use list of an accredited organization; these items are highlighted with a double asterisk (**).

Abbreviations	Intended Meaning	Misinterpretation	Correction
µg	Microgram	Mistaken as "mg"	Use "mcg"
AD, AS, AU	Right ear, left ear, each ear	Mistaken as OD, OS, OU (right eye, left eye, each eye)	Use "right ear," "left ear," or "each ear"
OD, OS, OU	Right eye, left eye, each eye	Mistaken as AD, AS, AU (right ear, left ear, each ear)	Use "right eye," "left eye," or "each eye"
BT	Bedtime	Mistaken as "BID" (twice daily)	Use "bedtime"
Cc	Cubic centimeters	Mistaken as "u" (units)	Use "mL"
D/C	Discharge or discontinue	Premature discontinuation of medication if D/C (intended to mean "discharge") has been misinterpreted as "discontinued" when followed by a list of discharge medications	Use "discharge" and "discontinue"
IJ	Injection	Mistaken as "IV" or "intrajugular"	Use "injection"
IN	Intranasal	Mistaken as "IM" or "IV"	Use "intranasal" or "NAS"
HS	Half-strength	Mistaken as bedtime	Use "half-strength"
hs	At bedtime, hour of sleep	Mistaken as half-strength	Use "bedtime"
IU**	International unit	Mistaken as IV (intravenous) or 10 (ten)	Use "units"
o.d. or OD	Once daily	Mistaken as "right eye" (OD—*oculus dexter*), leading to oral liquid medications administered in the eye	Use "daily"
OJ	Orange juice	Mistaken as OD or OS (right or left eye); drugs meant to be diluted in orange juice may be given in the eye	Use "orange juice"
Per os	By mouth, orally	The "os" can be mistaken as "left eye" (OS—*oculus sinister*)	Use "PO," "by mouth," or "orally"
q.d. or QD**	Every day	Mistaken as q.i.d., especially if the period after the "q" or the tail of the "q" is misunderstood as an "i"	Use "daily"
qhs	Nightly at bedtime	Mistaken as "qhr" or every hour	Use "nightly"
qn	Nightly or at bedtime	Mistaken as "qhr" or every hour	Use "nightly" or "at bedtime"
q.o.d. or QOD**	Every other day	Mistaken as q.d. (daily) or q.i.d. (4 times daily) if the "o" is poorly written	Use "every other day"
q.d.	Daily	Mistaken as q.i.d. (4 times daily)	Use "daily"
q6PM, etc.	Every evening at 6 PM	Mistaken as every 6 hours	Use "6 PM nightly" or "6 PM daily"
SC, SQ, sub q	Subcutaneous	SC mistaken as SL (sublingual); SQ mistaken as "5 every"; the "q" in "sub q" has been mistaken for "every" (e.g., a heparin dose ordered "sub q 2 hours before surgery" misunderstood as every 2 hours before surgery)	Use "subcut" or "subcutaneously"
ss	Sliding scale (insulin) or ½; (apothecary)	Mistaken as "55"	Spell out "sliding scale"; use "one-half" or "½"
SSRI	Sliding scale regular insulin	Mistaken as selective-serotonin reuptake inhibitor	Spell out "sliding scale (insulin)"
SSI	Sliding scale insulin	Mistaken as Strong Solution of Iodine (Lugol's)	Spell out "sliding scale (insulin)"
i/d	One daily	Mistaken as "tid"	Use "1 daily"
TIW or tiw	3 times a week	Mistaken as "3 times a day" or "twice a week"	Use "3 times weekly"

TABLE 20-7	Institute for Safe Medication Practice List of Error-Prone Abbreviations—cont'd		
Abbreviations	**Intended Meaning**	**Misinterpretation**	**Correction**
U or u**	Unit	Mistaken as the number 0 or 4, causing a 10-fold overdose or greater (e.g., 4U seen as 40 or 4u seen as 44); mistaken as "cc" so dose given in volume instead of units (e.g., 4u seen as 4cc)	Use "unit"
UD	As directed ("ut dictum")	Mistaken as unit dose (e.g., diltiazem 125 mg IV infusion "UD" misinterpreted as meaning to give the entire infusion as a unit [bolus] dose)	Use "as directed"

Used with permission, Institute for Safe Medication Practice (ISMP), Institute for Safe Medication Practices (ISMP): *ISMP's list of error-prone abbreviations, symbols, and dose designations*, 2010, available at http://www.ismp.org/Tools/error-proneabbreviations.pdf, accessed January 18, 2012.
**These abbreviations are included on The Joint Commission "minimum list" of dangerous abbreviations, acronyms, and symbols that must be included on the "Do Not Use" list of an organization, effective January 1, 2011.

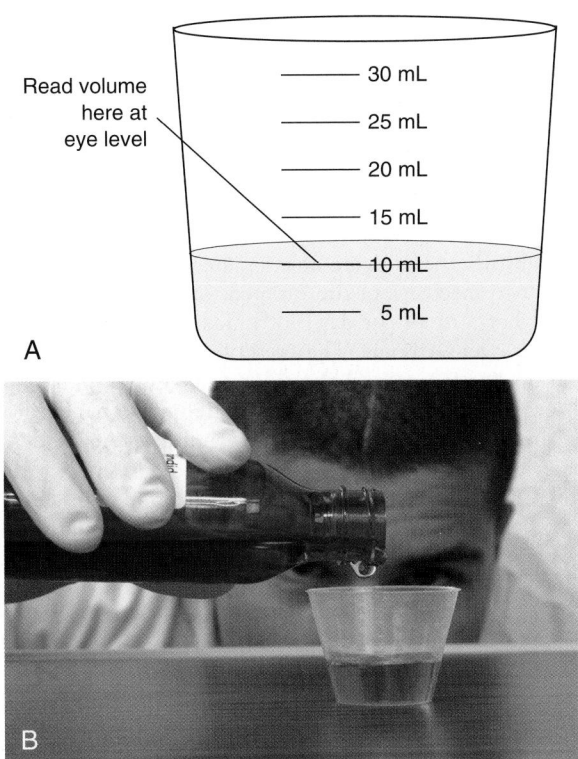

FIG 20-4 **A,** Pour desired volume of liquid so base of meniscus is level with line on scale. **B,** Place cup on flat surface and read at eye level to confirm volume poured.

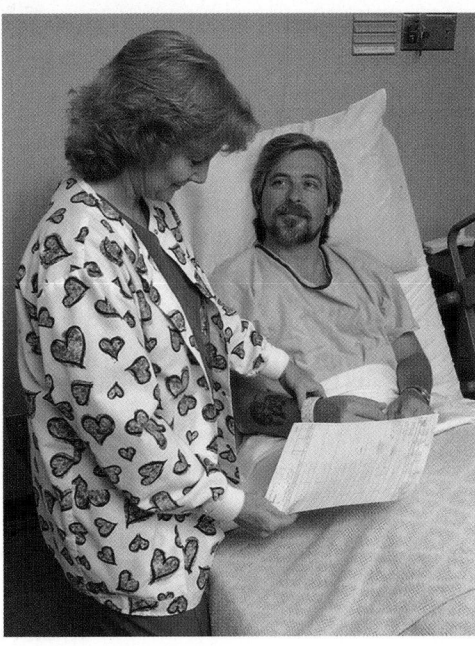

FIG 20-5 Before administering any medications, check patient's identification and allergy bracelets.

the patient's desire for them. This is especially a concern for pediatric patients. Always check to determine whether a medication can be crushed (see Chapter 21). Some medications (e.g., enteric-coated or slow-release) have special coatings to prevent them from being absorbed too quickly. These medications should not be crushed. Refer to the "Do Not Crush List" (ISMP, 2010c) to ensure that a medication is safe to crush.

Right Patient
Medication errors often occur because one patient gets a drug intended for another patient. Therefore a key step in administering medications safely is being sure that you give the right medication

to the right patient. It is difficult to remember every patient's name and face. Before giving a medication to a patient, always use at least two patient identifiers (TJC, 2012a). Acceptable patient identifiers include the patient's name, an identification number assigned by a health care agency, or date of birth. Do not use the patient's room number as an identifier. TJC (2012b) requires use of two patient identifiers when nurses administer medications. The required identification process mandates collecting patient identifiers reliably when a patient is first admitted to a health care agency. Once identifiers are assigned to a patient (e.g., putting identifiers on an armband and placing the armband on the patient), a nurse uses them to match the patient with the patient name on the MAR.

To identify a patient correctly in an acute care setting, at the patient's bedside compare the patient identifiers on the MAR with those on his or her identification bracelet (Fig. 20-5). Asking patients to state their full names and identification information

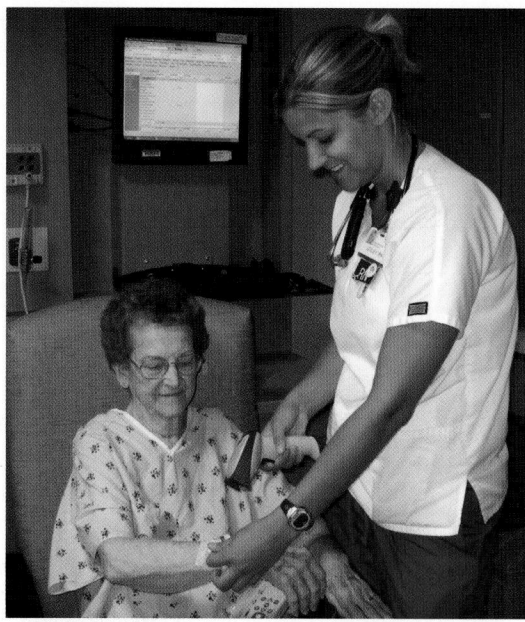

FIG 20-6   Nurse using bar-code scanner to identify patient during medication administration.

provides a third way to verify that you are giving medications to the right patient. If an identification bracelet becomes smudged or illegible or is missing, get a new one for the patient. In health care settings that are not acute care settings, TJC (2008) does not require the use of armbands for identification. However, nurses must use a system to verify the patient's identification with at least two identifiers before administering medications.

In addition to using two identifiers, some agencies use a wireless bar-code scanner to help identify the right patient (Fig. 20-6). This system requires the nurse to scan a personal bar code that is commonly placed on the nurse's name badge first. Then a bar code is scanned from the single-dose medication package. Finally the nurse scans the patient's armband. All of this information is stored in the computer for documentation purposes. The system helps prevent medication errors because it provides another step to ensure that the right patient receives the right medication.

Right Route

The prescriber's order must designate a route of administration. If the route of administration is missing or if the specified route is not the recommended route, consult the prescriber immediately. Recent evidence shows that medication errors involving the wrong route are common. For example, enteral and parenteral medications may become confused in the pediatric setting where liquid medications are frequently given orally. When oral medications are prepared in parenteral syringes, there is an increased risk of giving an oral medication through the parenteral route (ISMP, 2010d). The injection of a liquid intended for oral use produces local complications such as sterile abscess or fatal systemic effects. Medication companies label parenteral medications "for injectable use only." Label the syringe after preparing the medication and always use different syringes for enteral and parenteral medication administration (ISMP, 2010d).

Right Time

Safe medication administration involves adherence to prescribed doses and dosage schedules. Some agencies set schedules for medication administration. However, nurses are able to alter this schedule based on knowledge about a medication. For example, at some agencies medications that are taken once a day are given at 9:00 AM. However, if a medication works best when given at bedtime, the nurse administers it before the patient goes to sleep. In addition, acute care agencies use guidelines from the ISMP and Centers for Medicaid and Medicare Services (CMS, 2011; ISMP, 2011b) to determine safe, effective, and timely administration of scheduled medications. According to ISMP (2011b) and CMS (2011) guidelines, hospitals need to determine which medications are not eligible for scheduled dosing times and must be given at precise times (e.g., stat doses, first-time or loading doses, one-time doses). In addition, hospitals must determine which medications are time-critical scheduled and which are non–time-critical scheduled. With time-critical medications (e.g., antibiotics, anticoagulants, insulin, immunosuppresives), early or delayed administration of maintenance doses of more than 30 minutes before or after the scheduled dose will most likely cause harm or result in subtherapeutic responses in a patient. Non–time-critical medications include medications in which the timing of administration most likely will not affect the desired effect of the medication if the medication is given 1 to 2 hours before or after its scheduled time. Thus you administer time-critical–scheduled medications at a precise time or within 30 minutes before or after the scheduled time. You administer medications identified as non–time-critical within 1 to 2 hours of their scheduled time. Know your agency policies about the timing of medications to ensure that you administer medications at the right time (ISMP, 2011b,c).

Always know why a medication is ordered for a certain time of the day and whether you are able to alter the time schedule. For example, two medications are ordered, one q8h (every 8 hours) and the other 3 times per day. Both medications are scheduled 3 times a day over 24 hours. The prescriber intends for you to give the q8h medication around the clock to maintain its therapeutic blood levels. In contrast, you need to give the other medication during the waking hours. Each agency has a recommended time schedule for medications ordered at frequent intervals. You can alter these recommended times if necessary or appropriate.

A medication may also be ordered for special circumstances. A preoperative medication may be ordered stat (to be given immediately); now (as soon as available), usually within an hour; or on call, which means that the operating room or procedure room personnel will notify you when it is the appropriate time. Also, a medication may be given before or after meals.

Give priority to medications that must act at certain times. For example, give insulin at a precise interval before a meal. Give antibiotics on time around the clock to maintain therapeutic blood levels. Some medications require a nurse's clinical judgment in determining the proper time for administration. Administer a prn sleeping medication when the patient is ready for bed. You always document whenever there is a call to the patient's health care provider to obtain a change in a medication order.

Before discharging patients from a hospital, evaluate their medication regimen, especially if they were admitted to the hospital because of a problem with medication self-administration. A strategy to reduce medication errors at transition points is the process of medication reconciliation. Patients often leave the hospital with a basic knowledge of their medications but are unable to safely self-administer them once they return home. Help patients plan schedules based on preferred medication intervals, pharmacokinetics of the medication, and the patient's daily schedule. For patients who have difficulty remembering when to take medications, make a chart that lists the times when the patient should take each medication or prepare a special container to hold each timed dose.

Right Documentation

Accurate documentation allows nurses and other health care providers to communicate with one another and improves medication safety. Many medication errors result from inaccurate documentation. Therefore always document accurately at the time of administration and verify any inaccurate documentation before administering medications. To ensure the right documentation, first make sure that the information on your patient's MAR corresponds exactly with the prescriber's order and the label on the medication container. Written orders and medication forms must include the patient's name; the name of the ordered medication; and the medication dosage, route, and frequency. If there is any question about a medication order because it is incomplete, illegible, vague, or not understood, contact the health care provider before administering the medication.

Never document that you have administered a medication until you have actually given it. Document the name of the medication, the dose, the time of administration, and the route on the patient's MAR. Also document the site of any injections and the patient's response to medications. Your efforts to ensure proper documentation help provide safe care (Box 20-3).

MEDICATION PREPARATION

It is legally advisable to administer only the medications that you prepare. Administering a medication prepared by another nurse

BOX 20-3	Nurse's Six Rights for Safe Medication Administration
1	The right to a complete and clearly written order that clearly specifies the drug, dose, route, and frequency
2	The right to have the correct drug route and dose dispensed
3	The right to have access to drug information
4	The right to have policies on safe medication administration
5	The right to administer medications safely and identify problems in the system
6	The right to stop, think, and be vigilant when administering medications

From Hughes R: *Patient safety and quality: an evidence-based handbook for nurses,* Rockville, Md, 2008, Agency for Healthcare Research and Quality.

increases the opportunity for errors. You must perform several steps before actual administration of medications, including interpreting medication labels, converting measurement units within a system or between systems, and calculating medication doses. The importance of checking similar names and verifying the correct drug cannot be overemphasized.

Interpreting Medication Labels

Medication labels include several basic pieces of information: the trade name of the drug in large letters, the generic name in smaller letters, the form of the drug, the dosage, the expiration date, the lot number, and the name of the manufacturer (Fig. 20-7). The trade name given by the manufacturer suggests the action of the drug, and the generic name is the chemical name.

Clinical Calculation

To administer medications safely, use your mathematics skills to safely calculate dosages and mix solutions. This skill is important because medications are not always dispensed in the unit of measure in which they are ordered. Medication companies package and bottle medications in standard dosages. For example, a patient's health care provider orders 20 mg of a medication that is packaged in 40-mg vials. You are responsible for converting available units of volume and weight to the desired doses. Therefore be aware of approximate equivalents in all major measurement systems and make use of conversion tables. In addition to medication administration, nurses use volume and weight conversions in a variety of other nursing activities, including converting fluid ounces to milliliters to measure intake and output (I&O) or converting volume equivalents to calculate IV flow rates.

EVIDENCE-BASED PRACTICE

Many medication errors occur when nurses become distracted or lose focus during medication administration or fail to follow best-practice protocols and procedures related to medication administration. Research reveals that 43% of medication errors are a result of workplace distraction (Trbovich et al., 2010). Areas for medication administration preparation are highly visible locations with high levels of staff traffic (ISMP, 2009). Nurses become interrupted

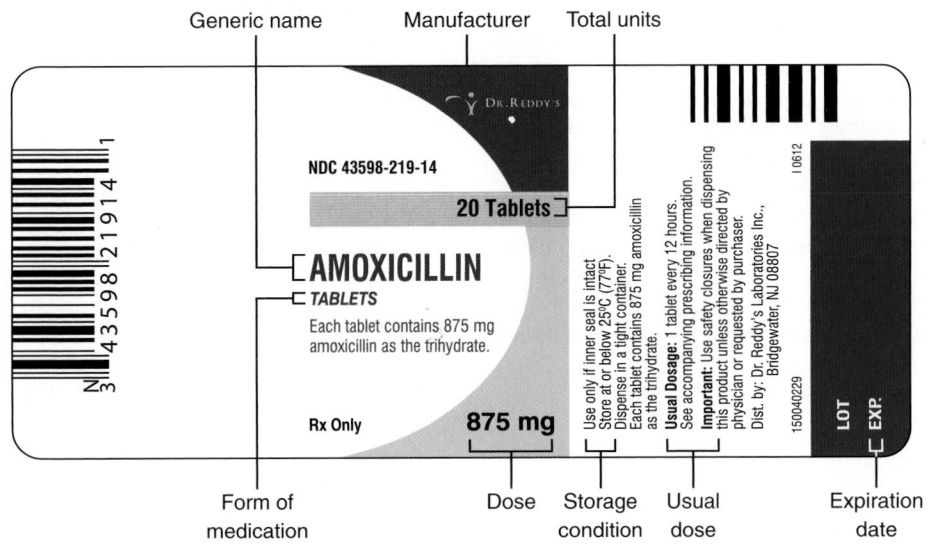

FIG 20-7   Interpreting medication label. (*Courtesy Dr. Reddy's Laboratories, Inc.*)

while accessing dispensing systems, depositing medications into delivery containers, and confirming orders on computer screens. The majority of distractions have been identified as questions from staff or family, equipment alarms, and personal conversations (Trbovich et al., 2010). Nurses need systems in place to avoid distractions to help prevent medication errors, including:

- Raising awareness of health care team members to avoid discussion during medication preparation and administration (Relihan et al., 2010).
- Reducing the number of distractions and interruptions around the automated medication dispensing machines (Anderson et al., 2010).
- Ensuring that all medication supplies are adequately stocked before the preparation phase (Relihan et al., 2010).
- In areas where medications are being prepared, using a brightly colored sign to alert staff and family to avoid interrupting the nurse who is preparing medications.
- Avoiding initiating any conversations while preparing medications and redirecting questions to another nurse or health care provider.

Conversions Within One System

Converting measurements within one system is relatively easy; simply divide or multiply in the metric system. For example, to change milligrams to grams, divide by 1000 or move the decimal three points to the left.

$$1000 \text{ mg} = 1 \text{ g}$$

$$350 \text{ mg} = 0.35 \text{ g}$$

To convert liters to milliliters, multiply by 1000 or move the decimal three points to the right.

$$1 \text{ L} = 1000 \text{ mL}$$

$$0.25 \text{ L} = 250 \text{ mL}$$

To convert units of measurement within the household system, consult an equivalency table. For example, when converting fluid ounces to quarts, you first need to know that 32 ounces is the equivalent of 1 quart. To convert 8 ounces to a quart measurement, divide 8 by 32 to get the equivalent, ¼ or 0.25 quart.

Conversion Between Systems

You will frequently determine the correct dose of a medication by converting weights or volumes from one system of measurement to another. For example, often you will convert metric units to equivalent household measures for use at home. To convert from one measurement system to another, use equivalent measurements. Tables of equivalent measurements are available in all health care agencies. The pharmacist is also a good resource.

Before making a conversion, compare the measurement system available with that ordered. For example, a prescriber orders Robitussin 30 mL, but the patient only has tablespoons at home. To provide proper instruction to the patient, you convert milliliters to tablespoons, which requires you to know the equivalency or refer to a table such as Table 20-6.

Dosage Calculations

Dosage calculations are necessary when the dose on the medication label differs from the dose ordered. There are several dose-calculation methods, including formula (Box 20-4) and dimensional analysis (Box 20-5). The most common methods are ration-proportion or use of a formula.

Example 1: When the dose ordered has the same label as the dose available

Dose ordered: 0.5 g
Tablets available: 0.25 g per tablet
Step 1. The starting factor is 0.5 g.
The answer label is tablets (i.e., how many tablets should be given?)
Step 2. Formulate the conversion equation:
The equivalent needed is 1 tablet = 0.25 g.

$$\frac{0.5 \text{ g}}{1} \times \frac{1 \text{ tab}}{0.25 \text{ g}} = \text{tabs}$$

Cancel labels (g). **Note:** If properly written, all labels except the answer label will cancel.
Step 3. Solve the equation. Reduce the numerical values and multiply the numerators and denominators.

$$\frac{^2 0.5 \text{ g}}{1} \times \frac{1 \text{ tab}}{0.25 \text{ g}} = 2 \text{ tabs}$$

BOX 20-4 | **Formula Method**

$$\frac{D}{H} = V = \text{Amount to give}$$

D is the desired dose or the dose ordered by the health care provider for the patient (e.g., 250 mg of penicillin PO 4 times daily).
H is the drug dose on hand or available for use. The dose is on the drug label (e.g., penicillin tablets 250 mg each).
V is the volume (liquid) or vehicle (number of tablets, capsules) that delivers the available dose.

Note: The desired dose (D) and the on-hand dose (H) must be in the same unit of measurement. If they are in different units, you must convert before completing the formula.

BOX 20-5 | **Dimensional Analysis**

Use the following steps to solve medication problems using dimensional analysis:
1. Identify the unit of measure that you need to administer. For example, if you are giving a pill, you will usually be giving a tablet or a capsule; for parenteral or oral medications, the unit is milliliters.
2. Estimate the answer in your mind.
3. Place the name or appropriate abbreviation for x on the left side of the equation (e.g., x tab, x mL).
4. Place available information from the problem in a fraction format on the right side of the equation. Place the abbreviation or unit that matches what you are going to administer (determined in Step 1) in the numerator.
5. Look at the medication order and add other factors into the problem. Set up the numerator so it matches the unit in the previous denominator.
6. Cancel out like units of measurement on the right side of the equation. You should end up with only one unit left in the equation, and it should match the unit on the left side of the equation.
7. Reduce to the lowest terms if possible and solve the problem or solve for x. Label your answer.
8. Compare your estimate from Step 1 with your answer in Step 2.

Example 2: When the dose ordered has a different label than the dose available

Dose ordered: 0.5 g

Tablets available: 250 mg per tablet

Step 1. The starting factor is 0.5 g.

The answer label is tablets (i.e., how many tablets should be given?)

Step 2. Formulate the conversion equation:

The equivalents needed are 1 g = 1000 mg and 1 tab = 250 mg.

$$\frac{0.5 \text{ g}}{1} \times \frac{1000 \text{ mg}}{1 \text{ g}} \times \frac{1 \text{ tab}}{250 \text{ mg}} = \text{tabs}$$

Cancel labels (g, mg).

Step 3. Solve the equation.

Reduce the values and multiply the numerators and the denominators.

$$\cancel{0.5 \text{ g}} \times \frac{{}^{4}\cancel{1000 \text{mg}}}{\cancel{1\text{g}}^{2}} \times \frac{1 \text{ tab}}{\cancel{250 \text{ mg}}} = \frac{4}{2} = 2 \text{ tabs}$$

Example 3: When the dose ordered is available in a liquid form

Dose ordered: Keflex 250 mg PO

Available: 125 mg per 5 mL

Step 1. The starting factor is 250 mg.

The answer label is mL.

Step 2. Formulate the conversion equation:

The equivalent needed is 125 mg = 5 mL.

$$\frac{250 \text{ mg}}{1} \times \frac{5 \text{ mL}}{125 \text{ mg}} = \text{mL}$$

Cancel labels (mg).

Step 3. Solve the equation.

Reduce and multiply.

$$\frac{{}^{2}\cancel{250 \text{ mg}}}{1} \times \frac{5 \text{ mL}}{\cancel{125 \text{ mg}}} = 10 \text{ mL}$$

Pediatric Doses

Calculating children's medication doses requires caution (Hockenberry and Wilson, 2011). Evidence shows that children are 3 times more at risk for experiencing an ADE than adults (Potera, 2011). Factors contributing to errors include workload, distractions, lack of knowledge, and the need to dilute medications (Ozkan et al., 2011). The child's age, weight, and maturity of body systems all affect the ability to metabolize and excrete medication. Other factors that influence medication dosages in children include the difficulty in evaluating the desired effect and the hydration status of the child. In most cases the prescriber will calculate the dose for a child before ordering the medication. However, it is your responsibility to be aware of the safe dosage range for any medication administered. Different formulas and methods are used to calculate drug doses in children. The two most common methods of calculating pediatric dosages are based on the child's weight or body surface area (BSA). Refer to a pediatric pharmacology resource, a pharmacist, or the health care provider if you have to calculate a medication based on BSA. Most of the time you calculate medications based on the child's weight. An example using body weight for dosage calculation is as follows:

$$\text{Body weight} \times \text{Amount/kg} = X \text{ mg of drug}$$

For example: Prescriber orders 1 mg/kg/day of prednisone orally in two divided doses for a child weighing 55 pounds. To convert pounds to kilograms use the following formula:

$$\text{Patient's weight in pounds} \times 1 \text{ kg/2.2 pounds} = \\ \text{Patient's weight in kilograms}$$

Step 1. Convert the child's weight to kilograms.

$$55 \text{ lbs} \times 1 \text{ kg/2.2 lbs} = 25 \text{ kg}$$

Step 2. Solve the equation.

$$25 \text{ kg} \times 1 \text{ mg/kg} = 25 \text{ mg}$$

The patient should receive 25 mg of prednisone orally per day in two divided doses.

Older Adult Dosages

Older adults also require special consideration during medication administration (Table 20-8). The changes of aging alter pharmacokinetics. In addition to physiologic changes of aging, behavioral and economic issues influence the older adult's use of medications.

A common problem for older adults is polypharmacy. There is no consensus definition for polypharmacy, although the common definitions include six or more concurrent drugs, one or more potentially inappropriate drugs, two or more medications from the same chemical class, two or more medications to treat the same illness, or the mixing of nutritional or herbal supplements with medications (Reamer et al., 2008; Maggiore et al., 2010; Meiner, 2011). Older adults experience polypharmacy when they seek relief from a variety of symptoms (e.g., constipation, insomnia, pain) by using OTC preparations. Polypharmacy increases the risk of adverse effects and interactions with other medications.

The nurse, prescriber, and pharmacist share the responsibility of reducing or eliminating the risk factors associated with medication regimens that older adults receive by assessing the patient's health status, current medication regimen (including OTC drugs and herbal products), the reason for existing and proposed medications, and any environmental factors that influence accurate and safe medication administration by the patient and caregivers.

TABLE 20-8	Safe Medication Administration in Older Adults

- Consult with the prescriber to keep the medication plan as simple as possible (Lehne, 2010).
- Keep instructions clear and simple and provide written materials in large print (Lehne, 2010).
- Teach the complications and interactions of all over-the counter medications (Meiner, 2011).
- Teach the older adult to set up a daily or weekly schedule for medications using memory aids such as a calendar (Meiner, 2011).
- Monitor patient's response to medications to assess for overuse or underuse of the medication and anticipate possible dosage modifications (Meiner, 2011).
- Reduce the chance of errors by color coding or labeling medication bottles (Meiner, 2011).
- Include patient's family caregiver in any type of instruction.

NURSING PROCESS

Application of the nursing process ensures that critical thinking and clinical judgment are integrated into a patient's care. As a nurse your role extends beyond simply giving drugs to a patient. You are responsible for monitoring patients' responses to medications; providing education to the patient and family; and informing the health care provider when medications are effective, ineffective, or no longer necessary.

Assessment

Before administering medications, perform a physical assessment, which will reveal physical findings for any indications or contraindications for medication therapy. Continue your assessment by determining if the patient has a history of medication allergies. When assessing for medication allergies, you must differentiate between actual allergic reactions, which can be life threatening, and drug intolerances, which are uncomfortable side effects. In an acute care setting patients with allergies wear identification bands that list each medication allergy. All allergies and types of reactions are noted on the patient's admission notes, medication records, and history and physical examination. *Never give a patient a medication when there is a known allergy.*

Your assessment also involves identifying medications that the patient takes every day at home, including prescriptions, OTC preparations, and herbal supplements. Determine how long the patient has taken each medication, current dosage schedule, and whether he or she has had any adverse effects to any of the medications. The patient should know the name, purpose, dosage, route, and side effects of medications and supplements that are being taken. Often patients take many medications and carry a list that includes this information. Patients have different levels of understanding. One patient may describe a diuretic as a "water pill," whereas another describes it as a drug to minimize swelling and lower blood pressure. By assessing the patient's level of knowledge, you determine the need for teaching. If a patient is unable to understand or remember pertinent information, it may be necessary to involve a family member.

Complete appropriate assessments, which may include vital signs, laboratory data, and the nature and severity of symptoms. If data contraindicate medication administration, hold the drug and notify the prescriber. When in doubt about medication information, check available medication references or the pharmacy.

Planning

During planning organize nursing activities to ensure the safe administration of medications. Current evidence shows that distractions or hurrying during preparation for medication administration increases the risk of medication errors (Relihan et al., 2010). The following are general goals of medication administration:

1 Patient achieves therapeutic effect of the prescribed medication
2 There are no patient complications related to the prescribed medication
3 Patient and/or family understand medication therapy
4 Patient and family self-administer medication safely (when appropriate)

Implementation

Nursing interventions focus on safe and effective drug administration. This includes careful medication preparation, accurate and timely administration, and patient education.

Pre-administration Activities

1 Identify the medication action, purpose, side effects, and nursing implications for administering and monitoring. Ensure that the medication order has not expired. Follow agency policy for medication order renewal.
2 Minimize distractions during medication preparation (e.g., discussion with staff, phone call, pager), close the door of the medication room or post "Do Not Disturb" signage, and do not perform other tasks while preparing a medication.
3 Make sure that the information on the medication computer sheet or MAR corresponds exactly with the prescriber's written order and with the medication container label. Do not interpret illegible handwriting; clarify with prescriber.
4 Read the label on the medication container and compare it with the MAR at least 3 times: before removing the container from the supply drawer, when placing the medication in an administration cup/syringe, and just before administering the medication to the patient.
5 Double-check all calculations and other high-risk medication administration processes (e.g., patient-controlled analgesia) and verify with another nurse.
6 Review any pre-administration assessments (e.g., vital signs, review of laboratory results).
7 Use good hand-hygiene technique. Avoid touching tablets and capsules. Use sterile technique for parenteral medications. Wear clean gloves when administering parenteral medications and certain topical medications.
8 Administer only those medications that you personally prepare. Do not ask another person to administer medications that you prepare. Keep medications secure.
9 When preparing medications, be sure that the label is clear and legible and that the drug is mixed properly; has not changed in color, clarity, or consistency; and has not expired.
10 Keep tablets and capsules in their wrappers and open them at the patient's bedside. This allows you to review each medication with the patient. If a patient refuses medication, there will be no question which one was withheld.

Medication Administration

1 Follow the *six rights* of medication administration.
2 Inform the patient of the name, purpose, action, and common side effects of each medication. Evaluate his or her knowledge of the medication and provide appropriate teaching.
3 Stay with the patient until the medication is taken. Provide assistance as necessary. Do not leave medication at the bedside without a prescriber order. For example, some patients may take their own vitamins while in the hospital.
4 Respect the patient's right to refuse a medication. If the medication wrapper remains intact, return the medication to the patient's unit-dose drawer. When medication is refused, determine the reason and take action accordingly.

Post-administration Activities

1 Record medications immediately after administration (see agency policy). Include the drug name, dose, route, time, and your signature.
2 Document data pertinent to patient's response. This is especially important when giving prn drugs.
3 If a patient refuses a medication, document that it was not given, the reason for refusal, and when you notified the health care provider.

Evaluation

After you administer a medication, consider how the medication is expected to affect the patient and evaluate his or her condition and response to it. Look for therapeutic and adverse effects. If adverse effects develop, you need to recognize the clinical signs and respond quickly.

1. Monitor for evidence of therapeutic effects, side effects, and adverse reactions. This includes monitoring physical response (e.g., heart rhythm, blood pressure, urine output, or laboratory results).
2. When a medication is given for relief of symptoms, ask the patient to report if symptoms have diminished or been relieved.
3. Observe injection sites for bruises, inflammation, localized pain, numbness, or bleeding.
4. Evaluate patient's and family caregiver's understanding of medication therapy and ability to self-administer medication.

SPECIAL HANDLING OF CONTROLLED SUBSTANCES

As a nurse, you are responsible for following legal regulations when administering controlled substances (medications with potential for abuse). Violations of the Controlled Substances Act may result in fines, imprisonment, and loss of license. Health care agencies have policies for the proper storage and distribution of controlled substances, including opioids (Box 20-6). Many agencies use computerized systems for medication access and distribution.

REPORTING MEDICATION ERRORS

Medication errors often harm patients because of inappropriate medication use. Errors include inaccurate prescribing; administering the wrong medication, by the wrong route, and in the wrong time interval; and administering extra doses or failing to administer a medication. Medication errors are related to professional practice, health care product design, or procedures and systems such as product labeling and distribution. When an error occurs, the patient's safety and well-being become the top priority. The nurse assesses and examines the patient's condition and notifies the health care provider of the incident as soon as possible. Once the patient is stable, the nurse reports the incident to the appropriate person in the agency (e.g., manager or supervisor).

The nurse is also responsible for preparing a written incident or occurrence report that must be filed usually within 24 hours of an incident (see Chapter 4). The incident report is an internal audit tool and not a permanent part of the medical record. To legally protect the health care professional and agency, do not refer to an incident report in the nurses' notes or electronic health record (EHR). Agencies use incident reports to track incident patterns and initiate performance improvement programs as needed. Depending on the circumstances and the severity of the outcome, the nurse or agency may be responsible for reporting the incident to TJC, MedWatch (FDA Medical Products Reporting Program), or USP Medication Errors Reporting Program.

It is good risk management to report all medication errors, including mistakes that do not cause obvious or immediate harm or near misses. You should feel comfortable in reporting an error and not fear repercussions from managerial staff. Even when a patient suffers no harm from a medication error, the agency can still learn why the mistake occurred and what to do in the future to avoid similar errors. There are strategies that you can implement to prevent medication errors (Box 20-7).

PATIENT AND FAMILY TEACHING

A well-informed patient is more likely to take medications correctly. However, many patients have limited health literacy, meaning that they do not understand how to read medication labels and calculate doses. Thus any education requires a thorough assessment of a patient's learning needs and abilities. Provide an individualized approach to teaching, using visual aids, instructional booklets, or even videotapes or DVDs. When teaching patients about their medications, include people identified as being significant to the patient's recovery (e.g., family caregivers or home care providers).

Begin instruction as soon as possible so you can have several teaching sessions. It is ideal to use instructional materials written no higher than a sixth-grade reading level. When providing

---

BOX 20-6 | Guidelines for Safe Narcotic Administration and Control

- All controlled substances are stored in a locked cabinet or container (computerized, locked cabinets are preferred).
- Authorized nurses carry a set of keys or computer entry code for the cabinet.
- An inventory record is used each time a narcotic is dispensed. Records are often kept electronically and provide an accurate ongoing account of the narcotics used, wasted, and remaining.
- Use the record to document a patient's name, date, name of medication, dose, time of medication administration, and signature of nurse dispensing the medication.
- A second nurse witnesses disposal of the unused portion, and the record is signed by both nurses. Computerized systems record the names of the nurses electronically. Follow agency policy for appropriate waste of narcotics.

BOX 20-7 | Steps to Prevent Medication Errors

- Follow the six rights of medication administration.
- Only prepare medications for one patient at a time.
- Be sure to read labels at least 3 times (comparing MAR with label): When removing medication from storage, before taking to patient's room, before giving medication.
- Use at least two patient identifiers (e.g., patient name, birth date, hospital number) whenever administering a medication.
- Do not allow any other activity to interrupt your administration of medication to a patient.
- Double-check all calculations and verify with another nurse.
- Do not interpret illegible handwriting; clarify with prescriber.
- Question unusually large or small doses.
- Document all medications as soon as they are given.
- When you have made an error, reflect on what went wrong and ask how you could have prevented it.
- Evaluate the context or situation in which a medication error occurred. This helps to determine if nurses have the necessary resources for safe medication administration.
- When repeated medication errors occur within a work area, identify and analyze the factors that may have caused the errors and take corrective action.
- Attend in-service programs on the medications you commonly administer.
- Follow agency policies and protocols during medication administration; do not take short cuts.

MAR, Medication administration record.

instruction, have the patient or family caregiver repeat the name and use for each medication plus the dosing instructions. Have the patient demonstrate preparation of each medication. Provide time to discuss problem scenarios (e.g., side effects develop or a syringe becomes contaminated) to test the patient's knowledge of what to do should something go wrong. Determine if the patient requires a compliance aid or memory cue. This is especially important in older adults. Medication dose containers organized by the hours and days of the week are very useful. In the event that patients miss a dose of medication, they need to know how to adjust their medication schedule safely.

Evaluating the effectiveness of teaching ensures that the patient can administer medications in a safe manner. One method of evaluating patient understanding is to create medication cards with the generic and trade names of the medication on the front of the card and all pertinent medication information on the back of the card. You can flash the card in front of the patient and ask him or her to read the name of the medication. Another method is to have patients read labels on prepared medications. Remember that medication bottles often have fine print and are difficult to read for the patient with impaired vision. If the patient correctly identifies the name of the medication, ask him or her the following questions:

- Why are you taking this medication?
- How often do you take this medication?
- What side effects can occur with this medication?
- If this side effect occurs, what are you going to do about it?

Be sure to also assess the patient's sensory, motor, and cognitive functions. Impairments may affect the patient's ability to safely self-administer medications, and family caregivers or home health aides may need to assist with medication administration. Many self-help devices are also available for purchase (e.g., pill boxes with times displayed and electronic dispensers).

Critical Thinking Exercises

Justin Brown is a 72-year-old patient who visits the medical clinic 1 month after a myocardial infarction (heart attack). He denies any chest pain since his angioplasty, which involved insertion of a stent into one of his coronary arteries to improve blood flow to the heart. He is currently taking an antidepressant, a thyroid supplement, a stool softener, and a cardiac drug (beta-adrenergic blocker). In addition, he takes melatonin, an herbal preparation for sleep. The physician has recently revised Mr. Brown's cardiac medication to metoprolol (Lopressor). He is now instructed to take 75 mg by mouth twice daily. The nurse notes that the drug is available in 150-mg tablets. Mr. Brown tells the clinic nurse that he has experienced some weakness and dizziness over the past week.

1 Which of the medications taken by Mr. Brown are likely to cause weakness and dizziness?
2 What might the health care provider who prescribed the medication do after receiving the nurse's report of Mr. Brown's weakness and dizziness?
3 As the nurse, what would be important to assess for Mr. Brown to take the 75-mg dose safely?

REVIEW QUESTIONS

1 An older adult is weak and malnourished. For what should the nurse be especially watching for after administering the patient's usual medications?
   1 Signs and symptoms of drug toxicity
   2 Increased dependence on the medication
   3 Side effects of the medication
   4 An allergic reaction
2 A nurse needs to draw a serum trough level of a medication. When should he or she obtain the blood sample?
   1 Right before the next dose of the drug is due
   2 Midpoint between the times the drug doses are given
   3 2 hours after the medication is given
   4 When the serum level is scheduled to plateau, usually early in the morning
3 A patient has asked for a pain medication to relieve the discomfort from her abdominal incision. She has experienced nausea since this morning after several bites of her soft-diet breakfast. She last received a dose of her ordered oral analgesic 4 hours ago. The medication, hydrocodone 10 mg PO, is ordered q4h prn. Which of the following rights of drug administration will most likely challenge the nurse caring for this patient?
   1 Right route
   2 Right patient
   3 Right dose
   4 Right time
4 A medication order is for 0.5 g PO every 12 hours. The medication is available in 250-mg tablets. How many tablets should the nurse administer?
   1 ½ tablet
   2 1 tablet
   3 1½ tablets
   4 2 tablets
5 A patient has been having enemas until clear for an upcoming intestinal surgery. He is on several oral medications. What effect do enemas have on the absorption of medications?
   1 They increase the rate of excretion of the medications.
   2 They decrease the rate of excretion of the medications.
   3 They prolong the effects of the medications.
   4 It is unknown because the mechanism of medication excretion is not stated.
6 A nurse is administering multiple medications to multiple patients on a very busy unit.
   Which action by the nurse requires an intervention?
   1 The nurse performs dosage calculations and has them checked by another nurse as needed.
   2 The nurse keeps unit-dose medications closed in their wrappers until arriving at the patient's bedside.
   3 The nurse administers clear liquid medication containing sediment at the bottom of the bottle.
   4 The nurse checks medications at least 3 times before administering them to the patient.
7 The home health nurse notes that an elderly patient uses mouthwash 3 or 4 times every day and that he periodically swallows some of it.
   Which action is most appropriate for the nurse to take?
   1 Tell the patient not to use the mouthwash as often
   2 Ask the patient if he smokes
   3 Obtain a dietary history from the patient from the past 2 days
   4 Check the patient's medications and the mouthwash label

8 The nurse is reviewing the medication order sheet and finds an order for MSO4 8 mg IM q 3-4h prn.
What is the appropriate initial nursing action?
   1 Contact the pharmacist to approve the order
   2 Ask another nurse if she can give the medication
   3 Contact the prescriber for clarification, including a "read-back"
   4 Administer the medication as ordered by the health care provider

9 The nurse administered lorazepam (Ativan), an antianxiety medication, to an 84-year-old patient who now is agitated and experiencing delirium.
What are the nurse's primary responsibilities?
   1 Administer naloxone (Narcan) and prepare to call a "code"
   2 Assess the patient's oxygen saturation and prepare to administer oxygen
   3 Monitor the patient and have another nurse call the prescriber
   4 Contact the nursing supervisor and the pharmacist

10 During the admission history the nurse determines that his 80-year-old patient is currently taking a salmon-colored blood pressure pill, a yellow "muscle relaxing" pill, a pink liquid to calm his stomach, and a green and yellow "joint" pill. Which action should the nurse take first?
   1 Ask the patient if he brought the medications with him
   2 Check the patient's armband before administering any medications
   3 Try to identify the medications by the patient's descriptions
   4 Call the pharmacist to see if she can figure out what the medications are

REFERENCES

Agrawal A: Medication errors: prevention using information technology systems, *Br J Clin Pharmacol* 67(6):681, 2009.

American Nurses Association (ANA): *Nursing scope and standards of practice*, ed 2, Silver Springs, Md, 2010, The Association.

Anderson P, Townsend T: Medication errors: don't let them happen to you, *Am Nurse Today* 5(3):23, 2010.

Bennett WL, et al: Comparative effectiveness and safety of medications for type 2 diabetes: an update including new drugs and 2-drug combinations, *Ann Intern Med* 154(9):602, 2011.

Centers for Medicare & Medicaid (CMS): *Medication administration guidance update*, 2011, CMS, available at https://www.cms.gov/Surveycertificationgeninfo/downloads/SCLetter12_05.pdf, accessed January 19, 2012.

Greene JA, et al: Why do the same drugs look different? Pills, trade dress, and public health, *N Engl J Med* 365(1):83, 2011.

Hockenberry MJ, Wilson D: *Wong's nursing care of infants and children*, ed 9, St Louis, 2011, Mosby.

Institute of Medicine (IOM): *Report brief, to err is human: building a safer health system*, 2000, available at http://www.iom.edu/~/media/Files/Report%20Files/1999/To-Err-is-Human/To%20Err%20is%20Human%201999%20%20report%20brief.pdf, accessed July, 2012.

Institute for Safe Medication Practices (ISMP): *Improving medication safety in community pharmacy: assessing risk and opportunities for change*, 2009, ISMP, available at http://www.ismp.org, accessed August 23, 2011.

Institute for Safe Medication Practices (ISMP): *ISMP's list of confused drug names*, 2010a, ISMP, available at http://www.ismp.org/Tools/confuseddrugnames.pdf, accessed January 18, 2012.

Institute for Safe Medication Practices (ISMP): *ISMP's list of error-prone abbreviations, symbols, and dose designations*, 2010b, ISMP, available at http://www.ismp.org/Tools/error-proneabbreviations.pdf, accessed January 18, 2012.

Institute for Safe Medication Practices (ISMP): *Oral doses that should not be crushed*, 2010c, ISMP, http://www.ismp.org/Tools/DoNotCrush.asp, accessed January 18, 2012.

Institute for Safe Medication Practices (ISMP): *Never use parenteral syringes for oral medications*, 2010d, available at http://www.accessdata.fda.gov/psn/transcript.cfm?show=94#9, accessed January 18, 2012.

Institute for Safe Medication Practices (ISMP): *Improving medication safety with anticoagulant therapy*, 2011a, available at http://www.ismp.org/tools/anticoagulantTherapy.asp, accessed January 18, 2012.

Institute for Safe Medication Practices (ISMP): *Acute care guidelines for timely administration of scheduled medications*, 2011b, available at http://www.ismp.org/Tools/guidelines/acutecare/tasm.pdf, accessed August 23, 2011.

Institute for Safe Medication Practices (ISMP): *Guidelines for timely medication administration: response to the CMS "30 minute" rule*, 2011c, available at http://www.ismp.org/Newsletters/acutecare/articles/20110113.asp, accessed January 18, 2012.

Kim KS, et al: Nurses' perceptions of medication errors and their contributing factors in South Korea, *J Nurs Manage* 19:346, 2011.

LaMantia M, et al: Interventions to improve transitional care between nursing homes and hospitals: a systematic review, *J Am Geriatr Soc* 58:77, 2010.

Lehne R: *Pharmacology for nursing care*, ed 7, St Louis, 2010, Saunders.

Macdonald M: Examining the adequacy of the 5 rights of medication administration, *Clin Nurse Specialist* 24(4):197, 2010.

Maggiore R, et al: Polypharmacy in older adults with cancer, *Oncologist* 15(5):507, 2010.

Meiner S: *Gerontologic nursing*, ed 4, St Louis, 2011, Mosby.

National Quality Forum (NQF): *National voluntary consensus report, standards for public reporting of patient safety information: a consensus report*, Washington, DC, 2010, NQF.

Ozkan S, et al: Frequency of pediatric medication administration errors and contributing factors, *J Nurse Care Qual* 26(2):136, 2011.

Poon EG, et al: Effect of bar-code technology on the safety of medication administration, *N Engl J Med* 362:1698, 2010.

Potera C: Collaboration reduces pediatric adverse drug events, *Pediatrics* 111(10):116, 2011.

Reamer LB, et al: Polypharmacy: misleading but manageable, *Clin Interv Aging* 3(2):383, 2008.

Relihan E, et al: The impact of a set of interventions to reduce interruptions and distractions to nurses during medication administration, *Qual Safe Health Care* 19(52):1, 2010.

Shane R: Current status of administration of medicines, *Am J Health Syst Pharm* 66(3):s42, 2009.

Sowan A, et al: Impact of computerized orders for pediatric continuous drug infusions on detecting infusion pump programming errors: a simulated study, *J Pediatr Nurs* 25(2):108, 2010.

The Joint Commission (TJC): Standards FAQ details: two patient identifiers, 2008, available at http://www.jointcommission.org/standards_information/jcfaqdetails.aspx?StandardsFAQId=145&StandardsFAQChapterId=77, accessed July 2012.

The Joint Commission (TJC): *Comprehensive accreditation manual for hospitals*, Oakbrook Terrace, Ill, 2012a, The Commission.

The Joint Commission (TJC): *National Patient Safety Goals*, Oakbrook Terrace, Ill, 2012b, The Commission, available at http://www.jointcommission.org/standards_information/npsgs.aspx.

Trbovich P, et al: Interruptions during the delivery of high-risk medications, *J Nurs Adm* 40(5):211, 2010.

US Food and Drug Administration (FDA): MedWatch, the FDA safety information and adverse event reporting program, 2010, available at http://www.fda.gov/Safety/MedWatch/default.htm, accessed January 18, 2012.

Oral and Topical Medications

MEDIA RESOURCES

- evolve http://evolve.elsevier.com/Perry/skills
  - Review Questions
  - ▶ Video Clips
  - Audio Glossary
- NSO Nursing Skills Online

KEY TERMS

Antianginal	Mydriatics	Ophthalmic	Suspension
Buccal medication	Nasal	Otic	Sympathomimetic
Cycloplegic	Nebulizer	Pruritus	Topical
Dermatologic	Nitroglycerin	Sublingual medication	Transdermal
Dry powder inhaler (DPI)	Ointment	Suppository	Vertigo
Metered-dose inhaler (MDI)			

OBJECTIVES

Mastery of content in this chapter will enable the nurse to:
- Correctly administer a medication by oral, enteral, and topical routes.
- Correctly administer medications for irrigation and instillation.
- Identify guidelines for administering oral, enteral, and topical medications.
- Describe factors to assess before administering medications.
- Differentiate types of topical administrations that require sterile technique and those that require clean medical aseptic technique.

- Instruct patients in the proper use of a metered-dose inhaler (MDI), a dry powder inhaler (DPI), and small-volume nebulizer.
- Identify conditions contraindicating the administration of medications by various oral and topical routes.
- Prepare a teaching plan regarding medication use for a selected patient.

Nonparenteral medications include those that are not given by injection such as oral medications, eardrops, and eyedrops. The route chosen depends on the properties and desired effects of the medication and the physical and mental condition of a patient. The oral route (by mouth) is the easiest and most desirable way to administer medications. There are many reasons why it may be necessary to change from one route to another. When this occurs, you are responsible for consulting with a health care provider for an order or conferring with the pharmacist to safely meet a patient's needs.

Topical administration of medications involves applying drugs directly to skin or mucous or tissue membranes. You apply medications to the skin by spraying, painting, or spreading medication over a localized area. Transdermal patches (adhesive-backed medicated disks), which are applied to the skin, provide a continuous release of medication over several hours or days. Topical administration avoids puncturing the skin and decreases the risk for infection and tissue injury that may occur with injections. When applying a disk, it is essential to rotate the site of application to decrease the incidence of a localized reaction.

Medications applied to membranes such as the cornea of the eye or the rectal mucosa are absorbed quickly because of the vascularity of the membrane. When drug concentrations are high, systemic effects can occur. For example, bradycardia and hypotension may occur after instillation of ophthalmic beta blockers such as timolol (Timoptic). Mucous and tissue membranes differ in their sensitivity to medications. For example, the cornea of the eye is very sensitive. Patients commonly experience burning sensations during administration of eyedrops and nose drops. Medications applied to vaginal or rectal mucosa are generally less irritating.

You can administer medications for topical use in the following ways:

1. *Direct application of liquid*: Eyedrops, gargling, swabbing the throat
2. Inserting *drug into a body cavity*: Rectal or vaginal suppositories, vaginal creams, or foams
3. Instillation *of fluid into body cavity (fluid is retained)*: Eardrops, nose drops, bladder and rectal instillation
4. *Irrigation of body cavity (fluid is not retained)*: Flushing eye, ear, vagina, bladder, or rectum with medicated fluid
5. *Spraying*: Instillation into nose or throat.
6. *Inhalation of medicated aerosol spray*: Distributes medication throughout the nasal passages and the tracheobronchial airway; two types of devices designed for this purpose: metered-dose inhalers (MDIs) and small-volume nebulizers
7. *Inhalation of dry powder medication*: Distributes medication in powder form throughout the tracheobronchial airway; device designed for this purpose: dry powder inhaler (DPI)
8. *Direct application to skin or mucosa*: Lotion, ointment, cream, powder, foam, spray, patch, and disk
9. *Sublingual*: Medication placed under the tongue; is dissolvable
10. *Buccal*: Medication placed between the upper or lower molar teeth and cheek area; is dissolvable

EVIDENCE-BASED PRACTICE

Nurses play an essential role in all phases of the medication administration process. Medication competency is a skill that all nurses must possess to improve the quality and safety of medication administration. Increasing safety is important in improving the quality of patient care (Popescu et al., 2011). An integrative review of the literature identifies the competencies that nurses can implement to increase patient safety and promote best practices (Sulosaari et al., 2011):

- Maintain current knowledge of anatomy and physiology and pharmacology.
- Maintain mathematics and calculation skills through practice and validation of correct medication doses.

- Communicate with the interdisciplinary team to ensure that the six rights of medication administration are followed.
- Assess patients before administration of medications and evaluate responses to achieve best practices.
- Accuracy of documentation is necessary to maintain patient safety.
- Best-practice guidelines for safe medication administration include clinical decision-making competency, theoretic competency, and clinical practice competency.

PATIENT-CENTERED CARE

An excellent time to provide patient education is during medication administration. Most patients discharged from hospitals continue on previously ordered medications and are placed on new medications. The goal of patient education is to improve patient adherence to medication regimens. Patients fail to adhere to medication regimens because of patient, medication, and provider issues (Berben et al., 2011; Shearer, 2009). Patient issues include cognitive impairment, depression, physical limitation, financial issues, and lack of knowledge. Medication issues include complex medication regimens and medication discrepancies. Provider issues include poor instruction, inappropriate prescriptions, and lack of provider knowledge about adherence. Patients need explanations about the purpose of medications, benefits, expected effects, and how to plan a daily schedule. Print materials should be developed to meet individual patient needs such as health literacy, visual impairment, or cognitive impairment. Be sure to involve family caregivers in the education sessions since they may be the ones administering medications.

Health beliefs vary by culture and influence how patients manage and respond to medication therapy. Differences in values, attitudes, and beliefs affect a patient's adherence to medication therapy. Herbal remedies and alternative therapies may be common practice in some cultures and interfere with prescribed medications. Some cultures discontinue their medication when symptoms are resolved, even if medications are still needed to manage the disease (Qureshi, 2010). It is also important to consider cultural influences on drug response, metabolism, and side effects if a patient is not responding to drug therapy as expected. A change in the medication may be necessary by the prescriber.

Safety Guidelines

1. Assess patient's sensory function, including sight, hearing, touch, and physical coordination. Sensory function and coordination deficits impair patient's ability to see medications, open prescription bottles, and read labels at home.
2. Patients often receive more than one oral medication at a time. Evaluate each medication for potential drug-drug or drug-food interactions. Always consult with a pharmacist to reduce the risk of an interaction.
3. Always assess for drug allergies. If patient reports having an allergy, ask about the type of reaction that occurred.
4. Evaluate if patient can take medication with food. In most cases the presence of food in the stomach delays drug absorption; however, some drugs irritate the stomach lining and need to be taken with food.
5. For all medications administered, review the order for patient's name, drug, dosage, route, and time of administration.
6. For all medications administered, gather information pertinent to the drug(s) ordered: purpose, normal dosage and route,

common side effects, time of onset and peak, contraindications, and nursing implications.

7 Determine if medications require any specific nursing actions (e.g., vital signs, drug levels, or electrolytes) before administration.

8 If patients are mentally and physically able, prepare them for discharge by instructing them in self-administration techniques. Include family caregivers if possible.

9 Check the expiration date for all medications.

SKILL 21-1 Administering Oral Medications

NSO *Safe Medication Administration Module / Lesson 5*

Patients are usually able to ingest or self-administer oral medications with few problems. If oral medications are contraindicated (e.g., inability to swallow, gastric suction) take precautions to protect patients from aspiration. Nurses usually prepare medications in areas designed for medication preparation or at unit-dose carts.

Delegation and Collaboration

The skill of administering oral medications cannot be delegated to nursing assistive personnel (NAP). The nurse directs the NAP about:

- Potential side effects of medications and to report their occurrence.

 Video Clip

- Informing nurse if patient condition changes or worsens (e.g., pain, itching, or rash) after medication administration.

Equipment

- ❏ Automated, computer-controlled drug dispensing system or medication cart
- ❏ Disposable medication cups
- ❏ Glass of water, juice, or preferred liquid and drinking straw
- ❏ Device for crushing or splitting tablets (*optional*)
- ❏ Paper towels
- ❏ Medication administration record (MAR) (electronic or printed)
- ❏ Clean gloves (if handling an oral medication)

STEP	RATIONALE

ASSESSMENT

1 Check accuracy and completeness of each medication administration record (MAR) with health care provider's medication order. Check patient's name and drug name, dosage, and route and time of administration Clarify incomplete or unclear orders with health care provider before administration.

2 Review pertinent information related to medication, including action, purpose, normal dose and route, side effects, time of onset and peak action, and nursing implications.

3 Assess for any contraindications to patient receiving oral medication, including being on NPO status, inability to swallow, nausea/vomiting, bowel inflammation, reduced peristalsis, recent gastrointestinal (GI) surgery, gastric suction, and decreased level of consciousness (LOC). Notify health care provider if any contraindications are present.

4 Assess risk for aspiration using a dysphagia screening tool if available (see Skill 30-3). Protect patient from aspiration by assessing swallowing ability (Box 21-1).

The health care provider's order is the most reliable source and only legal record of drugs that patient is to receive. Ensures that patient receives correct medication. Handwritten MARs are a source of medication errors (Poon et al., 2010; Jones and Treiber, 2010).

Allows you to anticipate effects of drug and observe patient's response.

Alterations in GI function can interfere with drug absorption, distribution, and excretion. Giving oral medications to patients with impaired swallowing or decreased LOC increases their risk for aspiration.

Aspiration occurs when food, fluid, or medication intended for GI administration is inadvertently administered into the respiratory tract. Patients with altered ability to swallow are at higher risk for aspiration (Kelly et al., 2011; Edmiaston et al., 2010).

BOX 21-1 | Protecting the Patient from Aspiration

- Assess patient's ability to swallow and cough and check for presence of gag reflex.
- Prepare oral medication in form that is easiest to swallow.
- Allow patient to self-administer medications if possible.
- If patient has unilateral (one-sided) weakness, place medication in stronger side of mouth.
- Administer pills one at a time, ensuring that each medication is properly swallowed before next one is introduced.

- Thicken regular liquids or offer fruit nectars if patient cannot tolerate thin liquids.
- Avoid straws because they decrease control patient has over volume intake, which increases risk of aspiration.
- Have patient hold and drink from a cup if possible.
- Time medications to coincide with mealtimes or when patient is well rested and awake if possible.
- Administer medications using another route if risk of aspiration is severe.

STEP	RATIONALE
5 Assess patient's medical history, history of allergies, medication history, and diet history. List any drug allergies on each page of the MAR and prominently display on patient's medical record. When allergies are present, patient should wear an allergy bracelet.	These factors influence how certain drugs act. Information reveals previous problems with medication administration.
6 Gather and review physical assessment findings and laboratory data that influence drug administration such as vital signs and results of renal and liver function studies.	Physical examination findings or laboratory data may contraindicate drug administration. Renal and liver function status affects metabolism and excretion of medications (Lewis et al., 2011).
7 Assess patient's knowledge regarding health and medication use, medication schedule, and ability to prepare medications.	Determines patient's need for medication education and guidance needed to achieve drug adherence.
8 Assess patient's preference for fluids and determine if medications can be given with these fluids. Maintain fluid restrictions as prescribed.	Some fluids interfere with medication absorption (e.g., dairy products affect tetracycline). Offering fluids during drug administration is an excellent way to increase patient's fluid intake. Fluids ease swallowing and facilitate absorption from the GI tract. However, fluid restrictions must be maintained.

NURSING DIAGNOSES

- Deficient knowledge: medication administration
- Impaired swallowing
- Noncompliance
- Readiness for enhanced self-health management
- Nausea
- Risk for aspiration

Related factors are individualized based on patient's condition or needs.

PLANNING

1 Expected outcomes following completion of procedure:	
• Patient responds appropriately to desired medication effect.	Drug has exerted its therapeutic action.
• Patient denies any GI discomfort or symptoms of alterations.	Oral medications can irritate GI mucosa.
• Patient explains purpose of medication and drug dosage schedule.	Demonstrates understanding of drug therapy.
2 Explain procedure to patient. Be specific if patient wishes to self-administer medications.	Makes patient a participant in care, which minimizes anxiety. Begins patient teaching regarding medications. Enables patient to self-administer drug, which increases feelings of independence.

IMPLEMENTATION

1 Prepare medications.	
a Perform hand hygiene.	Reduces transfer of microorganisms.
b Plan medication administration to avoid interruptions, keep door to medication room closed, do not take phone calls, limit conversation with colleagues for only essential information; follow agency "No Interruption Zone" policy.	Interruptions contribute to medication administration errors (Hall et al., 2010; Popescu et al., 2011).
c Arrange medication tray and cups in medication preparation area or move medication cart to position outside patient's room.	Organization of equipment saves time and reduces error.
d Access automated dispensing system (ADS) or unlock medicine drawer or cart.	Medications are safeguarded when locked in cabinet, cart, or ADS.
e Prepare medications for *one patient at a time.* Follow the six rights of medication administration. Keep all pages of MARs or computer printouts for one patient together or look at only one patient's medication administration computer screen.	Prevents preparation errors.
f Select correct medication from ADS, unit-dose drawer, or stock supply. Compare name of medication on label with MAR or computer printout (see illustration). Exit ADS after removing drug(s).	Reading label and comparing it against transcribed order reduces errors. Exiting ADS ensures that no one else can remove medications using your identity. *This is the first check for accuracy.*
g Check or calculate drug dose as necessary. Double-check any calculation. Check expiration date on all medications and return outdated medication to pharmacy.	Double-checking pharmacy calculations reduces risk for error. Agency policy may require you to check calculations of certain medications such as insulin with another nurse. Expired medications may be inactive or harmful to patient.

STEP	RATIONALE
h If preparing a controlled substance, check record for previous medication count and compare current count with supply available. Controlled drugs may be stored in computerized locked cart (see Chapter 20).	Controlled substance laws require nurses to carefully monitor and count dispensed narcotics.
i Prepare solid forms of oral medications.	Wrappers maintain cleanliness and identify drug name and dose, which can facilitate teaching.
(1) To prepare unit-dose tablets or capsules, place packaged tablet or capsule directly into medication cup without removing wrapper. Administer medications only from containers with labels that are clearly marked.	
(2) When using a blister pack, "pop" medications through foil or paper backing into a medication cup.	Packs provide a 1-month supply, with each "blister" usually containing a single dose.
(3) If it is necessary to give half the dose of medication, pharmacy should split, label, package, and send medication to unit. If you must split medication, use clean, gloved hand to cut with clean pill-cutting device (see illustration). Only cut tablets that are prescored by the manufacturer (line transverses the center of the tablet).	In health care agencies, only pharmacy should split tablets to ensure patient safety (ISMP, 2008). Reduces contamination of tablet.
(4) Place all tablets or capsules that patient will receive in one medicine cup, except for those requiring pre-administration assessments (e.g., pulse rate or blood pressure). Place in separate additional cup with wrapper intact.	Keeping medications that require preadministration assessments separate from others serves as reminder and makes it easier to withhold drugs as necessary.
(5) If patient has difficulty swallowing and liquid medications are not an option, use a pill-crushing device. Clean device before using. Place medicine in between two cups, and grind and crush (see illustration). Mix ground tablet in small amount (teaspoon) of soft food (custard or applesauce).	Large tablets are often difficult to swallow. Ground tablet mixed with palatable soft food is usually easier to swallow.
j Prepare liquids.	
(1) Thoroughly mix by shaking gently before administration. If drug is in unit-dose container with correct volume, shaking is not needed. If drug is in multidose bottle, remove bottle cap from container and place cap upside down on work surface.	Mixing liquid suspensions just before pouring ensures that correct amount of medication, not just the solvent, is measured for the dose. Prevents contamination of inside of cap.
(2) Hold bottle with label against palm of hand while pouring.	Prevents spilled liquid from dripping and soiling label.
(3) Place medication cup at eye level on countertop and fill to desired level on scale. Scale should be even with fluid level at its surface or base of meniscus, not edges (see illustration).	Ensures accuracy of measurement.

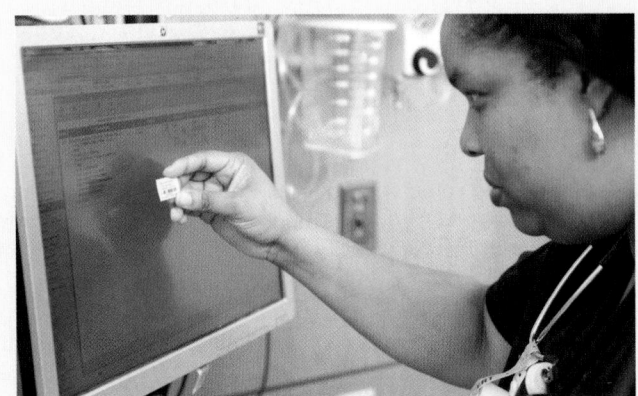

STEP 1f Nurse compares label of medication with transcribed medication order on computerized MAR.

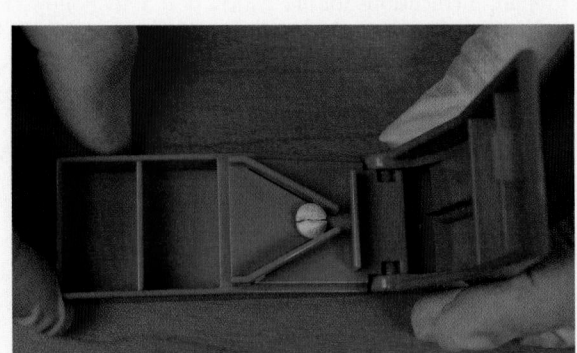

STEP 1i(3) Tablet is placed in pill-cutting device and cut in half.

STEP	RATIONALE
(4) Discard any excess liquid into sink or a place specially designated for wasting of medications. Wipe lip of bottle with paper towel and recap.	Prevents contamination of contents of bottle and prevents bottle cap from sticking.
(5) If giving less than 10 mL of liquid, prepare medication in oral syringe (see illustration). Do not use hypodermic syringe or syringe with needle or syringe cap.	Allows more accurate measurement of small amounts.

Clinical Decision Point *Only use syringes specifically designed for oral use when administering liquid medications. If using hypodermic syringes, the medication may be accidentally administered parenterally; or the syringe cap or needle, if not removed from the syringe before administration, may become dislodged and accidentally aspirated during administration of oral medications (ISMP, 2010).*

STEP	RATIONALE
(6) Administer liquid medication packaged in single-dose cup directly from the single-dose cup. Do not pour into a medicine cup.	Avoids unnecessary manipulation of dose.
k Before going to patient's room, compare patient's name and name of medication on label of prepared drugs with MAR.	Reading labels a second time reduces errors. *This is the second check for accuracy.*
l Return stock containers or unused unit-dose medications to shelf or drawer. Label medication cups and poured medications with patient's name before leaving medication preparation area. Do not leave drugs unattended.	Ensures that correct medications are prepared for correct patient.

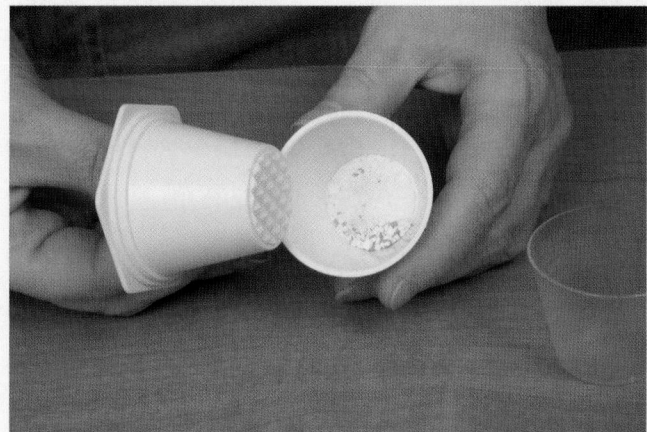

STEP 1i(5)   Crushing tablet with pill-crushing device.

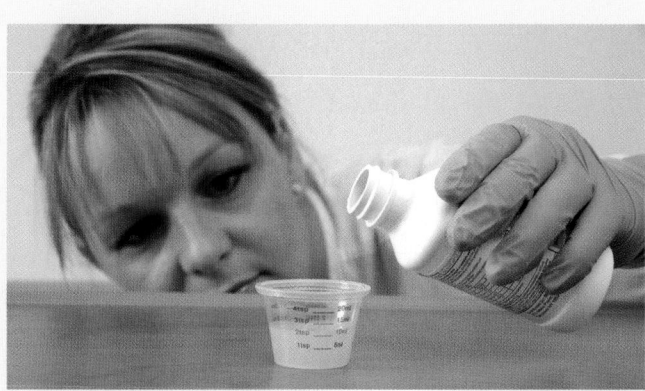

STEP 1j(3)   Measuring liquid medication. Look at meniscus at eye level.

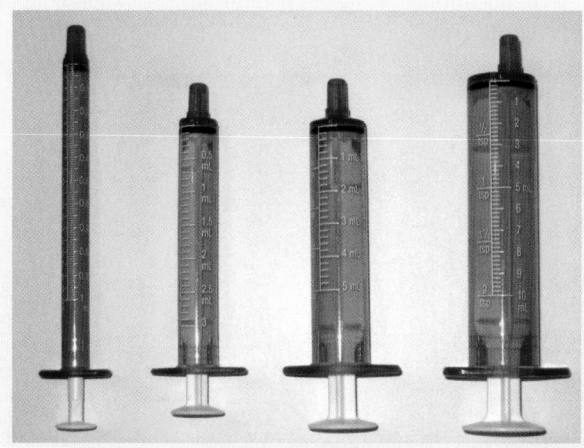

STEP 1j(5)   Use special oral medication syringes to prepare small amounts of liquid medications.

STEP	RATIONALE

2 Administer medications.

a Take medication(s) to patient at correct time (see agency policy). Medications that require exact timing include stat, first-time or loading doses, and one time doses. Give time-critical scheduled medications (e.g., antibiotics, anticoagulants, insulin, anticonvulsants, immunosuppressive agents) at exact time ordered (no later than 30 minutes before or after scheduled dose). Given non–time-critical scheduled medications within a range of 1 or 2 hours of scheduled dose (ISMP, 2011). During administration, apply six rights of medication administration.

Hospitals must adopt medication administration policy and procedure for timing of medication administration that considers nature of the prescribed medication, specific clinical application, and patient needs (DHHS, 2011; ISMP, 2011). Time-critical scheduled medications are those for which early or delayed administration of maintenance doses of greater than 30 minutes before or after the scheduled dose may cause harm or result in substantial suboptimal therapy or pharmacologic effect. Non–time-critical medications are those for which early or delayed administration within a specified range of either 1 or 2 hours should not cause harm or result in substantial suboptimal therapy or pharmacologic effect (ISMP, 2011; DHHS, 2011).

b Identify patient using two identifiers (i.e., name and birthday or name and account number) according to agency policy. Compare identifiers in MAR/medical record with information on patient's identification bracelet and/or ask patient to state name.

Ensures correct patient. Complies with The Joint Commission standards and improves patient safety (TJC, 2012).

Some agencies are now using a bar-code system to help with patient identification.

c At patient's bedside again compare MAR or computer printout with names of medications on medication labels and patient name. Ask patient if he or she has allergies.

This is the third check for accuracy and ensures that patient receives correct medication. Confirms patient's allergy history.

d Perform necessary preadministration assessment (e.g., blood pressure, pulse) for specific medications. Ask patient if he or she has allergies.

Determines whether specific medications should be withheld at that time. Confirms patient's allergy history.

e Discuss purpose of each medication, action, and possible adverse effects. Allow patient to ask any questions about drugs.

Patient has right to be informed, and patient's understanding of purpose of each medication improves adherence to drug therapy.

Clinical Decision Point *If patient expresses concern regarding accuracy of a medication, do not give the medication. Explore patient's concern and verify prescriber's order before administering. Listening to patient's concerns may prevent a medication error.*

f Help patient to sitting or Fowler's position. Use side-lying position if he or she is unable to sit. Have patient stay in this position for 30 minutes after administration.

Decreases risk for aspiration during swallowing.

g *For tablets:* Patient may wish to hold solid medications in hand or cup before placing in mouth. Offer water or preferred liquid to help patient swallow medications.

Patient can become familiar with medications by seeing each drug. Choice of fluid can improve fluid intake.

h *For orally disintegrating formulations (tablets or strips):* Remove medication from packet just before use. Do not push tablet through foil. Place medication on top of patient's tongue. Caution against chewing it.

Orally disintegrating formulations begin to dissolve when placed on tongue. Water is not needed. Careful removal from packaging is necessary because tablets and strips are thin and fragile.

i *For sublingually administered medications:* Have patient place medication under tongue and allow it to dissolve completely (see illustration). Caution patient against swallowing tablet or saliva.

Drug is absorbed through blood vessels of undersurface of tongue. If swallowed, drug is destroyed by gastric juices or rapidly detoxified by liver, preventing therapeutic blood level.

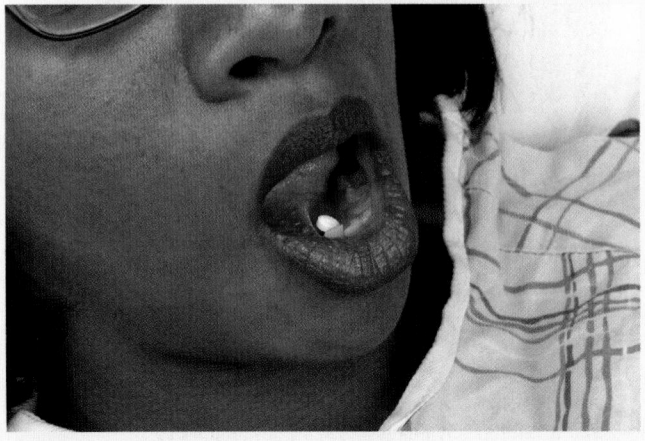

STEP 2i   Proper placement of sublingual tablet in sublingual pocket.

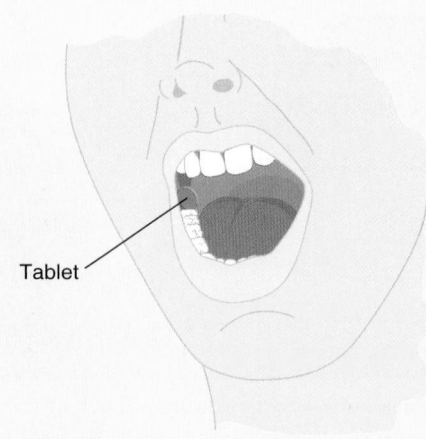

Tablet

STEP 2j   Buccal administration of tablet.

STEP	RATIONALE
j *For buccal administered medications:* Have patient place medication in mouth against mucous membranes of cheek and gums until it dissolves (see illustration).	Buccal medications act locally or systemically as they are swallowed in saliva.

Clinical Decision Point *Avoid administering anything by mouth until orally disintegrating buccal or sublingual medication is completely dissolved.*

STEP	RATIONALE
k *For powdered medications:* Mix with liquids at bedside and give to patient to drink.	When prepared in advance, powdered drugs thicken and some even harden, making swallowing difficult.
l *For crushed medications mixed with food:* Give each medication separately in teaspoon of food.	Ensures that patient swallows all of medicine.
m Caution patient against chewing or swallowing lozenges.	Lozenges act through slow absorption through oral mucosa, not gastric mucosa.
n Give effervescent powders and tablets immediately after dissolving.	Effervescence improves unpleasant taste and often relieves GI problems.
o If patient is unable to hold medications, place medication cup to lips and gently introduce each drug into mouth one at a time. A spoon can also be used to place pill in patient's mouth. Do not rush or force medications.	Administering a single tablet or capsule eases swallowing and decreases risk for aspiration.

Clinical Decision Point *If tablet or capsule falls to the floor, discard it and repeat preparation. Drug is contaminated.*

STEP	RATIONALE
p Stay until patient swallows each medication completely or takes it by the prescribed route. Ask patient to open mouth if uncertain whether medication has been swallowed.	Ensures that patient receives ordered dose. If left unattended, patient may not take dose or may save drugs, causing health risks.
q For highly acidic medications (e.g., aspirin), offer patient a nonfat snack (e.g., crackers) if not contraindicated by his or her condition.	Reduces gastric irritation. Fat content of foods may delay drug absorption.
r Help patient return to position of comfort.	Maintains patient's comfort.
s Dispose of soiled supplies and perform hand hygiene. Return cart to medication room if used. Clean work area.	Reduces spread of microorganisms.

EVALUATION

1 Return within an appropriate time to evaluate patient's response to medications, including therapeutic effects, side effects or allergy, and adverse reactions.	Evaluates therapeutic benefit of drug and helps to detect onset of side effects or allergic reactions. Sublingual medications act in 15 minutes; most oral medications act in 30 to 60 minutes.
2 Ask patient or family caregiver to identify drug name and explain purpose, action, dose schedule, and potential side effects.	Determines level of knowledge gained by patient and family.

Unexpected Outcomes

1 Patient exhibits adverse effects (e.g., side effect, toxic effect, allergic reaction).

2 Patient is unable to explain drug information.

3 Patient refuses medication.

Related Interventions

- Withhold further doses.
- Assess vital signs.
- Notify health care provider and pharmacy.
- Symptoms such as urticaria, rash, pruritus, rhinitis, and wheezing may indicate an allergic reaction and need for emergency medications.
- Add allergy information to patient's medical record.

- Further assess patient's or family caregiver's knowledge of medications and guidelines for drug safety.
- Further instruction or different approach to instruction is necessary.

- Assess why patient is refusing medication.
- Do not force patient to take medications.
- Notify health care provider.
- Record refused medication and patient's stated reason.

Recording and Reporting

- Record drug, dose, route, and time administered on patient's MAR immediately after administration, not before. Include initials or signature. Record patient teaching and validation of understanding in nurses' notes and electronic health record (EHR).
- If drug is withheld, record reason in nurses' notes and EHR and follow agency policy for noting withheld doses.
- Report adverse effects/patient response and/or withheld drugs to nurse in charge or health care provider. Depending on medication, immediate health care provider notification may be required.

Special Considerations

Teaching

- Instruct patient and family caregiver about specific information pertaining to drug regimen (purpose, action, dose, dosage intervals, side effects, foods to avoid or take with drugs).
- All patients should learn the basic guidelines for drug safety in the home (see Skill 42-6).

Pediatric

- Liquid forms of medication are safer to swallow to avoid aspiration of small pills.
- Children refuse bitter or distasteful oral preparations. Mix the drug with a small amount (about 1 teaspoon) of a sweet-tasting substance such as jam, applesauce, sherbet, ice cream, or fruit puree. Do not use honey for infants because of the risk of botulism. Offer the child juice or a flavored ice pop after medication administration. Do not place medication in an essential food item such as milk or formula; the child may refuse the food at a later time.
- Measure small amount of liquid medications using a plastic calibrated oral dosing syringe or a hollow-handled medicine spoon. Amounts less than a teaspoon are impossible to measure accurately with a molded medicine cup (Hockenberry and Wilson, 2011).

Gerontologic

- Physiologic changes of aging influence how oral medications are distributed, absorbed, and excreted. Common changes include loss of elasticity in oral mucosa; reduction in parotid gland secretion, causing dry mouth; delayed esophageal clearance, impaired swallowing; reduction in gastric acidity and stomach peristalsis, increased susceptibility to highly acidic drugs; reduced liver function, resulting in altered drug metabolism; and reduced renal function and colon motility, slowing drug excretion. Both altered drug metabolism and excretion may lead to drug toxicity (Lehne, 2010).
- Give medications with a full glass of water (unless restricted) to aid passage of the drug. Give patient time to swallow.
- Patients may have several health problems or chronic conditions requiring the use of multiple drugs, often prescribed by different health care providers. Polypharmacy creates a high risk for drug interactions and adverse reactions (Lehne, 2010).

Home Care

- When measuring liquid medications at home, patients should use measuring spoons, not eating utensil spoons that vary in volume.
- See Skills 41-3, Medication and Medical Device Safety, and Skill 42-6, Teaching Medication Self-Administration.

SKILL 21-2 Administering Medications Through an Enteral Feeding Tube

NSO *Enteral Nutrition Module / Lesson 5*

Patients who have enteral feeding tubes are unable to receive food or medications by mouth. Nasogastric feeding tubes generally are small-bore tubes that are inserted into the stomach via one of the nares (see Chapter 31). For long-term enteral feedings, a percutaneous endoscopic gastrostomy (PEG) tube or a jejunostomy tube may be inserted surgically. Do not administer medications into nasogastric tubes that are inserted for decompression.

Preferably medications administered by enteral tubes should be in liquid form. If a medication is not available in liquid, you will need to prepare an oral medication tablet or capsule by crushing or dissolving it. However, you cannot crush sublingual, sustained-release, chewable, long-acting, or enteric-coated medications. Consult with the hospital pharmacist about whether you can crush or dissolve a medication. Always verify correct placement of a nasogastric tube before administering medications (see Skill 31-2).

Delegation and Collaboration

The skill of administering medications by enteral feeding tubes cannot be delegated to nursing assistive personnel (NAP). The nurse directs the NAP to:

- Keep the patient's head of the bed elevated a minimum of 30 degrees (preferably 45 degrees) for 1 hour (follow agency policy) after medication administration.
- Report immediately to the nurse signs of aspiration such as coughing, choking, gagging, or drooling of liquid or dissolved pills.

Equipment

- ❏ Medication administration record (MAR) (electronic or printed)
- ❏ 60-mL syringe, catheter tip for large-bore tubes, Luer-Lok tip for small-bore tubes
- ❏ Gastric pH test strip (scale of 0 to 11.0)
- ❏ Graduated container
- ❏ Medication to be administered
- ❏ Pill crusher if medication in tablet form
- ❏ Water
- ❏ Tongue blade or straw to stir dissolved medication
- ❏ Clean gloves
- ❏ Stethoscope (for evaluation)

STEP	RATIONALE

ASSESSMENT

1 Check accuracy and completeness of each medication administration record (MAR) with health care provider's medication order. Check patient's name, drug name and dosage, route of administration, and time for administration. Clarify incomplete or unclear orders with health care provider before administration.

The health care provider's order is the most reliable source and only legal record of drugs that patient is to receive. Ensures that patient receives correct medication. Handwritten MARs are a source of medication errors (ISMP, 2010; Jones and Treiber, 2010).

2 Review pertinent information related to medication, including action, purpose, normal dose and route, side effects, time of onset and peak action, and nursing implications.

Allows you to anticipate effects of drug and observe patient's response.

3 Assess for any contraindications to receiving medications enterally, including presence of bowel inflammation, reduced peristalsis, recent gastrointestinal (GI) surgery, and gastric suction that cannot be turned off.

Alterations in GI function can interfere with drug absorption, distribution, and excretion. Patients with GI suction do not benefit from medication because it may be suctioned from the GI track before it is absorbed.

4 Assess patient's medical history, history of allergies, medication history, and diet history. If you identify contraindications, withhold medication and inform health care provider.

History reveals past problems with medication tolerance and response. Historical data allows you to anticipate how certain drugs act.

5 For postoperative patient, review postoperative orders for type of enteral tube care.

Manipulation and irrigation of tube or instillation of medications may be contraindicated.

6 Gather and review physical assessment data (e.g., bowel sounds, abdominal distention) and laboratory data (e.g., renal and liver function) that may influence drug administration.

Physical examination findings or laboratory data may contraindicate drug administration.

7 Assess for potential drug-food interactions.

Some drugs may require tube feeding to be stopped for an hour before and 2 hours after dose (Lehne, 2010).

8 Check with pharmacy for availability of liquid preparation for patient's medications. Prescriber may need to change dosage form.

9 Before administration of medications verify placement of feeding tube (see Skill 31-2).

Reduces risk for aspiration.

NURSING DIAGNOSES

- Feeding self-care deficit
- Impaired swallowing
- Risk for aspiration

Related factors are individualized based on patient's condition or needs.

PLANNING

1 Expected outcomes following completion of procedure:
- Patient experiences desired medication effect within period of onset of medication.

Drug has exerted its therapeutic action.

- Patient's feeding tube remains patent after administration of medication.

Patent enteral tube indicates passage of medication into stomach, ensuring proper absorption. If tube becomes blocked, administration of other medications and feedings will not be possible.

- Patient does not aspirate during or after medication administration.

Patient safety in medication administration is maintained.

2 Explain procedure to patient, including description of medication to be instilled into enteric tube.

Helps patient be a participant in care, which minimizes anxiety. Begins patient teaching regarding medications.

IMPLEMENTATION

1 Determine if medication interacts with enteral feeding. If interaction occurs, hold feeding for 30 minutes before medication administration (see agency policy or consult with pharmacist).

Facilitates absorption of medication (Phillips and Endacott, 2011).

2 Perform hand hygiene. Prepare medications for instillation into feeding tube (see Skill 21-1). Check medication label against MAR 2 times. Fill graduated container with 50 to 100 mL of tepid water. Use sterile water for immunocompromised or critically ill patients (Bankhead et al., 2009).

These are the first and second checks for accuracy. Preparation process ensures that right patient receives right medication. Tepid water prevents abdominal cramping, which can occur with cold water.

STEP	RATIONALE

Clinical Decision Point *Whenever possible, use liquid medications instead of crushed tablets; but, if you have to crush tablets, the tubing must be flushed before and after the medication to prevent the drug from adhering to the inside of the tube. In addition, make sure that concentrated medications are thoroughly diluted. Never add crushed medications directly to a tube feeding (Phillips and Endacott, 2011).*

a *Tablets:* Crush each tablet into a fine powder, using pill-crushing device or two medication cups (see Skill 21-1). Dissolve each tablet in separate cup of 30 mL of warm water.	Fine powder dissolves more easily, reducing chance of occluding feeding tube.
b *Capsules:* Ensure that contents of capsule (granules or gelatin) can be expressed from covering (consult with pharmacist). Open capsule or pierce gel cap with sterile needle and empty contents into 30 mL of warm water (or solution designated by drug company). Gel caps dissolve in warm water, but this may take 15 to 20 minutes.	Ensures that contents of capsules are in solution to prevent occlusion of tube.
c Prepare liquid medication according to Skill 21-1.	
3 Take medication(s) to patient at correct time (see agency policy). Medications that require exact timing include stat, first-time or loading doses, and one time doses. Give time-critical scheduled medications (e.g., antibiotics, anticoagulants, insulin, anticonvulsants, immunosuppressive agents) at exact time ordered (no later than 30 minutes before or after scheduled dose). Give non–time-critical scheduled medications within a range of 1 or 2 hours of scheduled dose (ISMP, 2011). During administration, apply six rights of medication administration.	Hospitals must adopt medication administration policy and procedure for timing of medication administration that considers nature of the prescribed medication, specific clinical application, and patient needs (DHHS, 2011; ISMP, 2011). Time-critical scheduled medications are those for which early or delayed administration of maintenance doses of greater than 30 minutes before or after the scheduled dose may cause harm or result in substantial suboptimal therapy or pharmacologic effect. Non–time-critical medications are those for which early or delayed administration within a specified range of either 1 or 2 hours should not cause harm or result in substantial suboptimal therapy or pharmacologic effect (ISMP, 2011; DHHS, 2011).
4 Identify patient using two identifiers (i.e., name and birthday or name and account number) according to agency policy. Compare identifiers in MAR/medical record with information on patient's identification bracelet and/or ask patient to state name.	Ensures correct patient. Complies with The Joint Commission standards and improves patient safety (TJC, 2012). Some agencies are now using a bar-code system to help with patient identification.
5 At patient's bedside again compare MAR or computer printout with names of medications on medication labels and patient name. Ask patient if he or she has allergies.	*This is the third check for accuracy* and ensures that patient receives correct medication. Confirms patient's allergy history.
6 Discuss purpose of each medication, action, and possible adverse effects. Allow patient to ask any questions about the drugs.	Patient has right to be informed, and patient's understanding of each medication improves adherence to drug therapy.
7 Elevate head of bed to minimum of 30 degrees and preferably 45 degrees (unless contraindicated) or sit patient up in a chair (Bankhead et al., 2009).	Reduces risk for aspiration, keeping head above stomach.
8 If continuous enteral tube feeding is infusing, adjust infusion pump to hold tube feeding.	Feeding solution should not infuse while residuals are checked or medications are administered.
9 Apply clean gloves. Check placement of feeding tube (see Skill 31-2) by observing gastric contents and checking pH of aspirate contents. *Gastric pH for a patient who has fasted for 4 hours is usually 1.0 to 4.0.*	Ensures proper tube placement and reduces risk of introducing fluids into respiratory tract.
10 Check for gastric residual volume (GRV). Draw up 10 to 30 mL of air into a 60-mL syringe and connect syringe to feeding tube. Flush tube with air and pull back slowly to aspirate gastric contents (see illustration). Determine GRV using either scale on syringe or a graduate container. Return aspirated contents to stomach unless a single GRV exceeds 500 mL or if two measurements taken 1 hour apart each exceed 250 mL (Bankhead et al., 2009) (check agency policy). When GRV is excessive, hold medication and contact health care provider.	GRV categories have been identified in studies as significant when patients have two or more GRVs of at least 250 mL or one or more GRVs exceeding 500 mL (Bankhead et al., 2009). Large residuals indicate delayed gastric emptying and put patient at increased risk for aspiration (Metheney et al., 2010).

STEP	RATIONALE
11 Irrigate the tubing. **a** Pinch or clamp enteral tube and remove syringe. Draw up 30 mL of water into syringe. Reinsert tip of syringe into tube, release clamp, and flush tubing. Clamp tube again and remove syringe. **b** Some enteral tubes are connected to continuous-feeding tubing with stopcock apparatus such as a Lopez valve that contains a medication port (see illustration). Attach tip of syringe to medication port on stopcock; turn "off" setting of stopcock away from patient and toward infusion tubing. Flush tube and set stopcock "off" again to medication port. Remove syringe.	Pinching or clamping tubing prevents leakage or spillage of stomach contents. Flushing ensures that tube is patent.
12 Remove bulb or plunger of syringe and reinsert syringe into tip of feeding tube.	Removal of bulb or plunger prepares syringe for delivery of medications.
13 Administer first dose of liquid or dissolved medication by pouring into syringe (see illustration). Allow to flow by gravity.	

Clinical Decision Point *If medication does not flow freely, raise the height of the syringe to increase the rate of flow or try having the patient change position slightly because the end of the feeding tube may be against the gastric mucosa. If these measures do not improve the flow, a gentle push with bulb of Asepto syringe or plunger of the syringe may facilitate flow of fluid.*

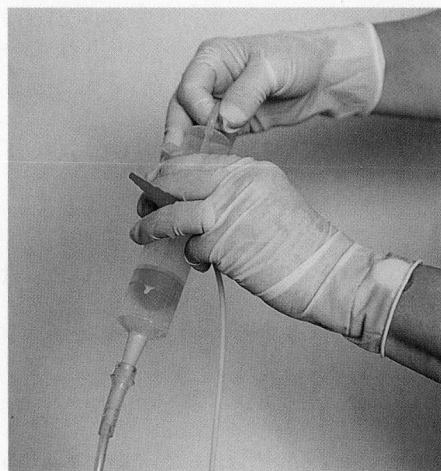
STEP 10 Aspirate stomach contents for residual volume.

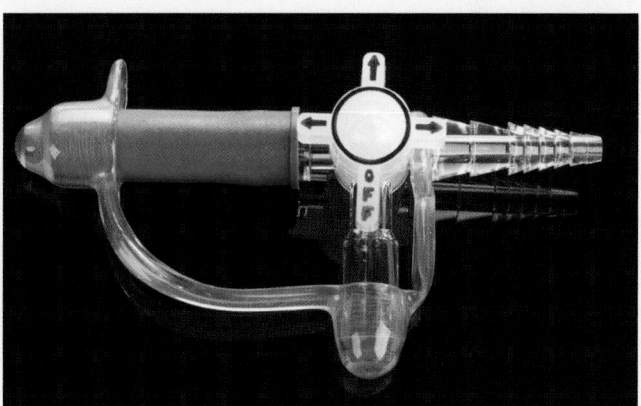
STEP 11b Lopez valve with medication port. *(Courtesy ICU Medical, Inc, San Clemente, Calif.)*

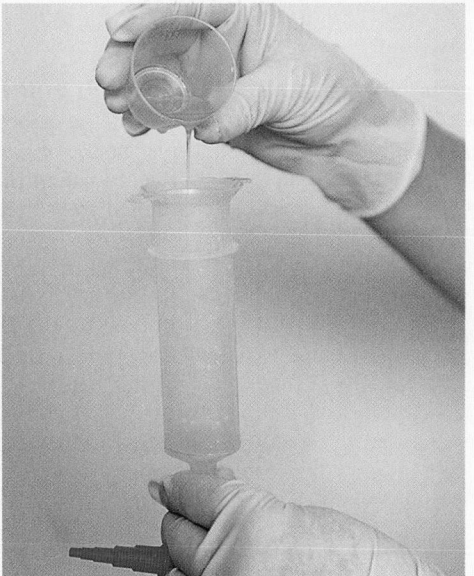
STEP 13 Pour liquid medication into syringe.

STEP	RATIONALE
a If giving only one dose of medication, flush with 30 mL of water after administration.	Maintains patency of enteral tube and ensures that medication passes through tube to stomach.
b To administer more than one medication, give each separately and flush between medications with 15 to 30 mL of water.	Allows for accurate identification of medication if dose is spilled. In addition, some medications may be incompatible (Boullata, 2009).
c Follow last dose of medication with 30 to 60 mL of water.	Maintains patency of enteral tube and ensures passage of medication into stomach (Boullata, 2009).
14 Clamp proximal end of feeding tube if tube feeding is not being administered and cap end of tube.	Prevents air from entering stomach between medication doses.
15 When continuous tube feeding is being administered by infusion pump, follow medication administration Steps 1 to 13. If medications are not compatible with feeding solution, hold feeding for additional 30 to 60 minutes.	Allows for adequate absorption of medication and avoids potential drug-food interaction between medication and enteral feeding.
16 Help patient to comfortable position and keep head of bed elevated for 1 hour (see agency policy).	Reduces risk of aspiration.
17 Dispose of soiled supplies, rinse graduated container and syringe with tap water, remove and dispose of gloves, and perform hand hygiene.	Reduces spread of microorganisms.

EVALUATION

1 Return within 30 minutes to evaluate patient's response to medications.	Monitoring patient's response evaluates therapeutic benefit of drug and helps detect onset of side effects or allergic reactions.

Unexpected Outcomes

1 Patient exhibits signs of aspiration, including respiratory distress, changes in vital signs, or changes in oxygen saturation.

2 Patient does not receive medication because of blocked enteral tube.

3 Patient exhibits adverse effects (side effect, toxic effect, allergic reaction).

Related Interventions

- Stop all medications/fluids through feeding tube.
- Elevate head of bed and stay with patient.
- Assess vital signs and breath sounds while another staff member notifies health care provider.
- For newly inserted tube, notify health care provider and obtain x-ray film confirmation of placement.
- Requires interventions to unclog tube to ensure drug delivery (Box 21-2).
- Withhold further doses.
- Always notify health care provider and pharmacy when patient exhibits adverse effects.
- Symptoms such as urticaria, rash, pruritus, rhinitis, and wheezing indicate allergic reaction.
- Enter patient allergy in medical record.

BOX 21-2   Unclogging a Blocked Feeding Tube

- Prevent tube from becoming blocked by flushing it with at least 15 to 30 mL of tepid water before and after administering each dose of medication, 30 to 60 mL after last dose of medication, before and after checking gastric residual volumes, and every 4 to 12 hours around-the-clock (refer to agency policies) (Bankhead et al., 2009).
- Gently flush tube with large-bore syringe and warm water. Do not use small-bore syringe because this exerts too much pressure and may rupture tube.
- If irrigation with water is not effective, obtain an order for a pancrelipase tablet (e.g., Viokase) and follow manufacturer guidelines for tube irrigation. In addition, a declogging stylus may be used (see agency policy).
- The tube may have to be removed, and a new one inserted if the medication is urgent.

Modified from Williams N: Medication administration through enteral feeding tubes: obstructed feeding tubes, *Am J Health System Pharmacy* 65(23):2347, 2008.

Recording and Reporting

- Record in nurses' notes and EHR the method used to check placement of enteral tube, GRV, and pH of stomach aspirate. Record actual time that each drug was administered on MAR immediately after administration, not before. Include initials or signature. Record patient teaching and validation of understanding in nurses' notes and EHR.
- Record total amount of water used for medication administration on proper intake and output (I&O) form.
- Report adverse effects, patient response, and/or withheld drugs to nurse in charge or health care provider.

Special Considerations
Teaching

- Teach patient or family caregiver how to store medications and tube-feeding supplements (see Chapter 31).
- Teach patient or family caregiver how to verify correct placement of tube before medication or tube feeding administration.

- Demonstrate to family caregiver how to prepare medications, including crushing them if appropriate.
- Teach family caregiver the importance of consistent flushing of feeding tube following medication administration.

Pediatric

- Volumes for instillation of medications or for irrigation of enteral tubes should be small enough to clear tubing (Hockenberry and Wilson, 2011; Williams, 2008).

SKILL 21-3 Applying Topical Medications to the Skin

NSO *Nonparenteral Medication Administration Module / Lesson 2*

 Video Clip

Topical administration of medication involves applying drugs locally to the skin, mucous membranes, or tissues. Topical drugs such as lotions, patches, pastes, and ointments primarily produce local effects; but they can create systemic effects if absorbed through the skin. Systemic effects are more likely to occur if the skin is thin, drug concentration is high, contact with the skin is prolonged, or the drug is applied to skin that is not intact. To protect from accidental exposure, apply topical drugs using gloves and applicators. Skin encrustations and dead tissue harbor microorganisms and block contact of medications with the affected tissue or membrane. Applying new medication over a previously applied medication does little to prevent infection or provide therapeutic benefit to a patient. Always clean the skin or wound thoroughly before applying a new dose of a topical medication. Apply each type of medication, whether an ointment, lotion, powder, or patch, in a specific way to ensure proper penetration and absorption.

Delegation and Collaboration

The skill of administering topical medications cannot be delegated to nursing assistive personnel (NAP). However, some agencies (e.g., long-term care) may allow NAP to apply some forms of topical agents (e.g., skin barriers) to irritated skin or for the protection of the perineum during morning or perineal care. Check agency policies. The nurse directs the NAP about:

- The expected therapeutic effects and potential side effects to report to the nurse.

Equipment

- ❏ Clean gloves (for intact skin) or sterile gloves (for nonintact skin)
- ❏ Option: Cotton-tipped applicators or tongue blades
- ❏ Ordered medication (powder, cream, lotion, ointment, spray, patch)
- ❏ Basin of warm water, washcloth, towel, nondrying soap
- ❏ Option: Sterile dressing, tape
- ❏ Felt-tip pen
- ❏ Medication administration record (MAR) (electronic or printed)
- ❏ Option: Plastic wrap, transparent dressing

STEP	RATIONALE

ASSESSMENT

1 Check accuracy and completeness of each medication administration record (MAR) with health care provider's medication order. Check patient's name, drug name and dosage, route of administration, and time for administration. Clarify incomplete or unclear orders with health care provider before administration.

The health care provider's order is the most reliable source and only legal record of drugs that patient is to receive. Ensures that patient receives correct medication. Handwritten MARs are a source of medication errors (ISMP, 2010; Jones and Treiber, 2010).

2 Review pertinent information related to medication, including action, purpose, normal dose and route, side effects, time of onset and peak action, and nursing implications.

Allows you to anticipate effects of drug and observe patient's response.

3 Assess condition of skin or membrane where medication is to be applied (see Chapter 6). If there is an open wound, perform hand hygiene and apply clean gloves. First wash site thoroughly with mild, nondrying soap and warm water, rinse, and dry. Be sure to remove any previously applied medication or debris. Also remove any blood, body fluids, secretions, or excretions. Assess for symptoms of skin irritation such as pruritus or burning. Remove gloves when finished.

Cleaning site thoroughly promotes proper assessment of skin surface. Assessment provides baseline to determine change in condition of skin after therapy. Application of certain topical agents can lessen or aggravate these symptoms.

4 Assess patient's medical history, history of allergies (including latex and topical agent), and medication history. Ask if patient has had reaction to a cream or lotion applied to skin.

Allergic contact dermatitis is relatively common and can worsen dermatologic (skin) condition. In addition, some patients may be allergic to preservatives or fragrances in topical medications. Latex allergy requires use of nonlatex gloves.

5 Determine amount of topical agent required for application by assessing skin site, reviewing health care provider's order, and reading application directions carefully (a thin, even layer is usually adequate).

An excessive amount of topical agent can chemically irritate skin, negate effectiveness of drug, and/or cause adverse systemic effects such as decreased white blood cell (WBC) counts.

STEP	RATIONALE
6 Assess patient's knowledge of action and purpose of medication being given, application schedule, and willingness to adhere to drug regimen.	Reveals patient's level of understanding and whether instruction is necessary.
7 Determine if patient or family caregiver is physically able to apply medication by assessing grasp, hand strength, reach, and coordination.	Necessary if patient is to self-administer drug at home.

NURSING DIAGNOSES

- Deficient knowledge regarding medication application
- Impaired skin integrity

- Pain (acute or chronic)
- Impaired physical mobility

- Readiness for enhanced self-health management
- Risk for infection

Related factors are individualized based on patient's condition or needs.

PLANNING

1 Expected outcomes following completion of procedure:	
• Patient is able to identify drug and describe action, purpose, dose, side effects, and schedule of medication.	Demonstrates learning.
• Patient is able to apply medication without assistance on prescribed schedule.	Demonstrates learning and compliance.
• With repeated applications, skin becomes clear, without inflammation or drainage from lesions.	Existing lesions heal and/or disappear as result of therapeutic action of medication.

IMPLEMENTATION

1 Prepare medications for application. Check label of medication against MAR 2 times (see Skill 22-1). Preparation usually involves taking bottle or tube of lotion, cream, ointment, or patch out of storage and to patient room. Check expiration date on container.	*These are the first and second checks for accuracy.* Process ensures that right patient receives right medication.
2 Take medication(s) to patient at correct time (see agency policy). Medications that require exact timing include stat, first-time or loading doses, and one time doses. Give time-critical scheduled medications (e.g., antibiotics, anticoagulants, insulin, anticonvulsants, immunosuppressive agents) at exact time ordered (no later than 30 minutes before or after scheduled dose). Give non–time-critical scheduled medications within a range of 1 or 2 hours of scheduled dose (ISMP, 2011). During administration, apply six rights of medication administration.	Hospitals must adopt medication administration policy and procedure for timing of medication administration that considers nature of the prescribed medication, specific clinical application, and patient needs (DHHS, 2011; ISMP, 2011). Time-critical scheduled medications are those for which early or delayed administration of maintenance doses of greater than 30 minutes before or after the scheduled dose may cause harm or result in substantial suboptimal therapy or pharmacologic effect. Non–time-critical medications are those for which early or delayed administration within a specified range of either 1 or 2 hours should not cause harm or result in substantial suboptimal therapy or pharmacologic effect (ISMP, 2011; DHHS, 2011).
3 Perform hand hygiene. Help patient to comfortable position.	
4 Identify patient using two identifiers (i.e., name and birthday or name and account number) according to agency policy. Compare identifiers in MAR/medical record with information on patient's identification bracelet and/or ask patient to state name.	Ensures correct patient. Complies with The Joint Commission standards and improves patient safety (TJC, 2012). Some agencies are now using a bar-code system to help with patient identification.
5 At patient's bedside again compare MAR or computer printout with names of medications on medication labels and patient name. Ask patient if he or she has allergies.	*This is the third check for accuracy* and ensures that patient receives correct medication. Confirms patient's allergy history.
6 Discuss purpose of each medication, action, and possible adverse effects. Allow patient to ask any questions about the drugs.	Patient has the right to be informed, and patient's understanding of each medication improves adherence to drug therapy.
7 If skin is broken, apply sterile gloves. Otherwise apply clean gloves.	Reduces spread of microorganisms.
8 **Apply topical creams, ointments, and oil-based lotions.**	
a Expose affected area while keeping unaffected areas covered.	Provides visualization for application and protects privacy.
b Wash, rinse, and dry affected area before applying medication (see Assessment, Step 3).	Cleaning removes microorganisms from remaining debris.

STEP	RATIONALE
c If skin is excessively dry and flaking, apply topical agent while skin is still damp.	Retains moisture within skin layers.
d Remove gloves, perform hand hygiene, and apply new clean or sterile gloves.	Sterile gloves are used when applying agents to open, noninfectious skin lesions. Changing gloves prevents cross-contamination of infected or contagious lesions and protects you from drug effects.
e Place required amount of medication in palm of gloved hand and soften by rubbing briskly between hands.	Softening topical agent makes it easier to spread on skin.
f Tell patient that initial application of agent may feel cold. Once medication is softened, spread it evenly over skin surface, using long, even strokes that follow direction of hair growth. Do not vigorously rub skin. Apply to thickness specified by manufacturer instructions.	Ensures even distribution and sufficient dosage of medication. Technique prevents irritation of hair follicles.
g Explain to patient that skin may feel greasy after application.	Ointments often contain oils.
9 Apply antianginal (nitroglycerin) ointment.	
a Remove previous dose paper. Fold used paper containing any residual medication with used sides together and dispose of it in biohazard trash container. Wipe off residual medication with tissue.	Prevents overdose that can occur with multiple-dose papers left in place. Proper disposal protects others from accidental exposure to medication.
b Write date, time, and nurse's initials on new application paper.	Label provides reference to prevent missing doses.
c Antianginal (nitroglycerin) ointments are usually ordered in inches and can be measured on small sheets of paper marked off in 1.25 cm (½-inch) markings. Unit-dose packages are available. Apply desired number of inches of ointment to paper-measuring guide (see illustration).	Ensures correct dose of medication.

Clinical Decision Point *Unit-dose packages are available.* NOTE: *One package equals 2.5 cm (1 inch); smaller amounts should not be measured from this package.*

d Select application site: Apply nitroglycerin to chest area, back, abdomen, or anterior thigh (Lehne, 2010). Do not apply on hairy surfaces or over scar tissue.	Application on hairy surfaces or scar tissue may interfere with absorption.
e Be sure to rotate application sites.	Minimizes skin irritation.
f Apply ointment to skin surface by holding edge or back of paper-measuring guide and placing ointment and wrapper directly on skin (see illustration). Do not rub or massage ointment into skin.	Minimizes chance of ointment covering gloves and later touching nurse's hands. Medication is designed to absorb slowly over several hours; massaging increases absorption rate.
g Secure ointment and paper with transparent dressing or strip of tape. Plastic wrap may be used as occlusive dressing.	Prevents staining of clothing or inadvertent removal of medication.
10 Apply transdermal patches (e.g., analgesic, nicotine, nitroglycerin, estrogen).	
a If old patch is present, remove it and clean area. Be sure to check between skinfolds for patch.	Failure to remove old patch can result in overdose. Many patches are small, clear, or flesh colored and can be easily hidden between skinfolds. Cleaning removes traces of previous patch.

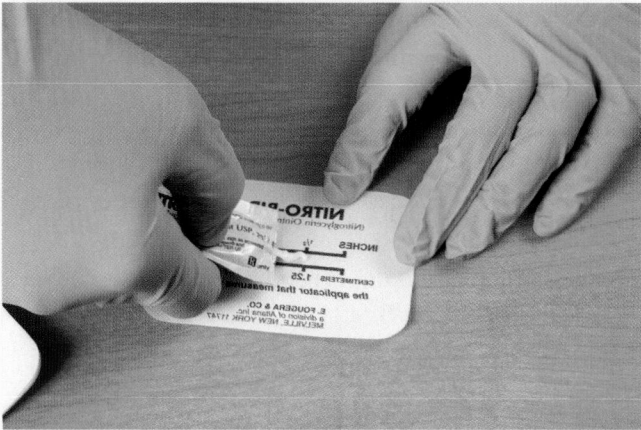

STEP 9c   Ointment spread in inches over measuring guide.

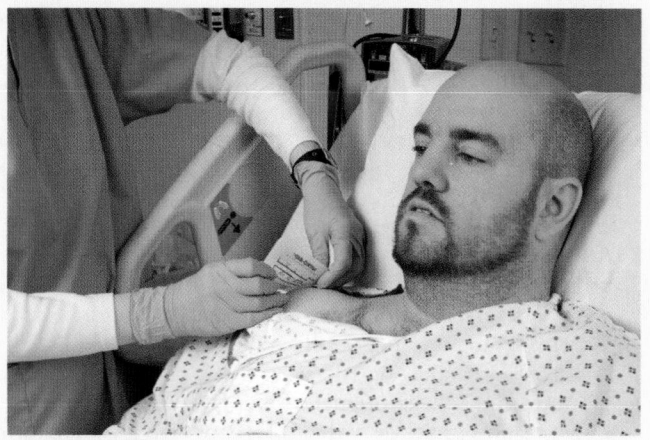

STEP 9f   Nurse applies wrapper with medication to patient's skin.

STEP	RATIONALE
b Dispose of old patch by folding in half with sticky sides together. Some agencies require patch to be cut before disposal (see agency policy). Dispose of it in biohazard trash bag.	Proper disposal prevents accidental exposure to medication.
c Date and initial outer side of new patch before applying it and note time of administration. Use soft-tip or felt-tip pen.	Visual reminder prevents missing or extra doses. Ballpoint pen damages patch and alters medication delivery.
d Choose a new site that is clean, dry, and free of hair. Some patches have specific instructions for placement locations (e.g., Testoderm patches are placed on scrotum; a scopolamine patch is placed behind the ear; never apply an estrogen patch to breast tissue or waistline). Do not apply patch on skin that is oily, burned, cut, or irritated in any way.	Ensures complete medication absorption.

Clinical Decision Point *Never apply heat such as with a heating pad over a transdermal patch because this results in an increased rate of absorption with potentially serious adverse effects.*

STEP	RATIONALE
e Carefully remove patch from its protective covering by pulling off liner. Hold patch by edge without touching adhesive edges.	Touching only edges ensures that patch will adhere and that medication dose has not changed. Removing protective covering allows medication to be absorbed through skin.
f Apply patch. Hold palm of one hand firmly over patch for 10 seconds. Make sure that it sticks well, especially around edges. Apply overlay if provided with patch.	Adequate adhesion prevents loss of patch, which results in decreased dose and effectiveness.
g Do not apply patch to previously used sites for at least 1 week.	Rotation of site reduces skin irritation from medication and adhesive.
h Instruct patient that transdermal patches are never to be cut in half; a change in dose would require prescription for new strength of transdermal medication.	Cutting transdermal patch in half would alter intended medication delivery of transdermal system, resulting in inadequate or altered drug levels.

Clinical Decision Point *It is recommended to have a daily "patch free" interval of 10 to 12 hours because tolerance develops if patches are used 24 hours a day every day (Lehne, 2010). Apply a new patch each morning, leave in place for 12 to 14 hours, and remove in the evening.*

STEP	RATIONALE
i Instruct patient to always remove old patch before applying new one. Patients should not use alternative forms of medication when using patches. For example, patients should not apply nitroglycerin ointment in addition to patch unless specifically ordered to do so by their health care provider.	Use of patch with additional or alternative drug preparation can result in toxicity or other side effects.
11 Administer aerosol sprays (e.g., local anesthetic sprays).	
a Shake container vigorously. Read container label for distance recommended to hold spray away from area, usually 15 to 30 cm (6 to 12 inches).	Mixing ensures delivery of fine, even spray. Proper distance ensures that fine spray hits skin surface. Holding container too close results in thin, watery distribution.
b Ask patient to turn face away from spray or briefly cover face with towel while spraying neck or chest.	Prevents inhalation of spray.
c Spray medication evenly over affected site (in some cases, time the spray for a period of seconds).	Ensures that affected area of skin is covered with thin spray.
12 Apply suspension-based lotion.	
a Shake container vigorously.	Mixes powder throughout liquid to form well-mixed suspension.
b Apply small amount of lotion to small gauze dressing or pad and apply to skin by stroking evenly in direction of hair growth.	Method of application leaves protective film of powder on skin after water base of suspension dries. Technique prevents irritation to hair follicles.
c Explain to patient that area will feel cool and dry.	Water evaporates to leave thin layer of powder.
13 Apply powder.	
a Be sure that skin surface is thoroughly dry. With your nondominant hand, fully spread apart any skinfolds such as between toes or under axilla and dry with towel.	Minimizes caking and crusting of powder. Fully exposes skin surface for application.
b If area of application is near face, ask patient to turn face away from powder or briefly cover face with towel.	Prevents inhalation of powder.
c Dust skin site lightly with dispenser so area is covered with fine, thin layer of powder. *Option:* Cover skin area with dressing if ordered by health care provider.	Thin layer of powder has slight lubricating properties to reduce friction and promote drying (Lilley et al., 2011).

STEP	RATIONALE
14 Help patient to comfortable position, reapply gown, and cover with bed linen as desired.	Provides for patient's sense of well-being.
15 Dispose of soiled supplies in receptacle especially designated for such articles, remove and dispose of gloves, and perform hand hygiene.	Keeps patient's environment neat and reduces spread of infection and residual medication to others.

EVALUATION

1 Ask patient or family caregiver to name the medication and its action, purpose, dose, schedule, and side effects.	Evaluates learning.
2 Have patient keep diary of doses taken.	Confirms adherence to prescribed therapy.
3 Observe patient or family caregiver apply topical medication.	Return demonstration measures learning.
4 Inspect condition of skin between applications.	Determines if skin condition improves.

Unexpected Outcomes

1 Skin site appears inflamed and edematous with blistering and oozing of fluid from lesions. These signs indicate subacute inflammation or eczema that can develop if skin lesions are getting worse.

2 Patient is unable to explain information about drug or does not administer as prescribed.

Related Interventions

- Hold medication
- Notify health care provider; alternative therapies may be needed.

- Identify possible reasons for noncompliance and explore alternative approaches or options.

Recording and Reporting

- Record actual time each drug that was administered, type of agent applied, strength, and site of application in nurses' notes/EHR and on MAR immediately after administration, not before. Include initials or signature. Record patient teaching and validation of understanding in nurses' notes. If you withhold a drug, record reason in nurses' notes and follow agency policy for noting withheld doses.
- Describe condition of skin before each application in nurses' notes and EHR.
- Report adverse effects/patient response and/or withheld drugs to nurse in charge or health care provider. Depending on medication, immediate health care provider notification may be required.

Special Considerations

Teaching

- If skin is inflamed, instruct patients to use only warm water rinse without soap for cleaning.

- Teach patient how to manage a transdermal patch that begins to peel off before the next dose is due. Rather than tape the patch or cover it, instruct patient to remove it, clean the skin, and apply a new patch to a different area (Ball and Smith, 2008).

Gerontologic

- Changes in the skin of an older adult patient include increased wrinkling, dryness, flaking, and increased tendency to bruise. Be aware of these changes when applying topical medications to ensure proper application. Older skin is often more fragile and must be handled gently when applying topical medications.

Home Care

- Instruct patient to wrap applicators, used patches, and similar materials and dispose of them into cardboard or plastic disposable containers. Careful disposal is necessary to ensure the safety of patient, other adults, pets, and children.

SKILL 21-4   Instilling Eye and Ear Medications

NSO *Nonparenteral Medication Administration Module / Lesson 3*

 Video Clip

Common eye (ophthalmic) medications are in the form of drops and ointments, including over-the-counter preparations such as artificial tears and vasoconstrictors (e.g., Visine® and Murine®). However, many patients receive prescribed ophthalmic drugs for eye conditions such as glaucoma, infection, and following cataract extraction. In addition, there is a third type of delivery system, the intraocular disk. Medications delivered by disk resemble a contact lens; but the disk is placed in the conjunctival sac, not on the cornea, and it remains in place for up to 1 week.

The eye is the most sensitive organ to which you apply medications. The cornea is richly supplied with sensitive nerve fibers. Care must be taken to prevent instilling medication directly onto the cornea. The conjunctival sac is much less sensitive and thus a more appropriate site for medication instillation.

Any patient receiving topical eye medications should learn correct self-administration of the medication, especially patients with glaucoma, who must often undergo lifelong medication administration for control of their disease. You can easily instruct patients while administering medications. Family caregivers often administer eye medications when patients are unable to manipulate applicators (e.g., arthritis or neurologic condition), immediately after eye surgery, and when a patient's vision is so impaired that it is difficult to assemble needed supplies and handle applicators correctly.

Ear (otic) medications are usually in a solution and instilled by drops. When administering ear medications, be aware of certain safety precautions. Internal ear structures are very sensitive to temperature extremes; administer eardrops at room temperature. Instilling cold drops can cause vertigo (severe dizziness) or nausea and debilitate a patient for several minutes. Although structures of the outer ear are not sterile, use sterile drops and solutions in case the eardrum is ruptured. A final safety precaution is to avoid forcing any solution into the ear. Do not occlude the ear canal with a medicine dropper because this can cause pressure within the canal during instillation and subsequent injury to the eardrum. If you follow these precautions, instillation of eardrops is a safe and effective therapy.

Delegation and Collaboration

The skill of administering eyedrop/eardrops cannot be delegated to nursing assistive personnel (NAP). The nurse directs the NAP about:

- Potential side effects of medications and to report their occurrence.
- The potential for temporary visual impairment or hearing changes after administration of eye medications.

Equipment

- ❏ Appropriate medication (eyedrops with sterile eyedropper, ointment tube, medicated intraocular disk, or eardrops)
- ❏ Clean gloves
- ❏ Medication administration record (MAR) (electronic or printed)

Eyedrops/Ointment

- ❏ Cotton ball or tissue
- ❏ Washbasin filled with warm water and washcloth
- ❏ Eye patch and tape (optional)

Eardrops

- ❏ Cotton-tipped applicator, cotton balls

STEP	RATIONALE

ASSESSMENT

1 Check accuracy and completeness of each medication administration record (MAR) with health care provider's medication order. Check patient's name, drug name and dosage, route (eye [s] or ear [s]), and time for administration. Clarify incomplete or unclear orders with health care provider before administration.

The health care provider's order is the most reliable source and only legal record of drugs that patient is to receive. Ensures that patient receives correct medication. Handwritten MARs are a source of medication errors (ISMP, 2010; Jones and Treiber, 2010).

2 Review pertinent information related to medication, including action, purpose, normal dose and route, side effects, time of onset and peak action, and nursing implications.

Allows you to anticipate effects of drug and observe patient's response.

3 Assess condition of external eye or ear structures (see Chapter 6). This may be done just before drug instillation (if drainage is present, apply clean gloves).

Provides baseline to determine if local response to medications occurs. Also indicates need to clean eye before drug application.

4 Determine whether patient has any symptoms of eye or ear discomfort or visual or hearing impairment.

Certain eye medications act to either lessen or increase these symptoms. Occlusion of external ear canal by swelling, drainage, or cerumen can impair hearing acuity and cause pain.

5 Assess patient's medical history, history of allergies (including latex), and medication history.

Factors influence how certain drugs act. Reveals patient's need for medication.

6 Assess patient's level of consciousness (LOC) and ability to follow directions.

If patient becomes restless or combative during procedure, greater risk for accidental eye injury exists.

7 Assess patient's knowledge regarding drug therapy and desire to self-administer medication.

Indicates need for health teaching. Motivation influences teaching approach.

8 Assess patient's ability to manipulate and hold dropper or ocular disk.

Reflects patient's ability to learn to self-administer drug.

NURSING DIAGNOSES

- Deficient knowledge regarding drug and self-administration
- Readiness for enhanced self-health management
- Impaired physical mobility
- Pain (acute or chronic)
- Risk for injury

Related factors are individualized based on patient's condition or needs.

STEP	RATIONALE

PLANNING

1 Expected outcomes following completion of procedure:
- Patient experiences desired effect of medication.
- Patient denies discomfort.
- Patient experiences no side effects, and symptoms (e.g., irritation) are relieved.
- Patient is able to discuss information about medication and technique correctly.
- Patient demonstrates self-instillation of eyedrops.

2 Explain procedure to patient.

Drug is administered correctly without injury to patient.
Drug is administered correctly without injury to patient.
Drug is distributed and absorbed properly.

Demonstrates learning.

Demonstrates learning.
Relieves anxiety and promotes patient participation.

IMPLEMENTATION

1 Prepare medications for instillation. Check label of medication against MAR 2 times (see Skill 22-1). Preparation usually involves taking eyedrops/eardrops out of refrigerator and rewarming to room temperature before administering to patient. Check expiration date on container.

These are the first and second checks for accuracy. Process ensures that right patient receives right medication.

2 Take medication(s) to patient at correct time (see agency policy). Medications that require exact timing include stat, first-time or loading doses, and one time doses. Give time-critical scheduled medications (e.g., antibiotics, anticoagulants, insulin, anticonvulsants, immunosuppressive agents) at exact time ordered (no later than 30 minutes before or after scheduled dose). Give non–time-critical scheduled medications within a range of 1 or 2 hours of scheduled dose (ISMP, 2011). During administration, apply six rights of medication administration.

Hospitals must adopt medication administration policy and procedure for timing of medication administration that considers nature of the prescribed medication, specific clinical application, and patient needs (DHHS, 2011; ISMP, 2011). Time-critical scheduled medications are those for which early or delayed administration of maintenance doses of greater than 30 minutes before or after the scheduled dose may cause harm or result in substantial suboptimal therapy or pharmacologic effect. Non–time-critical medications are those for which early or delayed administration within a specified range of either 1 or 2 hours should not cause harm or result in substantial suboptimal therapy or pharmacologic effect (ISMP, 2011; DHHS, 2011).

3 Perform hand hygiene and arrange supplies at bedside.

Reduces spread of microorganisms; ensures smooth, orderly procedure.

4 Identify patient using two identifiers (i.e., name and birthday or name and account number) according to agency policy. Compare identifiers in MAR/medical record with information on patient's identification bracelet and/or ask patient to state name.

Ensures correct patient. Complies with The Joint Commission standards and improves patient safety (TJC, 2012).

Some agencies are now using a bar-code system to help with patient identification.

5 At patient's bedside again compare MAR or computer printout with names of medications on medication labels and patient name. Ask patient if he or she has allergies.

This is the third check for accuracy and ensures that patient receives correct medication. Confirms patient's allergy history.

6 Discuss purpose of each medication, action, and possible adverse effects. Allow patient to ask any questions about the drugs. Patients who self-instill medications may be allowed to give drops under nurse's supervision (check agency policy). Tell patients receiving eyedrops (mydriatics) that vision will be blurred temporarily and sensitivity to light may occur.

Patient has right to be informed, and patient's understanding of each medication improves adherence to drug therapy.

7 Instill eye medications.

a Apply clean gloves. Ask patient to lie supine or sit back in chair with head slightly hyperextended, looking up.

Position provides easy access to eye for medication instillation and minimizes drainage of medication into tear duct.

Clinical Decision Point *Do not hyperextend the neck of a patient with cervical spine injury.*

b If drainage or crusting is present along eyelid margins or inner canthus, gently wash away. Soak any dried crusts with warm, damp washcloth or cotton ball over eye for several minutes. Always wipe clean from inner to outer canthus (see illustration). Remove gloves and perform hand hygiene.

Soaking allows easy removal of crusts without applying pressure to eye. Cleaning from inner to outer canthus avoids entrance of microorganisms into lacrimal duct (Lilley et al., 2011).

STEP	RATIONALE
c Explain there might be temporary burning sensation from drops.	Corneas are highly sensitive.
d Instill eyedrops.	
(1) Apply clean gloves. Hold cotton ball or clean tissue in nondominant hand on patient's cheekbone just below lower eyelid.	Cotton or tissue absorbs medication that escapes eye.
(2) With tissue or cotton resting below lower lid, gently press downward with thumb or forefinger against bony orbit, exposing conjunctival sac. Never press directly against patient's eyeball.	Prevents pressure and trauma to eyeball and prevents fingers from touching eye.
(3) Ask patient to look at ceiling. Rest dominant hand on patient's forehead; hold filled medication eyedropper approximately 1 to 2 cm (½ to ¾ inch) above conjunctival sac.	Action moves cornea up and away from conjunctival sac and reduces blink reflex. Prevents accidental contact of eyedropper with eye and reduces risk of injury and transfer of microorganisms to dropper (ophthalmic medications are sterile).
(4) Drop prescribed number of drops into conjunctival sac (see illustration).	Conjunctival sac normally holds 1 or 2 drops. Provides even distribution of medication across eye.
(5) If patient blinks or closes eye, causing drops to land on outer lid margins, repeat procedure.	Therapeutic effect of drug is obtained only when drops enter conjunctival sac.
(6) When administering drops that may cause systemic effects, apply gentle pressure to patient's nasolacrimal duct with clean tissue for 30 to 60 seconds over each eye, one at a time (see illustration). Avoid pressure directly against patient's eyeball.	Prevents overflow of medication into nasal and pharyngeal passages. Prevents absorption into systemic circulation.

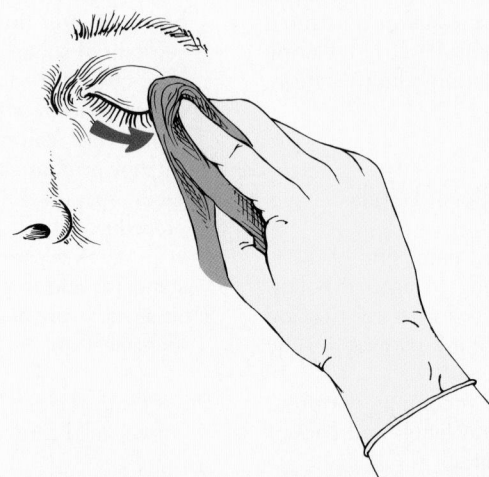

STEP 7b Clean eye, washing from inner to outer canthus before administering drops or ointment.

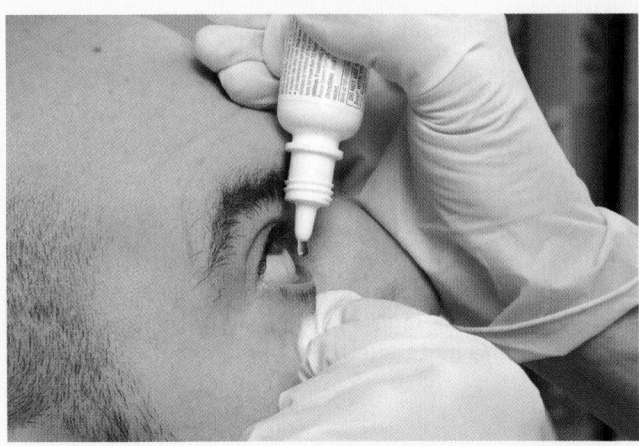

STEP 7d(4) Hold eyedropper over lower conjunctival sac.

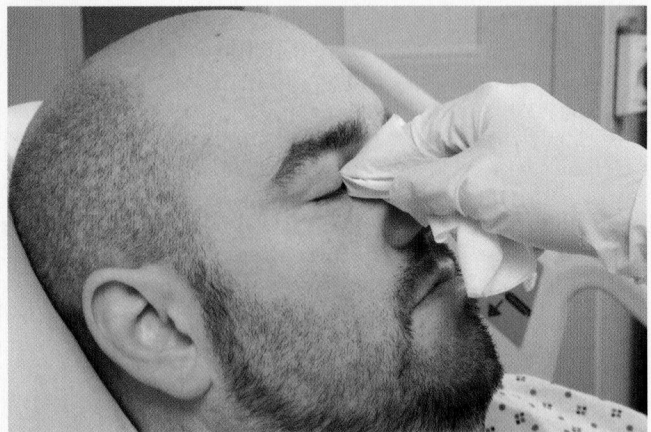

STEP 7d(6) Apply gentle pressure against nasolacrimal duct after giving eye medications.

STEP	RATIONALE
(7) After instilling drops, ask patient to close eyes gently.	Helps distribute medication. Squinting or squeezing eyelids forces medication from conjunctival sac.
e Instill eye ointment.	
(1) Holding applicator above lower lid margin, apply thin ribbon of ointment evenly along inner edge of lower eyelid on conjunctiva (see illustration) from inner to outer canthus.	Distributes medication evenly across eye and lid margin.
(2) Have patient close eye and rub lid lightly in circular motion with cotton ball if not contraindicated. Avoid placing pressure directly against patient's eyeball.	Further distributes medication without traumatizing eye.
(3) If excess medication is on eyelid, gently wipe it from inner to outer canthus.	Promotes comfort and prevents trauma to eye.
(4) If patient needs an eye patch, apply clean one by placing it over affected eye so entire eye is covered. Tape securely without applying pressure to eye.	Clean eye patch reduces risk of infection.
f Apply intraocular disk.	
(1) Open package containing disk. Gently press your fingertip against disk so it adheres to your finger. It may be necessary to moisten gloved finger with sterile saline. Position convex side of disk on your fingertip.	Allows you to inspect disk for damage or deformity.
(2) With your other hand gently pull patient's lower eyelid away from eye. Ask patient to look up.	Prepares conjunctival sac for receiving medicated disk and moves sensitive cornea away.
(3) Place disk in conjunctival sac so it floats on sclera between iris and lower eyelid (see illustration).	Ensures delivery of medication.
(4) Pull patient's lower eyelid out and over disk (see illustration). You should not be able to see disk at this time. Repeat if you can see disk.	Ensures accurate medication delivery.
8 After administering eye medications remove and dispose of gloves and soiled supplies, perform hand hygiene.	Reduces spread of microorganisms

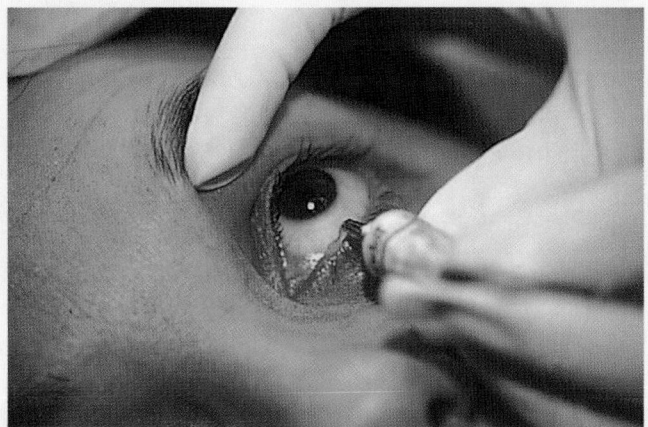

STEP 7e(1) Nurse applies ointment along inner edge of lower eyelid from inner to outer canthus.

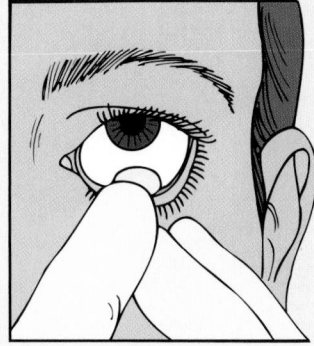

STEP 7f(3) Place intraocular disk in conjunctival sac between iris and lower eyelid.

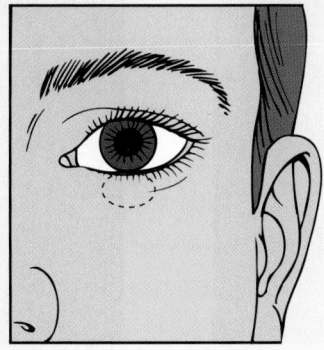

STEP 7f(4) Gently pull patient's lower eyelid over disk.

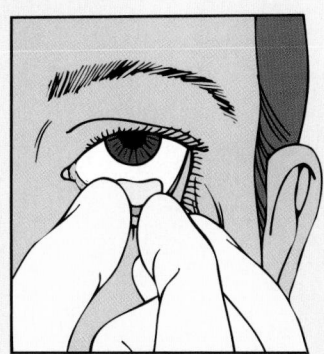

STEP 9b Carefully pinch disk to remove it from patient's eye.

STEP	RATIONALE
9 Remove intraocular disk.	
a Perform hand hygiene and apply clean gloves. Gently pull downward on lower eyelid using your nondominant hand.	Exposes disk.
b Using forefinger and thumb of your dominant hand, pinch disk and lift it out of patient's eye (see illustration).	
c Remove and dispose of gloves, perform hand hygiene.	Reduces spread of microorganisms.
10 Instill eardrops.	
a Perform hand hygiene. Apply clean gloves (only if drainage is present).	Reduces spread of microorganisms.
b Warm medication to room temperature by running warm water over bottle (make sure not to damage label or allow water to enter bottle).	Ear structures are very sensitive to temperature extremes. Cold may cause vertigo and nausea.
c Position patient on side (if not contraindicated) with ear to be treated facing up, or patient may sit in chair or at bedside. Stabilize patient's head with his or her own hand.	Facilitates distribution of medication into ear.
d Straighten ear canal by pulling pinna up and back to 10 o'clock position (adult or child older than age 3) or down and back to 6 to 9 o'clock position (child under age 3) (see illustrations).	Straightening ear canal provides direct access to deeper ear structures. Anatomic differences in younger children and infants necessitate different methods of positioning canal (Hockenberry and Wilson, 2011).
e If cerumen or drainage occludes outermost portion of ear canal, wipe out gently with cotton-tipped applicator (see illustration). Take care not to force cerumen into canal.	Cerumen and drainage harbor microorganisms and can block distribution of medication into canal. Occlusion blocks sound transmission.

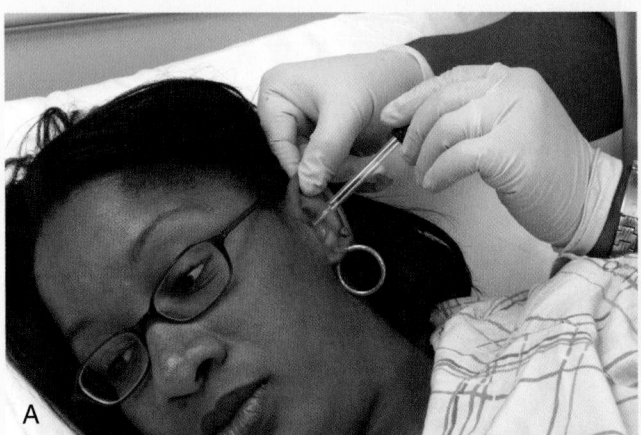
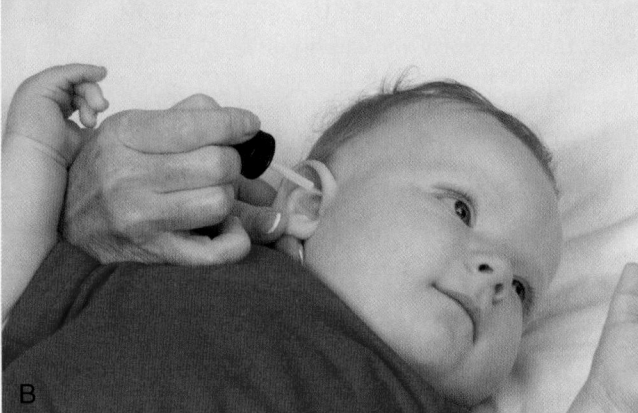

STEP 10d   A, Pull pinna up and back for adults and children older than 3 years. **B,** Pull pinna down and back for children under age 3.

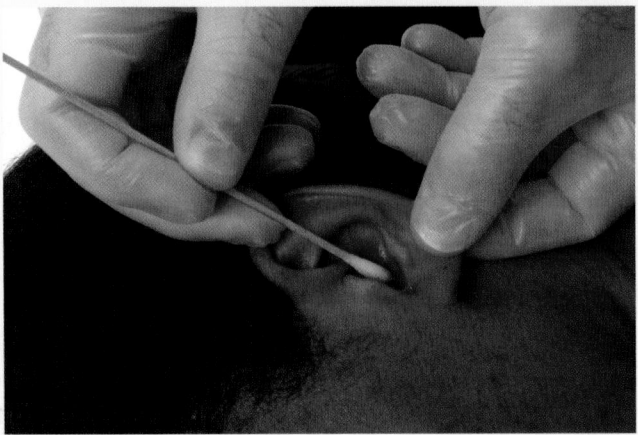
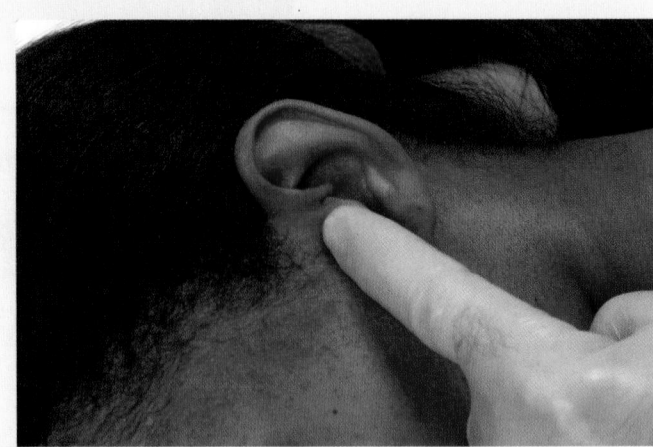

STEP 10e   Always clean only outer canal. Do not push cerumen or secretions into ear.

STEP 10g   Nurse applies gentle pressure to tragus of ear after instilling drops.

STEP	RATIONALE
f Instill prescribed drops holding dropper 1 cm ($\frac{1}{2}$ inch) above ear canal.	Avoiding contact prevents contamination of dropper, which could contaminate medication in container.
g Ask patient to remain in side-lying position for a few minutes. Apply gentle massage or pressure to tragus of ear with finger (see illustration).	Allows complete distribution of medication. Pressure and massage move medication inward.
h If ordered, gently insert portion of cotton ball into outermost part of canal. Do not press cotton into canal.	Prevents escape of medication when patient sits or stands.
i Remove cotton after 15 minutes. Help patient to comfortable position after drops are absorbed.	Allows time for drug distribution and absorption.
j Dispose of soiled supplies in proper receptacle, remove and dispose of gloves, and perform hand hygiene.	Reduces spread of microorganisms

EVALUATION

1 Observe response to medication by assessing visual or hearing changes, asking if symptoms are relieved, and noting any side effects or discomfort felt.	Evaluates effects of medication.
2 Ask patient to discuss purpose of drug, action, side effects, and technique of administration.	Determines patient's level of understanding.
3 Have patient or family caregiver demonstrate self-administration of next dose.	Provides feedback regarding competency with skill.

Unexpected Outcomes

1 Patient complains of burning or pain or experiences local side effects (e.g., headache, bloodshot eyes, local eye irritation). Drug concentration and patient's sensitivity both influence chances of side effects developing.

2 Patient experiences systemic effects from drops (e.g., increased heart rate and blood pressure from epinephrine, decreased heart rate and blood pressure from timolol).

3 Ear canal remains inflamed, swollen, tender to palpation. Drainage is present.

4 Patient's hearing acuity continues to be reduced.

5 Patient is unable to explain drug information or steps for taking eyedrops/eardrops and/or has trouble manipulating dropper.

Related Interventions

- Eyedrops may have been instilled onto cornea, or dropper touched surface of eye.
- Notify health care provider for possible adjustment in medication type and dosage.

- Notify health care provider immediately.
- Remain with patient. Assess vital signs.
- Withhold further doses.

- Notify health care provider for possible adjustment in medication type and dosage.

- Notify health care provider.
- Cerumen may be impacted requiring ear irrigation.

- Repeat instructions and include family caregiver as appropriate. Include return demonstration.

Recording and Reporting

- Record drug, concentration, dose or strength, number of drops, site of application (left, right, or both eye/ear), and time of administration on MAR immediately after administration, not before. Include initials or signature. Record patient teaching and validation of understanding in nurse's notes and EHR.
- Record objective data related to tissues involved (e.g., redness, drainage, irritation), any subjective data (e.g., pain, itching, altered vision or hearing), and patient's response to medications. Note any side effects experienced in nurses' notes and EHR.
- Report adverse effects/patient response and/or withheld drugs to nurse in charge or health care provider. Depending on medication, immediate health care provider notification may be required.

Special Considerations
Teaching

- Warn patients that mydriatics (agent used to dilate the pupils) temporarily blur vision. Wearing sunglasses reduces photophobia. If necessary, make arrangements for someone else to drive patient home from an office or clinic visit.
- Patients who receive medications that paralyze the ciliary muscles of the eye (e.g., scopolamine [Isopto-Hyoscine], atropine [Isopto Atropine], and cycloplegics) should not drive or attempt to perform any activity that requires acute vision after receiving medication.

Pediatric

- Infants often clench the eyes tightly to avoid eyedrops. Place the drops at the nasal corner where the lids meet with the infant supine. When the infant opens the eye, the medication will flow into it.

- When both eyedrops and ointment are ordered, administer the drops first, wait 3 minutes, and then administer the ointment. This allows time for each medication to have an effect.
- If the eye ointment is to be given once a day, administer at bedtime because it will blur the child's vision (Hockenberry and Wilson, 2011).
- Insert cotton pledgets loosely into ear canal to prevent medication from flowing out. To prevent cotton from absorbing medication, premoisten it with a few drops of medication (Hockenberry and Wilson, 2011).

Gerontologic
- Before discharging an older adult, evaluate patient's ability to perform all the necessary steps for the administration of eyedrops and ointments.
- Many older adults accumulate cerumen in the ear. This should be removed by irrigation before administering medication (see Chapter 19).

Home Care
- When using over-the-counter (OTC) eyedrops, patients should not share medications with other family caregivers. Risk for infection transmission is high. In addition, instruct patients to follow manufacturer instructions carefully for dosing.

SKILL 21-5 Administering Nasal Instillations

Patients with nasal sinus problems may receive drugs by spray, drops, or tampons. The most commonly administered form of nasal instillation is a decongestant spray or drops used to relieve sinus congestion and cold symptoms. Many over-the-counter (OTC) nasal preparations contain sympathomimetic drugs (e.g., Afrin or Neo-Synephrine). These drugs are relatively safe when administered nasally because only small doses are needed. However, the drugs can enter the systemic circulation by way of the nasal mucosa or by the gastrointestinal tract if an excess amount is swallowed, causing restlessness, nervousness, tremors, or insomnia in some patients. Long-term use of decongestant nasal spray can actually worsen nasal congestion because of a rebound effect. Nasal sprays are easy for a patient to self-administer. Health care providers treat severe nosebleeds by placing nasal packing or tampons, which are treated with epinephrine to slow bleeding.

Delegation and Collaboration
The skill of administering nasal instillations cannot be delegated to nursing assistive personnel (NAP). The nurse directs the NAP about:
- Potential side effects of medications and to report their occurrence to the nurse.
- Reporting any bloody nasal drainage.

Equipment
❑ Prepared medication with clean dropper or spray container
❑ Facial tissue
❑ Small pillow *(optional)*
❑ Washcloth *(optional)*
❑ Clean gloves
❑ Medication administration record (MAR) (electronic or printed)

STEP	RATIONALE

ASSESSMENT

1 Check accuracy and completeness of each medication administration record (MAR) with health care provider's medication order. Check patient's name, drug name and dosage, route (which sinus), and time for administration. Clarify incomplete or unclear orders with health care provider before administration.

The health care provider's order is the most reliable source and only legal record of drugs that patient is to receive. Ensures that patient receives correct medication. Handwritten MARs are a source of medication errors (ISMP, 2010; Jones and Treiber, 2010).

2 Review pertinent information related to medication, including action, purpose, normal dose and route, side effects, time of onset and peak action, and nursing implications.

Allows you to anticipate effects of drug and observe patient's response.

3 Assess patient's history (e.g., hypertension, heart disease, diabetes, and hyperthyroidism) and for history of allergies.

These conditions contraindicate use of decongestants that stimulate central nervous system.

4 Perform hand hygiene. Use penlight and inspect condition of nose and sinuses. Palpate sinuses for tenderness. Note type of drainage if present.

Provides baseline to monitor effects of medication. Presence of discharge interferes with drug absorption. Clear nasal discharge indicates sinus problem. Yellow or greenish discharge indicates infection.

5 Assess patient's knowledge regarding use of nasal instillations, technique for instillation, and willingness to learn self-administration.

Requires health teaching regarding use of drugs. Motivation influences teaching approach.

NURSING DIAGNOSES

- Deficient knowledge regarding drug action and purpose
- Readiness for enhanced self-health management
- Ineffective breathing pattern
- Pain (acute or chronic)
- Risk for injury

Related factors are individualized based on patient's condition or needs.

STEP	RATIONALE

PLANNING

1 Expected outcomes following completion of procedure:

- Patient is able to breathe without difficulty through nose.
- Patient's nasal sinuses are clear, moist, pink, without drainage after repeated instillations (applies to antiinfective medications).
- Patient is able to explain purpose of medication and administers nasal instillations correctly.

2 Explain procedure to patient and family caregiver regarding positioning and sensations to expect.

Rationale:

Nasal congestion has been relieved.
Inflammation of mucosa has been relieved.

Feedback reflects patient's learning.

Helps patient anticipate experience of procedure to reduce anxiety.

IMPLEMENTATION

1 Prepare medications for instillation. Check label of medication against MAR 2 times (see Skill 22-1). Preparation usually involves taking nasal drops or sprays out of storage and into patient room. Check expiration date on container.

These are the first and second checks for accuracy. Process ensures that right patient receives right medication.

2 Take medication(s) to patient at correct time (see agency policy). Medications that require exact timing include stat, first-time or loading doses, and one time doses. Give time-critical scheduled medications (e.g., antibiotics, anticoagulants, insulin, anticonvulsants, immunosuppressive agents) at exact time ordered (no later than 30 minutes before or after scheduled dose). Give non–time-critical scheduled medications within a range of 1 or 2 hours of scheduled dose (ISMP, 2011). During administration, apply six rights of medication administration.

Hospitals must adopt medication administration policy and procedure for timing of medication administration that considers nature of the prescribed medication, specific clinical application, and patient needs (DHHS, 2011; ISMP, 2011). Time-critical scheduled medications are those for which early or delayed administration of maintenance doses of greater than 30 minutes before or after the scheduled dose may cause harm or result in substantial suboptimal therapy or pharmacologic effect. Non–time-critical medications are those for which early or delayed administration within a specified range of either 1 or 2 hours should not cause harm or result in substantial suboptimal therapy or pharmacologic effect (ISMP, 2011; DHHS, 2011).

3 Identify patient using two identifiers (i.e., name and birthday or name and account number) according to agency policy. Compare identifiers in MAR/medical record with information on patient's identification bracelet and/or ask patient to state name.

Ensures correct patient. Complies with The Joint Commission standards and improves patient safety (TJC, 2012).
Some agencies are now using a bar-code system to help with patient identification.

4 At patient's bedside again compare MAR or computer printout with names of medications on medication labels and patient name. Ask patient if he or she has allergies.

This is the third check for accuracy and ensures that patient receives correct medication. Confirms patient's allergy history.

5 Discuss purpose of each medication, action, and possible adverse effects. Allow patient to ask any questions about drugs. Patients who self-instill medications may be allowed to give drops under nurse's supervision (check agency policy). Tell patients receiving nasal instillation that they may experience burning or stinging of mucosa or choking sensation as medication trickles into throat.

Patient has right to be informed, and patient's understanding of each medication improves adherence to drug therapy.

6 Perform hand hygiene. Arrange supplies and medications at bedside. Apply clean gloves (if drainage is present).

Reduces spread of microorganisms; ensures smooth, orderly procedure.

7 Gently roll or shake container. Instruct patient to clear or blow nose gently unless contraindicated (e.g., risk of increased intracranial pressure or nosebleed).

Ensures distribution of medication. Allows medication to reach sinuses.

8 **Administer nose drops.**

a Help patient to supine position and position head properly.

(1) For access to posterior pharynx, tilt patient's head backward.

(2) For access to ethmoid or sphenoid sinus, tilt head back over edge of bed or place small pillow under patient's shoulder and tilt head back (see illustration).

Proper positioning provides access to specific nasal passages.

STEP	RATIONALE
(3) For access to frontal and maxillary sinus, tilt head back over edge of bed or pillow with head turned toward side to be treated (see illustration).	Position allows medication to drain into affected sinus.
b Support patient's head with nondominant hand.	Prevents straining neck muscles.
c Instruct patient to breathe through mouth.	Mouth breathing reduces chance of aspirating nasal drops into trachea and lungs.
d Hold dropper 1 cm (½ inch) above nares and instill prescribed number of drops toward midline of ethmoid bone.	Avoids contamination of dropper. Instilling toward ethmoid bone facilitates distribution of medication over nasal mucosa.
e Have patient remain in supine position 5 minutes.	Prevents premature loss of medication through nares.
f Offer facial tissue to blot runny nose but caution patient against blowing nose for several minutes.	Provide comfort but allows for absorption of medication.
9 Administer nasal spray.	
a Help patient into upright position with head tilted slightly forward.	Proper positioning permits medication spray to reach nasal passages.
b Help patient insert tip of nasal spray into appropriate nares and occlude other nostril with finger (see illustration). Point spray tip toward side and away from center of nose.	Allows for proper administration of medication.

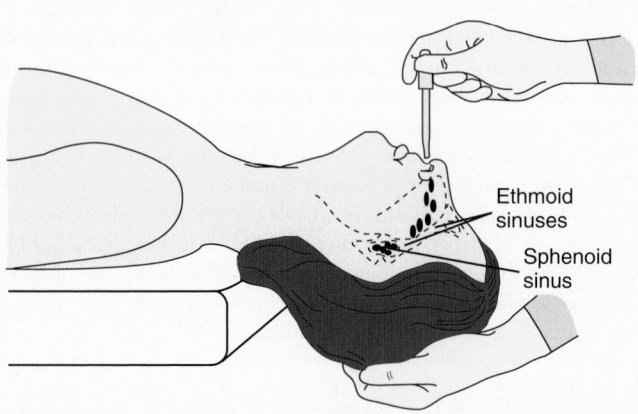

STEP 8a(2)   Position for instilling nose drops into ethmoid or sphenoid sinus.

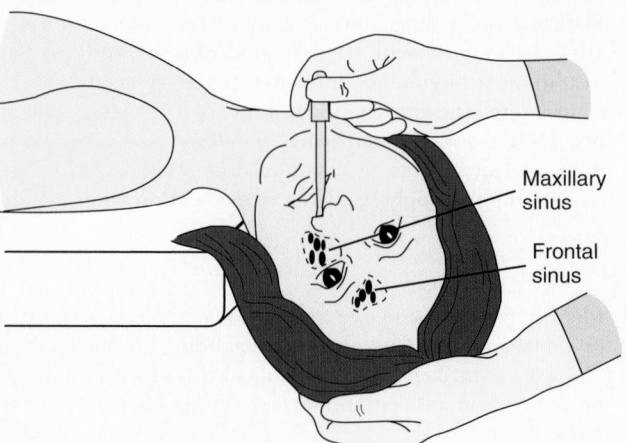

STEP 8a(3)   Position for instilling nose drops into frontal and maxillary sinus.

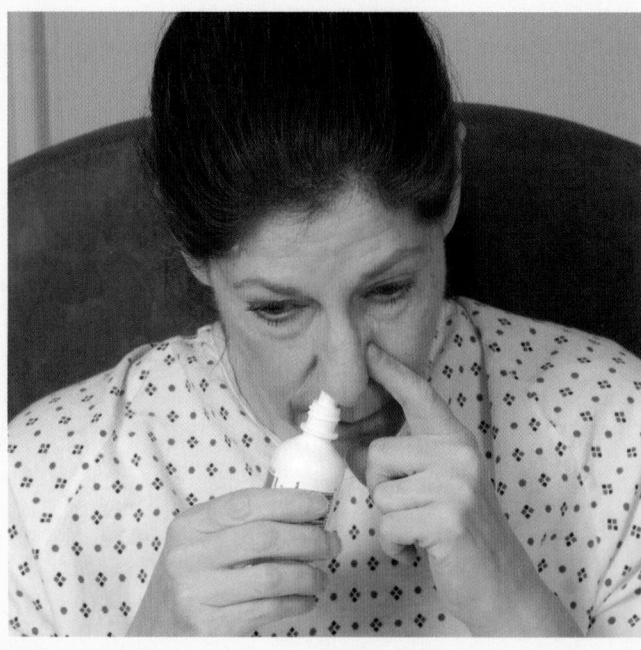

STEP 9b   Occlude the other nostril before self-administering nasal spray.

STEP	RATIONALE
c Have patient spray medication into nose while inhaling. Help him or her remove nozzle from nose and instruct to breathe out through mouth.	Allows for proper administration and distribution of nasal medication as high into nasal passages as possible.
d Offer facial tissue to blot runny nose but caution patient against blowing nose for several minutes.	Provides comfort but allows for absorption of medication.

Clinical Decision Point *Some medications are designed for one spray per dose. Examples include calcitonin (salmon), desmopressin (DDAVP, Stimate), and sumatriptan (Imitrex). It is essential to ensure that the patient understands the correct number of sprays to use per dose to prevent overdosing.*

10 Help patient to a comfortable position after medication is absorbed.	Restores comfort.
11 Dispose of soiled supplies, remove and dispose of gloves, and perform hand hygiene.	Reduces spread of microorganisms.

EVALUATION

1 Observe patient for onset of side effects 15 to 30 minutes after administration.	Drugs absorbed through mucosa can cause systemic reaction.
2 Ask if patient is able to breathe through nose after decongestant administration. May be necessary to have patient occlude one nostril at a time and breathe deeply.	Determines effectiveness of decongestant medication.
3 Reinspect condition of nasal passages between instillations.	Condition of mucosa reveals response to medication.
4 Ask patient to describe risks of overuse of decongestants and methods for administration.	Feedback ensures that patient can self-administer drugs properly.
5 Have patient demonstrate self-medication.	Feedback demonstrates learning.

Unexpected Outcomes

1 Patient is unable to breathe easily through nasal passages. Mucosa appears swollen, and congestion is unrelieved, due possibly to rebound effect.

2 Nasal mucosa remains inflamed and tender, with discharge from nares.

3 Patient complains of sinus headache. Sinuses remain congested.

4 Patient is unable to explain technique, risks of therapy, and self-administer medication.

Related Interventions

- Stop medication use.
- Notify health care provider and consider alternative therapy.

- Consider alternative therapy.

- Consider alternative therapy.

- Reinstruction is necessary.
- Include family caregiver when possible.

Recording and Reporting

- Record drug name, concentration, number of drops, nares into which drug was instilled, and actual time of administration on MAR immediately after administration, not before. Include initials or signature. Record patient teaching and validation of understanding in nurses' notes and EHR.
- Report any unusual systemic or adverse effects/patient response and/or withheld drugs to nurse in charge or health care provider.

Special Considerations

Teaching

- Instruct patients that each family caregiver should have a different dropper or spray applicator. Instruct patients to wash or rinse applicators after each use.

- Use OTC nasal sprays or nose drops for only one illness; bottles easily become contaminated with bacteria.

Pediatric

- Positioning child with head extended over edge of bed or pillow facilitates smooth instillation of nasal drops. Child should remain in this position for at least 1 minute to ensure that drops come in contact with affected tissue.
- Infants are nose breathers, and the possible congestion caused by nasal medications may inhibit their sucking. Administer nose drops if ordered 20 to 30 minutes before feedings (Hockenberry and Wilson, 2011).

SKILL 21-6   Using Metered-Dose Inhalers

NSO *Nonparenteral Medication Administration Module / Lesson 5*

Medications administered with handheld inhalers are dispersed through an aerosol spray, mist, or powder that penetrates the airways. Pressurized metered-dose inhalers (pMDIs), breath-actuated metered-dose inhalers (BAIs), and dry powder inhalers (DPIs) deliver medications that produce local effects such as bronchodilation. Some of these medications are absorbed rapidly through the pulmonary circulation and create systemic side effects (e.g., albuterol [Proventil] may cause palpitations, tremors, and tachycardia). Patients who receive drugs by inhalation frequently suffer from asthma and chronic respiratory disease. Drugs administered by inhalation provide control of airway hyperactivity or constriction. Because patients depend on these medications for disease control, they must learn about them and how to administer them safely.

An MDI is a small, handheld device that disperses medication into the airways through an aerosol spray or mist by activation of a propellant. Dosing is usually achieved with 1 or 2 puffs. DPIs deliver inhaled medication in a fine powder formulation to the respiratory tract (see Procedural Guideline 21-1). The deeper passages of the respiratory tract provide a large surface area for drug absorption, and the alveolar-capillary network absorbs medication rapidly.

An MDI delivers a measured dose of the drug with each push of a canister. Approximately 5 to 10 lbs of pressure is needed to activate the aerosol. This is difficult for some older patients because hand strength diminishes with age. Because use of an MDI requires coordination during the breathing cycle, many patients spray only the back of their throats and fail to receive a full dose. The inhaler must be depressed to expel medication just as the patient inhales. This ensures that medication reaches the lower airways. Poor coordination can be solved by the use of spacer devices (AeroChamber, InspirEase) or a breath-activated MDI such as the Maxair Autoinhaler. A spacer device decreases the amount of medication deposited into the oropharyngeal mucosa. Some spacers have a one-way valve that activates on inhalation, thereby removing the need for good hand-breath coordination (Lehne, 2010). Box 21-3 summarizes common problems that occur when using an inhaler.

Delegation and Collaboration

The skill of administering MDIs cannot be delegated to nursing assistive personnel (NAP). The nurse directs the NAP about:

- Potential side effects of medications and to report their occurrence to the nurse.
- Reporting breathing difficulty (e.g., paroxysmal coughing, audible wheezing).

Equipment

- ❏ Inhaler device with medication canister (MDI or DPI) (see Fig. 21-1, A to C)
- ❏ Spacer device such as AeroChamber or InspirEase (*optional*)
- ❏ Facial tissues (*optional*)
- ❏ Stethoscope
- ❏ Medication administration record (MAR) (electronic or printed)
- ❏ Pulse oximeter (*optional*)

BOX 21-3	**Common Problems in Using An Inhaler**

- *Not taking the medication as prescribed*: Taking either too much or too little.
- *Incorrect activation*: This usually occurs through pressing the canister *before* taking a breath. These actions should be done simultaneously so the drug can be carried down to the lungs with the breath.
- *Forgetting to shake the inhaler*: The drug is in a suspension; therefore particles may settle. If the inhaler is not shaken, it may not deliver the correct dose of the drug.
- *Not waiting long enough between puffs*: A delay between puffs is needed before taking a second puff; otherwise an incorrect dose may be delivered, or the drug may not penetrate into the lungs.
- *Failure to clean the valve*: Particles may jam the valve in the mouthpiece unless it is cleaned occasionally. This is a frequent cause of failure to get 200 puffs from one inhaler.
- *Failure to observe whether the inhaler is actually releasing a spray*: If it is not, this should be checked with the pharmacist.
- *Failure to recognize when the canister is empty*: This occurs when the metered-dose inhaler has no built-in dose counter or instructions in dose counting.

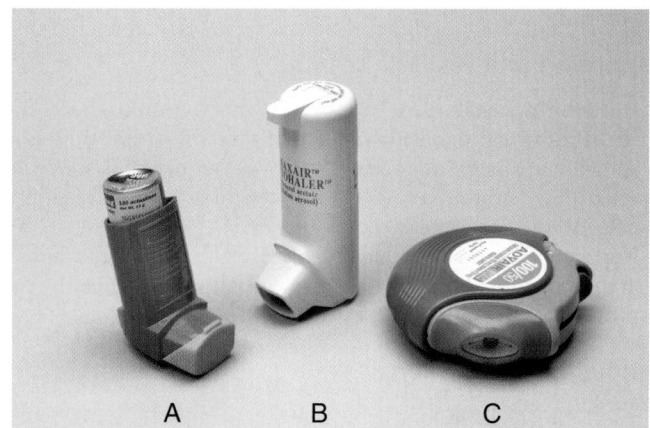

FIG 21-1 Types of inhalers. **A,** Metered-dose inhaler (MDI). **B,** Breath-activated inhaler (BAI). **C,** Dry powder inhaler (DPI).

STEP	RATIONALE

ASSESSMENT

1 Check accuracy and completeness of each medication administration record (MAR) with health care provider's medication order. Check patient's name, drug name and dosage, route, and time for administration. Clarify incomplete or unclear orders with health care provider before administration.

The health care provider's order is the most reliable source and only legal record of drugs that patient is to receive. Ensures that patient receives correct medication. Handwritten MARs are a source of medication errors (ISMP, 2010; Jones and Treiber, 2010).

2 Review pertinent information related to medication, including action, purpose, normal dose and route, side effects, time of onset and peak action, and nursing implications.

Allows you to anticipate effects of drug and observe patient's response.

3 Assess patient's medical history, history of allergies, and medication history.

Factors influence how certain drugs act. Reveals patient's need for medication.

4 Assess respiratory pattern and auscultate breath sounds.

Establishes baseline of airway status for comparison during and after treatment.

5 Assess patient's ability to hold, manipulate, and depress canister and inhaler.

Any impairment of grasp or presence of hand tremors interferes with patient's ability to depress canister within inhaler. Spacer device is often necessary.

6 Assess patient's readiness and ability to learn: asks questions about medication; is alert; participates in own care; is not fatigued, in pain, or in respiratory distress.

Mental or physical limitations affect patient's ability to learn and methods used for instruction.

7 Assess patient's knowledge and understanding of disease and purpose and action of prescribed medications.

Knowledge of disease is essential for patient to realistically understand use of inhaler.

NURSING DIAGNOSES

- Activity intolerance
- Anxiety
- Deficient knowledge regarding use of MDI

- Impaired gas exchange
- Ineffective breathing pattern

- Risk for injury
- Readiness for enhanced self-health management

Related factors are individualized based on patient's condition or needs.

PLANNING

1 Expected outcomes following completion of procedure:
  - Patient correctly self-administers metered dose.
  - Patient describes proper time during respiratory cycle to inhale and spray and number of inhalations for each administration.
  - Patient's breathing pattern improves, and lung sounds indicate airways are less restrictive.

Demonstrates learning.

Demonstrates learning and ensures correct administration of medication.

Demonstrates therapeutic effect of medication in improving gas exchange.

2 Explain procedure to patient. Be specific if patient wishes to self-administer drug. Explain where and how to set up at home.

Makes patient participant in care and minimizes anxiety.

IMPLEMENTATION

1 Prepare medications for inhalation. Check label of medication against MAR 2 times (see Skill 22-1). Preparation usually involves taking inhaler device out of storage and into patient room. Check expiration date on container.

These are the first and second checks for accuracy. Process ensures that right patient receives right medication.

2 Take medication(s) to patient at correct time (see agency policy). Medications that require exact timing include stat, first-time or loading doses, and one time doses. Give time-critical scheduled medications (e.g., antibiotics, anticoagulants, insulin, anticonvulsants, immunosuppressive agents) at exact time ordered (no later than 30 minutes before or after scheduled dose). Give non–time-critical scheduled medications within a range of 1 or 2 hours of scheduled dose (ISMP, 2011). During administration, apply six rights of medication administration.

Hospitals must adopt medication administration policy and procedure for timing of medication administration that considers nature of the prescribed medication, specific clinical application, and patient needs (DHHS, 2011; ISMP, 2011). Time-critical scheduled medications are those for which early or delayed administration of maintenance doses of greater than 30 minutes before or after the scheduled dose may cause harm or result in substantial suboptimal therapy or pharmacologic effect. Non–time-critical medications are those for which early or delayed administration within a specified range of either 1 or 2 hours should not cause harm or result in substantial suboptimal therapy or pharmacologic effect (ISMP, 2011; DHHS, 2011).

STEP	RATIONALE
3 Identify patient using two identifiers (i.e., name and birthday or name and account number) according to agency policy. Compare identifiers in MAR/medical record with information on patient's identification bracelet and/or ask patient to state name.	Ensures correct patient. Complies with The Joint Commission standards and improves patient safety (TJC, 2012). Some agencies are now using a bar-code system to help with patient identification.
4 At patient's bedside again compare MAR or computer printout with names of medications on medication labels and patient name. Ask patient if he or she has allergies.	*This is the third check for accuracy* and ensures that patient receives correct medication. Confirms patient's allergy history.
5 Discuss purpose of each medication, action, and possible adverse effects. Allow patient to ask any questions about the drugs. Explain what a metered-dose is and how to administer. Warn about overuse of inhaler and side effects.	Patient has right to be informed, and patient's understanding of each medication improves adherence to drug therapy.
6 Allow adequate time for patient to manipulate inhaler, canister, and spacer device (if provided). Explain and demonstrate how canister fits into inhaler.	Patient must be familiar with how to use equipment.

Clinical Decision Point *If using an MDI that is new or has not been used for several days, push a "test spray" into the air to prime the device before using. This ensures that the MDI is patent and the metal canister is positioned properly.*

STEP	RATIONALE
7 Explain steps for administering MDI without spacer (demonstrate when possible).	Simple step-by-step explanation allows patient to ask questions at any point during procedure.
a Remove mouthpiece cover from inhaler after inserting MDI canister into holder.	
b Shake inhaler well for 2 to 5 seconds (five or six shakes).	Ensures mixing of medication in canister.
c Hold inhaler in dominant hand.	
d Instruct patient to position inhaler in one of two ways:	
(1) Place mouthpiece in mouth with opening toward back of throat, closing lips tightly around it (see illustration).	
(2) Position mouthpiece 2 to 4 cm (1 to 2 inches) in front of widely opened mouth (see illustration), with opening of inhaler toward back of throat. Lips should not touch inhaler.	Directs aerosol spray toward airway. This is best way to deliver medication without a spacer.
e Have patient take deep breath and exhale completely.	Prepares airway to receive medication.
f With inhaler positioned, have patient hold it with thumb at mouthpiece and index and middle fingers at top. This is a three-point or bilateral hand position.	Hand position ensures proper activation of MDI (Lilley et al., 2011).
g Instruct patient to tilt head back slightly and inhale slowly and deeply through mouth for 3 to 5 seconds while depressing canister fully.	Medication is distributed to airways during inhalation.
h Have patient hold breath for about 10 seconds.	Allows tiny drops of aerosol spray to reach deeper branches of airways.

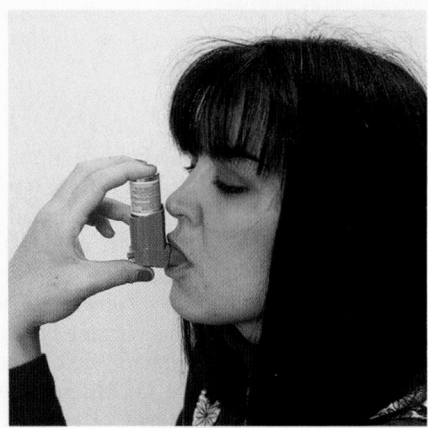

STEP 7d(1)   Patient opens lips and places inhaler mouthpiece in mouth with opening toward back of throat.

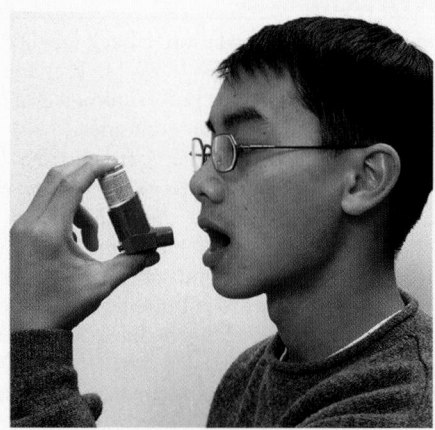

STEP 7d(2)   Patient positions inhaler mouthpiece 2 to 4 cm (1 to 2 inches) from widely open mouth. This is considered the best way to deliver medication without a spacer.

STEP	RATIONALE
i Remove MDI from mouth before exhaling and exhale slowly through nose or pursed lips.	Keeps small airways open during exhalation.
8 Explain steps to administer MDI using spacer device (demonstrate when possible).	
a Remove mouthpiece cover from MDI and mouthpiece of spacer device.	Inhaler fits into end of spacer device.
b Shake inhaler well for 2 to 5 seconds (five or six shakes).	Ensures mixing of medication in canister.
c Insert MDI into end of spacer device.	Spacer device traps medication released from MDI; patient then inhales drug from device. These devices improve delivery of correct dose of inhaled medication (Barrons et al., 2011).
d Instruct patient to place spacer device mouthpiece in mouth and close lips. Do not insert beyond raised lip on mouthpiece. Avoid covering small exhalation slots with the lips.	Medication should not escape through mouth.
e Have patient breathe normally through spacer device mouthpiece (see illustration).	Allows patient to relax before delivering medication.
f Instruct patient to depress medication canister, spraying one puff into spacer device.	Device contains fine spray and allows patient to inhale more medication.
g Patient breathes in slowly and fully (for 5 seconds).	Ensures that particles of medication are distributed to deeper airways.
h Instruct patient to hold full breath for 10 seconds.	Ensures full drug distribution.
9 Instruct patient to wait 20 to 30 seconds between inhalations (if same medication) or 2 to 5 minutes between inhalations (if different medications).	Drugs must be inhaled sequentially. Always administer bronchodilators before steroids so dilators can open airway passages (Lilley et al., 2011).
10 Instruct patient to not repeat inhalations before next scheduled.	Drugs are prescribed at intervals during day to provide constant drug levels and minimize side effects. Beta-adrenergic MDIs are used either on an "as needed" basis or regularly every 4 to 6 hours.
11 Warn patients that they may feel gagging sensation in throat caused by droplets of medication on pharynx or tongue.	This occurs when medication is sprayed and inhaled incorrectly.
12 About 2 minutes after last dose, instruct patient to rinse mouth with warm water and spit water out.	Inhaled bronchodilators may cause dry mouth and taste alterations. Steroids may alter normal flora of oral mucosa and lead to development of fungal infection (Lilley et al., 2011).
13 For daily cleaning, instruct patient to remove medication canister, rinse inhaler and cap with warm running water, and be sure that inhaler is completely dry before reuse. Do not get valve mechanism of canister wet.	Removes residual medication and reduces spread of microorganisms. Water damages valve mechanism of canister.
14 Ask if patient has any questions.	Clarifies misconceptions or misunderstanding.
15 Help patient to comfortable position and perform hand hygiene.	Reduces spread of microorganisms and promotes patient comfort.

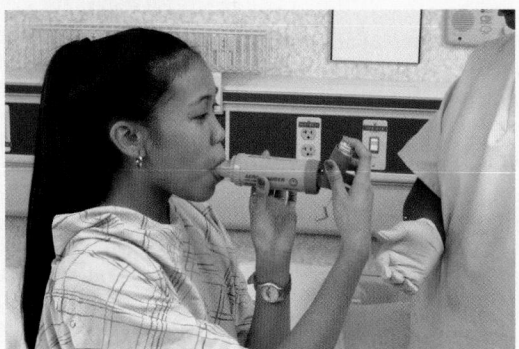

STEP 8e Using spacer device with an MDI.

STEP	RATIONALE

EVALUATION

1 Have patient explain and demonstrate steps in use and cleaning of inhaler.

2 Ask patient to explain drug schedule and dose of medication.

3 Ask patient to describe side effects of medication and criteria for calling health care provider.

4 After medication administration, assess patient's respirations, breath sounds, and peak flow measures if ordered.

Return demonstration provides feedback for measuring patient's learning.

Improves likelihood of adherence to therapy.

Allows patient to recognize signs of overuse and need to seek medical support when drugs are ineffective.

Determines status of breathing pattern and adequacy of ventilation/gas exchange.

Unexpected Outcomes	Related Interventions
1 Patient's respirations are rapid and shallow; breath sounds indicate wheezing.	• Evaluate vital signs and respiratory status. • Notify health care provider. • Reassess type of medication and/or delivery method.
2 Patient experiences paroxysms of coughing.	• Reassess patient's delivery method. • Notify health care provider.
3 Patient needs bronchodilator more than every 4 hours (may indicate respiratory problem).	• Reassess type of medication and delivery methods needed. • Notify health care provider.
4 Patient experiences cardiac dysrhythmias (light-headedness, syncope), especially if receiving beta-adrenergics.	• Withhold all further doses of medication. • Evaluate cardiac and pulmonary status (see Chapter 6). • Notify health care provider for reassessment of type of medication and delivery method.
5 Patient is not able to self-administer medication properly.	• Explore alternative delivery routes or devices.
6 Patient is unable to explain technique and risks of drug therapy.	• Further teaching is necessary. • Include family caregivers when possible.

Recording and Reporting

• Record drug administered, dose or strength, route, number of inhalations, and actual time administered on MAR immediately after administration, not before. Include initials or signature. Record patient teaching and validation of understanding in nurses' notes and EHR.

• Record in nurses' notes and EHR the patient's response to MDI (e.g., breath sounds), evidence of side effects (e.g., arrhythmia, feelings of anxiety), and patient's ability to use MDI.

• Report adverse effects/patient response and/or withheld drugs to nurse in charge or health care provider.

Special Considerations
Teaching

• Allow for supervised practice of the procedures. Patients may have difficulty timing an inhalation with activation of the medication canister without proper instruction (Lewis et al., 2011).

• Teach patient to keep track of the number of inhalations in the MDI (Box 21-4).

• Teach patients to use small, handheld peak flowmeters to monitor response to therapy when inhalers are prescribed (Barrons et al., 2011).

Pediatric

• A spacer is of benefit to young children because they have difficulty coordinating inhaler activation and inhaling (Hockenberry and Wilson, 2011).

• Educate child and parent about the need to use the inhaler during school hours. Help family find resources within the school or day care facility. Many school systems do not permit self-administration of MDIs. Follow school policy regarding

having the MDI available for use during school hours. A health care provider's order may be necessary.

Gerontologic

• Older adults may be unable to depress medication canisters because of weakened grasp or inability to coordinate actuation of the canister with inhalation. The use of a spacer device may be helpful.

Home Care

• Remind patients to carry prescribed inhalers to use as immediate treatment in case of an acute asthma attack.

BOX 21-4 | **Counting Doses in a Metered-Dose Inhaler**

Most metered-dose inhalers (MDIs) currently do not have automatic dose counters. Patients need to keep careful track of the number of inhalations used in their MDIs. Failure to do so may result in patients using an empty inhaler during an acute exacerbation of a respiratory problem. To track doses:

• Note first day of use on a calendar.
• Note number of inhalations in the canister (e.g., 200 inhalations per MDI).
• Note number of inhalations used per day (e.g., 2 inhalations a day, 3 times a day, equals 6 inhalations per day).
• Divide the total number of inhalations in the canister by the number of inhalations needed per day to determine the number of days that the inhaler should last (e.g., 200 inhalations divided by 6 inhalations per day equals approximately 33 days of 3-times-a-day dosing).
• Mark on a calendar the date the inhaler will be empty and obtain a refill of the inhaler a few days before this target date.

PROCEDURAL GUIDELINE 21-1 Using Dry Powder Inhaled Medications

Dry powder inhalers (DPIs) hold dry powdered medication and create an aerosol when the patient inhales through a reservoir that contains the medication. In contrast with the MDI, a DPI has no propellant. DPIs require less manual dexterity; and, because the device is breath activated, there is no need to coordinate puffs with inhalation. Compared with MDIs, DPIs deliver more medication to the lungs (Lehne, 2010). A DPI does not require a spacer. Medication inside a DPI can clump if the patient lives in a humid climate. Some patients cannot inhale fast enough to administer the entire dose of medication.

Delegation and Collaboration

The skill of administering DPI medications cannot be delegated to nursing assistive personnel (NAP). The nurse directs the NAP about:

- Potential side effects of medications and to report their occurrence to the nurse.
- Reporting paroxysmal coughing, audible wheezing, and patient's report of breathlessness or difficulty breathing.

Equipment

- ❏ Dry powder inhaler (see Fig. 21-1, C, p. 520)
- ❏ Stethoscope
- ❏ Washbasin or sink with warm water
- ❏ Medication administration record (MAR) (electronic or printed)
- ❏ Facial tissues (*optional*)

Procedural Steps

1 Check accuracy and completeness of each medication administration record (MAR) with health care provider's medication order. Check patient's name, drug name and dosage, route (which sinus), and time for administration. Clarify incomplete or unclear orders with health care provider before administration.

2 Review pertinent information related to medication, including action, purpose, normal dose and route, side effects, time of onset and peak action, and nursing implications.

3 Assess patient's medical history, history of allergies, and medication and diet history.

4 Assess respiratory pattern and auscultate breath sounds.

5 Assess patient's knowledge of medication and readiness to learn (e.g., asks questions about medication, requests education in use of DPI, is mentally alert, participates in own care).

6 Assess patient's ability to learn: Patient should not be fatigued, in pain, or in respiratory distress; assess level of understanding of technical vocabulary terms.

7 Determine patient's ability to hold, manipulate, and activate DPI.

8 If previously instructed in self-administration of DPI, assess patient's technique in using it.

9 Prepare medication for inhalation and check label on inhaler against MAR 2 times (see Skill 22-1). Preparation usually involves taking inhaler device out of storage and into patient room. *These are the first and second checks for accuracy. Check expiration date on container.*

10 Take medication to patient at correct time (see agency policy). Give medications that require exact or precise timing when ordered, give time-critical medications at time ordered (no later than 30 minutes before or after), and give non–time-critical medications within 1 or 2 hours of scheduled dose (DHHS, 2011; ISMP, 2011). During administration apply six rights of medication administration.

11 Identify patient using two identifiers (i.e., name and birthday or name and account number) according to agency policy. Compare identifiers in MAR/medical record with information on patient's identification bracelet and/or ask patient to state name.

12 At patient's bedside again compare MAR or computer printout with names of medications on medication labels and patient name. *This is the third check for accuracy.* Ask patient if he or she has allergies.

13 Discuss purpose of each medication, action, and possible adverse effects. Allow patient to ask any questions about the drugs. Explain what a DPI is and how to administer. Warn about overuse of inhaler and side effects.

14 If DPI has an external counter, note number indicated to determine doses remaining. Otherwise use technique in Box 21-4 for counting doses.

15 Prepare DPI for administration. Perform hand hygiene. Some DPIs require loading medication before administration; some require rotation of a lever to load medication or insertion of a capsule; and some require insertion of a disk into inhaler device. Follow manufacturer specific instructions.

Clinical Decision Point *The patient's inhaled breath pulls the drug into the airway. DPIs may differ as to how fast the patient should inhale the medication; consult specific instructions of manufacturer. In addition, do not shake DPI because powdered medication may spill out of device.*

16 Have patient place lips over mouthpiece of DPI and inhale quickly and deeply. Remove inhaler from mouth as soon as inhalation is complete but before exhalation. Instruct patients that, unlike with other inhaled medications, they may not taste or feel the dry powder or there may be a slight sweet taste.

17 Have patient hold breath for 10 seconds or as long as possible and then exhale. Do not exhale into DPI.

18 After using DPI, have patient rinse mouth with warm water and spit it out to reduce throat irritation and prevent oral candidiasis.

19 Return DPI to closed position or remove loaded capsule or disk if necessary. If an external counter is present, note number, which should be one less than the number in Step 14.

20 Have patient demonstrate use of DPI at next scheduled dose. Ask him or her to discuss purpose, action, and side effects of medication.

21 Auscultate breath sounds, evaluate respiratory rate, and ask patient about his or her breathing.

22 Record drug, dose or strength, route, number of inhalations, and time administered on MAR immediately after administration, not before. Include initials or signature. Record patient teaching and validation of understanding in nurses' notes and EHR.

SKILL 21-7   Using Small-Volume Nebulizers

Nebulization is a process of adding medications or moisture to inspired air by mixing particles of various sizes with air. Adding moisture to the respiratory system through nebulization improves clearance of pulmonary secretions. Medications such as bronchodilators, mucolytics, and corticosteroids are often administered by nebulization.

Small-volume nebulizers convert a drug solution into a mist that is then inhaled by a patient into their tracheobronchial tree. The droplets in the mist are much finer than those created by metered-dose inhalers (MDIs) or dry powder inhalers (DPIs). A face mask or a mouthpiece held between the teeth delivers a nebulized mist. A nebulized medication is designed to create a local effect, but it can be absorbed into the bloodstream through the alveoli. As a result, systemic effects from the medication may occur.

Delegation and Collaboration

In many health care agencies a respiratory therapist performs the skill of administering medications by nebulizer. The nurse must be aware of the type and actions of the inhaled medication that the patient is receiving. The skill of administering medications by nebulizer cannot be delegated to nursing assistive personnel (NAP). The nurse directs the NAP about:

- Potential side effects of medications and to report their occurrence to the nurse.
- Reporting paroxysmal coughing, ineffective breathing patterns, and other respiratory difficulties.

Equipment

- ❏ Medication ordered and diluent (if needed)
- ❏ Medicine dropper or syringe
- ❏ Nebulizer bottle and tubing assembly
- ❏ Small-volume nebulizer machine (often called *handheld nebulizer* or simply *nebulizer*)
- ❏ Pulse oximeter and peak flow device
- ❏ Stethoscope
- ❏ Medication administration record (MAR) (electronic or printed)

STEP	RATIONALE

ASSESSMENT

1 Check accuracy and completeness of each medication administration record (MAR) with health care provider's medication order. Check patient's name, drug name and dosage, route, and time for administration. Clarify incomplete or unclear orders with health care provider before administration.	The health care provider's order is the most reliable source and only legal record of drugs that patient is to receive. Ensures that patient receives correct medication. Handwritten MARs are a source of medication errors (ISMP, 2010; Jones and Treiber, 2010).
2 Review pertinent information related to medication, including action, purpose, normal dose and route, side effects, time of onset and peak action, and nursing implications.	Allows you to anticipate effects of drug and observe patient's response.
3 Assess patient's medical history, history of allergies, medication and diet history.	These factors influence how certain drugs act. Information also reflects patient's need for medications and risk for side effects.
4 Assess patient's grasp and ability to assemble, hold, and manipulate nebulizer equipment.	Any impairment of cognition or grasp or the presence of hand tremors affects patient's ability to use equipment.
5 Assess pulse, respirations, breath sounds, pulse oximetry, and peak flow measurement (if ordered) before beginning treatment.	Establishes baseline for comparison during and after treatment.
6 Assess patient's knowledge of medication and readiness to learn (e.g., patient asks questions about medication, requests education in use of nebulizer, is mentally alert, participates in own care).	Determines level of instruction needed to assume self-administration.

NURSING DIAGNOSES

• Activity intolerance	• Anxiety	• Risk for injury
• Impaired gas exchange	• Ineffective breathing pattern	• Readiness for enhanced self-health management
• Deficient knowledge regarding use of nebulizers		

Related factors are individualized based on patient's condition or needs.

PLANNING

1 Expected outcomes following completion of procedure:	
• Patient's breathing pattern is effective.	Demonstrates proper administration and therapeutic effect of medication.
• Patient's oxygen saturation level is adequate.	Demonstrates proper administration and therapeutic effect of medication.
• Patient describes side effects of medication and criteria for calling health care provider.	Increases likelihood of adherence to therapeutic regimen.

STEP	RATIONALE

- Patient demonstrates self-administration of nebulized dose of medication correctly.

Demonstrates learning.

2 Explain procedure to patient. Be specific if patient wishes to self-administer drug.

Makes patient participant in care and minimizes anxiety. Begins patient teaching regarding medications. Enables patient to self-administer drug if physically able and motivated.

IMPLEMENTATION

1 Prepare medications for inhalation. Check label of medication against MAR 2 times (see Skill 22-1). Preparation usually involves taking medication vial out of storage and taking to patient room. Check expiration date on container.

These are the first and second checks for accuracy. Process ensures that right patient receives right medication.

2 Take medication(s) to patient at correct time (see agency policy). Medications that require exact timing include stat, first-time or loading doses, and one time doses. Give time-critical scheduled medications (e.g., antibiotics, anticoagulants, insulin, anticonvulsants, immunosuppressive agents) at exact time ordered (no later than 30 minutes before or after scheduled dose). Give non–time-critical scheduled medications within a range of 1 or 2 hours of scheduled dose (ISMP, 2011). During administration, apply six rights of medication administration.

Hospitals must adopt medication administration policy and procedure for timing of medication administration that considers nature of the prescribed medication, specific clinical application, and patient needs (DHHS, 2011; ISMP, 2011). Time-critical scheduled medications are those for which early or delayed administration of maintenance doses of greater than 30 minutes before or after the scheduled dose may cause harm or result in substantial suboptimal therapy or pharmacologic effect. Non–time-critical medications are those for which early or delayed administration within a specified range of either 1 or 2 hours should not cause harm or result in substantial suboptimal therapy or pharmacologic effect (ISMP, 2011; DHHS, 2011).

3 Perform hand hygiene and arrange equipment needed.

Reduces transfer of microorganisms and saves time.

4 Identify patient using two identifiers (i.e., name and birthday or name and account number) according to agency policy. Compare identifiers in MAR/medical record with information on patient's identification bracelet and/or ask patient to state name.

Ensures correct patient. Complies with The Joint Commission standards and improves patient safety (TJC, 2012).

Some agencies are now using a bar-code system to help with patient identification.

5 At patient's bedside again compare MAR or computer printout with names of medications on medication labels and patient name. Ask patient if he or she has allergies.

This is the third check for accuracy and ensures that patient receives correct medication. Confirms patient's allergy history.

6 Discuss purpose of each medication, action, and possible adverse effects. Allow patient to ask any questions about the drugs. Explain how to assemble nebulizer and proper use.

Patient has right to be informed, and patient's understanding of each medication improves adherence to drug therapy.

7 Assemble nebulizer equipment per manufacturer directions.

Assembly may vary slightly with different manufacturers. Proper assembly ensures safe delivery of medication.

8 Add prescribed medication by pouring medicine into nebulizer cup. (Option, you may use a medicine dropper or syringe to instill medication.)

Ensures proper dose and delivery of ordered medication.

9 Attach top to the nebulizer cup and be sure it is secure. Then connect cup to mouthpiece or face mask..

Prevents loss of medication.

10 Connect tubing to both aerosol compressor and nebulizer cup.

11 Have patient hold mouthpiece between lips with gentle pressure, but be sure lips are sealed (see illustration).

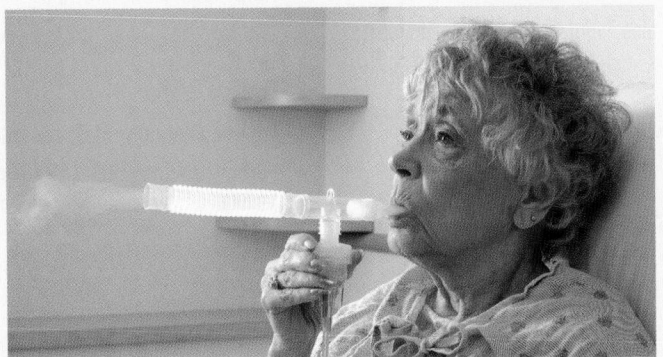

STEP 11 Nebulizer mouthpiece placed between patient's lips.

STEP	RATIONALE
a If patient is an infant, child, or fatigued adult or unable to follow instructions, use face mask.	Use of face mask does not require patient to remember to hold mouthpiece correctly. Correct delivery ensures sufficient deposition of medication.
b Use special adapters for patients with tracheostomy.	Promotes greater deposition of medication in airways.
12 Turn on small-volume nebulizer machine and ensure that a sufficient mist begins to flow.	Verifies that equipment is working properly during delivery of medication.
13 Have patient take deep breath, slowly, to a volume slightly greater than normal. Encourage brief, end-inspiratory pause for about 2 to 3 seconds, then have patient exhale passively.	Improves effectiveness of medication.
a If patient is dyspneic, encourage him or her to hold every fourth or fifth breath for 5 to 10 seconds.	Maximizes effectiveness of medication.
b Remind patient to repeat breathing pattern until drug is completely nebulized. This usually takes about 10 minutes.	Maximizes effectiveness of medication.
(1) Some health care providers set time limit as length of treatment rather than waiting for medication to completely nebulize.	
c Tap nebulizer cup occasionally during and toward end of treatment.	Releases droplets that are clinging to side of cup, thus allowing for renebulization of solution.
d Monitor patient's pulse during procedure, especially if beta-adrenergic bronchodilators are used.	Enables nurse to observe for potential side effects of medications.
14 When medication is completely nebulized, turn off machine. Rinse nebulizer cup per agency policy. Dry completely and store tubing assembly per agency policy.	Proper storage reduces transfer of microorganisms.
15 If steroids are nebulized, instruct patient to rinse mouth and gargle with warm water after nebulizer treatment.	Removes medication residue from oral cavity and helps to prevent oral candidiasis, a possible adverse effect of inhaled steroid therapy.
16 After nebulizer treatment is complete, have patient take several deep breaths and cough to expectorate mucus.	Nebulized medication is often ordered to open airways and promote expectoration of mucus.
17 Help patient to comfortable position and perform hand hygiene.	Reduces spread of microorganisms and promotes patient comfort.

EVALUATION

1 Assess patient's respirations, breath sounds, cough effort, sputum production, pulse oximetry, and peak flow measures if ordered.	Determines status of breathing pattern and adequacy of ventilation/gas exchange. Allows comparison with baseline data and evaluation of effectiveness of procedure.
2 Have patient explain and demonstrate steps in use of nebulizer.	Return demonstration provides feedback for measuring patient's learning.
3 Ask patient to explain drug schedule.	Improves likelihood of adherence to therapy.
4 Ask patient to describe side effects of medication and criteria for calling health care provider.	Allows patient to recognize signs of overuse and need to seek medical support when drugs are ineffective.

Unexpected Outcomes

1 Patient's breathing pattern is ineffective; respirations are rapid and shallow; breath sounds indicate wheezing.

2 Patient experiences paroxysms of coughing. Aerosolized particles can irritate posterior pharynx.

3 Patient experiences cardiac dysrhythmias (light-headedness, syncope), especially if receiving beta-adrenergics.

4 Patient is unable to self-administer medication properly.

5 Patient is unable to explain technique and risks of drug therapy.

Related Interventions

- Reassess type of medication and/or delivery method.
- Notify health care provider.

- Reassess type of medication and/or delivery method.
- Notify health care provider.

- Withhold all further doses of medication. Assess vital signs.
- Notify health care provider for reassessment of type of medication and delivery method.

- Explore alternative delivery routes or devices.

- Further teaching may be required.
- Include family caregivers when possible.

Recording and Reporting

- Record drug, dose and strength, route, length of treatment, and time administered on MAR immediately after administration, not before. Include initials or signature. Record patient teaching and validation of understanding in nurses' notes and EHR.
- Record patient's response to treatment in nurses' notes and EHR.
- Report adverse effects/patient response and/or withheld drugs to nurse in charge or health care provider.

Special Considerations

Teaching

- Teach patient not to store medication in nebulizer for later use.
- Advise patients taking long-acting beta-agonists about possible adverse effects, including nervousness, restlessness, tremor, headache, nausea, rapid or pounding heart, and dizziness.
- Teach patients to use small, handheld peak flowmeters to monitor response to therapy when inhaled drugs are prescribed (Barrons et al., 2011).

Pediatric

- Use a mask for the nebulizer treatment if child is too young to hold mouthpiece correctly for the duration of the treatment (Hockenberry and Wilson, 2011).
- Instruct child to breathe normally with mouth open to provide a direct route to the airways for the medication.
- Educate child and parent about the need to use the nebulizer during school or day care hours. Help family find resources within the school or day care facility. Follow school policy regarding having the nebulizer and medication available for use during school hours. A health care provider's order may be necessary.

Gerontologic

- Older adults with a weak grasp, hand tremors, or coordination problems may not be able to manipulate or hold a nebulizer.

Home Care

- When at home, rinse nebulizer parts after each use with clear water and air dry. In addition, clean parts (except for tubing and nebulizer compressor) daily with warm, soapy water; rinse; and allow to dry.

SKILL 21-8   Administering Vaginal Instillations

NSO *Nonparenteral Medication Administration Module / Lesson 6*

Female patients who develop vaginal infections often require topical application of antiinfective agents. Vaginal medications are available in foam, jelly, cream, or suppository form. Medicated irrigations or douches can also be given. However, their excessive use can lead to vaginal irritation.

Vaginal suppositories are oval shaped and come individually packaged in foil wrappers. They are larger and more oval than rectal suppositories (Fig. 21-2). Storage in a refrigerator prevents the solid suppositories from melting. You insert a suppository into the vagina with an applicator or a gloved hand. After insertion, body temperature causes the suppository to melt, and the medication is distributed. Foam, jellies, and creams are administered with an inserter or applicator. Patients often prefer administering their own vaginal medications, and you should give them privacy to do so. After instillation of a drug, a patient may wish to wear a perineal pad to collect excess drainage. Because vaginal medications are frequently given to treat infection, any discharge is often foul smelling. Follow good aseptic technique and offer a patient frequent opportunities for perineal hygiene (see Procedural Guideline 17-1).

Delegation and Collaboration

The skill of administering vaginal medications cannot be delegated to nursing assistive personnel (NAP). The nurse directs the NAP about:

- Potential side effects of medications and to report their occurrence to the nurse.
- Reporting any change in comfort level or new or increased vaginal discharge or bleeding to the nurse.

Equipment

- ❏ Vaginal cream, foam, jelly, tablet, suppository, or irrigating solution
- ❏ Applicators (Fig. 21-3) (if needed)
- ❏ Clean gloves
- ❏ Tissues
- ❏ Towels and/or washcloths
- ❏ Perineal pad; drape or sheet
- ❏ Water-soluble lubricants
- ❏ Bedpan
- ❏ Irrigation or douche container (if needed)
- ❏ Medication administration record (MAR) (electronic or printed)

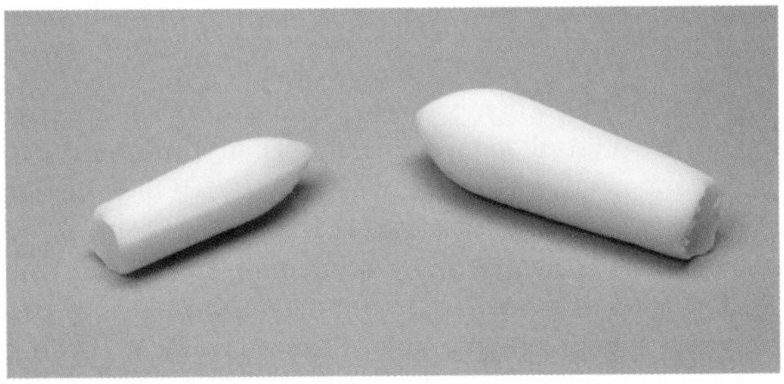

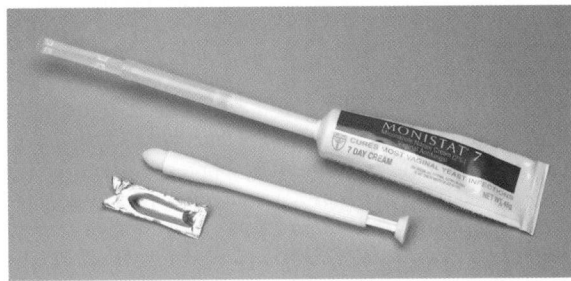

FIG 21-2 Vaginal suppositories (*right*) are larger and more oval than rectal suppositories (*left*).

FIG 21-3 From top: Vaginal cream with applicator, applicator, and vaginal suppository. (*From Lilley LL et al: Pharmacology and the nursing process, ed 6, St Louis, 2011, Mosby.*)

STEP	RATIONALE

ASSESSMENT

1 Check accuracy and completeness of each medication administration record (MAR) with health care provider's medication order. Check patient's name, drug name and dosage, route, and time for administration. Clarify incomplete or unclear orders with health care provider before administration.

2 Review pertinent information related to medication, including action, purpose, normal dose and route, side effects, time of onset and peak action, and nursing implications.

3 Assess patient's medical history, history of allergies, medication and diet history.

4 Perform hand hygiene and apply clean gloves. During perineal care inspect condition of vaginal tissues; note if drainage is present. Remove gloves and perform hand hygiene.

5 Ask if patient is experiencing any symptoms of pruritus, burning, or discomfort.

6 Review patient's knowledge of medication and readiness to learn (e.g., asks questions about medication, requests education in use of suppository).

7 Assess patient's ability to manipulate applicator, suppository, or irrigation equipment and to properly position self to insert medication (may be done just before insertion).

Rationale column:

The health care provider's order is the most reliable source and only legal record of drugs that patient is to receive. Ensures that patient receives correct medication. Handwritten MARs are a source of medication errors (ISMP, 2010; Jones and Treiber, 2010).

Allows you to anticipate effects of drug and observe patient's response.

These factors influence how certain drugs act. Information also reflects patient's need for medications and risk for side effects.

Prevents transmission of microorganisms. Identifies symptoms of vaginal irritation or infection.

Identifies symptoms of vaginal irritation or infection.

Indicates need for health teaching. Understanding influences adherence to therapy.

Presence of mobility restrictions indicates need for assistance.

NURSING DIAGNOSES

- Deficient knowledge regarding vaginal medication administration
- Sexual dysfunction
- Impaired physical mobility
- Pain (acute or chronic)

Related factors are individualized based on patient's condition or needs.

PLANNING

1 Expected outcomes following completion of procedure:
  - Vaginal tissues are pink and smooth. Genitalia are clear and without discharge.
  - Patient denies symptoms of discomfort and expresses relief from symptoms of infection/inflammation. Small amount of discharge that is color of medication is present.
  - Patient is able to discuss information about prescribed drug.
  - Patient demonstrates self-administration of suppository, medication, or irrigation.
2 Explain procedure to patient. Be specific if patient plans to self-administer medication.

Rationale column:

Tissues take on normal characteristics.

Inflammation or infection has resolved. When suppository or cream becomes distributed, small amount may escape from vaginal orifice.

Feedback reflects patient's learning.
Demonstrates learning.

Promotes patient's understanding. Enables patient to self-administer drug if physically able.

IMPLEMENTATION

1 Prepare suppository for administration. Check label of medication against MAR 2 times (see Skill 22-1). Preparation usually involves taking suppository out of refrigerator and taking to patient room. Check expiration date on container.

2 Take medication(s) to patient at correct time (see agency policy). Medications that require exact timing include stat, first-time or loading doses, and one time doses. Give time-critical scheduled medications (e.g., antibiotics, anticoagulants, insulin, anticonvulsants, immunosuppressive agents) at exact time ordered (no later than 30 minutes before or after scheduled dose). Give non–time-critical scheduled medications within a range of 1 or 2 hours of scheduled dose (ISMP, 2011). During administration, apply six rights of medication administration.

Rationale column:

These are the first and second checks for accuracy. Process ensures that right patient receives right medication.

Hospitals must adopt medication administration policy and procedure for timing of medication administration that considers nature of the prescribed medication, specific clinical application, and patient needs (DHHS, 2011; ISMP, 2011). Time-critical scheduled medications are those for which early or delayed administration of maintenance doses of greater than 30 minutes before or after the scheduled dose may cause harm or result in substantial suboptimal therapy or pharmacologic effect. Non–time-critical medications are those for which early or delayed administration within a specified range of either 1 or 2 hours should not cause harm or result in substantial suboptimal therapy or pharmacologic effect (ISMP, 2011; DHHS, 2011).

STEP	RATIONALE
3 Identify patient using two identifiers (i.e., name and birthday or name and account number) according to agency policy. Compare identifiers in MAR/medical record with information on patient's identification bracelet and/or ask patient to state name.	Ensures correct patient. Complies with The Joint Commission standards and improves patient safety (TJC, 2012). Some agencies are now using a bar-code system to help with patient identification.
4 At patient's bedside again compare MAR or computer printout with names of medications on medication labels and patient name. Ask patient if he or she has allergies.	*This is the third check for accuracy* and ensures that patient receives correct medication. Confirms patient's allergy history.
5 Discuss purpose of each medication, action, and possible adverse effects. Allow patient to ask any questions about the drugs. Explain procedure if patient plans to self-administer medication.	Patient has right to be informed, and patient's understanding of each medication improves adherence to drug therapy.
6 Perform hand hygiene, arrange supplies at bedside, and apply clean gloves. Close door or pull curtain.	Reduces transfer of microorganisms.
7 Have patient void. Help her lie in dorsal recumbent position. Patients with restricted mobility in knees or hips may lie supine with legs abducted.	Voiding prevents passing of urine during insertion of suppository. Position provides easy access to and good exposure of vaginal canal. Dependent position also allows suppository to completely dissolve in vagina.
8 Keep abdomen and lower extremities draped.	Minimizes patient's embarrassment by limiting exposure.
9 Be sure that vaginal orifice is well illuminated by room light. Otherwise position portable gooseneck lamp.	Proper insertion requires visualization of external genitalia if not self-administered.
10 **Insert vaginal suppository.**	
a Remove suppository from wrapper and apply liberal amount of water-soluble lubricant to smooth or rounded end (see illustration). Be sure that suppository is at room temperature. Lubricate gloved index finger of dominant hand.	Lubrication reduces friction against mucosal surfaces during insertion. Use of petroleum jelly may leave residue that harbors bacteria and yeast fungi.

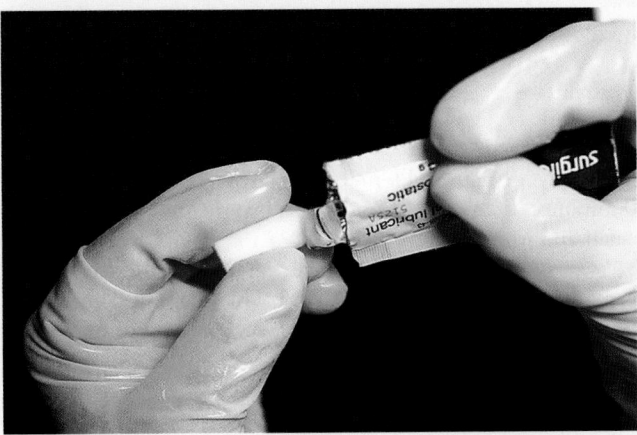

STEP 10a Lubricate tip of suppository.

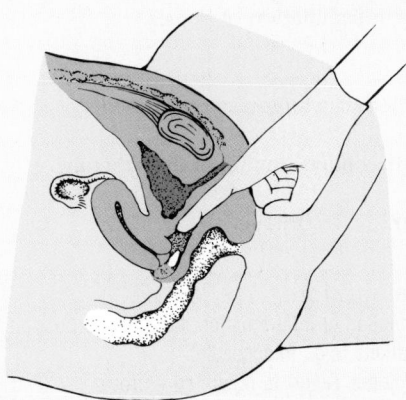

STEP 10c Angle of vaginal suppository insertion.

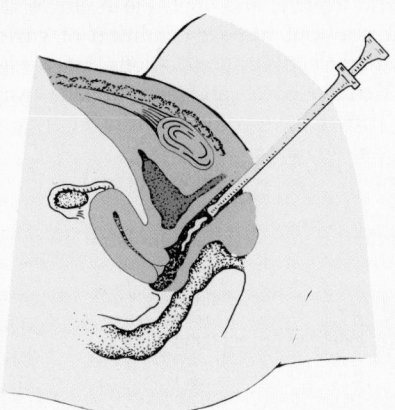

STEP 11c Applicator inserted into vaginal canal. Plunger pushed to instill medication.

STEP	RATIONALE
b With nondominant gloved hand gently separate labial folds in front-to-back direction.	Exposes vaginal orifice.
c With dominant gloved hand insert rounded end of suppository along posterior wall of vaginal canal the entire length of finger (7.5 to 10 cm [3 to 4 inches]) (see illustration).	Proper placement of suppository ensures equal distribution of medication along walls of vaginal cavity.
d Withdraw finger and wipe away remaining lubricant from around orifice and labia with tissue or cloth.	Maintains comfort.
11 Apply cream or foam.	
a Fill cream or foam applicator following package directions.	Dose is based on volume in applicator.
b With nondominant gloved hand gently separate labial folds.	Exposes vaginal orifice.
c With dominant gloved hand insert applicator approximately 5 to 7.5 cm (2 to 3 inches). Push applicator plunger to deposit medication into vagina (see illustration).	Allows equal distribution of medication along vaginal walls.
d Withdraw applicator and place on paper towel. Wipe off residual cream from labia or vaginal orifice with tissue or cloth.	Maintains patient comfort.
12 Administer irrigation or douche.	
a Place patient on bedpan with absorbent pad underneath.	Allows hips to be higher than shoulders and solution to reach posterior wall of vagina. Bedpan collects solution.
b Be sure that irrigation or douche fluid is at body temperature. Run fluid through container nozzle (priming the tubing).	Body temperature promotes patient comfort. Priming tubing removes air and moistens nozzle tip.
c Gently separate labial folds and direct nozzle toward sacrum, following floor of vagina.	Correct angle allows nozzle access into vagina.
d Raise container approximately 30 to 50 cm (12 to 20 inches) above level of vagina. Insert nozzle 7 to 10 cm (3 to 4 inches). Allow solution to flow while rotating nozzle. Administer all irrigating solution.	Rotating nozzle allows irrigation of all areas in vagina.
e Withdraw nozzle and help patient to comfortable sitting position.	Remaining solution drains by gravity.
f Allow patient to remain on bedpan for a few minutes. Clean perineum with soap and water.	Ensures all solution drains from vagina. Provides comfort for patient.
g Help patient off bedpan. Dry perineal area.	Provides comfort.
13 Instruct patient who received suppository, cream, or tablet to remain on her back for at least 10 minutes.	Allows melting and spreading of medication throughout vaginal cavity and prevents loss through vaginal orifice.
14 If using an applicator, wash with soap and warm water, rinse, and store for future use.	Vaginal cavity is not sterile. Soap and water help to remove bacteria and residual cream from applicator.
15 Offer perineal pad when patient resumes ambulation.	Provides patient comfort.
16 Discard gloves by turning them inside out and dispose of them and other soiled equipment in appropriate receptacle. Perform hand hygiene.	Reduces spread of microorganisms.

EVALUATION

1 Perform hand hygiene and apply clean gloves. Thirty minutes after administration, inspect condition of vaginal canal and external genitalia between applications. Assess vaginal discharge if present. Remove gloves and perform hand hygiene.	Determines whether vaginal medication effectively reduced irritation or inflammation of tissues.
2 Question patient regarding continued pruritus, burning, discomfort, or discharge.	Determines whether symptoms are relieved.
3 Ask patient to discuss purpose, action, and side effects of medication.	Reflects patient's understanding of drug therapy.
4 Observe patient demonstrate administration of next dose.	Reflects learning of technique.

Unexpected Outcomes	Related Interventions
1 Patient reports localized pruritus and burning.	• Results of infection or inflammation, but may be possible side effects of some medications (e.g., miconazole). • Monitor symptoms; report to health care provider.
2 Patient is unable to discuss drug therapy correctly.	• Repeat instructions or assess if patient is able to learn. • Include family caregiver when appropriate.
3 Patient is unable to self-administer medications.	• Reinstruction is necessary.

Recording and Reporting

- Record drug (or solution if vaginal instillation), dose, type of instillation, and time administered on MAR immediately after administration, not before. Include initials or signature. Record patient teaching and validation of understanding and ability to self-administer medication in nurses' notes and EHR.
- Report to health care provider if patient states that symptoms do not disappear or symptoms get worse.
- Report adverse effects/patient response and/or withheld drugs to nurse in charge or health care provider.

Special Considerations
Teaching

- Encourage patient to take *all* of the medication as prescribed, for the prescribed amount of time, to ensure effectiveness of the treatment.

- Women taking antifungal medications for the treatment of vaginal infections should abstain from sexual intercourse until the treatment is completed and the infection is resolved. Women should be told to continue to take the medication even if actively menstruating. Patients should notify the health care provider if symptoms persist past the treatment time period (Lilley et al., 2011).
- Many women prefer to self-administer vaginal irrigations and medications. These procedures may be self-administered while patient is sitting on the toilet. Ensure that patient is able to perform the procedure correctly.

Gerontologic

- Older adults may have difficulty manipulating suppository, applicator, or irrigating equipment. If so, a family caregiver may need instruction on how to insert the medication.

SKILL 21-9 Administering Rectal Suppositories

NSO *Nonparenteral Medication Administration Module / Lesson 6*

A rectal suppository is a form of medication that acts when it melts and is absorbed into the rectal mucosa. Rectal medications exert either local effects on gastrointestinal (GI) mucosa (e.g., promoting defecation) or systemic effects (e.g., relieving nausea or providing analgesia). The rectal route is not as reliable as oral or parenteral routes in terms of drug absorption and distribution. However, the medications are relatively safe because they rarely cause local irritation or side effects. Rectal medications are contraindicated in patients with recent surgery on the rectum, bowel, or prostate gland; rectal bleeding or prolapse; and very low platelet counts (Lilley et al., 2011).

Rectal suppositories are thinner and more bullet shaped than vaginal suppositories (see Fig. 21-2). The rounded end prevents anal trauma during insertion. When you administer a rectal suppository, placing it past the internal anal sphincter and against the rectal mucosa is important. Improper placement can result in expulsion of the suppository before the medication dissolves and is absorbed into the mucosa. If a patient prefers to self-administer a suppository, give specific instructions so the medication is deposited correctly. Do not cut the suppository into sections to divide the dosage; the active drug may not be distributed evenly within the suppository, and the result may be an inaccurate dose (Lilley et al., 2011).

Delegation and Collaboration

The skill of rectal medication administration cannot be delegated to nursing assistive personnel (NAP). The nurse directs the NAP about:

- Reporting expected fecal discharge or bowel movement to the nurse.
- Potential side effects of medications and to report their occurrence to the nurse.
- Informing nurse of any rectal discharge, pain, or bleeding.

Equipment

- ❏ Rectal suppository
- ❏ Water-soluble lubricating jelly
- ❏ Clean gloves
- ❏ Tissue
- ❏ Drape
- ❏ Medication administration record (MAR) (electronic or printed)

STEP	RATIONALE

ASSESSMENT

STEP	RATIONALE
1 Check accuracy and completeness of each medication administration record (MAR) with health care provider's medication order. Check patient's name, drug name and dosage, route, and time for administration. Clarify incomplete or unclear orders with health care provider before administration.	The health care provider's order is the most reliable source and only legal record of drugs that patient is to receive. Ensures that patient receives correct medication. Handwritten MARs are a source of medication errors (ISMP, 2010; Jones and Treiber, 2010).
2 Review pertinent information related to medication, including action, purpose, normal dose and route, side effects, time of onset and peak action, and nursing implications.	Allows you to anticipate effects of drug and observe patient's response.
3 Review patient's medical history for history of rectal surgery or bleeding, cardiac problems, history of allergies, and medication history.	Conditions may contraindicate use of suppository.
4 Review any presenting signs and symptoms of GI alterations (e.g., constipation or diarrhea).	Conditions indicate use of suppository.
5 Assess patient's ability to hold suppository and position self to insert medication.	Mobility restriction indicates need for nurse to help with drug administration.

STEP	RATIONALE
6 Review patient's knowledge of purpose of drug therapy and interest in self-administering suppository.	Indicates need for health teaching. Level of motivation influences teaching approach.

NURSING DIAGNOSES

• Constipation	• Deficient knowledge regarding	• Impaired physical mobility
• Readiness for enhanced self-health management	suppository administration	• Pain (acute or chronic)

Related factors are individualized based on patient's condition or needs.

PLANNING

1 Expected outcomes following completion of the procedure:	
• Patient reports relief or reduction in symptoms for which medication is prescribed.	Drug acts effectively.
• Patient describes purpose of medication.	Feedback reflects patient's learning.
• Patient demonstrates self-administration of rectal suppository.	Demonstrates learning.
2 Explain procedure to patient. Be specific if patient wishes to self-administer drug.	Promotes patient's understanding and cooperation. Enables patient to self-administer drug safely if physically able and motivated.

IMPLEMENTATION

STEP	RATIONALE
1 Prepare suppository for administration. Check label of medication against MAR 2 times (see Skill 22-1). Check expiration date on container.	*These are the first and second checks for accuracy.* Process ensures that right patient receives right medication.
2 Take medication(s) to patient at correct time (see agency policy). Medications that require exact timing include stat, first-time or loading doses, and one time doses. Give time-critical scheduled medications (e.g., antibiotics, anticoagulants, insulin, anticonvulsants, immunosuppressive agents) at exact time ordered (no later than 30 minutes before or after scheduled dose). Give non–time-critical scheduled medications within a range of 1 or 2 hours of scheduled dose (ISMP, 2011). During administration, apply six rights of medication administration.	Hospitals must adopt medication administration policy and procedure for timing of medication administration that considers nature of the prescribed medication, specific clinical application, and patient needs (DHHS, 2011; ISMP, 2011). Time-critical scheduled medications are those for which early or delayed administration of maintenance doses of greater than 30 minutes before or after the scheduled dose may cause harm or result in substantial suboptimal therapy or pharmacologic effect. Non–time-critical medications are those for which early or delayed administration within a specified range of either 1 or 2 hours should not cause harm or result in substantial suboptimal therapy or pharmacologic effect (ISMP, 2011; DHHS, 2011).
3 Identify patient using two identifiers (i.e., name and birthday or name and account number) according to agency policy. Compare identifiers in MAR/medical record with information on patient's identification bracelet and/or ask patient to state name.	Ensures correct patient. Complies with The Joint Commission standards and improves patient safety (TJC, 2012). Some agencies are now using a bar-code system to help with patient identification.
4 At patient's bedside again compare MAR or computer printout with names of medications on medication labels and patient name. Ask patient if he or she has allergies.	*This is the third check for accuracy* and ensures that patient receives correct medication. Confirms patient's allergy history.
5 Discuss purpose of each medication, action, and possible adverse effects. Allow patient to ask any questions about the drugs. Explain procedure if patient plans to self-administer medication.	Patient has right to be informed, and patient's understanding of each medication improves adherence to drug therapy.
6 Perform hand hygiene, arrange supplies at bedside, and apply clean gloves. Close room curtain or door.	Reduces transfer of microorganisms. Maintains privacy and minimizes embarrassment.
7 Help patient assume left side-lying Sims' position with upper leg flexed upward.	Position exposes anus and relaxes external anal sphincter. Left side-lying Sims' position lessens likelihood of suppository or feces being expelled.
8 If patient has mobility impairment, help into lateral position. Obtain assistance to turn patient and use pillows under upper arm and leg.	Provides support during procedure and patient comfort.
9 Keep patient draped with only anal area exposed.	Maintains privacy and facilitates relaxation.
10 Examine condition of anus externally. Option: Palpate rectal walls as needed (e.g., if impaction is suspected) (see Chapter 6). If you palpate rectal walls, dispose of gloves by turning them inside out and placing them in proper receptacle if they become soiled. Otherwise keep gloves on your hands.	Determines presence of active rectal bleeding. Palpation determines whether rectum is filled with feces, which interferes with suppository placement. Reduces spread of infection.

STEP	RATIONALE

Clinical Decision Point *Do not palpate patient's rectum if there is a recent history of rectal surgery. A suppository is contraindicated in the presence of active bleeding and diarrhea (Lilley et al., 2011).*

11 Apply new pair of clean gloves (if previous gloves were soiled and discarded).

Minimizes contact with fecal material to reduce transmission of infection.

12 Remove suppository from foil wrapper and lubricate rounded end with water-soluble lubricant. Lubricate gloved index finger of dominant hand. If patient has hemorrhoids, use liberal amount of lubricant and touch area gently.

Lubrication reduces friction as suppository enters rectal canal.

13 Ask patient to take slow, deep breaths through mouth and relax anal sphincter.

Forcing suppository through constricted sphincter causes pain.

14 Retract patient's buttocks with nondominant hand. With gloved index finger of dominant hand, insert suppository gently through anus, past internal sphincter, and against rectal wall, 10 cm (4 inches) in adults (see illustration) or 5 cm (2 inches) in infants and children. You should feel rectal sphincter close around your finger.

Suppository needs to be against rectal mucosa for eventual absorption and therapeutic action.

Clinical Decision Point *Do not insert suppository into a mass of fecal material; this will reduce effectiveness of medication.*

15 *Option:* A suppository may be given through a colostomy (not ileostomy) if ordered. Patient should lie supine. Use small amount of water-soluble lubricant for insertion.

16 Withdraw finger and wipe patient's anal area.

Provides comfort.

17 Ask patient to remain flat or on side for 5 minutes.

Prevents expulsion of suppository.

18 Discard gloves by turning them inside out and dispose of them and used supplies in appropriate receptacle. Perform hand hygiene.

Reduces transfer of microorganisms.

19 If suppository contains laxative or fecal softener, place call light within reach so patient can obtain assistance to reach bedpan or toilet.

Ability to call for assistance provides patient with sense of control over elimination.

20 If suppository was given for constipation, remind patient *not* to flush commode after bowel movement.

Allows staff to evaluate results of suppository.

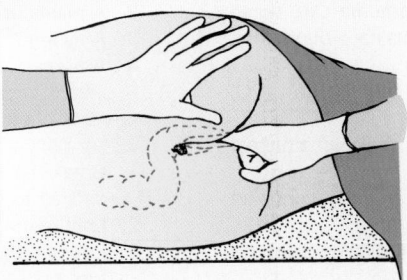

STEP 14 Insert rectal suppository past sphincter and against rectal wall.

EVALUATION

1 Return to bedside within 5 minutes to determine if suppository was expelled.

Determines if drug is distributed properly. Reinsertion may be necessary.

2 Ask if patient experienced localized anal or rectal discomfort during insertion.

Determines whether insertion of suppository was irritating.

3 Evaluate patient for relief of symptoms for which medication was prescribed (within time expected action of drug occurs).

Determines medication's effectiveness.

4 Ask patient to explain purpose of medication.

Reflects patient's understanding of drug therapy.

5 Have patient demonstrate self-administration of next dose of medication.

Demonstration measures learning.

Unexpected Outcomes

1 Patient's symptoms are unrelieved.

2 Patient experiences decreased heart rate during rectal suppository insertion.

3 Patient reports rectal pain during insertion.

4 Patient is unable to explain purpose of drug therapy.

Related Interventions

- Explore alternative therapy.
- Unintended vagal stimulation may occur, resulting in bradycardia in some patients.
- Monitor heart rate of patient. Rectal route may not be suitable for certain cardiac conditions.
- Suppository may need more lubrication.
- Rectal route may not be suitable; assess and notify health care provider.
- Reinstruction is necessary or patient is unwilling or unable to learn.

Recording and Reporting

- Record the drug, dosage, route, and actual time and date of administration on MAR immediately after administration, not before. Include initials or signature. Record patient teaching and validation of understanding and self-administration of suppository in nurses' notes.
- Report adverse effects/patient response and/or withheld drugs to nurse in charge or health care provider.

Special Considerations
Teaching

- Be certain that patient is aware that the foil wrapper must be removed before insertion and that the suppository is to be inserted rectally and not taken orally. If patient chooses to self-administer suppositories, or if a family caregiver plans to administer, teach principles and techniques of infection control to prevent contact with and spread of fecal material.

Pediatric

- With children it is often necessary to gently hold or tape the buttocks together for 5 to 10 minutes to relieve pressure on the anal sphincter until the urge to expel the suppository is gone (Hockenberry and Wilson, 2011).

Gerontologic

- Older adults with loss of sphincter control may have difficulty with retaining suppository.
- Older adults may have difficulty manipulating suppository, applicator, or irrigating equipment. If so, a family caregiver may need instruction on how to insert the medication

Critical Thinking Exercises

Mrs. Martin is a 75-year-old African-American homemaker hospitalized for 3 days with a diagnosis of dehydration. She has a history of hypertension, asthma, angina (heart pain), and osteoarthritis in her hands. She also has an abscess on her right calf that was caused by a bug bite that became infected. One week after her discharge, the home care nurse visits Mrs. Martin to review her medications and assess her wound. Mrs. Martin's medications include:

- Hydrochlorothiazide 25 mg every morning by mouth (PO) (diuretic)
- Diltiazem SR capsule, 60 mg twice a day PO (calcium channel blocker)
- Albuterol (Proventil) MDI 2 puffs 4 times a day (inhaled bronchodilator)
- Bacitracin topical ointment (500 units/g) applied topically to wound twice a day (antibiotic)
- Nitroglycerin transdermal patch (Nitro-Dur), 0.2 mg/hr, one each morning topically (nitrate)
- Nitrostat sublingual tablets, 400 mcg, as needed for chest pain (nitrate)

1 The nurse observes Mrs. Martin as she gives herself the inhaler. Mrs. Martin complains that she "just can't seem to breathe in at the same time as I press the inhaler." What action should the nurse take?

2 While inspecting Mrs. Martin's abscess, the nurse finds that there is a thick crust of old medication on the wound. Mrs. Martin explains, "I don't like to waste the medication that is already there, so I just put the new medicine on top of it." How should the nurse intervene?

3 While listening to Mrs. Martin's breath sounds, the nurse notes that she has three nitroglycerin transdermal patches on her chest. What should the nurse do?

REVIEW QUESTIONS

1 An infant is to receive 4 mL of an antibiotic by mouth. Which equipment would be most appropriate for preparation and administration?
   1 A teaspoon
   2 A plastic medication cup
   3 A syringe
   4 An oral-dosing syringe

2 A patient says that he has difficulty swallowing pills and would prefer to chew them. One of the medications is an extended-release tablet. Which is an appropriate action in response to his request?
   1 Break the tablet into halves or quarters so they are not as difficult to swallow
   2 Encourage the patient to chew the tablet instead
   3 Educate the patient on the purpose of extended-release tablets
   4 Crush the tablet and mix in applesauce

3 A patient is to receive medications through a gastrostomy. Which nursing actions are appropriate? (Select all that apply.)
   1 Verifying tube placement after medications are given
   2 Mixing all crushed medications together and give all at once
   3 Flushing tube with cold water after giving medications
   4 Flushing tube with 30 to 60 mL of water after the last dose of medication
   5 Checking for gastric residual before giving the medications
   6 Keeping the head of the bed elevated 30 to 60 minutes after the medications are given

4 An immunocompromised patient has an open wound that needs topical medication. Which nursing technique is most appropriate?
   1 Use clean gloves when applying the medication.
   2 Use sterile gloves when applying the medication.
   3 Previously applied medication should remain on the wound surface.
   4 Be sure to apply a thick layer of medication over the wound.

5 A patient is using transdermal patches to relieve his mild cardiac pain. Which patient statement demonstrates understanding of the use of transdermal patches?
  1 "I'll apply the patch to a different area each time."
  2 "I need to leave the old patch on to make sure I receive all the medicine."
  3 "If I get a headache from this medicine, I'll cut the patch in half."
  4 "It doesn't matter where I throw away the old patch because the medicine is gone."

6 The nurse is caring for a patient who is receiving nitroglycerin ointment. Which nursing intervention is most appropriate to protect the nurse against accidental exposure?
  1 Cleaning skin thoroughly before applying the next dose of medication
  2 Wearing gloves when applying the ointment
  3 Using the appropriate applicator to apply the medication
  4 Drawing blood to test for therapeutic drug values

7 The nurse is educating an adolescent about using a metered-dose inhaler (MDI) for exercise-induced asthma. The nurse knows that teaching was successful when the patient states:
  1 "I'll rinse my mouth thoroughly after I use my inhaler."
  2 "I'll wait 5 to 10 seconds between inhalations."
  3 "I'll position the inhaler between my lips and pointed toward the top of my mouth."
  4 "I should hold my breath 20 to 30 seconds after each inhalation."

8 A nurse is caring for an adult patient who is resistant to receiving his ear medication because last time it made him nauseated. Which nursing intervention will reduce the chance that this complication will happen again?
  1 Positioning the patient in supine position with his affected ear facing upward
  2 Pulling the pinna upward and outward
  3 Gently cleaning out any cerumen impaction before administering medication
  4 Running warm water over the medication bottle to warm the medication

9 The nurse is administering nasal drops for a maxillary sinus infection. How should the nurse position the patient to administer the drops?
  1 Tilt the patient's head over a pillow with the head turned to the affected side
  2 Tilt the patient's head backwards over the edge of the bed
  3 Place a small pillow under the patient's shoulder and tilt head back
  4 Lower the head of the bed and have the patient lie supine

10 A nurse is administering an ophthalmic ointment to a patient with conjunctivitis. Place the steps of the procedure in the correct order.
  1 Clean eye, washing from inner to outer canthus
  2 Assess condition of external eye structures
  3 Apply thin ribbon of ointment evenly along inner edge of lower eyelid on conjunctiva
  4 Have patient close eye and rub lid lightly in circular motion with cotton ball
  5 Ask patient to look at ceiling and explain steps to him or her

REFERENCES

Ball A, Smith K: Optimizing transdermal drug therapy, *Am J Health-System Pharmacy* 65(14):1337, 2008.

Bankhead R, et al: Enteral nutrition administration: ASPEN enteral nutrition practice recommendations, *J Parenter Enteral Nutr* 33(2):158, 2009.

Barrons R, et al: Inhaler device selection: Special considerations in elderly patients with chronic obstructive pulmonary disease, *Am J Health-System Pharmacy* 68(13):1221, 2011.

Berben L, et al: Which interventions are used by health care professionals to enhance medication adherence in cardiovascular patients? A survey of current clinical practice, *Eur J Cardiovasc Nurs* 10(1):14, 2011.

Boullata J: Drug administration through an enteral feeding tube, *Am J Nurs* 109(10):34, 2009.

Department of Health and Human Services: *Updated guidance on medication administration, Hospital Appendix A of the State Operations Manual (SOM)*, Baltimore, MD, 2011, Centers for Medicare & Medicaid Services, available at http://www.compass-clinical.com/hospital-accreditation/wp-content/uploads/2011/11/SCLetter12-pdfMedication-administration-guidance-Update-11182.pdf, accessed July 2012.

Edmiaston J, et al: Validation of a dysphagia screening tool in acute stroke patients, *Am J Crit Care* 19(4):357, 2010.

Hall LM, et al: Going blank: Factors contributing to interruptions to nurses' work and related outcomes, *J Nurs Manage* 18(8):1040, 2010.

Hockenberry M, Wilson D: *Wong's nursing care of infants Individualize related factors based on patient's condition or needs*, ed 9, St Louis, 2011, Mosby.

Institute for Safe Medication Practices (ISMP): *Splitting tablets challenges you and your patients*, 2008, available at http://www.ismp.org/newsletters/nursing/Issues/NurseAdviseERR200806.pdf, accessed February 3, 2012.

Institute for Safe Medication Practices (ISMP): *Never use parenteral syringes for oral medications*, 2010, available at http://www.accessdata.fda.gov/psn/transcript.cfm?show=94#9, accessed January 18, 2012.

Institute for Safe Medication Practices (ISMP): *Acute care guidelines for timely administration of scheduled medications*, 2011, available at http://www.ismp.org/Tools/guidelines/acutecare/tasm.pdf, accessed July 6, 2012.

Jones J, Treiber L: When 5 rights go wrong: medication errors from the nursing perspective, *J Nurs Care Qual* 25(3):240, 2010.

Kelly J, et al: An analysis of two incidents of medicine administration to a patient with dysphagia, *J Clin Nurs* 20(1-2):146, 2011.

Lehne RA: *Pharmacology for nursing care*, ed 7, Philadelphia, 2010, Saunders.

Lewis SM, et al: *Medical-surgical nursing: assessment and management of clinical problems*, ed 8, St Louis, 2011, Mosby.

Lilley LL, et al: *Pharmacology and the nursing process*, ed 6, St. Louis, 2011, Mosby.

Metheney A, et al: Effectiveness of an aspiration risk-reduction protocol, *Nurs Res* 59(1):18, 2010.

Phillips NM, Endacott R: Medication administration via enteral tubes: a survey of nurses' practices, *J Adv Nurs* 67(12):2586, 2011.

Poon EG, et al: Effect on bar-code technology on the safety of medication administration, *N Engl J Med* 362(18):1698, 2010.

Popescu A, et al: Multifactorial influences on and deviations from medication administration safety and quality in the acute medical/surgical context, *Worldviews Evidence-Based Nurs* 8(1):15, 2011.

Qureshi B: Cultural, religious, and ethnic issues in prescribing, *Practice Nurse* 39(5):35, 2010.

Shearer J: Improving oral medication management in the home health agencies, *Home Health Nurse* 27(3):184, 2009.

Sulosaari V, et al: An integrative review of the literature on registered nurses' medication competence, *J Clin Nurs* 20(3-4):464, 2011.

The Joint Commission (TJC): *National Patient Safety Goals*, Oakbrook Terrace, Ill, 2012, The Commission, available at http://www.jointcommission.org/standards_information/npsgs.aspx.

Williams N: Medication administration through enteral feeding tubes: obstructed feeding tubes, *Am J Health System Pharmacy* 65(23):2347, 2008.

Parenteral Medications

MEDIA RESOURCES

- **evolve** http://evolve.elsevier.com/Perry/skills
  learning system
  - Review Questions
  - ▶ Video Clips
  - Audio Glossary

- **NSO** Nursing Skills Online

KEY TERMS

Adverse reaction	Compatibility	Induration	Parenteral
Air embolus	Continuous subcutaneous	Infiltration	Phlebitis
Allergic reaction	infusion (CSQI or CSCI)	Infusion	Piggyback infusion
Ampule	Diluent	Injection	Saline lock
Anaphylactic reaction	Extravasation	Intradermal (ID) injection	Subcutaneous injection
Aqueous	Hematemesis	Intramuscular (IM) injection	Vial
Aspirate	Hematuria	Intravenous (IV) injection	Volume-control
Blunt-tip vial access cannula	Hypodermoclysis	Medication administration	administration set (Volutrol)
Bolus	Incompatibility	record (MAR)	Z-track method

OBJECTIVES

Mastery of content in this chapter will enable the nurse to:

- Correctly prepare injectable medications from a vial and an ampule.
- Identify advantages, disadvantages, and risks of administering medications by each injection route.
- Evaluate the effectiveness and outcomes of administering medications by each injection route.
- Explain the importance of selecting the proper-size syringe and needle for an injection.
- Discuss factors to consider when selecting injection sites.

- Discuss ways to promote patient comfort while administering an injection.
- Correctly administer intradermal, subcutaneous, and intramuscular injections.
- Compare the risks of three different intravenous routes.
- Correctly administer an intravenous infusion by intravenous piggyback, intermittent infusion, or bolus through a hanging intravenous line or saline lock.
- Initiate, maintain, and discontinue a continuous subcutaneous infusion.

The route of medication administration is the path by which a drug comes in contact with the body. *Parenteral* means administered in a manner other than through the digestive tract. Medications administered by the parenteral route enter body tissues and the circulatory system by injection. Injected medications are more quickly absorbed than oral medications; and parenteral routes are used when patients are vomiting, cannot swallow, and/or are restricted from taking oral fluids.

These medication administration procedures are invasive and thus pose greater risks than those associated with administering nonparenteral medications (see Chapter 21). Because infections originate from a variety of sources, you must use aseptic technique (Table 22-1). There are four routes for parenteral administration:

1 *Subcutaneous injection:* Injection into tissues just under the dermis of the skin
2 *Intramuscular (IM) injection:* Injection into the body of a muscle
3 *Intradermal (ID) injection:* Injection into the dermis just under the epidermis
4 *Intravenous (IV) injection or infusion:* Injection into a vein

Each type of injection requires a certain set of skills to ensure that the medication reaches the proper location. Failure to inject a medication correctly results in complications such as an inappropriate drug response (e.g., too rapid or too slow), nerve injury with associated pain, localized bleeding, tissue necrosis, and sterile abscess.

EVIDENCE-BASED PRACTICE

Currently there is increasing evidence that addresses practice guidelines for administration of injections. Over 16 billion preventive and curative injections are administered each year (Cocoman and Murray, 2010). In the past site selection was not evidence based, and needle selection was based on nursing preference. The literature has clearly identified the ventrogluteal site as best suited for intramuscular (IM) injection (Walsh and Brophy, 2010; Zimmermann, 2010). However, nurses were reluctant to use this site because of difficulty in anatomically locating it and their belief that it was not safe (Cocoman and Murray, 2010). There is now enough

consensual evidence to develop guidelines for administration of IM injections. Based on this evidence choose a muscle on the basis of its characteristics.

Ventrogluteal
- Deep and situated away from major nerves and blood vessels
- Easily identified by prominent bony landmarks
- Preferred site for medications that are larger in volume, more viscous, and irritating
- Less painful than vastus lateralis
- Recommended as pediatric IM injection site for children of all ages (Hockenberry and Wilson, 2011)

Vastus Lateralis
- Absence of major nerves and blood vessels
- Drug absorption rapid
- Site used for immunizations in children
- Recommended as pediatric IM injection site for infants up to 12 months of age (Hockenberry and Wilson, 2011)

Deltoid
- Easily accessible but not well developed in most patients
- Used for small volumes of medication
- Faster absorption rate
- May be used as a vaccination site for adults, based on development of muscle (Willcox, 2011)
- Recommended as pediatric IM injection site for children 18 months and older (Hockenberry and Wilson, 2011)

PATIENT-CENTERED CARE

Research shows that ethnicity, genetics, and culture influence drug response, pharmacokinetics, pharmacodynamics, and patient adherence and education (Giger, 2013; Groves, 2010). Knowledge about variations in therapeutic dose and adverse effects is essential in administering medications to different ethnic groups. Some patients experience a therapeutic response at a different dosage than recommended and require careful monitoring. For example, pediatric African patients do not respond well to attention deficit hyperactivity disorder (ADHD) medication (Malik et al., 2010). You need skill in communicating with and educating diverse patient populations. For example, if a patient's culture values patience and modesty, make your questions specific and take time when assessing his or her knowledge about adverse drug effects. Cultural assessment also yields information about dietary preferences, tobacco and alcohol use, and use of herbal remedies that affect drug action and response. Cultural context is essential in planning education for patients and families (Cherry and Stuart, 2011).

 Safety Guidelines

Patient safety in administering medication involves following the six rights of medication administration (see Chapter 20). When managing a patient's medications, communicate clearly with the interdisciplinary team, assess and incorporate the patient's priorities of care and preferences, and use the best evidence when making decisions about patient care. Follow these guidelines to ensure safe medication administration:

1 Be vigilant. Avoid distractions while preparing an injection. Be sure that your patients receive the appropriate medications. Know why your patient is receiving each medication; know what you need to do before, during, and after medication

TABLE 22-1	Preventing Infection During an Injection
Principle	**Technique**
Prevent contamination of solution	Ampules should not sit open, and medication should be removed quickly.
Prevent needle contamination	Avoid letting needle touch contaminated surface (e.g., outer edges of ampule or vial, outer surface of needle cap, your hands, countertop, or table surface). Avoid touching the length of the plunger or inner part of the barrel. Keep tip of syringe covered with cap or needle.
Prepare skin	Wash skin soiled with dirt, drainage, or feces with soap and water. Use friction and a circular motion while cleaning with an antiseptic swab. Swab from center of site and move outward in a 5-cm (2-inch) radius.
Reduce transfer of microorganisms	Perform hand hygiene for a minimum of 15 seconds.

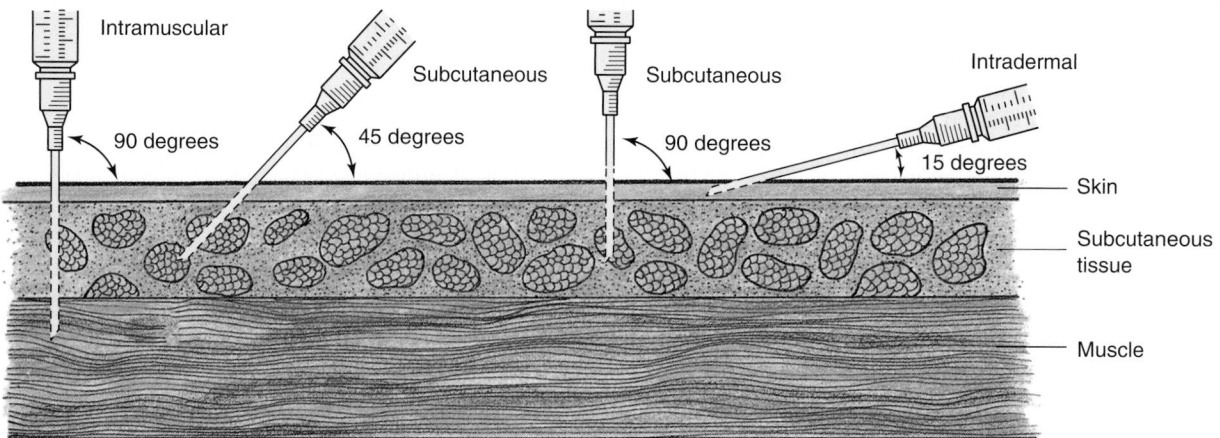

FIG 22-1   Comparison of angles of insertion of intramuscular (90 degrees), subcutaneous (45 to 90 degrees), and intradermal (15 degrees) injections.

administration; and evaluate the effectiveness of medications and any adverse effects after administration.

2   Verify that the medications have not expired.

3   Use at least two identifiers before administering medications and check against the medication administration record (MAR). Follow agency policy for patient identification.

4   Clarify unclear medication orders and ask for help whenever you are uncertain about an order or calculation. Consult with your peers, pharmacists, and other health care providers and be sure that you have resolved all concerns related to medication administration before preparing and giving medications.

5   Use technology (e.g., bar scanning, electronic MARs) that is available in your agency when preparing and giving medications. Follow all policies related to use of the technology and do not use "workarounds." A *workaround* bypasses a procedure, policy, or problem in a system. Nurses who use "workarounds" fail to follow agency protocols, policies, or procedures during medication administration in an attempt to administer medications to patients in a more timely manner.

6   Use strict aseptic technique during medication preparation and administration.

7   Educate patients about each medication that they take while you are administering it. Patients often are able to identify inappropriate medications. Make sure that you answer all of their questions before administering medications. Educate family caregivers if appropriate.

8   Most of the time you cannot delegate medication administration. Ensure that you follow standards set by the Nurse Practice Act in your state and guidelines established by your health care agency. Licensed practical nurses (LPNs) or licensed vocational nurses (LVNs) usually can administer medications via the oral (PO), subcutaneous, IM, and ID routes. Some states allow certified medication assistants (CMAs) to administer some types of medications (e.g., oral medication) in long-term care facilities.

9   No-interruption zones (NIZs) have been recommended by the Institute for Safe Medicine Practices. NIZs are created by placing red tape or tile borders on the floor around medication carts. Nurses standing in these zones are not to be interrupted (Anthony et al., 2010).

10 Minimize a patient's discomfort when giving an injection.

- Use sharp, beveled needles in the shortest length and smallest gauge possible.
- Change the needle if liquid medication coats its shaft.
- Position and flex a patient's limbs to reduce muscular tension.
- Divert a patient's attention away from the injection procedure.
- Apply a vapocoolant spray (e.g., Flouri-Methane spray or ethyl chloride) or topical anesthetic (e.g., EMLA cream) to an injection site before giving a medication when possible or place wrapped ice on the site for a minute before injection.
- Insert the needle at the proper angle, smoothly, and quickly (Fig. 22-1). Do not hesitate and slowly push the needle into tissue.
- Inject the medication slowly but smoothly.
- Hold the syringe steady once the needle is in the tissue to prevent tissue damage.
- Withdraw the needle smoothly at the same angle used for insertion.
- Gently apply an antiseptic pad (e.g., alcohol) or dry, sterile gauze pad to the site.
- Apply gentle pressure at the injection site.
- Rotate injection sites to prevent the formation of indurations and abscesses.

NEEDLESTICK PREVENTION

The most frequent route of exposure to bloodborne disease for health care workers is from needlestick injuries (American Nurses Association, 2010). Research has shown that most needlestick injuries occur in patient rooms and the operating room (American Nurses Association, 2010). These injuries occur when health care workers recap needles, mishandle intravenous (IV) lines and needles, or leave needles at a patient's bedside. However, the implementation of safe needle devices can prevent needlestick injuries (American Nurses Association, 2010). The Needlestick Safety and Prevention Act is a federal law that mandates health care agencies to use safe needle devices to reduce the frequency of needlestick injury (see Fig. 22-2, C). Employers must update their exposure control plans and seek employee input when evaluating and selecting safer medical devices (OSHA, 2012).

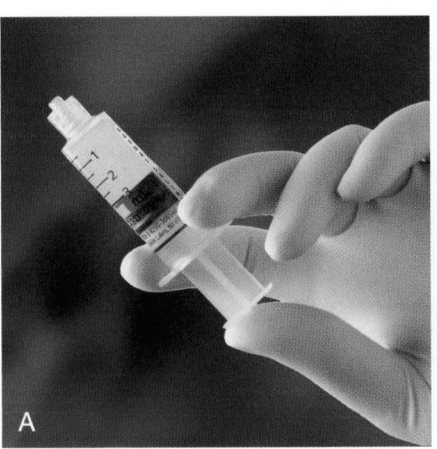 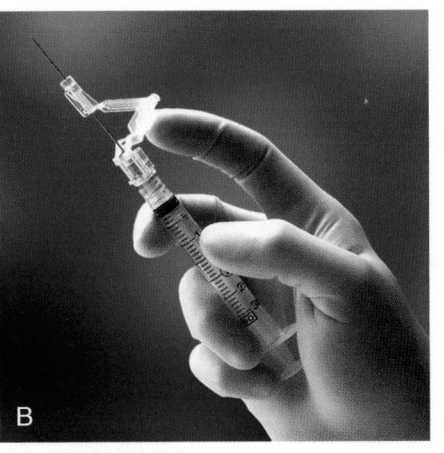 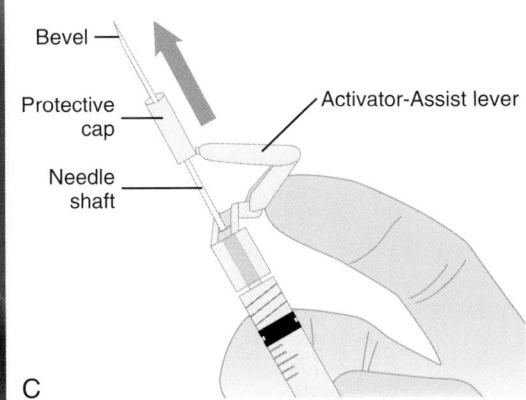

FIG 22-2 **A,** Needleless system. **B,** Safety needle system. **C,** Detail of safety needle system. (**A** and **B** *Courtesy and © Becton, Dickinson and Company.*)

BOX 22-1	Recommendations for the Prevention of Needlestick Injuries

1 Avoid using needles when effective needleless systems or SESIP safety devices are available.
2 Do not recap needles after medication administration.
3 Plan safe handling and disposal of needles before beginning a procedure that requires the use of a needle.
4 Immediately dispose of used needles, needleless systems, and SESIP into puncture- and leak-proof sharps disposal containers.
5 Maintain a sharps injury log (see agency policy).
6 Attend educational offerings regarding bloodborne pathogens and follow recommendations for infection prevention, including receiving the hepatitis B vaccine.
7 Report all needlestick and sharps-related injuries immediately according to agency policies.
8 Participate in the selection and evaluation of needleless systems of SESIP devices with safety features within your place of employment whenever possible.

Data from Occupational Safety and Health Administration (OSHA): *Bloodborne pathogens and needlestick injuries*, 77 FR 19934, 2012, available at http://www.osha.gov/pls/oshaweb/owadisp.show_document?p_table=STANDARDS&p_id=10051,accessed July 2012.
SESIP, Sharps with engineered sharps injury protection.

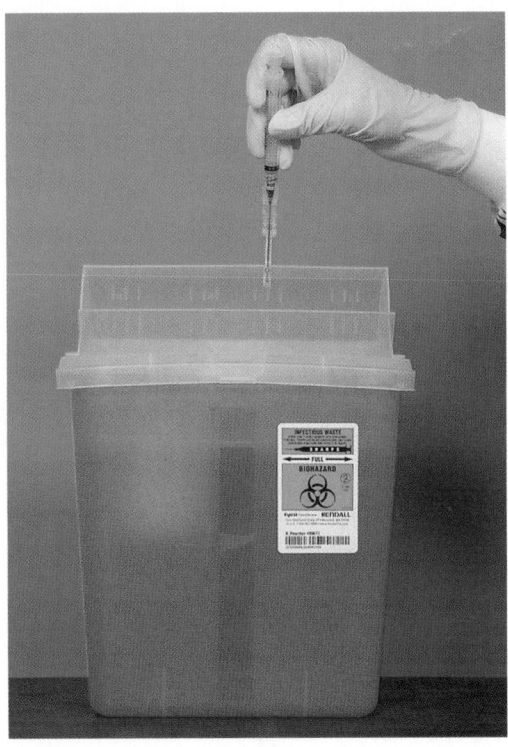

FIG 22-3　Sharps disposal using only one hand.

A sharp with engineered sharps injury protection (SESIP) is a device that is effective in preventing needlesticks. One type of SESIP is a blunt-end cannula; another is a safety syringe equipped with a plastic guard or sheath that slips over the needle as it is withdrawn from the skin (Fig. 22-2, A to C). The guard immediately covers the needle, eliminating the chance for a needlestick injury. A variety of other SESIP devices are found in needleless IV line connection systems (see Chapter 28). Box 22-1 lists recommendations for health care workers to use to reduce their risk of needlestick injuries.

Special puncture- and leak-proof containers are available in health care agencies for the disposal of sharps. Containers are made so only one hand needs to be used when disposing of an uncapped needle. In addition, containers must stand upright, not be allowed to overfill, and be colored red or labeled with a biohazard symbol (Fig. 22-3).

EQUIPMENT

Administer parenteral medication by using a needle and a syringe, available in a variety of sizes. Determine the appropriate size of syringe, length and gauge of needle, volume of solution, and medication route. These decisions are based on the quantity and type of medication prescribed and the body size of a patient. Most syringes come with needleless systems or safety needles that help prevent needlestick injuries. A variety of electronic infusion pumps deliver IV or continuous subcutaneous infusions. Infusion pumps ensure a constant and accurate delivery of medication.

SYRINGES

Syringes are single use, disposable, and either Luer-Lok or non–Luer-Lok. The design of the syringe tip influences the name. They are packaged separately, in a paper wrapper or rigid plastic container. Syringes come with or without a sterile needle and with a needleless SESIP device. The parts of a syringe are shown in (Fig. 22-4). Non–Luer-Lok syringes use needles or needleless devices that slip onto the tip. Luer-Lok syringes (Fig. 22-5, A) use standard needles or needleless devices that are twisted onto the tip and lock themselves in place. The Luer-Lok design prevents the accidental removal of a needle from the syringe.

Syringes come in a variety of sizes, ranging in capacity from 0.5 to 60 mL (see Fig. 22-5). When you select a syringe, choose the smallest syringe size possible to improve accuracy of medication preparation. In addition, avoid injecting a large volume of fluid into tissues. It is unusual to use a syringe larger than 5 mL for IM injections. Larger volumes create pain and discomfort for a patient. Syringes are most commonly marked in a scale of tenths of a milliliter (see Fig. 22-5, A). You use tuberculin (TB) syringes to prepare small amounts of medications, for intradermal (ID) and subcutaneous injections (see Fig. 22-5, B). Insulin syringes (see Fig. 22-5, C and D) hold 0.3 mL to 1 mL, and low-dose insulin syringes (30 units per 0.3 mL or 50 units per 0.5 mL) hold 0.3 mL to 1 mL. Both come with preattached needles and are calibrated in units. Most insulin syringes are U-100s, designed for use with U-100–strength insulin. Each milliliter of solution contains 100 units of insulin.

Use a larger syringe to administer some IV medications, add medications to IV solutions, and irrigate drainage tubes. Some syringes are packaged with their needle attached; and some syringes require you to change the needle based on the viscosity of the medication, route of administration, and size of the patient. Before use carefully examine the syringe to determine the measurement scale and ensure that you use the correct syringe for preparing the ordered medication.

NEEDLES

Some needles come attached to syringes. Others come packaged individually to allow flexibility in selecting the right needle for a patient. Needles are disposable, and most are made of stainless steel. A needle has three parts: the hub, which fits onto the tip of a syringe; the shaft, which connects to the hub; and the bevel, or slanted tip (Fig. 22-6). The needle hub, shaft, and bevel must remain sterile at all times. To prevent contamination, use gentle force to place the needle onto the syringe with the cap intact (Fig. 22-7, A and B). Some needles come with filters for preparation of medications. Never use filters when administering a medication.

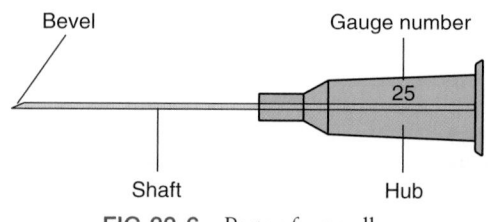
FIG 22-6 Parts of a needle.

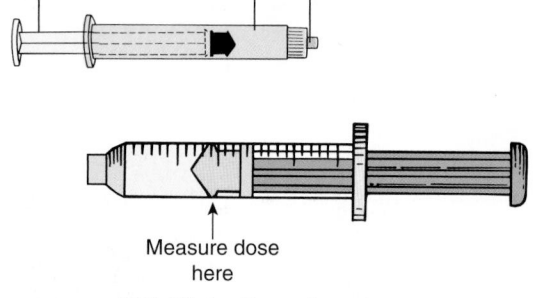
FIG 22-4 Parts of a syringe.

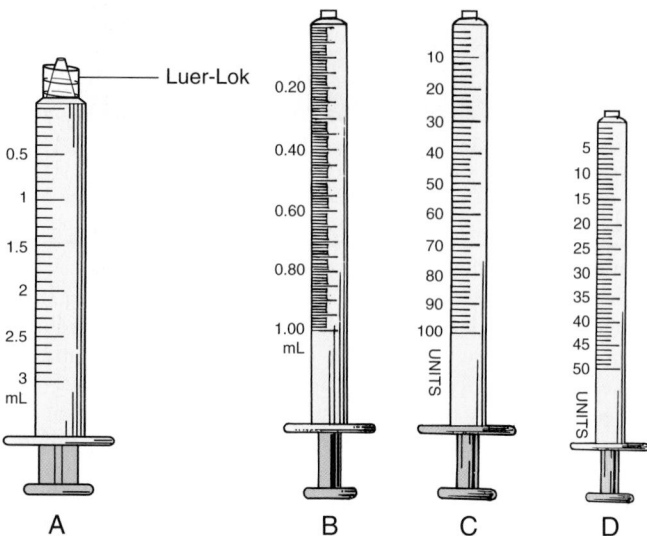
FIG 22-5 Examples of types of syringes. **A,** 3-mL Luer-Lok syringe marked in 0.1 (tenths). **B,** Tuberculin syringe marked in 0.01 (hundredths) for doses of less than 1 mL. **C,** Insulin syringe marked in units (100). **D,** Insulin syringe marked in units (50) for low dose.

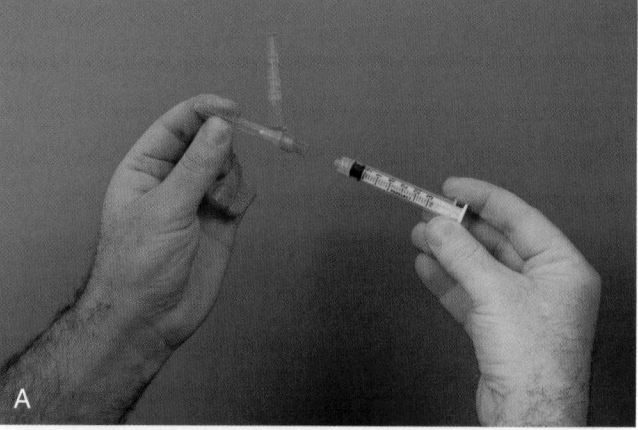

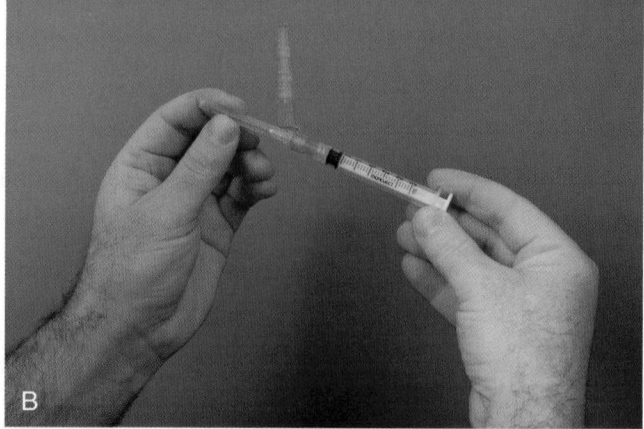
FIG 22-7 **A,** Capped needle placed on syringe tip. **B,** Needle secured.

The tip of a needle, or the bevel, is always slanted. The bevel creates a narrow slit when injected into tissue that quickly closes after the needle is removed to prevent leakage of medication, blood, or serum. Longer beveled tips are sharper and narrower, which minimizes tissue discomfort during a subcutaneous or IM injection.

Most needles vary in length from $\frac{3}{8}$ to 3 inches (Fig. 22-8). Use longer needles (1 inch to $1\frac{1}{2}$ inches) for IM injections and shorter needles ($\frac{3}{8}$ to $\frac{5}{8}$ inch) for subcutaneous injections. Choose the needle length according to a patient's size and weight, type of tissue to be injected, and route of administration. Children and small, thin adults generally require a shorter needle. The smaller the needle gauge, the larger the needle diameter. They are color coded for ease of selection. The selection of a gauge depends on the viscosity of fluid to be injected. For example, use a larger 22-gauge $1\frac{1}{2}$-inch needle for IM injections. Use a smaller 25-gauge $\frac{5}{8}$-inch needle for a subcutaneous injection.

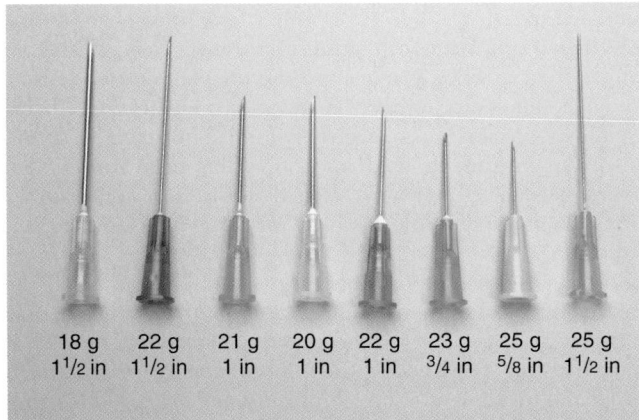

18 g 22 g 21 g 20 g 22 g 23 g 25 g 25 g
$1\frac{1}{2}$ in $1\frac{1}{2}$ in 1 in 1 in 1 in $\frac{3}{4}$ in $\frac{5}{8}$ in $1\frac{1}{2}$ in

FIG 22-8 Needles come in a variety of gauges and lengths. Choose correct needle, gauge and length, for the injection ordered. *(Lilley LL et al: Pharmacology for nurses, ed 6, St Louis, 2011, Mosby.)*

DISPOSABLE INJECTION UNITS

Single-dose, prefilled, disposable syringes are available for some medications. You do not need to prepare medication doses, except perhaps to expel unneeded portions of medication or air.

However, it is important to check the medication and concentration carefully because prefilled syringes appear very similar. Prefilled unit-dose systems such as Tubex and Carpuject injection systems include reusable plastic syringe holders and disposable, prefilled, sterile, glass cartridge units. To assemble a prefilled system, place the cartridge, barrel first, into the plastic syringe holder (Fig. 22-9, A). Following manufacturer instructions, turn the plunger rod to the left (counterclockwise) (see Fig. 22-9, B) and then lock to the right (clockwise) until it "clicks" (see Fig. 22-9, C). Finally remove the needle guard and advance the plunger (see Fig. 22-9, D) to expel air and excess medication as with a regular syringe. The cartridge may be used with SESIP needles. After giving the medication dispose of the glass cartridge safely in a puncture- and leak-proof container. This design reduces the risk for needlestick injury.

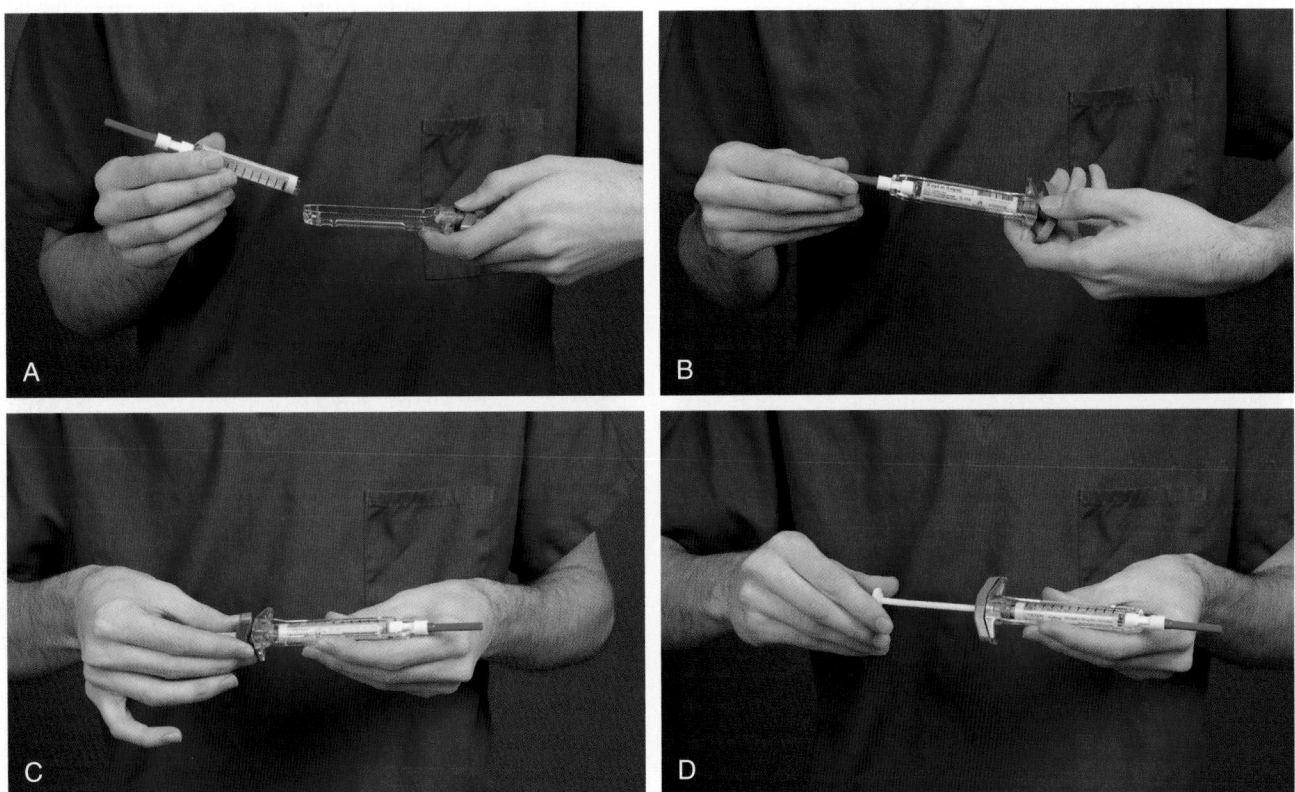

FIG 22-9 **A,** Carpuject syringe holder and prefilled sterile cartridge with needle. **B,** Assembling the Carpuject. **C,** The cartridge slides into the syringe barrel, turns, and locks at the needle end. **D,** The plunger screws into the cartridge end.

SKILL 22-1   Preparing Injections: Ampules and Vials

[NSO] *Injections Module / Lesson 2*

Ampules contain single doses of injectable medication in a liquid form and are available in sizes from 1 to 10 mL or more. An ampule is made of glass with a constricted, prescored neck that is snapped off to allow access to the medication (Fig. 22-10, A). A colored ring around the neck indicates where the ampule is prescored to be broken easily. Medication is easily withdrawn from the ampule by aspirating with a filter needle and syringe. Filter needles must be used when preparing medication from a glass ampule to prevent glass particles from being drawn into the syringe (Alexander et al., 2009; Nicholl and Hesby, 2002). *Do not* use the filter needle to administer the medication. Place an appropriate-size needle on the syringe after withdrawing the medication.

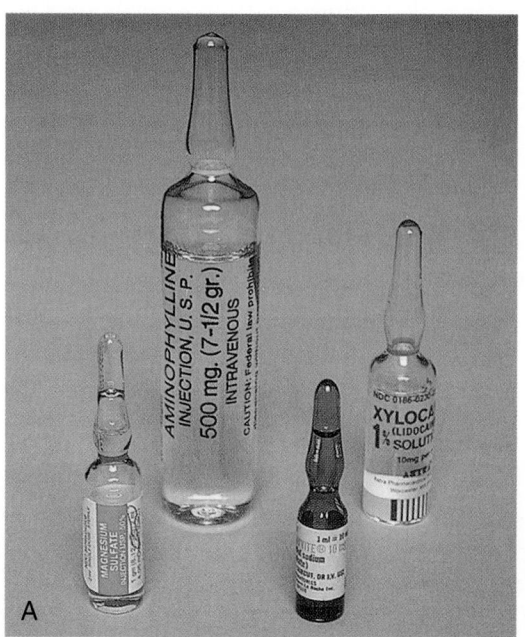

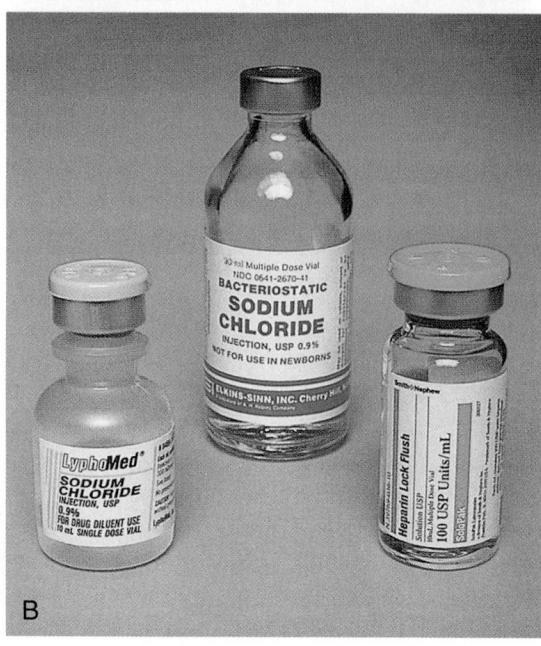

FIG 22-10   **A,** Medication in ampules. **B,** Medication in vials.

A vial is a single- or multi-dose plastic or glass container with a rubber seal at the top (see Fig. 22-10, B). After you open a single-dose vial discard it, regardless of the amount of medication used (Pugliese et al., 2010). A multi-dose vial contains several doses of a medication and thus can be used several times, although only for a single patient (Pugliese et al., 2010). When using a multi-dose vial, write the date that the vial is opened on the vial label. Verify with the agency how long an opened multi-dose vial may be used. Properly discard a multi-dose vial when the allowed time for being open has expired.

A metal or plastic cap protects a rubber seal of the vial. Remove the cap when you first prepare the vial for use. Vials may contain liquid or dry forms of medications; medications that are unstable in solution are packaged dry form. The vial label specifies the solvent or diluents used to dissolve the medication and the amount needed to prepare a desired medication concentration. Normal saline and sterile distilled water are the most common solutions.

Some vials have two chambers separated by a rubber stopper. One chamber contains the diluent solution; the other contains the dry medication. Before preparing the medication, push on the upper chamber to dislodge the rubber stopper and allow the powder and the diluent to mix. Unlike an ampule, a vial is a closed system. You must inject air into the vial to permit easy withdrawal of the solution. Some medications, even when in a vial, may need to be drawn up with a filter needle because of the nature of the medication. Agency policies and package inserts from the manufacturer indicate drugs that should be prepared with a filter needle.

Occasionally the prescriber orders an injectable medication that must be reconstituted because it comes in a powdered form. This frequently occurs with a time-sensitive injectable medication, which must be administered within a specific time period to guarantee full drug effectiveness.

Delegation and Collaboration
The skill of preparing injections from ampules and vials cannot be delegated to nursing assistive personnel (NAP).

Equipment
Medication in an Ampule
- Syringe, needle, and filter needle
- Small sterile gauze pad or unopened alcohol swab

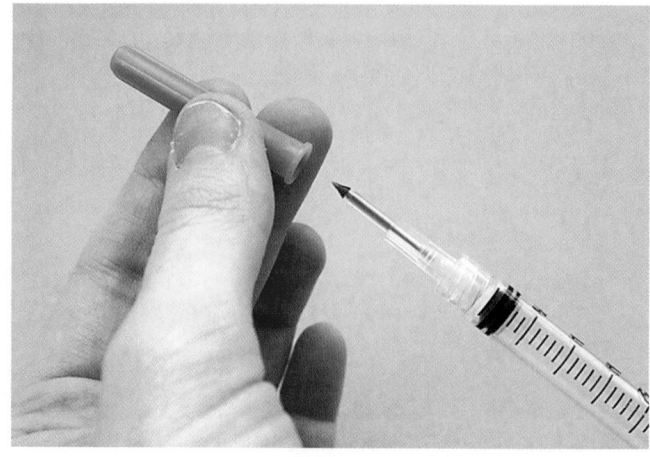

FIG 22-11   Syringe with needleless vial access adapter.

Medication in a Vial

❏ Syringe and two needles
❏ Needles:
  • Needleless blunt-tip vial access cannula (Fig. 22-11) or needle (with safety sheath) for drawing up medication (if needed)
  • Filter needle if indicated
❏ Small, sterile gauze pad or alcohol swab
❏ Diluent (e.g., 0.9% sodium chloride or sterile water if indicated)

Both

❏ Medication administration record (MAR) or computer printout
❏ Sharps with engineered sharps injury protection (SESIP) safety needle for injection
❏ Medication in vial or ampule
❏ Puncture-proof container for disposal of syringes, needles, and glass

STEP	RATIONALE

ASSESSMENT

1 Check accuracy and completeness of each MAR or computer printout with prescriber's written medication order. Check patient's name, medication name and dosage, route of administration, and time of administration. Recopy or reprint any portion of MAR that is difficult to read.

The prescriber's order is the most reliable source and legal record of patient's medications. Ensures that patient receives correct medications.
Handwritten MARs are a source of medication errors (ISMP, 2010; Jones and Treiber, 2010).

2 Assess patient's medical and medication history.

Determines need for medication or possible contraindications for medication administration.

3 Assess patient's history of allergies: Know type of allergies and normal allergic response.

Do not prepare medication if there is a known patient allergy.

4 Review medication reference information for action, purpose, side effects, and nursing implications.

Allows you to administer drug properly and monitor patient's response.

5 Assess patient's body build, muscle size, and weight if giving subcutaneous or intramuscular (IM) medication.

Determines type and size of syringe and needle for injection.

PLANNING

1 Expected outcomes following completion of procedure:
  • Proper dose is prepared. No air bubbles are in syringe barrel.

Ensures right dose. Air bubbles displace medication. Elimination of air ensures accuracy of medication dose.

IMPLEMENTATION

1 Perform hand hygiene and prepare supplies.

Reduces transmission of microorganisms.

2 Prepare medications.
  a If using a medication cart, move it outside patient's room.

Organization of equipment saves time and reduces error.

  b Unlock medication drawer or cart or log onto computerized medication dispensing system.

Medications are safeguarded when locked in cabinet, cart, or computerized medication dispensing system.

  c Follow agencies "No-Interruption Zone" policy. Prepare medications for one patient at a time. Keep all pages of MARs or computer printouts for one patient together or look at only one patient's electronic MAR at a time.

Preventing distractions reduces medication preparation errors (LePorte et al., 2009; Nguyen et al., 2010).
No-Interruption Zone has been shown to decrease interruptions during medication preparation (Anthony et al., 2010).

  d Select correct drug from stock supply or unit-dose drawer. Compare label of medication with MAR computer printout or computer screen.

Reading label and comparing it with transcribed order reduce errors. *This is the first check for accuracy.*

  e Check expiration date on each medication, one at a time.

Medications used past their expiration date are sometimes inactive, less effective, or harmful to patients.

  f Calculate drug dose as necessary. Double-check calculation. Ask another nurse to check calculations if needed.

Double-checking reduces error.

  g If preparing a controlled substance, check record for previous drug count and compare with supply available.

Controlled substance laws require careful monitoring of dispensed narcotics.

  h Do not leave drugs unattended.

Nurse is responsible for safekeeping of drugs.

3 **Prepare ampule.**
  a Tap top of ampule lightly and quickly with finger until fluid moves from its neck (see illustration).

Dislodges any fluid that collects above neck of ampule. All solution moves into lower chamber.

  b Place small gauze pad around neck of ampule (see illustration).

Protects fingers from trauma as glass tip is broken off. Do not use opened alcohol swab to wrap around top of ampule because alcohol may leak into ampule.

  c Snap neck of ampule quickly and firmly away from hands (see illustration).

Protects your fingers and face from shattering glass.

STEP	RATIONALE
d Draw up medication quickly, using filter needle long enough to reach bottom of ampule to access medication.	System is open to airborne contaminants. Filter needles filter out any fragments of glass (Alexander et al., 2009).
e Hold ampule upside down or set it on flat surface. Insert filter needle into center of ampule opening. Do not allow needle tip or shaft to touch rim of ampule.	Broken rim of ampule is considered contaminated. When ampule is inverted, solution dribbles out if needle tip or shaft touches rim of ampule.
f Aspirate medication into syringe by gently pulling back on plunger (see illustration).	Withdrawal of plunger creates negative pressure within syringe barrel, which pulls fluid into syringe.
g Keep needle tip under surface of liquid. Tip ampule to bring all fluid within reach of needle.	Prevents aspiration of air bubbles.
h If you aspirate air bubbles, do not expel air into ampule.	Air pressure forces fluid out of ampule, and medication will be lost.
i To expel excess air bubbles, remove needle from ampule. Hold syringe vertically with needle pointing up. Tap side of syringe to cause bubbles to rise toward needle. Draw back slightly on plunger and push plunger upward to eject air. Do not eject fluid.	Withdrawing plunger too far removes it from barrel. Holding syringe vertically allows fluid to settle in bottom of barrel. Pulling back on plunger allows fluid within needle to enter barrel so fluid is not expelled. You then expel air at top of barrel and within needle.

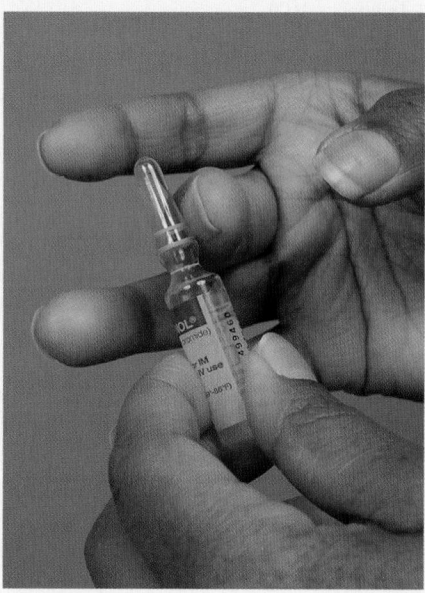

STEP 3a   Tapping ampule moves fluid down neck.

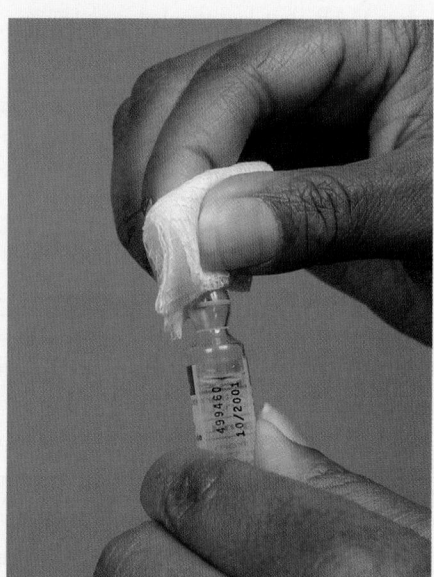

STEP 3b   Gauze pad placed around neck of ampule.

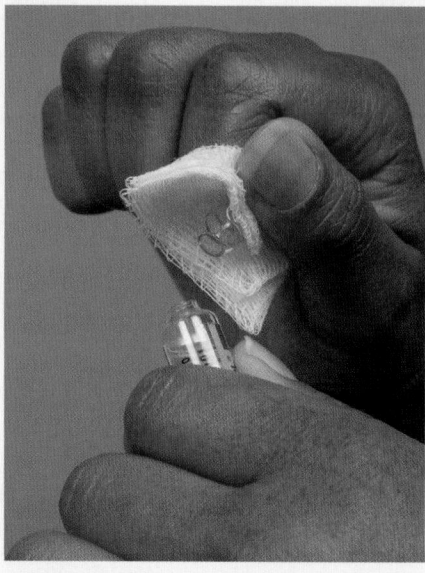

STEP 3c   Neck snapped away from hands.

STEP	RATIONALE
j If syringe contains excess fluid, use sink for disposal. Hold syringe vertically with needle tip up and slanted slightly toward sink. Slowly eject excess fluid into sink. Recheck fluid level in syringe by holding it vertically.	Safely disperses excess medication into sink. Position of needle allows you to expel medication without having it flow down needle shaft. Rechecking fluid level ensures proper dose.
k Cover needle with its safety sheath or cap. Replace filter needle with regular sharps with engineered sharps injury protection (SESIP) needle.	Minimizes needlesticks. Filter needles cannot be used for injection.

4 Prepare vial containing a solution.

STEP	RATIONALE
a Remove cap covering top of unused vial to expose sterile rubber seal. If a multi-dose vial has been used before, cap is already removed. Firmly and briskly wipe surface of rubber seal with alcohol swab and allow it to dry.	Vial comes packaged with cap that cannot be replaced after seal removal. Not all drug manufacturers guarantee that rubber seals of unused vials are sterile. Swabbing with alcohol reduces transmission of microorganisms. Allowing alcohol to dry prevents alcohol from coating needle and mixing with medication.
b Pick up syringe and remove needle cap or cap covering needleless access device. Pull back on plunger to draw amount of air into syringe equivalent to volume of medication to be aspirated from vial.	Injecting air into vial prevents buildup of negative pressure in vial when aspirating medication.

Clinical Decision Point *Some medications and agencies require use of a filter needle when preparing medications from vials. Check agency policy or medication reference. If you use a filter needle to aspirate medication, you need to change it to a regular SESIP needle of the appropriate size to administer medication (Alexander et al., 2009).*

STEP	RATIONALE
c With vial on flat surface, insert tip of needle or needleless device through center of rubber seal (see illustration). Apply pressure to tip of needle during insertion.	Center of seal is thinner and easier to penetrate. Using firm pressure prevents dislodging rubber particles that could enter vial or needle.
d Inject air into air space of vial, holding on to plunger. Hold plunger firmly; plunger is sometimes forced backward by air pressure within vial.	Injection of air creates vacuum needed to get medication to flow into syringe. Injecting into air space of vial prevents formation of bubbles and an inaccurate dose.
e Invert vial while keeping firm hold on syringe and plunger. Hold vial between thumb and middle fingers of nondominant hand (see illustration). Grasp end of syringe barrel and plunger with thumb and forefinger of dominant hand to counteract pressure in vial.	Inverting vial allows fluid to settle in lower half of container. Position of hands prevents forceful movement of plunger and permits easy manipulation of syringe.

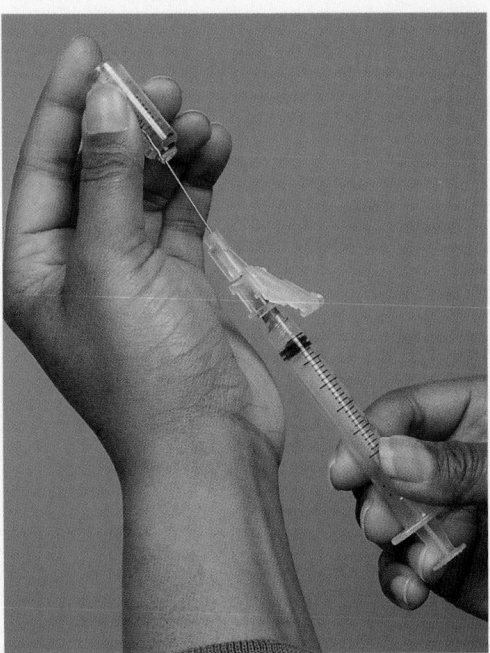

STEP 3f   Medication aspirated with ampule inverted.

STEP	RATIONALE
f Keep tip of needle or needleless device below fluid level.	Prevents aspiration of air.
g Allow air pressure from vial to fill syringe gradually with medication. If necessary, pull back slightly on plunger to obtain correct amount of medication.	Positive pressure within vial forces fluid into syringe.
h When you obtain desired volume, position needle in needleless device into air space of vial; tap side of syringe barrel gently to dislodge any air bubbles. Eject any air remaining at top of syringe into vial.	Forcefully striking barrel while needle is inserted in vial may bend needle. Accumulation of air displaces medication and causes dose errors.
i Remove needle or needleless access device from vial by pulling back on barrel of syringe.	Pulling plunger rather than barrel causes plunger to separate from barrel, resulting in loss of medication.
j Hold syringe at eye level at 90-degree angle to ensure correct volume and absence of air bubbles. Remove any remaining air by tapping barrel to dislodge any air bubbles (see illustration). Draw back slightly on plunger; then push it upward to eject air. Do not eject fluid. Recheck volume of medication.	Holding syringe vertically allows fluid to settle in bottom of barrel. Tapping dislodges air to top of barrel. Pulling back on plunger allows fluid within needle to enter barrel so you do not expel fluid. You then expel air at top of barrel and within needle.

Clinical Decision Point *When preparing medication from single-dose vial, do not assume that volume listed on label is total volume in vial. Some manufacturers provide small amount of extra liquid, expecting loss during preparation. Be sure to draw up only desired volume.*

k If you need to inject medication into patient's tissue, change needle to appropriate gauge and length according to route of medication administration.	Inserting needle through rubber stopper dulls beveled tip. New needle is sharper, and because no fluid is along shaft, does not track medication through tissues.
l For multi-dose vial, make label that includes date of opening, concentration of drug per milliliter, and your initials.	Ensures that nurses will prepare future doses correctly. You discard some drugs within a certain time frame after mixing.
5 Prepare vial containing powder (reconstituting medications).	
a Remove cap covering vial of powdered medication and cap covering vial of proper diluent. Firmly swab both rubber seals with alcohol swab and allow alcohol to dry.	Allowing alcohol to dry prevents it from coating needle and mixing with medication.
b Draw up manufacturer suggestion for volume of diluent into syringe following Steps 4b through 4j.	Prepares diluent for injection into vial containing powdered medication.
c Insert tip of needle or needleless device through center of rubber seal of vial of powdered medication. Inject diluent into vial. Remove needle.	Diluent begins to dissolve and reconstitute medication.
d Mix medication thoroughly. Roll in palms. Do not shake.	Ensures proper dispersal of medication throughout solution and prevents formation of air bubbles.

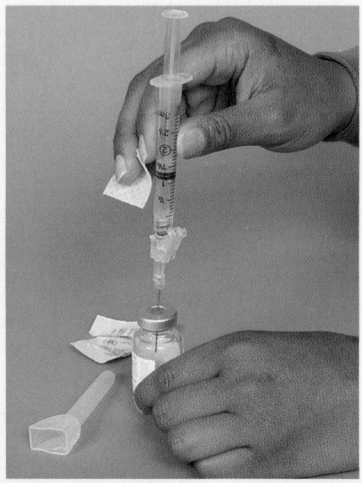

STEP 4c Insert safety needle through center of vial diaphragm (with vial flat on table).

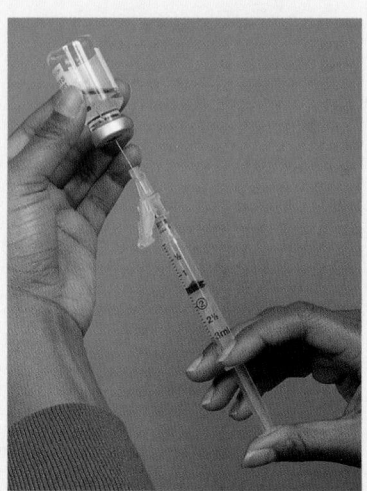

STEP 4e Withdraw fluid with vial inverted.

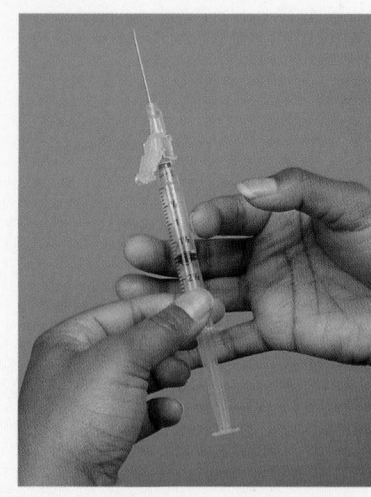

STEP 4j Hold syringe upright; tap barrel to dislodge air bubbles.

STEP	RATIONALE
e Reconstituted medication in vial is ready to be drawn into new syringe. Read label carefully to determine dose after reconstitution.	Once you add diluent, concentration of medication (mg/mL) determines dose you give. Reading medication label carefully decreases medication errors.
f Draw up reconstituted medication into syringe. Insert needleless device/needle into vial. Do not add air. Then follow Steps 4e through 4j.	Prepares medication for administration.

Clinical Decision Point *Some agencies require that you verify dose of certain medications (e.g., insulin and heparin) for accuracy with another nurse. Check guidelines before administering medication.*

6 Compare label of medication with MAR, computer screen, or computer printout.	*This is the second check for accuracy.*
7 Dispose of soiled supplies. Place broken ampule and/or used vials and used needle or needleless device in puncture- and leak-proof container. Clean work area and perform hand hygiene.	Proper disposal of glass and needle prevents accidental injury to staff. Controls transmission of infection.

EVALUATION

1 Just before administering drug to patient, compare MAR with label of prepared drug and compare dose in syringe with desired dose.	Ensures that dose is accurate. *This is the third check for accuracy.*

Unexpected Outcomes	Related Interventions
1 Air bubbles remain in syringe.	• Expel air from syringe and add medication to it until you prepare correct dose.
2 Incorrect dose of medication is prepared.	• Discard prepared dose. • Prepare correct new dose.

PROCEDURAL GUIDELINE 22-1   Mixing Parenteral Medications in One Syringe

Some medications need to be mixed from two vials or from a vial and an ampule. Mixing compatible medications avoids the need to give a patient more than one injection. Most nursing units have medication compatibility charts. Compatibility charts are in drug reference guides, posted within patient care areas, or available electronically. If you are uncertain about medication compatibilities, consult a pharmacist. When mixing medications, you must correctly aspirate fluid from each type of container. When using multi-dose vials, do not contaminate the contents of the vial with medication from another vial or ampule.

When you mix medications from a vial and an ampule, you prepare medications from the vial first. Then you withdraw medication from the ampule using the same syringe and a filter needle. When mixing medications from two vials, do not contaminate one medication with another, ensure that the final dose is accurate, and maintain aseptic technique.

Give special consideration to the proper preparation of insulin, which comes in vials. Insulin is the hormone used to treat diabetes mellitus. Insulin is classified by rate of action, including short duration, intermediate duration, and long duration. Often patients with diabetes mellitus receive a combination of different types of insulin to control their blood glucose levels. Before preparing insulin, gently roll all cloudy insulin preparations (Humulin-N) between the palms of your hands to resuspend the insulin (Lehne, 2010).

If more than one type of insulin is required to manage the patient's diabetes, you can mix them into one syringe if they are compatible. Always prepare the short- or rapid-acting insulin first to prevent it from being contaminated with the longer-acting insulin (Lehne, 2010). In some settings insulin is not mixed. Box 22-2 lists recommendations for mixing insulins.

Delegation and Collaboration

The skill of mixing medications in one syringe cannot be delegated to nursing assistive personnel (NAP). The nurse directs the NAP about:

- Potential side effects of medications and the need to report their occurrence to the nurse.

BOX 22-2	Recommendations for Mixing Insulins

- Patients whose blood glucose is well controlled on a mixed-insulin dose should maintain their individual routine when preparing and administering their insulin doses.
- No other medication or diluent should be mixed with any insulin product unless approved by the prescriber.
- Do not mix insulin glargine (Lantus) or insulin detemir (Levemir) with any other types of insulin and do not administer them intravenously.
- Inject rapid-acting insulins mixed with NPH insulin within 15 minutes before a meal.
- Verify insulin dosages during preparation with another nurse (if required by agency policy).

Data from American Diabetes Association (ADA): Standards of medical care in diabetes–2010: position statement, *Diabetes Care* 33(1):S11, 2010.

Continued

PROCEDURAL GUIDELINE 22-1   Mixing Parenteral Medications in One Syringe—cont'd

Equipment

- ❏ Single- or multi-dose vials and ampules containing medication
- ❏ Syringe and two needles
- ❏ Needles:
  - Needleless blunt-tip vial access cannula or needle for drawing up medication
  - Filter needle if indicated
  - Sharps with engineered sharps injury protection (SESIP) needle for injection
- ❏ Alcohol swab
- ❏ Puncture-proof container for disposing of syringes, needles, and glass
- ❏ Medication administration record (MAR) or computer printout
- ❏ Medication in vial or ampule

Procedural Steps

1 Check accuracy and completeness of MAR or computer printout with prescriber's written medication order. Check patient's name, medication name and dosage, route of administration, and time of administration. Recopy or reprint any portion of MAR that is difficult to read.

2 Review pertinent information related to medication, including action, purpose, side effects, and nursing implications.

3 Assess patient body build, muscle size, and weight if giving subcutaneous or (intramuscular) IM medication.

4 Consider compatibility of medications to be mixed and type of injection.

5 Check expiration date of medication printed on vial or ampule.

6 Perform hand hygiene.

7 Prepare medication for one patient at a time following the six rights of medication administration (see Chapter 20). Select an ampule or vial from the unit-dose drawer or automated dispensing system. Compare the label of each medication with the MAR or computer printout. In the case of insulin, ensure that correct type(s) of insulin are prepared. *This is the first check for accuracy.*

8 **Mixing medications from two vials (see illustration):**

   a Take syringe with needleless device or filter needle and aspirate volume of air equivalent to first medication dose (vial A).

   b Inject air into vial A, making sure that needle or needleless device does not touch solution (see illustration A).

   c Holding on to plunger, withdraw needle or needleless device and syringe from vial A. Aspirate air equivalent to second medication dose (vial B) into syringe.

   d Insert needle or needleless device into vial B, inject volume of air into vial B, and withdraw medication from vial B into syringe (see illustration B).

   e Withdraw needle or needleless device and syringe from vial B. Ensure that proper volume has been obtained.

   f Determine on syringe scale what the combined volume of medications should measure.

   g Insert needle or needleless device into vial A, being careful not to push plunger and expel medication within syringe into vial. Invert vial and carefully withdraw the desired amount of medication from vial A into syringe (see illustration C).

   h Withdraw needle or needleless device and expel any excess air from syringe. Check fluid level in syringe for proper dose. Medications are now mixed.

Clinical Decision Point *If too much medication is withdrawn from second vial, discard syringe and start over. Do not push medication back into either vial.*

   i Change needle or needleless device for appropriate-size needle if medication is being injected. Keep needle or needleless device capped until administration time.

9 **Mixing insulin:**

   a If patient takes insulin that is cloudy, roll bottle of insulin between hands to resuspend insulin preparation.

   b Wipe off tops of both insulin vials with alcohol swab.

   c Verify insulin dose against MAR.

   d If mixing rapid- or short-acting insulin with intermediate- or long-acting insulin, take insulin syringe and aspirate volume of air equivalent to dose to be withdrawn from intermediate- or long-acting insulin first (see illustration). If two intermediate- or long-acting insulins are mixed, it makes no difference which vial is prepared first.

Clinical Decision Point *If long-acting insulin glargine (Lantus) is ordered, note that this is a clear insulin, and it should not be mixed with other insulin preparations.*

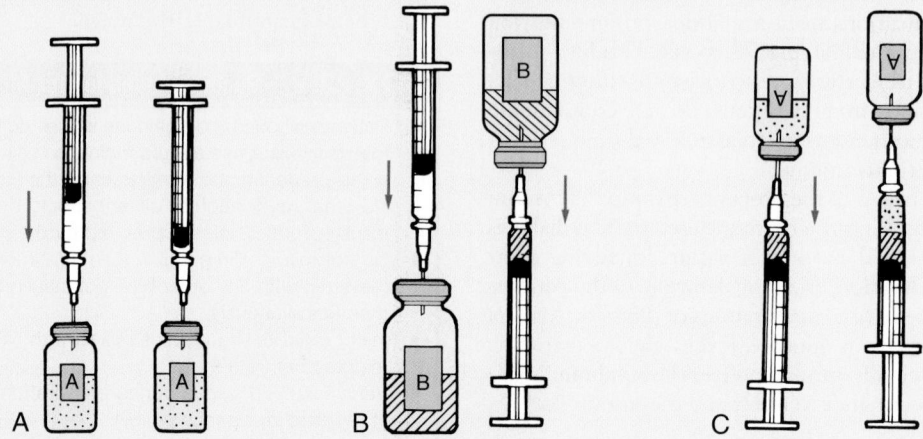

STEP 8   A, Injecting air into vial A. **B,** Injecting air into vial B and withdrawing dose. **C,** Withdrawing medication from vial A; medications are now mixed.

PROCEDURAL GUIDELINE 22-1 Mixing Parenteral Medications in One Syringe—cont'd

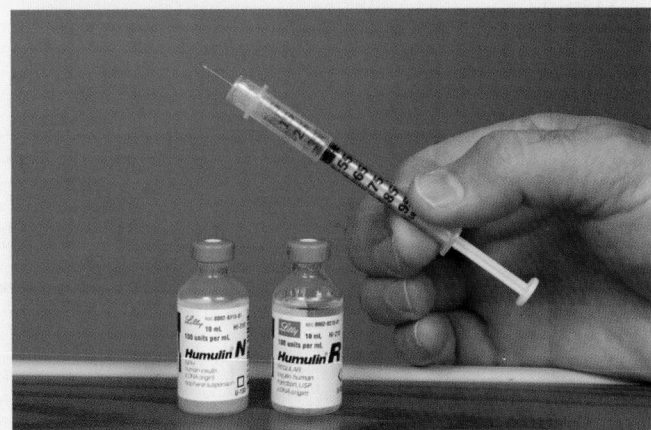

STEP 9d Aspirate air equivalent to dose to be withdrawn from intermediate insulin.

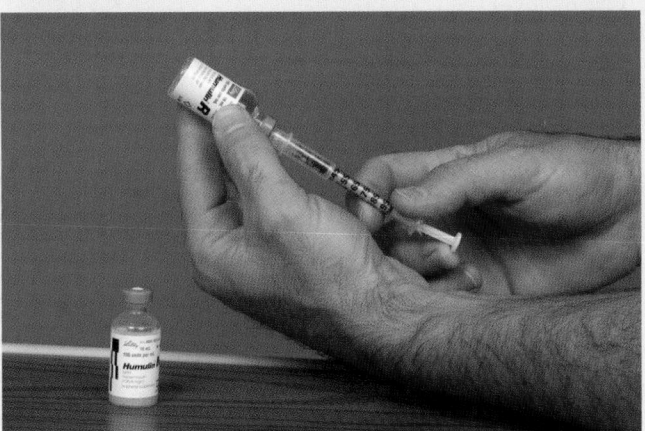

STEP 9g Withdrawal of short-acting insulin.

e Insert needle and inject air into vial of intermediate- or long-acting insulin. Do not let tip of needle touch solution.

f Remove syringe from vial of insulin without aspirating medication.

g With the same syringe, inject air equal to the dose of rapid- or short-acting insulin into vial and withdraw correct dose into syringe (see illustration).

h Remove syringe from rapid- or short-acting insulin and remove any air bubbles to ensure accurate dose.

i Verify short-acting insulin dosage with MAR and show insulin prepared in syringe to another nurse to verify that correct dosage of insulin was prepared. Determine which point on syringe scale the combined units of insulin should measure by adding the number of units of both insulins together (e.g., 4 units Regular +10 units NPH = 14 units total). Verify combined dosage.

j Place needle of syringe back into vial of intermediate- or long-acting insulin. Be careful not to push plunger and inject insulin in syringe into vial.

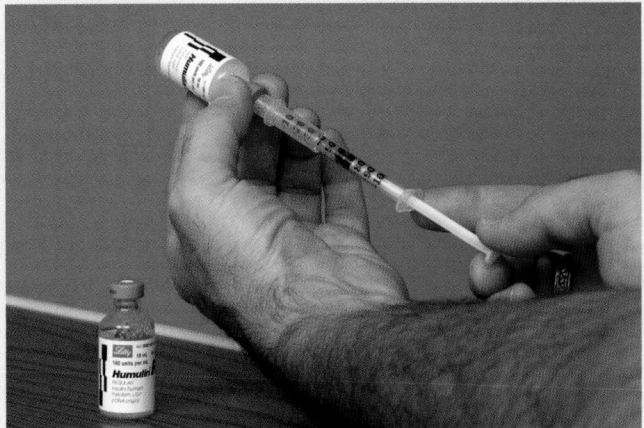

STEP 9k Withdrawal of intermediate insulin.

k Invert vial and carefully withdraw desired amount of insulin into syringe (see illustration).

l Withdraw needle and check fluid level in syringe. Keep needle of prepared syringe sheathed or capped until ready to administer medication.

10 **Mixing medications from a vial and an ampule:**

a Prepare medication from vial first, following Skill 22-1, Step 4.

b Determine on syringe scale what combined volume of medications should measure.

Clinical Decision Point *If needleless access device was used in preparing medication from vial, change needleless system to filter needle from ampule.*

c Next, using the same syringe, prepare second medication from ampule, following Step 3 in Skill 22-1.

d Withdraw filter needle from ampule and verify fluid level in syringe. Change filter needle to appropriate SESIP needle. Keep device or needle sheathed or capped until administering medication.

e Check syringe carefully for total combined dose of medications.

11 Compare MAR, computer screen, or computer printout with prepared medication and labels on vials/ampules. *This is the second check for accuracy.*

12 Dispose of soiled supplies. Place used ampules and/or vials and needle or needleless device in puncture- and leak-proof container.

13 Clean work area and perform hand hygiene.

14 Check syringe again carefully for total combined dose of medications.

15 *The third check for accuracy occurs at patient's bedside.*

SKILL 22-2 Administering Intradermal Injections

NSO *Injections Module / Lesson 4*

 Video Clip

You typically give intradermal (ID) injections for skin testing (e.g., tuberculosis screening and allergy tests). Because such medications are potent, you inject them into the dermis, where blood supply is reduced and drug absorption occurs slowly. A patient may have an anaphylactic reaction if the medications enter the circulation too rapidly. For patients with a history of multiple allergies, the physician may perform skin testing. Skin testing often requires you to visually inspect the test site; therefore make sure that the ID sites are free of lesions and injuries and relatively hairless. The inner forearm and upper back are ideal locations.

To administer an ID injection, use a tuberculin (TB) or small syringe with a short (⅜- to ⅝-inch), fine-gauge (25 to 27) needle. The angle of insertion for an ID injection is 5 to 15 degrees (see Fig. 22-1). Inject only small amounts of medication (0.01 to 0.1 mL) intradermally. Only administer amounts up to 0.1 mL to children (Hockenberry and Wilson, 2011). If a bleb does not appear or if the site bleeds after needle withdrawal, the medication may have entered subcutaneous tissues. In this situation skin test results will not be valid.

Delegation and Collaboration

The skill of administering ID injections cannot be delegated to nursing assistive personnel (NAP). The nurse directs the NAP about:

- Potential medication side effects and to report their occurrence to the nurse.
- Reporting any change in the patient's condition to the nurse.

Equipment

- ❏ Syringe: 1-mL TB syringe with preattached 25- or 27-gauge needle, ⅜- to ⅝-inch
- ❏ Small gauze pad
- ❏ Alcohol swab
- ❏ Vial or ampule of medication
- ❏ Clean gloves
- ❏ Medication administration record (MAR) or computer printout
- ❏ Puncture-proof container

STEP	RATIONALE

ASSESSMENT

1. Check accuracy and completeness of MAR or computer printout with prescriber's original medication order. Check patient's name, medication name and dosage, route of administration, and time of administration. Recopy or reprint any portion of MAR that is difficult to read.

    The prescriber's order is the most reliable source and legal record of patient's medications. Ensures that patient receives correct medications.
    Handwritten MARs are a source of medication errors (ISMP, 2010; Jones and Treiber, 2010).

2. Review medication reference information about expected reaction when testing skin with specific allergen or medication and appropriate time to read site.

    Type of reaction depends on patient's ability to mount a cell-mediated immune response. Knowledge of expected and adverse reactions to skin testing helps you determine for which symptoms to monitor, how frequently, and when to reassess patient.

3. Assess patient's history of allergies: known type of allergens and normal allergic reaction.

    You do not administer any medication if there is known patient allergy.

4. Assess for contraindication to ID injections, such as reduced local tissue perfusion. Assess for history of severe adverse reactions or necrosis that happened after previous ID injection.

    Medications are potent and can cause severe anaphylaxis.

5. Assess patient's knowledge of purpose and response to skin testing.

    Patients need to know when to return for follow-up reading of skin test and when and how to report any reaction.

6. Check date of expiration for medication.

    Dose potency increases or decreases when outdated.

NURSING DIAGNOSES

• Anxiety • Fear	• Deficient knowledge regarding skin testing	• Health-seeking behaviors regarding disease screening practices

Related factors are individualized based on patient's condition or needs.

PLANNING

1. Expected outcomes following completion of procedure:

    - Patient experiences very mild burning sensation during injection but no discomfort after injection.

        Normal reaction to medication deposited in dermis.

    - Small, light-colored bleb approximately 6 mm (¼ inch) in diameter forms at site and gradually disappears. Minimal bruising may be present.

        Medication is in dermis and eventually absorbed. Bruising is result of minor bleeding from capillaries.

    - Patient is able to identify signs of skin reaction and their significance.

        Demonstrates learning.

STEP	RATIONALE

IMPLEMENTATION

1 Prepare medications for one patient at a time using aseptic technique and avoiding distractions (see Skill 22-1). Check label of medication carefully with MAR or computer printout 2 times (see Skill 22-1 or Procedural Guideline 22-1) when preparing medication.

Ensures that medication is sterile. Preventing distractions reduces medication preparation errors (LePorte et al., 2009; Nguyen et al., 2010). *These are the first and second checks for accuracy* and ensure that correct medication is administered.

2 Take medication(s) to patient at correct time (see agency policy). Medications that require exact timing include stat, first-time or loading doses, and one time doses. Give time-critical scheduled medications (e.g., antibiotics, anticoagulants, insulin, anticonvulsants, immunosuppressive agents) at exact time ordered (no later than 30 minutes before or after scheduled dose). Give non–time-critical scheduled medications within a range of 1 or 2 hours of scheduled dose (ISMP, 2011). During administration, apply six rights of medication administration.

Hospitals must adopt medication administration policy and procedure for timing of medication administration that considers nature of the prescribed medication, specific clinical application, and patient needs (DHHS, 2011; ISMP, 2011). Time-critical scheduled medications are those for which early or delayed administration of maintenance doses of greater than 30 minutes before or after the scheduled dose may cause harm or result in substantial suboptimal therapy or pharmacologic effect. Non–time-critical medications are those for which early or delayed administration within a specified range of either 1 or 2 hours should not cause harm or result in substantial suboptimal therapy or pharmacologic effect (ISMP, 2011; DHHS, 2011).

3 Close room curtain or door.

Provides privacy.

4 Identify patient using two identifiers (i.e., name and birthday or name and account number) according to agency policy. Compare identifiers in MAR/medical record with information on patient's identification bracelet and/or ask patient to state name.

Ensures correct patient. Complies with The Joint Commission standards and improves patient safety (TJC, 2012). Some agencies are now using a bar-code system to help with patient identification.

5 At patient's bedside again compare MAR or computer printout with names of medications on medication labels and patient name. Ask patient if he or she has allergies.

This is the third check for accuracy and ensures that patient receives correct medication. Confirms patient's allergy history.

6 Discuss purpose of each medication, action, and possible adverse effects. Allow patient to ask any questions. Tell him or her that injection will cause a slight burning or sting.

Patient has right to be informed, and patient's understanding of each medication improves adherence to drug therapy. Helps minimize patient's anxiety.

7 Perform hand hygiene and apply clean gloves. Keep sheet or gown draped over body parts not requiring exposure.

Reduces transmission of infection.

8 Select appropriate site. Note lesions or discolorations of skin. If possible, select site three to four finger widths below antecubital space and one hand width above wrist. If you cannot use forearm, inspect upper back. If necessary, use sites appropriate for subcutaneous injections.

An ID injection site is free of discoloration or hair so you can see results of skin test and interpret them correctly (CDC, 2011b).

9 Help patient to comfortable position. Have him or her extend elbow and support it and forearm on flat surface.

Stabilizes injection site for easy accessibility.

10 Clean site with antiseptic swab. Apply swab at center of site and rotate outward in circular direction for about 5 cm (2 inches). *Option:* Use vapocoolant spray (e.g., ethyl chloride) before injection.

Mechanical action of swab removes secretions containing microorganisms.
Decreases pain at injection site.

11 Hold swab or gauze between third and fourth fingers of nondominant hand.

Gauze or swab remains readily accessible when withdrawing needle.

12 Remove needle cap from needle by pulling it straight off.

Preventing needle from touching sides of cap prevents contamination.

13 Hold syringe between thumb and forefinger of dominant hand with bevel of needle pointing up.

Smooth injection requires proper manipulation of syringe parts. With bevel up, you are less likely to deposit medication into tissues below dermis.

14 Administer injection.
   a With nondominant hand stretch skin over site with forefinger or thumb.

Needle pierces tight skin more easily.

   b With needle almost against patient's skin, insert it slowly at 5- to 15-degree angle until resistance is felt. Advance needle through epidermis to approximately 3 mm ($\frac{1}{8}$ inch) below skin surface. You will see bulge of needle tip through skin (see illustration).

Ensures that needle tip is in dermis. You will obtain inaccurate results if you do not inject needle at correct angle and depth (CDC, 2011b).

STEP	RATIONALE
c Inject medication slowly. Normally you feel resistance. If not, needle is too deep; remove and begin again.	Slow injection minimizes discomfort at site. Dermal layer is tight and does not expand easily when you inject solution.

Clinical Decision Point *It is not necessary to aspirate because dermis is relatively avascular.*

STEP	RATIONALE
d While injecting medication, note that small bleb (approximately 6 mm [¼ inch]) resembling mosquito bite appears on skin surface (see illustration).	Bleb indicates that you deposited medication in dermis.
e After withdrawing needle, apply alcohol swab or gauze gently over site.	Do not massage site. Apply bandage if needed.
15 Help patient to comfortable position.	Gives patient sense of well-being.
16 Discard uncapped needle or needle enclosed in safety shield and attached syringe in puncture- and leak-proof receptacle.	Prevents injury to patients and health care personnel. Recapping needles increases risk for a needlestick injury (OSHA, 2012).
17 Remove gloves and perform hand hygiene.	Reduces transmission of microorganisms.
18 Stay with patient for several minutes and observe for any allergic reactions.	Dyspnea, wheezing, and circulatory collapse are signs of severe anaphylactic reaction.

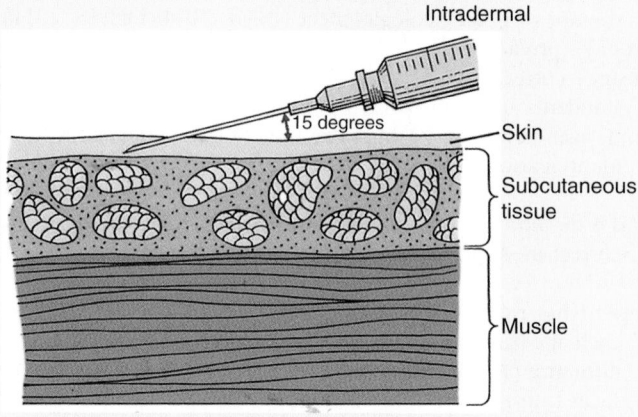

STEP 14b   Intradermal needle tip inserted into dermis.

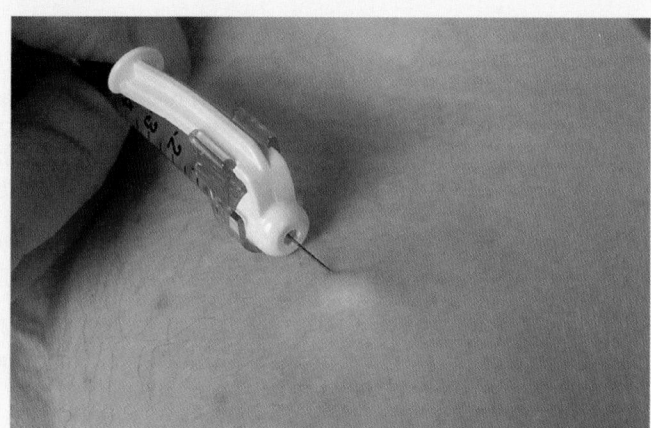

STEP 14d   Injection creates small bleb.

EVALUATION

1 Return to room in 15 to 30 minutes and ask if patient feels any acute pain, burning, numbness, or tingling at injection site.	Continued discomfort could indicate injury to underlying tissues.
2 Ask patient to discuss implications of skin testing and signs of hypersensitivity.	Patient's ability to recognize signs of skin testing helps to ensure timely reporting of results.
3 Inspect bleb. *Optional:* Use skin pencil and draw circle around perimeter of injection site. Read TB test site at 48 to 72 hours; look for induration (hard, dense, raised area) of skin around injection site of: • 15 mm or more in patients with no known risk factors for tuberculosis. • 10 mm or more in patients who are recent immigrants; injection drug users; residents and employees of high-risk settings; patients with certain chronic illnesses; children less than 4 years of age; and infants, children, and adolescents exposed to high-risk adults.	Determines if reaction to antigen occurs; indication positive for TB or tested allergens. Degree of reaction varies based on patient condition. Site must be read at various intervals to determine test results. Pencil marks make site easy to find. You determine results of skin testing at various times, based on type of medication used or type of skin testing completed. Manufacturer directions determine when to read test results.

STEP	RATIONALE

- 5 mm or more in patients who are human immunodeficiency virus (HIV) positive, have fibrotic changes on chest x-ray film consistent with previous tuberculosis infection, have had organ transplants, or are immunosuppressed (CDC, 2011b).

Unexpected Outcomes

1 Patient complains of localized pain or continued burning at injection site, indicating potential injury to nerve or vessels.

2 Raised, reddened, or hard zone (induration) forms around ID test site.

3 Patient has adverse reaction with signs of urticaria, pruritus, wheezing, and dyspnea.

4 Patient is unable to explain purpose or signs of skin testing.

Related Interventions

- Assess injection site.
- Notify patient's health care provider.

- Notify patient's health care provider.
- Document sensitivity to injected allergen or positive test if tuberculin skin testing was completed.

- Notify patient's health care provider.
- Follow agency policy for appropriate response to drug reactions (e.g., administration of antihistamine such as diphenhydramine [Benadryl] or epinephrine).
- Add allergy information to patient's record.

- Provide further teaching to patient or family caregiver.
- Recognize that patient is unable to learn at this time.

Recording and Reporting

- Record drug, dose, route, site, time, and date on MAR immediately after administration, not before. Correctly sign MAR according to agency policy.
- Record area of ID injection and appearance of skin in your notes.
- Report any undesirable effects from medication to patient's health care provider and document adverse effects according to agency policy.
- Record patient teaching, validation of understanding, and patient's response to medication.

Special Considerations

Teaching

- Instruct patient not to squeeze medication out of injection site.
- Teach patients that negative skin tests may not rule out allergies, especially when low concentrations of medication are used.

- Patient should wear medical identification band listing all allergies.
- Caution patient not to wash off pencil markings around injection site.
- Explain to patient how to observe for skin reactions.

Pediatric

- Children who are exposed to people with confirmed or suspected infectious tuberculosis should be tested for it immediately following exposure (Hockenberry and Wilson, 2011).
- Children with ongoing exposure to high-risk individuals (e.g., HIV-infected, homeless, incarcerated) should be tested for tuberculosis every 2-to-3 years (Hockenberry and Wilson, 2011).

Gerontologic

- The skin of the older adult is less elastic and must be held taut to ensure that ID injection is administered correctly.

SKILL 22-3 Administering Subcutaneous Injections

NSO *Injections Module / Lesson 3*

 Video Clip

Subcutaneous injections involve depositing medication into the loose connective tissue underlying the dermis. Because subcutaneous tissue does not contain as many blood vessels as muscles, medications are absorbed more slowly than with intramuscular (IM) injections. Physical exercise or application of hot or cold compresses influences the rate of drug absorption by altering local blood flow to tissues. Any condition that impairs blood flow is a contraindication for subcutaneous injections.

You give subcutaneous medications in small doses of less than 2 mL that are isotonic, nonirritating, nonviscous, and water soluble. Limited research indicates that volumes up to 2 mL may be given without tissue damage (Cocoman and Murray, 2008, 2010; Walker et al., 2010). In infants and children the recommendation is to administer amounts up to 0.5 mL in one site (Hockenberry and Wilson, 2011). Examples of subcutaneous medications

include epinephrine, insulin, allergy medications, opioids, and heparin. Because subcutaneous tissue contains pain receptors, the patient often experiences some discomfort.

The best subcutaneous injection sites include the outer aspect of the upper arms, the abdomen from below the costal margins to the iliac crests, and the anterior aspects of the thighs (Fig. 22-12). These areas are easily accessible and are large enough to allow rotating multiple injections within each anatomic location.

Choose an injection site that is free of skin lesions, bony prominences, and large underlying muscles or nerves. Site rotation prevents the formation of lipohypertrophy or lipoatrophy in the skin. The patient's body weight and amount of adipose tissue indicate the depth of the subcutaneous layer. Therefore base the needle length and angle of needle insertion on the patient's weight and estimate of subcutaneous tissue. Generally a 25-gauge ⅝-inch

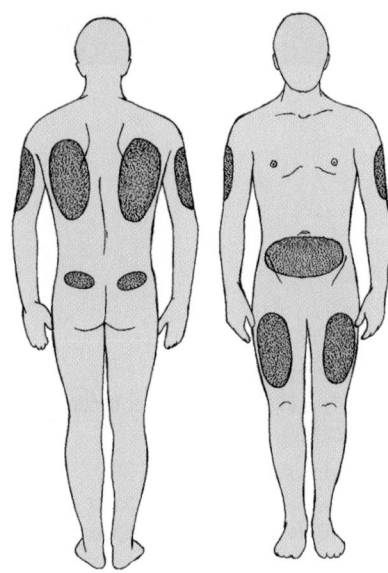

FIG 22-12 Common sites for subcutaneous injections.

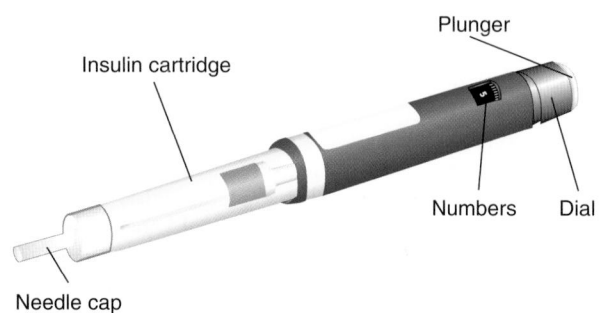

FIG 22-13 Insulin injection pen. (From *Lewis SL et al*: Medical-surgical nursing: assessment and management of clinical problems, *ed 8, St Louis, 2011, Mosby.*)

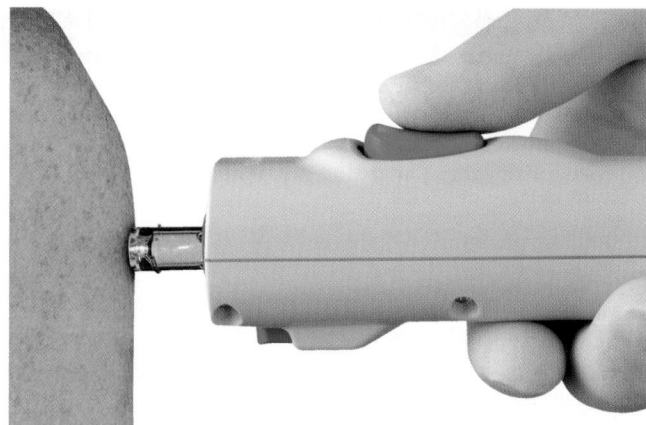

FIG 22-14 Jet injection system is held perpendicular to skin. (*Image courtesy Pharmajet. All rights reserved.*)

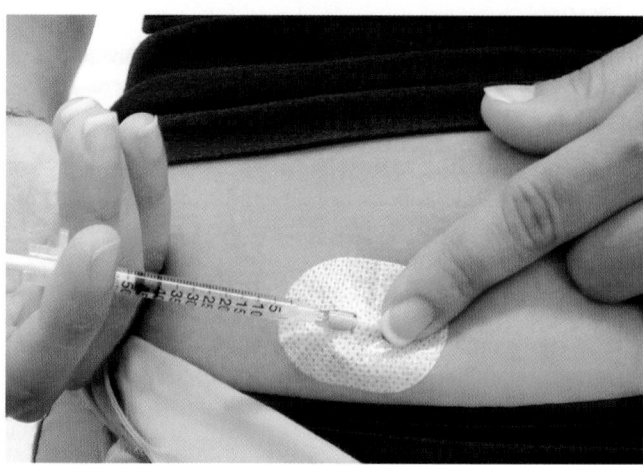

FIG 22-15 Subcutaneous device. (*Image courtesy IntraPump Infusion Systems. All rights reserved.*)

needle inserted at a 45-degree angle or a ½-inch needle inserted at a 90-degree angle deposits medications into the subcutaneous tissue of a normal-size patient. A child usually requires a 26- to 30-gauge ½-inch needle inserted at a 90-degree angle (Hockenberry and Wilson, 2011). If the patient is obese, pinch the tissue and use a needle long enough to insert through the fatty tissue at the base of the skinfold. Thin patients sometimes have insufficient tissue for injections. Therefore the upper abdomen is the best injection site for patients with little peripheral subcutaneous tissue. Aspiration after an injection, including heparin and insulin, is not necessary. Piercing a blood vessel and causing a hematoma formation are rare (Hunter, 2008b).

Several new technologies are available for administration of subcutaneous injections. *Injection pens* are a technology that patients can use to self-administer medications (e.g., epinephrine, insulin, or interferon) subcutaneously (Fig. 22-13). They offer a convenient delivery method using prefilled, disposable cartridges. The patient pinches the skin, inserts the needle, and injects a predetermined medication dose. Teaching is essential to ensure that patients use the correct injection technique and deliver the correct dose of medication. Patients need to be taught the importance of purging the pen before a dose is given. The disadvantages to this technology include increased risk for needlestick injury and

user's lack of knowledge and skill in administration technique and how to store the device (Aschenbrenner and Venable, 2009). One new technology is a *needleless injection system* that administers subcutaneous medications without the use of needles. Needle-free injections use high pressure to penetrate the skin with the medication into the subcutaneous tissue (Fig. 22-14). Another new advance in subcutaneous injection is the *subcutaneous injection device* (e.g., insuflon) (Fig. 22-15), which is inserted into the subcutaneous tissue; the needle is then removed, leaving the cannula in the tissue to provide an avenue for administering medications for up to 3 days without having to puncture the skin with each injection (Riley and Raup, 2010).

Special Considerations for Administration of Insulin

Most patients manage type 1 diabetes mellitus with injections. Anatomic injection site rotation is no longer necessary because newer human insulins carry a lower risk for hypertrophy. Patients choose one anatomic area (e.g., the abdomen) and systematically rotate sites within that region, which maintains consistent insulin absorption from day to day. Absorption rates of insulin vary based on the injection site. Insulin is most quickly absorbed in the abdomen and most slowly in the thighs (Lehne, 2010).

TABLE 22-2	Comparison of Insulin Preparations		
Insulin Type*	**Onset**	**Peak Effect (Hours)**	**Duration of Action (Hours)**
Rapid-Acting			
Insulin lispro (Humalog)	15-30 min	$\frac{1}{2}$-2$\frac{1}{2}$	3-6$\frac{1}{2}$
Insulin aspart (NovoLog)	10-20 min	1-3	3-5
Insulin glulisine (Apidra)	10-15 min	1-1$\frac{1}{2}$	3-5
Short-Acting			
Regular insulin† (e.g., Humulin R, Novolin R)	30-60 min	1-5	6-10
Intermediate-Acting			
Isophane insulin suspension (NPH)	1-2 hr	6-14	16-24
Long-Acting			
Insulin glargine (Lantus)‡	1 hr	Plateau	24
Insulin detemir (Levemir)‡	0.8-2 hr	Peakless	Up to 24

Data from Hodgson BB, Kizior RJ: *Saunders Nursing Drug Handbook 2013,* St Louis, 2013, Saunders.
*All above insulins are available in 100-unit strengths.
†This is the only insulin approved for intravenous or intramuscular use.
‡Cannot be mixed with other insulins.

BOX 22-3	General Guidelines for Insulin Administration

- Store vials of insulin in the refrigerator, not the freezer. Keep vials currently being used at room temperature. Do not inject cold insulin.
- Inspect vials before each use for changes in appearance (e.g., clumping, frosting, precipitation, change in clarity or color) indicating lack of potency.
- Do not interchange insulin types unless approved by the patient's prescriber.
- Preferred injection site includes the abdomen, avoiding a 5 cm (2-inch) radius around the umbilicus and the outer aspect of the thighs.
- Have patient self-administer insulin whenever possible. Generally children begin self-administration by adolescence.
- Patients who take insulin need to self-monitor their blood glucose.
- All patients who take insulin should carry at least 15 g carbohydrate (e.g., 4 ounces of fruit juice, 4 ounces of regular soft drink, 8 ounces of skim milk, 6 to 10 hard candies) in the event of a hypoglycemic reaction.

Adapted from American Diabetes Association: Standards in medical care of diabetes, 2011, *Am Diabetes Care* 34(S1):S11, 2011; Sheeja VS et al: Insulin therapy in diabetes management, *Int J Pharm Sci Rev Res* 2(2):98, 2010.

The timing of injections is critical to correct insulin administration. Health care providers plan insulin injection times based on blood glucose levels and when a patient will eat. Knowing the peak action and duration of the insulin is essential when developing an effective diabetes management plan. Table 22-2 compares a variety of insulin preparations. Box 22-3 provides general guidelines for insulin administration.

Special Considerations for Administration of Heparin

Heparin therapy provides therapeutic anticoagulation to reduce the risk for thrombus formation by suppressing clot formation. Therefore patients receiving heparin are at risk for bleeding, including bleeding gums, hematemesis, hematuria, or melena. Results from coagulation blood tests (e.g., activated partial thromboplastin time [aPTT] and partial thromboplastin time [PTT]) allow you to monitor the desired therapeutic range for intravenous (IV) heparin therapy.

Before administering heparin, assess for preexisting conditions that contraindicate its use, including cerebral or aortic aneurysm, cerebrovascular hemorrhage, severe hypertension, and blood dyscrasias. In addition, assess for conditions in which increased risk for hemorrhage is present: recent childbirth; severe diabetes and renal disease; liver disease; severe trauma; and active ulcers or lesions of the gastrointestinal (GI), genitourinary (GU), or respiratory tract. Assess the patient's current medication regimen, including use of over-the-counter (OTC) and herbal medications (e.g., garlic, ginger, ginkgo, horse chestnut, or feverfew), for possible interaction with heparin. Other medications that interact with heparin include aspirin, nonsteroidal antiinflammatory drugs (NSAIDs), cephalosporins, antithyroid agents, probenecid, and thrombolytics.

You administer heparin subcutaneously or intravenously. Low-molecular-weight heparins (LMWHs) (e.g., enoxaparin [Lovenox]) are more effective than heparin in some patients. The anticoagulant effects are more predictable (Lehne, 2010). LMWHs have a longer half-life and require less laboratory monitoring but are expensive. To minimize the pain and bruising associated with LMWH, it is given subcutaneously on the right or left side of the abdomen, at least 5 cm (2 inches) away from the umbilicus (the patient's "love handles"). Administer LMWH in its prefilled syringe with the attached needle and do not expel the air bubble in the syringe before giving the medication (Sanofi-Aventis, 2010).

Delegation and Collaboration

The skill of administering subcutaneous injections cannot be delegated to nursing assistive personnel (NAP). The nurse directs the NAP about:

- Potential medication side effects and to report their occurrence to the nurse.

Equipment

❑ Proper size syringe with engineered sharps injury protection (SESIP) needle:
- Subcutaneous: syringe (1- to 3-mL) and needle (25- to 27-gauge, $\frac{3}{8}$- to $\frac{5}{8}$-inch)
- Subcutaneous U-100 insulin: insulin syringe (1 mL) with preattached needle (28- to 31-gauge, $\frac{5}{16}$- to $\frac{1}{2}$-inch)
- Subcutaneous U-500 insulin: 1 mL tuberculin (TB) syringe with needle (25- to 27-gauge, $\frac{1}{2}$- to $\frac{5}{8}$-inch)

❏ Small gauze pad *(optional)*
❏ Alcohol swab
❏ Medication vial or ampule
❏ Clean gloves

❏ Medication administration record (MAR) or computer printout
❏ Puncture-proof container

STEP	RATIONALE

ASSESSMENT

1 Check accuracy and completeness of each MAR or computer printout with prescriber's written medication order. Check patient's name, medication name and dosage, route of administration, and time of administration. Recopy or reprint any portion of MAR that is difficult to read.

The prescriber's order is the most reliable source and legal record of the patient's medications. Ensures that patient receives correct medications.
Handwritten MARs are a source of medication errors (ISMP, 2010; Jones and Treiber, 2010).

2 Assess patient's medical and medication history.

Determines need for medication or possible contraindications for medication administration.

3 Assess patient's history of allergies: known type of allergies and normal allergic reaction.

Do not prepare medication if there is a known patient allergy.

4 Review medication reference information for medication action, purpose, normal dose, side effects, time and peak of onset, and nursing implications.

Allows you to administer medication safely and monitor patient's response to therapy.

5 Observe patient's previous verbal and nonverbal responses toward injection.

Anticipating patient's anxiety allows you to use distraction to reduce pain awareness.

6 Assess for contraindication to subcutaneous injections such as circulatory shock or reduced local tissue perfusion.

Reduced tissue perfusion interferes with drug absorption and distribution.

7 Assess patient's symptoms before initiating medication therapy.

Provides information to evaluate desired effect of medication.

8 Assess adequacy of patient's adipose tissue.

Adipose tissue influences methods for administering injections.

9 Assess relevant laboratory results (e.g., blood glucose, partial thromboplastin).

Provides baseline for measuring drug response.

10 Assess patient's knowledge of medication.

Poses implications for patient education.

NURSING DIAGNOSES

- Acute pain
- Anxiety

- Deficient knowledge regarding medication administration or drug therapy

- Fear
- Ineffective health maintenance

Related factors are individualized based on patient's condition or needs.

PLANNING

1 Expected outcomes following completion of procedure:
- Patient experiences no pain or mild burning at injection site.
- Patient achieves desired effect of medication with no signs of allergies or undesired effects.
- Patient explains purpose, dosage, and effects of medication.

Medications may cause minor tissue irritation.
Medication administered without patient injury.

Demonstrates learning.

IMPLEMENTATION

1 Perform hand hygiene and prepare medication using aseptic technique. Check label of medication carefully with MAR or computer printout 2 times (see Skill 22-1 or Procedural Guideline 22-1) when preparing medication.

Ensures that medication is sterile. *These are the first and second checks for accuracy* and ensure that correct medication is administered.

2 Take medication(s) to patient at correct time (see agency policy). Medications that require exact timing include stat, first-time or loading doses, and one time doses. Give time-critical scheduled medications (e.g., antibiotics, anticoagulants, insulin, anticonvulsants, immunosuppressive agents) at exact time ordered (no later than 30 minutes before or after scheduled dose). Give non–time-critical scheduled medications within a range of 1 or 2 hours of scheduled dose (ISMP, 2011). During administration, apply six rights of medication administration.

Hospitals must adopt medication administration policy and procedure for timing of medication administration that considers nature of the prescribed medication, specific clinical application, and patient needs (DHHS, 2011; ISMP, 2011). Time-critical scheduled medications are those for which early or delayed administration of maintenance doses of greater than 30 minutes before or after the scheduled dose may cause harm or result in substantial suboptimal therapy or pharmacologic effect. Non–time-critical medications are those for which early or delayed administration within a specified range of either 1 or 2 hours should not cause harm or result in substantial suboptimal therapy or pharmacologic effect (ISMP, 2011; DHHS, 2011).

STEP	RATIONALE
3 Close room curtain or door.	Provides privacy.
4 Identify patient using two identifiers (i.e., name and birthday or name and account number) according to agency policy. Compare identifiers in MAR/medical record with information on patient's identification bracelet and/or ask patient to state name.	Ensures correct patient. Complies with The Joint Commission standards and improves patient safety (TJC, 2012). Some agencies are now using a bar-code system to help with patient identification.
5 At patient's bedside again compare MAR or computer printout with names of medications on medication labels and patient name. Ask patient if he or she has allergies.	*This is the third check for accuracy* and ensures that patient receives correct medication. Confirms patient's allergy history.
6 Discuss purpose of each medication, action, and possible adverse effects. Allow patient to ask any questions. Tell patient that injection will cause slight burning or sting.	Patient has right to be informed, and patient's understanding of each medication improves adherence to drug therapy. Helps minimize patient's anxiety.
7 Perform hand hygiene and apply clean gloves. Keep sheet or gown draped over body parts not requiring exposure.	Reduces transmission of infection. Respects dignity of patient while exposing injection area.
8 Select appropriate injection site. Inspect skin surface over sites for bruises, inflammation, or edema. Do not use an area that is bruised or has signs associated with infection.	Injection sites are free of abnormalities that interfere with drug absorption. Sites used repeatedly become hardened from lipohypertrophy (increased growth in fatty tissue).

Clinical Decision Point *Applying ice to the injection site for 1 minute before the injection may decrease the patient's perception of pain (Hockenberry and Wilson, 2011).*

STEP	RATIONALE
9 Palpate sites and avoid those with masses or tenderness. Be sure that needle is correct size by grasping skinfold at site with thumb and forefinger. Measure fold from top to bottom. Make sure that needle is one-half length of fold.	You can mistakenly give subcutaneous injections in muscle, especially in abdomen and thigh sites. Appropriate size of needle ensures that you inject medication into subcutaneous tissue (Gibney et al., 2010; Hunter, 2008b).
a When administering insulin or heparin, use abdominal injection sites first, followed by thigh injection site.	Risk for bruising is not affected by site (Aschenbrenner and Venable, 2009).
b When administering LMWH subcutaneously, choose site on right or left side of abdomen, at least 5 cm (2 inches) away from umbilicus.	Injecting LMWH on side of abdomen helps decrease pain and bruising at injection site (Sanofi-Aventis, 2010).
c Rotate insulin site within an anatomic area (e.g., abdomen) and systematically rotate sites within that area.	Rotating injection sites within same anatomic site maintains consistency in day-to-day insulin absorption (Sheeja et al., 2010).
10 Help patient into comfortable position. Have him or her relax arm, leg, or abdomen, depending on site selection.	Relaxation of site minimizes discomfort.
11 Relocate site using anatomic landmarks.	Injection into correct anatomic site prevents injury to nerves, bone, and blood vessels.
12 Clean site with antiseptic swab. Apply swab at center of site and rotate outward in circular direction for about 5 cm (2 inches) (see illustration).	Mechanical action of swab removes secretions containing microorganisms.

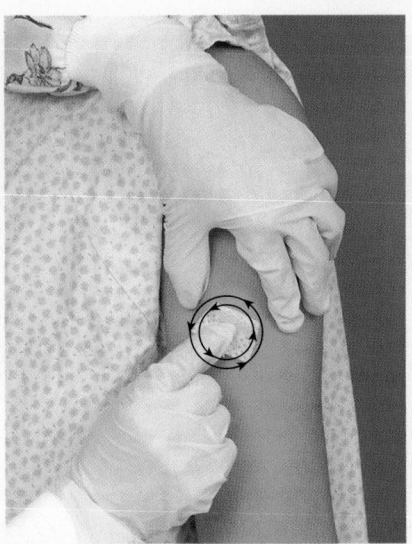

STEP 12 Cleaning site with circular motion.

STEP	RATIONALE
13 Hold swab or gauze between third and fourth fingers of nondominant hand.	Swab or gauze remains readily accessible for use when withdrawing needle after the injection.
14 Remove needle cap or protective sheath by pulling it straight off.	Preventing needle from touching sides of cap prevents contamination.
15 Hold syringe between thumb and forefinger of dominant hand; hold as dart (see illustration).	Quick, smooth injection requires proper manipulation of syringe parts.
16 Administer injection:	
a For average-size patient, hold skin across injection site or pinch skin with nondominant hand.	Needle penetrates tight skin more easily than loose skin. Pinching elevates subcutaneous tissue and desensitizes area.
b Inject needle quickly and firmly at 45- to 90-degree angle (see illustration). Release skin if pinched. *Option:* When using injection pen or giving heparin, continue to pinch skin while injecting medicine.	Quick, firm insertion minimizes discomfort. (Injecting medication into compressed tissue irritates nerve fibers.) Correct angle prevents accidental injection into muscle.
c For obese patient pinch skin at site and inject needle at 90-degree angle below tissue fold.	Obese patients have fatty layer of tissue above subcutaneous layer.
d After needle enters site, grasp lower end of syringe barrel with nondominant hand to stabilize it. Move dominant hand to end of plunger and slowly inject medication over several seconds (Hunter, 2008b) (see illustration). Avoid moving syringe.	Movement of syringe may displace needle and cause discomfort. Slow injection of medication minimizes discomfort.

Clinical Decision Point *Aspiration after injecting a subcutaneous medication is not necessary. Piercing a blood vessel in a subcutaneous injection is very rare (Hunter, 2008b). Aspiration after injecting heparin and insulin is not recommended (Aschenbrenner and Venable, 2009).*

e Withdraw needle quickly while placing antiseptic swab or gauze gently over site.	Supporting tissues around injection site minimizes discomfort during needle withdrawal. Dry gauze may minimize patient discomfort associated with alcohol on nonintact skin.
17 Apply gentle pressure to site. Do *not massage site.* (If heparin is given, hold alcohol swab or gauze to site for 30 to 60 seconds.)	Aids absorption. Massage can damage underlying tissue. Time interval prevents bleeding at site.
18 Help patient to comfortable position.	Gives patient sense of well-being.
19 Discard uncapped needle or needle enclosed in safety shield (see illustrations) and attached syringe into puncture- and leak-proof receptacle.	Prevents injury to patients and health care personnel. Recapping needles increases risk for needlestick injury (OSHA, 2012).

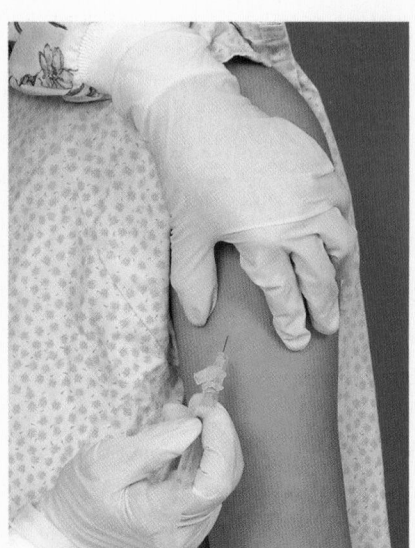

STEP 15 Holding syringe as if grasping a dart.

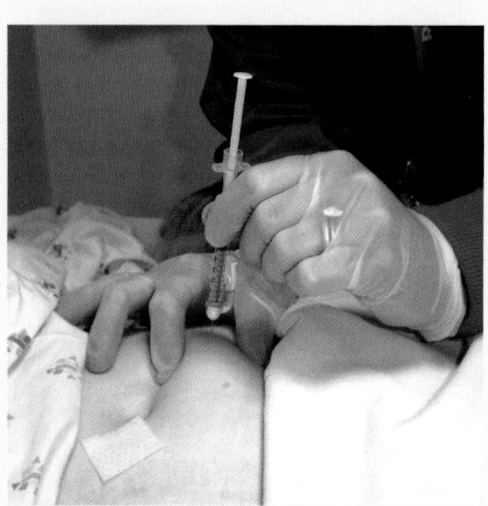

STEP 16b Subcutaneous injection. Angle and needle length depend on thickness of skinfold.

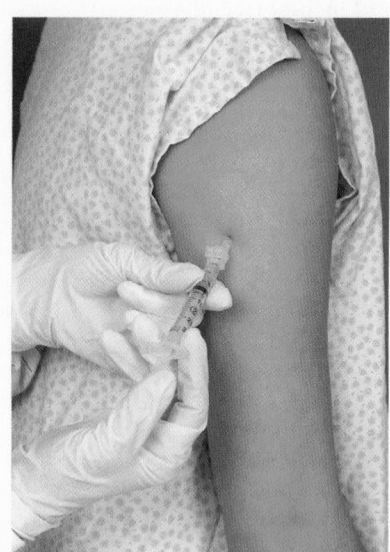

STEP 16d Inject medication slowly.

STEP	RATIONALE
20 Remove gloves and perform hand hygiene.	Reduces transmission of microorganisms.
21 Stay with patient for several minutes and observe for any allergic reactions.	Dyspnea, wheezing, and circulatory collapse are signs of severe anaphylactic reaction.

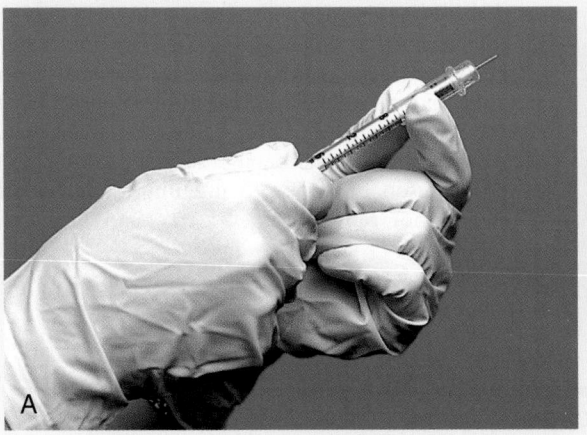 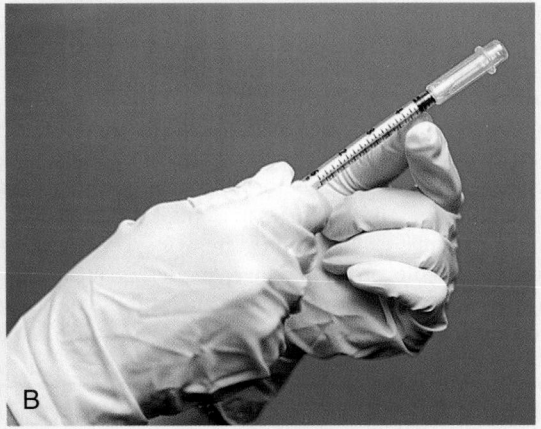

STEP 19 Needle with plastic guard to prevent needlesticks. **A,** Position of guard before injection. **B,** After injection guard locks in place, covering needle.

EVALUATION

1 Return to room in 15 to 30 minutes and ask if patient feels any acute pain, burning, numbness, or tingling at injection site.	Continued discomfort may indicate injury to underlying bones or nerves.
2 Inspect site, noting bruising or induration. Provide warm compress to site.	Bruising or induration indicates complication associated with injection.
3 Observe patient's response to medication at times that correlate with onset, peak, and duration of medication. Review laboratory results as appropriate (e.g., blood glucose, partial thromboplastin).	Adverse effects of parenteral medications develop rapidly. Evaluate effect of medication based on onset, peak, and duration of action.
4 Ask patient to explain purpose and effects of medication.	Evaluates patient's understanding of information taught.

Unexpected Outcomes

1 Patient complains of localized pain, numbness, tingling, or burning at injection site.

2 Patient displays adverse reaction with signs of urticaria, eczema, pruritus, wheezing, and dyspnea.

3 Hypertrophy of skin develops from repeated subcutaneous injection.

Related Interventions

- Assess injection site; may indicate potential injury to nerve or tissues.
- Notify patient's health care provider and do not reuse site.
- Monitor patient's heart rate, respirations, blood pressure, and temperature.
- Follow agency policy or guidelines for appropriate response to allergic reactions (e.g., administration of antihistamine such as diphenhydramine [Benadryl] or epinephrine) and notify patient's health care provider immediately.
- Add allergy information to patient's record.
- Do not use site for future injections.
- Instruct patient not to use site for 6 months.

Recording and Reporting

- Immediately after administration, record medication, dose, route, site, time, and date given on MAR. Correctly sign MAR according to agency policy.
- Record patient teaching, validation of understanding, and patient's response to medication in nurses' notes and electronic health record (EHR).
- Report any undesirable effects from medication to patient's health care provider and document adverse effects in record.

Special Considerations

Teaching

- Instruct patient to wear medical identification bracelet indicating important medical information, including bleeding tendencies, illnesses (e.g., diabetes) and allergies.
- Patients who require daily injections need to learn techniques of self-administration (see Skill 42-6). Teach injection techniques to a family caregiver.

Pediatric
- Administer only amounts up to 0.5 mL subcutaneously to small children (Hockenberry and Wilson, 2011).

Gerontologic
- Aging patients have less elastic skin and reduced subcutaneous skinfold thickness. The upper abdominal site is the best site to use when the patient has little subcutaneous tissue.

Home Care
- Improper disposal of used needles and sharps in the home setting poses a health risk to the public and waste workers. Several options for safe sharps disposal at home exist, including allowing patients to transport their own sharps containers from home to collection sites (e.g., doctor's office, a hospital, or a pharmacy); mailing their used syringes to a collection site (mail-back programs); syringe exchange programs; or special devices that destroy the needle on the syringe, rendering it safe for disposal. If the patient cannot implement any of these options, have him or her dispose of needles and other sharps in a hard plastic or metal container with a tightly sealed lid (e.g., empty detergent bottle or coffee can). Pamphlets for safe home disposal of sharps are on the Environmental Protection Agency (EPA) website (2004).
- Most insulin preparations have bacteriostatic properties that inhibit bacterial growth on the skin. Therefore patients with diabetes may reuse their syringes at home if they can safely recap the needles. Syringes should be discarded when the needles become dull or bent or contact any surface other than the skin. Wiping the needle off with alcohol is not recommended because the silicon coating on the needle is removed, making injections more painful. Immunocompromised patients and patients with poor personal hygiene, acute illness, or open hand wounds should not reuse syringes (American Diabetes Association, 2011).
- Teach injection techniques that minimize patient discomfort to patient and family caregiver.

SKILL 22-4   Administering Intramuscular Injections

NSO *Injections Module / Lesson 5*

 Video Clip

The intramuscular (IM) injection route deposits medication into deep muscle tissue, which has a rich blood supply, allowing medication to absorb faster than by the subcutaneous route. However, there is an increased risk for injecting drugs directly into blood vessels. Any factor that interferes with local tissue blood flow affects the rate and extent of drug absorption.

An IM injection requires a longer and larger-gauge needle to penetrate deep muscle tissue (see Fig. 22-1). The viscosity of the medication, injection site, patient's weight, and amount of adipose tissue influence needle size selection. Determine needle gauge by the medication to be administered. For example, administer immunizations and parenteral medications in aqueous solutions with a 20- to 25-gauge needle. Give viscous or oil-based solution with an 18- to 21-gauge needle. Use a small-gauge (22- to 25-gauge) needle for children. The CDC (2011a) current recommendations for needle length are based on patient weight and body mass index (BMI). An adult patient who is thin requires a needle length of 5/8 to 1 inch; whereas an average patient requires a 1-inch needle; patients over 70 kg require a 1- to 1½-inch needle, and those over 90 kg require a 1½-inch needle (CDC, 2011a). Evidence-based practice recommends needle lengths for adults based on site selection: vastus lateralis, 16- to 25-mm (5/8- to 1-inch); ventrogluteal, 38 mm (1½-inch); and deltoid, 25- to 38-mm (1- to 1½-inch) (Nicholl and Hesby, 2002). Recommendations for needle length include 25 mm (1 inch) for infants; 25- to 32- mm (1- to 1¼-inch) in toddlers; and 38-mm (1½-inch) needle in older children (Hockenberry and Wilson, 2011). Preterm and small, emaciated infants may require a shorter needle based on weight and muscle mass. Obese children may require a longer needle up to 38 mm (1½ inch) (Middleman et al., 2010). Based on the evidence, the recommendation for pediatric IM injection sites includes use of the anterolateral thigh for infants up to 12 months of age, deltoid in children 18 months and older, and ventrogluteal for children of all ages (Hockenberry and Wilson, 2011).

Muscle is less sensitive to irritating and viscous medication. A normal, well-developed adult can safely tolerate 2 to 5 mL of medication in larger muscles such as the ventrogluteal (Hunt, 2008; Nicholl and Hesby, 2002). However, clinically it is unusual to administer over 3 mL of medication in a single injection because the body does not absorb it well. Older adults and thin patients often tolerate only 2 mL in a single injection. The muscles of older infants and small children can tolerate 1 mL of medication in a single site. Children with larger muscles are able to tolerate a maximum volume of 2 mL of medication (Hockenberry and Wilson, 2011).

Administer IM injections so the needle is perpendicular to the patient's body and as close to a 90-degree angle as possible (Zimmerman, 2010). Rotate IM injection sites to decrease the risk for hypertrophy. Emaciated or atrophied muscles absorb medication poorly; thus avoid their use when possible. The Z-track method, a technique for pulling the skin during an injection, is recommended for IM injections (Nicholl and Hesby, 2002). It prevents leakage of medication into subcutaneous tissues, seals medication in the muscle, and minimizes irritation. To use the Z-track method, apply the appropriate-size needle to the syringe and select an IM site, preferably in a large, deep muscle such as the ventrogluteal. Pull the overlying skin and subcutaneous tissues approximately 2.5 to 3.5 cm (1 to 1½ inches) laterally to the side with the ulnar side of the nondominant hand. Hold the skin in this position until you have administered the injection (Fig. 22-16, A). After cleaning a site, inject the needle deeply into the muscle. To reduce injection site discomfort, there is no longer any need to aspirate after the needle is injected when *administering vaccines* (CDC, 2011a). It is the nurses' responsibility to follow agency policy for aspirating after injecting the needle. Keep the needle inserted for 10 seconds to allow the medication to disperse evenly. Release the skin after withdrawing the needle. This leaves a zigzag path that seals the needle track wherever tissue planes slide across one another see (Fig. 22-16, B). The medication is sealed in the muscle tissue.

Injection Sites

When selecting an IM site, determine that the site is free of pain, infection, necrosis, bruising, and abrasions. Also consider the location of underlying bones, nerves, and blood vessels and the volume of medication that you will administer. Because of the sciatic nerve location, the dorsogluteal muscle is not recommended as an injection site. If a needle hits the sciatic nerve, the patient may experience partial or permanent paralysis of the leg (Hunter, 2008a; Zimmerman, 2010).

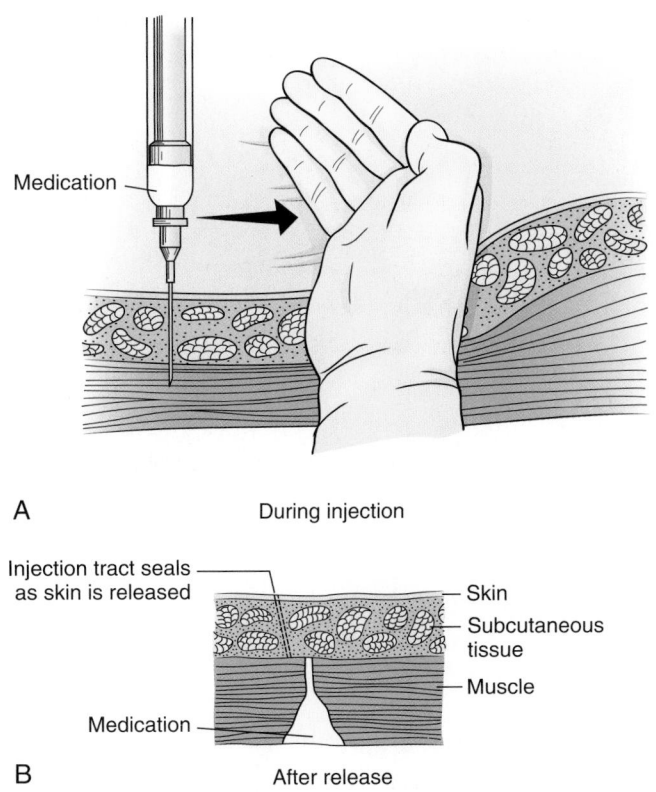

FIG 22-16 **A,** Pulling on overlying skin with dorsum of hand during IM injection moves tissue to prevent later tracking. **B,** Z-track left after injection prevents deposit of medication through sensitive tissue.

Ventrogluteal Site

The ventrogluteal muscle involves the gluteus medius and minimus and is a safe injection site for adults and children (Hockenberry and Wilson, 2011; Zimmerman, 2010). Research has shown that pain and nerve and tissue injury are associated with inappropriate site selection (Hunt, 2008; Hunter, 2008a; Zimmerman, 2010).

To locate the ventrogluteal muscle, have a patient lie in either the supine or lateral position; place the heel of your hand over the greater trochanter of the patient's hip with the wrist almost perpendicular to the femur. Use your right hand for the left hip and the left hand for the right hip. Point the thumb toward the patient's groin; point the index finger to the anterior superior iliac spine; and extend the middle finger back along the iliac crest toward the buttock. The index finger, the middle finger, and the iliac crest form a V-shaped triangle. The injection site is the center of the triangle (Fig. 22-17, A) (Nicholl and Hesby, 2002). To relax this muscle, patients lie on their side or back, flexing the knee and hip (see Fig. 22-17, B).

Vastus Lateralis Muscle

The vastus lateralis muscle is another injection site used in adults and is the preferred site for administration of biologics (e.g., immunizations) to infants, toddlers, and children (Hockenberry and Wilson, 2011). The muscle is thick and well developed; it is located on the anterior lateral aspect of the thigh. It extends in an adult from a hand breadth above the knee to a hand breadth below the greater trochanter of the femur (Fig. 22-18, A) (Nicholl and Hesby, 2002). Use the middle third of the muscle for injection. The width of the muscle usually extends from the midline of the thigh to the midline of the outer side of the thigh. With young children or

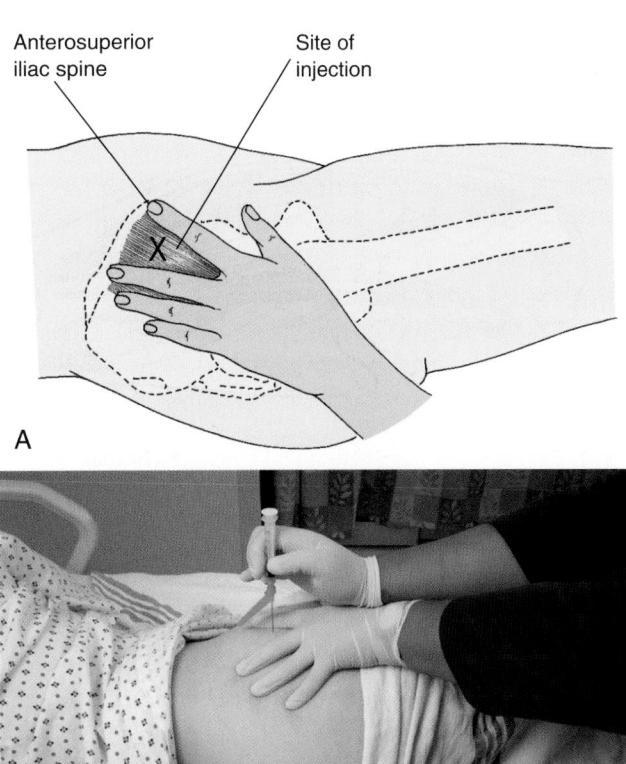

FIG 22-17 **A,** Anatomic view of ventrogluteal injection site. **B,** Injection at ventrogluteal site avoids major nerves and blood vessels.

cachectic patients, it helps to grasp the body of the muscle during injection to be sure that the medication is deposited in muscle tissue. To help relax the muscle, ask the patient to lie flat with the knee slightly flexed and foot externally rotated or assume a sitting position (Fig. 22-18, B).

Deltoid Muscle

Although the deltoid site is easily accessible, the muscle is not well developed in many adults. There is potential for injury because the axillary, radial, brachial, and ulnar nerves and the brachial artery lie within the upper arm under the triceps and along the humerus. Use this site for small medication volumes (2 mL or less) (Nicholl and Hesby, 2002). *Carefully assess the condition of the deltoid muscle; consult medication references for suitability of medication; and carefully locate the injection site using anatomic landmarks.* Use this site for small medication volumes; for administration of routine immunizations in toddlers, older children, and adults; or when other sites are inaccessible because of dressings or casts.

Locate the deltoid muscle by fully exposing the patient's upper arm and shoulder and asking him or her to relax the arm at the side or by supporting the patient's arm and flexing the elbow. Do not roll up any tight-fitting sleeve. Allow the patient to sit, stand, or lie down. Palpate the lower edge of the acromion process, which forms the base of a triangle in line with the midpoint of the lateral aspect of the upper arm. The injection site is in the center of the triangle, about 3 to 5 cm (1 to 2 inches) below the acromion process (Fig. 22-19, A) (Nicholl and Hesby, 2002). You

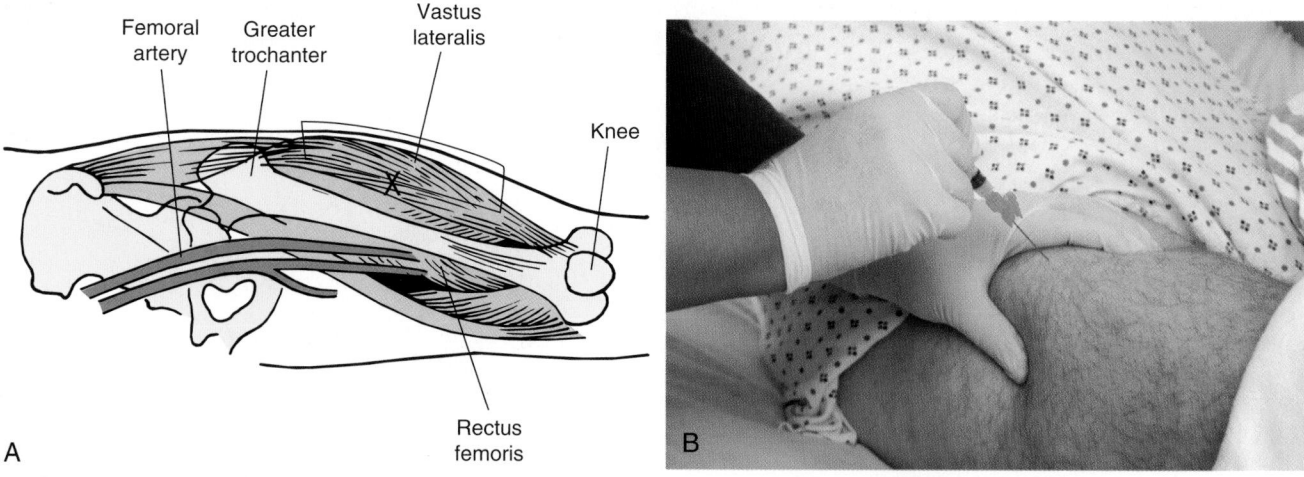

FIG 22-18   **A,** Landmarks for vastus lateralis site. **B,** Giving IM injection in vastus lateralis site.

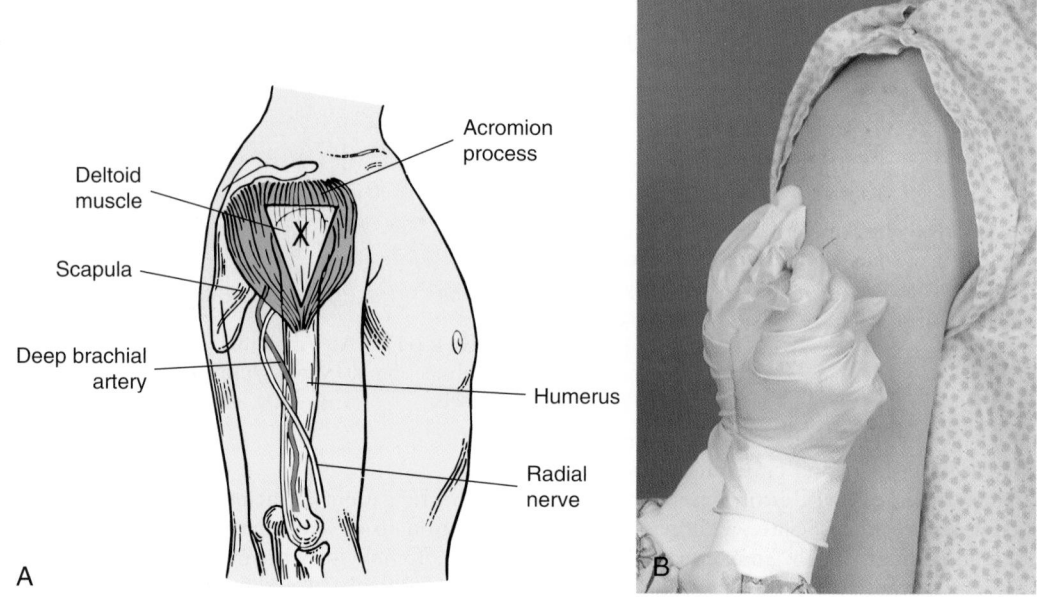

FIG 22-19   **A,** Landmarks for deltoid site. **B,** Giving IM injection in deltoid site.

locate the apex of the triangle by placing four fingers across the deltoid muscle with the top finger along the acromion process. The injection site is three finger widths below the acromion process (see Fig. 22-19, *B*).

Delegation and Collaboration

The skill of administering intramuscular injections cannot be delegated to nursing assistive personnel (NAP). The nurse directs the NAP about:

- Potential medication side effects and to report their occurrence to the nurse.
- Reporting any change in the patient's condition to the nurse.

Equipment

❑ Proper-size syringe and SESIP needle:
- 2- to 3-mL for adult
- 0.5- to 1-mL for infants and small children

❑ Needle length corresponds to site of injection and age and size of patient
❑ Needle gauge often depends on length of needle; administer biologic and medication in aqueous solution with a 20- to 25-gauge needle
❑ Alcohol swab
❑ Small gauze pad
❑ Vial or ampule of medication
❑ Clean gloves
❑ Medication administration record (MAR) or computer printout
❑ Puncture-proof container

STEP	RATIONALE

ASSESSMENT

1 Check accuracy and completeness of each MAR or computer printout with prescriber's written medication order. Check patient's name, medication name and dosage, route of administration, and time of administration. Recopy or reprint any portion of MAR that is difficult to read.

The prescriber's order is the most reliable source and legal record of patient's medications. Ensures that patient receives the correct medications.
Handwritten MARs are a source of medication errors (ISMP, 2010; Jones and Treiber, 2010).

2 Assess patient's medical and medication history.

Determines need for medication or possible contraindications for medication administration.

3 Assess patient's history of allergies: known type of allergies and normal allergic reaction.

Do not prepare medication if there is a known patient allergy.

4 Review medication reference information for medication action, purpose, normal dose, side effects, time of peak onset, and nursing implications.

Allows you to administer medication safely and monitor patient's response to therapy.

5 Observe patient's previous verbal and nonverbal responses toward injection.

Anticipating patient's anxiety allows you to use distraction to reduce pain awareness.

6 Assess for contraindication to IM injections such as muscle atrophy, reduced blood flow, or circulatory shock.

Atrophied muscle absorbs medication poorly. Factors interfering with blood flow to muscles impair drug absorption.

7 Assess patient's symptoms before initiating medication therapy.

Provides information for nurse to evaluate desired effects of medication.

Clinical Decision Point *Because of the documented adverse effects of IM injections, other routes of medication injection are preferred. Consider contacting health care provider for alternative route of medication administration.*

8 Assess patient's knowledge regarding medication to be received.

Poses implications for patient education.

NURSING DIAGNOSES

- Acute pain
- Anxiety
- Deficient knowledge regarding medication administration or drug therapy
- Fear

Related factors are individualized based on patient's condition or needs.

PLANNING

1 Expected outcomes following completion of procedure:
- Patient experiences no pain or mild burning at injection site.
- Patient achieves desired effect of medication with no signs of allergies or undesired effects.
- Patient explains purpose, dosage, and effects of medication.

Medications may cause minor tissue irritation.
Medication administered without patient injury.

Demonstrates learning.

IMPLEMENTATION

1 Prepare medications for one patient at a time using aseptic technique. Keep all pages of MARs or computer printouts for one patient together or look at only one patient's electronic MAR at a time. Check label of medication carefully with MAR or computer printout 2 times (see Skill 22-1 and Procedural Guideline 22-1) when preparing medication.

Ensures that medication is sterile. Preventing distractions reduces medication preparation errors (LePorte et al., 2009; Nguyen et al., 2010). *These are the first and second checks for accuracy* and ensure that correct medication is administered.

2 Take medication(s) to patient at correct time (see agency policy). Medications that require exact timing include stat, first-time or loading doses, and one time doses. Give time-critical scheduled medications (e.g., antibiotics, anticoagulants, insulin, anticonvulsants, immunosuppressive agents) at exact time ordered (no later than 30 minutes before or after scheduled dose). Give non–time-critical scheduled medications within a range of 1 or 2 hours of scheduled dose (ISMP, 2011). During administration, apply six rights of medication administration.

Hospitals must adopt medication administration policy and procedure for timing of medication administration that considers nature of the prescribed medication, specific clinical application, and patient needs (DHHS, 2011; ISMP, 2011). Time-critical scheduled medications are those for which early or delayed administration of maintenance doses of greater than 30 minutes before or after the scheduled dose may cause harm or result in substantial suboptimal therapy or pharmacologic effect. Non–time-critical medications are those for which early or delayed administration within a specified range of either 1 or 2 hours should not cause harm or result in substantial suboptimal therapy or pharmacologic effect (ISMP, 2011; DHHS, 2011).

STEP	RATIONALE
3 Close room curtain or door.	Provides privacy.
4 Identify patient using two identifiers (i.e., name and birthday or name and account number) according to agency policy. Compare identifiers in MAR/medical record with information on patient's identification bracelet and/or ask patient to state name.	Ensures correct patient. Complies with The Joint Commission standards and improves patient safety (TJC, 2012). Some agencies are now using a bar-code system to help with patient identification.
5 At patient's bedside again compare MAR or computer printout with names of medications on medication labels and patient name. Ask patient if he or she has allergies.	*This is the third check for accuracy* and ensures that patient receives correct medication. Confirms patient's allergy history.
6 Discuss purpose of each medication, action, and possible adverse effects. Allow patient to ask any questions. Tell patient that injection will cause a slight burning or sting.	Patient has right to be informed, and patient's understanding of each medication improves adherence to drug therapy. Helps minimize patient's anxiety.
7 Perform hand hygiene and apply clean gloves. Keep sheet or gown draped over body parts not requiring exposure.	Reduces transmission of infection. Respects patient's dignity while exposing injection site.
8 Select appropriate site. Note integrity and size of muscle. Palpate for tenderness or hardness. Avoid these areas. If patient receives frequent injections, rotate sites. Use ventrogluteal if possible.	Ventrogluteal is preferred injection site for adults. It is also preferred site for children of all ages (Hockenberry and Wilson, 2011; Hunt, 2008; Zimmerman, 2010).
9 Help patient to comfortable position. Position patient depending on chosen site (e.g., sit, lie flat, on side, or prone).	Reduces strain on muscle and minimizes injection discomfort.

Clinical Decision Point *Ensure that medical condition (e.g., circulatory shock) does not contraindicate patient's position for injection.*

10 Relocate site using anatomic landmarks.	Injection into correct anatomic site prevents injury to nerves, bone, and blood vessels.
11 Clean site with antiseptic swab. Apply swab at center of site and rotate outward in circular direction for about 5 cm (2 inches).	Mechanical action of swab removes secretions containing microorganisms.
a *Option:* Apply EMLA cream on injection site at least 1 hour before IM injection or use vapocoolant spray (e.g., ethyl chloride) just before injection.	Decreases pain at injection site.
12 Hold swab or gauze between third and fourth fingers of nondominant hand.	Swab or gauze remains readily accessible for use when withdrawing needle after injection.
13 Remove needle cap or sheath by pulling it straight off.	Preventing needle from touching sides of cap prevents contamination.
14 Hold syringe between thumb and forefinger of dominant hand; hold as dart, palm down.	Quick, smooth injection requires proper manipulation of syringe parts.
15 Administer injection.	
a Position ulnar side of nondominant hand just below site and pull skin laterally approximately 2.5 to 3.5 cm (1 to 1½ inches). Hold position until medication is injected. With dominant hand inject needle quickly at 90-degree angle into muscle (see Fig. 22-16, A).	Z-track creates zigzag path through tissues that seals needle track to avoid tracking medication. A quick dartlike injection reduces discomfort. Z-track injections can be used for all IM injections (Hunter, 2008a; Nicholl and Hesby, 2002).
b *Option:* If patient's muscle mass is small, grasp body of muscle between thumb and forefingers.	Ensures that the medication reaches muscle mass (CDC, 2011a; Hockenberry and Wilson, 2011).
c After needle pierces skin, still pulling on skin with nondominant hand, grasp lower end of syringe barrel with fingers of nondominant hand to stabilize it. Move dominant hand to end of plunger. Avoid moving syringe.	Smooth manipulation of syringe reduces discomfort from needle movement. Skin remains pulled until after medication is injected to ensure Z-track administration.
d Pull back on plunger 5 to 10 seconds. If no blood appears, inject medication slowly at rate of 10 sec/mL (Nicholl and Hesby, 2002).	Aspiration of blood into syringe indicates possible placement into a vein. Slow injection reduces pain and tissue trauma. The CDC no longer recommends aspiration for blood after administering vaccine (CDC, 2011a).

Clinical Decision Point *If blood appears in syringe, remove needle, dispose of medication and syringe properly, and prepare another dose of medication for injection.*

e Wait 10 seconds, smoothly and steadily withdraw needle, release skin, and apply gauze gently over site (Nicholl and Hesby, 2002) (see Fig. 22-16, B).	Allows time for medication to absorb into muscle before removing syringe. Dry gauze minimizes discomfort associated with alcohol on nonintact skin.

STEP	RATIONALE
16 Apply gentle pressure to site. Do not massage site. Apply bandage if needed.	Massage damages underlying tissue.
17 Help patient to comfortable position.	Gives patient sense of well-being.
18 Discard uncapped needle or needle enclosed in safety shield and attached syringe into puncture- and leak-proof receptacle.	Prevents injury to patients and health care personnel. Recapping needles increases risk for needlestick injury (OSHA, 2012).
19 Remove gloves and perform hand hygiene.	Reduces transmission of microorganisms.
20 Stay with patient for several minutes and observe for any allergic reactions.	Dyspnea, wheezing, and circulatory collapse are signs of severe anaphylactic reaction.

EVALUATION

1 Return to room in 15 to 30 minutes and ask if patient feels any acute pain, burning, numbness, or tingling at injection site.

Continued discomfort may indicate injury to underlying bones or nerves.

2 Inspect site; note any bruising or induration. Apply warm compress to site.

Bruising or induration indicates complication associated with injection. Document findings and notify health care provider.

3 Observe patient's response to medication at times that correlate with onset, peak, and duration of medication.

Intramuscular medications are absorbed rapidly. Adverse effects of parenteral medications develop rapidly. Evaluate effect of medication based on onset, peak, and duration of actions of medication.

4 Ask patient to explain purpose and effects of medication.

Evaluates patient's understanding of information taught.

Unexpected Outcomes

1 Patient complains of localized pain or continued burning at injection site, indicating potential injury to nerve or vessels.

2 During injection blood is aspirated.

3 Patient displays adverse reaction with signs of urticaria, eczema, pruritus, wheezing, and dyspnea.

Related Interventions

- Assess injection site.
- Notify patient's health care provider.

- Immediately stop injection and remove needle.
- Prepare new syringe of medication for administration.

- Follow agency policy or guidelines for appropriate response to allergic reactions (e.g., administration of antihistamine such as diphenhydramine [Benadryl] or epinephrine).
- Notify patient's health care provider immediately.
- Add allergy information to patient's record.

Recording and Reporting

- Immediately after administration, record medication, dose, route, site, time, and date given on MAR. Correctly sign MAR according to agency policy.
- Record patient teaching, validation of understanding, and patient's response to medication in nurse's notes and electronic health record (EHR).
- Report any undesirable effects from medication to patient's health care provider and document adverse effects in record.

Special Considerations
Teaching

- Patients who require regular injections (e.g., vitamin B$_{12}$) need to learn techniques of self-administration. Teach a family member or significant other injection techniques and the importance of rotating sites to decrease the risk for hypertrophy.
- Instruct patient and family member or significant other to observe injection sites for complications and immediately report complications to the health care provider.
- Instruct patient and family member or significant other to observe for effectiveness of medication and adverse reactions

and report ineffectiveness of medication and adverse reactions to the health care provider.
- Have patient perform several return demonstrations of medication preparation to validate that learning has taken place.

Pediatric

- Children can be very anxious or fearful of needles. Help with proper positioning and holding the child is sometimes necessary. Distraction such as blowing bubbles and pressure at the injection site before giving the injection can help alleviate anxiety (Hockenberry and Wilson, 2011).
- If possible apply EMLA cream on injection site at least 1 hour before IM injection or use a vapocoolant spray (e.g., ethyl chloride) just before injection to decrease pain (Hockenberry and Wilson, 2011).

Gerontologic

- Older patients may have decreased muscle mass, which reduces drug absorption from IM injections. In addition, older adults may have loss of muscle tone and strength that impairs mobility, placing them at high risk for falls from guarding an injection site.

Home Care

• Self-administration of an IM injection is difficult, especially in the vastus lateralis. Teach a significant other to identify and administer injections in this site.

• Instruct adult patients who require frequent injections to apply EMLA cream to the injection site before administration.

• Patients need instruction in safe disposal of syringes and needles (see Skill 22-3, Home Care Considerations).

• See Skill 41-1 for information about modifying safety risks in the home.

SKILL 22-5   Administering Medications by Intravenous Bolus

NSO *IV Medication Administration Module I Lesson 4*

In the past nurses often mixed medications into large volumes of intravenous (IV) fluids (500 to 1000 mL). However, today's safety standards and evidence-based practice no longer support this practice on a routine basis (Infusion Nurses Society [INS], 2011; ISMP, 2011; TJC, 2012). Many patient safety risks such as incorrect calculation, poor aseptic technique, incorrect labeling, pump programming errors, lack of medication knowledge, and mix-up with another medication occur when nurses have to prepare medications in IV containers on patient care units. There are a number of current best practices for preparation and administration of IV medication (Box 22-4).

An IV bolus is one method of medication administration currently practiced on patient care units. It introduces a concentrated dose of a medication directly into a vein by way of an existing IV access. An IV bolus or "push" usually requires small volumes of fluid, which is an advantage for patients who are at risk for fluid overload. Administering medications by IV bolus is common in emergencies when you need to deliver a fast-acting medication quickly. Because these medications act quickly, it is essential that you monitor patients closely for adverse reactions. Agencies have policies and procedures that identify the medications that nurses are allowed to administer by IV push and other IV routes. These policies are based on the medication, compatibility and availability of staff, and type of monitoring equipment available. There are advantages and disadvantages to administering IV push medications (Box 22-5).

The IV bolus is a dangerous method to administer medications because it allows no time to correct errors. Administering an IV push medication too quickly can cause death. Therefore be very careful in calculating the correct amount of the medication to give. In addition, a bolus may cause direct irritation to the lining of blood vessels; thus always confirm placement of the IV catheter or needle. Never give an IV bolus if the insertion site appears edematous or reddened or if the IV fluids do not flow at the ordered rate. Accidental injection of some medications into tissues surrounding a vein can cause pain, sloughing of tissues, and abscesses.

Verify the rate of administration of IV push medication using agency guidelines or a medication reference manual. The Institute for Safe Medication Practices (ISMP, 2011) has identified the

BOX 22-4	Best Practices for Administration of Intravenous Solutions and Medications

• Use standardized concentrations and dosages of medication.
• Use standardized procedures for ordering, preparing, and administering intravenous (IV) medications.
• Administer solutions and medications prepared and dispensed from the pharmacy or as commercially prepared when possible.
• Never prepare high-alert medications (e.g., heparin, dopamine, dobutamine, nitroglycerin, potassium, antibiotics, or magnesium) on a patient care unit.
• Use standardized infusion concentrations of "high-alert" medications.
• Standardize the storage of IV medications.
• Use the mnemonic CATS PRRR to help remember safety checks for administering IV medications: *C*, compatibilities; *A*, allergies; *T*, tubing correct; *S*, site checked; *P*, pump safety checked; *R*, right rate; *R*, release clamps; *R*, return and reassess the patient (Billings & Kowalski, 2005).
• Use standardized label practices. Bold patient name, generic drug name, and patient-specific dose.
• Correctly use technology such as intelligent-infusion devices, bar code–assisted medication administration, and electronic medication administration record.

Adapted from American Society of Health-System Pharmacists [ASHP]: Preventing patient harm and death, *Am J Health-Syst Pharm*; 65:2367, 2008; Infusion Nurses Society: Infusion nursing standards of practice, *J Intraven Nurs* 34(1S), 2011; Institute for Safe Medication Practices (ISMP): *Guidelines for standard order sets*, 2010, available at http://www.ismp.org/tools/guidelines/StandardOrderSets.pdf, accessed July 2011; Institute for Safe Medication Practices (ISMP): *Principles of designing a medication label for intravenous piggyback medication for patient specific, inpatient use*, 2011, available at http://www.ismp.org/tools/guidelines/labelFormats/IVPB.asp, accessed July 5, 2012; and The Joint Commission: 2011 *National Patient Safety Goals hospital program*, 2012, available at http://www.jointcommission.org, accessed July 2012.

BOX 22-5	Advantages and Disadvantages of the Intravenous Push Method

Advantages	Disadvantages
• There is rapid onset of medication effects, which is useful in patients experiencing critical or emergent health problems.	• *Not all medications can be delivered by IV push.*
	• There is higher risk for infusion reactions; some are mild to severe because the medication action peaks quickly.
• Medications can be prepared quickly and given over a shorter time than by intravenous (IV) piggyback.	• When giving medication quickly (e.g., less than 1 minute), there is very little opportunity to stop the injection if an adverse reaction occurs.
• Doses of short-acting medications can be titrated based on a patient's needs and responses to the drug therapy. This is important for infants, children, and older patients.	• Risk for infiltration and phlebitis is increased, especially if a highly concentrated medication, a small peripheral vein, or a short venous access device is used.
• Method provides a more accurate dose of medication delivered because no medication is left in intravenously.	• Hypersensitivity reaction can cause an immediate or delayed systemic reaction to a medication, requiring supportive measures.

following four strategies to reduce harm from rapid IV push medications:

1 Make sure that information regarding rate of administration of IV push medication is readily available.
2 Use less concentrated solutions whenever possible.
3 Avoid using terms in orders such as *IV push, IVP,* or *IV bolus* with medications that should be administered over 1 minute or longer. Use more descriptive terms such as *IV over 5 minutes.*
4 Consider alternatives such as a syringe pump to administer medication that has a high risk for adverse effects. If this is not an alternative to IV push, have pharmacy dilute the medication and administer in a piggyback.

Verify the rate of administration of IV push medication using agency guidelines or a medication reference manual. Review the amount of medication that a patient will receive each minute, the recommended concentration, and rate of administration. For example, if a patient is to receive 6 mL of a medication over 3 minutes, give 2 mL of the IV bolus medication every minute. Understand the purpose of the medication and any potential adverse reactions related to the rate and route of administration. Some IV medications can only be given IV push safely when a patient is being continuously monitored for dysrhythmias, blood pressure changes, or other adverse effects. Therefore you can push some medications only in specific areas within a health care agency (e.g., critical care unit). Confirm agency guidelines regarding requirements for special monitoring.

IV push medications are given through either an existing continuous IV infusion or an intermittent venous access (commonly called a *saline lock*). A saline lock is an IV catheter with a small "well" or chamber covered by a rubber cap. An IV catheter can be converted into a lock by inserting a special rubber-seal injection cap into the end of the catheter (see Chapter 28). Use of a lock saves time by eliminating constant monitoring of an IV line. It also offers better mobility, safety, and comfort for patients by eliminating the need for a continuous IV line. After you administer an IV bolus through an intermittent venous access, flush with a normal saline solution to keep it patent.

Delegation and Collaboration

The skill of administering medications by IV bolus cannot be delegated to nursing assistive personnel (NAP). The nurse directs the NAP about:

- Potential actions and side effects of the medications and to report their occurrence to the nurse.
- Reporting any patient complaints of moisture or discomfort around insertion site.
- Obtaining any required vital signs and reporting them to the nurse.

Equipment

- ❏ Watch with second hand
- ❏ Clean gloves
- ❏ Antiseptic swab
- ❏ Medication in vial or ampule
- ❏ Proper-size syringes for medication and saline flush with needleless device or SESIP needle (21- to 25-gauge)
- ❏ Intravenous lock: Vial of normal saline flush solution (saline recommended [INS, 2011]); if agency continues to use heparin flush, the most common concentration is 10 units/mL; check agency policy.
- ❏ Medication administration record (MAR) or computer printout
- ❏ Puncture-proof container

STEP	**RATIONALE**

ASSESSMENT

1 Check accuracy and completeness of each MAR or computer printout with prescriber's written medication order. Check patient's name, medication name and dosage, route of administration, and time of administration. Recopy or reprint any portion of MAR that is difficult to read.	The prescriber's order is the most reliable source and legal record of patient's medications. Ensures that patient receives correct medications. Handwritten MARs are a source of medication errors (ISMP, 2010; Jones and Treiber, 2010).
2 Assess patient's medical and medication history.	Identifies need for medication.
3 Review medication reference information for medication action, purpose, side effects, normal dose, time of peak onset, how slowly to give medication, and nursing implications such as need to dilute medication or administer it through a filter.	Knowledge of medication allows you to give it safely and monitor patient's response to therapy.
4 If you give medication through an existing IV line, determine compatibility of medication with IV fluids and any additives within IV solution.	IV medication is not always compatible with IV solution and/or additives, and a new site may need to be initiated.
5 Perform hand hygiene. Assess condition of IV needle insertion site for signs of infiltration or phlebitis.	Do not administer medication if site is edematous or inflamed.
6 Assess patency of patient's existing IV infusion line or saline lock (see Chapter 28).	For medication to reach venous circulation effectively, IV line must be patent, and fluids must infuse easily.
7 Check patient's history of medication allergies: known allergens and normal allergic response.	IV bolus delivers medication rapidly. Allergic response is immediate.
8 Assess patient's symptoms before initiating medication therapy.	Provides information to evaluate the desired effects of medication.
9 Assess patient's understanding of purpose of drug therapy.	Poses implication for education.

STEP	RATIONALE

NURSING DIAGNOSES

- Acute pain
- Deficient knowledge regarding medication therapy

Related factors are individualized based on patient's condition or needs.

PLANNING

1 Expected outcomes following completion of procedure:
- Patient experiences no medication side effects or adverse reactions.
- IV site remains intact, without signs of swelling or inflammation or symptoms of tenderness at site.
- Patient explains purpose and side effects of medication.

Medication administered safely with desired therapeutic effect achieved.

Medication infuses without complications to IV site and surrounding tissues.

Demonstrates learning.

IMPLEMENTATION

1 Prepare medications for one patient at a time using aseptic technique. Keep all pages of MARs or computer printouts for one patient together or look at only one patient's electronic MAR at a time. Check label of medication carefully with MAR or computer printout 2 times (see Skill 22-1 and Procedural Guideline 22-1) when preparing medication.

Ensures that medication is sterile. Preventing distractions reduces medication preparation errors (LePorte et al., 2009; Nguyen et al., 2010). *These are the first and second checks for accuracy and ensure that correct medication is administered.*

Clinical Decision Point *Some IV medications require dilution before administration. Verify with agency policy or pharmacy. If a small amount of medication is given (e.g., less than 1 mL), dilute medication in small amount (e.g., 5 mL) of normal saline or sterile water so the medication does not collect in the "dead spaces" (e.g., Y-site injection port, IV cap) of the IV delivery system.*

2 Take medication(s) to patient at correct time (see agency policy). Medications that require exact timing include stat, first-time or loading doses, and one time doses. Give time-critical scheduled medications (e.g., antibiotics, anticoagulants, insulin, anticonvulsants, immunosuppressive agents) at exact time ordered (no later than 30 minutes before or after scheduled dose). Give non–time-critical scheduled medications within a range of 1 or 2 hours of scheduled dose (ISMP, 2011). During administration, apply six rights of medication administration.

Hospitals must adopt medication administration policy and procedure for timing of medication administration that considers nature of the prescribed medication, specific clinical application, and patient needs (DHHS, 2011; ISMP, 2011). Time-critical scheduled medications are those for which early or delayed administration of maintenance doses of greater than 30 minutes before or after the scheduled dose may cause harm or result in substantial suboptimal therapy or pharmacologic effect. Non–time-critical medications are those for which early or delayed administration within a specified range of either 1 or 2 hours should not cause harm or result in substantial suboptimal therapy or pharmacologic effect (ISMP, 2011; DHHS, 2011).

3 Close room curtain or door.

Provides privacy.

4 Identify patient using two identifiers (i.e., name and birthday or name and account number) according to agency policy. Compare identifiers in MAR/medical record with information on patient's identification bracelet and/or ask patient to state name.

Ensures correct patient. Complies with The Joint Commission standards and improves patient safety (TJC, 2012).

Some agencies are now using a bar-code system to help with patient identification.

5 At patient's bedside again compare MAR or computer printout with names of medications on medication labels and patient name. Ask patient if he or she has allergies.

This is the third check for accuracy and ensures that patient receives correct medication. Confirms patient's allergy history.

6 Discuss purpose of each medication, action, and possible adverse effects. Allow patient to ask any questions. Explain that you will give medication through existing IV line. Encourage patient to report symptoms of discomfort at IV site.

Keep patient informed of planned therapies, minimizing anxiety. Patients who verbalize pain at IV site help detect IV infiltrations early, lessening damage to surrounding tissues.

7 Perform hand hygiene and apply clean gloves.

Reduces transmission of infection.

8 **IV push (existing IV line):**
   a Select injection port of IV tubing closest to patient. Use needleless injection port.

Follows provisions of Needle Safety and Prevention Act of 2001 (OSHA, 2012).

Clinical Decision Point *Never administer IV medications through tubing that is infusing blood, blood products, or parenteral nutrition solutions.*

STEP	RATIONALE
b Clean injection port with antiseptic swab. Allow to dry.	Prevents transfer of microorganisms during blunt cannula insertion.
c *Connect syringe to IV line*: Insert needleless tip of syringe containing drug through center of port (see illustration).	Prevents introduction of microorganisms. Prevents damage to port diaphragm and possible leakage from site.
d Occlude IV line by pinching tubing just above injection port (see illustration). Pull back gently on plunger of syringe to aspirate for blood return.	Final check ensures that medication is being delivered into bloodstream.

Clinical Decision Point *In the case of smaller-gauge IV needles, blood return sometimes is not aspirated even if IV line is patent. If IV site does not show signs of infiltration and IV fluid is infusing without difficulty, give IV push.*

e Release tubing and inject medication within amount of time recommended by agency policy, pharmacist, or medication reference manual. Use watch to time administrations (see illustration). You can pinch IV line while pushing medication and release it when not pushing medication. Allow IV fluids to infuse when not pushing medication.	Ensures safe medication infusion. Rapid injection of IV drug can be fatal. Allowing IV fluids to infuse while pushing IV drug enables medication to be delivered to patient at prescribed rate.

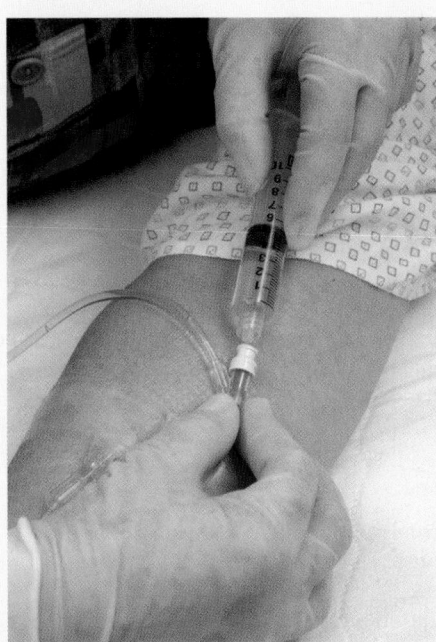

STEP 8c Connecting syringe to IV line with needleless blunt cannula tip.

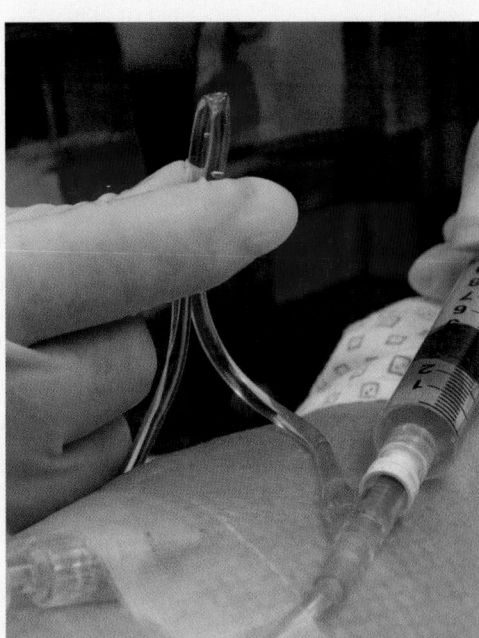

STEP 8d Occluding IV tubing above injection port.

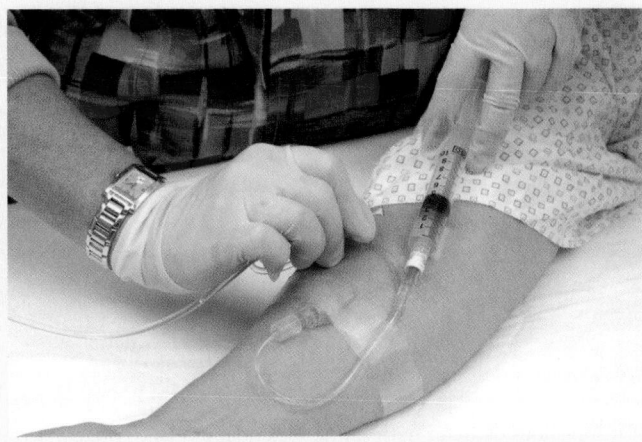

STEP 8e Using watch to time IV push medication.

STEP	RATIONALE
f After injecting medication, withdraw syringe and recheck IV fluid infusion rate.	Injection of bolus may alter rate of fluid infusion. Rapid fluid infusion can cause circulatory fluid overload.
g If IV medication is incompatible with IV fluids, stop IV fluids, clamp IV line, and flush with 10 mL of normal saline or sterile water (see agency policy). Then give IV bolus over appropriate amount of time and flush with another 10 mL of normal saline or sterile water at *same rate* as medication was administered.	Allows IV bolus to be administered without risks associated with IV incompatibilities. Ensure that agency guidelines permit flushing lines with incompatible medications. A new site may need to be initiated.
h If IV line that is currently hanging is a medication, disconnect it and administer IV push medication as outlined in Step 9. Verify agency policy for stopping IV fluids or continuous IV medications. If unable to stop IV infusion, start new IV site (see Chapter 28) and administer medication using IV push (IV lock) method.	Avoids giving patient sudden bolus of medication in existing IV line.

9 IV push (IV lock):

a Prepare flush solutions according to agency policy.	
(1) *Saline flush method (preferred method):* Prepare two syringes filled with 2 to 3 mL of normal saline (0.9%). Many agencies do not provide prefilled normal saline syringes for flushing IV lines.	Normal saline is effective in keeping IV locks patent and is compatible with wide range of medications.
(2) *Heparin flush method (not recommended; refer to agency policy).*	
b Administer medication:	
(1) Clean injection port with antiseptic swab.	Prevents transfer of microorganisms during needle insertion.
(2) Insert needleless tip of syringe with normal saline 0.9% through center of injection port of IV lock (see illustrations).	
(3) Pull back gently on syringe plunger and check for blood return.	Indicates if needle or catheter is in vein.
(4) Flush IV site with normal saline by pushing slowly on plunger.	Clears needle and reservoir of blood. Flushing without difficulty indicates patent IV line.

Clinical Decision Point *Carefully observe the area of skin above the IV catheter. Note any puffiness or swelling as the IV site is flushed, which could indicate infiltration into the vein, requiring removal of catheter.*

(5) Remove saline-filled syringe.	
(6) Clean injection port with antiseptic swab.	Prevents transmission of microorganisms.
(7) Insert needleless tip of syringe containing prepared medication through injection port of IV lock.	Allows administration of medication.
(8) Inject medication within amount of time recommended by agency policy, pharmacist, or medication reference manual. Use watch to time administration.	Many medication errors are associated with IV pushes being administered too quickly. Following guidelines for IV push rates promotes patient safety.
(9) After administering bolus, withdraw syringe.	
(10) Clean injection port with antiseptic swab.	Prevents transmission of microorganisms.

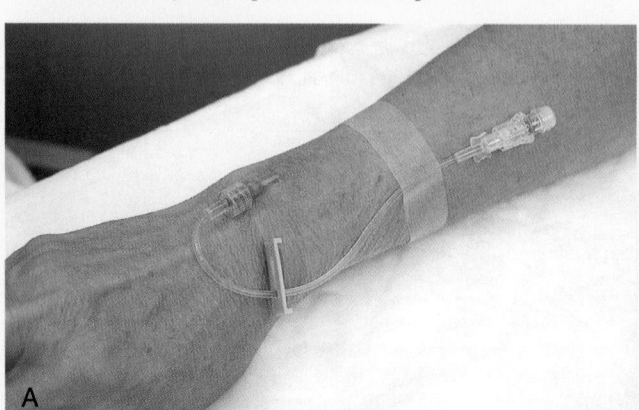 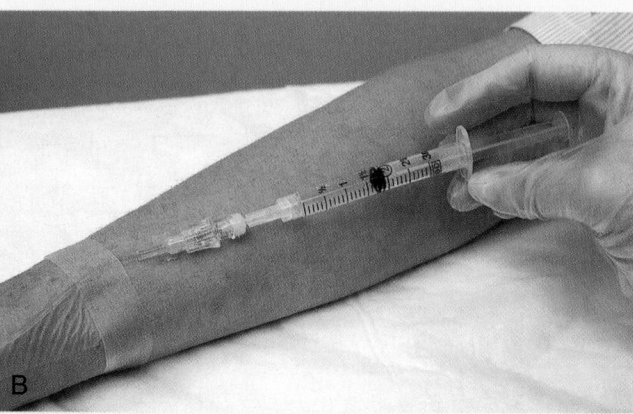

STEP 9b(2) **A,** Intravenous catheter with saline lock adapter. **B,** Syringe inserted into injection port.

STEP	RATIONALE
(11) Flush injection port. (a) Attach syringe with normal saline and inject flush at same rate that medication was delivered.	Flushing IV line with saline prevents occlusion of IV access device and ensures that all medication is delivered. Flushing IV site at same rate as medication ensures that any medication remaining within IV needle is delivered at the correct rate.
10 Dispose of SESIP covered needles and syringes in puncture- and leak-proof container.	Prevents accidental needlestick injuries and follows CDC guidelines for disposal of sharps (OSHA, 2012).
11 Stay with patient for several minutes and observe for any allergic reactions.	Dyspnea, wheezing, and circulatory collapse are signs of anaphylactic reaction.
12 Remove clean gloves and perform hand hygiene.	Reduces transmission of microorganisms.

EVALUATION

1 Observe patient closely for adverse reactions during administration and for several minutes thereafter.	IV medications act rapidly.
2 Observe IV site during injection for sudden swelling and for 48 hours after IV push.	Swelling indicates infiltration into tissues surrounding vein. Signs of infiltration may not occur for 48 hours.
3 Assess patient's status after giving medication to evaluate effectiveness of the medication.	Some IV bolus medications can cause rapid changes in patient's physiologic status. Some medications require careful monitoring and assessment and possibly future laboratory testing (e.g., vasopressors and antiarrhythmics require blood pressure and heart rate monitoring, and heparin requires laboratory studies after administration to determine therapeutic levels).
4 Ask patient to explain purpose and side effects of medication.	Evaluates learning.

Unexpected Outcomes	Related Interventions
1 Patient develops adverse reaction to medication.	• Stop delivering medication immediately and follow agency policy or guidelines for appropriate response to allergic reaction (e.g., administration of antihistamine such as diphenhydramine [Benadryl] or epinephrine) and reporting of adverse drug reactions. • Notify patient's health care provider of adverse effects immediately. • Add allergy information to patient's record.
2 IV medication is incompatible with IV fluids (e.g., IV fluid becomes cloudy in tubing) (see agency policy).	• Stop IV fluids and clamp IV line. • Flush IV line with 10 mL of 0.9% sodium chloride or sterile water. • Give IV bolus over appropriate amount of time. • Flush with another 10 mL of 0.9% sodium chloride or sterile water at same rate as medication was administered. • Restart IV fluids with new tubing at prescribed rate. • If unable to stop IV infusion, start a new IV site (see Chapter 28) and administer medication using IV push (IV lock) method.
3 IV site shows symptoms of infiltration or phlebitis (see Chapter 28).	• Stop IV infusion immediately or discontinue access device and restart in another site. • Determine how much damage IV medication can produce in subcutaneous tissue. • Provide IV extravasation care (e.g., injecting phentolamine [Regitine] around IV infiltration site) as indicated by agency policy, use a medication reference, and consult pharmacist to determine appropriate follow-up care.
4 Patient is unable to explain medication information.	• Provide patient with additional information, or patient is unable to learn at this time.

Recording and Reporting

- Immediately record medication administration, including drug, dose, route, time instilled, and date and time administered on MAR. Include initials or signature.
- Report any adverse reactions to patient's health care provider. Patient's response sometimes indicates need for additional medical therapy.
- Record patient's medication response in nurses' notes and electronic health record (EHR).

Special Considerations
Teaching

- Teach patient and/or significant other that effects of IV push medications occur rapidly. Explain reasons for giving medication slowly and teach signs of adverse effects.

Pediatric

- The therapeutic dosage of IV push medications for infants and children is often small and difficult to prepare accurately, even with a tuberculin syringe. You need to infuse these medications slowly and in small volumes because of the risk for fluid volume overload (Hockenberry and Wilson, 2011). To maintain pediatric patient safety, carefully follow agency policies when administering medications via IV bolus.

Gerontologic

- The renal and metabolic systems do not function as efficiently because of the aging process. To reduce the risk for adverse effects of IV push medications, have good drug knowledge about adverse effects and drug interactions (Aschenbrenner and Venable, 2009). Older patients may tolerate IV push medications if they are given over longer periods of time.

Home Care

- IV push medications are frequently given in the home. Nurses, pharmacists, and health care providers need to collaborate closely in the care of these patients. Patients and families who are independently responsible for managing IV medications need to understand all aspects of administration safety. Adequate eyesight and manual dexterity are necessary to manipulate the syringe. Patients need to understand their venous access device, rate to give medications, and how to flush their access device. Patients need to safely store their medications and dispose of their IV supplies, and they should know whom to contact in case of an emergency.

SKILL 22-6 Administering Intravenous Medications by Piggyback, Intermittent Infusion Sets, and Mini-Infusion Pumps

NSO *IV Medication Administration Module / Lesson 2*

One method of administering intravenous (IV) medications uses small volumes (25 to 250 mL) of compatible IV fluids infused over a desired period of time. This method reduces the risk for rapid dose infusion and provides independence for patients. Patients must have an established IV line that is kept patent by either a continuous infusion or intermittent flushes of normal saline. You can administer intermittent infusion of medication with any of the following methods.

Piggyback. A piggyback is a small (25- to 250-mL) IV bag or bottle connected to a short tubing line that connects to the *upper* Y-port of a primary infusion line or to an intermittent venous access such as a saline lock. The IV container that holds the medication is labeled following the IV piggyback medication format of the Institute for Safe Medication Practices (ISMP, 2011). The piggyback tubing is a microdrip or macrodrip system (see Chapter 28). The set is called a *piggyback* because the small bag or bottle is set *higher* than the primary infusion bag or bottle. In the piggyback setup the main line does not infuse when a compatible piggybacked medication is infusing. The port of the primary IV line contains a back-check valve that automatically stops the flow of the primary infusion once the piggyback infusion flows. After the piggyback solution infuses and the solution within the tubing falls below the level of the primary infusion drip chamber, the back-check valve opens, and the primary infusion starts to flow again.

Volume-Control Administration. Volume-control administration sets (e.g., Volutrol, Buretrol, Pediatrol) are small (50- to 150-mL) containers that attach just below the primary infusion bag or bottle. The set is attached and filled in a manner similar to that used with a regular IV infusion. However, the priming filling of the set is different, depending on the type of filter (floating valve or membrane) within the set. Follow package directions for priming sets.

Mini-Infusion Pump. The mini-infusion pump is battery operated and delivers medication in very small amounts of fluid (5 to 60 mL) within controlled infusion times using standard syringes (Fig. 22-20).

Needle Safety

The Needle Safety and Prevention Act of 2001 mandates that health care agencies use safe needle devices and manufactured needleless systems to reduce needlestick injury. Systems with catheter ports or Y-connector sites are designed to contain a needle housed in a protective covering. Needleless infusion lines allow a direct connection with the IV line via a recessed connection port, a blunt-ended cannula, or shielded-needle device, eliminating the risk for exposure to an IV needle (OSHA, 2012).

Delegation and Collaboration

The skill of administering IV medications by piggyback, intermittent infusion sets, and mini-infusion pumps cannot be delegated to nursing assistive personnel (NAP). The nurse directs the NAP about:

- Potential medication actions and side effects and to report their occurrence to the nurse.
- Reporting any patient complaints of moisture or discomfort around IV insertion site.
- Reporting any change in patient's condition or vital signs to the nurse.

Equipment

- ❑ Adhesive tape *(optional)*
- ❑ Antiseptic swab
- ❑ Clean gloves

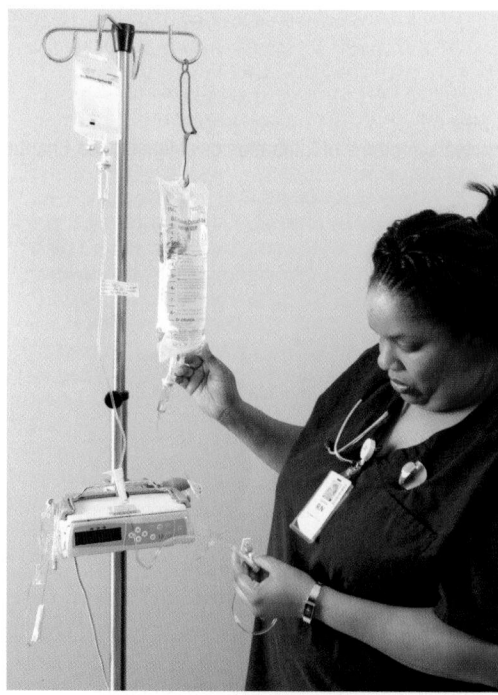

FIG 22-20 Mini-infusion pump.

❏ IV pole
❏ Medication administration record (MAR) or computer printout
❏ Puncture-proof container

Piggyback or Mini-infusion Pump
❏ Medication prepared in 50- to 250-mL labeled infusion bag or syringe
❏ Prefilled syringe of normal saline flush solution (for saline lock only)

❏ Short microdrip, macrodrip, or mini-infusion IV tubing set with blunt-ended (needleless) cannula attachment
❏ Needleless device
❏ Mini-infusion pump if indicated

Volume-Control Administration Set
❏ Volutrol or Buretrol
❏ Infusion tubing with needleless system attachment
❏ Syringe (1 to 20 mL)
❏ Vial or ampule of ordered medication

STEP	RATIONALE

ASSESSMENT

1 Check accuracy and completeness of each MAR or computer printout with prescriber's written medication order. Check patient's name, medication name and dosage, route of administration, and time of administration. Recopy or reprint any portion of MAR that is difficult to read.

2 Assess patient's medical and medication history.

3 Assess patient's history of allergies: known type of allergens and normal allergic reaction.

4 Review medication reference information for medication action, purpose, normal dose, side effects, time and peak of onset, how slowly to give medication, and nursing implications (e.g., need to dilute medication, administer through filter).

5 If you give medication through existing IV line, determine compatibility of medication with IV fluids and any additional additives within IV solution.

The prescriber's order is the most reliable source and legal record of patient's medications. Ensures that patient receives correct medications.
Handwritten MARs are a source of medication errors (ISMP, 2010; Jones and Treiber, 2010).
Determines need for medication or possible contraindications for medication administration.
IV administration of medication may cause rapid response. Allergic response is immediate.
Allows you to administer medication safely and monitor patient's response to therapy.

IV medication is sometimes not compatible with IV solution and/or additives.

> **Clinical Decision Point** *Never administer IV medications through tubing that is infusing blood, blood products, or parenteral nutrition solutions.*

6 Assess patency and placement of patient's existing IV infusion line or saline lock (see Chapter 28).

Do not administer medication if site is edematous or inflamed.

> **Clinical Decision Point** *If patient's IV site is saline locked, clean the port with alcohol and assess the patency of the IV line by flushing it with 2 to 3 mL of sterile sodium chloride.*

7 Assess patient's symptoms before initiating medication therapy.

8 Assess patient's knowledge of medication.

Provides information to evaluate desired effects of medication.
Poses implications for education.

NURSING DIAGNOSES

- Deficient knowledge regarding medication therapy
- Risk for imbalanced fluid volume
- Risk for ineffective health maintenance

Related factors are individualized based on patient's condition or needs.

PLANNING

1 Expected outcomes following completion of procedure:
   - Patient experiences no adverse reactions.
   - Medication infuses within desired time frame.
   - IV site remains intact without signs of swelling, inflammation, or symptoms of tenderness at site.
   - Patient explains medication purposes, action, side effects, and dosage.

Medication was administered safely with desired therapeutic effect.
IV line remains patent.
Fluid infuses into vein, not tissues.

Demonstrates learning.

STEP	RATIONALE

IMPLEMENTATION

1 Prepare medications for one patient at a time using aseptic technique. Check label of medication carefully with MAR or computer printout 2 times (see Skill 22-1 and Procedural Guideline 22-1) when preparing medication. Pharmacy prepares piggyback and prefilled syringes. You will prepare medication for Volutrol.

Ensures that medication is sterile. Preventing distractions reduces medication preparation errors (LePorte et al., 2009; Nguyen et al., 2010). *These are the first and second checks for accuracy* and ensure that correct medication is administered.

2 Take medication(s) to patient at correct time (see agency policy). Medications that require exact timing include stat, first-time or loading doses, and one time doses. Give time-critical scheduled medications (e.g., antibiotics, anticoagulants, insulin, anticonvulsants, immunosuppressive agents) at exact time ordered (no later than 30 minutes before or after scheduled dose). Give non–time-critical scheduled medications within a range of 1 or 2 hours of scheduled dose (ISMP, 2011). During administration, apply six rights of medication administration.

Hospitals must adopt medication administration policy and procedure for timing of medication administration that considers nature of the prescribed medication, specific clinical application, and patient needs (DHHS, 2011; ISMP, 2011). Time-critical scheduled medications are those for which early or delayed administration of maintenance doses of greater than 30 minutes before or after the scheduled dose may cause harm or result in substantial suboptimal therapy or pharmacologic effect. Non–time-critical medications are those for which early or delayed administration within a specified range of either 1 or 2 hours should not cause harm or result in substantial suboptimal therapy or pharmacologic effect (ISMP, 2011; DHHS, 2011).

3 Close room curtain or door. Perform hand hygiene and apply clean gloves.

Provides privacy. Reduces infection transmission.

4 Identify patient using two identifiers (i.e., name and birthday or name and account number) according to agency policy. Compare identifiers in MAR/medical record with information on patient's identification bracelet and/or ask patient to state name.

Ensures correct patient. Complies with The Joint Commission standards and improves patient safety (TJC, 2012).

Some agencies are now using a bar-code system to help with patient identification.

5 At patient's bedside again compare MAR or computer printout with names of medications on medication labels and patient name. Ask patient if he or she has allergies.

This is the third check for accuracy and ensures that patient receives correct medication. Confirms patient's allergy history.

6 Discuss purpose of each medication, action, and possible adverse effects. Allow patient to ask any questions. Explain that you will give medication through existing IV line. Encourage patient to report symptoms of discomfort at site.

Keep patient informed of planned therapies, minimizing anxiety. Patients who verbalize pain at IV site help detect IV infiltrations early, lessening damage to surrounding tissues.

7 Administer infusion.

  a **Piggyback infusion:**

    (1) Connect infusion tubing to medication bag (see Chapter 28). Fill tubing by opening regulator flow clamp. Once tubing is full, close clamp and cap end of tubing.

Filling infusion tubing with solution and freeing air bubbles prevent air embolus.

    (2) Hang piggyback (see illustration) medication bag above level of primary fluid bag. (Use hook to lower main bag.)

Height of fluid bag affects rate of flow to patient.

    (3) Connect tubing of piggyback infusion to appropriate connector on upper Y-port of primary infusion line:

Connection allows IV medication to enter main IV line.

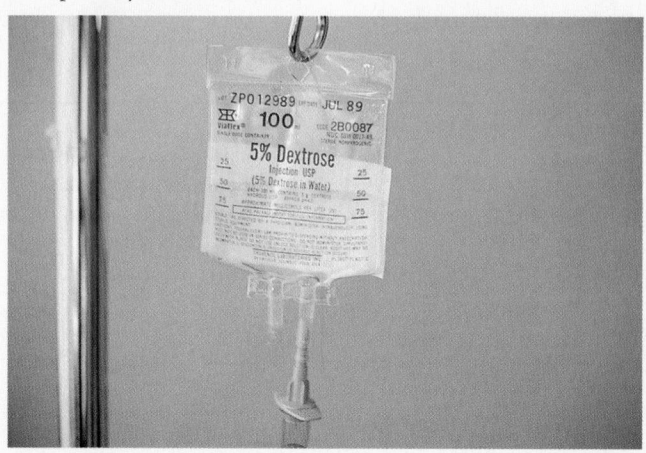

STEP 7a(2) Small-volume minibag for piggyback infusion.

STEP	RATIONALE
(a) *Needleless system:* Wipe off needleless port of main IV line with alcohol swab, allow to dry, and insert cannula tip of piggyback infusion tubing (see illustration).	Use needleless connections to prevent accidental needlestick injuries (INS, 2011; OSHA, 2012).
(4) *Option:* Normal saline lock: Follow Steps 9a(1) through 9b(6) in Skill 22-5 to flush and prepare lock. Wipe off port with alcohol swab, let dry, and insert tip of piggyback infusion tubing via needleless access.	Flushing of lock ensures patency.
(5) Regulate flow rate of medication solution by adjusting regulator clamp or IV pump infusion rate. Infusion times vary. Refer to medication reference or agency policy for safe flow rate.	Provides slow, safe, intermittent infusion of medication and maintains therapeutic blood levels.
(6) Once medication has infused:	
(a) Continuous infusion: Check flow rate of primary infusion. Primary infusion automatically begins after piggyback solution is empty.	Back-check valve on piggyback prevents flow of primary infusion until medication infuses. Checking flow rate ensures proper administration of IV fluids.
(b) Normal saline lock: Disconnect tubing, clean port with alcohol, and flush IV line with 2 to 3 mL of sterile 0.9% sodium chloride. Maintain sterility of IV tubing between intermittent infusions.	
(7) Regulate continuous main infusion line to ordered rate	Infusion of piggyback sometimes interferes with main line infusion rate.
(8) Leave IV piggyback and tubing in place for future drug administration (see agency policy) or discard in puncture- and leak-proof container.	Establishment of secondary line produces route for microorganisms to enter main line. Repeated changes in tubing increase risk for infection transmission.
b Volume-control administration set (e.g., Volutrol):	
(1) Fill Volutrol with desired amount of IV fluid (50 to 100 mL) by opening clamp between Volutrol and main IV bag (see illustration).	Small volume of fluid dilutes IV medication and reduces risk of fluid infusing too rapidly.
(2) Close clamp and check to be sure that clamp on air vent Volutrol chamber is open.	Prevents additional leakage of fluid into Volutrol. Air vent allows fluid in Volutrol to exit at regulated rate.
(3) Clean injection port on top of Volutrol with antiseptic swab.	Prevents introduction of microorganisms during needle insertion.
(4) Remove needle cap or sheath and insert needleless syringe or syringe needle through port and inject medication (see illustration). Gently rotate Volutrol between hands.	Rotating mixes medication with solution to ensure equal distribution in Volutrol.
(5) Regulate IV infusion rate to allow medication to infuse in time recommended by agency policy, pharmacist, or medication reference manual.	For optimal therapeutic effect, medication should infuse in prescribed time interval.
(6) Label Volutrol with name of medication; dosage, total volume, including diluent; and time of administration following ISMP (2011) safe medication label format.	Alerts nurses to medication being infused. Prevents other medications from being added to Volutrol.

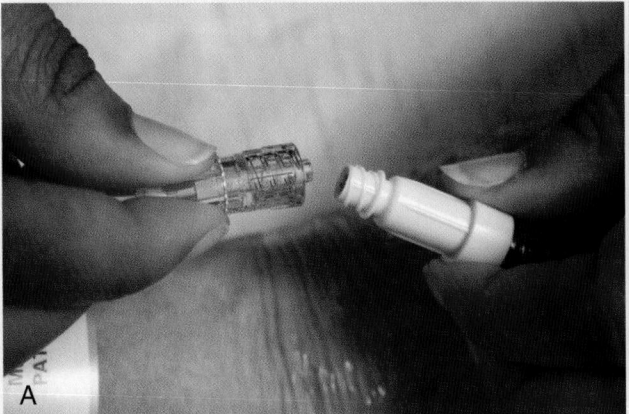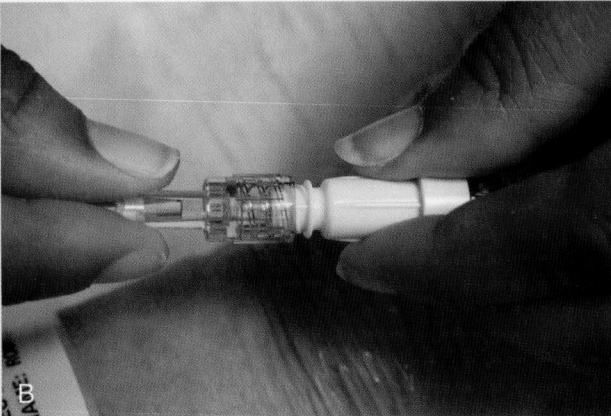

STEP 7a(3)(a) **A,** Needleless lock cannula system. **B,** Blunt-ended cannula inserts into port and locks.

STEP	RATIONALE
(7) If patient is receiving continuous IV infusion, check infusion rate after Volutrol infusion is complete.	Ensures appropriate rate of administration.
(8) Dispose of uncapped needle or needle enclosed in safety shield and syringe in puncture- and leak-proof container. Discard supplies in appropriate container. Perform hand hygiene.	Prevents accidental needlesticks (OSHA, 2012). Reduces transmission of microorganisms.

c Mini-infusion administration:

STEP	RATIONALE
(1) Connect prefilled syringe to mini-infusion tubing; remove end cap of tubing.	Special tubing designed to fit syringe delivers medication to main IV line.
(2) Carefully apply pressure to syringe plunger, allowing tubing to fill with medication.	Ensures that tubing is free of air bubbles to prevent air embolus.
(3) Place syringe into mini-infusion pump (follow product directions) and hang on IV pole. Be sure that syringe is secured (see illustration).	Secure placement is needed for proper infusion.
(4) Connect end of mini-infusion tubing to main IV line or saline lock:	Establishes route for IV medication to enter main IV line.
(a) *Existing IV line:* Wipe off needleless port on main IV line with alcohol swab, allow to dry, and insert tip of mini-infusion tubing through center of port.	Needleless connections reduce risk for accidental needlestick injuries (OSHA, 2012).
(b) *Normal saline lock:* Follow Steps 9a(1) through 9b(6) in Skill 22-5 to flush and prepare lock. Wipe off port with alcohol swab, allow to dry, and insert tip of mini-infusion tubing.	
(5) Set pump to deliver medication within time recommended by agency policy, pharmacist, or medication reference manual. Press button on pump to begin infusion.	Pump automatically delivers medication at safe, constant rate based on volume in syringe.
(6) Once medication has infused:	
(a) *Main IV infusion:* Check flow rate. Infusion automatically begins to flow once pump stops. Regulate infusion to desired rate as needed.	Maintains patent primary IV fluids.
(b) *Normal saline lock:* Disconnect tubing, clean port with alcohol, and flush IV line with 2 to 3 mL of sterile 0.9% sodium chloride. Maintain sterility of IV tubing between intermittent infusions.	

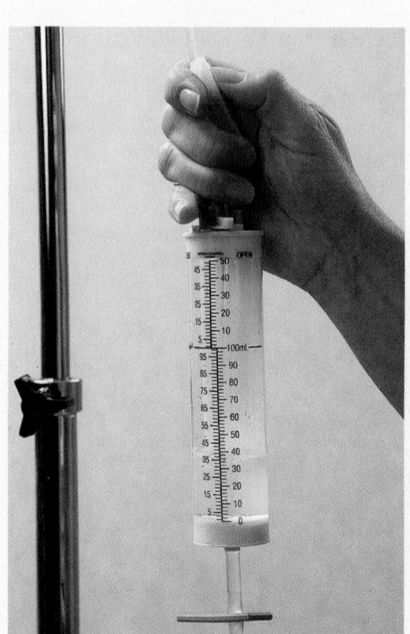

STEP 7b(1) Filling volume-control administration device.

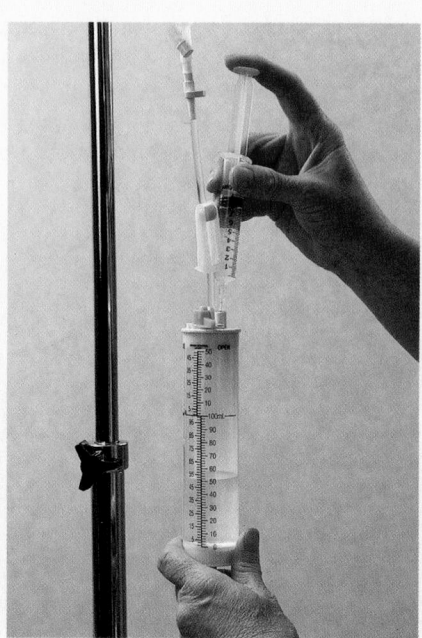

STEP 7b(4) Medication injected into device.

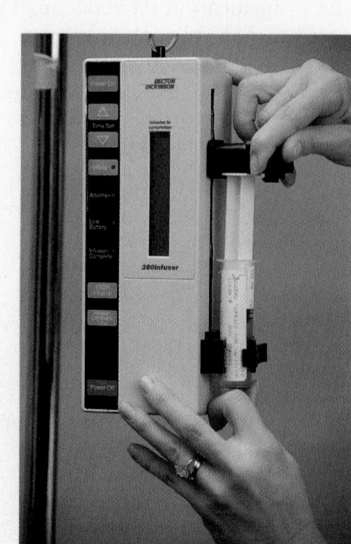

STEP 7c(3) Ensure that syringe is secure after placing it into mini-infusion pump.

STEP	RATIONALE
8 Dispose of supplies in puncture- and leak-proof container.	Prevents accidental needlesticks (OSHA, 2012).
9 Remove gloves and perform hand hygiene.	Reduces transmission of microorganisms.
10 Stay with patient for several minutes and observe for any allergic reactions.	Dyspnea, wheezing, and circulatory collapse are signs of severe anaphylactic reaction.

EVALUATION

1 Observe patient for signs or symptoms of adverse reaction.	IV medications act rapidly.
2 During infusion periodically check infusion rate and condition of IV site.	IV must remain patent for proper drug administration. Infiltration of IV site requires discontinuing infusion.
3 Ask patient to explain purpose and side effects of medication.	Evaluates patient's understanding of instruction.

Unexpected Outcomes

1 Patient develops adverse or allergic reaction to medication.

2 Medication does not infuse over established time frame.

3 IV site shows signs of infiltration or phlebitis (see Chapter 28).

Related Interventions
- Stop medication infusion immediately.
- Follow agency policy or guidelines for appropriate response to allergic reaction (e.g., administration of antihistamine such as diphenhydramine [Benadryl] or epinephrine) and reporting of adverse medication reactions.
- Notify patient's health care provider of adverse effects immediately.
- Add allergy information to patient record per agency policy.
- Determine reason (e.g., improper calculation of flow rate, poor positioning of IV needle at insertion site, infiltration).
- Take corrective action as indicated.
- Stop IV infusion and discontinue access device.
- Treat IV site as indicated by agency policy.
- Insert new IV catheter if therapy continues.
- For infiltration determine how harmful IV medication is to subcutaneous tissue. Provide IV extravasation care (e.g., injecting phentolamine [Regitine] around IV infiltration site) as indicated by agency policy or consult pharmacist to determine appropriate follow-up care.

Recording and Reporting
- Immediately record medication, dose, route, infusion rate, and date and time administered on MAR or computer printout. Include initials or signature.
- Record volume of fluid in medication bag or Volutrol on intake and output (I&O) form.
- Report any adverse reactions to patient's health care provider.

Special Considerations
Teaching
- Review all IV medications with patient and significant others, including why patient is receiving the medication and potential adverse effects, including allergic responses.
- Teach patient and/or significant others not to alter the ordered rate of infusion without consulting the prescriber. IV medications need to be infused at a specified rate to achieve their desired effect and avoid adverse effects.
- Teach patient and/or significant others to report any adverse effects immediately.

Pediatric
- Infants and young children are more vulnerable to alterations in fluid balance and do not adjust quickly to changes in fluid balance. Therefore, to assess fluid balance, monitor I&O carefully when infusing IV medications (Hockenberry and Wilson, 2011).

Gerontologic
- Altered pharmacokinetics of medications and the effects of polypharmacy place older adults at risk for medication toxicity. Carefully monitor the response of older adults to IV medications (Touhy and Jett, 2010).
- Older adults are at risk for developing fluid volume overload and require careful assessment for signs of overload and heart failure.

Home Care
- Patients or significant others who administer IV medications at home require education about the steps of medication administration. The patient or significant other needs to perform several return demonstrations of IV medication administration before performing this skill independently. In addition, patients and significant others need to know signs of IV medication administration complications such as phlebitis and infiltration and what to do for any problems.

SKILL 22-7   Administering Continuous Subcutaneous Medications

The continuous subcutaneous infusion (CSQI or CSCI) route of medication administration is used for selected medications (e.g., opioids, insulin). The route is also effective with medications to stop preterm labor (e.g., terbutaline [Brethine]) and to treat pulmonary hypertension (e.g., treprostinil sodium [Remodulin]). One factor that determines the infusion rate of CSQI is the rate of medication absorption. Most patients can absorb 3 to 5 mL/hr of medication (INS, 2011; Justad, 2009).

With CSQI, patients are able to manage their illness and/or pain without the risks and expenses involved with intravenous (IV) medication administration. The route is relatively easy for patients and families to learn and understand in the home setting. CSQI improves oncologic and postoperative pain control in infants, children, and adults (Cope et al., 2008; Justad, 2009). Box 22-6 summarizes benefits associated with the use of CSQI for pain management.

Patients with diabetes mellitus using CSQI for management of blood glucose levels receive intense diabetes self-management education from qualified diabetes educators and insulin pump trainers. The newest system integrates an insulin pump with real-time continuous glucose monitoring (Fig. 22-21) (Medtronic MiniMed, 2011). Patients with diabetes mellitus using insulin pumps generally require less insulin because it is absorbed and used more efficiently (Cummins et al., 2010; Jakisch et al., 2008). Box 22-7 lists criteria for selecting insulin pumps for patient use.

The procedure to initiate and discontinue CSQI therapy is similar, regardless of the type of medication being delivered.

However, nursing assessment and interventions vary, depending on the type of medication administered. For example, if the medication is for diabetes glucose management, you evaluate the patient's blood glucose levels and monitor episodes of hypoglycemia or hyperglycemia (Carchidi et al., 2011).

Use a small-gauge (25 to 27) winged butterfly IV needle or special commercially prepared Teflon cannula to deliver medications. Although Teflon cannulas are generally more expensive, they are more comfortable for the patient and have lower rates of complications than winged IV needles. The cannulas are associated with fewer needlestick injuries. Base the choice of needle type on agency guidelines or patient preference. Use the needle with the shortest length and the smallest gauge necessary to establish and maintain the infusion.

Use the same anatomic sites for subcutaneous injections and the upper chest. Site selection depends on a patient's activity level and the type of medication delivered. For example, pain medications given to ambulatory patients are best delivered in the upper chest, which allows a patient to move freely. Insulin is absorbed most consistently in the abdomen; thus choose a site in the abdomen away from the waistline. Always avoid sites where the tubing of the pump could be disturbed. Rotate sites used for medication administration at least every 2 to 7 days or whenever complications such as leaking occur (INS, 2011).

The CSQI route requires a computerized pump with safety features, including lockout intervals and warning alarms. Ideally medication pumps are individualized based on the medication being delivered and a patient's needs. You also need to consider the availability and cost of the pump and its supplies. When possible, have patients select the pump that fits their individual and home needs and is easiest to use.

Delegation and Collaboration

The skill of administering CSQI medications cannot be delegated to nursing assistive personnel (NAP). The nurse directs the NAP about:

BOX 22-6	Pain Management Benefits with Use of Continuous Subcutaneous Infusion

- Benefits patients with poor venous access
- Provides pain relief to patients who are unable to tolerate oral pain medications
- Allows patients greater mobility
- Onset of action about 20 minutes
- Better pain control than intramuscular injections
- Costs almost half of those associated with intravenous infusions

Modified from Ellershaw and Wilkinson: *Care of the dying*, ed 2, Oxford, 2010, Oxford University Press.

BOX 22-7	Patient Selection Criteria for Use of Insulin Pumps

- Possesses strong motivation and commitment to use diabetes management skills
- Requires or desires improved control of blood glucose levels
- Requires greater flexibility than allowed by traditional insulin injection schedules
- Is willing to participate in a formal diabetes education program
- Possesses strong critical thinking and problem-solving skills
- Accepts responsibilities associated with the self-management of diabetes
- Is able to perform self-blood glucose monitoring and operate the insulin pump
- Displays evidence of effective coping patterns
- Has support systems available
- Secures financial resources to cover costs associated with CSQI

Data from American Diabetes Association: Standards of medical care in diabetes, 2011, *Diabetes Care* 34(S1):S11, 2011; Cummins E et al: Clinical effectiveness and cost-effectiveness of continuous subcutaneous insulin infusion for diabetes: systematic review and economic evaluation, *Health Technol Assess* 14(11):iii, 2010.
CSQI, Continuous subcutaneous infusion.

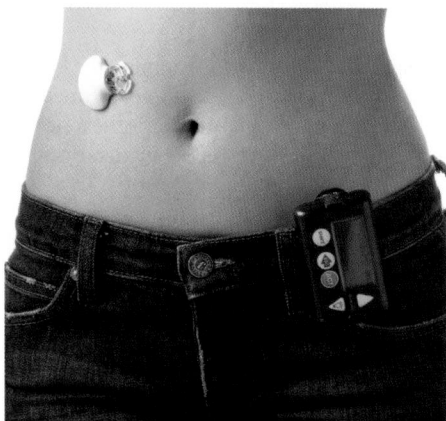

FIG 22-21   Mini-Med Paradigm REAL-Time Insulin CSQI Pump and Continuous Glucose Monitoring System. (*Courtesy Medtronic, Inc., North-ridge, Calif.*)

- Potential medication side effects or reactions and to report their occurrence to the nurse.
- Reporting complications (e.g., leaking, redness, discomfort) at the CSQI needle insertion site to the nurse.
- Obtaining any required vital signs and reporting them to the nurse.

Equipment
Initiation of CSQI
❑ Clean gloves
❑ Alcohol swab
❑ Antibacterial skin preparation such as chlorhexidine
❑ Small (25- to 27-)–gauge winged IV catheter with attached tubing or CSQI designed catheter (e.g., Sof-Set)

❑ Infusion pump
❑ Occlusive, transparent dressing
❑ Tape
❑ Medication in appropriate syringe or container
❑ Medication administration record (MAR) or computer printout
Discontinuing CSQI
❑ Clean gloves
❑ Small, sterile gauze dressing
❑ Tape or adhesive bandage
❑ Alcohol swab and chlorhexidine (*optional*)
❑ Puncture-proof container

STEP	RATIONALE

ASSESSMENT

1 Check accuracy and completeness of each MAR or computer printout with prescriber's written medication order. Check patient's name, medication name and dosage, route of administration, and time of administration. Recopy or reprint any portion of MAR that is difficult to read.

The prescriber's order is the most reliable source and legal record of patient's medications. Ensures that patient receives correct medications.
Handwritten MARs are a source of medication errors (ISMP, 2010; Jones and Treiber, 2010).

2 Assess patient's medical and medication history.

Determines need for medication or possible contraindications for medication administration.

3 Assess patient's history of allergies: known type of allergens and normal allergic reaction.

CSQI administration of medications may cause rapid response. Allergic response is immediate.

4 Collect drug reference information necessary to administer drug safely, including action, purpose, side effects, normal dose, time of peak onset, how slowly to give medication, and nursing implications.

Knowledge of medication allows you to give medication safely and monitor patient's response to therapy.

5 Assess patient's previous verbal and nonverbal response to needle insertion.

Injections are sometimes painful. Anticipating patient's anxiety allows you to use distraction to reduce pain awareness.

6 Assess for contraindications to CSQI (e.g., thrombocytopenia or reduced local tissue perfusion).

Reduced tissue perfusion interferes with medication absorption and distribution.

7 Assess adequacy of patient's adipose tissue to determine appropriate site.

Physiologic changes of aging or patient illness influence amount of subcutaneous tissue, which affects choice of catheter insertion site.

8 Assess patient's knowledge regarding medication to be received and use of medication pump.

Information poses implications for patient education.

9 Assess patient's symptoms before initiating medication therapy. Determine severity of pain (if using analgesia) or measure blood glucose level (if using insulin).

Provides information to evaluate desired effects of CSQI medication.

NURSING DIAGNOSES

• Anxiety	• Fear	• Risk for infection
• Deficient knowledge regarding CSQI therapy	• Ineffective health maintenance	• Risk for injury
	• Pain (acute, chronic)	

Related factors are individualized based on patient's condition or needs.

PLANNING

1 Expected outcomes following completion of procedure:
- Needle insertion site remains free from infection.

Risk for infection at needle insertion site is potential complication of CSQI therapy.

- Patient achieves desired effect of medication with no signs of adverse reactions.

Medication is delivered safely with desired therapeutic effect achieved.

- Patient explains purpose, dosage, and effects of medication and verbalizes understanding of CSQI therapy.

Demonstrates learning.

STEP	RATIONALE

IMPLEMENTATION

1 Review manufacturer directions for pump.

Ensures proper use of equipment.

2 Perform hand hygiene. Prepare medication using aseptic technique or check dose on prefilled syringe. Connect syringe and prime tubing with medication, being careful not to lose any medication. Compare label of medication with MAR or computer printout 2 times.

Ensures that medication is sterile. Checking label of medication with transcribed order reduces error. *This is the first check for accuracy* and ensures that correct medication is administered.

3 Obtain and program medication administration pump. Place syringe in pump.

Ensures that medication dose administered is accurate.

4 Read label on prefilled syringe and compare with MAR or computer printout.

This is the second check for accuracy.

5 Identify patient using two identifiers (i.e., name and birthday or name and account number) according to agency policy. Compare identifiers in MAR/medical record with information on patient's identification bracelet and/or ask patient to state name.

Ensures correct patient. Complies with The Joint Commission standards and improves patient safety (TJC, 2012).
Some agencies are now using a bar-code system to help with patient identification.

6 At patient's bedside again compare MAR or computer printout with names of medications on medication labels and patient name. Ask patient if he or she has allergies.

This is the third check for accuracy and ensures that patient receives correct medication. Confirms patient's allergy history.

7 Discuss purpose of each medication, action, and possible adverse effects. Allow patient to ask any questions. Tell patient that needle insertion will cause slight burning or stinging.

Patient has right to be informed, and patient's understanding of each medication improves adherence to drug therapy.

8 Position patient supine, drape, and provide for privacy.

Respects patient's dignity.

9 Initiate CSQI.

  a Be sure patient is comfortable, sitting or lying down.

Eases pain associated with insertion of needle.

  b Select appropriate injection site free of irritation and away from bony prominences and waistline. Most common sites used are subclavicular and abdomen.

Ensures proper medication absorption.

  c Perform hand hygiene and apply clean gloves. Clean injection site with alcohol using circular motion, followed by antiseptic, using straight cleaning strokes. Allow both agents to dry.

Reduces risk for infection at insertion site.

  d Hold needle in dominant hand and remove needle guard.

Prepares needle for insertion.

  e Gently pinch or lift up skin with nondominant hand.

Ensures that needle will enter subcutaneous tissue.

  f Gently and firmly insert needle at 45- to 90-degree angle (see illustration). Some shorter prepackaged needles (e.g., Sof-Set, Subcutaneous-Set) are inserted at a 90-degree angle. Refer to manufacturer directions.

Decreases pain related to insertion of needle.

  g Release skinfold and apply tape over "wings" of needle.

Secures needle.

Clinical Decision Point *Some cannulas have a sharp needle covered with a plastic catheter. In this case remove the needle and leave the plastic catheter in the skin.*

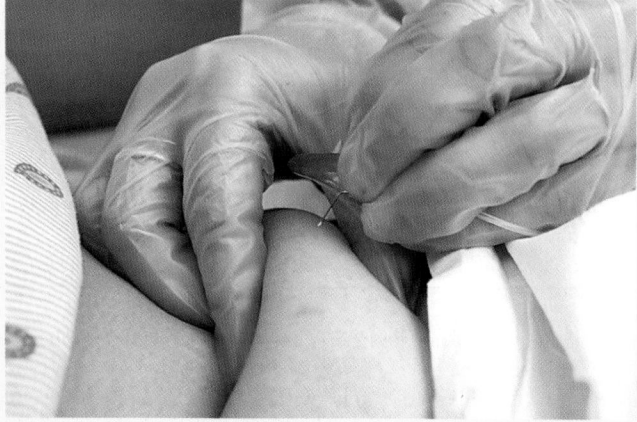

STEP 9f   Insertion of butterfly needle into subcutaneous tissue of abdomen.

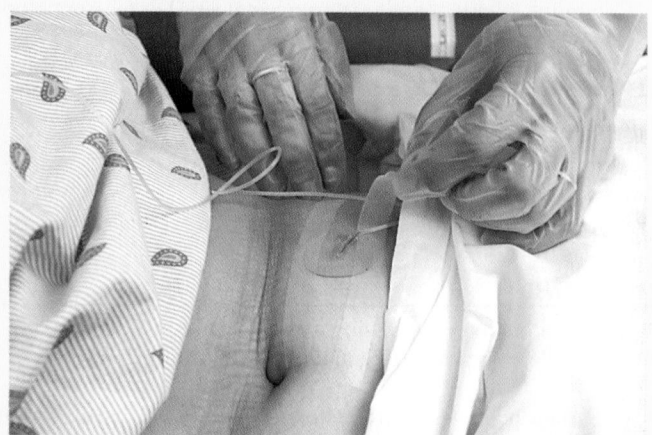

STEP 9h   Placement of transparent dressing over insertion site.

STEP	RATIONALE
h Place occlusive, transparent dressing over insertion site (see illustration).	Protects site from infection and allows you to assess site during medication infusion.
i Attach tubing from needle to tubing from infusion pump and turn pump on.	Allows you to administer medication.
j Dispose of any sharps in appropriate leak- and puncture-proof container. Discard used supplies, remove gloves, and perform hand hygiene.	Prevents accidental needlestick injuries and follows CDC guidelines for disposal of sharps (OSHA, 2012).
k Inspect site before leaving patient and instruct patient to inform you if site becomes red or begins to leak.	Initiate new site with new needle whenever erythema or leaking occurs. If site is free from complications, rotate needle every 2 to 7 days (INS, 2011).
l Stay with patient for several minutes and observe for any allergic reactions.	Dyspnea, wheezing, and circulatory collapse are signs of severe anaphylactic reaction.
10 Discontinue CSQI.	
a Verify order and establish alternative method for medication administration if applicable.	If medication will be required after discontinuing CSQI, a different medication and/or route is often necessary to continue to manage patient's illness or pain.
b Stop infusion pump.	Prevents medication from spilling.
c Perform hand hygiene and apply clean gloves.	Follows CDC recommendations to prevent accidental exposure to blood and body fluids (OSHA, 2012).
d Remove dressing without dislodging or removing needle. Discard properly.	Exposes needle.

Clinical Decision Point *If site is infected, clean it with alcohol and antiseptic. Apply triple antibiotic cream to site if it is excoriated (abraded).*

STEP	RATIONALE
e Remove tape from wings of needle and pull needle out at same angle at which it was inserted.	Minimizes patient discomfort.
f Apply gentle pressure at site until no fluid leaks out of skin.	Dressing adheres to site if skin remains dry.
g Apply small sterile gauze dressing or adhesive bandage to site.	Prevents bacterial entry into puncture site.
11 Dispose of uncapped needles and syringes in puncture- and leak-proof container.	Prevents accidental needlestick injuries and follows CDC guidelines for disposal of sharps (OSHA, 2012).
12 Remove and dispose of gloves and perform hand hygiene.	Reduces transmission of microorganisms.

EVALUATION

1 Evaluate patient's response to medication.	Determines effect of therapy. Decreased or absent response to medication may indicate that patient is not receiving medication into subcutaneous tissue (e.g., pump malfunction, medication leaking at site).
2 Assess site at least every 4 hours for redness, pain, drainage, or swelling.	Indicates infection at insertion site.
3 Ask patient to verbalize understanding of medication and CSQI therapy.	Demonstrates learning.

Unexpected Outcomes

1 Patient complains of localized pain or burning at insertion site; or site appears red or swollen or is leaking, indicating potential infection or needle dislodgement.

2 Patient displays signs of allergic reaction to medication.

3 CSQI becomes dislodged.

Related Interventions

- Remove needle and place new needle in different site.
- Continue to monitor original site for signs of infection and notify health care provider if you suspect infection.
- Stop delivering medication immediately and follow agency policy or guidelines for appropriate response to allergic reaction (e.g., administration of antihistamine such as diphenhydramine [Benadryl] or epinephrine) and reporting of adverse drug reactions.
- Notify patient's health care provider of adverse effects immediately.
- Add allergy information to medical record.
- Stop infusion, apply pressure at site until no fluid leaks out of skin, cover site with gauze dressing or adhesive bandage, and initiate new site.
- Assess patient to determine effects of not receiving medication (e.g., assess patient's pain level using age-appropriate pain scale, obtain blood glucose level).

Recording and Reporting

- After initiating CSQI, immediately chart medication, dose, route, site, time, date, and type of medication pump in patient's medical record. Use initials or signature.
- If medication is an opioid, follow agency policy to document waste.
- Record patient's response to medication and appearance of site every 4 hours or according to agency policy in nurses' notes and electronic health record (EHR).
- Report any adverse effects from medication or infection at insertion site to patient's health care provider and document according to agency policy. Patient's condition often indicates need for additional medical therapy.

Special Considerations

Teaching

- Instruct patient to wear medical alert bracelet along with medical information, including disease (e.g., diabetes), allergies, and a contact phone number for the pump manufacturer for technical support.
- Instruct patients to carry back-up batteries and extra medication if they are going to be away from home.
- Patients receiving insulin require intensive diabetes management education (Box 22-8).
- Never immerse pumps in water or expose them to x-ray films or magnetic resonance imaging.

Pediatric

- CSQI improves glycemic control in children and adolescents. There is a decreased rate of severe hypoglycemia, catheter-site infection, and weight gain (Cope et al., 2008; Hockenberry and Wilson, 2011).
- Insulin pumps offer more flexibility for adolescents, placing the responsibility of diabetes management on the child. Extensive child and family education is needed in using CSQI (Hockenberry and Wilson, 2011).
- Clean and change CSQI sites in children every 48 to 72 hours or at the first signs of inflammation (Hockenberry and Wilson, 2011).

Gerontologic

- CSQI delivers isotonic IV solutions to dehydrated older adults, known as *hypodermoclysis therapy*. This method of providing

---

BOX 22-8	Education Topics for Patients Receiving Insulin with Continuous Subcutaneous Infusion

- Blood glucose monitoring
- Meal planning and food choices
- Incorporating exercise into daily routine
- How to program and use the insulin pump
- Illness guidelines and management
- Management of hypoglycemia
- Prevention and management of hyperglycemia
- Prevention of infection, especially at CSQI infusion site
- Problem-solving and decision-making skills
- Special considerations and precautions (e.g., what to do with pump when showering and sleeping)

Modified from Dalton M et al.: Safety issues: use of continuous subcutaneous insulin infusion pumps (CSII) in hospitalized patients, *Hosp Pharm* 41(10):956, 2006.
CSQI, Continuous subcutaneous infusion.

---

hydration avoids the need to transfer a patient from home or long-term care facility to an acute care hospital. Infuse fluids slowly (e.g., 30 mL/hr) during the first hour of therapy. If the patient remains comfortable, you can increase the rate of infusion. Usually infusion rates do not exceed 60 mL/hr. Hypodermoclysis is an easy-to-use, safe, and cost-effective alternative to IV hydration for older adults (Gorski, 2009; Scales, 2011).

Home Care

- Patients in the home using CSQI need a responsible family caregiver if available. Educate the patient, family, and/or significant others about the desired effect of the medication, side effects and adverse effects of the medication, operation of the pump, how to evaluate the effectiveness of the medication, when and how to assess and rotate injection sites, and when to call a health care provider for problems. Patients need to know where and how to obtain and dispose of all required supplies.
- Patients managing CSQI at home may use an antibacterial soap (e.g., Hibiclens, pHisoHex) instead of alcohol and chlorhexidine to clean insertion site.

? Critical Thinking Exercises

The nurse is preparing to care for a patient newly diagnosed with thrombophlebitis who is scheduled to receive heparin 5000 units subcutaneously now and every 8 hours. The heparin comes from the pharmacy as a multi-dose vial.

1 Which information does the nurse need to know about the medication and vial before administering?
2 Which information does the nurse need to know about the patient before administering the heparin?
3 The patient weighs 100 kg (220 pounds). The drug calculation has determined that 1 mL of heparin needs to be administered. What size syringe and needle will be used to administer the injection? Which site is most appropriate to administer the medication?
4 In addition to the subcutaneous heparin, the patient is also receiving morphine sulfate 1 mg intravenous (IV) push every 6 hours as needed for pain. The patient has no allergies, and the nurse has reviewed the medication references and the health care provider's order. Which additional factors does the nurse need to assess before administering the morphine?

✓ REVIEW QUESTIONS

1 The nurse needs to reconstitute a medication for an intramuscular injection. Which action would indicate that the procedure was completed correctly?
  1 The nurse shakes the vial after the fluid is injected into it to mix it completely.
  2 The nurse determines the amount of prepared medication and concentration needed before adding the appropriate diluent.
  3 The powder is injected slowly into the vial of diluent.
  4 The nurse evaluates the concentration after the diluent and powder are mixed.
2 The nurse is mixing two medications in one syringe. One medication is in a vial, and the other is in an ampule. Which sequence of preparation is correct?
  1 The nurse withdraws the medication from the vial first.
  2 The nurse prepares the medication from the ampule first.
  3 The nurse draws all the medication out of both the ampule and the vial.
  4 The nurse inserts air into the ampule first.

3 An average-size 30-year-old woman is to have an intramuscular injection in the ventrogluteal site. Which needle is appropriate for administering the aqueous-based medication?
1 26 gauge, ⅝ inch
2 20 gauge, 1½ inch
3 25 gauge, 1 inch
4 22 gauge, 1½ inch

4 Before administration of an intravenous (IV) push medication, the nurse notes that the patient's IV site is cool, pale, and swollen. The nurse should take which action?
1 Stop the current IV infusion and change it to another site
2 Slow the rate of the IV infusion
3 Flush the IV line with a normal saline flush
4 Take off the IV dressing and place a new one on that is not as tight

5 Which action is the most important for the nurse to implement before giving an intravenous (IV) push medication?
1 Diluting the medication to minimize vein irritation
2 Stopping the primary (maintenance) fluid infusion
3 Assessing the IV insertion site
4 Ensuring that the correct filter needle is used to withdraw the medication from the vial

6 Which of the following assessment findings indicates a positive tuberculin reaction in a patient with no known risk factors for tuberculosis?
1 A large area of redness and swelling at the injection site
2 An induration of 18 mm
3 Frequent, productive cough accompanied by a fever
4 Sudden onset of shortness of breath and wheezing

7 Which of the following symptoms may indicate that a patient has sustained an injury to a nerve after an intramuscular (IM) injection?
1 Pain, numbness, and tingling at the injection site 2 hours after the injection
2 Pain experienced during the injection
3 Urticaria, eczema, wheezing, and dyspnea
4 Nausea, vomiting, and diarrhea

8 Match the needle size to use when administering an injection in each situation listed.
1 25-gauge, ⅝- to 1-inch
2 22-gauge, 1½-inch
3 27-gauge, ⅝-inch
a Intradermal Mantoux test
b Children older than 1 year
c Average-size female receiving intramuscular injection

9 A patient with diabetes is experiencing low blood glucose levels. The nurse teaches the patient to use which of the following when he or she experiences low blood glucose.
1 Drink 4 ounces of sugar-free juice
2 Eat several saltine crackers with peanut butter
3 Eat one or two hard candies
4 Drink at least 4 ounces of fruit juice

10 _____, _____, and _____ are symptoms of an anaphylactic reaction.

REFERENCES

Alexander M, et al: *Infusion nursing: an evidence-based approach*, ed 3, St Louis, 2009, Elsevier.

American Diabetes Association (ADA): Standards of medical care in diabetes, 2011, *Am Diabetes Care* 34(S1):S11, 2011.

American Nurses Association (ANA): *Preventing needlestick injuries: healthcare workers checklist*, 2010, available at http://www.nursingworld.org/Document Vault/OccupationalEnvironment/Needles/Checklist.aspx, accessed July, 2011.

Anthony K, et al: No interruption please: impact of a no-interruption zone on medication safety in intensive care units, *Crit Care Nurse* 30(3):21, 2010.

Aschenbrenner D, Venable S: *Drug therapy in nursing*, ed 3, Philadelphia, 2009, Lippincott, Williams & Wilkins.

Billings D, Kowalski K: Do your CATS PRRR? A mnemonic device to teach safety checks for administering intravenous medications, *J Contin Educ Nurs* 36(3):104, 2005.

Carchidi C, et al: Clinical effectiveness and cost-effectiveness of continuous subcutaneous insulin infusion for diabetes: systematic review and economic evaluation, *Am J Matern Child Nurs* 36(1):32, 2011.

Centers for Disease Control and Prevention (CDC): *Epidemiology and prevention of vaccine-preventable diseases*, ed 12, Washington, DC, 2011a, Public Health Foundation.

Centers for Disease Control and Prevention (CDC): *Tuberculin skin test fact sheet*, 2011b, http://www.cdc.gov/tb/publications/factsheets/testing/skintesting.htm, retrieved July 11, 2011.

Cherry C, Stuart J: *Pocket guide to culturally sensitive health care*, Philadelphia, 2011, FA Davis.

Cocoman A, Murray J: Intramuscular injections: a review of best practices for mental health nurses, *J Psychiatric Mental Health Nurs* 15:424, 2008.

Cocoman A, Murray J: Recognizing the evidence and changing practice on injection sites, *Br J Nurs* 19(18):1170, 2010.

Cope J, et al: Adolescent use of insulin and patient-controlled analgesia pump technology: a 10-year food and drug administration retrospective study of adverse events, *Pediatrics* 121(5):1133, 2008.

Cummins E, et al: Clinical effectiveness and cost-effectiveness of continuous subcutaneous insulin infusion for diabetes: systematic review and economic evaluation, *Health Technol Assess* 14(11):iii, 2010.

Department of Health and Human Services, Centers for Medicare & Medicaid Services: *Updated guidance on medication administration, Hospital Appendix A of the State Operations Manual*, Baltimore, MD, 2011, Department of Health and Human Services.

Environmental Protection Agency (EPA): New information about disposing of medical sharps, October 2004, http://www.epa.gov/osw/nonhaz/industrial/medical/med-govt.pdf, Accessed July 5, 2012.

Gibney M, et al: Skin and subcutaneous adipose layer thickness in adults with diabetes at sites used for insulin injections: implications for needle length recommendation, *Curr Med Res Opin* 26(6):1520, 2010.

Giger JN: *Transcultural nursing: assessment and intervention*, ed 6, St Louis, 2013, Mosby.

Gorski L: Speaking of standards: continuous subcutaneous access devices, *J Infusion Nurs* 32(4):185, 2009.

Groves A: Cultural competency at the bedside, *Med Surg Matters* 19(4):4, 2010.

Hockenberry MJ, Wilson D: *Wong's nursing care of infants and children*, ed 9, St Louis, 2011, Mosby.

Hunt C: Which site is best of an IM injection? *Nursing2008* 38(11):62, 2008.

Hunter K: Intramuscular injection technique, *Nurs Stand* 22(24):35, 2008a.

Hunter K: Subcutaneous injection technique, *Nurs Stand* 22(21):41, 2008b.

Infusion Nurses Society (INS): Infusion nursing standards of practice, *J Intraven Nurs* 34(1S), 2011.

Institute for Safe Medication Practices (ISMP): *Guidelines for standard order sets*, 2010, available at http://www.ismp.org/tools/guidelines/StandardOrderSets.pdf, accessed July 2011.

Institute for Safe Medication Practices (ISMP): *Principles of designing a medication label for intravenous piggyback medication for patient-specific inpatient use*, 2011, available at http://www.ismp.org/Tools/guidelines/labelFormats/Piggyback.asp, accessed July 5, 2012.

Institute for Safe Medication Practices (ISMP): *Acute care guidelines for timely administration of scheduled medications*. 2011, http://www.ismp.org/Tools/guidelines/acutecare/tasm.pdf, accessed July 11 2012.

Jakisch B, et al: Comparison of continuous subcutaneous insulin (CSII) and multiple daily injections (MDI) in pediatric type I diabetes: a multicenter matched-pair cohort analysis over 3 years, *Diabetic Med* 25(1):80, 2008.

Jones J, Treiber L: When 5 rights go wrong: medication errors from the nursing perspective, *J Nurs Care Qual* 25(3):240, 2010.

Justad M: Continuous subcutaneous infusion: an efficacious, cost-effective analgesia alternative at the end of life, *Home Healthc Nurse* 27(3):140, 2009.

Lehne R: *Pharmacology for nursing care*, ed 7, St Louis, 2010, Saunders.

LePorte L, et al: Effect of distraction-free environment on medication errors, *Am J Health-System Pharmacy* 66(9):795, 2009.

Malik M, et al: Culturally adapted pharmacotherapy and integrative formulation, *Child Adolesc Psychiatric Clin North Am* 19(4):791, 2010.

Medtronic MiniMed: *MiniMed Paradigm REAL-Time Insulin Pump and Continuous Glucose Monitoring System*, 2011, available at http://www.minimed.com/products/index.html, accessed July 2011.

Middleman A, et al: Effect of needle length when immunizing obese adolescents with hepatitis B vaccine, *Pediatrics* 125(3):508, 2010.

Nicholl L, Hesby A: Intramuscular injection: an integrative research review and guideline for evidence-based practice, *Appl Nurs Res* 16(2):159, 2002.

Nguyen E, et al: Medication safety initiative in reducing medication errors, *J Nurs Care Qual* 25(3):224, 2010.

Occupational Safety and Health Administration (OSHA): *Bloodborne pathogens and needlestick injuries*, 77 FR 19934, 2012, available at http://www.osha.gov/pls/oshaweb/owadisp.show_document?p_table=STANDARDS&p_id=10051, accessed July 2012.

Pugliese G, et al: Injection practices among clinicians in United States health care settings, *Am J Infect Control* 38:789, 2010.

Riley D, Raup G: Impact of subcutaneous injection device on improving patient care, *Nurs Manage* 41(6):49, 2010.

Sanofi-Aventis: *Lovenox injections at home*, 2010, available at http://www.lovenox.com/consumer/prescribed-lovenox/lovenox-at-home.aspx, accessed July 5, 2012.

Scales K: Use of hypodermoclysis to manage dehydration, *Nurs Older People* 23(5):16, 2011.

Sheeja VS, et al: Insulin therapy in diabetes management, *Int J Pharm Sci Rev Res* 2(2):98, 2010.

The Joint Commission (TJC): *National Patient Safety Goals*, Oakbrook Terrace, Ill, 2012, The Commission, available at http://www.jointcommission.org/standards_information/npsgs.aspx.

Touhy T, Jett K: *Gerontological nursing & healthy aging*, ed 3, St Louis, 2010, Mosby.

Walker J, et al: Evidence-based practice guidelines: a survey of subcutaneous dexamethasone administration, *Int J Palliative Nurs* 16(10):494, 2010.

Walsh L, Brophy K: Staff nurses' site choice for administering intramuscular injections to adult patients in the acute care setting, *J Adv Nurs* 12:1034, 2010.

Willcox A: Principles and practice of vaccination, *Pract Nurs* 22(2):192, 2011.

Zimmermann PG: Revisiting IM injections, *Am J Nurs* 110(2):60, 2010.

Oxygen Therapy

SKILLS AND PROCEDURES

MEDIA RESOURCES

- **evolve** http://evolve.elsevier.com/Perry/skills
  - Review Questions
  - ▶ Video Clips
  - Audio Glossary

- **NSO** Nursing Skills Online

KEY TERMS

Circumoral cyanosis
Hypercapnia
Hypoxemia
Hypoxia

Incentive spirometry
Nasal cannula
Noninvasive positive-
  pressure ventilation

Oxygen mask
Oxygen therapy
Peak expiratory flow rate
  (PEFR)

Positive-pressure ventilation
T tube
Tidal volume
Tracheostomy collar

OBJECTIVES

Mastery of content in this chapter will enable the nurse to:
- Discuss indications for oxygen therapy.
- Describe methods for administering oxygen therapy.
- Demonstrate applying a nasal cannula and an oxygen mask.
- Demonstrate administering oxygen therapy to a patient with an artificial airway.
- Demonstrate proper peak expiratory flow rate (PEFR) measurements.

- Demonstrate proper use of incentive spirometry.
- Demonstrate use of noninvasive positive-pressure ventilation using continuous positive airway pressure (CPAP) or bi-level positive airway pressure (BiPAP).
- Demonstrate care of a patient receiving mechanical ventilation.

NSO *Airway Management Module / Step 1*

Oxygen therapy is the administration of supplemental oxygen (O_2) to a patient to prevent or treat hypoxia. Hypoxia is a condition in which there is insufficient oxygen to meet the metabolic demands of the tissues and cells. Hypoxia results from hypoxemia, a deficiency of arterial blood oxygen. Hemoglobin is the carrier of respiratory gases, oxygen, and carbon dioxide (CO_2). It combines with a gas to carry it to and from the cells. Decreased hemoglobin levels reduce the amount of oxygen transported to the cells and carbon dioxide transported away from the cells. Hemoglobin levels and acid-base status directly affect oxygenation. Acidemia increases the ability of hemoglobin to release oxygen to the tissues.

Alkalemia decreases the ability of hemoglobin to release oxygen to the tissues.

Various diseases (e.g., pneumonia, chronic bronchitis) require the use of oxygen therapy. Pneumonia results in impaired gas exchange because of fluid and secretions in the lung, which decrease the diffusion of oxygen from the lungs to the arterial blood supply. Some patients with chronic bronchitis, a form of chronic obstructive pulmonary disease (COPD), have normal arterial oxygen levels during the day but oxygen desaturation, a reduction in the arterial oxygen level, during sleep. Frequently these patients require daytime and nocturnal oxygen therapy to prevent hypoxemia (Tiep et al., 2010).

- Apprehension, anxiety, behavioral changes
- Decreased level of consciousness, confusion, drowsiness, altered concentration
- Increased pulse rate
- Increased rate and depth of respiration or irregular respiratory patterns
- Decreased lung sounds, adventitious lung sounds (e.g., crackles, wheezes)
- Elevated blood pressure evolving to decreased blood pressure
- Pulse oximetry (SpO$_2$) less than 90%
- Dyspnea
- Use of accessory muscles of respiration, rib retractions
- Cardiac dysrhythmias
- Pallor, cyanosis
- Increased fatigue
- Dizziness
- Clubbing of nails resulting from prolonged, chronic hypoxia

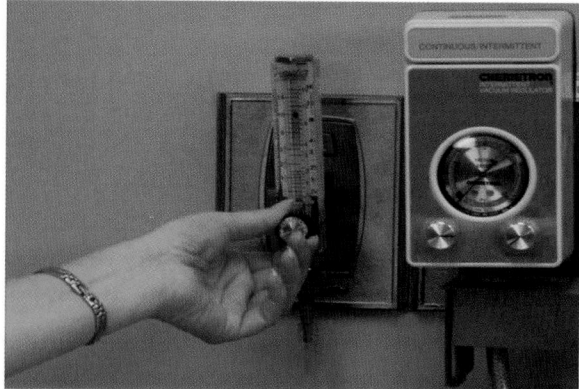

FIG 23-1 Flowmeter attached to oxygen source.

Oxygen by mask or nasal prongs is used in a wide variety of acute care settings. Usually no harm occurs with short-term use of oxygen. However, acute respiratory failure from COPD is a special case because uncontrolled administration of oxygen in this condition may cause acute hypoventilation and carbon dioxide retention with dire consequences. The recommendation is to limit oxygen administration to the minimum needed to raise arterial oxygen saturation to a level that provides adequate oxygen delivery to tissues (88% to 92%) and no higher (Austin et al., 2010).

Patients with cardiovascular disease such as left ventricular failure are not always able to supply oxygen to the tissues because of decreased cardiac output. Supplemental oxygen helps decrease the work of the left ventricle and increase oxygen delivery to the tissues.

The nursing assessment of a patient requiring supplemental oxygen therapy may reveal findings associated with hypoxia (Box 23-1). Presenting symptoms of hypoxia depend on the patient's age, level of health, present disease process, and presence of chronic illnesses. Anxiety, confusion, and restlessness are early signs (Carbery, 2008). In early stages of hypoxia, blood pressure is elevated; and, if the hypoxia remains uncorrected, hypotension develops. As hypoxia worsens, the patient's activity tolerance decreases, vital signs worsen, and the patient's level of consciousness decreases.

Cyanosis, a bluish discoloration of the skin and mucous membranes, is a late sign of hypoxia. Vasoconstriction of the peripheral blood vessels or decreased oxyhemoglobin causes cyanosis. Cyanosis is present in patients who have decreased level of oxyhemoglobin, are very cold, or have decreased peripheral circulation because of vascular disease. Never assume that a lack of cyanosis means adequate oxygenation. Cyanosis caused by hypoxia is observed in the oral mucosa; the conjunctiva of the eye; and around the lips, known as *circumoral cyanosis*.

OXYGEN DELIVERY SYSTEMS

Oxygen therapy is inexpensive, widely available, and used in a variety of settings. Patients with decreased tissue oxygenation benefit from controlled oxygen administration. Long-term oxygen treatment is one of the few interventions that improve survival in COPD (Stoller et al., 2010). Treat oxygen as a medication. As with any drug, continuously monitor the dosage or concentration of oxygen and routinely check the health care provider's orders to verify that the patient is receiving the prescribed oxygen

concentration. Follow the six rights of medication administration when administering oxygen (see Chapter 20).

Selection of the type of oxygen delivery system is based on the level of oxygen support that the patient needs, the severity of the hypoxia, and the disease process. Consider other factors such as the patient's age, level of health and orientation, presence of an artificial airway, whether the setting is in the hospital or the home, type of home environment, and type of support and care given after discharge.

Oxygen delivery devices fall into one of two categories, high flow or low flow, depending on their ability to provide enough flow to match the patient's spontaneous minute volume. Matching a patient's spontaneous minute volume is imperative for patient comfort and adequate oxygen delivery. High-flow devices discourage entraining room air, which dilutes the inspired oxygen percentage (FiO$_2$). High-flow devices include venturi-mask, large-volume nebulizer, and blender masks. Low-flow devices include nasal cannula and simple, nonrebreather, and partial rebreather masks. Common oxygen delivery devices include nasal cannula, various types of face masks, and tracheostomy mask.

Oxygen is available in a number of systems. In a hospital or institutional setting it is available in a bulk liquid oxygen system designed to store it at a precise and safe temperature and deliver it as a gas through wall outlets in a patient's room. An oxygen flowmeter regulates the flow rate in liters per minute (Fig. 23-1).

Oxygen is also available as compressed gas in various-size cylinders and exists as a nonliquid gas stored at a precise temperature under high pressure and measured as pounds per square inch (psi). Oxygen cylinders used in hospital and institutional care settings include large cylinders and smaller E cylinders (Fig. 23-2). In addition, still smaller, easily transported cylinders are available for use in the home. Patients using home oxygen commonly use concentrators, some of which are portable.

EVIDENCE-BASED PRACTICE

Oxygen remains one of the most effective therapeutic agents available (Tiep et al., 2010). Although this therapy benefits hypoxemic patients with pulmonary problems and those with acute exacerbations of COPD, it also relieves pulmonary vasoconstriction and right-sided heart workload and decreases myocardial ischemia. As a result, cardiac output improves. In addition, there is evidence that improved oxygen delivery to the lungs through oxygen administration decrease the work of breathing. These effects on oxygen ventilation and work of breathing may help prevent respiratory muscle fatigue (Jardins and Burton, 2011; Kim et al., 2008).

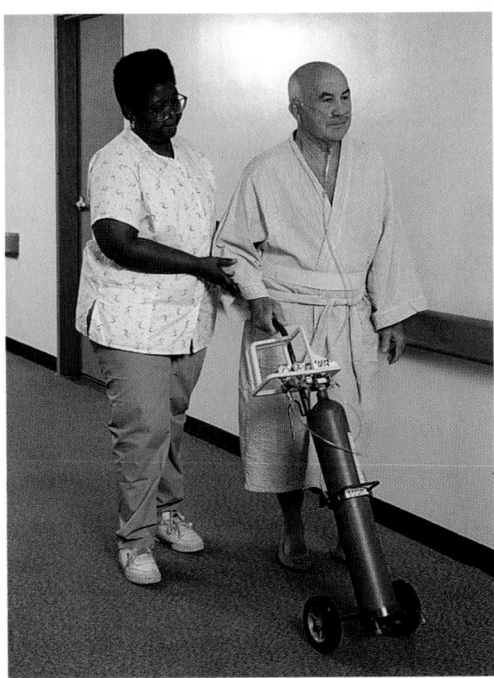

FIG 23-2   Smaller E tank for portability.

Oxygen is like any other "drug" and should be administered cautiously and observed closely for side effects:

- Initiate oxygen protocols when patients with respiratory conditions are hypoxic.
- Ensure that there are no contraindications to oxygen therapies (e.g., some patients with elevated $PaCO_2$ [hypercarbia] are at risk for increased respiratory failure).
- Assess physiologic gas exchange parameters when therapy is initiated and as indicated by patient's condition. This should be done within 2 hours for any patient diagnosed with COPD.
- Check all oxygen equipment for safety and function at least once per shift.
- Check oxygen systems more frequently when oxygen concentration can vary (e.g., hood, high-flow device).
- Avoid interruption of oxygen therapy during patient transport.
- When patient has a tracheostomy and is being transported off the floor, notify respiratory therapy.

PATIENT-CENTERED CARE

Orient patients and family members to the oxygen setup and necessary precautions needed when oxygen is in use. Patients and visitors with limited English proficiency may not be able to understand signs posted in the room. Safely accommodate valued practices of cultural groups when using oxygen. For example, some cultures burn incense, which does not have a flame, to promote healing of ill members (Galanti, 2008). When oxygen is used in the home, designate areas where patients can safely burn incense and encourage family members to bring the ashes to the bedside. Some cultures light candles to celebrate or honor holidays and may accept the use of battery-operated candles while in the hospital (Spector, 2008). Collaborate with family members and religious leaders on how to accommodate these practices during illness and recovery.

Safety Guidelines

1 Know a patient's normal range of vital signs and pulse oximetry (SpO_2) values. Hypoxia affects a patient's vital signs and SpO_2 values.

2 Be aware of environmental conditions. Patients with chronic respiratory diseases have difficulty maintaining optimal oxygen levels in polluted environments. If a patient is to receive home oxygen therapy, complete an environmental assessment to determine respiratory hazards in the home such as the use of gas stoves or kerosene space heaters or the presence of smokers in the home.

3 Document a patient's smoking history. Smoking damages the mucociliary clearance mechanism of the lungs and paralyzes the ciliary action, resulting in a decreased ability to clear mucus from the airways. Chronic bronchitis is caused primarily by smoking and results in pooling of mucus in the airways, creating an environment for the development of infections. Long-term chronic bronchitis ultimately results in hypoxia.

4 Know a patient's most recent hemoglobin values and past and current arterial blood gas (ABG) values.

5 Oxygen is a medication. Increasing the oxygen liter flow rate for shortness of breath is similar to doubling heart, asthma, or other medications.

6 Provide education to patient and family about home oxygen therapy so they understand proper use of the equipment. Safety measures for oxygen use are very important (see Chapter 42) (Box 23-2).

7 All oxygen delivery devices fall into three categories, depending on their ability (or inability) to provide enough flow to match a patient's spontaneous minute volume.

8 All oxygen delivery devices are supplemental, high flow, and/or positive pressure.

SKILL 23-1   Applying a Nasal Cannula or Oxygen Mask

Video Clip

Nasal Cannula

A nasal cannula is a simple, effective, and comfortable device for delivering oxygen to a patient (Fig. 23-3). It allows a patient to breathe through the mouth or nose, is available for all age-groups, and is adequate for short- or long-term use. Cannulas are inexpensive, disposable, and easily accepted by most patients. The two tips of the cannula, about 1.5 cm ($\frac{1}{2}$ inch) long, protrude from the center of a disposable tube and are inserted into the nostrils. Oxygen is delivered via the cannula at a flow rate from 1 to 6 L/min. Higher flow rates dry airway mucosa and do not increase the inspired oxygen concentration (FiO_2). You do not use humidification for rates less than 4 L/min. At flow rates greater than 4 L/min, humidification helps prevent drying of nasal and oral mucous membranes. You can estimate approximate FiO_2 by the flow rate (Table 23-1). The delivered oxygen percentage varies, depending on the rate and depth of a patient's breathing.

Oxygen Mask

The simple face mask (Fig. 23-4) is for short-term oxygen therapy. It fits loosely and delivers oxygen concentrations from 40% to 60%. The mask is contraindicated for patients with carbon dioxide retention because it makes the retention worse. The percentage of oxygen delivered with a simple face mask depends on the liter flow and depth of respirations (see Table 23-1).

A plastic face mask with a reservoir bag (Fig. 23-5) and a Venturi mask deliver higher concentrations of oxygen. When used as a nonrebreather, the plastic face mask with a reservoir bag delivers 60% to 90% oxygen at appropriate flow rates (see Table 23-1). This oxygen mask maintains a high-concentration oxygen supply in the reservoir bag. Frequently inspect the bag to make sure that it is fully inflated. If it is *not fully inflated*, the patient breathes in large amounts of exhaled carbon dioxide.

A Venturi mask is a cone-shaped high-flow device with entrainment ports of various sizes at the base of the mask (Fig. 23-6). The entrainment ports adjust to permit regulation of FiO_2 from 24% to 60%. This mask is useful because it delivers a more precise concentration of oxygen to a patient (see Table 23-1).

The face tent is a shieldlike device that fits under a patient's chin and sweeps around the face (Fig. 23-7). It is used primarily for humidification and for oxygen only when a patient cannot or will not tolerate a tight-fitting mask. Because it is so close to a patient's face, there is no way to estimate how much oxygen is delivered to him or her.

Oxygen hoods and tents are commonly used in the pediatric setting. These devices are able to provide high concentrations of humidified oxygen. This is particularly useful in the child with airway inflammation, epiglottitis (croup), or other respiratory tract infections.

Delegation and Collaboration

The skill of applying a nasal cannula or oxygen mask (not adjusting oxygen flow rate) can be delegated to nursing assistive personnel (NAP). The nurse is responsible for assessing the patient's

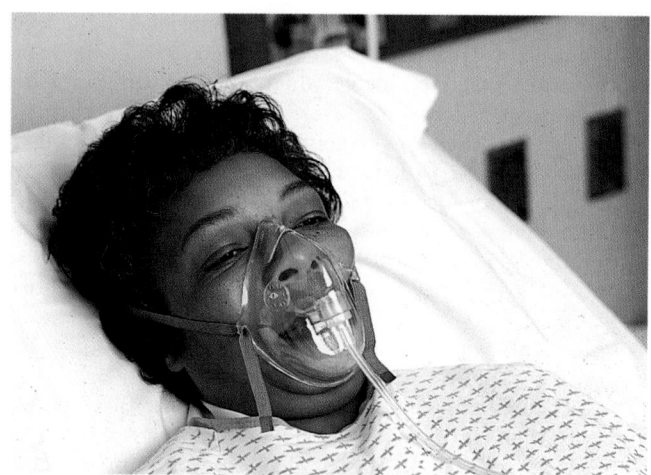
FIG 23-4   Simple face mask.

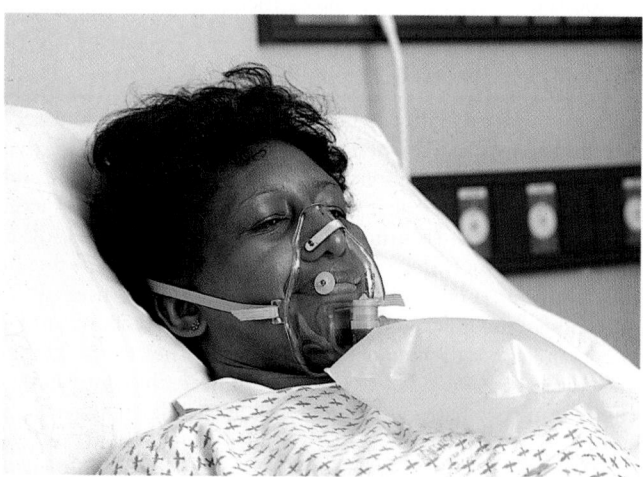
FIG 23-5   Plastic face mask with reservoir bag.

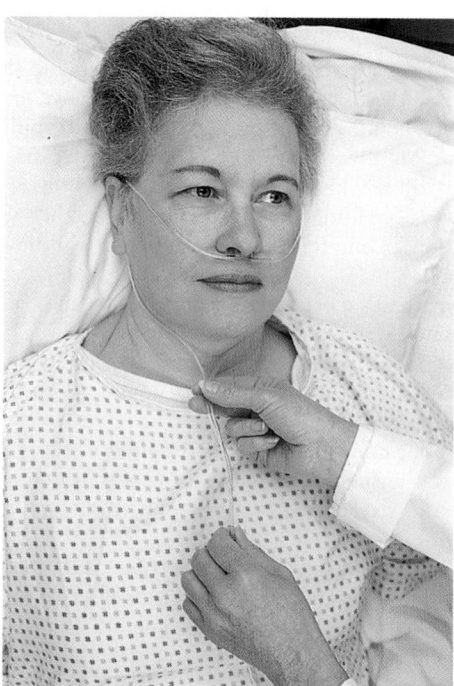
FIG 23-3   Nasal cannula adjusted for proper fit.

TABLE 23-1 | Oxygen Delivery Systems

Delivery System	FiO₂ Delivered	Advantages	Disadvantages
Nasal cannula	1 L/min: 24% 2 L/min: 28% 3 L/min: 32% 4 L/min: 36% 5 L/min: 40% 6 L/min: 44%	Safe and simple Easily tolerated Delivers low concentrations while allowing patient to eat, speak, and drink Does not impede eating or talking Inexpensive, disposable	Unable to use with nasal obstruction Drying to mucous membranes Can dislodge easily May cause skin irritation or breakdown Patient's breathing pattern will affect exact FiO₂
Oxymizer	1-15 L/min: 24%-60%	Higher concentrations without mask Releases O₂ only on inhalation Conserves O₂, increased portability Does not require humidification	Nasal reservoir may interfere with drinking from cup May be cosmetically unappealing Potential reservoir membrane failure Patient's breathing pattern affects exact FiO₂
Simple face mask	5-6 L/min: 40% 6-7 L/min: 50% 7-8 L/min: 60%	Can help to provide humidified O₂	Exact FiO₂ level difficult to estimate Requires high FiO₂ levels to prevent rebreathing of CO₂ Patient inhales room air through side holes in mask
Venturi mask	4 L/min: 24%-28% 8 L/min: 35%-40% 12 L/min: 50%-60%	Controls amount of specified oxygen concentration Delivers percentage of FiO₂ from 24%-60% Does not dry mucous membranes Delivers humidity with oxygen concentration	Hot and confining; increased levels of humidification may irritate skin A specific flow rate is necessary to deliver a specific FiO₂, and the FiO₂ is decreased if the mask does not fit properly Interferes with eating and talking
Partial nonrebreather—Bag should always remain partially inflated. Therefore flow rate must be high enough to prevent collapse of bag.	10-12 L/min: 80%-90%	Delivers increased FiO₂ Useful for patients requiring high concentration of O₂	No inspiratory valve; thus exhaled air mixes with inspired air Hot and confining; may irritate skin; tight seal necessary Interferes with eating and talking Bag may twist and kink
Nonrebreathing mask	15 L/min: 60%-90%	Valve closes during expiration; thus exhaled air does not enter reservoir and mix with inhaled air	Requires tight seal; difficult to maintain and uncomfortable May irritate skin *Bag should not totally deflate*
Face tent	8-12 L/min: 28%-100%	Alternative to aerosol mask Provides high humidity with O₂	Difficult to keep in place, and FiO₂ cannot be controlled
Oxygen hood—usually pediatric use	5-8 L/min: 28%-40% 8-12 L/min: 49%-85%	Provides warmed humidified oxygen at a specific temperature	Flow rate of less than 5 L/min may lead to CO₂ narcosis
Oxygen tent—usually pediatric use	10-15 L/min: up to 50%	Provides humidified O₂ and can provide cool environment to control body temperature	Can be isolating for the child because every time tent is opened the O₂ and humidity levels change

Data from Cairo JM, Pilbeam SP: *Mosby's respiratory care equipment*, ed 8, St Louis, 2010, Mosby; and British Thoracic Society Guidelines: Guideline for emergency oxygen use in adult patients: Executive summary, 2008, available at http://www.brit-thoracic.org.uk/Portals/0/Guidelines/Emergency oxygen guideline/Emergency Oxygen Supplement_web.pdf, accessed August 31, 2012.
FiO₂, Fraction of inspired oxygen concentration.

respiratory system, response to oxygen therapy, and setup of the oxygen therapy and liter flow, including the adjustment of oxygen flow rate. The nurse directs the NAP by:
- Informing how to safely place or adjust the device (e.g., loosening the strap on the oxygen cannula or mask).
- Instructing to inform the nurse immediately about any changes in vital signs; changes in level of consciousness (LOC); skin irritation from the cannula, mask, or straps; or patient complaints of pain or breathlessness.
- Having personnel provide skin care around patient's ears and nose.

Equipment
- ❏ Oxygen delivery device as ordered by health care provider
- ❏ Oxygen tubing (consider extension tubing)
- ❏ Humidifier, if indicated
- ❏ Sterile water for humidifier
- ❏ Oxygen source
- ❏ Oxygen flowmeter
- ❏ Appropriate room signs

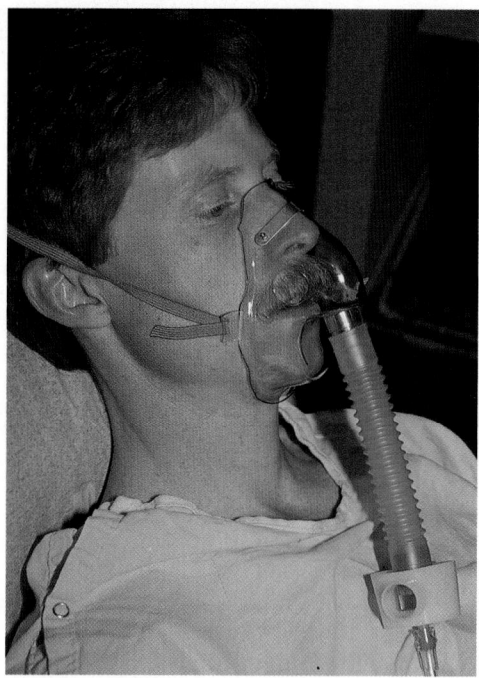

FIG 23-6 Venturi mask.

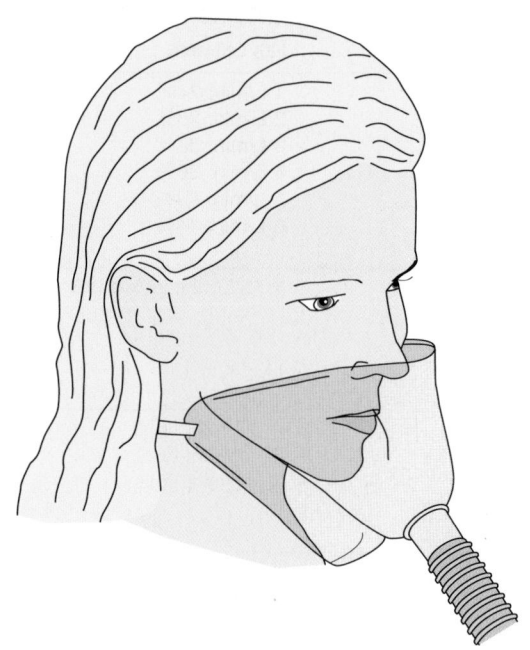

FIG 23-7 Face tent for oxygen delivery.

STEP	RATIONALE

ASSESSMENT

1 Assess patient's respiratory status, including symmetry of chest wall expansion, chest wall abnormalities (e.g., kyphosis), temporary conditions (e.g., pregnancy, trauma) affecting ventilation, respiratory rate and depth, sputum production, and lung sounds (see Chapter 6) and for signs and symptoms associated with hypoxia (see Box 23-1).

Changes in ventilation and gas exchange resulting in hypoxia require oxygen therapy.

> **Clinical Decision Point** *Patients with sudden changes in their vital signs, LOC, or behavior may be experiencing profound hypoxia. Patients who demonstrate subtle changes over time may have worsening of a chronic or existing condition or a new medical condition (Kaul et al., 2009).*

2 Observe for patent airway and remove airway secretions by having patient cough and expectorate mucus or by suctioning (see Chapter 25).

Secretions plug the airway, decreasing the amount of oxygen that is available for gas exchange in lungs.

3 If available, note patient's most recent arterial blood gas (ABG) results or pulse oximetry (SpO_2) value.

Objectively documents patient's pH, arterial oxygen, arterial carbon dioxide, or arterial oxygen saturation.

4 Review patient's medical record for medical order for oxygen, noting delivery method, flow rate, and duration of oxygen therapy.

Ensures safe and accurate oxygen administration. Safe oxygen delivery includes the six rights of medication administration (see Chapter 20).

NURSING DIAGNOSES

- Impaired gas exchange
- Ineffective airway clearance
- Ineffective breathing pattern

Related factors are individualized based on patient's condition or needs.

PLANNING

1 Expected outcomes following completion of procedure:
   - Patient's signs of hypoxia are reduced or eliminated.
   - Patient's vital signs remain stable or return to baseline.

Patient demonstrates improved oxygenation.

When there is no underlying cardiovascular disease, patients adapt to decreased oxygen levels by increasing pulse and blood pressure. This is a short-term adaptive response. Once signs of hypoxia are reduced or controlled, patient's vital signs usually return to normal.

   - Patient's work of breathing decreases.

Pulmonary conditions such as pneumonia or asthma cause varying degrees of airway narrowing. With improved oxygenation, patient's airways are open, and work of breathing decreases.

STEP	RATIONALE
• Patient experiences increased lung expansion.	Improved oxygenation helps to resolve collapsed and constricted airways, improves the work of breathing, and thus improves lung expansion.
• Patient's LOC returns to baseline.	Improvement in oxygenation relieves hypoxia and improves patient's mental status.
• ABG values or SpO_2 returns to normal or baseline.	Documents physiologic response to oxygen therapy.
• Patient's nares and nasal mucosa remain intact.	Oxygen cannula applied and monitored correctly.
2 Explain procedure to patient and family.	Increases compliance and cooperation of patient and family.

IMPLEMENTATION

STEP	RATIONALE
1 Perform hand hygiene. Apply face shield if risk of exposure to splashing mucus exists.	Reduces transmission of microorganisms.
2 Identify patient using two identifiers (i.e., name and birthday or name and account number) according to agency policy. Compare identifiers in MAR/medical record with information on patient's identification bracelet and/or ask patient to state name.	Ensures correct patient. Complies with The Joint Commission standards and improves patient safety (TJC, 2012).
3 Attach oxygen delivery device (e.g., cannula, mask) to oxygen tubing and attach end of tubing to humidified oxygen source adjusted to prescribed flow rate (see Fig. 23-1).	Humidity prevents drying of nasal and oral mucous membranes and airway secretions. Ensures correct O_2 delivery.
4 Apply oxygen device:	Directs flow of oxygen into patient's upper respiratory tract. Patient is more likely to keep device in place if it fits comfortably.
a Place the two tips of the cannula into patient's nares. If the tips are curved, they should point downward inside the nostrils. Then loop the cannula tubing up and over patient's ears. Adjust the lanyard so the cannula fits snugly but not too tightly (see Fig. 23-3).	
b Apply a mask by placing it over patient's mouth and nose. Then bring the straps over patient's head and adjust to form a comfortable but tight seal (see Fig. 23-4).	
5 Maintain sufficient slack on oxygen tubing and secure to patient's clothes.	Allows patient to turn head without causing mask to shift position or dislodge nasal cannula.
6 Observe for proper function of oxygen delivery device:	Ensures patency of delivery device and accuracy of prescribed oxygen flow rate.
a *Nasal cannula:* Cannula is positioned properly in nares; oxygen flows through tips.	Provides prescribed oxygen rate and reduces pressure on tips of nares.
b *Reservoir nasal cannula* OXYMIZER: Fit as for nasal cannula. Reservoir is positioned under patient's nose or worn as pendant.	Delivers higher flow of oxygen with nasal cannula. Delivers a 2:1 ratio (e.g., 6 L/min nasal cannula is approximately equivalent to 3.5 L/min with OXYMIZER device).
c *Nonrebreathing mask* (see Fig. 23-5): Apply as regular mask. Valves on mask close; thus exhaled air does not enter reservoir bag.	Does not allow exhaled air to be rebreathed. Valves on mask side ports permit exhalation but close during inhalation to prevent inhaling room air.
d *Venturi mask* (see Fig. 23-6): Apply as regular mask. Select appropriate flow rate (see Table 23-1).	It is used when high-flow device is desired.
e *Face tent* (see Fig. 23-7): Apply tent under patient's chin and over mouth and nose. It will be loose, and a mist is always present.	Excellent source of humidification; however, you cannot control oxygen concentrations, and patient who requires high oxygen cannot use this device.
7 Verify setting on flowmeter and oxygen source for proper setup and prescribed flow rate.	Ensures delivery of prescribed oxygen therapy in conjunction with specific cannula/mask.
8 Check cannula/mask every 8 hours. Keep humidification container filled at all times.	Ensures patency of cannula and oxygen flow. Oxygen is a dry gas; when it is administered via nasal cannula of 4 L/min or more, you must add humidification so patient inhales humidified oxygen (American Thoracic Society, 2012).
9 Post "Oxygen in use" signs on wall behind bed and at entrance to room.	Alerts visitors and care providers that oxygen is in use.
10 Perform hand hygiene.	Reduces transmission of microorganisms.

STEP	RATIONALE

EVALUATION

1 Monitor patient's response to changes in oxygen flow rate with SpO_2. NOTE: Monitor ABGs when ordered; however, obtaining ABG measurement is an invasive procedure, and ABGs are not measured frequently.

Continual monitoring with SpO_2 is required for patients on oxygen therapy. Base changes in supplemental oxygen on individual patient's oxygen saturation levels.

2 Perform a physical assessment, listening to lung sounds, palpating chest excursion, inspecting color of skin, and observing for decreased anxiety, improved LOC and cognitive abilities, decreased fatigue, and absence of dizziness. Measure vital signs.

Evaluates patient's response to supplemental oxygen. As patient's oxygen level improves, physical signs and symptoms improve.

3 Assess adequacy of oxygen flow each shift.

Ensures patency of oxygen delivery device.

4 Observe patient's external ears, bridge of nose, nares, and nasal mucous membranes for evidence of skin breakdown.

Oxygen therapy sometimes causes drying of nasal mucosa. The delivery device can cause skin breakdown where device comes in contact with face, neck, and ears.

Unexpected Outcomes

1 Patient experiences skin irritation or breakdown (e.g., at ears, bridge of nose, nares, other pressure areas), drying of nasal and oral mucosa, sinus pain, or epistaxis.

2 Patient experiences continued hypoxia.

3 Patient experiences nasal and upper airway mucosa drying.

Related Interventions

- Increase humidification to oxygen delivery system.
- Provide appropriate skin care. Do not use petroleum-based gel around oxygen because it is flammable (American Lung Association, 2012).
- Notify health care provider.
- Obtain health care provider's orders for follow-up SpO_2 monitoring or ABG determinations.
- Consider measures to improve airway patency, coughing techniques, and oropharyngeal or orotracheal suctioning.
- If oxygen flow rate is greater than 4 L/min, use humidification. When oxygen flow is less than 4 L/min, the humidification system of the body is sufficient (British Thoracic Society Guidelines, 2008).
- Assess patient's fluid status and increase fluids if appropriate.
- Provide frequent oral care.
- Obtain health care provider order for use of sterile nasal saline intermittently.

Recording and Reporting

- Record the respiratory assessment findings; method of oxygen delivery, flow rate, patient's response; any adverse reactions or side effects; or change in health care provider's orders.
- Report any unexpected outcome to health care provider or nurse in charge.

Special Considerations

Teaching

- If oxygen therapy continues after discharge, teach patient and family the importance of and rationale for it, how to use the oxygen delivery device, how to contact the supplier of medical equipment, and when to contact the health care provider (see Chapter 42).
- Discuss safety precautions for oxygen use (see Box 23-2) with patient and family.
- Discuss signs of oxygen toxicity and carbon dioxide retention (e.g., confusion, headache, decreased LOC, somnolence, carbon dioxide narcosis, respiratory arrest) that patient needs to report to the health care provider.

Pediatric

- Some infants and small children are able to tolerate a nasal cannula. Secure the prongs of the cannula with Dermiclear tape or strips of transparent dressing over the child's cheek.
- Typically infants receive oxygen therapy via an oxygen hood. Place the hood over patient's head (sometimes over the

shoulders of a small infant). Sufficient room must exist between the curve of the hood and patient's neck to allow carbon dioxide to escape.

- Inspect toys placed in the tent for safety and suitability. Any source of sparks (e.g., from mechanical or electrical toys) is a potential fire hazard (Hockenberry and Wilson, 2011).
- Provide comfort and reassurance to the child. Make sure that child is able to see someone nearby (Hockenberry and Wilson, 2011).

Gerontologic

- Because of the fragility of older adults' skin and mucous membranes, offer oral hygiene and skin care more frequently. Water-based gels such as Aquagel are useful but also dry quickly and need more frequent application.
- Older adults often have a reduced oxygen-carrying capacity if they have a decreased hemoglobin level as a result of cardiac or other underlying illnesses.

Home Care

- Obtain appropriate referrals to determine if patient meets the standards for third-party reimbursement (e.g., PaO_2 55 mm Hg or less during sleep or exercise). If patients have dependent edema, pulmonary hypertension, or hematocrit greater than 56%, they are eligible with a PaO_2 of 56 to 59 mm Hg (American Thoracic Society, 2012).

- Oxygen tubing in the home setting is available in lengths of 15 m (50 feet).
- Provide information about a reliable oxygen therapy equipment vendor within the community to determine if patient and family are able to use a home-fill system with an oxygen concentrator, which provides patient opportunity to fill portable canister as needed (Stoller et al., 2010).
- Consider using oxygen-conserving devices (e.g., OXYMIZER) that administer oxygen in a pulse-dosed flow during inhalation only. These reduce the use and cost of long-term oxygen therapy.

SKILL 23-2 Administering Oxygen Therapy to a Patient with an Artificial Airway

Patients with an artificial airway require constant humidification to the airway (see Chapter 25). An artificial airway bypasses the normal filtering and humidification process of the nose and mouth. The two devices that supply humidified gas to an artificial airway are a T tube and a tracheostomy collar.

The T tube, also called a *Briggs adaptor*, is a T-shaped device with a 15-mm (⅗-inch) connection that connects an oxygen source to an artificial airway such as an endotracheal (ET) tube or tracheostomy (Fig. 23-8). The recommended flow rate is 10 L/min with a nebulizer set to the appropriate FiO_2.

A tracheostomy collar is a curved device with an adjustable strap that fits around a patient's neck (Fig. 23-9). There are two ports: an exhalation port that remains patent at all times and the port that connects to the oxygen source with large-bore tubing.

The flow rate is set at 10 L/min with a nebulizer set to the appropriate FiO_2 that provides humidification to the lower airways via the tracheostomy tube opening.

Delegation and Collaboration

The skill of administering oxygen therapy to a patient with an artificial airway cannot be delegated to the nursing assistive personnel (NAP). The nurse directs the NAP about:

- Patient-specific variations for application or adjustment of the T tube or tracheostomy collar (e.g., methods to avoid pressure or pulling on the artificial airway, methods for handling accumulated secretions in devices).
- Immediately reporting to the nurse unexpected outcomes such as increase in anxiety, change in vital signs, and increased secretions associated with the oxygen delivery device.

Equipment

- ❏ T tube or tracheostomy collar
- ❏ Large-bore oxygen tubing
- ❏ Nebulizer
- ❏ Sterile water for nebulizer
- ❏ Oxygen or gas source
- ❏ Clean gloves
- ❏ Goggles (if splash risk exists)
- ❏ Flowmeter

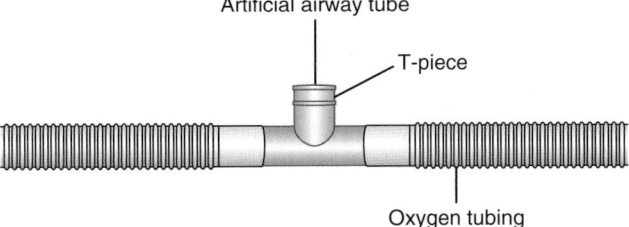

FIG 23-8 T tube.

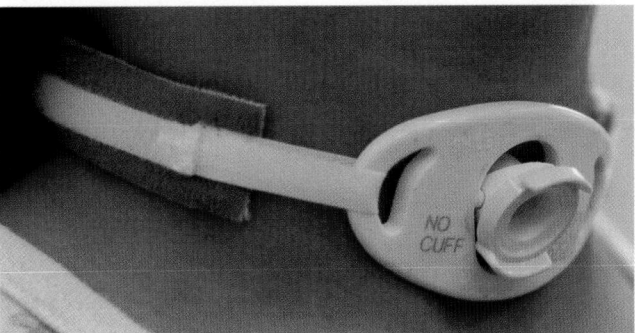

FIG 23-9 Tracheostomy collar.

STEP	RATIONALE

ASSESSMENT

1 Assess patient's respiratory status, including symmetry of chest wall expansion, respiratory rate and depth, sputum production, and lung sounds (see Chapter 6); and assess for signs and symptoms associated with hypoxia (see Box 23-1).

Changes in ventilation and gas exchange resulting in hypoxia require oxygen therapy.

2 Observe for patent airway and remove airway secretions by having patient cough and by suctioning (see Chapter 25).

Secretions plug airway, decreasing amount of oxygen available for gas exchange in lung. Secretions also occlude T tube or tracheostomy collar, impeding oxygen delivery to patient.

3 Monitor pulse oximetry (SpO_2) and, if available, note patient's most recent arterial blood gas (ABG) results.

Objectively documents patient's pH, arterial oxygen, arterial carbon dioxide, or arterial oxygen saturation.

4 Review patient's medical record for medical order for oxygen, noting delivery method, flow rate, and duration of oxygen therapy.

Ensures safe and accurate oxygen administration.

NURSING DIAGNOSES

- Impaired gas exchange
- Ineffective airway clearance
- Ineffective breathing pattern

Related factors are individualized based on patient's condition or needs.

PLANNING

1 Expected outcomes following completion of procedure:
- Signs of hypoxia are reduced or eliminated.

Patient experiences improved oxygenation.

- Patient's vital signs return to baseline.

When there is no underlying cardiovascular disease, patient adapts to decreased oxygen levels by increasing pulse and blood pressure. This is a short-term adaptive response. Once signs of hypoxia are reduced or controlled, patient's vital signs usually return to normal.

- Patient's work of breathing decreases.

With improved oxygenation, tissue oxygen demand is met and work of breathing decreases.

- Patient experiences increased lung expansion.

Improved oxygenation helps to resolve collapsed and constricted airways, improve work of breathing, and thus improve lung expansion.

- Patient's level of consciousness (LOC) returns to baseline.

Improvement in oxygenation relieves hypoxia and improves patient's mental status.

- ABG values or arterial oxygen saturation returns to normal or baseline.

Documents physiologic response to oxygen therapy.

- Tracheal stoma remains intact without irritation or peristomal skin breakdown.

Tension on tracheal stoma from oxygen therapy equipment has potential to cause pressure on stoma and surrounding skin.

2 Explain purpose of T tube or tracheostomy collar to patient and family.

Explanation decreases patient's anxiety and reduces oxygen consumption.

IMPLEMENTATION

1 Perform hand hygiene, apply clean gloves, goggles; consider use of barrier gown.

Reduces transmission of microorganisms by preventing contact with pulmonary secretions. Patients with excessive secretions or forceful productive coughs place caregiver at risk for splash contact.

2 Identify patient using two identifiers (i.e., name and birthday or name and account number) according to agency policy. Compare identifiers in MAR/medical record with information on patient's identification bracelet and/or ask patient to state name.

Ensures correct patient. Complies with The Joint Commission standards and improves patient safety (TJC, 2012).

3 Attach T tube or tracheostomy collar to large-bore oxygen tubing and to humidified room air or oxygen source as indicated.

Provides supplemental humidification to avoid drying of airway.

4 If health care provider orders oxygen, adjust flow rate to 10 L/min or as ordered. Adjust nebulizer to proper FiO_2 setting. Attach T tube to ET or tracheostomy tube. Place tracheostomy collar over tracheostomy tube and adjust straps so it fits snugly.

Flow rate ensures humidification; nebulizer regulates FiO_2.

STEP	RATIONALE
5 Observe that T tube does not pull on ET or tracheostomy tube. Observe for secretions within T tube or tracheostomy collar and suction as necessary (see Chapter 25).	Pulling effect increases patient's discomfort and causes pressure to side of patient's mouth or tracheal stoma. Maintains patent airway.
6 Observe oxygen tubing frequently for accumulation of fluid. If fluid is present, drain tube away from patient, disconnect from collar or T tube, and discard fluid in proper receptacle.	Excess water is medium for bacterial growth. Draining contaminated water into proper receptacle prevents contamination of entire humidifying unit.
7 Set up suction equipment at patient's bedside.	Some patients experience increased airway secretions resulting from humidification.
8 Remove gloves and goggles; perform hand hygiene.	Reduces transmission of microorganisms.

EVALUATION

1 Monitor patient's ABG levels or measure SpO_2.	Monitoring with SpO_2 allows for noninvasive, cost-effective trending of patient's arterial oxygen saturation and pulse rate.
2 Observe position of oxygen delivery device to ensure that it is not pulling on artificial airway.	Pulling on artificial airway results in damage to oral cavity or stoma.
3 Measure patient's vital signs, palpate chest excursion, and observe patient's behavior.	Indicates if hypoxia has been relieved.

Unexpected Outcomes

1 Patient experiences tracheal stoma irritation; thick, tenacious secretions; pressure areas on neck or near stoma site.

2 Patient experiences continued hypoxia.

Related Interventions

- Implement measures to maintain skin integrity (see Chapter 18).
- Increase frequency of airway care.
- Suction secretions from artificial airway and lungs as indicated.
- Determine if cause of continued hypoxia is oxygen delivery device, plugging of airway, oxygen flow rate, or a new clinical problem.
- Notify health care provider of continued or worsening hypoxia.

Recording and Reporting

- Record the respiratory assessment findings; method of oxygen delivery, flow rate, condition of tracheal stoma, patient's response; any adverse reactions or side effects; and change in health care provider's orders.
- Report any unexpected outcome to health care provider or nurse in charge.

Special Considerations
Teaching
- See Teaching Considerations for Skill 23-1.

Home Care
- Some patients who are at home have both a permanent tracheostomy and a T tube or a tracheostomy collar. The patient or caregiver needs to be physically able to perform tracheostomy care and suctioning techniques, as well as understand how to manage oxygen (see Chapter 25).

SKILL 23-3 Using Incentive Spirometry

Incentive spirometry helps a patient deep breathe. An incentive spirometer (IS) is most often used following abdominal or thoracic surgery to reduce the incidence of postoperative pulmonary atelectasis. The use of an IS is especially important in patients with underlying pulmonary diseases because of their risk for postoperative pneumonia. Studies demonstrate that, although postoperative deep breathing and coughing are as effective as incentive spirometry, the use of an IS in combination with coughing and other methods for lung expansion (e.g., chest physiotherapy) lowers rates of postoperative pneumonia (Agostini and Singh, 2009).

Incentive spirometry provides visual feedback to patients about the depth of their breaths. The two types of ISs are flow oriented and volume oriented. Flow-oriented ISs have one or more plastic chambers with freely movable, colored balls. As a patient inhales slowly, the balls are elevated to a premarked area (Fig. 23-10). A patient's goal is to keep the balls elevated for as long as possible to ensure maximal sustained inhalation; not to snap the balls to the top of the chamber with a rapid, very brief, low-volume breath. Even if a very slow inspiration does not elevate the balls, this pattern helps a patient improve lung expansion. The advantage of a flow-oriented IS is the slow, steady expansion of the lung.

Volume-oriented devices use a bellows that a patient must raise to a predetermined volume by inhaling slowly (Fig. 23-11). An achievement light or counter provides feedback to the patient. Some devices have a marker that moves up as a patient inhales. The advantage of the volume-oriented IS is that a patient can achieve a known inspiratory volume and measure it with each breath.

Incentive spirometry encourages patients to breathe deeply and achieve their normal inspiratory capacity. Before surgery it is helpful to determine a patient's baseline inspiratory capacity. An inspiratory volume half to three quarters of baseline is an acceptable postoperative volume. Patients benefiting from incentive spirometry include those using it before surgery, especially before

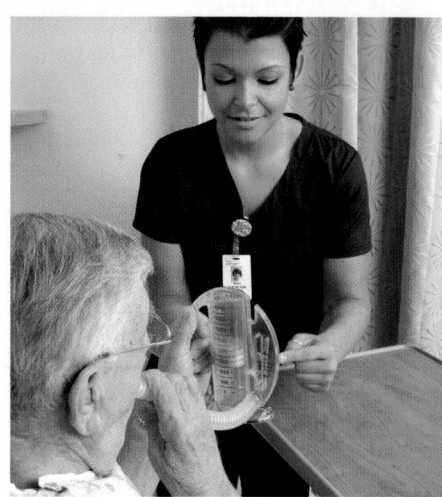

FIG 23-10   Flow-oriented incentive spirometer.

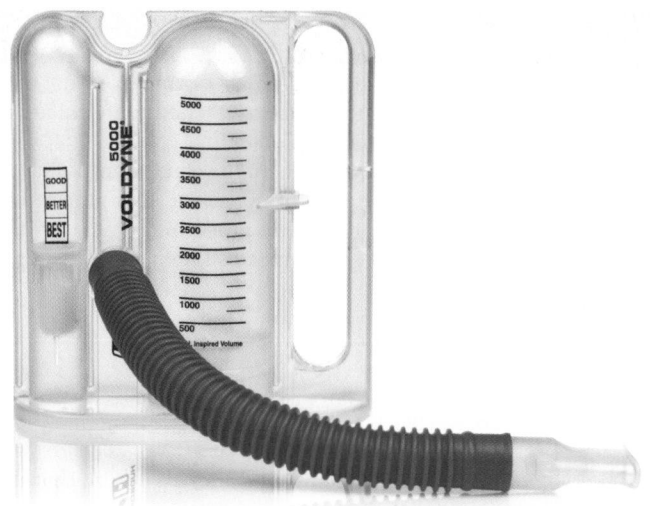

FIG 23-11   Volume-oriented incentive spirometer.

abdominal, cardiac, or orthopedic surgery; patients with a history of smoking, pneumonia, or chronic respiratory disease; and patients with atelectasis (Agostini and Singh, 2009).

Delegation and Collaboration

The skill of assisting a patient to use incentive spirometry can be delegated to nursing assistive personnel (NAP). The nurse is responsible for patient assessment, monitoring, and evaluating the patient response. The nurse directs the NAP by:

- Informing about the patient's target goal for incentive spirometry.
- Informing to immediately notify the nurse about any unexpected outcomes such as chest pain, excessive sputum production, and fever.

Equipment
❏ Flow- or volume-oriented IS

STEP	RATIONALE

ASSESSMENT

1 Identify patients who will benefit from incentive spirometry: those who have existing pulmonary disease, are overweight, or have other debilitating chronic illnesses (Agostini and Singh, 2009).

Alerts health care personnel to patients at risk for respiratory complications during illness or after surgery.

2 Assess patient for confusion, malnutrition, cognitive impairment, and decreased necessary motor skills.

Determines risks for difficulty performing incentive spirometry.

3 Assess patient's respiratory status, including symmetry of chest wall expansion, respiratory rate and depth, sputum production, and lung sounds (see Chapter 6).

Decreased chest wall movement, crackles or decreased lung sounds, increased respiratory rate, or increased sputum production can indicate a need for incentive spirometry to improve lung expansion.

4 Assess level of pain at rest and during activity (e.g., coughing) using a 0-to-10 scale.

Pain decreases effective incentive spirometry by restricting chest expansion.

5 Review health care provider's order for incentive spirometry.

Health care agencies often require a medical order for incentive spirometry to receive third-party reimbursement.

NURSING DIAGNOSES

- Acute pain
- Impaired gas exchange
- Ineffective airway clearance
- Ineffective breathing pattern

Related factors are individualized based on patient's condition or needs.

PLANNING

1 Expected outcomes following completion of procedure:
   - Patient demonstrates correct use of IS.
   - Patient achieves target volume and number of repetitions per hour.
   - Patient has improved breath sounds.

Demonstrates learning.
Demonstrates increased lung expansion.

Incentive spirometry helps patient in deep breathing and managing airway secretions.

STEP	RATIONALE
2 Explain procedure to patient and family.	Understanding purpose of incentive spirometry and its proper use improves compliance with use.
3 Indicate to patient where target volume is on IS. NOTE: If possible, demonstrate use of IS.	Encourages patients to "do better" with each breath and meet or exceed target volume. When patients have a visual target, they can gauge their improvement.

IMPLEMENTATION

1 Perform hand hygiene.	Reduces transmission of microorganisms.
2 Position patient in most erect position (e.g., high-Fowler's if tolerated) (Smeltzer et al., 2009).	Promotes optimal lung expansion during respiratory maneuver.
3 Instruct patient to exhale completely through mouth and place lips tightly around mouthpiece.	Showing patient how to correctly place mouthpiece is reliable technique for teaching psychomotor skill and enables patient to ask questions.
4 Instruct patient to take a slow, deep breath and maintain constant flow, like pulling through a straw. When patient cannot inhale any more, he or she has reached maximal inspiration. Have patient hold breath for at least 3 seconds and then exhale normally.	Maintains maximal inspiration; reduces risk for progressive collapse of individual alveoli.

> **Clinical Decision Point** *Some patients with chronic obstructive pulmonary disease (COPD) are able to hold their breath for only 2 to 3 seconds. Encourage them to do their best and try to extend the duration of breath holding. Allow patients to rest between IS breaths to prevent hyperventilation and fatigue.*

5 Have patient repeat maneuver, encouraging him or her to reach prescribed goal.	Ensures correct use of IS and patient's understanding of use.
6 Remind patient to perform IS exercises 5 to 10 times followed by controlled coughing every hour while awake or as directed by health care provider. Keep IS within patient's reach.	Repeated use of IS improves lung expansion and promotes clearing of airways, especially in patients with underlying lung disease (Wilkins et al., 2009). Using controlled cough techniques reduces risk for coughing spasms.
7 Perform hand hygiene.	Reduces transmission of microorganisms.

EVALUATION

1 Observe patient's ability to use incentive spirometry by return demonstration.	Determines patient's ability to perform breathing exercise correctly.
2 Assess if patient is able to achieve target volume or frequency.	Measures adherence to therapy and lung expansion.
3 Auscultate chest during respiratory cycle.	Documents lung expansion, identifies any abnormal lung sounds, and determines if airways are clear.

Unexpected Outcomes	Related Interventions
1 Patient is unable to achieve incentive spirometry target volume.	• Encourage patient to attempt incentive spirometry more frequently, followed by rest periods. • Teach cough-control exercises. • Teach patient how to splint and protect incision sites during deep breathing. • Administer ordered analgesic if acute pain is inhibiting use of IS.
2 Patient has decreased lung expansion and/or abnormal breath sounds.	• Teach patient cough-control exercises. • Provide assistance with suctioning if patient cannot effectively cough up secretions. • Teach patient to examine sputum for consistency, amount, and color changes.

Recording and Reporting

• Record the lung sounds before and after incentive spirometry, the frequency of use, the volumes achieved, and any adverse effects.
• Report any changes in respiratory assessment or patient's inability to use IS to health care provider.

Special Considerations
Teaching

• Do not let patient use the device if he or she cannot understand or demonstrate proper use.

Pediatric

• Incentive spirometry is not typically used in pediatrics except for school-age children; a pediatric patient needs the fine-motor skills and ability to follow instructions to effectively use an IS (Hockenberry and Wilson, 2011).
• Allowing a child to play with and try out the IS helps to decrease his or her anxiety and encourages participation in care.

- Use games or bubbles and balloons to encourage small children to take deep breaths. These activities help achieve the same goals as incentive spirometry in some children.

Gerontologic

- Older adults with chronic illnesses or arthritis have difficulty coordinating the use of the IS. They require additional time to demonstrate the procedure (Sieber and Barnett, 2011).
- COPD, common in the older-adult population, is an important patient-related risk factor; in addition, heart failure, cigarette use, obesity, obstructive sleep apnea, and decreased cognitive status are also risks for developing postoperative pulmonary complications. Using an IS before and after surgery has the potential to reduce these risks.
- Weakened respiratory muscles and decreased elastic recoil properties of the lungs affect a patient's ability to cough and deep breathe. Therefore it takes an older adult longer to achieve the target volume (Sieber and Barnett, 2011).

SKILL 23-4 Care of a Patient Receiving Noninvasive Positive-Pressure Ventilation

Noninvasive positive-pressure ventilation (NIPPV) maintains positive airway pressure and improves alveolar ventilation without the need for an artificial airway. In addition, this mechanical ventilation alternative reduces and reverses atelectasis, improves oxygenation, reduces pulmonary edema, and improves cardiac function (Frace, 2008). Continuous positive airway pressure (CPAP) keeps the terminal airways (alveoli) partially inflated, reducing the risk for atelectasis; and, if atelectasis has occurred, positive pressure helps in reinflation. Because the alveoli remain partially inflated, there is continued exchange of respiratory gases, and as a result a patient's oxygenation improves (Hoo, 2011). In a cardiac patient NIPPV reduces pulmonary edema because the increased alveolar pressure forces interstitial fluid out of the lungs and back into the pulmonary circulation. In patients with altered cardiac function secondary to sleep apnea, NIPPV provides improved myocardial oxygenation and function.

In selected patients such as those with postpolio syndrome and other neuromuscular diseases, heart failure, sleep disorders, and pulmonary diseases, NIPPV is often the treatment of choice to support ventilation without the hazards associated with endotracheal intubation (Frace, 2008). In addition, there is a reduced risk for pneumonia, gastric aspiration, and ventilator dependency when using NIPPV.

NIPPV delivers both inspiratory positive airway pressure (IPAP) and expiratory positive airway pressure (EPAP) (Hoo, 2011). Thus NIPPV has the option of providing CPAP or bi-level positive airway pressure (BiPAP). For most patients it is recommended to try CPAP initially. If this delivery mechanism is not effective, BiPAP is tried.

CPAP maintains a set positive airway pressure measured by centimeters of water (cm H_2O) throughout the patient's inspiratory and expiratory breathing cycles (Fig. 23-12). A CPAP of 5 cm H_2O provides 5 cm of pressure during inspiration and expiration. It is beneficial in patients who retain carbon dioxide such as with obstructive sleep apnea (OSA) or acute exacerbations of chronic

TABLE 23-2	Problems Associated with Continuous Positive Airway Pressure and Bi-level Positive Airway Pressure
Problem	**Cause**
Discomfort	Mask that fits over patient's nose is tight fitting. Oxygen flow rate causes dry mucous membranes.
Psychosocial	Relationship with sleep partner is difficult. There are possible sensations of claustrophobia.
Risks to skin integrity	Tight fit of mask causes diaphoresis, pressure, and increased risk for skin breakdown. Patients need to remove mask to relieve pressure.
Hypercapnia	Although CPAP improves alveolar function, which increases carbon dioxide clearance from the blood, it also causes air trapping. In some patients this causes a rise in carbon dioxide levels. Initially you need to monitor patient's ABG levels.
Gastric distention	CPAP/BiPAP forces more air into the stomach, which causes distention and discomfort.
Noise	Some patients find the older machines very noisy, interfering with sleep and leisure activities such as watching television or listening to music.

Data from Frace M: Noninvasive ventilation: CPAP and BiPAP on the medical-surgical unit, *Med-Surg Matters* 17(3):12, 2008; and Hoo G: Noninvasive ventilation, June 2011, available at http://emedicine.medscape.com/article/304235-overview, accessed March 2, 2012.
ABG, Arterial blood gas; *BiPAP,* bi-level positive airway pressure; *CPAP,* continuous positive airway pressure.

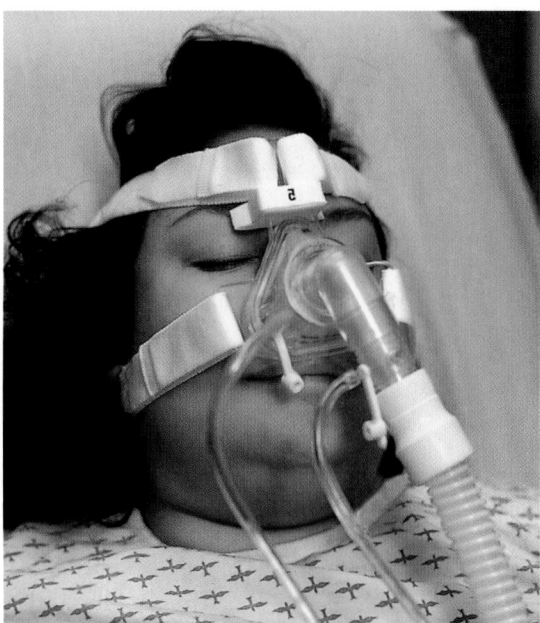

FIG 23-12 Mask suitable for continuous positive airway pressure (CPAP).

obstructive pulmonary disease (COPD) (Hoo, 2011). CPAP keeps the airway open and prevents upper airway collapse. As a result, a patient breathes more normally, sleeps better, and has markedly reduced snoring. In OSA the upper airway collapses during sleep and prevents normal airflow. When the airflow is interrupted, the patient's oxygen saturation drops, and frequent awakenings occur. The usual CPAP pressure is 4 to 10 cm H_2O (Frace, 2008), but it should be determined by a formal sleep study and prescribed accordingly (Table 23-2).

BiPAP is delivered via face mask; thus some patients find it uncomfortable and noisy (see Table 23-2). It works by providing assistance during inspiration and preventing airway closure during expiration. It uses two modes of pressure: one for inspiration and one for expiration. The health care provider designates the pressure during inspiration. BiPAP generates a preset positive-pressure support during inspiration, which increases the patient's tidal volume and ultimately alveolar ventilation. This inspiratory pressure support ends when the patient initiates the expiratory phase. As a result there is an increase in the functional residual capacity (the amount of air remaining in the lungs at the end of expiration), reduced airway closure, reexpansion of atelectatic areas, and improved oxygenation. During expiration BiPAP delivers sufficient expiratory pressure to keep the airways open (Frace, 2008).

The goals for NIPPV include improved oxygenation, decreased carbon dioxide retention, improved sleep, enhanced quality of life, reduced morbidity, improved physical and physiologic function, and cost-effectiveness (Frace, 2008). Patients and families who are candidates for NIPPV are prepared for discharge by a multidisciplinary team, including representatives of nursing, respiratory care, medicine, dietary service, and social service; the home care nurse; and the home care durable medical equipment company.

Delegation and Collaboration

The skill of caring for a patient receiving noninvasive ventilation cannot be delegated to nursing assistive personnel (NAP). The nurse directs the NAP by:

- Informing about the need to immediately report to the nurse any changes in patient's vital signs, oxygen saturation, mental status, or skin color.
- Instructing on how to modify care such as how long the mask can be removed, oral care, or any special skin care needs.
- Informing about the prescribed settings on the NIPPV equipment and notifying nurse of any change in settings or patient comfort.

Equipment

(NOTE: When device is used in the home, the home care equipment vendor provides the equipment.)

- ❏ Nasal mask/full face mask (with quick-release straps), or nasal pillows
- ❏ Oxygen source and tubing
- ❏ CPAP/BiPAP per health care provider order
- ❏ Humidification source, if needed
- ❏ BiPAP and CPAP machines may be used for NIPPV in some critical care areas.
- ❏ Delivery tubing
- ❏ Pulse oximetry
- ❏ Clean gloves
- ❏ Gown, mask, and goggles (if splash risk exists)

STEP	RATIONALE

ASSESSMENT

	STEP	RATIONALE
1	Assess patient's respiratory status, including symmetry of chest wall expansion, respiratory rate and depth, oxygen saturation, sputum production, and lung sounds (see Chapter 6). When possible, ask patient about dyspnea and observe for signs and symptoms associated with hypoxia (see Box 23-1).	Decreased chest wall movement, crackles or decreased lung sounds, increased respiratory rate, increased sputum production, or signs of worsening hypoxia may make patient a candidate for noninvasive positive pressure ventilation or changes in NIPPV settings.
2	Observe patient's skin over bridge of nose, around external ears, back of head.	The mask can place pressure on skin and increase risk for skin breakdown.
3	Observe patient's ability to clear and remove airway secretions by coughing.	Secretions plug the airway, decreasing amount of oxygen that is available for gas exchange in the lung.
4	Obtain pulse oximetry results; when available, note patient's most recent arterial blood gas (ABG) results.	Objectively documents patient's pH, arterial oxygen, arterial carbon dioxide, or arterial oxygen saturation.
5	Obtain vital signs and pulse oximetry before initiation of therapy.	Provides baseline data to compare desired or untoward vital sign changes resulting from therapy.

Clinical Decision Point *NIPPV is contraindicated in cardiac or respiratory arrest, nonrespiratory organ failure, facial surgery or trauma, inability to protect the airway and/or high risk for aspiration, and inability to clear secretions. Controversy surrounding the use of NIPPV in "do-not-resuscitate" or "do not intubate" patients has been addressed by a task force of the Society of Critical Care Medicine, which recommends that it be applied only after careful discussion of goals of care and parameters of treatment with patients and their families (Matzo and Sherman, 2010).*

	STEP	RATIONALE
6	Review patient's medical record for medical order for CPAP/BiPAP and appropriate settings.	Health care provider's order is necessary for this therapy.

NURSING DIAGNOSES

- Activity intolerance
- Impaired gas exchange
- Sleep deprivation

Related factors are individualized based on patient's condition or needs.

STEP	RATIONALE

PLANNING

1 Expected outcomes following completion of procedure:

- Patient has increased lung expansion.

  Patient experiences improved oxygenation.

- Patient maintains ABG levels or oxygen saturation within normal range or at baseline.

  NIPPV delivered appropriately based on patient assessment data.

Clinical Decision Point *When first initiating CPAP/BiPAP, it is important to monitor gas exchange, especially in patients with COPD, cardiogenic pulmonary edema, or acute respiratory failure. You do this to observe for carbon dioxide retention. If patient has "do not resuscitate" orders (for comfort measures only), careful consideration is given before starting noninvasive ventilation (Hoo, 2011).*

- Patient experiences reduction in feelings of dyspnea and work of breathing.

  In patients with acute conditions there is usually an improvement in dyspnea (Filippatos, Mebazaa, and Masip, 2008).

  Patients with chronic pulmonary diseases often require nocturnal CPAP/BiPAP indefinitely to achieve long-term benefits.

- Patient's vital signs and respiratory assessment parameters improve.

  Reduced pulse and respiratory rate, improved mental status, improved skin color, and decreased use of accessory and abdominal muscles occur because patient's work of breathing decreases as level of oxygenation improves (Frace, 2008).

- Patient's skin around bridge of nose, ears, and back of head remains clear without breakdown.

  Mask applied properly and monitored for pressure occurrence.

2 Explain to patient and family the purpose and reasons for CPAP/BiPAP.

  Helps reduce sense of claustrophobia from mask. In addition, information reduces anxiety and increases cooperation and adherence to therapy.

IMPLEMENTATION

1 Perform hand hygiene; apply clean gloves. Apply mask, gown, and goggles if secretions are projectile.

  Reduces transmission of microorganisms and exposure to pulmonary secretions.

2 Identify patient using two identifiers (i.e., name and birthday or name and account number) according to agency policy. Compare identifiers in MAR/medical record with information on patient's identification bracelet and/or ask patient to state name.

  Ensures correct patient. Complies with The Joint Commission standards and improves patient safety (TJC, 2012).

3 Determine correct mask size. Use a masking chart to determine the correct size (S, M, L, XL). NOTE: *It is imperative that mask have quick-release straps.*

  Mask should fit snugly over patient's nose (CPAP) or nose and/or mouth (BiPAP) to create a tight seal for delivering positive pressure. In case of emergency (e.g., vomiting, respiratory arrest), quick-release straps allow mask to be removed quickly. This system also allows patient to remove mask quickly as needed (Frace, 2008).

4 Connect CPAP/BiPAP device delivery tubing to pressure generator.

  Ensures that patient is receiving proper NIPPV as ordered.

5 Connect patient to pulse oximetry.

  It is important to continually monitor patient's level of oxygenation when initiating NIPPV (Hoo, 2011).

6 Set CPAP/BiPAP initial settings:

  These settings allow health care team to determine initial patient response.

  a CPAP: 4 to 8 cm H_2O

  CPAP provides single positive pressure throughout breathing cycle, which helps to keep alveoli open at end-expiration.

  b BiPAP: Inspiratory pressure usually set at 10 to 15 cm H_2O; expiratory pressure usually set at 4 to 10 cm H_2O (Frace, 2008)

  BiPAP supplies pressures at both inhalation and exhalation. The inhalation pressure is set according to health care provider's order and helps to prevent airway closure. Expiratory pressure is set according to health care provider's order and keeps alveoli open at end-expiration (Frace, 2008).

7 Perform frequent skin assessment to determine presence of pressure, skin irritation, or skin breakdown.

  Mask that is too tight increases risk for skin breakdown over bridge of nose.

8 Dispose of supplies as appropriate, remove gloves and other personal protective equipment, and perform hand hygiene.

  Reduces transmission of microorganisms.

STEP	RATIONALE

EVALUATION

1 Observe for decreased anxiety; improved level of consciousness and cognitive abilities; decreased fatigue; absence of dizziness. Measure vital signs, palpate chest excursion, observe skin color, and ask patient to describe sense of dyspnea.

Determines patient's response to NIPPV. As hypoxia and hypercapnia are reduced or corrected, the patient's physical assessment parameters improve.

2 Monitor pulse oximetry.

Documents patient's level of oxygenation. When first initiating NIPPV, it is important to obtain ABG levels in patients in whom abnormal gas exchange is suspected, after the first hour, and per agency protocol.

3 Observe skin integrity over bridge of patient's nose.

Mask that is too tight causes skin breakdown, and frequent skin assessment is necessary.

4 If NIPPV is planned for use in home, observe and monitor patient's and family's ability to manipulate device and face mask.

Determines patient's ability to perform self-care and adhere to CPAP/BiPAP plan. Success of noninvasive ventilation depends largely on patient acceptance and adherence (Hoo, 2011).

Unexpected Outcomes	Related Interventions
1 Patient experiences hypoxia.	• Notify health care provider. • Reassess patient. • Determine correct settings and integrity of NIPPV.
2 Patient experiences hypercapnia.	• Notify health care provider. • Reassess patient. • Determine correct settings and integrity of NPPV.
3 Patient states sense of smothering or claustrophobia.	• Explain system to patient again. • Demonstrate use of quick-release straps. • Have patient demonstrate use of quick-release straps.

Recording and Reporting

• Record respiratory assessment findings, CPAP/BiPAP settings, vital signs and pulse oximetry, patient response, patient teaching outcomes.

• Report to charge nurse or health care provider: sudden change in patient's respiratory status and any decline in ABG levels or pulse oximetry values.

Special Considerations

Teaching

• Teach patient and family the best hours to use the machine (e.g., bedtime, watching television); usually patient receives 6 to 8 hours of continual CPAP/BiPAP.

• Teach patient and family how to apply the mask, connect it to the machine, and add oxygen if ordered.

• Instruct family to bring the machine, along with a list of correct settings, to the hospital any time patient is admitted.

• When patients require home NIPPV, instruct in complete care of the CPAP/BiPAP system. Skills include assembling the system, cleaning it, and daily equipment maintenance.

Home Care

• The durable medical equipment provider, the home care nurse, and the primary care nurse develop a teaching plan to ensure that patient and family have working knowledge of the system before discharge.

• Instruct patient and primary caregiver in what to do in case of respiratory distress or power failure.

• Notify appropriate power company so, in the event of a power outage, the home is on priority for restoring power.

PROCEDURAL GUIDELINE 23-1   Use of a Peak Flow Meter

For patients who have measurable changes in the flow of their airways such as patients with asthma or reactive airways disease, peak expiratory flow rate (PEFR) measurements are useful. The PEFR is the maximum flow that a patient forces out during one quick, forced expiration and is measured in liters. Use these measurements as an objective indicator of a patient's current status or the effectiveness of treatment. Decreased PEFR may indicate the need for further interventions such as increased doses of bronchodilators or antiinflammatory medications. Normal PEFR values vary according to a person's age, gender, and size.

Patients with asthma perform PEFR measures in the home to monitor the status of their airways. Health care providers usually recommend that patients measure their PEFR during the following times: every morning, before taking asthma medicines, during asthma symptoms or an asthma attack, after taking medicine for an asthma attack, and other times recommended by their healthcare provider. The health care provider will explain how to know if a person's asthma is controlled. A system of asthma zones—green, yellow and red—are commonly used for patients to gauge if their PEFR is well controlled.

Delegation and Collaboration

Initial assessment of a patient's condition cannot be delegated. The skill of follow-up PEFR measurements can be delegated to nursing assistive personnel (NAP).

Equipment

❏ Peak flow meter
❏ Patient diary/action plan (if appropriate)

Procedural Steps

1 Assess previous PEFR readings and the target set by patient's health care provider.
2 Instruct patient about the purpose and rationale.
3 Patient should be standing. If patient cannot stand, help him or her to high-Fowler's position or any other position that promotes optimum lung expansion.
4 Slide the mouthpiece into base of the numbered scale to zero position.
5 Instruct patient to take a deep breath.
6 Have patient place meter mouthpiece in the mouth and close lips, making a firm seal.
7 Have patient blow out as hard and fast as possible through the mouth only in one single breath.
8 Repeat maneuver two additional times. Record the highest number in the chart or patient's diary.
9 If patient is to record PEFR at home, have him or her demonstrate PEFR technique independently and assess ability to record PEFR accurately on chart using "traffic light" pattern. Green zone (80% to 100% of personal best number) indicates that no asthma symptoms are present. Yellow zone (50% to 80% of personal best number) signals caution. Red zone (less than 50% of personal best number) signals a medical alert, and patient should call health care provider immediately (Grad et al., 2009).
10 Help patient implement an appropriate action plan as prescribed by health care provider.
11 Instruct patient to clean unit weekly following manufacturer instructions.

SKILL 23-5   Care of a Patient on a Mechanical Ventilator

Patients requiring mechanical ventilation need support for ventilation and/or oxygenation. Clinical problems such as respiratory failure, exacerbation of chronic obstructive lung disease (COPD), spinal cord trauma, respiratory muscle paralysis, and pneumonia require mechanical ventilation support (Roca et al., 2010). Patients receiving mechanical ventilation are most often in an intensive care unit.

An artificial airway such as an endotracheal (ET) tube or tracheostomy tube is necessary for mechanical ventilation (see Chapter 25). There are two types of mechanical ventilation: positive pressure and negative pressure. Positive-pressure ventilation is the usual method of ventilation that delivers a positive pressure to inflate the lungs. Multiple complications are associated with positive-pressure ventilation: decreased cardiac output, aspiration, tension pneumothorax (see Chapter 25), bronchospasm, laryngeal trauma, sinusitis, and ventilator-associated pneumonia. In addition, as the length of time needed for mechanical ventilation increases, there is an increased risk of failure to wean from the ventilator (Carbery, 2008). Be alert for these side effects. Negative-pressure ventilation is a noninvasive, negative-pressure ventilation technique. It is used for patients with primary neuromuscular illnesses that interfere with normal respiratory muscle function such as multiple sclerosis and muscular dystrophy. You fit a patient with a poncho or shell that is connected to the ventilator. Air is removed from between the patient's chest wall and the interior wall of the poncho or shell, causing the patient to inhale. A patient using negative-pressure ventilation does not need an artificial airway.

The skill described in this chapter focuses on positive-pressure mechanical ventilation frequently used in acute, subacute, and some selective home care settings. Many types of positive-pressure mechanical ventilators are available for acute care use (Fig. 23-13).

Modes of Ventilation

There are many different modes of mechanical ventilation to support different conditions and physiologic processes. Mechanical ventilation controls or assists a patient's respirations when he or she is unable to maintain adequate gas exchange because of respiratory or ventilatory failure (Table 23-3). The ventilator takes over the physical work of moving air into and out of the lungs, but it does not replace or alter the physiologic function of the lung. Mechanical ventilation maintains or improves ventilation, oxygenation, and breathing pattern. Patients with impaired ventilation have low oxygen level (hypoxemia), retain carbon dioxide (hypercapnia), and have difficulty breathing. Invasive mechanical ventilation requires an artificial airway (see Chapter 25).

It is important that patients remain on mechanical ventilation only as long as necessary because there is an increased mortality risk associated with positive-pressure ventilation. Caring for a patient on mechanical ventilation and weaning from it require interdisciplinary collaboration. Nursing care includes providing emotional support, preventing complications (e.g., pneumothorax, atelectasis, decreased cardiac output, pulmonary barotraumas, stress ulcer, or infection), promoting optimal respiratory gas exchange, and monitoring for equipment failure.

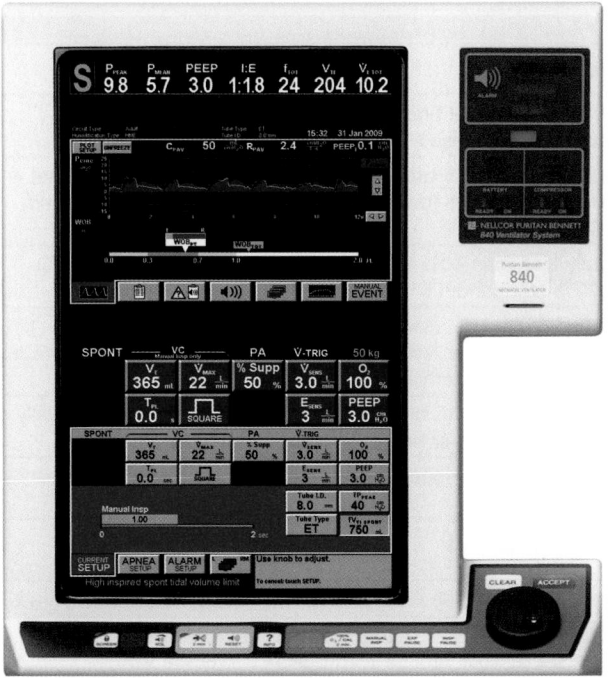

FIG 23-13 840 Series ventilator system. (*Reprinted by permission from Nellcor Puritan Bennet LLC, Boulder, Colo, Part of Covidien.*)

Alarms and Settings

The mechanical ventilator has a number of settings to adjust the amount of oxygen delivered, the amount of tidal volume, the time for inspiration and expiration, and the pressure at which each breath is delivered. The tidal volume, the amount of air per breath, is usually set by the patient's ideal body weight (5 to 8 mL/kg). If the patient has a restrictive lung disease such as pulmonary fibrosis, a flail chest, or recent thoracic surgery, the tidal volumes are usually set lower.

The respiratory rate is usually set at 10 to 16 breaths/min. Initially the FiO_2 is usually set at 100% and is quickly reduced to less than 40% based on patient arterial blood gas (ABG) levels. The goal of providing oxygenation is to maintain a PaO_2 of >60 mm Hg using an FiO_2 of 40% or less. Table 23-4 lists the ventilator parameters with which you need to become familiar to care for a patient on mechanical ventilation.

There are several alarms on the ventilator to ensure patient safety. Each ventilator is a little different; however, the basic alarms are similar. Alarms common to all ventilators include high-pressure, low-pressure, low-exhaled volume, and oxygen alarms (Table 23-5). You need to know how to respond to the ventilator alarms and which nursing actions are required to preserve the patient's respiratory status. The two most frequent alarms are the

TABLE 23-3	Overview of Mechanical Ventilation	
Types	**Description**	**Nursing Considerations**
Continuous positive airway pressure (CPAP)	Applies positive pressure during entire respiratory cycle.	Used for patients who breathe spontaneously but have hypoxemic respiratory failure; useful during weaning. Patients with COPD may tire after long hours of CPAP and require increased pressure support.
Positive end-expiratory pressure (PEEP)	Applies positive pressure during expiration.	Used for treating hypoxemic respiratory failure.
Volume-targeted	Delivers a preset volume to patient; peak inspiratory pressure varies.	Use in short-term ventilation and with ventilator weaning.
Pressure-targeted	Delivers flow to patient until a preset pressure is reached; tidal volume varies.	Useful when excessive inspiratory pressures could damage lungs, as in neonates; tidal volume varies with airway resistance and lung compliance.
High-Frequency		
High-frequency jet ventilation (HFJV)	Delivers gas rapidly under low pressure via special injector cannula. Delivers 100-200 breaths/min with tidal volume of 50-400 mL.	Patient on any mode of high-frequency ventilation requires continuous sedation and neuromuscular blocking agent administration.
High-frequency oscillatory ventilation (HFOV)	Delivers over 200 breaths/min with very small tidal volumes. Airway pressure controlled.	Most common of high-frequency types: maintains alveolar ventilation with low airway pressure; useful for treating esophageal or bronchopleural fistulas; helps avert barotraumas in high-risk patients if used early in treatment.
Mode of Use		
Assist-control	Patient initiates breathing, but backup control delivers preset number of breaths at set volume.	
Synchronized intermittent mandatory ventilation (SIMV)	Ventilator delivers set number of breaths at specified volume. Some patients breathe spontaneously between SIMV breaths at volumes differing from those set on the machine.	Requires frequent monitoring during weaning from mechanical ventilation.

COPD, Chronic obstructive pulmonary disease.

TABLE 23-4 | Ventilator Parameters

Parameter	Definition	Ventilator Setting
Tidal volume (V_T)	Amount of air inspired and expired with each breath	5-8 mL/kg of ideal body weight (patients with nonrestrictive pulmonary diseases) (Weigand, 2011).
Respiratory rate (R or RR)	Number of breaths delivered per minute	Usual rate is 10-16 breaths/min. However, the rate can be set 4-20 breaths/min, with lower rates used during weaning (Weigand, 2011).
Fraction of inspired oxygen (FiO_2)	Amount of oxygen that patient receives	Ideally less than 40% to maintain PaO_2 >60 mm Hg and SpO_2 >90% (Weigand, 2011).
Positive end-expiratory pressure (PEEP) (see also Table 23-3)	Positive pressure applied at end-expiration to improve oxygenation	5 cm H_2O may be used to approximate physiologic PEEP. May require higher levels (10-20 cm H_2O) in respiratory failure (e.g., refractory hypoxemia).
Sighs	Larger-than-normal breath to provide hyperinflation; helps prevent atelectasis	Usually twice the V_T breath; about 10-15 mL/kg. Rate is usually set at 10-15 times per hour. *Sighs are not always used.*
Sensitivity	Determines inspiratory effort required to trigger the ventilator	A breath can be triggered by a change in either flow or pressure.
Peak airway pressure	Maximal pressure level achieved during a breath	<40 cm H_2O.
I:E ratio	Comparison of inspiratory (I) to expiratory (E) time	Example: Inspiration 0.5 seconds, expiration 1 second, then I:E = 1:2 (Weigand, 2011).
Exhaled minute ventilation (V_E)	Measures the exhaled minute ventilations in liters	Alarm set at 15% greater than patient's average V_E.

PEEP, Positive End Expiratory Pressure.

TABLE 23-5 | Troubleshooting Mechanical Ventilation

Ventilator Alarm	Possible Causes	Nursing Interventions
Sudden increase in peak airway pressure (high-pressure alarm)	Coughing Airway plugging Changes in patient position Pneumothorax Incorrect ET tube position Kinked ventilator circuit Excessive water in ventilator circuit	Clear secretions by suctioning. Reposition patient. Assess breath sounds and chest wall movement. Verify placement of ET tube. Assess breath sounds. Verify centimeter level of ET tube. Check circuit; unkink tubing. Drain ventilator tubing.
Gradual increase in peak airway pressure	Decreasing lung compliance Exacerbation of acute process	Evaluate breath sounds; suction. Check for reversible causes: airway plugging, bronchospasm.
Sudden decrease in peak airway pressure (low-pressure alarm)	Patient disconnected from ventilator Leak in ventilator circuit	Check for disconnection. Evaluate circuit connections; tighten loose connections.
Change in minute ventilation or tidal volume	Leak in ET cuff	Check cuff seal.
Decrease	Airway secretions System leak Increased respiratory rate	Suction excessive secretions. Check circuit connections. Evaluate respiratory rate.
Increase	Hypoxia	Evaluate for signs of hypoxia. Evaluate need to obtain ABG sample or monitor pulse oximetry.
Change in respiratory rate	Patient anxiety Increased metabolic demand Hypoxia	Reassure patient. Evaluate body temperature, heart rate, and rhythm. Monitor pulse oximetry.

ABG, Arterial blood gas; *ET*, endotracheal.

high-pressure and low-pressure alarms. The high-pressure alarm is usually set at 10 to 15 cm greater than the peak airway pressure. When this alarm sounds, it indicates that the ventilator has met resistance to delivering the tidal volume and requires more pressure to inflate the lungs. Some patients have coughed during the inspiratory cycle; some need suctioning or have changed position. More acute problems that require immediate nursing intervention include the development of a pneumothorax or displacement of the ET or tracheostomy tube. The low-pressure alarm sounds when the ventilator has no resistance to inflating the lung. The patient may be disconnected from the ventilator, or a leak has developed in the ventilator circuit (Weigand, 2011).

Home Mechanical Ventilation

A patient on mechanical ventilation can be managed successfully in the home. Neuromuscular disease such as amyotrophic lateral sclerosis (ALS), muscular dystrophy, brain and spinal cord diseases, chest wall disease, central hypoventilation syndrome, and advanced chronic obstructive pulmonary disease (COPD) are a few of the diseases that can be managed at home on mechanical ventilators. Many factors determine if a patient and family are candidates for home ventilation. Assessment criteria include the desire of the patient and family, the patient's acceptance of ventilator dependence, the patient's and family's ability to understand and perform daily care procedures, the home environment, personal and monetary resources, and technologies for support in the community.

The goals of long-term ventilator care include extension of life, enhancement of the quality of life, provision of an environment that enhances individual potential, reduction of morbidity, improvement of physical and physiologic function, and cost-effectiveness. Patients who are candidates for home mechanical ventilation are prepared for discharge by a multidisciplinary team, including representatives of nursing, medicine, dietary service, and social service; the home care nurse; and the home care durable medical equipment company. The nurse in the hospital needs to be familiar with the home ventilator to help the patient and family with discharge planning and education (Ballangrud et al., 2009).

Delegation and Collaboration

The skill of caring for a patient on a mechanical ventilator cannot be delegated to nursing assistive personnel (NAP). The nurse directs the NAP to:

- Report immediately to the nurse any change in the patient's respiratory status, vital signs, oxygen saturation and if patient indicates breathlessness.
- Inform the RN immediately if any of the ventilator alarms sound.

Equipment

- ❏ Appropriate mechanical ventilator
- ❏ Oxygen source
- ❏ Pulse oximetry (SpO_2) probe and monitor
- ❏ Capnography ($EtCO_2$) window and monitor (if available)
- ❏ Stethoscope
- ❏ 10-mL syringe
- ❏ Oral airway/bite block
- ❏ Manual resuscitation bag (bag-valve-mask) with oxygen connecting tubing and flowmeter
- ❏ Clean gloves
- ❏ Goggles (if splash risk exists)
- ❏ Suction equipment at bedside (in-line/individual catheters)
- ❏ Chlorhexidine solution and toothbrush for oral care
- ❏ Method for patient communication
- ❏ Ventilator flow sheet to document ventilator changes and settings

STEP	RATIONALE

ASSESSMENT

	STEP	RATIONALE
1	Assess patient's level of consciousness (LOC) and ability to cooperate with mechanical ventilation and need for special positioning such as head of bed at 30 degrees.	Determines patient's ability to cooperate and understand aspects of care. Anxious and combative patients may require sedation to tolerate mechanical ventilation.
2	Assess patient's need for sedation (check agency policy).	Sedation is sometimes used in mechanically ventilated patients to reduce respiratory efforts, decrease oxygen demand, and improve ABG and oxygen saturation levels.

Clinical Decision Point *When patients on mechanical ventilation become excessively anxious or combative or try to override the ventilator, sedation is often used. Check agency policy for the specific indications for sedation and the specific protocol for administering and monitoring sedation levels for these patients.*

	STEP	RATIONALE
3	Assess patient's respiratory status, including symmetry of chest wall expansion, respiratory rate and depth, sputum production, and lung sounds (see Chapter 6), and assess for signs and symptoms associated with hypoxia (see Box 23-1).	Decreased chest wall movement, crackles or decreased lung sounds, increased respiratory rate, increased sputum production, or signs of worsening hypoxia indicate need for mechanical ventilation or changes in current ventilator settings to improve oxygenation.
4	Check ventilator, $EtCO_2$ (if available), SpO_2, and ventilator and cardiac alarms at beginning of each shift and periodically throughout care and compare with health care provider's orders.	Verifies that ventilator settings are as ordered by health care provider.
5	Apply clean gloves and verify placement of artificial airway through auscultation of lung sounds and verification of distal tip marking on ET tube. Determine that tube is placed securely (see Chapter 25).	Prevents migration of tube into right or left bronchus and accidental extubation.
	a Auscultate over trachea for presence of air leak. When air leak is present, you will hear movement of air over trachea.	
	b Using minimal occlusive pressure, check inflation of cuff of artificial airway (see Chapter 25).	Cuff of artificial airway needs to be inflated to create a seal for positive-pressure ventilation to occur.

Clinical Decision Point *When patients have periodic chest x-ray film examinations, also verify placement of the artificial airway.*

STEP	RATIONALE
6 Observe for patent airway and, if necessary, remove airway secretions by suctioning (see Chapter 25). Remove and dispose of gloves and perform hand hygiene.	Secretions plug airway, decreasing amount of oxygen that is available for gas exchange in lung. Secretions also occlude T tube or tracheostomy collar, impeding oxygen delivery to the patient.
7 If available, note patient's most recent ABG results or SpO_2. Determine if any factors have changed during mechanical ventilation.	Objectively documents patient's pH, arterial oxygen, arterial carbon dioxide, or arterial oxygen saturation.
8 Determine method for communication with patient. If possible, review previous communication techniques with patient and family.	Patients with an artificial airway and mechanical ventilation cannot communicate verbally. In addition, some of these patients are too weak to use a note pad to communicate their needs. Therefore assessing for and determining communication needs before instituting mechanical ventilation is ideal. However, each time patient has a new caregiver, assess communication preferences.
9 Review patient's medical record for medical order for mechanical ventilation, noting mode of ventilation, respiratory rate, oxygen setting, and tidal volume.	Mechanical ventilation and changes in ventilator settings require health care provider's order.

NURSING DIAGNOSES

- Dysfunctional ventilatory weaning response
- Impaired gas exchange
- Impaired spontaneous ventilation
- Impaired verbal communication
- Ineffective airway clearance
- Ineffective breathing pattern
- Risk for infection

Related factors are individualized based on patient's condition or needs.

PLANNING

1 Expected outcomes following completion of procedure:	
• Patient has improved lung expansion.	As patient's lungs and lung mechanics improve, lung expansion increases.
• Patient maintains ABG levels and oxygen saturation within normal range or at patient baseline.	Verifies that ventilator settings are effective in improving or maintaining patient's level of oxygenation.
• Patient's vital signs and respiratory assessment parameters improve.	Reduced pulse and respiratory rate, improved mental status, improved skin color, and decreased use of accessory and abdominal muscles occur because patient's work of breathing decreases as level of oxygenation improves (Carbery, 2008).
• Patient experiences reduction in feelings of dyspnea and work of breathing.	As pulmonary problem resolves, patient's perceptions of dyspnea and actual work of breathing decline (Hoo, 2011).
• Patient uses communication board, paper and pencil, or computer to state needs.	Appropriate communication system matches patient's abilities.
2 Explain ventilator system to patient and family and be sure to include purpose of and reasons for initiation of mechanical ventilation.	Helps patient express fears and wishes. Plays role in weaning process (Smeltzer et al., 2009).
3 Position patient with head of bed elevated at an angle of 30 to 45 degrees (unless contraindicated). Compare identifiers with information on patient's identification bracelet.	Positioning patients with head of bed elevated at 30 to 45 degrees or higher significantly reduces gastric reflux, thereby decreasing risk for aspiration and ventilator-associated pneumonia (VAP) (AACN, 2011).

IMPLEMENTATION

1 Perform hand hygiene; apply clean gloves. Apply mask, gown, and goggles if secretions are projectile.	Reduces transmission of microorganisms and exposure to pulmonary secretions.
2 Identify patient using two identifiers (i.e., name and birthday or name and account number) according to agency policy. Compare identifiers with information on patient's identification bracelet.	Ensures correct patient. Complies with The Joint Commission standards and improves patient safety (TJC, 2012).
3 Attach mechanical ventilator to ET or tracheostomy tube. Observe for proper functioning of mechanical ventilator.	Connects artificial airway to ventilator and ensures closed system, which enables ventilator to exert appropriate pressure or volume to meet patient's oxygen demands.

Clinical Decision Point *The mechanical ventilator requires programming of accurate settings before attaching to the patient. This is most often the responsibility of the respiratory therapist; however, it is usually a collaborative responsibility of the nurse.*

STEP	RATIONALE
4 Verify that ET or tracheostomy tube is properly positioned during an inspiratory and expiratory cycle by listening to both lungs and assessing chest wall symmetry.	Properly placed artificial airway ensures that both lungs are equally ventilated. Improper airway placement leads to unilateral lung ventilation.
5 Observe patient for synchronization with mechanical ventilation and response to therapy.	Ensures that patient is comfortable using ventilator and has not experienced any adverse hemodynamic effects.
6 Monitor heart rate, blood pressure, respiratory rate, and cardiac rhythm.	Implementation of mechanical ventilation results in decreased venous return and associated hemodynamic changes (Manthous, 2010).
7 Reassess and mark level of ET tube at lips or nares (see Chapter 25).	Provides measure to compare with baseline for depth of tube placement. ET tube must be placed through vocal cords into trachea. Ensures that tube is not too close to carina or in right main stem bronchus.
8 Set up suction equipment, including oral suctioning (see Chapter 25).	Need to provide airway care and suctioning of ET or tracheostomy tube as needed to prevent plugging of airway and reduce risk for infection.
9 Reposition patient regularly to promote best oxygenation and ventilation. This position can be high-Fowler's, lateral, or even prone. Monitor SpO_2 levels during and after positioning.	Positioning affects oxygenation and ventilation. SpO_2 drops during position change and recovers once patient is completely positioned. In other patients a change in position (e.g., high-Fowler's to lateral) results in sustained drop in SpO_2, thus indicating that patient in unable to tolerate that particular position at that time.

10 Collaborate with health care provider frequently about status of patient, response to therapy, and ongoing monitoring.
  a Monitor SpO_2 continuously.
  b Monitor $EtCO_2$ continually and with serial ABG levels to detect possible overventilation or inadequate alveolar ventilation.
 	
  c Obtain ABG levels with changes in patient's condition or ventilator changes.
	Assesses oxygenation status and continued need for mechanical ventilation.
	Provides ability to continually assess oxygenation levels.
	Overventilation causes respiratory alkalosis from decreased carbon dioxide. Inadequate alveolar ventilation causes respiratory acidosis from increased carbon dioxide retention (Carbery, 2008; Wilkins et al., 2009).
	Provides more accurate measure of oxygen saturation and partial pressures of oxygen and carbon dioxide.

11 Perform hourly safety checks on patient and ventilator system:
  a Make sure that patient can reach call light.
  b Check security of all ventilator connections; make sure that alarms are all turned on, including both high- and low-pressure alarms and volume alarms.
  c Verify that all ventilator settings are correct and correspond to health care provider's orders (Kallus, 2009).
  d Check and refill humidifier as needed. Check corrugated tubing for condensation; drain and appropriately discard liquid.
  e When present, observe temperature gauges on panel of mechanical ventilator, making sure that gas is delivered at correct temperature. Desired temperature of inspired gas is 98.6° F (37° C).
	
	Provides mechanism for patient to contact health care personnel.
	Ensures continuous safe and proper functioning of ventilator system. Enables you to identify and correct problems in a timely manner.
	Maintains integrity of the system and ensures that all settings are consistent with health care provider's orders.
	Ensures continuous humidification. Condensation that returns to humidifier can cause possible bacterial contamination.
	
	The temperature of inspired gas artificially alters patient's body temperature.

12 Perform mouth care at least 4 times per 24 hours (see Chapter 17). Use toothbrush and solution such as chlorhexidine, which is effective in reducing oral bacteria and risk for ventilator-associated pneumonia (Munro et al., 2009).	VAP is common, and it is associated with microaspiration of oropharyngeal secretions. Frequent mouth care reduces patient's risk for VAP. Oral care at least 4 times per 24 hours helps reduce risk for pneumonias (AACN, 2009).
13 Perform nursing activities to prevent hazards of immobility (e.g., help patient change position, perform range-of-joint motion exercise, and encourage independence and activity as tolerated).	Maintaining activity avoids complications associated with decreased mobility such as pressure ulcers, pneumonia, deep vein thrombosis (DVT), and activity intolerance. Patients receiving mechanical ventilation need help with activity.
14 Keep patient informed on progress and plan for weaning from mechanical ventilator.	Apprehension and anxiety occur when patient is not properly informed about progress, changes in care, or changes in ventilator setting. Patients need information and emotional support to successfully tolerate and wean from mechanical ventilation (Carbery, 2008).
15 Remove gloves and goggles; perform hand hygiene.	Reduces transmission of microorganisms and exposure to pulmonary secretions.

STEP	RATIONALE

EVALUATION

1 Reassess and monitor patient's response to mechanical ventilation every 2 to 4 hours.

   a *Neurologic assessment:* LOC, orientation, sleepiness, changes in anxiety

   b *Pulmonary assessment:* Lung sounds, airway clearance, work of breathing, breathing pattern, rate of respirations, SpO_2, $EtCO_2$

   c *Cardiovascular assessment:* Vital signs, heart rhythm, heart sounds, lower-extremity edema

2 Observe SpO_2 and monitor gas exchange.

3 Observe integrity of patient ventilator system.

4 Observe and evaluate effectiveness of communication methods:

   a Ask patient if needs and concerns are addressed.

   b Observe for signs of frustration (e.g., patient shaking head in irritation, crying, withdrawal).

   c Observe patient/family and health care personnel use communication methods.

Rationale column:

Patients requiring mechanical ventilation have unstable physiologic status. It is important to perform key focused evaluation measures frequently as patient's condition warrants.

Documents patient's level of oxygenation and ventilation.

Ensures adequate delivery of mechanical ventilation.

Communication, or lack of it, increases patient's frustration, sense of powerlessness, and confusion during mechanical ventilation and weaning process (Carbery, 2008).

Unexpected Outcomes

1 Patient experiences stiff, noncompliant lung; alveolar edema; pulmonary congestion; chest pain; intraalveolar hemorrhage; substernal chest pain; pneumothorax; continued decrease in blood pressure related to use of positive pressure.

2 Patient experiences hypoxia, hypercapnia.

3 Patient experiences self-extubation.

4 Patient experiences tension pneumothorax, as evidenced by sudden respiratory distress: air hunger, distended neck veins, tracheal/mediastinal shift, hypotension, and tachycardia.

5 Pressure alarm sounds.

6 Low-volume alarm sounds.

Related Interventions

- Notify health care provider.
- Remain with patient.
- Conduct complete cardiac and pulmonary assessment.

- Notify health care provider.
- Reassess patient.
- Assess integrity of ventilator system.
- Expect ventilator change (increase positive end-expiratory pressure [PEEP] levels).

- Maintain patent airway by suctioning and inserting oral airway.
- Provide oxygen.
- Assess patient's respiratory status and level of oxygenation and ventilation.
- Notify health care provider.

- Remain with patient, remove patient from ventilator, and ventilate with bag-valve-mask (see Chapter 27).
- Notify health care provider.
- Ask NAP to obtain chest tube insertion kit.
- Ask additional personnel to obtain patient's vital signs.

- Assess for airway obstruction (e.g., secretions, patient biting on ET tube).
- Remove obstruction (e.g., ET suctioning, inserting oral airway/bite block).

- Assess integrity of ventilator tubing and reconnect if disconnected.
- Check for airway displacement (e.g., extubation).
- Assess integrity of airway cuff (e.g., deflate and reinflate and determine if seal is present) (see Chapter 25).
- Remain with patient, remove him or her from ventilator, and ventilate with bag-valve-mask.

Recording and Reporting

- Record in progress notes: respiratory assessment findings; mode of mechanical ventilation, oxygen level, actual patient tidal volume, actual patient respiratory rate, peak airway pressure, patient's response to mechanical ventilation, level of the ET, any adverse reactions or side effects.
- Report to nurse in charge or health care provider: sudden change in patient's respiratory status, ventilator-associated problems.

Special Considerations

Teaching

- Teach patient and family about the rationale for mechanical ventilation and the alarms and what they mean.
- Teach patient and family alternative communication techniques to reduce frustration and fear.

Pediatric

- Increasing numbers of children are on home mechanical ventilation. For this reason it is important to include the parent in the child's care as appropriate. Parents also need to be prepared that, when a readmission to a hospital occurs, because of the chronic nature of the illness the child may not be readmitted to an intensive care unit but rather may remain on the general medical or surgical area.

- Once the child is stable on the mechanical ventilator, promote normal or near-normal activities as the child's condition warrants (e.g., promote play, resume school activities, encourage mobility).

Gerontologic

- Presence of underlying chronic illnesses increase patient's risk for longer intensive care, hospital stays.
- Older adults are usually not able to tolerate the usual sedative, antianxiety medications ordered. The prescribed dose is based on patient's baseline kidney and liver functions (Lehne, 2010).

Home Care

- Patients requiring home mechanical ventilation need to learn complete care of the mechanical ventilator system, suctioning, and artificial airway care. Skills include assembling the ventilator circuit, cleaning the circuit, and daily equipment maintenance.
- Use a checklist for ensuring consistency of care for patient on a ventilator.

- Evaluate the following areas during each visit: oxygen flow, alarm system, inspiratory pressure, high-pressure alarm, tidal volume setting, humidifier, respiratory rate, tubing, temperature, resuscitation bag, tracheostomy care, breath sounds, suctioning, and tubing changes.
- The durable medical equipment provider, the home care nurse, and the primary care nurse develop a teaching plan to ensure that patient and family have a complete working knowledge of the ventilator before discharge.
- Teach patient and family caregiver what to do in case of respiratory distress or power failure. Check to determine availability of emergency batteries.
- Instruct family in use of the bag-valve-mask (see Chapter 27).
- Patients who require long-term mechanical ventilation are transferred to a chronic ventilator facility or a long-term ventilator dependency floor within the hospital when they are medically stable. The purpose of such a transfer is to aggressively rehabilitate patient through physical, occupational, and speech therapy. The overall goal is to effectively wean patient from the mechanical ventilator. However, not all patients can be weaned from the ventilator.

Critical Thinking Exercises

You are caring for Mr. Landon, who has a history of chronic obstructive pulmonary disease (COPD) that is well controlled. However, 2 weeks ago he developed an upper respiratory tract infection and was treated with antibiotics. He completed his full course of antibiotics, but his symptoms continued. He has a 4-day history of fever greater than 102.8° F (39.4° C) fatigue, productive cough, worsening dyspnea, and decreased activity tolerance. His health care provider does a complete examination, orders a chest x-ray film examination, and obtains a sputum specimen. Preliminary chest x-ray film results indicate right lower lobe pneumonia. Mr. Landon is admitted to a general medicine floor for treatment with intravenous (IV) antibiotics, supplemental oxygen, and pulmonary hygiene measures.

1   You observe Mr. Landon and notice that he is fatigued, has difficulty speaking, and in general looks very uncomfortable. You decide to do a focused assessment. Which systems will you assess, and what information will you obtain? State your rationale for choosing these systems.
2   Mr. Landon is started on oxygen therapy via nasal cannula at 2 L/min. What is the approximate FiO_2 level, and what are the hazards for oxygen therapy in this patient?
3   Mr. Landon begins to remove the cannula because of discomfort at the nares and ears from the device. What are the causes of this discomfort? What are your interventions to reduce the discomfort?
4   One of the nurses suggests a partial rebreather mask for Mr. Landon's oxygen therapy. You do not think this is a good idea, and the rationale for your decision is:
    a   Increased inspired oxygen percentage
    b   Decreased carbon dioxide retention
    c   Decreased oxygen percentage
    d   Increased carbon dioxide retention

REVIEW QUESTIONS

1   A patient arrives on the nursing unit because of a sudden onset of dyspnea. Which assessment data would the nurse expect to find?
    1   A respiratory rate of 24 breaths/min
    2   Cyanosis
    3   Clubbing of the fingers
    4   A regular breathing pattern
2   A patient with an oxygen mask with a reservoir bag is seen while making initial rounds. Which problem might the patient experience if the reservoir bag becomes deflated?
    1   Elevated oxygen levels
    2   Elevated carbon dioxide levels
    3   Drying of the nasal mucous membranes
    4   Decrease in the number of respirations
3   You are preparing to observe a patient with COPD perform incentive spirometry exercises. With which of the following steps is the patient likely to have difficulty?
    1   Placing the mouthpiece correctly
    2   Being able to hold breath for 3 seconds after inhalation
    3   Being able to blow quickly into the device
    4   Performing incentive spirometry three times for each reading
4   Humidification is added to a nasal cannula when the flow is set at:
    1   1 L/min.
    2   2 L/min.
    3   3 L/min.
    4   4 L/min.
5   A patient needs an FiO_2 of 80%. Which of these oxygen delivery devices can deliver oxygen at this FiO_2 level? (Select all that apply.)
    1   Nasal cannula at 6 L/min
    2   Venturi mask at 12 L/min
    3   Nonrebreathing mask at 6 L/min
    4   Partial rebreathing mask at 6 L/min
6   In assessing the adequacy of oxygen therapy, which of the following is most effective?
    1   Checking the color of mucous membranes
    2   Counting the respiratory rate
    3   Measuring pulse oximetry
    4   Auscultating lung sounds

7 A patient is receiving oxygen by nasal cannula. Which statement by the patient indicates that teaching regarding oxygen therapy has been effective?
   1 "I was feeling better, so I removed my oxygen."
   2 "I asked my spouse not to put Vaseline on my lips."
   3 "I can take off my oxygen to walk to the bathroom."
   4 "I do not want to be oxygen dependent, so I need continuous pulse oximetry."

8 Noninvasive positive-pressure ventilation (NIPPV) _____ and _____ without the need for an artificial airway. Fill in the blank.

9 Patients are unable to speak when they have an ET tube in place. What is the recommended method to communicate with these patients?
   1 Talk to patients as if they have a hearing loss by speaking very loudly.
   2 Leave a pen and paper within reach to allow them to write comments.
   3 Provide a communication board such as an alphabet board for family to communicate with patient.
   4 Ask family members to explain the plan of care to the patient.

10 A patient with a tracheostomy tube and humidification collar also has an underlying diagnosis of chronic obstructive pulmonary disease. The nurse hears a bubbling sound on approaching the patient, although the patient is lying calmly and quietly. What is the appropriate action for the nurse to take?
    1 Suction the patient's tracheostomy tube
    2 Liquefy the patient's pulmonary secretions
    3 Check the oxygen tubing for fluid accumulation
    4 Elevate the patient's head slightly to improve oxygenation

REFERENCES

Agostini P, Singh S: Incentive spirometry following thoracic surgery: what should we be doing? *Physiotherapy* 95(2):76, 2009.

American Association of Critical Care Nurses (AACN): *Practice alert: Prevention of aspiration*, 2011, available at http://www.aacn.org/WD/practice/docs/practicealerts/aacn-aspiration-practice-alert.pdf, accessed July 21, 2012.

American Association of Critical-Care Nurses (AACN): *Practice alert—oral care in the critically ill*, Mission Viejo, Calif, 2009, The Association.

American Lung Association: *Supplemental oxygen*, 2012, available at http://www.lung.org/lung-disease/copd/living-with-copd/supplemental-oxygen.html, accessed July 19, 2012.

American Thoracic Society: Home oxygen therapy, 2012, available at http://www.thoracic.org/clinical/copd-guidelines/for-health-professionals/management-of-stable-copd/long-term-oxygen-therapy/home-oxygen-therapy.php, accessed September 1, 2012.

Austin MA et al: Effect of high-flow oxygen on mortality in chronic obstructive pulmonary disease patients in prehospital setting: randomized controlled trial, *Br Med J* 341:c5462, 2010.

Ballangrud R, et al: Clients' experiences of living at home with a mechanical ventilator, *J Adv Nurs* 65(2):425, 2009.

British Thoracic Society Guidelines: *Thorax* 63(suppl VI), 2008: doi:10.1136/thx.2008/102947.

Carbery C: Basic concepts in mechanical ventilation, *J Perioperative Pract* 18(3):106, 2008.

Filippatos F, Mebazaa A, Masip J: Noninvasive ventilation improved dyspnea but did not reduce short-term mortality in acute cardiogenic pulmonary edema, *Ann Intern Med* 149:JC6, 2008.

Frace M: Noninvasive ventilation: CPAP and BiPAP on the medical-surgical unit, *Med-Surg Matters* 17(3):12, 2008.

Galanti GA: *Caring of patients from different cultures*, ed 3, Philadelphia, 2008, University of Pennsylvania Press.

Grad R et al: Peak flow measurements in children with asthma: what happens at school? *J Asthma* 946(6):535, 2009.

Hockenberry MJ, Wilson D: *Wong's clinical manual of pediatric nursing*, ed 8, St Louis, 2011, Mosby.

Hoo G: *Noninvasive ventilation*, 2011, available at http://emedicine.medscape.com/article/304235-overview, accessed March 2, 2012.

Jardins TD, Burton GG: *Clinical manifestations and assessment of respiratory disease*, ed 5, St Louis, 2011, Elsevier.

Kallus C: Building a solid understanding of mechanical ventilation, *Nursing2009* 39(6):22, 2009.

Kaul S et al: Non-invasive ventilation (NIPPV) in the clinical management of acute COPD in 233 UK hospitals: results from the RCP/BTS 2003 National COPD audit, *J Chronic Obstruct Pulmon Dis* 6(3):171, 2009.

Kim V et al: Oxygen therapy in chronic obstructive pulmonary disease, *Proc Am Thoracic Soc* 5(4):513, 2008.

Lehne R: *Pharmacology for nursing care*, ed 7, St Louis, 2010, Mosby.

Manthous C: Avoiding circulatory complications during endotracheal intubation and initiation of positive-pressure ventilation, *J Emerg Med* 38(5):622, 2010.

Matzo M, Sherman D: *Palliative care nursing: quality care to the end of life*, ed 3, New York, 2010, Springer Publishing.

Munro C et al: Chlorhexidine toothbrushing, and preventing ventilator-associated pneumonia in critically ill adults, *Am J Crit Care* 18(5):428, 2009.

Roca O et al: High-flow oxygen therapy in acute respiratory failure, *Respir Care* 55(4):408, 2010.

Sieber F, Barnett S: Preventing postoperative complications in the elderly, *Anesthesiol Clin* 29(1):83, Philadelphia, 2011, Saunders.

Smeltzer SC et al: *Brunner & Suddharth's textbook of medical-surgical nursing*, ed 12, Philadelphia, 2009, Lippincott, Williams & Wilkins.

Spector R: *Cultural diversity in health and illness*, Upper Saddle River, NJ, 2008, Prentice Hall.

Stoller JK et al: Oxygen therapy for COPD: current evidence and the long-term oxygen treatment trial, *Chest* 138(1):179, 2010.

The Joint Commission (TJC): *National Patient Safety Goals*, Oakbrook Terrace, Ill, 2012, The Commission, available at http://www.jointcommission.org/standards_information/npsgs.aspx.

Tiep BL et al: Long-term management of COPD via a clinical guidance system: an update on a continuous care model, *Am J Respir Crit Care Med* 181:A1217, 2010.

Weigand D: *AACN procedure manual for critical care*, ed 6, St Louis, 2011, Mosby.

Wilkins R et al: *Egan's fundamentals of respiratory care*, ed 9, St Louis, 2009, Mosby.

Performing Chest Physiotherapy

SKILLS AND PROCEDURES

MEDIA RESOURCES

- evolve *learning system* http://evolve.elsevier.com/Perry/skills

  - Review Questions
  - Audio Glossary

KEY TERMS

Chest physiotherapy (CPT)	Percussion	Shaking
Mucociliary transport	Postural drainage (PD)	Vibration

OBJECTIVES

Mastery of content in this chapter will enable the nurse to:

- Assess for the need to perform chest physiotherapy (CPT) maneuvers.
- Determine the need to modify or discontinue CPT maneuvers, including contraindications and individual variations.
- Explain how to prepare a patient and family for the performance of each CPT maneuver.

- Perform the outlined CPT maneuvers, including standard and modified versions.
- Describe expected and unexpected outcomes of each CPT maneuver.
- Describe discharge teaching and planning related to the use of each CPT maneuver in the home setting.
- Describe approach for use of an acapella device and a vest airway clearance system.

Chest physiotherapy (CPT) is used to mobilize pulmonary secretions. CPT includes physical chest wall maneuvers such as percussion, vibration and shaking, and postural drainage (PD), followed by productive coughing or suctioning. Percussion is a rhythmic force that a caregiver provides by clapping cupped hands against a patient's thorax. It helps to loosen retained secretions from the airway. The maneuvers of vibration and shaking move secretions from the smaller distal airways into the larger central airways. Vibration is a fine, shaking pressure applied to the chest wall only during exhalation. Shaking is a stronger bouncing maneuver supplying a concurrent, compressive force to the chest wall.

Careful patient assessment is a prerequisite for administering any CPT maneuver because the therapy is usually targeted to the affected areas as opposed to all the lung fields (Fleming and Morgan, 2010). PD requires positioning a patient so the position of the lung segment to be drained allows gravity to have its greatest effect. CPT maneuvers move secretions into the large central airways; then these secretions are removed through coughing or suctioning. Coughing occurs when a patient takes a deep breath, closing the glottis to build up a back pressure, and then forcefully exhales. During the expiratory phase of a cough, the airways compress, causing them to narrow. Airway narrowing and forced exhalation increase the force of airflow in the large central airways, and mucus moves up and out of the trachea. CPT and coughing maneuvers assist with airway clearance of mucus in patients with retained tracheobronchial secretions (Allan et al., 2009).

Secretions accumulate in the airways of patients with bronchitis, asthma, cystic fibrosis (CF), pneumonia, and bronchiectasis. Surgical patients in the postoperative period sometimes have excess secretions because of the effects of anesthesia and ineffective coughing because of incision pain (Allan et al., 2009). Mucus plugs, atelectasis, and lobular collapse occur when secretions accumulate in the airways.

CPT is often used in combination with other therapies, including antibiotics, bronchodilators, mucolytic agents, and systemic hydration. These therapies along with CPT reduce mucus production and promote airway clearance. The goals of these therapies are (1) to clear the airways of excessive secretions to reduce the work of breathing, and (2) to improve a patient's ability to cough up secretions (Morrison and Agnew, 2011).

In the normal lung the mucociliary transport system clears the airways of excessive mucus and inhaled particles. This system lines the internal lumen of the entire tracheobronchial tree and consists of a thin layer of mucus that is constantly being propelled toward the larynx by cells that have hairlike projections called *cilia*. Inhaled particles are trapped on the mucus, and the cilia act as a conveyor belt to sweep the mucus toward the throat, where it is swallowed or removed by coughing. Airways normally remain clear, and mucus is constantly being cleared almost as fast as it is made. Normal mucus remains thin, white, and watery. When disease causes excessive sputum production, therapeutic interventions help natural airway clearance mechanisms (cough and mucociliary transport) clear the airways of obstructing mucus.

In various disease states mucus clearance slows down, or the cilia are overwhelmed by production of large quantities of mucus. The lungs no longer clear the mucus as fast as it is produced. Secretions stagnate in the airways, change color, and become thick and sticky. The cilia cannot remove large amounts of thick mucus from the lungs. In addition, many people with lung disease cannot cough effectively to clear airways. Therefore it is important to use other maneuvers to aid in clearing excess lung secretions and provide adequate hydration.

The impact of a patient's hydration status on airway clearance remains unclear. However, in some situations an increased fluid intake helps to thin oral secretions so they are easily coughed up and expectorated after CPT. The frequency of CPT depends on patients' conditions (e.g., during an acute pulmonary illness it often takes three or four CPT treatments per day and 2 L or more of fluid a day to clear and thin secretions.

EVIDENCE-BASED PRACTICE

CPT maneuvers are effective in selected patients such as those with CF, bronchiectasis, other chronic pulmonary diseases, and some surgeries (Lester and Flume, 2009). Recent studies compare the effectiveness of newer airway clearance methods (oscillating positive expiratory pressure devices such as the Acapella device [see Procedural Guideline 24-1], high-frequency chest wall oscillators such as the Vest airway clearance system (see Procedural Guideline 24-2) and intrapulmonary compression ventilators with standard manual CPT (Lester and Flume, 2009; Silva et al., 2009). These studies demonstrate that CPT and the newer devices are safe and effective modalities to aid sputum clearance for a variety of adult and pediatric lung diseases. Although there are few studies on the effectiveness of CPT in adults with chronic obstructive pulmonary disease (COPD) and pneumonia, CPT does help to clear some airway secretions in these patients (Fleming and Morgan, 2010):

- Use assessment findings to determine which lung field(s) require CPT maneuvers.
- Involve patients and families in the CPT plan and selection of mechanical devices. The use of the Acapella device or the Vest often improves patient satisfaction and adherence to CPT (Lester and Flume, 2009; Morrison and Agnew, 2011).
- Patients and families require detailed instructions regarding the mechanical device because it is often self-administered in the home settings (Lester and Flume, 2009).
- Reinforce to patients and families that these devices are easy to use and do not cause any discomfort.

PATIENT-CENTERED CARE

Patients who often require CPT maneuvers are those with chronic illness, postsurgical respiratory complications, or acute respiratory illnesses. Often these patients' physiologic capacities are weakened; they are often anxious because of their illness or surgery; and they may be in pain. Before initiating any CPT maneuvers, it is important to be sure that the patient is comfortable and as pain free as possible. Therefore preprocedure pain assessment and interventions are a priority.

In addition, CPT maneuvers are fatiguing for the acutely ill person, for the person with cardiac disease, and when there is an underlying chronic condition. As a result it is important to plan CPT during short periods interspersed with rest periods, at a time when the patient is rested, and not immediately after a meal. Because these patients are so acutely ill, everything in the hospital setting is new to them, and patient education about the procedure is essential and must be individualized to their needs.

The patient with chronic pulmonary illnesses poses different challenges. Often these patients must devote several hours of their day to activities to assist in airway clearance. As a result CPT maneuvers need to be timed with the patient's routine, personal goals, and social activities (Lester and Flume, 2009). When dealing with patients who have CF, skipping CPT maneuvers is not an option. Often these patients get tired of the daily routine and need assistance in designing an individualized plan for airway clearance.

The skills in this chapter include a great deal of patient touching. Asian and Muslim cultures consider it very poor taste to touch in public. In addition, the skills of physical therapy sometimes involve a gentle percussion or shaking of a patient's rib cage. Patients and families from cultures where violence is an everyday occurrence need detailed information about the procedure so they do not misunderstand the intent and objective of CPT. Always explain which type of touching is involved and what a patient may feel during the treatment, and provide an opportunity for a patient to temporarily stop and rest during the procedure.

BOX 24-1	Contraindications for Postural Drainage

- Increased intracranial pressure
- Head and neck injury until stabilized
- Active hemorrhage with hemodynamic instability
- Recent spinal surgery (e.g., laminectomy) or acute spinal injury
- Active hemoptysis
- Empyema
- Bronchopleural fistula
- Pulmonary edema associated with heart failure
- Large pleural effusions
- Pulmonary embolism
- Aged, confused, or anxious patients who are unable to tolerate position change
- Rib fracture, with or without flail chest
- Surgical wound or healing tissue

Trendelenburg's Position Is Contraindicated for the Following:
- Uncontrolled hypertension
- Distended abdomen
- Esophageal surgery
- Recent gross hemoptysis
- Uncontrolled airway at risk for aspiration

Modified from White G: *Basic clinical lab competencies for respiratory care: an integrated approach*, ed 5, Clifton Park, NY, 2012, Cengage Learning.

Safety Guidelines

1 Know a patient's normal range of vital signs. Conditions such as atelectasis and pneumonia requiring CPT can affect a patient's vital signs. The degree of change is related to the level of hypoxia, overall cardiopulmonary status, and tolerance to the procedure.

2 Know a patient's current medications. Some medications, particularly diuretics and antihypertensives, cause fluid and hemodynamic changes. These changes affect a patient's tolerance of the positional changes. Steroid medications, age, and malnutrition increase a patient's risk for pathologic rib fractures and often contraindicate rib shaking.

3 Know a patient's medical and surgical history. Certain conditions such as increased intracranial pressure, spinal cord injuries, abdominal aneurysm resection, bone metastases, or severe osteoporosis contraindicate the positional changes of postural drainage (Box 24-1). Thoracic trauma contraindicates percussion, vibration, and shaking.

4 Know a patient's level of cognitive function. Alteration in mental status often makes it difficult or impossible for a patient to understand the procedure and participate in coughing and expectorating secretions.

5 Have suction machine equipment available to assist in clearing airway secretions (see Chapter 25).

6 Know a patient's activity tolerance because, when patients are not used to physical activity, their ability to tolerate CPT maneuvers decreases. However, with gradual increases in activity and planned CPT, their tolerance improves.

SKILL 24-1 Performing Postural Drainage

Postural drainage is the use of positioning techniques to drain secretions from specific segments of the lungs and bronchi into the trachea. Each position drains a specific corresponding section of the tracheobronchial tree from the upper, middle, or lower lung field into the trachea. Coughing or suctioning helps remove secretions from the trachea. Fig. 24-1 shows the anatomy of the upper, middle, and lower lobe bronchi. The images in Table 24-1 show the body position used for the corresponding lung segment.

Use patient history and physical assessment findings to select which lung segments require postural drainage. In addition, use knowledge of a patient's condition and disease process, chest x-ray film examination results, and the extent of the pathologic condition to individualize the postural drainage therapy.

Delegation and Collaboration

The skill of chest physiotherapy (CPT) can be delegated to nursing assistive personnel (NAP). It is the nurse's responsibility to assess the patient, review laboratory and x-ray film examination results, and determine that the patient is stable and able to tolerate the procedure. The nurse directs the NAP to:

• Immediately report to the nurse changes in patient's comfort level, changes in breathing pattern, and tolerance of the procedure.

• Use specific patient precautions related to disease, mobility status, position restrictions, or treatment.

Equipment

☐ Stethoscope
☐ Pulse oximeter
☐ Trendelenburg's hospital bed or tilt table (more common in pediatric agencies)
☐ Water in pitcher and glass
☐ Tissues and paper bag
☐ Chair (for draining upper lobes)
☐ Extra pillows
☐ Clear graduated screw-top container
☐ Oral hygiene care: toothbrush, toothpaste, mouthwash, or chlorhexidine oral rinse if ordered
☐ Suction equipment (if patient unable to cough and clear own secretions)
☐ Clean gloves (*when there is risk of exposure to patient's respiratory secretions*)
☐ Patient education materials

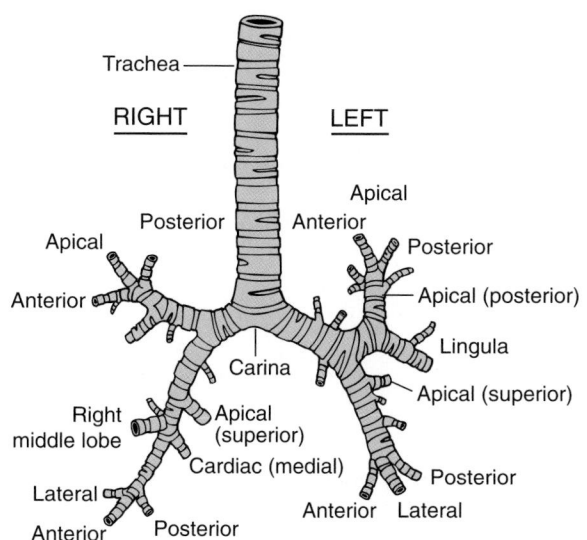

FIG 24-1 Tracheobronchial tree. (*Modified from Frownfelter DL, Dean E: Principles and practice of cardiopulmonary therapy, ed 43, St Louis, 2006, Mosby.*)

TABLE 24-1	Positions and Procedures for Drainage, Percussion, Vibration, and Shaking

Area and Procedure	Position of Patient
Left and Right Upper Lobe Anterior Apical Bronchi Position patient in chair or high-Fowler's, leaning back. Percuss and vibrate with heel of hands at shoulders and fingers over collarbones (clavicles) in front; do both sides at same time. Position hands for CPT over left and right upper lobe anterior apical bronchi.	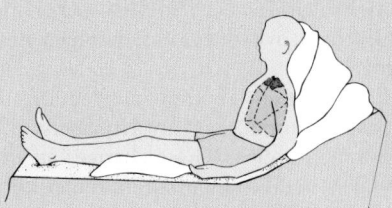
Left and Right Upper Lobe Posterior Apical Bronchi Position patient in chair, leaning forward on pillow or table. Percuss and vibrate with hands on either side of upper spine. Do both sides at same time. Position hands for CPT over left and right upper lobe posterior apical bronchi.	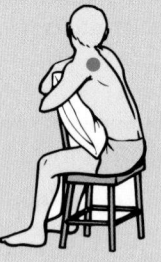
Right and Left Anterior Upper Lobe Bronchi Position patient flat on back with small pillow under knees. Percuss and vibrate just below clavicle on either side of sternum. Position hands for CPT over right and left anterior upper lobe bronchi.	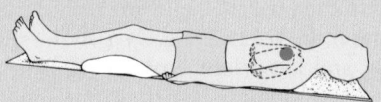
Left Upper Lobe Lingular Bronchus Position patient on right side with arm overhead in Trendelenburg's position, with foot of bed raised 30 cm (12 inches), as tolerated.* Place pillow behind back and roll patient one-quarter turn onto it. Percuss and vibrate lateral to left nipple below axilla. Position hands for CPT over left upper lobe lingular bronchus.	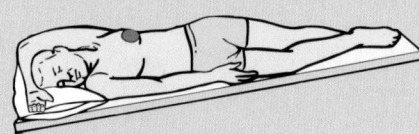
Left and Right Anterior Lower Lobe Bronchi Position patient on back, with foot of bed elevated 45 to 50 cm (18 to 20 inches). Have knee bent on pillow. Percuss and vibrate over lower anterior ribs on both sides. Position hands for CPT over left and right anterior lower lobe bronchi.	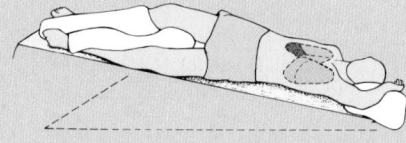
Right Lower Lobe Lateral Bronchi Position patient on abdomen in Trendelenburg's position with foot of bed raised 45 to 50 cm (18 to 20 inches) as tolerated. Percuss and vibrate on left and right side of chest below shoulder blades (scapulas) posterior to midaxillary line. Position hands for CPT over right lower lobe lateral bronchus.	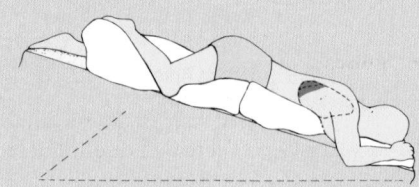
Left Lower Lobe Lateral Bronchi Position patient on right side in Trendelenburg's position with foot of bed raised 45 to 50 cm (18 to 20 inches) as tolerated. Percuss and vibrate on left side of chest below scapulas posterior to midaxillary line. Position hands for CPT over left lower lobe lateral bronchus.	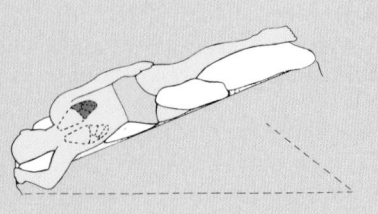
Right and Left Lower Lobe Superior Bronchi Position patient flat on stomach with pillow under stomach. Percuss and vibrate below scapulas on either side of spine. Position hands for CPT over right and left lower superior bronchi.	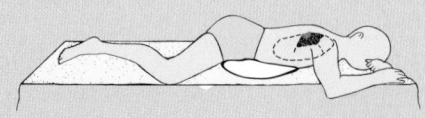

CPT, Chest physiotherapy.
*In adult settings Trendelenburg's position is not used as frequently. Verify use with agency policy and health care provider's order.

STEP	RATIONALE

ASSESSMENT

1 Assess patient for history of decreased level of consciousness and muscle weakness or disease processes such as pneumonia and chronic obstructive pulmonary disease (COPD) (see Box 24-1).

Conditions that pose risk for impaired airway clearance require CPT.

> **Clinical Decision Point** *If the use of Trendelenburg's position or other postures causes severe hypertension, severe hypoxemia, or severe shortness of breath, therapy is contraindicated (see Box 24-1). In addition, when patients have a risk for or a history of gastroesophageal reflux (GER), which is regurgitation of stomach contents into the esophagus, the head-down positions should not be used (Lester and Flume, 2009).*

2 Review medical record and assess patient for signs and symptoms, including x-ray film changes consistent with atelectasis, lobar collapse pneumonia, or bronchiectasis; ineffective coughing; thick, sticky, tenacious, and discolored secretions that are difficult to cough up.

Indicates need to perform postural drainage. X-ray film data and signs and symptoms indicate accumulation of pulmonary secretions and ineffective airway clearance.

3 Auscultate all lung fields for decreased breath sounds and adventitious lung sounds.

Findings identify bronchial segments needing drainage. Areas of lung congestion and postures for drainage vary, depending on disease process, patient condition, and clinical problems.

4 Assess vital signs and pulse oximetry before postural drainage treatment.

Provides baseline to evaluate patient's response to therapy.

5 Determine patient's and family caregiver's understanding of and ability to perform home postural drainage.

Identifies potential areas for instruction. Home care CPT is indicated in patients with chronic conditions such as those with cystic fibrosis, chronic bronchitis, or bronchiectasis (Lester and Flume, 2009).

6 Use a 0-to-10 pain scale to determine patient's level of comfort.

Determines patient's level of pain and if preprocedure analgesia is needed.

NURSING DIAGNOSES

- Acute pain
- Deficient knowledge regarding postural drainage and airway clearance

- Impaired gas exchange
- Ineffective airway clearance

- Ineffective breathing pattern

Related factors are individualized based on patient's condition or needs.

PLANNING

1 Expected outcomes following completion of procedure:
   - Lung sounds improve or become clear.
   - Sputum is more easily coughed and expectorated or suctioned out.
   - Secretions appear more normal in color and consistency.

   - Pulse oximetry (SpO$_2$) levels increase and dyspnea decreases.

   - Chest x-ray film shows improvements: lobar collapse and atelectasis are decreased or eliminated.

Clearing of airways documents effectiveness of procedure.
CPT provides mechanical stimulus to loosen secretions from wall of airway; thus secretions are easier to expectorate.
When infection is present, returning to normal indicates resolving infection.
As secretions are removed, patient exchange of respiratory gases improves, and dyspnea gradually declines.
CPT improves atelectasis and facilitates removal of secretions from airways. As a result there is visual improvement on chest x-ray film.

2 Prepare patient for procedure:
   a If patient's pain rating is 4 or greater on assessment, administer analgesia 20 minutes before CPT maneuvers.
   b Explain purpose and rationale for procedure. Explain positioning, sensations, how long it will take, and any discomforts or side effects.
   c Encourage high fluid intake program (minimum of 1500 mL) unless contraindicated by other diseases and if health care provider approves. Maintain record of fluid intake and output.
   d Plan treatments so they do not overlap with meals or tube feeding. Avoid postural drainage 1 to 2 hours before or 1 to 2 hours after meals or bolus tube feedings. Stop all continuous gastric tube feedings for 30 to 45 minutes before postural drainage. Check for residual feeding in patient's stomach; if greater than 100 mL, hold treatment.

Pain control is essential for patient to actively participate in CPT maneuvers and cough forcefully to clear airways.
Helps promote cooperation. Well-prepared patient is usually more relaxed and comfortable, which is essential for effective drainage.

Fluids thin secretions and make them easier to cough up. Patients need close monitoring and encouragement when first starting high fluid intake program (DeTurk and Cahalin, 2010).
Performing postural drainage when patient's stomach is empty helps avoid gastric reflux or vomiting and aspiration of stomach contents.

STEP	RATIONALE
e Schedule treatments at appropriate times during day (e.g., coordinate with any bronchodilator therapy, which is usually administered 20 minutes before CPT).	Scheduling of CPT avoids conflict with other interventions and/or diagnostic testing.

Clinical Decision Point *If patient is receiving inhaled bronchodilator, nebulizers, or aerosol treatment, provide postural drainage 20 minutes after such therapy.*

STEP	RATIONALE
f Have patient remove any tight or restrictive clothing.	Helps patient relax and promotes deep breathing.

IMPLEMENTATION

STEP	RATIONALE
1 Close room door or pull curtains around patient's bed. Perform hand hygiene and apply clean gloves as indicated.	Maintains privacy. Reduces transmission of microorganisms.
2 Identify patient using two identifiers (i.e., name and birthday or name and account number) according to agency policy. Compare identifiers with information on patient's identification bracelet.	Ensures correct patient. Complies with The Joint Commission standards and improves patient safety (TJC, 2012).
3 Use findings from physical assessment and chest x-ray film to select congested areas for draining. Consult with primary health care provider as needed.	Individualized treatment helps relieve specific areas of congestion identified during patient assessment.
4 Help patient to desired position to drain congested areas (see Table 24-1). Place pillows for support and comfort. Drape patient appropriately.	Proper patient positioning promotes drainage of pulmonary secretions.
5 Have patient maintain posture for 10 to 15 minutes.	In adults draining each area takes time.
6 During 10 to 15 minutes of drainage in selected postures, perform chest percussion and vibration and shaking (see Procedural Guideline 24-2) over affected lung region. Table 24-1 shows all postures and hand placement for percussion and vibration and shaking.	Provides mechanical forces to help move airway secretions.
7 After 10 to 15 minutes of drainage in first posture, have patient sit up and cough. If indicated, save expectorated secretions in clear container. If patient cannot cough, suctioning is necessary (see Chapter 25, Skill 25-2).	Any secretions moved to central airways are removed by cough or suctioning before placing patient into next drainage position. Coughing is most effective when patient is sitting up and leaning forward.

Clinical Decision Point *Sometimes patients experience transient dyspnea and fatigue because of airway irritation and bronchospasm from the secretions. These patients often benefit from an oscillating or vibrating device such as an Acapella device (see Procedural Guideline 24-1).*

STEP	RATIONALE
8 Have patient rest briefly if necessary. Note pulse oximeter readings.	Short rest periods between postures prevent fatigue and increase tolerance. Pulse oximeter values may fall slightly.
9 Have patient take sips of water.	Keeping mouth moist aids in expectoration of secretions.
10 Repeat Steps 4 to 9 until all congested areas selected are drained. Make sure that each treatment does not exceed 30 to 60 minutes.	Postural drainage is used only to drain areas involved and is based on individual assessment.
11 Offer to help patient with oral hygiene.	Promotes comfort and reduces bad breath.
12 Remove gloves and perform hand hygiene.	Reduces transmission of microorganisms.

EVALUATION

1 Auscultate lung fields.	Clearance of secretions usually relieves gurgling, early inspiratory crackles, and palpable crepitus.
2 Inspect character and amount of sputum.	Determines if there are more secretions coughed up and if they are adequately thinned.
3 Review diagnostic reports, including sputum collections/cultures, chest x-ray films, and blood gas levels.	Provides objective data on improvements in lung function.
4 Obtain vital signs, pulse oximetry.	Procedure can result in dysrhythmias and decreases in oxygen saturation in some patients.

Unexpected Outcomes

1 Patient experiences severe dyspnea, bronchospasm, hypoxemia, or hypercarbia and/or is unable to tolerate treatment.

2 No improvement in chest assessment or chest x-ray film examination results.

3 Hemoptysis occurs; or patient develops acute hypotension, severe chest pain, vomiting, aspiration, and/or dysrhythmias.

Related Interventions

- Discontinue, modify, or shorten treatments.
- Administer bronchodilator or nebulizer therapy 20 minutes before CPT.
- Suction and ventilate with bag-valve-mask as needed and closely monitor arterial blood gas (ABG) levels, O_2 saturation, and vital signs.
- Initially increase treatments and encourage and teach coughing exercises.
- Increase hydration.
- Notify health care provider because patient may need sputum culture, change in antibiotics, mucolytics, or a bronchoscopy to remove thick mucus plugs.
- Stop therapy, place patient in high-Fowler's position, and obtain vital signs.
- Call for help and notify health care provider.
- Remain with patient; keep patient comfortable, calm, warm, and quiet.
- If patient vomits or aspirates, suction airway and place him or her on his or her side.
- Prepare for possible oxygen administration.

Recording and Reporting

- Record pretherapy and posttherapy assessment findings and chest x-ray film results; frequency and duration of treatment; postures used and bronchial segments drained; cough effectiveness; need for suctioning; color, amount, and consistency of sputum; hemoptysis or other unexpected outcomes; and patient's tolerance and reactions.
- If patient and family caregiver receive instruction in home care, chart instructions given, understanding of therapy, demonstration of skill, patient acceptance of home care, barriers to learning and implementation, and referrals for home care or rehabilitation.

Special Considerations
Teaching

- Best times for treatments are (1) in the morning before breakfast, when patient can clear secretions that accumulate overnight; and (2) about 1 hour before bedtime, so lungs are clear before sleeping and patient has time after treatment to cough up any mobilized secretions. Frequency depends on need and patient's tolerance and varies from once daily to every 2 to 4 hours in an acute situation.
- Instruct patient's family or caregiver in recognizing when patient's respiratory status requires breathing exercises or postural drainage.

- Teach patient and family caregiver how to assume postures at home. Some postures need modification to meet patient needs. For example, if the patient is very short of breath, place him or her in a supine, side-lying semi-Fowler's or side-lying Trendelenburg's position to drain lateral lower lobes.

Pediatric

- In a child with cystic fibrosis CPT is a cornerstone therapy and is usually performed at least twice daily, on rising in the morning and in the evening (Hockenberry and Wilson, 2011).
- Many cystic fibrosis patients benefit from the use of the Vest airway clearance system (see Procedural Guideline 24-2) (Hockenberry and Wilson, 2011).

Gerontologic

- Take extra care and thoroughly assess when using postural drainage in older adults. Change positions more slowly and closely assess for any changes in oxygen saturation or vital signs with position changes.
- Older adults with chronic cardiac and pulmonary conditions do not always tolerate a supine or side-lying position for CPT. In these positions patients experience decline in forced vital capacity (FVC) and subsequent decline in oxygen saturation.

Home Care

- If specialized home or outpatient follow-up is needed, refer patient to pulmonary nurse specialist, pulmonary rehabilitation team, or home care personnel (Lester and Flume, 2009).
- Obtain foam wedge or multiple pillows for correct positioning.

PROCEDURAL GUIDELINE 24-1   Using an Acapella Device

The Acapella device is a respiratory rehabilitation device designed to aid sputum clearance (Silva et al., 2009). This device is easy to use as patients are able to perform airway clearance independently. The Acapella is a handheld airway clearance device (Fig. 24-2). It provides positive expiratory pressure (PEP) with oral airway oscillations. PEP stabilizes airways and improves aeration of the distal lung areas. During exhalation pressure from the airways is transmitted to the Acapella device, which helps mucus dislodge from the airway walls and as a result prevents airway collapse, accelerates expiratory flow, and moves mucus toward the trachea.

This device combines resistive features of PEP and vibration to mobilize airway secretions. Patients with chronic conditions such as cystic fibrosis appear to receive the greatest benefit from this type of treatment.

Delegation and Collaboration

The skill of using an Acapella device can be delegated to nursing assistive personnel (NAP). The nurse is responsible for performing respiratory assessment, determining that the procedure is appropriate and that a patient is able to tolerate it, and evaluating a patient's response to it. The nurse directs the NAP to:

- Be alert for patient's tolerance of procedure such as comfort level and changes in breathing pattern and immediately report changes to the nurse.

Continued

PROCEDURAL GUIDELINE 24-1   Using an Acapella Device—cont'd

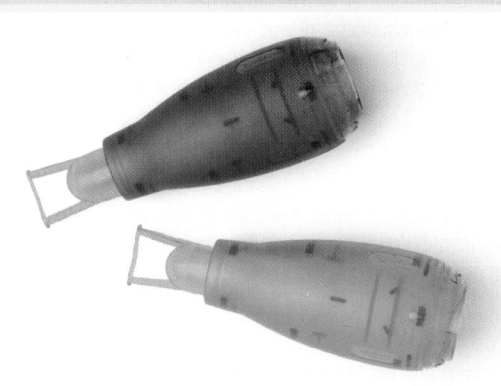

FIG 24-2   Acapella device. (Used with permission, Smithsmedical. com.)

- Use specific patient precautions such as positioning restrictions related to disease or treatment.

Equipment
- ❏ Stethoscope
- ❏ Pulse oximeter
- ❏ Water and glass
- ❏ Chair
- ❏ Tissues and paper bag
- ❏ Clear graduated screw-top container
- ❏ Suction equipment (if patient unable to cough and clear own secretions)
- ❏ Acapella device (see Fig. 24-2)
- ❏ Clean gloves (optional)
- ❏ Patient education materials

Procedural Steps
1 Verify the need for a health care provider's order per agency policy.
2 Identify patient using two identifiers (i.e., name and birthday or name and account number) according to agency policy. Compare identifiers with information on patient's identification bracelet (TJC, 2012).

3 Assess respirations and auscultate lung sounds for signs and symptoms indicating the need for this treatment.
4 Assess patient's and family's understanding of the device and procedure and explain and clarify procedure as needed.
5 Prepare Acapella device:
   a Initial setting: turn Acapella frequency adjustment dial counterclockwise to lowest resistance setting.
   b As patient improves or is more proficient, adjust the proper resistance level upward by turning the dial clockwise. This initial setting helps patient to adjust to the device.

Clinical Decision Point *Determine if aerosol drug therapy is ordered. If so, attach a nebulizer to the end of the Acapella valve.*

6 Instruct patient to:
   a Sit comfortably.
   b Take in a breath that is larger than normal but not to fill lungs completely. Instruct patient to inhale to about 75% of inspiratory capacity.
   c Place mouthpiece into the mouth, maintaining a tight seal.
   d Hold breath for 2 to 3 seconds.
   e Try not to cough and to exhale slowly for 3 to 4 seconds through the device while it vibrates.

Clinical Decision Point *If patient cannot maintain an exhalation for this length of time, adjust the dial clockwise. Clockwise adjustment increases the resistance of the vibrating opening, which allows the patient to exhale at a lower flow rate.*

   f Repeat cycle for 5 to 10 breaths as tolerated.
   g Remove mouthpiece and perform one to two forceful exhalations and "huff" coughs.
   h Repeat Steps a to g as ordered.
7 Auscultate lung fields.
8 Obtain vital signs, pulse oximetry.
9 Inspect color, character, and amount of sputum.
10 Help patient with oral hygiene.
11 Review Unexpected Outcomes for Skill 24-1.
12 Document procedure and patient's tolerance.

PROCEDURAL GUIDELINE 24-2   Performing Percussion, Vibration, and Shaking

During postural drainage a nurse, respiratory therapist, or trained family member sometimes uses physical maneuvers such as percussion, vibration, and shaking on the rib cage over lung tissue. The clinician uses techniques on specific parts of the rib cage over each affected lung region. Normally the mucociliary escalator and cough transport of the body can effectively clear airway secretions. However, when a patient's ability to clear the airways is reduced, the techniques of percussion, vibration, and shaking are combined with postural drainage.

Percussion involves clapping a patient's chest wall with cupped hands. If done correctly, it painlessly sets up vibrations in the chest to dislodge retained secretions. Vibration is a sustained co-contraction of the upper extremities by the caregiver to produce a vibratory force that is transmitted to the thorax over the involved lung region. Vibration is only done during exhalation, with the flat part of the palm over the area. It requires all muscles in the caregiver's arm and shoulder to contract and tremble.

Shaking is a more vigorous downward rocking motion on the rib cage done with the flat part of the hand during exhalation. Shaking requires a caregiver to apply controlled pressure from the shoulder and back while slightly leaning on a patient's chest; a rocking motion is created by flexing and extending elbows using the triceps.

Vibration and shaking augment the natural movement of the rib cage during exhalation and help with secretion clearance. Never use the clavicles, breast tissue, sternum, spine, waist, and abdomen for percussion, vibration, and shaking; only perform these maneuvers over the ribs.

PROCEDURAL GUIDELINE 24-2 Performing Percussion, Vibration, and Shaking—cont'd

High-Frequency Chest Wall Oscillation (Compression)

High-frequency chest wall oscillation (HFCWO) or compression consists of a vest linked to an air-pulse generator. One HFCWO devise is the Vest airway clearance system, which assists removal of secretions from the lungs (Fig. 24-3). This system is beneficial for patients with neuromuscular diseases, cystic fibrosis, obstructive and restrictive pulmonary diseases, and ineffective coughing ability. In addition, patients with sputum production of 25 to 30 mL/day also benefit from this device because HFCWO decreases the viscosity of mucus, making it easier to cough productively.

Delegation and Collaboration

The skill of performing percussion, vibration, and shaking can be delegated to nursing assistive personnel (NAP). The nurse is responsible for the respiratory assessment and review of the patient's chest x-ray film (with a physician) to determine patient stability, which areas of the lungs are affected, and specific positions for the patient to assume. The nurse directs the NAP to:

- Be alert for patient's tolerance of the procedure, monitor vital signs, and be alert to any patient precautions related to disease or treatment.
- Report any problems with tolerance of the procedure, pain, dyspnea, or changes in vital signs.

Equipment

- Stethoscope
- Hospital bed (tilt table placed in Trendelenburg's position, optional, check agency policy)
- Chair (for upper lobes)
- One-to-four pillows
- Water pitcher and glass
- Tissues and paper bag
- Clear graduated screw-top container
- Mechanical vibrator or percussor (*optional*)
- HFCWO device such as the Vest airway clearance system
- Single layer of clothing

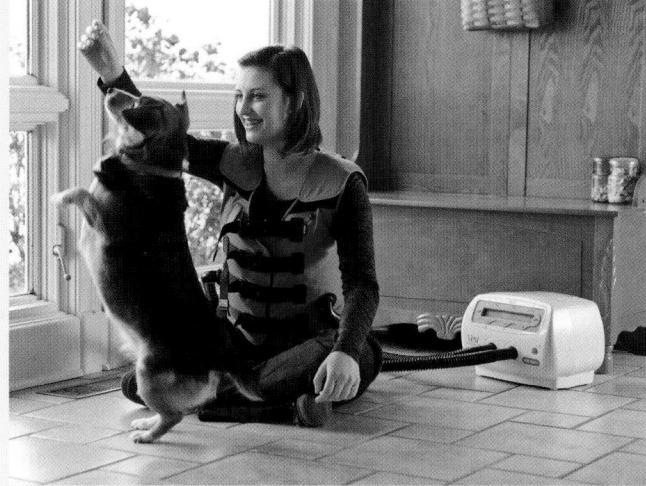

FIG 24-3 High-frequency chest wall oscillation vest for home use. (*Copyright © 2012 Hill-Rom Services, Inc. Reprinted with permission. All rights reserved.*)

- Clean gloves (if there is a risk for exposure to patient's respiratory secretions)
- Oral hygiene care: toothbrush, toothpaste, mouthwash, or chlorhexidine oral rinse if ordered
- Suction equipment (*optional*)
- Stethoscope, pulse oximeter

Procedural Steps

1 Identify patient using at least two identifiers (i.e., name and birthday or name and account number) according to agency policy. Compare identifiers with information on patient's identification bracelet (TJC, 2012).
2 Assess breathing pattern, including muscles used for breathing, respiratory rate and depth, extent of excursion, and chest wall movement.
3 Assess patient and review medical record for signs, symptoms, and conditions that indicate need to perform these skills (see Skill 24-1, Assessment).

Clinical Decision Point *Percussion, vibration, and shaking are contraindicated with rib fracture, fracture of other rib cage structures such as clavicle or sternum, pain, severe dyspnea, and severe osteoporosis. Thin, frail patients with osteoporosis are most susceptible to injury and are taught other secretion control measures (e.g., forceful coughing, humidification).*

4 Identify and assess area of rib cage over affected bronchial segment for pain, tenderness, abnormal configuration, abnormal excursion or chest wall movement during breathing, and muscle tension. Percussion, vibration, or shaking is contraindicated if one of these assessment findings are present since the treatment has the potential to cause further injury and impair chest wall motion.
5 Determine patient's understanding and assess ability to cooperate with therapy, both in hospital and at home.
6 Explain procedure in detail: patient's positioning, sensations, how it will be done, how long it will take, and any discomforts or side effects.
7 Help patient to relax and deep breathe during procedure. Have patient practice exhaling slowly through pursed lips while relaxing chest wall muscles. Instruct patient to blow out using abdominal muscles, not rib cage muscles.
8 Perform hand hygiene and apply clean gloves as appropriate.
9 Elevate bed to comfortable working height and stand close to bed with arms directly in front and knees slightly bent.
10 Use findings from physical assessment and chest x-ray film to select congested areas of lung. Position patient in appropriate drainage position (see Table 24-1). If a vest airway clearance system (HFCWO) is ordered, progress to Step 15. Place pillows for support and comfort.
11 Perform percussion for 3 to 5 minutes in each position as tolerated. Begin on appropriate part of chest wall over draining area (see Table 24-1). Always ask if patient is experiencing any discomfort such as undue pressure or stinging of the skin.
   a Place hands side by side on chest wall over area to be drained. Cup hands with fingers and thumbs held tightly together. Make sure that entire outer portion of hand makes contact with chest wall to avoid air leaks (see illustration).

Continued

PROCEDURAL GUIDELINE 24-2   Performing Percussion, Vibration, and Shaking—cont'd

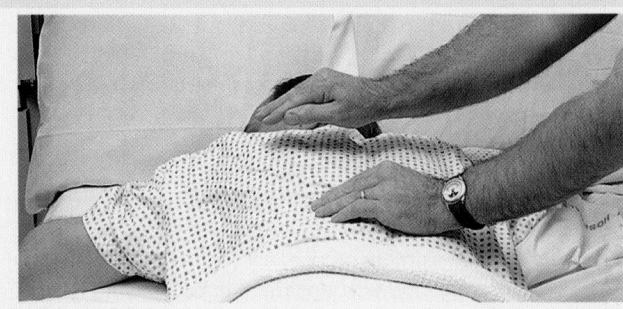

STEP 11a   Chest wall percussion, alternating hand clapping against patient's chest wall.

b   When clapping, most arm movement comes from the elbow and wrist joints. Clapping is often done for 5 minutes without stopping or for 2 to 3 minutes, alternating with vibration and shaking.

c   Alternately clap chest with cupped hands to create rhythmic popping sound resembling galloping horse. Perform clapping at moderate or fast speed, whichever is most comfortable and effective.

12   Perform chest wall vibration and shaking over each affected area (see Table 24-1). Perform vibrations in sets of three followed by coughing so any loosened secretions are expectorated.

a   Place flat portion of hand over area and have patient take slow, deep breath through nose.

b   Gently resist chest wall as it rises during inhalation.

c   Have patient hold breath for 2 to 3 seconds and exhale through pursed lips, while contracting abdominal muscles and relaxing chest wall muscles. Chest wall relaxes and falls.

d   While patient is exhaling, gently push down and vibrate chest wall with flat part of hand.

e   Repeat vibration 3 times and have patient cascade cough by taking deep breath and doing series of small coughs until end of breath. Instruct patient not to inhale between coughs. Vibrate chest wall as patient coughs. When applying pressure to ribs, always follow natural movement of rib cage. Allow patient to sit up and cough as needed.

Clinical Decision Point *When a patient has excessive pulmonary secretions, which occur with cystic fibrosis, a mechanical vibrator instead of manual vibration is more effective in removing them.*

f   Monitor patient's tolerance of vibration and ability to relax chest wall and breathe properly as instructed.

13   Perform shaking with vibration:

a   Place flat part of hand over area and have patient inhale slowly through nose.

b   During inhalation apply light pressure on ribs and stretch skin so it is tight.

c   Have patient hold breath for 2 to 3 seconds.

d   As patient exhales increase pressure. Maintain pressure while applying intermittent rocking motion on ribs. Pressure is directed toward following natural expiratory rib cage movement.

e   Instruct patient to exhale through pursed lips and relax chest wall muscles as much as possible.

f   Repeat shaking 3 times, have patient inhale deeply, and then do rib shaking during cascade cough.

14   Perform a total of three or four sets of three vibrations or shaking with vibration followed by coughing over each lung segment as tolerated. Strength and frequency of vibration and shaking will vary.

15   Vest Airway Clearance System (HFCWO) device:

a   Position patient in a comfortable body position.

b   Explain procedure and equipment to patient and family caregiver.

c   Place Vest on patient and assess for proper fit.
   (1)   With Vest deflated, adjust the closures so it fits comfortably.
   (2)   Vest should rest on the shoulder and extend to the top of the hip bone.
   (3)   Assess chest wall motion. Breathing should not be restricted when Vest is deflated.

d   Connect the tubing to the generator and the ports of the Vest. Turn on power.

e   Adjust pressure control as ordered; usually pressure is between 5 and 6.

f   Adjust frequency; usually set between 10 and 15 Hz.

g   Administer any aerosol therapy as prescribed.

h   Depress and maintain pressure on the hand/foot control to initiate Vest therapy.

i   After 5 to 10 minutes, release hand/foot control.

16   Instruct patient to cough or suction if he or she is unable to cough up mucus (see Chapter 25).

17   Continue with treatment; usually 15 to 30 minutes.

18   Help patient with oral hygiene.

19   Remove gloves and perform hand hygiene.

20   If long-term therapy is needed, teach patient and significant others the procedure for home use for Acapella or HFCWO devices. If they cannot learn or use, refer for outpatient or home care follow-up.

21   Auscultate lung fields.

22   Obtain vital signs, pulse oximetry.

23   Inspect color, character, and amount of sputum.

24   Document procedure and patient's response.

Critical Thinking Exercises

Mr. Meyersohn is a 29-year-old college student with a history of cystic fibrosis. He was admitted to the hospital 3 days ago for pneumonia, with a respiratory rate of 30 beats/min and 90% saturation on 2 L of oxygen via nasal cannula. He has a fever of 38.8° C (101.8° F). Chest x-ray film showed bilateral lower lobe pneumonia and lobar collapse of his right middle lobe.

1 Chest physiotherapy (CPT) was ordered. Which positions would you use?

2 Based on the chest x-ray film findings, what would you expect to find on physical examination of the chest, and which additional signs and symptoms would you expect to see?

3 After 24 hours of aggressive CPT a chest x-ray film examination was repeated. It showed improvement with good expansion of the right middle lobe and improved aeration of the lower lobes. Were the improvements in the x-ray film examination a result of the CPT? What other clinical improvement would you expect?

4 What would you document regarding the CPT and clinical assessment?

REVIEW QUESTIONS

1 A nurse is caring for the following group of patients who are receiving postural drainage with percussion. Which patient needs the most monitoring for potential side effects as a result of the procedure?
1 A 76-year-old elementary school teacher with diabetes
2 A 42-year-old year stockbroker on long-term steroids
3 A 66-year-old female who plays tennis twice weekly
4 A 58-year-old African-American male businessman

2 A patient with pneumonia has a major significant accumulation of thick secretions and requires chest physiotherapy (CPT). Which action by the nurse will help the patient clear respiratory secretions following CPT?
1 Set up a fluid intake schedule with a goal of 1500 mL/day
2 Have patient use his incentive spirometer twice each shift
3 Ambulate patient as much as possible to prevent stasis
4 Encourage patient to take several warm showers every day

3 During chest physiotherapy (CPT) the patient's oxygen saturation goes from 96 to 90. Which action should the nurse take initially?
1 Check patient's vital signs
2 Stop the CPT session for that time
3 Stop and ask patient how he feels
4 Listen to patient's lungs

4 A patient with continuous gastric tube feedings is due for postural drainage. After aspirating 125 mL residual feeding from the stomach, which action should the nurse take?
1 Elevate the head of the bed
2 Hold the postural drainage treatment
3 Listen to patient's lungs
4 Prepare patient for postural drainage

5 A patient with heart failure requires postural drainage. Which intervention should the nurse anticipate to meet patient needs?
1 Providing short rest periods between positions
2 Having patient take sips of water frequently during the treatment
3 Providing mouth care after the postural drainage is finished
4 Listening to each of the lung fields for 1 minute

6 A patient is hospitalized with respiratory failure caused by exacerbation of severe emphysema and bronchiectasis. Chest x-ray film examination revealed good lung expansion except for left lower lobe collapse. In which position should you place the patient for the ordered chest physiotherapy?
1 Right side-lying Trendelenburg's
2 Left side-lying Trendelenburg's
3 Right side-lying flat
4 Right side-lying Trendelenburg's with one-quarter turn back onto a pillow

7 A patient was admitted with recurrence of bilateral upper lobe lung abscesses caused by tuberculosis. Chest computed tomography examination showed fluid- and air-filled abscesses in bilateral upper lobes anteriorly. How should you position the patient to drain these areas?
1 Sitting up in a chair and leaning backward onto a pillow
2 Sitting up in a chair and leaning forward onto a pillow or table
3 Lying on back flat in bed
4 Lying prone with bed flat

8 A patient needing chest physiotherapy finished his lunch at 1 PM. When is the soonest that he should receive postural drainage?
1 30 minutes later
2 At 2 PM
3 Before his next snack
4 Right after dinner

9 A frail older adult needs chest physiotherapy because during assessment adventitious lung sounds revealed retained respiratory secretions. Which approach would be most appropriate to help this patient get rid of these secretions?
1 Encouraging him to increase his oral fluid intake
2 Teaching him how to forcefully cough
3 Performing postural drainage on the affected lobes
4 Using vibration and shaking over the affected lobes

10 A patient experiences severe dyspnea and hemoptysis during a session of chest physiotherapy (CPT). After stopping the CPT, what is the initial appropriate nursing intervention?
1 Notifying the health care provider
2 Administering a bronchodilator to ease the dyspnea
3 Assessing patient
4 Elevating the head of patient's bed

REFERENCES

Allan JS, et al: High-frequency chest-wall compression during the 48 hours following thoracic surgery, *Respir Care* 54(3):340, 2009.

DeTurk W, Cahalin L: *Cardiovascular and pulmonary physical therapy: An evidence-based approach,* ed 2, New York, 2010, McGraw-Hill.

Fleming S, Morgan G: Insufficient evidence to recommend routine adjuvant chest physiotherapy for adults with pneumonia, *Evidence-Based Nurs* 13(3):73, 2010.

Hockenberry MJ, Wilson D: *Wong's nursing care of infants and children,* ed 9, St Louis, 2011, Mosby.

Lester MK, Flume PA: Airway clearance therapy guidelines and implementation, *Respir Care* 54(6):733, 2009.

Morrison L, Agnew J: *Oscillating devices for airway clearance in people with cystic fibrosis (Review),* The Cochrane Library, Issue 1, Cochrane Collaboration, London, 2011, John Wiley and Sons, available at www.theconchranelibrary.com, accessed February 2011.

Silva CEA, et al: Laboratory evaluation of the Acapella device: pressure characteristics under different conditions and a software tool to optimize its practical use, *Respir Care* 54(11):1480, 2009.

The Joint Commission (TJC): *National Patient Safety Goals,* Oakbrook Terrace, Ill, 2012, The Commission, available at http://www.jointcommission.org/standards_information/npsgs.aspx.

25

Airway Management

MEDIA RESOURCES

- Evolve http://evolve.elsevier.com/Perry/skills
  - Review Questions
  - Video Clips
  - Audio Glossary

- NSO Nursing Skills Online

KEY TERMS

Artificial airway	Endotracheal (ET) tube	Intubation	Respiratory distress
Atelectasis	Hypercapnia	Laryngospasm	Suction
Bronchospasm	Hyperventilation	Obturator	Suction catheter
Closed-system suction catheter	Hypoxemia	Outer and inner cannula	Tracheostomy
	Hypoxia	Preoxygenation	Yankauer suction

OBJECTIVES

Mastery of content in this chapter will enable the nurse to:
- Identify guidelines for managing a patient's airway.
- Describe the nursing interventions for airway management.
- Discuss the indications for airway suctioning.
- Discuss the indications for tracheostomy care.

- Correctly perform oropharyngeal suctioning, tracheal suctioning, endotracheal care, and tracheostomy tube care.
- Correctly inflate a cuff on an endotracheal or tracheostomy tube.
- Change a tracheostomy tube or inner cannula.

Airway management involves maintaining the patency of a patient's nose, upper airway, trachea, and lower airway of the respiratory system. The primary goal is to maintain adequate tissue oxygenation. Many courses of action are available to promote an open or patent airway, which has the potential to become obstructed by mucus, mechanical obstruction (i.e., soft tissue in upper airway), or a foreign body. These actions do not always require a health care provider's order. Consult a health care provider if there are any concerns about the appropriateness of an intervention or when an airway obstruction is present, even when treatment relieves the obstruction. Hydration, positioning, nutrition, chest physiotherapy techniques,

suctioning, deep breathing, coughing, humidity, incentive spirometry, and aerosol therapy are noninvasive techniques that are helpful in maintaining a patent airway.

When patients are unable to clear airway secretions with coughing, chest physiotherapy, or other noninvasive techniques, more invasive measures such as suctioning or inserting an artificial airway are needed. An artificial airway is a plastic or rubber device (such as a tracheostomy or endotracheal tube) that is inserted into the upper or lower respiratory tract to facilitate ventilation or the removal of secretions. These additional measures are necessary, especially in weak, confused, or critically ill patients.

EVIDENCE-BASED PRACTICE

Preoxygenation and deep breathing, sometimes referred to as *hyperventilation*, help to reduce suction-induced hypoxemia (AARC, 2010). Hyperinflation is the process of providing 100% oxygen to a patient before airway suctioning:

- Preoxygenation provides a patient with a short-term increase in supplemental oxygen. Techniques include increasing oxygen flow rate on a nasal cannula or oxygen mask, increasing the percent of inspired oxygen of breaths delivered by a mechanical ventilator, or increasing oxygen flow rates to artificial airways.
- Not all patients require preoxygenation unless they are hypoxemic before suctioning.
- Following suctioning, return a patient's oxygen level to presuctioning levels to avoid increased risk for oxygen toxicity (AARC, 2010).

The practice of normal saline instillation (NSI) into artificial airways is no longer recommended as standard practice. Initially this instillation was believed to improve secretion removal. However, the research on this practice is inconclusive. The following items identify the lack of evidence for support or the potential side effects of the practice:

- Clinical studies comparing the results of suctioning using NSI with those of standard suctioning do not show any clinical or significant results (AARC, 2010; Halm and Krisko-Hagel, 2008).
- Suctioning with or without isotonic normal saline (INS) produces similar amounts of secretions and significant decreases in oxygen saturation.
- Potential side effects are increases in heart rate for 4 to 5 minutes after suctioning with INS as opposed to dry suctioning.
- Level of a patient's dyspnea after suctioning with or without INS was not significantly different.
- Use of INS with suctioning has the potential to increase ventilator-associated pneumonia because INS can dislodge bacteria from the upper airway to the lower portions of the airway (AARC, 2010; Halm and Krisko-Hagel, 2008).

PATIENT-CENTERED CARE

Artificial airways alter patients' ability to communicate, possibly causing feelings of fear, frustration, and vulnerability. Recommendations to improve communication for patients with an altered airway include developing alternate means of communication and to "acknowledge the lack of voice to the patient" (Foster, 2010). If nurses identify anger and frustration in their patients, they need to consider the need for improved communication methods. Nurses also need to thoroughly educate patients and make sure that they understand any procedures or tests. Regular pain medication administration for tracheostomy site soreness and before suctioning or dressing changes is helpful in promoting comfort and trust.

Collaboration with families is essential when providing alternative means of communication for patients. Patients and families who have English as their second language or do not speak English require additional attention from nurses and other health care providers to prevent misunderstanding treatment options. As a nurse, obtain translators or other communication aids so patients and families understand the need for an artificial airway and the subsequent treatments. Once communication is established, a patient and family will have more trust in the care provided, which will promote cooperation and rapport (Gill et al., 2009).

 Safety Guidelines

1. Know a patient's normal range of vital signs and oxygen saturation levels. Baseline physiologic measures serve as a means to identify individual abnormalities and recognize the worsening of an illness.
2. Know a patient's medical history. Smoking alters normal mucociliary clearance. Certain disorders such as chronic obstructive pulmonary disease (COPD), asthma, cystic fibrosis, pneumonia, thoracic surgery, chest trauma, and abdominal surgery place patients at increased risk for an obstructed airway.
3. Identify conditions that increase a patient's risk for aspiration of gastric contents into the lung, resulting in airway obstruction. These include the presence of enteral feeding tubes or other nasal or oral gastric tubes, a decreased level of consciousness, and a decreased swallowing ability.
4. Use caution when suctioning patients with a head injury. The suction procedure causes an elevation in intracranial pressure (ICP). Reduce this risk by presuctioning hyperventilation, which results in hypocarbia. This in turn induces vasoconstriction, thereby reducing the risk of ICP.
5. Determine if a patient has a history of nasal problems such as nasal trauma, nasal polyps, deviated nasal septum, or chronic sinusitis. Allergy problems may cause mucosal swelling that narrows nasal passages, which affects the ability to easily pass a suction catheter.
6. Review a patient's respiratory assessments from the past 12 or 24 hours. These are relative baseline measurements that help to distinguish between gradual and acute changes in a patient's status.
7. Perform a systematic respiratory assessment of upper and lower airways, including identifying respiratory rate, respiratory pattern, respiratory muscles used, breath sounds, ability to cough effectively, integrity of the rib cage, and the characteristics of sputum production.
8. Identify and become familiar with the use of equipment available at the agency. Many types of artificial airways, suction catheters, and suction machines are available. Knowing how to operate the equipment before use promotes positive outcomes.
9. Test all equipment before use. Have adequate supplies on hand at the bedside. Equipment must work properly to provide safe nursing care. Determine that the suction machine is generating adequate negative suction pressure and that there are suction catheters and appropriate equipment at the bedside.
10. Know the side effects of medications and other therapies. Some medications such as beta-adrenergic blockers have the side effect of bronchospasm. An adverse effect of opioids and sedatives is respiratory depression. Similarly, too much oxygen reduces the drive to breathe in patients with chronic hypercapnia (elevated arterial carbon dioxide tension). Some position changes affect a patient adversely. For example, in patients with impaired spinal cord innervations of the respiratory muscles, supine positions place the diaphragm at a mechanical disadvantage and increase the risk for aspiration.

SKILL 25-1 Performing Oropharyngeal Suctioning

NSO *Airway Management Module / Lesson 3*

 Video Clip

A Yankauer, or tonsillar tip, suction device is used for oropharyngeal suctioning (i.e., the removal of pharyngeal secretions through the mouth) (Fig. 25-1). A Yankauer suction catheter is made of rigid, minimally flexible plastic. The tip of this suction catheter usually has one large and several small openings through which the mucus enters with application of negative pressure. The Yankauer suction catheter is angled to facilitate removal of secretions through a patient's mouth. This catheter is used instead of a standard suction catheter when oral secretions are extremely copious and thick because it handles large volumes of secretions better than a standard suction catheter. The Yankauer catheter is not used to suction the nares or trachea because of its size.

The Yankauer suction device is useful in the removal of secretions from the mouth. Yankauer suctioning is used when the patient is able to cough effectively but is unable to clear secretions. In addition, patients who benefit most are those who have had oral and maxillofacial surgery, trauma to the mouth, neurovascular injury, and cerebrovascular accident causing hemiparesis and

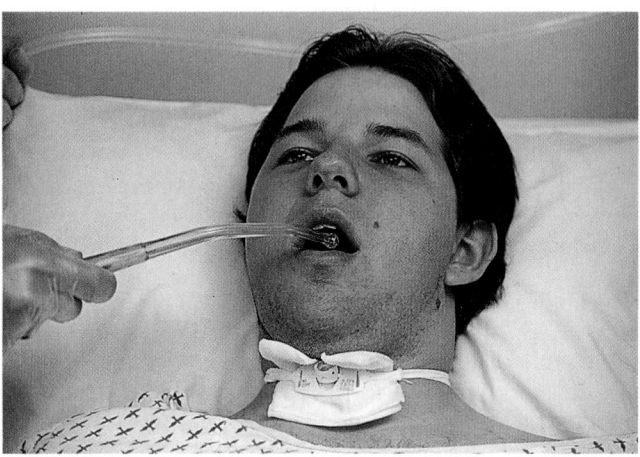

FIG 25-1 Oropharyngeal suctioning.

drooling or impaired swallowing. Patients with artificial airways and impaired swallowing require use of the Yankauer suction device to provide oral hygiene.

Delegation and Collaboration
The skill of performing oropharyngeal (Yankauer) suctioning can be delegated to nursing assistive personnel (NAP). Do not routinely delegate this skill for patients with oral or neck surgery in the immediate postoperative period. The nurse is responsible for assessing the patient's respiratory status. The nurse directs the NAP about:

- Appropriate suction limits for oropharyngeal suctioning for a particular patient (e.g., the appropriate suction pressure, expected frequency of suctioning, and expected color and volume of secretions).
- The risks of applying excessive or inadequate suction pressure.
- Avoiding mouth sutures, applying suction against sensitive tissues, and dislodging tubes in the patient's nose or mouth.
- Avoiding stimulation of the gag reflex.
- Immediately reporting to the nurse change in vital signs, pulse oximetry, sputum (i.e., bloody), difficulty breathing, or discomfort during or after the procedure.

Equipment
- ❑ Yankauer or tonsillar tip suction catheter
- ❑ Clean gloves
- ❑ Towel, cloth, or disposable paper drape
- ❑ Mask, goggles, or face shield
- ❑ Disposable cup or nonsterile basin
- ❑ Tap water or normal saline (about 100 mL)
- ❑ Suction machine or wall suction device
- ❑ Connecting tubing (6 feet)
- ❑ Oral airway (if indicated)
- ❑ Washcloth (if indicated)
- ❑ Pulse oximeter, stethoscope

STEP	RATIONALE

ASSESSMENT

1 Identify risk factors for airway obstruction: impaired cough or gag reflex, weakened respiratory muscles, impaired swallowing, and decreased level of consciousness.	Risk factors prevent patient from protecting airway from aspiration or clearing secretions safely.
2 Assess for signs and symptoms of hypoxia (low oxygen use at cellular or tissue level), hypoxemia (low oxygen tension in blood), or hypercapnia (elevated carbon dioxide tension in blood): apprehension, anxiety, decreased ability to concentrate, lethargy, decreased level of consciousness (especially acute), increased fatigue and dizziness, behavioral changes (e.g., irritability and restlessness), tachycardia, tachypnea, decreased depth of breathing, elevated blood pressure, cardiac dysrhythmias, pallor, cyanosis, dyspnea, and use of accessory muscles for breathing.	Suctioning of airways is indicated with alterations in oxygenation associated with secretion accumulation.
3 Obtain patient's oxygen saturation level via pulse oximetry (SpO_2) (see Chapter 5). Keep oximeter in place.	Provides an objective baseline measure of oxygen saturation and an early indication of changes in oxygenation status.

STEP	RATIONALE
4 Determine patient's ability to hold or manipulate catheter and his or her knowledge about use of suction catheter and procedure.	Encourages cooperation; minimizes risks and anxiety. Identifies teaching needs. Physical factors such as impaired mobility of upper extremities prevent patient from using catheter to help control oral secretions.
5 Assess for signs and symptoms of upper airway obstruction: gurgling on inspiration or expiration, restlessness, obvious excessive oral secretions, drooling, gastric secretions or vomitus in mouth, or coughing without clearing secretions from upper airway.	Secretions pool in upper airway, which can cause total airway obstruction and hypoxia. The risk for aspiration of gastric contents and airway obstruction is increased in patients with vomiting, delayed gastric emptying, and impairment in esophageal sphincter control, cough, swallowing, or gag reflex.
6 Auscultate for presence of adventitious sounds (see Skill 25-2).	Determines if lower airway secretions are present and establishes baseline.

NURSING DIAGNOSES

- Deficient knowledge regarding use of suction
- Impaired gas exchange

- Impaired swallowing
- Ineffective airway clearance
- Ineffective breathing pattern

- Risk for aspiration
- Risk for infection

Related factors are individualized based on patient's condition or needs.

PLANNING

1 Expected outcomes following completion of procedure:	
• No gurgling sounds are heard in patient's pharynx on inspiration and expiration.	Suctioning is effective. Secretions are removed from large upper airway.
• Drooling is diminished or absent.	Excessive drooling indicates that patient is unable to handle oral secretions.
• Vomitus or gastric secretions are absent from mouth.	Gastric secretions retained in oral cavity increase patient's risk for aspiration pneumonia.
• SpO$_2$ improves or remains the same.	Removal of secretions helps to improve oxygen saturation level.

Clinical Decision Point *In patients with chronic pulmonary disease, the SpO$_2$ value may remain the same after oropharyngeal suctioning.*

2 Explain to patient how procedure helps clear airway secretions and relieves some breathing problems. Explain that coughing, gagging, or (less commonly) sneezing is normal and lasts only a few seconds. Encourage patient to cough out secretions and show how to splint painful areas during procedure. Practice coughing if able.	Gagging or coughing occurs when posterior pharynx is suctioned or as a result of excess secretions. Coughing secretions out of lower airway or posterior pharynx decreases amount of suctioning required. Splinting reduces abdominal incision discomfort during coughing or gagging.
3 Position patient in semi-Fowler's or sitting position. Place towel, cloth, or paper drape across patient's neck and chest.	Promotes patient comfort and removal of airway secretions. Towel protects gown and bed linen from contamination by secretions.

IMPLEMENTATION

1 Identify patient using two identifiers (i.e., name and birthday or name and account number according to agency policy). Compare identifiers with information on patient's identification bracelet.	Ensures correct patient. Complies with The Joint Commission standards and improves patient safety (TJC, 2012).
2 Perform hand hygiene and apply clean gloves. Apply mask or face shield if splashing is likely.	Reduces transmission of microorganisms.
3 Fill cup or basin with approximately 100 mL of water or normal saline.	Aids in cleaning catheter after suctioning and assesses that equipment functions.
4 Connect one end of connecting tubing to suction machine and other to Yankauer suction catheter. Turn on suction machine; set vacuum regulator to appropriate setting (see manufacturer instructions).	Prepares suction apparatus. Elevated pressure settings increase risk for trauma to oral mucosa.
5 Check that suction machine is functioning properly by placing tip of catheter in water or saline and suctioning small amount from cup or basin.	Ensures equipment function and lubricates catheter.
6 Remove patient's oxygen mask if present. Nasal cannula may remain in place. Keep oxygen mask near patient's face.	Allows access to mouth. Reduces chance of hypoxia.

STEP	RATIONALE

Clinical Decision Point *Be prepared to quickly reapply supplemental oxygen if SpO₂ value falls below 90% or respiratory distress develops during or at the end of oropharyngeal suctioning.*

STEP	RATIONALE
7 Insert catheter into mouth along gum line to pharynx. Move catheter around mouth until secretions have cleared. Encourage patient to cough. Replace oxygen mask.	Movement of catheter prevents suction tip from invaginating oral mucosal surfaces and causing trauma. Coughing moves secretions from lower airway into mouth and upper airway.

Clinical Decision Point *Be careful using a Yankauer tip with a patient who had recent oral or head/neck surgery.*

STEP	RATIONALE
8 Rinse catheter with water in cup or basin until connecting tubing is cleared of secretions. Turn off suction. Wash face if secretions are present on patient's skin.	Rinses catheter and reduces probability of transmission of microorganisms. Clean suction tubing enhances delivery of set suction pressure. Prevents skin breakdown.
9 Observe respiratory status. Repeat procedure if indicated. May need to use standard suction catheter to reach into trachea if respiratory status not improved (see Skill 25-2).	Directs nurse to continue or cease intervention or choose another intervention.
10 Remove towel, cloth, or disposable drape and place in trash or in laundry if soiled. Reposition patient; Sims' position encourages drainage and should be used if patient has decreased level of consciousness.	Reduces transmission of microorganisms. Facilitates drainage of oral secretions.
11 Discard remainder of water into appropriate receptacle. Rinse basin in warm soapy water and dry with paper towels. Discard disposable cup into appropriate receptacle. Place catheter in clean, dry area.	Reduces transmission of microorganisms and maintains medical asepsis. Moist environment encourages microorganism growth.

Clinical Decision Point *Keep catheter in nonairtight container such as brown paper or plastic bag attached to bedrail or in suction canister area. Do not store the catheter where it will come in contact with secretions or excretions, which promote bacterial growth.*

STEP	RATIONALE
12 Remove gloves, mask, or face shield and dispose of in appropriate receptacle. Perform hand hygiene.	Reduces transmission of microorganisms to other patients and equipment.
13 Position patient and provide oral hygiene as needed.	Promotes patient's comfort.

EVALUATION

1 Compare assessment findings before and after procedure.	Identifies physiologic response to suction procedure.
2 Auscultate chest and airways for adventitious sounds.	Presence of lower airway adventitious sounds suggests need for lower airway suctioning.
3 Inspect mouth for any vomitus.	Clear oral airway is necessary to prevent aspiration.
4 Obtain postsuction SpO₂ measure. Compare with presuction level.	Provides objective measure of effectiveness of suction procedure (AARC, 2004).
5 Observe patient or family perform Yankauer suctioning.	Demonstrates learning.

Unexpected Outcomes

1 Patient's respiratory distress increases.

2 Bloody secretions are suctioned.

Related Interventions

- Suction further or implement nasal or tracheal suctioning.
- Evaluate need for other means to protect airway (e.g., oral intubation, oral airway, positioning).
- Provide supplemental oxygen.
- Notify health care provider.

- Assess oral cavity for trauma or lesions.
- Reduce amount of suction pressure used.
- Observe catheter tip for nicks, which cause mucosal trauma.
- Increase frequency of oral hygiene.

Recording and Reporting

- Record the amount, consistency, color, and odor of secretions; number of times suctioned, patient's response to suctioning; and presuction and postsuction cardiopulmonary assessment findings (see Chapter 6).
- Record instructions given to caregivers and note their ability to correctly perform procedure.
- Report any unresolved outcomes such as worsening respiratory distress to the health care provider.

Special Considerations

Teaching
- Instruct patient and family caregiver not to allow catheter to fall to the floor. If this occurs, teach patient and caregiver how to clean or obtain a clean catheter (see Home Care Considerations).
- Provide information regarding signs and symptoms of worsening respiratory status.

Pediatric
- Airways of infants and children are smaller than those of an adult; even small amounts of mucus cause airway obstruction.
- Position infants with breathing problems or excessive vomitus in supine or side-lying position (Hockenberry and Wilson, 2011).
- Suction should be completed for only 5 seconds because of risk of deoxygenation. Allow 30 to 60 seconds for patient to reoxygenate (Hockenberry and Wilson, 2011).

- Complete oral suctioning first and then nasal suctioning to decrease the risk of aspiration (Hockenberry and Wilson, 2011).
- Use bulb syringe. Compress syringe before insertion to prevent forcing secretions into infant's bronchi. Within the hospital replace the bulb every 24 hours (Hockenberry and Wilson, 2011).

Gerontologic
- Patients with dysphagia may benefit from oral suctioning before, during, and after meals.
- Oral mucosa in older adults is fragile; use a lower suction pressure.
- Older adults are prone to aspiration of oral secretions because of decreased cough and gag reflexes (Meiner and Lueckenotte, 2011).

Home Care
- Make sure that patient and family caregiver know how to clean and disinfect or change the secretion collection container every 24 hours according to home care protocol. Many agencies seal and dispose of the entire disposable secretion collection canister as biohazardous material.
- Assess knowledge level of patient and family caregiver to determine amount of instruction required and frequency of home health visits necessary to reach goals.
- Assess home for the presence of respiratory irritants, including cigarette smoke, dust, pollen, animal dander, mold, and chemicals.

SKILL 25-2 Airway Suctioning

NSO Airway Management Module / Lessons 1, 5, and 6

 Video Clip

The major differences between oropharyngeal and tracheal airway suctioning are the depth suctioned, the potential for complications, and the need for it to be a sterile procedure. Oropharyngeal suctioning only removes secretions from the back of the throat. Tracheal airway suctioning extends into the lower airway and is indicated to remove respiratory secretions and maintain optimum ventilation and oxygenation in patients who are unable to independently remove these secretions. When a patient's oxygen saturation falls below 90%, this is a good indicator of the need for suctioning. Assess patients to determine frequency and depth of suctioning. Some patients require suctioning every hour or two, whereas others need it only once or twice a day (AARC, 2004).

If the secretions are only in the nose and mouth, only the pharynx requires suctioning. However, in most instances you will suction both the pharynx and the trachea. Suction secretions from the pharynx as often as necessary using oropharyngeal or nasopharyngeal suctioning. Secretions that are not removed are more likely to be aspirated into the lungs, increasing the risk for infection and respiratory failure. This requires tracheal suction.

Tracheal suctioning has many risks, including hypoxemia, which often results in cardiac dysrhythmias, laryngeal spasm, or bradycardia. Bradycardia is associated with stimulation of the vagus nerve. Nasal trauma and bleeding can develop from trauma from a suction catheter introduced through the nares (AARC, 2004).

Nasopharyngeal and Nasotracheal Suctioning

Nasopharyngeal and nasotracheal suctioning help to maintain a patent airway by removing secretions from the nares, pharynx, throat, and trachea by introducing a suction catheter through the nares. This type of suctioning is used when oral suctioning (see Skill 25-1) is ineffective or inappropriate or when the lower airway requires removal of secretions. It involves inserting a small rubber or soft plastic tube into the nares to the pharynx or trachea and applying negative pressure to withdraw mucus.

Artificial Airway Suctioning

Endotracheal (ET) tubes and tracheostomy tubes (TTs) are artificial airways inserted to relieve airway obstruction, provide a route for mechanical ventilation, permit easy access for secretion removal, and protect the airway from gross aspiration in patients with impaired cough or gag reflexes.

Endotracheal Tubes

NSO Airway Management Module / Lesson 7

ET intubation is a procedure performed by a health care provider or specially trained personnel (e.g., certified registered nurse anesthesiologist, respiratory therapist, or rescue personnel). An ET tube is inserted through the nares (nasal ET tube) or the mouth (oral ET tube) past the epiglottis and vocal cords into the trachea (Fig. 25-2, A and B).

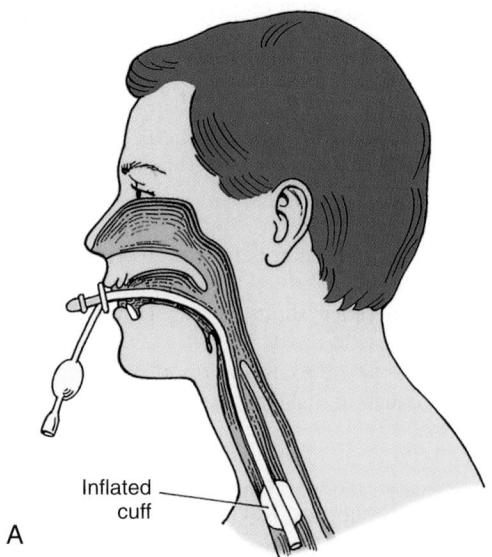

Inflated cuff

A

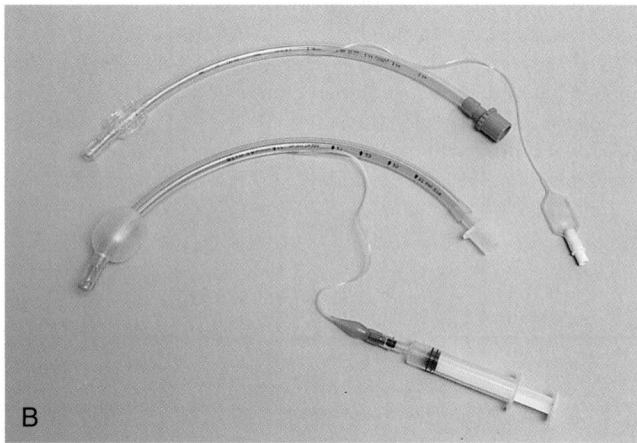

B

FIG 25-2   **A,** Endotracheal (ET) tube with inflated cuff. **B,** ET tubes with uninflated and inflated cuffs and syringe for inflation.

The length of time that an ET tube remains in place is somewhat controversial; however, in most cases after 2 to 4 weeks, if a patient still requires an artificial airway, a TT is inserted (AARC, 2010). Oral ET tubes are usually made of plastic or rubber. Adult sizes of ET tubes have a cuff molded onto the tube to prevent the aspiration of oral secretions or gastric contents into the lung and/or to obstruct the escape of air from mechanical ventilator breaths through the upper airway.

Tracheostomy Tubes

A TT can be temporary or permanent, depending on a patient's condition. It is inserted directly into the trachea through a small incision made in a patient's neck. TTs are made of several different materials, including polyvinyl chloride– or silicone-based plastics and stainless steel or metallic compounds. Metal tracheostomy tubes are thermal sensitive and must be protected from extreme heat and cold to prevent tissue injury in the patient. Most metal and plastic TTs contain an inner cannula that is temporarily withdrawn for cleaning airway-occluding mucus without removing the entire TT (see Skill 25-4) (White et al., 2010).

A cuff on a TT serves the same purpose as one on an ET tube. Cuffs are made of a balloonlike inflatable plastic; usually you manually inflate one with air (see Skill 25-5). Plastic-covered foam cuffs are self–air inflating if the inflation port is left open to the atmosphere (Frace, 2010; Regan and Dallachiesa, 2009).

Some agencies use a closed suction catheter system or in-line suction catheter device to minimize infections, especially in critically ill or immunosuppressed patients (Pedersen et al., 2009). Use of a closed-system catheter (in-line) allows quicker lower airway suctioning without applying sterile gloves or a mask and does not interrupt ventilation and oxygenation in critically ill patients (see Procedural Guideline 25-1). With a closed-system method the patient's artificial airway is not disconnected from the mechanical ventilator (Jongerden et al., 2011).

Delegation and Collaboration

The skills of nasotracheal and new artificial airway suctioning cannot be delegated to nursing assistive personnel (NAP). When the patient has an established tracheostomy and you determine that he or she is stable, you can delegate suctioning. The nurse directs the NAP about:

- Any unique modifications of the skill such as the need for supplemental oxygen or the use of a clean-versus-sterile suction technique.
- Appropriate suction limits for suctioning TT and risks of applying excessive or inadequate suction pressure.
- Signs and symptoms of hypoxemia such as change in patient's respiratory status, confusion, and restlessness and to report these signs immediately to the nurse.
- Reporting any change in secretion quality, quantity, and color.

Equipment

- ❏ Appropriate-size suction catheter (smallest diameter that will remove secretions effectively)
- ❏ Nasal or oral airway (if indicated)
- ❏ Two sterile gloves or one sterile and one clean glove
- ❏ Clean towel or paper drape
- ❏ Suction machine/source
- ❏ Mask, goggles, or face shield
- ❏ Connecting tubing (6 feet)
- ❏ Small Y-adapter (if catheter does not have a suction control port)
- ❏ Water-soluble lubricant
- ❏ Sterile basin
- ❏ Sterile normal saline solution or water, about 100 mL
- ❏ Pulse oximeter and stethoscope

STEP	RATIONALE

ASSESSMENT

1 Assess for risk factors for upper or lower airway obstruction, including obstructive lung disease, pulmonary infections, impaired mobility, sedation, decreased level of consciousness, seizures, presence of feeding tube, decreased gag or cough reflex, and decreased swallowing ability.

Presence of these risk factors can impair patient's ability to clear secretions from airway, increase risk for retaining secretions, and necessitate nasopharyngeal or nasotracheal suctioning.

2 Determine presence of apprehension, anxiety, decreased ability to concentrate, lethargy, decreased level of consciousness (especially acute), increased fatigue, dizziness, behavioral changes (especially irritability), pallor, cyanosis, dyspnea, or use of accessory muscles.

Signs and symptoms indicate hypoxia (low oxygen at cellular or tissue level), hypoxemia, or hypercapnia. Anxiety and pain consume oxygen and in turn worsen signs of hypoxia. Patients with conditions such as acute respiratory distress syndrome, pulmonary edema, and heart failure are at particular risk. for hypoxia.

3 Assess vital signs, including pulse oximetry (SpO_2) and, if on ventilator, peak inspiratory pressure and tidal volume.

Establishes baseline. Signs of hypoxia include decreased oxygen saturation, increased pulse rate, increased rate of breathing, decreased depth of breathing, elevated blood pressure, and cardiac dysrhythmias.

4 Assess signs and symptoms of upper and lower airway obstruction requiring airway suctioning, including wheezing, crackles, or gurgling on inspiration or expiration; restlessness; ineffective coughing; absent or diminished breath sounds; tachypnea; hypertension or hypotension; cyanosis; decreased level of consciousness, especially acute; or excess nasal secretions, drooling, or gastric secretions or vomitus in mouth (AARC, 2004).

Physical signs and symptoms result from decreased oxygen to tissues and pooling of secretions in upper and lower airways. Assessment is necessary before and after suction procedure (AARC, 2004).

5 Assess for additional factors that anatomically influence upper or lower airway function: recent surgery; head, chest, or neck tumors; facial or nasal trauma; and neuromuscular diseases.

Abnormal anatomy impairs normal drainage of secretions (e.g., nasal swelling, deviated septum, or facial fractures). Tumors in or around lower airway impair secretion removal by occluding or externally compressing lumen of airway.

6 Assess factors that affect volume and consistency of secretions.
   a Fluid balance

Thickened or copious secretions increase risk for airway obstruction.
Fluid overload increases amount of secretions.
Dehydration promotes thicker secretions.

   b Lack of humidity

The environment influences secretion formation and gas exchange. Airway suctioning is needed when patient cannot clear secretions effectively.

   c Infection (e.g., pneumonia)

Patients with respiratory infections are prone to increased secretions that are thicker and sometimes more difficult to expectorate.

   d Allergies, sinus drainage

Increases volume of secretions in pharynx.

7 For endotracheal suctioning assess patients' peak inspiratory pressure when on volume-controlled ventilation or tidal volume during pressure-controlled ventilation.

Increased peak inspiratory pressure or decreased tidal volume may indicate airway obstruction (AARC, 2010).

8 Weigh a patient's need for suction and consider contraindications to nasotracheal suctioning (AARC, 2004):
   a Facial or neck trauma/surgery
   b Acute head injuries
   c Bleeding disorders
   d Nasal bleeding
   e Epiglottitis or croup
   f Laryngospasm
   g Irritable airway
   h Gastric surgery

Consider these conditions only if suctioning appears to be hazardous. Passage of catheter through nasal route causes additional trauma, increases nasal bleeding, or causes severe bleeding in presence of bleeding disorders. In presence of epiglottitis, croup, laryngospasm, or irritable airway, entrance of suction catheter via nasal route causes intractable coughing, hypoxemia, and severe bronchospasm; this may necessitate emergency intubation or tracheostomy.

Clinical Decision Point *ET suctioning is necessary for patients with artificial airways. Most contraindications are relative to a patient's risk of developing adverse reactions or a worsening clinical condition as a result of the procedure. The decision to withhold suctioning to avoid a possible adverse reaction may in fact be lethal (AARC, 2010).*

9 Examine sputum microbiology data.

Certain bacteria are easier to transmit or require isolation because of virulence or antibiotic resistance.

10 Assess patient's understanding of procedure.

Reveals need for instruction.

STEP	RATIONALE

NURSING DIAGNOSES

- Deficient knowledge regarding suctioning
- Fatigue
- Impaired gas exchange
- Impaired spontaneous ventilation
- Impaired swallowing
- Ineffective airway clearance
- Ineffective breathing pattern
- Risk for aspiration
- Risk for infection

Related factors are individualized based on patient's condition or needs.

PLANNING

STEP	RATIONALE
1 Expected outcomes following completion of procedure: • Upper and lower airways demonstrate absent or diminished adventitious sounds, including gurgles, crackles, wheezes on inspiration and expiration.	Airways are cleared of secretions.
• Heart rate, blood pressure, respiratory rate and effort, and SpO_2 readings are within normal range.	When airway secretions are removed and oxygenation improves, patient's vital signs, SpO_2 readings, and respiratory assessment findings improve as well (AARC, 2004).
• Absence of drooling, gastric secretions, or vomitus in mouth; nasal secretions.	Secretions retained in oral cavity increase patient's risk for pneumonia.
• Patient verbalizes easier breathing if able.	Patent airway reduces work of breathing.
2 Explain to patient how procedure will help clear airway and relieve breathing difficulty. Explain that temporary coughing, sneezing, gagging, or shortness of breath is normal during procedure.	Encourages cooperation and minimizes risks, anxiety, and pain of procedure.
3 Explain importance of and encourage coughing to remove secretions during procedure. Practice coughing, using splinting if appropriate (see Chapter 36).	Facilitates secretion removal and reduces frequency and duration of future suctioning.
4 Have patient assume position comfortable for nurse and patient (usually semi-Fowler's or sitting upright with head hyperextended unless contraindicated).	Reduces stimulation of gag reflex, promotes patient comfort and secretion drainage, and prevents aspiration. Reduces strain on nurse's back. Hyperextension facilitates insertion of catheter into trachea.
5 Place pulse oximeter on patient's finger. Take reading and leave oximeter in place.	Provides continuous SpO_2 value to determine patient's response to suctioning.

IMPLEMENTATION

STEP	RATIONALE
1 Identify patient using two identifiers (i.e., name and birthday or name and account number) according to agency policy. Compare identifiers with information on patient's identification bracelet.	Ensures correct patient. Complies with The Joint Commission standards and improves patient safety (TJC, 2012).
2 Perform hand hygiene and apply mask, goggles, or face shield if splashing is likely.	Reduces transmission of microorganisms.
3 Connect one end of connecting tubing to suction machine and place other end in convenient location near patient. Turn suction device on and set suction pressure to as low a level as possible and yet able to effectively clear secretions (AARC, 2010). Occlude end of suction tubing to check pressure.	Excessive negative pressure damages nasal pharyngeal and tracheal mucosa and induces greater hypoxia. Lowest possible suction pressure is recommended; less than 150 mm Hg in adults (AARC, 2010; Pedersen et al., 2009).

Clinical Decision Point *After suctioning, readjust ventilator settings to preprocedural levels to avoid increased risk for oxygen toxicity and absorption, atelectasis from prolonged administration of high concentrations of oxygen, and increased carbon dioxide retention in patients with chronic obstructive lung disease (Pedersen et al., 2009).*

STEP	RATIONALE
4 Prepare suction catheter. **a *One-time-use* catheter:** (1) Using aseptic technique, open suction kit or catheter. If sterile drape is available, place it across patient's chest or on over-bed table. Do not allow suction catheter to touch any nonsterile surfaces.	Prepares catheter, maintains asepsis, and reduces transmission of microorganisms. Provides sterile surface on which to lay catheter between passes.
(2) Unwrap or open sterile basin and place on bedside table. Be careful not to touch inside of basin. Fill with about 100 mL sterile normal saline solution or water (see illustration).	Saline or water is used to clean tubing after each suction pass.

STEP	RATIONALE
(3) Open lubricant. Squeeze small amount onto open sterile catheter package without touching package. NOTE: *Lubricant is not necessary for artificial airway suctioning.*	Prepares lubricant while maintaining sterility. Using water-soluble lubricant helps avoid lipoid aspiration pneumonia. Excessive lubricant occludes catheter.
b *Closed (in-line) suction* **catheter: see Procedural Guideline 25-1.**	
5 Apply sterile glove to each hand or apply nonsterile glove to nondominant hand and sterile glove to dominant hand.	Reduces transmission of microorganisms and maintains sterility of suction catheter.
6 Pick up suction catheter with dominant hand without touching nonsterile surfaces. Pick up connecting tubing with nondominant hand. Secure catheter to tubing (see illustration).	Maintains catheter sterility. Connects catheter to suction.
7 Check that equipment is functioning properly by suctioning small amount of normal saline solution from basin.	Ensures equipment function. Lubricates internal catheter and tubing.
8 Suction airway:	
a **Nasopharyngeal and nasotracheal suctioning:**	
(1) Increase oxygen flow rate for face masks as ordered by health care provider (Lewis et al., 2011). Have patient deep breathe slowly, if possible.	Hyperoxygenation is recommended, especially in patients who are hypoxemic (AARC, 2010). May help reduce suction-induced decline in oxygenation.
(2) Lightly coat distal 6 to 8 cm (2.4 to 3.2 inches) of catheter with water-soluble lubricant.	Lubricates catheter for easier insertion.
(3) Remove oxygen delivery device, if applicable, with nondominant hand. Without applying suction and using dominant thumb and forefinger, gently but quickly insert catheter into nares. Instruct patient to deep breathe and insert catheter following natural course of nares. Slightly slant catheter downward or through mouth. Do not force through nares (see illustration).	Application of suction pressure while introducing catheter into trachea increases risk for damage to mucosa and increases risk for hypoxia. Passing catheter during inhalation improves likelihood of entering trachea.

Clinical Decision Point *Be sure to insert catheter during patient inhalation, especially if inserting it into trachea, because epiglottis is open. Do not insert during swallowing or catheter will most likely enter esophagus. Never apply suction during insertion. Patient should cough. If patient gags or becomes nauseated, catheter is most likely in esophagus, and you need to remove it.*

(a) *Nasopharyngeal* (without applying suction): In adults insert catheter about 16 cm (6.4 inches); in older children, 8 to 12 cm (3 to 5 inches); in infants and young children, 4 to 7.5 cm (1.6 to 3 inches). Rule of thumb is to insert catheter distance from tip of nose (or mouth) to angle of mandible.	Ensures that catheter tip reaches pharynx for suctioning.
(i) Apply intermittent suction for no more than 15 seconds by placing and releasing nondominant thumb over catheter vent. Slowly withdraw catheter while rotating it back and forth between thumb and forefinger.	Intermittent suction removes pharyngeal secretions.

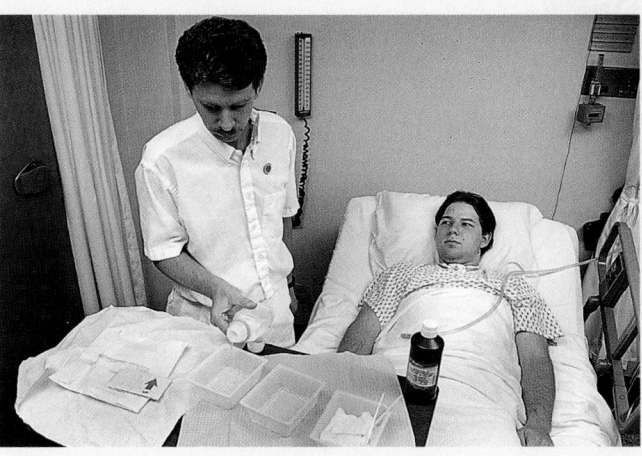

STEP 4a(2) Pouring sterile saline into tray.

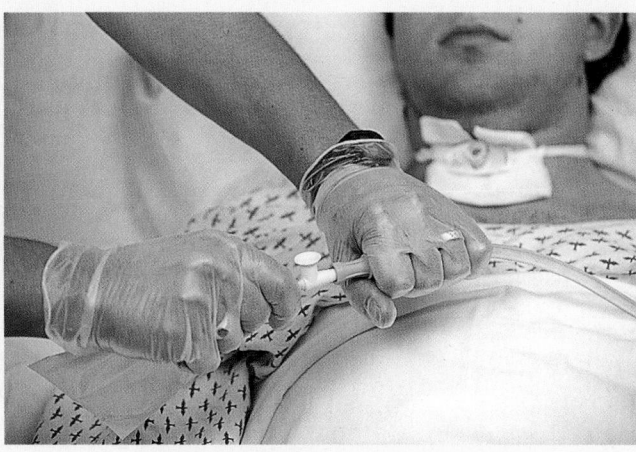

STEP 6 Attaching catheter to suction.

STEP	RATIONALE
(b) *Nasotracheal* (without applying suction): In adults insert catheter about 20 cm (8 inches); in older children about 16 to 20 cm (6 to 8 inches); and in young children and infants, 8 to 14 cm (3 to 5½ inches).	Ensures that catheter tip reaches trachea.

Clinical Decision Point *When using the nasal approach, perform tracheal suctioning before pharyngeal suctioning whenever possible. The mouth and pharynx contain more bacteria than the trachea. If copious oral secretions are present before beginning the procedure, suction mouth with oral suction device first.*

Clinical Decision Point *When there is difficulty passing the catheter, ask patient to cough or say "ahh" or try to advance the catheter during inspiration. Both measures help to open the glottis to permit passage of the catheter into the trachea.*

STEP	RATIONALE
(i) Apply intermittent or continuous suction for no more than 10 seconds by placing non-dominant thumb over vent of catheter and slowly withdrawing catheter while rotating it back and forth between dominant thumb and forefinger. Encourage patient to cough. Replace oxygen device, if applicable, and have patient deep breathe.	Both intermittent and continuous suction can cause tracheal tissue damage (Lynn-McHale Wiegand, 2011; Pederson et al., 2009). Suctioning longer than 10 seconds causes cardiopulmonary compromise, usually from hypoxemia or vagal overload (AARC, 2010).
(4) Positioning: In some instances turning patient's head helps you suction more effectively. If you feel resistance after insertion of catheter, use caution; it has probably hit carina. Pull catheter back 1 to 2 cm (0.4 to 0.8 inches) before applying suction (AARC, 2004).	Turning patient's head to side elevates bronchial passage on opposite side. Turning head to right helps with suctioning of left main-stem bronchus; turning head to left helps you suction right main-stem bronchus. Suctioning too deep may cause tracheal mucosa trauma.

Clinical Decision Point *Monitor patient's vital signs and oxygen saturation throughout suction procedure. If the patient's pulse drops more than 20 beats/min or increases more than 40 beats/min or if SpO₂ falls below 90% or 5% from baseline, stop suctioning.*

STEP	RATIONALE
(5) Rinse catheter and connecting tubing with normal saline or water until cleared.	Secretions that remain in suction catheter or connecting tubing decrease suctioning efficiency.
(6) Assess for need to repeat suctioning procedure. Do not perform more than two passes with catheter. Observe for alterations in cardiopulmonary status. When possible, allow adequate time (at least 1 minute) between suction passes for ventilation and oxygenation. Encourage patient to deep breathe with oxygen mask in place (if ordered) and cough.	Suctioning can induce hypoxemia, dysrhythmias, laryngospasm, and bronchospasm. Deep breathing ventilates and reoxygenates alveoli. Repeated passes clear airway of excessive secretions but can also remove oxygen and may induce laryngospasm (Higgins, 2009a).

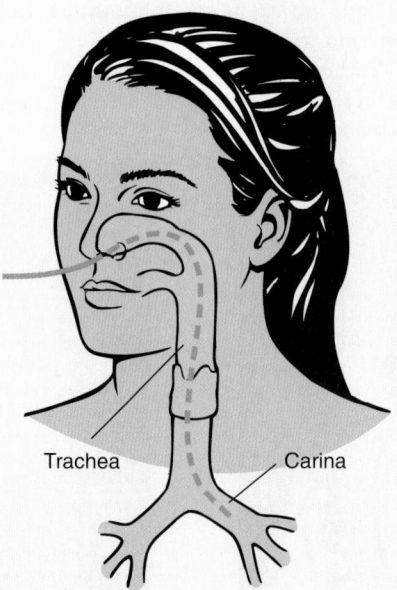

STEP 8a(3) Pathway for nasotracheal catheter progression.

STEP	RATIONALE

b Artificial airway suctioning:

(1) Hyperoxygenate patient with 100% oxygen for 30 to 60 seconds before suctioning by adjusting fractional inspired oxygen (FiO_2) setting on a mechanical ventilator or using an oxygen-enrichment program on microprocessor ventilators (AARC, 2010). Manual ventilation of a patient is not recommended; it is ineffective for providing FiO_2 of 1.0 (AARC, 2010).

Preoxygenation converts large proportion of resident lung gas to 100% oxygen to offset amount used in metabolic consumption while ventilation or oxygenation is interrupted and volume is lost during suctioning (Lewis et al., 2011; Pedersen et al., 2009).

Clinical Decision Point *Suctioning can cause elevations in intracranial pressure (ICP) in patients with head injuries. Reduce this risk by presuction hyperoxygenation, which results in hypocarbia, which in turn induces vasoconstriction. Vasoconstriction reduces the potential for an increase in ICP. Limit suctioning to 2 times with each suctioning procedure (AARC, 2004).*

(2) If patient is receiving mechanical ventilation, open swivel adapter or, if necessary, remove oxygen or humidity delivery device with nondominant hand.

Exposes artificial airway.

(3) Without applying suction, gently but quickly insert catheter into artificial airway using dominant thumb and forefinger (it is best to try to time catheter insertion into artificial airway with inspiration) until you meet resistance or patient coughs; then pull back 1 cm (0.4 inch) (Pedersen et al., 2009).

Application of suction pressure while introducing catheter into trachea increases risk for damage to tracheal mucosa and increased hypoxia. Pulling back stimulates cough and removes catheter from mucosal wall so catheter is not resting against tracheal mucosa during suctioning. Shallow suctioning is recommended to prevent tracheal mucosa trauma (AARC, 2010).

Clinical Decision Point *If unable to insert catheter past the end of the ET tube, the catheter is probably caught in the Murphy eye (i.e., side hole at the distal end of the ET tube that allows for collateral airflow in the event of tracheal main-stem intubation). If this happens, rotate the catheter to reposition it away from the Murphy eye or withdraw it slightly and reinsert with the next inhalation. Usually the catheter meets resistance at the carina. One indication that the catheter is at the carina is acute onset of coughing because the carina contains many cough receptors. Pull the catheter back 1 cm (0.4 inch) (AARC, 2004).*

(4) Apply continuous suction by placing nondominant thumb over vent of catheter; slowly withdraw catheter while rotating it back and forth between dominant thumb and forefinger (see illustration). Encourage patient to cough. Watch for respiratory distress.

Continuous suction and rotation of catheter are recommended because studies show that tracheal tissue damage from intermittent and continuous suctioning is similar (Pedersen et al., 2009). If catheter "grabs" mucosa, remove thumb to release suction.

Clinical Decision Point *If patient develops respiratory distress during the suction procedure, immediately withdraw catheter and supply additional oxygen and breaths as needed. In an emergency, administer oxygen directly through the catheter. Disconnect suction and attach oxygen at prescribed flow rate through the catheter.*

(5) If patient is receiving mechanical ventilation, close swivel adapter or replace oxygen delivery device.

Reestablishes artificial airway.

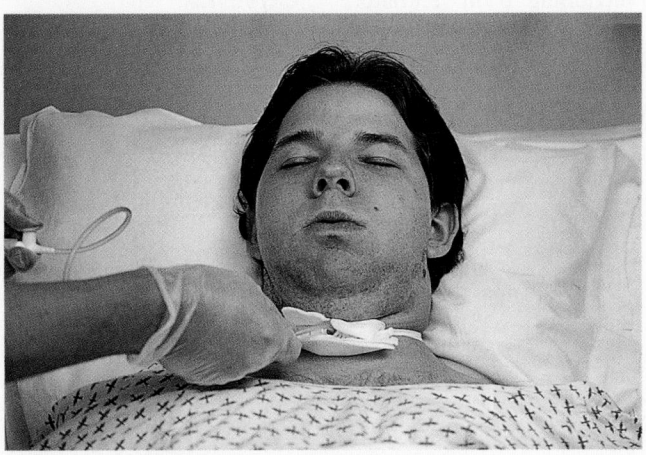

STEP 9b(4) Suctioning tracheostomy.

STEP	RATIONALE
(6) Rinse catheter and connecting tubing with normal saline until clear. Use continuous suction.	Removes catheter secretions. Secretions left in tubing decrease suctioning efficiency and provide environment for microorganism growth.
(7) Assess patient's vital signs, cardiopulmonary status, and ventilator measures for secretion clearance. Repeat Steps (1) through (6) once or twice more to clear secretions. Allow adequate time (at least 1 full minute) between suction passes.	Suctioning can induce dysrhythmias, hypoxia, and bronchospasm and impair cerebral circulation or adversely affect hemodynamic stability (Higgins, 2009a).
(8) Encourage patient to deep breathe if able. Hyperoxygenate for at least 1 minute following same technique used to preoxygenate (AARC, 2010).	Reoxygenates and reexpands alveoli. Suctioning causes hypoxemia and atelectasis. Hyperventilation should not be used routinely (AARC, 2010).
(9) When pharynx and trachea are sufficiently cleared of secretions, perform oropharyngeal suctioning to clear mouth of secretions. Do not suction nose again after suctioning mouth.	Removes upper airway secretions. More microorganisms generally are present in mouth. Upper airway is considered "clean," and lower airway is considered "sterile." You can use same catheter to suction from sterile to clean areas (e.g., tracheal suctioning to oropharyngeal suctioning) but not from clean to sterile areas.
9 When suctioning is complete, disconnect catheter from connecting tubing. Roll catheter around fingers of dominant hand. Pull glove off inside out so catheter remains coiled in glove. Pull off other glove over first glove in same way. Discard in appropriate receptacle. Turn off suction device.	Seals contaminants in gloves. Reduces transmission of micro-organisms (Higgins, 2009a).
10 Remove towel, place in laundry or appropriate receptacle, and reposition patient. (Apply clean gloves to continue personal care.)	Reduces transmission of microorganisms. Promotes comfort.
11 If indicated, readjust oxygen to original level because patient's blood oxygen level should have returned to baseline.	Prevents absorption atelectasis (i.e., tendency for airways to collapse if proximally obstructed by secretions). Prevents oxygen toxicity while allowing patient time to reoxygenate blood.
12 Discard remainder of normal saline into appropriate receptacle. If basin is disposable, discard into appropriate receptacle. If basin is reusable, rinse it out and place it in soiled utility room.	Reduces transmission of microorganisms.
13 Remove face shield and discard into appropriate receptacle. Perform hand hygiene.	Reduces transmission of microorganisms.
14 Place unopened suction kit on suction machine table or at head of bed.	Provides immediate access to suction catheter for next procedure.
15 Help patient to a comfortable position and provide oral hygiene as needed.	

EVALUATION

1 Compare patient's vital signs, cardiopulmonary assessments, and SpO$_2$ values before and after suctioning. If on ventilator, compare FiO$_2$ and tidal volumes.	Identifies physiologic effects of suction procedure to restore airway patency.
2 Ask patient if breathing is easier and if congestion is decreased.	Provides subjective confirmation that suctioning procedure has relieved airway.
3 Observe character of airway secretions.	Provides data to document presence or absence of respiratory tract infection or thickened secretions.

Unexpected Outcomes

1 Patient's respiratory status does not improve.

2 Bloody secretions are returned after suctioning.

3 Unable to pass suction catheter through naris at first attempt.

4 Patient has paroxysms of coughing.

5 No secretions obtained during suctioning.

Related Interventions

- Limit length of suctioning.
- Determine need for more frequent suctioning, possibly of shorter duration.
- Determine need for supplemental oxygen. Supply oxygen between suctioning passes.
- Notify health care provider.

- Determine amount of suction pressure used. May need to be decreased.
- Ensure that suction is completed correctly using intermittent suction and catheter rotation.
- Evaluate suctioning frequency.
- Provide more frequent oral hygiene.

- Try other naris or oral route.
- Increase lubrication of catheter.
- Insert nasal airway, especially if suctioning through patient's nares frequently.
- If obstruction is mucus, apply suction to relieve obstruction but not to mucosa. If you think obstruction is a blood clot, consult with health care provider.

- Administer supplemental oxygen.
- Allow patient to rest between passes of suction catheter.
- Consult with health care provider regarding need for inhaled bronchodilators or topical anesthetics.

- Evaluate patient's fluid status and adequacy of humidification on oxygen delivery device.
- Assess for signs of infection.
- Determine need for chest physiotherapy (see Chapter 24).

Recording and Reporting

- Record the amount, consistency, color, and odor of secretions; size of catheter; route of suctioning; and patient's response to suctioning.
- Document patient's presuctioning and postsuctioning vital signs, cardiopulmonary status, and ventilation measures (see Chapter 6).

Special Considerations

Teaching

- Instruct patient that coughing increases during the procedure.
- Explain why supplemental oxygen is given before and after suctioning if indicated.

Pediatric

- Small-diameter suction catheters required in pediatrics should be half the diameter of the child's TT (Gardner and Shirland, 2009; Hockenberry and Wilson, 2011).
- Hyperoxygenate with 100% oxygen in pediatric patients and 10% increase of baseline in neonates before suctioning (AARC, 2010).
- Perform ET suctioning only when clinically indicated in infants and neonates. Clinical signs are notable changes in respiratory rate and breath sounds, increased secretions, bradycardia, or restlessness (Gardner and Shirland, 2009).
- Thick secretions are more difficult to remove because of small diameter of suction catheter.
- Make sure that distance suctioned is not greater than 0.5 cm (0.2 inches) beyond the tip of the artificial airway. To determine distance, place catheter near a sample artificial airway (Hockenberry and Wilson, 2011).
- Infant airways have less cartilage and may collapse easily, especially in premature infants or those with reactive airways.
- Suctioning should not last beyond 5 seconds (Hockenberry and Wilson, 2011), and negative pressure should not exceed 100 mm Hg (AARC, 2010; Gardner and Shirland, 2009).

Gerontologic

- Older adults lose some properties of elastic recoil and gas exchange.
- Capillaries of older adults are often fragile, predisposing patient to bleeding problems.
- Patients with coronary artery disease are at greater risk for cardiopulmonary compromise.

Home Care

- Although most patients with airway clearance problems at home have a tracheostomy, some require nasal pharyngeal suctioning. Catheters are often used for a 24-hour period and then cleaned and disinfected; or they are cleaned with soapy water after each use and discarded after 24 hours.
- Instruct patient and family caregiver to clean and disinfect or change the secretion collection container every 24 hours according to home care or agency protocol.
- In the home setting stress the importance of brief intervals of applying suction pressure. Instruct those performing suctioning to hold their breath during the application of negative suction pressure to help them remember to not suction too long.

PROCEDURAL GUIDELINE 25-1   Closed (In-Line) Suction

NSO *Airway Management Module / Lesson 6*

Delegation and Collaboration

The skill of airway suction with a closed (in-line) suction catheter cannot be delegated to nursing assistive personnel (NAP). In special situations such as suctioning a permanent tracheostomy, this procedure may be delegated to NAP. The nurse is responsible for cardiopulmonary assessment and evaluation of patient. The nurse directs the NAP about:

- Any individualized aspects of patient care that pertain to suctioning (e.g., position, duration of suction, pressure settings).
- Expected quality, quantity, and color of secretions and to inform the nurse immediately if there are changes.
- Patient's anticipated response to suction and to immediately report to the nurse changes in vital signs, complaints of pain, shortness of breath, confusion, or increased restlessness.

Equipment

- ❏ Closed-system or in-line suction catheter
- ❏ Suction machine
- ❏ Connecting tubing (6 feet)
- ❏ Two clean gloves (*optional*)
- ❏ Mask, goggles, or face shield
- ❏ Pulse oximeter and stethoscope

Procedural Steps

1. Perform assessment as in Skill 25-2.
2. Identify patient using two identifiers (i.e., name and birthday or name and account number) according to agency policy. Compare identifiers with information on patient's identification bracelet.
3. Explain the procedure to patient and the importance of coughing during the suctioning procedure. Even if patients cannot speak, they deserve to have information regarding the procedure.
4. Help patient assume a position of comfort for both patient and nurse, usually semi- or high-Fowler's position. Place towel across patient's chest.
5. Perform hand hygiene, apply clean gloves and face shield, and attach suction.
   a. In many agencies a respiratory therapist attaches the catheter to the mechanical ventilator circuit. If catheter is not already in place, open suction catheter package using aseptic technique and attach closed suction catheter to ventilator circuit by removing swivel adapter and placing closed suction catheter apparatus on ET or TT. Connect Y on mechanical ventilator circuit to closed suction catheter with flex tubing (see illustrations A and B).
   b. Connect one end of connecting tubing to suction machine; connect other end to the end of a closed-system or in-line suction catheter. Turn suction device on, set vacuum regulator to appropriate negative pressure, and check pressure. Many closed-system suction catheters require slightly higher suction pressures (consult manufacturer guidelines).
6. Hyperoxygenate patient (usually 100% oxygen) by adjusting the FiO_2 setting on the ventilator or by using a temporary oxygen-enrichment program available on microprocessor

ventilators (AARC, 2010). Manual ventilation is not recommended.

7. Pick up suction catheter enclosed in plastic sleeve with dominant hand.
8. Wait until patient inhales to insert catheter. Use a repeating maneuver of pushing catheter and sliding (or pulling) plastic sleeve back between thumb and forefinger until resistance is felt or patient coughs. Pull back 1 cm (0.5 inches) before applying suction to avoid tissue damage to carina.
9. Encourage patient to cough and apply suction by squeezing on suction control mechanism while withdrawing catheter. Apply continuous suction for no longer than 10 seconds as you remove the suction catheter. Be sure to withdraw catheter completely into plastic sheath so it does not obstruct airflow.
10. Reassess cardiopulmonary status, including pulse oximetry and ventilator measures, to determine need for subsequent suctioning or complications. Repeat Steps 5 to 9 one more time to clear secretions. Allow adequate time (at least 1 full minute) between suction passes for ventilation and reoxygenation.
11. When airway is clear, withdraw catheter completely into sheath. Be sure that colored indicator line on catheter is visible in the sheath. Squeeze vial or push syringe while applying suction to rinse inner lumen of catheter. Use at least 5- to 10-mL of saline to rinse the catheter until it is clear of retained

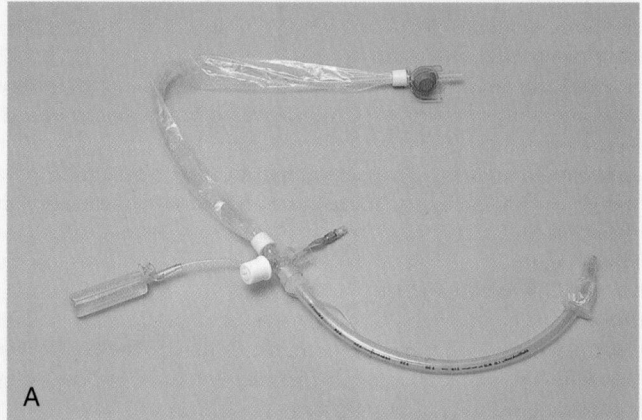

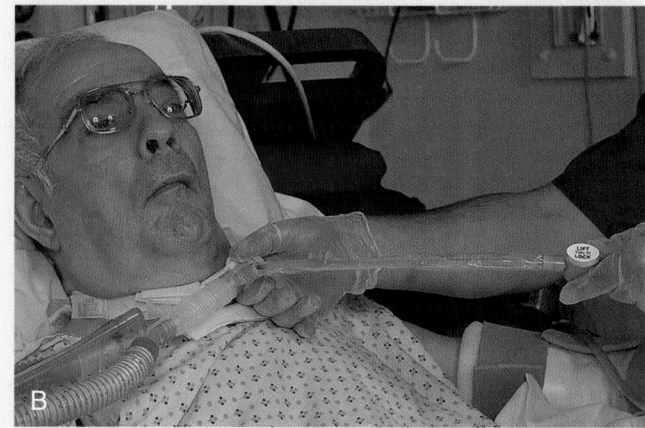

STEP 5a A, Closed-system suction catheter attached to endotracheal tube. **B,** Suctioning tracheostomy with closed-system suction catheter.

PROCEDURAL GUIDELINE 25-1   Closed (In-Line) Suction—cont'd

secretions, which can cause bacterial growth and increase the risk for infection. Lock suction mechanism if applicable and turn off suction.

12 Hyperoxygenate for at least 1 minute by following the same technique used to preoxygenate (AARC, 2010).

13 If patient requires oral or nasal suctioning, perform Skill 25-1 or 25-2 with separate standard suction catheter.

14 Reposition patient. Remove gloves and face shield, discard into appropriate receptacle, and perform hand hygiene.

15 Compare patient's respiratory assessments before and after suctioning, observe airway secretions, and document findings.

Clinical Decision Point *Based on research, closed (in-line) suctioning does not decrease the risk of ventilator-associated pneumonia (VAP) when compared to open suctioning (Jongerden et al., 2011; Subirana et al., 2010).*

SKILL 25-3   Performing Endotracheal Tube Care

NSO *Airway Management Module / Lesson 7*

Endotracheal (ET) tubes are flexible, plastic tubes placed in the mouth or through the nose and advanced down into the trachea to establish short-term artificial airways to administer mechanical ventilation, relieve upper airway obstruction, protect against aspiration, and clear secretions. Routine care maintains correct position of the tube and good hygiene.

After insertion of an ET tube, the cuff is inflated. Preventing cuff-related problems is a critical component of nursing care and depends on securing the tube and inflating the cuff properly. In many agencies these functions are shared by nursing and respiratory therapy staff. Allowing an ET tube to slip lower into the airway can prevent ventilation of a lung, usually the left lung. Allowing it to slide too far up the tracheobronchial tree can allow air to escape through or damage the vocal cords. Properly securing an ET tube prevents incidental extubation from coughing or pulling on the tube. Additional risks of movement of an artificial airway are tracheal stenosis, tracheomalacia, erosion of the innominate artery, and tracheoesophageal fistula, particularly when the cuff is overinflated. Proper nursing care reduces risks for each of these complications (Stonecypher, 2010).

Once a tube is inserted, confirmation of placement is achieved using a chest x-ray film or capnography. Capnography is the noninvasive measurement of the partial pressure of carbon dioxide (CO_2) in exhaled breath expressed as the CO_2 concentration over time. It is recommended as a reliable way to validate the correct placement of an ET tube (AARC, 2011). The carbon dioxide monitor measures CO_2 directly from the airway, with the sensor located on the airway adapter at the hub of the ET.

After a tube is inserted and secured and the cuff is inflated (see Skill 25-5), your chief concern is to maintain patency of the ET tube. In patients who cannot clear their secretions, periodic suctioning of the artificial airway achieves airway patency.

Ventilator-associated pneumonia (VAP) occurred in 10% to 20% of ventilated patients who ventilated for more than 2 days (Browne et al., 2011; Scherzer, 2010). VAP causes 90% of health care–acquired infections in ventilated patients and causes an increase in hospital length of stay by 5 to 7 days and a 50% higher mortality rate (Oleska & Muscedere, 2011; Scherzer, 2010). VAP is defined as developing after 48 hours following intubation (Niël-Weise et al., 2011). Best-practice guidelines indicate that the following interventions are advantageous in preventing VAP:

- Elevate the head of the bed at 30 to 45 degrees to prevent aspiration (Selvaraj, 2010; Stonecypher, 2010).
- Change patient position every 2 hours to decrease risk for atelectasis, pulmonary infections, pressure ulcers, discomfort, and urinary stasis (Winkelman and Chiang, 2010).
- Provide oral care with chlorhexidine by swab every 8 hours. If chlorhexidine is contraindicated, a toothbrush can be used to remove dental plaque organisms. Toothettes are not adequate to clean the dental plaque, but they may be used between brushing for comfort (Ames, 2011; Browne et al., 2011; Rewa and Muscedere, 2011).
- Maintain the ET cuff pressures at 20 cm H_2O to decrease movement of secretions to the lower airways (Stonecypher, 2010).
- Carefully monitor patient for aspiration when enteral feedings are infusing.
- Change ventilator circuits every 48 hours because of potential bacteria within tubing condensation (Stonecypher, 2010).
- Remove subglottal secretions every 4 to 6 hours or before position changes (Browne et al., 2011; Scherzer, 2010; Stonecypher, 2010).

Delegation and Collaboration

This skill of performing ET care cannot be delegated to nursing assistive personnel (NAP). NAP may assist the nurse with ET care. The nurse directs the NAP to:

- Immediately report any signs of respiratory problems or increased airway secretions.
- Immediately report if the ET tube appears to have moved or become obstructed or dislodged.
- Immediately report changes in patient's mood, level of consciousness, irritability, vital signs, or decreased pulse oximetry value.

Equipment

- ❏ Towel
- ❏ ET and oropharyngeal suction equipment
- ❏ 1- or 1½-inch-wide adhesive or waterproof tape (do not use paper or silk tape) or commercial ET tube holder and mouth guard (follow manufacturer instructions for securing)
- ❏ Clean gloves (two pairs)
- ❏ Adhesive remover swab or acetone on cotton ball
- ❏ Chlorhexidine swabs, nonalcohol mouthwash or toothpaste
- ❏ Toothbrush, toothette, and shaving supplies

❏ One wet and one soapy washcloth or paper towels
❏ Clean 2 × 2–inch gauze
❏ Tincture of benzoin, liquid adhesive, or skin preparation pads

❏ Tongue blade (*optional*)
❏ Mask, goggles, face shield (if indicated)
❏ Stethoscope

STEP	RATIONALE
ASSESSMENT	
1 Auscultate lungs and observe respiratory rate and depth.	Provides baseline measure of ventilation.
2 Observe for soiled or loose tape; pressure sore on nares, lips, or corner of mouth; excess nasal or oral secretions; patient moving tube with tongue, biting tube or tongue; tube repositioned by health care provider or other specially trained personnel; foul-smelling mouth.	Presence of ET tube impairs ability of patient to swallow oral secretions. Patient is at increased risk for developing pressure areas from impaired circulation as tube is pulled or pressed against mucosal tissues.
3 Observe for factors that increase risk for complications from ET tube: type and size of tube, movement of tube up and down trachea (in and out), cuff overinflation or underinflation, duration of tube placement, presence of facial trauma, malnutrition, and neck or thoracic radiation.	Tube rotating from side to side can cause pressure sores. Tube moving up and down trachea predisposes patient to develop tracheoesophageal fistula or tracheomalacia. Tube can become dislodged from lower airway (incidental extubation), or it can enter main-stem bronchus. Cuff underinflation increases risk for aspiration, whereas overinflation may cause ischemia or necrosis of tracheal tissue from obstruction of capillary bed. Patient can "tongue" oral tube easily and dislodge it. Longer duration of intubation is associated with increased risk for lower airway complications, as in facial trauma.
4 Determine proper ET tube depth as noted by centimeters at lip or gum line. This line is marked on tube and recorded in patient's record at time of intubation.	Ensures that tube is proper depth to adequately ventilate both lungs and that it is not too high, which causes vocal cord damage, or too low, which results in right main-stem intubation, in which only the right lung is ventilated.
5 Assess patient's knowledge of procedure.	Encourages cooperation, minimizes risks and anxiety. Identifies teaching needs.

NURSING DIAGNOSES

- Deficient knowledge regarding ET care
- Fatigue
- Impaired gas exchange

- Impaired skin integrity
- Impaired spontaneous ventilation
- Impaired swallowing
- Ineffective airway clearance

- Ineffective breathing pattern
- Risk for aspiration
- Risk for infection

Related factors are individualized based on patient's condition or needs.

PLANNING	
1 Expected outcomes following completion of procedure:	
• ET tube remains in correct position in patient's trachea evidenced by depth of tube same as when started or as ordered (same centimeter marking at gums or lips); bilateral breath sounds are equal.	Maintaining ET position promotes adequate ventilation of lungs. Complications of lower airway and vocal cord trauma prevented.
• Patient's skin around mouth and oral mucous membranes does not have pressure areas or other injury from biting.	ET tube does not place undue pressure against corners of mouth, causing pressure area. Patient is not able to bite inner cheeks or tongue.
2 Explain procedure and patient's need to participate, including not biting or moving ET tube with tongue; trying not to cough when tape is off ET tube; keeping hands down and not pulling on tubing.	Reduces anxiety, encourages cooperation, and reduces risks.

IMPLEMENTATION	
1 Identify patient using two identifiers (i.e., name and birthday or name and account number) according to agency policy. Compare identifiers with information on patient's identification bracelet.	Ensures correct patient. Complies with The Joint Commission standards and improves patient safety (TJC, 2012).
2 Perform hand hygiene. Apply clean gloves and mask, goggles, or face shield if indicated.	Reduces transmission of microorganisms.

STEP	RATIONALE
3 Administer endotracheal, nasopharyngeal, or oropharyngeal suction (see Skills 25-1 and 25-2 and Procedural Guideline 25-1).	Removes secretions. Diminishes patient's need to cough during procedure.
4 Connect oral suction catheter to suction source. Help patient to comfortable position.	Prepares patient for oropharyngeal suctioning.
5 Prepare securement option:	
a *Tape method*: Cut piece of tape long enough to go completely around patient's head from naris to naris plus 15 cm (6 inches): adult, 30 to 60 cm (12 to 24 inches). Lay tape adhesive-side up on bedside table. Cut and lay 8 to 15 cm (3 to 6 inches) of second piece of tape, adhesive sides together, in center of the long strip to prevent tape from sticking to hair. Smaller strip of tape should cover area between ears around back of head.	Preparing tape ahead allows you to have one hand positioned on ET tube throughout procedure. Adhesive tape needs to encircle head below ears with sufficient tape left to wrap around tube.
b *Commercially available ET tube holder*: Open package per manufacturer instructions. Set device aside with head guard in place and Velcro strips open.	Commercial devices are latex free, fast, and convenient. These devices avoid need for tape and resultant skin breakdown and are easily applied in presence of facial hair.
6 Instruct assistant to apply pair of gloves and hold ET tube firmly at patient's lips or nares. Note number marking on ET tube at gum line or lips.	Reduces transmission of microorganisms. Maintains proper tube position and prevents incidental extubation.

Clinical Decision Point *Do not allow assistant to hold the tube away from the lips or nares. Doing so allows too much "play" in the tube and increases the risk for tube movement and accidental extubation. Never let go of the ET tube because it could become dislodged.*

STEP	RATIONALE
7 Remove old tape or device.	Provides access to skin under tape for assessment and hygiene. Reduces transmission of microorganisms.
a *Tape*: Carefully remove tape from ET tube and patient's face. If tape is difficult to remove, moisten with (soapy) wet washcloth, water, or adhesive tape remover. Discard tape in appropriate receptacle if nearby.	
b *Commercially available device*: Remove Velcro strips from ET tube and remove ET tube holder from patient.	Velcro adhesive strips hold ET tube in place and provide marker to measure distance to patient's lips or gums. These devices all permit access to patient's mouth and lips for ease in oropharyngeal suctioning and oral hygiene.
8 Remove any secretions or adhesive from patient's face.	Promotes hygiene. Adhesive causes damage to skin. Prevents poor adhesion of new tape.
a Use adhesive remover swab to remove excess adhesive left on face after tape removal. Wash adhesive remover from face.	
9 Remove oral airway or bite block, if present, and place on towel.	Provides access to and complete observation of patient's oral cavity.

Clinical Decision Point *Do not remove oral airway if patient is actively biting ET tube. Wait until tape is partially or completely secured to ET tube.*

STEP	RATIONALE
10 Clean mouth, gums, and teeth opposite ET tube with 5 mL of 0.12% chlorhexidine swabs every 8 hours unless contraindicated; brush teeth thoroughly and rinse with nonalcohol mouthwash. Administer oropharyngeal suctioning with Yankauer suction catheter during brushing and rinsing.	Promotes hygiene and reduces risk for VAP. Chlorhexidine swabs provide oral decontamination associated with lower risk of VAP (Browne et al., 2011). Alcohol-based mouthwashes dry oral mucosa (Lewis et al., 2011). Suctioning removes pooled secretions.
11 *Oral ET tube only*: Remembering "cm" ET tube marking at level of gums or lips, with help of assistant move ET tube to opposite side or center of mouth. Do not change tube depth. Reposition tube on opposite side or center of mouth at least every 24 to 48 hours according to agency protocol (oral ET tube only).	Prevents formation of pressure sores at sides of patient's mouth. Ensures correct position of tube. Measuring tube at lip line can be distorted from edema, trauma, or disease process.
12 Repeat oral cleaning as in Step 10 on opposite side of mouth.	Removes secretions from mouth and oral pharynx.
13 Clean face and neck with soapy washcloth, rinse, and dry. Shave male patient as necessary.	Moisture and beard growth prevent adhesive tape adherence.
14 Pour small amount of skin protectant or liquid adhesive on clean 2 × 2–inch gauze and dot on upper lip (oral ET tube) or across nose (nasal ET tube) and cheeks to ear. Allow to dry completely.	Protects skin from tape burns and makes more adherent.

STEP	RATIONALE
15 Secure ET tube.	
a Tape method:	
(1) Slip tape under patient's head and neck, adhesive side up. Take care not to twist tape or catch hair. Do not allow tape to stick to itself. It helps to gently stick end of tape to tongue blade, which serves as guide. Then slide tongue blade under patient's neck. Center tape so double-faced tape extends around back of neck from ear to ear.	Positions tape to secure ET tube in proper position.
(2) On one side of face secure tape from ear to nares (nasal ET tube) or over lip to ET tube (oral ET tube). Tear remaining tape in half lengthwise, forming two pieces that are 2 cm (0.8 inch) wide. Secure bottom half of tape across upper lip (oral ET tube) or across top of nose (nasal ET tube) to opposite ear (see illustration A). Wrap top half of tape around tube and up from bottom (see illustration B). Tape should encircle tube at least 2 times for security.	Secures tape to face. Using top tape to wrap prevents downward drag on ET tube.
(3) Gently pull other side of tape firmly to pick up slack and secure to opposite side of face and ET tube same as first piece (see illustration). NOTE: ET tube is secured. Assistant can release hold. (You may want assistant to help reinsert oral airway.)	Secures tape to face and tube. ET tube should be at same depth at lips or gum line. Check earlier assessment for verification of tube depth in centimeters.

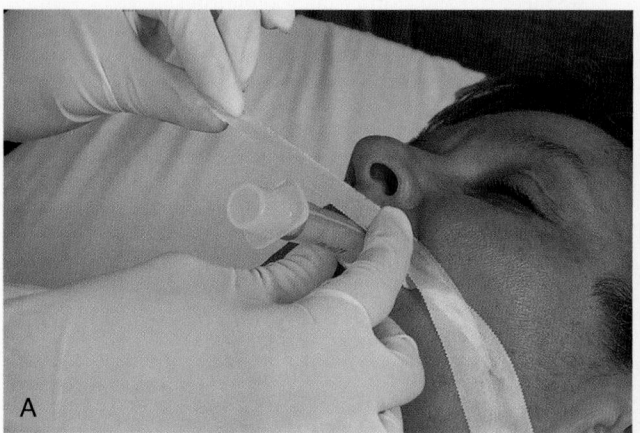 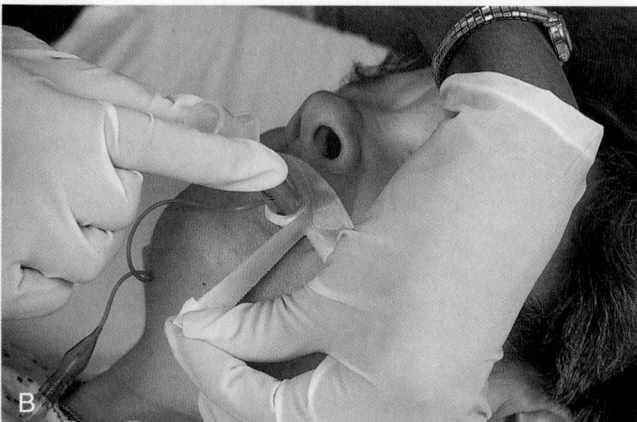

STEP 15a(2)   **A,** Securing bottom half of tape across patient's upper lip. **B,** Securing top half of tape around tube.

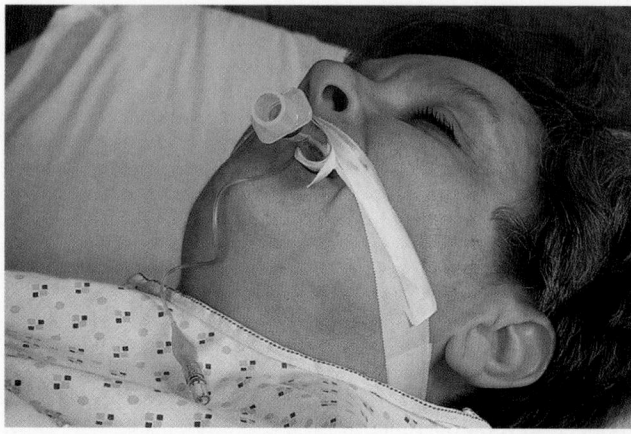

STEP 15a(3)   Tape securing endotracheal tube.

STEP	RATIONALE
b Commercially available device:	
(1) Thread ET tube through opening designed to secure it. Be sure that pilot balloon is accessible.	Commercially available holders have a slit in front of holder designed to secure ET tube.
(2) Place strips of ET holder under patient at occipital region of head.	
(3) Verify that ET tube is at established depth using lip or gum line marker as guide.	Ensures that ET tube remains at correct depth as determined during assessment.
(4) Attach Velcro strips at base of patient's head. Leave 1 cm (0.5 inch) slack in strips (see illustration).	
(5) Verify that tube is secure, it does not move forward from patient's mouth or backward down into patient's throat, and there are no pressure areas on oral mucosa or occipital region of head.	Tube must be secure so it remains at correct depth. It can be secured without being tight and causing pressure.
16 Remove and clean oral airway in warm soapy water and rinse well. Half hydrogen peroxide and half normal saline solution aids in removal of crusted secretions. Nonalcohol mouthwash freshens patient's mouth. Shake excess water from oral airway. Be sure to rinse hydrogen peroxide mixture from airway.	Promotes hygiene. Reduces transmission of microorganisms.
17 Reinsert oral airway without pushing tongue into oropharynx and secure with tape (see Chapter 27).	Prevents patient from biting ET tube and allows access for oropharyngeal suctioning.
18 Discard soiled items in appropriate receptacle. Remove towel and place in laundry.	Reduces transmission of microorganisms.
19 Reposition patient.	Promotes comfort.
20 Remove gloves and mask, goggles, or face shield; discard in receptacle; and perform hand hygiene. (Assistant performs same steps.) Place clean items (e.g., tincture of benzoin, mouthwash, excess swabs) in place of storage.	Reduces transmission of microorganisms. Ensures that contaminated gloves and hands do not touch clean items.

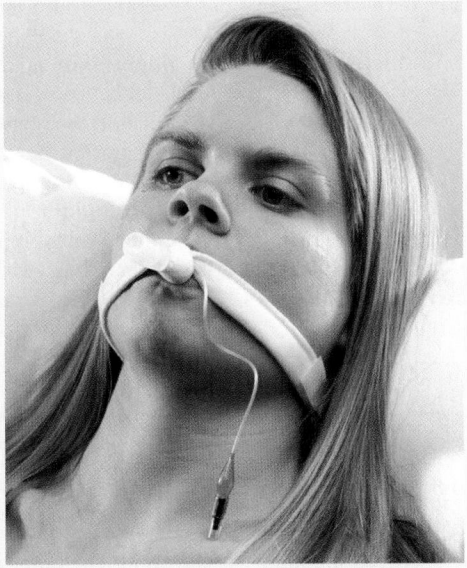

STEP 15b(4) Endotracheal tube holder in place with pilot balloon accessible and Velcro strips secured. (*Courtesy Dale Medical Products, Plainesville, Mass.*)

EVALUATION

1 Compare respiratory assessments before and after ET tube care.	Identifies any changes in presence and quality of breath sounds after procedure.
2 Observe depth and position of ET tube according to health care provider recommendation.	Position of ET tube should not be altered.
3 Assess security of tape by gently tugging at tube.	Tape should remain attached to face. Patient may cough during tugging.
4 Assess skin around mouth and oral mucous membranes for intactness and pressure sores.	Tape should not tear skin. Pressure areas should be absent.

Unexpected Outcomes

1 Patient is accidentally extubated.

2 ET tube moves in airway.

3 Patient has unequal breath sounds.

4 Patient has pressure sores from tube.

5 Air escapes around tube.

Related Interventions

- Remain with patient while calling for assistance.
- Ventilate with bag-valve-mask as needed.
- Assess patient for airway patency, spontaneous breathing, and vital signs.
- Prepare for reintubation.

- Repeat taping or securing procedure.
- In very active patients without facial injury who are at risk for self-extubation, consider applying second piece of tape around back of head.

- Evaluate ET tube for proper depth before and after tube care. If it is deeper or shallower, notify health care provider, who may order a chest x-ray film. Then reposition tube only if allowed by agency and you have received appropriate instructions.
- Suction patient.

- Increase frequency of ET tube care.
- Apply antimicrobial ointment per agency protocol.
- Align oxygen and humidity supply tubing so they do not pull ET tube, creating pressure sores.
- Monitor for infection. If skin tear is present on cheeks or over nose or upper lip, apply protective barrier such as stoma adhesive patch or hydrocolloid dressing and apply tape to this.

- Verify position of tube and check for proper cuff inflation. If tube position is incorrect, reposition according to protocol or notify health care provider (see Skill 25-5).

Recording and Reporting

- Document respiratory assessments before and after care, patient's tolerance of procedure, ordered and actual depth of ET tube, frequency of ET tube care, integrity of oral and nasal mucosa, pressure sore care, and frequency and extent of ET tube care.
- Report unequal breath sounds, accidental extubation, or respiratory distress to the health care provider.

Special Considerations
Teaching

- Instruct patient and family caregivers not to manipulate the ET tube, tape, or ET tube holder. If patient is complaining or appears uncomfortable, instruct family caregiver to ask for the nurse.

- Instruct patient and family caregiver to inform the nurse if the tube causes gagging. Repositioning of the tube and/or sedation are options for reducing gagging.

Pediatric

- Neonatal and pediatric procedures for securing ET tubes and suctioning airways vary (Hockenberry and Wilson, 2011).
- Infant skin is more prone to tearing when removing tape (Hockenberry and Wilson, 2011).
- Because of infants' delicate skin, you will not always use skin preparation before securing ET tube. ET tube holders are best used in this population.

Gerontologic

- Older adult skin is more prone to tearing when removing tape.
- Older adults with tendency toward inadequate nutrition are more prone to complications (e.g., infection, breakdown of oral mucosa).

SKILL 25-4   Performing Tracheostomy Care

NSO *Airway Management Module / Lesson 8*

 Video Clip

A tracheostomy is a 51- to 76-mm (2- to 3-inch) curved metal or plastic tube inserted into a stoma through the neck and into the trachea to maintain a patent airway. It is placed in patients who require long-term airway management because of airway obstruction, airway clearance needs, and long-term intubation (Regan and Dallachiesa, 2009). A tracheostomy offers advantages over long-term endotracheal (ET) tube placement such as decreased laryngeal and tracheal tissue injury, ease of breathing, and access for better oral hygiene (White et al., 2010). Some patients with a tracheostomy tube are able to cough secretions out of the tube completely, whereas others are only able to cough secretions up into it.

A tracheostomy tube has a flange that fits against a patient's neck and an outer cannula or primary airway. It may have a removable inner cannula for cleaning and an inflatable cuff that surrounds the outer cannula (Fig. 25-3, A). An inflation tube and valve connect to the cuff for inflation. The pilot balloon expands and contracts on inflation and deflation. An inflated cuff keeps the tube stable within the trachea.

Standards for care include properly securing the tube, inflating the cuff to an appropriate pressure, maintaining patency by suctioning, and providing oral hygiene. A tracheostomy tube can cause granulation tissue to form on the vocal cords, epiglottis, or trachea secondary to inappropriate cuff inflation. (See Cuff inflation in Skill 25-5.)

An intubated patient is unable to speak because of placement of a tracheostomy tube which prevents normal airflow over and vibration of the vocal cords. Use verbal and nonverbal communication skills when you care for an intubated patient. Alphabet

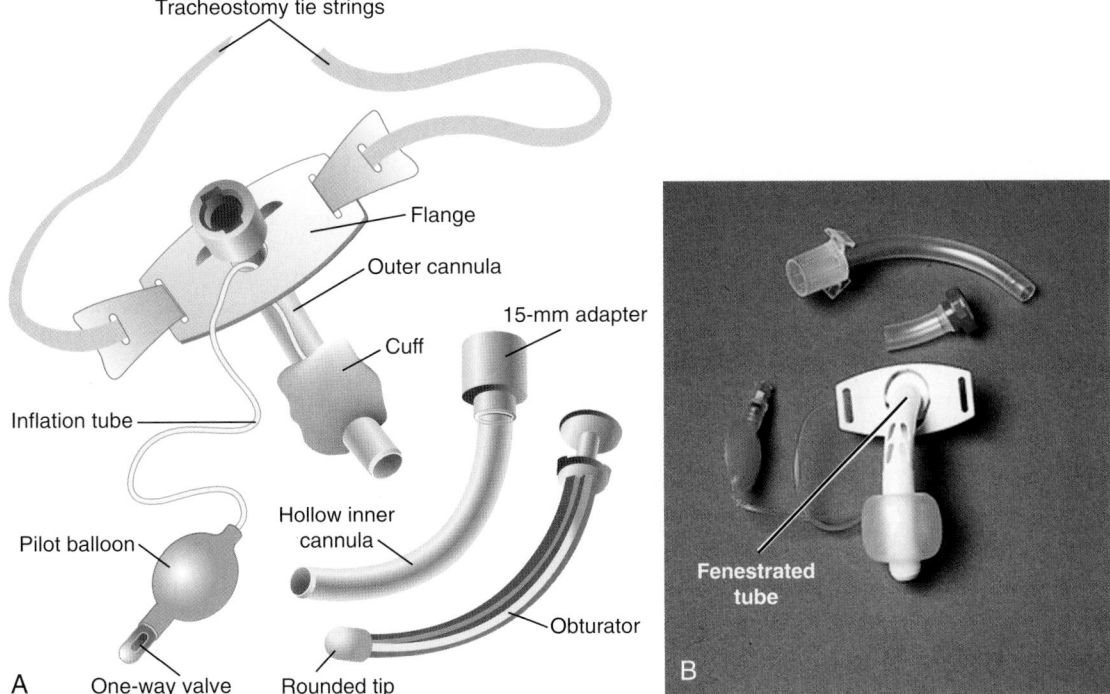

Tracheostomy tie strings

Flange

Outer cannula

15-mm adapter

Cuff

Inflation tube

Pilot balloon

Hollow inner cannula

Obturator

A One-way valve Rounded tip

B

Fenestrated tube

FIG 25-3 A, Parts of tracheostomy tube. B, Fenestrated tracheostomy tube with cuff, inner cannula, decannulation plug, and pilot balloon. (*From Lewis SL: Medical-surgical nursing: assessment and management of clinical problems, ed 8, St Louis, 2011, Mosby.*)

charts, pen and paper, slates or chalkboards, or magnetic pen doodle boards are some common communication tools. You may place a speaking valve over some tracheostomy tubes, which allows a patient to speak (Regan and Dallachiesa, 2009). One type of tracheostomy tube is fenestrated, which means that the outer cannula has precut openings (see Fig. 25-3, *B*). When the inner cannula is removed and the cuff is deflated, patients can speak. A speech pathologist must evaluate patients for aspiration risk before cuff deflation and inner cannula removal.

Delegation and Collaboration

The skill of performing tracheostomy care is not routinely delegated to nursing assistive personnel (NAP). In some settings patients who have well-established tracheostomy tubes may have the care delegated to NAP. The nurse is responsible for assessing a patient and evaluating for proper artificial airway care. The nurse directs the NAP to:

- Immediately report any changes in patient's respiratory status, level of consciousness, confusion, restlessness or irritability, or in level of comfort.
- Immediately report any dislodgement or excessive movement of the tracheostomy tube.

- Immediately report abnormal color of the tracheal stoma and drainage.

Equipment

- ❏ Bedside table
- ❏ Towel
- ❏ Tracheostomy suction supplies (see Skill 25-2)
- ❏ Sterile tracheostomy care kit, if available (be sure to collect supplies listed that are not available in kit), or two sterile 4 × 4–inch gauze pads
  - Sterile cotton-tipped applicators
  - Sterile tracheostomy dressing (precut and sewn surgical dressing)
  - Sterile basin
  - Normal saline
  - Small sterile brush (pipe cleaner) (or disposable inner cannula)
  - Roll of twill tape, tracheostomy ties, or tracheostomy holder
  - Scissors
- ❏ Pulse oximeter
- ❏ Clean gloves (two pair)
- ❏ Mask, goggles, or face shield

STEPS	RATIONALE

ASSESSMENT

1 Observe for excess peristomal secretions, excess intratracheal secretions, soiled or damp tracheostomy ties, soiled or damp tracheostomy dressing, diminished airflow through tracheostomy tube, or signs and symptoms of airway obstruction requiring suctioning (see Skill 25-2).

Indicate need for tracheostomy care caused by presence of secretions at stoma site or within tracheostomy tube.

STEPS	RATIONALE
2 Assess patient's hydration status, humidity delivered to airway, status of existing infection, patient's nutritional status, and ability to cough.	Determines factors that affect amount and consistency of secretions in tracheostomy and patient's ability to clear airway.
3 Assess vital signs, oxygen saturation, lung sounds, and patient's ability to clear airway.	Provides baseline to determine patient response to therapy.
4 Assess patient's understanding of and ability to perform own tracheostomy care.	Allows you to identify potential need for instruction.
5 Check when tracheostomy care was last performed.	Tracheostomy care is provided at least every 4 to 8 hours and more often if indicated (e.g., increased airway or stoma secretions, infection [airway or stoma]) (Regan and Dallachiesa, 2009).

NURSING DIAGNOSES

- Deficient knowledge regarding tracheostomy care
- Impaired gas exchange
- Impaired spontaneous ventilation

- Ineffective airway clearance
- Ineffective breathing pattern
- Risk for aspiration

- Risk for impaired skin integrity
- Risk for infection

Related factors are individualized based on patient's condition or needs.

PLANNING

1 Expected outcomes following completion of procedure:	
• Inner and outer cannulas of tracheostomy tube are free of secretions; ties are clean, secured snugly, and tied in double square knot.	Tracheostomy tube is patent and secure, optimizing amount of oxygen delivered to patient and limiting risk of infection from retained secretions.
• Stoma site is pink, does not bleed, and is free of secretions and signs of infection.	Indicates absence of infection at stoma site. Dry, intact tracheostomy stoma reduces risk for subsequent systemic infection.
2 Have another nurse or NAP assist in this procedure (Lewis et al., 2011).	Prevents accidental extubation of tracheostomy tube.
3 Explain procedure and patient's participation.	Encourages cooperation, minimizes risks, and reduces anxiety.
4 Help patient to position comfortable for both nurse and patient (usually supine or semi-Fowler's).	Promotes patient comfort and prevents nurse muscle strain.
5 Place towel across patient's chest.	Reduces transmission of microorganisms.

IMPLEMENTATION

1 Identify patient using two identifiers (i.e. name and birthday or name and account number) according to agency policy. Compare identifiers with information on patient's identification bracelet.	Ensures correct patient. Complies with The Joint Commission standards and improves patient safety (TJC, 2012).
2 Perform hand hygiene. Apply clean gloves and face shield if applicable.	Reduces transmission of microorganisms.
3 Apply pulse oximeter sensor.	Provides monitoring for oxygen desaturation during procedure.
4 Suction tracheostomy (see Skill 25-2). Before removing gloves, remove soiled tracheostomy dressing and discard in glove with coiled catheter.	Removes secretions to avoid occluding outer cannula while inner cannula is removed. Reduces need for patient to cough.
5 Perform hand hygiene. Prepare equipment on bedside table.	Prepares equipment and allows for smooth, organized completion of tracheostomy care.
a Open sterile tracheostomy kit. Open two 4 × 4–inch gauze packages using aseptic technique and pour normal saline on one package. Leave second package dry. Open two cotton-tipped swab packages and pour normal saline on one package. Do not recap normal saline.	
b Open sterile tracheostomy dressing package.	
c Unwrap sterile basin and pour about 0.5 to 2 cm (½ to 1 inch) of normal saline into it.	
d Open small sterile brush package and place aseptically into sterile basin.	
e Prepare length of twill tape long enough to go around patient's neck 2 times, about 60 to 75 cm (25 to 30 inches) for an adult. Cut ends on diagonal. Lay aside in dry area.	Cutting ends of tie on diagonal aids in inserting tie through eyelet.

STEPS	RATIONALE
f If using commercially available tracheostomy tube holder, open package according to manufacturer directions.	
6 Hyperoxygenate patient using ventilator settings or by applying oxygen source loosely over tracheostomy.	Required if patient has oxygen saturation levels below 92% (Higgins, 2009b). Helps to reduce amount of oxygen desaturation.
7 Apply sterile gloves. Keep dominant hand sterile throughout procedure.	Reduces transmission of microorganisms.

Clinical Decision Point *For tracheostomy tube with no inner cannula or Kistner button, continue with Step 9.*

STEPS	RATIONALE
8 **Care of tracheostomy with inner cannula:**	
a While touching only outer aspect of tube, unlock and remove inner cannula with nondominant hand following line of tracheostomy. Drop inner cannula into normal saline basin.	Removes inner cannula for cleaning. Normal saline loosens secretions from inner cannula.
b Replace tracheostomy collar, T tube, or ventilator oxygen source over outer cannula. (NOTE: May not be able to attach T tube and ventilator oxygen devices to all outer cannulas when inner cannula is removed.)	Maintains supply of oxygen to patient as needed.
c To prevent oxygen desaturation in affected patients, quickly pick up inner cannula and use small brush to remove secretions inside and outside inner cannula (see illustration).	Tracheostomy brush provides mechanical force to remove thick or dried secretions.
d Hold inner cannula over basin and rinse with normal saline, using nondominant (clean) hand to pour normal saline.	Removes secretions and normal saline from inner cannula.
e Replace inner cannula (see illustration) and secure "locking" mechanism. Reapply ventilator after hyperoxygenating patient if needed.	Secures inner cannula and reestablishes oxygen supply.
9 **Tracheostomy with disposable inner cannula:**	
a Remove new cannula from manufacturer packaging.	
b While touching only outer aspect of tube, withdraw inner cannula and replace with new cannula. Lock into position.	
c Dispose of contaminated cannula in appropriate receptacle and reconnect to ventilator or oxygen supply.	Prevents transmission of infection. Restores oxygen delivery.
10 Using normal saline-saturated cotton-tipped swabs and 4 × 4–inch gauze, clean exposed outer cannula surfaces and stoma under faceplate extending 5 to 10 cm (2 to 4 inches) in all directions from stoma (see illustration). Clean in circular motion from stoma site outward using dominant hand to handle sterile supplies.	Aseptically removes secretions from stoma site. Moving in outward circle pulls mucus and other contaminants from stoma to periphery.
11 Using dry 4 × 4–inch gauze, pat lightly at skin and exposed outer cannula surfaces.	Dry surfaces prohibit formation of moist environment for microorganism growth and skin excoriation (Higgins, 2009b).
12 Secure tracheostomy.	

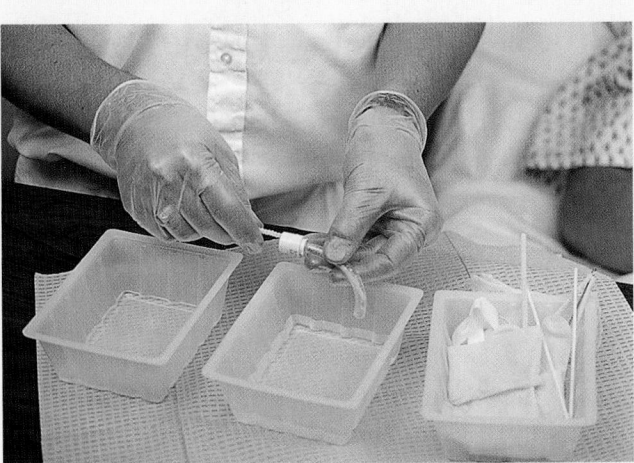

STEP 8c Cleaning tracheostomy inner cannula.

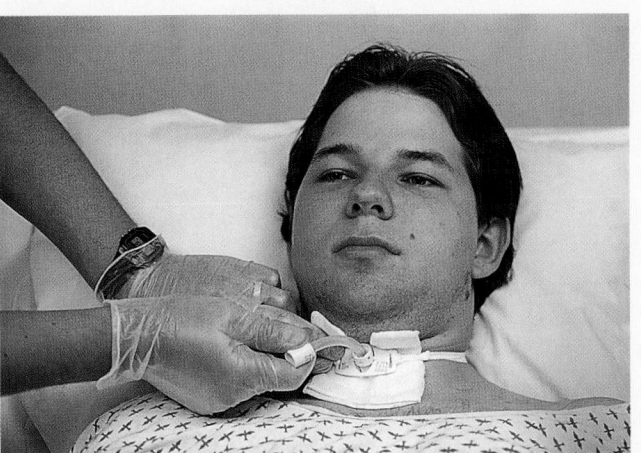

STEP 8e Reinserting inner cannula.

STEPS	RATIONALE

a Tracheostomy tie method:

(1) Instruct assistant, if available, to apply clean gloves and securely hold tracheostomy tube in place. With assistant holding tracheostomy tube, cut old ties.

Promotes hygiene and reduces transmission of microorganisms. Secures tracheostomy tube to prevent incidental extubation.

Clinical Decision Point *Assistant must not release hold on tracheostomy tube until new ties are firmly tied. If working without an assistant, do not cut old ties until new ties are in place and securely tied (Lewis et al., 2011).*

(2) Take prepared tie, insert one end of tie through faceplate eyelet, and pull ends even (see illustration).

(3) Slide both ends of tie behind head and around neck to other eyelet and insert one tie through second eyelet.

(4) Pull snugly.

Secures tracheostomy tube.

(5) Tie ends securely in double square knot, allowing space for only one loose or two snug finger widths in tie (see illustration).

One finger width of slack prevents ties from being too tight when tracheostomy dressing is in place and also prevents movement of tracheostomy tube into lower airway (Frace, 2010).

Critical Decision Point *Do not use scissors to cut gauze pads as they may shed fibers that could be inhaled by patient. Use a manufactured pad for this purpose (Frace, 2010; Higgins, 2009b).*

(6) Insert fresh 4 × 4–inch tracheostomy dressing under clean ties and faceplate (see illustration).

Absorbs drainage. Dressing prevents pressure on clavicle heads (Frace, 2010; Regan and Dallachiesa, 2009).

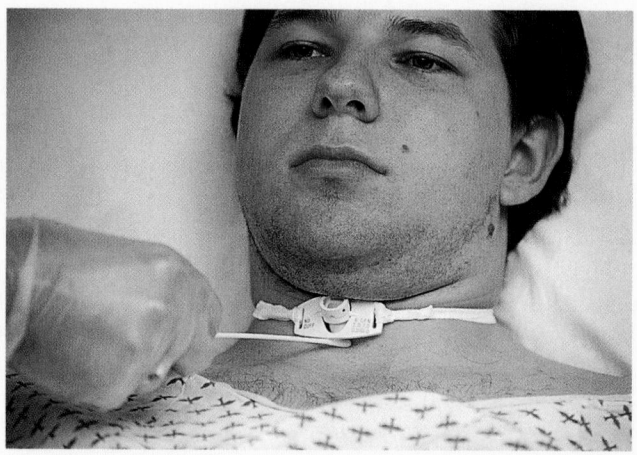

STEP 10   Cleaning around stoma.

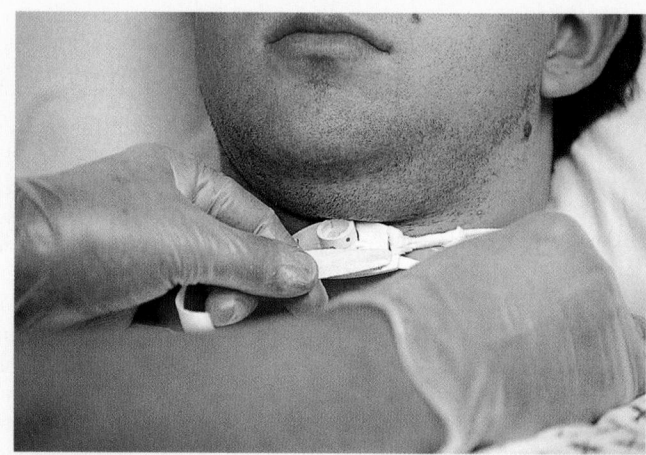

STEP 12a(2)   Replacing tracheostomy ties. Do not remove old tracheostomy ties until new ones are secure.

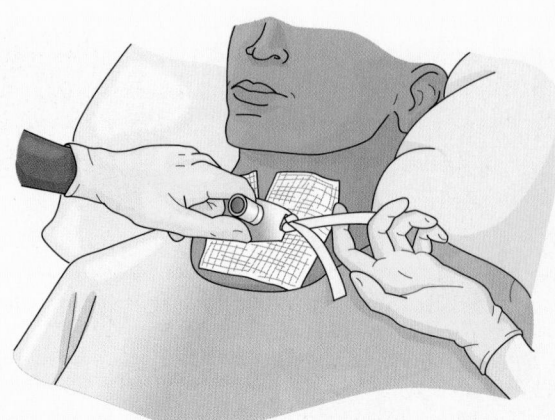

STEP 12a(5)   Tracheostomy ties properly placed. (*From Sorrentino SA: Mosby's textbook for nursing assistants, ed 8, St Louis, 2013, Mosby.*)

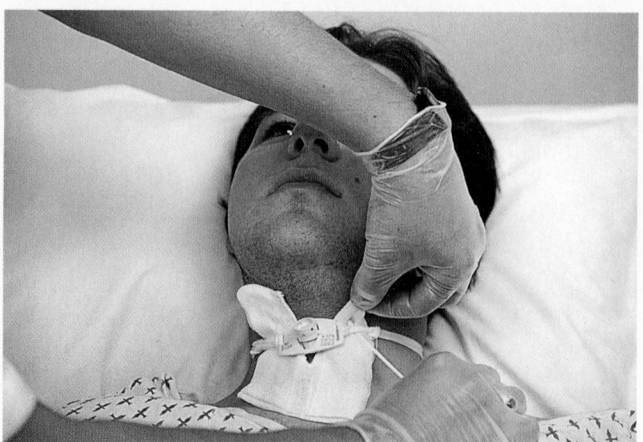

STEP 12a(6)   Applying tracheostomy dressing.

STEPS	RATIONALE
b Tracheostomy tube holder method:	Prevents incidental dislodgement of tube.
(1) While wearing gloves, maintain secure hold on tracheostomy tube. This can be done with an assistant; or, when an assistant is not available, leave old tracheostomy tube holder in place until new device is secure.	
(2) Align strap under patient's neck. Be sure that Velcro attachments are on either side of tracheostomy tube.	
(3) Place narrow end of ties under and through faceplate eyelets. Pull ends even and secure with Velcro closures (see illustration).	
(4) Verify that there is space for only one loose or two snug finger widths under neck strap.	
13 Position patient comfortably and assess respiratory status.	Promotes comfort. Some patients require posttracheostomy care suctioning.
14 Be sure that oxygen or humidification delivery sources are in place and set at correct levels.	Humidification provides moisture for airway, makes it easier to suction secretions, and decreases risk of mucus plugs (Frace, 2010; Regan and Dallachiesa, 2009).
15 Remove gloves and face shield and discard in appropriate receptacle.	Reduces transmission of microorganisms.
16 Replace cap on normal saline bottles. Store reusable liquids, date container, and store unused supplies in appropriate place.	Once opened, normal saline is considered free of bacteria for 24 hours.
17 Perform hand hygiene.	Reduces transmission of microorganisms among patients.

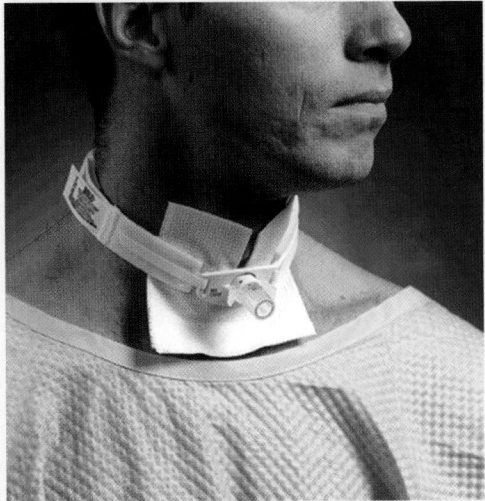

STEP 12b(3)   Tracheostomy tube holder in place. (*Courtesy Dale Medical Products, Plainesville, Mass.*)

EVALUATION

1 Compare assessments before and after tracheostomy care.	Determines effectiveness of tracheostomy care.
2 Assess fit of new tracheostomy ties and ask patient if tube feels comfortable.	Tracheostomy ties are uncomfortable and place patient at risk for tissue injury when they are too loose or too tight.
3 Inspect inner and outer cannulas for secretions.	Presence of secretions on cannulas indicates need for more frequent tracheostomy care.
4 Assess stoma for inflammation, edema, or discolored secretions.	Broken skin places patient at risk for infection.
	Stoma infection requires change in tracheostomy skin care plan.

Unexpected Outcomes

1   Excessively loose or tight tracheostomy ties/tracheostomy holder.

2   Inflammation of tracheostomy stoma.

3   Patient has pressure area around tracheostomy tube.

4   Accidental decannulation.

5   Respiratory distress from mucus plug in cannula.

Related Interventions

- Adjust ties or apply new ties/tracheostomy holder.

- Increase frequency of tracheostomy care.
- Apply topical antibacterial solution, allow it to dry, and apply bacterial barrier.
- Apply hydrocolloid or transparent dressing just under stoma to protect skin from breakdown. Consult with skin care specialist.

- Increase frequency of tracheostomy care and keep dressing under face-plate at all times.
- Consider using double dressing or applying hydrocolloid or stoma adhesive dressing around stoma.

- Call for assistance.
- Replace old tracheostomy tube with new tube. Some experienced nurses or respiratory therapists may be able to quickly reinsert tracheostomy tube.
- Keep spare tracheostomy tube of same size and kind at bedside in event of emergency replacement (Weber-Jones, 2010).
- Same-size ET tube can be inserted in stoma in an emergency.
- Insert suction catheter to confirm that new tube is in trachea.
- Be prepared to manually ventilate patients in whom respiratory distress develops with Ambu bag until tracheostomy is replaced.
- Notify health care provider.

- Remove inner cannula if applicable for cleaning or suction cannula.
- Notify health care provider if tracheostomy tube requires replacement (Weber-Jones, 2010).

Recording and Reporting

- Record respiratory assessments before and after care; type and size of tracheostomy tube; frequency and extent of care; type, color, and amount of secretions; patient tolerance and understanding of procedure; and special care in event of unexpected outcomes.
- Report accidental decannulation or respiratory distress to the health care provider.

Special Considerations

Teaching

- Different types of tracheostomy tubes have different faceplates. Some are rigid; others are not. Instruct caregivers not to lift up rigid faceplates or they will dislodge tube.
- Some commercial tracheostomy tube holders require removal of excess tie material to fit properly.
- If you anticipate long-term placement of tracheostomy, plan to teach patient and family tracheostomy care.

- Patients with new tracheostomy frequently have bloody secretions for 2 to 3 days after procedure and for 24 hours after each tracheostomy tube change (Frace, 2010).

Pediatric

- Children generally have shorter necks, making the stoma more difficult to clean.
- Pediatric tracheostomy tubes (smaller than size 4) do not contain an inner cannula.
- Nurses perform routine tracheostomy tube changes weekly after a tract has formed, generally 5 days (Hockenberry and Wilson, 2011).

Gerontologic

- Some older adults may have more fragile skin and are more prone to skin breakdown from secretions or pressure (Meiner and Lueckenotte, 2011).
- Some older adults with impaired nutrition do not heal well.

SKILL 25-5   Inflating the Cuff on an Endotracheal or Tracheostomy Tube

A cuff on a tracheal tube prevents the escape of air between the tube and the walls of the trachea and reduces aspiration when a patient is receiving mechanical ventilation. The goals of correctly inflating the cuff on an artificial airway are to promote lung inflation for mechanical ventilation, prevent aspiration of gastric contents, and at the same time allow drainage of secretions that accumulate between the epiglottis and the cuff (Box 25-1). The amount of air inserted in a cuff is based on several factors (i.e., the size of the patient's trachea and the external diameter of the artificial airway). If the cuff pressures are too high, permanent damage to the tracheal mucosa occurs (Frace, 2010). Maintain cuff pressures between 20 and 25 mm Hg or less (Lewis et al., 2011).

No recommendation exists for a preferred method for cuff inflation. Most patients have a low-pressure cuff with a cuff manometer. The manometer allows for accurate monitoring of cuff pressures by respiratory therapists.

Delegation and Collaboration

The skill of inflating the cuff on an endotracheal or tracheostomy tube cannot be delegated to nursing assistive personnel (NAP). The nurse directs the NAP to:

- Immediately report any change in vital signs, respiratory status, confusion, restlessness, or discomfort.

BOX 25-1	Indications for Cuff Inflation

Mechanical Ventilation
- Continuous airway pressure
- Positive end expiratory pressure (PEEP)
- Inability to meet ventilatory requirements with cuff down
- Inability to meet oxygen requirements with cuff down

Risk of Aspirating Gastric Contents
- Feeding tube, especially large bore, in stomach
- Gastroesophageal reflux disease
- Hiatal hernia
- During and after meals
- Impaired gastric emptying
- Decreased gag reflex
- Impaired swallowing

- Immediately report any indication of the artificial airway moving or appearing loose.

Equipment
- ❏ Endotracheal (ET)/tracheostomy suction equipment (see Skill 25-2)
- ❏ Stethoscope
- ❏ 5- or 10-mL syringe
- ❏ Alcohol wipe
- ❏ Mask, goggles, face shield (if indicated)
- ❏ Clean gloves (if indicated)

STEP	RATIONALE

ASSESSMENT

1 Observe for signs and symptoms of gurgling on expiration, decreased exhaled tidal volume (mechanically ventilated patient), spasmodic coughing, tense test balloon on tube, flaccid test balloon on tube, and unexpected phonation.

Partially deflated cuff allows secretions to enter trachea and permits vocalization. High cuff pressure can result in necrosis, tracheomalacia, or tracheoesophageal fistula. Overinflated cuff may cause patient to cough (Frace, 2010).

2 Assess vital signs; respiratory effort; and, if on ventilator, tidal volume.

Assesses respiratory status and provides baseline to determine response to therapy.

3 If patient is to be discharged with cuffed tracheostomy tube, determine family caregiver's understanding of and ability to perform procedure.

Identifies teaching needs.

NURSING DIAGNOSES

- Deficient knowledge about cuff inflation
- Impaired spontaneous ventilation
- Ineffective breathing pattern
- Risk for infection
- Risk for aspiration

Related factors are individualized based on patient's condition or needs.

PLANNING

1 Expected outcomes following completion of procedure:
- Mechanically ventilated patient receives prescribed tidal volume.

Proper inflation of cuff ensures that ventilator delivers correct tidal volume.

- Minimal leak is auscultated at end of inspiration.

Allows drainage of secretions during inhalation when airway is at widest but prevents gross aspiration during exhalation when airway is narrower. Prevents continuous contact of tracheal mucosa with cuff.

- No evidence of excessive phonation, aspiration of gastric or mouth contents, tracheoesophageal fistula, or tracheomalacia is present.

Proper level of cuff inflation is maintained consistently. Aspiration and phonation occur when cuff is underinflated. Tracheoesophageal fistula and tracheomalacia occur when cuff is overinflated (Frace, 2010).

2 Explain procedure and how patient can participate. Explain that some coughing during procedure is normal.

Encourages cooperation, minimizes risks, and reduces anxiety.

IMPLEMENTATION

1 Identify patient using two identifiers (i.e., name and birthday or name and account number) according to agency policy. Compare identifiers with information on patient's identification bracelet.

Ensures correct patient. Complies with The Joint Commission standards and improves patient safety (TJC, 2012).

2 Perform hand hygiene. Apply clean gloves and a face shield if indicated.

Reduces transmission of microorganisms.

3 Help patient to position of comfort (generally semi-Fowler's).

Promotes patient comfort and facilitates drainage.

STEP	RATIONALE
4 Suction secretions through ET or tracheostomy tube and also mouth (see Skills 25-1 and 25-2 or Procedural Guideline 25-1).	Ensures patent airway and facilitates hearing airflow with stethoscope. Prevents aspiration of oral secretions during cuff deflation.
5 Connect syringe to pilot balloon.	Allows immediate access to equipment for adjusting cuff pressure.
6 Place stethoscope in sternal notch or above tracheostomy tube and listen for minimal amount of air leak at end of inspiration (see illustration).	Assesses proper cuff inflation.

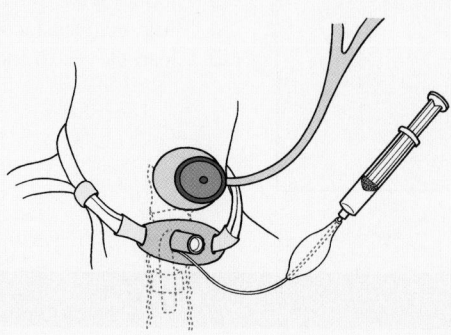

STEP 6   Inflating cuff on tracheostomy while listening with stethoscope.

STEP	RATIONALE
7 If you do not hear an air leak, remove all air from cuff.	Releases excessive cuff pressure, which can reduce capillary blood flow and increase tissue necrosis.
8 Reinflate cuff according to agency policy.	Inflates cuff to minimal leak. If air leak is audible with ear, it is too large. If you do not hear an air leak, cuff is overinflated.
9 If you hear excessive air leak, slowly add air as in Step 8.	Excess air leak may prevent adequate lung expansion and increase risk for aspiration.
10 Remove stethoscope and wipe diaphragm with alcohol wipe.	Reduces transmission of microorganisms.
11 Remove syringe and discard into appropriate receptacle or store per policy. Do not leave attached to pilot balloon valve.	Reduces transmission of microorganisms. Prevents accidental deflation of cuff.
12 Reposition patient.	Promotes comfort.
13 Remove gloves and face shield. Discard into appropriate receptacle. Perform hand hygiene.	Reduces transmission of microorganisms.

EVALUATION

1 Compare respiratory assessments before and after cuff care.	Determines effectiveness of cuff care procedure and patient tolerance.
2 Observe exhaled tidal volume from mechanical ventilator. Exhaled tidal volume should not be less than 50 mL of delivered tidal volume.	Ensures appropriate ventilation of lungs.
3 Auscultate for audible air leak.	Air leak should be heard only with stethoscope.
4 Observe for excessive phonation, presence of gastric secretions in airway secretions, or tracheoesophageal fistula.	Occurs with inadequate or excessive cuff inflation.

Unexpected Outcomes

1 Cuff pressure is excessive.

2 Excessive volume is required to inflate cuff.

3 Excessive air leak is present.

4 Cuff requires increased amounts of air to maintain minimal leak.

Related Interventions

- Remove air from cuff.
- Reinflate with appropriate minimal leak technique.
- Notify health care provider.
- Patient may need insertion of larger tube.
- Reposition patient or tubing.
- Reinflate cuff per protocol.
- Prepare for insertion of new tube by health care provider or trained personnel if cuff ruptures.
- Prepare to manually ventilate patient if needed.
- Reassess position of tube.
- Cuff of ET tube is sometimes higher in trachea (where airway is wider) than previously.
- Withdraw all air from cuff so pilot balloon is completely deflated (flat).
- Remove syringe from pilot balloon. Watch to see if air reenters pilot balloon (cuff). If so, the cuff is leaking, and tube requires replacement.
- Fill cuff appropriately.

Recording and Reporting

- Document presence of minimal leak at end of inspiration, volume of air injected into cuff, secretions obtained when suctioning, frequency of cuff care, patient tolerance of procedures, and safe cuff pressure levels.

Pediatric

- Pediatric tracheostomy tubes and neonatal and many pediatric ET tubes do not contain cuffs.

? Critical Thinking Exercises

You are assigned to care for Mrs. Karlowski, a 55-year-old bank manager. You receive the following information in report: Past medical history—she has a history of chronic lung disease with a long history of smoking. She has no medication allergies. She complains of occasional bouts of bronchitis, which are treated with antibiotics on an outpatient basis. Current complaint includes a 1-week history of upper respiratory symptoms with increasing shortness of breath; and a 2-day history of fever, cough, malaise, nausea, and worsening shortness of breath. Focused assessment: Alert and oriented; VS: 140/86, 110, 34, temp orally 39.2°C (102.6°F). Oxygen saturation baseline is 89%; now at 86%. Respiratory assessment: decreased breath sounds with crackles throughout the lower lobes.

1 Mrs. Karlowski complains of thick secretions in her mouth. She feels that she can cough up the pulmonary secretions, but the secretions still remain in her mouth, and they make her nauseous. Which intervention would you select to help her clear oral secretions? Explain your choice.
   1 Yankauer suctioning
   2 Nasotracheal suctioning
   3 Orotracheal suctioning

2 When you are performing airway management interventions, the risk for health care–associated pneumonia is always present. What can you do to reduce this risk when using a suction technique to clear tracheal secretions? (Select all that apply.) Explain your choice(s).
   1 Perform hand hygiene
   2 Use sterile suction technique
   3 Use clean suction technique
   4 Use humidified oxygen

3 While suctioning Mrs. Karlowski, you observe that the returned sputum is thicker and brown tinged. This is very different from earlier sputum. Which action would you take? (Select all that apply.) Explain your choice(s).
   1 Notify health care provider or nurse in charge
   2 Decrease humidification
   3 Increase fluids
   4 Obtain artificial airway
   5 Obtain sputum specimen

✓ REVIEW QUESTIONS

1 A patient hospitalized for acute pneumonia has a 10-year history of chronic lung disease and cannot clear her respiratory secretions from the posterior pharynx even with coughing. Which suctioning intervention is appropriate?
   1 Oropharyngeal
   2 Nasopharyngeal
   3 Endotracheal
   4 Tracheal

2 A patient needs both the trachea and the oral pharynx suctioned. In which order should the nurse suction these areas and why? Place in correct order.
   1 Suction the oral cavity last
   2 Suction the oral cavity first
   3 Suction nasotracheally first
   4 Suction nasotracheally last

3 A patient is in the intensive care unit after a thoracotomy and has subsequent hypoxia. Which of the following manifestations is an associated symptom of hypoxia?
   1 Increased mentation
   2 Feeling of calm
   3 Normal heart rate and rhythm
   4 Lethargy

4 The nurse is caring for a patient with an artificial airway whose pulse oximeter reading drops from 90% to 85%. What is the priority nursing action?
   1 Check for the presence of a pulse
   2 Assess for an adequate blood pressure
   3 Check for a patent airway
   4 Check the connections of the oxygen supply

5 A patient with an endotracheal tube has unequal breath sounds, even after being suctioned and repositioned. Which nursing intervention is indicated at this time?
   1 Notify the health care provider
   2 Call for help
   3 Suction the airway
   4 Reposition patient's endotracheal tube deeper

6 You are assigned a patient with a tracheostomy, and you need to change the patient's dressing because you note that the dressing is moist. Place the following steps to secure the tracheostomy in the correct order.
   1 Slide both ends of tie behind head and around neck to other eyelet and insert one tie through second eyelet.
   2 Ask for assistance from the NAP to hold the tracheostomy tube.
   3 Secure ties.
   4 Cut old ties.
   5 Take prepared tie and insert one end of tie through faceplate eyelet and pull ends even.
   6 Insert fresh dressing under clean ties and faceplate.

7 Mr. Stone has a tracheostomy with an inner cannula that needs to be cleaned. He is receiving 40% humidified oxygen via a tracheotomy mask. Which intervention should the nurse take to prevent desaturation?
   1 Have Mr. Stone sit upright.
   2 Use hydrogen peroxide on the 4×4s to clean Mr. Stone's inner cannula.
   3 Quickly clean Mr. Stone's inner cannula.
   4 Reinsert the inner cannula; you do not have to lock it down after the initial cleaning.

8 Place the steps for securing an oral endotracheal (ET) tube with tape in the correct order after completing suctioning.
   1 Remove old tape from patient's face.
   2 Apply clean gloves.
   3 Cut piece of tape long enough to go completely around patient's head from naris to naris plus 15 cm (6 inches).
   4 Remove any secretions or adhesive from patient's face.
   5 Instruct helper to apply pair of gloves and hold ET tube firmly at patient's lips or nares.

9 Which of the following intervention(s) help to preventing ventilator-associated pneumonia? (Select all that apply.)
1 Elevating the head of the bed at 10 degrees to prevent aspiration
2 Changing patient position every 4 hours to decrease risk for atelectasis, pulmonary infections, pressure ulcers, discomfort, and urinary stasis
3 Providing oral care with chlorhexidine by swab every 8 hours
4 Maintaining endotracheal cuff pressures at 20 cm H_2O to decrease movement of secretions to the lower airways

10 Managing a patient's airway requires several safety guidelines. Which of the following statements is (are) true in maintaining airways safely? (Select all that apply.)
1 Respiratory assessment only needs to include the respiratory rate and oxygen saturation levels.
2 The risk of aspiration is important to assess when enteral feeding tubes are present.
3 Evaluate all airway equipment for functionality before use.
4 Review of baseline or previous shift information is not necessary to your care of the patient.

REFERENCES

American Association of Respiratory Care (AARC): AARC clinical practice guidelines: nasotracheal suctioning—2004 revision and update, 2004, available at http://www.rcjournal.com/cpgs/pdf/09.04.1080.pdf, accessed August 13, 2011.

American Association of Respiratory Care (AARC): AARC clinical practice guidelines: endotracheal suctioning of mechanically ventilated patients with artificial airways, Respir Care 55(6):758, 2010, available at http://www.guideline.gov/content.aspx?id=23992, accessed February 18, 2012.

American Association of Respiratory Care (AARC): AARC clinical practice guidelines: capnography/capnometry during mechanical ventilation, Respir Care 56(4):503, 2011.

Ames N: Evidence to support tooth brushing in critically ill patients, Am J Crit Care 20(3):242, 2011.

Browne JA, et al: Pursuing excellence: development of an oral hygiene protocol for mechanically ventilated patients, Crit Care Nurs Q 34(1):25, 2011.

Foster A: More than nothing: the lived experience of tracheostomy while acutely ill, Intensive Crit Care Nurs 26(1):33, 2010.

Frace M: Tracheostomy care on the medical-surgical unit, Medsurg Nurs 19(1):58, 2010.

Gardner D, Shirland L: Evidence-based guideline for suctioning the intubated neonate and infant, Neonatal Netw 28(5):281, 2009.

Gill P, et al: Access to interpreting services in England: secondary analysis of national data, BMC Public Health 9:12, 2009, DOI:10.1186/1471-2458-9-12.

Halm M, Krisko-Hagel K: Instilling normal saline with suctioning: beneficial technique or potentially harmful sacred cow? Am J Crit Care 17(5):469, 2008.

Higgins D: Tracheostomy care: Part one—using suction, Nurs Times 105(4):16, 2009a.

Higgins D: Tracheostomy care: Part three—dressing, Nurs Times 105(6):12, 2009b.

Hockenberry MJ, Wilson D: Wong's nursing care of infants and children, ed 9, St Louis, 2011, Mosby.

Jongerden I, et al: Effect of open and closed endotracheal suctioning on cross-contamination with gram-negative bacteria: a prospective crossover study, Crit Care Med 39(6):1313, 2011.

Lewis SL, et al: Medical-surgical nursing: assessment and management of clinical problems, ed 8, St Louis, 2011, Mosby.

Lynn-McHale Wiegand D: AACN procedure manual for critical care, ed 6, St Louis, 2011, Saunders.

Meiner SE, Lueckenotte AG: Gerontologic nursing, ed 5, St Louis, 2011, Mosby.

Niël-Weise B, et al: An evidence-based recommendation on bed head elevation for mechanically ventilated patients, Crit Care 15(2):R111, 2011.

Oleska R, Muscedere J: Ventilator-associated pneumonia: update on etiology, prevention, and management, Curr Infect Rep 13:287, 2011.

Pedersen C, et al: Endotracheal suctioning of the adult intubated patient—what is the evidence? Intensive Crit Care Nurs 25:21, 2009.

Regan E, Dallachiesa L: How to care for a patient with a tracheostomy, Nursing 09 39(8):34, 2009.

Rewa O, Muscedere J: Ventilator-associated pneumonia: update on etiology, prevention, and management, Curr Infect Dis Rep 13(3):287, 2011.

Scherzer R: Subglottic secretion aspiration in the prevention of ventilator-associated pneumonia: a review of the literature, Dimens Crit Care Nurs 29(6):276, 2010.

Selvaraj N: Artificial humidification for the mechanically ventilated patient, Nurs Stand 25(8):41, 2010.

Stonecypher K: Ventilator-associated pneumonia: the importance of oral care in intubated adults, Crit Care Nurs Q 33(4):339, 2010.

Subirana M, et al: Closed tracheal suction systems versus open tracheal suction systems for mechanically ventilated adult patients (review), Cochrane Collaboration 7, 2010, DOI: 10.1002/14651858.CD004581.pub2.

The Joint Commission (TJC): National Patient Safety Goals, Oakbrook Terrace, Ill, 2012, The Commission, available at http://www.jointcommission.org/standards_information/npsgs.aspx.

Weber-Jones J: Obstructed tracheostomy tubes: clearing the air, Nursing 2010 40(1):49, 2010.

White AC, et al: When to change a tracheostomy tube, Respir Care 55(8):1069, 2010.

Winkelman C, Chiang L: Manual turns in patients receiving mechanical ventilation, Crit Care Nurs 30(4):36, 2010.

Closed Chest Drainage Systems

SKILLS AND PROCEDURES

MEDIA RESOURCES

- **evolve** learning system http://evolve.elsevier.com/Perry/skills
  - Review Questions
  - Audio Glossary

- **NSO** Nursing Skills Online

KEY TERMS

Air leak	Intrapleural pressure	Pneumothorax	Tension pneumothorax
Atmospheric pressure	Mediastinal shift	Positive pressure	Tidaling
Chest tube	Negative pressure	Subcutaneous emphysema	Visceral pleura
Hemothorax	Parietal pleura		

OBJECTIVES

Mastery of content in this chapter will enable the nurse to:
- Explain the physiology of normal respiration.
- List three common sites for chest tube placement.
- List three conditions requiring chest tube insertion.
- Describe closed chest drainage systems: water-seal and waterless systems.
- Describe principles and mechanisms of chest tube suction.

- Discuss measures to maintain patient safety during chest tube insertion, maintenance, and removal.
- Describe methods of troubleshooting chest tube systems.
- Discuss the nursing principles in caring for patients with chest tubes.
- Describe autotransfusion.

The chest cavity is a closed structure bound by muscle, bone, connective tissue, vascular structures, and the diaphragm. This cavity has three distinct sections, each sealed from the others: one section for each lung and a third section for the mediastinum, which surrounds structures such as the heart, esophagus, trachea, and great vessels.

The lungs are covered with a membrane called the *visceral pleura*. The interior chest wall is lined with a membrane called the *parietal pleura* (Fig. 26-1). The space between the visceral and parietal pleura is called the *pleural space* and is filled with approximately 7-to-20 mL of lubricating fluid to help the pleura slide during respiration (Twedell, 2009). During inspiration the intercostal muscles pull outward, and the diaphragm contracts and pulls downward, thereby increasing the size of the chest cavity. As a result an increase in the amount of negative pressure (vacuum effect) is exerted in the intrapleural space.

During inspiration increased negative pressure pulls the lungs against the expanded chest cavity, increasing their size.

The expanding lungs cause the intrapulmonic (alveolar) pressure to fall lower than atmospheric pressure, thus increasing the negative pressure within the lungs. This change in pressure causes air to rush into the lungs until the intrapulmonic pressure is equal to the pressure in the atmosphere. When the chest cavity stops expanding and the lungs are full of air, the respiratory muscles and diaphragm relax and return the chest cavity to its resting stage. Expiration (exhalation) is a passive process that results from relaxation of the inspiratory muscles that decrease the space in the chest cavity.

Trauma, disease, or surgery can result in air, blood, pus, or lymph fluid leaking into the intrapleural space, creating a positive pressure that collapses lung tissue (Durai et al., 2010). Small leaks (24% or less) are sometimes absorbed spontaneously and may not require a chest tube. The usual intervention for larger leaks is a chest tube to remove air and fluid from the pleural space, prevent air and/or fluid from reentering the pleural space, and reestablish normal intrapleural and intrapulmonary pressures.

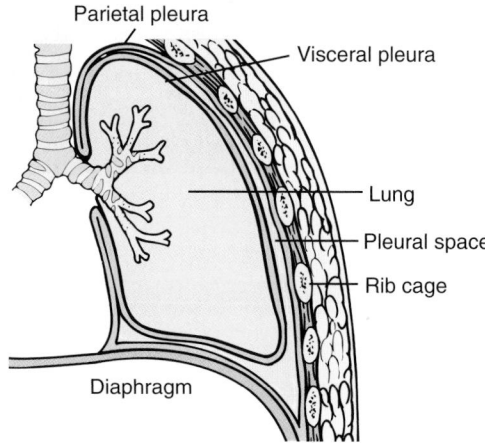

Parietal pleura

Visceral pleura

Lung

Pleural space

Rib cage

Diaphragm

FIG 26-1 Partial structures of lungs.

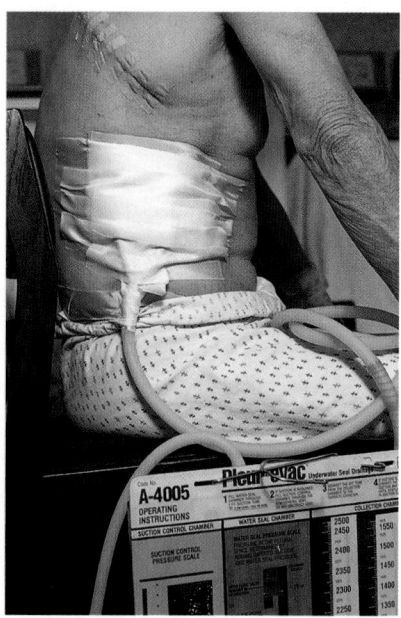

FIG 26-2 Pleural chest tube in place following thoracic surgery.

A number of clinical conditions such as cancer, infection, pancreatitis, connective tissue disease, autoimmune diseases, asbestos exposure, certain drugs, or collagen vascular diseases increase pleural fluid entry or decrease fluid exit from the lung. This is called a *pleural effusion;* and, when present, a patient usually needs a diagnostic thoracentesis and pleural fluid analysis to determine the cause of the exudate (see Chapter 44) (Twedell, 2009). Patients usually need one or more chest tubes to promote drainage of the excess fluid and lung expansion (Mertin et al., 2009; Twedell, 2009).

A pneumothorax is collapse of the lung caused by a collection of air in the pleural space. The loss of negative intrapleural pressure causes the lung to collapse. A variety of mechanisms cause a pneumothorax. A traumatic pneumothorax develops as a result of penetrating chest trauma such as a stabbing (open) or the chest striking the steering wheel in an automobile accident (closed). A spontaneous or primary pneumothorax sometimes occurs from the rupture of a small bleb (blister) on the surface of the lung or an invasive procedure such as insertion of a subclavian intravenous (IV) line. Secondary pneumothorax occurs because of underlying disease such as emphysema. A patient with a pneumothorax usually feels sharp chest pain that worsens on inspiration or coughing because atmospheric air irritates the parietal pleura. As a pneumothorax worsens, a patient will experience easy fatigue, a rapid heart rate, and low blood pressure (U.S. National Library of Medicine, 2011).

A tension pneumothorax, a life-threatening situation, occurs from rupture in the pleura when air accumulates in the pleural space more rapidly than it is removed. The pleural space functions as a one-way valve, causing an increase in the amount of air and pressure. If left untreated, the lung on the affected side collapses; and the mediastinum shifts to the opposite (unaffected side), leading to tracheal deviation, reduced venous return, and subsequent decrease in cardiac output. Tracheal deviation is a late sign and may be absent in some cases (Bethel, 2008). A patient has sudden chest pain, a fall in blood pressure, tachycardia, acute pleuritic pain, diaphoresis, dry cough, and cardiopulmonary arrest can occur. Patients with chest trauma, fractured ribs, invasive thoracic bedside procedures (e.g., insertion of central lines), and those on high-pressure mechanical ventilation are at risk for tension pneumothorax (Bethel, 2008). If emergent treatment is required, a needle decompression is achieved with a large-gauge needle (14 or 16 gauge) inserted into the second intercostal space, midclavicular line. A "hissing" sound is noted, followed by a rapid stabilization of the patient's vital signs and respiratory status (Briggs, 2010).

A hemothorax is collapse of the lung caused by an accumulation of blood and fluid in the pleural cavity between the chest wall and the lung, usually as a result of trauma. It produces a counterpressure and prevents the full expansion of the lung. A hemothorax is also caused by rupture of small blood vessels from inflammatory processes such as pneumonia or tuberculosis. In addition to pain and dyspnea, signs and symptoms of shock can develop if blood loss is severe (Mertin et al., 2009).

Chest tube insertion is the treatment for most types of effusions, pneumothorax, hemothorax, and postoperative chest surgery or trauma. A chest tube is a large catheter inserted through the thorax to remove fluid (effusions), blood (hemothorax), and/or air (pneumothorax). Small-bore chest tubes (12 to 20 Fr) are sufficient to remove air, and large-bore (24 to 32 Fr) tubes are needed to remove fluid and blood. In some settings the traditional reusable glass three-bottle system is still used but rarely. Clear, plastic, disposable containers are most common (Durai et al., 2010). The newest system available is the mobile chest drain, which allows a patient to move about with less restriction. Regardless of the system used, the principles of patient management are the same. A pleural chest tube (Fig. 26-2) is inserted when air or fluid enters the pleural space, compromising oxygenation or ventilation. A closed chest drainage system with or without suction is attached to the chest tube to promote drainage of air and fluid. Lung reexpansion occurs as the fluid or air is removed from the pleural space (Briggs, 2010; Twedell, 2009).

The location of the chest tube indicates the type of drainage expected. Apical (second or third intercostal space) and anterior chest tube placement promotes removal of air. Because air rises, these chest tubes are placed high, allowing evacuation of air from the intrapleural space and lung reexpansion (Fig. 26-3). The air is discharged into the atmosphere, and there is little or no drainage in the collection chamber.

Chest tubes placed low (usually in the fifth or sixth intercostal space) and posterior or lateral drain fluid (see Fig. 26-3). Fluid in the intrapleural space is affected by gravity and localizes in the lower portion of the lung cavity. Tubes placed in these positions drain blood and fluid. Frequently applying suction helps with this

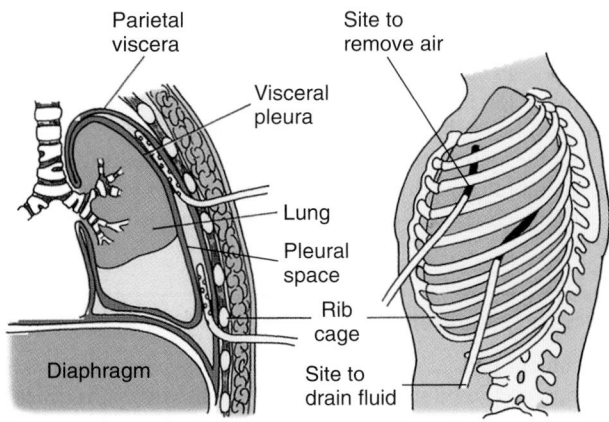

FIG 26-3 Diagram of sites for chest tube placement.

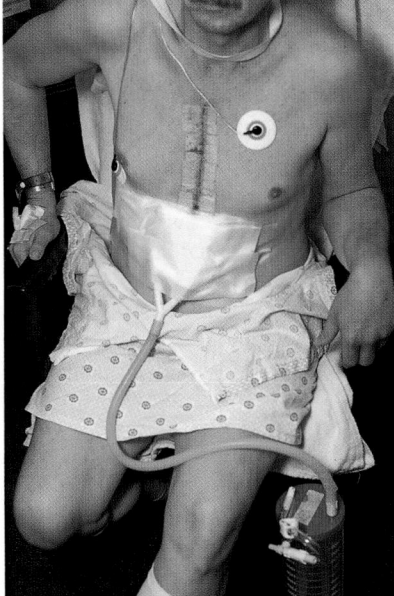

FIG 26-4 Mediastinal chest tube.

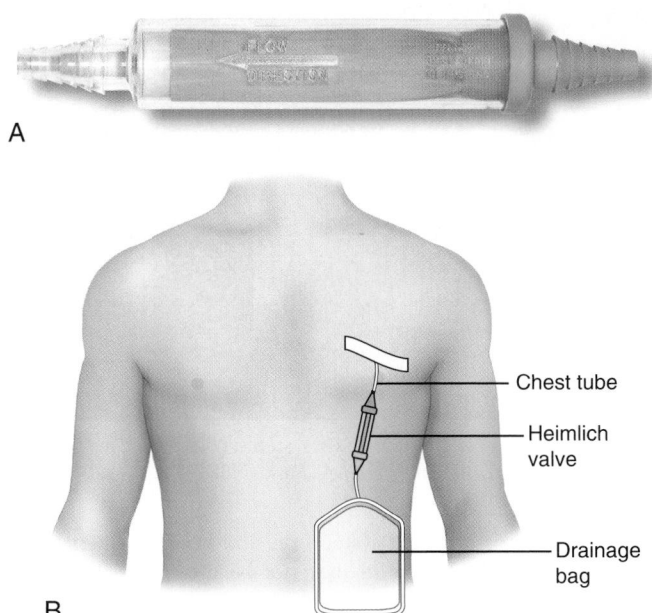

FIG 26-5 **A,** Heimlich chest drain valve is a specially designed flutter valve that is used in place of a chest drainage unit for small uncomplicated pneumothorax with little or no drainage and no need for suction. The valve allows for escape of air but prevents reentry of air into the pleural space. (*Image courtesy Becton, Dickenson and Company, Franklin Lakes, New Jersey. All rights reserved.*) **B,** Placement of valve between chest tube and drainage bag, which can be worn under clothing.

drainage. Fluid drainage is expected after open-chest surgery and with some chest trauma (Briggs, 2010).

A mediastinal chest tube is placed in the mediastinum, just below the sternum (Fig. 26-4), and is connected to a drainage system. This tube drains blood or fluid, preventing its accumulation around the heart. A mediastinal tube is commonly used after open-heart surgery.

Occasionally in emergency situations and for a small pneumothorax a catheter is inserted through the chest wall, and a rubber flutter one-way valve (e.g., a Heimlich valve) is attached to the catheter (Fig. 26-5, A and B). As a patient exhales, the positive pressure generated by the air leaving the chest enters the tubing, causing the valve to open so air is released. During inspiration the tube collapses on itself, preventing air from reentering the chest. No drainage chamber is used with this device; therefore it is not used when patients need fluid drained such as from a hemothorax or a pleural effusion (Lewis et al., 2011).

Smaller "pigtail catheters" are also used and are less traumatic than the large-bore tubes. In addition, if they occlude the health care provider can irrigate them with sterile water. However, because these tubes are small, the size of the tube lumen does not promote

drainage of blood, and they are not used for chest trauma (Lewis et al., 2011).

Mobile chest drains are devices that are lighter and self-contained and allow patients to move with less restriction. As a result there is a decreased risk for deep vein thrombosis, pulmonary embolism, and other complications associated with immobility. In addition, because the system is lighter, a patient has less pain. These mobile systems rely on gravity or dry suction for drainage. They are ideal for patients with persistent drainage or air leaks requiring prolonged need for a chest tube (Varela et al., 2010). Patients who require a mobile chest drainage system at home need sufficient discharge planning and patient teaching directed toward safe operation of the system (see Home Care Considerations for Skill 26-1).

The disposable systems such as an Atrium or Pleur-Evac chest drainage system are one-piece molded plastic units that provide for a single- or multiple-chamber closed drainage system (Fig. 26-6). A single-chamber system allows air from a pneumothorax to bubble out of the water seal and escape through the air outlet while preventing air from reentering the intrapleural space. This system is not recommended for the evacuation of fluid because drainage would raise the level of the water-seal liquid. An increased height of fluid in the water seal increases the resistance to drainage on expiration and eventually stops the drainage entirely.

A two- or three-chamber system drains both a hemothorax and a pneumothorax effectively. The two-chamber system permits liquid to flow into the collection chamber, and air flows into the water-seal chamber. A three-chamber system promotes the drainage of fluid and air with controlled suction. In both systems the first chamber provides a compartment for fluid or blood drainage, and a second compartment for either a water seal or a one-way

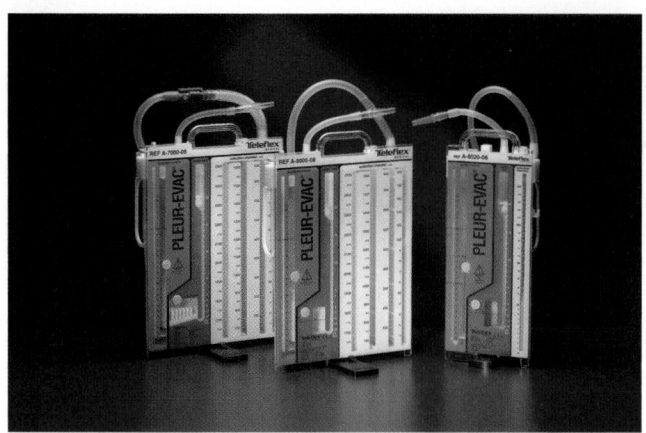

FIG 26-6 Disposable chest drainage systems. (*Pleur-Evac images courtesy Teleflex Medical, Research Triangle Park, NC.*)

valve. In the three-chamber system, the third compartment is for suction control, which may or may not be used. The disposable units appear to be the system of choice because they are cost-effective and some facilitate autotransfusion, a common practice in open-heart surgeries.

EVIDENCE-BASED PRACTICE

Small chest tubes often become blocked by blood clots and fibrin. Milking and stripping a chest tube are processes used to clear the clots. Milking is the manual compression of a chest tube in an attempt to move the chest tube drainage toward the collection device. Milking involves squeezing the chest tube back and forth intermittently with the hands along the length of the tube. Stripping a chest tube involves using continuous pressure on the tube while running the hands down from the site of insertion to the drainage container.

The evidence has changed related to the use of stripping. It causes a dangerous increase in intrathoracic pressure, which damages the lung tissue (Durai et al., 2010). Milking does not alter intrathoracic pressure as much as stripping (Briggs, 2010). However, it is used only in select situations (e.g., when chest tube drainage becomes acutely occluded from multiple clots).

Careful management of chest tube drainage prevents the need to milk chest tubes:

- Avoid dependent loops of the drainage tube; or, when these loops cannot be avoided (such as when the patient is sitting), lift and clear the tube every 15 minutes.
- Tailor the length of the drainage tube to a patient. The tubing must be long enough to allow a patient to move but not so long that dependent loops hang down the side of the bed. If the tubing is coiled, looped, or clotted, the drainage is impeded and can result in a tension pneumothorax (Briggs, 2010).

PATIENT-CENTERED CARE

Health care–acquired infections (HAIs) occur at the rate of 13 per 1000 patient days in U.S. intensive care units (ICUs). As patient advocates, nurses need to know the factors leading to infections. HAIs often cost over $40,000 per patient and burden patients and families with higher mortality rates and prolonged hospitalizations. Invasive procedures such as mechanical ventilation, central venous catheters, and chest tubes can all increase the risk for HAIs. Oldfield et al. (2009) studied 120 ICU patients who had one or more chest tubes to identify their risk for HAIs. The researchers found that patients with chest tubes for longer than 20 days had a six-times greater risk of developing an HAI than those with chest tubes for fewer than 20 days. Based on this information, nurses must be vigilant for patient assessment findings that indicate the need for a chest tube and encourage deep-breathing exercises and early mobility, use of appropriate analgesia to promote activity, and patient education regarding these practices (Oldfield et al., 2009).

Safety Guidelines

1 Document patient's baseline vital signs, oxygen saturation, lung sounds, and respiratory status. Changes in vital signs or respiratory status often indicate a malfunction of a chest drainage system.

2 Observe the water seal for intermittent bubbling from its U tube or a rise and fall of fluid that is synchronous with respirations (Briggs, 2010). For example, in a nonmechanically ventilated patient the fluid level rises during inspiration and falls during expiration. When a patient is on a mechanical ventilator, the opposite occurs.

  a Constant bubbling in the water seal or a sudden, unexpected stoppage of water-seal activity is considered abnormal and requires immediate attention (Briggs, 2010).

  b Unexpected stoppage of activity may indicate a blockage or reexpansion. In these situations immediate attention and correction are indicated. After 2 to 3 days, tidaling or bubbling on expiration is expected to stop, indicating that the lung has reexpanded (Briggs, 2010).

3 In a waterless system look for a rise and fall of fluid in the diagnostic air-leak indicator synchronous with respirations. Constant left-to-right bubbling (when facing the indicator) or violent rocking is considered abnormal and indicates an air leak.

4 Note the expected amount of chest tube drainage, and monitor drainage on a regular basis (e.g., every hour initially and then every 4 hours). At the end of the shift, make a mark to indicate the fluid level with the date and time on the side of the drainage collection chamber. Note the drainage amount as output.

  a A sudden decrease in the amount of chest tube drainage can indicate a possible clot or obstruction in the chest tube.

  b Notify a health care provider when there is a sudden increase of more than 250 mL of drainage over 1 hour, which can indicate fresh bleeding from the thorax (Durai et al., 2010).

  c Drainage from a pneumothorax is generally limited. Any fluid buildup is caused by chest tube insertion trauma. The chest tubes promote the removal of air from the intrapleural space.

5 Know the expected color of the drainage. Drainage from recent open-chest surgery is initially bright red and gradually becomes serous as the postoperative course continues. Blood-tinged fluid usually indicates malignancy, pulmonary infarction, or severe inflammation. Frank blood indicates a hemothorax. Pus indicates an empyema, which is a collection of pus in the pleural cavity (Briggs, 2010).

6 In the water-seal system observe for constant, gentle bubbling in the suction control chamber when it is connected to suction. In the waterless system a designated amount of suction is maintained by setting the suction source and dialing the prescribed suction level in the float ball column.

7 Assess both types of systems for air leaks. If an air leak exists, determine whether it is in the patient (patient-centered air

leak) or in the chest tube system (system-centered air leak). To rule out an air leak as patient-centered, you assess the patient's respiratory status. Document and report any changes in lung sounds, pulse oximetry, respiratory rate, or mentation.

Remember that continuous bubbling in the water-seal chamber with an absence of bubbles in the suction control chamber indicates that there is a leak in the system (Briggs, 2010). Ensure that all tubing connections are tight.

SKILL 26-1 Managing Closed Chest Drainage Systems

NSO Chest Tubes Module / Lessons 1 and 3

There are two types of commercial drainage systems: the water-seal and the waterless systems (Table 26-1). This skill reviews the nursing responsibilities and interventions related to the safe management of chest tubes. Review the roles and responsibilities of the health care provider for chest tube placement (Table 26-2).

Water-Seal Systems

NSO Chest Tubes Module / Lesson 2

Two-Chamber Water-Seal System

On expiration fluid or air is forced out of the intrapleural space. Suction pulls air or fluid through the chest tube into the drainage collection chamber. On entering the drainage collection chamber, this fluid or air displaces the air present in the chamber by pushing it through the water seal and out of the system into the atmosphere. The water-seal chamber is left open to air to drain. If the tubing is clamped, there is no mechanism for air to vent. To maintain the water-seal system, the chest tube system must remain upright. When it is tipped or overturned, the water seal is disrupted.

Three-Chamber Water-Seal System

If suction is used, the three-chamber water-seal system (Fig. 26-7) is set up with the suction control chamber added. A prescribed amount of sterile fluid (e.g., 20 cm of water) is poured into the suction control chamber, which is then attached to a suction source by tubing. The amount of sterile water added depends on manufacturer recommendations. The chamber is filled to the set volume for the prescribed amount of suction. Sterile water is added several times a day because of evaporation. As the fluid level decreases, the amount of suction also declines. The wall or portable suction device is turned up until the water in the suction control bottle exhibits a continuous, gentle bubbling. This provides the prescribed amount of suction (negative pressure).

If the suction source delivers more negative pressure than the suction control chamber water level allows, there is no danger because atmospheric air is pulled into the suction control chamber through an inlet, causing the excess suction to dissipate. The extra

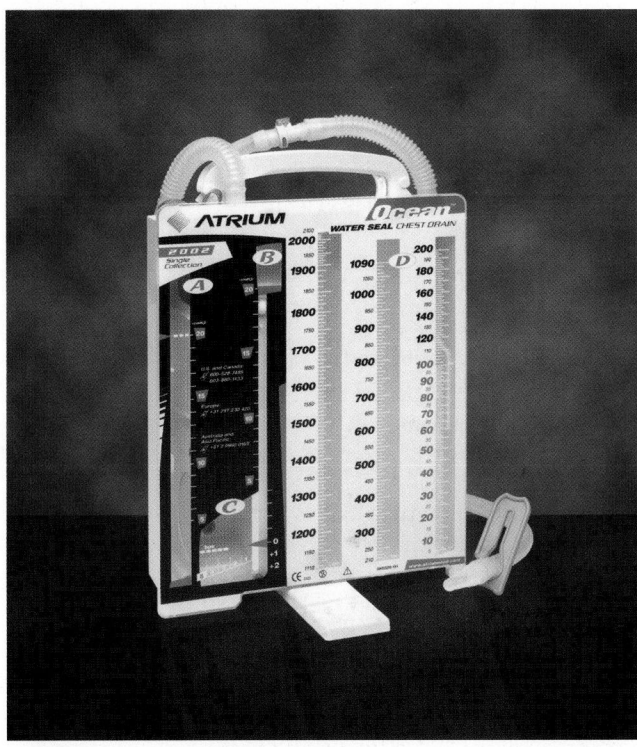

FIG 26-7 Disposable water-seal chest drainage system with suction. *(Used with permission, Atrium Medical Corp.)*

| TABLE 26-1 | Comparison of Chest Tube Drainage Systems |

Drainage System Type	Function	Advantage	Disadvantage
Water-seal system (see Fig. 26-7)	Two-chamber provides one-way valve for chest drainage. Water seal prevents reentry of air into lung. Three-chamber adds a chamber to aid evacuation of chest drainage.	Easy set-up and use Cost-effective	System must be kept upright to maintain seal. Drainage chamber may fill up quickly if patient has large amount of drainage. Sterile water must be added several times a day to maintain suction and water seal because of evaporation.
Waterless system (see Fig. 26-8)	Also provides three chambers, but no water is required to establish a seal.	Water seal maintained even if system is knocked over More space provided for drainage	Water must be added to system if patient requires evaluation of an air leak.
Dry suction system (see Fig. 26-9)	Also provides three chambers, but no water is required to establish a seal.	Easy set up Quiet operation Can be used when higher levels of suction are required	Sterile water must be added to system if patient requires suction.

air pulled into the chamber causes vigorous bubbling. If this occurs, lower the suction source setting to reduce noise and evaporation of the fluid. The absence of bubbling indicates that no suction is being exerted into the system. Raise the suction setting to restore gentle bubbling.

The middle chamber of a traditional chest drainage system is the water seal. The water seal allows air to exit from the pleural space on exhalation and prevent it from entering the pleural cavity or mediastinum on inhalation. When the appropriate amount of sterile water is added, a 2-cm water seal is established. To maintain effective water seal the chest drainage unit must remain upright, and you must monitor the water level in the water-seal chamber to check for evaporation. Bubbling in the water-seal chamber indicates an air leak.

Waterless Systems
Two-Chamber Waterless System

The principles of the waterless system are similar to those of the water-seal system except that fluid is not required for setup. Because water is not used, accidentally tipping the system does not compromise the patient's condition.

The water seal is replaced by a one-way valve (Fig. 26-8) located near the top of the system. Most of the container serves as the drainage chamber. The suction chamber does not depend on water. Instead it contains a float ball, which is set by a suction control dial after the suction source is turned on. A diagnostic air-leak indicator is located on the face of the unit. It requires the addition of 15 mL of fluid for visualization. The function of the indicator is to identify one of the following:

TABLE 26-2	Process for Insertion of Chest Tubes
Role	**Purpose**
Explain purpose, procedure, and possible complications to patient and have patient sign consent form.	Provides informed consent.
Have pain medication available to administer before or immediately after chest tube insertion as appropriate according to patient's condition.	Analgesia improves patient comfort throughout procedure and helps patient take appropriate deep breaths to promote lung reexpansion and drainage of fluid in pleural space.
Perform hand hygiene. Clean chest wall with antiseptic.	Reduces transmission of microorganisms.
Apply mask and gloves.	Maintains surgical asepsis.
Drape area of chest tube insertion with sterile towels. Inject local anesthetic and allow time to take effect.	Maintains surgical asepsis. Decreases pain during procedure.
Make a small incision over the rib space where tube is to be inserted. Thread a clamped chest tube through the incision. Health care provider clamps chest tube until system is connected to water seal.	Inserts chest tube into intrapleural space. Clamping prevents entry of atmospheric air into chest and worsening of pneumothorax.
Suture chest tube in place if suturing is policy or health care provider preference.	Secures chest tube in place.
Cover chest tube insertion site with sterile 4 × 4–inch gauze and large dressing to form an occlusive dressing supported with an elastic bandage (Elastoplast). Sterile petrolatum gauze is used around the tube.	Holds chest tube in place and occludes site around it. Helps stabilize chest tube and holds dressing tightly in place. Sterile petrolatum gauze helps prevent air leak.
Water-Seal System Remove connector cover from patient's end of chest drainage tubing with sterile technique. Secure drainage tubing to chest tube and drainage system.	Health care provider is responsible for making certain that system is set up properly, proper amount of water is in the water seal, dressing is secure, and chest tube is securely connected to drainage system.
Water-Seal Suction Connect system to suction or supervise a nurse connecting it to suction if suction is to be used.	Health care provider is responsible for determining and checking amount of fluid that is to be added to suction control chamber and prescribing suction setting.
Waterless System Remove connector cover from patient's end of chest drainage tubing with sterile technique. Secure drainage tubing to chest tube and drainage system.	Health care provider is responsible for making certain that system is set up properly and chest tube is securely connected to drainage system.
Waterless Suction Turn on suction source. Set float ball level to prescribed setting.	Health care provider is responsible for prescribing level of float ball and suction setting.
Health care provider or nurse adds sterile water or normal saline to diagnostic indicator.	Allows quick assurance that system is functioning properly. Connects chest tube to drainage.
Unclamp chest tube.	Verifies correct chest tube placement.
In both systems health care provider orders and reviews chest x-ray film studies.	

1 The lung is expanding normally. This is indicated by a gentle tidaling of the fluid in the diagnostic indicator.

2 The lung is probably reexpanded if after 2 or 3 days the tidaling has stopped.

3 There is an air leak in the system if, when facing the system, the observer sees the fluid bubbling left to right. Locate and correct the source of the air leak.

FLOW PATTERN

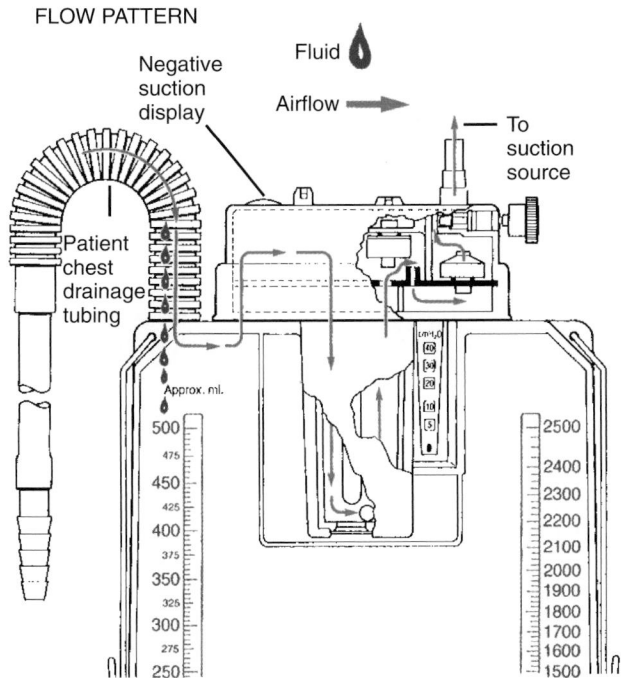

FIG 26-8 Disposable waterless chest drainage system with suction.

Three-Chamber Waterless System

When suction is ordered, attach the suction chamber port to the suction source by tubing, turn the suction on, and set the float ball to the prescribed setting. If the float ball does not rise to the prescribed level, increase the suction source setting until it does. The system is now functioning with suction.

There are usually two suction settings: one at either the suction control chamber or the float ball setting and the other at the suction source. The chamber or float ball setting is a safety factor to reduce the possibility that the intrapleural tissues receive too much suction, causing injury.

Dry Suction System

Dry suction control systems provide many advantages (Fig. 26-9), including higher suction pressure levels, easy setup, and the lack of continuous bubbling, which provides for quiet operation. There is no fluid to evaporate, which decreases the amount of suction necessary. A self-compensating regulator controls dry suction units. A dial is set to the prescribed suction control setting. These units are preset to −20 cm of water pressure, but they are adjustable from −10 to −40 cm. However, the dry suction control systems require or have pre-sealed sterile water in the water-seal chamber (Atrium, 2010).

Delegation and Collaboration

The skill of chest tube management cannot be delegated to nursing assistive personnel (NAP). The nurse directs the NAP about:

- Proper positioning of the patient with chest tubes to facilitate chest tube drainage and optimal functioning of the system.
- How to ambulate and transfer patient with chest drainage.
- Measuring vital signs and reporting any abnormal changes in vital signs, complaints of chest pain or sudden shortness of breath, or excessive bubbling in water-seal chamber to the nurse immediately.

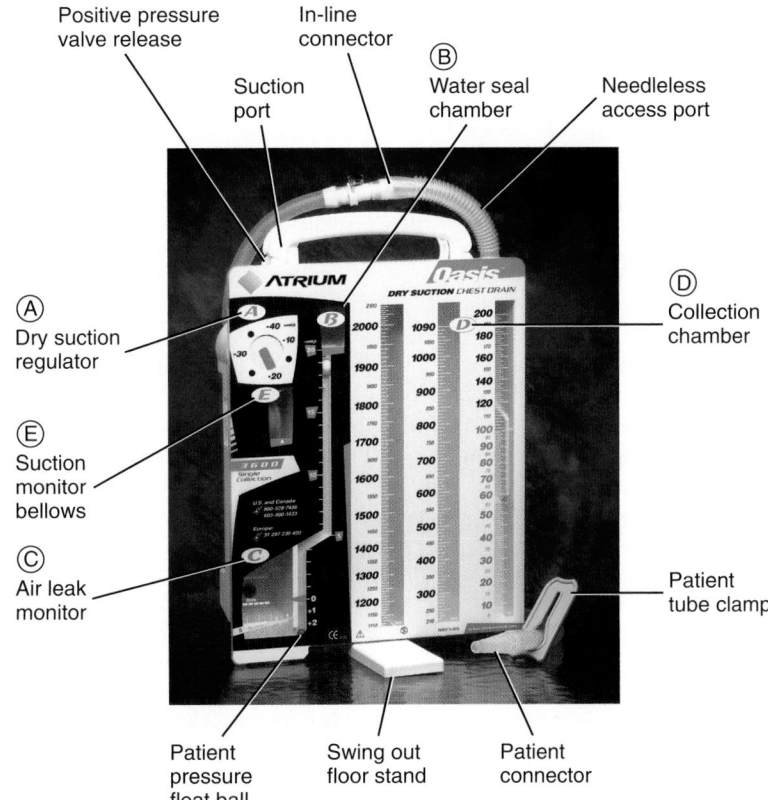

FIG 26-9 Dry suction chest drainage system. (*Used with permission, Atrium Medical Corp.*)

- The danger of any disconnection of system, change in type and amount of drainage, sudden bleeding, or sudden cessation of bubbling. Notify the nurse immediately.

Equipment

❏ Prescribed chest drainage system
❏ Suction source and setup (wall canister or portable)
  - *Water-seal system:* Add sterile water or normal saline (NS) solution to cover the lower 2.5 cm (1 inch) of the water-seal U tube. Or pour sterile water or NS into the suction control chamber if suction is to be used (see manufacturer directions)
  - *Waterless system:* Add vial of 30- to 45-mL sterile sodium chloride or water (for diagnostic air-leak indicator), 20-mL syringe, 21-gauge needle, and antiseptic swab
  - Dry suction system
❏ Clean gloves
❏ Sterile gauze sponges

❏ Local anesthetic, if not an emergent procedure
❏ Chest tube tray (all items are sterile): Knife handle (1), chest tube clamp, small sponge forceps, needle holder, knife blade No. 10, 3-0 silk sutures, tray liner (sterile field), curved 8-inch Kelly clamps (2), 4 × 4–inch sponges (10), suture scissors, hand towels (3), sterile gloves
❏ Dressings: Petrolatum gauze, split chest-tube dressings, several 4 × 4–inch gauze dressings, large gauze dressings (2), and 4-inch tape or elastic bandage (Elastoplast)
❏ Head cover
❏ Facemask/face shield
❏ Sterile gloves
❏ Two rubber-tipped hemostats (shodded) for each chest tube
❏ 1-inch adhesive tape for taping connections or plastic zip ties
❏ Stethoscope, sphygmomanometer, and pulse oximeter

STEP	RATIONALE
ASSESSMENT	
1 Measure vital signs and pulse oximetry.	Provides baseline to determine patient's response to chest tube.
2 Perform a complete respiratory assessment.	Patients in need of chest tubes have impaired oxygenation and ventilation.
a Signs and symptoms of increased respiratory distress and hypoxia (e.g., decreased breath sounds over affected and nonaffected lungs, marked cyanosis, asymmetric chest movements, displaced trachea, shortness of breath, and confusion).	Signs and symptoms associated with respiratory distress are related to type and size of pneumothorax, hemothorax, or preexisting illness. Signs of hypoxia are related to inadequate oxygen to tissues.
b Assess for sharp, stabbing chest pain or chest pain on inspiration, hypotension, and tachycardia. If possible, ask patient to rate level of comfort on a scale of 0 to 10.	Sharp stabbing chest pain with or without decreased blood pressure and increased heart rate may indicate tension pneumothorax. Presence of pneumothorax or hemothorax is painful, frequently causing sharp inspiratory pain. In addition, there is discomfort associated with presence of a chest tube, not just with its insertion. As a result, patients tend to not cough or change position in an effort to minimize this pain (Durai et al., 2010).
3 Assess patient for known allergies. Ask patient if he or she has had a problem with medications, latex, or anything applied to skin.	Povidone-iodine or chlorhexidine are antiseptic solutions used to clean skin before tube insertion (Durai et al., 2010). Lidocaine is a local anesthetic administered to reduce pain. The chest tube will be held in place with tape.
4 Review patient's medication record for anticoagulant therapy, including aspirin, warfarin (Coumadin), heparin, or platelet aggregation inhibitors such as ticlopidine (Ticlid) or dipyridamole (Persantine).	Anticoagulation therapy can increase procedure-related blood loss.
5 Review patient's hemoglobin and hematocrit levels.	Parameters reflect if blood loss is occurring, which may affect oxygenation.
6 For patients who have chest tubes, observe:	
a Chest tube dressing and site surrounding tube insertion.	Ensures that dressing is intact and occlusive seal remains without air or fluid leaks and that area surrounding insertion site is free of drainage or skin irritation.
b Tubing for kinks, dependent loops, or clots.	Maintains patent, freely draining system, preventing fluid accumulation in chest cavity. Subcutaneous emphysema can occur if tubing is blocked or kinked. When tubing is coiled, looped, or clotted, drainage is impeded, and there is an increased risk for a tension pneumothorax or surgical emphysema (Briggs, 2010). If chest tube remains in place for some time, patient's risk for infection increases (Oldfield et al., 2009).
c Chest drainage system should remain upright and below level of tube insertion.	An upright drainage system facilitates drainage and maintains water seal.
7 Assess patient's knowledge of procedure.	Encourages cooperation, minimizes risks and anxiety. Identifies teaching needs.

STEP	RATIONALE

NURSING DIAGNOSES

- Anxiety
- Acute pain
- Impaired gas exchange
- Risk for Infection

Related factors are individualized based on patient's condition or needs.

PLANNING

STEP	RATIONALE
1 Expected outcomes following completion of procedure: • Patient is oriented and less anxious. • Vital signs are stable. • Patient reports no chest pain. • Breath sounds are auscultated in all lobes. Lung expansion is symmetric, pulse oximetry (SpO$_2$) is stable or improved, and respirations are nonlabored. • Chest tube remains in place, and chest drainage system remains airtight. • Gentle tidaling (fluctuations or rocking) is evident in water-seal or diagnostic indicator.	Hypoxia is relieved. Decreased hypoxia improves vital sign measures. Reexpansion of lung reduces chest pain. Reexpansion of lung promotes normal respirations. Indicates correct placement and patency of chest tube drainage system. Indicates that system is functioning normally. Reflects changes in intrapleural pressure.

IMPLEMENTATION

STEP	RATIONALE
1 Identify patient using two identifiers (i.e., name and birthday or name and account number) according to agency policy. Compare identifiers with information on patient's identification bracelet.	Ensures correct patient. Complies with The Joint Commission standards and improves patient safety (TJC, 2012).
2 Check agency policy and determine whether informed consent is needed.	Invasive medical procedures typically require informed consent.
3 Review health care provider's order for chest tube placement.	Insertion of a chest tube requires health care provider order.
4 Perform hand hygiene.	Maintains sterility of system for use under sterile operating room conditions.
5 Set up water-seal system (or dry system with suction); see manufacturer guidelines.	
a Obtain chest drainage system. Remove wrappers and prepare to set up a two- or three-chamber system.	
b While maintaining sterility of drainage tubing, stand system upright and add sterile water or NS to appropriate compartments.	Reduces possibility of contamination.
(1) *Two-chamber system (without suction):* Add sterile solution to water-seal chamber (second chamber), bringing fluid to required level as indicated.	Water-seal chamber acts as one-way valve so air cannot enter pleural space (Briggs, 2010).
(2) *Three-chamber system (with suction):* Add sterile solution to water-seal chamber (middle chamber). Add amount of sterile solution prescribed by health care provider to suction control (third chamber), usually 20 cm water pressure. Connect tubing from suction control chamber to suction source. Tailor length of drainage tube to patient (see illustration).	Depth of rod below fluid level dictates highest amount of negative pressure that can be present within system. For example, 20 cm of water is approximately 20 cm of water pressure. Any additional negative pressure applied to the system is vented into the atmosphere through suction control vent. This safety device prevents damage to pleural tissues from an unexpected surge of negative pressure from suction source. Excessively long drainage tube may result in occlusions.
(3) *Dry suction system:* Fill water-seal chamber with sterile solution. Adjust suction control dial to prescribed level of suction; suction ranges from −10 to −40 cm of water pressure. Suction control chamber vent is never occluded when suction is used. NOTE: On a dry suction system, *DO NOT* obstruct positive-pressure relief valve. This allows air to escape.	Automatic control valve on dry suction control device adjusts to changes in patient air leaks and fluctuation in suction source and vacuum to deliver the prescribed amount of suction.
6 Set up waterless system (see manufacturer guidelines).	
a Remove sterile wrappers and prepare to set up.	Maintains sterility of system for use under sterile operating room conditions.
b For two-chamber system (without suction), nothing is added or needs to be done to system.	Waterless two-chamber system is ready for connecting to patient's chest tube after opening wrappers.

STEP	RATIONALE
c For three-chamber system (with suction), connect tubing from suction control chamber to suction source.	Suction source provides additional negative pressure to system.
d Instill 15 to 45 mL of sterile water or NS into diagnostic indicator injection port located on top of system.	Allows observation of rise and fall in water in diagnostic air leak window. Constant left-to-right bubbling or rocking is abnormal and indicates an air leak. This is not necessary for mediastinal drainage because there is no tidaling. In an emergency, system *does not* require water for set up.
7 Secure all tubing connections with tape in double-spiral fashion using 2.5-cm (1-inch) adhesive tape or use zip ties (nylon cable) with a clamp (Bauman and Handley, 2011). Check system for patency by:	Prevents atmospheric air from leaking into system and patient's intrapleural space. Provides chance to ensure airtight system before connection to patient.

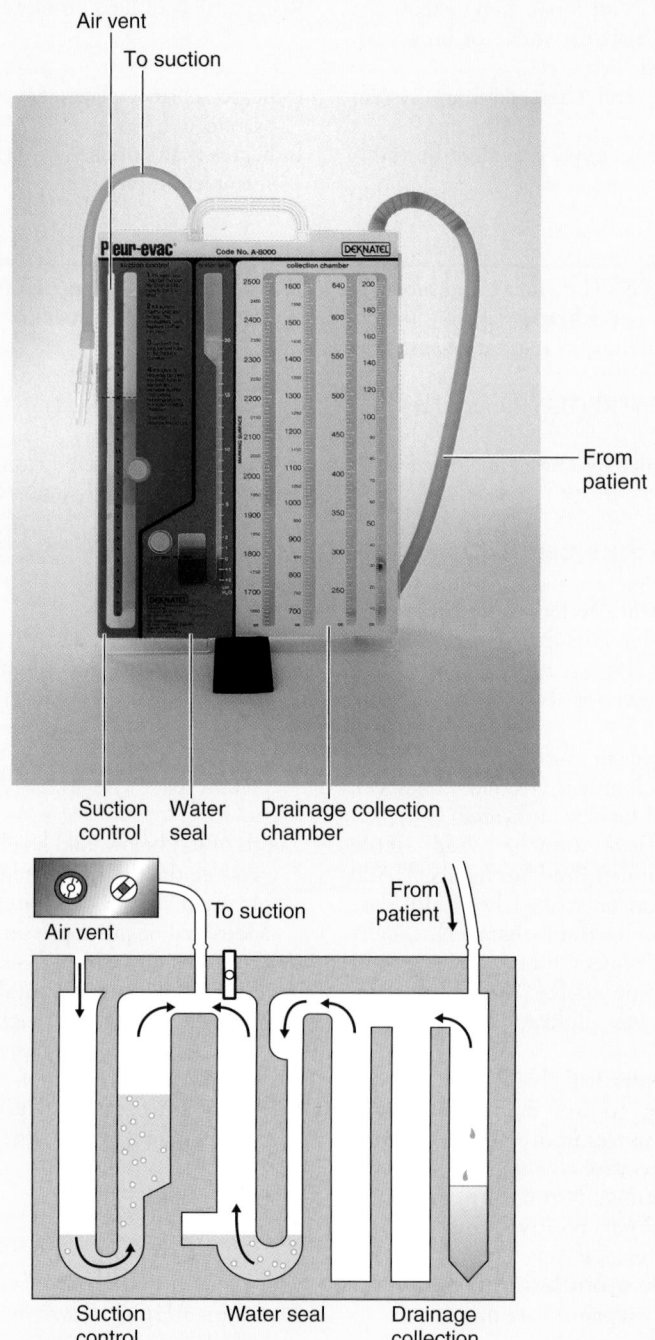

STEP 5b(2) *Top,* Pleur-Evac drainage system, a commercial three-chamber chest drainage device. *Bottom,* Schematic of drainage device.

STEP	RATIONALE
a Clamping drainage tubing that will connect to patient's chest tube.	
b Connecting tubing from float ball chamber to suction source.	
c Turning on suction to prescribed level.	
8 Turn off suction source and unclamp drainage tubing before connecting patient to system. Make a second check to be sure that drainage tubing is not excessively long. Suction source is turned on again after patient is connected.	Having patient connected to suction when it is initiated could damage pleural tissues from sudden increase in negative pressure. Tubing that is coiled or looped may become clotted and cause a tension pneumothorax.
9 Administer premedication such as sedatives or analgesics as ordered.	Reduces patient anxiety and pain during procedure.

Clinical Decision Point *During procedure carefully monitor patient for changes in level of sedation.*

STEP	RATIONALE
10 Provide psychological support to patient (Durai et al., 2010). **a** Reinforce preprocedure explanation. **b** Coach and support patient throughout procedure.	Reduces patient anxiety and helps complete procedure efficiently.
11 Perform hand hygiene and apply clean gloves. Position patient for tube insertion so side in which tube is to be inserted is accessible to health care provider.	Reduces transmission of microorganisms.
12 Help health care provider with chest tube insertion by providing needed equipment and local analgesic. Health care provider will anesthetize skin over insertion site, make a small skin incision, insert a clamped tube, suture it in place, and apply occlusive dressing.	Ensures smooth insertion.
13 Help health care provider attach drainage tube to chest tube; remove clamp. Turn on suction to prescribed level.	Connects drainage system and suction (if ordered) to chest tube.
14 Tape or zip-tie all connections between chest tube and drainage tube. (NOTE: Chest tube is usually taped by health care provider at time of tube placement; check agency policy).	Secures chest tube to drainage system and reduces risk for air leak that causes breaks in airtight system.
15 Check systems for proper functioning. Health care provider will order a chest x-ray film.	Verifies intrapleural placement of tube.
16 After tube placement position patient: **a** Use semi-Fowler's or high-Fowler's position to evacuate air (pneumothorax). **b** Use high-Fowler's position to drain fluid (hemothorax).	Permits optimum drainage of fluid and/or air.
17 Check patency of air vents in system. **a** Water-seal vent must have no occlusion. **b** Suction control chamber vent is not occluded when suction is used. **c** Waterless systems have relief valves without caps.	Permits displaced air to pass into atmosphere. Provides safety factor of releasing excess negative pressure into atmosphere. Provides safety factor of releasing excess negative pressure.
18 Position excess tubing horizontally on mattress next to patient. Secure with clamp provided so it does not obstruct tubing.	Prevents excess tubing from hanging over edge of mattress in dependent loop. Drainage collected in loop can occlude drainage system, which predisposes patient to a tension pneumothorax (Briggs, 2010).
19 Adjust tubing to hang in straight line from chest tube to drainage chamber.	Promotes drainage and prevents fluid or blood from accumulating in pleural cavity.

Clinical Decision Point *Frequent gentle lifting of the drain allows gravity to assist blood and other viscous material to move to the drainage bottle. Patients with recent chest surgery or trauma need to have the chest drain lifted based on assessment of the amount of drainage; some patients might need chest tube drains lifted every 5 to 10 minutes until drainage volume decreases. However, when coiled or dependent looping of tubing is unavoidable, the tubing is lifted every 15 minutes at a minimum to promote drainage (Briggs, 2010).*

STEP	RATIONALE
20 Place two rubber-tipped hemostats (for each chest tube) in an easily accessible position (e.g., taped to top of patient's headboard). These should remain with patient when ambulating.	Chest tubes are double clamped under specific circumstances: (1) to assess for an air leak (Table 26-3), (2) to empty or quickly change disposable systems, or (3) to assess if patient is ready to have tube removed.

Clinical Decision Point *In the event of a chest tube disconnection and risk of contamination, submerge the tube 2 to 4 cm (1 to 2 inches) below the surface of a 250-mL bottle of sterile water or NS until a new chest tube unit can be set up (Bauman and Handley, 2011).*

STEP	RATIONALE
21 Dispose of sharps in proper container, dispose of used supplies, then perform hand hygiene.	Reduces transmission of microorganisms.
22 Care of patient after chest tube insertion:	
a Perform hand hygiene and apply clean gloves. Assess vital signs, oxygen saturation; skin color; breath sounds; rate, depth, and ease of respirations; and insertion site every 15 minutes for the first 2 hours, then at least every shift (see agency policy).	Provides immediate information about procedure-related complications such as respiratory distress and leakage.
b Monitor color, consistency, and amount of chest tube drainage every 15 minutes for first 2 hours. Indicate level of drainage fluid, date, and time on write-on surface of chamber.	Provides baseline for continuous assessment of type and quantity of drainage. Ensures early detection of complications.
(1) Expect less than 100 mL/hr from a mediastinal tube immediately after surgery and no more than 500 mL in first 24 hours.	Sudden gush of drainage may result from coughing or changing patient's position, releasing pooled/collected blood rather than indicating active bleeding.
(2) Expect between 100 and 300 mL in the first 3 hours after insertion of posterior chest tube, with total of 500 to 1000 mL expected in first 24 hours. Drainage is grossly bloody during first several hours after surgery and changes to serous.	Acute bleeding indicates hemorrhage. Health care provider should be notified if there is more than 250 mL of bloody drainage in an hour (Durai et al., 2010).
(3) Expect little or no output from anterior chest tube that is inserted for a pneumothorax.	
c Observe chest dressing for drainage.	Drainage around tube may indicate blockage.
d Palpate around tube for swelling and crepitus (subcutaneous emphysema) as noted by crackling.	Indicates presence of air trapping in subcutaneous tissues. Small amounts are commonly absorbed. Large amounts are potentially dangerous.
e Check tubing to ensure that it is free of kinks and dependent loops.	Promotes drainage.
f Observe for fluctuation of drainage in tubing and water-seal chamber during inspiration and expiration. Observe for clots or debris in tubing.	If fluctuation or tidaling stops, it means that either the lung is fully expanded or system is obstructed (Bauman and Handley, 2011). In nonmechanically ventilated patient, fluid rises in water-seal or diagnostic indicator (waterless system) with inspiration and falls with expiration. The opposite occurs in patient who is mechanically ventilated. This indicates that system is functioning properly (Lewis et al., 2011).
g Keep drainage system upright and below level of patient's chest.	Promotes gravity drainage and prevents backflow of fluid and air into pleural space.
h Check for air leaks by monitoring bubbling in water-seal chamber: Intermittent bubbling is normal during expiration when air is being evacuated from pleural cavity, but continuous bubbling during both inspiration and expiration indicates leak in system.	Absence of bubbling may indicate that lung is fully expanded in patient with a pneumothorax. Check all connections and locate sources of air leak as described in Table 26-3.
i Remove gloves and dispose of used soiled equipment in appropriate biohazard container. Perform hand hygiene.	Prevents accidents involving contaminated equipment.

EVALUATION

1 Evaluate patient for decreased respiratory distress and chest pain. Auscultate patient's lungs and observe chest expansion.	Determines status of lung expansion.
2 Monitor vital signs and pulse oximetry.	Determines if level of oxygenation has improved.
3 Reassess patient's level of comfort on scale of 0 to 10, comparing level with comfort before chest tube insertion.	Indicates need for analgesia. Patient with chest tube discomfort hesitates to take deep breaths and as a result is at risk for pneumonia and atelectasis.
4 Evaluate patient's ability to use deep-breathing exercises while maintaining comfort.	Indicates patient's ability to promote lung expansion and prevent complications.
5 Monitor continued functioning of system as indicated by reduction in amount of drainage, resolution of air leak, and complete reexpansion of the lung.	Detects early signs of system complications or indicates possible removal of chest tube.

TABLE 26-3	Problem Solving with Chest Tubes

Assessment	Intervention
Air leak can occur at insertion site, at connection between tube and drainage device, or within drainage device itself. Determine when air leak occurs during respiratory cycle (e.g., inspiration or expiration). Continuous bubbling is noted in water-seal chamber that is attached to suction (Briggs, 2010). If water-seal unit is not attached to suction, a total absence of bubbling and drainage would indicate a leak.	Check all connections between chest tube and drainage system. Locate leak by clamping tube at different intervals along the tube. Leaks are corrected when constant bubbling stops. If present on a chest drainage system such as the Sahara S 1100a Pleur-Evac, observe the air-leak meter to determine the size of the leak.
Assess for location of leak by clamping chest tube with two rubber-shod or toothless clamps close to chest wall. If bubbling stops, air leak is inside patient's thorax or at chest insertion site.	Unclamp tube, reinforce chest dressing, and notify health care provider immediately. Leaving chest tube clamped can cause collapse of lung, mediastinal shift, and eventual collapse of other lung from buildup of air pressure within the pleural cavity.
If bubbling continues with the clamps near the chest wall, gradually move one clamp at a time down drainage tubing away from patient and toward suction control chamber. When bubbling stops, leak is in section of tubing or connection between clamps.	Replace tubing or secure connection and release clamps.
If bubbling still continues, it indicates that leak is in the drainage system.	Change the drainage system.
Assess for tension pneumothorax: • Severe respiratory distress • Low oxygen saturation • Chest pain • Absence of breath sounds on affected side • Tracheal shift to unaffected side • Hypotension and signs of shock • Tachycardia	Make sure that chest tubes are patent: remove clamps, eliminate kinks, or eliminate occlusion. Notify health care provider immediately and prepare for another chest tube insertion. A one-way flutter (Heimlich) valve or large-gauge needle may be used for short-term emergency release of pressure in the intrapleural space. Have emergency equipment, oxygen, and code cart available because condition is life threatening.
Water-seal tube is no longer submerged in sterile fluid because of evaporation.	Add sterile water to water-seal chamber until distal tip is 2 cm (1 inch) under surface level.

Unexpected Outcomes

1 Patient develops respiratory distress. Chest pain, a decrease in breath sounds over affected and nonaffected lungs, marked cyanosis, asymmetric chest movements, presence of subcutaneous emphysema around tube insertion site or neck, hypotension, tachycardia, and/or mediastinal shift, are critical and indicate a severe change in patient status such as excessive blood loss or tension pneumothorax.

2 Air leak is unrelated to patient's respirations.

3 There is no chest tube drainage.

4 Chest tube is dislodged.

5 Substantial increase in bright red drainage is observed.

Related Interventions

• Notify health care provider immediately.
• Collect set of vital signs and pulse oximetry.
• Prepare for chest x-ray.
• Provide oxygen as ordered.

• See Table 26-3 for determining source of an air leak and problem solving.
• Notify health care provider.

• Observe for kink in chest drainage system.
• Observe for possible clot in chest drainage system.
• Observe for mediastinal shift or respiratory distress (medical emergency).
• Notify health care provider.

• Immediately apply pressure over chest tube insertion site.
• Have assistant obtain sterile petroleum gauze dressing. Apply as patient exhales. Secure dressing with tight seal.
• Notify health care provider.

• Obtain vital signs.
• Monitor drainage.
• Assess patient's cardiopulmonary status.
• Notify health care provider.

Recording and Reporting

- Record respiratory assessment, type of drainage device, amount of suction if used, amount of drainage in chamber, and presence of absence of an air leak. Record patient teaching and validation of understanding in nurses' notes and electronic health record (EHR).
- Record level of patient comfort and baseline vital signs, including oxygen saturation. If postoperative patient, record vital signs and oxygen saturation every 15 minutes for at least 2 hours after surgery.
- Record integrity of dressing and presence of drainage on dressing.
- Report any unexpected outcomes immediately to nurse in charge or health care provider.

Special Considerations

Teaching

- Instruct patient and family caregivers regarding proper functioning of chest tube and drainage system.
- Inform patient to remain in bed if chest tube is attached to suction (Maliakal, 2011).
- Instruct patient to not lie on the tubing or allow it to get kinked to promote drainage (Maliakal, 2011).
- Instruct patient to immediately report any changes in chest comfort.

Pediatric

- If possible, using pictures and special dolls, familiarize child and family with equipment before inserting chest drainage system (Hockenberry and Wilson, 2011).

- Chest tube drainage greater than 3 mL/kg/hr for more than 3 consecutive hours is excessive and may indicate postoperative hemorrhage. Notify the health care provider immediately (Hockenberry and Wilson, 2011).

Gerontologic

- Fragility of the older adult's skin requires special care and planning for management of chest tube dressing. Frequently assess surrounding skin for signs of skin breakdown.

Home Care

- Patients with chronic conditions (e.g., uncomplicated pneumothorax, effusions, empyema) that require long-term chest tube may be discharged with smaller mobile drains (Varela et al., 2010).
- Instruct patient how to ambulate and remain active with a mobile chest tube drainage system.
- Instruct patient and family caregivers about when to contact health care provider regarding changes in the drainage system (e.g., chest pain, breathlessness, change in color or amount of drainage, leakage on the dressing around the chest tube).
- Provide patient and family caregiver information specific to the type of drain; when possible have patient demonstrate proper maintenance of the mobile drainage system. Most of these systems do not have a suction control chamber and use a mechanical one-way valve instead of a water-seal chamber (Varela et al., 2010).

SKILL 26-2 Assisting with Removal of Chest Tubes

[NSO] *Chest Tubes Module / Lesson 4*

Actual removal of a chest tube is most often the function of a physician or health care provider such as a physician's assistant or nurse practitioner. If you are to remove a chest tube, this procedure must be part of agency policy and procedure standards, and you must be competent in the skill. You will complete a designated number of removals under the observation of the health care provider. This skill details nursing responsibilities and health care provider actions for chest tube removal (Briggs, 2010).

Prepare a patient for chest tube removal by assessing the need for pre-removal analgesia, obtaining the required medication orders, and instructing a patient about the process and what will be requested of him or her. During removal of the chest tube, it is important to instruct a patient to take a deep breath and hold it (Valsalva maneuver) until the tube is removed. This maneuver prevents air from being sucked into the chest as the tube is pulled out and an occlusive dressing is applied (Bauman and Handley, 2011; Briggs, 2010; Durai et al., 2010).

Delegation and Collaboration

The skill of assisting with removal of chest tubes cannot be delegated to nursing assistive personnel (NAP). The nurse directs the NAP to:

- Immediately report to the nurse any patient sensations of shortness of breath, increased chest pain, dizziness, or increased anxiety.
- Report to the nurse any drainage on the dressing placed over the chest tube site.

Equipment

- ❏ Suture set
- ❏ Sterile scissors
- ❏ Sterile forceps
- ❏ Clean gloves
- ❏ Sterile gloves
- ❏ Facemask/face shield
- ❏ Prepared sterile dressing: petrolatum-impregnated gauze, 4 × 4 inch–gauze dressings, and large dressings
- ❏ 4-inch adhesive tape or elastic bandage (Elastoplast) cut into strips
- ❏ Stethoscope, sphygmomanometer, pulse oximeter
- ❏ Disposable bed pad

STEP	RATIONALE

ASSESSMENT

1 Assess status of patient's lung re-expansion.

   a Provide health care provider with results of chest x-ray film. — Reveals position of lung tissue in chest cavity and whether sufficient lung reexpansion has occurred (Briggs, 2010; Durai et al., 2010).

   b Note trend in water-seal fluctuation over last 24 hours. Determine if bubbling is present. — Pleura of expanded lung seals holes on internal tip of chest tube, halting fluctuation in water seal. Halt in fluctuation for 24 hours indicates that lung is expanded. When bubbling is present, it usually indicates that lung has not fully expanded (Briggs, 2010; Durai et al., 2010).

   c Confirm that drainage has decreased to less than 100-to-150 mL/day (Briggs, 2010; Hunter, 2008). — Pleural drainage was removed, allowing lung to reexpand.

   d Percuss lung for resonance (see Chapter 6). — Normal resonance occurs with reexpansion.

   e Auscultate lung sounds. — Normal breath sounds are heard bilaterally with reexpansion.

2 Assess patient's level of comfort using a scale of 0 to 10 and determine when last analgesic medication was given. — Chest tube removal is painful; additional analgesia or breathing exercises are often necessary (Briggs, 2010; Durai et al., 2010).

3 Determine patient's understanding of chest tube removal procedure. — Encourages cooperation and minimizes risks and anxiety. Identifies teaching needs.

4 Do not clamp chest tube before removal. Assess for changes in vital signs, oxygen saturation, chest pain, apprehension, and symptoms of tension pneumothorax. — Clamping chest tube before removal to assess patient's tolerance is no longer recommended because there is no benefit to the practice. If a chest tube that was continuing to bubble is clamped, a tension pneumothorax may occur (Briggs, 2010; Hunter, 2008).

NURSING DIAGNOSES

- Acute pain
- Anxiety
- Risk for impaired gas exchange

Related factors are individualized based on patient's condition or needs.

PLANNING

1 Expected outcomes following completion of procedure:
- Lung reexpansion is maintained. — Source of air or fluid loss is sealed or has healed.
- Patient does not experience discomfort. — Pain management is achieved.
- Spontaneous healing of chest tube insertion site occurs after removal of tube without infection or other complications. — Large, nonporous occlusive dressing at puncture site promotes uncomplicated healing.

2 Explain procedure to patient. — Reduces anxiety and promotes patient cooperation.

IMPLEMENTATION

1 Identify patient using two identifiers (i.e., name and birthday or name and account number) according to agency policy. Compare identifiers with information on patient's identification bracelet. — Ensures correct patient. Complies with The Joint Commission standards and improves patient safety (TJC, 2012).

2 Administer prescribed medication for pain relief about 30 minutes before procedure. — Reduces discomfort and relaxes patient. Medication reaches peak effect at time of tube removal. Patients report sensations ranging from pain to pulling when chest tube is removed (Durai et al., 2010; Hunter, 2008).

3 Perform hand hygiene and apply clean gloves and face shield if needed. — Reduces transmission of microorganisms.

4 Help patient to sitting position on edge of bed, lying supine or on side without chest tubes. Place pad under chest tube site. — Health care provider prescribes patient's position to facilitate tube removal. Pad absorbs any drainage associated with tube removal.

5 Health care provider prepares an occlusive dressing of petrolatum-impregnated gauze on a pressure dressing, sets it aside on sterile field, and applies sterile gloves. — Essential to prepare in advance for quick application to wound on tube withdrawal.

6 Support patient physically and emotionally while health care provider removes dressing and clips sutures. — Patients state that, when they know that the tube is being pulled, they can mentally prepare themselves for the procedure. Support from health care team reduces anxiety and promotes cooperation.

STEP	RATIONALE
7 Health care provider asks patient to perform Valsalva maneuver (take deep breath and hold it) or exhale completely and hold it.	Prevents air from being sucked into chest as tube is removed (Bauman and Handley, 2011; Durai et al., 2010). A complication associated with removal of chest tubes is recurrent pneumothorax, which results from atmospheric air reentering pleural cavity. This occurs when patient inhales during tube removal.
8 Health care provider quickly pulls out chest tube and tightens and ties purse-string suture if present, after which patient is instructed to breathe normally.	This forms an airtight seal and prevents entry of air through chest wound. Sutures aid in skin closure (Briggs, 2010; Durai et al., 2010; Hunter, 2008).
9 Health care provider applies sterile occlusive dressing over wound and firmly secures it in position with elastic bandage (Elastoplast) or wide tape.	Keeps wound aseptic. Prevents entry of air into chest. Wound closure occurs spontaneously.
10 Help patient to upright position supported by pillows.	Restores patient's comfort. Patients report that proper positioning following chest tube removal helps to relieve procedure-related sensations of pain and pulling (Hunter, 2008).
11 Remove used equipment from bedside. Dispose in appropriate receptacle.	Prevents spread of microorganisms.
12 Remove gloves and perform hand hygiene.	Reduces transmission of microorganisms.

EVALUATION

1 Auscultate lung sounds.	Helps to confirm lung remains expanded.
2 Palpate skin over area where tube was inserted for subcutaneous emphysema.	Subcutaneous emphysema results from entrance of air into subcutaneous space. It is painful, and as a result patients may not take full lung expansion (Briggs, 2010; Durai et al., 2010).
3 Evaluate for signs of respiratory distress immediately after tube removal and during first few hours after removal.	Provides for early notification of health care provider if adverse symptoms occur. Chest tubes may need reinsertion.

Critical Decision Point *If air is heard escaping from the chest tube site, reinforce the occlusive dressing and immediately notify health care provider.*

4 Evaluate patient's vital signs, oxygen saturation, pulmonary status, and psychological status.	Detects early signs and symptoms of complications.
5 Review chest x-ray film.	Identifies early signs of incomplete lung expansion. If complications are noted, a computed tomography (CT) scan, which is better at identifying chest tube location, should be recommended (Lewis et al., 2011).
6 Ask about patient's level of pain or comfort. Observe for nonverbal cues of pain and assess level of discomfort on scale of 0 to 10.	Indicates that wound did not close well. Determines patient's tolerance of procedure.
7 Check chest dressing for drainage and patency. When changing dressing, note wound for signs of healing.	Ensures occlusion and proper healing of chest wound.

Unexpected Outcomes

1 Dyspnea and labored respirations noted after chest tube removal; potential recurrence of pneumothorax, hemothorax, or effusion.

2 Infection is noted at insertion site.

Related Interventions

- Notify health care provider.
- Obtain vital signs and oxygen saturation.
- Stay with patient.

- Prepare for possible chest tube reinsertion.
- Assess patient's vital signs for elevated temperature, tachypnea, and tachycardia. Assess wound for drainage, odor, erythema, or increased pain.

Recording and Reporting

- Record removal of tube, amount and appearance of drainage in the collection bottle, appearance of wound and dressing, and patient's response in nurses' notes and EHR.
- Record vital signs and respiratory assessment on flow sheet.
- Record patient teaching and validation of understanding in nurses' notes and EHR.

- Report unexpected outcomes to nurse in charge or health care provider.

Special Considerations
Teaching

- Instruct patient and family caregiver to immediately report signs of chest pain, shortness of breath, or sensations of chest discomfort.

Pediatric
- Pediatric patients usually require analgesia (e.g., morphine sulfate 0.1 mg/kg in combination with midazolam [Versed]) before chest tube removal (Hockenberry and Wilson, 2011).

- EMLA (locally applied anesthetic patch) placed under the occlusive dressing at the chest tube insertion site 1 hour before tube removal reduces pain of procedure. However, child may still feel the "pulling" sensation (Hockenberry and Wilson, 2011).

SKILL 26-3 Autotransfusion of Chest Tube Drainage

In autotransfusion blood lost from trauma, injury, or surgery is infused back into a patient's circulatory system. When reinfusion is linked with chest drainage, it is a relatively risk-free, inexpensive, and easy method of replacing blood. Benefits of autotransfusion include an immediate blood supply, no risk of transfusion reaction, and more oxygen supplied to vital organs (Bauman and Handley, 2011). Patients must also have a patent intravenous (IV) line in place (see Chapter 28). Reinfusion is contraindicated in patients with coagulation disorders, infections, cancer, and pre-existing liver or kidney dysfunction (Atrium, 2010; Bauman and Handley, 2011).

Delegation and Collaboration
The skill of reinfusion of chest tube drainage cannot be delegated to nursing assistive personnel (NAP). The nurse directs the NAP to:
- Immediately inform nurse of changes in patient's vital signs or pulse oximetry (SpO₂) levels.
- Immediately inform nurse about increased or decreased drainage from chest tube.

Equipment
- ❏ Adult/pediatric single-use chest drainage and autotransfusion unit (Fig. 26-10)
- ❏ *Optional:* Continuous autotransfusion system (ATS) with a blood-compatible infusion pump (check agency policy)
- ❏ Microaggregate blood filter (40-μm filter, see manufacturer instructions)

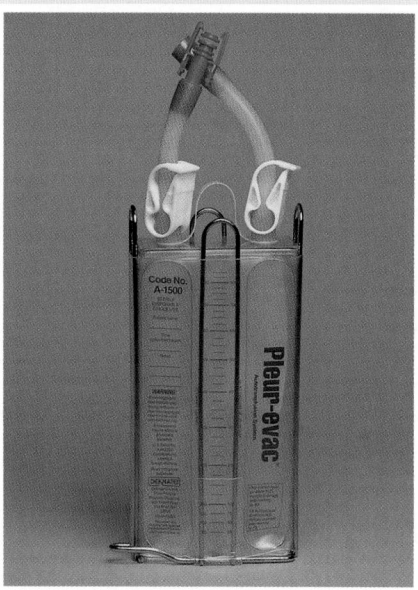

FIG 26-10 Example of autotransfusion unit.

- ❏ Nonvented blood-compatible IV administration set
- ❏ Antiseptic swab
- ❏ Infusion pump (see manufacturer instructions)
- ❏ Replacement bag
- ❏ Gown, clean gloves, and mask as needed

STEP	RATIONALE

ASSESSMENT

1 See Assessment for Skill 26-1.
2 Determine presence of active bleeding (at least 50-to-100 mL/hr), through chest tube. | Indicates need for possible reinfusion of chest tube drainage. |

Clinical Decision Point *Collected blood never remains in the chest drain or ATS blood bag for more than 6 hours before autotransfusion. Immediate use is preferred (Atrium, 2010; Bauman and Handley, 2011).*

3 Assess IV site (see Chapter 28); note size of IV catheter. 18-gauge angiocatheter preferred. | Determines presence of adequate and patent IV site for administration of blood products. |
4 Obtain baseline laboratory data (e.g., hemoglobin and hematocrit). | Provides data to measure effectiveness of reinfusion of chest drainage on patient's circulating blood volume. |

NURSING DIAGNOSES

- Decreased cardiac output
- Ineffective peripheral tissue perfusion
- Risk for infection

Related factors are individualized based on patient's condition or needs.

STEP	RATIONALE

PLANNING

1 Expected outcomes following completion of procedure:

- Vital signs, hematocrit, and hemoglobin stabilize.

  Reinfusion reduces significant blood loss associated with closed chest drainage.

- Drainage system functions correctly and lung reexpands in 48 to 72 hours.

  Negative pressure is reestablished in intrapleural space.

- IV line remains patent.

  Patent IV is necessary for reinfusion of cleansed mediastinal tube drainage.

2 Explain procedure to patient.

Reduces anxiety and promotes patient cooperation.

IMPLEMENTATION

1 System setup:

a Set up ATS according to technique that maintains sterility of unit and following the three steps printed on front of unit.

Contamination of unit provides ready source of infection to patient.

b Make certain that all connections are tight and all clamps are open.

Tight connections ensure an airtight system, and open clamps allow chest drainage to enter ATS bag.

c A 200-μm double-sided mesh filter is located in ATS bag to filter drainage.

Filtering drainage removes extraneous materials and microemboli.

d ATS collection bag has capacity of 1000 mL marked in increments of 25 mL and an area for marking times and amounts.

Dark-red drainage is expected only during immediate postoperative period. This drainage turns serous over time.

Clinical Decision Point *Continuous ATS is prescribed following cardiac surgery. This is a closed system with a specific infusion pump and IV circuit. This system requires specific education and is used in selected situations (Atrium, 2010). Check agency policy.*

2 Identify patient using two identifiers (i.e., name and birthday or name and account number) according to agency policy. Compare identifiers in MAR/medical record with information on patient's identification bracelet and/or ask patient to state name.

Ensures correct patient. Complies with The Joint Commission standards and improves patient safety (TJC, 2012).

3 Perform hand hygiene and apply clean gloves.

Reduces transmission of microorganisms.

4 Prepare chest drainage for reinfusion.

a Following manufacturer directions, open replacement bag and close the two white clamps.

Contamination of unit provides ready source of contamination to patient. Closed clamps maintain closed system during replacement.

b Use high-negativity relief valve to reduce excessive negativity.

This eases removal of initial collection bag from metal support stand.

c *Bag transfer:*

  (1) Close clamp on chest drainage tubing.

Prevents air from entering chest cavity through tube and collapsing lung.

  (2) Close clamps on top of initial ATS collection bag.

Maintains closed system for reinfusion, preventing contamination of the blood.

  (3) Connect chest drainage tube to new ATS bag.

Establishes new ATS.

  (4) Make certain that all connections are tight.

Ensures an airtight system.

  (5) Open all clamps on chest drainage tube and replacement bag.

Reestablishes an autotransfusion collection system.

d Connect connectors on top of initial collection bag and remove bag by lifting it from the side hook and then from the foot hook.

Maintains closed system within bag and removes it for use in autotransfusion.

e Secure replacement bag by connecting the foot hook, replacing the metal frame into the side hook of the chest drainage unit, and pushing down to secure the frame onto the hook.

Provides safe attachment of replacement bag to chest drainage unit.

f Place thumbs on top of metal frame and push up with fingers to slide bag out; remove replacement bag.

5 Reinfuse chest drainage.

a Use new microaggregate filter to reinfuse each autotransfusion bag.

Prevents infusion of microemboli and provides maximal filtration for each bag.

STEP	RATIONALE
b Access bag by inverting it, wiping off port with antiseptic swab, and spiking through the port with the microaggregate filter and twisting.	Connects autotransfusion bag to transfusion tubing.
c With bag upside down, gently squeeze it to remove air and prime filter with blood.	Gentle pressure is used to prevent hemolysis.
d Hang bag on an IV pole and continue to prime tubing until all air is gone. Clamp tubing, attach it to patient's IV access, and adjust clamp to deliver reinfusion at appropriate rate.	Removes all air from transfusion tubing. Reinfusion is delivered either by gravity, application of a blood cuff (not to exceed 150 mm Hg pressure), or blood-compatible IV pump (see Chapter 29).
e If ordered, anticoagulants (Anticoagulant Citrate Dextrose Solution-A or Citrate Phosphate Dextrose Solution, USP) are added to reinfusion through self-sealing port in autotransfusion connector.	Prevents clotting in autotransfusion. Reversing heparin with protamine to preoperative levels or collection of nonheparinized blood following emergency chest trauma may require a citrate anticoagulant (Atrium, 2010).
f Monitor patient's vital signs and SpO$_2$ according to patient condition and agency policy. For some patients this may be as frequent as every 15 minutes; for other patients it may be every hour.	Patients who require autotransfusion usually have complex physiologic needs, and their vital signs change quite rapidly. Consistent, frequent monitoring allows for timely identification of changes and initiation of appropriate interventions to restore physiologic stability.
6 Discontinue autotransfusion.	
a Clamp chest drainage tube only briefly and only if ordered by health care provider and connect it directly to chest drainage unit with red and blue connectors.	Clamping chest tube for any length of time can cause a tension pneumothorax (Hunter, 2008; Lewis et al., 2011).
b Open chest drainage tube clamp.	All drainage will be collected directly in drainage unit and appropriately discarded.
7 Discard used supplies and perform hand hygiene.	Reduces transmission of microorganisms.

EVALUATION

1 Monitor vital signs, hematocrit, and hemoglobin.	Helps determine effects of treatment.
2 Monitor chest drainage system and patient's lung sounds.	Helps determine proper functioning of system and its effectiveness.
3 Evaluate IV infusion site for infiltration and phlebitis.	Patent IV infusion site is maintained.

Unexpected Outcomes	Related Interventions
1 Chest tube is dislodged.	• Immediately apply pressure over chest tube insertion site.
	• Have assistant apply sterile petrolatum-impregnated occlusive dressing.
	• Notify health care provider.
2 Patient has dyspnea, chest pain, and labored respirations.	• Verify that chest tube is patent and draining.
	• Obtain vital signs.
	• Notify health care provider.
3 Patient has signs of infection, fever, and chills.	• Obtain wound cultures as ordered.
	• Obtain vital signs.

Recording and Reporting

• Record drainage and reinfusion with times and amounts of each; include patient's response to reinfusion. Describe condition of IV infusion site. Record patient teaching and validation of understanding in nurses' notes and EHR.

Special Considerations
Teaching

• Prepare patient and family caregivers for the procedure so they will understand when the patient's blood is reinfused. Patients and their families may have had this instruction before surgery but need reinforcement.

Critical Thinking Exercises

Mr. Moberly is in his first postoperative day following open heart surgery. He has a right pleural and mediastinal chest tube to drainage. His last vital signs were blood pressure (BP) 110/64 mm Hg; pulse 126 beats/min; respirations on mechanical ventilator 16 breaths/min; SpO_2, 90%; temperature, 99.0° F (rectally). The last hourly chest tube drainage was 75 mL from the pleural tube and 100 mL from the mediastinal tube.

1 Why is it important to check vital signs, check for air leaks, and note the amount of chest drainage every 15 to 30 minutes for at least 2 hours after Mr. Moberly returns from surgery?

2 Mr. Moberly's chest tube drainage ranged from 75 to 100 mL from both chest tubes over the last 3 hours. Which measures do you take to maintain chest tube patency?

3 It is now 12 hours after surgery, and Mr. Moberly is transferred from bed to chair. Immediately following this transfer you note drainage of 50 mL of dark red fluid. What are your actions?

REVIEW QUESTIONS

1 The nurse is caring for a patient with a new chest tube. The patient is anxious and fearful of taking pain medications because he knows that he needs to be active, take deep breaths, and cough. Which action is the best for the nurse to take to address this fear?
   1 Tell him that the medication will make him sleepy
   2 Explain that by controlling pain he will be able to be active and cough well
   3 Notify the health care provider
   4 Give him the medication anyway

2 A postoperative thoracotomy patient complains of increased sharp chest pain. The nurse's assessment reveals an increased respiratory rate, increased pulse rate, and increased anxiety. When assessing the chest tube system, the nurse notes that the water-seal chamber of the collection tubing is empty. What is causing the patient's chest pain?
   1 Improper function of the chest tube system
   2 Improved pneumothorax
   3 Tension pneumothorax
   4 Incisional pain

3 Patients with chest tubes that remove bloody drainage from the chest cavity usually are at risk for respiratory problems. These patients have many care priorities. What are two important priorities related to management of the chest tube system?
   1 Monitoring chest tube drainage and maintaining chest tube patency
   2 Monitoring chest tube drainage and promoting activity
   3 Promoting airway clearance and maintaining chest tube patency
   4 Promoting activity and airway clearance

4 Patients who have a pneumothorax have which type of chest tube?
   1 Pleural tubes placed in the second or third intercostal space
   2 Pleural tubes placed in the fifth or sixth intercostal space
   3 Pleural tubes placed laterally
   4 Pleural tubes placed posteriorly

5 The nurse is caring for a patient with a chest tube to treat a pneumothorax. The tube and occlusive dressing become dislodged. What should be the nurse's immediate action?
   1 Call for help and take vital signs
   2 Take vital signs and perform a pulmonary assessment
   3 Secure an occlusive dressing over chest tube site and take vital signs
   4 Notify the health care provider and prepare to insert a new chest tube

6 When caring for a patient with a chest tube, which activities can a nurse delegate to nursing assistive personnel (NAP)? (Select all that apply.)
   1 Caring for a patient with a chest tube connected to a disposable drainage system
   2 Helping to remove chest tubes
   3 Reinfusion of chest tube drainage
   4 None of the above

7 A patient comes through the emergency department after an automobile accident 6 hours ago. He has had a chest tube inserted at a small community hospital. He is transferred immediately to the intensive care unit. The nurse's assessment finds that the 18 Fr chest tube is draining serosanguineous fluid, with approximately 75 mL draining over the last hour. The medical record indicates the patient has a hemothorax. The patient's SpO_2 is 90, and respirations are 18 per minute. Based on the nurse's findings the most important action would be:
   1 Monitoring the patient's vital signs
   2 Notifying the health care provider about the appearance of the drainage
   3 Providing analgesic for the patient's pain
   4 Frequently checking the position of the chest drainage tube and note if it stays patent

8 The nurse is assisting the health care provider with removal of a chest tube. Which of the following statements is incorrect?
   1 The patient must be in a prone position to complete the chest tube removal.
   2 The nurse administers the ordered analgesia 30 minutes before the procedure.
   3 The nurse provides emotional support during tube insertion.
   4 The nurse has suction available.

9 Mr. Rifas is a 39-year-old who presented to the emergency department with a tension pneumothorax following a motorcycle accident. He is now on your medical-surgical floor with a chest tube in place at 20 cm of suction. The prior shift reported that Mr. Rifas had a total of 180 mL serous drainage. When you go to assess Mr. Rifas, you notice 250 mL of bright red blood in the chest drainage system. You assess his vital signs: blood pressure, 102/56; heart rate, 142; respiratory rate, 28/min; and oxygen saturation, 89%. In addition, Mr. Rifas is complaining of dyspnea. Which of the following actions is the priority?
   1 Do nothing; this is normal for a patient following a tension pneumothorax.
   2 Continue to monitor Mr. Rifas' vital signs.
   3 Notify the health care provider immediately.
   4 Notify the charge nurse to let her know that you will need to have a new canister ordered.

10 Stripping the chest tube is no longer best practice because it causes increased_____, which can lead to lung tissue injury.

REFERENCES

Atrium: *Managing chest drainage–autotransfusion*, Hudson, NH, 2010, Atrium, Welcome to Atrium, available at http://www.atriummed.com/pdf/ats%20ifu.pdf, accessed August 13, 2011.

Atrium: *Oasis™ Dry Suction Water Seal Drain*, Hudson, NH, 2010, Atrium, available at http://www.atriummed.com/EN/chest_drainage/oasis.asp, accessed August 9, 2012.

Bauman A, Handley C: Chest-tube care: the more you know the easier it gets, *Am Nurse Today* 6(9):27, 2011.

Bethel J: Tension pneumothorax, *Emerg Nurs* 16(4):26, 2008.

Briggs D: Nursing care and management of patients with interpleural drains, *Nurs Stand* 24(21):47, 2010.

Durai R, et al: Managing a chest tube and drainage system, *Nurs Stand* 91(2):275, 2010.

Hockenberry MJ, Wilson D: *Nursing care of infants and children*, ed 9, St Louis, 2011, Mosby.

Hunter J: Chest drain removal, *Nurs Stand* 22(45):35, 2008.

Lewis ML, et al: *Medical-surgical nursing: assessment and management of clinical problems*, ed 8, St Louis, 2011, Mosby.

Maliakal M: Chest tubes, *Nursing 2011* 7:33, 2011.

Mertin S, et al: Getting to the heart of pleural effusions: a case study, *J Am Acad Nurse Pract* 21:506, 2009.

Oldfield M, et al: Examining the association between chest tube–related factors and the risk of developing health care–associated infections in the ICU of a community hospital: a retrospective case-control study, *Intensive Crit Care Nurs* 25:38, 2009.

The Joint Commission (TJC): *National Patient Safety Goals,* Oakbrook Terrace, Ill, 2012, The Commission, available at http://www.jointcommission.org/standards_information/npsgs.aspx.

Twedell D: Pleural effusions: etiology, diagnosis, and management, *J Contin Educ Nurs* 40(6):248, 2009.

U.S. National Library of Medicine: PubMed Health: Collapsed Lung, 2011, available at http://www.ncbi.nlm.nih.gov/pubmedhealth/PMH0001151/, accessed 7.25.2012.

Varela G, et al: Portable chest drainage systems and outpatient chest tube management, *Thorac Surg Clin* 20:421, 2010.

Emergency Measures for Life Support

MEDIA RESOURCES

- **evolve** *learning system* http://evolve.elsevier.com/Perry/skills
  - Review Questions
  - Audio Glossary

KEY TERMS

Advance directive	Bag-mask device	Code event	Endotracheal intubation
Automated external defibrillator (AED)	Cardiopulmonary resuscitation (CPR)	Do not resuscitate (DNR)	Manual defibrillator
		Dysrhythmia	Oral airway

OBJECTIVES

Mastery of content in this chapter will enable the nurse to:
- Discuss indications for oral airway insertion.
- Identify need for automated external defibrillator (AED) application and indications for use.
- State indications for cardiopulmonary resuscitation (CPR).
- Discuss code management.
- State the end points for CPR.
- Demonstrate in a laboratory or clinical situation: insertion of an oral airway, use of an AED, and performance of CPR.

Cardiopulmonary arrests are emergency situations that you must be prepared to handle at any time. Cardiac arrest is the cessation of circulating blood flow, which eliminates oxygen transport and perfusion. Many cardiac arrests are caused by irregular heart rhythms known as dysrhythmias. The causes of dysrhythmias may include electrolyte disturbances (potassium, magnesium, or calcium), heart damage, and certain prescribed or recreational medications. A dysrhythmia causes symptoms that vary in severity from minor to lethal. Lethal dysrhythmias include ventricular tachycardia (VT) and ventricular fibrillation (VF) and require a medically delivered electrical shock for treatment. Early defibrillation or shock may quickly return the heart to normal without further deterioration of a patient's status. The majority of arrests involve the collapse of both the respiratory and cardiovascular systems. This is defined as a *cardiopulmonary arrest*. Unless otherwise indicated within a patient's advance directive or a do-not-resuscitate (DNR) health care provider's order, all patients receive cardiopulmonary resuscitation (CPR) in the event of an arrest.

In addition to initiating CPR, you must anticipate and recognize prearrest indications such as tachycardia, hypotension, tachypnea, decreasing oxygen saturation below 90% despite provision of supplemental oxygen, and a decreasing urine output of less than 50 mL in 4 hours (Ehlenbach et al., 2009). Each agency has policies for initiating the rapid-response team before a code occurs.

You will learn to approach a resuscitation attempt in a systematic and organized fashion to ensure the most expeditious care. Within most hospitals this arrest situation is referred to as a "code" (e.g., "code blue," "code 7"). Each agency has a specific code or signal to summon immediate assistance in the event of a cardiac and/or respiratory arrest. The goal is to provide resuscitation in a timely manner to restore cardiopulmonary function and avoid poor neurologic outcomes or death. Most nurses and nursing students are required to be certified in basic life support (BLS) measures.

EVIDENCE-BASED PRACTICE

The Committee on Emergency Cardiac Care (Berg et al., 2010a) reviews and conducts research on cardiac arrest treatment and outcomes and has created evidence-based guidelines for both initial care (BLS) and ongoing measures (advanced cardiovascular life support [ACLS]) (Neumar et al., 2010). The 2010 American Heart Association (AHA) resuscitation guidelines emphasize the importance of high-quality CPR, which includes continuous chest compression for bystanders, a new emergency medical services (EMS) algorithm, and aggressive postresuscitation care (AHA, 2010). These new methods have shown to dramatically improve survival in patients with witnessed arrest and shockable rhythm (Ewy and Kern, 2009). The method suggests use of continuous chest compression without mouth-to-mouth ventilations for witnessed cardiac arrest. For bystanders with access to automated external defibrillators (AEDs) and EMS personnel who arrive during the first 4 to 5 minutes of the arrest, the delivery of a defibrillator shock is recommended. The updated CPR guidelines from the AHA include a hands-only approach (continuous chest compressions) for the untrained lay rescuer. The sequence of actions has changed from A B C (airway, breathing, circulation) to C A B (circulation, airway, breathing). Methods to improve survival after cardiopulmonary arrest include:

- Immediate recognition and activation of emergency medical response.
- Early CPR that emphasizes chest compressions.
- Rapid defibrillation if indicated.
- Effective advanced cardiac life support
- Integrated postcardiac care such as cooling to preserve neurologic function (Peberdy et al., 2010). Many hospitals have developed protocols for using external cooling techniques and intravascular cooling devices.

Many hospitals now allow family members and significant others to remain in a patient's room during resuscitative efforts and invasive procedures. Evaluation of these programs confirms a remarkable level of approval and gratitude by participating family members (AACN, 2010). Survey of family members noted a significant reduction in posttraumatic stress and self-reports of a greater sense of resolution and fulfillment among witnesses of resuscitative efforts compared with nonwitnesses.

PATIENT-CENTERED CARE

Whenever a patient requires resuscitation, his or her family is also a prime nursing concern. When caring for patients from diverse cultures and religions, consider an individual's meaning and interpretation of life support and resuscitation. You can perform many interventions to help families during emergency situations. Use a professional language interpreter to explain the patient's status to them. In addition, use cultural and religious support personnel to facilitate understanding of the events by family members and accommodate the patient's religious and cultural practices. Be prepared to handle large numbers of visitors who may remain at the bedside to provide support for the family and/or pray for the patient. Collaborate with the family decision maker and leader to plan rotating visits at the bedside. It is helpful to designate a waiting area to accommodate the group.

Advance directives offer valuable information concerning a patient's resuscitation status and individual patient decisions regarding resuscitation efforts. Although advance directives are often addressed before or during a patient's hospitalization, you play an important role in encouraging patients to complete the document.

Although individuals may be part of a specific cultural or religious group, an individual may not follow all aspects of that culture or religion. Therefore it is essential that you consider each individual's interpretation and wishes to ensure the right of self-determination.

Safety Guidelines

1. Know a patient's baseline vital signs, noting any irregularities in cardiac rhythm. Dysrhythmias can precipitate a cardiopulmonary arrest. Cardiovascular conditions that place a patient at risk for dysrhythmias include coronary artery disease, myocardial infarction, open-heart surgeries, acid-base imbalances, and toxicities.

2. Know a patient's most recent serum electrolyte values. Electrolyte imbalances (e.g., potassium, magnesium, and calcium) can precipitate cardiopulmonary arrest.

3. When a patient has been exposed to a chemical or drug, attempt to determine the type and amount of the substance involved. Certain chemicals (e.g., ethanol, tranquilizers, opiates) depress the respiratory center and can result in a respiratory arrest. Oversedation involving the use of patient-controlled analgesia (PCA) pumps or epidural administration can also contribute to respiratory depression. Overdoses of some drugs can cause ventricular dysrhythmias and cardiopulmonary arrest.

SKILL 27-1   Inserting an Oropharyngeal Airway

An oropharyngeal airway is a semicircular, minimally flexible, curved piece of hard plastic (Fig. 27-1). When inserted, it extends from just outside the lips, over the tongue, and to the pharynx (Fig. 27-2). Oral airways allow you to suction through a central core or along the side of the airway and maintain airway patency in an unconscious patient.

Oral airways vary in length and width (Table 27-1). Choose the size of an oral airway based on a patient's age and the width and length of his or her mouth. Size is correct if, when the flange is held parallel to the front teeth with the airway against the patient's cheek, the end of the curve reaches the angle of the jaw.

Delegation and Collaboration

The skill of inserting an oropharyngeal airway cannot be delegated to nursing assistive personnel (NAP). Respiratory therapists have the training to insert an oral airway. The nurse directs the NAP to:

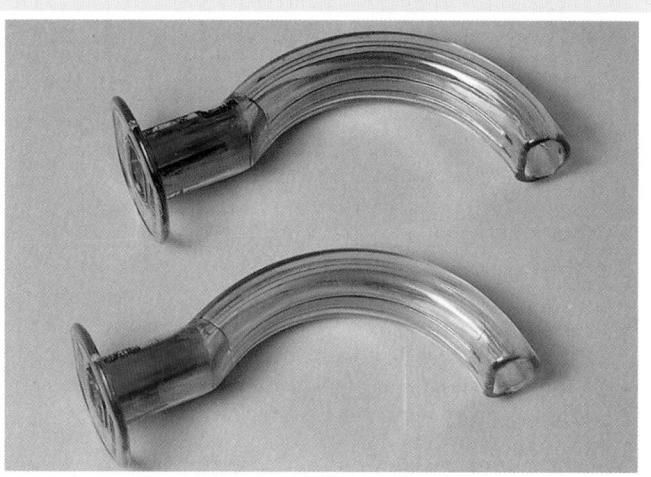

FIG 27-1 Oral airways.

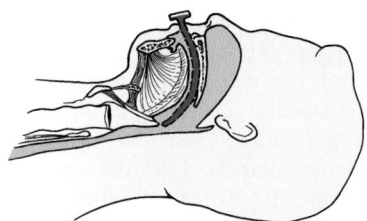

FIG 27-2 Placement of oral airway.

- Immediately report to the nurse any signs of airway distress, vomiting, or change in level of consciousness.

Equipment
- ❏ Appropriate-size oral airway (see Table 27-1)
- ❏ Clean gloves
- ❏ Tissues or washcloths
- ❏ Suction equipment if indicated
- ❏ Nonallergenic tape (optional)
- ❏ Face shield if indicated
- ❏ Tongue blade
- ❏ Stethoscope

TABLE 27-1	Oral Airway Guidelines for Size* by Age
Size	**Age**
30-34 mm or size 000	Premature neonates
40 mm or size 00	Newborn
50 mm or size 0	Newborn to 1 yr
60 mm or size 1	1 to 2 yr
70 mm or size 2	2 to 6 yr
80 mm or size 3	6 to 18 yr
90 mm or size 4	Adult medium
100 mm or size 5	Adult large
110 mm or size 6	Adult extra large

*Measure from the corner of the mouth to the angle of the jaw just below the ear for size estimation.

STEP	RATIONALE

ASSESSMENT

1 Identify need to insert an oral airway. Signs and symptoms include upper airway gurgling with breathing, absent cough or gag reflex, increased oral secretions, excessive drooling, grinding teeth, clenched teeth, biting of orotracheal or gastric tubes, labored respirations, and increased respiratory rate.

These conditions place patient at risk for obstruction of the upper airway. Use oral airways only in unconscious patients. They may stimulate vomiting or laryngospasm if inserted in a semiconscious or conscious patient.

2 Determine factors that may contribute to upper airway obstruction such as age (children have a proportionally larger tongue) or presence of a nasal or oral airway and drainage tubes (swallowing is more difficult with tubes in place).

Allows you to accurately assess need for oral airway placement. Patients at greater risk for upper airway obstruction are infants, children, and adults with upper airway congestion, loss of consciousness, seizure disorders, neuromuscular diseases, increased oral secretions, or facial trauma.

3 Assess for presence of gag reflex; gently place tongue blade on back of patient's tongue.

Provides guide as to when oral airway can be safely removed in postoperative patient.

4 Ensure that patient does not have dentures in place before attempting an oral airway insertion.

Oral airway insertion can dislodge dentures and cause worsening airway obstruction.

Clinical Decision Point *Never insert an oral airway in a conscious patient or a patient with recent oral trauma, oral surgery, or loose teeth. Never force an airway into place.*

5 Assess family member's knowledge of procedure.

Identifies learning needs of family. Patient will be unconscious.

NURSING DIAGNOSES

- Ineffective airway clearance
- Risk for aspiration

Related factors are individualized based on patient's condition or needs.

PLANNING

1 Expected outcomes following completion of procedure:
  - Patient's respiratory status improves, as evidenced by respirations with normal rate, easier removal of secretions, and lack of gurgling noise in throat with respirations.

Airway is clear of secretions.

  - Patient is not able to grind teeth or bite tubes.
  - Patient's tongue does not obstruct airway.

Oral airway prevents tooth contact with other teeth or with tubes.
Oral airway keeps tongue in correct position to maintain patent airway.

2 Family members can verbalize understanding of need for oropharyngeal airway.

Teaching was successful.

STEP	RATIONALE
IMPLEMENTATION	
1 Position unconscious patient in semi-Fowler's position if possible.	Provides easy access to oral cavity.
2 Perform hand hygiene and apply clean gloves and face shield (when possible).	Reduces transmission of microorganisms.
3 Whenever possible, use padded tongue blade to open patient's mouth; if necessary, use thumb and forefinger of nondominant hand to open jaws and teeth.	Provides access to oral cavity. To avoid a bite, do not insert your fingers into patient's mouth. Use extreme caution if manually opening patient's jaw and teeth.
4 Insert oral airway.	When inserting airway, take care not to push patient's tongue into pharynx.
a Hold oral airway with curved end up and insert distal end until airway reaches back of throat; then turn airway over 180 degrees and follow natural curve of tongue. *Option:* Hold airway sideways, insert halfway, and then rotate airway 90 degrees while gliding it over natural curvature of tongue. Make sure that outer flange is just outside patient's lips.	Proper insertion of airway prevents displacement of patient's tongue into posterior oropharynx.

Clinical Decision Point *In a **pediatric patient,** **DO NOT** **rotate** the oral airway on insertion because the airway tip will damage the soft palate.*

STEP	RATIONALE
5 Suction secretions as needed.	Removes secretions; maintains patent airway.
6 Reassess patient's respiratory status; auscultate lungs.	Verifies respiratory status and patent airway.
7 Clean patient's face with soft tissue or washcloth.	Promotes hygiene.
8 Discard tissue into appropriate receptacle, place washcloth in dirty or soiled linen bag, remove gloves and face shield and discard in appropriate receptacle; perform hand hygiene.	Reduces transmission of microorganisms.
9 Administer mouth care frequently.	Increases patient comfort and removes debris. It also provides moisture to oral mucosal tissues.

Clinical Decision Point *Do not use lemon glycerin swabs for oral care because they are drying to mucosal tissues and promote bacterial growth. Oral airway will need to be removed, cleaned or discarded, and replaced in patients with excessive oral secretions. Frequent suctioning of the oral cavity may be required. Oral airways are not a long-term solution. They can cause significant lip and tongue erosion.*

STEP	RATIONALE
EVALUATION	
1 Observe patient's respiratory status and compare respiratory assessments before and after insertion of oral airway.	Identifies patient's response to insertion of airway.
2 Evaluate that airway is patent and that patient's tongue does not obstruct airway.	Ensures route for oxygen delivery to patient.
3 Observe for patient pushing airway out with tongue or coughing.	Patient's ability to clear his or her own airway may have returned. Indicates reassessment of need for an oral airway.

Unexpected Outcomes	Related Interventions
1 Patient continually coughs and gags when airway is inserted.	• Do not continue inserting airway if patient begins to gag. Stimulation of gag reflex can cause vomiting and aspiration. • Remove oral airway and position patient on side. • Reassess need for artificial airway prn.
2 Airway obstruction not relieved.	• Obtain immediate assistance. • Reinsert airway or determine from physician if another form of airway is needed. • Assess for other causes of obstruction.
3 Patient pushes airway out of place or out of mouth.	• Patient may be at point where he or she is able to breathe on own. Reassess patient's need for oral airway.
4 Unable to insert oral airway; patient is combative or you are unable to pry mouth open.	• Obtain assistance. • Reassess patient's need for oral airway. • Provide sedation as ordered.

Recording and Reporting
- Record in nurses' notes and electronic health record (EHR) assessment findings while inserting oral airway; size of oral airway; other interventions performed at same time, especially positioning and suctioning; and patient's response to procedure.

Special Considerations
Pediatric
- Oral airways are seldom used in treatment of airway obstruction in infants and children. Because the airway is narrow, they are often more occlusive than beneficial (Hockenberry and Wilson, 2011).

SKILL 27-2 Use of an Automated External Defibrillator

Defibrillation is the electrical attempt to stop a lethal arrhythmia such as ventricular fibrillation. An automated external defibrillator (AED) allows for individuals trained only in basic life support to defibrillate. AEDs eliminate the need for training in rhythm interpretation and make early defibrillation practical and achievable. The AED is a defibrillator that incorporates a rhythm analysis system. The device attaches to a patient by two adhesive pads and connecting cables. Most AEDs are stand-alone boxes with a very simple three-step function (Fig. 27-3) and verbal prompts to guide the responder. All AEDs offer automated rhythm analysis, whereby the rhythm is compared to thousands of other rhythms stored in the AED computer software. On rhythm identification, some AEDs automatically provide the electrical shock after a verbal warning (fully automated). Other AEDs recommend a shock, if needed, and then prompt the responder to press the shock button.

Delegation and Collaboration
Basic life support certification provides hands-on training with an AED for laypersons, nursing assistive personnel (NAP), and licensed health care professionals. Most hospitals using AEDs have given the authority to use an AED to all cardiopulmonary resuscitation (CPR)–certified personnel, including NAP. Refer to specific hospital policies for use of the AED.

Equipment
- ❏ AED
- ❏ Pair of AED adhesive pads

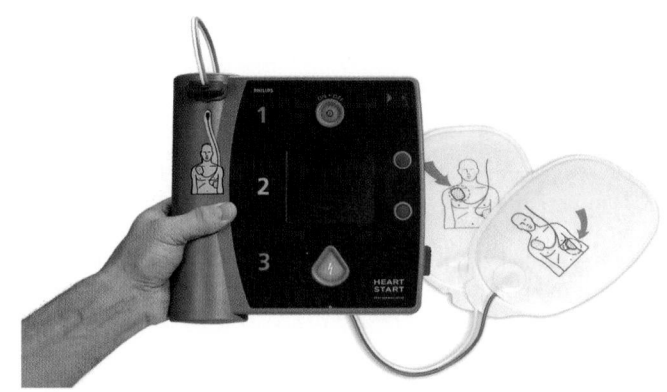

FIG 27-3 Automated external defibrillator device. (*Courtesy Philips Medical Systems.*)

STEP	RATIONALE

ASSESSMENT

1 Establish person's unresponsiveness and call for help. (In community settings have someone call 9-1-1.)	This information helps to determine if the individual is unresponsive rather than asleep, intoxicated, hearing impaired, or postictal. Rapid response by qualified professionals ensures ongoing resuscitation support.
2 Establish absence of respirations and lack of circulation: no pulse, no respirations, no movement.	Indicates need for emergency measures, including AED.

Clinical Decision Point *An AED should be applied only to a patient who is unconscious, not breathing, and pulseless. For children younger than 8 years old, AED pads designed for children should be used. When child pads are not available, use adult AED pads (Berg et al., 2010b).*

NURSING DIAGNOSES

- Decreased cardiac output
- Impaired spontaneous ventilation
- Ineffective breathing pattern
- Ineffective tissue perfusion

Related factors are individualized based on patient's condition or needs.

PLANNING

1 Expected outcomes following completion of procedure:
  • Patient's cardiac rhythm is converted back to stable rhythm.
 	
  • Patient regains pulse and respirations.
	Defibrillation provides electrical shock to convert a lethal dysrhythmia.
	CPR and defibrillation were successful.

STEP	RATIONALE

IMPLEMENTATION

1 Assess patient for unresponsiveness, not breathing and pulselessness.

These are indicators of cardiopulmonary arrest.

2 Activate code team in accordance with hospital policy and procedure.

First available person brings resuscitation cart and AED.

3 Start chest compressions and continue until AED is attached to patient and verbal prompt of device advises you, "Do not touch the patient."

To minimize interruption time of chest compressions, continue CPR while AED is being applied and turned on.

4 Place AED next to patient near chest or head.

Ensures easy access to device.

Clinical Decision Point *If the AED is immediately available, attach it to patient as soon as possible. The faster defibrillation is delivered, the better the survival rate (Ewy and Kern, 2009).*

5 Turn on power (see illustration).

Turning on the power will begin the verbal prompts to guide you through the next steps.

6 Attach the device. Place the first AED pad on the upper right sternal border directly below the clavicle. Place the second AED pad lateral to the left nipple with the top of the pad a few inches below the axilla (see illustration). Ensure that cables are connected to the AED.

Alternative pad placement of AED pads is not recommended. AEDs analyze most heart rhythms using lead II. If the AED pads are placed as directed, patient's heart rhythm will be analyzed in lead II.

Patients with large amounts of chest hair may require shaving to obtain adequate pad contact.

Clinical Decision Point *Do not attach pads to a wet surface, over a medication patch, or over a pacemaker or implanted defibrillator. Wet surfaces, implanted defibrillators, and medication patches reduce the effectiveness of the defibrillation attempt and result in complications.*

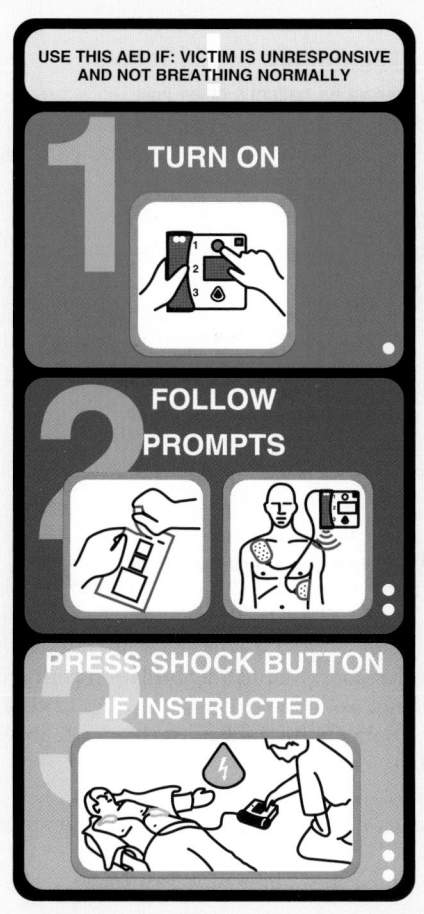

STEP 5 Power panel with AED prompts. *(Courtesy Philips Medical Systems.)*

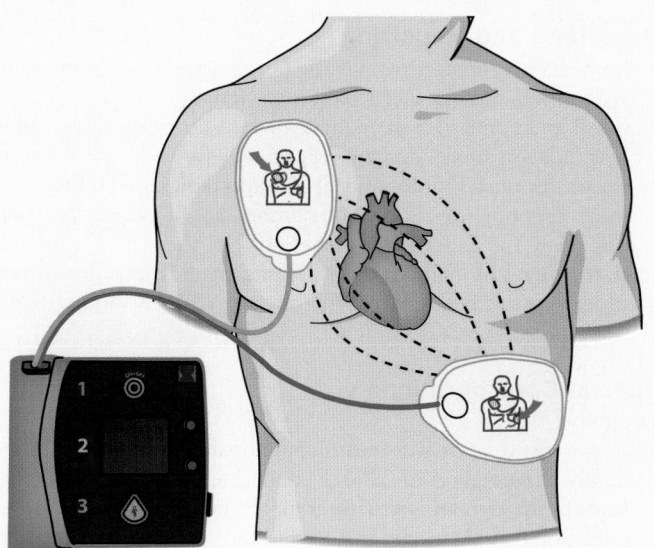

STEP 6 Placement of AED pads with device next to patient.

STEP	RATIONALE
7 Do *NOT* touch patient when AED prompts you. Direct rescuers and bystanders to avoid touching patient by announcing "Clear!" Allow the AED to analyze the rhythm. Some devices require that an analysis button be pressed. The AED takes approximately 5 to 15 seconds to analyze the rhythm.	Each brand of AED is different; thus familiarity with the specific model that you are using is important. Not touching patient when directed prevents artifact errors, avoids all movement during analysis (Link et al., 2010), and prevents shock from being delivered to bystanders.
8 Before pressing the shock button, announce loudly to clear the victim and perform a visual check to ensure that no one is in contact with him or her.	Clearing patient ensures safety for those involved in rescue efforts.
9 Immediately begin chest compression after the shock and continue for 2 minutes. Do *NOT* remove the pads.	Continues cardiac perfusion.
10 Deliver two breaths using mouth-to-mouth with barrier device or mouth-to-mask device or bag-mask device. Watch for chest rise and fall. Deliver 10-to-12 breaths/min.	In a hospital setting where protected methods of artificial ventilation are available, mouth-to-mouth without a barrier device is not recommended because of risk for microbial contamination.
11 After 2 minutes of CPR, the AED will prompt you not to touch patient and will resume analysis of patient's rhythm. This cycle will continue until patient regains a pulse or physician determines death.	

EVALUATION

1 Inspect pad adhesion to chest wall. If pads are not in good contact with chest wall, remove them and apply a new set. Attach new set of pads to the AED.	Poor pad-skin contact reduces the effectiveness of the shock, causes skin burns, or increases chance of shocking those involved in the rescue efforts. Always apply a new set of pads. Do *NOT* reuse.
2 Check for a palpable pulse. Continue resuscitative efforts until patient regains pulse or the physician determines death.	

Unexpected Outcomes

1 Patient's heart rhythm does not convert into a stable rhythm with pulse after defibrillation.

2 Patient's skin has burns under AED pads.

Related Interventions

- Assess pad contact on patient's chest wall.
- Do not touch patient during AED rhythm analysis.
- Avoid placing AED pads over medication patches, pacemaker, or implantable defibrillator generators.
- Assess AED pad contact on chest.
- Ensure that chest is dry before applying pads to chest.
- Apply skin care as indicated if patient is resuscitated successfully.

Recording and Reporting

- Immediately report arrest via the hospital-wide communication system, indicating exact location of victim.
- Cardiopulmonary arrest requires precise documentation. Most hospitals use a form designed specifically for in-hospital arrests.
- Record in nurses' notes and EHR or on designated CPR worksheet: onset of arrest, time and number of AED shocks (you will not know the exact energy level used by the AED), time and energy level of manual defibrillations, medications given, procedures performed, cardiac rhythm, use of CPR, and patient's response.

Special Considerations
Teaching

- If patient is at risk for cardiopulmonary arrest, instruct the family or caregivers in CPR or encourage them to obtain certification through an instructor from the hospital, American Red Cross, or American Heart Association.

- Patient and family should keep emergency numbers taped to the phone or consider programming them into speed dial function on both home and mobile phones. Stress the use of 9-1-1.
- It is extremely helpful if family has list of medications that patient is presently taking.

Pediatric

- Most AEDs are specifically designed for adult use only and are therefore not recommended for use in children younger than 8 years old or less than 25 kg body weight (Link et al., 2010). Adult pads can be used if child pads are not available; be sure not to overlap pads. Manual defibrillation performed by health care personnel using lower energy settings (2 to 4 joules/kg) is the most common method of pediatric defibrillation (Link et al., 2010).

Home Care

- AEDs are available for use in the community and home setting.

SKILL 27-3 Code Management

All who respond to cardiopulmonary arrests should follow a simple, standardized, easy-to-remember approach. Initially a code is managed by the first responder performing the basic skills of cardiopulmonary resuscitation (CPR), which includes the primary survey of C (circulation), A (airway), B (breathing), D (early defibrillation). These interventions continue until the code team arrives. The initial process also includes notification of the hospital resuscitation or code team. Most of the code team members have been trained in the advanced cardiac life support (ACLS) guidelines and the performance of the secondary survey: C (rhythm analysis of cardiac rhythm), A (airway intubation), B (confirmation of airway and ventilation) and D (differential diagnosis of the cause). Both surveys must be reassessed continually and managed as appropriate throughout the code situation.

The hospital response team usually includes a physician, intensive care nurse, respiratory therapy personnel, anesthesiology personnel, and possibly radiology and laboratory technologists. A pastoral care representative is often available to be with the family.

The ability of a non-ACLS–certified nurse to initiate resuscitative efforts can prevent lethal dysrhythmias such as ventricular fibrillation from deteriorating to asystole (absence of cardiac electrical activity) and provide a chance for the heart to return to its normal rhythm. Table 27-2 summarizes basic cardiac arrhythmias. Early CPR and defibrillation delivered within the primary survey optimizes heart and brain function, leading to improved survivability. Equipment may be readily available at the bedside or in a designated area of the hospital unit. It is the nurse's responsibility to know how to use this equipment and to know its location and the contents of the resuscitation or crash cart.

CPR certification is a requirement of nurses and nursing students. Therefore CPR will not be covered in detail within this chapter. Table 27-3 summarizes some points regarding CPR skills, including differences in adult, child, and infant techniques.

Delegation and Collaboration

The skill of code management cannot be delegated to nursing assistive personnel (NAP). However, NAP who are certified in basic life support (BLS) techniques can perform the basic skills of CPR. Most NAP are certified in BLS and can use an automated external defibrillator (AED). Most hospitals reserve the skill of manual defibrillation for licensed personnel who are ACLS certified or have received competency validation to perform manual

TABLE 27-2	Common Cardiac Dysrhythmias
Rhythm Characteristics and Etiology	**Clinical Significance and Management**

Sinus Tachycardia

Rhythm Characteristics and Etiology	Clinical Significance and Management
Regular rhythm, rate 100-180 beats/min (higher in infants), normal P wave, normal QRS complex.	Some patients with heart disease are unable to increase their heart rate to meet increased oxygen demands.
Rate increase is often normal response to exercise, emotion, or stressors such as pain, fever, pump failure, hyperthyroidism, and certain drugs (e.g., caffeine, nitrates, epinephrine, nicotine).	Correct underlying factors; discontinue drugs producing the side effect.

Sinus Bradycardia

Rhythm Characteristics and Etiology	Clinical Significance and Management
Regular rhythm, rate less than 60 beats/min, normal P wave, normal PR interval, normal QRS complex.	No clinical significance unless associated with signs and symptoms of reduced cardiac output such as dizziness or syncope or presence of chest pain.
Rate decrease is normal response to sleep or in well-conditioned athlete; diminished blood flow to SA node, vagal stimulation, hypothyroidism, increased intracranial pressure, or pharmacologic agents (e.g., digoxin, propranolol, quinidine, procainamide) sometimes cause abnormal drops in rate.	Bradycardia with hypotension and decreased cardiac output is treated with atropine; pacemaker is sometimes necessary.

Continued

TABLE 27-2	Common Cardiac Dysrhythmias—cont'd

Rhythm Characteristics and Etiology	**Clinical Significance and Management**

Atrial Fibrillation (A-fib)

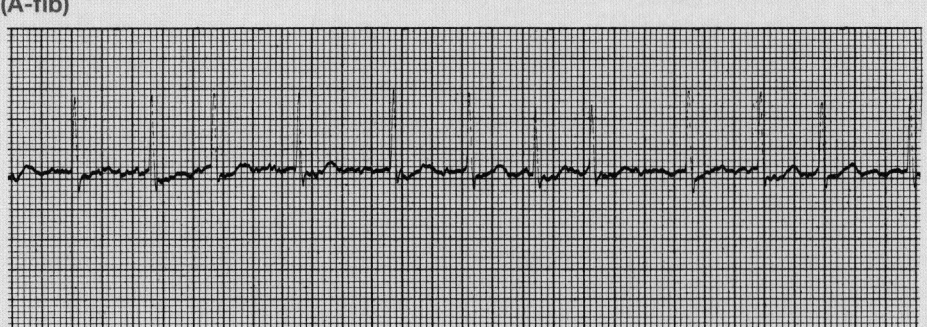

Chaotic, irregular atrial activity resulting in an irregular ventricular response. No identifiable P waves. Irregular ventricular response resulting in an irregular cardiac rate and rhythm. The conduction of the multiple atrial impulses across the atrioventricular (AV) node determines the rate. Caused by aging, calcification of the sinoatrial (SA) node, or changes in myocardial blood supply.	There is loss of the atrial kick (portion of the cardiac output squeezed in the ventricles with a coordinated atrial contraction), pooling of blood in the atria, and development of microemboli. The patient often complains of fatigue, a fluttering in the chest, or shortness of breath if the ventricular response is rapid. Commonly occurring dysrhythmia in the aging and older adult.

Ventricular Tachycardia

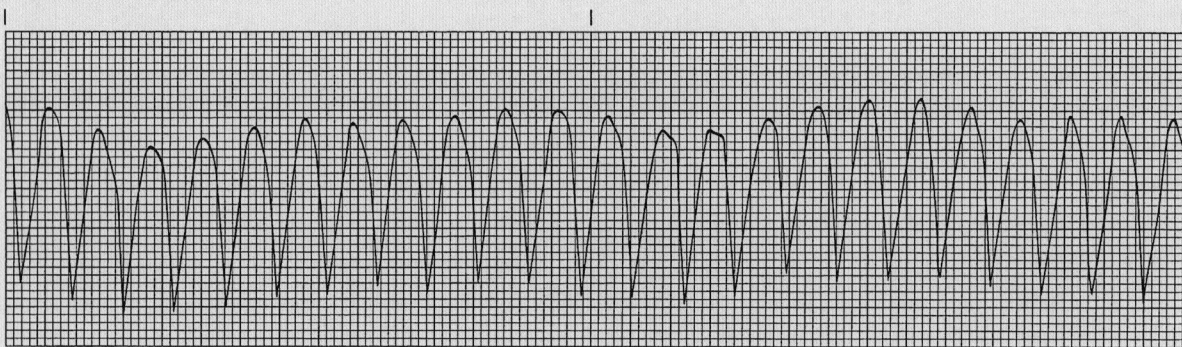

Rhythm slightly irregular, rate 100-200 beats/min, P wave absent, PR interval absent, QRS complex wide and bizarre, >0.12 second.	Results in decreased cardiac output caused by decreased ventricular filling time; often leads to severe hypotension and loss of pulse and consciousness.
Caused by changes in the normal pacemaker of the heart such as decrease in blood flow, ischemia, or embolus.	Acute loss of pulse and respiration. Immediate chest compressions and defibrillation are required.

Ventricular Fibrillation

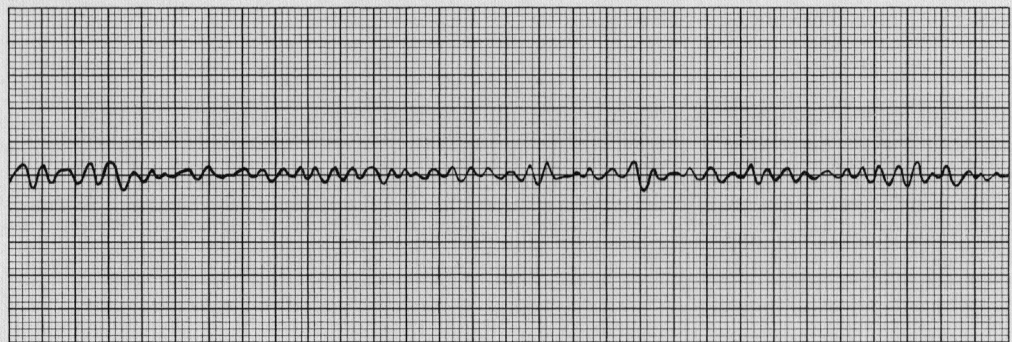

Uncoordinated electrical activity. No identifiable P, QRS, or T wave. Causes include sudden cardiac death, electrical shock, acute myocardial infarction, drowning, or trauma.	Acute loss of pulse and respiration. Immediate chest compressions and defibrillation are required. Availability of AED is recommended in public and/or private places where large numbers of people gather or where people who are at high risk for heart attack live.

Modified from Berg RA et al: 2010 American Heart Association Guidelines for cardiopulmonary resuscitation and emergency cardiovascular care. Part 5: Adult basic life support, *Circulation* 122(suppl 3):S685, 2010a.

TABLE 27-3	Adult, Child, and Infant Cardiopulmonary Resuscitation Techniques (Health Care Providers)		
Technique	**Adult**	**Child (1-8 Years Old)**	**Infant (Under 1 Year) Does Not Include Newborns**
Chest compressions: Push hard and fast to allow complete recoil	Begin compressions if no pulse Lower half of sternum, between nipples 3.75 to 5 cm (1½ to 2 inches) One to two rescuers: 100/min at a rate of 30 compressions to 2 breaths (30:2)	Begin compressions if no pulse or pulse <60/min Lower half of sternum, between nipples Heel of one hand or as for adults At least ⅓ depth of chest One rescuer: 30 compressions, 2 breaths (30:2) Two rescuers: 15 compressions, 2 breaths (15:2)	Begin compressions if no pulse or pulse <60/min Just below nipple line (lower half of sternum) Two fingers, two thumbs (encircling hands) One rescuer: 30 compressions, 2 breaths (30:2) Two rescuers: 15 compressions, 2 breaths (15:2)
Defibrillation using AED	Use adult pads Provide 5 cycles of CPR before shock if response time is greater than 4 to 5 minutes and arrest was not witnessed Otherwise, AED should be applied as soon as available, and shock as soon as advised Resume compressions immediately after shock	Use child pads whenever possible If none, use adult pads but do not overlap them Apply AED as soon as available, and shock as soon as advised	If there is a shockable rhythm, manual defibrillation is used
Airway	Head tilt–chin lift (HCP: Suspected trauma, use jaw thrust)	Head tilt–chin lift (HCP: Suspected trauma, use jaw thrust)	Head tilt–chin lift (HCP: Suspected trauma, use jaw thrust)
HCP: Rescue breathing mouth-to-mask or bag-mask without chest compressions	10 to 12 breaths/min (approximately 1 breath every 5-6 seconds)	12 to 20 breaths/min (approximately 1 breath every 3 seconds)	12 to 20 breaths/min (approximately 1 breath every 3 seconds)
HCP: Rescue breaths for CPR with advanced airway (endotracheal tube/tracheotomy)	8 to 10 breaths/min (approximately 1 breath every 6-8 seconds)	8 to 10 breaths/min (approximately 1 breath every 6-8 seconds)	8 to 10 breaths/min (approximately 1 breath every 6-8 seconds)
Foreign body airway obstruction	Abdominal thrusts	Abdominal thrusts	Back slaps and chest thrusts

Data from Berg RA et al: 2010 American Heart Association Guidelines for cardiopulmonary resuscitation and emergency cardiovascular care. Part 5: Adult basic life support, *Circulation* 122(suppl 3):S685, 2010a; and Berg MD et al: 2010 American Heart Association Guidelines for cardiopulmonary resuscitation and emergency cardiovascular care. Part 13: Pediatric basic life support, *Circulation* 122(suppl 3):S862, 2010b.
AED, Automated external defibrillator; *CPR,* cardiopulmonary resuscitation; *HCP,* health care provider.

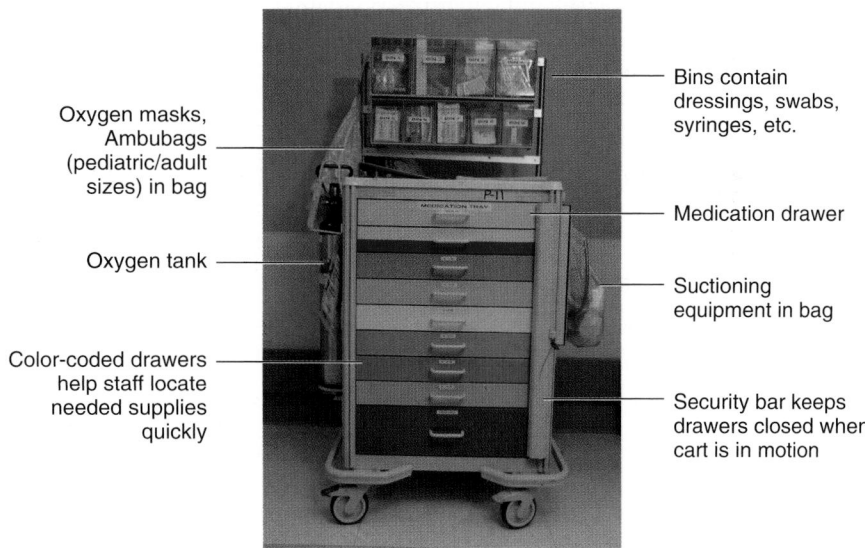

FIG 27-4   Emergency resuscitation cart.

defibrillation. All other skills in the code situation are directed by the code team leader and performed by nurses, respiratory therapists, and other health care professionals.

Equipment

❑ Crash cart (Fig. 27-4)—Most adult carts have the following equipment:
- Clean and sterile gloves, gown, protective eyewear
- Oxygen source
- Bag-mask device or resuscitation bag
- Oral airways
- Laryngoscope, handle, and laryngoscope blades, straight and curved
- Endotracheal (ET) tubes, various sizes (5-to-9 mm for adults; 0-to-4 mm for pediatrics)

- Carbon dioxide detector to confirm ET tube placement
- Tape or commercial ET tube holder
- Backboard
- AED and/or manual defibrillator with AED/defibrillator pads
- Intravenous (IV) needles (sizes for adults and pediatrics)
- Central vascular access kit
- IV tubing and fluids (normal saline [NS] and 5% dextrose in water [D₅W])
- Syringes
- Laboratory specimen tubes
- Arterial blood gas kit
- Emergency medications
- ACLS guidelines or algorithms

❑ Suction source and suction equipment if not with crash cart

STEP	RATIONALE

ASSESSMENT

1 Determine if patient is unconscious by shaking him or her and shouting, "Are you OK?" Assess patient unresponsiveness.

Confirms that patient is unresponsive rather than intoxicated, sleeping, or hearing impaired. Substance abuse, hypoglycemia, toxicities, seizures, trauma, ketoacidosis, and shock can also cause unconsciousness.

Clinical Decision Point *If an unresponsive person has adequate respirations and pulse, remain until further assistance is present. Place victim in a modified lateral recovery position (see illustration). Continue to assess for the presence of respirations and pulse because a recurrent arrest may develop.*

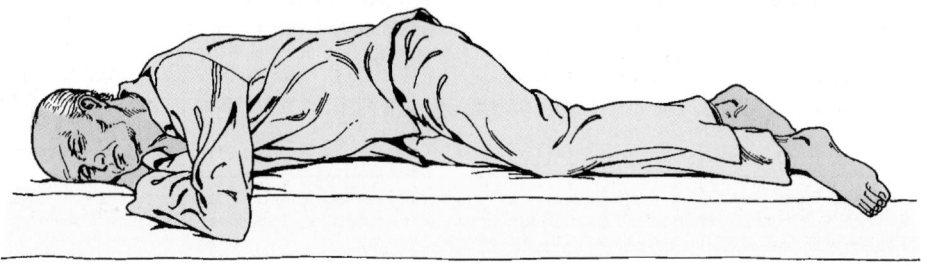

STEP 1   Recovery position.

NURSING DIAGNOSES

- Decreased cardiac output
- Impaired gas exchange
- Impaired spontaneous ventilation
- Ineffective breathing pattern
- Ineffective tissue perfusion

Related factors are individualized based on patient's condition or needs.

PLANNING

1 Expected outcomes following completion of procedure:
- Patient regains pulse and respirations.
- Patient receives postresuscitation care:
  - Transport to intensive care unit (ICU).
  - Continue ongoing care in the ICU.

2 Immediately activate the hospital code team or emergency medical services (EMS). Tell co-workers to bring AED (if available) and crash cart to bedside.

CPR was successful.
Ongoing treatment and support needed.

Ensures timely application of defibrillation, CPR, and ACLS to arrest victim.

STEP	RATIONALE

IMPLEMENTATION

Primary survey: *C* (Circulation)

1 Check carotid pulse on adult or child; use brachial or femoral pulse in an infant. Palpate for no more than 10 seconds (Berg et al., 2010a).

2 Place victim on hard surface such as floor, ground, or backboard. Victim must be flat. Logroll victim to flat, supine position using spine precautions if trauma is suspected.

Carotid pulse is the easiest to locate in adults and children. Femoral pulse may also be palpated in a child or infant.

External compression of heart is facilitated. Heart is compressed between sternum and spinal vertebrae, which must be on hard and firm surface. Do *NOT* delay the start of CPR. Positioning patient on hard surface may take more than one or two rescuers. You may need to wait to safely move him or her. Place backboard or position patient as soon as appropriate assistance is present.

Primary survey: *A* (Airway)

3 Apply clean gloves and face shield.

4 Open airway.

   a Head tilt–chin lift (no trauma) (see illustration) *or*

   b Jaw thrust (cervical trauma is suspected) (see illustration)

Reduces transmission of microorganisms.

Determine if patient has spontaneous respirations. Tongue is most common cause of blocked airway in unresponsive patient.

Suspect spinal cord injury in patients with trauma. Jaw-thrust maneuver prevents head extension and neck movement and further paralysis or spinal cord injury. Apply rigid cervical collar and immobilize patient as soon as possible to reduce cervical spine motion.

Primary survey: *B* (Breathing)

5 Attempt to ventilate patient with slow breaths using one of these methods.

   a Mouth-to-mouth using barrier device.

   b Mouth-to-mask using pocket mask (see illustration).

   c Bag-mask device (see illustrations).

6 If available, insert oral airway (see Skill 27-1).

7 Suction secretions if necessary or turn victim's head to one side unless trauma is suspected.

Slow breaths deliver air at low pressure to reduce risk of gastric distention.

Forms airtight seal to prevent air from escaping through nose.

Provides secure seal and permits use of supplemental oxygen.

Gives breaths with enough force to make the chest rise.

Maintains tongue on anterior floor of mouth and prevents obstruction of posterior airway by tongue.

Suctioning prevents airway obstruction. Turning patient's head to one side allows gravity to drain any secretions, decreasing risk of aspiration.

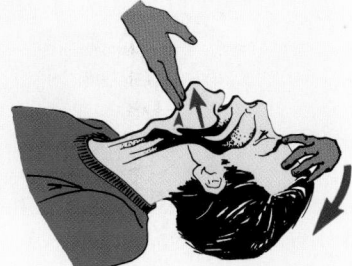

STEP 4a Head tilt–chin lift. (*From Sorrentino S: Mosby's textbook for nursing assistants, ed 7, St Louis, 2008, Mosby.*)

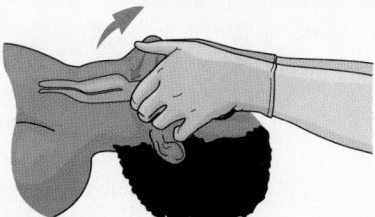

STEP 4b Jaw thrust without head tilt.

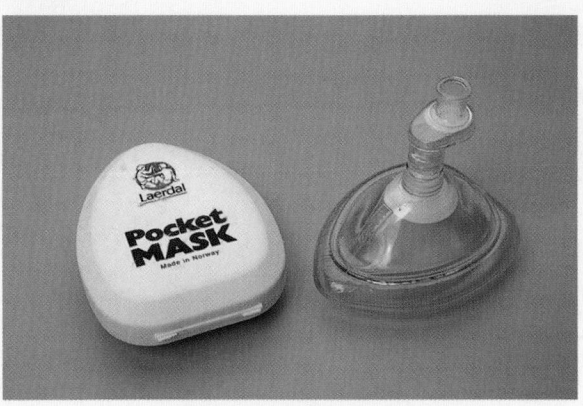

STEP 5b Pocket mask.

STEP	RATIONALE

Primary survey: *D* (Defibrillation)

8 If pulse is absent and AED is available, apply AED immediately as appropriate.

Most successful defibrillation rates occur when AED is applied and used within 5 minutes following collapse. Survival rates decline when defibrillation is delayed.

   a After one shock, resume CPR for 5 cycles and begin rhythm analysis and shock sequence again.

One shock followed by chest compressions for 5 cycles provides sufficient blood flow and perfusion before another set of shocks is delivered (Berg et al., 2010a).

9 If pulse is absent and an AED is unavailable, immediately initiate chest compressions.

   a Assume correct hand position and compression ratio for patient (see illustrations).

Specific hand position, compression depth, and ratio are different for adults, children, and infants to avoid injury to heart, lung, or liver (see Table 27-3).

Clinical Decision Point *Ensure that fingers are off the ribs and lowermost part of the xiphoid process. This minimizes the chance of rib fracture that could result in punctured lung or liver laceration, which further compromises cardiopulmonary status. Continue chest compressions, ventilation, and AED use.*

Secondary survey: Implementation

1 Give code leader brief verbal report on events performed before code team's arrival (i.e., code, vital signs, medical diagnosis, and code intervention).

This information is critical in selection of appropriate treatment for patient.

2 On arrival of sufficient personnel, delegate tasks as appropriate while core group continues with resuscitation efforts.

Delegation of duties is essential to meet critical needs of patient and his or her family in timely matter.

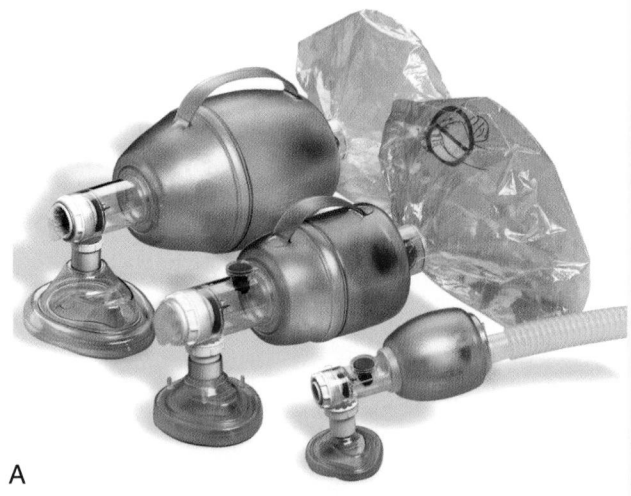 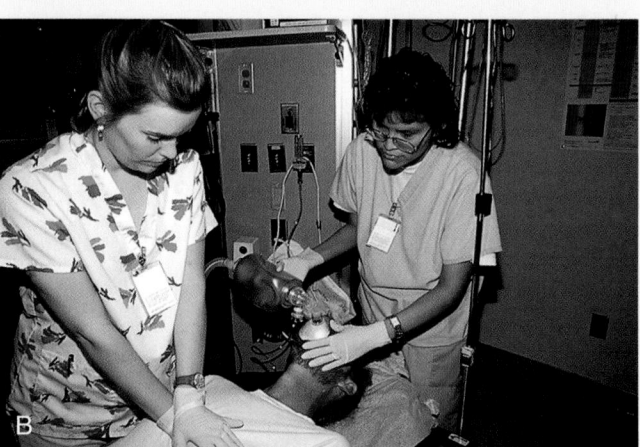

STEP 5c **A,** Bag-mask device. **B,** Two-rescuer breathing with bag-mask device. (*Courtesy Ambu USA.*)

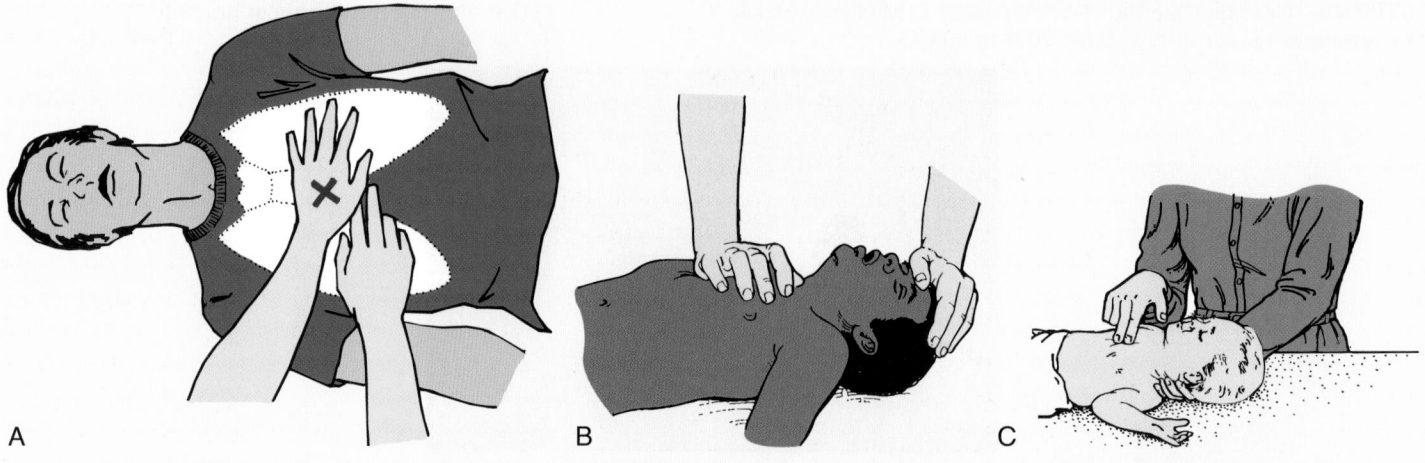

STEP 9a **A,** Proper hand position—adult. **B,** Proper hand position—child. **C,** Proper hand position—infant.

STEP	RATIONALE

a Assist victim's roommate or visitors away from code scene. Assign pastoral care or other nurses to communicate with family.

b Delegate someone to remove excess furniture or equipment from room.

c Have someone bring patient's chart to bedside or have access to patient's electronic health record (EHR).

Clarifies patient's medical condition, code status, and presence of any allergies.

d Assign nurse as recorder to record/document events of code.

Ensures accurate documentation of events of code, medications, and treatments administered.

e Assign another nurse to get medications and supplies from crash cart to hand off to code team members. The bedside nurse is involved in tasks such as medication administration, vital signs, and helping with procedures.

Provides code personnel with appropriate medication and equipment in timely fashion.

Secondary survey: *C* (Analysis of cardiac rhythm)

3 Attach manual defibrillator/monitor to patient using electrocardiogram (ECG) electrodes, quick-look paddles with gel pads, or "hands-off" defibrillation electrode to visualize cardiac rhythm (see illustration).

Cardiac rhythm monitor devices provide immediate rhythm display for analysis without disruption of rescue breathing and chest compression.

4 If cardiac rhythm is "shockable," continue CPR and assist code team with manual defibrillation.

Manual defibrillation is performed by ACLS-certified personnel.

a Turn on defibrillator and select proper energy level following agency policy and equipment directions.

Energy is delivered in prescribed doses. Manual biphasic devices deliver shocks at a lower level (200 joules); monophasic waveforms use 360 joules.

b Apply conductive gel or gel pads to patient's chest where defibrillator paddles will be placed. Some defibrillators use "hands-off pads" that are applied to patient's chest and directly connect to manual defibrillator.

Good skin-to-paddle/pad contact ensures appropriate discharge of current and decreases chance of skin burns (Link, 2010).

c Place paddles or pads on patient's chest wall.

Ensures appropriate discharge of current.

d Verify that no one is in physical contact with patient, bed, or any item contacting patient during defibrillation. A warning must be called out before initiating charge.

Prevents accidental delivery of shock or injury to personnel.

5 Establish IV access with large-bore IV needle (14- to 22-gauge) and begin infusion of 0.9% NS.

Provides a route for rapid drug administration and access for blood samples and fluid administration. Physiologic saline is isotonic. Rapid fluid infusion facilitates dispersal of medication throughout cardiovascular system.

a If you cannot obtain peripheral IV access, physician may pursue central venous access.

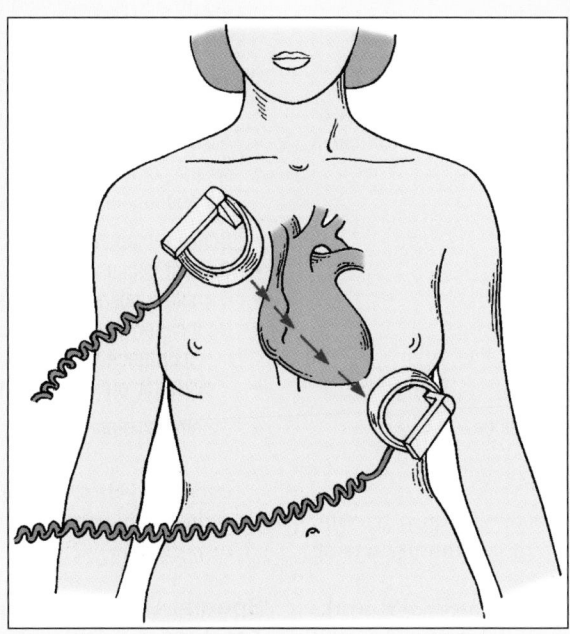

STEP 3 Paddle placement for defibrillation.

STEP	RATIONALE
6 Help with procedures as needed.	Most equipment needed for special procedures during code is on the crash cart. Knowledge of crash cart contents is very helpful in the code to provide personnel with the appropriate equipment.
7 Continue CPR until relieved, until victim regains spontaneous pulse and respiration, rescuer is exhausted and unable to perform CPR effectively, or physician discontinues CPR.	Interruptions in CPR are planned and organized. They usually occur during change of CPR personnel, defibrillation, and intubation. An interruption should not exceed 10 seconds (Berg et al., 2010a).

Secondary survey: *A* (Intubate airway)

STEP	RATIONALE
8 If respirations are absent, help the code team with ET intubation.	Intubation provides a patent airway and facilitates pulmonary ventilation. Laryngeal mask airway or esophageal-tracheal Combitube can also be used to provide advanced airway support.
a Have available laryngoscope handle, laryngoscope blades, curved and straight blades, ET tubes, stylet, suction, and tape or ET tube holder. Ensure that light source on laryngoscope is functional.	Light is necessary on laryngoscope to visualize vocal cords and intubate trachea. Batteries may need to be changed.

Secondary survey: *B* (Confirmation of airway and ventilation)

STEP	RATIONALE
9 Assist in confirmation of ET tube placement or advanced airway support by auscultating lungs for bilateral breath sounds. Carbon dioxide (CO_2) detector or esophageal detector devices are used as secondary methods to confirm correct airway placement (Neumar et al., 2010).	Auscultation of lungs and exhaled CO_2 monitoring or esophageal detector device further verifies correct airway placement and adequacy of ventilation and gas exchange.
10 Ventilate using bag device on intubation.	Chest x-ray film is usually obtained after patient has been stabilized to confirm placement of ET tube and central venous catheters. Avoid hyperventilation. Increased intrathoracic pressure caused by incomplete exhalation results in reduced cardiac output (Neumar et al., 2010).

Secondary survey: *D* (Differential diagnosis)

STEP	RATIONALE
11 Help physician obtain laboratory and diagnostic studies.	Helps in determining cause of the arrest.

EVALUATION

1 Reassess primary and secondary surveys throughout the code event.	This keeps the process organized and addresses immediate needs of the patient.
2 Palpate carotid pulse at least every 5 minutes after first minute of CPR.	Documents adequacy of external cardiac compressions.
3 Observe for spontaneous return of respirations or heart rate every 2 minutes.	Assessment of pulse, respiration, heart rate, and cardiac rhythm can occur after chest compressions and ventilation have been interrupted briefly every 2 minutes.
4 Ensure that interruptions in CPR are minimized.	Interruptions are associated with reduced coronary artery perfusion pressure and lower mean coronary perfusion pressure (Berg et al., 2010a).

Unexpected Outcomes

1 Patient develops skeletal injury such as fractured ribs or sternum or internal organ injury such as lacerated lung or liver as a result of chest compressions.

2 Patient's CPR is unsuccessful.

3 Rescuer is unassisted, tires, and is unable to continue.

Recording and Reporting

- Immediately report arrest, indicating exact location of victim. In hospital setting follow hospital policy. In community setting activate the emergency response system.
- Record in nurses' notes and EHR or on designated CPR worksheet: onset of arrest, time and number of AED shocks (you will not know the exact energy level used by the AED), time and

Related Interventions

- Obtain appropriate diagnostic tests to document injuries.
- Assess patient's postarrest breathing for symmetry and pain.
- Assess for intrathoracic or intraabdominal bleeding (hematomas, increasing abdominal girth).
- Contact chaplain services.
- Contact social worker.
- Complete postmortem care on patient (see Chapter 16).
- Notification of coroner and organ procurement agency needs to be made in accordance with local hospital or state law.
- Provide for privacy for patient's family to say their good-byes to patient.
- Obtain assistance.

energy level of manual defibrillations, medications given, procedures performed, cardiac rhythm, use of CPR, and patient's response.

Special Considerations
Teaching

- See Skill 27-2 for teaching considerations.

Pediatric

- All persons involved in administering CPR must understand different breathing/compression ratios, hand (fingers) placement, and depth of compression in children and infants compared with adults.
- Infants and children experience respiratory arrest much more frequently than full cardiopulmonary arrest.
- Quick reference, color-coded guides are frequently used in pediatric codes to quickly determine appropriate drug doses and equipment sizes.

Gerontologic

- In older adults compressions often result in rib or cartilage fractures.
- Remove loose-fitting dentures to avoid obstructing the airway. If dentures fit securely, leave them in to provide a tight seal when providing ventilations.

Home Care

- In the community and long-term care settings, patients may have implanted cardioverter defibrillators (ICDs) and/or pacemakers. For these patients, families need to know how to administer CPR and the specific capabilities of the patient's ICD/pacemaker. Placement of defibrillator or AED pads/paddles may need to be altered to avoid placement directly on top of an ICD or pacemaker generator. Remove medication patches from chest.
- Soft surfaces such as a mattress, car seat, or grassy surface decrease efficiency of external cardiac compressions.

? Critical Thinking Exercises

You are the charge nurse for night shift on a general medical floor. On your rounds you find your patient, Ethel Waters, lying unresponsive on the floor of the bathroom. She is 85 years old and was admitted with heart failure. An automated external defibrillator (AED) is available down the hall.

1 What should you do first? Explain your choice.
  1 Apply the AED
  2 Call for help
  3 Check for a pulse
  4 Open airway and provide two breaths

2 Your co-worker arrives to Mrs. Water's room with the AED. What is your next step? Explain your choice.
  1 Check for a pulse
  2 Start chest compressions
  3 Apply the AED
  4 Continue with 8 to 10 breaths/min

3 Your co-worker has started chest compressions on Mrs. Waters. Under which of the following circumstances should you interrupt performance of the chest compressions? Explain your choice.
  1 Arrival of the code team
  2 AED advises, "Do NOT touch the patient."
  3 Initiation of bag-mask ventilation
  4 Intravenous (IV) line insertion

4 Cardiopulmonary resuscitation (CPR) continues for Mrs. Waters. Which of the following action(s) should occur every 2 minutes?
  1 Checking IV fluids
  2 Interrupting chest compression to assess for spontaneous pulse/respirations
  3 Continuing chest compression uninterrupted
  4 AED reanalyzing the cardiac rhythm

5 The code team has arrived to continue resuscitation attempts on Mrs. Waters. Which activities will be involved in the code team's work? How can you participate?

✓ REVIEW QUESTIONS

1 Which of the following is(are) the goal(s) of resuscitation?
  1 Return of pulse
  2 Providing oxygen to the victim as soon as possible
  3 Restoring cardiopulmonary function and avoid poor neurologic outcomes
  4 Restoring cardiopulmonary function or avoid poor neurologic outcomes

2 The primary purpose of a hospital team is/are to: (Select all that apply.)
  1 Intervene early to prevent cardiac arrest.
  2 Transfer the patient to the intensive care unit (ICU).
  3 Reduce hospital mortality rate.
  4 Remove the need for the code team.

3 Which of the following is a nursing concern for the family of an arrest victim?
  1 Accommodate families' religious and cultural practices.
  2 Do not allow family in patient's room at any time.
  3 Question families' reasons for refusing organ donation.
  4 Have multiple health care providers speak to the family.

4 A nurse is reviewing the procedure for insertion of an oropharyngeal airway. Which of the following is true about an oral airway?
  1 It eliminates the need to position the head of the unconscious patient.
  2 It eliminates the possibility of an upper airway obstruction.
  3 It needs to be inserted even when a patient has had recent oral trauma.
  4 It may stimulate vomiting or laryngospasm if inserted in the semiconscious patient.

5 A visitor suffers a cardiac arrest, and resuscitation is begun. The nurse would be correct doing CPR and operating an AED if which of the following sequence of steps were followed?
  1 Check for a pulse, provide chest compressions until the AED arrives, attach the AED, open the airway, provide two breaths if needed.
  2 Wait for the AED, open the airway, provide two breaths if needed, check for a pulse, and attach the AED if no pulse.
  3 Call for help, get the AED, open the airway, provide two breaths if needed, check for a pulse, continue compressions if no pulse is present, attach the AED.
  4 Provide two breaths, check for a pulse, call for the AED, provide chest compressions until the AED arrives, attach the AED.

6 You need to open the airway of a suspected trauma victim. Which technique would you use to open the airway in this patient?
  1 Head tilt
  2 Chin lift
  3 Jaw thrust
  4 Lateral lying position

7 Which of the following are appropriate personnel to use an AED?
  1 Only licensed providers
  2 Any basic life support (BLS) provider
  3 Only physicians
  4 Only charge nurses

8 The nurse is participating in a code on an adult and waiting for the AED to arrive. At what rate should the compressions and breaths be delivered?
  1 60/min at a ratio of 30 compressions to 2 breaths
  2 60/min at a ratio of 15 compressions to 2 breaths
  3 80/min at a ratio of 15 compressions to 2 breaths
  4 100/min at a ratio of 30 compressions to 2 breaths
9 The nurse is involved in resuscitating a patient. The AED has just delivered a shock. What should be done immediately after the shock has been delivered?
  1 Continue CPR for another minute until the AED recharges
  2 Start an IV line of normal saline with a large-size IV catheter
  3 Reposition patient's head for better respiratory effort
  4 Continue CPR for 2 minutes
10 Which of the following indicates that your artificial breaths are adequate?
  1 The seal on the barrier device leaks air whenever the breath is given.
  2 The bag-mask device is connected to oxygen.
  3 The oral airway is in place.
  4 Artificial breathing has enough force to make the chest rise.

REFERENCES

AACN Practice Alert: *Family presence during resuscitation and invasive procedures,* 2010, American Association of Critical Care Nurses, The Association, available at http://www.aacn.org/WD/Practice/Docs/PracticeAlerts/Family%20Presence%2004-2010%20final.pdf, accessed July 19, 2012.

American Heart Association (AHA): Part I: Executive Summary: 2010 American Heart Association guidelines for cardiopulmonary resucitation and emergency vascular care, *Circulation* 122(suppl):S640, 2010.

Berg RA, et al: 2010 American Heart Association Guidelines for cardiopulmonary resuscitation and emergency cardiovascular care. Part 5: Adult basic life support, *Circulation* 122(suppl 3):S685, 2010a.

Berg MD, et al: 2010 American Heart Association Guidelines for cardiopulmonary resuscitation and emergency cardiovascular care. Part 13: Pediatric basic life support, *Circulation* 122(suppl 3):S862, 2010b.

Ehlenbach W, et al: Epidemiologic study of in-hospital cardiopulmonary resuscitation in the elderly, *N Engl J Med* 36(1):22, 2009.

Ewy G, Kern K: Recent advances in cardiopulmonary resuscitation, *J Am Coll Cardiol* 53:149, 2009.

Hockenberry MJ, Wilson D: *Wong's nursing care of infants and children,* ed 9, St Louis, 2011, Mosby.

Link MS, et al: American Heart Association Guidelines for cardiopulmonary resuscitation and emergency cardiovascular care. Part 6: Electrical therapies: automated external defibrillators, defibrillation, cardioversion, and pacing, *Circulation* 122(suppl 3):S706, 2010.

Neumar RW, et al: 2010 American Heart Association Guidelines for cardiopulmonary resuscitation and emergency cardiovascular care. Part 8: Adult advanced cardiovascular life support, *Circulation* 122(suppl 3):S729, 2010.

Peberdy MA, et al: 2010 American Heart Association Guidelines for cardiopulmonary resuscitation and emergency cardiovascular care. Part 9: Postcardiac arrest care, *Circulation* 122(suppl 3):S768, 2010.

Intravenous and Vascular Access Therapy

SKILLS AND PROCEDURES

MEDIA RESOURCES

- evolve learning http://evolve.elsevier.com/Perry/skills
  - Review Questions
  - ▶ Video Clips
  - Audio Glossary
- NSO Nursing Skills Online

KEY TERMS

Biohazard container
Catheter
Catheter-related
  bloodstream infection
  (CRBSI)
Central vascular access
  device (CVAD)
Central line–associated
  bloodstream infection
  (CLABSI)
Drop factor

Electrolyte
Electronic infusion device
  (EID)
Embolus (emboli)
Exit site
Fluid volume deficit (FVD)
Fluid volume excess
  (FVE)
Heparin lock
Hypertonic
Hypotonic

Implanted venous port
Infiltration
Infusion pump
Injection cap
Isotonic
Noncoring needle
Nontunneled central
  vascular catheters
Over-the-needle catheter
  (ONC)
Percutaneous

Peripherally inserted central
  catheter (PICC)
Phlebitis
Saline lock
Sharps container
Smart pump
Subcutaneous tunnel
Thrombosis
Tunneled central vascular
  catheter
Venipuncture

OBJECTIVES

Mastery of content in this chapter will enable the nurse to:

- Discuss patient conditions requiring intravenous (IV) therapy.
- Explain how to prepare a patient and family caregiver for IV therapy.
- Discuss complications of IV therapy.
- Identify individualized outcomes for patients requiring IV therapy.
- Explain techniques for preventing transmission of infection for a patient receiving IV therapy.

- Demonstrate initiating IV therapy, regulating IV flow rate, changing IV solutions, changing IV tubing, changing IV dressings, and discontinuing a short peripheral IV.
- Identify common types of central vascular access devices (CVADs) and describe their care and maintenance.
- Identify the educational needs of patients with CVADs.

The goal of intravenous (IV) therapy is to maintain or prevent fluid and electrolyte imbalances, administer continuous or intermittent solutions or medications, replenish blood volume, and assist in pain management. Assessments of a patient's anatomy and physiology of the circulatory system, fluid and electrolyte balance, disease pathophysiology, type and duration of prescribed therapy, allergies, and patient's response to illness play a key role in decision making to ensure safe delivery of infusion solutions or medications. Evidence-based practice guides the safe, efficient, quality care necessary to provide infusion therapy. For the skills in this chapter, follow the six rights of administrating parenteral solutions or medications: *Right* drug/solution, *Right* dose/concentration, *Right* patient, *Right* route, *Right* date/time, and *Right* documentation (Alexander et al., 2010; INS, 2011; Policy and Procedures INS, 2011). Defined further, these rights include knowledge of the correct solution and equipment; and how to initiate an infusion, regulate infusion rate, care for and maintain the infusion equipment, identify and correct any infusion-related complications, and discontinue an infusion. To safely and correctly provide infusion therapy, you need astute clinical management and specialized IV therapy skills in addition to your knowledge and professional accountability.

INTRAVENOUS SOLUTIONS

The use of IV therapy for a patient with an alteration in fluid and electrolyte balance is common in nursing practice. Many prepared IV solutions are available for use (Table 28-1). IV solutions fall into several categories: isotonic, hypotonic, and hypertonic. Isotonic fluids have the same osmolality as body fluids and are used to replace extracellular volume (e.g., prolonged vomiting). They effectively mimic the fluid loss of the body in the absence of an electrolyte imbalance. Hypotonic solutions are those that have an effective osmolality less than that of body fluids and are used most often to hydrate cells (e.g., hypertonic dehydration, required water replacement). Hypertonic solutions are those that have an effective osmolality greater than body fluids and are used most often to increase extracellular fluid volume (e.g., replace electrolytes, treat shock). A patient's specific fluid and electrolyte imbalance and serum electrolyte values guide the need for administration of the appropriate IV fluid (Alexander et al., 2010).

Administer all IV fluids carefully; isotonic solutions could cause increased fluid overload in patients with renal or cardiac disease; hypotonic solutions could exacerbate a hypotensive state in a patient with low blood pressure; and hypertonic solutions are irritating to the vein and have the potential to cause increased risk of heart failure and pulmonary edema.

Premixed solutions are available in which medications or electrolytes have been added by the manufacturer. Advantages are the increased stability of the solution, selection of the correct medication, and diluents. Disadvantages are that admixtures come in more than one dosage, leading to potential medication errors. As the choices of premixed solutions increase, so does the risk of related complications. Conduct a complete assessment of a patient's history, physical assessment, and review of laboratory findings before initiating any solutions or medications. When initiating IV therapy you must verify that the order is complete. Elements of a complete order include patient identification, type of solution or medication, volume, rate of infusion, frequency of infusion, route, dosage (medication), and any special considerations. The nurse administering IV solutions or medications should be aware of the indications for the prescribed therapy, any adverse reactions,

TABLE 28-1	Intravenous Solutions		
Solution	**Concentration**	**Other Names**
Dextrose in Water Solutions		
Dextrose 5% in water*	Isotonic	D_5W
Dextrose 10% in water	Hypertonic	$D_{10}W$
Dextrose 50% in water	Hypertonic	$D_{50}W$
Saline Solutions		
0.45% sodium chloride (half NS)	Hypotonic	½ NS 0.45% NS
0.33% sodium chloride (one-third NS)	Hypotonic	⅓ NS
0.9% sodium chloride† (NS)	Isotonic	NS 0.9% NS 0.9% NaCl
3%-5% sodium chloride	Hypertonic	3%-5% NS 3%-5% NaCl
Dextrose in Saline Solutions		
Dextrose 5% in 0.9% sodium chloride	Hypertonic	$D_5$0.9%NaCl $D_5$0.9%NS D_5NS
Dextrose 5% in 0.45% NaCl sodium chloride	Hypertonic	$D_5$0.45%NaCl $D_5$0.45%NS D_5½NS
Multiple Electrolyte Solutions		
Lactated Ringer's‡	Isotonic	LR
Dextrose 5% in Lactated Ringer's	Hypertonic	D_5LR

LR, Lactated Ringer's; *NS*, normal saline.
*Dextrose is quickly metabolized, leaving free water to be distributed evenly in all fluid compartments (Alexander et al., 2010).
†Although it is isotonic because the total concentration of electrolytes equals plasma concentration, it contains 154 mEq of both sodium and chloride, which is a higher concentration of these electrolytes than is found in the plasma, which can cause fluid volume excess (Alexander et al., 2010).
‡Contains sodium, potassium, calcium, chloride, and lactate.

special monitoring (laboratory values, vital signs, intake and output [I&O]), and appropriate interventions (INS, 2011).

INTRAVENOUS CATHETERS

To administer IV solutions and medications, a venous access device (VAD) is inserted into a vein with the final tip residing in a location that is appropriate for the pH and osmolarity of the solution or medication (INS, 2011). Solutions and medications with a pH of less than 5.0 or greater than 9.0 and an osmolarity greater than 600 mOsm/L are infused with a central vascular access device (CVAD) with final tip placement in the superior or inferior vena cava. Solutions and medications with a pH between 5.0 and 9.0 and an osmolarity less than 600 mOsm/L may be infused via a short peripheral or midline catheter (Alexander et al., 2010; INS, 2011). Solutions or medications with low or high pH and high osmolarity have the potential to cause infusion-related complications such as phlebitis when administered with a short peripheral or midline catheter (Alexander et al., 2010). Table 28-2 outlines the vascular access device (VAD) options for peripheral administration.

The choice of VADs can be overwhelming because there are a variety of sizes, number of lumens, and materials used to

TABLE 28-2	Peripheral Vascular Access Device Options	
Type	**Use**	**Types of Infusions**
Winged infusion butterfly needle	One-time infusion, IV push administration	Solutions or medications with pH between 5.0 and 9.0 Osmolarity less than 600 mOsm/L (INS, 2011)
Short, over-the-needle catheter (ONC) (7.5 cm [less than 3 inches])	Continuous infusion, intermittent infusion, short-term duration (INS, 2011)	Solutions or medications with pH between 5.0 and 9.0 Osmolarity less than 600 mOsm/L (INS, 2011)
Midline peripheral catheters (7.5 to 20 cm [3 to 8 inch])	Continuous infusion and intermittent infusion (1 to 4 weeks) (INS, 2011)	Solutions or medications with pH between 5.0 and 9.0 Osmolarity less than 600 mOsm/L (INS, 2011)

IV, Intravenous.

TABLE 28-3	Recommendations for Short Peripheral Catheter Selection
Catheter Size (Gauge)	**Clinical Indication**
14, 16, 18	Trauma, surgery, blood transfusion
20	Continuous or intermittent infusions, blood transfusion
22	Continuous or intermittent infusions, children and elderly patients Administration of blood or blood product in pediatrics and neonates
24	Fragile veins for intermittent or continuous infusions; administration of blood or blood production in pediatrics or neonates

Modified from Alexander M et al: *Infusion nursing evidence based approach,* ed 3, St Louis, 2010, Mosby.

manufacture the devices (Fig. 28-1). When selecting the appropriate VAD, consider a patient's prescribed therapy, length of treatment, duration the device remains in place, vascular integrity, patient preference, and resources available to care for the device (INS, 2011). Table 28-3 indicates the appropriate uses for the more common catheter sizes.

EVIDENCE-BASED PRACTICE

Research suggests that a dedicated, nurse-driven IV team that implements the most current technologies, maintains infusion therapy knowledge, uses infection-prevention practices, and incorporates current standards and guidelines will improve patient outcomes and reduce complications (Ackley et al., 2008; Alexander et al., 2010; INS, 2011).

Evidence-based practice (EBP) in the prevention of infusion-related complications such as catheter-related bloodstream infections (CRBSIs) and central line–associated bloodstream infections (CLABSIs) could significantly reduce patient morbidity and mortality (Alexander et al., 2010; Policy and Procedures INS, 2011). Placement of a VAD, infusion of solutions and medications, and manipulation of infusion equipment all contribute to an increased risk of infection. It is imperative that you follow established infection-prevention strategies.

- Perform hand hygiene before or after touching a patient, before handling an invasive device, before donning and after removing gloves, and after contact with inanimate objects near a patient.
- Clean skin site before venipuncture with an appropriate single-use antiseptic solution.
- Routine site care and dressing changes are not required on short peripheral catheters unless the dressing is soiled or not intact.
- Chlorhexidine solution is preferred for skin antisepsis (INS, 2011). Povidone-iodine, 70% alcohol, or tincture of iodine (1% or 2%) may also be used. Chlorhexidine is not recommended for infants under 2 months of age.
- Use a catheter stabilization device that allows for visual inspection of an insertion site.

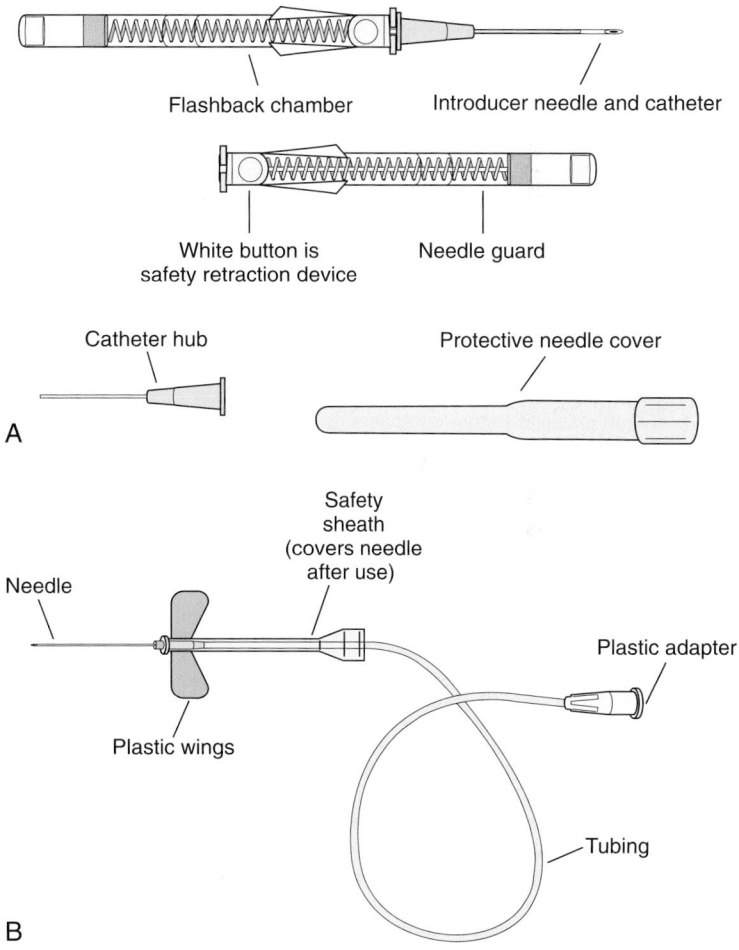

FIG 28-1 Intravenous access device options. **A,** Over-the-needle catheter (ONC) device. **B,** Steel butterfly needle.

- Primary and secondary continuous administration sets used to administer fluids other than lipid, blood, or blood products should be changed no more often than every 96 hours.

PATIENT-CENTERED CARE

Communication, comfort, and education are essential components of patient-centered care when delivering infusion therapy.

Educating patients and family caregivers about the prescribed IV therapy and goals of therapy may be difficult unless you give attention to patients' cultural and linguistic needs. Education includes clear and concise terms for all aspects of IV therapy and individualized training that include self-care practices (INS, 2011). Nursing interventions used during the insertion of the VAD to help alleviate anxiety and fear would include preparing a patient before insertion of the short peripheral IV catheter by placing him or her in a comfortable position, speaking directly to him or her, and answering questions as honestly as possible. Ask patients if they have had IV therapy in the past. Know what are their concerns and expectations. When you prepare for insertion, use techniques that minimize discomfort. Your ability to recognize diversity in patients, whether it is cultural, linguistic, or religious or caused by past experiences, will prepare you to be confident in providing infusion therapy to patients.

Safety Guidelines

1 Know a patient's baseline vital signs before initiating IV therapy. Fluid and electrolyte imbalances affect vital signs. Dehydration sometimes produces hypotension and tachycardia. Fluid overload results in hypertension and bounding pulses.

2 Know a patient's medical history, current medications, and therapies. Medications affect fluid and electrolyte balance (e.g., diuretics or steroids). Determine his or her previous experience with IV therapy.

3 Beware of prolonged environmental conditions that affect a patient's fluid status (e.g., exposure to hot, humid weather), leading to fluid and electrolyte imbalances, particularly in the infant, older adult, and chronically ill.

4 Ensure that an IV system is intact and there is no evidence of phlebitis or infiltration. An intact system ensures that you have maintained sterility and that no fluid or medication has been lost.

5 Note the date of the last IV administration set and dressing change (Box 28-1).

6 Maintain sterility of a patent IV system using INS standards (see Box 28-1).

7 Know the standard precautions for infection control and the Occupational Safety and Health Administration (OSHA) standards for occupational exposure to bloodborne pathogens (Box 28-2).

BOX 28-1	INS Standards to Decrease Intravascular Infection Related to Intravenous Therapy

- Palpate catheter insertion site for tenderness daily through the intact dressing.
- Directly inspect a catheter site if patient develops tenderness at site, fever without obvious source, or symptoms of local or bloodstream infection.
- Perform hand hygiene before and after palpating, inserting, replacing, or dressing any intravascular device.
- Clean skin site before venipuncture with an appropriate single-use antiseptic solution.
- Allow site to air-dry before proceeding with procedure: 2% chlorhexidine 30 seconds, povidone-iodine at least 2 minutes.
- Do not palpate insertion site after skin has been cleaned with single-use antiseptic solution.
- Use catheter stabilization device that allows visual inspection of access site.
- Change gauze dressings that cover a catheter site every 48 hours.
- Intravenous tubing administration sets can remain sterile for 96 hours.
- Replace dressing over peripheral venous catheters when replacing catheter or when dressing becomes damp, loosened, or soiled.
- Clean injection ports with single-use antiseptic solution before accessing system.
- Replace short, peripheral venous catheters and rotate sites based on clinical assessment indicating signs or symptoms of IV-related complications.

Modified from Infusion Nurses Society: Infusion nursing standards of practice, *J Intraven Nurs* 34(suppl 1):S1, 2011.
INS, Infusion Nurses Society.

BOX 28-2	Standards for Reducing Occupational Exposure to Bloodborne Pathogens

1 Gloves are necessary when there is a reasonable expectation that the employee may contact blood (e.g., during vascular access procedures or while changing IV administration sets).

2 Immediately place contaminated needles, needleless devices, and other sharps in puncture-resistant, leak-proof containers properly labeled as a biohazard; when the containers are full, seal and dispose of them properly.

3 Do not bend, shear, recap, or remove contaminated needles from the syringe after use.

4 Occupational Safety and Health Administration (OSHA) requires reports of needlestick injuries, and the health care agency must provide medical evaluation and follow-up.

5 Hepatitis B vaccinations should be made available to all employees who have occupational exposure.

6 Training and education about exposure prevention and use of protective equipment must be offered to high-risk workers who initiate IV therapy.

7 Each agency must have an infection control plan, including methods to reduce health care worker's exposure to biohazardous wastes.

8 Agencies must have engineering and work practice controls to eliminate or minimize employee exposure. Controls may include sharps disposal containers and self-sheathing needles.

Modified from Occupational Safety and Health Administration (OSHA): Occupational exposure to bloodborne pathogens, needlestick, and other sharps injuries: final rule, CFR 29, part 1910, *Fed Reg* 66:5317, 2001, updated April 2011, available at http://www.osha.gov/pls/oshaweb/owadisp.show_document?p_table=FEDERAL_REGISTER&p_id=16265, accessed 8/21/12.

SKILL 28-1 Initiating Intravenous Therapy

NSO *IV Fluid Administration Module / Lessons 1 and 2*

 Video Clip

Infusion therapy provides access to the venous system to deliver solutions and medications or blood and blood products. Reliable venous access for infusion therapy administration is essential.

Your role is to select the appropriate vascular access device (VAD) needed to place a short peripheral intravenous (IV) catheter or to assist clinicians with placement of a midline or central vascular access device (CVAD). In addition, skills are needed to prepare the infusion equipment and become familiar with the various infusion systems used during an infusion. Some solutions and medications can be administered continuously, whereas others are given intermittently. Various types of administration sets, needleless devices, extension sets, flushes, and pumps and the knowledge and skills for their correct and safe use are required. Know and follow INS standards, your agency policy and procedures, and state or government practice guidelines when providing IV therapy.

Delegation and Collaboration

The skill of initiating IV therapy cannot be delegated to nursing assistive personnel (NAP). Delegation to licensed practical nurses (LPNs) varies by state Nurse Practice Act. The nurse instructs the NAP to:

- Inform the nurse if the patient complains of any IV site–related complications such as pain, redness, swelling, bleeding.
- Inform the nurse if the patient's IV dressing becomes wet.
- Inform the nurse if the solution of fluid in the IV bag is low or the electronic infusion device (EID) alarm is sounding.

Equipment

- ❑ Appropriate short peripheral IV catheter for venipuncture (see Table 28-3) (Select the smallest gauge and length possible to administer the prescribed therapy [INS, 2011].)
- ❑ IV start kit supplies (available in some agencies): May contain a sterile drape to place under patient's arm, tourniquet, tape, transparent dressing, cleansing agents(s) (2% chlorhexidine preferred or povidone-iodine and 70% alcohol) and 2 × 2–inch gauze pads
- ❑ Clean gloves (latex free for patients with latex allergy)
- ❑ Extension set with needleless connection device (also called saline lock, heparin lock, IV plug or adapter)
- ❑ Prefilled 5-mL syringe with flush agent (preservative-free normal saline [NS] 0.9% normal saline solution [NSS] [INS, 2011])
- ❑ Alcohol pads
- ❑ Stabilization device (optional) and skin protectant
- ❑ Prescribed intravenous solution
- ❑ Administration set, either macrodrip or microdrip, depending on prescribed rate; if using EID, appropriate administration set
- ❑ 0.2-micron filter for nonlipid (fat emulsions) solutions (may be incorporated into the infusion set)
- ❑ Protective equipment: Goggles and mask (optional, check agency policy)
- ❑ IV pole, rolling or ceiling mounted
- ❑ EID if available
- ❑ Watch with second hand to calculate drip rate
- ❑ Special patient gown with snaps at shoulder seams if available (makes removal with IV tubing easier)
- ❑ Needle disposal container (also called *sharps container* or *biohazard container*)

STEP	RATIONALE

ASSESSMENT

1 Review accuracy and completeness of health care provider's order for type and amount of IV fluid, medication additives, infusion rate, and length of therapy. Follow six rights of medication administration (see Chapter 20).

Before administering solutions or medications an order from a licensed independent practitioner (LIP) is needed (Alexander et al., 2010; INS, 2011; Policy and Procedures INS, 2011).

  a Check approved online database, drug reference book, or pharmacist about IV fluids composition, purpose, potential incompatibilities and side effects.

Ensures safe and correct administration of IV therapy and appropriate selection of vascular access device (VAD).

2 Assess patient's knowledge of procedure, reason for prescribed therapy, and arm placement preference.

Provides patient-centered care by determining level of emotional support and instruction needed (Policy and Procedures INS, 2011).

3 Assess for clinical factors/conditions that will respond to or be affected by administration of IV solutions.

Provides baseline to determine effectiveness of prescribed therapy. A systems approach is recommended to assess for fluid and electrolyte imbalances (Alexander et al., 2010; LeFever et al., 2010).

  a Body weight

Changes in body weight reflect fluid loss or gain. One kilogram or 2.2 lbs of body weight is equivalent to gain or loss of 1 L of fluid (Alexander et al., 2010).

  b Clinical markers of vascular volume:

STEP	RATIONALE
(1) Urine output (decreased, dark yellow).	Kidneys respond to extracellular volume (ECV) deficit by reducing urine production and concentrating urine. Kidney disease can also cause oliguria.
(2) Vital signs: Blood pressure, respirations, pulse, temperature.	Changes in blood pressure may be associated with fluid volume status (fluid volume deficit [FVD]) seen in postural hypotension. Respirations can be altered in presence of acid-base imbalances. Temperature elevations increase need for fluid requirements (a temperature of 101° F [38.3° C] and 103° F [39.4° C] requires at least 500 mL of fluid replacement within a 24-hr period) (Alexander et al., 2010).
(3) Distended neck veins. (Normally veins are full when person is supine and flat when person is upright.)	Indicator of fluid volume status: flat or collapsing with inhalation when supine with ECV deficit; full when upright or semi-upright with ECV excess.
(4) Auscultation of lungs.	Crackles or rhonchi in dependent portions of lung may signal fluid buildup caused by ECV excess.
(5) Capillary refill	Indirect measure of tissue perfusion (sluggish with ECV deficit).
c Clinical markers of interstitial volume	
(1) Skin turgor (Pinch skin over sternum or inside of forearm.)	Failure of skin to return to normal position within 3 seconds indicates ECV deficit. This is called *tenting* (Alexander et al., 2010).
(2) Dependent edema (pitting or nonpitting) 1+ indicates barely detectable edema; 4+ indicates deep pitting (see Chapter 6).	Pitting edema is seen with a weight gain of 10 to 15 lbs (4.5-6.8 kg) of retained fluid (Alexander et al., 2010).
(3) Oral mucous membrane between cheek and gum	More reliable indicator than dry lips or skin. Dry between cheek and gums indicates ECV deficit.
d Thirst	Occurs with hypernatremia and severe ECV deficit. Not a reliable indicator for older adults (Meiner, 2011).
e Behavior and level of consciousness:	
(1) Restlessness and mild confusion	Occurs with FVD or acid-base imbalance.
(2) Decreased level of consciousness (lethargy, confusion, coma)	Occurs with severe ECV deficit. May occur with osmolality and acid-base imbalances.
4 Determine if patient is to undergo any planned surgeries or procedures.	Allows anticipation and placement of appropriate VAD for infusion and avoids placement in an area that will interfere with medical procedures (INS 2011).
5 Assess laboratory data.	Helps determine priority assessments and establishes baseline for determining if therapy is effective.
6 Assess patient's history of allergies, especially to iodine, adhesive, or latex.	Equipment used during VAD insertion may contain substances to which patient is allergic.

NURSING DIAGNOSES

- Anxiety
- Deficient knowledge regarding IV therapy

- Risk for electrolyte imbalance

- Risk for injury

Related factors are individualized based on patient's condition or needs.

PLANNING

1 Expected outcomes following completion of procedure:	
• Fluid and electrolyte balance returns to normal.	Proper solution is infused at proper rate and monitored, resolving fluid and electrolyte imbalance (Alexander et al., 2010).
• Vital signs are stable and within normal limits for patient.	Demonstrates response of circulatory system to fluid and electrolyte replacement (Alexander et al., 2010).
• No redness, drainage, swelling, or pain present at venipuncture site.	Ensures that catheter is without infusion-related complications (INS, 2011).
• Patient is able to explain purpose and risks of IV therapy.	Demonstrates learning (Alexander et al., 2010; INS, 2011).

STEP	RATIONALE

IMPLEMENTATION

1 Identify patient using two identifiers (i.e., name and birthday or name and account number) according to agency policy. Compare identifiers in MAR/medical record with information on patient's identification bracelet and/or ask patient to state name.

Ensures correct patient. Complies with The Joint Commission standards and improves patient safety (TJC, 2012).

2 Instruct patient about rationale for infusion, including solution and medications ordered, procedure for initiating an IV, and signs and symptoms of complications.

Provides patient with information about procedure and promotes compliance (Policy and Procedures INS, 2011).

3 Help patient to comfortable sitting or supine position. Provide adequate lighting.

Promotes comfort and relaxation of patient. Aids in successful vein location.

4 Perform hand hygiene. Gather and organize equipment on clean, clutter-free bedside stand or over-bed table.

Reduces transmission of infection and contamination of equipment (INS, 2011).

5 Change patient's gown to more easily removed gown with snaps at shoulder if available.

Use of this gown decreases risk of inadvertently dislodging VAD or administration set when changing gown.

6 Open sterile packages using sterile aseptic technique (see Chapter 8).

Maintains sterility of equipment and reduces spread of microorganisms.

7 *Option*: Prepare short extension tubing with needleless connector or stand-alone saline lock (injection cap) to attach to VAD catheter hub.

Short extension tubing prevents traction on VAD. Many agencies use short extension tubing for continuous infusions and stand-alone saline locks (capped catheters).

Clinical Decision Point *Short extension sets may be used on short peripheral catheters. Will decrease potential contact with hub and reduce blood contact. Must be of Luer-Lok connection (Alexander et al., 2010; INS, 2011; Policy and Procedures INS, 2011).*

a Remove protective cap from needleless connector. Swab injection cap with antiseptic swab. Attach syringe with sterile 0.9% normal saline solution (NS) flush and inject through cap into short extension set, keeping syringe attached.

Removes air from tubing, preventing it from being introduced into vein (Alexander et al., 2010; Policy and Procedures INS, 2011).

b Maintain sterility of end of connector and set aside for attaching to catheter hub after successful venipuncture.

Prevents touch contamination.

8 Prepare IV tubing and solution for continuous infusion.

a Check IV solution using six rights of medication administration (see Chapter 20). If using bar code, scan code on patient's wristband and then on IV fluid container. Be sure that prescribed additives such as potassium and vitamins have been added. Check solution for color, clarity, and expiration date. Check bag for leaks.

IV solutions are medications and need to be checked carefully to reduce risk of error. Bar code system reduces medication errors (Poon et al., 2010). Do not use solutions that are discolored, contain particles, or are expired. Do not use leaking bags because the integrity has been compromised and they present an opportunity for infection (Alexander et al., 2010; Policy and Procedures INS, 2011; INS, 2011).

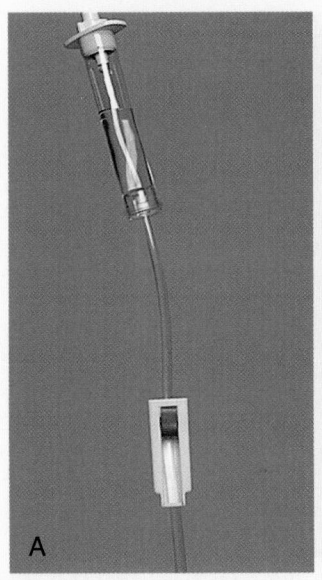 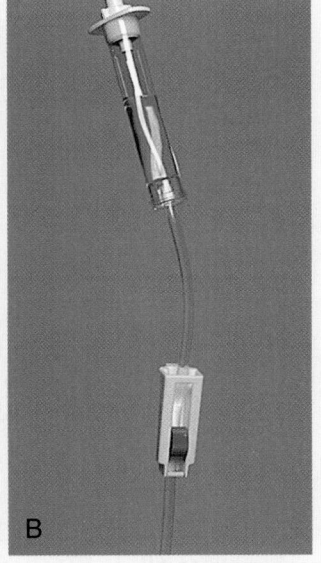

STEP 8d **A,** Roller clamp in open position. **B,** Roller clamp in closed position.

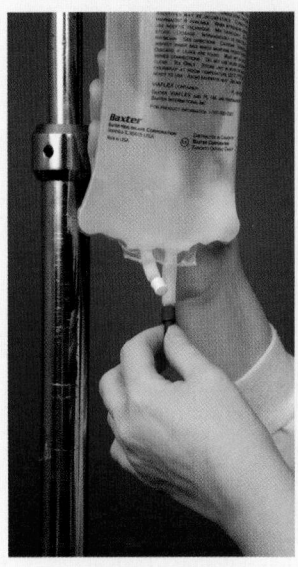

STEP 8e Removing protective sheath from IV bag port.

STEP	RATIONALE
b Open infusion set, maintaining sterility of both tubing ends. Electronic infusion devices (EIDs) sometimes have a special dedicated administration set.	Prevents touch contamination, which allows microorganisms to enter infusion equipment and bloodstream.
c Removing appropriate end caps, attach extension tubing (if used) with injection port to distal end of infusion set, maintaining sterility. Leave end cap on distal end of extension tubing.	Distal end of extension tubing with injection port attaches to IV catheter hub after venipuncture.
d Place roller clamp (see illustration A) about 2 to 5 cm (1 to 2 inches) below drip chamber and move roller clamp to "off" position (see illustration B).	Close proximity of roller clamp to drip chamber allows more accurate regulation of flow rate. Moving clamp to "off" prevents accidental spillage of IV solution during priming.
e Remove protective sheath over IV tubing port on plastic IV solution bag (see illustration) or top of bottle.	Provides access for insertion of infusion tubing into solution using sterile technique.
f Remove protective cap from tubing insertion spike (not touching spike) and insert spike into port of IV bag (see illustration). Clean rubber stopper on glass-bottled solution with single-use antiseptic and insert spike into black rubber stopper of IV bottle. Bottles need special vented tubing.	Flat surface on top of bottled solution may contain contaminants, whereas opening to plastic bag is recessed. Prevents contamination of bottled solution during insertion of spike.

Clinical Decision Point *Do not touch spike because it is sterile. If contamination occurs (e.g., spike is accidentally dropped on the floor), discard that IV tubing and obtain a new one.*

g Compress drip chamber and release, allowing it to fill one-third to one-half full (see illustration).	Creates suction effect; fluid enters drip chamber to prevent air from entering tubing.
h Prime infusion tubing by filling with IV solution: Remove protective cap on end of tubing (you can prime some tubing without removal) and slowly open roller clamp to allow fluid to travel from drip chamber through tubing to needle adapter. Invert Y connector to displace air. Return roller clamp to "off" position after priming tubing (filled with IV fluid). Replace protective cap on end of infusion tubing.	Priming ensures that tubing is clear of air before connection with VAD. Slow fill of tubing decreases turbulence and chance of bubble formation. Closing clamp prevents accidental loss of fluid. Maintains sterility.
i Be certain that tubing is clear of air and air bubbles. To remove small air bubbles, firmly tap IV tubing where air bubbles are located. Check entire length of tubing to ensure that all air bubbles are removed (see illustration).	Large air bubbles act as emboli.
j If using optional long extension tubing (not short tubing in Step 7), remove protective cap and attach it to distal end of IV tubing, maintaining sterility. Then prime long extension tubing.	Priming removes air from tubing so it does not enter patient's vascular system.

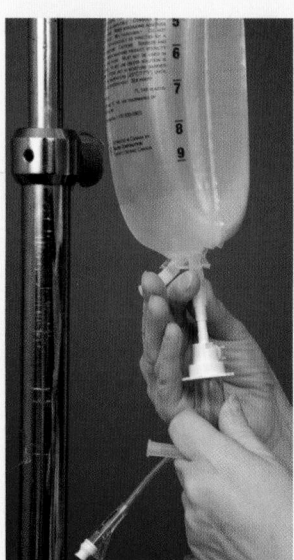

STEP 8f Inserting spike into IV bag.

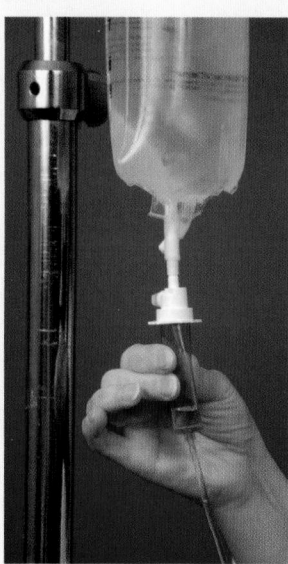

STEP 8g Squeezing drip chamber to fill with fluid.

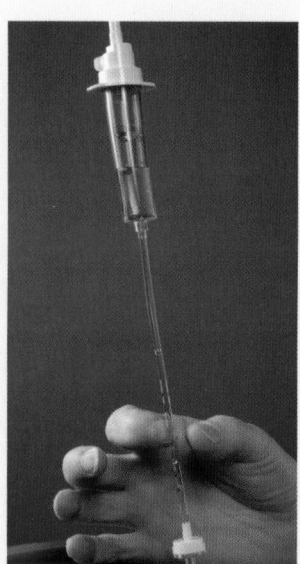

STEP 8i Removing air bubbles from tubing.

STEP	RATIONALE
9 Perform hand hygiene and apply clean gloves. Wear eye protection and mask (see agency policy) if splash or spray of blood is possible.	Reduces transmission of microorganisms. Decreases exposure to human immunodeficiency virus (HIV), hepatitis, and other bloodborne organisms (INS, 2011). Prevents spraying blood from contacting your mucous membranes.

Clinical Decision Point *Gloves are not necessary to locate vein but must be applied before preparing the site.*

STEP	RATIONALE
10 Apply tourniquet around arm above antecubital fossa 10 to 15 cm (4 to 6 inches) above proposed insertion site (see illustration). Do not apply tourniquet too tightly to avoid injury, bruising skin, or occluding artery. Check for presence of radial pulse. (Option a: Apply tourniquet on top of a thin layer of clothing such as a gown sleeve to protect fragile or hairy skin.) (Option b: Blood pressure cuff may be used in place of tourniquet: Inflate cuff to just below patient's diastolic pressure [less than 50 mg Hg].)	Tourniquet should be tight enough to impede venous return but not occlude arterial flow (Alexander et al., 2010; Policy and Procedures INS, 2011). If patient has fragile veins, tourniquet should be applied loosely or not at all to prevent damage to veins and bruising.
11 Select vein for VAD insertion (see illustration). Veins on dorsal and ventral surfaces of arms (e.g., cephalic, basilic, or median) are preferred in adults. Avoid lateral surface of wrist (10 to 12.5 cm [4 to 5 inches]) because of potential for nerve damage (INS, 2011). **a** Use most distal site in nondominant arm if possible.	Ensures adequate vein that is easy to puncture and less likely to rupture. Veins of lower extremities should not be used for routine IV therapy in adults because of risk of tissue damage and thrombophlebitis (INS, 2011). Patients with VAD placement in their dominant hand have decreased ability to perform self-care.

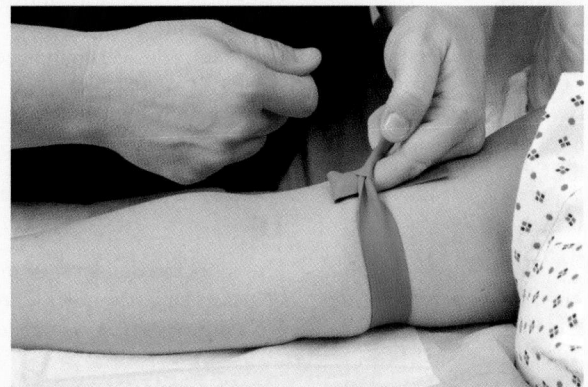

STEP 10   Tourniquet placed on arm for initial vein selection.

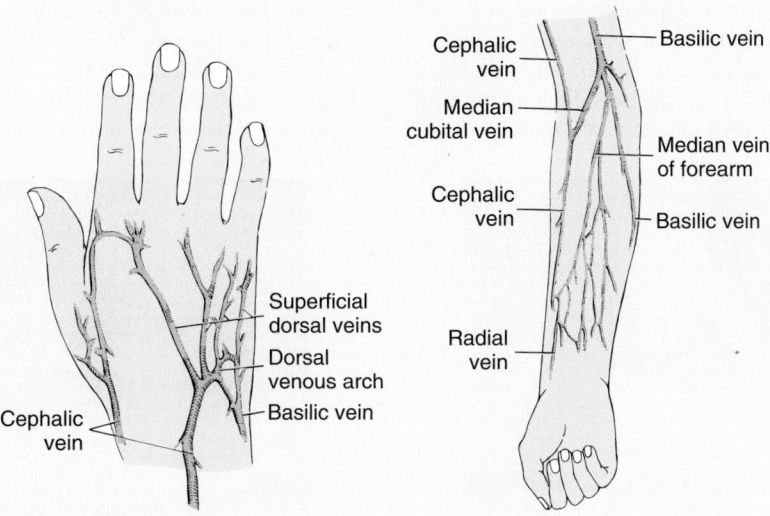

STEP 11   Cephalic, basilic, and median cubital veins are best for IV placement in adults.

STEP	RATIONALE

b Select a well-dilated vein.
Methods to improve venous distention:
  (1) Place extremity in dependent position and stroke from distal to proximal below proposed venipuncture site.
  (2) Apply warmth to extremity for several minutes (e.g., warm washcloth or dry heat).
	Increased volume of blood in vein at venipuncture site makes vein more visible.
	Promotes venous filling.
	
	Heat increases blood supply through vasodilation (INS, 2011).

Clinical Decision Point *Vigorous friction and multiple tapping of a vein, especially in older adults, causes hematoma and/or venous constriction.*

STEP	RATIONALE

12 Select a vein large enough for VAD insertion:
  a With your index finger, palpate vein by pressing downward. Note resilient, soft, bouncy feeling while releasing pressure (see illustration).
  b Avoid vein selection in:
    (1) Areas with tenderness, redness, rash, pain, or infection.
 	
    (2) Extremity affected by previous cerebrovascular accident (CVA), paralysis, dialysis shunt, or mastectomy.
    (3) Site distal to previous venipuncture site, sclerosed or hardened veins, infiltrate site, areas of venous valves, or phlebotic vessels.
    (4) Fragile dorsal veins in older adults.
  c Choose site that will not interfere with patient's activities of daily living (ADLs), use of assist devices, or planned procedures.
13 Release tourniquet temporarily and carefully.
 	
Option: Clip arm hair with scissors if necessary (explain to patient).
Option: You may apply topical local anesthetic to IV site 30 minutes before insertion. Monitor for allergic reaction.
	Fingertip is more sensitive and better for assessing vein location and condition.
	
	It would be difficult to assess for any signs or symptoms of complications if an IV device were inserted in an area already compromised (INS, 2011).
	Increases risk for complications such as infection, lymphedema, or vessel damage (INS, 2011).
	Such sites cause infiltration around newly placed VAD site and vessel damage.
	
	Veins have increased risk for infiltration.
	Keeps patient as mobile as possible.
	
	Restores blood flow and prevents venospasm when preparing for venipuncture.
	Hair impedes venipuncture or adherence of dressing.
	
	Local anesthetic reduces discomfort (must have health care provider order for use of local anesthetic).

Clinical Decision Point *If hair removal is needed, do not shave area with a razor. Shaving may cause microabrasions that increase risk of infection (INS, 2011).*

STEP	RATIONALE
14 Apply clean gloves if not done in Step 9. **15** Place adapter end of short infusion tubing (prepared in Step 7) or extension/injection cap for saline lock nearby in sterile package. **16** If area of insertion appears to need cleaning, use soap and water first and dry. Use chlorhexidine antiseptic swab or applicator to clean insertion site, using friction in a horizontal plane with first swab, in a vertical plane with second swab, and in a circular motion moving outward with third swab (see illustration). Allow to dry completely. Refrain from touching cleaned site unless using sterile technique. Allow drying time between agents if agents are used in combination (alcohol and betadine).	Reduces transmission of microorganisms. Permits smooth, quick connection of infusion to short peripheral catheter once vein is accessed. Mechanical friction in this pattern allows penetration of antiseptic solution to epidermal layer of the skin (Alexander et al., 2010; INS, 2011; Policy and Procedures INS, 2011). Allowing antiseptic solution to air-dry completely effectively reduces microbial counts (INS, 2011). 2% Chlorhexidine dries in 30 seconds (INS, 2011). Touching cleaned area introduces microorganisms from your finger to site. If this happens, prepare site again.

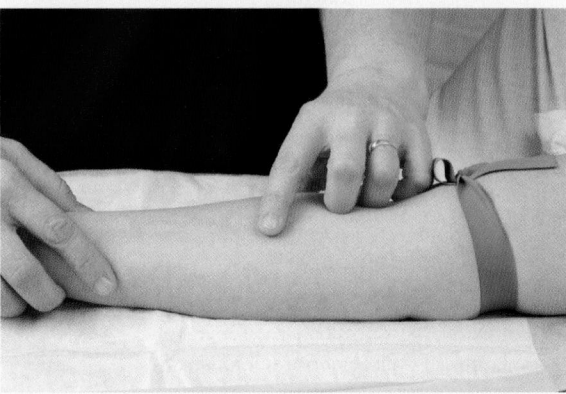

STEP 12a Palpate vein.

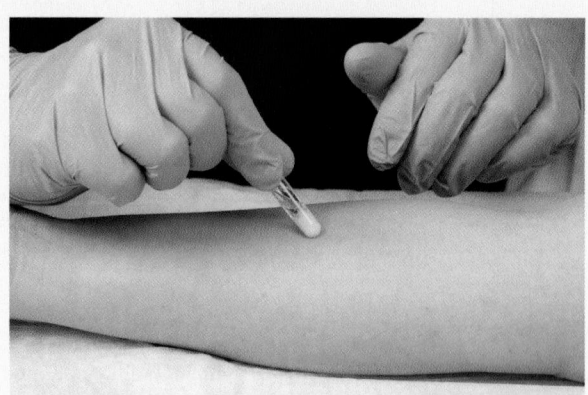

STEP 16 Clean site with 2% chlorhexidine.

STEP	RATIONALE
17 Reapply tourniquet 10 to 15 cm (4 to 6 inches) above anticipated insertion site. Check presence of radial pulse.	Diminished arterial flow prevents venous filling. Pressure of tourniquet causes vein to engorge.
18 Perform venipuncture. Anchor vein below site by placing thumb over vein and gently stretching skin against direction of insertion 4 to 5 cm (1½ to 2 inches) distal to the site (see illustration). Instruct patient to relax hand.	Stabilizes vein for needle insertion and prevents vein from rolling. Skin becomes taut, decreasing drag on insertion of device.
a Warn patient of a sharp, quick stick. Insert VAD with bevel up at 10- to 30-degree angle slightly distal to actual site of venipuncture in direction of vein (see illustration).	Places needle at a 10- to 30-degree angle to vein. When vein is punctured, risk for puncturing posterior vein wall is reduced. Superficial veins require smaller angle. Deeper veins require greater angle.

Clinical Decision Point *Use each VAD only once for each insertion attempt.*

19 Observe for blood return through flashback chamber of catheter, indicating that bevel of needle has entered vein (see illustration A). Lower catheter until almost flush with skin. Advance catheter approximately 0.6 cm (¼ inch) into vein and loosen stylet of over-the-needle catheter (ONC). Continue to hold skin taut while stabilizing needle and advance catheter off needle to thread just the catheter into vein until hub rests at venipuncture site (see illustration B). *Do not reinsert stylet once it is loosened.* Advance catheter while safety device automatically retracts stylet (technique will vary by product type). Follow manufacturer guidelines.	Increased venous pressure from tourniquet increases backflow of blood into catheter or tubing. Allows for full penetration of vein wall, placement of catheter in inner lumen of vein, and advancement of catheter off stylet. Reduces risk for introduction of microorganisms along catheter. Advancing entire stylet into vein may penetrate wall of vein, resulting in hematoma. Reinsertion of stylet causes catheter shearing in vein and potential catheter embolization (INS, 2011).

Clinical Decision Point *A single nurse should not make more than two attempts at initiating IV access (INS, 2011). After two attempts the nurse should have another nurse attempt the insertion.*

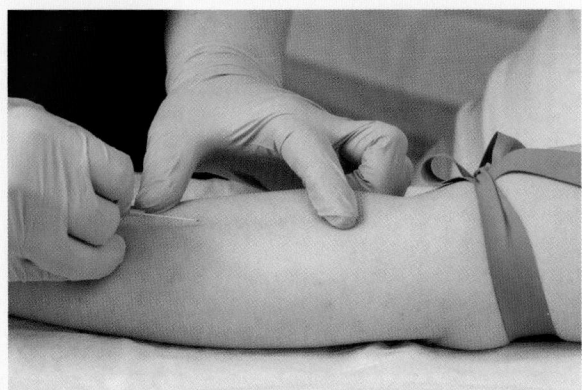

STEP 18 Stabilize vein below insertion site.

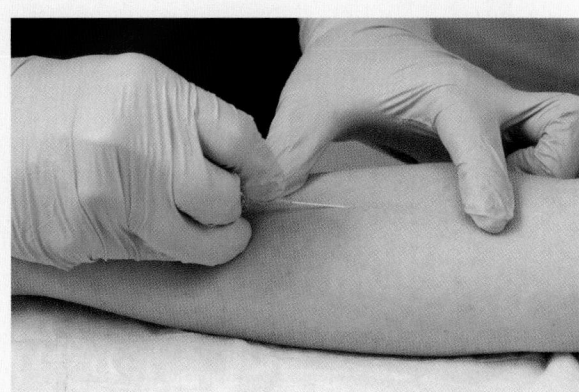

STEP 18a Puncture skin with catheter at 10- to 30-degree angle.

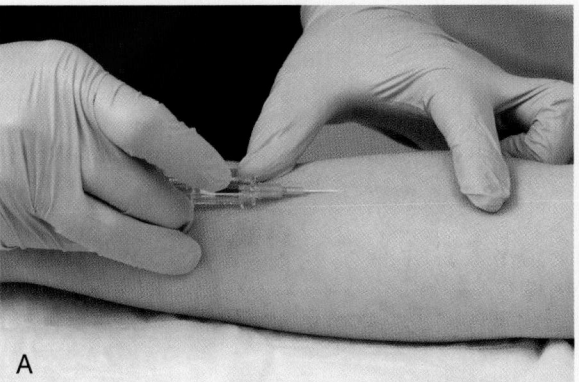

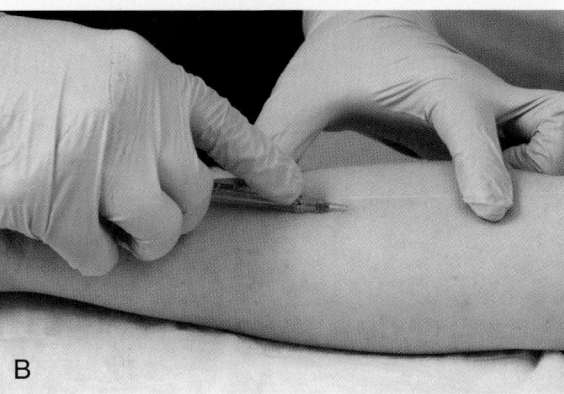

STEP 19 **A,** Observe for blood return in flashback chamber. **B,** Advance catheter into vein until hub rests at veinpuncture site.

STEP	RATIONALE
20 Stabilize catheter with nondominant hand and release tourniquet or blood pressure cuff with other. Apply gentle but firm pressure with middle finger of nondominant hand 3 cm (1¼ inches) above insertion site. Keep catheter stable with index finger.	Permits venous flow, reduces backflow of blood, and allows connection with administration set with minimal blood loss (INS, 2011).
21 Quickly connect Luer-Lok end of prepared extension set, or saline lock of primary administration set, to end of catheter. Do not touch point of entry of connection. Secure connection.	Prompt connection of infusion set maintains patency of vein and prevents risk of exposure to blood. Maintains sterility.
22 Flush VAD. Slowly flush a primed extension set with remaining saline from attached prefilled syringe (see illustration A) or begin a primary infusion by slowly opening slide clamp or adjusting roller clamp of IV tubing. Observe for swelling.	Positive-pressure flushing allows fluid to displace removed stylet, creates positive pressure in catheter, and prevents reflux of blood into catheter lumen (Policy and Procedures INS, 2011).
Option: Remove syringe. Attach distal end of primary IV tubing to needleless connector on short extension tubing that is attached to catheter (see illustration B).	Initiates flow of fluid through IV catheter, preventing clotting of device. Swelling indicates infiltration, and catheter would need to be removed.
23 Secure catheter (procedures differ; follow agency policy).	
a *Manufactured catheter stabilization device:* Wipe selected area with single-use skin protectant and allow to dry. Apply sterile adhesive strip over catheter hub. Slide device under catheter hub and center hub over device. Holding catheter in place, peel off half of liner, press to adhere to skin. Repeat on other side. Holding catheter in place, pull tab out from center of device to create opening, insert catheter into slit. This frames IV site (see illustration). Then apply dressing.	Use of manufactured stabilization device preserves integrity of access device, minimizes catheter movement at hub, and prevents catheter dislodgement or loss of access (INS, 2011).

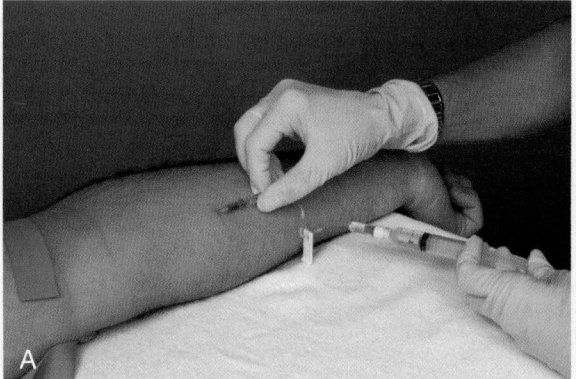 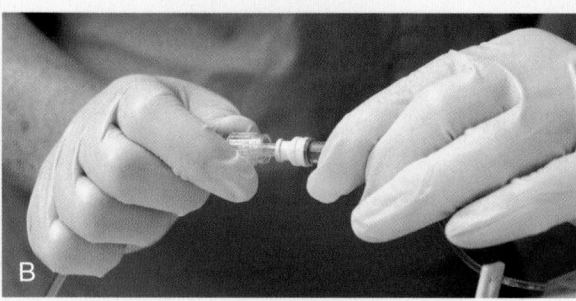

STEP 22 A, Flush primed end of extension set. **B,** Connect IV tubing to the short extension set that is attached to the catheter.

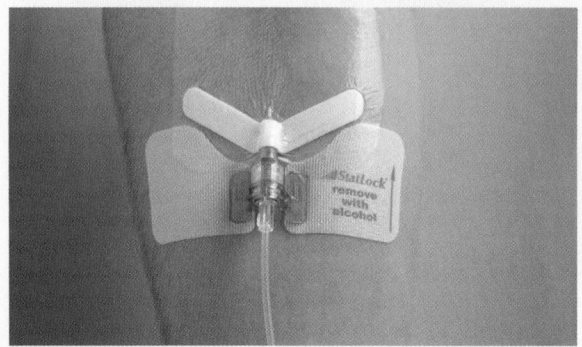

STEP 23a   Catheter stabilization device in place. (*Image Courtesy C.R. Bard, Inc., All rights reserved.*)

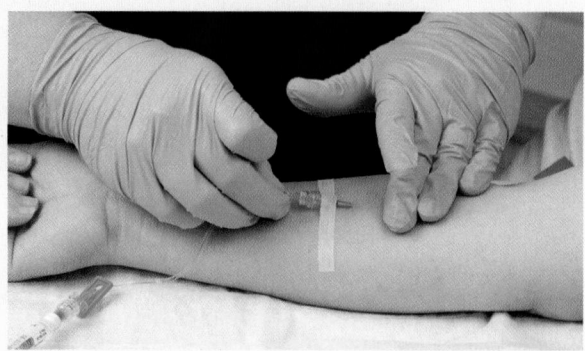

STEP 23c   Tape over catheter hub.

STEP	RATIONALE

b *Transparent dressing*: Secure catheter with nondominant hand while preparing to apply dressing.

c *Sterile gauze dressing*: Place narrow piece 1.27 cm (½ inch) of sterile tape over catheter hub (see illustration). Place tape only on catheter, *never* over insertion site. Secure site to allow easy visual inspection. Avoid applying tape or gauze around arm.

Prevents accidental dislodgement of catheter.

Use sterile tape under sterile dressing to prevent site contamination. Regular adhesive tape is potential source of pathogenic bacteria (INS, 2011).
Prevents back-and-forth motion of catheter.

24 Apply sterile dressing over site.

a Transparent dressing (TSM):

(1) Carefully remove adherent backing. Apply one edge of dressing and gently smooth remaining dressing over IV site, leaving connection between IV tubing and catheter hub uncovered. Remove outer covering and smooth dressing gently over site (see illustration).

(2) Take a 2.5 cm (1-inch) piece of tape and place it over extension or administration set tubing (see illustration). **Do not apply tape on top of transparent dressing.**

Occlusive dressing protects site from bacterial contamination. Allows for visualization of insertion site and surrounding area for signs and symptoms of IV-related complications (INS, 2011). Connection between administration set and hub needs to be uncovered to facilitate changing tubing if necessary.
Removal of tape from transparent dressing can cause accidental removal of catheter.
Tape on top of transparent dressing prevents moisture from being carried away from skin.

b Sterile gauze dressing:

(1) Place 2 × 2–inch gauze pad over insertion site and catheter hub. Secure all edges with tape. Do not cover connection between IV tubing and catheter hub (see illustration).

(2) Fold 2 × 2–inch gauze in half and cover with 2.5-cm (1-inch)–wide tape extending about an inch from each side. Place under tubing/catheter hub junction (see illustration).

Optional method of securing device if patient is allergic to transparent dressing. It is not the preferred method to cover and secure IV device because gauze prevents visualization of insertion site (INS, 2011).
Tape on top of gauze makes it easier to access hub/tubing junction. Gauze pad elevates hub off skin to prevent pressure area.

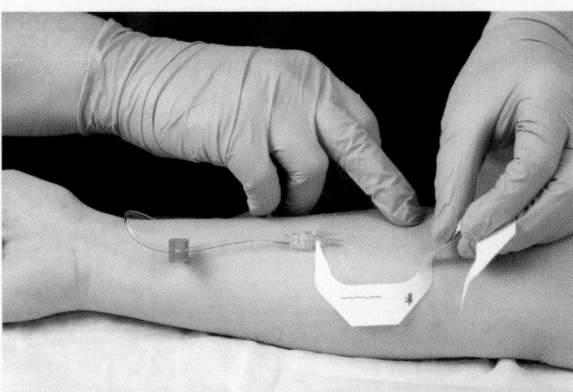

STEP 24a(1) Apply transparent dressing.

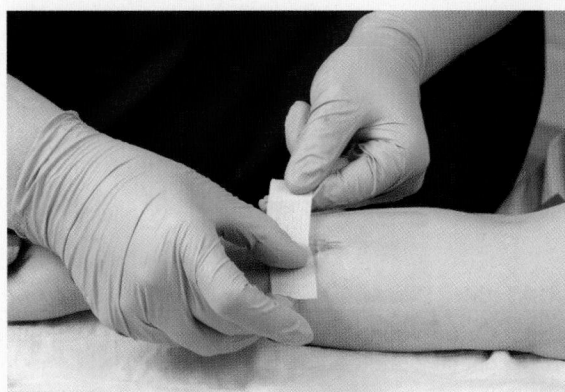

STEP 24a(2) Place tape over administration set tubing.

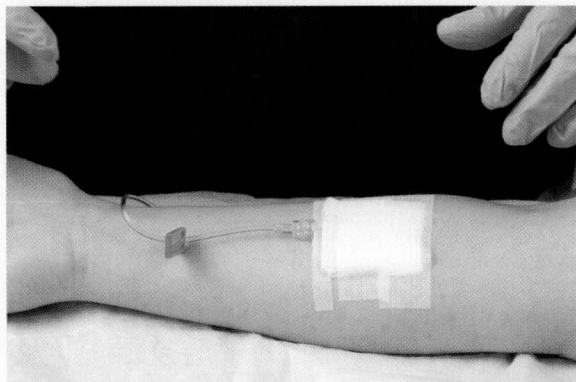

STEP 24b(1) Place 2 × 2–inch gauze over insertion site and catheter hub.

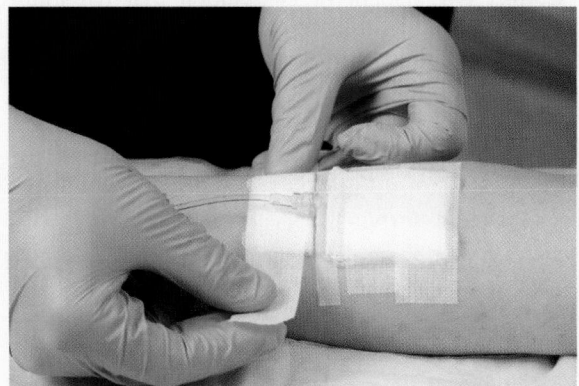

STEP 24b(2) Apply 2 × 2–inch gauze dressing under tubing junction.

STEP	RATIONALE
25 Loop the short extension tubing or the continuous infusion administration tubing alongside arm and place second piece of tape directly over tubing and secure (see illustration).	Securing administration set or extension set reduces risk for dislodging catheter if IV tubing is pulled (i.e., loop comes apart before catheter dislodges).
26 For continuous infusion, insert tubing of IV administration set into electronic infusion device (EID). Check ordered rate of infusion, then turn on EID, program it, and begin infusion at correct rate. If infusing by gravity drip, adjust flow rate to correct drops per minute (see Skill 28-2)	Manipulation of catheter during dressing application alters flow rate. EID maintains correct rate of flow for IV solution. Flow fluctuates; thus it must be checked at intervals for accuracy.
27 Label dressing per agency policy. Include date and time of IV insertion, VAD gauge size and length, and your initials (see illustration).	Allows for recognition of type of device and length of time that device has been in place.
28 Dispose of used stylet or other sharps in appropriate sharps container. Discard supplies. Remove gloves and perform hand hygiene.	Reduces transmission of microorganisms; prevents accidental needlestick injuries.
29 Instruct patient in how to move or turn without dislodging VAD.	Prevents accidental dislodgement of catheter.

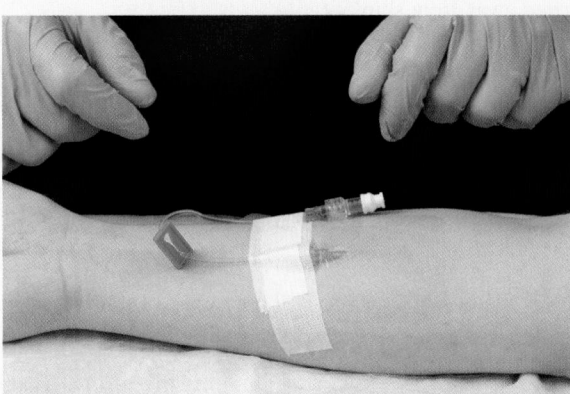

STEP 25   Loop and secure tubing.

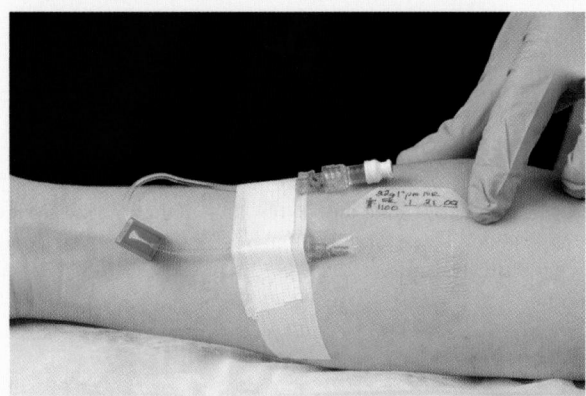

STEP 27   Label IV dressing.

EVALUATION

1   Routine site care and dressing changes are not performed on short peripheral catheters unless dressing is soiled or no longer intact.

An occlusive transparent dressing is changed at time of site rotation (Alexander et al., 2010; INS, 2011; Policy and Procedures INS, 2011). Gauze dressings are changed every 48 hours (INS, 2011).

2   Observe patient every 1 to 2 hours or at established intervals per agency policy and procedure for the following:

  a   Correct type/amount of IV solution that has infused by observing fluid level in IV container.

Correct administration of fluid volume prevents fluid imbalance.

  b   Check infusion rate on EID or count drip rate (if gravity drip).

Accurate monitoring of drip rate further ensures correct volume administration.

  c   Check patency of VAD.

Flow rate is slowed or stopped.

Clinical Decision Point   *If IV is positional, fluid will run slowly or stop, depending on position of patient's arm; if this continues, you may have to restart IV.*

  d   Observe patient during palpation of vessel (over TSM) for signs of discomfort.

Tenderness is an early sign of phlebitis (INS, 2011).

STEP	RATIONALE
e Inspect insertion site, note color (e.g., redness or pallor). Inspect site for presence of swelling (which is sign of infiltration) or pain and tenderness (which is a sign of phlebitis) (Table 28-4). Palpate temperature of skin above dressing.	Redness, inflammation, tenderness, and warmth indicate vein inflammation or phlebitis. Use a standard scale for assessing and documenting infiltration (INS, 2011).
3 Observe patient to determine response to therapy (e.g., laboratory values, I&O, weights, vital signs, postprocedure assessments).	IV fluids and additives maintain or restore fluid and electrolyte balance. Early recognition of complications leads to prompt treatment.

Unexpected Outcomes

Related Interventions

1 FVD as manifested by decreased urine output, dry mucous membranes, decreased capillary refill, a disparity in central and peripheral pulses, tachycardia, hypotension, shock.

- Notify health care provider.
- Requires readjusting infusion rate.

2 FVE as manifested by crackles in lungs, shortness of breath, edema.

- Reduce IV flow rate if symptoms appear.
- Notify health care provider.

3 Electrolyte imbalances indicated by abnormal serum electrolyte levels, changes in mental status, alterations in neuromuscular function, cardiac arrhythmias, and changes in vital signs.

- Notify health care provider.
- Adjust additives in IV or type of IV fluid per order.

4 Infiltration is indicated by slowing of infusion; insertion site is cool to touch, pale, and painful.

- Stop infusion and discontinue IV (see (Procedural Guideline 28-1).
- Elevate affected extremity.
- Restart new IV above previous location of infiltrate or opposite extremity if continued therapy is necessary.
- Document degree of infiltration and nursing intervention.

5 Phlebitis is indicated by pain and tenderness at IV site with erythema at site or along path of vein. Insertion site is warm to touch, and rate of infusion may be altered.

- Stop infusion immediately and discontinue IV (see (Procedural Guideline 28-1).
- Restart new IV if continued therapy is necessary in area above previous location or opposite extremity.
- Place moist warm compress over area of phlebitis.
- Continue to monitor site for 48 hours after catheter is removed for postinfusion phlebitis (INS, 2011).
- Document degree of phlebitis and nursing interventions per agency policy and procedure (see Table 28-4).

6 Bleeding occurs at venipuncture site.

- Verify that system is intact and replace dressing if loosened.
- Restart new IV if bleeding from site does not stop or if IV is dislodged.

7 IV site infection. Monitor site for signs and symptoms of infection, which may include redness, pain, edema, induration, temperature, and drainage.

- Notify health care provider for appropriate interventions such as culturing of device or site.
- Restart new IV if continued therapy is necessary in area above location or opposite extremity.
- Document presence and severity of infection and interventions.

TABLE 28-4	Phlebitis Scale
Grade	**Clinical Criteria**
0	No symptoms
1	Erythema at access site with or without pain
2	Pain at access site with erythema and/or edema
3	Pain at access site with erythema and/or edema Streak formation Palpable venous cord
4	Pain at access site with erythema and/or edema Streak formation Palpable venous cord >1 inch (2.5 cm) in length Purulent drainage

From Infusion Nurses Society: Infusion nursing standards of practice, *J Intraven Nurs* 34(1S):S65, 2011.

Recording and Reporting

- Record in nurses' notes and electronic health record (EHR) the number of attempts and sites of insertion; precise description of insertion site (e.g., cephalic vein on dorsal surface of right lower arm, 2.5 cm [1 inch] above wrist); flow rate; method of infusion (gravity or EID), size and type, length, and brand of catheter; and time infusion started and patients response to insertion. Use an infusion therapy flow sheet when available.
- If using an EID, document type and rate of infusion and device identification number.
- Record patient's status, IV fluid, amount infused, and integrity and patency of system according to agency policy.
- Report to oncoming nursing staff: type of fluid, flow rate, status of VAD, amount of fluid remaining in present solution, expected time to hang subsequent IV container, and patient condition.

- Report to health care provider any signs and symptoms of IV-related complications.

Special Considerations
Teaching
- Instruct patient in signs and symptoms of IV-related complications (e.g., infiltration, phlebitis, and inflammation).
- Instruct patient to inform nurse or NAP if rate slows or stops or if patient sees blood in the tubing or on the dressing.
- Teach patient how to ambulate with IV pole or stand.
- Instruct patient to protect IV when performing hygiene activities.

Pediatric
- Perform venipuncture in a neutral space to allow the child's room to be a safe place.
- In addition to the usual venipuncture sites, the four scalp veins and dorsum of the foot are used in infants.
- Needle selection is based on age: 26- to 24-gauge for neonates, 24- to 22-gauge for children (Hockenberry and Wilson, 2011; INS, 2011).
- Use local anesthetics and distraction strategies to minimize distress associated with venipuncture (Alexander et al., 2010).
- Apply latex-free tubing or rubber band or use a blood pressure cuff inflated to just below diastolic blood pressure. In accessing scalp veins aim the catheter downward toward the heart so the flow of infusion can follow venous return (INS, 2011).
- Allow older children to select IV site to increase cooperation so they believe that they have some control over their treatment.
- To maintain safety in positioning, have extra help when starting an IV on a child. Use therapeutic hugging, usually in a sitting position, to provide close contact (Hockenberry and Wilson, 2011). NAP can help with positioning.
- Choose age-appropriate activities compatible with the maintenance of the IV infusion to maintain normal growth and development.

Gerontologic
- Veins of the older population are very fragile; they have less subcutaneous support tissue, and their skin is thinning (Alexander et al., 2010). Avoid sites that are easily moved or bumped. Use a commercial protective device to protect the site and reduce manipulation (Fig. 28-2).
- In older patients the use of a 22- or 24-gauge catheter is appropriate for most therapies. Smaller-gauge catheters are less traumatizing to the vein but still allow blood flow to provide increased hemodilution of the IV fluids or medications (Alexander et al., 2010).

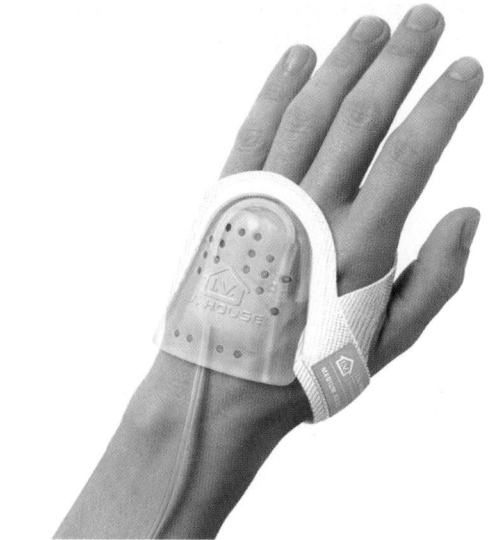

FIG 28-2 I.V. House Protective Device. (*Courtesy I.V. House.*)

- If possible, avoid the back of the older adult's hand or the dominant arm for venipuncture because use of these sites interferes with their independence.
- As older adults lose subcutaneous tissue, the veins lose stability and roll away from the needle. To stabilize the vein, pull the skin taut and toward you with your nondominant hand and anchor the vein with your thumb.
- Reduce the angle of insertion (e.g., 5 to 15 degrees on insertion) to accommodate more superficial veins.
- Some older adults do not complain of pain at the insertion site; however, a large amount of fluid may infiltrate before a patient experiences discomfort.

Home Care
- Ensure that a patient is able and willing to self-administer IV therapy or that there is a reliable family caregiver to provide IV therapy care at home.
- Ensure that all sharps and equipment contaminated by blood are disposed of in puncture-resistant containers with lids. Some suppliers provide sharps containers for needle disposal. Teach patient and family to dispose of any open and sheathed needles into sharps container.
- Instruct patient and family caregiver about procedures of IV therapy, including hand hygiene and aseptic technique while handling syringes and other supplies.
- Ensure availability of 24-hour assistance with provider of home infusion therapy pharmaceuticals and equipment.
- Teach patient about activity restrictions (e.g., avoiding strenuous exercise of the arm with the IV).

SKILL 28-2 Regulating Intravenous Flow Rate

NSO *Intravenous Fluid Therapy Management Module / Lesson 2*

 Video Clip

After initiating an infusion and ensuring that the line is patent, regulate the rate of infusion according to the health care provider's order. Accurate infusion rates are essential in the delivery of solutions and medications. Appropriate regulation of fluid rates reduces complications (e.g., phlebitis, infiltration, fluid overload,

or clotting of the VAD) associated with IV therapy (Policy and Procedures INS, 2011). Changes in patient position, flexion of the IV site extremity, and occlusion of the IV device influence infusion rates. Vasospasm of the vein, venous trauma, or manipulation of the device also affects infusion rates. A patient achieves therapeutic outcomes and fewer complications when an IV system and flow rate are assessed systematically (Alexander et al., 2010).

There are a variety of methods for calculating infusion rates. Electronic infusion devices (EIDs) maintain correct flow rates and catheter patency and prevent an unexpected bolus of IV infusion. Many EIDs provide a record of the volume of fluid infused over a period of time.

An EID delivers a measured amount of fluid over a period of time (e.g., 100 mL/hr) using positive pressure. Infusion pumps are necessary for patients requiring low hourly rates, at risk for volume overload, with impaired renal clearance, or receiving solutions or medications that require a specific hourly volume (Alexander et al., 2010). EIDs use an electronic sensor and an alarm that signals if the pressure in the system changes and the desired flow rate alters. For example, when an infiltration occurs in the subcutaneous tissue or a patient's position obstructs IV flow, pressure builds up, and the alarm sounds. An infiltration is sometimes extensive before a positive-pressure EID alarm responds. The use of an EID does not absolve a nurse from checking to ensure that the pump is functioning and infusing at the prescribed rate (INS, 2011).

Non-EIDs such as a volume-control device deliver small fluid volumes with the aid of gravity. Patient and mechanical factors (e.g., height of the IV fluid container, IV tubing size, or fluid viscosity) affect an IV gravity controller. One example of a volume-control device is a calibrated chamber placed between the IV container and the insertion spike and drip chamber of an administration set (Fig. 28-3). You place a small volume of IV fluid in the chamber and regulate it for administration. The advantage of this system is that only the smaller volume of fluid infuses if the rate of the IV is inadvertently increased. Volume-control devices are beneficial when administering fluids to neonates, very young children, and older adults (Alexander et al., 2010). With either type of device, a patient requires consistent monitoring to verify the accurate infusion of the IV solution and detect and prevent complications.

The capabilities of EID have increased over the years, allowing for enhanced patient safety (Alexander et al., 2010). Multifunctional EIDs are designed to be a final step in preventing errors that relate directly to administration of IV medications. These "smart pumps" have built-in software programmed from health care pharmacy databases with unit-specific profiles (Fig. 28-4). The pump has an audible and visual alert when its setting does not match the medication administration guidelines, helping to prevent infusion errors. Each pump has the potential to use add-on syringe pumps, permit multiple infusions, and administer patient-controlled analgesia. The potential reduction in serious medication errors and the improved patient outcomes have prompted many organizations to implement this technology (Alexander et al., 2010; INS, 2011). Know and follow your agency and manufacturer recommendations for selection and use of EIDs, alarm settings, pump controls, and features. Diligence is necessary on your part to assess and monitor patients since use of any EID or controller is not without the risk of malfunction, placing a patient at risk for harm or injury.

Patients in alternative care settings (e.g., home care, long-term care) can receive infusion therapy with ambulatory pumps, which promote independence and improved quality of life. Most pumps weigh less than 6 lbs and range from palm size to fitting in a backpack. Programming capabilities range from rate adjustments, remote site adjustments, and therapy-specific settings.

Delegation and Collaboration

The skill of regulating IV flow rate cannot be delegated to nursing assistive personnel (NAP). Delegation to licensed practical nurses (LPNs) varies by state Nurse Practice Act. The nurse instructs the NAP to:

- Inform the nurse when the EID alarm signals.
- Inform the nurse when the fluid container is empty.
- Report any patient complaints of discomfort related to infusion such as pain, burning, bleeding, or swelling.

Equipment

- ❏ Watch with second hand
- ❏ Calculator, paper, and pencil
- ❏ Tape
- ❏ Label
- ❏ IV administration set: EID (optional), volume-control device (*optional*)

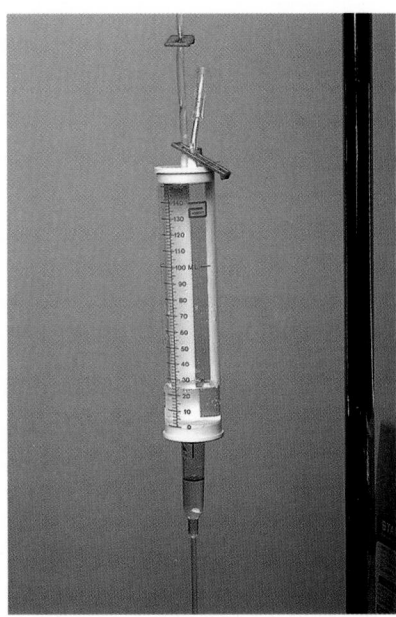

FIG 28-3   Volume-control device.

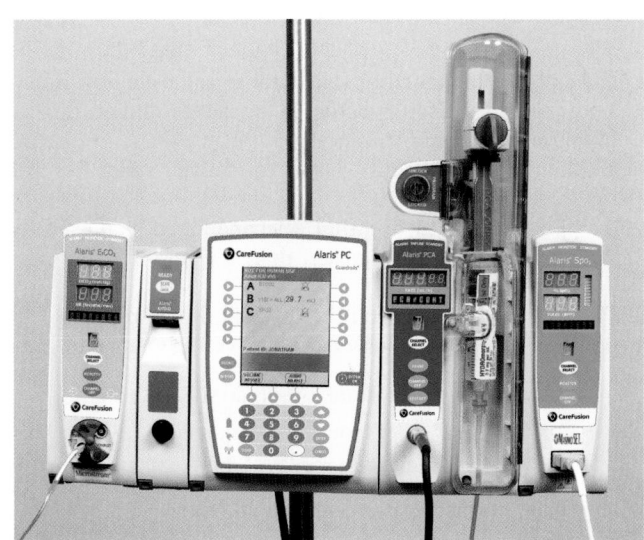

FIG 28-4   Smart pump. (*Photo courtesy Cardinal Health, Dublin, Ohio.*)

STEP	RATIONALE

ASSESSMENT

1 Review accuracy and completeness of health care provider order in patient's medical record for patient name and correct solution: type, volume, additives, rate, and duration of IV therapy. Follow six rights of drug administration (see Chapter 20).

Ensures that correct IV fluid is administered.

2 Assess patient's knowledge of how positioning of IV site affects flow rate.

Fosters patient participation in maintaining most effective position of arm with IV equipment. Nurse is responsible for positioning control clamp or setting infusion device rate.

3 Perform hand hygiene. Inspect IV site for signs and symptoms of IV-related complications such as pain, swelling, or redness.

Observation or reports of any IV-related complications indicate need to reestablish patent IV access.

4 Observe for patency of IV tubing and VAD.

IV line and VAD must be free of kinks, knots, and clots for fluid to infuse at proper rate.

5 Identify patient risk for fluid and electrolyte imbalance, given type of IV fluid (e.g., neonate, history of cardiac or renal disease).

Helps prioritize assessments. Volume control needs to be strict. Guides choice of infusion device.

NURSING DIAGNOSES

- Deficient fluid volume
- Risk for infection
- Excess fluid volume
- Risk for injury

Related factors are individualized based on patient's condition or needs.

PLANNING

1 Expected outcomes following completion of procedure:
- Serum electrolyte levels remain within normal limits.
- Patient receives prescribed volume of solution over desired time interval.
- No signs or symptoms of IV-related complications (e.g., infiltration, infection).

IV fluid helps to maintain fluid and electrolyte levels.
Patient achieves therapeutic outcomes.

Patient completes therapy without complications.

IMPLEMENTATION

1 Identify patient using two identifiers (i.e., name and birthday or name and account number) according to agency policy. Compare identifiers in MAR/medical record with information on patient's identification bracelet and/or ask patient to state name.

Ensures correct patient. Complies with The Joint Commission standards and improves patient safety (TJC, 2012).

Clinical Decision Point *It is common for health care providers to write an abbreviated IV order such as: "D$_5$W with 20 mEq KCl 125 mL/hr continuous." This order implies that the IV should be maintained at this rate until order has been written for IV to be discontinued or changed to another order.*

2 Have paper and pencil or calculator to calculate flow rate.

Use mathematic calculations to obtain correct rate.

3 Know calibration (drop factor) in drops per milliliter (gtt/mL) of infusion set used by agency:

a Microdrip: 60 gtt/mL: Used to deliver rates less than 100 mL/hr.

Microdrip tubing universally delivers 60 gtt/mL. Used when small or very precise volumes are to be infused.

b Macrodrip: 10 to 15 gtt/mL (depending on manufacturer): Used to deliver rates greater than 100 mL/hr.

There are different commercial parenteral administration sets for macrodrip tubing. Used when large volumes or fast rates are necessary. Know drip factor for tubing being used.

4 Determine how long each liter of fluid should run. Calculate milliliters per hour (hourly rate) by dividing volume by hours:

Basis of calculation to ensure infusion of fluid over prescribed hourly rate.

$$mL/hr = \frac{Total\ infusion\ (mL)}{Hours\ of\ infusion}$$

1000 mL/8 hr = 125 mL/hr

or if 3 L is ordered for 24 hours:

3000 mL/24 hr = 125 mL/hr

STEP	RATIONALE

5 Select one of the following formulas to calculate minute flow rate (drops per minute) based on drop factor of infusion set:

$$\text{a} \quad \text{mL/hr}/60 \text{ min} = \text{mL/min}$$

$$\text{Drop factor} \times \text{mL/min} = \text{Drops/min}$$

or

$$\text{b} \quad \text{mL/hr} \times \text{Drop factor}/60 \text{ min} = \text{Drops/min}$$

Calculate minute flow rate for a bag 1 : 1000 mL with 20 mEq KCl @ 125 mL/hr.

Microdrip:

$$125 \text{ mL/hr} \times 60 \text{ gtt/mL} = 7500 \text{ gtt/hr}$$

$$7500 \text{ gtt} \div 60 \text{ minutes} = 125 \text{ gtt/min}$$

Macrodrip:

$$125 \text{ mL/hr} \times 15 \text{ gtt/mL} = 1875 \text{ gtt/hr}$$

$$1875 \text{ gtt} \div 60 \text{ minutes} = 31\text{–}32 \text{ gtt/min}$$

Once you determine hourly rate, these formulas compute correct flow rate.

When using microdrip, milliliters per hour (mL/hr) always equals drops per minute (gtt/min).

Multiply volume by drop factor and divide product by time (in minutes).

6 *For gravity infusions:* Confirm hourly rate and minute rate based on drop factor of infusion set. Using formula (see Step 5), calculate flow rate.

   a Ensure that IV container is 36 inches above the IV site for adults.

   b Regulate flow rate by counting drops in drip chamber for 1 minute by watch; adjust roller clamp to increase or decrease rate of infusion.

7 *For use of EID for infusion:* Follow manufacturer guidelines for setup of EID.

   a Insert IV tubing into chamber of control mechanism (see manufacturer directions) (see illustration).

   b Turn on power button, select required drops per minute or volume per hour, close door to control chamber, and press start button (see illustration).

Calculates minute flow rate for regulation of infusion.

Pressure caused by gravity is necessary to overcome venous pressure and resistance from tubing and catheter (INS, 2011).
Regulates flow to prescribed rate.

Most electronic infusion pumps use positive pressure to infuse. Infusion pumps propel fluid through tubing by compressing and milking IV tubing.

Clinical Decision Point *An anti–free flow safeguard (preventing bolus infusion in the event of machine malfunction or when tubing is removed from machine) is an important element of an EID and is required. Always check manufacturer recommendations for specific device features.*

---

   c Open drip regulator completely while EID is in use.

   d Monitor infusion rate and IV site for complications according to agency policy. Use watch to verify rate of infusion, even when using EID.

Ensures that pump freely regulates infusion rate.
Infusion controllers or pumps are not perfect and do not replace frequent, accurate nursing evaluation. EIDs continue to infuse IV fluids after a complication has developed (INS, 2011).

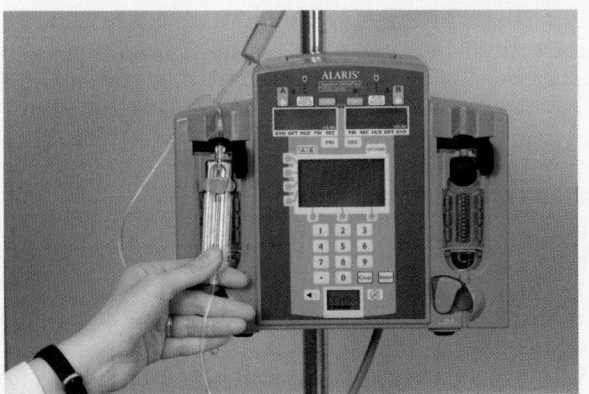

STEP 7a Insert IV tubing into chamber of control mechanism.

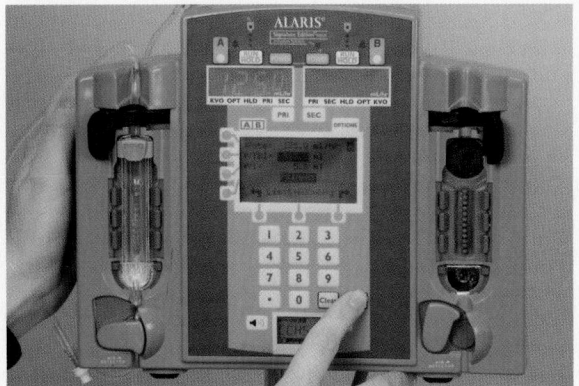

STEP 7b Select rate and volume to be infused and press start button.

STEP	RATIONALE
e Assess patency of system when alarm signals.	Alarm indicates some blockage in system. Empty solution container, tubing kinks, closed clamp, infiltration, clotted catheter, air in the tubing, and/or low battery will all trigger EID alarm.
8 *For volume-control device:*	
a Place volume-control device between IV container and insertion spike of infusion set using aseptic technique.	Delivers small fluid volumes but needs refilling as volume becomes low. Reduces risk for sudden fluid infusion.
b Place no more than a 2-hour allotment of fluid into device by opening clamp between IV bag and device.	Allows for continuous infusion of fluid if you do not return in exactly 60 minutes to refill volume. If infusion rate accidentally increases, patient receives only a 2-hour allotment of fluid.
c Assess system at least hourly; add fluid to volume-control device. Regulate flow rate.	Maintains patency of system and patient monitoring.
9 Attach label to IV fluid container with date and time container changed (check agency policy).	Provides reference to determine next time for container change, especially with keep vein open (KVO) rate.
10 Instruct patient in purpose of alarms, to avoid raising hand or arm that affects flow rate, and to avoid touching control clamp.	Information allows patient to protect IV site and informs him or her about rationale for not altering control rate.

EVALUATION

1 Monitor IV infusion at least every hour, noting volume of IV fluid infused and rate.	Ensures that correct volume infuses over prescribed time period.
2 Observe patient for signs of fluid volume excess or deficit and signs of fluid and electrolyte imbalance.	Determines response to therapy. Signs and symptoms of dehydration, overhydration, or electrolyte imbalance warrant changing rate of fluid infused.
3 Evaluate for signs of IV-related complications (e.g., infiltration, phlebitis, occluded venous access device [VAD], kink or knot in infusion tubing).	Prevents complications that decrease or stop flow rate.

Unexpected Outcomes

1 Sudden infusion of large volume of solution occurs with patient having symptoms of dyspnea; crackles in lung; and increased urine output, indicating fluid overload.

2 IV fluid container empties with subsequent loss of IV line patency.

3 IV infusion is slower than ordered.

Related Interventions

- Slow infusion rate: KVO rates must have specific rate ordered by licensed independent practitioner (LIP) (Policy and Procedures INS, 2011).
- Notify health care provider immediately.
- Place patient in high-Fowler's position.
- Anticipate new IV orders.
- Administer diuretics if ordered.
- Discontinue present IV and restart new short peripheral catheter in new site.
- Check for positional change that affects rate, height of IV container, kinking of tubing or obstruction.
- Check VAD site for complications.
- Consult health care provider for new order to provide necessary fluid volume.

Recording and Reporting

- Record rate of infusion in drops per minute or milliliters per hour in nurses' notes and EHR or on parenteral administration form according to agency policy.
- Document use of any EID or control device and identification number on that device.
- At change of shift or when leaving on break, report rate of and volume left in infusion to nurse in charge or next nurse assigned to care for patient.

Special Considerations
Teaching

- Instruct patient to notify nurse if any signs or symptoms of IV complications are noted (e.g., swelling or pain).
- Patient using an EID should know the significance of alarms and when to notify nursing.
- Teach patient about factors affecting flow rate, to protect IV site, and importance of not altering rate control.

Pediatric

- Consider physiologic differences in children, particularly focusing on total body weight (85% to 90% water). Dehydration is a common cause of fluid and electrolyte imbalance; assessment of fluid needs includes meter square weight or caloric method (Alexander et al., 2010; Hockenberry and Wilson, 2011).
- Infusion pumps (especially syringe pumps) are almost always used in pediatrics because they infuse very small amounts of fluids and accurately provide the prescribed volume of IV solution.
- Use only small-volume containers for infusions (250 mL for children younger than 12 months, 500 mL for older children) (Alexander et al., 2010). Microdrip tubing is recommended for children.

Gerontologic

- Renal changes in older adults reduce the ability of the kidney to concentrate and dilute urine in response to water or salt excess. Combined with cardiac deficiencies and decreased blood flow to organs, an older patient balances between dehydration and fluid overload. Use an EID and microdrip tubing to administer fluids. Monitor electrolyte levels, blood urea nitrogen (BUN), creatinine, urine output, and daily weight (Alexander et al., 2010).
- Some older patients easily develop cerebral edema from rapid dextrose infusions. Older patients with impaired renal function often develop hypernatremia from normal saline infusions.

Home Care

- Ensure that patient is able and willing to operate an infusion pump and administer IV therapy. If patient is unable to provide self-care, be sure that a reliable family caregiver is available in the home.
- Discuss proper EID function with patient. Consider use of an ambulatory-type device.
- Teach patient and family caregiver what EID alarms mean, methods to troubleshoot them, and how to disconnect the tubing from the EID pump in the event of a pump failure.
- Provide patient with a contact phone number that he or she can access 24 hours a day for problems.
- If using gravity infusion, teach patient and family caregiver to time drops per minute using watch with second hand.
- Ensure that patient's electrical outlets are properly grounded.

SKILL 28-3 Changing Intravenous Solutions

NSO *Intravenous Fluid Therapy Management Module / Lesson 3*

Patients receiving intravenous (IV) therapy over time require periodic changes of IV solutions. IV containers include plastic bags and glass bottles. You change a container when there is an order for a new solution or when it becomes time to add a sequential container to avoid exceeding hang time (Alexander et al., 2010). It becomes clinically appropriate to change the type of solution depending on a patient's fluid and electrolyte balance, response to therapy (e.g., therapeutic drug monitoring), and goals of therapy. The Infusion Nurses Society (INS) recommends changing a fluid container within 24 hours after adding a medication or an administration set (INS, 2011). The use of ambulatory infusion devices may remain longer than 24 hours if you use aseptic technique, if the system remains closed without injection ports or add-on tubing, and if the medication is stable for a longer time period. Organizational skills are necessary to complete this task in a manner that decreases the risk of infusion-related complications such as infusion container becoming empty or clotting off of a venous access device (VAD).

Delegation and Collaboration

The skill of changing an IV solution cannot be delegated to nursing assistive personnel (NAP). Delegation to licensed practical nurses (LPNs) varies by state Nurse Practice Act. The nurse instructs the NAP to:

- Inform the nurse when an IV container is near completion.
- Report any cloudiness or precipitate in the IV solution.
- Report alarm sounding on electronic infusion device (EID).
- Report that insertion site appears with IV-related complications (e.g., red, swollen, or patient complaints of discomfort).

Equipment

❑ IV solution as ordered by health care provider

STEP	RATIONALE

ASSESSMENT

1 Review accuracy and completeness of health care provider's order in patient's medical record for patient name and correct solution: type, volume, additives, rate, and duration of IV therapy. Follow six rights of drug administration (see Chapter 20).

Ensures that correct IV fluid is administered (Policy and Procedures INS, 2011).

2 Note date and time when IV tubing and solution were last changed.

Ensures correct change of tubing and dressings.

3 Check the IV solution for integrity including, but not limited to, discoloration, cloudiness, leakage, expiration date. Determine compatibility of all IV fluids and additives by consulting approved online database, drug reference, or pharmacist.

If there has been a break in the integrity of the solution container, a new bag is needed. Incompatibilities cause physical, chemical, and therapeutic changes with adverse patient outcomes (INS, 2011).

STEP	RATIONALE
4 Determine patient's understanding of need for continued IV therapy.	Indicates need for any patient education.
5 Assess patency of current venous access device (VAD) site, observing for any signs or symptoms of complications such as redness, swelling, complaints of discomfort.	New IV access site is necessary if IV is not patent.
6 Assess IV tubing for puncture, contamination, or occlusions.	Indicates need for tubing change.
7 Check laboratory data, such as potassium level.	Compare data with baseline to determine ongoing response to IV solution administration.

NURSING DIAGNOSES

- Deficient fluid volume
- Deficient knowledge regarding IV infusion
- Risk for injury

Related factors are individualized based on patient's condition or needs.

PLANNING

1 Expected outcomes following completion of procedure:
- IV solution is correct.
- VAD remains patent.
- Patient and family caregiver can explain purpose of IV solution change.

Patient receives solution ordered for treatment of diagnosis.
Ensures infusion of fluid into intravascular space.
Demonstrates learning.

IMPLEMENTATION

1 Collect equipment. Have next solution prepared at least 1 hour before needed. If solution is prepared in pharmacy, ensure that it has been delivered to patient care unit. Allow solution to warm to room temperature if it has been refrigerated. Check that solution is correct and properly labeled. Check solution expiration date. Ensure that any light sensitivity restrictions are followed.

Adequate planning reduces risk for clot formation in vein caused by empty IV container. Checking that solution is correct prevents medication error.

2 Identify patient using two identifiers (i.e., name and birthday or name and account number) according to agency policy. Compare identifiers with information in MAR/medical record with information on patient's identification bracelet and/or ask patient to state name.

Ensures correct patient. Complies with The Joint Commission standards and improves patient safety (TJC, 2012).

3 Change solution when fluid remains only in neck of container (about 50 mL) or when new type of solution has been ordered.

Prevents waste of solution.

4 Prepare patient and family caregiver by explaining procedure, its purpose, and what is expected of patient.

Decreases anxiety and promotes cooperation.

5 Perform hand hygiene.

Reduces transmission of microorganisms.

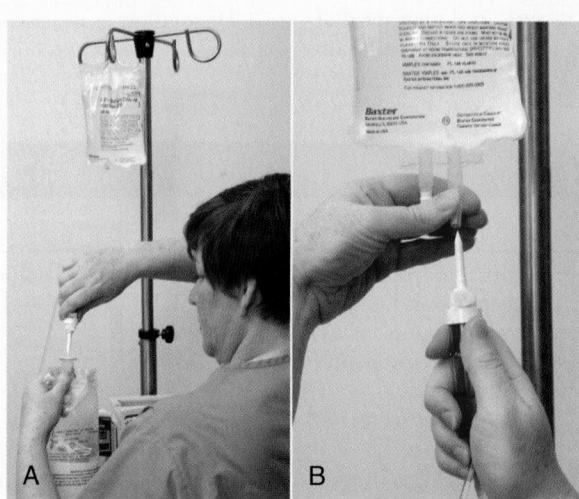

STEP 8   A, Quickly remove spike from old solution container. **B,** Without touching tip, insert spike into new container.

STEP	RATIONALE
6 Prepare new solution for changing. If using plastic bag, hang on IV pole and remove protective cover from IV tubing port. If using glass bottle, remove metal cap and metal and rubber disks.	Permits quick, smooth, and organized change from old to new solution.
7 Close roller clamp on existing solution to stop flow rate. Remove tubing from EID (if used). Then remove old IV fluid container from IV pole. Hold container with tubing port pointing upward.	Prevents solution remaining in drip chamber from emptying while changing solutions. Prevents solution in bag from spilling.
8 Quickly remove spike from old solution container and, without touching tip, insert spike into new container (see illustration).	Reduces risk for solution in drip chamber becoming empty and maintains sterility.

Clinical Decision Point *If spike is contaminated, you will need a new IV tubing set.*

9 Hang new container of solution on IV pole.	Gravity helps with delivery of fluid into drip chamber.
10 Check for air in tubing. If air bubbles have formed, remove them by closing roller clamp, stretching tubing downward, and tapping tubing with finger (bubbles rise in fluid to drip chamber) (see illustration).	Reduces risk for air entering tubing. Use of an air-eliminating filter also reduces risk.
11 Make sure drip chamber is one-third to one-half full. If drip chamber is too full, level can be decreased by removing bag from IV pole, pinching off tubing below drip chamber, inverting container, squeezing drip chamber (see illustration), releasing and turning solution container upright, and releasing pinch on tubing.	Reduces risk for air entering tubing. If chamber is completely filled, you cannot observe or regulate drip rate.
12 Regulate flow to ordered rate by using roller clamp on tubing or programming EID.	Maintains measures to restore fluid balance and deliver IV fluid as ordered.
13 Place time label on side of container and label with time hung, time of completion, and appropriate intervals. If using plastic bags, mark only on label and not container.	Provides visual comparison of volume infused compared with prescribed rate of infusion. Ink on container sometimes leaks into plastic bags (INS, 2011).

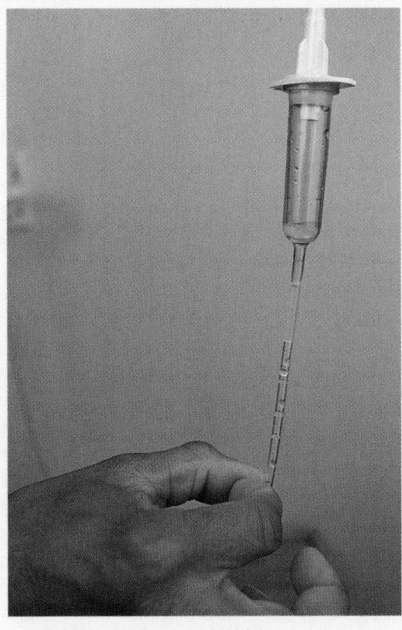

STEP 10 Tap tubing to cause air bubbles to rise up to drip chamber.

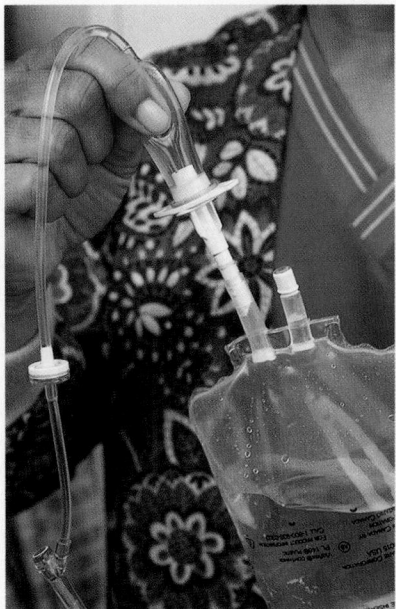

STEP 11 Squeeze drip chamber to fill with fluid. Be sure to leave chamber one-third to one-half full.

STEP	RATIONALE

EVALUATION

1 Observe functioning, intactness, and patency of IV system and flow rate.

Ensures proper fluid administration.

2 Observe patient for signs of fluid volume deficit (FVD) or fluid volume excess (FVE) to determine response to IV therapy.

Provides ongoing evaluation of patient's fluid status.

3 Assess patient for signs and symptoms of IV-related complications. Palpate skin for temperature, edema, or tenderness.

Provides ongoing evaluation of VAD patency.

Unexpected Outcomes

1   Flow rate is incorrect; patient receives too little or too much fluid.

Related Interventions

- Notify health care provider if patient's anticipated infusion is 100 to 200 mL less than or greater than anticipated (follow agency policy).
- Evaluate patient for adverse effects of infusion.
- Determine and correct the cause of incorrect flow rate (e.g., change in position, tubing kink).
- Use EID when accurate flow rate is critical.

Recording and Reporting

- Record amount and type of solution infused, amount and type of solution started, and flow rate according to agency policy.
- Record solution and tubing change on patient's record. Use parenteral (IV) therapy flow sheet, if available.

Special Considerations
Teaching
- Inform patient of new solution, additives, flow rate, and potential side effects.

Home Care
- Teach patient and family caregiver how to perform an IV solution change. Observe them performing procedure.

SKILL 28-4   Changing Infusion Tubing

NSO *Intravenous Fluid Therapy Management Module / Lesson 3*

An important component of patient care is maintaining the integrity of the intravenous (IV) system through the conscientious use of infection-prevention principles. Administration sets are the primary method to carry a solution or medication to a patient. These administration sets are considered the primary set. In addition, patients may have add-on devices (e.g., filters, extension sets), which you connect to the primary set as indicated by the prescribed therapy. Secondary sets may be used as a method to administer additional medications in conjunction with the primary infusion (e.g., antibiotics). Depending on the solution or medication being infused and the method for administration (i.e., primary set with or without add-on device, secondary sets), adherence to infection-prevention principles must be followed to ensure positive patient outcomes. Luer-Lok connections should be used to prevent accidental disconnection and needlestick injury (INS, 2011). When the short peripheral site is rotated, the administration set should be changed (INS, 2011). Follow agency policy and procedures for specific requirements (Table 28-5).

Administration sets used for parenteral nutrition (see Chapter 32) and blood or blood products (see Chapter 29) have specific criteria with which you need to be familiar when administering these advanced therapies (see agency policy). Whenever possible, schedule tubing changes when it is time to hang a new IV container (see Skill 28-1). To prevent entry of bacteria into the bloodstream, maintain sterility during tubing and solution changes. If the tubing becomes damaged, is leaking, or becomes contaminated, it must be changed, regardless of the tubing change schedule.

TABLE 28-5 | **Administration Set Changes**

Primary and Secondary Continuous Infusions	Primary Intermittent Infusions	Use of Add-on Devices
• Every 96 hours for fluids *other* than lipid, blood, or blood products. • Extending to every 7 days may be considered if an antiinfective CVAD is being used and if fluids that enhance microbial growth are not administered (less than 10% dextrose solutions). • If the secondary set is removed from the primary set, the secondary set is now considered an intermittent set and should be changed every 24 hours.	• Should be changed every 24 hours because of increased risk of infection with repeatedly disconnecting and reconnecting administration set. • Aseptically attach a covering device to the end of the administration set after each intermittent use. *Avoid* attaching the exposed end of the administration set to port on the same set (e.g., looping).	• Should be minimized since each is a potential source of contamination and disconnection. • Use of administration sets with devices as part of the set is preferred. • Aseptically change with insertion of new short peripheral catheter or with each administration set replacement.

CVAD, Central vascular access device.
Modified from Infusion Nurses Society: Infusion nursing standards of practice, *J Intraven Nurs* 30(suppl 1):S1, 2011.

Delegation and Collaboration

The skill of changing infusion tubing cannot be delegated to nursing assistive personnel (NAP). Delegation to licensed practical nurses (LPNs) varies by state Nurse Practice Act. The nurse instructs the NAP to:

- Report to the nurse any leakage from or around the IV tubing.
- Report if tubing has become contaminated (lying on the floor).

Equipment

- ❏ Clean gloves
- ❏ Antiseptic wipes (alcohol wipes)
- ❏ Label

Continuous IV Infusion

- ❏ Microdrip or macrodrip administration set infusion tubing as appropriate
- ❏ Add-on device as necessary (e.g., filters, extension set, needleless connector)
- ❏ Tubing label

Intermittent Extension Set

- ❏ 3- to 5-mL syringe filled with preservative-free normal saline (NS) 0.9% normal saline solution (NSS)
- ❏ Short extension tubing (if necessary), injection cap

STEP	RATIONALE

ASSESSMENT

1 Note date and time when IV tubing was last changed (see Table 28-5 for recommendations on administration set changes).	Decreases risk of infection.
2 Assess tubing for puncture, contamination, or occlusion that requires immediate change.	Compromised tubing results in fluid leakage and bacterial contamination.
3 Determine patient's understanding of need for continued IV therapy.	Reinforces need for further instruction.

NURSING DIAGNOSIS

- Deficient knowledge regarding IV therapy
- Risk for infection

Related factors are individualized based on patient's condition or needs.

PLANNING

1 Expected outcomes following completion of procedure:	
• Patient's IV site is free from signs and symptoms of IV-related complications (e.g., infection, redness, swelling, or pain).	Adherence to administration set changes decreases risk of complications.
• Patient experiences no leakage of solution from or around IV tubing.	Intact system decreases risk for microbial contamination.
• Patient's IV tubing is patent.	Brief interruption of IV infusion does not result in occlusion of venous access device (VAD).
• Patient and family caregiver explain procedure, purpose, and patient expectations.	Demonstrates learning.

IMPLEMENTATION

1 Identify patient using at least two identifiers (i.e., name and birthday or name and account number) according to agency policy. Compare identifiers with information on patient's identification bracelet.	Ensures correct patient. Complies with The Joint Commission standards and improves patient safety (TJC, 2012).
2 Prepare patient by explaining procedure, its purpose, and what is expected of him or her.	Decreases anxiety; promotes cooperation; and prevents sudden movement of extremity, which could dislodge IV catheter.
3 Coordinate tubing changes with solution changes when possible.	Decreases number of times system is open.
4 Perform hand hygiene.	Reduces transmission of microorganisms.
5 Open new infusion set and connect add-on pieces (e.g., filters, extension tubing). Keep protective coverings over infusion spike and distal adapter. Secure all connections.	Securing connections reduces risk later of air emboli and infection. Protective covers reduce entrance of microorganisms. All connections should be of Luer-Lok type (INS, 2011).
6 Apply clean gloves. If patient's IV cannula hub is not visible, remove IV dressing (see Skill 28-5). Do not remove tape securing cannula to skin.	Cannula hub must be visible to provide smooth transition when removing old and inserting new tubing. Infections related to IV therapy are most often caused by catheter hub contamination (INS, 2011).
7 Prepare infusion tubing with new bag. (See Skill 28-1, Step 8.)	

STEP	RATIONALE
8 Prepare infusion tubing with existing continuous IV infusion bag.	
a Move roller clamp on new IV tubing to "off" position.	Prevents fluid spillage.
b Slow rate of infusion through old tubing to KVO rate, using EID or roller clamp.	Prevents occlusion of VAD.
c Compress and fill drip chamber of old tubing.	Ensures that fluid chamber remains full until new tubing is changed.
d Invert container and remove old tubing. Keep spike sterile and upright. *Optional:* Tape old drip chamber to IV pole without contaminating spike.	Fluid in drip chamber will continue to run and maintain catheter patency.
e Place insertion spike of new tubing into solution container. Hang solution bag on IV pole, compress and release drip chamber on new tubing, and fill drip chamber one-third to one-half full.	Permits drip chamber to fill and promotes rapid, smooth flow of solution through tubing.
f Slowly open roller clamp, remove protective cap from adapter (if necessary), and prime new tubing with solution. Stop infusion and replace cap. Place end of adapter near patient's IV site.	Removes air from tubing and replaces it with IV solution. Equipment is positioned for a quick connection of new tubing.
g Stop EID or turn roller clamp on old tubing to "off" position.	Prevents fluid spillage.
9 Prepare tubing with extension set or saline lock.	
a If short extension tubing is needed, use sterile technique to connect new injection cap to new extension set or tubing.	Prepares extension set for connecting with IV.
b Swab injection cap with antiseptic swab. Insert syringe with 3 to 5 mL of saline solution and inject through injection cap into extension set.	Maintains patency of catheter. Prevents introduction of microorganisms.
10 Reestablish infusion.	
a Gently disconnect old tubing from extension tubing (or from IV catheter hub) and quickly insert adapter of new tubing or saline lock into extension tubing connection (or IV catheter hub) (see illustrations for example of connecting tubing to short extension set).	Allows smooth transition from old to new tubing, minimizing time system is open.

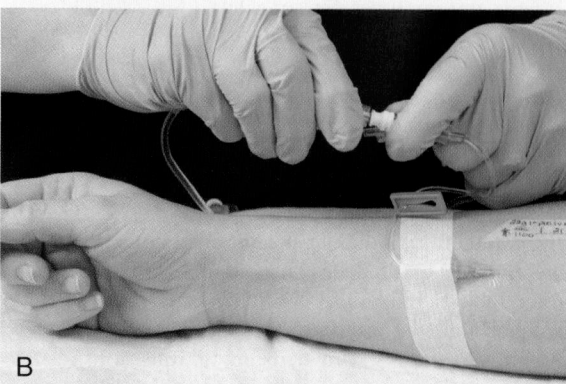

STEP 10a **A,** Disconnect old tubing. **B,** Insert adapter of new tubing.

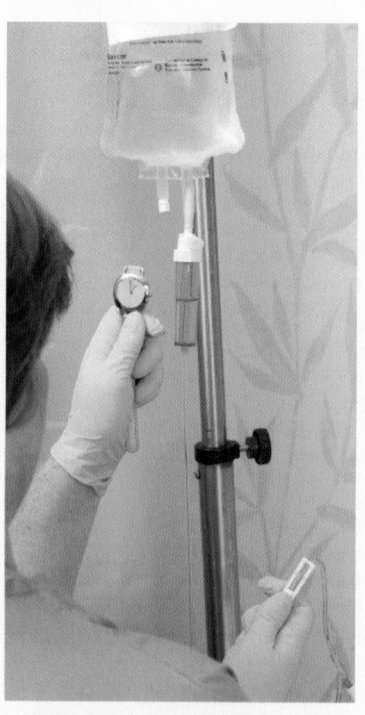

STEP 10b Regulate flow of IV.

STEP	RATIONALE
b For continuous infusion, open roller clamp on new tubing and regulate drip rate using roller clamp (see illustration) or EID.	Ensures catheter patency and prevents occlusion.
c Attach piece of tape or preprinted label with date and time of tubing change onto tubing below drip chamber.	Provides reference to determine next time for tubing change.
d Form loop of tubing and secure it to patient's arm with strip of tape.	Avoids accidental pulling against site and stabilizes catheter.
11 Remove and discard old IV tubing. If necessary, apply new dressing (see Skill 28-5). Remove and dispose of gloves. Perform hand hygiene.	Reduces transmission of microorganisms.

EVALUATION

1 Evaluate flow rate hourly and observe connection site for leaking.	Ensures proper fluid administration.
2 Observe patient for signs of fluid volume deficit (FVD) or fluid volume excess (FVE) to determine response to IV therapy.	Provides ongoing evaluation of patient's fluid and electrolyte status.
3 Check entire IV system for patency, starting with solution bag hanging and working all the way down system to patient's IV access insertion site.	Prevents improper fluid infusion.

Unexpected Outcomes
1 IV infusion is slower than ordered.

Related Interventions
- Check for positional change that affects rate, height of IV container, kinking of tubing, or obstruction.
- Check for patency by opening roller clamp.
- Check VAD site for complications.
- Consult health care provider for new order to provide necessary fluid volume.

Recording and Reporting
- Record tubing change, type of solution, volume, and rate of infusion on patient's record. Use a special IV therapy flow sheet for parenteral fluids per agency protocol.

Special Considerations
Teaching
- Instruct patient to notify nurse if fluid leaks from or around IV site or tubing or if tubing separates from catheter.

Home Care
- Instruct patient or family caregiver in procedure for performing a sterile IV tubing change.
- Ensure that patient is able and willing to perform tubing change and maintain IV access site or that there is a reliable person at home to provide this IV therapy care.

SKILL 28-5   Changing a Short Peripheral Intravenous Dressing

NSO *Intravenous Fluid Therapy Management Module / Lesson 4*

Administration of solutions via the parenteral route is not without complications, which can be either systemic or local (Alexander et al., 2010). Systemic complications occur within the vascular system and are usually remote to the infusion site (e.g., septicemia, circulatory overload, and embolism). Local complications result from trauma to the inner layer of the vein (tunica intima) as a direct result of many factors such as poor insertion technique, inappropriate size of short peripheral device (see Table 28-3), infusing a solution or medication with a pH or osmolarity not within required ranges (see Table 28-2), and poor assessment and incorrect technique for short peripheral dressing changes (Alexander et al., 2010; Policy and Procedures INS, 2011). Short peripheral intravenous (IV) catheters require strict adherence to infection-prevention measures to avoid complications associated with these devices. The skin insertion site is the most common source of colonization and infection for IV catheters. Therefore you need to securely apply catheter dressings and change dressings when wet, soiled, or loosened. You may stabilize short peripheral IV catheters with a manufactured stabilization device, sterile tapes, or surgical strips and cover the site with a transparent semipermeable membrane (TSM) dressing or sterile gauze (INS, 2011). You change a transparent dressing during catheter site rotation of a short peripheral device and immediately if integrity of the dressing is compromised.

Change gauze dressings every 48 hours and immediately if integrity is compromised. When using gauze under a transparent dressing (although not recommended), it is considered a gauze dressing and should be changed every 48 hours (INS, 2011).

Delegation and Collaboration

The skill of changing a short peripheral IV dressing cannot be delegated to nursing assistive personnel (NAP). The nurse instructs the NAP to:

- Report to the nurse if a patient complains of moistness or loosening of an IV dressing.
- Protect the IV dressing during hygiene and activities of daily living (ADLs).

Equipment

- ❏ Antiseptic swabs (2% chlorhexidine preferred or 70% alcohol, povidone-iodine)
- ❏ Adhesive remover (*optional*)
- ❏ Skin protectant swab
- ❏ Clean gloves
- ❏ Strips of sterile, precut tape (or roll of sterile tape), or stabilization device
- ❏ Commercially available IV site protection (*optional*) (see Fig. 28-2)
- ❏ Sterile transparent semipermeable dressing

or

- ❏ Sterile 2 × 2– or 4 × 4–inch gauze pad

STEP	RATIONALE
ASSESSMENT	
1 Determine when dressing was last changed. Dressing should be labeled to include date and time applied, size and type of venous access device (VAD), and date VAD was inserted.	Provides information regarding length of time that present dressing has been in place. In addition, you are able to plan for dressing change (INS, 2011).
2 Perform hand hygiene. Observe present dressing for moisture and intactness. Determine if moisture is from site leakage or external source.	Moisture is medium for bacterial growth and renders dressing contaminated. Nonadhering dressing increases risk for bacterial contamination to venipuncture site or displacement of IV catheter.
3 Observe IV system for proper functioning or complications (e.g., current flow rate, tubing, or catheter kinks). Palpate catheter site through intact dressing for complaints of tenderness, pain, or burning. (**Note:** Apply clean gloves if gauze dressing is moist.)	Unexplained decrease in flow rate indicates problems with VAD placement and patency. Pain is associated with phlebitis and infiltration.
4 Monitor body temperature.	Elevated temperature can be related to infection at VAD site or systemic complication.
5 Assess patient's understanding of need for continued IV infusion.	Reveals need for patient instruction.

NURSING DIAGNOSES

- Acute pain
- Deficient knowledge regarding IV therapy
- Risk for infection

Related factors are individualized based on patient's condition or needs.

PLANNING	
1 Expected outcomes following completion of procedure:	
• IV insertion site remains free of IV-related complications (redness, swelling, tenderness, or exudate).	Proper care maintains IV site.
• Patient and family caregiver can explain procedure and purpose of VAD dressing change.	Demonstrates learning.

IMPLEMENTATION	
1 Explain procedure and purpose to patient and family caregiver. Explain that patient will need to hold affected extremity still. Explain how long procedure will take.	Decreases anxiety, promotes cooperation, and gives patient time frame around which to plan personal activities.
2 Perform hand hygiene. Collect equipment. Apply clean gloves.	Reduces transmission of microorganisms. Infections related to IV therapy are most often caused by catheter hub contamination; thus you need to use careful technique throughout dressing change (INS, 2011).

STEP	RATIONALE
3 Identify patient using two identifiers (i.e., name and birthday or name and account number) according to agency policy. Compare identifiers with information on patient's identification bracelet.	Ensures correct patient. Complies with The Joint Commission standards and improves patient safety (TJC, 2012).
4 Remove dressing. *For transparent semipermeable dressing:* Remove by pulling up one corner and pulling side laterally while holding catheter hub with nondominant hand (see illustration). Repeat on other side. Leave tape or catheter stabilization device that secures IC catheter in place. *For gauze dressing:* Stabilize catheter hub while loosening tape and removing old dressing one layer at a time by pulling toward insertion site. Leave tape that secures VAD to skin intact. Be cautious if IV tubing becomes tangled between two layers of dressing.	Technique minimizes discomfort during removal. Use alcohol swab on transparent dressing next to patient's skin to loosen dressing.
5 Observe insertion site for signs and symptoms of IV-related complications (tenderness, redness, swelling, exudate, or complaints of pain). If complication exists or if ordered by health care provider, discontinue infusion (see Procedural Guideline 28-1).	Presence of complication indicates need to remove VAD at current site.
6 Prepare new sterile tape strips for use. If IV is infusing properly, gently remove tape or stabilization device securing VAD. Stabilize VAD with one finger. Use adhesive remover to clean skin and remove adhesive residue if necessary.	Exposes venipuncture site. Stabilization prevents accidental displacement of VAD. Adhesive residue decreases ability of new tape to adhere securely to skin.

Clinical Decision Point *Keep one finger over catheter at all times until tape or dressing secures placement. If patient is restless or uncooperative, it is helpful to have another staff member help with procedure.*

7 While stabilizing IV, clean insertion site with chlorhexidine antiseptic swab, using friction vertically and horizontally and moving from insertion site outward with a third swab (see illustration). Allow antiseptic solution to dry completely.	Allowing antiseptic solutions to air-dry completely effectively reduces microbial counts (INS, 2011). 2% Chlorhexidine takes 30 seconds to dry (INS, 2011).
8 *Optional:* Apply skin protectant solution to area where you will apply tape or dressing. Allow to dry.	Coats skin with protective solution to maintain skin integrity, prevents irritation from adhesive, and promotes adhesion of dressing.
9 While securing catheter, apply a sterile dressing over site (procedures differ; follow agency policy). **a** *Manufactured catheter stabilization device:* Apply catheter stabilization device as directed in Skill 28-1, Step 23a.	Manufactured catheter stabilization device preserves integrity of VAD and minimizes catheter movement at hub (INS, 2011). Must be placed under transparent dressing and is a sterile device.

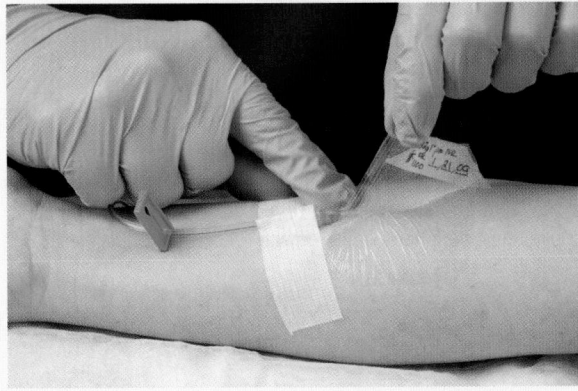

STEP 4 Remove transparent dressing by pulling side laterally.

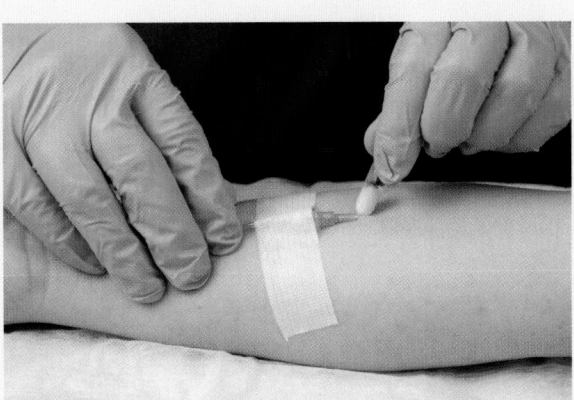

STEP 7 Clean peripheral insertion site with antiseptic swab.

STEP	RATIONALE
b *Transparent dressing*: Apply transparent dressing as directed in Skill 28-1, Step 23b.	Prevents accidental dislodgement of catheter. Allows continuous inspection of insertion site (Alexander et al., 2010). Occlusive dressing protects site from bacterial contamination. Connection between administration set and hub needs to be uncovered to facilitate changing tubing if necessary.
c *Sterile gauze dressing*: Apply sterile gauze dressing as directed in Skill 28-1, Step 23c.	Only use sterile tape under sterile dressing to prevent site contamination. Gauze dressing obscures observation of insertion site and is changed every 48 hours (INS, 2011).

Clinical Decision Point *Because Band-Aids are not occlusive and nonsterile tape increases the risk for insertion site infection, do not use either over catheter insertion points.*

10 Remove and discard gloves.	Prevents transmission of microorganisms.
11 *Optional*: Apply site protection device (e.g., I.V. House Ultra Protective Dressing®).	Reduces risk for phlebitis and infiltration from mechanical motion.
12 Anchor IV tubing with additional pieces of tape if necessary. When using transparent dressing, avoid placing tape over the dressing.	Prevents accidental displacement of VAD.
13 Label dressing per agency policy. Information on label includes date and time of IV insertion, VAD gauge size and length, and your initials.	Communicates type of device and time interval for dressing change and site rotation (INS, 2011).
14 Discard equipment and perform hand hygiene.	Reduces transmission of microorganisms.

EVALUATION

1 Observe function, patency of IV system, and flow rate after changing dressing.	Validates that IV is patent and functioning correctly. Manipulation of catheter and tubing will affect rate of infusion.
2 Inspect condition of short peripheral site for signs and symptoms of IV-related complications (e.g., redness, complaints of pain, swelling, or exudate).	Complications such as phlebitis and infiltration require removal of short peripheral catheter and insertion of new catheter at new site above area of complication or other extremity.
3 Monitor patient's body temperature.	Elevated temperature indicates infection that can be associated with contamination of venipuncture site or septicemia.

Unexpected Outcomes

1 Short peripheral catheter is infiltrated, as evidenced by decreased flow rate or edema, pallor, or decreased temperature around insertion site.

2 Phlebitis is present (see Table 28-4).

3 Short peripheral catheter is accidentally removed or dislodged.

4 Patient has an elevated temperature.

5 Insertion site is red, edematous, and/or painful and/or has presence of exudate, indicating infection at venipuncture site.

Related Interventions

- Stop infusion and remove catheter (see Procedural Guideline 28-1).
- Restart new short peripheral catheter in other extremity or above previous insertion site if continued therapy is necessary.
- Stop infusion and remove short peripheral catheter (see Procedural Guideline 28-1).
- Restart new catheter in other extremity if continued therapy is necessary.
- Restart new short peripheral catheter if continued therapy needed.
- Notify health care provider.
- Prepare to obtain blood culture or culture of IV site to evaluate source of infection.
- Notify health care provider. Culture of catheter tip and/or exudate may be ordered (confirm before removal of IV).
- Remove short peripheral catheter (see Procedural Guideline 28-1).

Recording and Reporting

- Record time short peripheral dressing was changed, reason for change, type of dressing material used, patency of system, and description of venipuncture site.
- Report to nurse in charge or oncoming nursing shift that dressing was changed and any significant information about integrity of system.
- Report to health care provider and document any complications.

Special Considerations

Teaching

- Instruct patient to notify nurse if site appears red or swollen, has drainage, or is painful.

Pediatric

- Pediatric patients are not always able to fully understand explanations. Presence of parent or security toy during procedure helps to decrease fear and increase cooperation. Perform procedure on patient's toy or doll first.
- Assistance is necessary to keep patient still and protect IV catheter from dislodgement.

- Use commercially available IV site protectors to cover and protect the IV site in young active children.
- Dried povidone-iodine should be removed with saline wipes or sterile water in infants under 2 months or pediatric patients with compromised skin integrity (INS, 2011).

Gerontologic

- Some older adults have fragile skin; thus prevent skin tears by minimizing the use of tape directly on the skin and applying skin protectant before applying tape.
- Infiltration may go unnoticed because of the decreased elasticity of skin and loose skinfolds. Because of decreased tactile sensation, a large amount of fluid may infiltrate before pain occurs.

Home Care

- Instruct patient and family caregiver about the signs and symptoms of IV-related complications.
- Have patient or family caregiver demonstrate hand hygiene.
- Teach patient to keep site dry during bath or shower by wrapping in plastic bag and taping occlusively.
- Teach patient and family caregiver what to do if dressing becomes compromised or if catheter comes out. If catheter comes out, apply gauze pressure dressing at site and notify home health agency nurse.

PROCEDURAL GUIDELINE 28-1 Discontinuing a Short Peripheral Intravenous Access

NSO *Intravenous Fluid Administration Module / Lesson 4*

You discontinue a short peripheral intravenous (IV) catheter when the prescribed length of therapy is completed or a complication occurs (e.g., phlebitis, infiltration, or catheter occlusion). The technique for discontinuing a short peripheral IV catheter follows infection-prevention guidelines to minimize the chance of the patient's acquiring an infection. Care must also be taken because the risk of catheter emboli may occur if the catheter breaks off during removal.

Delegation and Collaboration

The skill of discontinuing a short peripheral intravenous line cannot be delegated to nursing assistive personnel (NAP). Delegation to licensed practical nurses (LPNs) varies by state Nurse Practice Act. The nurse instructs the NAP to:

- Report to the nurse any bleeding at the site after catheter has been removed.
- Report any complaints by patient of pain or observations of redness at the site.

Equipment

- ❑ Clean gloves
- ❑ Sterile 2 × 2– or 4 × 4–inch gauze sponge
- ❑ Antiseptic swab
- ❑ Tape

Procedural Steps

1 Observe existing IV site for signs and symptoms of IV-related complications (pain, infiltration, phlebitis, exudate).
2 Assess if patient is receiving an anticoagulant or has a history of a coagulopathy.
3 Review accuracy and completeness of health care provider's order for discontinuation of IV therapy.
4 Assess patient's understanding of the need for IV to be discontinued.

5 Identify patient using two identifiers (i.e., name and birthday or name and account number) according to agency policy. Compare identifiers with information on patient's identification bracelet.
6 Explain procedure to patient before you remove catheter. Explain that patient needs to hold affected extremity still.
7 Turn IV tubing roller clamp to "off" position or turn electronic infusion device (EID) off and roller clamp to "off" position.
8 Perform hand hygiene and apply clean gloves.
9 Carefully remove IV site dressing and stabilize IV device (see Skill 28-5). Then remove tape securing catheter.

Clinical Decision Point *Never use scissors to remove the tape or dressing because you may accidentally cut the catheter.*

10 Place clean sterile gauze above insertion site and withdraw catheter, using slow, steady motion. Keep hub parallel to skin (see illustration).

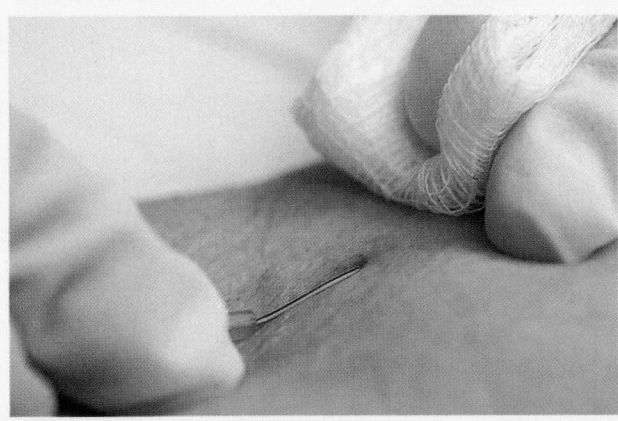

STEP 10 IV catheter is removed slowly, keeping catheter parallel to vein.

Continued

PROCEDURAL GUIDELINE 28-1   Discontinuing a Short Peripheral Intravenous Access—cont'd

Clinical Decision Point *Do not raise or lift catheter before it is completely out of the vein to avoid trauma or hematoma formation.*

11 Apply pressure to site for a minimum of 30 seconds until bleeding has stopped.
    NOTE: Apply pressure for at least 5 to 10 minutes if patient is on anticoagulants.
12 Inspect catheter for intactness after removal; note tip integrity and length.

13 Observe site for evidence of any complications such as bleeding, pain, exudate, or swelling.
14 Apply clean, folded gauze dressing over insertion site and secure with tape.
15 Discard used supplies, remove gloves, and perform hand hygiene.
16 Document procedure in patient's medical record.

SKILL 28-6   Caring for Central Vascular Access Devices

The need for safe and convenient intravenous (IV) therapy has led to the development of vascular access devices (VADs) designed for long-term access to the venous or arterial systems. Physicians or credentialed advanced practice nurses place these devices into the central vascular system. A central vascular access device (CVAD) differs from short peripheral or midline catheters related to the final catheter tip location. A CVAD has a final tip location in the lower third of the superior vena cava and the junction of the right atrium (Fig. 28-5) (INS, 2011). For CVADs placed in the femoral region the final tip placement should be in the inferior vena cava above the level of the diaphragm (INS, 2011). Many factors are considered before placement of a CVAD such as the pH and osmolarity of the solution or medication (pH less than 5.0 or greater than 9.0, osmolarity greater than 600 mOsm/L) to be administered, duration of therapy (greater than 7 days), status of veins for short peripheral access, and disease process (e.g., cancer, pain management). Your role is to help the health care provider place a CVAD, care for and maintain the device, administer solutions or medications, and assess for signs and symptoms of complications (Alexander et al., 2010). CVADs can be categorized as short- or long-term devices with various types within each category (Table 28-6).

Each of these devices has similarities and differences of which as a nurse you need to be aware because they will impact care and maintenance of each CVAD and patient education. These devices are composed of silicone or polyurethane and can be coated with heparin, antibiotics, or chlorhexidine (Alexander et al., 2010). Tip configuration can be either open ended or closed (valved) ended.

Open-ended devices are those in which the catheter tip is open like a "straw." These devices carry a higher risk for complications (e.g., hemorrhage, air embolism, and occlusion from fibrin or clots) (Alexander et al., 2010). Valve-tipped devices are those in which the tip is configured with a three-way pressure-activated valve (e.g.,

TABLE 28-6	Central Vascular Access Devices
Short-Term Devices	**Long-Term Devices**
Nontunneled Percutaneous	*External Tunneled (Hickman, Broviac, Groshong)*
• Length of dwell: days to several weeks	• Length of dwell: Considered permanent
• Insertion sites: subclavian, external/internal jugular, and femoral veins	• Insertion sites: Chest region through subclavian or jugular vein
• Insertion technique: Not surgically placed, can be done at bedside, direct puncture into intended vein without passing through subcutaneous tissue	• Insertion technique: Surgery required: Tunneling of the proximal end subcutaneously from insertion site and bringing it out through skin at an exit site (Fig. 28-7)
• Held in place with sutures or manufactured securement device	• Held in place by a Dacron cuff coated in antimicrobial solution; in approximately 2-3 weeks scar tissue forms around cuff, fixing catheter in place
Peripherally Inserted Central Catheters (PICCs) (Fig. 28-6)	*Implanted Venous Ports*
• Length of dwell: as long as they function properly with no evidence of intravenous (IV)-related complications	• Length of dwell: considered permanent
• Insertion sites: Antecubital fossa or upper arm (basilic or cephalic vein) and advanced until catheter tip reaches superior vena cava (SVC)	• Insertion sites: Chest, abdomen, or inner aspect of forearm
• Insertion technique: Not surgically placed, can be done at bedside, in home setting, or in radiology setting	• Insertion techniques: Requires surgery; catheter placed via subclavian or jugular vein and attached to reservoir located within a subcutaneous pocket (Fig. 28-8)
• Held in place with sutures or manufactured securement device	• Held in place within reservoir pocket and accessed using a noncoring needle (Fig. 28-9)

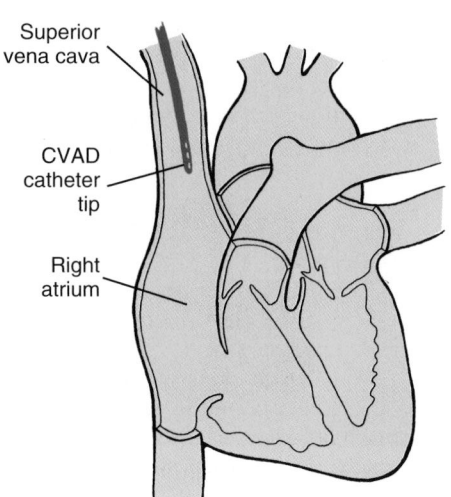

FIG 28-5   Catheter tip from CVAD lies in superior vena cava.

Superior vena cava

CVAD catheter tip

Right atrium

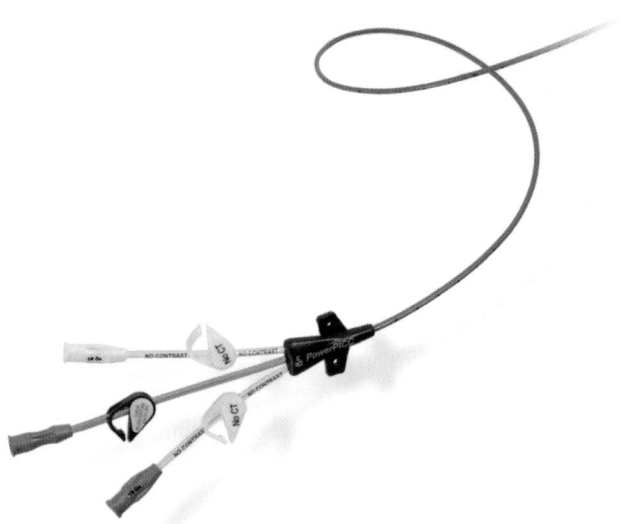

FIG 28-6 Peripherally inserted central catheter (PICC). *(Courtesy and copyright © Bard Access Systems.)*

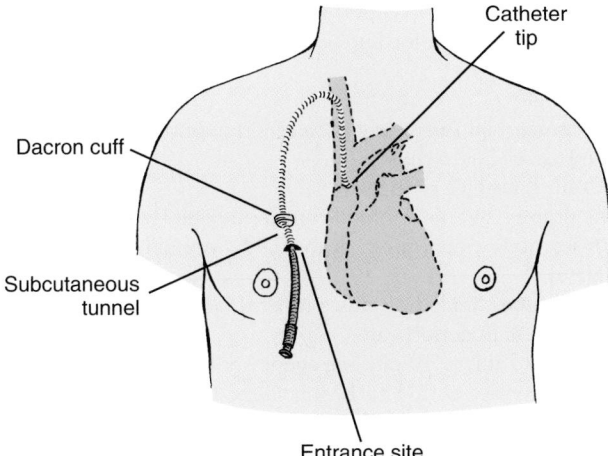

FIG 28-7 Tunneled catheter is in place, threaded into superior vena cava.

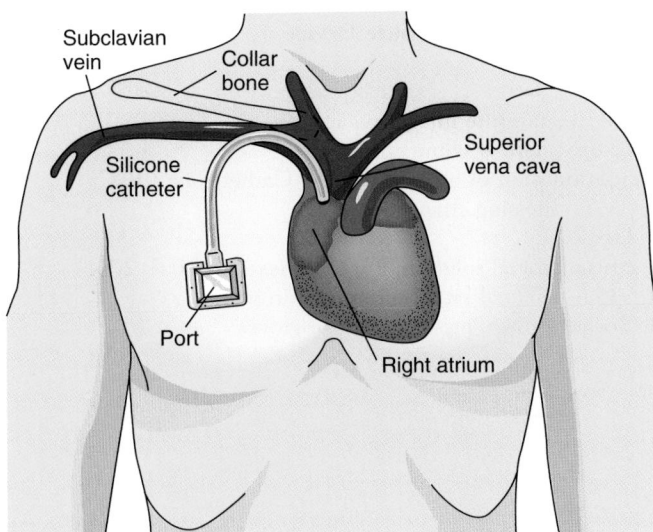

FIG 28-8 Implanted port and catheter.

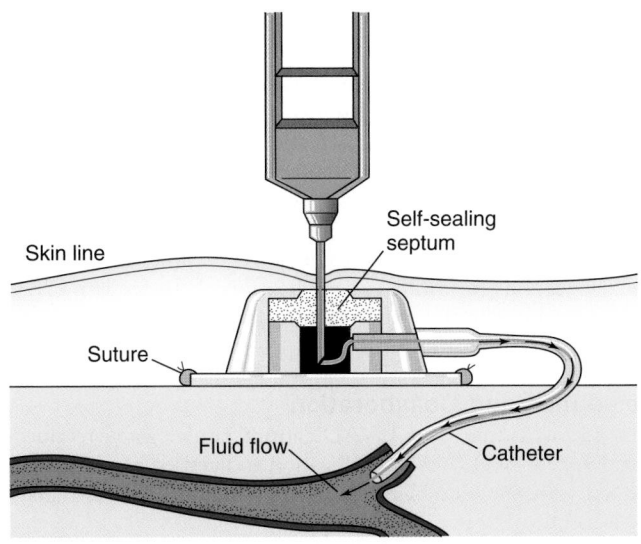

FIG 28-9 Cross section of implantable port showing access of port with noncoring needle.

Groshong); or the hub of the device has a pressure-activated valve (e.g., PAS V), which reduces the risk of hemorrhage, air embolism, and occlusion. CVADs can have single or multiple lumens. The choice of the number of lumens depends on a patient's condition and prescribed therapy. Patients requiring numerous infusions and blood samplings may have a device placed with more than one lumen allowing simultaneous administration of solutions and medications. In addition, multilumens allow for administration of incompatible solutions or medications. With the exception of the implanted venous port, each of these devices is accessed using the hub of the device located on the end of each of the external lumen(s). Implanted venous ports are located within the reservoir pocket; therefore there are no external lumen(s) to which to attach administration sets or flush syringes. To use the implanted venous port the septum is palpated; and, using sterile technique, a special noncoring needle is inserted through the skin into a self-sealing injection port (see Fig. 28-9). When a port is not in use, no external catheter is present. According to the *INS Flushing Protocols,* implanted venous ports should be flushed monthly with 3 to 5 mL of heparin (100 units/mL) to maintain patency (INS, 2011).

Primary complications associated with CVADs are usually related to infection commonly referred to as *central line–associated bloodstream infections (CLABSIs)* caused by contamination of the catheter from the skin of the patient or poor infection-prevention practices during insertion or care and maintenance (Alexander et al., 2010). According to the National Quality Forum a list of serious reportable event (SRE) (Safe Practice 21) actions should be taken to prevent CLABSIs by implementing evidence-based intervention practices (NQF, 2011). The Institute for Healthcare Improvement (2011) recently introduced a CLABSI bundle. Care bundles are groupings of best practices with respect to a disease process or condition that individually improve care, but result in substantially greater improvement when applied together. The science supporting the bundle components is sufficiently established to be considered the standard of care. The IHI Central Line Bundle is a group of evidence-based interventions for patients with intravascular central catheters that, when implemented together, result in better outcomes than when implemented individually (IHI, 2011).

The key components of the IHI Central Line Bundle are:
• Hand hygiene
• Maximal barrier precautions on insertion
• Chlorhexidine skin antisepsis
• Optimal catheter site selection, with avoidance of the femoral vein for central venous access in adult patients
• Daily review of line necessity with prompt removal of unnecessary lines

Care of CVADs requires knowledge of the purpose and function of the devices and prevention of complications. Patients with CVADs require health education and teaching about infection-prevention practices and skin care.

Delegation and Collaboration

The skill of caring for a CVAD cannot be delegated to nursing assistive personnel (NAP). Delegation to licensed practical nurses (LPNs) varies by state Nurse Practice Act. The nurse instructs the NAP to:
• Report the following to the nurse immediately: patient's dressing becomes damp or soiled, catheter line appears to be pulled out farther than original insertion position, IV line becomes disconnected, patient has a fever, patient complains of pain at the site.
• Help with positioning patient during insertion and care.

Equipment

Insertion and Dressing Care
❑ Hair clippers
❑ Central vascular access insertion tray (Fig. 28-10)
❑ Caps
❑ Sterile gowns
❑ Sterile drapes
❑ Masks and protective eyewear
❑ Nonsterile gloves
❑ Sterile gloves (powder free)
❑ Gauze pads

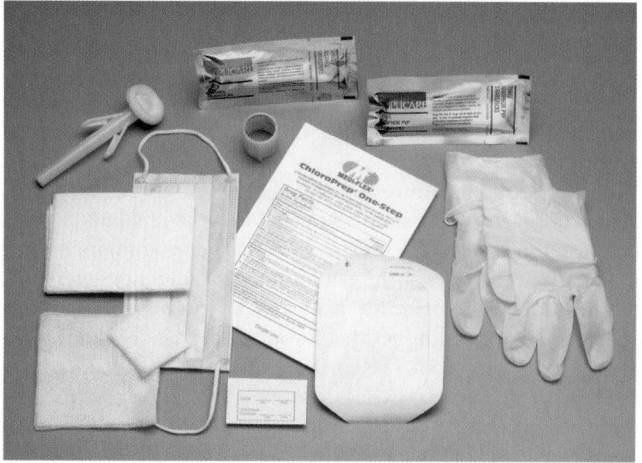

FIG 28-10 CVAD insertion tray.

❑ Surgical towels
❑ Antimicrobial solutions: 2% chlorhexidine (IHI, 2011)
❑ 1% lidocaine (Xylocaine)
❑ Sterile drapes
❑ 10-mL syringe
❑ Transparent dressing (transparent semipermeable membrane [TSM]) or gauze 4 × 4 dressing for catheter insertion site
❑ Tape
❑ IV infusion pump
❑ Tincture of benzoin (*optional*)

Site Care and Dressing Change
❑ CVAD dressing change kit, which includes:
  • Sterile gloves
  • Mask
  • Antimicrobial swabs (e.g., 2% chlorhexidine [IHI, 2011] [see agency policy])
  • Transparent antimicrobial dressing (TSM)
  • 4 × 4 Gauze pads
  • Tape measure
  • Sterile tape
  • Label
❑ Catheter stabilization device (if not sutured) for peripherally inserted central catheter (PICC) or nontunneled catheters
❑ Needleless injection cap(s) for each lumen(s)
❑ Noncoring needle for implanted venous port

Blood Sampling
❑ Clean gloves
❑ Antimicrobial swabs (e.g., 2% chlorhexidine, alcohol)
❑ 5-mL Luer-Lok syringes
❑ 10-mL Luer-Lok syringes
❑ Vacutainer system or blood transfer device (see agency policy)
❑ Preservative-free saline flush 0.9% normal saline solution (NSS)
❑ Blood tubes, including waste tubes, labels
❑ Needleless injection cap
❑ Syringe (5 mL or 10 mL; see agency policy) for discarded blood
❑ 10-mL syringe with 5 to 10 mL saline flush
❑ 10-mL syringe with 3 mL heparin flush (100 units/mL)
❑ Clean gloves

Changing the Injection Cap
❑ Clean gloves
❑ Antimicrobial swabs (e.g., 2% chlorhexidine)
❑ Needleless injection cap(s)
❑ 10-mL syringe with 10 mL normal saline (NS) flush 0.9% NSS

Flushing a Positive-Pressure Device
❑ Clean gloves
❑ Alcohol swabs
❑ Positive-pressure injection cap
❑ 10-mL prefilled saline syringe

Discontinuation of a Nontunneled Catheter or PICC
❑ CVAD dressing change kit
❑ Tape
❑ Antimicrobial solution: 2% chlorhexidine (IHI, 2011)
❑ Suture removal kit (if sutures are in place)
❑ Goggles, gown, mask, and clean gloves

STEP	RATIONALE

ASSESSMENT

1 Review accuracy and completeness of health care provider's order for insertion of CVAD for size and type. Assess treatment schedule: times for administration of IV solutions, medications, and blood sampling. Follow six rights of medication administration (see Chapter 20).

Identifies patient's need for vascular access, evaluates response to therapy, and determines education needs. Insertion of central catheter requires informed consent (INS, 2011).

2 Assess patient's hydration status: Skin turgor, dryness of mouth, skin texture, and fluid intake and output.

Provides baseline. In addition, dehydration is depletion of fluid volume and makes insertion of central vascular catheter more difficult.

3 Assess patient for any surgical procedures of upper chest or anatomic irregularities of proposed insertion site.

Previous surgical procedures or central vascular catheterizations indicate that you should not use a particular site. Spinal deformities and contractions make positioning difficult.

4 Assess CVAD placement site for skin integrity (open lesions) and signs of infection (i.e., redness, swelling, tenderness, exudate).

Compromised skin integrity contraindicates catheter insertion and can lead to secondary complications.

5 Assess patient for allergy to iodine, lidocaine (Xylocaine), latex, or chlorhexidine.

Medications, solutions used during catheter insertion, and use of gloves and tape can cause serious allergic reactions.

6 Assess type of CVAD intended for placement. Review manufacturer directions concerning catheter and maintenance.

Care and management depends on type and size of catheter or port, number of lumens, purpose of therapy.

7 Assess for proper function of existing CVAD before therapy: integrity of catheter, ability to flush or infuse fluid, ability to aspirate blood.

Blood return should be obtained before infusion of solutions or medications (INS, 2011). If resistance is met and/or no blood return is noted, patency must be established before infusing solutions or medications (INS, 2011).

8 Assess if any catheter lumens require flushing or if CVAD site needs dressing change by referring to medical record, nurses' notes, agency policies, and manufacturer-recommended guidelines for use.

Provides guidelines for maintaining catheter patency and preventing infection.

9 Assess patient's understanding of CVAD and knowledge of purpose, care, and maintenance. For long-term use ask patient to discuss steps in care and perform procedure (e.g., catheter site cleaning or dressing change).

Determines patient's level of understanding.
Provides opportunity to educate patient for home care of CVAD.

NURSING DIAGNOSES

- Deficient fluid volume
- Deficient knowledge regarding care of CVAD
- Excess fluid volume
- Impaired skin integrity
- Risk for infection
- Risk for injury

Related factors are individualized based on patient's condition or needs.

PLANNING

1 Expected outcomes following completion of procedure:

- Insertion occurs without complication.

Placement of CVAD carries risks such as pneumothorax, hematoma, air embolism, thrombosis, and infection.

- Placement of catheter tip is in superior vena cava near junction of right atrium or inferior vena cava above level of diaphragm (femoral approach).

Confirmation of tip location is required before use of CVAD (INS, 2011).

- CVAD site is intact, with no evidence of signs or symptoms of postinsertion complications (e.g., catheter migration, redness, swelling, aching or pain).

Catheter is patent, properly placed, and without evidence of complications.

- Prescribed solutions and medications infuse without difficulty.

Catheter remains patent.

- Patient and family caregiver are able to explain purpose of CVAD therapy and perform required catheter care and infusion of solutions and medications.

Demonstrates that patient and family caregiver have understanding and competency in caring for CVAD.

STEP	RATIONALE

IMPLEMENTATION

1 Explain procedure and purpose to patient and family caregiver. Explain to patient that he or she must not move during procedure. Offer opportunity at this time to toilet and offer pain medication (if needed). | Decreases anxiety, promotes cooperation, and prevents sudden movement during sterile procedure.

2 Identify patient using two identifiers (i.e., name and birthday or name and account number) according to agency policy. Compare identifiers in MAR/medical record with information on patient's identification bracelet and/or ask patient to state name. | Ensures correct patient. Complies with The Joint Commission standards and improves patient safety (TJC, 2012).

3 Catheter insertion: nontunneled device

  a Physician, with assistance of nurse, positions patient in Trendelenburg's or supine position for jugular or subclavian placement. | Opens angle between clavicle and first rib; dilates veins to facilitate eventual catheter insertion.

  Nurse places rolled towel or bath blanket between patient's shoulder blades, rotating them slightly to 10-degree angle. Turn patient's head away from insertion site. | Head down, below heart, promotes maximum filling and distention with increase in diameter of subclavicular vein (Phillips, 2010; Policy and Procedures, INS 2011); 10-degree tilt effectively achieves increase in diameter of vein.

  b Perform hand hygiene using antiseptic soap for 60 seconds.

  c If necessary, use scissors or electric clippers to remove any hair around insertion site. Explain rationale to patient. | Transient microorganisms reside in body hair. Clippers do not cause microabrasions, which harbor microorganisms (INS, 2011).

  d Nurse positions drape underneath area to be cannulated. | Barrier protection to prevent infection.

  e Physician and nurse apply cap, mask, eyewear, surgical gown, and powder-free sterile gloves. | Maximum barrier precautions needed when inserting central vascular catheter (INS, 2011).

  f Physician opens central vascular access kit and adds any sterile equipment to kit for use during insertion (see Chapter 8). | Maintains sterile field.

  g Site preparation.
    (1) Use 2% Chlorhexidine: Use scrubbing motion back and forth (vertically and horizontally) for 30 seconds and allow to air-dry for 30 seconds. | 2% Chlorhexidine is preferred for skin antisepsis. Is not recommended for infants under 2 months of age (INS, 2011).

  h After cleansing site, physician and nurse remove gloves. Physician changes into second pair of sterile gloves and nurse performs hand hygiene. (Check agency policy because some agencies require strict precaution.) | Gloves become contaminated from surface bacteria picked up in solution.

  i Physician uses large sterile drape and sterile towels to create sterile field. Physician finds anatomic landmarks and places fenestrated drape appropriately over proposed insertion site. | Provides sterile work space for catheter insertion (INS, 2011).

  j Physician arranges equipment in kit in preparation for catheter insertion. | Ensures smooth, orderly procedure.

  k Nurse sets up IV bag, fills tubing, and covers end of tubing with sterile cap (see Skill 28-1). | IV tubing is ready to be connected to IV catheter.

Clinical Decision Point *Trendelenburg's position is contraindicated in patients with head injuries, increased intracranial pressure, certain respiratory conditions, and spinal cord injuries.*

  l Nurse wipes off top of 1% lidocaine bottle with alcohol swabs and holds bottle upside down. *Optional:* Topical transdermal anesthetic agents can be applied before insertion. | Removes surface bacteria; allows physician to withdraw lidocaine while maintaining asepsis. Lidocaine has potential for creating allergic reaction and tissue damage.

  m Physician injects needle into bottle and withdraws approximately 3 to 4 mL lidocaine. He or she injects needle into site for subclavian puncture and anesthetizes venipuncture site, waiting 1 to 2 minutes for effect to take place. | Minimizes discomfort patient feels during venipuncture.

Clinical Decision Point *Just before time of insertion, ask patient to hold breath and strain. This is a Valsalva maneuver, which increases central venous pressure to prevent entry of air into the catheter. The Valsalva maneuver is the preferred method, although breath holding and humming may be a necessary option in uncooperative patients. In addition, if patient is unable to perform maneuvers, compress patient's abdomen gently.*

STEP	RATIONALE
n Physician inserts IV catheter into subclavian vein. Usually he or she does this by locating vein with large-bore cannula, removing needle from cannula, threading wire into cannula and vein, removing cannula over wire, and threading central vein catheter over wire to appropriate location (Seldinger technique) (Alexander et al., 2010).	Large vein is selected because it will be less irritated by hypertonic solutions or medications.
o Physician determines patency of line by withdrawing blood with 5-mL syringe, flushing with 0.9% sodium chloride solution, and placing caps on hubs.	Determines patency of device.
p Physician applies catheter securement device (e.g., manufactured stabilization device, sutures, sterile tape, or surgical Steri-Strips) to secure central vascular catheter in place. Cover with transparent dressing.	Suturing catheter to skin at insertion site increases risk for infection. Catheter securement devices are noninvasive and preferred for preventing catheter dislodgement (INS, 2011).
q Physician removes sterile drapes and completes procedure.	
r Nurse adjusts IV infusion to prescribed rate and connects to electronic infusion pump once chest x-ray film study is obtained.	Central line cannulations increase risk for pneumothorax (entrance of air into pleural space). Chest x-ray film examination verifies absence of pneumothorax and confirms location of IV catheter before solutions are administered at rapid flow (INS, 2011).
4 Insertion site care and dressing change	
a Position patient in comfortable position with head slightly elevated or, in the case of a PICC or midline device, have arm extended.	Provides access to patient.
b Prepare dressing materials. *Transparent dressing*: Provide insertion site care every 5 to 7 days and as needed. *Gauze dressing*: Provide insertion site care every 48 hours and as needed.	Transparent semipermeable membrane dressings have the advantage of being able to visualize the IV site. Gauze is preferable to TSM if the patient is diaphoretic or if the site is oozing or bleeding (INS, 2011).
c Perform hand hygiene and apply mask.	Reduces transfer of microorganisms; prevents spread of airborne microorganisms over CVAD insertion site.
d Apply clean gloves. Remove old dressing by lifting and removing either TSM or tape and gauze in direction of catheter insertion. Discard in appropriate biohazard container.	Stabilizes catheter as you remove dressing.
e Remove catheter stabilization device if used. Must be removed with alcohol.	Allows clear visualization of insertion site and surrounding skin (INS, 2011).

Clinical Decision Point *If sutures are used for initial catheter stabilization and become loosened or are no longer intact, alternative stabilization measures should be used (INS, 2011). Recent recommendations include use of a stabilization device because of the increased risk for infection when the catheter is sutured (Alexander et al., 2010).*

STEP	RATIONALE
f Inspect catheter, insertion site, and surrounding skin. Measure mid-arm circumference above insertion site.	Insertion sites require regular inspection for early detection of signs and symptoms of IV-related complications (infection, pain, redness, swelling, drainage, or bleeding) (INS, 2011). Measurement of mid-arm circumference assesses for thrombosis.
g Remove and discard clean gloves, perform hand hygiene. Open CVAD dressing kit using sterile technique, and *apply sterile gloves*. Area to be cleaned should be same size as dressing.	Sterile technique is required to apply new dressing.
h Cleanse site: (1) 2% Chlorhexidine (preferred). Apply using back-and-forth motion vertically and horizontally for at least 30 seconds; allow to dry for 30 seconds. (2) Povidone-iodine may be used in some settings (see agency policy).	Allowing antiseptic solutions to air-dry completely effectively reduces microbial counts (INS, 2011). Drying allows time for maximum microbicidal activity of agents (Policy and Procedures INS, 2011).
i Apply skin protectant to entire area. Allow drying completely so skin is not tacky.	Protects irritated or fragile skin from dressing. It must be used if catheter stabilization device is used.
j *Option*: Use chlorhexidine-impregnated dressing for short-term CVADs.	These dressings should be considered for patients over 2 months of age to prevent catheter-related bloodstream infection (CRBSI) (INS, 2011).

STEP	RATIONALE
k Apply new catheter stabilization device per manufacturer instructions if catheter is not sutured in place.	Provides catheter stability to minimize dislodgement or migration.
l Apply sterile, transparent semipermeable dressing, or gauze dressing over insertion site (see Skill 28-1).	Transparent dressing allows for clear visualization of catheter site between dressing changes (Policy and Procedures INS, 2011).
m Apply label to dressing with date, time, and your initials.	Provides information about next dressing change.
n Dispose of soiled supplies and used equipment. Remove gloves and perform hand hygiene.	Reduces transmission of microorganisms.

5 Blood sampling

STEP	RATIONALE
a Perform hand hygiene and apply clean gloves.	Reduces transmission of microorganisms. Prevents transfer of body fluids.
b Turn off all infusions for at least 1 minute before drawing blood. Note: If you cannot stop infusion, draw blood from peripheral vein.	Prevents interruption of critical fluid therapy.
c When drawing through multilumen catheters, the distal lumen (or one recommended by manufacturer) is preferred.	Distal lumen typically is largest-gauge lumen (Alexander et al., 2010).
d Clean injection cap with antiseptic solution and allow to dry completely. Attach syringe and flush with 3 to 5 mL of preservative-free 0.9% sodium chloride.	Maximizes bactericidal effectiveness of antiseptic swab. Determines catheter patency and clears IV (Policy and Procedures INS, 2010).
e Syringe Method Note: Check agency policy for use of Vacutainer with CVADs.	
(1) Remove end of IV tubing or injection cap from catheter hub. Keep end of tubing sterile.	
(2) Disinfect catheter hub with antiseptic solution.	Reduces risk of microorganisms.
(3) Attach an empty 10-mL syringe, unclamp catheter (if necessary) and withdraw blood 1.5 to 2 times fill volume (4 to 5 mL) of catheter for the discard sample.	Discard sample reduces risk of drug concentrations or diluted specimen (Alexander et al., 2010).
(4) Reclamp catheter (if necessary); remove syringe with blood and discard in appropriate biohazard container.	Open and valved CVADs differ in recommendations for clamping before removal of injection cap and syringe(s) (e.g., Hickman versus Groshong) (INS, 2011).
(5) Clean hub with another antiseptic solution.	
(6) Attach second syringe(s) to obtain required volume of blood needed for specimen ordered.	Multiple syringes may be required, depending on specimens required and number of blood tubes needed.
(7) Unclamp catheter(if necessary) to withdraw blood.	
(8) Once specimens are obtained, reclamp catheter (if necessary) and remove syringe.	

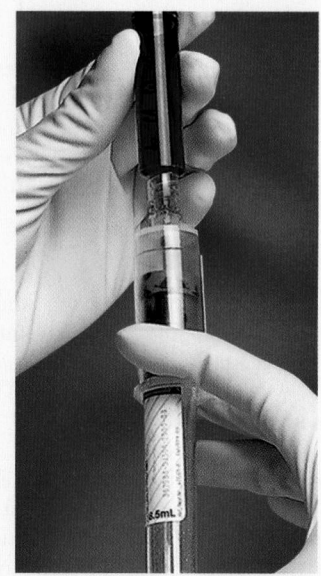

STEP 5f   Blood specimen transfer device. *(Courtesy and ©Becton Dickinson & Co.)*

STEP	RATIONALE
(9) Clean catheter hub with antiseptic solution.	
(10) Attach prefilled injection cap attached to 10-mL syringe with 10 mL of 0.9% sodium chloride to catheter, unclamp (if necessary), and flush. Reclamp catheter (if necessary).	Flushing with 10 mL of 0.9% sodium chloride after blood draw is minimum volume of solution recommended (INS, 2011). Reduces risk for catheter clotting after procedure.
(11) Remove syringe and discard into appropriate biohazard container.	Reduces transmission of microorganisms.
f Transfer blood using transfer vacuum device (see illustration).	Reduces risk of blood exposure.
g Flush catheter with syringe containing heparin solution (check agency policy).	Heparin flush volume and concentration vary by agency and type of catheter. Flush Groshong catheters with 0.9% sodium chloride only.

Clinical Decision Point *Always use a 10-mL syringe on central lines to minimize pressure during injection.*

STEP	RATIONALE
h Remove syringe. Attach new sterile cap (see Step 6) or IV tubing to hub of catheter. Cleanse end of IV tubing with antiseptic swab before reconnecting. Resume infusion as ordered or clamp catheter (if necessary).	Decreases risk of contamination.
i Dispose of soiled equipment and used supplies. Remove gloves and perform hand hygiene.	Reduces transmission of microorganisms.

6 Changing injection cap

STEP	RATIONALE
a Determine if injection caps should be changed.	Injection caps are usually changed with each administration set change, at least every 7 days for catheter maintenance, if residual blood is present, and when integrity is compromised (INS, 2011).
b Prepare new injection cap(s):	Understanding of the types of injection caps available is imperative as the flushing technique will vary based on the type of device (e.g., positive or neutral displacement valves).
(1) Perform hand hygiene. Remove cap from package and clean septum with antiseptic solution using friction.	
(2) Keep protective cap on tip of injection cap.	Maintains sterility.
(3) Prime injection cap by attaching prefilled syringe and flushing with 0.9% normal saline through cap until fluid is seen in protective cap. Keep syringe attached.	Removes air from system.
c If required based on device type, clamp catheter lumens one at a time by using slide or squeeze clamp.	Prevents air from entering system when opened. Patient can also perform Valsalva maneuver during cap changes.
d Remove old injection caps using aseptic technique.	Routine injection cap changes decrease catheter infections.
e Apply clean gloves. Clean catheter hub with antiseptic swab. Connect new injection cap(s) on catheter hub.	Allowing antiseptic solutions to air-dry completely effectively reduces microbial counts (INS, 2011). Drying allows time for maximum antimicrobial activity of agents.
f Flush catheter with 10-mL syringe of 0.9% sodium chloride followed by heparin solution as required by manufacturer.	Prevents clot formation.
g Dispose of all soiled supplies and used equipment. Remove gloves and perform hand hygiene.	Reduces spread of microorganisms.

7 Flushing a positive-pressure device

STEP	RATIONALE
a Perform hand hygiene and apply clean gloves.	Reduces transmission of microorganisms.
b Prepare positive-pressure device by attaching prefilled saline syringe. Prime through device and leave syringe attached.	Maintains sterility of device.
c Clamp catheter (if necessary). Remove injection cap and discard.	
d Connect positive-pressure device, unclamp catheter, and flush through with saline as ordered.	Do not add extension tubing, which negates positive-pressure action of valve.
e Reclamp after syringe has been removed.	If CVAD has a clamp, it needs to be engaged. If clamp is not engaged and device becomes loose and comes off, patient is exposed to possible air embolism or bleeding (INS, 2011).
f Dispose of all soiled supplies and used equipment. Remove gloves and perform hand hygiene.	Reduces spread of microorganisms.

STEP	RATIONALE
8 Discontinuing nontunneled catheters or PICCs	
a Verify health care provider's order to discontinue line. Check agency policy because most require physician to discontinue CVAD. In some settings advanced practice nurses or specially credentialed nurses can remove devices.	Verifies appropriateness of procedure. Only a competent health care professional can remove a CVAD.
b If IV fluids or medications are to continue, prepare to convert them to a short peripheral or midline before CVAD discontinuation. NOTE: Be aware of pH and osmolarity of solution or medication for appropriateness of conversion to short peripheral or midline catheter.	Prevents interruption of IV medication/fluid therapy.
c Position patient in 10-degree Trendelenburg's position.	Position promotes venous filling and prevents air embolus during catheter removal.
d Perform hand hygiene.	Prevents transmission of microorganisms.
e Turn off IV fluids infusing through central line.	Prevents fluid loss during CVAD removal.
f Place moisture-proof pad under site.	Minimizes soiling of bed linen. Provides clean environment.
g Apply gown, gloves, mask, and goggles.	Prevents transmission of microorganisms and exposure to bloodborne pathogens.
h Gently remove CVAD dressing. Discard in biohazard container. Inspect catheter and insertion site.	Prevents skin tears. Provides information about catheter and site before removal. Disposal prevents transmission of microorganisms.
i Remove gloves and perform hand hygiene; open CVAD dressing change kit and suture removal kit (if sutures in place). Add additional items to sterile field. Don sterile gloves.	Prevents transfer of organisms on soiled dressing to catheter insertion site.
j Clean CVAD site using combination antiseptic or chlorhexidine swabs (check agency policy). Begin at insertion site and move outward in circular motion or, with chlorhexidine only, use back-and-forth scrub method, vertical, horizontal and circular, for 30 seconds. Allow to dry completely.	Removes microorganisms from skin surrounding insertion site. Allowing antiseptic solutions to air-dry completely effectively reduces microbial counts (INS, 2011).
k If catheter securement device is present, carefully remove catheter from device and remove device with alcohol.	Alcohol aids in removal of securement device.
l To remove sutures with nondominant hand, grasp suture with forceps. Using dominant hand, carefully cut suture with sterile scissors; avoid damaging skin or catheter. Lift suture out and discard. Continue until all sutures are removed.	Technique prevents pulling contaminated end of suture through patient's skin.

Clinical Decision Point *All CVADs require measurements of external catheter and total length of catheter removed. PICC lines also require measurement of the upper-arm circumference.*

STEP	RATIONALE
m Using nondominant hand, apply sterile 4 × 4–inch gauze to site. Instruct patient to take deep breath and hold it as you withdraw catheter.	Valsalva maneuver reduces risk for air embolus by decreasing negative pressure in respiratory system.
n With dominant hand remove catheter in smooth, continuous motion an inch at a time. Note any resistance while removing catheter. Inspect catheter for intactness, especially along tip. Keeping fingers near insertion site, immediately apply pressure to site and continue until bleeding stops.	Gentle removal of catheter prevents stretching and breaking it. Damaged catheter may break off and leave a piece in patient's arm. Direct pressure reduces risk for bleeding and hematoma formation.

Clinical Decision Point *It is often necessary to apply pressure longer if patient is receiving anticoagulation therapy or has prolonged clotting times.*

STEP	RATIONALE
o Apply petroleum-based ointment to exit site (*optional:* see agency policy). Apply sterile occlusive dressing such as transparent dressing or sterile gauze to site. Change dressing every 24 hours until healed.	Reduces chance of air embolism and seals vein tract (INS, 2011). Inspect catheter removal site for bleeding and infection until it is healed (INS, 2011).
p Label dressing with date, time, and your initials.	Identifies date of catheter removal and need for dressing change.
q Inspect catheter integrity and discard in biohazard container. NOTE: Catheter cultures should be performed when catheter is removed for suspected CRBSIs. Catheter cultures should not be obtained routinely (INS, 2011; Mermel et al., 2009).	If catheter tip is broken or compromised, place in container and label for possible follow-up.

STEP	RATIONALE
r Return patient to comfortable position. Be sure that short peripheral IV or midline is infusing at correct rate.	Maintains IV fluid therapy.
s Dispose of soiled supplies; remove gloves and personal protective equipment. Perform hand hygiene.	Reduces transmission of microorganisms.

EVALUATION

1 Determine daily, in consultation with physician, the continued need for the CVAD.	Daily review of line necessity with prompt removal of unnecessary lines is a practice recommended in the IHI CLABSI bundle (IHI, 2011).
2 Observe patient for shortness of breath or pain in chest or shoulder after CVAD insertion. Auscultate for breath sounds.	Pain, shortness of breath, and absent breath sounds indicate complication of pneumothorax.
3 Observe patient for bleeding or swelling at insertion site or neck and occlusiveness of dressing.	Symptoms indicate infiltration of IV fluids into subcutaneous tissues or damage to vessel lumen. Dressing must remain occlusive to protect against entrance of microorganisms.
4 Monitor intake and output as directed by agency policy for fluid balance and monitor laboratory values for electrolyte balance as indicated.	Assesses patient's circulatory system and indicates fluid volume excess or deficit.
5 Routinely assess vital signs of patient, noting changes symptomatic of infection.	Catheter-related sepsis causes fever, chills, flushed skin, tachycardia.
6 Observe catheter insertion site and exit for erythema, warmth, tenderness, edema, or drainage.	Continual monitoring for signs of inflammation or infection is essential.
7 Observe all catheter connection points, being sure they are secure (see agency policy).	An intact system prevents accidental blood loss or entrance of air.
8 Inspect condition of catheter and connection tubing as directed by agency policy for leaks or tears, kinks or obstructions, or cracked hubs.	Break in integrity of system predisposes patient to hemorrhage, infection or air embolus.
9 Observe for clot formation in catheter, air embolism, infiltration/extravasation during infusions, and catheter migration.	Early detection of complications improves patient outcomes.
10 Consult x-ray film examination reports for catheter placement.	A routine chest x-ray film examination will confirm position of catheter tip.
11 Evaluate ability of patient and family caregiver to provide care and maintain catheter or infusion port through discussion and return demonstrations of dressing changes and skin care. Determine need for restrictions on daily activities.	Measures patient's ability to care for self and any additional learning needs.

Unexpected Outcomes
1 For catheter complications, see Table 28-7.

2 Patient or family caregiver is unable to explain or perform CVAD care.

Related Interventions
- See Table 28-7.

- Indicates need for home care referral or additional instruction.

Recording and Reporting
- Immediately notify health care provider of signs and symptoms of any complications.
- Document catheter site care in nurses' notes and EHR: size of catheter, change of injection caps, appearance of site, condition and type of securement device, date and time of dressing change.
- Document in nurses' notes and EHR the condition of exit site or port insertion site, including skin integrity, signs of complications, placement, integrity, external catheter length, mid-arm circumference, and functionality of catheter.
- Document in nurses' notes and EHR catheter removal: patient position, appearance of site, length of catheter removed, integrity of catheter after removal, dressing applied, patient's tolerance of procedure, presence/absence of bleeding from site every 15 minutes for 1 hour, and any problems with removal.
- Document in nurses' notes and EHR blood draw: date, time, sample drawn.

- Document in nurses' notes and EHR unexpected outcomes, health care provider notification, interventions, and patient response to treatment.

Special Considerations
Teaching
- Instruct patient to report discomfort around the site; discomfort in arms, shoulders, or side of the neck; or any shortness of breath.
- Discuss and provide written emergency measures and telephone numbers of health care personnel to be used in case of catheter damage, displacement, swelling, redness, or leakage at insertion site; occlusion of port or catheter; temperature above 100.4° F (38° C) (see agency policy); and shaking chills.
- Provide written instruction for dressing changes, inspection of insertion site, flushing, and tubing changes.
- Arrange for instruction and return demonstration of skills by patient or family caregiver.

TABLE 28-7	Complications of Vascular Access Devices		
Complication	**Assessment**	**Prevention**	**Intervention**
Catheter damage, breakage	Every shift observe for pinholes, leaks, tears. Assess for drainage from site after flushing.	Follow proper clamping procedure. Avoid sharp objects near catheter. Use needleless system device. Use only 10-mL syringe for flushing. Never flush against resistance.	Clamp catheter near insertion site and place sterile gauze over break or hole until repaired. Use only repair kit that is recommended by manufacturer. Remove catheter.
Occlusion: Thrombus, fibrin sheath, fibrin tail, precipitation, malposition	Assess insertion site and sutures. Assess for blood return. Assess for ability to infuse fluid. Assess equipment. If port is in place, reaccess and verify noncoring needle placement. Assess with syringe directly on catheter. Assess for discomfort or pain in shoulder, neck, ear, or arm at insertion site. Assess for neck or shoulder edema.	Follow routine flushing with positive pressure and/or use positive-pressure valve injection cap. Secure with catheter stabilization device to prevent tension on CVAD. Do not flush against resistance. Flush between medications. Flush vigorously after viscous solutions. Avoid mixing incompatible drugs. Avoid kinking catheter.	Reposition patient. Have patient cough and deep breathe. Raise patient's arm overhead. Obtain venogram if ordered. Administer thrombolytics if ordered. Remove catheter (CVAD requires order). Obtain x-ray film as ordered. Do not use a 1-mL syringe to instill saline because pressure exceeds 200 psi.
Infection and sepsis: Exit site, tunnel, thrombus, port pocket (CLABSI)	Assess exit site for redness, drainage, edema, or tenderness. Assess for signs of systemic infection. Monitor laboratory findings.	Use aseptic technique. Prevent contamination of catheter hub. Adhere to dressing change technique. Apply transparent semipermeable dressing over exit site.	Obtain blood cultures first from peripheral and CVAD if ordered. Remove catheter (CVAD requires order). Replace catheter.
Dislodgement	Assess length of catheter daily. Inform patient of possible catheter dislodgement. Identify edema at exit site or drainage. Palpate exit site and tunnel for coiling (catheter can feel cordlike underneath the skin). Assess for distended neck veins.	Loop and tape catheter securely. Use catheter stabilization device and transparent semipermeable dressing. Avoid pulling on CVAD. Avoid manipulating catheter by hand.	Insert new catheter. Secure with catheter stabilization device. Teach patient not to manipulate catheter.
Catheter migration (e.g., length of catheter moved from original position), pinch-off syndrome (e.g., compression of catheter between clavicle and first rib), port separation or catheter fracture (e.g., internal fracture or separation of catheter)	Assess for patient complaints of gurgling sounds. Assess for change in patency of catheter by evaluating change in flow rate, local irritation, swelling, occlusion, tenderness, pain, inability to aspirate fluid and/or blood. Pain at site when flushed or symptoms of embolus. Obtain x-ray film examination. Assess edema of arm and hand on side of insertion. Assess for distended neck veins. Assess for inability to infuse fluids. Assess length of catheter daily.	Avoid trauma. Avoid placement near site of local infection, scarring, or skin disorder.	Reposition under fluoroscopy as ordered. Remove catheter as ordered. Stop all fluid administration.
Skin erosion (e.g., mechanical loss of skin tissue), hematomas (e.g., local collection of blood), cuff extrusion (e.g., tissue at edges of insertion site separate), scar tissue formation over port	Assess for loss of viable tissue over septum site. Assess for separation of exit site edges. Assess for drainage at exit site. Assess for redness. Assess for edema, contusions. Note if tunneled catheter is exposed (Dacron cuff is visible).	Maintain nutritional status. Avoid pressure or trauma. Rotate with each port access. Do not reinsert a noncoring needle in the same "hole" of a previous insertion. This creates a permanent hole in the septum. Do not use standard needle to access port.	Remove CVAD as ordered. Improve nutrition. Provide appropriate skin care.

TABLE 28-7 | Complications of Vascular Access Devices—cont'd

Complication	Assessment	Prevention	Intervention
Infiltration, extravasation	Assess for erythema. Assess for edema. Assess for spongy feeling. Assess for swelling around IV site and at termination of catheter tip. Assess for labored breathing. Assess for aspiration of fluid and/or blood. Assess for complaints of pain with infusion of solutions or medications (e.g., burning). Assess for no free-flow IV drip.	Immediately stop vesicant administration. Administer antidote or therapeutic medications to maintain tissue integrity according to protocol.	Apply cold/warm compresses according to specific vesicant protocol. Provide emotional support. Obtain x-ray film if ordered. Use antidotes per protocol. Discontinue IV fluids.
Pneumothorax, hemothorax, air emboli, hydrothorax	Assess for subcutaneous emphysema by inspecting and palpating skin around insertion site and along arm. Inspection may reveal edema where air is located, and air may travel if skin is loose. Palpation reveals a crackling sensation such as popping plastic bubble wrap. Assess for chest pain. Assess for dyspnea, apnea, hypoxia, tachycardia, hypotension, nausea, confusion.	Use injection cap on distal end when not in use. Do not leave catheter open to air. If appropriate for device, be sure that clamps are engaged.	Administer oxygen as ordered. Elevate feet. Aspirate air, fluid. If air emboli suspected, place patient on left side with head down. Remove catheter as ordered. Help with insertion of chest tubes as ordered.
Incorrect placement	Assess for cardiac dysrhythmias. Assess for hypotension. Assess for neck distention. Assess for narrow pulse pressure. Assess for inadequate blood withdrawal. Assess for retrograde flow of blood (flow of blood back into tubing usually caused by decreased pressure gradient between venous system and access device unit [e.g., IV infusion, heparin lock]).	Obtain x-ray film examination after placement. Reposition catheter as warranted.	Stop all fluid administration until placement is confirmed. Discontinue catheter (requires order). Obtain x-ray film and electrocardiogram (for PICC and CVAD). Administer support medications as ordered.

CLABSI, Central line–associated bloodstream infection; *CVAD,* central vascular access device; *CVC,* central venous catheter; *IV,* intravenous; *PICC,* peripherally inserted central catheter.

- Have patient or family caregiver maintain a list of caregivers and telephone numbers (e.g., physician, nurse, social worker, pharmacist, dietitian).

Pediatric
- Central vein catheters that are of a smaller diameter and shorter length are available for children and infants.
- Take care to secure infant catheters in a manner that does not allow them to twist. Small-diameter catheters are fragile, and twisting them causes them to tear.
- Amount and dosage of flush solution (heparin/saline) vary with age and size. Record volume of blood draws on intake and output record.

Gerontologic
- Some older adults have difficulty with lying flat in bed, and a modification of the totally supine position during CVAD insertion is often necessary.
- PICC insertion may provide an alternative route of administration and reduce the risk of complications associated with subclavian or jugular insertion.

Home Care
- Initiate early referral for discharge planning to social service, counselor, or home care coordinator for assessment of resources.
- Provide patient with written list of providers for supplies and equipment.
- Instruct patient or family caregiver in flushing technique, site care and dressing change, and emergency interventions.
- Instruct patient and family caregiver in adaptations of hospital procedures that they can make at home (e.g., good hand hygiene instead of sterile gloves).
- Ongoing assessment by the home care provider is essential in the early detection of complications and preservation of CVADs.
- Assess home environment and determine suitable area for dressing changes, avoiding areas where contaminants are potential hazards.
- Provide appropriate information about home disposal of soiled dressings and equipment (see Chapter 42).

? Critical Thinking Exercises

A patient is admitted to the medical unit from the emergency department with a diagnosis of pneumonia and dehydration. The health care provider has ordered 1000 mL $D_5 \frac{1}{2}$ NS at 100 mL/hr to be started on admission. The patient has an intravenous (IV) infusion running in her left antecubital fossa that shows evidence of inadequate flow rate, and the patient complains of discomfort at the site.

1 Using microdrip tubing, what would be the correct drip rate for this IV? Using a 15 gtt/mL macrodrip tubing, what would be the correct drip rate for this IV?

2 When you obtain the IV fluids for the patient, which assessment steps are necessary before you change the solution?

3 Which assessments and interventions are required for the existing IV in the left arm?

4 Discuss the information to document after discontinuing the left antecubital IV.

✓ REVIEW QUESTIONS

1 A patient is receiving 1 L of D_5 lactated Ringer's (LR) every 12 hours using an administration set with a drop factor of 15 gtt/mL. At what rate should the nurse set this infusion?
  1 10 gtt/min
  2 21 gtt/min
  3 33 gtt/min
  4 83 gtt/min

2 A patient had an intravenous (IV) catheter inserted 48 hours ago to receive antibiotic therapy. During assessment of the IV site the nurse observes redness and tenderness on palpation. The nurse documents that the IV was discontinued and restarted because of which complication of IV therapy?
  1 Clotting of the IV catheter
  2 Infiltration
  3 Phlebitis
  4 Puncturing of the opposite side of the vein

3 Considerations for selecting an intravenous (IV) catheter for a patient include which of the following?
  1 Selecting the longest catheter with the largest gauge
  2 Selecting the longest catheter with the smallest gauge
  3 Selecting the shortest catheter with the smallest gauge
  4 Selecting the shortest catheter with the largest gauge

4 Place in correct order the following steps for changing a dressing over a short peripheral IV device:
  1 Clean insertion site with antiseptic swab.
  2 After removing tape, remove transparent dressing (transparent semipermeable membrane [TSM]).
  3 Apply new transparent dressing (TSM).
  4 Observe site for signs and symptoms of intravenous (IV)-related complications.

5 A midline catheter is considered a central vascular access device.
  1 True
  2 False

6 An obese patient who had a right mastectomy several years ago has better veins in her right hand but is left handed. Where should the nurse place the intravenous (IV) catheter?
  1 In her right hand
  2 In her left lower arm
  3 Wherever the patient wants
  4 In her right antecubital site

7 The health care provider discontinued a patient's anticoagulant therapy. Which nursing intervention is most appropriate after the nurse removes the intravenous (IV) catheter from his hand?
  1 Apply pressure to the IV site until the bleeding stops.
  2 Convert the catheter to an intermittent heparin lock for 24 hours.
  3 Encourage the patient to keep his hand elevated for 10 minutes.
  4 Use a warm compress at the site for several minutes.

8 A patient just had a peripherally inserted central catheter (PICC) placed in the right antecubital site. When reading the x-ray film report verifying correct placement of the catheter, the nurse knows that the tip of the PICC is located correctly if it is in which vessel?
  1 The inferior vena cava
  2 The basilic vein
  3 The cephalic vein
  4 The superior vena cava

9 Which of the following is a key component of the Central Line Bundle?
  1 Chlorhexidine skin antisepsis
  2 Soap and water skin preparation
  3 Alcohol skin antisepsis
  4 Hydrogen peroxide skin preparation

10 An order is received to provide a solution with an osmolarity greater than 600 mOsm/L to a patient. Which of the following intravenous (IV) devices is appropriate?
  1 Short peripheral in cephalic vein
  2 Midline in basilic vein
  3 Peripherally inserted central catheter (PICC) in subclavian vein
  4 Implanted venous port in superior vena cava (SVC)

REFERENCES

Ackley BJ, et al: *Evidence-based nursing care guidelines medical surgical interventions*, ed 3, St Louis, 2008, Mosby.

Alexander M, et al: *Infusion nursing evidence-based approach*, ed 3, St Louis, 2010, Elsevier.

Hockenberry M, Wilson D: *Wong's nursing care of infants and children*, ed 9, St Louis, 2011, Mosby.

Infusion Nurses Society: Infusion nursing standards of practice, *J Intraven Nurs* 30(suppl 1):S1, 2011.

Infusion Nurses Society: *Policy and procedures for infusion nursing*, ed 4, Norwood, Mass, 2011, Author.

Institute for Healthcare Improvement: Implement the IHI Central Line Bundle, Cambridge, Mass, 2011. available at http://www.ihi.org/knowledge/Pages/Changes/ImplementtheCentralLineBundle.aspx, accessed August 20, 2012.

LeFever J, et al: *Fluids and electrolytes with clinical applications a programmed approach*, ed 8, Clifton Park, NY, 2010, Delmar Cengage Learning.

Mermel L, et al: Clinical practice guidelines for the diagnosis and management of intravascular catheter-related infection: 2009 update by the Infectious Diseases Society of America, *Clin Infect Dis* 49:1, 2009.

Meiner SE: *Gerontologic nursing*, ed 4, St Louis, 2011, Mosby.

National Quality Forum: List of serious reportable events (SREs), updated 2011, available at http://www.qualityforum.org/Topics/SREs/List_of_SREs.aspx.

Phillips LD: *Manual of IV therapeutics: evidenced based practice for infusion therapy*, ed 5, Philadelphia, 2010, FA Davis.

Poon EG, et al: Effect of bar-code technology on the safety of medication administration, *New Engl J Med* 362(18):1698, 2010.

The Joint Commission (TJC): *National Patient Safety Goals*, Oakbrook Terrace, Ill, 2012, TJC, available at http://www.jointcommission.org, accessed October 2008.

29

Blood Transfusions

MEDIA RESOURCES

- **evolve** *learning system* http://evolve.elsevier.com/Perry/skills
  - Review Questions
  - ▶ Video Clips
  - Audio Glossary

- **NSO** Nursing Skills Online

KEY TERMS

Agglutinate
Allogeneic
Anemia
Autologous transfusion
Autotransfusion
Blood group

Blood transfusion
Blood type
Febrile nonhemolytic
  reaction (FNH)
Hemochromatosis
Hemolysis

Human leukocyte antigen
  (HLA)
Immune-mediated platelet
  refractoriness
Reinfusion
Thrombocytopenia

Transfusion reaction
Transfusion-related acute
  lung injury (TRALI)
Transfusion-associated
  graft-versus-host disease
  (TA-GVHD)

OBJECTIVES

Mastery of content in this chapter will enable the nurse to:
- Discuss indications for blood therapy.
- Describe various transfusion reactions.

- Demonstrate the following skills on selected patients: initiating blood therapy, implementing autotransfusion, and monitoring for adverse reactions to transfusion.

Since the first blood transfusion over 200 years ago, transfusion therapy has evolved to a much more complex process with many different blood components. A competent nurse must know not only the complexities of the ABO and Rh system, but also the numerous components of blood that can be transfused and the serious negative outcomes that can occur.

Transfusion therapy or blood replacement is the intravenous (IV) administration of whole blood (Fig. 29-1), its components (Fig. 29-2, A and B), or a plasma-derived product (Fig. 29-3) for therapeutic purposes (Alexander et al., 2010). Transfusions restore intravascular volume with whole blood or albumin, restore the oxygen-carrying capacity of blood with red blood cells, and provide clotting factors and/or platelets. The most common method of blood transfusion is allogeneic blood (blood donated from someone else). Despite precautions, transfusion therapy carries risks. Compatibility of the patient and donor is essential. Human-related errors (e.g., improper labeling, poor hand-off between nurses and the person transporting blood, or the method used to complete a blood requisition) that may lead to the administration of incompatible transfusions can occur in every step of the process. In addition, disease transmission is also a possibility (Alexander et al., 2010; Busch, 2008; Gabriel, 2008). Comprehensive screening and testing reduce these occurrences considerably; however, the administration of blood and blood products cannot be taken lightly since a majority of the complications result from human error during transfusion (Alexander et al., 2010). Complications resulting from immunologic response to blood or blood products can be reduced by modifications such as washed or irradiated red blood cells or leukocyte-reduced blood.

Autologous transfusion or autotransfusion is a method in which a patient's own blood is collected and reinfused for the purpose of intravascular volume replacement (Alexander et al., 2010; AABB, 2011). Patients who have a concern about transfusion-related reactions or transmission of disease find positive advantages to autologous transfusion. It is ideal for preoperative blood donation, intraoperative cell salvage, and postoperative blood salvage. Preoperative blood donation is the most commonly used type of autologous donation. In this process patients donate their own blood approximately 4 to 6 weeks before therapy via phlebotomy, which is performed weekly. The last donation must occur more than 72 hours

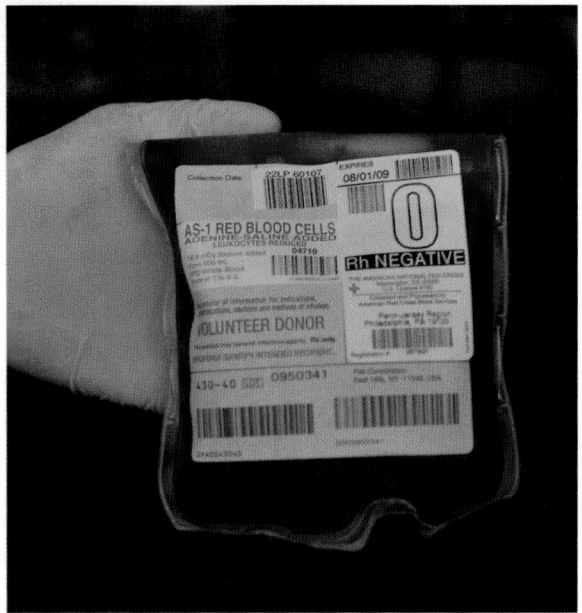

FIG 29-1 Unit of blood. (*Image courtesy American Red Cross.*)

TABLE 29-1	Types of Blood Preservatives	
Anticoagulant Preservative	**Composition**	**Shelf Life Provided (Days)**
CPD	Citrate, phosphate, and dextrose	21
CPDA-1	CPD plus adenine	35
CPDA-1 additive system	CPD plus various preservative combinations	35-42

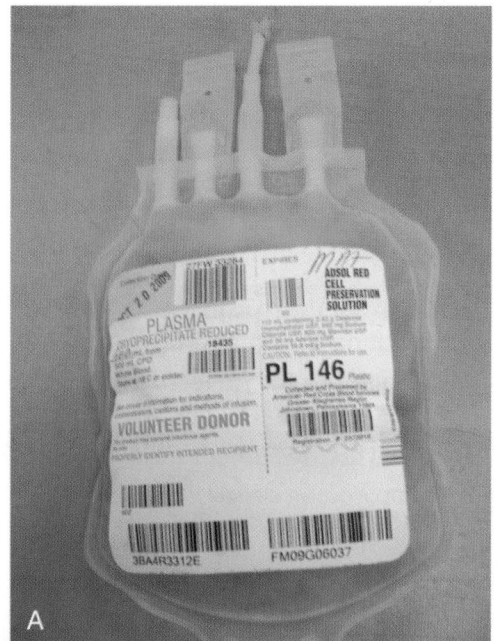

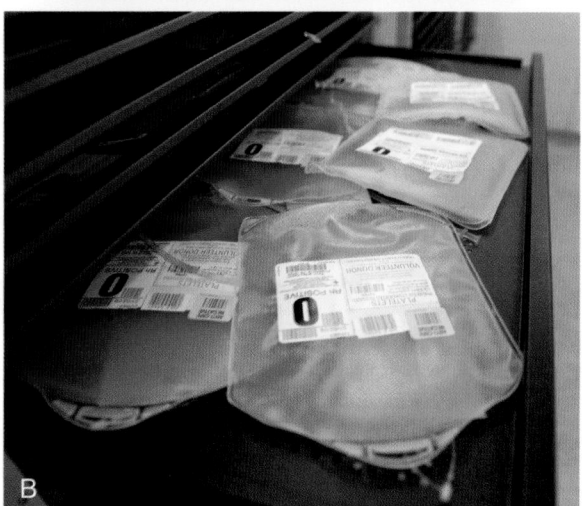

FIG 29-2 Bag of Cryo (**A**) and bag of platelets (**B**). (*Images courtesy American Red Cross.*)

before surgery. The donated blood is stored at 1° to 6° C (33.8° to 42.8° F) for 35 to 42 days (Alexander et al., 2010; AABB, 2011).

To decrease transfusion-related adverse events, blood and its components are treated and stored in controlled environments. Blood is a living tissue; and, once obtained via the donor, it must remain healthy before transfusion (Alexander et al., 2010). Various anticoagulants and preservatives are used to maintain the shelf life of donated blood. Citrate-phosphate-dextrose (CPD) and citrate-phosphate-dextrose-adenine (CPDA-1) are two commonly used anticoagulant preservatives (Table 29-1) (Alexander et al., 2010; AABB, 2011). Caution is needed when infusing an older unit of blood. When blood is stored, there is continual destruction of red blood cells, which releases potassium (K) from the cells into the plasma. Often a laboratory test of a patient's K level is ordered before administering a unit of blood.

As a nurse your role during a blood transfusion is to carry out the health care provider's order by safely administering the blood/blood products and assessing a patient before, during, and after the transfusion.

ABO SYSTEM

There are three blood-typing systems: ABO, Rh, and human leukocyte antigen (HLA). These systems ensure a close match between transfused products and a recipient's blood. The ABO system uses the presence or absence of specific antigens on the surface of red

blood cells to identify blood groups. When the type A antigen is present, the blood group is type A. When the type B antigen is present, the blood group is type B. When both A and B antigens are present, the blood group is type AB, and when neither A nor B antigens are present, the blood group is type O (Alexander et al., 2010; AABB, 2011) (Table 29-2).

Antibodies that react against the A and B antigens are naturally present in the plasma of people whose red blood cells do not carry the antigen. These antibodies (agglutinins) react against the foreign antigens (agglutinogens). Incompatible red blood cells agglutinate (clump together) and result in a life-threatening hemolytic transfusion reaction. People with type A blood have anti-B antibodies; people with type B blood have anti-A antibodies. People with type AB blood have neither antibody and can receive all blood types. People with type O blood have both A and B antibodies and can receive only type O blood (Alexander et al., 2010; AABB, 2011; Snyder et al., 2008).

TABLE 29-2 | ABO System

Patient Blood Type (Rh Factor)	Red Blood Cell Antigen	Transfuse with Type A	Transfuse with Type B	Transfuse with Type AB	Transfuse with Type O	Transfusion Options
A (+)	A	Yes	No	No	Yes	A+, A– O+, O–
A (–)	A	Yes	No	No	Yes	A–, O–
B (+)	B	No	Yes	No	Yes	B+, B– O+, O–
B (–)	B	No	Yes	No	Yes	B–, O–
AB (+)	AB	Yes	Yes	Yes	Yes	A+, A– B+, B– O+, O– Universal recipient
AB (–)	AB	Yes	Yes	Yes	Yes	A– B– O–
O (+)	None	No	No	No	Yes	O+, O–
O (–)	None	No	No	No	Yes	O– Universal donor

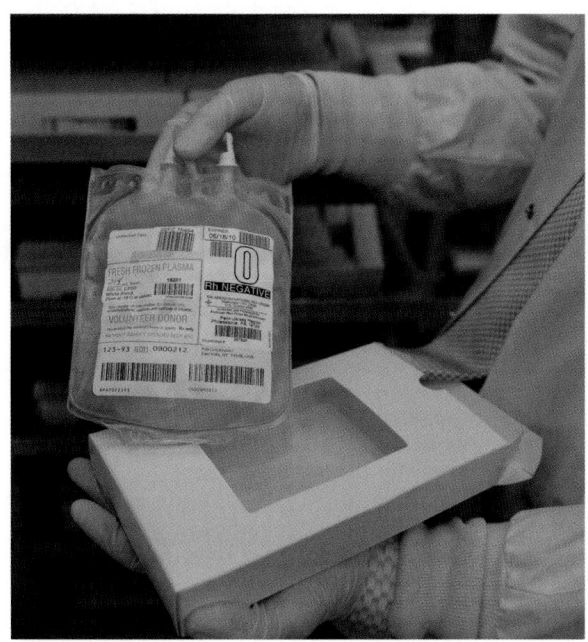

FIG 29-3 Bag of plasma. (*Image courtesy American Red Cross.*)

RH SYSTEM

Although nearly 50 types of Rh antigen may be present on the surface of red blood cells, the type D antigen is widely prevalent and is most likely to elicit an immune response. It is the presence or absence of the D antigen that determines a person's Rh type. A person with the D antigen is Rh positive, and a person without the D antigen is Rh negative (Alexander et al., 2010, AABB, 2011, Gabriel, 2008). Unlike the ABO antigens, there are not naturally occurring antibodies to the Rh(D) antigen. A person with Rh-negative blood must first be exposed to Rh-positive blood before any Rh antibodies are formed. A person with Rh-negative blood who is exposed to a large volume (200 mL or more) of Rh-positive blood will develop enough antibodies to cause a severe

transfusion reaction with repeat exposure. These antibodies take up to 2 weeks to form. Therefore, in the case of massive transfusion as used in trauma situations, Rh-positive blood may be used for a person with Rh-negative blood without adverse effect, provided that the person has not been previously exposed to Rh-positive blood (Alexander et al., 2010; AABB, 2011).

An Rh-negative mother previously exposed to Rh antigen can transfer Rh antibodies across the placenta to an Rh-positive fetus. This can result in severe fetal hemolysis (i.e., the breakdown of red blood cells, with resultant anemia and jaundice) and is often fatal to the infant. To prevent current or future fetal hemolysis, Rh(D) immune globulin (RhoGam) is given by intramuscular injection to the mother. RhoGam can suppress or destroy the fetal Rh-positive blood cells that have passed from the fetal to the maternal circulation.

HUMAN LEUKOCYTE ANTIGEN SYSTEM

Although most commonly linked to transplant rejection, human leukocyte antigens (HLA)s are highly immunogenic antigens that can cause serious transfusion complications. HLA antibodies are located on the cell surface of leukocytes. They may also be found on lymphocytes, granulocytes, monocytes, and platelets (Alexander et al., 2010; AABB, 2011; Gabriel, 2008). HLA complications most commonly seen are:

- Febrile nonhemolytic reaction (FNH).
- Immune-mediated platelet refractoriness.
- Transfusion-related acute lung injury (TRALI).
- Transfusion-associated graft-versus-host disease (TA-GVHD).

EVIDENCE-BASED PRACTICE

Compliance with standards and policies and ongoing education are essential to maintain patient safety and reduce potential errors. Safety and risk management are key factors in transfusion therapy. ABO incompatibilities are one of the most serious errors with transfusions and usually have fatal outcomes (Alexander et al., 2010; AABB, 2011; Gabriel, 2008). A human error most often involves misidentification of the patient or the unit of blood or mislabeling the pretransfusion blood sample. Advances in technology help to decrease transfusion-related errors:

- Bar-code technology helps prevent errors in the identification process between a patient and the compatible blood unit.
- Radiofrequency transponder microchips are used to standardize and document key steps in the blood collection and confirm the recipient–blood unit matching at a patient's bedside.

Advanced technologic laboratory screening procedures also help to ensure safe transfusions with regard to bloodborne pathogens:

- Screening identifies and thereby reduces pathogen transmission.
- Better assessment of blood and plasma cell integrity is available to avoid loss of blood component function.
- Blood alternative therapies with pharmacologic developments such as colloids, crystalloids, erythropoietin, antifibrinolytics, and hematinics reduce the risks associated with transfusing human blood.

PATIENT-CENTERED CARE

When administering blood products, you need to consider a patient's values and cultural beliefs about blood therapy. A person's perception of his or her disease or health condition affects how receptive he or she is to receiving blood. Blood transfusion is often equated to severity of illness. Allay patient anxieties when possible. Some religions do not allow blood transfusions. For example,

members of Jehovah's Witness do not allow blood transfusions or organ donation if it involves blood exchange (Snyder et al., 2008). It is helpful to consult a religious leader when caring for patients in need of blood therapy. Be familiar with agency policies and procedures to follow when patients refuse blood transfusion and inform the health care provider of a patient's decision.

Another aspect of patient-centered care is safety, specifically the prevention of transfusion-related complications. Transfusion-related reactions occur most commonly from clerical error. To ensure safe patient outcomes, the National Quality Forum (NQF) endorses a list of serious reportable events (SREs), which outlines 28 events that are preventable. Regarding transfusion therapy, any "patient death or serious disability associated with a hemolytic reaction due to the administration of ABO/HLA–incompatible blood or blood products" is considered a Care Management Event and must be reported (NQF, 2011).

 Safety Guidelines

1. Administration of blood and blood components requires meticulous attention to detail (e.g., preparation, administration, and monitoring) to prevent life-threatening transfusion reactions (Table 29-3).
2. Ensure that each blood unit is correctly labeled; check against patient's identification.
3. Review agency policy and procedure regarding administration of blood or blood products.
4. Two nurses should verify correct unit and correct patient before administration.

TABLE 29-3	Transfusion Reactions				
Reaction	**Mechanism**	**Onset**	**Signs and Symptoms**	**Prevention**	**Nursing Intervention**
Febrile, nonhemolytic (most common)	Accompanies less than 1% of transfusions; possible sensitivity of recipient to leukocytes or platelets in donor's blood	30 min after initiation to 6 hrs after completion of transfusion	Fever greater than 1°C above baseline, flushing, chills, headache, muscle pain; occurs most frequently in immunosuppressed patients	Use leukocyte-reduced blood products in patients who have experienced febrile nonhemolytic reactions in the past.	**Stop transfusion.** Administer antipyretics as ordered. Monitor temperature every 4 hrs.
Acute hemolytic transfusion reaction	ABO, Rh incompatibility; causes intravascular destruction of transfused RBCs as antibodies in recipient's plasma attach to antigens on donor RBCs.	Within 15 minutes of transfusion initiation	Severe pain in kidney area and chest; increased temperature (up to 41°C or 105°F), increased heart rate; sensation of heat and pain along vein receiving blood; chills, low back pain, headache, nausea, chest or back pain, chest tightness, dyspnea, bronchospasm, anxiety, hypotension, vascular collapse, disseminated intravascular coagulation, possibly death	Carefully identify patient and blood sample obtained for blood typing and compatibility screening. When blood is released from blood bank, match with patient information. Follow agency verification procedures at bedside before transfusion.	**Stop transfusion.** Remove blood product and tubing. Maintain IV access. Notify health care provider. Monitor vital signs at least every 15 min. Administer ordered therapy to correct arterial blood pressure and coagulopathy. Insert Foley catheter. Monitor intake and output hourly. Assess for shock. Dialysis may be required. Obtain blood and urine samples and send to laboratory with unused portion of unit of blood. Document reaction according to agency policy.

TABLE 29-3	Transfusion Reactions—cont'd				
Reaction	**Mechanism**	**Onset**	**Signs and Symptoms**	**Prevention**	**Nursing Intervention**
Delayed hemolytic transfusion reaction	Immune response mounted by recipient against non-ABO donor antigens; usually the result of destruction of transfused RBCs by alloantibodies not detected during cross-match	2-14 days	Unexplained fever, unexplained decrease in Hgb/Hct, increased bilirubin levels, jaundice	Careful cross-matching of donor and recipient blood. Has potential to be missed because it may occur several days after transfusion.	Monitor laboratory values for anemia. (Recognition is important because subsequent transfusions may cause an acute hemolytic reaction.) If detected, notify health care provider and blood bank. Most delayed hemolytic reactions require no treatment.
Allergic reaction (mild-to-moderate)	Caused by recipient allergy to a plasma protein in donor's blood	During transfusion to 1 hr after transfusion	Local erythema, hives, and urticaria, itching or pruritus	May administer antihistamines before transfusion if prescribed.	**Stop transfusion.** Notify health care provider and blood bank. Administer antihistamines as ordered. Monitor and document vital signs every 15 min. Transfusion may be restarted if fever, dyspnea, and wheezing are not present.
Allergic reaction (severe)	Caused by recipient allergy to a donor antigen (usually IgA) Agglutination of RBCs obstructing capillaries and blocking blood flow, causing symptoms to all major organ systems	Within 5-15 min of initiation of transfusion	Coughing, nausea, vomiting, respiratory distress, wheezing, hypotension, loss of consciousness, possible cardiac arrest	Transfusion of saline-washed or leukocyte-depleted RBCs.	This is a life-threatening reaction. **Stop transfusion.** Maintain IV access. Notify health care provider and blood bank. Administer antihistamines, corticosteroids, epinephrine, and antipyretics as ordered. Measure and document vital signs until stable. Initiate cardiopulmonary resuscitation if necessary.
Graft-versus-host disease	Donor lymphocytes are destroyed by recipient's immune system. In immunocompromised patients the donor lymphocytes are identified as foreign; however, patient's immune system is not capable of destroying, and in turn patient's lymphocytes are destroyed.	Days to weeks	Skin rash, fever, jaundice caused by liver dysfunction, bone marrow suppression	Administer irradiated blood and/or leukocyte-depleted RBC products as prescribed.	Administer methotrexate and corticosteroids as ordered.

Continued

TABLE 29-3	Transfusion Reactions—cont'd				
Reaction	**Mechanism**	**Onset**	**Signs and Symptoms**	**Prevention**	**Nursing Intervention**
Circulatory overload	Occurs with transfusion of excessive volume or excessively rapid rate; can lead to pulmonary edema.	Anytime during or within 1-2 hrs after transfusion	Dyspnea, cough, crackles at lung bases, tachypnea, headache, hypertension, tachycardia, increased central venous pressure, distended neck veins	Administer blood or component at prescribed rate, usually no greater than 2-4 mL/kg/hr; pay particular attention to rate and volume in older adults, young children, and patients with cardiac and renal disorders. Administer PRBCs instead of whole blood. Minimize amount of saline infused with transfusion.	Slow or stop transfusion as ordered. Elevate patient's head. Notify health care provider. Administer diuretics as ordered.
Infectious disease transmission	Microorganism contamination of infused product	During transfusion to 2 hrs after transfusion Complete transfusion within 4 hrs	High fever, chills, abdominal cramping, vomiting, diarrhea, profound hypotension, flushed skin, back pain	Proper care of blood or blood product from time of procurement through end of administration.	**Stop transfusion.** Remove blood product and tubing. Maintain IV access. Notify health care provider. Monitor and document vital signs. Obtain samples for blood culture and Gram stain from recipient. Administer IV fluids, broad-spectrum antimicrobials, vasopressors, and steroids as ordered.
Iron overload	Iron from donated blood binds to protein and is not eliminated	May occur with multiple transfusions or chronic transfusion therapy	Cardiac dysfunction, SOB, arrhythmias, heart failure, increased serum transferrin, increased liver enzymes, jaundice	Chelation, phlebotomy, monitor serum iron levels.	Monitor patient for heart failure, cardiac disorder, liver disorder, serum transferrin.

Data modified from Alexander M, et al.: *Infusion nursing: an evidence-based approach,* ed 3, St Louis, 2010, Mosby; and American Association of Blood Banks: *Standards for blood banks and transfusion services.* ed 27, Bethesoa, Md, 2011, The Association.
HF, Heart failure; *Hct,* hematocrit; *Hgb,* hemoglobin; *IV,* intravenous; *PRBCs,* packed red blood cells; *RBC,* red blood cell; *SOB,* shortness of breath.

SKILL 29-1   Initiating Blood Therapy

NSO *Blood Therapy Module / Lessons 1 & 2*

 Video Clip

Blood is administered for different clinical indications (Table 29-4). A patient's medical condition determines which blood component is indicated. A health care provider's order is required for the administration of a blood product. A nurse is responsible for understanding which components are appropriate in various situations. In addition, a nurse must ensure that a blood sample has been collected and sent to the laboratory within 72 hours for typing and compatibility screening. The blood sample collector must be meticulous when labeling the patient's identification information on the blood tube. This is the first step in the prevention of error (Alexander et al., 2010; Gabriel, 2008).

Blood is stored in a refrigerated environment. In emergency situations rapid transfusion of cold blood may lead to dysrhythmias and a reduction of core temperature. Sometimes a blood-warmer machine is used for large transfusions of greater than 50 mL/kg/hr or patients with cold agglutinins (Ackley et al., 2008) (Fig. 29-4).

Do not heat blood products in a microwave or with hot water because this is dangerous and may destroy blood cells.

Delegation and Collaboration

The skill of initiating transfusion therapy cannot be delegated to nursing assistive personnel (NAP). The skill of initiating transfusion therapy by a licensed practical nurse (LPN) varies by state Practice Acts. After the transfusion has been started and the patient is stable, monitoring of a patient by NAP does not relieve a registered nurse (RN) of the responsibility to continue to assess the patient during the transfusion. The nurse instructs the NAP about:

- Frequency of vital sign monitoring needed.
- What to observe such as complaints of shortness of breath, hives, and/or chills and reporting this information to the nurse.

TABLE 29-4	Blood and Blood Component Products*				
Blood Product and Source	**Volume and Infusion Time**	**Able to Transmit HIV/HBV**	**ABO/RH Testing Needed**	**Actions/Uses**
Whole blood—Single donor: allogeneic or autologous	300-550 mL Within 4 hrs	Yes	Yes—Must be ABO identical; Rh—Yes	Replaces red cell mass and plasma volume; expected to raise Hgb 1 g/100 mL and Hct by 3% in nonhemorrhaging adult.
Packed RBCs—Single donor: allogeneic or autologous	250-350 mL Within 4 hrs	Yes	Yes/Yes	Preferred method of replacing red blood cell mass; expected to raise Hgb/Hct level same as whole blood.
Leukocyte-poor RBCs— Single donor: allogeneic or directed	200-250 mL Within 4 hrs	Yes	Yes/Yes	Replaces RBCs while preventing febrile, nonhemolytic transfusion reactions; reduces risk for CMV transmission.
Irradiated RBCs—Single donor: allogeneic or directed	250-350 mL Within 4 hrs	Yes	Yes/Yes	Replaces RBCs while preventing transfusion-associated graft-versus-host disease; used in immunodeficient patients (any blood component can be irradiated).
Fresh frozen plasma— Single donor	200-250 mL Infuse within 24 hrs of thawing Within 4 hrs	Yes	Yes/No	Replaces plasma without RBCs or platelets; contains most coagulation factors and complement; used in control of bleeding when replacement of coagulation factors is needed (e.g., DIC, TTP).
Cryoprecipitate—Multiple donors, pooled	5-20 mL/unit; 1 unit/10 kg body weight 1-2 mL/min Infuse within 6 hrs of thawing or 4 hrs of pooling	Yes	No/No	Replaces factors VIII, XIII, von Willebrand's factor, and fibrinogen.
Platelets—Multiple/ random donor, pooled	40-70 mL/unit; 1 unit/10 kg body weight Within 6 hrs of pooling	Yes	Yes/Yes	Used in patients with thrombocytopenia. Certain microaggregate filters are not to be used with platelets—check manufacturer instructions.
Platelets—Single donor	200-500 mL Within 4 hrs	Yes	Yes/Yes	Single-donor platelets are most useful in immunologically refractory patients when given as HLA matched with recipient. Each unit expected to raise platelet count by 5000-10,000/mL in a 70-kg patient.
Colloid components— Albumin 5% pooled	250-500 mL 1-10 mL/min	No	No/No	Oncotically equivalent to plasma; used to treat hypoproteinemia in burns and hypoalbuminemia in shock and ARDs; used to support blood pressure in dialysis and acute liver failure.
Colloid components— Albumin 25% pooled	50-100 mL 0.2-0.4 mL/min	No	No/No	Increases circulating blood volume by increasing intravascular oncotic pressure.

Data modified from Alexander M et al.: *Infusion nursing: an evidence-based approach*, ed 3, St Louis, 2010, Mosby; American Association of Blood Banks (AABB): *Standards for blood banks and transfusion services*, ed 27, Bethesda, Md, 2011, The Association.
*Other less commonly used blood components include factors VIII and IX concentrates, granulocytes, immunoglobulin, and saline-washed RBCs.
ARD, Acute respiratory disease; *CMV*, cytomegalovirus; *DIC*, disseminated intravascular coagulation; *HBV*, hepatitis B virus; *Hct*, hematocrit; *Hgb*, hemoglobin; *HIV*, human immunodeficiency virus; *HLA*, human leukocyte antigen; *RBC*, red blood cell; *TTP*, thrombotic thrombocytopenic purpura.

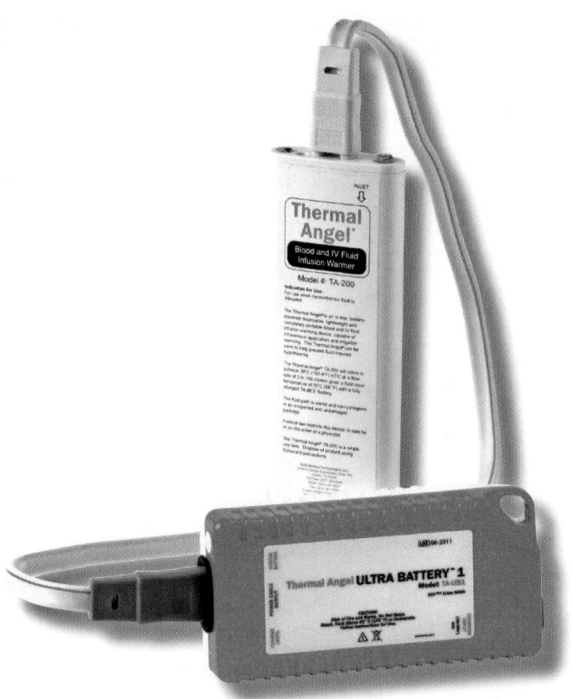

FIG 29-4 Blood-warming system. *(Used with permission of Estill Medical Technologies, Inc. All rights reserved.)*

- Obtaining blood components from the blood bank (check agency policy).

Equipment
❑ Y-type blood administration set (in-line filter) (NOTE: Depending on blood product, special tubing and filter are necessary.)
❑ Prescribed blood product
❑ 250-mL bag 0.9% NaCl (normal saline) intravenous (IV) solution
❑ Antiseptic wipes (chlorhexidine based)
❑ Clean gloves
❑ Tape
❑ Vital sign equipment: Thermometer, blood pressure cuff, and stethoscope
❑ Signed transfusion consent form

Optional Equipment
❑ Rapid infusion pump
❑ Electronic infusion device (EID) (Verify that pump can be used to deliver blood and blood products)
❑ Leukocyte-depleting filter
❑ Blood warmer
❑ Pressure bag
❑ Pulse oximeter

STEP	RATIONALE

ASSESSMENT

1 Verify health care provider's order for specific blood or blood product, date, time to begin transfusion, duration, and any pretransfusion or posttransfusion medications to administer.

A health care provider's order must be present before transfusing a blood product. Verifying order helps to ensure that appropriate blood component will be administered (Alexander et al., 2010; INS, 2011a). Premedications such as an antihistamine or antipyretic may be ordered, especially if patient demonstrated previous transfusion sensitivity.

2 Obtain patient's transfusion history and note known allergies and previous transfusion reactions. Verify that type and cross-match have been completed within 72 hours of transfusion.

Identifies patient's prior response(s) to transfusion of blood components. If patient has experienced reaction in the past, anticipate similar reaction and be prepared to rapidly intervene.

3 Verify that IV cannula is patent and without complications such as infiltration or phlebitis.

Patent IV ensures that transfusion will be infused within established time guidelines.

    a Administer blood or blood components to an adult, using a 14- to 24-gauge short peripheral catheter.

The gauge of the IV cannula should be appropriate for accommodating the infusion of blood and/or blood components (INS, 2011a). Large-gauge cannulas promote rapid flow of blood components.

    b Transfuse a neonate or pediatric patient using a 22- to 24-gauge device (INS, 2011a).
    c A 1.9 Fr is the smallest central venous access device (CVAD) that can be used (INS, 2011a).

Use of smaller cannula gauges such as 24 gauge often requires blood bank to divide the unit so each half can be infused within allotted time or pressure-assisted devices.

4 Assess laboratory values such as hematocrit, coagulation values, platelet count.

Provides baseline for later evaluation of patient response to transfusion.

5 Check that patient has properly completed and signed transfusion consent before retrieving blood.

Agencies require patients to sign consent forms before receiving blood component therapy because of inherent risks (INS, 2011a).

6 Know indications or reasons for transfusion (e.g., packed red blood cells [PRBCs] for patient with low hematocrit level from gastrointestinal bleeding or surgery blood loss).

Allows you to anticipate patient's response to therapy.

7 Obtain and record pretransfusion baseline vital signs (temperature, respirations, and blood pressure). If patient is febrile (temperature greater than 37.8°C [100°F]), notify health care provider before initiating transfusion.

Change from baseline vital signs during infusion alerts nurse to potential transfusion reaction or adverse effect of therapy (INS, 2011a).

STEP	RATIONALE
8 Assess patient's need for IV fluids or medications while transfusion is infusing.	If IV medications need to be administered during transfusion, second IV site is necessary. No other infusions are to be administered through same IV site as blood transfusion. Administer blood or blood components only with 0.9% normal saline solution (INS, 2011a).
9 Assess patient's understanding of procedure and rationale.	Alleviates some of the anxiety patient may have.

NURSING DIAGNOSES

- Activity intolerance
- Decreased cardiac output
- Deficient fluid volume

- Deficient knowledge regarding transfusion

- Excess fluid volume
- Ineffective peripheral tissue perfusion

Related factors are individualized based on patient's condition or needs.

PLANNING

1 Expected outcomes following completion of the procedure:	
• Patient verbalizes understanding of rationale for therapy.	Indicates patient's understanding and ability to make an informed decision for consent.
• Patient experiences improved activity tolerance.	Oxygenation is improved.
• Mucous membranes are pink and patient has brisk capillary refill.	Tissue perfusion is improved.
• Patient's cardiac output returns to baseline.	Intravascular volume is restored.
• Patient's systolic blood pressure improves, and urine output is 0.5 to 1 mL/kg/hr.	Parameters reflect optimal fluid status and adequate renal blood flow.
• Patient's laboratory values improve in targeted areas (e.g., hematocrit, coagulation values, platelet count).	Indicates that patient responds appropriately to blood or blood component infusion.
2 Explain procedure to patient and family caregiver.	Promotes patient's cooperation and ability to report complications.

IMPLEMENTATION

1 Preadministration protocol:	
a Obtain blood component from blood bank following agency protocol (see illustration). Blood transfusion must be initiated within 30 minutes after release from laboratory or blood bank (INS, 2011a).	Timely acquisition ensures that product is safe to administer. Agency protocol usually encompasses safeguards to ensure quality control throughout transfusion process.
b Check blood bag for any signs of contamination (i.e., clumping/clots, gas bubbles, purplish color) and presence of leaks.	Do not transfuse blood if integrity is compromised. Air bubbles, clots, and discoloration indicate bacterial contamination or inadequate anticoagulation of stored component and are contraindications for transfusion of that product (Alexander et al., 2010; AABB, 2011; Gabriel, 2008).
	Blood serves as medium for bacterial growth.

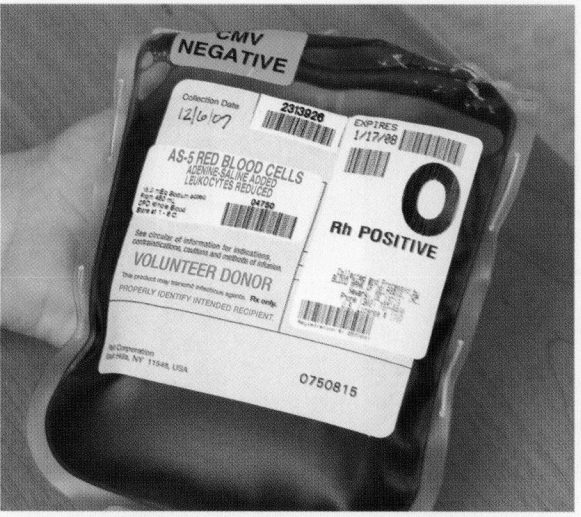

STEP 1a Unit of blood with label.

STEP	RATIONALE
c Verbally compare and correctly verify patient, blood product, and type with another person considered qualified by your agency (e.g., RN or LPN) before initiating transfusion. Check the following: (1) Identify patient using two identifiers (i.e., name and birthday or name and account number) according to agency policy. Compare identifiers in MAR/medical record with information on patient's identification bracelet and/or ask patient to state name. (2) Transfusion record number and patient's identification number match.	Strict adherence to verification procedures before administration of blood or blood components reduces risk for administering wrong blood to patient. Misidentification of patient is one of the most important factors in transfusion errors (INS, 2011a). Ensures correct patient. Complies with The Joint Commission standards and improves patient safety (TJC, 2012). Prevents accidental administration of wrong component.

Clinical Decision Point *If you notice a discrepancy during verification procedure, do not administer the product. Notify blood bank and appropriate personnel as indicated by agency policy. Return blood to blood bank until discrepancy is resolved (INS, 2011a).*

STEP	RATIONALE
(3) Patient's name is correct on all documents. Check identification number and date of birth on identification band and patient record. (4) Check unit number on blood bag with blood bank form to ensure that they are the same. (5) Blood type matches on transfusion record and blood bag. Verify that component received from blood bank is same component that health care provider ordered (e.g., packed red cells, platelets) (see illustration). (6) Check that patient's blood type and Rh type are compatible with donor blood type and Rh type (e.g., Patient A+: Donor A+ or 0+). (7) Check expiration date and time on unit of blood. (8) Just before initiating transfusion, check patient identification information with blood unit label information (see illustration). Do not administer blood to patient without an identification bracelet. (9) Both individuals verify patient and unit identification record process as directed by agency policy. **d** Review purpose of transfusion and ask patient to report any changes that he or she may feel during the transfusion. **e** Empty urine drainage collection container or have patient void.	Ensures that patient receives correct therapy. One of most common causes of patient receiving incorrect transfusion is obtaining wrong blood component from blood bank (Alexander et al., 2010; Gabriel, 2008; INS, 2011a). Verifies accurate donor blood type and compatibility. Never use expired blood because cell components deteriorate and may contain excess citrate ions (Alexander et al., 2010; AABB, 2011; INS, 2011a). Serves as last point of patient and blood confirmation and is most important step in verification process (Alexander et al., 2010; INS, 2011a; INS, 2011b). Documentation is the legal medical record. Signs and symptoms of transfusion reactions include chills, low back pain, shortness of breath, rash, hives, or itching (Alexander et al., 2010). Prompt notification aids in early intervention. If transfusion reaction occurs, urine specimen containing urine produced after initiation of transfusion will be sent to the laboratory (Alexander et al., 2010).

Clinical Decision Point *Initiate the blood transfusion within 30 minutes from time of release from blood bank. If this cannot be completed because of factors such as an elevated temperature, immediately return the blood to the blood bank and retrieve it when you can administer it.*

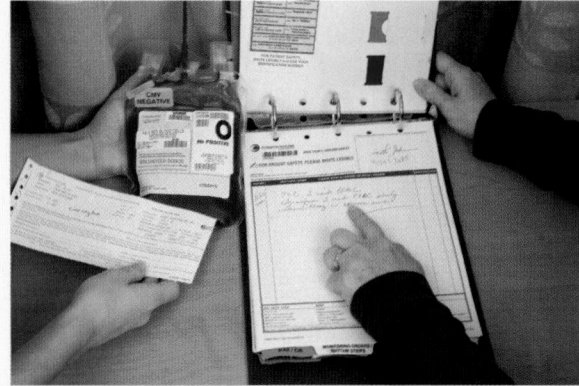

STEP 1c(5) Two clinicians verifying blood type with health care provider order.

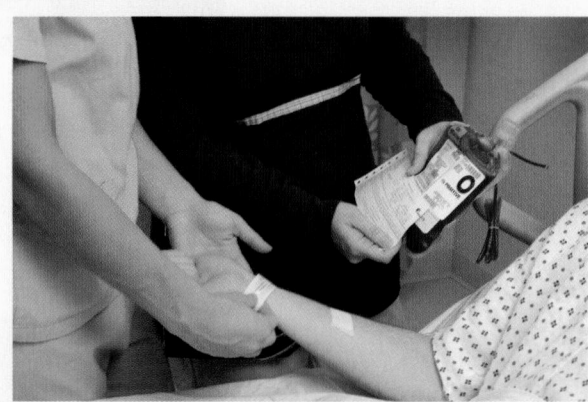

STEP 1c(8) Two clinicians verifying identification of patient and blood product.

STEP	RATIONALE
2 Administration:	
a Perform hand hygiene. Apply clean gloves.	Using standard precautions reduces risk for transmission of microorganisms.
b Open Y-tubing blood administration set for single unit. Use multiset if multiple units are to be transfused.	Y-tubing facilitates maintenance of IV access with normal saline in case patient will need more than 1 unit of blood.
c Set all clamp(s) to "off" position.	Setting clamps to "off" position prevents accidentally spilling and wasting product.
d Spike 0.9% normal saline IV bag with one of Y-tubing spikes. Hang bag on IV pole and prime tubing. Open upper clamp on normal saline side of tubing and squeeze drip chamber until fluid covers filter and one third to one half of drip chamber (see illustration).	Primes tubing with fluid to eliminate air in Y-tubing. Closing clamp prevents spillage and waste of fluid.
e Maintain clamp on blood product side of Y-tubing in "off" position. Open common tubing clamp to finish priming tubing to distal end of tubing connector. Close tubing clamp when tubing is filled with saline. All three tubing clamps should be closed. Maintain protective sterile cap on tubing connector.	This will completely prime tubing with saline, and IV line is ready to be connected to the patient's vascular access device (VAD).
f Prepare blood component for administration. Gently agitate blood unit bag, turning back and forth, upside down. Remove protective covering from access port. Spike blood component unit with other Y connection. Close normal saline clamp above filter, open clamp above filter to blood unit, and prime tubing with blood. Blood will flow into drip chamber (see illustration). Tap filter chamber to ensure that residual air is removed.	Gentle agitation suspends red blood cells in anticoagulant. Protective barrier drape may be used to catch any potential blood spillage. Tubing is primed with blood unit and ready for transfusion into patient.

Clinical Decision Point *Normal saline is compatible with blood products, unlike solutions that contain dextrose, which cause coagulation of blood. Only use 0.9% normal saline solution to administer blood. No other solutions are to be administered with blood (piggybacked) (INS, 2011a).*

g Maintaining asepsis, attach primed tubing to patient's VAD. Open common tubing clamp and regulate blood infusion to allow only 2 mL/min to infuse in initial 15 minutes.	This initiates infusion of blood product into patient's vein.

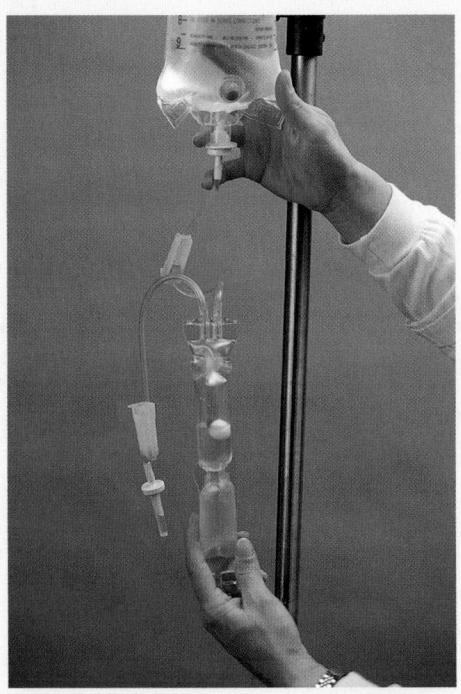

STEP 2d Blood administration set primed with normal saline.

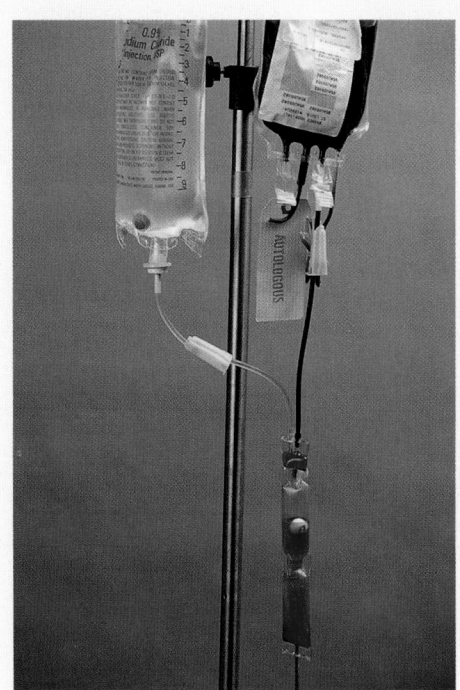

STEP 2f Unit of blood connected to Y-tubing setup.

STEP	RATIONALE
h Remain with patient during first 15 minutes of transfusion. Initial flow rate during this time should be 2 mL/min or 20 gtt/min (using macrodrip of 10 gtt/mL).	Most transfusion reactions occur within first 15 minutes of a transfusion (Snyder et al., 2008). Infusing small amount of blood component initially minimizes volume of blood to which patient is exposed, thereby minimizing severity of reaction.

Clinical Decision Point *If signs of a transfusion reaction occur, stop the transfusion, start normal saline with a new primed tubing directly to the VAD, and notify the health care provider immediately (see Skill 29-2). Do not infuse saline through existing tubing because it will cause blood in tubing to enter patient.*

i Monitor patient's vital signs at 5 minutes, 15 minutes, and every 30 minutes until 1 hr after transfusion (AABB, 2011) or per agency policy.	Frequently monitoring vital signs helps to quickly alert you to transfusion reaction (Alexander et al., 2010; Gabriel, 2008; INS, 2011a).
j If there is no transfusion reaction, regulate rate of transfusion according to health care provider's orders. Check drop factor for blood tubing.	Maintaining prescribed rate of flow decreases risk for fluid volume excess while restoring vascular volume. Drop factor for most blood tubing is 10 gtt/mL.

Clinical Decision Point *Do not let a unit of blood hang for more than 4 hours because of danger of bacterial growth. Administration sets should be changed at the completion of each unit or every 4 hours to reduce bacterial contamination (INS, 2011a). Never store blood in an agency refrigerator.*

Clinical Decision Point *Never inject medication into the same IV line with a blood component because of the risk for contaminating the blood product with pathogens and the possibility of incompatibility. Maintain a separate IV access if patient requires IV solutions or medications (INS, 2011a).*

k After blood has infused, clear IV line with 0.9% normal saline and discard blood bag according to agency policy. When consecutive units are ordered, maintain IV patency with 0.9% normal saline at keep vein open (KVO) rate and retrieve subsequent unit for administration.	Infusing IV saline solution infuses remainder of blood in IV tubing and keeps IV line patent for supportive measures in case of transfusion reaction (INS, 2011a).
l Appropriately dispose of all supplies. Remove gloves and perform hand hygiene.	Standard precautions during transfusion reduce transmission of microorganisms.

EVALUATION

1 Observe IV site and status of infusion each time vital signs are taken.	Detects presence of IV-related complications (e.g., infiltration, phlebitis) and verifies continuous and safe infusion of blood product.
2 Observe for any changes in vital signs and any signs of transfusion reactions such as chills, flushing, itching, dyspnea, or rash.	Compare presenting signs and symptoms to baseline assessment of patient before transfusion. These are early signs of transfusion reaction (see Table 29-3).
3 Observe patient and assess laboratory values to determine response to administration of blood component.	Aids in determining whether goals of therapy have been reached or if further blood component therapy will be required. Laboratory results may not reflect transfusion reaction for several hours.

Unexpected Outcomes

1 Patient displays signs and symptoms of transfusion reaction.

2 Patient develops infiltration or phlebitis at venipuncture site.

3 Rate of infusion slows in absence of infiltration.

4 Fluid overload occurs and/or patient exhibits difficulty breathing or has crackles on auscultation.

Related Interventions

- Stop transfusion immediately.
- Disconnect blood tubing at VAD hub and cap distal end with sterile connector to maintain sterile system.
- Connect normal saline-primed tubing at VAD hub to prevent any subsequent blood from infusing from tubing.
- Keep vein open with slow infusion of normal saline at 10 to 12 gtt/min to ensure venous patency and maintain venous access for medication or to resume transfusion.
- Notify health care provider.
- See Table 29-3 for interventions.
- Remove IV line and insert new VAD (above compromised site or in opposite extremity). Restart product if remainder can be infused within 4 hours of initiation of transfusion.
- Institute nursing measures to reduce discomfort at infiltrated or phlebotic area.
- Verify that IV catheter is patent and all clamps are open.
- Gently flush IV line with normal saline or use pressure bag or EID that permits blood transfusion.
- Slow or stop transfusion, elevate head of bed, and inform health care provider of physical findings.
- Administer diuretics, morphine, and/or oxygen as ordered by health care provider.
- Continue frequent assessments and closely monitor vital signs and intake and output.

Recording and Reporting

- Record pretransfusion medications, vital signs, location and condition of IV site, and patient education.
- Record the type and volume of blood component, blood unit/donor/recipient identification, compatibility, and expiration date according to agency policy, along with patient's response to therapy. Document on the transfusion record, nurses' notes, electronic health record (EHR), medication administration record, flow sheet, and/or intake and output sheet, depending on agency policy.
- Record volume of normal saline and blood component infused.
- Report signs and symptoms of a transfusion reaction immediately to the health care provider.
- Record amount of blood received by autotransfusion and patient's response to therapy.
- Report to health care provider any intratransfusion/posttransfusion deterioration in cardiac, pulmonary, and/or renal status.
- Record vital signs before, during, and after transfusion.

Special Considerations

Teaching

- Instruct patient regarding rationale for transfusion and anticipated amount of time for completion of transfusion.
- Discuss with patient and family caregiver the rationale for frequent vital sign monitoring throughout transfusion.
- Inform patient and family caregiver to notify nurse if patient experiences itching, swelling, dizziness, dyspnea, low back pain, and/or chest pain because these may indicate a transfusion reaction.
- Instruct patient to inform nurse if pain, swelling, or redness occurs at IV site because these indicate infiltration.

Pediatric

- Infuse the first 50 mL or 20% of volume (whichever is smaller) of a blood transfusion very slowly in a pediatric patient. Nurse should stay with the child during this time frame (Hockenberry and Wilson, 2011).

- Smaller portions of blood are often available for use with pediatric patients (AABB, 2011).
- A 27-, 26-, or 24-gauge cannula can be used to infuse PRBCs without significant hemolysis (Alexander et al., 2010; Hockenberry and Wilson, 2011).
- Umbilical catheters or catheters placed in the small saphenous veins are commonly used in infants and/or pediatric patients (Alexander et al., 2010).

Gerontologic

- Some older adults have decreased cardiac function, thus requiring a slower infusion time. Half units may be obtained if a patient is unable to tolerate the volume in a whole unit of blood or blood component.
- In older adults at risk for circulatory overload, regulate flow rate at 1 mL/kg/hr.

Home Care

- Patients who have had prior transfusion reactions, acute angina, or heart failure are not good candidates for home transfusion.
- Initiate the transfusion as soon as possible after component is obtained from blood bank. Transport blood in an insulated container with coolant to maintain temperature.
- Nursing personnel must be present during the entire transfusion process and for 30 to 60 minutes after transfusion.
- When blood sample is obtained for blood typing and crossmatching, attach identification band to patient with full name and identification number used by laboratory. This provides clear identification of patient when blood component transfusion is initiated.
- Instruct patient and family caregiver regarding signs and symptoms of a delayed hemolytic transfusion reaction (i.e., unexplained fever, decrease in hemoglobin and hematocrit levels 2 to 14 days after transfusion) so they can report them and receive treatment if necessary.
- Return the container, empty bags, and tubing to the home care agency after completion of the transfusion.

SKILL 29-2 Monitoring for Adverse Transfusion Reactions

NSO *Blood Therapy Module / Lesson 3*

Adverse transfusion reactions may occur any time during a transfusion of blood products. Life-threatening reactions usually occur within the first 15 minutes of transfusion. Remain with a patient during this time to monitor physiologic responses.

Several types of adverse reactions may result from a blood transfusion (see Table 29-3). A hemolytic reaction is a systemic response to the administration of a blood product that is incompatible with that of the recipient. The product contains allergens to which the recipient is sensitive or allergic, or it is contaminated with pathogens. Some patients who have a history of frequent transfusion may receive premedication with diphenhydramine (Benadryl) to combat acquired sensitivities.

Before a transfusion each blood unit undergoes extensive serologic testing to reduce the risk for patients acquiring a bloodborne disease. Symptoms that indicate an adverse reaction range from fever, chills, and skin rash to hypotension and cardiac arrest. Some patients also experience a delayed transfusion reaction, which sometimes does not occur for days or weeks after the transfusion (Alexander et al., 2010; AABB, 2011). Other possible adverse outcomes that result from transfusion therapy include transmission of diseases, circulatory overload, and transfusion-related acute lung injury (TRALI), characterized by noncardiogenic pulmonary edema with an onset within 6 hours of transfusion (Alexander et al., 2010; Busch, 2008). The most fatal risk for transfusion-associated death is the erroneous transfusion of ABO-incompatible allogeneic units (AABB, 2011; King, 2008). Agencies must report fatalities that occur as the result of a transfusion reaction to the Food and Drug Administration (NQF, 2011).

Delegation and Collaboration

The skill of monitoring for adverse blood transfusion reactions by a licensed practical nurse (LPN) varies by state Nurse Practice acts. After the transfusion has been started and the patient is stable, monitoring of a patient by nursing assistive personnel (NAP) does not relieve a registered nurse (RN) of the responsibility to continue to assess the patient during the transfusion. The nurse instructs the NAP about:

- Frequency of vital sign monitoring needed.
- The signs and symptoms of a transfusion reaction that patient may exhibit and to immediately report these to the nurse.

STEP	RATIONALE
ASSESSMENT	
1 With initiation of a transfusion, observe patient for fever with or without chills.	Fever indicates onset of an acute hemolytic reaction, febrile nonhemolytic reaction, or bacterial sepsis.
2 Assess patient for tachycardia and/or tachypnea and dyspnea.	Indicates acute hemolytic reaction or circulatory overload. In the case of circulatory overload, a cough may accompany these symptoms.
3 Observe patient for drop in blood pressure.	Hypotension indicates infectious disease transmission, an acute hemolytic reaction, and anaphylaxis.
4 Observe patient for hives or skin rash, including assessment of trunk and back.	These are early indications of an allergic reaction, anaphylaxis, or graft-versus-host disease, which occurs after transfusion.
5 Observe patient for flushing.	These are early indications of an acute hemolytic reaction or a febrile nonhemolytic reaction. Sometimes localized flushing presents with an allergic reaction.
6 Observe patient for gastrointestinal symptoms.	Nausea and vomiting are present in acute hemolytic transfusion reactions, anaphylactic reactions, or infectious disease transmission.

Clinical Decision Point *Report sepsis and other infections caused by a transfusion to the blood bank and an agency infection control department, which will communicate the information to the state health department and the Centers for Disease Control and Prevention (NQF, 2011).*

7 Observe patient for wheezing, chest pain, and possible cardiac arrest.	These are all indications of an anaphylactic reaction.
8 Be alert to patient complaints of headache or muscle pain in presence of fever.	Both indicate febrile nonhemolytic reaction.
9 Monitor patient for disseminated intravascular coagulation (DIC), renal failure, anemia, and hemoglobinemia/hemoglobinuria by reviewing laboratory test results (complete blood count [CBC] with differential, hemoglobin [Hgb], hematocrit [Hct]).	All are late signs of an acute hemolytic reaction.
10 Auscultate patient's lungs and monitor central venous pressure (CVP) if possible.	Crackles in bases of lungs and rising CVP are indications of circulatory overload.
11 Observe patient for jaundice and increased liver enzyme levels, indicating liver damage; and decreased red blood cells (RBCs), white blood cells (WBCs), and platelets, indicating bone marrow suppression.	These indicate graft-versus-host disease and would occur following transfusion.

STEP	RATIONALE
12 In patients receiving massive transfusions, observe for mild hypothermia, cardiac dysrhythmias, hypotension, hypocalcemia, and hemochromatosis (iron overload).	Cold blood products affect cardiac conduction system, resulting in ventricular dysrhythmias. Other cardiac dysrhythmias, hypotension, and tingling indicate hypocalcemia, which occurs when citrate (used as a preservative for some blood products) combines with patient's calcium. Iron overload may occur after 10 transfusions (see Table 29-3). It usually occurs in patients who require chronic transfusions.

NURSING DIAGNOSES

- Acute pain
- Anxiety
- Decreased cardiac output
- Excess fluid volume
- Hyperthermia
- Hypothermia
- Impaired gas exchange
- Risk for infection

Related factors are individualized based on patient's condition or needs.

PLANNING

1 Expected outcomes following completion of the procedure:	
• Patient's cardiac parameters (heart rate, blood pressure, CVP) return to baseline.	Intravascular volume is restored, reaction reversed.
• Patient maintains core body temperature of 36° to 37.2°C (97° to 99°F).	Helps to confirm absence of transfusion reaction, infection, and sepsis.
• Patient has urine output of 0.5 to 1 mL/kg/hr.	Reflects optimal fluid status.
• Patient maintains oxygen saturation of greater than 95%.	Improved tissue perfusion.
• Patient is comfortable and calm.	Absence of transfusion reaction. Appropriate nursing measures keeps patient at ease.
2 Explain treatment of reaction to patient and family caregiver.	Calms anxiety and helps patient/family caregiver anticipate nurse's actions.

IMPLEMENTATION

1 If you suspect transfusion reaction:	
a **Immediately stop transfusion.**	Severity of reaction is related to amount of blood component infused and cause of reaction. It is critical to prevent any more blood from infusing into patient.
b Remove blood component and tubing containing blood product. Replace them with new bag of 0.9% normal saline and tubing (see Chapter 28). Connect tubing to hub of intravenous (IV) catheter. *Exception:* If patient symptoms suggest mild allergic reaction, stop transfusion, administer antihistamine, and restart or discontinue transfusion per health care provider's order.	Prevents additional blood in tubing from being infused.
c Maintain patent IV line using 0.9% normal saline.	Normal saline keeps patent IV and provides route for emergency medications and fluids.
d Obtain vital signs. Remain with patient for continuous monitoring and assessment. Do not leave patient alone.	Vital signs are objective measure of patient's condition, which can deteriorate rapidly.
e Notify health care provider.	Transfusion reactions require immediate medical intervention. Follow protocol for emergency interventions for anaphylactic reactions.
f Notify blood bank.	Blood bank has procedure to follow when notified of transfusion reaction.
g Obtain blood samples (if needed) from extremity opposite extremity receiving transfusion. Check agency policy regarding number and type of tubes to be used.	Typically one tube of blood will be cross-matched to pretransfusion sample to ensure that correct blood was given to recipient. Blood will be checked for antibodies to determine type of reaction. A second sample will be checked for free hemoglobin in serum, indicating hemolysis, and bilirubin level should be obtained.
h Return remainder of blood component and attached blood tubing to blood bank according to agency policy.	A sample of this blood will be cross-matched to patient's pretransfusion and posttransfusion samples to determine if error in cross-matching occurred.

STEP	RATIONALE
i Monitor patient's vital signs every 15 minutes or more frequently if needed.	Maintains ongoing assessment of patient's cardiopulmonary status and response to treatment.
j Administer prescribed medications according to type and severity of transfusion reaction.	Follow medical protocol or health care provider's orders.
(1) Epinephrine	Stimulates sympathetic nervous system to relieve respiratory distress and combat vasodilation in anaphylaxis.
(2) Antihistamine	Diminishes some aspects of allergic response by blocking histamine receptors.
(3) Antibiotics	Administered when bacterial contamination/sepsis is suspected.
(4) Antipyretics/analgesics	Administered to relieve fever and discomfort in acute hemolytic reactions, febrile nonhemolytic reactions, graft-versus-host disease, and bacterial sepsis.
(5) Diuretics/morphine	Treats circulatory overload by reducing intravascular volume (diuresis) and decreasing vascular tone (opioid effect).
(6) Corticosteroids	Stabilizes cell membranes, decreasing histamine release. Administered in severe allergic reactions.
(7) IV fluids	Rapid administration of IV fluids counteracts some symptoms of anaphylactic shock.
k In the event of cardiac arrest, initiate cardiopulmonary resuscitation (see Chapter 27).	Anaphylaxis can quickly lead to cardio-pulmonary arrest. Prompt resuscitation may prevent further complications.
l Obtain first voided urine sample and send to laboratory. You may need to insert a Foley catheter to obtain the urine (see Chapter 33).	Hemoglobinuria occurs with acute hemolytic reactions. Degree of damage to kidneys is influenced by pH of urine and rate of urinary excretion. Attempts will be made to initiate diuresis and alkalinize urine. If kidney damage is severe, dialysis may be required.

EVALUATION

1 Continue monitoring patient for signs and symptoms of transfusion reactions.	Continued monitoring of patient's cardiopulmonary status and physiologic response will indicate if reaction has been reversed.

Unexpected Outcomes
1 Patient's physiologic status worsens.

Related Interventions
- Appropriate interventions depend on type of transfusion reaction. Table 29-3 provides general guidelines.

Recording and Reporting
- Document the exact time transfusion reaction was first noted, all vital signs and other physiologic assessments, treatments instituted, and patient response in medical record. Complete transfusion reaction report (see agency policy).
- Immediately report presence of transfusion reaction and patient's physical assessment findings to nurse in charge and health care provider.

Special Considerations
Teaching
- Teach patients and family caregiver signs and symptoms of transfusion reactions and steps to take if they occur.
Pediatric
- Irradiated RBCs and platelets are preferable in children under 6 years of age because of their immature immune systems and to avoid graft-versus-host disease.

Gerontologic
- Administer blood components cautiously to older adults, considering both rate and amount of infusion, because they are at risk for developing circulatory overload.
Home Care
- Certain adverse outcomes (development of hepatitis) or transfusion reactions (delayed hemolysis) occur days to weeks after patient has received transfusion and may become evident in the home setting. It is important that patient, family caregiver, and home care workers be aware of signs and symptoms of these adverse occurrences and steps to be taken should they occur.

Critical Thinking Exercises

Catherine Cooper is a 68-year-old woman scheduled for a right total knee replacement in 6 weeks. She has a history of previous injury from years of playing tennis and basketball. She states that she is concerned about the possibility of receiving a blood transfusion. She has read stories of people contracting diseases and viruses, and her friends have told her about someone who became very ill from a transfusion.

1 You are conducting Ms. Cooper's preoperative planning. How should you respond to her concerns?

2 Ms. Cooper decided to donate a unit of blood before her operation in the event that she needed transfusion therapy after surgery. She comments to you that she is so glad that she doesn't have to worry about any problems since she is receiving her own blood. What can you tell her about what to expect about her blood donation?

3 Following type and cross, it is determined that Mrs. Cooper has AB+ blood. Which type of blood can she receive? Which type of antigens does she carry on her red blood cells?

4 Describe your responsibilities associated with initiating and monitoring the transfusion.

5 The health care provider orders another transfusion of red blood cells. Because Ms. Cooper had only 1 unit of autologous blood, she consents to a unit of allogeneic blood. Within 15 minutes of the blood initiation, Ms. Cooper complains of itching. Which actions should you take?

REVIEW QUESTIONS

1 The nurse is preparing a blood transfusion infusion set. Which solution should be used to prime the tubing?
1 0.45% sodium chloride ($\frac{1}{2}$ NS)
2 Dextrose 5% in 0.45% sodium chloride ($D_5\frac{1}{2}$NS)
3 0.9% sodium chloride (normal saline [NS])
4 Dextrose 5% in 0.9% sodium chloride (D_5NS)

2 A patient with A– blood type needs a blood transfusion. Which blood types are appropriate for the patient to receive?
1 A+ or A–
2 A– or O+
3 A– or O–
4 A+ or AB–

3 A patient is to receive blood that has been stored for a long period of time. Which recent laboratory value should the nurse check before administering the unit?
1 Sodium
2 Hematocrit
3 Hemoglobin
4 Potassium

4 A patient is to receive a blood transfusion. Which nursing action has the greatest impact on preventing a potential transfusion reaction?
1 Administering an antihistamine 15 minutes before the transfusion
2 Comparing the patient's identification bracelet with the blood bag label number
3 Ensuring that the patient knows his or her blood type
4 Obtaining the patient's previous transfusion history

5 A patient receiving a blood transfusion begins having signs and symptoms of a transfusion reaction. In addition to stopping the transfusion and assessing vital signs, what else should the nurse do?
1 Hang a new infusion setup with D_5W to maintain an access for medications
2 Finish infusing the blood remaining in the tubing and flush the tubing with the normal saline hanging on the Y-tubing
3 Keep the existing tubing patent with a dextrose solution in case diphenhydramine is needed
4 Hang a new infusion setup with normal saline to maintain an intravenous (IV) access

6 Place the following steps for the administration of a unit of packed red blood cells (PRBCs) in the correct order.
1 Verbally compare and correctly verify patient and blood product
2 Check appearance of blood for leaks, bubbles, clots, or purplish color
3 Prepare Y-tubing administration set with 0.9% normal saline solution (NSS)
4 Obtain baseline vital signs

7 Anticoagulant preservative citrate-phosphate-dextrose-adenine (CPDA-1) maintains the shelf life for donated blood by how many days?
1 21
2 14
3 35
4 42

8 Human leukocyte antigen (HLA) complications include:
1 Fetal hemolysis.
2 Transfusion-related acute lung injury (TRALI).
3 Rh incompatibility.
4 No reaction.

9 During the administration of blood the health care provider orders intravenous (IV) antibiotics to be infused. The most appropriate intervention is to:
1 Stop the transfusion.
2 Piggyback into the transfusion.
3 Question the order.
4 Start a new IV site.

10 Administration of blood and blood products can be delegated to the nursing assistive personnel (NAP).
1 True
2 False

REFERENCES

Ackley B, et al: *Evidence-based nursing care guidelines*, St Louis, 2008, Mosby.

Alexander M, et al: *Infusion nursing: an evidence-based approach*, ed 3, St Louis, 2010, Mosby.

American Association of Blood Banks (AABB): *Standards for blood banks and transfusion services*, ed 27, Bethesda, Md, 2011, The Association.

Busch M: Transfusion-associated AIDS. In Rossi EC, editor: *Principles of transfusion medicine*, ed 4, 2008, Bethesda, Md, 2008, Wiley-Blackwell.

Gabriel J: Infusion therapy part two: prevention and management of complications, *Nurs Stand* 22(32):41, 2008.

Hockenberry MJ, Wilson D: *Wong's nursing care of infants and children*, ed 9, St Louis, 2011, Mosby.

Infusion Nurses Society (INS): Infusion nursing standards of practice, *J Infus Nurs* 34(suppl 1):S93, 2011a.

Infusion Nurses Society (INS): *Policy and procedures for infusion nursing*, ed 4, Norwood, Mass, 2011b, The Society.

King K: *Blood transfusion therapy: a physicians' handbook*, ed 9, Basel, Switzerland, 2008, Karger.

National Quality Forum (NQF): *National voluntary consensus standards for patient safety: a consensus report*, Washington, DC, 2011, NQF.

Snyder E, et al: *Rossi's principles of transfusion medicine*, ed 4, St Louis, 2008, Mosby.

The Joint Commission (TJC): *National Patient Safety Goals*, Oakbrook Terrace, Ill, 2012, The Commission, available at http://www.jointcommission.org/standards_information/npsgs.aspx.

Oral Nutrition

MEDIA RESOURCES

- **evolve** http://evolve.elsevier.com/Perry/skills
  - Review Questions
  - ▶ Video Clips
  - Audio Glossary

KEY TERMS

Albumin	Bolus	MyPlate Food Guidance	Nutritional risk
Anthropometrics	Dysphagia	system	Nutritional screening
Aspiration	Gag reflex	National Dysphagia Diet	Prealbumin
Body mass index (BMI)	Malnutrition		

OBJECTIVES

Mastery of content in this chapter will enable the nurse to:
- Perform accurate nutritional screening.
- Identify and refer patients for nutritional assessment to a registered dietitian.
- Assess a patient's ability to swallow.

- Identify risk factors for aspiration related to dysphagia.
- Evaluate a patient's tolerance of oral nutrition.
- Identify appropriate meals for a patient to receive.
- Demonstrate how to properly feed a patient who cannot self-feed.

Nutrition is a basic component of health that affects a patient's rate of recovery from short-term and chronic illness, surgery, and injury. Lack of attention to a patient's nutritional status leads to malnutrition. Malnutrition develops as a result of decreased intake of nutrients, increased nutrient requirements, or complications associated with a disease process such as poor nutrient absorption (Adams et al., 2008). Complications such as muscle wasting, delayed wound healing, increased susceptibility to skin breakdown, and infection result from malnutrition. Complications lead to prolonged hospitalization, increased cost, and possibly increased mortality rates (Adams et al., 2008; Fletcher, 2009; Grodner et al., 2012). Box 30-1 provides a list of risk factors for nutritional problems.

Nurses have a key role in assessing, planning, and initiating interventions to ensure that patients receive the support required to maintain optimal nutritional status (Jefferies et al., 2011). You collaborate with a variety of health care professionals regarding the nutritional health of patients and participate in nutritional screenings and assessments. You also assess and help patients with feeding and identify patients at risk for difficulty swallowing and aspiration during feeding.

SCREENING FOR NUTRITIONAL RISK

Nutrition screening, assessment, and intervention are key components of nutrition care (Mueller et al., 2011). Nutritional screening identifies individuals who are either malnourished or are at risk for malnutrition and can determine if a detailed nutritional assessment is indicated (Hammond and Litchford, 2012; Mueller et al., 2011). The Joint Commission (TJC) (2012) standards require the identification of patients who are nutritionally at risk by means of an initial screening mechanism. Nutritional screening must be completed within 24 hours of admission to a hospital, within 14 days of admission to a long-term care facility, or within a facility-defined period of time in ambulatory and home care settings (TJC, 2012). In addition, TJC also requires education and training of patients regarding nutritional intervention and modified diets.

- Clear- or full-liquid diets for more than 3 days without nutrient supplementation or with inappropriate or insufficient nutrient supplementation
- Intravenous feeding (dextrose or saline) or NPO for more than 3 days without supplementation
- Low intakes of prescribed diet or tube feedings
- Weight 20% above or 10% below desirable body weight (accounting for edema)
- Pregnancy weight gain deviating from normal patterns
- Diagnoses that increase nutritional needs or decrease nutrient intake (or both): Cancer, malabsorption, diarrhea, hyperthyroidism, excessive inflammation, postoperative status, hemorrhage, infected or draining wounds, burns, infection, major trauma
- Chronic use of drugs, especially alcohol, which affects nutritional intake
- Alterations in chewing, swallowing, appetite, taste, and smell
- Body temperature consistently above 37° C (98.6° F) for more than 2 days
- Hematocrit: <43% in men, <37% in women; hemoglobin <14 g/dL in men, <12 g/dL in women
- Absolute decrease in lymphocyte count (<1500 cells/mm^3)
- Elevated (>250 mg/dL) or decreased (<130 mg/dL) total plasma cholesterol
- Serum albumin <3 g/dL in patients without renal or liver disease, generalized dermatitis, overhydration

Modified from Grodner M et al: *Foundations and clinical applications of nutrition: a nursing approach,* ed 5, St Louis, 2012, Mosby.
NPO, Nothing by mouth.

Nurses screen for actual and potential nutritional alterations by focusing on the effects of an illness or disease on a patient's nutritional status such as recent weight loss and decreased oral intake (Jefferies et al., 2011). Assessment determines presence of physical limitations and psychosocial factors that might affect a patient's nutritional intake (Fletcher, 2009). Findings will determine the need for consultation with a registered dietitian (RD) to complete a more in-depth assessment of a patient's current nutritional status. In addition, assessment findings can lead to a medical referral for a speech-language pathologist (SLP) if the patient has swallowing difficulties. Recommendations for improving nutritional status such as change in diet, alternative feeding methods, or further medical assessment and intervention stem from nutritional assessments (Mueller et al., 2011).

NUTRITION SCREENING AND ASSESSMENT TOOLS

A variety of screening tools standardize the nutrition assessment process, including the Subjective Global Assessment (SGA), which is commonly used to evaluate the presence of malnutrition in patients with different disease conditions. In contrast, The Malnutrition Universal Screening Tool (MUST) was developed to assess older adults in various clinical settings, including acute care, long-term care, and the community (Fig. 30-1). It is a five-step screening tool that identifies adults who are malnourished, at risk for malnutrition, or obese. MUST also provides management guidelines if an individual is found to be malnourished (Raymond, 2010).

The Mini Nutritional Assessment (MNA) (Fig. 30-2) is a nutritional screening tool also used with the elderly (Bauer et al., 2010).

It is a simple, well-validated nutrition screening and assessment tool designed as a first step in providing comprehensive, coordinated nutritional services for persons 65 years and older residing in the assisted-living community long-term care facilities (Skates and Anthony, 2009). It quickly identifies those who are at risk for malnutrition or are malnourished at an early stage so treatment can be initiated early (Skates and Anthony, 2009). The screening includes questions related to change in oral intake, weight loss, mobility, stress, and body mass index (BMI). The assessment component includes arm and calf circumference, specific questions related to eating habits, and questions related to medical history. After a screening, refer any patients at risk so their nutritional status can be improved (Phillips et al., 2010).

Nutritional Assessment by a Registered Dietitian

Nurses and dietitians work closely together to provide comprehensive nutritional care to patients. Dietitians use a problem-solving method, the nutrition care process (NCP), to think critically and make decisions regarding nutrition therapy (Charney and Escott-Stump, 2012). The process is similar to the nursing process. There are four interrelated steps: nutrition assessment, nutrition diagnosis, nutrition intervention, and nutrition monitoring and evaluation (ADA, 2008; Charney and Escott-Stump, 2012). The dietitian first performs a comprehensive assessment of a patient's nutritional status, including medical, social, nutritional, and medication history; physical examination; anthropometric measurements; and laboratory data. The goal of the assessment is to develop an effective nutritional plan of care that addresses patients' nutritional problems. The RD then makes a nutritional diagnosis that describes alterations in a patient's nutritional status that a dietitian can treat independently (ADA, 2008). The nutritional intervention is a purposely planned activity with the intent to resolve the nutrition diagnosis (i.e., to change a nutrition-related alteration). Nutrition monitoring and evaluation identifies patient progress, including patient understanding and adherence.

FOUNDATIONS OF NUTRITION

Dietary guidelines are reviewed regularly and modified based on the most current evidence related to nutrition, physical activity, and health. *Dietary Guidelines for Americans* was released in January 2011 and targets individuals 2 years and older (USDA and US DHHS, 2010). The intent is to promote health, reduce the risk of chronic diseases, and prevent and reverse obesity through improved nutrition and physical activity. The 2010 guidelines stress maintaining calorie balance over time, staying within a personal calorie limit, and choosing physical activities that fit within an individual's lifestyle.

In addition, the guidelines focus on consumption of nutrient-dense foods and sugar-free beverages that include vegetables, fruits, whole grains, seafood, eggs, beans, unsalted nuts and seeds, lean meats, poultry, and fat-free and low-fat milk products (Kennedy et al., 2011; USDA and USDHHS, 2010). The guidelines accommodate food preferences, cultural traditions, and customs of diverse individuals (USDA, 2010b).

The MyPlate Food Guidance System (Fig. 30-3) replaces MyPyramid (USDA, 2010a). The new symbol was developed in an effort to promote healthy eating by reminding individuals to make healthy food choices. It illustrates the five food groups using a familiar visual of a plate and includes only the five food groups in an effort to help individuals prioritize their choices and focus on the entire meal (Center for Nutrition Policy, 2011). The names of the five food groups have been modified to grains, vegetables, fruit,

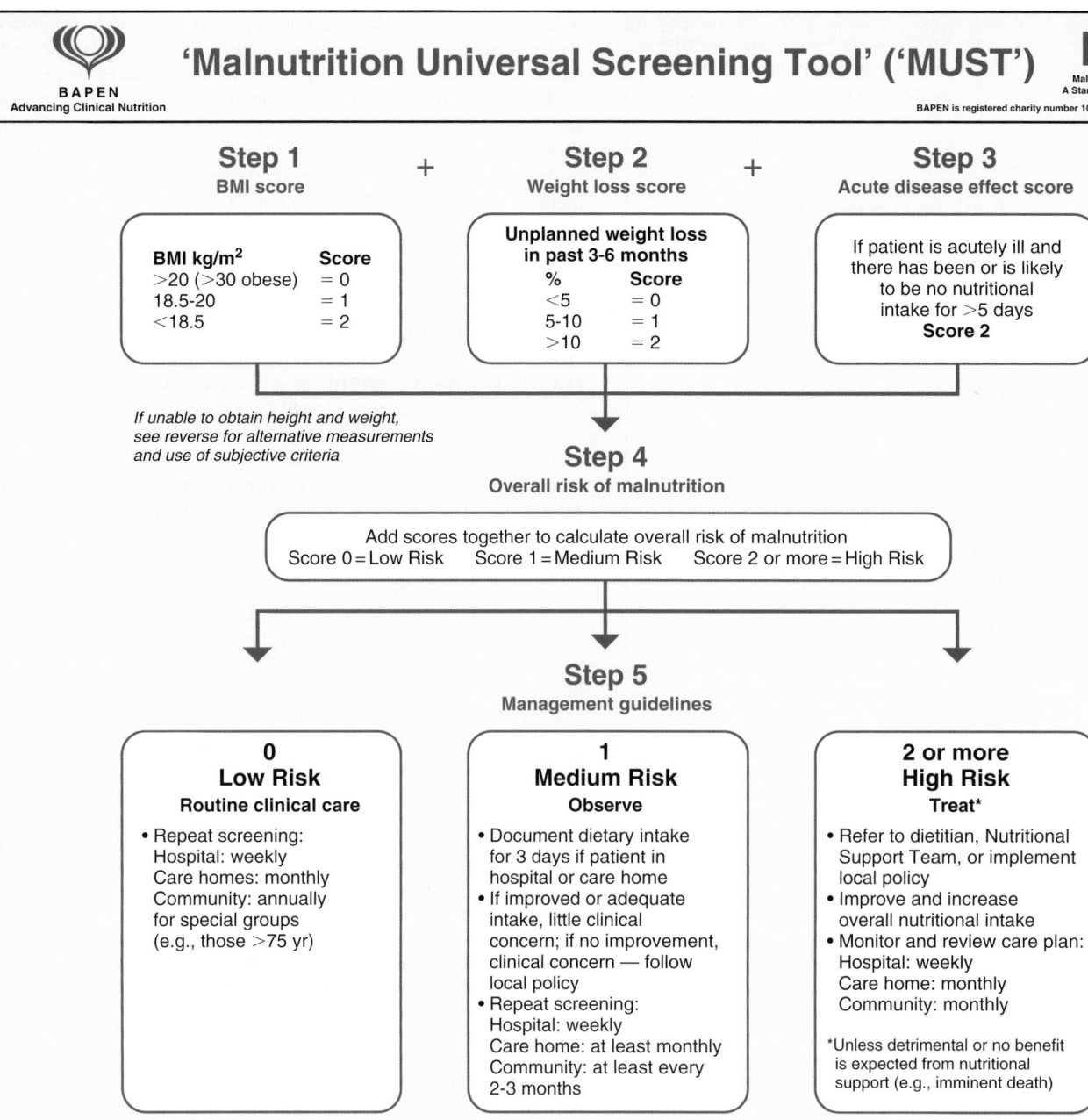

FIG 30-1   Malnutrition Universal Screening Tool (MUST). (*Courtesy BAPEN.*)

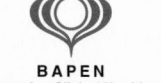

'Malnutrition Universal Screening Tool' ('MUST')

BAPEN
Advancing Clinical Nutrition

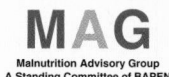

Malnutrition Advisory Group
A Standing Committee of BAPEN
BAPEN is registered charity number 1023927   www.bapen.org.uk

Alternative measurements and considerations

Step 1: BMI (body mass index)

If height cannot be measured
- Use recently documented or self-reported height (if reliable and realistic).
- If the subject does not know or is unable to report their height, use one of the alternative measurements to estimate height (ulna, knee height, or demispan).

If height and weight cannot be obtained
- Use mid–upper arm circumference (MUAC) measurement to estimate BMI category.

Step 2: Recent unplanned weight loss

If recent weight loss cannot be calculated, use self-reported weight loss (if reliable and realistic).

Subjective criteria

If height, weight, or BMI cannot be obtained, the following criteria that relate to them can assist your professional judgment of the subject's nutritional risk.

1. BMI
- Clinical impression: thin, acceptable weight, overweight. Obvious wasting (very thin) and obesity (very overweight) can also be noted.

2. Unplanned weight loss
- Clothes and/or jewelry have become loose fitting (weight loss).
- History of decreased food intake, reduced appetite, or swallowing problems over 3-6 months and underlying disease or psychosocial/physical disabilities likely to cause weight loss.

3. Acute disease effect
- No nutritional intake or likelihood of no intake for more than 5 days.

FIG 30-1, cont'd

dairy, and protein food groups. Each group contains a variety of foods with similar nutrient content and reflects the way food is used by consumers (Center for Nutrition Policy and Promotion, 2011). Recommendations for building a healthy plate include making half of the plate fruits and vegetables; adding lean protein, including seafood twice a week and whole grain; and including dairy such as a cup of fat-free or low-fat milk. Soy milk or fat-free or low-fat yogurt can be used alternatively in the meal.

EVIDENCE-BASED PRACTICE

Malnutrition is a serious and debilitating condition that is prevalent yet not fully identified. Consequently it may remain untreated in hospitals, the community, and long-term care (Adams et al., 2008; Gout et al., 2009). It is important that all health care workers understand factors associated with inadequate nutritional intake. Patients have identified barriers to adequate nutritional intake, including pain, decreased appetite, nausea, and side effects of medications (Adams et al., 2008; Holst et al., 2010).

As a primary caregiver you are in the ideal position to monitor a patient's nutritional status. Barriers to effective nutritional care by nurses include lack of interest and inadequate nutritional knowledge, resulting in inconsistencies in nutritional screening and documentation (Holst et al., 2010; Mowe et al., 2008). After screening and assessment, you need to collaborate with other health team members to design and implement actions that optimize patients' nutritional health (Fletcher and Carey, 2011):

- Nutritional care of patients is a primary responsibility of registered nurses and is essential to prevent complications associated with malnutrition.
- Regular and ongoing nutritional screening and assessment are imperative for early detection and improvement of outcomes for high-risk and malnourished patients (Gout et al., 2009).
- Failure of nurses to identify and refer malnourished patients for evaluation can result in adverse clinical outcomes (Gout et al., 2009).

Mini Nutritional Assessment
MNA®

Last name:	First name:	Sex:	Date:

Age:	Weight, kg:	Height, cm:	I.D. number:

Complete the screen by filling in the boxes with the appropriate numbers.
Add the numbers for the screen. If score is 11 or less, continue with the assessment to gain a Malnutrition Indicator Score.

Screening

A Has food intake declined over the past 3 months due to loss of appetite, digestive problems, chewing or swallowing difficulties?
0 = Severe loss of appetite
1 = Moderate loss of appetite
2 = No loss of appetite ☐

B Weight loss during the last 3 months
0 = Weight loss greater than 3 kg (6.6 lb)
1 = Does not know
2 = Weight loss between 1 and 3 kg (2.2 and 6.6 lb)
3 = No weight loss ☐

C Mobility
0 = Bed or chair bound
1 = Able to get out of bed/chair but does not go out
2 = Goes out ☐

D Has suffered psychological stress or acute disease in the past 3 months
0 = Yes   2 = No ☐

E Neuropsychological problems
0 = Severe dementia or depression
1 = Mild dementia
2 = No psychological problems ☐

F Body mass index (BMI) (weight in kg)/(height in m)²
0 = BMI less than 19
1 = BMI 19 to less than 21
2 = BMI 21 to less than 23
3 = BMI 23 or greater ☐

Screening score (subtotal max. 14 points) ☐☐

12 points or greater Normal–not at risk–no need to complete assessment
11 points or below Possible malnutrition–continue assessment

Assessment

G Lives independently (not in a nursing home or hospital)
0 = No   1 = Yes ☐

H Takes more than 3 prescription drugs per day
0 = Yes   1 = No ☐

I Pressure sores or skin ulcers
0 = Yes   1 = No ☐

Ref.: Vellas B, Villars H, Abellan G, et al. Overview of the MNA®: Its History and Challenges. *J Nutr Health Aging* 2006;10:456–465.

Rubenstein LZ, Harker JO, Salva A, Guigoz Y, Vellas B. Screening for Undernutrition in Geriatric Practice Developing the Short-Form Mini Nutritional Assessment (MNA-SF). *J Geront* 2001;56A: M366–377.

Guigoz Y. The Mini-Nutritional Assessment (MNA®) Review of the Literature: What does it tell us? *J Nutr Health Aging* 2006;10:466–487.

J How many full meals does the patient eat daily?
0 = 1 meal
1 = 2 meals
2 = 3 meals ☐

K Selected consumption markers for protein intake
• At least one serving of dairy products
  (e.g., milk, cheese, yogurt) per day? Yes☐ No☐
• Two or more servings of legumes
  or eggs per week?   Yes☐ No☐
• Meat, fish, or poultry every day   Yes☐ No☐
0.0 = If 0 or 1 yes
0.5 = If 2 yes
1.0 = If 3 yes ☐.☐

L Consumes two or more servings of fruits or vegetables per day?
0 = No   1 = Yes ☐

M How much fluid (e.g., water, juice, coffee, tea, milk) is consumed per day?
0.0 = Less than 3 cups
0.5 = 3 to 5 cups
1.0 = More than 5 cups ☐.☐

N Mode of feeding
0 = Unable to eat without assistance
1 = Self-fed with some difficulty
2 = Self-fed without any problem ☐

O Self-view of nutritional status
0 = Views self as being malnourished
1 = Is uncertain of nutritional state
2 = Views self as having no nutritional problem ☐

P In comparison with other people of the same age, how does the patient consider his/her health status?
0.0 = Not as good
0.5 = Does not know
1.0 = As good
2.0 = Better ☐.☐

Q Mid-arm circumference (MAC) in cm
0.0 = MAC less than 21
0.5 = MAC 21 to 22
1.0 = MAC 22 or greater ☐.☐

R Calf circumference (CC) in cm
0 = CC less than 31   1 = CC 31 or greater ☐

Assessment (max. 16 points) ☐☐.☐

Screening score ☐☐

Total Assessment (max. 30 points) ☐☐.☐

Malnutrition Indicator Score
17 to 23.5 points   At risk of malnutrition ☐

Less than 17 points   Malnourished

FIG 30-2 Nestlé Mini Nutritional Assessment tool used to assess nutritional status of geriatric patients. (*Courtesy Nestlé Nutrition Institute.*)

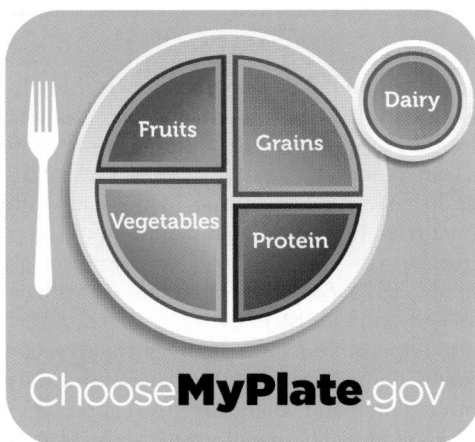

FIG 30-3 MyPlate showing the five essential food groups. (*From US Department of Agriculture [USDA]: Choose MyPlate, 2010, available at* http://chooseMYPlate.gov, *accessed July 26, 2012.*)

PATIENT-CENTERED CARE

Culture as related to nutrition is the shared knowledge, beliefs, values, and customs of a group around food and eating (Burns, 2009) (Box 30-2). Using a patient-centered approach to nutrition ensures a relevant and individualized nutritional plan for your patients. Make every attempt to provide patients with nutritional food that is familiar and congruent with their beliefs (O'Regan, 2009). Food preferences are a major factor in patient adherence to modifications of safe oral intake. A patient must be a part of the decision-making process when dietary modifications are required. Assess his or her willingness to accept diet modifications and be aware that patient and family members might have difficulty accepting dietary modifications that clash with personal meaning and values towards food (Burns, 2009). Alterations in the ability to safely self-feed and/or needing to consume an altered diet and fluids may impact a patient's perception of quality of life. Psychological reactions may include altered body image, embarrassment, depression, and feelings of social isolation (DeFabrizio and Rajappa, 2010).

Mealtime in a health care setting is the ideal time to interact with patients. During the meal continue your patient assessment, encourage decision making, and provide education. Use the time to teach patient, family, and significant others rationales for dietary modifications, including positioning during and after meals. Risk for aspiration increases if modifications are not followed (Garcia and Chambers, 2010). Maintain a patient's dignity as you implement individualized actions to correct, promote, or maintain nutritional health.

 Safety Guidelines

1 Assess for signs and symptoms of malnutrition and identify patients at risk.

BOX 30-2 | Cultural Considerations To Enhance Patient Nutrition

Understand the meaning of food and food preferences for patient and family. Avoid making value judgments about their food preferences and practices.

Food is often associated not only with caring and love but also with health promotion, maintenance, and restoration.

Assess religious and cultural influences on nutritional practices:
- African-Americans and Mexicans have large extended family networks. Eating food prepared by family members or loved ones can meet nutritional needs and serve as an expression of love.
- Buddhists and Hindus are generally vegetarians because of their respect for life and belief in transmigration of the soul.
- Vegetarians and vegans prefer meat substitutes.
- Hindus generally avoid eating beef, but some eat chicken and lamb, whereas some fast to obtain blessing from their gods.
- Muslims eat *halal* foods and avoid those that are classified such as *haram* (pork, alcohol).
- Orthodox Jews generally eat kosher foods and avoid serving meat and dairy at the same time. They eat fish with fins and scales (e.g., tuna), animals that chew their cud (e.g., cows), and nonpredatory birds (e.g., chicken). Shellfish cannot be eaten.
- Muslims fast all day, including from food and water, during the month of Ramadan. They eat before dawn and during evenings.

Collect information on the types of foods that are generally given for different types of conditions:
- Some African-Americans believe that certain foods build blood, thereby preventing anemia.
- Some pregnant Hispanic and African-American women have specific cravings and believe that they need to eat starch or red clay to promote a baby's health.
- Asians, Hispanics, Eastern Europeans, and Africans believe in the hot-and-cold theory of health and illness. Foods are classified as cold or hot based on their characteristics, independent of the temperature at which they are served. There is no universal agreement across cultures about which foods are hot or cold.

Understand food practice, and collaborate to develop healthy alternatives. Use cultural food guides developed for specific populations:
- Assess which ingredient or food content you need to reduce.
- A Chinese patient on a low-sodium diet needs to use low-sodium soy sauce and avoid shrimp paste and oyster sauce.

---

2 Identify patients at risk for dysphagia and collaborate with other members of the health care team to minimize complications such as aspiration pneumonia (NQF, 2010).
3 Ensure that patients receive the correct therapeutic diets.
4 Assess level of consciousness before feeding.

SKILL 30-1   Performing a Nutritional Assessment

Assessment of nutritional status is an essential part of patient care and is the foundation for diagnosing nutritional problems (Bauer et al., 2010; Mueller et al., 2011). It may lead to recommendations such as change in diet, need for alternative mode of nutrition intake, or improvement in a patient's nutritional status (Ukleja et al., 2010). There are four basic components of a holistic nutritional assessment: (1) patient history (psychological and social); (2) dietary history; (3) physical examination and anthropometric measurements; and (4) biochemical indices (Grodner et al., 2012).

History

Elements of a patient history such as appetite, psychosocial factors affecting intake, economics, and cultural issues provide a background for factors influencing current nutritional status (Burns, 2009). Collect the history by reviewing a patient's medical record and by direct interview. The medical history indicates medications, surgery, and coexisting medical conditions compromising nutrition. The psychological history includes screening for depression, alcohol abuse, or abnormal psychiatric behavior leading to decreased food intake. A social history provides important insight into poverty, avoidance of specific food groups, and food customs influencing nutritional education.

Physical Examination

A nutrition-focused physical examination can identify some nutritional deficiencies that may not be identified by other assessment approaches (Table 30-1) (Hammond and Litchford, 2012; Litchford, 2012). Conduct the examination in an organized manner and tailor it to each patient to ensure efficiency and thoroughness (see Chapter 6) (Hammond and Litchford, 2012).

Anthropometrics

Anthropometric measurements are commonly used to describe nutritional status because they reflect body composition (Kahn et al., 2009). Anthropometry involves taking body measurements using simple techniques that measure height and weight, skinfold thickness, and waist and muscle circumferences. Muscle circumferences include measuring the mid-arm and calf. Calf circumference is a sensitive indicator of nutritional status in the elderly because it indicates lean muscle changes (Portero-McLellan, 2010). Evaluation of results involves comparison of the data collected with predetermined reference points that determine if the patient falls into a nutritional risk category such as severity of malnutrition (Grodner et al., 2012). Registered dietitians typically measure circumferences and skinfold thickness.

Nurses are responsible for taking height and weight measurements. Height and weight are useful in determining the nutritional status of both children and adults. Length is important in evaluating growth in children. The use of length alone as an indicator of nutritional status is usually only used in children (Fletcher, 2009). The length and weight of a child are plotted on a growth chart and evaluated against standards based on the normal U.S. population. This information is essential to tracking the growth of children over time, which reflects nutritional adequacy.

Height is needed to assess weight and body size and calculate body mass index (BMI) in adults (Fletcher, 2009; Grodner et al., 2012; Perry, 2009). Direct measurement of height is done using a movable measuring arm on a clinical platform scale. In this case the individual must be able to stand erect. When a patient cannot stand, it is possible to obtain an accurate indirect height by measuring knee height in the lying position using special equipment.

Body weight is a simple, gross estimate of body composition. As a nutritional screening tool, weight is used to recognize changes that may suggest altered nutritional status, for predicting energy expenditure, and to calculate BMI (CDC, 2011; Grodner et al., 2012; Perry, 2009). When weight loss is expected, an assessment requires the collection of usual body weight (UBW) and actual body weight (ABW) to determine percent of weight change.

$$\% \text{ Weight change} = \frac{(\text{Usual weight} - \text{Actual weight})}{\text{Usual weight}}$$

TABLE 30-1	Clinical Signs of Nutritional Status	
Body Area	**Signs and Symptoms of Nutritional Risk**	**Nutritional Implications**
Hair	Dull, shedding, easily pluckable	Generalized protein calorie malnutrition
Face	Malar pigmentation (dark skin over cheeks and under eyes)	Niacin, B vitamins
	Bitemporal wasting	Malnutrition
	Nasolabial seborrhea	Niacin, riboflavin, vitamin B_6 deficiency
	Edematous	Protein deficiency
	Moon face	Corticosteroid impact
	Pallor	Inadequate Fe^{++}, undernutrition
Eyes	Pale eye membranes	Inadequate Fe^{++}
Lips	Cheilosis (red/swelling)	Inadequate niacin, vitamin B_6, riboflavin, Fe^{++}
	Angular fissures	
Gingiva	Spongy, bleeding, abnormal redness	Inadequate vitamin C
Tongue	Glossitis (red, raw, fissured)	Inadequate folate, niacin, riboflavin, Fe^{++}, vitamin B_6, vitamin B_{12}
	Pale, atrophic, smooth/slick (filiform papillary atrophy), magenta	Inadequate Fe^{++}, vitamin B_{12}, niacin, folate
		Inadequate riboflavin
Nails	Spoon shaped, brittle, ridged	Inadequate Fe^{++}
Back	Bony prominences along shoulder girdle	Malnutrition

Modified from Seidel H et al: *Mosby's guide to physical examination*, ed7, St Louis, 2011, Mosby.

Percent of weight change is a useful nutrition index. Table 30-2 summarizes weight changes as indicators of nutritional status. The magnitude and direction of weight change are more meaningful than standard weight references when dealing with sick or debilitated patients (Grodner et al., 2012). When evaluating fluctuations in weight, determine the period of time over which it occurred. Assess whether a patient has been dieting recently or following an exercise program. Also assess for signs of fluid volume deficit or excess, which can cause weight fluctuations (see Chapter 33). Fluid may be the cause if more than 1 pound (0.45 kg) is gained in a day (Grodner et al., 2012).

Measure an ambulatory patient's weight by using beam scales with movable but detachable weights or electronic scales (Grodner et al., 2012). Some agencies have hospital beds that have the capability to obtain weights on nonambulatory patients. Previously determined weight of the bed is deducted so the patient's precise weight is measured. Another alternative to weighing nonambulatory patients is a wheelchair scale. Platform scales are specifically designed to be installed on the floor so a wheelchair/chair or walker can be used. The weight of the wheelchair needs to be weighed separately if different wheel chairs are used. This type of scale ensures that a patient can remain safely in his or her wheelchair as an accurate weight is obtained.

BMI is a ratio of weight to height and is associated with overall mortality and nutritional risk (Nelms, 2010). The use of BMI allows people to compare their own weight status to that of the general population (Centers for Disease Control and Prevention, 2011) and is one of the best methods for assessing degree of underweight, excess weight, and obesity. Calculation requires only height and weight and is most easily done by referring to a standard BMI chart (Fig. 30-4).

However, BMI alone is not a perfect predictor of overweight or obesity because it is calculated from an individual's weight, which includes both muscle and fat. For example, highly trained athletes may have a high BMI because of increased muscularity rather than increased body fat (Centers for Disease Control and Prevention, 2011; Kravitz, 2010). As a result, some individuals may have a high BMI but not a high percentage of body fat. In addition, BMI may underestimate body fat in the elderly and in those who have lost muscle mass (National Heart, Lung and Blood Institute, 2008). It is a weak indicator of weight-related problems among certain ethic groups, such as African-Americans and Hispanic-American women (National Institute of Diabetes, Digestive and Kidney Diseases, 2008). Box 30-3 lists BMI by degree of body adiposity.

BMI and waist circumference provide useful estimates of body fat distribution (Kravitz, 2010). The location of excess fat on the body is important. If it is distributed around the waist, it is more likely that health problems will develop than if it is mainly in the hips and thighs. Abdominal fat (visceral or intraabdominal fat) is related to coronary heart disease, hypertension, diabetes, and sleep apnea (Kravitz, 2010). A circumference greater than 16 cm (40 inches) for men and greater than 14 cm (35 inches) in women corresponds with an increased cardiovascular risk (Kravitz, 2010).

TABLE 30-2	Weight Change As an Indicator of Nutritional Status	
Weight Change (%)	**Time Period**	**Nutritional Status**
1-2	1 week	Moderate weight loss
>2	1 week	Severe weight loss
5	1 month	Moderate weight loss
>5	1 month	Severe weight loss

From Grodner M, et al: *Foundations and clinical applications of nutrition: a nursing approach*, ed 4, St Louis, 2012, Mosby.

BODY MASS INDEX (BMI)

Height (ft/in)	Weight in Pounds													
	120	**130**	**140**	**150**	**160**	**170**	**180**	**190**	**200**	**210**	**220**	**230**	**240**	**250**
4'8	26.9	29.1	31.4	33.6	35.9	38.1	40.4	42.6	44.8	47.1	49.3	51.6	53.8	56.0
4'10	25.1	27.2	29.3	31.3	33.4	35.5	37.6	39.7	41.8	43.9	46.0	48.1	50.2	52.2
5'0	23.4	25.4	27.3	29.3	31.2	33.2	35.1	37.1	39.1	41.0	43.0	44.9	46.9	48.8
5'2	21.9	23.8	25.6	27.4	29.3	31.1	32.9	34.7	36.6	38.4	40.2	42.1	43.9	45.7
5'4	20.6	22.3	24.0	25.7	27.5	29.2	30.9	32.6	34.3	36.0	37.8	39.5	41.2	42.9
5'6	19.4	21.0	22.6	24.2	25.8	27.4	29.0	30.7	32.3	33.9	35.5	37.1	38.7	40.3
5'8	18.2	19.8	21.3	22.8	24.3	25.8	27.4	28.9	30.4	31.9	33.4	35.0	36.5	38.0
5'10	17.2	18.7	20.1	21.5	23.0	24.4	25.8	27.3	28.7	30.1	31.6	33.0	34.4	35.9
6'0	16.3	17.6	19.0	20.3	21.7	23.1	24.4	25.8	27.1	28.5	29.2	31.2	32.5	33.9
6'2	15.4	16.7	18.0	19.3	20.5	21.8	23.1	24.4	25.7	27.0	28.2	29.5	30.8	32.1
6'4	14.6	15.8	17.0	18.3	19.5	20.7	21.9	23.1	24.3	25.6	26.8	28.0	29.2	30.4
6'6	13.9	15.0	16.2	17.3	18.5	19.6	20.8	22.0	23.1	24.3	25.4	26.6	27.7	28.9
6'8	13.2	14.3	15.4	16.5	17.6	18.7	19.8	20.9	22.0	23.1	24.2	25.3	26.4	27.5

Key

	Obese (30+)
	Overweight (25.0-29.9)
	Normal (18.5-24.9)
	Underweight (below 18.5)

FIG 30-4 Body mass index grid. *Data from Centers for Disease Control and Prevention (CDC): Healthy weight—it's not a diet, it's a lifestyle, August 16, 2011, available at http://www.cdc.gov/ healthyweight/index.html, accessed May 5, 2012.*

BOX 30-3 | Body Mass Index

To calculate body mass index (BMI):

$$BMI = Weight\ (kg)/Height\ (m)^2$$

or

$$BMI = \frac{Weight\ (lb)}{Height\ (inches) \times Height\ (inches)} \times 703$$

Classification of BMI in Adults

Degree of Adiposity	BMI
Underweight	<18.5 kg/m²
Normal weight	18.5-24.9 kg/m²
Overweight	25-29.9 kg/m²
Obesity (class 1)	30-34.9 kg/m²
Obesity (class 2)	35-39.9 kg/m²
Extreme obesity (class 3)	≥40 kg/m²

From Expert Panel on the Identification, Evaluation, and Treatment of Overweight and Obesity in Adults: *The practical guide: identification, evaluation, and treatment of overweight and obesity in adults,* Bethesda, Md, 2000, National Institutes of Health.
BMI, Body mass index.

Biochemical Markers of Nutritional Status

Laboratory-based nutritional testing provides objective data along with nutritional-based physical assessment, dietary intake assessment, and anthropometric data to determine nutrition-related health conditions (Grodner et al., 2012; Litchford, 2012). Laboratory data show variations in nutritional status before clinical or anthropometric changes are detected (Litchford, 2012). Results can be influenced by inflammation, diseases, medication trauma, or stress (Portero-McLellan et al., 2010) and fluid balance alterations (Prins, 2010). There is lack of consensus about which biochemical marker clearly assesses nutritional status (Beghetto et al., 2009). Traditionally serum albumin and prealbumin levels are used because they measure visceral proteins (proteins other than muscle tissue). Normal serum albumin values are within 3.5 to 5.0 g/dL. For nutritional analysis values between 2.8 and 3.5 g/dL may indicate compromised protein status (Grodner et al., 2012). Prealbumin also provides a measure of visceral protein status and normally ranges from 20 to 50 mg/dL. The test is useful in monitoring short-term changes in visceral protein (Grodner et al., 2012). It often is used to monitor nutritional interventions (Barbosa-Silva, 2008). A patient has compromised protein status when levels are between 10 and 15 g/dL. Red blood cells should be assessed for nutritional-based anemias. Assess iron, vitamin B₁₂, and folate levels to confirm a nutritional anemia diagnosis (Prins, 2010).

It is important to remember that no one component of the nutritional assessment directly measures nutritional status or determines nutritional problems or needs. Each part of the process must be used to interpret the patient's nutritional health. Once the nutritional assessment is complete, analysis of all data is completed. Interpreting the data in a meaningful and relevant way allows nutritional nursing diagnoses to be identified and goals to be determined followed by appropriate and individualized interventions.

Delegation and Collaboration

The skill of performing and interpreting a nutritional assessment cannot be delegated to nursing assistive personnel (NAP). However, measurement of a patient's height and weight can be delegated. The nurse directs the NAP to:

- Measure patient's weight after voiding, at the same time of day and wearing same clothing.
- Use the internal bed scale according to guidelines (if applicable).
- Report inability to measure height if patient is nonambulatory.

Equipment

- ❏ Scale (beam, electronic, bed with scale, wheelchair/chair)
- ❏ Assessment sheet and pen or computerized assessment form

STEP	RATIONALE

ASSESSMENT

STEP	RATIONALE
1 Assess patient's knowledge of procedure.	Encourages cooperation, minimizes risks and anxiety. Identifies teaching needs.
2 Ask patient to report usual body weight (UBW), noting recent changes in weight. Ask if weight loss was intentional or unintentional.	In adults weight is usually stable. A loss of 10 lbs (4.5 kg) during a 6-month period whether intentional or unintentional, is a critical indicator for further assessment, especially in the older adult (Dimaria-Ghalili, 2008).
3 Obtain complete and thorough nursing history (see Chapter 6), including social, economic, and psychological factors affecting nutrition. Determine patients' current nutritional habits.	Identifies patients who are at nutritional risk (Burns, 2009). Determines teaching needs related to nutritional health.
4 Perform physical assessment (see Chapter 6), including condition of skin, hair, nails, oral mucosa, muscle mass, and strength. Note any mental changes.	The most obvious signs of malnutrition on physical examination are apparent in the skin, mouth, muscles, and central nervous system (Lewis et al., 2011).
5 Review results of relevant laboratory tests (e.g., albumin, prealbumin).	Test data provide clues about nutritional status.
6 Determine medications and other dietary supplements that patient is taking (over-the-counter and prescribed). Be aware of common drug-drug and drug-nutrient interactions.	Certain medications inhibit or increase action of other medications. Some nutrients interact with medications. For example, vitamin K–rich foods (green leafy vegetables) interfere with action of warfarin (Coumadin) (anticoagulant). Medications such as mineral oil laxatives impair nutrient use.

STEP	RATIONALE
7 Measure ABW.	Women tend to underestimate their weight more than men, and for both sexes extent of underreporting increases as actual weight increases (Grodner et al., 2012).
a Have patient void. Be sure that he or she is wearing underwear or hospital gown. Make sure that patient is weighed either barefoot or with same shoes. Weigh at same time of day.	Improves accuracy of actual weight for comparison over time.
b Make sure that beam scale has been calibrated. If ambulatory, help patient to stand still on scale with weight evenly distributed on both feet.	Accurate measurement requires regularly calibrated and maintained scales (Perry, 2009). Standing still with equal weight distribution aids in obtaining accurate weight (Grodner et al., 2012).
c If patient is unable to stand, use wheelchair or bed scale.	Ensures accurate measurement of weight while maintaining patient's safety.
d Record weight to the nearest 0.25 lb (0.1 kg).	Provides precise measurement of weight used to calculate BMI.
8 Measure actual height.	On average, when asked, people report being slightly taller than they actually are (Grodner et al., 2012).
a Help patient to standing position; have him or her stand erect with weight equally distributed on both feet.	Ensures accurate height (Grodner et al., 2012).
b Instruct patient to let arms hang free at sides with palms facing thighs.	Prevents movement of shoulders, which will result in inaccurate measurement.
c Have patient look straight ahead, take a deep breath, and hold position while bringing horizontal bar firmly on top of head. Measure to nearest 0.1 cm ($\frac{1}{8}$ inch). Make sure that your eyes are level with bar to read measurement.	Steady position ensures accurate measurement. Provides precise measurement of height used to calculate BMI.
9 Calculate IBW.	
a Calculate via standard height and weight chart. IBW range for normal is 10% above and 10% below IBW.	Use IBW to compare with patient's actual weight to determine if he or she is at risk for nutritional alteration.
b Use the following formulas: *Male*: 106 lbs (48.1 kg) for first 5 feet, then add 6 lbs (2.7 kg) per additional 2.5 cm (inch). *Female*: 100 lbs (45.4 kg) for the first 5 feet, then add 5 lbs (2.25 kg) per additional 2.5 cm (inch).	
10 Calculate BMI: $$BMI = \frac{Weight\ (kg)}{Height^2\ (m^2)}$$	Assesses patient's adiposity (obesity) against national standards (Centers for Disease Control and Prevention, 2011).
a Divide weight in pounds by 2.2.	Converts pounds into kilograms.
b Convert height to inches. Multiply inches by 2.54.	Converts height in inches to centimeters.
c Divide height in centimeters by 100.	Converts height to meters.
d Divide weight in kilograms by the square of height in meters (m^2).	Computes BMI.
11 Assess patient's diet history, including current diet, food choices/preferences, appetite, explanations for any restrictions, food allergies, and food intolerances.	Assesses factors affecting diet adequacy and appetite (Burns, 2009).
12 Have patient provide 24-hour diet recall. Ask him or her to report all food and beverages consumed over past 24 hours.	Estimated or measured food records can provide a more realistic picture of patient's intake (Grodner et al., 2012).
13 Determine patient's ability to manipulate eating utensils and self-feed.	Difficulty in self-feeding creates significant risk for malnutrition (Meiner, 2011).
14 Explain to patient that nutritional assessment is complete.	Allows time for patient to ask questions about assessment.
15 Report diet restrictions and preferences to food and nutrition department.	Ensures that an inpatient or resident will receive appropriate diet.

NURSING DIAGNOSES

• Deficient knowledge regarding nutritional recommendations	• Imbalanced nutrition: more than body requirements	• Imbalanced nutrition less than body requirements

Related factors are individualized based on patient's condition or needs.

EVALUATION

1 Review history and physical findings. Note abnormal findings or areas of concern.	Permits prompt identification of risk for malnutrition and need for nutritional interventions.
2 Compare patient's weight for height with IBW. Compare BMI with recommended BMI for height/weight.	Determines nutritional risk factors and health-related conditions (National Heart, Lung and Blood Institute, 2008).

STEP	RATIONALE
3 Compare normal laboratory test levels with patient's levels.	When considered with other nutritional parameters, abnormal values can indicate malnutrition (Grodner et al., 2012; Litchford, 2012).

Unexpected Outcomes

1 Body weight is below or above UBW and/or IBW.

Related Interventions

- Ensure that patient is receiving correct diet.
- Identify trends in weight loss/gain.
- Check that patient is being weighed on same scale, with same type of clothing/shoes, and at same time of day.
- Report changes to registered dietitian (RD) or health care provider so RD can conduct a nutritional assessment, calculate patient's caloric needs (calories per kilogram), and determine amount of protein that patient requires and route of nutrition (enteral versus parenteral) (see Chapters 31 and 32).

Recording and Reporting

- Record assessment finding results on nutritional screening form. Notify health care provider of abnormal findings.
- Make referral to the RD.

Special Considerations

Gerontologic

- The "normal" anthropometric standards are based on a healthy middle-age population. However, there are methods of comparing anthropometric measurements over time for older adults (Meiner, 2011).

Pediatric

- Anthropometric data include measurement of length, weight, and head circumference in children. Compare these measurements with standard growth charts to determine percentiles. The most commonly used growth charts are from the National Center for Health Statistics (Hockenberry and Wilson, 2011). These charts now include BMI for age and weight for stature percentiles.

SKILL 30-2   Assisting an Adult Patient with Oral Nutrition

Hospitalized patients receive a number of different oral diets that require a health care provider's order. A therapeutic diet treats many illness and disease states (Table 30-3). For specific information about special diets see the agency dietary manual or contact a registered dietitian (RD). You can modify a regular diet in two ways: quantitatively or qualitatively (Grodner et al., 2012). Qualitative diets include modifications in consistency, texture, or nutrients such as clear or full liquid. Quantitative diets include modifications in number or size of meals served or amounts of specific nutrients such as six small feedings or kcalorie diets. You can supplement any diet with oral nutrition supplements. You prepare a patient so he or she can be comfortable and not interrupted during a meal. You may be asked to maintain a calorie count. Usually the percentage of each food that a patient eats is recorded next to the food choice directly on the menu for each meal. The RD is able to determine caloric intake and need for nutrition supplements or dietary change. Liquid supplements with or between meals can significantly increase protein and calorie intake (O'Regan, 2009).

Helping adults with oral nutrition requires time, patience, knowledge, and understanding. Most people eat without assistance. However, the older adult commonly loses some fine-motor skills required to get food from the plate and into the mouth. When they are ill, many patients require assistance either to feed themselves or, if necessary, to be fed by another person if unable to eat independently (Webster and Healy, 2009; Wright et al., 2008). Altered dentition, improperly fitted dentures, oral lesions or infections, or diseases causing impaired digestion limit the types and consistencies of foods tolerated. Hemiplegia, fractured arm, quadriplegia,

debilitating illness, or generalized weakness limits self-feeding ability and appetite. The presence of intravenous (IV) catheters or tubing, dressings, and bandages also limits mobility needed for self-feeding. Consult an occupational therapist (OT) for collaboration on assessing patients' ability to self-feed and for recommendations for adaptive equipment and supplies for self-feeding. An adult who needs help to eat needs compassion and understanding. Use common sense when feeding an adult and provide a socially meaningful mealtime experience.

Delegation and Collaboration

The skill of assisting a patient with oral nutrition can be delegated to nursing assistive personnel (NAP). However, the nurse is responsible to determine if a patient is able to receive oral nutrition, including swallowing ability and restrictions. The nurse directs the NAP by:

- Explaining any specific swallowing strategies/techniques unique to the patient.
- Reviewing when to stop feeding and report immediately to the nurse incidences of coughing, gagging, or difficulty swallowing.

Equipment

- ❑ Stethoscope and tongue blade for assessment
- ❑ Washcloths and towels
- ❑ Tongue blade
- ❑ Adaptive utensils as necessary for self-feeding
- ❑ Oral hygiene supplies

TABLE 30-3 | Progressive and Therapeutic Diets

Diet	Description
Clear-liquid	Foods that are clear and liquid at room or body temperature (e.g., water, apple or cranberry juice, gelatin, Popsicles), that leave little residue, and are easily absorbed; commonly ordered for short-term use (24 to 48 hours) after surgery, before diagnostic tests, and after episodes of diarrhea and vomiting
Full-liquid	Includes foods on clear-liquid diet plus addition of smooth-textured dairy products (e.g., milk and ice cream), strained soups and custard, refined cooked cereals, vegetable juice, and pureed vegetables; commonly ordered before or after surgery for patients who are acutely ill from infection or for patients who cannot chew or tolerate solid foods; must verify that patients are able to tolerate lactose before providing dairy products
Pureed	Includes foods on clear- and full-liquid diet plus easily swallowed foods that do not require chewing (e.g., scrambled eggs, pureed meats, vegetables, and fruits; mashed potatoes); ordered for patients with head and neck abnormalities or who have had oral surgery; can be modified for low sodium, fat, or calorie count
Mechanical or dental-soft	Consists of all previous diets plus addition of lightly seasoned ground or finely diced meats, flaked fish, cottage cheese, cheese, rice, potatoes, pancakes, light breads, cooked vegetables, cooked or canned fruit, bananas, and peanut butter; avoid tough meats, nuts, bacon, and fruits with tough skins or membranes; ordered for patients who have chewing problems or mild GI problems; used as a transition diet from liquids to regular
Soft/low-residue	Addition of low-fiber, easily digested foods such as pastas, casseroles, moist tender meats, and canned cooked fruits and vegetables; includes foods that are easy to chew and simply cooked; does not permit fatty, rich, and fried foods; is sometimes referred to as *low fiber*
High-fiber	Addition of fresh uncooked fruits, steamed vegetables, bran, oatmeal and dried fruits; includes sufficient amounts of indigestible carbohydrates to relieve constipation, increase GI motility, and increase stool weight
Regular or diet as tolerated	No restrictions; permits patient preferences and allows for postoperative diet progression
Sample Therapeutic Diets Restricted fluids	Required in severe heart failure or kidney failure
Sodium-restricted	Allows low levels of sodium and may include a 4-g (no added salt), 2-g (moderate), 1-g (strict), or 500-mg (very strict) diet; may be ordered for patients with heart failure, renal failure, cirrhosis, or hypertension
Fat-modified	Low total and saturated fat and low cholesterol intake limited to less than 300 mg daily, and fat intake 30% to 35%; eliminates or reduces fatty foods for hypercholesterolemia, malabsorption disorders, and diarrhea
Diabetic	Essential treatment for patients with diabetes mellitus; provide patient with a diet recommended by the American Diabetes Association, which allows for patients to select set amount of food from basic food groups.

Grodner M et al: *Foundations and clinical applications of nutrition: a nursing approach*, ed 4, St Louis, 2012, Mosby.
GI, Gastrointestinal.

STEP	RATIONALE

ASSESSMENT

1 Assess patient's knowledge of procedure.

2 Assess if patient passes flatus and is without nausea. Auscultate bowel sounds.

3 Review health care provider's diet order.

4 Assess presence and condition of teeth. Determine if dentures are poorly fitted.

5 Assess a neurologic patient's cranial nerve function. Assess cranial nerves V, VII, IX, and X (see Chapter 6).

6 Determine to what extent patient is able to self-feed. Assess physical motor skills (e.g., ability to grasp utensils, hold cup and move to mouth). Evaluate level of consciousness, visual acuity and peripheral vision, and mood.

7 Assess patient's appetite, tolerance of foods, recent fluid intake, cultural and religious preferences, and food likes and dislikes.

8 Assess patient's ability to swallow (see Skill 30-3).

Encourages cooperation, minimizes risks and anxiety. Identifies teaching needs.

Determines if gastrointestinal tract is functioning normally (see Chapter 6).

Awareness of specific diet order ensures that patient gets appropriate meal tray.

Absence of teeth and ill-fitting dentures inhibit normal chewing and preparation of food for safe swallowing. This places patient at risk for dysphagia (Kyle, 2011) (see Skill 30-3).

Intact cranial nerves are necessary for safe swallowing. As a chronic neurologic disease progresses, cranial nerves become damaged, leading to dysphagia (Remig and Weeden, 2012).

Patients with any level of independence should be encouraged to feed self as much as possible. Thorough understanding of patient's physical and cognitive limitations alerts you to type of assistance patient needs. Visual impairments make it difficult to see food and utensils (Chang and Roberts, 2011).

Determines type of foods and size of meals that can potentially improve oral intake.

Determines aspiration risk, influencing food selection.

STEP	RATIONALE

NURSING DIAGNOSES

- Feeding self-care deficit
- Impaired swallowing
- Risk for aspiration
- Risk for deficient fluid volume
- Risk for imbalanced nutrition less than body requirements

Related factors are individualized based on patient's condition or needs.

PLANNING

1 Expected outcomes following completion of procedure:

- Patient's weight is maintained or trends toward desired level.
- Patient's nutrition-related laboratory values trend toward normal.
- Patient demonstrates increased ability to self-feed or open items on tray as appropriate.
- Patient coughs appropriately with no indication of respiratory compromise.

Nutritional intake meets daily needs.

Biochemical markers along with nutritional assessment indicate nutritional status.

Indicates increased strength, improved mental status, and increased well-being.

Ineffective cough and respiratory compromise are indicators of dysphagia and aspiration.

IMPLEMENTATION

1 Prepare patient's room for mealtime.

   a Perform hand hygiene. Clear over-bed table.

   b Help patient to comfortable sitting position in chair or place bed in high-Fowler's position. If patient is unable to sit, turn him or her on side with head of bed elevated.

2 Prepare patient for meal.

   a Help patient with pain relief and elimination needs and help him or her perform hand hygiene before meals.

   b Help patient put in dentures and put on eyeglasses or insert contact lenses if used.

3 Ask in which order patient would like to eat his or her meal. Ask about desired seasonings. Help patient to cut food in bite size pieces if unable to do independently.

4 Use adaptive eating and drinking aids as needed according to your assessment (e.g., two-handled cup with lid, plate with plate guard, utensils with splints, utensils with enlarged handles) (see illustration).

5 Identify food placement for disoriented, visually impaired, or easily fatigued patients by locating on plate as if plate were a clock (see illustration).

Reduces transmission of microorganisms and prepares room for food tray.

Upright position facilitates swallowing, reducing aspiration risk.

Conditions such as pressure ulcer, traction, or spinal surgery prevent positioning with head elevated.

Increases patient's comfort and enjoyment of meal, which helps increase patient's nutritional intake.

Enhances patient's ability to see, bite, chew, and swallow food.

Allows patient more independence and control. Small pieces are easier to chew and minimize risk for aspiration.

Eating and drinking aids help to place, direct, and control food bolus (saliva-softened mass of chewed food) and liquid and to maintain proper head posture while eating (Ney et al., 2009).

Helps patient locate food items; may be able to feed self if given adequate information about food placement on tray.

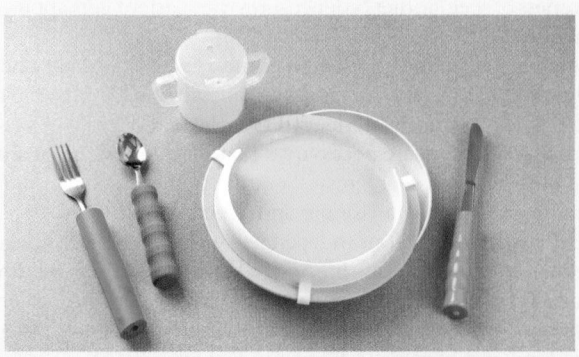

STEP 4 Mealtime equipment. *Clockwise from upper left:* Two-handled cup with lid, plate with plate guard, utensils with splints, and utensils with enlarged handles.

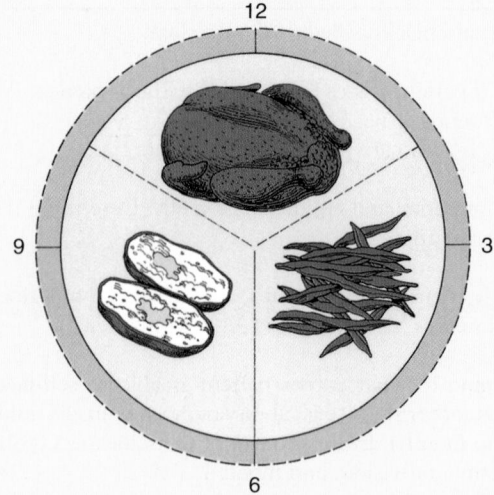

STEP 5 Clock setup to prepare food on a plate for the visually impaired patient.

STEP	RATIONALE
6 Feed patient in manner that facilitates chewing and swallowing.	
a *Older adult*: Feed small amounts at a time, observing biting, chewing, swallowing, and fatigue between bites; be sure that patient has swallowed food.	Chewing and sitting up for feeding accelerates onset of fatigue (Ebersole et al., 2008).

Clinical Decision Point *If you suspect that patient is aspirating, stop feeding immediately and suction airway (see Skill 30-3).*

STEP	RATIONALE
b *Neurologically impaired patient*: Feed small amounts at a time and assess for ability to chew, manipulate tongue to form bolus, and swallow. Check for food left inside cheeks (pocketing).	Some patients with limited tongue strength and control are unable to move food to back of mouth for swallowing. Checking for "pocketed" food in mouth prevents aspiration (Remig and Weeden, 2012).
7 Provide fluids as requested. Encourage patients not to drink all liquid at beginning of meal.	Helps with swallowing. Prevents patient from filling up on liquids.
8 Talk with patient during meal.	Meal should be a pleasant event. Conversation promotes socialization. Involve family if possible.
9 Use meal as opportunity to educate patient (e.g., topics related to nutrition, postoperative exercises, discharge plans).	Education can occur whenever nurse and patient are together.
10 Help patient with hand hygiene and performing mouth care.	Maintains comfort.
11 Help patient to resting position, leave head elevated 30-45 degrees for 30-60 minutes after meal.	Patient may feel tired after full meal. Elevation of head reduces risk for aspiration.
12 Return patient's tray to appropriate place and perform hand hygiene.	Reduces spread of microorganisms.

EVALUATION

1 Monitor body weight daily or weekly.	Determines nutritional status.
2 Monitor laboratory values as indicated.	Biochemical markers such as albumin and prealbumin aid in identifying changes in nutritional status.
3 Monitor intake and output (I&O) (see Chapter 6) and percentage of food on tray after meal.	
4 Observe patient's ability to self-feed, including ability to feed certain items, part, or all of meal.	Helps to determine what assistance patient needs with feeding.
5 Observe patient for choking, coughing, gagging, or food left in mouth during eating.	Indicates dysphagia and possible aspiration.

Unexpected Outcomes

1 Patient is unable to eat entire meal or refuses to eat.

2 Patient chokes on food.

Related Interventions

- Determine why patient is unable to finish meal (e.g., inadequate personnel for feeding assistance, ingestion of large volume of liquids immediately before meal). Also clarify if patient has food preferences, culture influences, or religious restrictions.
- Determine if patient is in pain or nauseated or if he or she has constipation.
- Perform oral assessment; provide oral care as needed.
- If inability to eat meal is a repeated problem, collaborate with health care provider and RD.

- Stop feeding immediately; place on side with head pointing down, suction food and secretions from mouth and airway.
- Contact health care provider if choking occurs repeatedly.
- Suggest appropriate referrals (e.g., speech-language pathologist, RD) (see Skill 30-3).

Recording and Reporting

- Document in patient's chart tolerance of diet and amount eaten. Record percentage of the meal eaten by the patient (e.g., 25% of food consumed at breakfast).
- If patient is on calorie counts, record caloric intake on appropriate form; if evaluating I&O, record fluid intake on appropriate form.
- If patient is receiving oral nutritional supplements (e.g., Ensure, Boost), record the amount taken and communicate patient

tolerance (likes or dislikes, supplements to fill or replace meals) to the health care team.
- Report any swallowing difficulties, food dislikes, refusal to eat.

Special Considerations
Teaching

- Discuss dietary concerns of patient's illness. Explain why specific foods are not included in a meal or why only limited amounts are allowed (Grodner et al., 2012).

- Instruct patient and family to maintain a balanced diet and monitor intake of fluids and percent or amount of meals and snacks consumed. If intake falls below 75% for any length of time, refer patient to an RD for medical nutrition therapy.
- Teach family caregivers techniques to safely help patient in feeding. Have family encourage patient to do as much as possible to feed self.

Pediatric
- Human milk is the most desirable complete diet for infants during the first 6 months. Infants who are breastfed or bottle-fed do not require additional fluids, especially water or juice, during the first 4 months of life. Excessive intake of water causes water intoxication, failure to thrive, and hyponatremia. Typically infants do not consume solid foods until 6 months of age. Iron-fortified infant cereal is usually the first solid food to offer. A common sequence for introducing solid food is one new food every 5 to 7 days. Strained fruits followed by vegetables and

finally meats is the usual pattern (Hockenberry and Wilson, 2011).
- Do not mix solid foods in a bottle and feed through a nipple with a larger hole (Hockenberry and Wilson, 2011).

Gerontologic
- Some older adults have diminished appetite because of loss of taste and smell and decreased number of taste buds (Chang and Roberts, 2011).
- Interactions between nutrients and medications affect taste of foods or metabolism, absorption, digestion, or excretion of drugs.

Home Care
- Assess financial resources of patient and family to determine if they are able to purchase nutritionally complete foods for patient.
- Help patient and family identify ways to make meals in the home pleasant and enjoyable experiences.

SKILL 30-3 Aspiration Precautions

 Video Clip

The ability to swallow effectively and safely is a basic human need. Safe transport of food and fluid through the mouth, pharynx, and esophagus to the stomach requires a complex and fine coordination of cranial nerves and the muscles of the tongue, pharynx, larynx, and jaw. Any alteration or delay in the swallowing process causes dysphagia (difficulty swallowing). People with dysphagia have difficulty holding food and fluid in their mouths or experience difficulty in the movement of food and fluids into the esophagus (Nazarko, 2009). Dysphagia can occur at any age, but is most common in the elderly because the likelihood of diseases associated with swallowing alterations increases with age (Garcia and Chambers, 2010; Palmer and Metheny, 2008). Approximately 40% of individuals older than age 60 experience dysphagia (Ney et al., 2009).

Almost any condition that produces general muscle weakness or any condition associated with neurologic impairment of the swallowing mechanism and altered mental status places patients at risk for dysphagia (e.g., brain injury, stroke) (Leder et al., 2011; Thomas, 2008) (Box 30-4). These patients may also have altered swallowing reflexes such as difficulty knowing what to do when food is placed in the mouth and holding food in the mouth for prolonged periods (Brady, 2008).

Be aware that patients without primary neurologic diagnoses such as myocardial infarction (heart attack), pneumonia, and chronic obstructive pulmonary disease are also at risk for dysphagia (DeFrabrizio and Rajappa, 2010; Garon, et al., 2009). Structural obstructions and medication side effects cause difficulty swallowing (DeFabrizio and Rajappa, 2010; Ney et al., 2009). Symptoms of dysphagia vary, depending on the swallowing alteration (Garcia and Chambers, 2010). You should suspect dysphagia if a patient has frequent drooling, loss of food from the mouth during eating, pocketing food (holding food in the cheek), and spitting pieces of food out. In addition, a patient might experience choking or coughing during or following meals and a gurgling or wet-sounding voice quality (Brady, 2008; Kyle, 2011). He or she may complain about the sensation of food sticking in his or her throat or make multiple attempts to swallow.

Inability to coordinate the complex, sequential swallowing mechanism slows eating, results in food being left in the mouth, and may lead to failure to adequately protect the airway (Thomas, 2008). Gastric material and secretions in the mouth and pharynx and pathogenic bacteria enter the trachea and lungs (Eisenstadt, 2010). The aspirated material may be food, water, vomitus, or oral contents. Aspiration pneumonia can be a fatal complication of dysphagia, especially in older adults (Garcia and Chambers, 2010;

BOX 30-4	Causes of Dysphagia

Neurogenic
Stroke
Cerebral palsy
Guillain-Barré syndrome
Multiple sclerosis
Amyotrophic lateral sclerosis (Lou Gehrig's disease)
Diabetic neuropathy
Parkinson's disease

Myogenic
Myasthenia gravis
Aging
Muscular dystrophy
Polymyositis

Obstructive
Benign peptic stricture
Lower esophageal ring
Candidiasis
Head and neck cancer
Inflammatory masses
Trauma/surgical resection
Anterior mediastinal masses
Cervical spondylosis

Other
Gastrointestinal or esophageal resection
Rheumatologic disorders
Connective tissue disorders
Vagotomy

Lewis et al., 2011). Tachypnea (respirations above 26) is an early clue of aspiration (Eisenstadt, 2010). Other signs include cough; dyspnea (trouble breathing); decreased breath sounds; and abnormal breath sounds such as wheezing, rales, and rhonchi (see Chapter 6). A wet-sounding vocal quality is a clinical indicator that the patient may be silently aspirating saliva (Brady, 2008).

Silent or asymptomatic aspiration refers to passage of foods or liquids into the trachea and lungs without producing a productive cough or other signs consistent with aspiration (Garon et al., 2009). The condition often results from sensory damage to the pharynx and muscle weakness in the throat and mouth that produces a lack of protective cough reflex (Garon et al., 2009). Lack of outward signs such as coughing reduces awareness by the patient, family, and health team members that aspiration is occurring. This can result in longer periods of ingestion of food and liquids into the lungs and places the patient in a higher-risk group for the development of pneumonia (Garon et al., 2009). The more subtle signs associated with silent aspiration are easy to miss and include lack of speech, depressed alertness, wet quality to voice, drooling, difficulty controlling secretions, and absence of gag reflex.

Dysphagia Evaluation

The goal of dysphagia evaluation and management is to ensure that a patient will be able to swallow oral fluids and food safely (Brady, 2008). You are in close contact with patients and are in a key position to identify swallowing difficulties and make referrals to appropriate health care professionals as needed. When your assessment shows that a patient is at risk for dysphagia and aspiration, referral for a more comprehensive examination is necessary (Box 30-5). At-risk patients must be assumed to have difficulty swallowing and

---

BOX 30-5 | **Criteria for Dysphagia Referral**

Before Referral:
If the answer is yes to either of the following two questions, referral at this time is not appropriate.
- Is patient unconscious or drowsy?
- Is patient unable to sit in an upright position for a reasonable length of time?

Please Consider the Next Two Questions Before Making the Referral:
- Is the patient near the end of life?
- Does the patient have an esophageal problem that will require surgical intervention?

When Observing the Patient or Giving Mouth Care, Look for the Following:
- Open mouth (weak lip closure)
- Drooling liquids or solids
- Poor oral hygiene/thrush
- Facial weakness
- Tongue weakness
- Difficulty with secretions
- Slurred, indistinct speech
- Change in voice quality
- Poor posture or head control
- Weak involuntary cough
- Delayed cough (up to 2 minutes after swallow)
- General frailty
- Confusion/dementia
- No spontaneous swallowing movements

If any of the above is present, the patient may have swallowing problems and need referral to a speech-language pathologist.

---

be at risk for choking and aspiration. (Hollin, 2011; Tanner, 2010). The single most important measure to prevent aspiration is to place the patient on NPO until a swallowing evaluation determines that dysphagia poses no substantial risk (Tanner, 2010). Any patient who is at risk for aspiration needs to be formally referred for a dysphagia evaluation by a speech-language pathologist (SLP). Early screening and intervention are crucial in the prevention of aspiration and pneumonia (Hines et al., 2011). The Joint Commission mandates that patients admitted with a stroke diagnosis be screened before they can ingest an oral diet (TJC, 2012). Use simple orientation questions and single-step commands to determine the potential for both aspiration and safe oral intake before dysphagia screening (Leder et al., 2009). Dysphagia screening is a minimally invasive evaluation procedure that initially documents the likelihood that dysphagia is present, the need for further swallowing assessment, and the safety of patient intake.

Bedside screening for dysphagia includes giving patient water or foods with different textures and observing for coughing, gagging, choking, and voice alteration. Individuals who have a weak spontaneous cough are not able to ingest water without clinical signs of aspiration (Garon et al., 2009; Marques et al., 2008). However, bedside assessment is not sufficient for evaluating the frequency of silent aspiration because it does not have specific symptoms (Garon et al., 2009; Nam-Jong Paik, 2011; Thomas, 2008). Recommendations include accompanying fluid administration with pulse oximetry measurement. Normal oxygen saturation (SpO_2) is greater than 95%. A drop in oxygen saturation greater than or equal to 2% is used to determine aspiration (Bours et al., 2009; Marques et al., 2008; Weinhardt, 2008).

Dysphagia Management

Dysphagia management includes dietary modification by altering the consistency of foods and liquids and is most effective when implemented using a multidisciplinary approach (Garcia and Chambers, 2010). The SLP and registered dietitian (RD) are central to dysphagia management. An SLP specializes in swallowing disorders and makes treatment recommendations to the health care provider that may include texture modifications for food and liquids. The RD ensures that recommendations are balanced with the nutritional and caloric needs of patients. Appropriate food choices and consistency of liquids are individualized and based on which phase of swallowing is dysfunctional (Bottino-Bravo and Thomas, 2008). Changes in food and/or liquid consistencies, elimination of oral intake, and initiation of tube feedings are common diet modifications.

In October 2002 the American Dietetic Association published the National Dysphagia Diet. The diet standards provide guidelines and standard terminology for food and texture modifications. The diet comprises four levels: dysphagia puree, dysphagia mechanically altered, dysphagia advanced, and regular (Table 30-4). There are also four levels of liquid consistencies used simultaneously with diet modification. These include thin liquids (low viscosity) such as water, coffee, tea and anything that liquefies in the mouth at room temperature. Swallowing thin liquids requires the most coordination and control (Remig and Weeden, 2012). Thin liquids create safety risks in swallowing because of their speed and decreased texture for patients with impaired oral motor control (Garcia et al., 2010).

Thickened liquids are commonly prescribed to prevent aspiration pneumonia (Frey and Ramsberger, 2011). Nectarlike liquids (medium viscosity) are liquids such as peach or apricot nectar that are thickened but drip off a spoon at a slower rate than thin liquids. Honeylike liquids (high viscosity) are thickened so the liquid drips

TABLE 30-4 | National Dysphagia Diet Stages

Stage	Description	Examples
NDD 1: Dysphagia pureed	Uniform, pureed, cohesive, pudding-like texture	Smooth hot cereals cooked to a "pudding" consistency; mashed potatoes; pureed meat and vegetables; pureed pasta on rice; yogurt
NDD 2: Dysphagia mechanically altered	Moist, soft textured. Easily forms a bolus	Cooked cereals; dry cereals moistened with milk; canned fruit (except pineapple); moist ground meat; well-cooked noodles in sauce/gravy; well cooked, diced vegetables
NDD 3: Dysphagia advanced	Regular foods (except very hard, sticky, or crunchy foods)	Moist breads (e.g., butter, jelly); well-moistened cereals, peeled soft fruits (peach, plum, kiwi); tender, thin-sliced meats; baked potato (without skin); tender, cooked vegetables
Regular	All foods	No restrictions

Modified from National Dysphagia Task Force (NDDTF): *National dysphagia diet: standardization for optimal care*, Chicago, 2002, American Dietetic Association.

off a spoon at a much slower rate. A thickening agent alters flavor and texture qualities (Garcia et al., 2010). There are often complaints about their taste and thickness, which increase nonadherence (Brady, 2008; Frey and Ramsberger, 2011). There are spoon-thick viscosity liquids that include foods that do not easily drip off a spoon. It is important to remember that the desired thickness of a liquid depends on the patient's swallowing deficit. Always read the label directions when modifying liquids to prepare the desired thickness (Garcia et al., 2010). If a patient's diagnostic tests reveal aspiration with all food and liquid consistencies, intravenous fluids (parenteral nutrition) (see Chapter 32) may be initiated short term to maintain hydration (see Chapter 28) until alternatives for oral nutrition are discussed and accepted by the patient for nutritional support. Enteral nutrition (tube feeding) is used for long-term nutritional support (see Chapter 31).

Consequences Of Dysphagia
Physiologic consequences of dysphagia include decreased appetite, weight loss, dehydration, malnutrition, and pneumonia (DeFabrizio and Rajappa, 2010; Garcia and Chambers, 2010). Dietary intake may be affected for long periods of time; and the malnutrition that occurs is secondary to insufficient protein, calorie, and micronutrient intake (Meiner, 2011). Dysphagia may affect a patient's quality of life. Understand the emotional impact of losing the ability to eat and drink safely. A patient's normal nutritional intake is altered because he or she either is unable to consume oral nutrition or has to make diet modifications to swallow without risk of aspiration. Emotional responses may include altered body image,

embarrassment, social isolation, and depression (DeFrabrizio and Rajappa, 2010). In addition, a patient may feel as though he or she is a burden to family members or caregivers (DeFrabrizio and Rajappa, 2010).

Delegation and Collaboration
The assessment of a patient's risk for aspiration and determination of positioning cannot be delegated to nursing assistive personnel (NAP). However, NAP may feed patients after receiving instruction on aspiration precautions. The nurse directs the NAP to:
- Position patient upright or according to medical restrictions during and after feeding.
- Use aspiration precautions while feeding patients who need assistance.
- Immediately report any onset of coughing, gagging, or a wet voice or pocketing of food.

Equipment
- Upright chair or bed in high-Fowler's position
- Thickening agents as designated by SLP (rice, cereal, yogurt, gelatin, commercial thickener)
- Tongue blade
- Penlight
- Oral hygiene supplies (see Chapter 17)
- Pulse oximeter
- Suction equipment (see Chapter 25)
- Clean gloves

STEP	RATIONALE

ASSESSMENT

1 Assess patient's knowledge of aspiration risks.

2 Perform a nutritional assessment (see Skill 30-1).

3 Assess mental status, including alertness, orientation, and ability to follow simple commands (e.g., open your mouth; stick out your tongue).

4 Determine if patient has an increased risk for aspiration and assess for signs and symptoms of dysphagia (see Box 30-4). Use dysphagia screening tool if available.

5 Assess patient's oral health. Check level of dental hygiene, missing teeth or poorly fitting dentures (apply clean gloves if needed).

Encourages cooperation, minimizes anxiety. Identifies teaching needs.

Patients with dysphagia alter their eating patterns or choose foods that do not provide adequate nutrition (White et al., 2008).

If orientation and command-following are impaired, there is a higher risk of aspiration than with patients who are oriented and can follow commands (Leder et al., 2009).

Performing an assessment before feeding determines when referral to SLP is necessary. Interventions to minimize aspiration and possible pneumonia can be implemented.

Poor oral hygiene can result in decayed teeth, plaque, and periodontal disease and cause growth of bacteria in the mouth, which can be aspirated (Eisenstadt, 2010).

STEP	RATIONALE
6 Observe patient during mealtime for signs of dysphagia such as coughing, dyspnea, or drooling. Note during and at end of meal if patient tires.	Indicates swallowing impairment and possible aspiration. Chewing and sitting up for feeding accelerate onset of fatigue (Meiner, 2011). Fatigue increases risk for aspiration (White et al., 2008).

NURSING DIAGNOSES

- Impaired swallowing
- Risk for aspiration

Related factors are individualized based on patient's condition or needs.

PLANNING

1 Expected outcomes following completion of procedure: • Patient does not exhibit signs or symptoms of aspiration. • Patient maintains stable weight.	Interventions for preventing aspiration are successful. Patient is able to maintain adequate oral nutrition.

IMPLEMENTATION

1 Perform hand hygiene.	Prevents transmission of microorganisms.
2 Indicate on patient's chart and Kardex that dysphagia/aspiration risk is present. *Option:* Some agencies use different-colored meal trays to signify patients at risk for aspiration.	Identifying patient as dysphagic reduces risk that he or she will receive oral nutrition without supervision.
3 Apply pulse oximeter to patient's finger during feeding.	A decrease in oxygen saturation may indicate aspiration (Weinhardt, 2008).
4 Position patient in an upright (90 degrees) or highest position allowed by medical condition during mealtimes.	Uses gravity to facilitate safe swallowing and enhances esophageal motility (Grodner et al., 2012; Ney et al., 2009). Side-lying position is an option if patient cannot have head elevated.
5 Using penlight and tongue blade, gently inspect mouth for pockets of food.	Pockets of food found inside cheeks occur when patient has difficulty moving food from mouth into pharynx; may lead to aspiration (Remig and Weeden, 2012). Patient is usually unaware of pocketing (Chang and Roberts, 2011).
6 Have patient assume chin-tuck position.	Chin-tuck or chin-down position helps reduce aspiration by positioning epiglottis in more forward position, allowing for airway protection during swallowing (Brady, 2008). Position also slows movement of food and liquid through mouth and pharynx, minimizing risk of aspiration (Ney et al., 2009).
a Have patient swallow twice or repeatedly and monitor swallowing and for any respiratory difficulty.	Double- or repeat-swallowing requires patient to use additional swallows to help clear any remaining food from an unprotected airway (Garcia and Chambers, 2010).
7 Add thickener to thin liquids to create desired consistency per SLP evaluation.	Increasing viscosity or thickness of liquid slows movement through mouth and pharynx and protects airway (Brady, 2008).
8 Encourage patient to feed himself or herself.	Promotes independence and may help patient to initiate more natural swallow (Brady, 2008).
9 Tell patient not to tilt head backward when eating or while drinking out of a glass or cup.	Backward head tilt extends neck; thus food and liquid are more likely to be misdirected into airway (Ney et al., 2009).
10 If patient is unable to feed self, place ½ to 1 teaspoon of food on unaffected side of mouth, allowing utensils to touch mouth or tongue.	Small bites help patient's ability to swallow (Grodner et al., 2012). Provides tactile cue to begin eating; avoids pocketing of food on weaker side, which may increase risk of aspiration (Brady, 2008).
11 Provide verbal cues while feeding. Remind patient to chew and think about swallowing.	Helps to elicit normal swallow and prevent aspiration (Brady, 2008).
12 Avoid mixing food of different textures in same mouthful. Alternate liquids and bites of food.	Single textures are easier to swallow than multiple textures. Alternating solids with liquids helps to remove food residue in mouth (Ney et al., 2009).
13 Minimize distractions and do not rush patient. Allow time for adequate chewing and swallowing.	Environmental distractions and conversations during mealtime increase risk for aspiration (Chang and Roberts, 2011).
14 Use sauces, condiments, and gravies to facilitate cohesive food bolus formation.	Cohesive food bolus helps to prevent pocketing or small food particles from entering the airway (Ney et al., 2009).
15 Report signs and symptoms of dysphagia or aspiration to health care provider.	Communication with members of health care team regarding high-risk patients may prevent adverse outcomes in dysphagic patients (Tanner, 2010). Identifies need to have an assessment performed by radiologist or SLP (White et al., 2008).

STEP	RATIONALE
16 Ask patient to remain sitting upright for at least 30 to 60 minutes after meals.	Remaining upright after meals or snack reduces chance of aspiration by allowing food particles remaining in pharynx to clear (Frey and Ramsberger, 2011).
17 Provide thorough oral hygiene after meals (see Chapter 17).	Oral hygiene reduces plaque and secretions containing bacteria that can cause pneumonia, especially in patients with decreased immunity (Eisenstadt, 2010; Frey and Ramsberger, 2011).
18 Perform hand hygiene.	Reduces spread of microorganisms

EVALUATION

1 Continually evaluate at-risk patient's ability to cough and manage oral secretions. Also monitor ability to swallow food and fluids of different textures and viscosities without choking.	Indicates improvement with swallowing and absence of signs related to aspiration (DeFabrizio and Rajappa, 2010). Ability to swallow can improve or deteriorate (Nazarko, 2009).
2 Weigh patient daily or weekly.	Determines if weight is stable and reflects nutritional status.
3 Monitor patient's intake and output (I&O), calorie count, and food intake.	Aids in detection of malnutrition and dehydration resulting from dysphagia.
4 Monitor pulse oximetry readings for high-risk patients when eating.	Deteriorating oxygen saturation levels indicate aspiration.

Unexpected Outcomes

1   Patient coughs, gags, complains of food "stuck in throat," and has wet quality to voice when eating.

2   Patient experiences weight loss.

Related Interventions

- Stop feeding immediately and place patient on NPO. Notify health care provider and suction as needed.
- Anticipate consultation with SLP for swallowing exercises and techniques to improve swallowing.
- Consult with health care provider and RD about increasing frequency of meals or providing oral nutritional supplements or alternative feeding methods such as tube feedings.

Recording and Reporting

- Document in patient's medical record assessment findings, patient's tolerance of liquids and food textures, amount of assistance required, position during meal, absence or presence of any symptoms of dysphagia during feeding fluid intake, and amount eaten.
- Report any coughing, gagging, choking, or swallowing difficulties to health care provider.

Special Considerations

Pediatric

- Monitor growth, hydration, and nutritional status in children with dysphagia (Hollin, 2011).
- Families and caregivers caring for children with dysphagia require support, information, reassurance, and appreciation for their efforts (Hollin, 2011).
- Be aware that silent aspiration has been reported in children with dysphagia before, during, and after swallowing (Hollin, 2011).

Gerontologic

- The risk for aspiration pneumonia is higher in older adults because of an increased incidence of dysphagia and gastroesophageal reflux (Meiner, 2011; White et al., 2008).
- Malnutrition occurs rapidly in older adults with dysphagia. Enteral feedings are sometimes necessary, but there is still a risk for aspiration (Meiner, 2011).

Home Care

- Educate patient and family caregivers about aspiration precautions used to prevent pneumonia (Bottino-Bravo and Thomas, 2008).
- Determine patient's and family caregiver's knowledge of appropriate food choices, strategies to increase caloric intake, and food and liquid texture modifications.
- Dysphagia in home care is best managed with a multidisciplinary approach that includes patient, family caregivers, health care provider, nurse occupational therapist, and speech therapist (Bottino-Bravo and Thomas, 2008).

Critical Thinking Exercises

Mr. Jasper is a 73-year-old patient with Alzheimer's disease. He is receiving medication that leaves him with a dry mouth. Results of a nutritional screening indicate difficulty swallowing. Symptoms include frequent coughing during the meal. The speech-language pathologist (SLP) recommended a dysphagia mechanically altered diet with thickened liquids. He currently weighs 138 lbs (62.7 kg) and is 180 cm (6 feet) tall. His daughter visits frequently. Although he can feed himself, she usually feeds him during scheduled mealtimes in the busy dining room. She frequently gives him sips of her coffee and bites of his favorite oatmeal cookies. The daughter encourages him to bend his head backward to make sure that he drinks all of the liquids in a cup or glass.

1 Determine Mr. Jasper's body mass index (BMI) and rate his nutritional status.

2 Develop a teaching plan related to decreasing Mr. Jasper's aspiration risk. Include rationales for your actions.

3 The SLP recommends a soft/low-residue diet. Identify three foods to include.

REVIEW QUESTIONS

1 An older adult is admitted to the hospital, where the Mini Nutritional Assessment (MNA) is done and a score of 19 is obtained. Which priority measure should be included in this patient's care?
1 Evaluation of potential interactions between drugs and foods consumed
2 Having the registered dietitian talk with the patient about which foods could be eaten more easily
3 Obtaining a weight every day at the same time and on the same scale
4 Assessing what the patient understands related to nutritional health

2 The nurse is feeding a patient at risk for aspiration. The patient's oxygenation status is being monitored by pulse oximetry. Before feeding, oxygenation level is 95%. The nurse suspects that the patient may be silently aspirating. The pulse oximetry reading would be:_____. (Fill in the blank.)

3 Which of the following should not be delegated by the nurse to nursing assistive personnel (NAP)?
1 Nutritional screening
2 Aspiration precautions
3 Feeding
4 Pulse oximetry

4 Which statement made by a patient during a nutritional assessment requires follow-up by the nurse?
1 "My weight changed from 195 to 185 in 1 month."
2 "I've increased my intake of fruits and vegetables."
3 "I'm trying to exercise, but I don't have the time."
4 "I try to eat 3 meals a day."

5 A patient is unable to eat more than 25% of any meal because of pain and nausea. Which of the following interventions would be most important for the nurse to perform?
1 Encourage the patient to eat small amounts several times during the day
2 Ask the patient which foods and beverages cause the least amount of nausea
3 Record a chronology of what the patient has been eating for the past 2 days
4 Determine strategies to decrease the pain and nausea

6 The nurse performs a physical assessment on a newly admitted patient and notes a diminished gag reflex. The health care provider has written an order for the patient to have a full liquid diet ordered. What is the most appropriate nursing action?
1 Place the patient on NPO status
2 Observe the patient while eating
3 Elevate the head of patient's bed to prepare him or her for the meal
4 Change the diet order to clear liquids to see how the patient tolerates the fluids

7 Which of the following foods is the safest for the patient with dysphagia?
1 Applesauce
2 Shredded wheat and milk
3 Jell-O
4 Orange sherbet

8 Which finding assessed on physical examination of an adult patient is a potential indicator of malnutrition?
1 Pink, spongy gums
2 Soft and toned muscles
3 Shiny, sparse hair
4 Smooth and swollen tongue

9 Which statement made by a patient receiving a clear liquid diet indicates a need for further teaching?
1 "I'll order ice tea for lunch."
2 "I drank my coffee with cream and sweetener."
3 "I really want grape popsicles with each meal."
4 "I really like beef bouillon with lunch."

10 The nurse is caring for a patient who is of the Orthodox Jewish faith. In keeping with their religious practices, the patient will not eat:
1 Duck.
2 Shrimp.
3 Ham.
4 Hamburger.

REFERENCES

American Dietetic Association (ADA): Part 1: The 2008 update, J Am Diet Assoc 108(7):1113, 2008.

Adams N, et al: Recognition by medical and nursing professionals of malnutrition and risk of malnutrition in elderly hospitalized patients, Nutr Diet 65:144, 2008.

Barbosa-Silva M: Subjective and objective nutritional assessment methods: what do they really assess? Curr Opin Clin Nutr Metabol Care 11:248, 2008.

Bauer JM, et al: Evaluation of nutritional status in older persons: nutritional screening and assessment, Curr Opin Clin Nutr Metabol Care 13:8, 2010.

Beghetto MG, et al: Accuracy of nutritional assessment tools for predicting adverse outcomes, Nutricion Hospitalaria 24(1):56, 2009.

Bottino-Bravo P, Thomas J: When it's a hard act to swallow: dysphagia in home care, Home Healthc Nurse 26(4):244, 2008.

Bours G, et al: Bedside screening tests vs. videofluoroscopy or fiberoptic endoscopic evaluation of swallowing to detect dysphagia in patients with neurological disorders, J Adv Nurs 65(3):477, 2009.

Brady A: Managing the patient with dysphagia, Home Healthc Nurse 26(1):41, 2008.

Burns C: Seeing food through older eyes: the cultural implications of dealing with nutritional issues in aged and aging, Nutr Diet 66:200, 2009.

Center for Nutrition Policy and Promotion: 2011, International Food Information Counsel Foundation, 2011, available at http://www.foodinsight.org/Resources/Detail.aspx?topic=Questions_and_Answers_About_the_Dietary_Guidelines_For_Americans, accessed July 26, 2012.

Centers for Disease Control and Prevention (CDC): Healthy weight, 2011, available at http://www.cdc.gov/healthyweight/assessing/index.html, accessed July 26, 2011.

Chang C, Roberts B: Strategies for feeding patients with dementia, Am J Nurs 111(4):36, 2011.

Charney P, Escott-Stump S: Overview of nutrition diagnosis and intervention. In Mahan LK, Escott-Stump S, Raymond JL, editors: Krause's food nutrition and the nutrition care process, ed 13, Philadelphia, 2012, Saunders.

DeFabrizio M, Rajappa A: Contemporary approach to dysphagia management, J Nurse Pract 6(9):625, 2010.

DiMaria-Ghalili RA: Nutrition. In Capezuti E, et al, editors: Evidenced-based geriatric nursing protocols for best practice, New York, 2008, Springer.

Ebersole P, et al: Toward healthy aging: Human needs and nursing response, ed 7, St Louis, 2008, Mosby.

Eisenstadt E: Dysphagia and aspiration pneumonia in older adults, *J Acad Nurse Pract* 22:17, 2010.

Fletcher J: Identifying patients at risk of malnutrition: nutrition screening and assessment, *Gastrointest Nurs* 7(5):12, 2009.

Fletcher A, Carey E: Knowledge, attitudes and practices in the provision of nutritional care, *Br J Nurs* 20(10):615, 2011.

Frey K, Ramsberger G: Comparison of outcomes before and after implementation of a water protocol for patients with cerebrovascular accident and dysphagia, *J Neurosci Nurs* 43(3):165, 2011.

Garcia J, Chambers E: Managing dysphagia through diet modifications, *Am J Nurs* 110(11):26, 2010.

Garcia J, et al: Quality of care issues for dysphagia: modifications involving oral fluids, *J Clin Nurs* 19:1618, 2010.

Garon B, et al: Silent aspiration: results of 2,000 video fluoroscopic evaluations, *J Neurosci Nurs* 41(4):178, 2009.

Gout BS, et al: Malnutrition identification, diagnosis and dietetic referrals: are we doing a good enough job? *Nutr Diet* 66:206, 2009.

Grodner M, et al: *Foundations and clinical applications of nutrition: a nursing approach,* ed 4, St Louis, 2012, Mosby.

Hammond K, Litchford M: Dietary and clinical assessment. In Mahan LK, Escott Stump S, Raymond JL, editors: *Krause's food nutrition and the nutrition care process,* ed 13, Philadelphia, 2012, Saunders.

Hines S, et al: Identification and nursing management of dysphagia in individuals with acute neurological impairment, *Br J Evid Based Healthc* 9:148, 2011.

Hockenberry MJ, Wilson D: *Wong's nursing care of infants and children,* ed 9, St Louis, 2011, Mosby.

Hollin R: Identification and management of dysphagia in children with neurological impairments, *Aust Nurs J* 18(10):31, 2011.

Holst M, et al: Can the patient perspective contribute to quality of nutritional care? *Scand J Caring Sci* 25(1):176, 2010.

Jefferies D, et al: Nuturing and nourishing: the nurses' role in nutritional care, *J Clin Nurs* 20:317, 2011.

Kahn MS, et al: Malnutrition, anthropometric, biochemical abnormalities in patients with diabetic nephropathy, *J Renal Med* 19(4):275, 2009.

Kennedy ET, et al: The 2010 dietary guidelines: what Americans should be eating, *J Nurse Pract* 7(5):425, 2011.

Kravitz L: Waist to hip ratio, waist circumference, and BMI: what to use for health risk indication and why, *IDEA Fitness J* 7(9):18, 2010.

Kyle G: Managing dysphagia in older people with dementia, *Br J Commun Nurs* 16(1):6, 2011.

Leder S, et al: Answering orientation questions and following single-step verbal commands: effect on aspiration status, *Dysphagia* 24:290, 2009.

Leder S, et al: Initiating safe oral feeding in critically ill intensive care and step-down unit patients based on passing a 3-ounce (90 milliliters) water swallow challenge, *J Trauma: Injury Infect Crit Care* 70(5):1201, 2011.

Lewis SL, et al: *Medical-surgical nursing,* ed 8, St Louis, 2011, Mosby.

Litchford M: Clinical: biochemical assessment. In Mahan LK, Escott-Stump S, Raymond JL, editors: *Krause's food nutrition and the nutrition care process,* ed 13, Philadelphia, 2012, Saunders.

Marques C, et al: Bedside assessment of swallowing in stroke: water tests are not enough, *Topics Stroke Rehabil* 15(4):378, 2008.

Meiner S: *Gerontologic nursing,* ed 4, St Louis, 2011, Mosby.

Mowe M, et al: Insufficient nutritional knowledge among health care workers? *Clin Nutr* 27(2):196, 2008.

Mueller C, et al: ASPEN: Clinical guidelines: nutrition, assessment, and interventions in adults, *J Parenter Enter Nutr* 35(1):16, 2011.

Nam-Jong Paik: *Dysphagia,* 2011, available at http://emedicine.medscape.com/article/324096-overview, accessed July 26, 2012.

National Heart, Lung and Blood Institute (NHLBI): *Obesity education initiative,* 2008, available at http//www.nhlbi.n:ih.gov/health/public/heart/obesity/lose_wt/risk.htm, accessed August 16, 2011.

National Institute of Diabetes, Digestive and Kidney Diseases: *Weight and waist measurements: tools for adults,* 2008, available at http://win.niddk.nih.gov/publications/tools.htm, accessed July 26, 2012.

National Quality Forum (NQF): *National voluntary consensus standards for patient safety: a consensus report,* Washington, DC, 2010, NQF.

Nazarko L: Nutrition. Part 5: Dysphagia, *Br J Healthc Assist* 3(5):228, 2009.

Nelms M: Assessment of nutritional status and risk. In Nelms MN, et al, editors: *Understanding nutrition therapy and pathophysiology,* ed 2, Belmont, Calif, 2010, Wadsworth.

Ney D, et al: Senescent swallowing: impact, strategies, and interventions, *Nutr Clin Practice* 24:395, 2009.

O'Regan P: Nutrition for patients in hospital, *Nurs Stand* 23(23):35, 2009.

Palmer J, Metheny N: How to try this: preventing aspiration in older adults with dysphagia, *Am J Nurs* 108(2):40, 2008.

Perry L: Using height, weight and other body measurements in nutritional assessments, 2009, available at http://www.nursingtimes.net/using-height-weight-and-other-body-measurements-in-nutritional-assessments/1958313.article, accessed July 26, 2012.

Phillips M, et al: Nutritional screening in community-dwelling older adults: a systematic review. *Asia Pac J Clin Nutr* 19(3):440, 2010.

Portero-McLellan K, et al: The use of calf circumference measurement as an anthropometric tool to monitor nutritional status in elderly inpatients, *J Nutr Health Aging* 14(4):266, 2010.

Prins A: Nutritional assessment of the critically ill patient, *S Afr Clin Nurs* 23(1):11, 2010.

Raymond A: Recognizing and managing undernutrition, *Pract Nurse* 40(9):15, 2010.

Remig V, Weeden A: Medical nutrition therapy for neurologic disorders. In Mahan LK, Escott-Stump S, Raymond JL, editors: *Krause's food nutrition and the nutrition care process,* ed 13, Philadelphia, 2012, Saunders.

Skates J, Anthony P: The mini nutritional assessment: an integral part of geriatric assessment, *Nutrition Today* 44(1):21, 2009.

Tanner D: Lessons from nursing home dysphagia malpractice litigation, *J Gerontol Nurs* 36(3):41, 2010.

The Joint Commission (TJC): *2012 Comprehensive accreditation manual for hospitals: the official handbook,* Oakbrook Terrace, Ill, 2012, TJC.

Thomas D: Hard to swallow: management of dysphagia in nursing home residents, *Am Medical Directors Assoc* 9(7):455, 2008.

Ukleja A, et al: Standards for nutrition support: adult hospitalized patients, *Nutr Clin Pract* 25:403, 2010.

US Department of Agriculture (USDA): *Choose MyPlate,* 2010a, available at http://chooseMYPlate.gov, accessed July 26, 2012.

US Department of Agriculture (USDA): *Executive summary,* 2010b, available at http://www.cnpp.usda.gov/publications/DietaryGuidelines/2010/PolicyDoc/ExecSumm.pdf accessed August 7, 2012.

US Department of Agriculture (USDA) and US Department of Health and Human Services (USDHHS): *Dietary guidelines for Americans,* 2010, available at http://health.gov/dietaryguidelines/dga2010/dietaryguidelines2010.pdf, accessed July 26, 2012.

Webster J, Healy J: Continuing professional development: nutrition in hospitalized patients, *Nurs Older People* 21:31, 2009.

Weinhardt J: Accuracy of a bedside dysphagia screening: a comparison of registered nurses and speech therapists. *Rehabil Nurs* 33(6):247, 2008.

White G, et al: Dysphagia: cause, assessment, treatment, and management, *Geriatrics* 63(5):15, 2008.

Wright L, et al: The effectiveness of targeted feeding assistance to improve the nutritional intake of elderly dysphagic patients in hospital, *J Human Nutr Diet* 21:555, 2008.

31

Enteral Nutrition

SKILLS AND PROCEDURES

Skill 31-1   Inserting and Removing a Small-Bore Nasogastric or Nasoenteric Feeding Tube, p. 777
Skill 31-2   Verifying Feeding Tube Placement, p. 782
Skill 31-3   Irrigating a Feeding Tube, p. 786
Skill 31-4   Administering Enteral Nutrition: Nasoenteric, Gastrostomy, or Jejunostomy Tube, p. 788
Procedural
Guideline 31-1 Care of a Gastrostomy or Jejunostomy Tube, p. 793

MEDIA RESOURCES

- **evolve** http://evolve.elsevier.com/Perry/skills
  - Review Questions
  - Audio Glossary

- **NSO** Nursing Skills Online

KEY TERMS

Enteral nutrition
Gastrostomy feeding tube

Jejunostomy feeding
tube

Nasogastric (NG) feeding
tube

Pulmonary aspiration
Residual volume

OBJECTIVES

Mastery of content in this chapter will enable the nurse to:
- Assess patients who are to receive enteral tube feedings.
- Demonstrate the ability to correctly insert a small-bore feeding tube.
- Discuss the rationale for methods to determine nasogastric or nasoenteric feeding tube placement.

- Discuss the reasons for risks for pulmonary complications during the insertion and maintenance of a feeding tube.
- Demonstrate the appropriate technique for irrigating a feeding tube.
- Demonstrate three appropriate techniques for administering enteral formulas.
- Evaluate a patient's tolerance of enteral feeding.

Enteral nutrition, commonly called *tube feeding*, refers to the delivery of nutritional formulas through a tube that has been placed into the gastrointestinal (GI) tract. Candidates for tube feeding include patients who have adequate digestion and absorption but cannot ingest, chew, or swallow food safely or in adequate amounts. A tube feeding is administered into the stomach or small intestine. The selection of the type of tube and placement method depends on the anticipated duration of feeding and other patient-related factors such as gastric emptying and risk for pulmonary aspiration, the most serious complication of tube feeding. For short-term feeding nasal or oral feeding tubes are appropriate. Terms used to describe these types of tubes include *nasogastric (NG)*, *orogastric (OG)*, and *nasoenteric*. When the duration of tube feeding extends beyond 4 weeks or in situations in which access to the GI tract through the nose or mouth is contraindicated, direct enteral access through the abdominal wall is the optimal choice. The

stomach (gastrostomy tube) and jejunum (jejunostomy tube) are the usual sites for long-term feeding tubes.

Besides inserting a tube, nursing responsibilities include verifying and maintaining proper position of a tube, keeping it patent, administering the nutrient formula, and preventing complications. A nurse, dietitian, and health care provider collaborate to select an enteral feeding formula based on a patient's protein and calorie requirements and digestive ability. Liquid formulas in the United States are sterile and lactose free. Disease-specific formulas are available, but research does not always support their efficacy (Chen and Peterson, 2009).

EVIDENCE-BASED PRACTICE

Safe and effective enteral nutrition depends on knowledgeable nurses and high-quality nursing care. A multidisciplinary approach with adherence to evidence-based protocols or

775

algorithms enhances the quality and safety of enteral nutrition (Bankhead et al., 2009; Kenny and Goodman, 2010). Follow these evidence-based guidelines to ensure correct placement of enteral feeding tubes:

- NG feeding tubes are often inserted at the bedside, without technologic assistance, in a procedure commonly referred to as *blind* placement. More sophisticated aids such as fluoroscopy or electromagnetic tracking may be required to successfully direct a tube into the small bowel (Bankhead et al., 2009).
- The most serious complication of NG tube insertion is inadvertent pulmonary intubation. Researchers estimate that 1% to 2% of NG tubes placed blindly enter the airway undetected, which can lead to serious pulmonary injury (Krenitsky, 2011).
- Feeding tubes are positioned into the small bowel to reduce the incidence of pulmonary aspiration of stomach contents. Research has not consistently demonstrated this benefit, but newer techniques for detecting aspiration provide some evidence that small intestine feeding does reduce the incidence of pulmonary aspiration (Metheny et al., 2011).
- Variation in the color and pH of fluid withdrawn from feeding tubes can help to differentiate tubes positioned in the stomach from those that rest in the small intestine. However, these indicators are not consistently reliable for distinguishing between placement in the GI tract and tracheobronchial system. X-ray film confirmation of correct tube placement is mandatory before enteral feeding or medication is administered through a blindly placed feeding tube (Bankhead et al., 2009).
- Carbon dioxide (CO_2) detectors can help locate the position of tubes during insertion and potentially reduce insertion-related pulmonary injury. A sensor attached to the end of the feeding tube changes color in the presence of CO_2, thus indicating that the tube may have entered the airway. However, capnography cannot accurately identify tubes that terminate in the esophagus, a situation that can lead to reflux and pulmonary aspiration of enteral formula (Bankhead et al., 2009; Munera-Seeley et al., 2008).
- Maintaining and monitoring tube location during feeding and keeping the head-of-bed elevation at a minimum of 30 degrees (preferably 45 degrees) effectively reduces aspiration and subsequent pneumonia (Kenny and Goodman, 2010).
- Measurement of gastric residual volumes (GRVs) is done routinely during tube feeding to identify risk for regurgitation and pulmonary aspiration of gastric contents. This technique involves withdrawing and measuring the contents of the stomach at regular intervals during tube feeding. Feeding is stopped when GRVs exceed a specified level; however, studies have failed to demonstrate a consistent relationship between GRV and risk of pulmonary aspiration (DeLegge, 2011; Metheny et al., 2008). Recommendations for stopping tube feeding for elevated GRVs range from 250 to 500 mL (Bankhead et al., 2009; DeLegge, 2011; Metheny et al., 2008). Researchers agree that decisions to stop tube feeding must not rely solely on GRV but should also include an assessment of a patient's clinical condition (Metheny et al., 2008).

PATIENT-CENTERED CARE

The insertion and use of a feeding tube often raises emotional and psychological concerns. A patient and family caregiver need reassurance and encouragement throughout the insertion procedure and once the tube feeding is underway. Nursing interventions such as oral hygiene and care of the nasal passage or tube insertion site promote patient comfort during tube feeding and can reduce complications.

Although tube feeding may offer life-sustaining treatment, artificial nutrition can never replace the social and symbolic benefits of sharing meals. Many social, religious, and cultural events involve food; and patients requiring long-term tube feeding may feel a sense of loss regarding their ability to participate in life activities. Studies show that many patients associate tube feeding with low quality of life (Bozetti, 2008). In these cases a multidisciplinary team, including a speech pathologist (to evaluate the ability to swallow safely), can help patients and family caregivers use strategies to preserve or enhance quality of life. If oral intake is not contraindicated, encourage tube-fed patients to partake of food for the pleasurable sensations associated with eating. Support groups such as the Oley Foundation can serve as valuable sources of information and practical advice for patients who require long-term tube feeding.

Enteral nutrition therapy is not obligatory in cases of futile care or end-of-life situations. However, some clinical circumstances, as in cases of advanced dementia or degenerative neurologic disease, can raise ethical concerns about the role of enteral nutrition. Although a convincing body of evidence demonstrates a link between poor clinical outcomes and tube feeding in patients with progressive neurologic disease, not all patients or their family caregivers are willing to forgo nutritional support in this situation. Patients with a living will or other advance directive may specifically refuse the use of artificial feeding by tube. Decisions about whether tube feeding should be started or continued demand a multidisciplinary approach that considers cultural, spiritual, and psychological dimensions of the issue. Situations such as this require effective communication with the patients and their family caregiver, realistic goals, and respect for patient autonomy (Baroccas et al., 2010).

Safety Guidelines

1 Be aware of factors that increase risk for complications related to feeding tube insertion: altered level of consciousness, abnormal clotting, impaired gag or cough reflex.
2 Know the purpose of the feeding and the intended location of the tip of the feeding tube.
3 Take precautions to prevent microbial contamination of enteral formulas.
4 Be aware of safety measures to prevent pulmonary aspiration of gastric contents and accidental tube displacement by patients.
5 Consult with a pharmacist regarding a patient's medications and their route of delivery to determine if administration via feeding tube is appropriate.
6 Be vigilant when manipulating components of enteral feeding systems for procedures such as medication administration or tube irrigation to avoid tubing misconnections with intravenous systems or other medical devices (NQF, 2011).

SKILL 31-1   Inserting and Removing a Small-Bore Nasogastric or Nasoenteric Feeding Tube

NSO *Enteral Nutrition Module / Lessons 1 and 2*

Throughout this chapter nasally placed feeding tubes (8 to 12 Fr) are referred to as *nasogastric (NG) tubes*; but some types of NG tubes, which are larger and more rigid, are used for gastric decompression instead of feeding (see Chapter 34). Because feeding tubes are soft and flexible, many use a removable guidewire or stylet to provide stiffness during tube insertion. Although these wires facilitate placement of a tube, they also add to the risk of pulmonary or esophageal injury during insertion. Nurses can also pass feeding tubes through the mouth, especially in critical care when the patient is also intubated or when contraindications to nasal placement such as a basilar skull fracture or facial trauma exist.

Placement of a feeding tube requires a health care provider's order. All candidates for NG or nasoenteric tube placement require an assessment of their coagulation status. Because anticoagulation and bleeding disorders pose a risk for epistaxis during nasal tube placement, the health care provider may order platelet transfusion or other corrective measures before tube insertion.

Delegation and Collaboration
The skill of feeding tube insertion cannot be delegated to nursing assistive personnel (NAP). However, NAP may help with patient positioning and comfort measures during tube insertion.

Equipment
❑ Small-bore NG or nasoenteric tube with or without stylet (select the smallest diameter possible to enhance patient comfort) (Fig. 31-1)
❑ 60-mL Luer-Lok or catheter-tip syringe
❑ Stethoscope and pulse oximeter
❑ Hypoallergenic tape, semipermeable (transparent) dressing, or tube fixation device
❑ Tincture of benzoin or other skin barrier protectant
❑ pH indicator strip (scale 0.0 to 11.0)
❑ Cup of water and straw or ice chips (for patients able to swallow)
❑ Emesis basin
❑ Towel or disposable pad
❑ Facial tissues
❑ Clean gloves
❑ Suction equipment in case of aspiration
❑ Penlight to check placement in nasopharynx
❑ Tongue blade

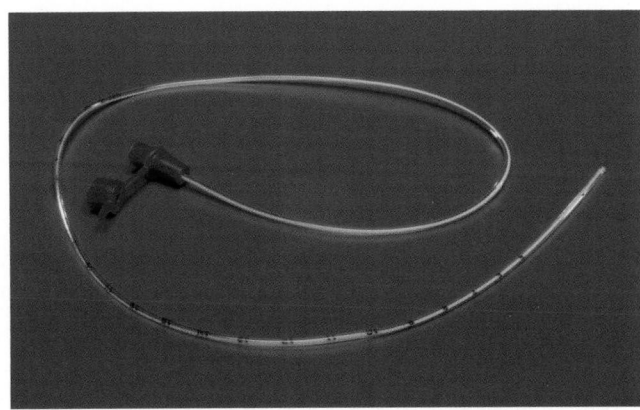

FIG 31-1   Small-bore feeding tube. (*Courtesy Kendall Brands, Mansfield, Mass.*)

STEP	RATIONALE

ASSESSMENT

1 Verify health care provider's order for type of tube and enteric feeding schedule.

Health care provider's order is needed to intubate patient with feeding tube.

2 Assess patient's knowledge of procedure.

Encourages cooperation, reduces anxiety, and minimizes risks. Identifies teaching needs.

3 Have patient close each nostril alternately and breathe. Examine each naris for patency and skin breakdown.

Sometimes nares are obstructed or irritated, or a septal defect or facial fractures are present. Place tube in most patent nostril.

4 Review patient's medical history (e.g., for basilar skull fracture, nasal problems, nosebleeds, facial trauma, nasal-facial surgery, deviated septum, anticoagulant therapy, coagulopathy).

History of these problems may require you to consult with health care provider to change route of nutritional support. Passage of tube intracranially can cause neurologic injury.

> **Clinical Decision Point** *If a patient is at risk for intracranial passage of the tube, avoid the nasal route. Oral placement or placement under medical supervision using direct visualization is preferable. Insertion of a gastrostomy or jejunostomy tube is another alternative.*

5 Assess patient's mental status (ability to cooperate with procedure, sedation), presence of cough and gag reflex, ability to swallow, critical illness, and presence of an artificial airway.

These are risk factors for inadvertent tube placement into tracheobronchial tree (Krenitsky, 2011).

> **Clinical Decision Point** *Recognize situations in which blind placement of a feeding tube poses an unacceptable risk for placement. Devices designed to detect pulmonary intubation such as CO_2 sensors or electromagnetic tracking devices enhance patient safety. Alternatively, to avoid insertion complications from blind placement in high-risk situations, clinicians trained in the use of visualization or imaging techniques should place tubes (AACN, 2010; Krenitsky, 2011).*

6 Perform physical assessment of abdomen (see Chapter 6).

Absent bowel sounds, abdominal pain, tenderness, or distention may indicate medical problem contraindicating feedings.

STEP	RATIONALE

NURSING DIAGNOSES

- Imbalanced nutrition: less than body requirements
- Readiness for enhanced nutrition
- Risk for aspiration

Related factors are individualized based on patient's condition or needs.

PLANNING

1 Expected outcomes following completion of procedure:
- Tube is verified as placed in stomach or intestine.

  Correct technique ensures placement in intended location (Bourgault and Halm, 2009).
- Feeding tube remains patent.

  Proper irrigation clears tube of formula residue (Bankhead et al., 2009).
- Patient has no respiratory distress (e.g., increased respiratory rate, coughing, poor color) or signs of discomfort or nasal trauma.

  Correctly placed tube causes no interference with airway.

2 Explain procedure to patient, including sensations that will be felt during insertion.

Increases patient's cooperation with intubation procedure and helps lessen anxiety.

3 Explain to patient how to communicate during intubation by raising index finger to indicate gagging or discomfort.

Patient must have way of communicating to alleviate stress and enhance cooperation.

IMPLEMENTATION

1 Identify patient using two identifiers (i.e., name and birthday or name and account number) according to agency policy. Compare identifiers with information on patient's identification bracelet.

Ensures correct patient. Complies with The Joint Commission standards and improves patient safety (TJC, 2012).
Some agencies are now using a bar-code system to help with patient identification.

2 Perform hand hygiene.

Reduces transmission of microorganisms.

3 Position patient upright in high Fowler's position unless contraindicated. If patient is comatose, raise head of bed as tolerated in semi-Fowler's position with head tipped forward, chin to chest. If necessary have an assistant help with positioning of confused or comatose patients. If patient is forced to lie supine, place in reverse Trendelenburg's position.

Reduces risk for pulmonary aspiration in event patient should vomit. Forward head position assists with closure of airway and passage of tube into esophagus.

4 Apply pulse oximeter and measure vital signs.

Permits objective assessment of respiratory status during tube insertion.

5 Determine length of tube to be inserted and mark location with tape or indelible ink.
- **a** Measure distance from tip of nose to earlobe to xyphoid process of sternum (see illustration).

  Length approximates distance from nose to stomach.

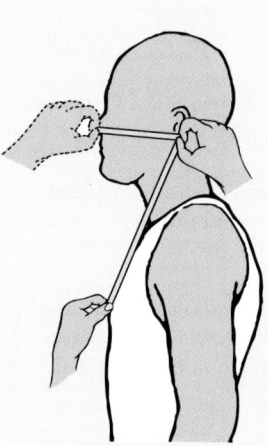

STEP 5a Determine length of tube to be inserted.

STEP	RATIONALE

Clinical Decision Point *Tip of tube must reach stomach to avoid the risk for pulmonary aspiration, which occurs when tubes terminate in the esophagus.*

6 Prepare NG or nasoenteric tube for intubation.

   a Inject 10 mL of water from 30- to 60-mL Luer-Lok or catheter-tip syringe into the tube.

Ensures that tube is patent. Avoid using non–Luer-Lok syringes and connectors to reduce risk of tubing misconnection (Simmons et al., 2011).

   b If using stylet, make certain that it is positioned securely within tube.

Promotes smooth passage of tube into gastrointestinal (GI) tract. Improperly positioned stylet can cause tube to kink or injure patient.

7 Cut hypoallergenic tape 10 cm (4 inches) long or prepare membrane dressing or other tube fixation device.

Used to secure tubing after insertion.

8 Apply clean gloves.

Reduces transmission of microorganisms.

9 Dip tube with surface lubricant into glass of room-temperature water or apply water-soluble lubricant (see manufacturer directions).

Activates lubricant to facilitate passage of tube into naris and GI tract.

10 Explain the step and gently insert tube through nostril to back of throat (posterior nasopharynx). This may cause patient to gag. Aim back and down toward ear (see illustration).

Natural contours facilitate passage of tube into GI tract.

11 Have patient flex head toward chest after tube has passed through nasopharynx.

Closes off glottis and reduces risk for tube entering trachea.

12 Encourage patient to swallow by giving small sips of water or ice chips. Advance tube as patient swallows.

Swallowing facilitates passage of tube past oropharynx. Distinct tug may be felt as patient swallows, indicating that tube is following expected path.

13 Reemphasize need to mouth breathe and swallow during procedure.

Helps facilitate passage of tube and alleviates patient's fears during procedure.

14 When tip of tube reaches carina (approximately 25 to 30 cm [10 to 12 inches] in an adult), stop and listen for air exchange from distal portion of tube.

Audible breath sounds may indicate that tube is in respiratory tract; remove and start over. Some agency policies require radiograph at 30 to 35 cm (12 to 14 inches) to rule out airway position before proceeding with tube insertion (Krenitsky, 2011).

15 Advance tube each time patient swallows until desired length has been passed (see illustration).

Reduces discomfort and trauma to patient.

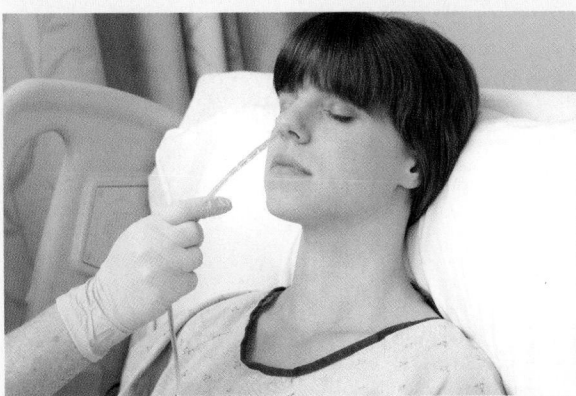

STEP 10 Insert tube through nostril to back of throat.

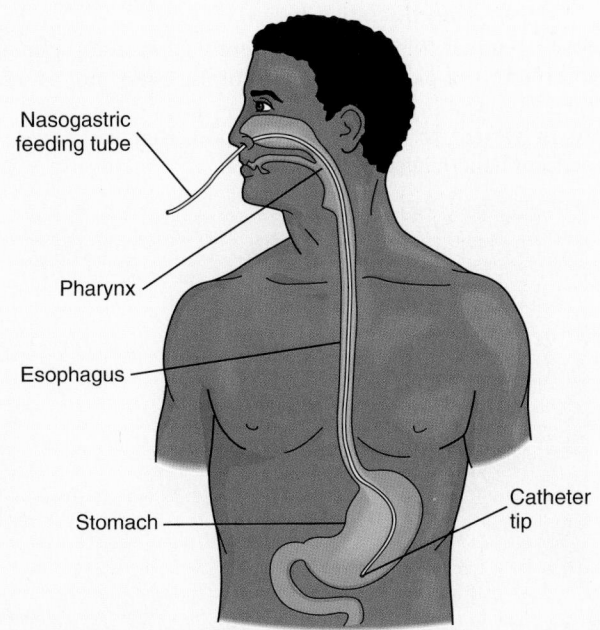

STEP 15 NG feeding tube inserted through nose and esophagus into stomach.

STEP	RATIONALE

Clinical Decision Point *Do not force the tube or push against resistance. If patient starts to cough, experiences a drop in oxygen saturation, or shows other signs of respiratory distress, withdraw the tube into the posterior nasopharynx until normal breathing resumes.*

16 Check for position of tube in back of throat with penlight and tongue blade.	Tube may be coiled, kinked, or entering trachea.
17 Temporarily anchor tube to nose with small piece of tape.	Movement of tube stimulates gagging. Assesses general position before anchoring tube more securely.
18 Keep tube secure and check placement of tube by aspirating stomach contents to measure gastric pH (see Skill 31-2).	Proper tube position is essential before initiating feeding.

Clinical Decision Point *Insufflation of air into tube while auscultating abdomen is not a reliable means to determine position of feeding tube tip (AACN, 2010; Bourgault and Halm, 2009; Kenny and Goodman, 2010).*

19 Anchor tube to patient's nose, avoiding pressure on nares. Mark exit site on tube with indelible ink. Select one of the following options for anchoring:	Properly secured tube allows patient more mobility and prevents trauma to nasal mucosa.
a Apply tape:	Prevents pulling of tube. May require frequent change if tape becomes soiled.
(1) Apply tincture of benzoin or other skin adhesive on tip of patient's nose and allow it to become "tacky."	Helps tape adhere better. Protects skin.
(2) Remove gloves and split one end of tape lengthwise 5 cm (2 inches).	
(3) Place intact end of tape over bridge of patient's nose. Wrap each of the 5-cm strips in opposite directions around tube as it exits nose (see illustration).	Secures tube firmly.
b Apply membrane dressing or tube fixation device:	Permits longer securement without need to change dressing.
(1) Membrane dressing:	
(a) Apply tincture of benzoin or other skin protector to patient's cheek and area of tube to be secured.	
(b) Place tube against patient's cheek and secure tube with membrane dressing, out of patient's line of vision.	Decreases risk for patient's inadvertent extubation.
(2) Tube fixation device:	
(a) Apply wide end of patch to bridge of nose (see illustration).	
(b) Slip connector around feeding tube as it exits nose (see illustration).	
20 Fasten end of NG tube to patient's gown using clip (see illustration) or piece of tape. Do not use safety pins to secure tube to gown.	Reduces traction on naris if tube moves. Safety pins become unfastened and cause injury to patients.
21 Assist patient to comfortable position. Remove gloves and perform hand hygiene.	

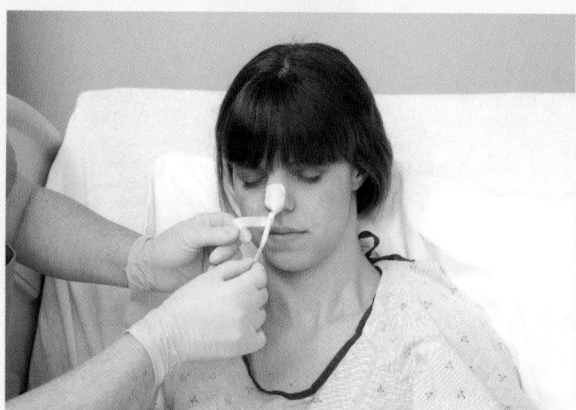

STEP 19a(3) Wrap first strip of tape down length of feeding tube. Bring second strip down around length of tube, wrapping in opposite direction.

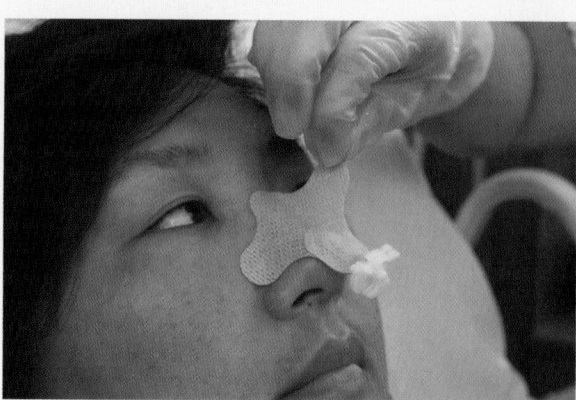

STEP 19b(2)(a) Apply tube fixation patch to bridge of nose.

STEP	RATIONALE

Clinical Decision Point *Leave stylet in place until correct position is verified by x-ray film. Never try to reinsert a partially or fully removed stylet while feeding tube is in place. This can cause perforation of tube and injure patient.*

22 Obtain x-ray film of chest/abdomen.

X-ray film examination is most accurate method to determine feeding tube placement (Bankhead et al., 2009).

23 Apply clean gloves and administer oral hygiene (see Chapter 17). Clean tubing at nostril with washcloth dampened in mild soap and water.

Promotes patient comfort and integrity of oral mucous membranes.

24 Remove gloves, dispose of equipment, and perform hand hygiene.

Reduces transmission of microorganisms.

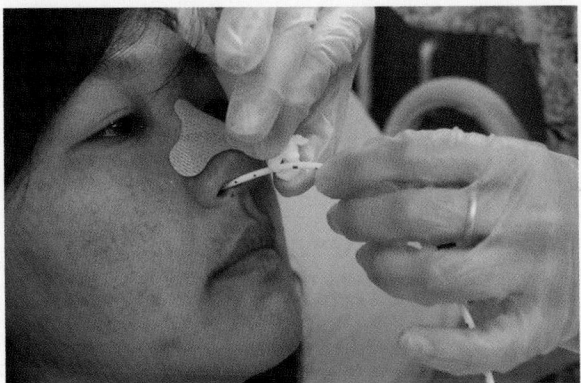

STEP 19b(2)(b) Slip connector around feeding tube.

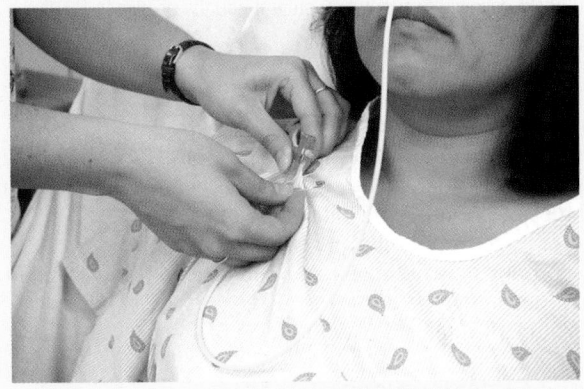

STEP 20 Fastening feeding tube to patient's gown.

Tube Removal

1 Verify health care provider's order for type of tube and enteric feeding schedule.

Health care provider's order is needed to remove feeding tube.

2 Gather equipment: Disposable pad, tissues, clean gloves, disposable plastic bag or receptacle.

3 Explain procedure to patient.

Encourages cooperation, reduces anxiety, and minimizes risks. Identifies teaching needs.

4 Perform hand hygiene. Apply clean gloves.

Reduces transmission of microorganisms.

5 Position patient in high Fowler's position unless contraindicated.

Reduces risk for pulmonary aspiration in event patient should vomit.

6 Place disposable pad or towel over patient's chest.

Prevents mucus and gastric secretions from soiling patient's clothing.

7 Disconnect tube from feeding administration set if present.

Prevents formula from spilling from tube as it is removed.

8 Remove tape or tube fixation device from patient's nose. Unclip tube from patient's gown.

Allows tube to be removed easily.

9 Instruct patient to take deep breath and hold it.

Prevents inadvertent aspiration of gastric contents while tube is removed.

10 Kink end of tube securely by folding it over on itself.

Keeps any residual fluid in tube from flowing out.

11 Completely withdraw tube by pulling it out steadily and smoothly. Dispose of it into appropriate receptacle.

Prevents transmission of microorganisms.

12 Offer tissues to patient to blow nose.

Clears nasal passages of remaining secretions.

13 Offer mouth care.

Promotes patient's comfort.

14 Remove gloves; perform hand hygiene.

Reduces transmission of microorganisms.

EVALUATION

1 Observe patient's response to intubation. Have patient speak. Check vital signs. *Option:* You may use capnography in critical care settings to determine if tip of tube is in trachea or lung.

Abnormal lung sounds may indicate aspiration. Assists with confirmation of tube placement.

2 Confirm x-ray results with health care provider

Verifies position of tube before initiating enteral feeding.

3 Remove the stylet (if used) after x-ray film verification of correct placement.

If placement needs adjustment, stylet is still in place.

STEP	RATIONALE
4 Routinely check location of external exit site marking on the tube and color and pH of fluid aspirated from tube.	Routine evaluation ensures correct placement of tube and reduces the risk of aspiration.
5 After removal, assess patient's level of comfort.	Provides for continued comfort of the patient.

Unexpected Outcomes

1 Aspiration of stomach contents into respiratory tract (delayed response or small-volume aspiration), evidenced by auscultation of crackles or wheezes, dyspnea, or fever.

2 Displacement of feeding tube to another site (e.g., from duodenum to stomach) possibly occurs when patient coughs or vomits.

Related Interventions

- Report change in patient condition to health care provider; if there has not been a recent chest x-ray film, suggest ordering one.
- Position patient on side.
- Suction nasotracheally and orotracheally
- Prepare for possible initiation of antibiotics.

- Aspirate GI contents and measure pH.
- Remove displaced tube and insert and verify placement of new tube.
- If there is a question of aspiration, obtain chest x-ray film.

Recording and Reporting

- Record and report type and size of tube placed, location of distal tip of tube, patient's tolerance of procedure, and confirmation of tube position by x-ray film examination.
- Record removal of tube and patient's tolerance.
- Report any type of unexpected outcome and the interventions performed.
- Tube removal: record patient's level of comfort.

Special Considerations

Teaching

- Instruct patient or family caregiver to offer oral hygiene frequently and keep patient's lips lubricated.
- Teach patient or family caregiver to report tension on feeding tube or displacement of tape or tube fixation device; instruct patient or caregiver to stabilize the tube and call for help.

Pediatric

- The distance from nose-to-ear-to–mid-umbilicus better predicts insertion length for gastric tube placement in neonates and children than traditional nose-to-ear-to-xyphoid measurements (Cirgin Ellett et al., 2011).

- X-ray film confirmation of tube position is not routinely performed because of the radiation risk.
- Routine flushing of tubes is not recommended in pediatric patients.
- When inserting a feeding tube in an infant, observe for vagal stimulation evidenced by a decreased heart rate.

Gerontologic

- Ensure adequate lubrication of tube to decrease discomfort for the older adult because of the potential for decreased oral or nasopharyngeal secretions.

Home Care

- Assess patient or primary caregiver's ability to maintain a tube for a feeding program.
- Assess the environmental safety and sanitation of patient's home to determine potential for infection or injury.
- Teach patient or primary caregiver how to assess tube placement (see Skill 31-2).
- Teach the family caregiver correct method for securing a feeding tube.

SKILL 31-2 Verifying Feeding Tube Placement

NSO *Enteral Nutrition Module / Lesson 3*

Nurses insert small-bore feeding tubes nasally for intermittent or continuous feeding. It is possible for the tip of a feeding tube to move or migrate into a different location (e.g., from the stomach into the intestine or esophagus, from the intestine into the stomach). Although all tubes should be marked to document correct position, tube dislocation can sometimes occur without any external evidence that the tube has moved. The risk of aspiration of regurgitated gastric contents into the respiratory tract increases when the tip of the tube accidentally dislocates upward into the esophagus.

Following initial x-ray film verification of correct feeding tube position, you must monitor the tube to ensure that the tube tip remains in the intended site. Based on a patient's clinical condition and agency policies, you check feeding tube position at regular intervals (often every 4 to 6 hours) and before administering formula or medications through the tube. Radiographic verification is impractical every 4 to 6 hours, but the reports of routine chest and abdominal films should be monitored for reference to the feeding tube location. Because no single bedside method of monitoring tube position during feeding is completely reliable, there are a number of techniques to use in combination to detect feeding tube dislocation:

- Monitor the external length of the tube and observe the appearance, volume, and pH of fluid aspirated through it. The color of the fluid can help differentiate gastric from intestinal placement. Because most intestinal aspirates are stained by bile to a distinct yellow color and most gastric aspirates are not, the difference in color can often distinguish the sites (Fig. 31-2).
- Testing the pH of an aspirate at the bedside using pH paper offers some information regarding the position of a feeding tube, but results are not reliable during continuous feeding and should be used in combination with other indicators with careful assessment of a patient in the clinical setting (AACN, 2010; Bankhead et al., 2009; Renner, 2010).
- Obtain repeat x-ray film confirmation if bedside methods create any doubt regarding the location of the tube.

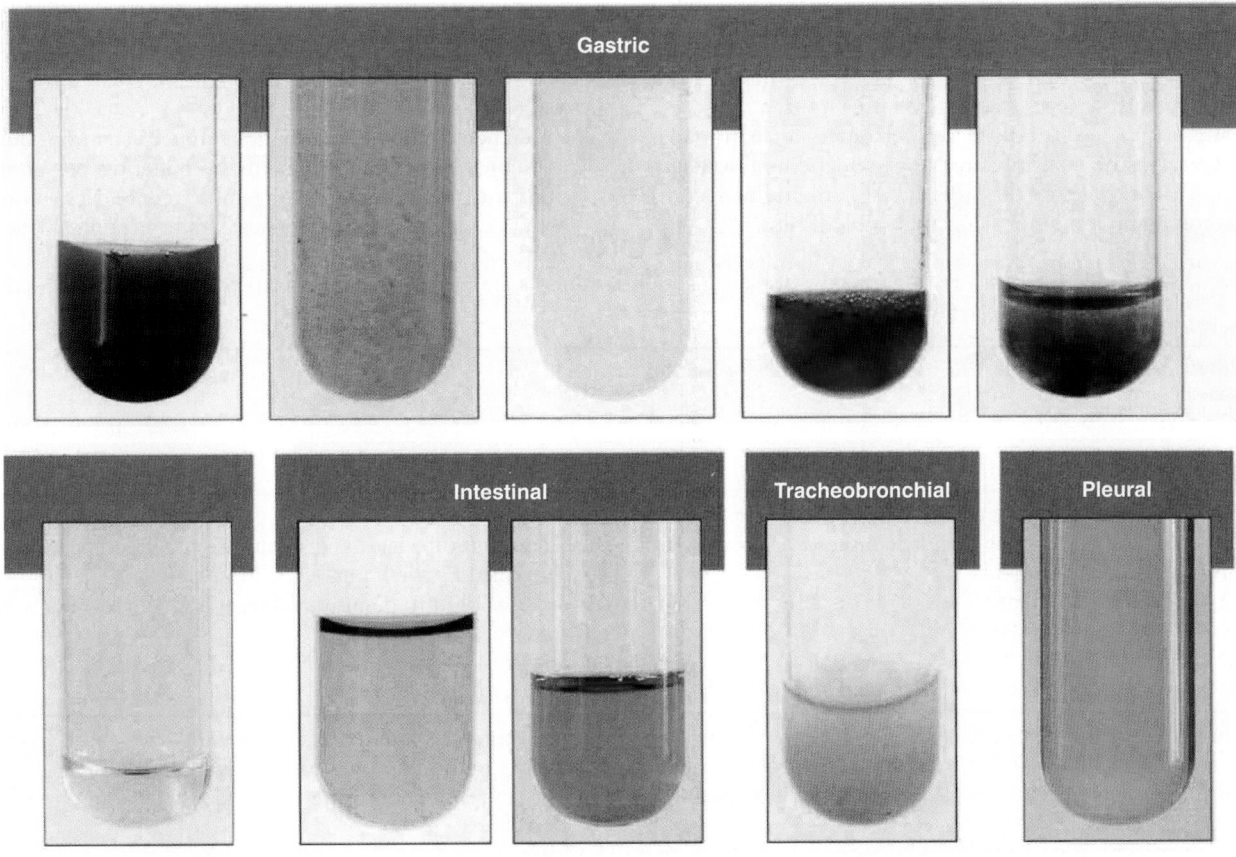

FIG 31-2   Typical color of aspirates from stomach, intestine, and airway. (*Used with permission from Metheny NA, et al: pH, color, and feeding tubes, RN 61:25, 1998.*)

Delegation and Collaboration

The verification of tube placement is the responsibility of the nurse and cannot be delegated to nursing assistive personnel (NAP). The nurse directs the NAP to:

- Immediately inform the nurse if patient's respirations change or patient complains of shortness of breath, coughing, or choking.
- Immediately inform the nurse if the patient vomits or the NAP notices vomitus in patient's mouth during oral hygiene.
- Immediately inform the nurse if nasal skin irritation is present.

- Immediately inform the nurse if a change in the external length of the tube occurs, which could indicate displacement of the tube.

Equipment

- ❑ 60-mL catheter-tip syringe
- ❑ Stethoscope
- ❑ Clean gloves
- ❑ pH indicator strip (scale of 0.0 to 11.0)
- ❑ Small medication cup

STEP	RATIONALE

ASSESSMENT

1 Review agency policy and procedures for frequency and method of checking tube placement. Do not insufflate air into tube to check placement.

Maintains quality of patient care. Listening for air instilled through tube is unreliable (AACN, 2010; Bankhead et al., 2009).

2 Observe for signs and symptoms of respiratory distress during feeding: coughing, choking, or reduced oxygen saturation.

Once the tube has been correctly placed into gastrointestinal (GI) tract, movement into pulmonary system is unlikely. However, a tube that has been pulled back into esophagus can lead to regurgitation and aspiration of formula.

3 Identify conditions that increase risk for spontaneous tube migration or dislocation:
   a Altered level of consciousness, agitation.
   b Retching/vomiting/coughing.
   c Nasotracheal suction.

Feeding tubes may become dislocated by increases in intraabdominal pressure or coughing, but most frequently they are displaced when patient moves or during pulls on tube.

STEP	RATIONALE
4 Observe external portion of tube for movement of ink mark away from mouth or naris (see Skill 31-1).	Increased external length of tube indicates that distal tip is no longer in correct position.
5 Review patient's medication record for orders for continuous feeding or a gastric acid inhibitor (e.g., cimetidine [Tagamet], ranitidine [Zantag], famotidine [Pepcid AC], nizatidine [Axid]) or a proton pump inhibitor (e.g., omeprazole [Prilosec]).	The presence of enteral formula in aspirated secretions diminishes usefulness of pH measurements by buffering pH of stomach. Similarly, H_2 receptor antagonists reduce acid content of secretions, also raising pH value (Bankhead et al., 2009; Renner, 2010).
6 Review patient's record for history of prior tube displacement.	Patients are at increased risk for repeated tube displacement.

NURSING DIAGNOSES

- Impaired gas exchange
- Risk for aspiration

Related factors are individualized based on patient's condition or needs.

PLANNING

1 Expected outcomes following completion of procedure: • Color, pH, and appearance of gastric aspirate are consistent with initial tube placement.	Indicates that tube has likely remained in correct location, initially confirmed by x-ray film (AACN, 2010).
2 Explain procedure to patient.	Patient has right to be informed regarding all procedures. Relieves anxiety.

IMPLEMENTATION

1 Identify patient using two identifiers (i.e., name and birthday or name and account number) according to agency policy. Compare identifiers with information on patient's identification bracelet.	Ensures correct patient. Complies with The Joint Commission standards and improves patient safety (TJC, 2012). Some agencies are now using a bar-code system to help with patient identification.
2 Prepare equipment at patient's bedside, perform hand hygiene, and apply clean gloves.	Reduces transmission of microorganisms.
3 Verify tube placement at the following times: **a** For intermittently tube-fed patients, test placement immediately before each feeding and before medications. **b** Follow agency policy regarding pH testing for patients receiving continuous tube feeding. AACN (2010) recommends that continuous feedings be stopped for several hours to obtain reliable pH readings. **c** Wait to verify placement at least 1 hour after medication administration by tube or mouth.	Each administration of feeding/medication can lead to pulmonary aspiration if tube is displaced. pH testing is of minimal value during continuous tube feeding. Feedings should not be stopped for purpose of pH testing, but pH testing may be helpful when feedings are interrupted for procedures or diagnostic studies (AACN, 2010). Premature withdrawal of contents will remove unabsorbed medication, reducing dose delivered to patient.
4 Draw up 30 mL of air into a 60-mL syringe and attach to end of feeding tube. Flush tube with 30 mL of air before attempting to aspirate fluid. Repositioning patient from side to side is helpful. In some cases more than one bolus of air is necessary.	Burst of air aids in aspirating fluid more easily. Smaller syringes generate unnecessarily high pressures inside tube. It is often more difficult to aspirate fluid from small intestine than from stomach or smaller-size tube (AACN, 2010).
5 Draw back on syringe slowly and obtain 5 to 10 mL of gastric aspirate (see illustration). Observe appearance of aspirate (see Fig. 31-2).	Drawing back quickly or with a smaller syringe may cause tube to collapse. Quantity is sufficient for pH testing. Appearance of aspirate helps to assess position of tube. Aspirates from nasogastric (NG) tubes of continuously tube-fed patients often look like curdled enteral formula. Gastric aspirates from intermittently tube-fed patients are not typically bile stained (unless intestinal fluid has refluxed into stomach) (AACN, 2010).
6 Gently mix aspirate in syringe. Expel few drops into clean medicine cup. Measure pH of aspirated GI contents by dipping pH strip into fluid or by applying a few drops of fluid to strip. Compare color of strip with color on chart (see illustration) provided by manufacturer.	Mixing ensures equal distribution of contents for testing. Most-accurate readings of gastric pH levels are provided by pH paper covering a minimal range of from 0 to 11.0.
a Gastric fluid from patient who has fasted for at least 4 hours usually has pH range of 5.0 or less.	A pH reading of 5.0 or less is reliable indicator of stomach placement, especially when gastric acid inhibitor is not being used (AACN, 2010; Bankhead et al., 2009).
b Fluid from tube in small intestine of fasting patient usually has pH greater than 6.0 (AACN, 2010; Bankhead et al., 2009).	Intestinal contents are more basic than stomach contents.

STEP	RATIONALE
c Patient with continuous tube feeding may have pH of 5.0 or higher (AACN, 2010; Bankhead et al., 2009).	Formulas contain solutions that are basic.
d pH of pleural fluid from tracheobronchial tree is generally greater than 6.0 (AACN, 2010).	
7 If after repeated attempts it is not possible to aspirate fluid from a tube that was confirmed by x-ray film to be in desired position and if there are no risk factors for tube dislocation, monitor external length of tube and observe patient for evidence of respiratory distress (AACN, 2010; Bankhead et al., 2009).	Reports of routine chest or abdominal x-ray films can be used to monitor tube location. Repeat radiographic confirmation of tube position is indicated if external length of tube changes, tape holding tube comes loose, or patient coughs forcefully or vomits (Bankhead et al., 2009).
8 Irrigate tube (see Skill 31-3).	Keeps tube patent.
9 Remove and dispose of gloves and supplies in appropriate receptacle. Perform hand hygiene.	Reduces transmission of microorganisms.

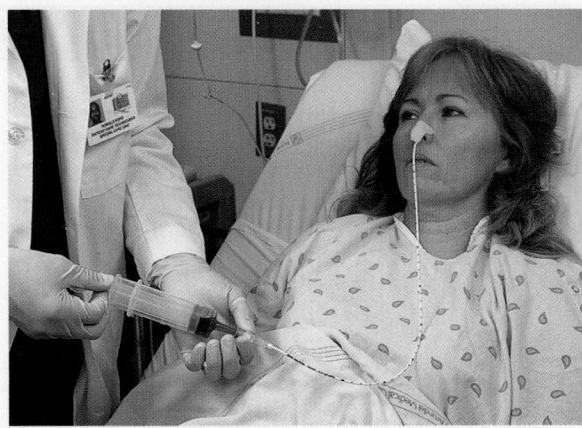

STEP 5   Obtaining gastric aspirate.

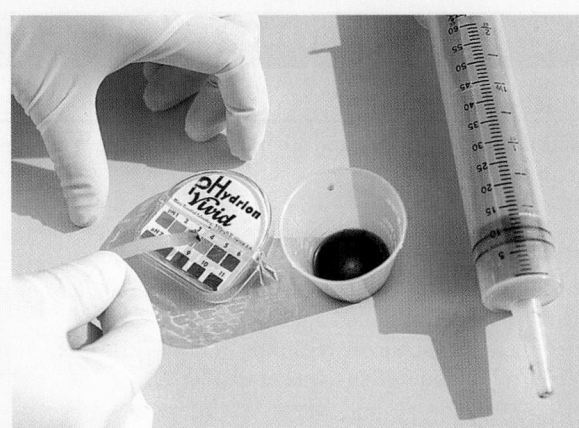

STEP 6   Compare color on test strip with color on pH chart.

EVALUATION

1 Observe patient for respiratory distress: persistent gagging, paroxysms of coughing, drop in O_2 saturation, respiratory patterns (e.g., rate and depth) that are inconsistent with baseline measures.	Feeding enters airways.
2 Verify that external length of tube, pH, and appearance of aspirate are consistent with initial tube placement.	Indicates that tip of tube is likely to be positioned in same place as it was following x-ray film confirmation.

Unexpected Outcomes

1 Red or brown coloring (coffee grounds appearance) of fluid aspirated from feeding tube indicates new or old blood, respectively, in GI tract.

2 Patient develops severe respiratory distress (e.g., dyspnea, decreased oxygen saturation, increased pulse rate) as a result of aspiration or tube displacement into lung.

3 Abdomen becomes distended.

Related Interventions

• If color is not related to medications recently administered, notify health care provider.

• Stop any enteral feedings.
• Notify health care provider.
• Obtain chest x-ray film as ordered.

• Notify health care provider.
• Stop enteral feedings.

Recording and Reporting

• Record and report pH and appearance of aspirate.

Special Considerations
Teaching

• Instruct patient to not pull or alter position of enteral tube.

Pediatric

• Decrease the amount of air insufflated according to the size of patient (e.g., an infant may only need 1 mL of air, a small child 5 mL) before withdrawal of gastric secretions.

Home Care

• Instruct patient or primary caregiver not to proceed with feedings or medication administration via the tube if there is any doubt as to its proper placement.

SKILL 31-3 Irrigating a Feeding Tube

Feeding tubes must remain patent to ensure that liquid nutritional formulas can pass through easily. All types of feeding tubes require routine irrigation to keep a tube patent. Inability to instill air or fluid suggests that a tube is occluded. Curdled enteral formula and improperly crushed medications are the most common causes of feeding tube occlusion.

Delegation and Collaboration

The skill of irrigating a feeding tube cannot be delegated to nursing assistive personnel (NAP).

The nurse directs the NAP to:
- Report when a continuous tube feeding stops infusing.

Equipment
- ❏ 60-mL catheter-tip syringe
- ❏ Water (tap water or sterile [see agency policy], dated and initialed container at patient's bedside)
- ❏ Towel
- ❏ Clean gloves
- ❏ Stethoscope

STEP	RATIONALE
ASSESSMENT	
1 Inspect volume, color, and character of gastric aspirates (if obtainable).	Excess volume of secretions (more than 250 mL) may indicate delayed gastric emptying.
2 Assess bowel sounds.	Determines if peristalsis is present.
3 Note ease with which tube feeding infuses through tubing.	Failure of formula to infuse as desired may indicate developing obstruction.
4 Monitor volume of enteral formula administered during a shift and compare with ordered amount.	Indicates whether sufficient volume of feeding is infusing.
5 Refer to agency policies regarding routine irrigation, usually every 4 to 12 hours (Bankhead et al., 2009).	Determines frequency of irrigations.

NURSING DIAGNOSES

- Deficient fluid volume
- Excess fluid volume
- Imbalanced nutrition: less than body requirements

Related factors are individualized based on patient's condition or needs.

PLANNING	
1 Expected outcomes following completion of procedure:	
• Feeding tube remains patent.	Irrigation fluid clears inner lumen of feeding tube of solids and secretions.
• Patient receives prescribed caloric intake.	Feeding infuses without interruption.
2 Explain procedure to patient.	Decreases patient anxiety.
3 Position patient in high-Fowler's (if tolerated) or semi-Fowler's position.	Reduces reflux and risk for pulmonary aspiration during irrigation.

IMPLEMENTATION	
1 Identify patient using two identifiers (i.e., name and birthday or name and account number) according to agency policy. Compare identifiers with information on patient's identification bracelet.	Ensures correct patient. Complies with The Joint Commission standards and improves patient safety (TJC, 2012). Some agencies are now using a bar-code system to help with patient identification.
2 Perform hand hygiene, prepare equipment at patient's bedside, and apply clean gloves.	Reduces transmission of microorganisms. Ensures an organized approach to irrigation.
3 Verify tube placement (see Skill 31-2) if fluid can be aspirated for pH testing.	With tip of tube correctly placed in stomach, irrigation will not increase risk for pulmonary aspiration.
4 Irrigate routinely before, between, and after final medication (before feedings are reinstituted); and before an intermittent feeding is administered.	Certain formulas have properties that predispose to tube clogging. Irrigation prevents mixing of medications in tube, which may cause clogging.
5 Draw up 30 mL of water in syringe (see illustration). Do not use irrigation fluids from bottles that are used on other patients. Patient should have an individual bottle of solution.	This amount of solution will flush length of tube. Water is most effective agent for preventing tube clogging. Alternative flushing solutions such as cola and fruit juices increase clogging of tubes because of acidity of these fluids (Bankhead et al., 2009; Dandeles and Lodolce, 2011).

STEP	RATIONALE
6 Change irrigation bottle every 24 hours. Irrigation trays, which hold both irrigation fluid and syringe, are considered open systems and may be more easily contaminated than sterile water bottles.	Ensures sterile solution. Sterile water is required for neonates and patients who are immune suppressed or critically ill (Bankhead et al., 2009). Tap water may be appropriate in some clinical settings and in home care if municipal water supply is safe (Bankhead et al., 2009).
7 Kink feeding tube while disconnecting it from administration tubing or while removing plug at end of tube (see illustration).	Prevents leakage of gastric secretions.
8 Insert tip of syringe into end of feeding tube. Release kink and slowly instill irrigation solution (see illustration).	Infusion of fluid clears tubing.

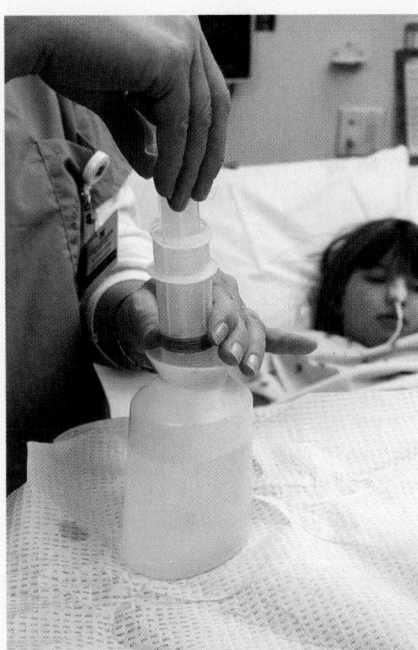

STEP 5   Draw up 30 mL of water into syringe.

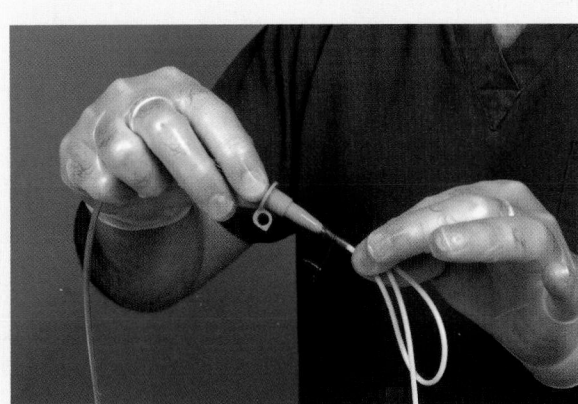

STEP 7   Kink tubing while unplugging feeding tube.

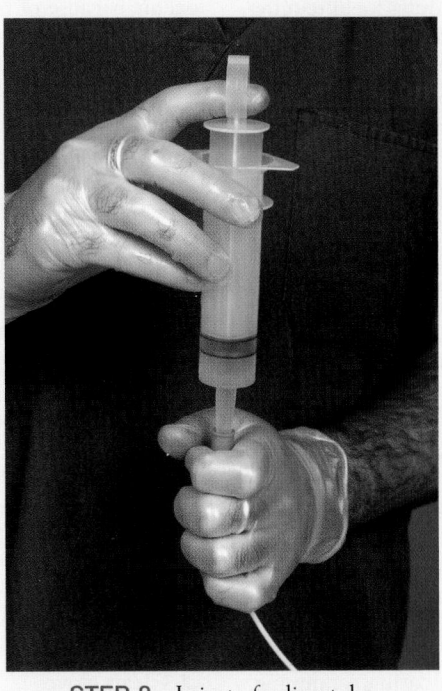

STEP 8   Irrigate feeding tube.

STEP	RATIONALE
9 If unable to instill fluid, reposition patient on left side and try again.	Tip of tube may be against stomach wall. Changing patient's position may move tip away from stomach wall.
10 When water has been instilled, remove syringe. Reinstitute tube feeding or administer medication as ordered. Flush each medication completely through tube (see Skill 21-2).	Tubing is clear and patent. Ensures that full dose reaches stomach and medications do not mix with formula.
11 Remove and discard gloves; dispose of supplies in appropriate receptacle. Perform hand hygiene.	Reduces transmission of microorganisms.

EVALUATION

1 Observe ease with which tube feeding instills through tubing.	A successfully irrigated tube is patent, allowing for free flow of solution.
2 Monitor patient's caloric intake.	Total enteral nutrition infuses without difficulty.

Unexpected Outcomes
1 Tube cannot be irrigated and remains obstructed.

2 Fluid and electrolyte imbalances occur. Insufficient irrigation can cause water deficiency; excessive irrigations can cause fluid volume excess.

Related Interventions
- Repeat irrigation; if unsuccessful, notify health care provider. Tube may need to be removed, and a new tube placed.
- Notify health care provider of abnormal electrolyte levels or imbalanced intake and output.

Recording and Reporting
- Record time of irrigation, amount and type of fluid instilled.
- Report if tubing has become clogged.

Special Considerations
Pediatric
- Irrigation of a tube requires a smaller volume of solution in children: 1 to 3 mL for neonates and 3 to 5 mL for pediatric patients (Bankhead et al., 2009).

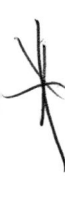

SKILL 31-4 Administering Enteral Nutrition: Nasoenteric, Gastrostomy, or Jejunostomy Tube

NSO *Enteral Nutrition Module / Lesson 4*

Enteral nutrition, or tube feeding, is a method for providing nutrients to patients who are not able to meet their nutritional requirements orally. As a rule, candidates for enteral nutrition must have a sufficiently functional gastrointestinal (GI) tract to absorb nutrients. Examples of indications for enteral feeding include the following:

1 Situations in which normal eating is not safe because of high risk for aspiration: Altered mental status, swallowing disorders, impaired gag reflex, dependence on mechanical ventilation, certain esophageal conditions (strictures, or dysmotility), and delayed gastric emptying.
2 Clinical conditions that interfere with normal ingestion or absorption of nutrients or create hypermetabolic states: Surgical resection of oropharynx, proximal intestinal obstruction or fistula, pancreatitis, burns, and severe pressure ulcers.
3 Conditions in which disease or treatment-related symptoms reduce oral intake: Anorexia, nausea, pain, fatigue, shortness of breath, or depression.

Gastric feedings are the most common type of enteral nutrition, allowing tube-feeding formulas to enter the stomach and then pass gradually through the intestinal tract to ensure absorption. In contrast, small bowel feeding occurs beyond the pyloric sphincter of the stomach, which theoretically reduces the risk for pulmonary aspiration, provided that feedings do not reflux back into the stomach (Metheny et al., 2011). To avoid bloating, cramping, and diarrhea, an enteral infusion pump is used to control the

administration rate of small bowel feedings and many continuous gastric feedings. Inadequate delivery of nutrients, potentially leading to caloric deficit or electrolyte disturbances, sometimes occurs because of frequent interruptions in feeding.

Delegation and Collaboration

The skill of administration of nasoenteric tube feeding can be delegated to nursing assistive personnel (NAP). (Refer to agency policy.) However, a registered nurse (RN) or licensed practical nurse (LPN) must first verify tube placement and patency. The nurse directs the NAP to:

- Elevate head of bed to a minimum of 30 degrees (preferably 45 degrees) or sit patient up in bed or a chair.
- Not adjust feeding rate; infuse the feeding as ordered.
- Report any difficulty infusing the feeding or any discomfort voiced by patient.
- Report any gagging, paroxysms of coughing, or choking.
- Provide frequent oral hygiene.

Equipment
- ❑ Disposable feeding bag, tubing, or ready-to-hang system
- ❑ 60-mL or larger catheter-tip syringe
- ❑ Stethoscope
- ❑ Enteral infusion pump for continuous feedings
- ❑ pH indicator strip (scale 0.0 to 11.0)
- ❑ Prescribed enteral formula
- ❑ Clean gloves

STEP	RATIONALE

ASSESSMENT

1 Assess patient's clinical status to determine potential need for tube feedings: Decreased level of consciousness, nutritional deficits, head or neck surgery, facial trauma, or impaired swallow. Consult with nutrition support team or health care provider.	Identify candidates for enteral nutrition before they become nutritionally depleted.
2 Assess patient for food allergies.	Prevents patient from developing localized or systemic allergic responses to feeding.
3 Perform physical assessment of abdomen, including auscultation for bowel sounds before feeding (see Chapter 6).	Absent bowel sounds are not a contraindication to feeding; but a change from baseline in abdominal examination, particularly if tenderness or distention is present, should be reported to ordering health care provider to determine if tube feeding can proceed safely (Bankhead et al., 2009; McClave et al., 2009).
4 Obtain baseline weight and review serum electrolytes and blood glucose measurement. Assess patient for fluid volume excess or deficit, electrolyte abnormalities, and metabolic abnormalities (e.g., hyperglycemia).	Enteral feedings should restore or maintain patient's nutritional status. Measures provide objective data and baseline to determine selection of formula and measure effectiveness of feedings.
5 Verify health care provider's order for type of formula, rate, route, and frequency.	Ensures that correct formula will be administered in appropriate volume. Enteral formulas are not interchangeable.

NURSING DIAGNOSES

- Imbalanced nutrition: less than body requirements
- Impaired swallowing
- Readiness for enhanced nutrition
- Risk for aspiration

Related factors are individualized based on patient's condition or needs.

PLANNING

1 Expected outcomes following completion of procedure:	
• Patient achieves established target for body weight over time.	Indicates that patient's nutritional status is maintained or improved.
• Patient has no sign of respiratory distress.	Feeding tube does not enter airway, and patient does not aspirate feeding.
• Patient remains or returns to fluid/electrolyte balance.	Scheduled feedings are administered as ordered.
• Patient is free of abdominal cramping.	Feeding administered without abdominal distention.
2 Explain procedure to patient.	Decreases patient anxiety.

IMPLEMENTATION

1 Identify patient using two identifiers (i.e., name and birthday or name and account number) according to agency policy. Compare identifiers with information on patient's identification bracelet.	Ensures correct patient. Complies with The Joint Commission standards and improves patient safety (TJC, 2012). Some agencies are now using a bar-code system to help with patient identification.
2 Perform hand hygiene. Apply clean gloves (Bankhead et al., 2009).	Reduces transmission of microorganisms and potential contamination of enteral formula.
3 Obtain formula to administer:	
a Verify correct formula and check expiration date; note condition of container.	Ensures that correct therapy is to be administered and checks integrity of formula.
b Provide formula at room temperature.	Cold formula causes gastric cramping and discomfort because liquid is not warmed by mouth and esophagus.
4 Prepare formula for administration:	
a Use aseptic technique when manipulating components of feeding system (e.g., formula, administration set, connections).	Bag, connections, and tubing must be free of contamination to prevent bacterial growth (Bankhead et al., 2009).
b Shake formula container well. Clean top of canned formula with alcohol swab before opening it (Bankhead et al., 2009).	Ensures integrity of formula; prevents transmission of microorganisms.
c For closed systems, connect administration tubing to container. If using open system, pour formula from brick pack or can into administration bag (see illustration).	Formulas are available in closed-system containers that contain a 24- to 48-hour supply of formula or in an open system, in which formula must be transferred from brick packs or cans to a bag before administration.

STEP	RATIONALE
5 Open roller clamp and allow administration tubing to fill. Clamp off tubing with roller clamp. Hang container on intravenous (IV) pole.	Prevents introduction of air into stomach once feeding begins.
6 Place patient in high-Fowler's position or elevate head of bed at least 30 degrees (preferably 45 degrees). For patient forced to remain supine, place in reverse Trendelenburg's position.	Elevated head helps prevent pulmonary aspiration.
7 Verify tube placement (see Skill 31-2). Observe appearance of aspirate and note pH measure.	Verifies if tip of tube is in stomach or intestine based on pH value.
8 Check gastric residual volume (GRV) before each feeding (for bolus and intermittent feedings) and every 4 to 6 hours (for continuous feedings) (Metheny et al., 2008; Bankhead et al., 2009).	GRV determines if gastric emptying is delayed. Intestinal residual is usually very small. If residual volume is greater than 10 mL, displacement of tube into stomach may have occurred.
a Draw up 10 to 30 mL air into syringe and connect to end of feeding tube.	
b Inject air into tube. Pull back slowly and aspirate total amount of gastric contents (see illustration).	
c Return aspirated contents to stomach unless volume exceeds 250 mL (see agency policy) (Metheny, 2010).	Prevents loss of nutrients and electrolytes in discarded fluid. Some questions exist regarding safety of returning high volumes of fluid into stomach (Metheny, 2010).
d Do not administer feeding when a single GRV measurement exceeds 500 mL or when two measurements taken 1 hour apart each exceed 250 mL (Bankhead et al., 2009) (check agency policy).	Some controversy exists regarding ability of elevated GRVs to identify risk for pulmonary aspiration. However, frequent interruptions of feeding based on GRV levels is a well-recognized reason for failure to meet nutritional goals (Bankhead et al., 2009; DeLegge, 2011; Metheny et al., 2008).
e Flush feeding tube with 30 mL water (see Skill 31-3).	Prevents clogging of tubing.
9 Before attaching feeding administration set to feeding tube, trace tube to its point of origin. Label administration set, "Tube Feeding Only."	Avoids misconnections between feeding set and IV systems or other medical tubing or devices (Bankhead et al., 2009; Simmons et al., 2011).
10 Intermittent gravity drip:	
a Pinch proximal end of feeding tube and remove cap. Connect distal end of administration set tubing to feeding tube and release tubing.	Prevents excessive air from entering patient's stomach and leakage of gastric contents.
b Set rate by adjusting roller clamp on tubing or attach tubing to feeding pump. Allow bag to empty gradually over 30 to 45 minutes (see illustration). Label bag with tube-feeding type, strength, and amount. Include date, time, and initials.	Gradual emptying of tube feeding reduces risk for abdominal discomfort, vomiting, or diarrhea induced by bolus or too-rapid infusion of tube feedings.

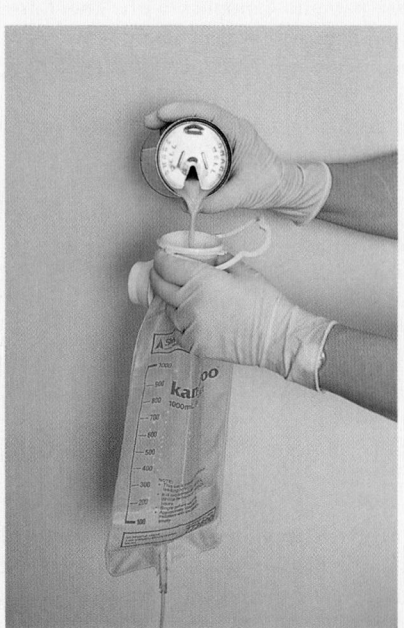

STEP 4c   Pour formula into open feeding container.

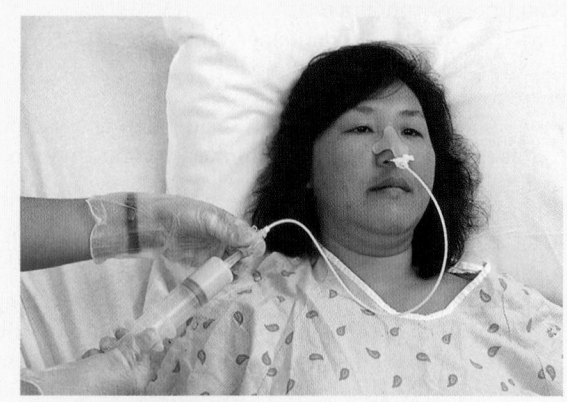

STEP 8b   Check for GRV.

STEP	RATIONALE

Clinical Decision Point *Use pumps designated for tube feeding, not IV fluids.*

c Change bag every 24 hours.	Decreases risk for bacterial colonization.
11 Continuous drip method:	Continuous feeding method is designed to deliver prescribed hourly rate of feeding and reduce risk for abdominal discomfort.
a Connect distal end of administration set tubing to feeding tube as in Step 10a.	
b Thread tubing through feeding pump; set rate on pump and turn on (see illustration).	Delivers continuous feeding at steady rate and pressure. Feeding pump alarms for increased resistance.

Clinical Decision Point *Maximum hang time for formula is 12 hours in an open system; 24 to 48 hours in closed, ready-to-hang system (if it remains closed). Refer to manufacturer guidelines.*

12 Advance rate of tube feeding gradually, as ordered.	Tube feeding can usually begin with full-strength formula. Gradual advancement to goal rates helps to prevent diarrhea and gastric intolerance to formula (Bankhead et al., 2009).
13 Flush tubing with 30 mL water every 4 hours during continuous feeding (see agency policy), before and after an intermittent feeding. Have registered dietitian recommend total free water requirement per day and obtain health care provider's order (see Skill 31-3).	Provides patient with source of water to help maintain fluid and electrolyte balance. Clears tubing of formula.
14 When patient is receiving intermittent tube feeding, cap or clamp end of feeding tube when not being used.	Prevents air from entering stomach between feedings and limits microbial contamination of system.
15 Rinse bag and tubing with warm water whenever feedings are interrupted. Use new administration set every 24 hours.	Rinsing bag and tubing with warm water clears old tube feedings and reduces bacterial growth.
16 Dispose of supplies and perform hand hygiene.	Reduces transmission of microorganisms.

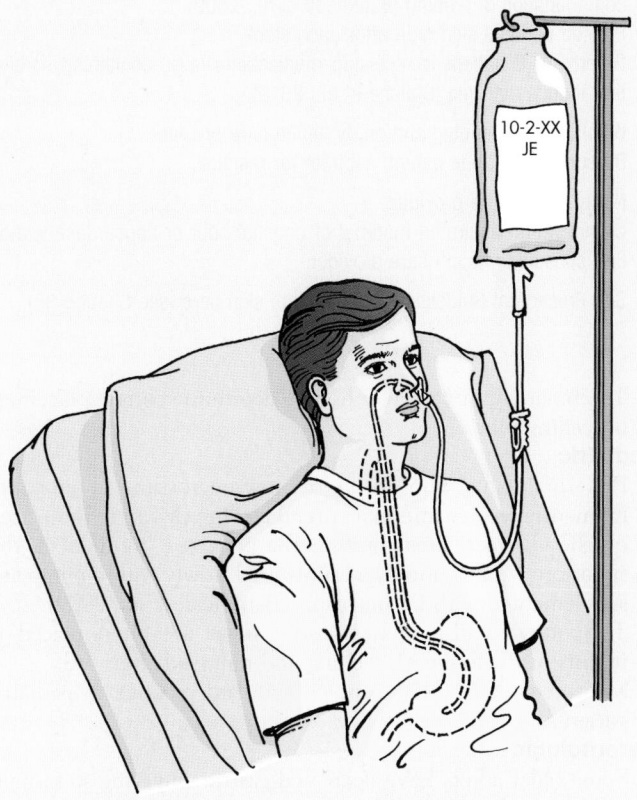

STEP 10b Administer intermittent feeding.

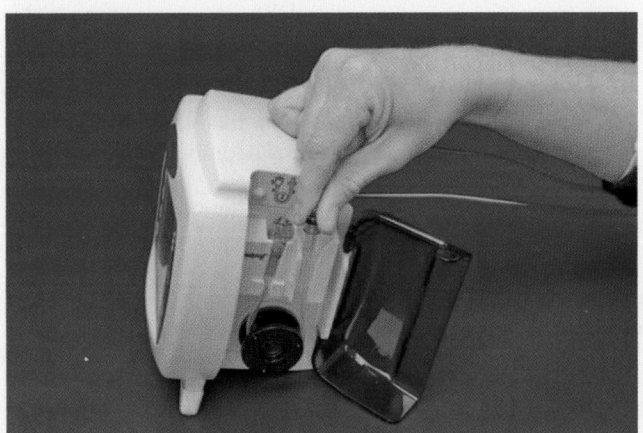

STEP 11b Connect tubing through infusion pump. *(Image used with permission Covidien. All rights reserved.)*

STEP	RATIONALE

EVALUATION

1 Measure GRV per policy, usually every 4 to 6 hours, and ask if nausea or abdominal cramping is present.	GI tolerance of tube feedings must be closely monitored to avoid complications.
2 Monitor intake and output at least every 8 hours and calculate daily totals every 24 hours.	Intake and output are indications of balance or fluid volume excess or deficit.
3 Weigh patient daily until maximum administration rate is reached and maintained for 24 hours; then weigh patient 3 times per week.	Slow weight gain is indicator of improved nutritional status; however, sudden gain of more than 2 lbs (0.9 kg) in 24 hours usually indicates fluid retention.
4 Monitor laboratory values.	Determines correct administration of formula rate and strength.
5 Observe patient's respiratory status.	Change in respiratory status indicates aspiration of tube feeding into respiratory tract.
6 Auscultate bowel sounds.	Evaluates status of gastric peristalsis.
7 For tubes placed through abdominal wall, inspect site for signs of impaired skin integrity.	Enteral tubes often cause pressure and excoriation at insertion site.

Unexpected Outcomes	**Related Interventions**
1 Feeding tube becomes clogged.	• Attempt to flush tube with water.
	• Special products are available for unclogging feeding tubes; do not use soda and juice.
	• Hold feeding and notify health care provider.
	• Maintain patient in semi-Fowler's position.
2 GRV exceeds 250 mL or cutoff per agency policy.	• Recheck residual in 1 hour (see agency policy).
	• Notify health care provider if GRV remains high (typically hold feeding if residual >250 mL two consecutive checks).
3 Patient aspirates formula.	• See Related Interventions for Skill 31-1.
4 Patient develops large amount of diarrhea (more than three loose stools in 24 hours).	• Notify health care provider. Consult dietitian about need to change formula.
	• Consider other causes such as *Clostridium difficile* infection or bacterial contamination of feeding (Bankhead et al., 2009).
	• Provide perianal skin care after each stool.
	• Determine if patient is receiving medications (e.g., containing sorbitol) that induce diarrhea (Btaiche et al., 2010).
5 Patient develops nausea and vomiting, which may indicate paralytic ileus.	• Withhold tube feeding and notify health care provider.
	• Be sure that tube is patent; aspirate for residual.
6 Fluid withdrawn through tube has foul odor or unusual appearance.	• Notify health care provider.
	• Do not return aspirated material of unusual odor or appearance without first consulting health care provider.
7 Skin around gastrostomy or jejunostomy site breaks down.	• See Procedural Guideline 31-1. Institute skin care (see Chapter 38).

Recording and Reporting

- Record and report amount and type of feeding, method of infusion, patient's response to tube feeding (e.g., GRV, cramping), patency of tube, condition of skin at tube site.
- Record volume of formula and any additional water on intake and output form.
- Report type of feeding, status of feeding tube, patient's tolerance, and adverse outcomes.

Special Considerations
Teaching

- Instruct patients and family caregivers not to reconnect lines that have separated but to seek clinical assistance.
- Teach patient and caregiver that, if tolerated, patient should remain upright for 1 hour after feedings.
- Instruct patient or caregiver that patient may express feelings of fullness, increased gas, belching, or diarrhea.

- Teach patient or caregiver how to determine correct placement of feeding tube.

Pediatric

- Preterm infants who are at risk for necrotizing enterocolitis frequently receive minimal enteral feeding (MEF) to limit stress on the GI tract. Breast milk is the preferred "formula" in this situation. MEF is usually administered slowly with a pump and supplemented with IV nutrition (Bankhead et al., 2009).
- Temporary small-bore nasogastric tubes are often placed in infants just before each feeding and removed afterward.
- Measurement of GRV is not a standard practice in pediatric patients.

Gerontologic

- Some older adults have decreased gastric emptying so formula remains in the stomach longer than for younger patients. GRV checks are especially important in patients with impaired cognition to decrease the risk for pulmonary aspiration.

Home Care

• Ask patient or family caregiver about any symptoms or discomfort during enteral feedings. Reinforce instruction to contact nurse if symptoms of discomfort occur.

• Teach patient or caregiver how to perform skin care around the gastrostomy or jejunostomy tube and signs and symptoms of infection at insertion site (see Procedural Guideline 31-1).

PROCEDURAL GUIDELINE 31-1   Care of a Gastrostomy or Jejunostomy Tube

Feeding tubes can be placed directly into the gastrointestinal (GI) tract through the abdominal wall in patients who cannot tolerate nasoenteric feeding tubes or require long-term enteral nutrition. The stomach (gastrostomy tube) and jejunum (jejunostomy tube) are the most common sites for long-term feeding tubes. Long-term tubes require endoscopic, radiologic, or surgical placement. The insertion method used to place tubes may call for specific nursing interventions in the postinsertion period, but otherwise these tubes are used in a similar way to other feeding tubes. Feedings delivered via a gastrostomy tube are relatively safe to administer, provided the patient has normal gastric emptying. Gastrostomy tubes are often called G *tubes*; but they are also commonly referred to as percutaneous endoscopic gastrostomy *(PEG) tubes*, a term used to describe tubes placed endoscopically. Gastrostomy tubes range in size from 16 Fr to 28 Fr and exit through an incision in the upper left quadrant of the abdomen, where an internal bumper or balloon and an external bumper or disk hold the tube in place (Fig. 31-3).

Jejunostomy tubes are indicated when the risk of regurgitation and aspiration is especially high, as in cases of severely delayed gastric emptying or conditions such as pancreatitis that limit the use of the stomach for feeding. Jejunostomy tubes can be placed directly into the small intestine in a surgical procedure or threaded through the stomach into the jejunum under fluoroscopy. Some jejunal tubes inserted through this transgastric approach are dual-channel devices that have openings in both the stomach and the small intestine portion of the tube. These *combination tubes*, as they are called, allow simultaneous gastric decompression and intestinal feeding for patients with impaired gastric emptying or upper-GI cancers. Each lumen of a combination tube is clearly labeled to distinguish between the gastric and the jejunal ports (Fig. 31-4). Sometimes a jejunostomy tube may be placed through an existing PEG tube. The percutaneous endoscopic jejunostomy

(PEJ) tube is passed through the PEG and advanced into the jejunum (Fig. 31-5). Because the PEJ tube occupies the lumen of the PEG tube, this tube-through-a-tube design does not allow drainage of the stomach during small-intestine feeding. In the case of both combination tubes and PEJ tubes, you must know whether

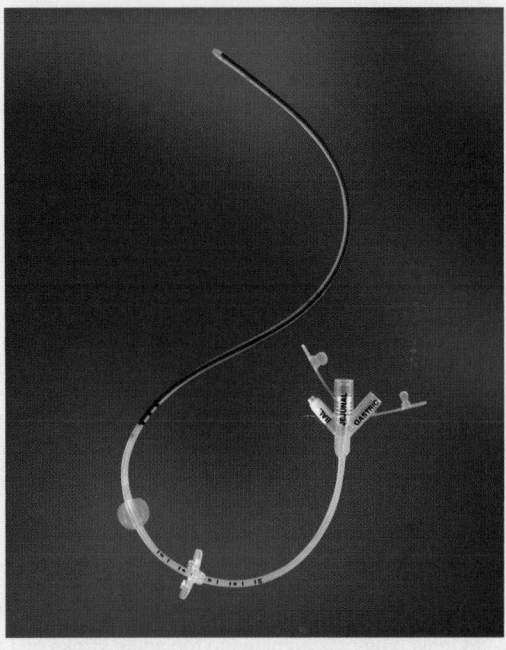

FIG 31-4 Dual lumen "combination tube" to allow jejunal feeding and gastric decompression. *(Image used with permission Kimberly-Clark Health Care. All rights reserved.)*

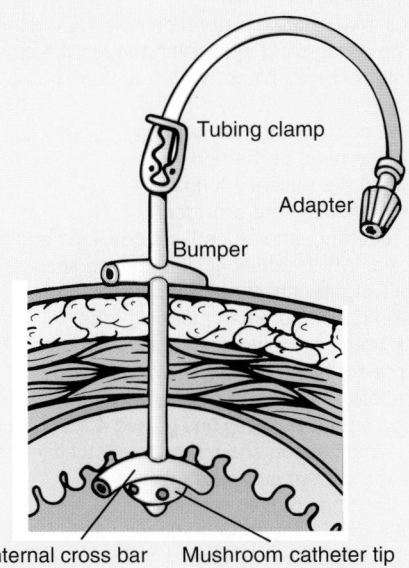

FIG 31-3 Placement of PEG tube into stomach.

Tubing clamp

Adapter

Bumper

Internal cross bar   Mushroom catheter tip

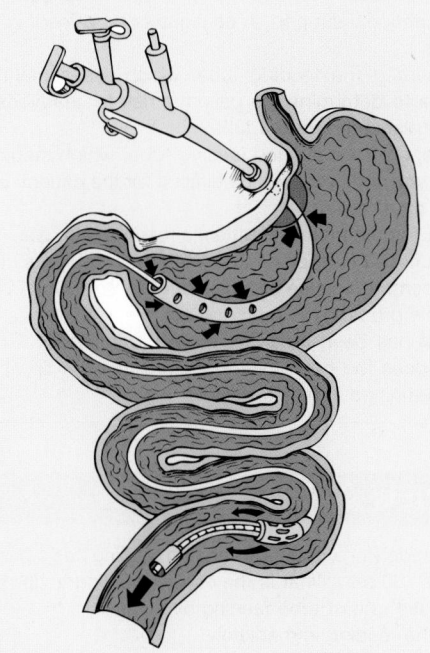

FIG 31-5 Endoscopic insertion of jejunostomy tube.

Continued

PROCEDURAL GUIDELINE 31-1   Care of a Gastrostomy or Jejunostomy Tube—cont'd

the intended site for formula delivery is gastric or jejunal to ensure safe and effective nutritional care.

Delegation and Collaboration

Care of a PEG or PEJ tube cannot be delegated to nursing assistive personnel (NAP). However, there may be some exceptions (refer to nurse practice acts and agency policy). The nurse directs the NAP to:

- Inform the nurse of any patient complaints of discomfort at the insertion site.
- Inform the nurse of any drainage on the insertion site dressing.

Equipment

- ❏ Normal saline, dated and initialed container at patient's bedside
- ❏ 4 × 4–inch gauze
- ❏ Prepared drain-gauze dressing
- ❏ Tape
- ❏ Clean gloves

Procedural Steps

1. Determine whether exit site is left open to air or if a dressing is indicated. Check health care provider's order or verify agency policy.
2. Identify patient using two identifiers (i.e., name and birthday or name and account number) according to agency policy.

Compare identifiers with information on patient's identification bracelet.

3. Perform hand hygiene and apply clean gloves.
4. Remove old dressing. Fold dressing with drainage contained inside; remove gloves inside out over dressing. Discard in appropriate container.
5. Assess exit site for evidence of excoriation, drainage, infection, or bleeding.
6. Clean skin around site with warm water and mild soap or saline (according to agency policy) using 4 × 4–inch gauze. (If drainage is present, apply clean gloves.)
7. Dry site completely.
8. Apply thin layer of protective skin barrier to exit site if indicated (e.g., site excoriated).
9. If dressing is ordered, place a drain-gauze dressing over external bar or disc. NOTE: Do not place dressing under external bar; this can cause gastric tissue erosion or internal abdominal wall pressure.
10. Secure dressing with tape.
11. Place date, time, and initials on new dressing.
12. Remove gloves and dispose of supplies in appropriate receptacle. Perform hand hygiene.
13. Document in nurse' notes and electronic health record (EHR) appearance of exit site, drainage noted, and dressing application.
14. Report to health care provider any exit site complications.

? Critical Thinking Exercises

A 72-year-old male patient is admitted to the acute stroke unit following a cerebral hemorrhage. As a result of his stroke, he has left-sided paralysis and is sometimes not responsive to verbal commands. He recognizes his family and at times has spoken a few words. The nutrition support team has recommended that he have a small-bore feeding tube inserted for nutritional support. A continuous tube-feeding formula has been ordered.

1. Before inserting the feeding tube, which assessments would be appropriate to determine the patient's risk for inadvertent tracheopulmonary placement of the tube?
2. As you prepare to insert the feeding tube, which steps of the procedure do you anticipate will be difficult for the patient, and how can you adapt as a result?
3. Twenty-four hours after the patient's feeding tube was inserted, the nurse has difficulty withdrawing any stomach contents from the tube. What is a common cause of tube clogging, and what could be done to avoid this problem?
4. The patient has been receiving enteral nutrition for 3 days. Which measures does the nurse use to ensure that the tip of the feeding tube has remained in his stomach?

✓ REVIEW QUESTIONS

1. A patient receiving continuous gastric feeding has a gastric residual volume of 150 mL. What is the correct nursing action?
   1. Decrease rate of tube feeding by 50%
   2. Stop the feeding immediately
   3. Continue tube feeding as ordered
   4. Discard the fluid withdrawn through the tube

2. A nurse caring for a neutropenic patient prepares to irrigate the feeding tube. Which of the following steps are included in this procedure? (Select all that apply.)
   1. Identify correct patient by checking name and room number
   2. Position patient flat in bed
   3. Perform hand hygiene and apply clean gloves
   4. Use 30 mL sterile water as a flushing agent
   5. Insert tip of syringe into end of feeding tube and slowly instill irrigation solution
   6. Flush tube every 4 hours and before and after medication administration

3. A patient's oxygenation saturation level has gone from 97% to 90% during a coughing spell even though the small-bore feeding tube seems to be in place. Which action should the nurse take initially?
   1. Stop the continuous tube feeding
   2. Elevate the head of the bed
   3. Auscultate the patient's lungs
   4. Notify the health care provider

4. A patient receiving enteral feedings develops abdominal cramping and diarrhea. Which additional information should the nurse check before notifying the health care provider?
   1. The patency of the enteral feeding tube
   2. If the formula or medications contain sorbitol
   3. If the patient has a history of a latex allergy
   4. A complete assessment of the gastrointestinal system

5. A patient on enteral nutrition has gained 4 lbs (1.8 kg) over the past 48 hours. Which action should the nurse take initially?
   1. Check the current laboratory values
   2. Check for signs of fluid retention
   3. Slow the rate of the tube feeding by 20%
   4. Ask the patient how he feels

6 Which of the following is the most reliable method of verifying the location of blindly inserted feeding tubes?
   1 pH testing of fluid withdrawn through the tube
   2 Auscultating over the epigastrium while instilling air through the tube
   3 Observing the color and appearance of fluid aspirated through the tube
   4 An x-ray film image of the entire course of the tube

7 As a result of a motor vehicle accident, a patient has had multiple facial fractures and suffered a stroke. Based on these facts, which route is the safest and most likely for feeding tube placement?
   1 Nasoenteric
   2 Gastrostomy tube
   3 Jejunostomy tube
   4 Percutaneous endoscopic gastrostomy (PEG)

8 What is the most important intervention that a nurse can perform to prevent health care–associated infections related to enteral nutrition?
   1 Inserting nasogastric tubes using sterile technique
   2 Keeping formula cold at all times
   3 Using aseptic technique when handling the feeding system
   4 Changing the feeding bags and liquid on time

9 The nurse is checking placement of a feeding tube of a patient who is receiving enteral medications. Which of the following techniques is correct in this situation?
   1 The nurse attaches a 20-mL syringe to the tube and pulls back quickly while watching for facial grimacing.
   2 The nurse places the patient flat in bed 30 minutes before checking for gastric residual volume.
   3 The nurse attaches syringe and pulls the plunger slowly to obtain 10 mL of gastric juice at least an hour after medications were given.
   4 The nurse flushes the tube with 60 mL of air through the syringe while watching for abdominal distention.

10 In assessing an elderly patient who is receiving a nasogastric (NG) tube feeding, it is noted that the patient has a history of constipation. The nurse notes that bowel sounds are diminished. What is the most appropriate nursing action?
   1 Assess for nausea, abdominal pain, tenderness, or distention
   2 Consult with health care provider to obtain an order for cathartic medications
   3 Weigh the patient
   4 Stop the feeding immediately

REFERENCES

American Association of Critical Care Nurses (AACN): *Verification of feeding tube placement (blindly inserted)*, 2010, AACN, available at http://www.aacn.org/WD/Practice/Docs/PracticeAlerts/Verification_of_Feeding_Tube_Placement_05-2005.pdf, accessed August 1, 2012.

Bankhead R, et al: Enteral nutrition practice recommendations, *JPEN J Parenter Enteral Nutr* 33:122, 2009.

Baroccas A, et al: ASPEN ethics position paper, *Nutr Clin Pract* 6:672, 2010.

Btaiche IF, et al: Critical illness, gastrointestinal complications, and medication therapy during enteral feeding in critically ill adult patients, *Nutr Clin Pract* 25:32, 2010.

Bourgault AM, Halm MA: Feeding tube placement in adults: safe verification method for blindly inserted tubes, *Am J Crit Care* 18:73, 2009.

Bozetti F: Quality of life and enteral nutrition, *Curr Opin Clin Nutr Metab Care* 11:661, 2008.

Chen Y, Peterson SJ: Enteral nutrition formulas: Which formula is right for your adult patient? *Nutr Clin Pract* 24:344, 2009.

Cirgin Ellett ML, et al: Predicting the insertion length for gastric tube placement in neonates, *J Obstet Gynecol Neonatal Nurs* 40:412, 2011.

Dandeles LM, Lodolce AE: Efficacy of agents to prevent and treat enteral feeding tube clogs, *Ann Pharmacother* 45:676, 2011.

Delegge DH: Managing gastric residual volumes in the critically ill patient: an update, *Curr Opin Nutr Metab Care* 14:193, 2011.

Kenny DJ, Goodman P: Care of the patient with enteral feeding: an evidence-based protocol, *Nurs Res* 59(suppl):S22, 2010.

Krenitsky J: Blind bedside placement of feeding tubes: treatment or threat? *Practical Gastroenterol* XXXV:32, 2011.

McClave SA, et al: Guidelines for the provision and assessment of nutrition support therapy in the adult critically ill patient, *JPEN J Parenter Enteral Nutr* 33:277, 2009.

Metheny NA, et al: Gastric residual volume and aspiration in critically ill patients receiving gastric feeding, *Am J Crit Care* 17:512, 2008.

Metheny NA: Inconclusive evidence regarding the volume of gastric aspirate that can be safely reintroduced following residual volume measurements, *Evidence-based Nurs* 13:71, 2010.

Metheny NA, et al: Relationship between feeding tube site and respiratory outcomes, *JPEN J Parenter Enteral Nutr* 35:346, 2011.

Munera-Seeley V, et al: Use of a colorimetric carbon dioxide sensor for nasoenteric feeding tube placement in critical care patients compared with clinical methods and radiography, *Nutr Clin Pract* 23:318, 2008.

National Quality Forum (NQF): *National voluntary consensus standards for patient safety: a consensus report*, Washington, DC, 2010, NQF.

Renner M: Far from reliable: pH testing in the neonatal intensive care unit, *J Pediatr Nurs* 25:580, 2010.

Simmons D, et al: Tubing misconnections: normalization of deviance, *Nutr Clin Pract* 26:28, 2011.

The Joint Commission (TJC): *National patient safety goals*, Oakbrook Terrace, III, 2012, The Commission, available at http://www.jointcommission.org/standards_information/npsgs.aspx.

Parenteral Nutrition

MEDIA RESOURCES

- e**volve** http://evolve.elsevier.com/Perry/skills
  - Review Questions
  - ▶ Video Clips
  - Audio Glossary

- Mosby's Nursing Video Skills, 4th edition

KEY TERMS

Amino acid
Bacteremia

Lipid emulsion
Parenteral nutrition (PN)

Peripherally inserted central
catheter (PICC)

Glucose monitoring

OBJECTIVES

Mastery of content in this chapter will enable the nurse to:
- Describe the purpose and components of parenteral nutrition (PN).
- Identify patients who are candidates for PN.
- Discuss risks associated with PN.

- List the monitoring procedures used for patients receiving PN.
- Identify measures used to prevent complications of PN.
- Demonstrate appropriate nursing care and use of safe precautions when caring for a patient receiving PN.

Parenteral nutrition (PN) is a specialized form of nutritional support that is given intravenously by an infusion pump to patients who have significant gastrointestinal (GI) dysfunction. PN is intended to meet the nutritional needs of patients until their GI function has improved enough to allow adequate intake using the oral or tube feeding route. In addition, PN meets long-term nutritional needs with infusions at home if GI dysfunction is expected to be long term (months to years) (Box 32-1). PN is an adjunctive therapy to enteral tube feeding in critically ill patients with larger nutrient requirements than can be provided with tube feeding because of limited GI function. Clinically stable, well-nourished adults can be maintained on peripheral IV therapy for up to 2 weeks without difficulty (Worthington and Gilbert, 2012). The goal for patients with short-term GI dysfunction is to provide nutritional requirements while minimizing PN-related complications until patients can resume full oral diets or meet their needs with enteral tube feedings (ASPEN, 2007; Worthington and Gilbert, 2012). Long-term nutritional management goals include ensuring that nutrient requirements are met while avoiding toxicity and minimizing complications.

RISKS ASSOCIATED WITH PARENTERAL NUTRITION

Although the use of PN has been an important technologic advance that allowed improved care for patients with GI disorders, a number of complications have been associated with the therapy, the most frequent of which is catheter-related bloodstream infection (CRBSI), a risk that is found in both hospitalized patients and those with PN at home (Table 32-1). Hospitalized patients who are allowed nothing by mouth (NPO) and have PN have a risk of sludge accumulating in the gallbladder; and some cases result in acute cholecystitis, a problem that most often resolves once patients are able to eat again and PN is stopped. PN has also been associated with liver disease, particularly in patients with multiple bloodstream infections, very severe GI disease, and longer PN duration (Worthington and Gilbert, 2012). In-home PN patients with severe GI disease and long-term PN have been reported to develop metabolic bone disease (Worthington and Gilbert, 2012). There is also a risk of allergic reaction when PN is administered, although the incidence of allergy is low.

VENOUS ACCESS FOR ADMINISTRATION OF PARENTERAL NUTRITION

The type of catheter to use for administration of PN depends on patient factors and the expected length of PN therapy. The location of the catheter is defined based on where the distal tip of the catheter lies. Concentrated PN solutions are quickly diluted when infused into a large-diameter central vein (Fig. 32-1). PN should not be infused into a peripheral intravenous (IV) or midline catheter because of the increased risk for phlebitis. If only peripheral lines are available, the orders

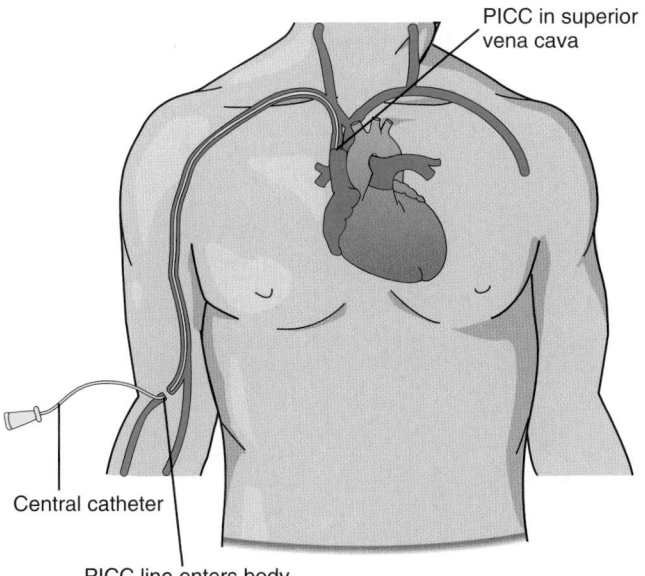

FIG 32-2 Peripherally inserted central catheter.

BOX 32-1 | Indications for Parenteral Nutrition

Short-term (Less Than 1 month) Gastrointestinal Dysfunction
- Small intestinal surgery
- Intestinal obstruction
- Intolerance to adequate rates of enteral tube feeding
- Severe mucositis or gastrointestinal (GI) tract pain after cancer therapy
- High-output GI fistula
- Severe acute pancreatitis and inability to tolerate enteral tube feeding
- Anastomotic leak or severe GI bleed after obesity surgery
- Severe malnutrition before surgery

Long-term Gastrointestinal Dysfunction
- Short-bowel syndrome
- Dysmotility syndromes
- Radiation enteritis
- Permanent bowel obstruction caused by tumor

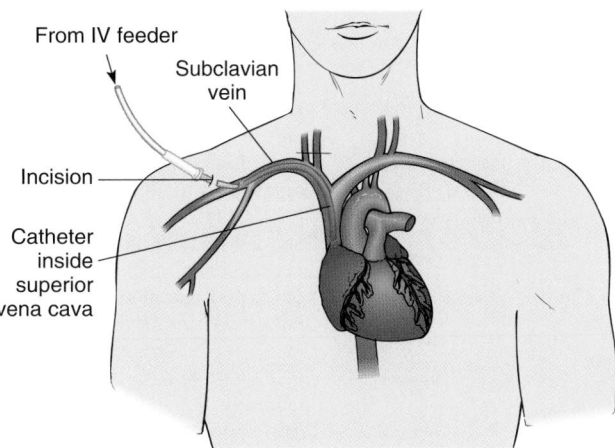

FIG 32-1 Placement of central venous catheter inserted into subclavian vein. *IV*, Intravenous. *(Courtesy Rolin Graphics.)*

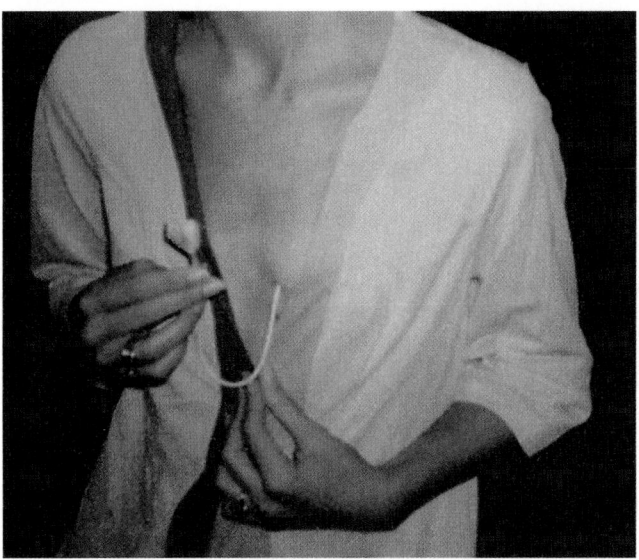

FIG 32-3 Tunneled catheter used for home central parenteral nutrition. *(From Morgan SL, Weinsier RL: Fundamentals of clinical nutrition, ed 2, St Louis, 1998, Mosby.)*

should state clearly that the administration route will be a peripheral IV line so the compounding pharmacy will prepare the PN with a lower osmolarity (Table 32-2), which will require added fluid volume. Patients who cannot tolerate larger volumes of fluid intake such as those with renal, cardiac, or hepatic failure or those with severe malnutrition should be considered candidates for central lines if PN is needed. Many hospitals use peripherally inserted central catheters, termed *PICC lines* (Fig. 32-2), that are placed by specially trained nurses or radiologists. The catheter is threaded through a peripheral vein (such as the antecubital vein) until the tip reaches a central vein. These catheters may be inserted at the patient's bedside. Following central venous catheter insertion, do not initiate PN until placement of venous catheter tip is confirmed by a radiograph. Lipid emulsions may be administered through a separate peripheral line, through a central line by a Y-connector tubing (see Chapter 22), or as an admixture to the PN solution. Patients who will self-administer their PN solutions at home will require a central catheter, most typically a tunneled device (Fig. 32-3; see Chapter 28). They may also require special tubing to enable them to access the catheter without assistance. Patients who require IV access have a risk of CRBSI. The risk of CRBSI is increased with multilumen catheters, use of PN, multiple

IV therapies, and central venous access handling by multiple caregivers. Careful handling of the central line, dressings, tubing, and PN port is essential (see Skill 28-6).

COMPONENTS OF A PARENTERAL NUTRITION SOLUTION

A PN solution is produced using sterile technique in a laminar airflow hood in a pharmacy to reduce the risk of microbial and pyrogen contamination. The components of the PN solution are amino acids, glucose, and lipid as energy sources, with the addition of electrolytes, minerals, trace elements, vitamins, and water. The addition of lipid emulsion to the PN solution results in a preparation called *a 3:1, 3-in-1,* or *total nutrition admixture (TNA).* The advantage to a 3:1 mixture is that it allows lipid infusion over 24 hours, decreasing the risk of hypertriglyceridemia from more rapid lipid infusion. Although PN without lipid can be infused using tubing with a 0.22-μm filter, a larger 1.2-μm filter is needed when

TABLE 32-1	Complications of Parenteral Nutrition			
Problem	**Cause**	**Symptoms**	**Immediate Action**	**Prevention**
Pneumothorax	Tip of catheter enters pleural space during insertion, causing lung to collapse	Sudden chest pain, difficulty breathing, decreased breath sounds, cessation of normal chest movement on affected side, tachycardia	Per health care provider's order, the proper professional (CRNP, PA-C, or MD) may remove the central catheter. Administer oxygen via nasal cannula. Insert chest tube to remove air under water seal drainage or dry one-way valve system	Medical personnel should be properly trained to insert central catheters. Researchers suggest use of ultrasound when placing CVCs (Lamperti et al., 2012). Catheter should be secured properly to prevent migration, movement.
Air embolism	IV tubing disconnected; part of catheter system open or removed without being clamped	Sudden respiratory distress; decreased oxygen saturation levels, shortness of breath, coughing, chest pain, decreased blood pressure	Clamp catheter; position patient in left Trendelenburg's position; call health care provider; administer oxygen as needed	Make sure that all catheter connections are secure; clamp catheter when not in use. Never use a stopcock with a CVC. Instruct patient in Valsalva maneuver for tubing changes.
Localized infection (exit site or tunnel)	Poor aseptic technique in removal of skin flora during site preparation and dressing care	*Exit site*: Erythema, tenderness, induration, or purulence within 2 cm (0.8 inches) of skin at exit site *Tunnel*: Same as above but extends beyond 2 cm from exit site	Call health care provider *Exit*: Warm compress, daily site care, oral antibiotics *Tunnel*: Remove catheter	Provide catheter site care using aseptic technique; include cleaning of site, application of new stabilization device, and application of sterile dressing (INS, 2011). Change transparent dressings every 7 days, gauze dressings every 48 hours (INS, 2011). Change dressing if damp, loosened, or soiled or when inspection of site is necessary (INS, 2011). Clean site with chlorhexidine, tincture of iodine, iodophor, or 70% alcohol solution for a minimum of 3 to 5 min. Routine use of antibiotic ointment not recommended (INS, 2011).
Catheter-related sepsis or bacteremia (In 2009 U.S. incidence in ICU patients is down more than 50% from 2001 levels, but 41,000 patients have CRBSI each year [CDC, 2011].)	Catheter hub contamination; contamination of infusate; spread of bacteria through bloodstream from distant site	*Systemic*: Isolation of same microorganism from blood culture and catheter segment, with patient showing fever, chills, malaise, elevated white blood cell count	*Systemic*: Antibiotics intravenously, removal of catheter by proper professional (CRNP, PA-C, or MD).	Use full sterile-barrier precautions during catheter insertion and dressing change. Use antibiotic-impregnated catheters. Do not disconnect tubing unnecessarily. Replace IV tubing and filter every 72 hours for standard PN (INS, 2011).
Hyperglycemia	Possible blood-draw error, confirm with bedside glucose device; patient receiving too little insulin in PN solution	Excessive thirst, urination, blood glucose >160 mg/100 dL, confusion	Call health care provider; may need to slow infusion rate (health care provider order)	Review medical history for blood drawn through central line with PN infusing (repeat peripheral blood draw), glucose intolerance or diabetes, new infection, new medication such as steroids; keep rate as ordered; never increase PN to "catch up." Maintain blood glucose in range of 90-130 mg/100 dL or within range ordered by health care provider. Use aseptic technique and routine blood glucose monitoring.

TABLE 32-1	Complications of Parenteral Nutrition—cont'd			
Problem	Cause	Symptoms	Immediate Action	Prevention
Hypoglycemia	PN abruptly discontinued; too much insulin	Patient shaky, dizzy, nervous, anxious, hungry, blood glucose level <80 mg/100 dL	Call health care provider; if PN discontinued abruptly, may need to restart $D_{10}W$ at previous PN rate. If patient has oral intake, give ½ cup fruit juice. Perform blood glucose monitoring; retest in 15 to 30 min.	Decrease PN, "tapering" gradually until discontinued; blood glucose monitoring is used to ensure adequate insulin.

CRBSI, Catheter-related bloodstream infection; *CVC,* central venous catheter; *PN,* Central parenteral nutrition; *CRNP,* certified registered nurse practitioner; *ICU,* intensive care unit; *IV,* intravenous; *MD,* medical doctor; *PA-C,* physician's assistant-certified.

TABLE 32-2	Comparison of Central versus Peripheral Parenteral Nutrition Orders	
	Central Parenteral Nutrition	Peripheral Parenteral Nutrition
Osmolality	>600 mOsm	<600 mOsm
Route of administration	Central venous catheter	Small peripheral vein
Usual daily caloric intake	20-35 kcal/kg/day	5-10 kcal/kg/day
Usual daily volume (mL)	1000-2000	2000-3000
Fat emulsion	Minor caloric source	Major caloric source

lipid is infused. A filter is necessary because it prevents particulate matter or large droplets of lipid from reaching a patient, which could potentially result in a pulmonary embolism.

Patients who receive PN solutions containing glucose and amino acids but no lipids are at risk for essential fatty acid deficiency (EFAD). EFAD can appear within 3 weeks of fat-free PN administration when no oral or enteral fat intake is provided (Worthington and Gilbert, 2012). EFAD is characterized by scaly dermatitis, hair loss, impaired wound healing, decreased resistance to stress, increased susceptibility to respiratory tract infections, anemia, thrombocytopenia, and liver function abnormalities.

MEDICATIONS

In some patients regular insulin is added to a PN admixture to maintain blood glucose control. In addition, some hospital policies also permit the addition of medications that reduce gastric acidity. However, the routine addition of any medications is discouraged when the compatibility and stability of the components are not known. Bedside addition of any medication is prohibited by most hospital policies because of the risk of solution contamination.

ADMINISTRATION OF PARENTERAL NUTRITION

Nurses collaborate with nutrition support teams and health care providers in administering PN and monitoring patients' response

to PN therapy. Although practice patterns vary across hospitals, typically dietitians or pharmacists provide advice on nutrition support goals and/or write PN orders. Nurses at the bedside administer the ordered PN with care regarding accuracy of PN label versus orders, with attention to obtaining blood glucose, laboratory panels, intake/output measures, body weight, vital signs, and food intake if the patient has a diet order.

LABORATORY MONITORING

Because hyperglycemia has been linked with increased infection rates, monitoring blood glucose levels during a PN infusion is an important procedure (see Skill 43-9). Typical orders may be to monitor blood glucose levels every 6 hours (4 times daily) until it is within optimal limits (i.e., 70 to 180 mg/dL) or as defined by unit protocols for 48 hours. Then you monitor blood glucose daily for the duration of PN therapy. When the goal is to prepare a patient for home infusion of PN, it is very important to monitor glucose levels approximately 2 hours after an infusion begins (peak level) and 2 hours after it ends (trough level) to evaluate the need for adding regular human insulin to the infusion bag.

Patients who require PN infusions do so for medical or surgical conditions that are often associated with electrolyte instability. Thus a typical laboratory panel relative to PN infusions would include a baseline assessment of electrolytes, serum proteins, and complete blood count (Box 32-2). Nutrients in a PN infusion may alter serum levels. In very malnourished patients, during a process termed *refeeding syndrome,* some electrolytes (e.g., potassium [K], magnesium [Mg] and phosphorus) may shift intracellularly with glucose provided in the PN, potentially resulting in low serum levels with risk for arrhythmias and muscle weakness. If refeeding syndrome is predicted based on the degree of malnutrition or if it occurs, electrolyte panels may be ordered 2 or 3 times daily to permit adequate electrolyte repletion.

MONITORING PATIENT STATUS AND OUTCOMES

Since a PN solution is typically provided in response to GI dysfunction and to support nutritional needs, it is important for you to monitor data that describes patient progress. Measurement of intake and output is very important to document when a patient's GI function is changing and to provide information regarding the adequacy of fluid intake from the PN solution. The patient's body weight is a second sign of whether hydration needs are being met and, over a longer term, whether energy needs are adequate. Since there is a risk of bloodstream infection in patients with catheters, monitoring temperature regularly is important. Most typically intake and output are measured every 8 hours, vital signs every 4 hours, and body weight at least 3 times weekly (see Box 32-2).

EVIDENCE-BASED PRACTICE

When critically ill patients cannot tolerate enteral nutrition, PN alone provides beneficial effects and decreases patient infection rates when it is initiated early versus later in their care (Kutsogiannis et al., 2011; Thibault and Pichard, 2010). Patterns of practice regarding blood glucose control in hospitalized patients who receive PN are controversial and may change over time. In some instances there is lower mortality when critically ill patients receive insulin to maintain tight blood glucose control (Pasquel et al., 2010). A clinical trial documented 10% higher mortality in patients who were not overfed but were treated with insulin to achieve tight blood glucose control (NICE-SUGAR, 2009). Because of concern about the risks of hypoglycemia, several professional organizations recommend more relaxed goals for glycemic control (Worthington and Gilbert, 2012).

- Early nutritional assessment is crucial to determine a patient's need for PN as a single or adjunct nutritional therapy (Worthington and Gilbert, 2012).
- When PN is the only nutritional therapy for critically ill patients, a patient who was healthy and well-nourished before the illness can wait 7 days for its initiation (Worthington and Gilbert, 2012).
- Patients with preexisting nutritional deficits and catabolic illnesses require earlier PN intervention.

- Blood glucose should be maintained in a range of 70 to 180 mg/dL (Moghissi et al., 2009).
  - Hypoglycemia with blood glucose level <70 mg/dL should be avoided (Moghissi et al., 2009).
- The ideal method for delivering PN is through a central venous catheter, which allows for a higher concentration of nutrients (Kutsogiannis et al., 2011; Worthington and Gilbert, 2012).

PATIENT-CENTERED CARE

Patients needing PN are usually quite ill and at times require a lengthy stay in a health care agency. In addition, some patients receive PN in their home setting. Regardless of the reason or duration for PN, each patient has individual care needs that extend beyond the nutritional support that PN offers. Remember that your patients have individual preferences related to their hygiene practices; these preferences should never be overlooked because a patient requires PN. Include patient and family in decisions to maintain patient control, activity level, personal decision making, and socialization with friends and family.

PN may pose concerns for members of ethnic groups or people with philosophic beliefs that include restriction of animal products. Consider the following guidelines:

- Accommodate religious and cultural beliefs that require avoidance of animal products.
  - The components of PN are largely synthetic and do not contain pork.
  - The lipid emulsion contains egg phospholipid, a product that may be objectionable to vegan patients.
- Even though people who are ill are exempt from expectations of fasting during Ramadan, some devout Muslim patients may prefer to fast from dawn to dusk.
  - If this is the case, the patient's PN may be gradually cycled to begin the infusion at dusk and take it down at dawn the next morning.
- The use of mechanical devices such as infusion pumps may be objectionable for Orthodox Jews on the Sabbath.
  - If this is the case, discuss the possibility of running the pump with a fully charged battery rather than having it plugged in to an electrical outlet.

Safety Guidelines

1. Know the complications associated with PN, including metabolic disturbances, fluid imbalance, technical management of catheter system, and infections.
2. Monitor a patient's vital signs, electrolyte levels, glucose levels, triglyceride levels, weight, and fluid intake and output and compare baseline with treatment values. Some patients who receive PN have rapid changes in these values.
3. Know the patient's recent temperature range. Patients with peripheral or central IV lines are susceptible to CRBSIs; an elevated temperature is an early indicator of a bacterial infection.
4. Routinely assess the site of a central venous access device for signs of infection.
5. Use strict aseptic technique in the care and maintenance of central venous catheters and PICC lines.

SKILL 32-1   Administering Parenteral Nutrition Through a Central Line

Administration of parenteral nutrition through a central line (CPN) requires the use of strict aseptic technique and application of critical thinking. Because of the composition of CPN fluids, patients can experience metabolic and fluid balance changes quickly. In addition, the clinical condition of patients receiving CPN is usually poor, especially when they have alterations in host defenses, severe underlying illnesses, and extremes of age. You will need to anticipate changes in a patient's condition that signal developing complications. Similarly, you need to use good judgment to maintain the intravenous (IV) system and ensure that it is functioning properly.

Delegation and Collaboration

The skill of administering CPN cannot be delegated to nursing assistive personnel (NAP). The nurse directs the NAP to:

- Report when the pump alarms, catheter dressings are wet, temperature is elevated, or a patient has any complaints.
- Perform fingerstick blood glucose monitoring as directed and report any abnormal results to the nurse.

- Report vital signs that are out of range to nurse.
- Weigh patient as directed.

Equipment

❑ IV infusion tubing with Luer-Lok tip
❑ Parenteral (PN) solution
❑ IV filter (1.2-μm filter for three-in-one solutions or lipids containing a membrane that is particulate retentive and air eliminating; 0.22-μm filter for solutions that do not contain lipids) (INS, 2011)
❑ IV infusion pump
❑ Bedside glucose monitoring kit
❑ Adhesive tape or tubing label
❑ Clean gloves
❑ Stethoscope
❑ Medication administration record (MAR) or computer printout

STEP	RATIONALE

ASSESSMENT

1 Assess indications of and risks for protein/calorie malnutrition: weight loss from baseline or ideal, muscle atrophy/weakness, edema, lethargy, failure to wean from ventilatory support, chronic illness, and nothing by mouth for more than 6 days. Confer with nutritional support team.	Clinical indications for PN. These baseline details provide a baseline from which change can be noted.
2 Inspect condition of central vein access site for presence of inflammation, edema, and tenderness. Inspect tubing of access device for patency and kinking.	Identifies early signs of infection, infiltration, or disruption in system integrity. Development of complication contraindicates infusion of fluids and indicates need to establish new IV site.
3 Assess levels of serum albumin, total protein, transferrin, prealbumin, and triglycerides and check blood glucose level by fingerstick (see Chapter 43).	Provides baseline for measuring patient's nutritional status. In addition, nutritional baseline identifies patient's unique requirements, and PN admixture is tailored to patient's specific needs (Worthington and Gilbert, 2012). Serum glucose determines patient's baseline and tolerance to high levels of glucose in CPN solution.
4 Assess patient's medical history for factors influenced by PCN administration: electrolyte levels; renal, cardiac, and hepatic function. Assess for history of allergies.	Some patients require that CPN therapy be adapted by composition or volume (requires health care provider order) based on medical history. CPN includes constituents (e.g., medications) to which patient may be allergic.
5 Assess vital signs, auscultate patient's lung sounds, and measure weight.	Provides baseline for monitoring patient's response to fluid infusion and nutrients. Crackles in lungs are early indication of fluid volume excess.
6 Consult with health care provider and dietitian on calculation of calorie, protein, and fluid requirements for patient.	Provides multidisciplinary plan for patient's nutritional support.
7 Verify order for nutrients, minerals, vitamins, trace elements, electrolytes, added medications, and flow rate. Check for compatibility of added medications.	CPN is often ordered daily in hospital setting after review of laboratory values. In home setting orders may be obtained less frequently (e.g., weekly). Pharmacies that prepare parenteral solutions will check medication compatibility.

NURSING DIAGNOSES

- Deficient fluid volume
- Excess fluid volume
- Imbalanced nutrition: less than body requirements
- Risk for infection
- Risk for unstable blood glucose level

Related factors are individualized based on patient's condition or needs.

STEP	RATIONALE

PLANNING

1 Expected outcomes following completion of procedure:

- Patient's ideal weight gain is between 1 and 2 lbs (0.5 to 1 kg) per week.

  Weight is an indicator of patient's nutritional status and determines fluid volume. Weight gain greater than 1 lb (0.5 kg)/day indicates fluid retention.

- Serum glucose levels are less than 180 mg/dL or maintained between 70 and 140 mg/dL. Check health care provider's order for desired glucose range.

  The benefits of tight glucose control have not been determined; thus a glucose range should be individualized to a patient's specific health care need (Worthington and Gilbert, 2012). Both high and low blood glucose levels have been associated with morbidity and complications (Moghissi et al., 2009).

- Central venous access device is patent; and site is free of pain, swelling, redness, or inflammation.

  Ensures that CPN is infusing into vein rather than into surrounding tissues and that there are no signs of an access device infection.

- Patient is afebrile.

  Absence of systemic infection.

2 Explain purposes of CPN to patient.

  Promotes understanding and reduces anxiety.

3 If CPN solution is refrigerated, remove from refrigeration 1 hour before infusion.

  Solution should be at room temperature for administration (INS, 2011).

IMPLEMENTATION

1 Perform hand hygiene.

  Reduces transmission of microorganisms.

2 Review transcriber's order against MAR and ensure that solution is correct and properly labeled.

  Prevents medication error. *This is the first check for accuracy.*

3 Compare label of CPN bag with MAR or computer printout; check for correct additives and solution expiration date. Also check patient's name against label of CPN bag.

  This is the second check for accuracy.

4 Inspect 2 : 1 CPN solution for particulate matter; inspect 3 : 1 CPN solution for separation of solution.

  Deterioration of three-in-one solution results in breakdown of emulsion.

Clinical Decision Point *Do not use CPN solution if it has coalesced (thick, dense layer of fat droplets at surface, appearing 10 cm [4 inches] in thickness) or oiled out (fat droplets separate from solution that appear as a clear layer at surface) or appears abnormal in any way. Notify the pharmacy and request a new solution (Hardy and Puzovic, 2009).*

5 Identify patient using two identifiers (i.e., name and birthday or name and account number) according to agency policy. Compare identifiers in MAR/medical record with information on patient's identification bracelet and/or ask patient to state name.

  Ensures correct patient. Complies with The Joint Commission requirements and improves patient safety (TJC, 2012). *This is the third check for accuracy.*

6 Apply clean gloves. Attach appropriate filter to IV tubing. Prime tubing with CPN solution, making sure that no air bubbles remain, and turn off flow with roller clamp (see Chapter 28). Scrub hub of appropriate catheter port with alcohol swab. Connect end of tubing to central catheter and label port. Open roller clamp to rate that maintains patency of line.

  Air introduced into central circulation can result in an air embolus, a fatal complication. Labeling of high-risk catheters prevents connection with inappropriate tube or catheter (TJC, 2012).

7 Place IV tubing into IV infusion pump, open roller clamp completely, and regulate flow rate on pump as ordered (see Chapter 28) (see illustration). In some agencies, infusion rate is immediately set at the ordered rate. In other agencies an initial rate of 40 to 60 mL/hr is established, and the rate is gradually increased until patient's nutritional needs are supplied (refer to agency policy).

  PN flow rates are ordered to meet patient's metabolic and electrolyte needs. Maintaining rates prevents electrolyte imbalances.

Critical Decision Point *Increase rate of infusion gradually to prevent metabolic and electrolyte abnormalities because central PN is hyperosmolar and patients usually tolerate it when it is increased incrementally. If PN must be discontinued suddenly, hang infusion of 5% dextrose in water at same infusion rate to prevent hypoglycemia. PN solution, including lipids, should be infused within 24 hours (INS, 2011).*

8 Infuse all IV medications or blood through an alternative IV line. Do not obtain blood samples or central venous pressure readings through same lumen or port used for CPN.

  Prevents drug incompatibility. Prevents occlusion of central line and reduces risk for transmission of infection.

STEP	RATIONALE

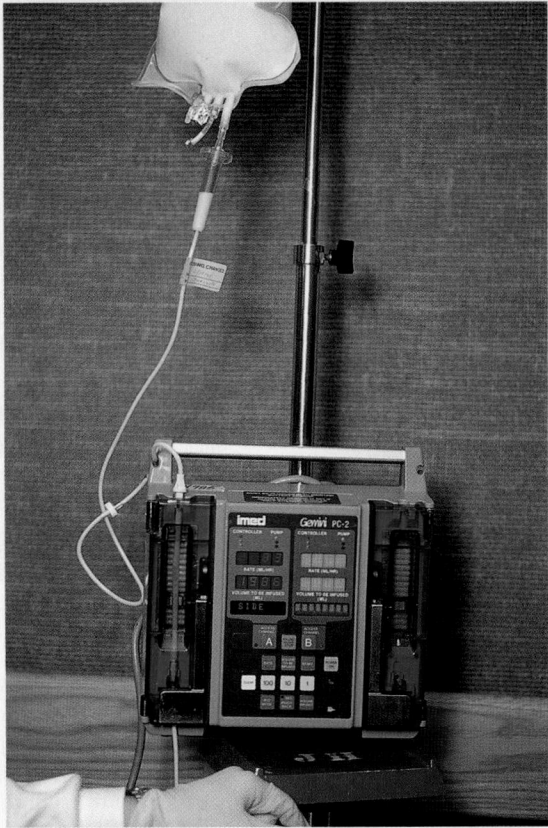

STEP 7 Parenteral nutrition solution infusing via infusion pump.

9 Do not interrupt PN infusion (e.g., during showers, transport to procedure, blood transfusion) and be sure that rate does not exceed ordered rate.

Maintains continuous infusion of nutrients; prevents hypoglycemic reaction. Never attempt to catch up on a delayed infusion.

10 Change infusing tubing and filter using strict aseptic technique. Change IV administration sets for CPN every 24 hours and immediately on suspected contamination (INS, 2011).

Prevents development of catheter-related bacteremia (Worthington and Gilbert, 2012).

11 Discard used supplies and perform hand hygiene.

Reduces transmission of infection.

EVALUATION

1 Monitor flow rate routinely, at least hourly.

Too-rapid or too-slow infusion could result in metabolic disturbances such as hyperglycemia and fluid overload.

2 Monitor fluid intake and urine and gastrointestinal fluid output every 8 hours.

Prevents fluid imbalance from too-slow or too-rapid infusion.

3 Obtain daily weights or weights as ordered.

Routine measurement of weights will reflect a gain/loss resulting either from caloric intake or fluid retention. Gradual weight gain, if weight gain is the goal, indicates adequate tolerance.

4 Assess for fluid retention; palpate skin of extremities; auscultate lung sounds.

Weight gain in excess of 1 lb (0.5 kg)/day, dependent edema, lung crackles, and intake greater than output per each 24-hour period indicate fluid retention.

5 Monitor patient's glucose level every 6 hours or as ordered and other laboratory parameters daily or as ordered.

Maintenance of normal electrolyte levels, satisfactory fluid balance, acceptable serum glucose levels, and improvement in serum proteins indicate adequate tolerance to PN.

6 Inspect central venous access site.

Determines IV patency and absence of infection, infiltration, or phlebitis.

7 Monitor for temperature, elevated white blood cell count, and malaise.

Signs of systemic infection.

Unexpected Outcomes

1 There is redness, swelling, and tenderness around venous access site, indicating possible exit site infection.

2 Patient develops fever, malaise, and chills, indicating systemic infection.

3 Infusion stops flowing or flows at rate slower than ordered.

4 Patient experiences weight gain greater than 1 lb (0.5 kg)/day. Taut skin turgor is also present. Crackles auscultated over lung fields.

5 Serum glucose level is greater than 180 mg/dL or target set by health care provider.

6 Serum electrolyte levels are out of normal range.

Related Interventions

- Notify health care provider.
- Apply warm compress and initiate daily site care as ordered.
- Systemic antibiotic therapy may begin.

- Check exit site for signs of infection.
- Notify health care provider and consult about need to obtain cultures of exit site or blood.
- Systemic antibiotic therapy may begin.

- Venous access device is possibly occluded with fibrin or particulate matter. Report occlusion to health care provider.
- If device is a surgically placed device or peripherally inserted central catheter (PICC), thrombolytic agent may be ordered.

- Notify health care provider.
- Anticipate need to reduce IV infusion rate.

- Notify health care provider.
- Indicates intolerance to glucose load in CPN solution.
- Possible need for addition of insulin to CPN, modification of CPN solution, or sliding-scale insulin coverage.

- Indicates movement of electrolytes in response to infusion of fluids and glucose or excess requirements caused by medications or gastrointestinal losses. May need to adjust electrolyte levels in solution.

Recording and Reporting

- Record condition of central venous access device, rate and type of infusion, catheter lumen used for infusion, intake and output (I&O) every 8 hours, blood glucose levels, vital signs, and weights.
- If signs of infection, occlusion, fluid retention, or infiltration occur, notify the health care provider.

Special Considerations

Teaching

- Instruct patient and family in the purpose and goals of CPN. Keep them informed about daily care of central line.

Pediatric

- Consider children's developmental needs when they are on long-term CPN. Perform regular assessments of development to determine child's progress. Implement interventions to encourage expected milestones (Hockenberry and Wilson, 2011).

Gerontological

- Some older adults have impaired ability to tolerate higher fluid volumes because of cardiac or renal impairment.

Home Care

- Patients requiring long-term CPN benefit from a referral to a home nutrition therapy team.

- Patients receiving home CPN usually have a tunneled or implanted catheter inserted into the subclavian vein (see Fig. 32-3) to reduce the possibility of infection. Patients or family members need to learn to perform catheter site care, dressing changes, and techniques for connecting and disconnecting PN solutions.
- Some patients receive home CPN at night during sleep (cyclic CPN) to allow the freedom to leave home or work during the day. Most patients also take oral diet as tolerated, although their impaired gastrointestinal function limits nutrient absorption.
- Teach patient and family caregiver to monitor patient's weight, oral intake, I&O, and serum glucose level.
- Teach patient and family caregiver about actions to take in case of emergency or unexpected outcomes such as telephoning the health care provider or going to the hospital, depending on the circumstances.
- If home CPN patients require insulin in their CPN, they will need a home glucose monitoring device and instruction in its use.
- Patient teaching for home CPN administration will be given by home infusion nurses after discharge or may be initiated in the hospital and continued at home.

SKILL 32-2 Administering Parenteral Nutrition Through a Peripheral Line

 Video Clip

The administration of parenteral nutrition (PN) via peripheral veins (PPN) requires a lower nutrient content and is more appropriate for preventing malnutrition than for correcting nutritional deficits. Patients with elevated nutritional requirements from hypermetabolic illnesses or conditions and patients with fluid restrictions are not suitable candidates (Worthington and Gilbert, 2012). This therapy is for short-term use, usually for 2 weeks or less. The PPN solution uses lower concentrations

of dextrose and amino acids to reduce the osmolality (see Table 32-2 on p. 799) and decrease the risk for phlebitis. Adding lipid emulsion adds a source of calories with minimal impact on the osmolality. A lipid emulsion must be administered through vented intravenous (IV) tubing as a primary IV or as a piggyback.

This skill describes a piggyback administration of PN. Administration sets (including piggybacks) used for fat emulsions are changed every 24 hours and immediately on suspected contamination (INS, 2011). The administration set must have a Luer-Lok design. Indications for PPN include the following:

1 *Adequate peripheral access:* Despite its lower osmolality, PPN tends to cause phlebitis and often requires frequent changes in the access location.

2 *Ability to tolerate larger volumes of fluid:* Because of the lower concentration of dextrose in PPN, a larger volume of fluid is required to attain adequate calories. Some patients with impaired renal or cardiac function do not tolerate PPN.

3 *Ability to tolerate lipid emulsions:* Lipid is the most calorically dense nutrient. One liter of 10% dextrose without lipid provides only 340 kcal. A 250-mL amount of 20% lipid solution provides 500 kcal.

Delegation and Collaboration

The skill of administering PPN through a peripheral IV line cannot be delegated to nursing assistive personnel (NAP). The nurse directs the NAP to:

- Report patient complaint of burning, pain, or redness at peripheral IV site.

- Report to nurse infusion pump alarms or moist IV site dressing.
- Report to nurse patient complaints of shortness of breath and change in vital signs.

Equipment

- ❏ PPN solution
- ❏ Lipid emulsion in glass container or in a separate chamber of the PN bag
- ❏ IV tubing for PPN with 0.22-μm filter for amino acid/dextrose solution
- ❏ Nonphthalate vented IV tubing infusion set for fat emulsion
- ❏ Needleless cannula
- ❏ Bedside glucose monitoring kit
- ❏ Antimicrobial swab
- ❏ Infusion pump
- ❏ Clean gloves
- ❏ Medication administration record (MAR) or computer printout

STEP	RATIONALE

ASSESSMENT

1 Assess patient for hypertriglyceridemia. Obtain orders for serum triglyceride level before initiation of PPN and weekly.	Determines patient's ability to metabolize lipid.
2 Select or initiate appropriate functional IV site (18-gauge catheter) to administer PPN and lipid emulsion. Assess its patency and function (see Chapter 28).	Large-gauge catheter ensures more efficient flow of infusion.
3 Check health care provider's order against MAR for volume of fat emulsion, PPN solution, and administration time for fat emulsion.	Health care provider must order fat emulsions and PPN. Fat emulsions may cause adverse symptoms if infused too rapidly as separate infusion. Infusion time is normally at least 8 hours. Fat emulsions should hang no longer than 12 hours as separate infusion from original container. *This is the first check for accuracy.*
4 Read label of fat emulsion solution.	Lipid emulsions are white and opaque; thus make sure to avoid confusing enteral tube feeding formula with parenteral lipids.
5 Assess blood glucose level by fingerstick (see Skill 43-9).	Provides baseline to determine tolerance to glucose infusion.
6 Assess patient's fluid status by monitoring for edema, shortness of breath, or fluid intake greater than fluid output.	The fluid intake that is given with PPN may cause fluid overload in patients who are elderly or have impaired renal or cardiac function (Worthington and Gilbert, 2012).
7 Obtain patient's weight and vital signs before beginning infusion.	Provides baseline information to determine effectiveness and tolerance to PPN solution.

NURSING DIAGNOSES

- Excess fluid volume
- Imbalanced nutrition: less than body requirements
- Risk for infection
- Risk for unstable blood glucose level

Related factors are individualized based on patient's condition or needs.

PLANNING

1 Expected outcomes following completion of procedure:	
• Triglyceride level is <250 mg/dL in most patients.	Indicates adequate clearance of lipid.
• Venipuncture site is free of phlebitis, pain, swelling, redness, and inflammation.	Ensures proper administration and monitoring of PPN with lipids.
• Patient does not show signs of systemic infection (e.g., elevated temperature).	Temperature is indication of possible systemic infection related to PN.
• Patient does not show signs of allergy to lipids.	Monitoring of infusion requires observation for allergic response to infusion.
2 Explain purposes of PPN and fat emulsion.	Promotes understanding and reduces anxiety.

STEP	RATIONALE
3 Place patient in comfortable position for IV insertion or initiation of infusion.	When patients are comfortable, they tolerate procedures more readily.
4 If PPN solution is refrigerated, remove from refrigeration 1 hour before infusion.	Solution should be at room temperature for administration (INS, 2011).

IMPLEMENTATION

1 Perform hand hygiene.	Reduces transmission of microorganisms.
2 Compare label of PPN bag and lipid emulsion bottle with MAR or computer printout; check for correct additives and solution expiration date. Also check patient's name.	Prevents medication error. *This is the second check for accuracy.*
3 Examine lipid solution for separation of emulsion into layers or fat globules or presence of froth.	Do not administer if these elements appear.
4 Identify patient using two identifiers (i.e., name and birthday or name and account number) according to agency policy. Compare identifiers in patient's MAR/medical record with information on patient's identification bracelet and/or ask patient to state name.	Ensures patient identity. Complies with The Joint Commission requirements and improves patient safety (TJC, 2012). *This is the third check for accuracy.*
5 Measure patient's vital signs.	Provides baseline assessment. Immediate allergic reaction can develop once infusion begins.
6 Apply clean gloves. Prepare IV tubing for PPN solution (see Skill 28-3); run solution through tubing to remove excess air. Turn roller clamp to "off" position. Add sterile capped needle or place sterile cap on end of tubing. Follow same procedure with separate infusion set for lipid infusion.	To prevent air from entering vascular system, clear all tubing.
7 Connect PPN solution to patient's functional peripheral IV (see Skill 22-6). Gently disconnect old PPN tubing from IV site and insert adapter of new PPN infusion tubing. Open roller clamp on new tubing. Allow solution to run to ensure that tubing is patent; then regulate IV drip rate using electronic infusion pump.	Prevents disruption of existing IV and ensures patent infusion. Pump will deliver infusion at prescribed rate.
8 Clean needleless peripheral line tubing injection port with antimicrobial swab.	Removes surface organisms at injection site and prevents organisms from entering blood system.
9 Insert needleless valve at end of fat emulsion infusion tubing into injection port of main IV, closest to patient but below infusion filter on main parenteral nutrition line. Label tubing.	Fat emulsions cannot infuse through a 0.22-μm IV filter. Refer to agency policy; if larger, 1.2-μm filter is used, lipids may be infused above filter (INS, 2011). Labeling of high-risk catheters prevents connection with an inappropriate tube or catheter (TJC, 2012). Height of solution prevents backup into main infusion tubing.
10 Open roller clamp completely on fat emulsion infusion and check flow rate on infusion pump.	Initial slow infusion allows you to observe for allergic response.
11 Infuse lipids initially at 1 mL/min for adults and 0.1 mL/min for child for first 15 to 30 minutes; increase rate as ordered.	Up to 2.5 g fat/kg per day may be infused, but current practice is generally to give <1 g fat/kg body weight per day in adults.
12 Begin PPN at ordered rate. 20% fats are infused over at least 8 hours. All lipids can hang for 12 hours as a separate infusion.	The rate of PPN administration does not need to be increased gradually. The lower concentration of dextrose allows most patients to tolerate the full administration rate without difficulty.
13 Discard supplies and perform hand hygiene.	Reduces transmission of microorganisms.

EVALUATION

1 Monitor flow rate routinely hourly or more frequently if necessary.	Too-rapid or too-slow infusion could result in metabolic disturbances such as hyperglycemia.
2 Measure vital signs and patient's general comfort level every 10 minutes for first 30 minutes.	Monitors patient for lipid allergy.

STEP	RATIONALE
3 Monitor patient's laboratory values (e.g., triglycerides, liver function tests) daily and perform blood glucose monitoring as ordered. Measure serum lipids 4 hours after discontinuing infusion.	Provides objective data to measure response to therapy (e.g., ability of liver to metabolize lipids). Measurement of lipids too soon after an infusion will yield incorrect blood values.
4 Monitor temperature every 4 hours and regularly inspect venipuncture site for signs of phlebitis or infiltration.	Determines onset of fever, a complication of intolerance to fat emulsion or sepsis. Determines integrity of IV system.
5 Assess patient's weight, intake and output (I&O), condition of peripheral extremities (for edema), and breath sounds.	Weight gain, I&O imbalance, peripheral edema, and crackles in lungs indicate fluid retention.

Unexpected Outcomes

1 There is intolerance to fat emulsion, as evidenced by increased triglyceride levels, increased temperature (3° to 4°F), chills, flushing, headache, nausea and vomiting, diaphoresis, muscle ache, chest and back pain, dyspnea, pressure over the eyes, vertigo.

2 See Unexpected Outcomes and Related Interventions for Skill 32-1.

Related Interventions

- Turn PN infusion off.
- Inform health care provider.
- Prepare to treat anaphylactic reaction according to health care provider's orders.
- Record lipid allergy in patient's medical record.

Recording and Reporting

- Record condition of IV site, type of solutions, rate and status of infusion, catheter lumen used for infusion, I&O every 8 hours, blood glucose levels, vital signs, weights, and other assessment findings in nurses' notes and electronic health record (EHR) or appropriate flow sheets.
- Record any adverse reactions in nurses' notes and EHR.
- If signs of fat intolerance, infection, occlusion, fluid retention, or infiltration occur, notify the health care provider.

Special Considerations
Teaching
- PPN administration does not occur in the home.

Pediatric
- See Skill 32-1.

Gerontologic
- Some older adults may have fragile peripheral veins or poor fluid tolerance because of cardiac or renal dysfunction, making PPN undesirable.

Home Care
- See Skill 32-1.

? Critical Thinking Exercises

Mr. Giles is a 43-year-old patient admitted to the hospital with a severe exacerbation of Crohn's disease. He lost 4.5 kg (10 lbs) in the last 3 weeks and suffers recurrent abdominal pain, cramping, and loose stools. He is unable to tolerate food orally, becoming easily nauseated. He is to receive bowel rest and nutritional support with parenteral nutrition (PN). The health care provider inserted a central line for 3:1 PN therapy.

1 Identify four physical parameters that can change quickly and should be part of your baseline assessment before initiating PN.

2 Explain why it is necessary to assess blood glucose measurement before a patient receives PN.

3 On the third day after central line insertion, the patient develops a fever and fatigue, preferring to stay in bed. What might the fever indicate, and what could be its source?

4 Two days after beginning PN infusion, Mr. Giles experiences a 2-kg (5-lb) weight gain. He comments, "This stuff is great. I'm gaining back some of the weight I lost." What would be your response? What would you include in a nursing assessment?

✓ REVIEW QUESTIONS

1 A patient is being switched from a standard intravenous (IV) solution to PN. What should the nurse tell the patient about why a large-diameter vein needs to be used for the infusion? (Select all that apply.)
   1 The fluid is very hyperosmolar.
   2 The fluid cannot flow through smaller veins.
   3 Peripheral veins become very irritated because of the content of the fluid.
   4 The patient will have the infusion for a long time; he will have use of both of his hands without an IV in them.

2 A patient is receiving an infusion of lipids through his central line. What symptoms might suggest that he or she is experiencing a lipid allergy?
   1 Elevated temperature, chills, nausea, and chest pain
   2 Respiratory distress, shortness of breath, chest pain, and decreased blood pressure
   3 Increased temperature, chills, malaise, and elevated white blood cell count
   4 Nausea and vomiting and bleeding and swelling at the insertion site

3 A patient is receiving a 3:1 PN infusion. How often should the IV infusion tubing be changed?
   1 Once a week
   2 Every 24 hours
   3 Every 72 hours
   4 After each solution is administered

4   What is the main purpose of PN?
   1   To provide full nutrient requirements while oral intake is precluded
   2   To replace enteral tube feedings
   3   To cure metabolic alterations from cancer
   4   To obtain additional caloric intake during hospitalization

5   What are the components of PN?
   1   Trace elements and electrolytes
   2   Vitamins
   3   Glucose, amino acids, lipids, and water
   4   All of the above

6   Which size filter should be used with a lipid-containing PN infusion?
   1   No filter required
   2   0.22-μm filter
   3   1.2-μm filter
   4   2-μm filter

7   Which of the following is the most frequent risk associated with PN?
   1   Bowel obstruction
   2   Pneumonia
   3   High albumin levels
   4   Catheter-related bloodstream infections

8   Which of the following risks is more common with long-term use of PN than short-term PN?
   1   Hyperglycemia
   2   Hypercholesterolemia
   3   Hepatic disease
   4   Renal disease

9   A patient with which of the following is a good candidate for short-term PN?
   1   Anastomotic leak
   2   Intestinal obstruction
   3   Severe mucositis
   4   Severe malnutrition before surgery
   5   All of the above

10   Which of the following patients is a good candidate for long-term PN in the home?
   1   Short-bowel syndrome or dysmotility
   2   Inadequate food intake
   3   Personal preference
   4   Limited use of upper extremities because of disease process

REFERENCES

American Society for Parenteral and Enteral Nutrition (ASPEN): Standards of practice: nutrition support nurses, *Nutr Clin Pract* 22(4):458, 2007.

Centers for Disease Control and Prevention: Vital signs: central line—associated blood stream infections—United States, 2001, 2008, and 2009, *MMWR* 60(08):243, 2011, available at http://www.cdc.gov/mmwr/preview/mmwrhtml/mm6008a4.htm?s_cid=mm6008a4_w, accessed March 19, 2012.

Hardy G, Puzovic M: Formulation, stability, and administration of parenteral nutrition with new lipid emulsions, *Nutr Clin Pract* 24(5):616, 2009.

Hockenberry MJ, Wilson D: *Wong's nursing care of infants and children*, ed 9, St Louis, 2011, Mosby.

Infusion Nurses Society (INS): Infusion nursing standards of practice, *J Intraven Nurs* 34(suppl 1S):S91, 2011.

Kutsogiannis J, et al: Early use of supplemental parenteral nutrition in critically ill patients: results of an international multicenter observational study, *Crit Care Med* 39(12):2691, 2011.

Lamperti M, et al: International evidence-based recommendations on ultrasound-guided vascular access, *Intens Care Med* 38(7):1105, 2012.

Moghissi ES, et al: American Association of Clinical E, American Diabetes A: American Association of Clinical Endocrinologists and American Diabetes Association consensus statement on inpatient glycemic control, *Diabetes Care* 32:1119, 2009.

NICE-SUGAR Study Investigators: Intensive versus conventional glucose control in critically ill patients, *N Engl J Med* 360:1283, 2009.

Pasquel FJ, et al: Hyperglycemia during total parenteral nutrion: an important marker of poor outcome and mortality in hospitalized patients, *Diabetes Care* 33(4):738, 2010.

The Joint Commission (TJC): *National patient safety goals*, Oakbrook Terrace, Ill, 2012, The Commission, available at http://www.jointcommission.org/standards_information/npsgs.aspx.

Thibault R, Pichard C: Parenteral nutrition in critical illness: Can it safely improve outcomes? *Crit Care Clin* 26:467, 2010.

Worthington PH, Gilbert KA: Parenteral nutrition: risks, complications, and management, *J Infusion Nurs* 35(1):52, 2012.

Urinary Elimination

MEDIA RESOURCES

- evolve http://evolve.elsevier.com/Perry/skills
  learning system
  - Review Questions
  - ▶ Video Clips
  - Audio Glossary
- NSO Nursing Skills Online
- Mosby's Nursing Video Skills, 4th edition

KEY TERMS

Catheterization
Micturition
Postvoid residual (PVR)

Urinary retention
Urinary tract infection

OBJECTIVES

Mastery of content in this chapter will enable the nurse to:
- Discuss nursing interventions that promote normal micturition when toilet access is compromised or after a catheter is removed.
- Discuss the relationship between fluid balance and urinary elimination.
- Identify factors that increase risk for catheter-associated urinary tract infection (CAUTI).

- Perform the following skills: place and remove urinal, insert urinary catheter, care for an indwelling urinary catheter, measure postvoid residual (PVR) with catheterization and bladder scan, irrigate a catheter, remove an indwelling catheter, apply a condom catheter, and care for a suprapubic catheter.

A key nursing responsibility is to support patients as they respond to threats to their health. A basic human function is urinary elimination, a function that can be compromised by a wide variety of illnesses and conditions. It is the role of a nurse to support bladder emptying as needed by helping a patient to a toilet or bedside commode, assist with a urinal, or perform catheterization. During acute illness a patient may require urinary catheterization for close monitoring of urine output or to facilitate bladder emptying when bladder function is compromised. Some patients require long-term indwelling catheters, urethral or suprapubic, when the bladder fails to empty effectively. The nurse also implements measures to minimize risk for infection when bladder function is impaired or urinary drainage tubes are required.

EVIDENCE-BASED PRACTICE

In 2009 the Centers for Medicare and Medicaid Services (CMS) enacted policies that addressed expensive and potentially preventable conditions. One of those conditions included the use of indwelling urinary catheters in the acute care setting (CMS, 2009). The CMS policies included a major focus on preventing complications such as catheter-associated urinary tract infection (CAUTI). Soon after, the Centers for Disease

Control and Prevention (CDC) published its revised evidence-based guidelines for the prevention of CAUTI (Gould et al., 2009). Other major organizations such as Shea and Infectious Disease Society of America (Lo et al., 2008); Association for Professionals in Infection Control and Epidemiology (APIC) (Green et al., 2008); International Consultation on Continence (Cottenden et al., 2009); and the Wound Ostomy Continence Nursing Society (WOCN) (Parker et al., 2009; Willson, 2009) have all published evidenced-based documents related to catheterization and catheter care. The Joint Commission (TJC) has included in its 2012 National Patient Safety Goals (2012) those that require the implementation of evidenced-based practices related to urinary catheterization to reduce CAUTI. All of these evidenced-based guidelines/goals contain common practices that nurses should incorporate when performing urinary catheterization and/or caring for patients with indwelling catheters. The practices for preventing CAUTI include:

- Aseptic insertion of urinary catheters (Gould et al., 2009; Green et al., 2008; Lo et al., 2008).
- Limiting the use of indwelling catheters to essential conditions and removing them as soon as medically indicated (Gould et al., 2009; Green et al., 2008; Nazarko, 2008). Examples of appropriate indications for catheterization include acute urinary retention, accurate intake and output measurement in critically ill patients, perioperative preparation for select surgeries, healing of open sacral or perineal wounds in incontinent patients, patients requiring prolonged bedrest, and comfort for end-of-life care (Gould et al., 2009).
- Using the smallest catheter possible (Gould et al., 2009; Lo et al., 2008; Parker et al., 2009).
- Daily cleansing of the urethral meatus with soap and water or perineal cleanser (Gould et al., 2009).
- Maintaining a closed urinary drainage system (Gould et al., 2009; Green et al., 2008; Lo et al., 2008).
- Maintaining a free flow of urine through the catheter (Gould et al., 2009, Green et al., 2008; Lo et al., 2008).
- Avoiding urethral trauma by securing a catheter (Gould et al., 2009; Green et al., 2008; Lo et al., 2008).
- Antiseptics applied to the urinary meatus are not effective and should not be applied (Willson et al., 2009).
- Antiseptic solutions placed in drainage bags and complex urinary drainage systems have not been found to be effective (Gould et al., 2009).

PATIENT-CENTERED CARE

The personal level of touch required when you assist patients with problems in urinary elimination requires you to understand their values and preferences. Determine how patients feel about having to undergo procedures such as catheterization. Try to adapt procedures to minimize the invasive nature of catheterization and maintain a patient's dignity and respect.

When caring for patients from divergent cultures, it is important to incorporate into the plan of care sensitivity and awareness of factors that may impact how you deal with urinary elimination problems. Variations within a cultural group are common. Assess each patient and care for him or her as an individual. Many cultures have specific beliefs and practices related to elimination, privacy, and gender-specific care. For example:

- Provide for a same-gender caregiver for cultures that emphasize female modesty and prohibit nonrelated males and females from touching, such as Iranian, Jewish Orthodox, Korean, Hindu, and Vietnamese (Purnell, 2009).

- Hispanic families tend to emphasize interdependence over independence; thus family presence at the bedside for important decision making is common (D'Avanzo, 2008).
- Privacy is important in many cultures; thus careful attention to draping is important.
- Some cultures continue to practice female genital circumcision, which can include removal of all or part of the clitoris; complete removal of the clitoris; part or complete removal of the labia minora; or in its most severe form the total removal of the clitoris and labia and sewing together the labia majora, leaving only a small opening for urine and menses (AAP, 2010).

Safety Guidelines

1 Regularly assess and determine patients' functional status, such as their ability to safely stand and/or transfer to a toilet or commode, their ability to follow and understand directions, and their motivation to help in self-care activities, such as using a toilet, commode, or urinal.
2 Evaluate a patient's normal pattern of micturition. Patients taking diuretic medications should have a toilet, commode, and/or urinal close to their bed or chair. Respond to any request for toileting assistance in a prompt manner to lessen the chance of patients falling as they try to reach a toilet.
3 Consider a patient's age when assessing voiding habits. Toilet training and enuresis are concerns for toddlers and preschoolers. Frail older adults are at higher risk for incontinence because of multiple health care problems and associated physiologic changes.
4 Patients who need assistance with elimination should have a call bell within easy reach and the offer for assistance at regular

TABLE 33-1	Signs of Fluid Volume Deficit and Fluid Volume Excess
Eyes	*FVD:* Sunken eyes, dry conjunctivae, decreased or absence of tearing *FVE:* Periorbital edema, blurred vision, papilledema
Mouth	*FVD:* Sticky, dry mucous membrane; dry, cracked lips; decreased saliva; increased viscosity of saliva; furrowed, shrunken tongue *FVE:* Excessive salivation
Skin	*FVD:* Increased skin temperature; dry, scaly skin; poor turgor *FVE:* Edema, anasarca
Cardiovascular	*FVD:* Increased pulse rate, weak pulse, hypotension, decreased pulse volume/pressure, decreased capillary filling, increased hematocrit, flat neck veins *FVE:* Bounding pulse rate, blood pressure normal with or without orthostatic changes, third heart sound (S_3), distended neck veins
Gastrointestinal	*FVD:* Sunken abdomen *FVD* or *FVE:* Vomiting, diarrhea, abdominal cramps
Renal	*FVD:* Oliguria or anuria, urine specific gravity increased (normal, 1.010 to 1.030) *FVE:* Decreased urine specific gravity, diuresis (if kidneys are normal)

FVD, Fluid volume deficit; *FVE,* fluid volume excess.

intervals, especially in the morning after awakening, after meals, and before bedtime.

5 Adequate oral intake is essential for bladder health, especially if a patient has an indwelling urinary catheter. Some patients with urinary problems limit fluid intake in fear of incontinence and/or increased urinary frequency. Explain the importance of fluid intake in maintaining urinary health.

6 Evaluate urinary output.

  a Know the average output range for a patient. Adult urinary output averages 2200 to 2700 mL in 24 hours. An hourly output of less than 30 mL/hr for 2 hours identifies the need for further evaluation.

  b Know the signs of dehydration and fluid overload (Table 33-1). Start measurement of intake and output (I&O) when there is an actual or anticipated change in fluid balance.

  c Assess a patient's most recent serum electrolyte measurements. Abnormal values reflect alterations in fluid balance that can lead to deterioration in patients' health.

  d Weigh a patient to determine fluid status. Ask him or her to empty the bladder. Weigh with the same scale; at the same time of day; and with comparable articles of clothing, including bed linen if bed weights are necessary.

7 Maintain aseptic technique when catheterizing a patient to prevent CAUTI (NQF, 2011).

PROCEDURAL GUIDELINE 33-1   Assisting with Use of a Urinal

 Video Clip

A urinal is a container used to hold urine when access to a toilet is restricted. Patients who may need a urinal include those who have compromised mobility, severe dyspnea, or other illnesses that make walking to a bathroom impossible or excessively painful. In some instances a male patient may be able to stand at the bedside and use a urinal. Most urinals are used by men, but there are specially designed urinals for women (Fig. 33-1). The female urinal has a larger opening at the top with a defined rim, which helps position the urinal closely against the genitalia.

Delegation and Collaboration

The skill of assisting a patient in using a urinal can be delegated to nursing assistive personnel (NAP). The nurse directs the NAP to:

- Adjust for any special needs or adaptations such as a need to hold a urinal for a patient.
- Provide personal hygiene as necessary after urination.
- Report immediately any changes in urine color, clarity, and odor; development of incontinence (involuntary loss of urine); patient reports of dysuria, which could indicate an infection; and any changes in the frequency and amount of urine.
- Explain the procedure to patient and family to promote understanding and participation in care.

Equipment

- ❏ Urinal
- ❏ Clean gloves
- ❏ Graduated cylinder (used for measuring volume if urinal is not marked)
- ❏ Supplies for diagnostic urine tests and specimen collection (see Chapter 43)
- ❏ Washbasin, washcloths, towels, and soap
- ❏ Toilet tissue

Procedural Steps

1 Assess patient's normal urinary elimination habits, including any episodes of incontinence.
2 Determine how much assistance is needed to place and remove the urinal.
3 Determine if a urine specimen is to be collected.
4 Explain procedure to patient.
5 Provide privacy by closing bedside curtain and room door.
6 Assess for a distended bladder by inspecting the lower one third of the abdomen or palpating gently above symphysis pubis.
7 Perform hand hygiene and apply clean gloves.
8 Help patient into appropriate position: *for a male patient*: on side, back, sitting with head of bed elevated, or in standing position; *for a female patient*: lying supine. If needed, place an absorbent pad under patient's buttocks to protect bed linens from accidental spills.

Clinical Decision Point *Before having a patient stand to void, assess lower-extremity strength and mobility and for orthostatic hypotension, especially if he has been on prolonged bed rest.*

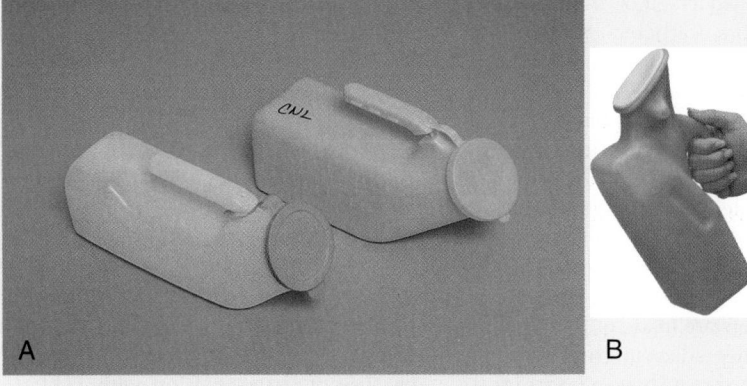

FIG 33-1   **A,** Male. **B,** Female urinals. (**B** *Courtesy Briggs Medical Service Co.*)

Continued

PROCEDURAL GUIDELINE 33-1   Assisting with Use of a Urinal—cont'd

9   If possible, a male patient should hold urinal and position penis in urinal. If needed, help patient by positioning penis completely in urinal and holding urinal in place or by helping him hold urinal. Ensure that the urinal is placed dependent of the flow of urine.

10   Help a female patient by positioning the urinal against the genitalia and stabilizing it to keep it in position and dependent of urine flow.

11   Cover patient with bed linens and place the call bell within reach. If possible, give patient further privacy by leaving the bedside after ensuring that he or she is in a safe and comfortable position.

12   After patient has finished voiding, remove urinal and assess characteristics of the urine for color, clarity, odor, and amount. Help him or her wash and dry penis or genitalia.

13   Measure urine and record output on intake and output (I&O) record, if needed (see Chapter 6).

14   Empty and clean urinal. Return urinal to patient for future use.

15   Help patient perform hand hygiene as needed.

16   Remove and dispose of gloves; perform hand hygiene.

SKILL 33-1   Insertion of a Straight or an Indwelling Urinary Catheter

NSO *Urinary Catheterization Module / Lessons 1 and 2*

Urinary catheterization is the placement of a tube through the urethra into the bladder to drain urine. This is an invasive procedure that requires a medical order and aseptic technique in institutional settings (Gould et al., 2009; Lo et al., 2008). Urinary catheterization may be short term (2 weeks or less) or long term (more than 1 month) (Parker et al., 2009). There are a limited number of conditions in which the use of a short- or long-term urinary catheter is appropriate (see Evidence-Based Practice). Excessive accumulation of urine in the bladder is painful for a patient; increases the risk for urinary tract infection (UTI); and can cause backward flow of urine up the ureters to the kidneys, causing kidney damage. Urinary incontinence, an involuntary leakage of urine, may require indwelling catheterization if the leaking urine interferes with wound healing (Cottenden et al., 2009). Intermittent catheterization is used to measure postvoid residual (PVR) when a bladder scanner is not available or as a way to manage chronic urinary retention.

The steps for inserting an indwelling and a single-use straight/intermittent catheter are the same. The difference lies in the inflation of a balloon to keep the indwelling catheter in place and the presence of a closed drainage system. Urinary catheters are made with one to three lumens (Fig. 33-2). Single-lumen catheters (see Fig. 33-2, A) are used for intermittent catheterization (i.e., the insertion of a catheter for one-time bladder emptying). Double-lumen catheters, designed for indwelling catheters, provide one lumen for urinary drainage and a second lumen to inflate a balloon that keeps the catheter in place (see Fig. 33-2, B). Triple-lumen catheters (see Fig. 33-2, C) are used for continuous bladder irrigation or when it becomes necessary to instill medications into the bladder. One lumen drains the bladder, a second lumen is used to inflate the balloon, and a third lumen delivers irrigation fluid into the bladder.

A health care provider chooses a catheter on the basis of factors such as latex allergy, history of catheter encrustation, and susceptibility to infection. Indwelling catheters are made of latex or silicone. Latex catheters with special coatings reduce urethral irritation (Cottenden et al., 2009). All silicone catheters have a larger internal diameter and may be helpful in patients who require frequent

catheter changes because of encrustation (Newman and Wein, 2009). Antimicrobial catheters are coated with silver or an antibiotic. These coated catheters have been shown to reduce the incidence of catheter-associated urinary tract infection (CAUTI) for short-term use, but to date there are insufficient data to support their use in long-term catheter users (Drekonja et al. 2008; Parker et al. 2009; Schumm and Lam, 2008). Straight or intermittent catheters are made of rubber (softer and more flexible) or polyvinylchloride (PVC). Patients who self-catheterize have a large selection of catheters, some with special coatings that do not require lubrication and some that are self-contained systems consisting of a catheter prelubricated and packaged with a preconnected drainage bag.

The size of a urinary catheter is based on the French (Fr) scale, which reflects the internal diameter of the catheter. Most adults with an indwelling catheter should have a size 14 to 16 Fr to minimize trauma and risk for infection. Larger catheter diameters increase the risk for urethral trauma (Parker et al., 2009). However, larger sizes are used in special circumstances such as after urologic surgery or in the presence of gross hematuria. Smaller sizes are needed for children (i.e., 5-6 Fr for infants, 8-10 Fr for children, and 12 Fr for young girls).

Indwelling catheters come in a variety of balloon sizes from 3 mL (for a child) to 30 mL for continuous bladder irrigation (CBI). The size of the balloon is usually printed on the catheter port (Fig. 33-3). The recommended balloon size for an adult is a 5-mL balloon (filled with 10 mL). Long-term use of larger balloons (30 mL) has been associated with increased patient discomfort, irritation, and trauma; increased risk of catheter expulsion; and incomplete emptying of the bladder because of urine that pools below the level of the catheter drainage lumen (Cottenden et al., 2009; Newman and Wein, 2009).

For patients with urinary retention or critical illness and who require long-term catheterization, catheter changes should be individualized, not routine (Gould et al., 2009; Green et al., 2008; Willson et al., 2009). They should be changed for leaking, for blockage, and before obtaining a sterile specimen for urine culture (Smith et al., 2008). Long-term catheterization should be avoided because of its association with UTI (Green, et al., 2008). Make every attempt to remove catheters as soon as a patient can void.

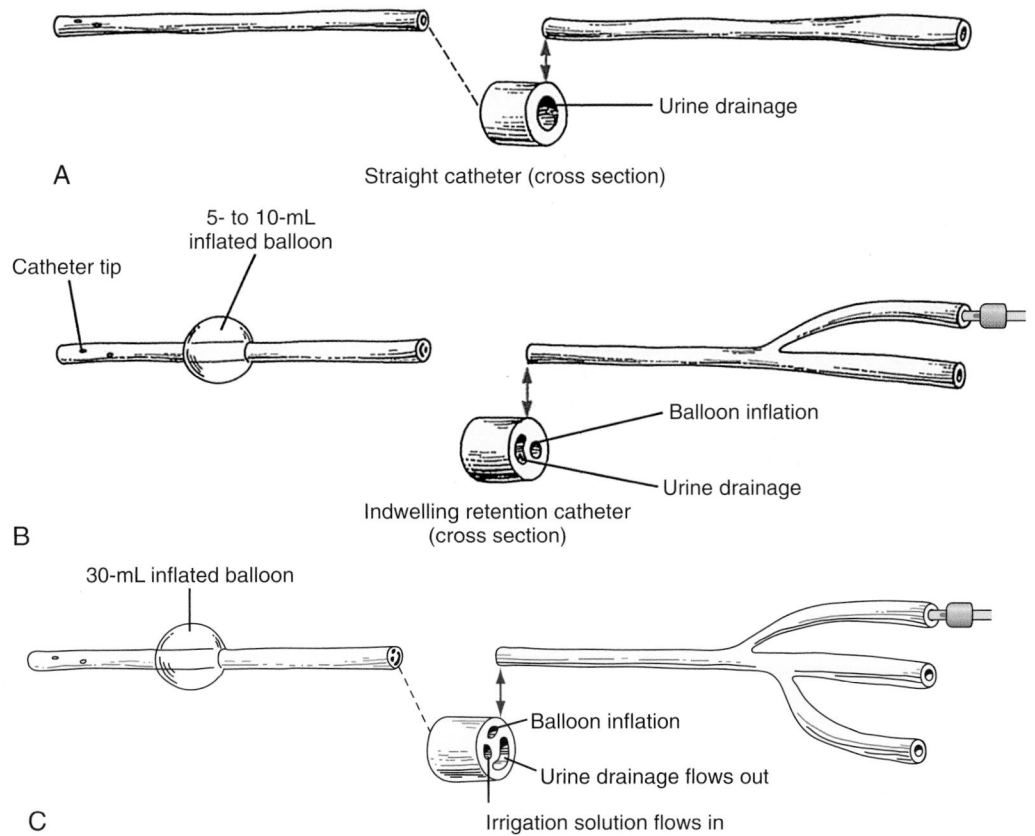

FIG 33-2 **A,** Single-lumen or straight catheter (cross section). **B,** Double-lumen or indwelling retention catheter (cross section). **C,** Triple-lumen catheter for continuous closed irrigation (cross section).

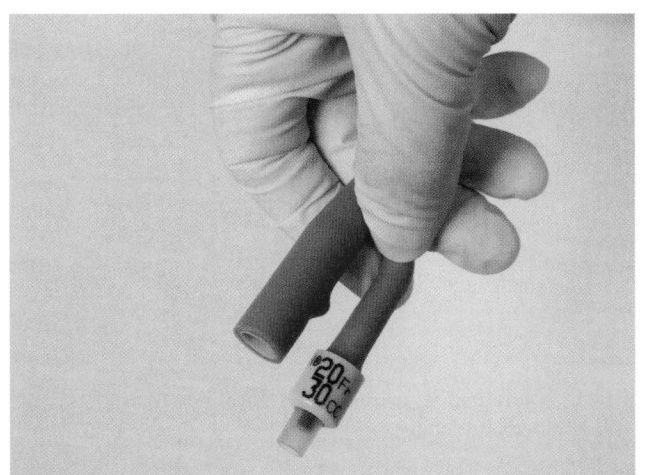

FIG 33-3 Size of catheter and balloon printed on catheter inflation valve.

An indwelling catheter is attached to a urinary drainage bag to collect the continuous flow of urine. Always hang the bag below the level of the bladder on the bed frame or a chair so urine drains down, out of the bladder. The bag should never touch the floor. When a patient ambulates, carry the bag below the level of his or her bladder. The only exception to this rule is when a catheter is attached to a specially designed drainage bag (belly bag) that is worn across the abdomen. A one-way valve prevents the back flow of urine into the bladder.

Delegation and Collaboration

The skill of inserting a straight or indwelling urinary catheter cannot be delegated to nursing assistive personnel (NAP). The nurse directs the NAP to:

- Help with patient positioning, focus lighting for the procedure, maintain privacy, empty urine from collection bag, and help with perineal care.
- Report postprocedure patient discomfort or fever to the nurse.
- Report abnormal color, odor, amount of urine in drainage bag, and if the catheter is leaking or causes pain.

Equipment

❑ Catheter kit (Fig. 33-4) containing the following sterile items: (Catheter kits vary; thus it is important to check the list of contents on the package.)
- Catheter of correct size and type for procedure or patient condition (i.e., indwelling [double lumen 14 or 16 Fr] or intermittent [usually 12 to 14 Fr]). Some kits contain a catheter with attached drainage bag; others contain only a catheter; others have no catheter.
- Drapes (one fenestrated—has an opening in the center)
- Sterile gloves
- Lubricant
- Antiseptic cleaning solution such as chlorhexidine or povidone-iodine incorporated in an applicator or to be added to cotton balls (forceps to pick up cotton balls)
- Specimen container
- Prefilled syringe with sterile water for balloon inflation of an indwelling catheter

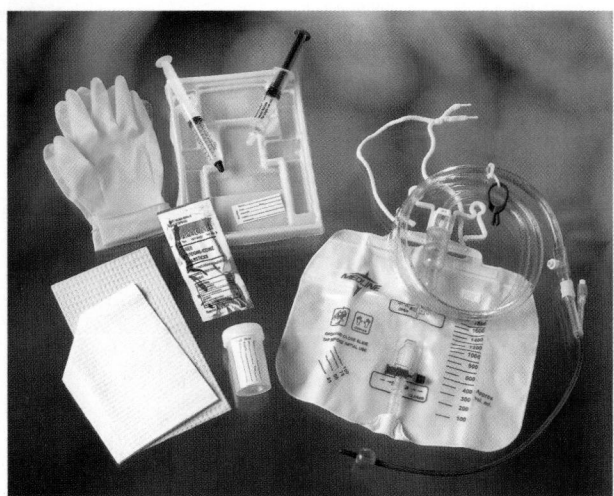

FIG 33-4 Indwelling catheterization kit includes drainage device, specimen cup, sterile drapes, sterile gloves, indwelling catheter, cleaning solution, sterile saline, sterile cotton balls, forceps, and lubricant. (*Image used with permission Medline Industries. All rights reserved.*)

- Sterile drainage tubing and collection bag (Some kits come preconnected; others do not, and a separate package is required.)
❏ Sterile drainage tubing and bag (if not included in the kit)
❏ Device to secure catheter (i.e., strap)
❏ Extra sterile gloves and catheter (optional)
❏ Bath blanket
❏ Waterproof absorbent pad
❏ Clean gloves; basin with warm water, soap or perineal cleaner, washcloth; and towel for perineal care
❏ Additional lighting as needed (such as a flashlight or procedure light)
❏ Measuring container for urine

STEP	RATIONALE

ASSESSMENT

1 Review patient's medical record, including health care provider's order and nurses' notes. Note previous catheterization, including catheter size, response of patient, and time of catheterization.	Identifies purpose of inserting catheter (such as for measurement of PVR, preparation for surgery, or specimen collection) and potential difficulty with catheter insertion.
2 Review medical record for any pathologic condition that may impair passage of catheter (e.g., enlarged prostate gland in men, urethral strictures).	Obstruction of urethra may prevent passage of catheter into bladder.
3 Ask patient and check chart for allergies.	Identifies allergy to antiseptic, tape, latex, and lubricant.
4 Assess patient's weight, level of consciousness, developmental level, ability to cooperate, and mobility.	Determines positioning for catheterization; indicates how much assistance is needed to properly position patient, ability of patient to cooperate during procedure, and level of explanation needed.
5 Assess patient's gender and age.	Determines catheter size.
6 Assess patient's knowledge, prior experience with catheterization, and feelings about the procedure.	Reveals need for patient instruction and/or support.

Clinical Decision Point *Large catheters can damage the urethra and urinary meatus, increase bladder irritability, and cause urine to leak around the catheter because of spasm (Cottenden et al., 2009). Use the smallest-size catheter possible to minimize trauma and patient discomfort (Gould et al., 2009; Lo et al., 2008).*

7 Assess for pain and bladder fullness. Palpate bladder over symphysis pubis or use bladder scanner (if available) (see Procedural Guideline 33-2).	Palpation of full bladder causes pain and/or urge to void, indicating full or overfull bladder.
8 Perform hand hygiene and apply clean gloves. Inspect perineal region, observing for perineal anatomic landmarks, erythema, drainage or discharge, and odor. Remove gloves and perform hand hygiene.	Assessment of female perineal landmarks improves accuracy and speed of catheter insertion.

NURSING DIAGNOSES

- Acute pain
- Anxiety
- Deficient knowledge regarding catheterization
- Impaired urinary elimination
- Risk for infection
- Urinary retention

Related factors are individualized based on patient's condition or needs.

STEP	RATIONALE
PLANNING	
1 Expected outcomes following completion of procedure:	
• Patient's bladder is not palpable.	Bladder successfully emptied.
• Patient verbalizes absence of abdominal discomfort or bladder pressure/fullness.	Catheterization and free flow of urine through catheter relieve bladder distention and discomfort.
• Patient has urine output of at least 30 mL/hr as measured in urinary drainage bag.	Verifies presence of catheter in bladder, catheter patency, and adequate kidney function.
• Patient verbalizes purpose and expectations about procedure.	Reflects patient understanding of procedure.
2 Explain procedure to patient.	Promotes cooperation.
3 Arrange for extra personnel to help as necessary.	Some patients are unable to assume positioning independently for procedure.
IMPLEMENTATION	
1 Identify patient using two identifiers (i.e., name and birthday or name and account number) according to agency policy. Compare identifiers with information on patient's identification bracelet.	Ensures correct patient. Complies with The Joint Commission standards and improves patient safety (TJC, 2012).
2 Check patient's plan of care for size and type of catheter (if this is a reinsertion). Use smallest-size catheter possible. Collect all required equipment.	Ensures that patient receives correct size and type of catheter. Larger catheter diameters increase the risk for urethral trauma (Parker et al., 2009). Small catheter allows for adequate drainage of periurethral glands.
3 Perform hand hygiene.	Reduces transmission of microorganisms.
4 Provide privacy by closing room door and bedside curtain.	Promotes comfort and protects patient confidentiality.
5 Raise bed to appropriate working height. If side rails in use, raise side rail on opposite side of bed and lower side rail on working side.	Promotes good body mechanics. Use of side rails in this manner promotes patient safety.
6 Place waterproof pad under patient.	Prevents soiling of bed linen.

Clinical Decision Point *Obtain assistance to position and support weak, frail, obese, or confused patients from a co-worker.*

STEP	RATIONALE
7 Position patient:	
a Female patient:	
(1) Help to dorsal recumbent position (on back with knees flexed). Ask patient to relax thighs so you can rotate hips.	Exposes perineum and allows hip joints to be externally rotated.
(2) Alternate female position: Position side-lying (Sims') position with upper leg flexed at knee and hip. Support patient with pillows if necessary to maintain position.	Alternate position is more comfortable if patient cannot abduct leg at hip joint (e.g., patient has arthritic joints or contractures).
b Male patient:	
(1) Position supine with legs extended and thighs slightly abducted.	Comfortable position for patient aids in visualization of penis.
8 Drape patient.	Protects patient dignity by avoiding unnecessary exposure of body parts.
a Female patient	
(1) Drape with bath blanket. Place blanket diamond fashion over patient, with one corner at patient's midsection, side corners over each thigh and abdomen, and last corner over perineum (see illustration).	
b Male patient	
(1) Drape patient by covering upper part of body with small sheet or towel; drape with separate sheet or bath blanket so only perineum is exposed (see illustration).	
9 Apply clean gloves. Wash perineal area with soap and water, rinse, and dry (see Chapter 17). Use gloves to examine patient and identify urinary meatus. Remove and discard gloves.	Hygiene before initiating aseptic catheter insertion removes secretions, urine, and feces that could contaminate sterile field and increase risk for CAUTI.
10 Position light to illuminate genitals or have assistant available to hold light source to visualize urinary meatus.	Adequate visualization of urinary meatus helps with speed and accuracy of catheter insertion.
11 Perform hand hygiene.	Reduces transmission of microorganisms.

STEP	RATIONALE
12 Open outer wrapping of catheterization kit. Place inner wrapped catheter kit tray on clean, accessible surface such as bedside table or, if possible, between patients' open legs. Patient size and positioning dictate exact placement.	Provides easy access to supplies during catheter insertion.
13 Open inner sterile wrap covering tray containing catheterization supplies, using sterile technique (see Chapter 8). Fold back each flap of sterile covering one at a time, with last flap opened toward patient.	Sterile wrap serves as sterile field.
a Indwelling catheterization open system: Open separate package containing drainage bag, check to make sure that clamp on drainage port is closed, and place drainage bag and tubing in an easily accessible location. Open outer package of sterile catheter, maintaining sterility of inner wrapper (see Chapter 8).	Open drainage bag systems have separate sterile packaging for sterile catheter, drainage bag and tubing, and insertion kit.
b Indwelling catheterization closed system: All supplies are in sterile tray and are arranged in sequence of use.	Closed drainage bag systems have catheter preattached to drainage tubing and bag.
c Straight catheterization: All needed supplies are in sterile tray that contains supplies and can be used for urine collection.	
14 Put on sterile gloves. (Or apply sterile drape with ungloved hands when drape is packed as first item. Touch only edges of drape. Then apply clean gloves.)	Maintains surgical asepsis.
15 Drape perineum, keeping gloves sterile.	Sterile drapes provide sterile field over which you will work during catheterization.
a *Drape female:*	
(1) Pick up square sterile drape touching only edges (2.5 cm [1 inch]).	When creating the cuff over sterile gloved hands, sterility of gloves and workspace is maintained.
(2) Allow drape to unfold without touching unsterile surfaces. Allow top edge of drape (2.5 to 5 cm [1 to 2 in]) to form cuff over both hands.	
(3) Place drape with shiny side down on bed between patient's thighs. Slip cuffed edge just under buttocks as you ask patient to lift hips. Take care not to touch contaminated surfaces with sterile gloves	
(4) Pick up fenestrated sterile drape out of tray. Allow drape to unfold without touching unsterile surfaces. Allow top edge of drape to form cuff over both hands. Apply drape over perineum, exposing labia (see illustration).	Opening in drape creates sterile field around labia.

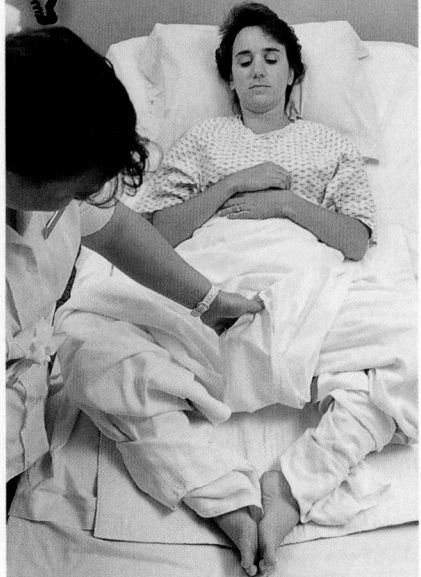

STEP 8a(1)   Female patient draped and in dorsal recumbent position.

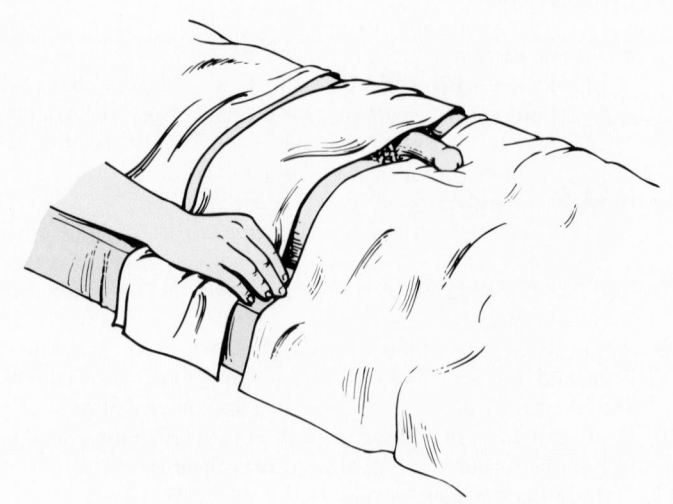

STEP 8b(1)   Draping male patient with blankets.

STEP	**RATIONALE**

b *Drape male:*

   (1) Use of square drape is optional; you may apply fenestrated drape instead.

   (2) Pick up edges of square drape and allow to unfold without touching unsterile surfaces. Place over thighs, with shiny side down, just below penis.

   (3) Place fenestrated drape with opening centered over penis (see illustration).

16 Move tray closer to patient. Arrange remaining supplies on sterile field, maintaining sterility of gloves. Place sterile tray with cleaning medium (premoistened swab sticks or cotton balls, forceps, and solution) lubricant, catheter, and prefilled syringe for inflating balloon (indwelling catheterization only) on sterile drape.

Provides easy access to supplies during catheter insertion and helps to maintain aseptic technique. Appropriate placement is determined by size of patient and position during catheterization.

   a If kit contains sterile cotton balls, open package of sterile antiseptic solution and pour over cotton balls. Some kits contain a package of premoistened swab sticks. Open end of package for easy access (see illustration and Fig. 33-4).

Use of sterile supplies and antiseptic solution reduces risk of CAUTI (Gould et al., 2009; Lo et al., 2008).

   b Open sterile specimen container if specimen to be obtained (see Chapter 43).

Makes container accessible to receive urine from catheter if specimen is needed.

   c For indwelling catheterization, open sterile wrapper of catheter and leave catheter on sterile field. If part of a closed system kit, remove tray with catheter and pre-attached drainage bag and place on sterile drape. Make sure that clamp on drainage port of bag is closed. If needed and if part of sterile tray, attach catheter to drainage tubing.

Indwelling catheterization trays vary. Some have preattached catheters; others need to be attached but are part of the sterile tray; others do not have catheter or drainage system as part of tray.

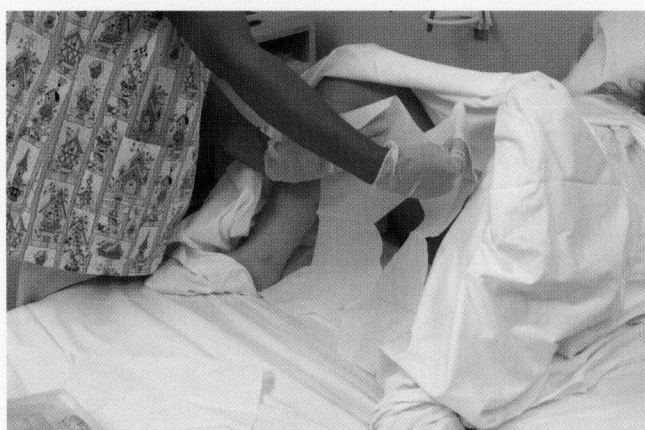

STEP 15a(4) Place sterile fenestrated drape (with opening in center) over female's perineum.

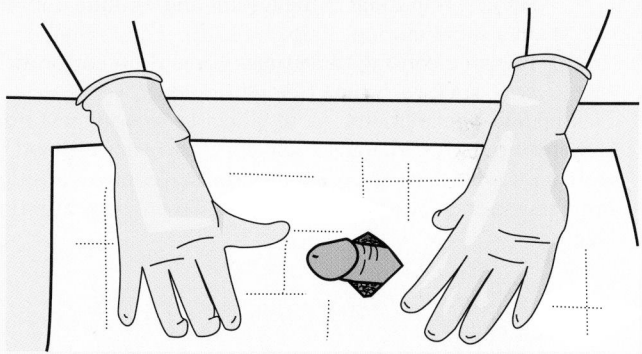

STEP 15b(3) Draping male with fenestrated drape.

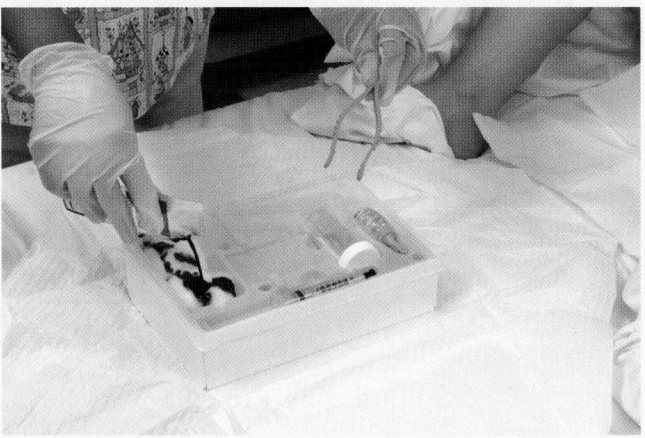

STEP 16a Sterile kit includes antiseptic swabs.

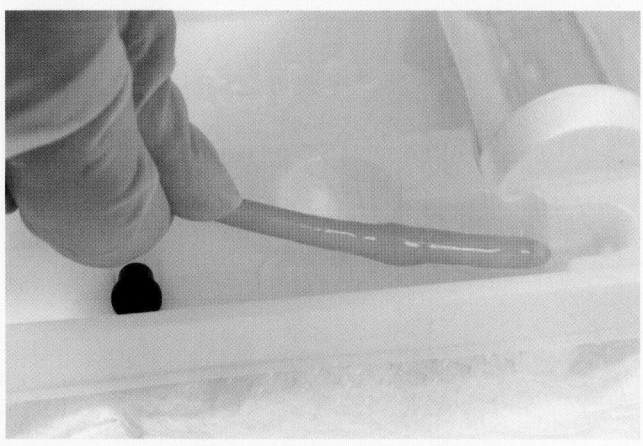

STEP 16d Lubricating catheter.

STEP	RATIONALE
d Open packet of lubricant and squeeze out on sterile field. Lubricate catheter tip by dipping it into water-soluble gel 2.5 to 5 cm (1 to 2 inches) for women and 12.5 to 17.5 cm (5 to 7 inches) for men (see illustration).	Lubrication minimizes trauma to urethra and discomfort during catheter insertion. Male catheter needs enough lubricant to cover length of catheter inserted.

Clinical Decision Point *Pretesting a balloon on an indwelling catheter by injecting fluid from the prefilled sterile water syringe into the balloon port is no longer recommended. Testing the balloon may distort and stretch it and lead to damage, causing increased trauma on insertion.*

17 Clean urethral meatus:	
a Female patient:	
(1) Separate labia with fingers of nondominant hand (now contaminated) to fully expose urethral meatus.	Optimal visualization of urethral meatus is possible.
(2) Maintain position of nondominant hand throughout procedure.	Closure of labia during cleaning means that area is contaminated and requires cleaning procedure to be repeated.
(3) Holding forceps in dominant hand, pick up one moistened cotton ball or pick up one swab stick at a time. Clean labia and urinary meatus from clitoris toward anus. Use new cotton ball or swab for each area that you clean. Clean by wiping far labial fold, near labial fold, and directly over center of urethral meatus (see illustration).	Front-to-back cleaning moves from area of least contamination toward highly contaminated area. Follows principles of medical asepsis (see Chapter 7). Dominant gloved hand remains sterile.
b Male patient:	
(1) With nondominant hand (now contaminated) retract foreskin (if uncircumcised) and gently grasp penis at shaft just below glans. Hold shaft of penis at right angle to body. This hand remains in this position for remainder of procedure.	When grasping shaft of penis, avoid pressure on dorsal surface to prevent compression of urethra. Losing grasp during cleaning means that area is contaminated and requires cleaning procedure to be repeated.
(2) Using uncontaminated dominant hand, clean the meatus with cotton balls/swab sticks, using circular strokes, beginning at the meatus and working outward in a spiral motion.	Circular cleaning pattern follows principles of medical asepsis (see Chapter 7).
(3) Repeat cleansing three times using clean cotton ball/swab stick each time (see illustration).	
18 Pick up and hold catheter 7.5 to 10 cm (3 to 4 inches) from catheter tip with catheter loosely coiled in palm of hand. If catheter is not attached to drainage bag, make sure to position urine tray so end of catheter can be placed there once insertion begins.	Holding catheter near tip allows for its easier manipulation during insertion. Coiling catheter in palm prevents distal end from striking nonsterile surface.

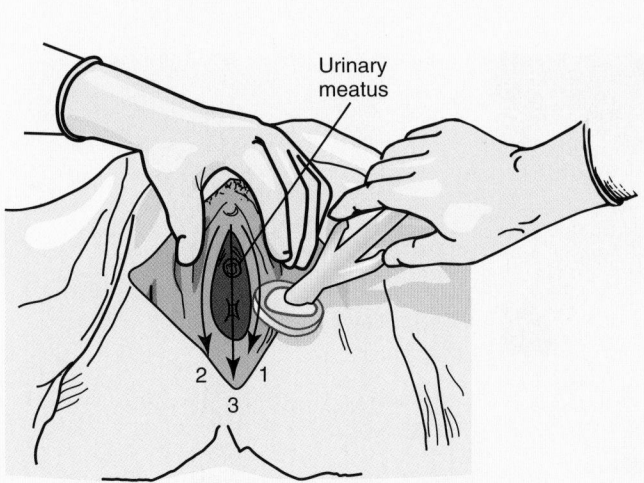

STEP 17a(3)   Cleaning female perineum.

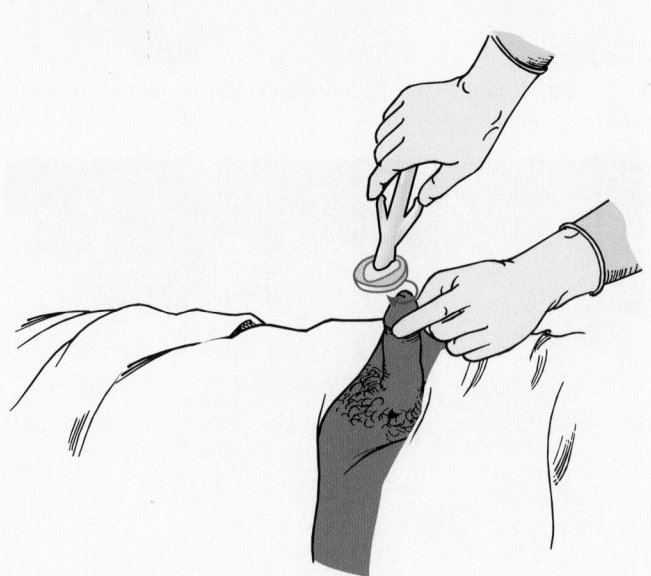

STEP 17b(3)   Cleaning male urinary meatus.

STEP	RATIONALE

19 Insert catheter:

a Female patient:

(1) Ask patient to bear down gently and slowly insert catheter through urethral meatus (see illustration).

Bearing down may help visualize urinary meatus and promotes relaxation of external urinary sphincter, aiding in catheter insertion.

(2) Advance catheter total of 5 to 7.5 cm (2 to 3 inches) or until urine flows out of catheter. When urine appears, advance catheter another 2.5 to 5 cm (1 to 2 inches). Do not use force to insert catheter.

Urine flow indicates that catheter tip is in bladder or lower urethra.

(3) Release labia and hold catheter securely with nondominant hand.

Clinical Decision Point *If no urine appears, catheter may be in vagina. If misplaced, leave catheter in vagina as landmark indicating where not to insert and insert another sterile catheter.*

b Male patient:

(1) Lift penis to a position perpendicular (90 degrees) to patient's body and apply gentle upward traction (see illustration).

Straightens urethra to ease catheter insertion.

(2) Ask patient to bear down as if to void and slowly insert catheter through urethral meatus.

Relaxation of external sphincter aids in insertion of catheter.

(3) Advance catheter 17 to 22.5 cm (7 to 9 inches) *or until urine flows out end of catheter.*

There are variations in length of male urethra. Flow of urine indicates that tip of catheter is in bladder or urethra but not necessarily that the balloon portion of an indwelling catheter is in bladder.

(4) Stop advancing with a straight catheter. When urine appears in an indwelling catheter, advance it to bifurcation (inflation and deflation ports exposed) (see illustration).

Further advancement of catheter to bifurcation of drainage and balloon inflation port ensures that balloon portion of catheter is not still in prostatic urethra (D'Cruz et al., 2009; Méndez-Probst et al., 2012; Newman and Wein, 2009).

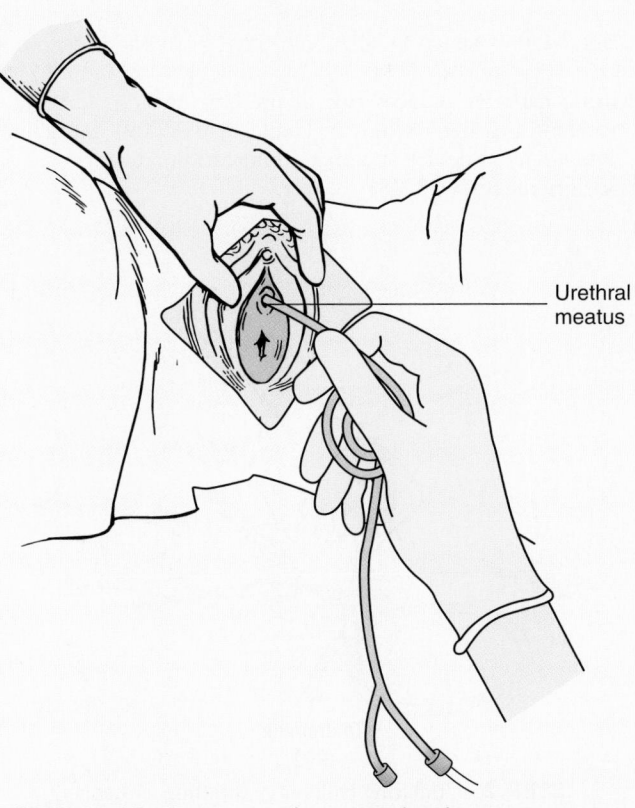

Urethral meatus

STEP 19a(1) Inserting catheter into female urinary meatus.

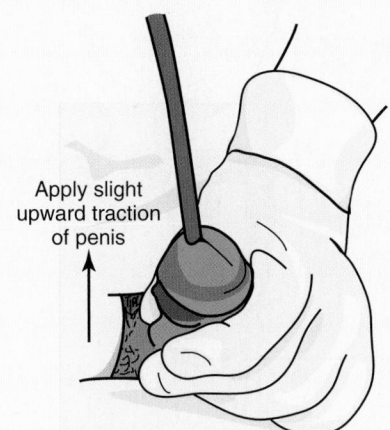

Apply slight upward traction of penis

STEP 19b(1) Inserting catheter into male urinary meatus.

STEP	RATIONALE

Clinical Decision Point *If there is resistance or pain when advancing the catheter in a male, do not use force and stop catheter advancement. Ask patient to take slow, deep breaths to promote relaxation. Hold catheter gently in place without forcing. After a few seconds the sphincter may relax, and the catheter can be advanced. An inability to advance a catheter may mean an enlarged prostate or some other obstruction of the urethra.*

STEP	RATIONALE
(5) Lower penis and hold catheter securely in nondominant hand.	Prevents accidental dislodgement of catheter.
20 Allow bladder to empty fully unless agency policy restricts maximum volume of urine drained (see agency policy).	There is no definitive evidence regarding whether there is benefit in limiting maximal volume drained.
21 Collect urine specimen as needed (see Chapter 43). Fill specimen container to 20 to 30 mL by holding end of catheter over cup.	Sterile specimen for culture analysis can be obtained.
a Label and bag specimen according to agency policy. Label specimen in front of patient (TJC, 2012). Send to laboratory as soon as possible.	Fresh urine specimen ensures more accurate findings. Labeling ensures that diagnostic results will be connected to correct patient.
22 Straight catheterization: When urine stops flowing, withdraw catheter slowly and smoothly until removed.	Minimizes trauma to urethra.
23 Inflate catheter balloon with amount of fluid designated by manufacturer.	Indwelling catheter balloons should not be underinflated. Underinflation causes balloon distortion and potential bladder damage (Newman and Wein, 2009).
a Continue to hold catheter with nondominant hand.	Holding on to catheter before inflating balloon prevents expulsion of catheter from urethra.
b With free dominant hand, connect prefilled syringe to injection port at end of catheter.	
c Slowly inject total amount of solution (see illustration).	

Clinical Decision Point *If patient complains of sudden pain during inflation of a catheter balloon or resistance is felt when inflating the balloon, stop inflation, allow the fluid from the balloon to flow back into the syringe, advance catheter further, and reinflate balloon. The balloon may have been inflating in the urethra. If pain continues, remove catheter and notify health care provider.*

STEP	RATIONALE
d After inflating catheter balloon, release catheter from nondominant hand. *Gently* pull catheter until resistance is felt. Then advance catheter slightly.	By moving catheter slightly back into bladder, pressure on bladder neck is avoided.
e Connect drainage tubing to catheter if it is not already preconnected.	
24 Secure indwelling catheter with catheter strap or other securement device. Leave enough slack to allow leg movement. Attach securement device at tubing just above catheter bifurcation.	Securing catheter reduces risk of urethral erosion, CAUTI, or accidental catheter removal (Gould et al., 2009). Attachment of securement device at catheter bifurcation prevents occlusion of catheter (Gray, 2008).

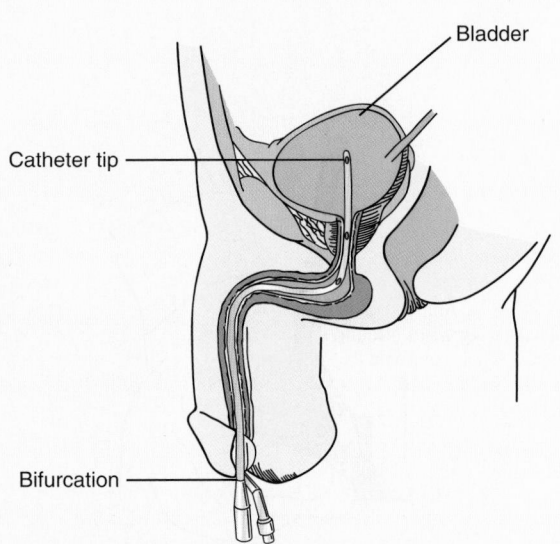

STEP 19b(4) Male anatomy with correct catheter insertion to bifurcation.

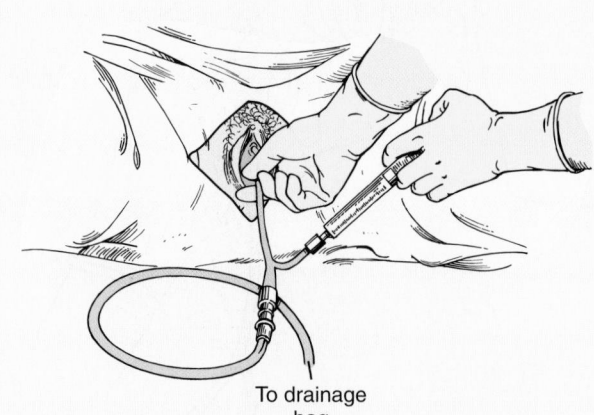

STEP 23 Inflating balloon (indwelling catheter).

STEP	RATIONALE

a Female patient:
Secure catheter tubing to inner thigh, allowing enough slack to prevent tension (see illustration).

b Male patient:

(1) Secure catheter tubing to upper thigh (see illustration) or lower abdomen (with penis directed toward chest). Allow slack in catheter so movement does not create tension on catheter.

Anchoring catheter reduces traction on urethra and minimizes urethral injury (Stoller, 2008).

(2) If retracted, replace foreskin over glans penis.

Leaving foreskin retracted can cause discomfort and dangerous edema.

25 Clip drainage tubing to edge of mattress. Position drainage bag lower than bladder by attaching to bed frame. Do not attach to side rails of bed (see illustration).

Drainage bags that are below level of bladder ensure free flow of urine, thus decreasing risk for CAUTI (Gould et al., 2009; Lo et al., 2008). Bags attached to movable objects such as a side rail increase risk for urethral trauma because of pulling or accidental dislodgement.

26 Check to make sure that there is no obstruction to urine flow. Coil excess tubing on bed and fasten to bottom sheet with clip or other securement device.

Obstruction to flow of urine increases risk for CAUTI (Gould et al., 2009; Lo et al., 2008).

27 Provide hygiene as needed. Help patient to comfortable position.

28 Dispose of supplies in appropriate receptacles.

29 Measure urine and record.

Provides baseline for urine output.

30 Remove gloves and perform hand hygiene.

Reduces transmission of infection.

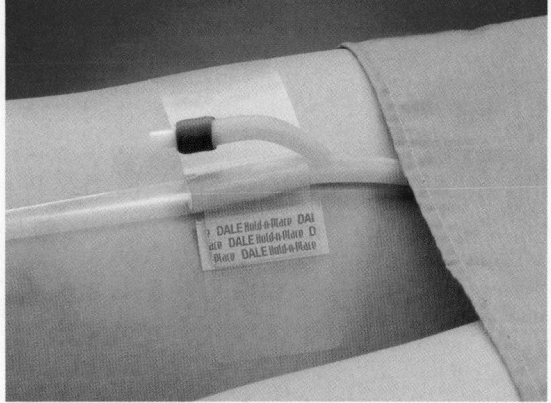

STEP 24a   Securing indwelling catheter on female with adhesive securement device.

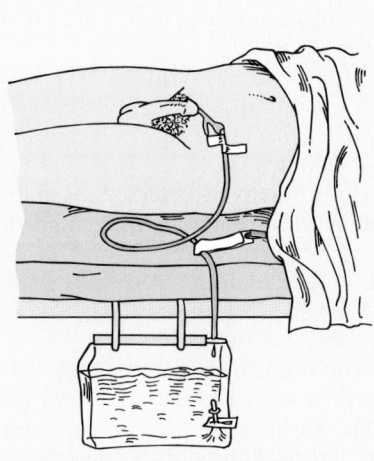

STEP 24b(1)   Securing indwelling catheter on male with tape.

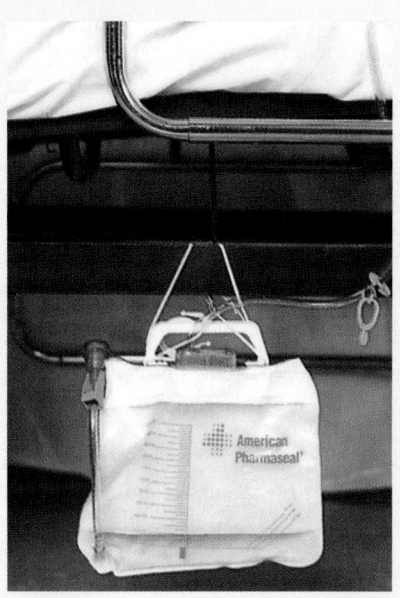

STEP 25   Drainage bag below level of bladder.

STEP	RATIONALE

EVALUATION

1 Palpate bladder for distention or use bladder scan.	Determines if distention is relieved.
2 Ask patient to describe level of comfort.	Determines if patient's sensation of discomfort or fullness has been relieved.
3 Indwelling catheter: Observe character and amount of urine in drainage system.	Determines if urine is flowing adequately.
4 Indwelling catheter: Determine that there is no urine leaking from catheter or tubing connections.	Prevents injury to patient's skin and ensures closed sterile system.

Unexpected Outcomes	Related Interventions
1 Catheter goes into vagina.	• Leave catheter in vagina.
	• Clean urinary meatus again. Using another catheter kit, reinsert sterile catheter into meatus (check agency policy). **NOTE:** If gloves become contaminated, start procedure over.
	• Remove catheter in vagina after successful insertion of second catheter.
2 Sterility is broken during catheterization by nurse or patient.	• Replace gloves if contaminated and start over.
	• If patient touches sterile field but equipment and supplies remain sterile, avoid touching that part of sterile field.
	• If equipment and/or supplies become contaminated, replace with sterile items or start over with new sterile kit.
3 Patient complains of bladder discomfort, and catheter is patent as evidenced by adequate urine flow.	• Check catheter to ensure that there is no traction on it.
	• Notify health care provider. Patient may be experiencing bladder spasms or symptoms of UTI.
	• Monitor catheter output for color, clarity, odor, and amount.

Recording and Reporting

- Record and report the reason for catheterization, type and size of catheter inserted, amount of fluid used to inflate balloon, specimen collection (if applicable), characteristics and amount of urine, patient's response to procedure, and any education in nurses' notes and electronic health record (EHR).
- Record amount of urine on intake and output (I&O) flow sheet record.
- Report persistent catheter-related pain, inadequate urine output, and discomfort to health care provider.

Special Considerations

Teaching

- Explain that a feeling of burning, pinching, and/or pressure may be experienced when the catheter is inserted into the urethra. This sensation is normal and will go away.
- Discuss with the patient routine care of the catheter and drainage system that includes avoiding any kinking in the drainage tubing, keeping the drainage bag dependent, avoiding pulling on the catheter, and daily hygiene.
- Explain that adequate fluid intake helps prevent catheter blockage.

Pediatric

- When caring for an infant or young child, explain procedures to parents. Describe procedure to child at level the child is able to understand (Hockenberry and Wilson, 2011).
- Children and adolescents will experience some discomfort during catheterization. Assistance and gentle holding may be necessary, especially with younger children. Most children prefer to have the parents remain with them during the procedure. Ask adolescents if they would like a parent to remain with them.
- Catheterization in infants and children may be made easier by use of an adequate amount of catheter lubricant containing 2% lidocaine (Xylocaine) (Hockenberry and Wilson, 2011).
- Teaching young children to blow into a straw or pinwheel can aid in relaxing pelvic muscles during catheter insertion (Hockenberry and Wilson, 2011).

Gerontologic

- The urethral meatus of an older woman may be difficult to identify because of urogenital atrophy.
- Symptoms of a UTI in an older adult may be difficult to recognize and may only be indicated by a change in mental status or fever (Smith et al., 2008).
- Older adults have an increased risk for UTI related to increased prevalence of chronic disease such as diabetes and prostatic hypertrophy and higher prevalence of incontinence (Robichard and Blondeau, 2008).
- The presence of a urinary catheter and its drainage tubing and bag can interfere with the already compromised mobility of the older adult.
- Catheter use in older adults has been associated with increased mortality (Srulevich and Chopra, 2008).

Home Care

- Patients who are at home may use a leg bag during the day and switch to a larger-volume bag at night. If a patient changes from a large-volume bag to a leg bag, instruct him or her in the importance of handwashing and cleaning the connection ports with alcohol before changing bags.

- Teach patients and/or caregivers how to properly position the drainage bag; empty the urinary drainage bag; and observe urine color, clarity, odor, and amount.
- Educate patients and/or caregivers about the signs of UTI and troubleshooting techniques for a leaking catheter.

- Arrange for home delivery of catheter supplies, always ensuring that there is at least one extra catheter, insertion kit, and drainage bag in the home.

SKILL 33-2 Care and Removal of an Indwelling Catheter

NSO *Urinary Catheterization Module / Lesson 5*

 Video Clip

Providing regular perineal hygiene, preventing catheter-related trauma, and removing indwelling catheters as soon as possible are important interventions to reduce risk of catheter-associated urinary tract infection (CAUTI) (Gould et al., 2009); Parker et al., 2009). Prolonged indwelling catheterization is a major risk factor for CAUTI. When removing an indwelling catheter, it is important to ensure that the catheter balloon is fully deflated to minimize trauma to the urethra. Often clinicians clamp catheter tubing before removal in the belief that the practice allows the bladder to fill and obtain bladder tone. However, evidence is unclear that the practice of clamping a catheter before removal will improve bladder function after removal (Gould et al., 2009; Nyman et al., 2010).

All patients should have their voiding monitored after catheter removal for at least 24 to 48 hours by using a voiding record or bladder diary. Record the time and amount of each voiding, including any incontinence, in the diary. Use a bladder scan to monitor bladder functioning by measuring postvoid residual (see Procedural Guideline 33-2). Abdominal pain and distention, a sensation of incomplete emptying, incontinence, constant dribbling of urine, and voiding in very small amounts can indicate inadequate bladder emptying requiring intervention.

The risk of urinary tract infection (UTI) increases with the use of an indwelling catheter (Parker et al., 2009). Symptoms of infection can develop 2 to 3 or more days after catheter removal. Inform patients of the risk for infection, prevention measures, and signs and symptoms that need to be reported to the primary care provider.

Delegation and Collaboration
The skill of performing routine catheter care can be delegated to nursing assistive personnel (NAP). The skill of removing an indwelling catheter can be delegated to NAP (see agency policy);

however, the nurse must first assess a patient's status and verify the order. The nurse directs the NAP to:

- Report characteristics of the urine (color, clarity, odor, and amount).
- Report the condition of the patient's genital area (e.g., color, rashes, open areas, odor, soiling from fecal incontinence, trauma to tissues around urinary meatus).
- Check size of balloon and syringe needed to deflate balloon and report if balloon does not deflate and if there is bleeding after removal.
- Report time and amount of first voiding after catheter is removed.
- Report patient complaints that might indicate a CAUTI: fever, chills, burning, flank pain, back pain, and blood in the urine (Hooton et al., 2010).
- Report patient complaints that might indicate a UTI after catheter removal: dysuria, hematuria, urgency, frequency, lower abdominal pain, change in mental status, lethargy (Hooton et al., 2010).

Equipment
Catheter Care
- ❏ Clean gloves
- ❏ Waterproof pad
- ❏ Bath blanket
- ❏ Soap, washcloth, towel, and basin filled with warm water

Removing a Catheter
- ❏ 10-mL or larger syringe without needle (Information on balloon size [mL] is printed directly on balloon inflation valve [see Fig. 33-3].)
- ❏ Graduated cylinder to measure urine
- ❏ Toilet, bedside commode, urine "hat," urinal, or bedpan
- ❏ Bladder scanner (if indicated)

STEP	RATIONALE

ASSESSMENT

1 Catheter care:

a Observe urinary output and urine characteristics.

Sudden decrease in urine output may indicate occlusion of catheter. Cloudy, foul-smelling urine associated with other systemic symptoms may indicate CAUTI.

b Assess for history or presence of bowel incontinence.

Most common bacteria to cause CAUTI are *Escherichia coli*, a major colonizer of the bowel; thus fecal incontinence increases risk for CAUTI (Gould et al., 2009; Jacobsen et al., 2008).

c Observe for any discharge, redness, bleeding, or presence of tissue trauma around urethral meatus (this may be deferred until catheter care).

Indicates inflammatory process, possible infection, or erosion of catheter through urethra.

d Assess patient's knowledge of catheter care.

Determine need for patient education related to catheter care.

STEP	RATIONALE
2 Catheter removal:	
a Review patient's medical record, including health care provider's order and nurses' notes. Note length of time catheter was in place.	Catheters in place for more than a few days cause higher risk for catheter encrustation and UTI (Jacobsen et al., 2008).
b Assess patient's knowledge and prior experience with catheter removal.	Reveals need for patient instruction and/or support.
c Assess urine color, clarity, odor, and amount. Note any urethral discharge, irritation of genital region, or trauma to urinary meatus (this may be deferred until just before removal).	May be an indicator of inflammation or UTI and a source of discomfort during catheter removal.
d Determine size of catheter inflation balloon by looking at balloon inflation valve.	Determines size of syringe needed to deflate balloon and amount of fluid expected in syringe after deflation.

NURSING DIAGNOSES

- Impaired urinary elimination
- Deficient knowledge related to catheter care
- Risk for infection

Related factors are individualized based on patient's condition or needs.

PLANNING

1 Expected outcomes following catheter care:	
• Genital area is free of secretions, fecal matter, and irritation.	Basic hygiene, especially after bowel movements, reduces risk for CAUTI (Gould et al., 2009).
• Patient verbalizes feeling of comfort.	Cleaning relieves local discomfort from irritation of catheter.
2 Expected outcomes after catheter removal:	
• Patient voids at least 150 mL with each voiding no more than 6 to 8 hours after removal.	Indicates return of voluntary bladder function without urinary retention.
• Patient verbalizes feeling of complete bladder emptying and absence of discomfort.	
• Patient identifies signs and symptoms of UTI.	Indicates patient learning.
3 Explain procedure to patient. Discuss signs and symptoms of UTI. If applicable, teach patient how to perform catheter hygiene.	Reduces anxiety and promotes cooperation. Self-care supports patient's sense of autonomy.

IMPLEMENTATION

1 Identify patient using two identifiers (i.e., name and birthday or name and account number) according to agency policy. Compare identifiers with information on patient's identification bracelet.	Ensures correct patient. Complies with The Joint Commission standards and improves patient safety (TJC, 2012).
2 Close room door and bedside curtain.	Provides patient privacy.
3 Perform hand hygiene.	Reduces transmission of microorganisms.
4 Raise bed to appropriate working height. If side rails are raised, lower side rail on working side.	Promotes use of proper body mechanics.
5 Organize equipment for perineal care and/or removal of catheter.	Increases efficiency of procedure.
6 Position patient with waterproof pad under buttocks and cover with bath blanket, exposing only genital area and catheter (see Skill 33-1).	Shows respect for patient dignity by only exposing genital area and catheter.
a Female in dorsal recumbent position.	
b Male in supine position.	
7 Apply clean gloves.	Reduces transmission of infection.
8 Remove catheter securement device while maintaining connection with drainage tubing.	Provides ability to easily clean around catheter or to remove it.
9 Catheter care:	
a *Female:* Use nondominant hand to gently separate labia to fully expose urethral meatus and catheter. Maintain position of hand throughout procedure.	Provides full visualization of urethral meatus. Full separation of labia prevents contamination of meatus during cleaning.
b *Male:* Use nondominant hand to retract foreskin if not circumcised and hold penis at shaft just below glans. Maintain hand position throughout procedure.	Retraction of foreskin provides full visualization of urethral meatus.

STEP	RATIONALE

Clinical Decision Point *Accidental closing of labia or dropping of penis during cleaning requires procedure to be repeated.*

c Grasp catheter with two fingers to stabilize it.

Prevents unnecessary traction on catheter.
Pulling on catheter is cause of discomfort for patient and can damage urethra and bladder neck.

d Assess urethral meatus and surrounding tissues for inflammation, swelling, discharge, or tissue trauma and ask patient if burning or discomfort is present.

Determines frequency and type of ongoing care required. Indicates possibility of CAUTI or catheter erosion through urethra.

e Provide perineal hygiene using mild soap and warm water (see Chapter 17).

Antiseptic cleaners have not been proven to decrease risk for CAUTI (Gould et al., 2009).

f Using clean washcloth, clean catheter.

(1) Starting close to urinary meatus, clean catheter in circular motion along its length for about 10 cm (4 inches), moving away from body (see illustration). Remove all traces of soap. *For male patients:* Reduce or reposition foreskin after care.

Reduces presence of secretions or drainage on outside catheter surface.

g Reapply catheter securement device. Allow slack in catheter so movement does not create tension on it.

Securing indwelling catheter reduces risk of urethral trauma, urethral erosion, CAUTI, or accidental removal (Cipa-Tatum et al., 2011; Gould et al., 2009).

10 Routinely check drainage tubing and bag.

a Catheter is secured to upper thigh (for women) or abdomen (for men).

Maintains unobstructed flow of urine out of bladder (Gould et al., 2009).

b Tubing is coiled and secured onto bed linen.

c Tubing is not looped or positioned above level of bladder.

d Tubing is not kinked or clamped.

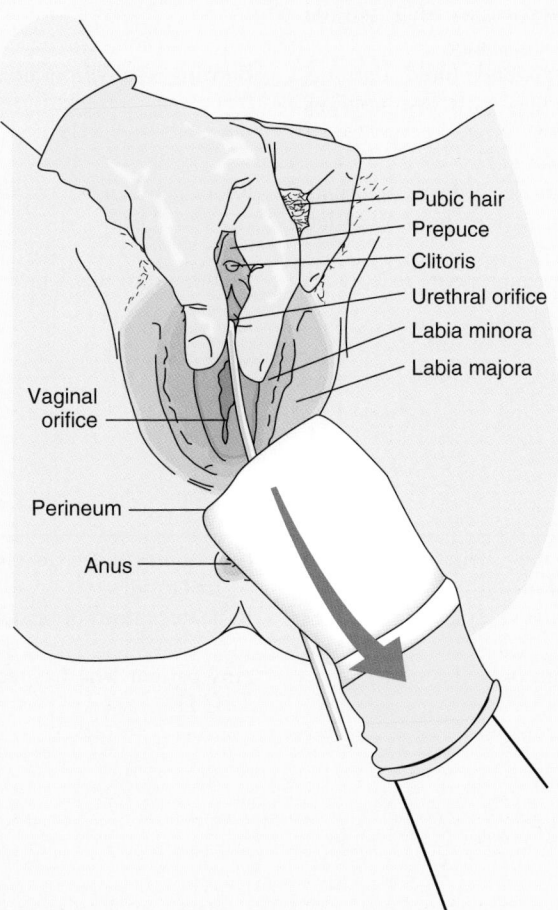

Pubic hair
Prepuce
Clitoris
Urethral orifice
Labia minora
Labia majora
Vaginal orifice
Perineum
Anus

STEP 9f(1) Catheter is cleaned starting at meatus and moving downward while holding it securely.

STEP	RATIONALE
e Drainage bag is positioned below level of bladder with urine flowing freely into bag.	
f Drainage bag is not overfull. Empty drainage bag when ½ full.	Overfull drainage bag creates tension and pulls on catheter, resulting in trauma to urethra and/or urinary meatus (Cipa-Tatum, 2011).
11 Catheter removal: (Follow Steps 1 to 10 before catheter removal.)	
a Move syringe plunger up and down to loosen and then pull back plunger to 0.5 mL. Insert hub of syringe into inflation valve (balloon port). Allow balloon fluid to drain into syringe by gravity. Syringe should fill. Make sure that entire amount of fluid is removed by comparing removed amount to volume needed for inflation.	Partially inflated balloon can traumatize urethral wall during removal. Passive drainage of catheter balloon prevents formation of ridges in balloon. These ridges can cause discomfort or trauma during removal.
b Pull catheter out smoothly and slowly. Examine it to ensure that it is whole. Catheter should slide out easily. Do not use force. If you note any resistance, repeat Step 11a to remove remaining water.	Nonwhole catheter means that pieces of catheter may still be in bladder. Notify health care provider immediately.
c Wrap contaminated catheter in waterproof pad. Unhook collection bag and drainage tubing from bed.	Promotes patient comfort and safety.
d Reposition patient as necessary. Provide hygiene as needed. Lower level of bed and position side rails accordingly.	Promotes patient comfort and safety.
e Empty, measure, and record urine present in drainage bag (see Chapter 6).	Documents urinary output.
f Encourage patient to maintain or increase fluid intake (unless contraindicated).	Maintains normal urine output.
g Initiate voiding record or bladder diary. Instruct patient to tell you when need to empty bladder occurs and that all urine needs to be measured. Make sure that patient understands how to use collection container.	Evaluates bladder function.
h Explain that many patients experience mild burning, discomfort, or small-volume voiding with first voiding, which soon subsides.	Burning results from urethral irritation.
i Inform patient to report any signs of UTI.	
j Ensure easy access to toilet, commode, bedpan, or urinal. Place urine "hat" on toilet seat if patient is using toilet. Place call bell within easy reach.	Reduces incidence of falls during toileting. Urine hat collects first voided urine.
12 Dispose of all contaminated supplies in appropriate receptacle, remove gloves, and perform hand hygiene.	Reduces transmission of microorganisms.

EVALUATION

1 Inspect catheter and genital area for soiling, irritation, and skin breakdown. Ask patient about discomfort.	Determines if area is cleaned properly and/or if patient has any irritation.
2 Observe time and measure amount of first voiding after catheter removal.	Indicates return of bladder function after catheter removal.
3 Evaluate patient for signs and symptoms of UTI.	Any patient who has recently had catheter removed is at risk for UTI.

Unexpected Outcomes

1 Water from inflation balloon does not return into syringe.

2 Patient has fever, chills, burning, flank pain, back pain, hematuria, painful urination, urgency, frequency, lower abdominal pain, change in mental status, and lethargy (Hooton et al., 2010).

3 Patient is unable to void after catheter removal, has sensation of not emptying, strains to void, or experiences small voiding amounts with increasing frequency.

Related Interventions

- Reposition patient; ensure that catheter is not pinched or kinked.
- Remove syringe. Attach new syringe and allow enough time for passive emptying.
- Attempt to empty balloon by gently pulling back on syringe plunger.
- If catheter balloon does not deflate, *do not* cut balloon inflation valve to drain water. Notify health care provider.

- Assess for bladder distention and tenderness.
- Monitor vital signs and urine output.
- Report findings to health care provider; signs and symptoms may indicate UTI.

- Assess for bladder distention.
- Help to normal position for voiding and provide privacy.
- Perform bladder ultrasound (see Procedural Guideline 33-2) to assess for excessive urine volume in bladder.
- If patient is unable to void within 6 to 8 hours of catheter removal and/or experiences abdominal pain, notify health care provider.

Recording and Reporting

- Record time for catheter care and appearance of urine; describe condition of meatus and catheter.
- Record and report time of catheter removal, amount of water removed from balloon, condition of urethral meatus and catheter, and the time, amount, and characteristics of first voided urine.
- Record teaching related to catheter care, catheter removal, and fluid intake.
- Report hematuria, dysuria, inability or difficulty voiding, and any new incontinence after a catheter is removed.

Special Considerations
Teaching

- Unless contraindicated, patients with a catheter should drink at least 2200 mL of fluid per day to promote continuous flushing of the bladder and prevent sediment from collecting in the catheter tubing.

- Instruct patient to hold collection bag below the level of the bladder when ambulating.
- Instruct patient not to disconnect the catheter from the collection tubing and bag.

Pediatric

- During catheter removal do not force catheter out of bladder if you meet resistance. When excessive tubing has been inserted in bladder, there have been occurrences of knotting of the tube (Hockenberry and Wilson, 2011).

Gerontologic

- Older adults may exhibit atypical signs and symptoms of CAUTI such as a change in mental status attributed to delirium. A change in mental status may include confusion, agitation, and/or lethargy.

Home Care

- Assess patient and primary caregiver for ability and motivation to participate in routine catheter care.

PROCEDURAL GUIDELINE 33-2 Bladder Scan and Catheterization to Determine Residual Urine

A bladder scanner (Fig. 33-5) is a noninvasive device that creates an ultrasound image of the bladder for measuring the volume of urine in the bladder. The device makes calculations to report accurate urine volumes, especially lower volumes (Al-Shaikh et al., 2009). Use a bladder scanner to assess bladder volume whenever inadequate bladder emptying is suspected such as after the removal of indwelling urinary catheters, in the evaluation of new-onset incontinence, and after urologic surgery. The most common use for the bladder scan is to measure postvoid residual (PVR), the volume of urine in the bladder after a normal voiding. To obtain the most reliable reading, measure PVR within 10 minutes of voiding (Newman and Wein, 2009). A volume less than 50 mL is considered normal. Two or more PVR measurements greater than 100 mL require further investigation (Newman and Wein, 2009). If a bladder scanner is not available, obtain a PVR by measuring urine emptied from the bladder after a straight catheterization.

first determine the timing and frequency of the bladder scan measurement and interpret the measurements obtained. The nurse also assesses the patient's ability to toilet before measuring PVR and the abdomen for distention if urinary retention is suspected. The nurse directs the NAP to:

- Follow manufacturer recommendations for the use of the device.
- Measure PVR volumes 10 minutes after helping the patient to void.
- Report and record bladder scan volumes.

Equipment

❏ Bladder scanner (follow manufacturer instructions for use)
❏ Ultrasound gel
❏ Cleaning agent for scanner head, such as an alcohol pad
❏ Urethral catheterization tray with single-use catheter for straight/intermittent catheterization (see Skill 33-1)

Delegation and Collaboration

The skill of measuring bladder volume by bladder scan can be delegated to nursing assistive personnel (NAP). The nurse must

Procedural Steps

1 Identify patient using two identifiers (i.e., name and birthday or name and account number) according to agency policy.

Continued

PROCEDURAL GUIDELINE 33-2   Bladder Scan and Catheterization to Determine Residual Urine—cont'd

Compare identifiers with information on patient's identification bracelet.

2 Assess intake and output (I&O) record to determine urine output trends and check the plan of care to verify correct timing of the bladder scan measurement.

3 Perform hand hygiene and apply clean gloves.

4 Provide privacy by closing room door and bedside curtain.

5 Discuss procedure with patient. If the measurement is for PVR, ask patient to void and measure voided urine volume. Measurement should be within 10 minutes of voiding.

6 Measurement of PVR with the bladder scan

   a Help patient to supine position with head slightly elevated. Raise bed to appropriate working height. If side rails are raised, lower side rail on working side.

   b Expose patient's lower abdomen.

   c Turn on scanner per manufacturer guidelines.

   d Set gender designation per manufacturer guidelines. Women who have had a hysterectomy should be designated as male.

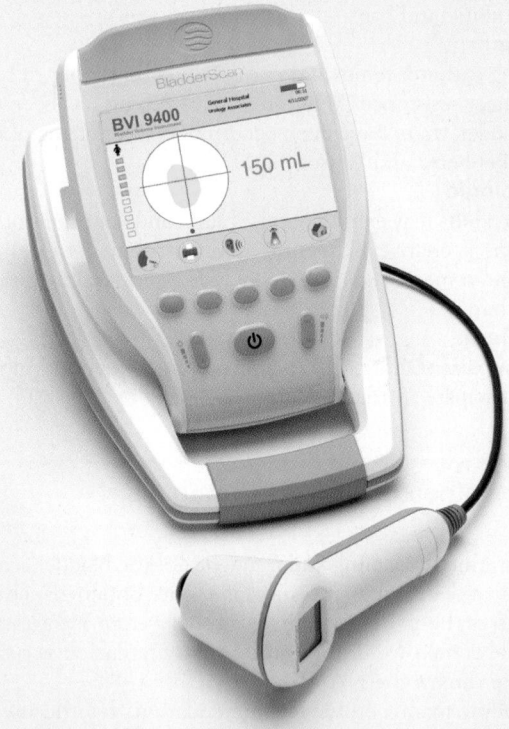

FIG 33-5   Bladder scanner with image.

e Wipe scanner head with alcohol pad or other cleaner and allow to air dry.

f Palpate patient's symphysis pubis (pubic bone). Apply generous amount of ultrasound gel (or if available a bladder scan gel pad) to midline abdomen 2.5 to 4 cm (1 to 1.5 inches) above symphysis pubis.

g Place scanner head on gel, ensuring that scanner head is oriented per manufacturer guidelines.

h Apply light pressure, keep scanner head steady, and point it slightly downward toward bladder. Press and release the scan button (see illustration).

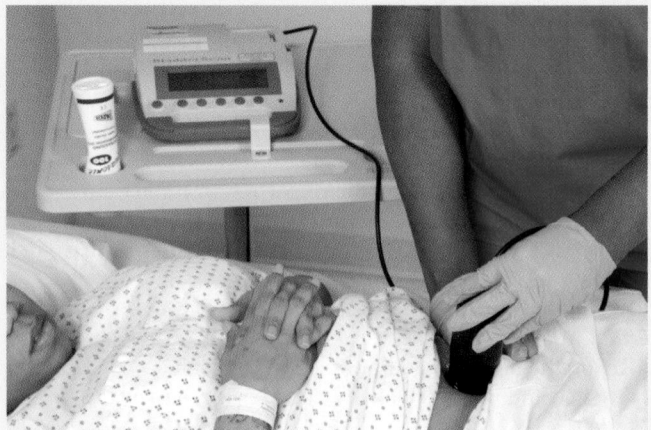

STEP 6h   Placement of bladder scan head.

i Verify accurate aim (refer to manufacturer guidelines). Complete scan and print image (if needed).

j Remove ultrasound gel from patient's abdomen with paper towel.

k Remove ultrasound get from scanner head and wipe with alcohol pad or other cleaner; allow to air-dry.

l Help patient to comfortable position. Lower bed and replace side rails accordingly.

m Remove gloves and perform hand hygiene.

7 Measurement of PVR using straight/intermittent catheterization (see Skill 33-1).

8 Review health care provider's order to determine how often to assess residual urine.

9 Review I&O record to determine urine output trends.

SKILL 33-3   Performing Catheter Irrigation

Urinary catheter irrigations are performed on an intermittent or a continuous basis to maintain catheter patency. There are two types of irrigation: closed catheter irrigation and open irrigation. Closed catheter irrigation provides intermittent or continuous irrigation of a urinary catheter without disrupting the sterile connection between the catheter and the drainage system (Fig. 33-6). Intermittent irrigation involves insertion of a sterile catheter into a catheter port to irrigate a bolus of fluid. Continuous bladder

irrigation (CBI) is a continuous infusion of a sterile solution into the bladder, usually using a three-way irrigation system with a triple-lumen catheter. It is often used after genitourinary surgery to keep the bladder clear and free of blood clots or sediment.

Open catheter irrigation is used only when intermittent irrigation of the catheter and bladder is required. The skill involves breaking or opening the closed drainage system at the connection between the catheter and the drainage system. **This procedure**

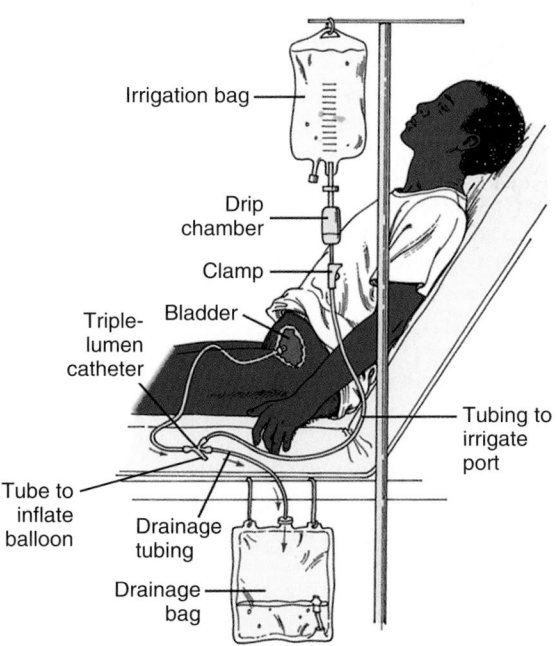

FIG 33-6 Closed continuous bladder irrigation.

should be avoided unless irrigation is needed to relieve or prevent obstruction (Senese et al., 2005). Strict asepsis is required throughout the procedure to minimize contamination and subsequent development of a urinary tract infection (UTI). Both open and closed irrigation can be used to irrigate the bladder with medication.

Delegation and Collaboration

The skill of catheter irrigation cannot be delegated to nursing assistive personnel (NAP). The nurse directs the NAP to:

- Report if the patient complains of pain, discomfort, or leakage of fluid around the catheter.
- Monitor and record intake and output (I&O); report immediately any decrease in urine output.
- Report any change in the color of the urine, especially the presence of blood clots.

Equipment

❑ Sterile irrigation solution at room temperature (as prescribed)
❑ Antiseptic swabs
❑ Clean gloves

Closed Intermittent Irrigation
❑ Sterile container
❑ Sterile 30- to 60-mL irrigation syringe (piston type)
❑ Syringe to access system (Luer-Lok syringe without needle for needleless access port per manufacturer directions)
❑ Screw clamp or rubber band (used to temporarily occlude catheter as irrigant is instilled)

Closed Continuous Irrigation
❑ Irrigation tubing with clamp to regulate irrigation flow rate
❑ Y-connector (optional) to connect irrigation tubing to double-lumen catheter
❑ Intravenous (IV) pole (closed continuous or intermittent)

Open Intermittent Irrigation
❑ Disposable sterile irrigation kit that contains solution container, collection basin, drape, sterile gloves, 30- to 60-mL irrigation syringe (piston type)
❑ Sterile catheter plug
❑ Sterile gloves *(optional)*

STEP	RATIONALE

ASSESSMENT

1 Verify in medical record:
   a Order for irrigation method (continuous or intermittent), type (sterile saline or medicated solution), and amount of irrigant.

   b Type of catheter in place (see Fig. 33-2).

Health care provider's order is required to initiate therapy. Frequency and volume of solution used for irrigation may be in the order or standardized as part of agency policy.

Single- and double-lumen catheters are used with open irrigation. Triple-lumen catheters are used for both intermittent and continuous closed irrigation.

2 Palpate bladder for distention and tenderness.

Bladder distention indicates that flow of urine may be blocked from draining.

3 Assess patient for abdominal pain or spasms, sensation of bladder fullness or catheter bypassing (leaking).

May indicate overdistention of bladder caused by catheter blockage. Offers baseline to determine if therapy is successful.

4 Observe urine for color, amount, clarity, and presence of mucus, clots, or sediment.

Indicates if patient is bleeding or sloughing tissue, which would require increased irrigation rate or frequency of catheter irrigation.

5 Monitor I&O. If CBI is being used, amount of fluid draining from bladder should exceed amount of fluid infused into bladder.

If output does not exceed irrigant infused, catheter obstruction (i.e., blood clots, kinked tubing) should be suspected, irrigation stopped, and prescriber notified (Lewis et al., 2011).

6 Assess patient's knowledge regarding purpose of performing catheter irrigation.

Reveals need for patient instruction/support.

NURSING DIAGNOSES

- Acute pain
- Impaired urinary elimination
- Deficient knowledge regarding catheter irrigation
- Risk for infection

Related factors are individualized based on patient's condition or needs.

STEP	RATIONALE

PLANNING

1 Expected outcomes following completion of this procedure:

- With CBI: Urine output is greater than volume of irrigating solution instilled.

Indicates patency of drainage system, allowing for drainage of urine and irrigating solution.

- Patient reports relief of bladder pain or spasms.

Indicates bladder emptying.

- Urine output has decreased with an absence of blood clots and sediment. (NOTE: Urine will be bloody following bladder/urethral surgery, gradually becoming lighter and blood tinged in 2 to 3 days.)

Indicates that catheter is at decreased risk for occlusion with blood clots.

- Absence of fever, lower abdominal pain, cloudy and/or foul-smelling urine.

Signs of UTI are not present.

- Patient can explain purpose of procedure and what to expect.

Demonstrates learning.

2 Explain procedure to patient.

Reduces anxiety and promotes cooperation.

IMPLEMENTATION

1 Identify patient using two identifiers (i.e., name and birthday or name and account number) according to agency policy. Compare identifiers in MAR/medical record with information on patient's identification bracelet and/or ask patient to state name.

Ensures correct patient. Complies with The Joint Commission standards and improves patient safety (TJC, 2012).

2 Perform hand hygiene.

Reduces transmission of microorganisms.

3 Provide privacy by closing room door and bedside curtain.

Protects patient comfort and self-esteem.

4 Raise bed to appropriate working height. If side rails are raised, lower side rail on working side.

Promotes use of good body mechanics.

Position provides access to catheter and promotes patient dignity as much as possible.

5 Position patient supine and expose catheter junctions (catheter and drainage tubing).

Position provides access to catheter and promotes patient dignity as much as possible.

6 Remove catheter securement device.

Eases access to catheter parts.

7 Organize supplies according to type of irrigation prescribed. Apply clean gloves.

Ensures an efficient procedure.

8 **Closed continuous irrigation:**

a Close clamp on new irrigation tubing and hang bag of irrigating solution on IV pole. Insert (spike) tip of sterile irrigation tubing into designated port of irrigation solution bag using aseptic technique (see illustration).

Prevents air from entering tubing. Air can cause bladder spasms. Technique prevents transmission of microorganisms.

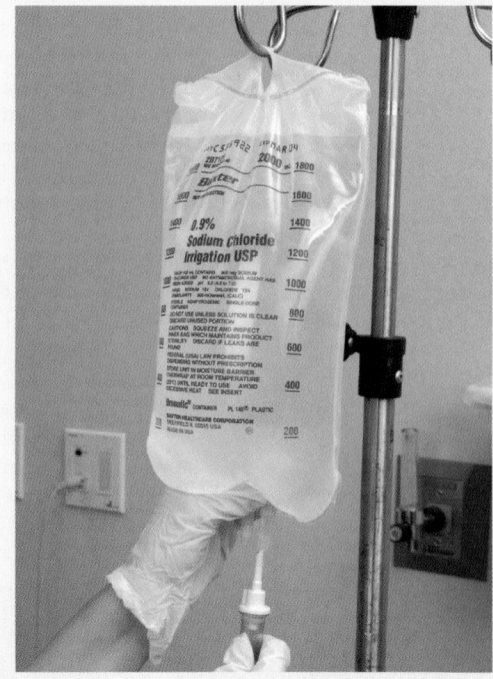

STEP 8a Spiking bag of sterile irrigation solution for continuous bladder irrigation.

STEP	RATIONALE
b Fill drip chamber half full by squeezing chamber; then open clamp and allow solution to flow (prime) through tubing, keeping end of tubing sterile. Once fluid has completely filled tubing, close clamp and recap end of tubing.	Priming tubing with fluid prevents introduction of air into bladder.
c Using aseptic technique, connect tubing securely to drainage port of Y-connector on double/triple–lumen catheter.	Reduces transmission of microorganisms.
d Adjust clamp on irrigation tubing to begin flow of solution into bladder. If set volume rate is ordered, calculate drip rate and adjust rate at roller clamp. If urine is bright red or has clots, increase irrigation rate until drainage appears pink (according to ordered rate or agency protocol).	Continuous drainage is expected. It helps to prevent clotting in presence of active bleeding in bladder and flushes clots out of bladder.
e Observe for outflow of fluid into drainage bag. Empty catheter drainage bag as needed.	Discomfort, bladder distention, and possible injury can occur from overdistention of bladder when bladder irrigant cannot adequately flow from bladder. Bag will fill rapidly and may need to be emptied every 1 to 2 hours.
9 Closed intermittent irrigation:	Fluid is instilled through catheter in a bolus, flushing system. Fluid drains out after irrigation is complete.
a Pour prescribed sterile irrigation solution into sterile container.	
b Draw prescribed volume of irrigant (usually 30 to 50 mL) into syringe using aseptic technique. Place sterile cap on tip of needleless syringe.	Ensures sterility of irrigating fluid.
c Clamp catheter tubing below soft injection port with screw clamp (or fold catheter tubing onto itself and secure with rubber band).	Occluding catheter tubing below point of injection allows irrigating solution to enter catheter and flow upward toward bladder.
d Using circular motion, clean catheter port (specimen port) with antiseptic swab.	Reduces transmission of microorganisms.
e Insert tip of needleless syringe using twisting motion into port.	Ensures that catheter tip enters lumen of catheter.
f Inject solution using slow, even pressure.	Gentle instillation of solution minimizes trauma to bladder mucosa.
g Remove syringe and remove clamp (or rubber band) allowing solution to drain into urinary drainage bag. (NOTE: Some medicated irrigants may need to dwell in bladder for prescribed period, requiring catheter to be clamped temporarily before being allowed to drain.)	Allows drainage to flow out by gravity. Medications must be instilled long enough to be absorbed by lining of bladder. Clamped drainage tubing and bag should not be left unattended.
10 Open intermittent irrigation:	
a Sterile gloves may be required (see agency policy).	Prevents introduction of microorganisms into urinary catheter and drainage system.
b Open sterile irrigation tray. Establish sterile field (see Chapter 8) and pour required amount of sterile solution into sterile solution container. Replace cap on large container of solution. Add sterile irrigation syringe (piston type) to sterile field. Have antiseptic wipe open and ready for use.	Maintains sterile field.
c Position sterile drape under catheter.	Creates sterile field on which to work and prevents soiling of bed linen.
d Aspirate prescribed volume of irrigation solution into irrigating syringe (usually 30 mL). Place syringe in sterile solution container until ready to use.	Prepares solution for instillation into catheter. Maintains sterility of irrigating syringe.
e Move sterile collection basin close to patient's thigh.	Prevents soiling of bed linen and reaching over sterile field.
f Wipe connection point between catheter and drainage tubing with antiseptic wipe before disconnecting.	Reduces transmission of microorganisms.
g Disconnect catheter from drainage tubing, allowing any urine to flow into sterile collection basin. Cover open end of drainage tubing with sterile protective cap and position tubing so it stays coiled on top of bed with end resting on sterile drape.	Maintains sterility of inner aspects of catheter lumen and drainage tubing. Reduces potential of infection by way of microorganism contamination.
h Insert tip of syringe into lumen of catheter and gently push plunger to instill solution (see illustration).	Gentle fluid instillation minimizes risk of trauma to bladder.

STEP	RATIONALE

Clinical Decision Point *When irrigating a catheter using the open method, do not force the irrigation. Catheter may be completely occluded and needs to be changed.*

i Remove syringe, lower catheter, and allow solution to drain into collection basin. Amount of drainage solution should be equal to or greater than amount instilled. If ordered, repeat sequence of instilling solution and draining until drainage is clear of clots and sediment.	If clot has been removed, solution will drain freely into basin.
j After irrigation is complete, remove protector cap from urinary drainage tubing end, clean end of tubing with antiseptic wipe, and reinsert into lumen of catheter.	Restores sterile system.
11 Anchor catheter with catheter securement device (see Skill 33-1).	Prevents trauma to urethral tissue caused by pulling catheter.
12 Help patient to safe and comfortable position. Lower bed and place side rails accordingly.	Promotes patient comfort and safety.
13 Dispose of all contaminated supplies in appropriate receptacle, remove gloves, and perform hand hygiene.	Reduces transmission of microorganisms.

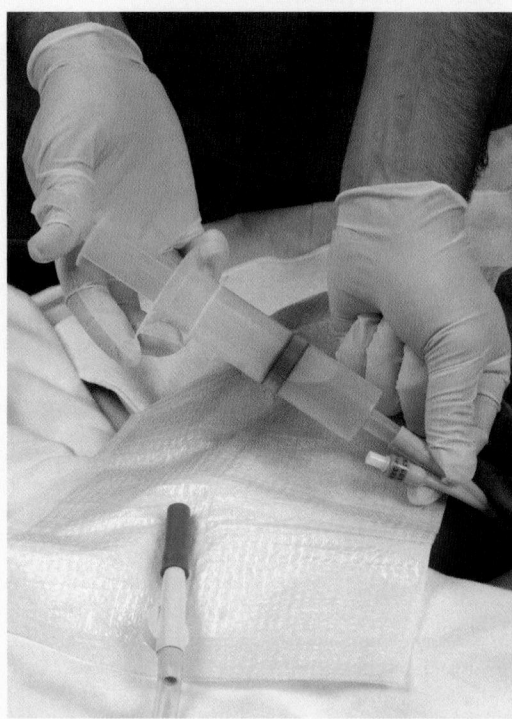

STEP 10h Gentle instillation of sterile irrigation solution.

EVALUATION

1 Measure actual urine output by subtracting total amount of irrigation fluid infused from total volume drained into basin.	Determines accurate urinary output.
2 Review I&O flow sheet to verify that hourly output into drainage bag is in appropriate proportion to irrigating solution entering bladder. Expect more output than fluid instilled because of urine production.	Determines urinary output in relation to irrigation.
3 Inspect urine for blood clots and sediment and be sure that tubing is not kinked or occluded.	Decrease in blood clots means that therapy is successful in maintaining catheter patency. System is patent.
4 Evaluate patient's comfort level.	Indicates catheter patency by absence of symptoms of bladder distention.
5 Monitor for signs and symptoms of infection.	Patients with indwelling catheters remain at risk for infection.

Unexpected Outcomes

1 Irrigating solution does not return (intermittent irrigation) or is not flowing at prescribed rate (CBI).

2 Drainage output is less than amount of irrigation solution infused.

3 Bright-red bleeding with the irrigation (CBI) infusion wide open.

4 Patient experiences pain with irrigation.

5 Fever; cloudy, foul-smelling urine; abdominal pain; change in mental status, indicating a possible infection.

Related Interventions

- Examine tubing for clots, sediment, and kinks.
- Notify health care provider if irrigant does not flow freely from bladder, patient complains of pain, or bladder distention occurs.

- Examine drainage tubing for clots, sediment, or kinks.
- Inspect urine for presence of or increase in blood clots and sediment.
- Evaluate patient for pain and distended bladder.
- Notify health care provider.

- Assess for hypovolemic shock (vital signs, skin color and moisture, anxiety level).
- Leave irrigation infusion wide open and notify health care provider.

- Examine drainage tubing for clots, sediment, or kinks.
- Evaluate urine for presence of or increase in blood clots and sediment.
- Evaluate for distended bladder.
- Notify health care provider.

- Notify health care provider.
- Monitor vital signs and character of urine.

Recording and Reporting

- Record irrigation method, amount of and type of irrigation solution, amount returned as drainage, characteristics of output, urine output, and patient tolerance to procedure in nurses' notes.
- Report catheter occlusion, sudden bleeding, infection, or increased pain to health care provider.
- Record I&O on appropriate flow sheet.

Special Considerations

Teaching

- Instruct patient and family caregiver to observe urine daily for changes in color, presence of mucus or blood, and odor.
- Inform patients that bleeding is common after many urologic procedures and to expect bright red-tinged urine during the first

48 hours after surgery, followed by a change in urine ranging from pink-tinged to clear.
- Instruct patient to maintain adequate oral intake of 2 L/day (unless contraindicated).

Home Care

- Patients and/or caregivers can be taught to perform catheter irrigations with adequate support, demonstration/return demonstration, and written instructions.
- Teach patients and/or caregivers to observe urine color, clarity, odor, and amount.
- Arrange for home delivery and storage of catheter/irrigation supplies.
- Teach patients and/or caregivers signs of catheter obstruction or UTI.

SKILL 33-4 Applying a Condom-Type External Catheter

NSO *Urinary Catheterization Module / Lesson 3*

The external urinary catheter, also called a *condom catheter* or *penile sheath*, is a soft, pliable condom-like sheath that fits over the penis, providing a safe and noninvasive way to contain urine. Most external catheters are made of soft silicone that reduces friction. The silicone is clear, allowing for easy visualization of skin under the catheter. Latex catheters are still available and used by some patients. It is important to verify that a patient does not have a latex allergy before applying this type of catheter.

Condom-type external catheters are held in place by either an adhesive coating of the internal lining of the sheath, a double-sided self-adhesive strip, brush-on adhesive applied to the penile shaft, or in rare cases an external strap. The catheter may be attached to a small-volume (leg) drainage bag or a large-volume (bedside) urinary drainage bag, both of which need to be kept lower than the level of the bladder. The condom-type external catheter is suitable for incontinent patients who have complete and spontaneous bladder emptying. The catheters come in a variety of styles and sizes. For the best fit and correct application it is important to refer to manufacturer guidelines. Condom-type external catheters are

associated with less risk for urinary tract infection (UTI) than indwelling catheters; thus they are an excellent option for the male with urinary incontinence (Newman and Wein, 2009). Other externally applied catheters are available for men who cannot be fitted for a condom-type external catheter. One type attaches to the glans penis using hydrocolloid strips (Wells, 2008) that stay in place for multiple days and allows straight catheterization. Another option available is a reusable condom-like device that is held in place by specially designed underwear.

Delegation and Collaboration

Assessment of the skin of a patient's penile shaft and determination of a latex allergy are done by a nurse before catheter application. The skill of applying a condom catheter can be delegated to nursing assistive personnel (NAP). The nurse directs the NAP to:

- Follow manufacturer directions for applying the condom catheter and securing device.
- Monitor urine intake and output (I&O) and record if applicable.
- Immediately report any redness, swelling, or skin irritation or breakdown of glans penis or penile shaft.

Equipment

- ❑ Condom catheter kit (condom sheath of appropriate size, securement device [internal adhesive or strap], skin preparation solution [per manufacturer directions])
- ❑ Urinary collection bag with drainage tubing or leg bag and straps
- ❑ Basin with warm water and soap
- ❑ Towels and washcloth(s)
- ❑ Bath blanket
- ❑ Clean gloves
- ❑ Scissors, hair guard, or paper towel

STEP	RATIONALE

ASSESSMENT

1 Assess urinary pattern, ability to empty bladder effectively, and degree of urinary continence.

2 Assess skin of penis for rashes, erythema, and/or open areas. (This may be deferred until just before catheter application.)

3 Assess patient's mental status, knowledge of purpose of using condom-type catheter, and ability to apply device. It may be appropriate to include family members in assessment.

4 Verify patient's size and type of condom catheter on plan of care or use manufacturer measuring guide to measure length and diameter of penis in flaccid state.

Incontinent patients are at risk for skin breakdown and thus candidates for condom catheter.

Provides baseline to compare changes in condition of skin after application of condom catheter. **Condom catheters can be applied only to intact skin** (Newman and Wein, 2009).

Identifies patient learning needs and if self-application can be taught or if family member needs to be included in instruction.

Identifies proper size of catheter needed. Penile shaft should be at least 2 cm (5 inches) in length to ensure successful application. If too small, condom catheter may fall off and compress urethra, stopping urine flow or causing local tissue trauma; if too big the catheter may leak or fall off (Kyle, 2011).

NURSING DIAGNOSES

- Deficient knowledge regarding catheter application
- Risk for impaired skin integrity
- Stress urinary incontinence (male)
- Total urinary incontinence

Related factors are individualized based on patient's condition or needs.

PLANNING

1 Expected outcomes following completion of procedure:
- Patient's skin is free from urine wetness.
- Glans and penile shaft are free of skin irritation or breakdown.
- Patient explains purpose of procedure and what to expect.

2 Explain procedure to patient.

Catheter is applied correctly.
Catheter is secure and not too tight.
Helps to minimize anxiety and promotes cooperation.
Reduces anxiety and promotes cooperation.

IMPLEMENTATION

1 Identify patient using two identifiers (i.e., name and birthday or name and account number) according to agency policy. Compare identifiers with information on patient's identification bracelet.

2 Perform hand hygiene.

3 Provide privacy by closing room door and bedside curtain.

4 Raise bed to appropriate working height. Lower side rail on working side.

5 Prepare urinary drainage collection bag and tubing (large-volume drainage bag or leg bag). Clamp off drainage bag port. Place nearby ready to attach to condom after applied.

6 Help patient into supine position or sitting position. Place bath blanket over upper torso. Fold sheets so only penis is exposed.

7 Apply clean gloves. Provide perineal care (see Chapter 17). Dry thoroughly before applying device. In uncircumcised male ensure that foreskin has been replaced to normal position before applying condom catheter. Do not apply barrier cream.

Ensures correct patient. Complies with The Joint Commission standards and improves patient safety (TJC, 2012).

Reduces transmission of microorganisms.
Promotes patient comfort and self-esteem.
Promotes use of good body mechanics.

Provides easy access to drainage equipment after applying condom catheter.

Respects patient dignity; draping prevents unnecessary exposure of body parts.

Prevents skin breakdown from exposure to secretions. Removes any residual adhesives. Perineal care minimizes skin irritation and promotes adhesion of new external catheter. Barrier creams prevent sheath from adhering to penile shaft (Pomfret, 2008).

STEP	RATIONALE
8 Clip hair at base of penis as necessary before application of condom sheath. Some manufacturers provide a hair guard that is placed over penis before applying device. Remove hair guard after applying catheter. An alternative to hair guard is to tear a hole in a paper towel, place it over penis, and remove after application of device.	Hair adheres to condom and is pulled during condom removal or may get caught in adhesive as external catheter is applied.

Clinical Decision Point *The pubic area should not be shaved because it may increase risk for skin irritation (Pomfret, 2008).*

STEP	RATIONALE
9 Apply condom catheter. With nondominant hand grasp penis along shaft. With dominant hand, hold rolled condom sheath at tip of penis with head of penis in the cone. Smoothly roll sheath onto penis. Allow 2.5 to 5 cm (1 to 2 inches) of space between tip of glans penis and end of condom catheter (see illustration).	Excessive wrinkles or creases in external catheter sheath after application may mean that patient needs smaller size (Newman and Wein, 2009).
10 Apply appropriate securement device as indicated in manufacturer guidelines.	Condom must be secured firmly so it is snug and stays on but not tight enough to cause constriction of blood flow. Application of gentle pressure ensures adherence of adhesive with penile skin.
a Self-adhesive condom catheters: After application apply gentle pressure on penile shaft for 10 to 15 seconds to secure catheter.	
b Outer securing strip-type condom catheters: Spiral wrap penile shaft with strip of supplied elastic adhesive. Strip should not overlap itself. Elastic strip should be snug, not tight (see illustration).	Using spiral wrap technique allows supplied elastic adhesive to expand so blood flow to penis is not compromised.
11 Remove hair guard if used. Connect drainage tubing to end of condom catheter. Be sure that condom is not twisted. If using large drainage bag, place excess tubing on bed and secure to bottom sheet.	Allows urine to be collected and measured. Keeps patient dry. Twisted condom obstructs urine flow, causing urine pooling, skin irritation; and weakening and deterioration of adhesive, causing catheter to come off (Pomfret, 2008).
12 Help patient to safe, comfortable position. Lower bed and place side rails accordingly.	Promotes safety and comfort.
13 Dispose of contaminated supplies, remove gloves, and perform hand hygiene.	Reduces spread of microorganisms.
14 Remove and reapply daily following Steps 9 to 11 unless an extended-wear device is used. To remove condom, wash penis with warm, soapy water and gently roll sheath and adhesive off penile shaft.	Prevents trauma and irritation to penile sheath.

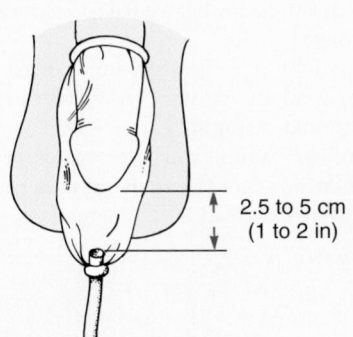

STEP 9 Condom catheter.

2.5 to 5 cm
(1 to 2 in)

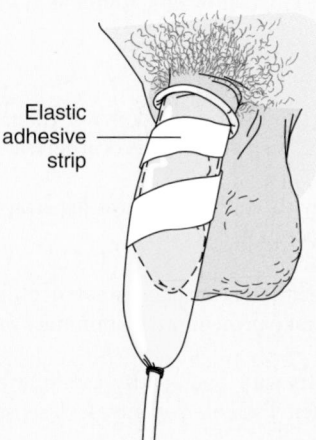

Elastic adhesive strip

STEP 10b Spiral application of adhesive strip.

STEP	RATIONALE

EVALUATION

1 Observe urinary drainage.
2 Inspect penis with condom catheter in place within 15 to 30 minutes after application. Assess for swelling and discoloration and ask patient if there is any discomfort.
3 Inspect skin on penile shaft for signs of breakdown or irritation at least daily, when performing hygiene, and before reapplying condom.

Twisted condom prevents urine from draining into collection bag. Determines if condom is applied too tightly, impeding circulation to penis.

Changing external catheter will decrease the chance of infection.

Unexpected Outcomes

1 Skin around penis is erythematous, ulcerated, or denuded.

Related Interventions

- Check for latex allergy or allergy to skin preparation or adhesive device.
- Remove condom and notify health care provider.
- Do not reapply until penis and surrounding tissue are free from irritation.
- Ensure that condom is not twisted and urine flow is unobstructed after application.

2 Penile swelling or discoloration occurs.

- Remove external catheter.
- Notify health care provider.
- Reassess current condom size. See manufacturer size chart.

3 Condom catheter does not stay on.

- Ensure that catheter tubing is anchored and that patient understands to not pull or tug on catheter.
- Reassess condom catheter size. Refer to manufacturer guidelines for sizing.
- Observe whether condom catheter outlet is kinked and urine is pooling at tip of condom, bathing penis in urine; reapply as necessary and avoid catheter obstruction.
- Assess need for another brand of external catheter (i.e., one that is self-adhesive).

4 Frequency and amount of urination reduced.

- Check for bladder distention.
- Observe whether urine is pooling at tip of condom and bathing penis in urine; reapply as necessary.
- Check for kinks in tubing or in condom catheter.

Recording and Reporting

- Record condom application; condition of penis, skin, and scrotum; urinary output; and voiding pattern in nurses' notes and EHR.
- Report penile erythema, rashes, and/or skin breakdown.

Special Considerations

Teaching

- Teach about signs of skin breakdown or trauma.
- Teach patient to keep condom and catheter kink free and positioned below level of bladder.
- Teach patient with leg bag to assess leg straps periodically for tightness and loosen as necessary.

Pediatric

- Use of condom catheters are uncommon in children. When used in adolescents, take precautions to minimize embarrassment.

Gerontologic

- Evaluate patients with neuropathy carefully before applying a condom catheter. Patient may not feel sensation of pressure

from condom device. Assess penile skin at more frequent intervals, at least twice daily.
- Condom catheters are not recommended in patients with prostatic obstruction.

Home Care

- Teach patient and family caregivers appropriate assessments such as signs and symptoms of UTI, signs of skin irritation, or poor-fitting catheter sheath.
- Loose-fitting clothing may be needed to accommodate the catheter and drainage system.
- Ensure that patient and caregiver understand correct steps in applying the condom catheter. Manufacturers often supply patient educational materials.
- Teach patient or family caregiver to empty drainage bag frequently when one-half full to avoid unnecessary tension on the catheter that can lead to problems keeping the catheter intact.

SKILL 33-5 Suprapubic Catheter Care

A suprapubic catheter is a urinary drainage tube inserted surgically into the bladder through the abdominal wall above the symphysis pubis (Fig. 33-7). The catheter may be sutured to the skin, secured with an adhesive material, or retained in the bladder with a fluid-filled balloon similar to an indwelling catheter.

Suprapubic catheters are placed when there is blockage of the urethra (e.g., enlarged prostate, urethral stricture, after urologic surgery) and in situations when a long-term urethral catheter causes irritation or discomfort or interferes with sexual functioning.

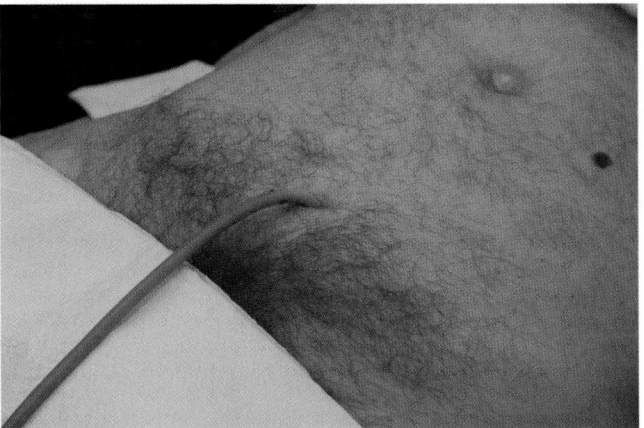

FIG 33-7 Suprapubic catheter without a dressing.

Delegation and Collaboration
The skill of caring for a newly established suprapubic catheter cannot be delegated to nursing assistive personnel (NAP); however, care of an established suprapubic catheter may be delegated (refer to agency policy). The nurse directs the NAP to:
- Report patient's discomfort related to the suprapubic catheter.
- Empty drainage bag and document urinary output on intake and output (I&O) record.
- Report any change in the amount and character of the urine.
- Report any signs of redness, foul odor, or drainage around catheter insertion site.

Equipment
- Clean gloves (sterile may be needed in some cases, see agency policy)
- Cleaning agent (sterile normal saline solution)
- Sterile cotton-tipped applicators
- Sterile surgical drainage gauze (split gauze)
- Sterile gauze dressing
- Washcloth, towel, soap, and water
- Tape
- Velcro tube holder or tube stabilizer (optional)

STEP	RATIONALE

ASSESSMENT

1 Assess urine in drainage bag for amount, clarity, color, odor, and sediment.

Abnormal findings indicate potential complications such as urinary tract infection (UTI), decreased urinary output, and catheter occlusion.

2 Observe dressing for drainage and intactness.

Drainage indicates potential complication such as infection. Dressing may become nonocclusive because of tape choice or drainage.

3 Assess catheter insertion site (may be deferred until you clean site) for signs of inflammation (i.e., pain, erythema, edema, and drainage) and for the growth of overgranulation tissue. Ask patient if there is any pain at site; if so, have him or her rate on scale of 0 to 10.

If insertion is new, slight inflammation may be expected as part of normal wound healing but can also indicate infection. Overgranulation tissue can develop at insertion site as reaction to catheter. In some instances intervention may be needed (Rigby, 2009).

4 Assess for elevated temperature and chills.

Increased temperature may indicate UTI or skin site infection.

5 Assess patient's knowledge of purpose of catheter and its care.

Determines level of instruction/support required.

6 Check for allergies.

Patient may be sensitive to tape, latex, or antiseptic solution.

NURSING DIAGNOSES
- Acute pain
- Deficient knowledge regarding catheter care
- Risk for infection
- Impaired skin integrity
- Impaired urinary elimination

Related factors are individualized based on patient's condition or needs.

PLANNING

1 Expected outcomes following completion of procedure:
- Patient verbalizes no pain or discomfort at insertion site and over bladder.

Patent catheter system keeps bladder empty and patient comfortable.
- Urine output is 30 mL or greater per hour.

Indicates that catheter is patent.
- Urine remains clear without foul odor, and patient is afebrile.

Indicates that patient is free of catheter-associated urinary tract infection (CAUTI).

STEP	RATIONALE

- Catheter exit site is free of infection (i.e., erythema, edema, drainage, tenderness). | Indicates absence of infection and irritation of skin.
- Patient can explain the purpose and expected outcome of procedure. | Helps to minimize anxiety.
- 2 Explain procedure to patient. | Reduces anxiety and promotes cooperation.

IMPLEMENTATION

1 Perform hand hygiene. — Reduces transmission of infection.

2 Provide privacy by closing room door and bedside curtain. — Promotes comfort and patient's self-esteem.

3 Raise bed to appropriate working height. If side rails are raised, lower side rail on working side. — Promotes use of good body mechanics.

4 Prepare supplies and open gauze packets in same manner as for applying dry dressing (see Chapter 39). — Keeps dressing sterile until application.

5 Apply clean gloves. Loosen tape and remove existing dressing. Note type and presence of drainage. Remove gloves and perform hand hygiene. — Provides baseline for condition of suprapubic wound. Reduces transmission of infection from dressing.

6 Clean insertion site using sterile aseptic technique for newly established catheter (option used less frequently; review agency policy or consider individual patient need). — Catheter site is made surgically and therefore is treated similarly to other incisions as designated by agency policy as either using aseptic or sterile technique.

  a Apply sterile gloves.

  b Without creating tension, hold catheter up with nondominant hand while cleaning. Use sterile gauze moistened in saline and clean skin around insertion site in circular motion, starting near insertion site and continuing in outward widening circles for approximately 5 cm (2 inches) (see illustration). — Moves from area of least contamination to area of most contamination. Tension on catheter may cause discomfort or damage to wall of bladder or catheter to slip out of place.

  c With fresh, moistened gauze, gently clean base of catheter, moving up and away from site of insertion (proximal to distal). — Removes microorganisms that reside on any drainage that adheres to tubing.

  d Once insertion site is dry, use sterile gloved hand to apply drain dressing (split gauze) around catheter (see illustration). Tape in place. — Collects drainage that develops around catheter insertion site.

7 Clean using medical aseptic technique for new or established catheter:

  a Apply clean gloves.

  b Without creating tension, hold catheter up with nondominant hand while cleaning. Clean with soap and water in circular motion, starting near catheter insertion site and continuing in outward widening circles for approximately 5 cm (2 inches). — Cleansing and drying suprapubic insertion site requires general hygienic measures; dressing is an option if drainage is not present (Newman and Wein, 2009).

  c With a fresh washcloth or gauze, gently clean base of catheter, moving up and away from site of insertion (proximal to distal). — Removes microorganisms that reside in any drainage that adheres to tubing.

  d *Option:* Apply drain dressing (split gauze) around catheter and tape in place.

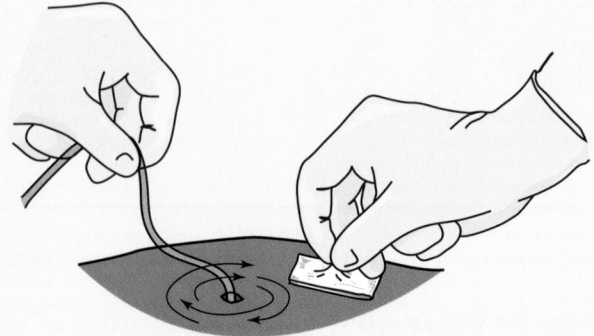

STEP 6b   Cleaning around suprapubic catheter in circular pattern.

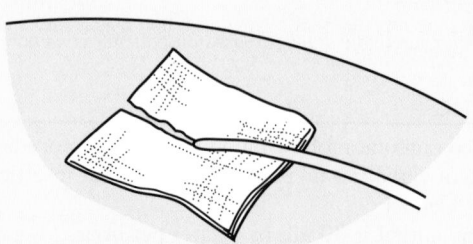

STEP 6d   Split drain dressing for superpubic catheter.

STEP	RATIONALE
8 Secure catheter to lateral abdomen with tape or Velcro multipurpose tube holder.	Secures catheter and reduces risk of excessive tension on suture and/or catheter.
9 Coil excess tubing on bed. Keep drainage bag below level of bladder at all times.	Maintains free flow of urine, thus decreasing risk for CAUTI (Gould et al., 2009).
10 Dispose of all contaminated supplies in appropriate receptacle, remove gloves, and perform hand hygiene.	Reduces transmission of microorganisms.

EVALUATION

1 Ask patient to rate pain or discomfort from suprapubic catheter on scale of 0 to 10.	Determines if bladder is draining and patient is free of infection.
2 Monitor for signs of infection. (e.g., fever, elevated white blood count) and observe urine for clarity, sediment, unusual color, or odor.	Suprapubic catheters increase risk for UTI.
3 Observe catheter insertion site for erythema, edema, discharge, tenderness. Check dressing at minimum of every 8 hours.	Indicators of a site infection.

Unexpected Outcomes	Related Interventions
1 Patient develops symptoms of UTI or catheter site infection.	• Increase fluid intake to at least 2200 mL in 24 hours (unless contraindicated). • Monitor vital signs, I&O; observe amount, color, consistency of urine; assess site. • Notify health care provider.
2 Urine leaks around catheter.	• Check catheter and drainage tubing for kinks or other causes of occlusion. • Monitor vital signs; assess urine for signs of infection. • Change dressing frequently; protect skin from moisture. • Notify health care provider.
3 Suprapubic catheter becomes dislodged.	• Cover site with sterile dressing. • Notify health care provider. If newly established catheter, it will need to be reinserted immediately.
4 Skin surrounding catheter exit site becomes red or irritated and/or develops open areas.	• Notify health care provider. • Change dressing (if used) more frequently to keep site dry. • Consult with wound care nurse.

Recording and Reporting

• Record and report character of urine and type of dressing change, including assessments of insertion site and patient's comfort level with the catheter and dressing change in nurses' notes and EHR.
• Record urine output on I&O flow sheet. When there is both a suprapubic and urethral catheter, record outputs from each catheter separately.

Special Considerations
Teaching

• If not contraindicated, encourage patients to consume a minimum of 2200 mL of fluids daily.
• Teach patient to keep the drainage bag lower than the bladder and to keep tubing free of kinks.

Home Care

• Teach patients and/or family caregivers how to clean and apply a dressing (if applicable) using a clean technique.
• Caution patients and/or family caregivers about avoiding the use of powders or creams around the catheter unless specifically instructed to do so (Newman and Wein, 2009).
• Teach patients and/or family caregivers how to properly position the drainage bag; empty the urinary drainage bag; and observe urine color, clarity, odor, and amount.
• Arrange for home delivery of catheter supplies, always ensuring that there is at least one extra catheter and drainage bag in the home.
• Teach patients and/or family caregivers signs of catheter obstruction, UTI, and wound infection.

Critical Thinking Exercises

You are caring for an 80-year-old woman of Middle Eastern heritage with a history of a stroke, type 2 diabetes, urinary retention, urinary incontinence, and recurrent urinary tract infections (UTIs). The health care provider has ordered measurement of postvoid residual (PVR) by either straight catheterization or bladder scan. There is also an order for an indwelling catheter if the PVR exceeds 400 mL.

1. Which assessments would be pertinent for this patient?
2. Explain why an assessment of PVR is important for this patient?
3. When measuring PVR, should the nurse use the bladder scanner, or should a straight catheterization be performed? Give the rationale for your answer.
4. Explain the teaching that would be appropriate when assessing PVR urine.

✓ REVIEW QUESTIONS

1. The nurse is applying an external condom-type catheter. Which nursing intervention minimizes the risk of skin irritation and infection?
    1. Applying the condom sheath so the end of the catheter is 7 to 12.5 cm (3 to 5 inches) from the tip of the penis
    2. Shaving the pubic area so hair does not adhere to the condom or is pulled during removal
    3. Providing hygiene before applying the condom-type catheter
    4. Applying tape to the condom sheath to keep it securely in place

2. Place the following steps for insertion of an indwelling catheter in a female patient in appropriate order.
    a. Insert and advance catheter.
    b. Lubricate catheter.
    c. Inflate catheter balloon.
    d. Clean urethral meatus with antiseptic.
    e. Drape patient with the sterile square and fenestrated drapes.
    f. When urine appears, advance another 2.5 to 5 cm (1 to 2 inches).
    g. Prepare sterile field and supplies.
    h. Gently pull catheter until resistance is felt.
    i. Attach drainage tubing.
       1. g, d, e, b, a, f, c, h, i
       2. e, g, b, d, a, f, c, h, i
       3. g, e, b, d, f, a, c, h, i
       4. d, e, g, b, a, f, h, c, i

3. What is a critical step when inserting an indwelling catheter into a male patient?
    1. Quickly inflate the catheter balloon with sterile saline.
    2. Secure the catheter drainage tubing to the bed sheets.
    3. Advance to the bifurcation of the drainage and balloon ports.
    4. Advance until urine flows and then insert ¼ inch (0.6 cm) more.

4. The nurse is preparing to remove an indwelling urinary catheter. Which nursing interventions should the nurse implement? (Select all that apply.)
    1. Attach a 5-mL syringe to the inflation port.
    2. Allow the balloon to drain into the syringe by gravity.
    3. Initiate a voiding record/bladder diary.
    4. Pull catheter quickly.
    5. With steady force, pull back on the syringe plunger.

5. Which nursing interventions are appropriate in the care of a patient with an established suprapubic catheter? (Select all that apply.)
    1. Using sterile technique, clean the skin close to the catheter with a circular motion.
    2. Wipe away any drainage on the catheter by wiping down the catheter toward the insertion site.
    3. Inspect the insertion site for erythema, edema, discharge, or tenderness.
    4. Secure catheter to abdomen with tape or a tube-holder device.
    5. Apply tension to the catheter when cleaning the site and tubing.

6. The urine flow has stopped in a patient's indwelling urinary catheter, and the nurse assesses tenderness and distention over the lower abdomen. What would be an initial nursing action?
    1. Irrigating the catheter with sterile water or saline
    2. Assessing the catheter drainage tubing for kinking
    3. Encouraging fluid intake
    4. Removing the catheter

7. Which instructions should the nurse give the nursing assistive personnel (NAP) concerning an ambulatory patient who has had an indwelling urinary catheter removed that day?
    1. Limit oral fluid intake to avoid urinary incontinence.
    2. Expect patient complaints of suprapubic fullness and discomfort.
    3. Report the time and amount of first voiding.
    4. Have patient stay in bed and use a urinal or bedpan until first voiding.

8. Which patient condition is appropriate for the insertion of an indwelling urinary catheter?
    1. Stage I pressure ulcer exposed to leaking urine
    2. Patient unable to independently toilet
    3. Elevated postvoid residual
    4. Urinary incontinence

9. Which size indwelling urinary catheter is best for an adult female patient?
    1. 18 Fr, 5-mL balloon
    2. 16 Fr, 30-mL balloon
    3. 14 Fr, 5-mL balloon
    4. 12 Fr, 30-mL balloon

10. A patient with hematuria has a three-way indwelling urinary catheter with continuous bladder irrigation (CBI) and is complaining of lower abdominal pain. What should be the nurse's first action?
    1. Increasing the rate of the CBI
    2. Checking urine flow to the drainage bag
    3. Decreasing the rate of the CBI
    4. Taking the patient's temperature

REFERENCES

Al-Shaikh G, et al: Accuracy of bladder scanning in the assessment of postvoid residual volume, *J Obstet Gynecol Can* 31(6):526, 2009.

American Academy of Pediatrics (AAP): Ritual genital cutting of female minors, *Pediatrics* 125(5):1088, 2010.

Centers for Medicare & Medicaid Services (CMS): Hospital-acquired conditions (present on admission indicator), 2009, available at http://www.cms.hhs.gov/HospitalAcqCond/06_Hospital-Acquired_Conditions.asp, accessed June 30, 2011.

Cipa-Tatum J, et al: Urethral erosion: a case for prevention, *J Wound, Ostomy, Continence Nurs* 38(5):581, 2011.

Cottenden A, et al: Management using continence products. In Abrams P, et al, editors: *Incontinence*, 2009, ed 4, Paris, France, 2009, Health Publications, p 1521.

D'Avanzo CE: *Mosby's Cultural health assessment*, ed 4, St Louis, 2008, Mosby.

D'Cruz R, et al: Catheter balloon-related urethral trauma in children, *J Paediatr Child Health* 45:564, 2009.

Drekonja DM, et al: Antimicrobial urinary catheters: a systemic review, *Expert Rev Med Devices* 5(4):495, 2008.

Gould CV, et al: *Guideline for prevention of catheter-associated urinary tract infections*, Healthcare Infection Control Practices Advisory Committee, 2009, available at http://www.cdc.gov/hicpac/cauti/001_cauti.html, accessed August 2012.

Gray M: Securing the indwelling catheter, *Am J Nurs* 108(12):44, 2008.

Green L, Marx J, Oriola S: Guide to the elimination of catheter-associated urinary tract infections, *APIC*, 2008, available at www.apic.org/Resource_/Elimination GuideForm/c0790db8-2aca-4179-a7ae-676c27592de2/File/APIC-CAUTI-Guide.pdf, accessed October 1, 2011.

Hockenberry MJ, Wilson D: *Wong's Nursing care of infants and children*, ed 10, St Louis, 2011, Mosby.

Hooton TM, et al: Diagnosis, prevention, and treatment of catheter-associated urinary tract infection in adults: 2009 international clinical practice guidelines from the Infectious Diseases Society of America, *Clin Infect Dis* 50:625, 2010.

Jacobsen SM, et al: Complicated catheter-associated urinary tract infections due to *Escherichia coli* and *Proteus mirabilis*, *Clin Microbiol Rev* 21(1):26, 2008.

Kyle G: The use of urinary sheaths in male incontinence, *Br J Nurs* 20(6):338, 2011.

Lewis SL, et al: *Medical surgical nursing: assessment and management of clinical problems*, ed 5, St Louis, 2011, Mosby.

Lo E, et al: Strategies to prevent catheter-associated urinary tract infections in acute care hospitals, *Infect Control Hospital Epidemiol* 19(suppl 1):S41, 2008.

Méndez-Probst CE, et al: Fundamentals of instrumentation and urinary tract drainage. In Wein A, et al, editors: *Campbell-Walsh Urology*, ed 10, Philadelphia, 2012, Saunders.

National Quality Forum (NQF): *National voluntary consensus standards for public reporting of patient safety event information: a consensus report*, Washington, DC, 2011, NQF.

Nazarko L: Reducing the risk of catheter-related urinary tract infection, *Br J Nurs* 17(16):1002, 2008.

Newman, DK, Wein AJ: *Managing and treating urinary incontinence*, ed 2, Baltimore, 2009, Health Professions Press.

Nyman MH, Johansson J, Gustafsson M: A randomized controlled trial on the effect of clamping the indwelling urinary catheter in patients with hip fracture, *J Clin Nurs* 19: 405, 2010.

Parker D, et al: Evidence-based report card: nursing interventions to reduce the risk of catheter-associated urinary tract infection. Part 1: Catheter selection, *J Wound, Ostomy, Continence Nurs* 36(1):23, 2009.

Pomfret I: The use of sheaths in male urinary incontinence, *Continence Essentials* (1):70, 2008.

Purnell LD: *Guide to culturally competent heath care*, ed 2, Philadelphia, 2009, FA Davis.

Rigby D: An overview of suprapubic catheter care in community practice, *Br J Commun Nurs* 14(7):278, 2009.

Robichard S, Blondeau JM: Urinary tract infections in older adults: current issues and new therapeutic options, *Geriatr Aging* 11(1):582, 2008.

Schumm K, Lam TBL: Types of urethral catheters for management of short-term voiding problems in hospitalized adults, *Cochrane Database of Syst Rev 2*: CD004013, 2008.

Senese V, et al: *SUNA clinical practice guidelines: care of the patient with an indwelling catheter*, Pitman, NJ, 2005, Society of Urologic Nurses and Associates, available at http://www.suna.org/resources/indwellingCatheter.pdf, accessed February 27, 2012.

Smith PW, et al: SHEA/APIC guideline: infection prevention and control in the long-term care facility, *Am J Infect Control* 36:504, 2008.

Srulevich M, Chopra A: Voiding disorders in long-term care, *Ann Long-Term Care* 16(12):1, 2008.

Stoller ML: Retrograde instrumentation of the urinary tract. In Tanagho EA, McAnanch JW, editor: *Smith's General urology*, ed 17, New York, 2008, Lange McGraw Hill, p 155.

The Joint Commission (TJC): *National Patient Safety Goals*, Oakbrook Terrace, Ill, 2012, The Commission, available at http://www.jointcommission.org/standards_information/npsgs.aspx.

Willson M, et al: Evidence-based report card: nursing interventions to reduce the risk of catheter-associated urinary tract infection. Part 2: Staff education, monitoring, and care techniques, *J Wound Ostomy Continence Nurs* 36(2):137, 2009.

Wells M: Managing urinary incontinence with BioDerm external continence device, *Br J Nurs Continence Suppl* 17(9):S24, 2008.

Bowel Elimination and Gastric Intubation

MEDIA RESOURCES

- evolve http://evolve.elsevier.com/Perry/skills
  - Review Questions
  - ▶ Video Clips
  - Audio Glossary

- NSO Nursing Skills Online

KEY TERMS

Bowel management system	Decompression	Hemorrhoids	Obstipation
Cathartic	Defecation	Impaction	Occult blood
Cleansing enema	Enema	Medicated enema	Oil-retention enema
Constipation	Fracture pan		

OBJECTIVES

Mastery of content in this chapter will enable the nurse to:
- Describe factors that promote and impede normal bowel elimination.
- Discuss methods to relieve constipation or impaction.
- Describe precautions to follow in administering an enema.

- Describe approaches for managing a patient's comfort during nasogastric tube insertion.
- Implement the following skills: helping a patient use a bedpan, digitally removing stool, administering an enema, and inserting a nasogastric tube.

Regular elimination of bowel waste products is essential for normal body functioning. Because bowel function depends on the balance of physical and psychological factors; elimination patterns and habits vary among individuals. When patients' functional status changes or they become ill, they may not be able to maintain normal elimination habits. They require assistance such as the use of a bedpan or enema administration. To manage patients' elimination problems, you need to understand normal elimination and factors that promote, impede, or alter elimination such as constipation, diarrhea, and fecal incontinence.

If left unrecognized, constipation can lead to fecal impaction, in which stool blocks the intestinal lumen. If a patient is constipated, you will likely administer enemas or digitally remove impacted stool (Kyle, 2009). When patients undergo surgery or experience an alteration in gastrointestinal (GI) peristalsis, the insertion of a nasogastric (NG) tube is needed for gastric decompression. Gastric decompression reduces nausea and vomiting by keeping the stomach empty.

EVIDENCE-BASED PRACTICE

Constipation is a symptom, not a disease (Box 34-1). The signs of constipation usually include infrequent bowel movements (fewer than 3 times a week), difficulty in evacuating feces, inability to defecate, and hard feces. When intestinal motility slows, the body absorbs additional fecal water. The passage of dry, hard stools occurs when little water remains to soften and lubricate the stool. Constipation has shown to be a side effect of opioid use, decreased mobility, and change in fluid and diet intake (Linari et al., 2011). Interventions for the control of constipation initially include changes in lifestyle such as increased dietary fiber, increased fluids, moderate exercise, and elimination of laxative use (Ostaszkiewicz et al., 2010). Use the following stepwise levels of interventions.

- Walk for 20 minutes, 3 times per week.
- Avoid skipping breakfast and increase intake of soluble and insoluble fiber by drinking one glass of a cloudy juice (e.g., pear) with breakfast and increasing fruit intake (e.g., pears, prunes, kiwi fruit).
- Increase fluid intake if less than 1200 mL per day.
- To promote optimal defecation sit on toilet with legs apart and elbows on knees. Support feet on a stool if unable to reach the floor.
- Respond to the urge to move bowels when the urge first occurs. Establish a bowel routine at the same time of day.
- Try an over-the-counter (OTC) bulk-forming laxative (e.g., psyllium [Metamucil] or methylcellulose [Citrucel]) if all other measures are unsuccessful.

| **BOX 34-1** | **Common Causes of Constipation** |

- Irregular bowel habits and ignoring the urge to defecate
- Chronic illnesses (e.g., Parkinson's disease, multiple sclerosis, rheumatoid arthritis, chronic bowel diseases, depression, eating disorders)
- Low-fiber diet high in animal fats (e.g., meats, dairy products, eggs), refined sugars (rich desserts), and low fluid intake that slow peristalsis
- Lengthy bed rest or lack of regular exercise
- Laxative misuse
- Older adults: Slowed peristalsis, loss of abdominal muscle elasticity, and reduced intestinal mucus secretion and often eating low-fiber foods (Touhy, 2010)
- Neurologic conditions that block nerve impulses to the colon (e.g., spinal cord injury, tumor)
- Colonic action slowed by medications such as anticholinergics, antispasmodics, anticonvulsants, antidepressants, antihistamines, antihypertensives, antiparkinsonism drugs, bile acid sequestrants, diuretics, antacids, iron supplements, calcium supplements, opioids

PATIENT-CENTERED CARE

Bowel elimination is a very private activity. It is important to show respect for a patient's privacy, provide necessary comfort and hygiene measures, and attend to his or her emotional needs when performing required skills. When caring for patients with elimination issues from other cultural and ethnic groups, modify nursing interventions to meet their elimination needs. Provide for culturally sensitive hygiene needs. For example, cultures such as Hindus and Muslims have distinct hygienic practices, which designate the left hand to perform unclean procedures such as cleansing after a bowel elimination. It is important to use the right hand to first touch a patient and then to use the left hand to handle the bedpan and help the patient to cleanse after bowel movement. When caring for a patient who speaks another language or for whom English is the second language, use an interpreter as needed. Provide gender-congruent care for patients from cultures that emphasize separate gender roles and female modesty.

To provide safe patient-centered care, you should determine a patient's normal pattern of bowel elimination and accommodate that pattern while the patient is in a health care setting. Determine the time a patient normally has a bowel movement and the amount of assistance needed. Consider developmental changes that affect bowel functioning throughout the life span. For example, an older adult who becomes less active and has decreased muscle tone and changes in eating patterns is at higher risk for experiencing constipation. Be aware of side effects of medications that impair normal elimination pattern by causing constipation or diarrhea. Also be aware of foods that promote normal peristaltic movement, including high-fiber foods such as raw fruit, whole grains, and green leafy vegetables. Make sure that these are consistent with a patient's prescribed diet and cultural preferences.

Safety Guidelines

1 Promote comfort when a patient uses a bedpan. Encourage patient to use the bathroom when able.
2 Answer the call light promptly to prevent a patient from attempting to get out of bed without assistance.

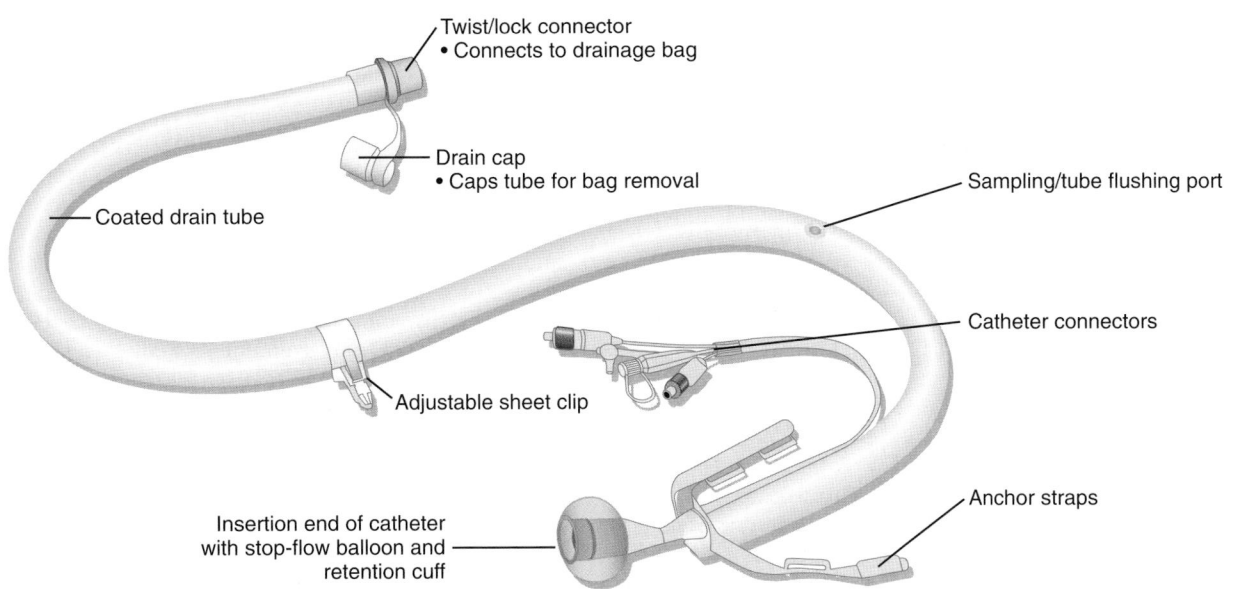

FIG 34-1 Actiflo bowel management system. (*Courtesy Hollister Incorporated, Libertyville, Ill.*)

3 When possible place patients on a toileting schedule and offer assistance with toileting at regular intervals.
4 When handling fecal matter, always use standard precautions (see Chapter 7).
5 Reduce transmission of the spores causing *Clostridium difficile* by using a bowel management system (Fig. 34-1). The system is comprised of an intrarectal catheter that has a retention cuff, an intraluminal balloon, an inflation port, silicone tubing, and a collection bag. The contraindications for use of a bowel management system are included on the package insert and should be considered carefully before insertion.

SKILL 34-1 Assisting a Patient in Using a Bedpan

A patient restricted to bed must use a bedpan for bowel elimination. Two types of bedpans are available (Fig. 34-2). The regular and most commonly used bedpan has a curved, smooth upper end and a tapered lower end. The upper end (wide end) of the regular pan fits under a patient's buttocks toward the sacrum, with lower end (tapered end) fitting just under the upper thighs toward the foot of the bed. A fracture pan, designed for patients with body or leg casts or those who are restricted from raising their hips (e.g., following total joint replacement), slips easily under a patient. The shallow upper end of the pan with a flat, wide rim fits under a patient's buttocks toward the sacrum, with the deep lower open end toward the foot of the bed.

Delegation and Collaboration
The skill of providing a bedpan can be delegated to nursing assistive personnel (NAP). The nurse directs the NAP about:
- Correct positioning guidelines for patients with mobility restrictions or for those who have therapeutic equipment such as wound drains, intravenous (IV) catheters, or traction.
- Providing perineal and hand hygiene for patient as necessary after using a bedpan.

Equipment
- ❑ Clean gloves
- ❑ Bedpan (regular or fracture) (see Fig. 34-2)
- ❑ Bedpan cover
- ❑ Toilet tissue
- ❑ Specimen container (if necessary), plastic bag clearly labeled with date, patient's name, and identification number
- ❑ Basin, washcloths, towels, and soap
- ❑ Waterproof, absorbent pads (if necessary)
- ❑ Clean drawsheet (if necessary)
- ❑ Stethoscope

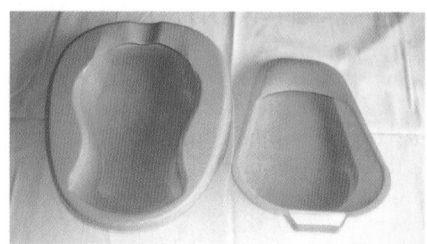

FIG 34-2 Types of bedpans. *Left,* Regular bedpan. *Right,* Fracture bedpan.

STEP	RATIONALE

ASSESSMENT

1 Assess patient's normal bowel elimination habits: routine pattern, character of stool, effect of certain foods/fluids and eating habits on bowel elimination, effect of stress and level of activity on normal bowel elimination patterns, current medications, and normal fluid intake.

Managing patient's elimination problems depends on thorough understanding of normal elimination and factors that create alterations. Peristalsis is strongest during the hour after first meal of the day. Anticipate when to offer bedpan.

2 Auscultate abdomen for bowel sounds and palpate lower abdomen for distention.

Normal bowel sounds occur irregularly at rate of 5 to 35 per minute. Presence of feces in colon, often mistaken for an abdominal mass, can be felt as a soft, rounded, boggy mass in the cecum and ascending, descending, or sigmoid colon (Seidel et al., 2011).

3 Assess patient to determine level of mobility, including ability to sit upright and lift hips or turn.

Determines if patient can help in positioning on bedpan or if assistance is needed. Determines whether to use regular or fracture bedpan. Older adults, obese patients, patients who have had hip or knee surgery or spinal injury, and debilitated patients often require assistance of two or more nurses to help them onto or off bedpan.

4 Assess patient's level of comfort. Ask about presence of rectal or abdominal pain, presence of hemorrhoids, or irritation of skin surrounding anus.

Pain limits patient's ability to help with positioning. Rectal or abdominal pain reduces patient's ability to bear down during defecation.

5 Determine need for stool specimen.

Provides opportunity to obtain specimen container before placing patient on bedpan.

STEP	RATIONALE

NURSING DIAGNOSES

- Acute pain
- Bowel incontinence
- Chronic pain
- Diarrhea
- Impaired physical mobility
- Perceived constipation
- Risk for constipation
- Toileting self-care deficit

Related factors are individualized based on patient's condition or needs.

PLANNING

1 Expected outcomes following completion of procedure: • Perianal skin is clean and intact.	Hygiene technique after defecation keeps perianal skin clear of fecal secretions.
• Patient eliminates without pain or discomfort.	Patient is positioned comfortably on bedpan.
2 Explain procedure to patient, including self-help tips (e.g., how to use a trapeze, how to move hips).	Promotes independence, reduces anxiety, and helps patient to assist during procedure.
3 Obtain assistance from additional nursing personnel as warranted.	Adequate personnel resources minimize muscle strain for you and patient. Reduces patient's discomfort.

IMPLEMENTATION

1 Perform hand hygiene.	Reduces transmission of microorganisms.
2 Provide privacy by closing curtains around bed or door of room.	Reduces embarrassment and promotes bowel elimination (Cohen, 2009).
3 Raise side rail on opposite side of bed.	Protects patient from falling out of bed. Patient can use side rail to grasp onto and help self move about in bed and onto bedpan.
4 Raise bed horizontally according to your height.	Promotes use of good body mechanics and minimizes muscle strain for you and patient.
5 Have patient assume supine position.	Position eases eventual pan placement.

Clinical Decision Point *Observe for the presence of drains, dressings, IV fluids, and traction. These devices make it difficult for a patient to assist with positioning, and you will likely need more personnel to help place him or her on a bedpan.*

6 Place patient who can help on a bedpan. **a** Apply clean gloves. Raise head of patient's bed 30 to 60 degrees.	Prevents hyperextension of back and provides support to upper torso when patient raises hips. Sitting position promotes defecation.
b Remove upper bed linens so they are out of the way but do not expose patient.	Prevents embarrassment to patient; demonstrates respect for patient's sense of dignity (Cohen, 2009).
c Teach patient how to flex knees and lift hips upward.	If legs, upper torso, and arms are supporting body weight, little effort should be required of patient.
d Place your hand, closest to patient's head, palm up under patient's sacrum to help lift. Ask patient to bend knees and raise hips. As patient raises hips, use other hand to slip bedpan under him or her (see illustrations). Be sure that open rim of bedpan is facing toward foot of bed. Do not force pan under patient's hips. (*Optional*: Have patient use overhead trapeze frame to raise hips.)	Positions bedpan high under buttocks so feces enters pan. Incorrect placement of bedpan causes discomfort for patient and spillage of contents. Forcing bedpan under patient increases risk for friction injury to underlying skin and tissues.
e *Optional*: If using fracture pan, slip it under patient as hips are raised (see illustration). Be sure that deep, open, lower end of bedpan is facing toward foot of bed.	Patient requires less maneuvering and does not have to lift hips.
7 Place patient who is immobile or has mobility restrictions on bedpan. **a** Apply clean gloves. Lower head of bed flat or raise head slightly (if tolerated by medical condition).	Helps patient who cannot lift hips, who must remain flat, or who medically is not permitted to lift hips to roll onto bedpan.
b Remove top linens as necessary to turn patient while minimizing exposure.	Prevents embarrassment to patient; demonstrates respect for patient's sense of dignity (Cohen, 2009).

STEP	RATIONALE
c Help patient roll onto side with back toward you. Place bedpan firmly against patient's buttocks and down into mattress. Be sure that open rim of bedpan is facing toward foot of bed (see illustrations).	Incorrect placement causes discomfort to patient and spillage of contents.

Clinical Decision Point *If patient has had total hip replacement, make sure that abduction pillow placed between the legs to prevent dislocation of the new joint remains in place. Use a fracture pan.*

STEP	RATIONALE
d Keep one hand against bedpan; place other around far hip of patient. Ask patient to roll back onto bedpan, flat in bed. Do not force pan under patient.	Using minimal exertion, this places patient squarely on pan. Avoid forcing bedpan under patient to decrease risk for friction injury to underlying skin and tissues.
e Raise patient's head 30 degrees or to a comfortable level (unless contraindicated).	Patient assumes sitting position unless condition necessitates maintaining flat position.
f Have patient bend knees or raise knee gatch (unless contraindicated).	Relieves stress on back.
8 Maintain patient's comfort and safety. Cover patient for warmth. Place small pillow or rolled towel under lumbar curve of back.	Provides added comfort. Pain reduces or eliminates urge to defecate, which will result in bowel elimination problems.
9 Have call bell and toilet tissue within reach for patient.	Promotes safety by preventing patient from reaching over edge of bed for objects out of reach.
10 Ensure that bed is in lowest position and raise upper side rails.	Promotes patient safety and enables patient to reposition pan as needed.
11 Remove and discard gloves and perform hand hygiene.	Reduces transmission of microorganisms.
12 Allow patient to be alone but monitor status and respond promptly.	Reassures patient. Removing bedpan in timely manner prevents pressure ulcers.
13 Perform hand hygiene and apply clean gloves.	Reduces transmission of microorganisms.

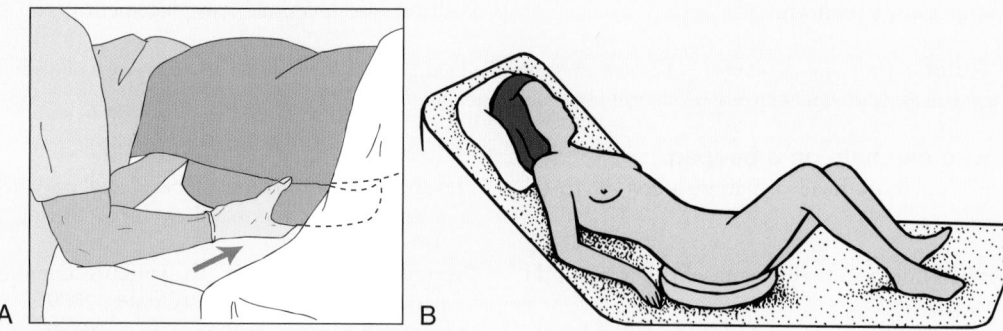

STEP 6d **A,** Placing bedpan under patient's hips. **B,** Correct positioning for placing mobile patient on bedpan.

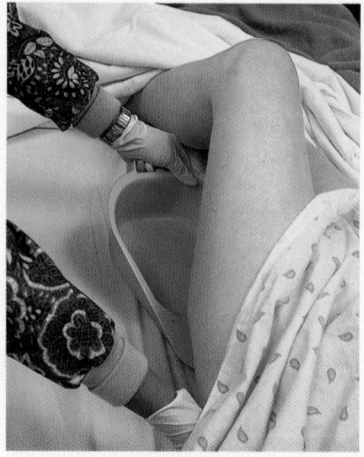

STEP 6e Patient lifts hips as fracture pan is positioned.

STEP	RATIONALE
14 *Remove bedpan:*	
a Place patient's bedside chair close to working side of bed.	Provides area to place bedpan and contents on chair after removal from patient to prevent accidental spilling of full bedpan on bed surface.
b Maintain privacy; determine if patient is able to wipe own perineal area. If you clean perineal area, use several layers of toilet tissue or disposable washcloths. For female patients clean from mons pubis toward rectal area.	Maintains respect for privacy. Cleanses from clean to dirty area of perineum.
c Deposit contaminated tissue in bedpan if no specimen or intake and output (I&O) is needed.	Toilet tissue will contaminate specimen and affect accurate output measurement.
d For mobile patient: Ask patient to flex knees, placing body weight on lower legs, feet, and upper torso; lift buttocks up from bedpan. At same time place hand farthest from patient on side of bedpan to support it (prevent spillage) and place other hand (closest to patient) under sacrum to help lift. Have patient lift and remove bedpan. Place bedpan on draped bedside chair and cover.	Avoids pulling or forcing pan from under hips because this action pulls skin and causes tissue injury.
e For immobile patient: Lower head of bed. Help patient roll onto side away from you and off bedpan. Hold bedpan flat and steady while patient is rolling off; otherwise spillage will occur. Place bedpan on draped bedside chair and cover.	Reduces spread of microorganisms. Reduces spread of offensive odors.
15 Allow patient to perform hand hygiene. Change soiled linens, remove and dispose of gloves, and return patient to comfortable position.	Reduces chance of skin breakdown when bedridden patient lies on dry, wrinkle-free linens.

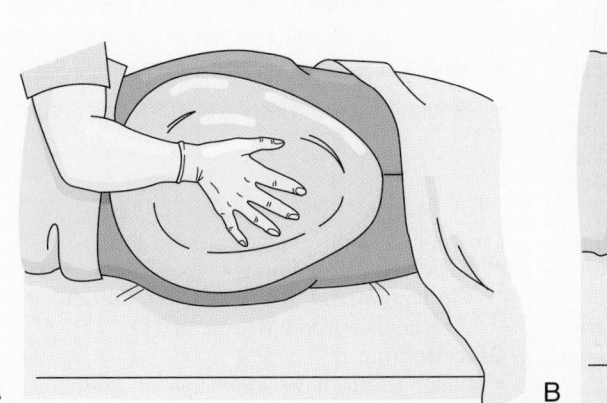 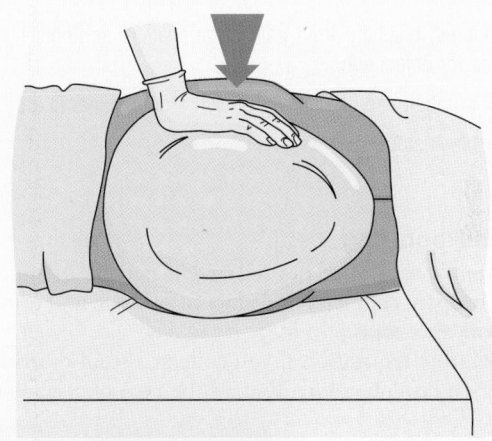

A

B

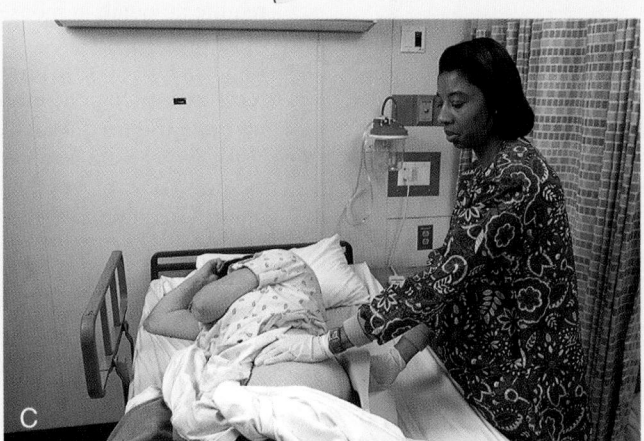

C

STEP 7c   A, Position patient on one side and place bedpan firmly against buttocks. **B,** Push down on bedpan and toward patient. **C,** Nurse places bedpan in position. (*A and B from Sorrentino SA: Mosby's textbook for nursing assistants, ed 7, St Louis, 2009, Mosby.*)

STEP	RATIONALE
16 Place bed in its lowest position. Ensure that call bell, phone, drinking water, and desired personal items (e.g., books) are within easy access.	Promotes comfort and reduces risk for injury to patient.
17 Option: Obtain stool specimen as ordered (see Chapter 43). Wear gloves when emptying contents of bedpan into toilet or in special receptacle in utility room. Use spray faucet attached to most institution toilets to rinse bedpan thoroughly. Use disinfectant if required by agency, then store pan. Remove gloves.	If bedpan becomes very soiled, replace with clean one and send soiled one for sterilization or properly dispose (see agency policy).
18 Perform hand hygiene.	Reduces transmission of microorganisms.

EVALUATION

1 Assess characteristics of stool. Note color, odor, consistency, frequency, amount, shape (see Fig. 34-3), and constituents. Assess characteristics of urine if patient voided in bedpan.	Helps to identify significant changes or findings.
2 Evaluate patient's ability to use bedpan.	Provides continual assessment of patient's self-toileting ability.
3 Inspect patient's perianal area and surrounding skin while removing bedpan.	Liquid stool predisposes patient to skin breakdown.
4 Evaluate patient's overall activity tolerance and comfort.	Defecation and use of bedpan are tiring.

Unexpected Outcomes	Related Interventions
1 Patient is unable to successfully use bedpan.	• If patient's mobility allows, obtain order for use of bedside commode.
2 Patient is incontinent of stool. Avoid use of adult briefs for bedridden patient.	• Establish regular schedule of offering bedpan. Adult briefs mask toileting needs and may potentiate skin breakdown. • Discuss with staff need to answer patient's request for toileting assistance promptly and use toileting schedule.
3 Patient is constipated, resulting from pain of defecation, immobility, or unnatural position for defecation.	• See evidence-based practice section, p. 842.
4 Patient develops irritation and breakdown of skin around perianal area.	• Administer perianal skin care using moisture barrier.
5 Blood in stool or black stool.	• Perform fecal occult blood test (FOBT) (see Chapter 43).

Recording and Reporting

• Record the type of assistance needed and if patient tolerates getting on/off bedpan, character and amount of stool, and urine output if patient also voids.
• Complete laboratory requisition if you collected stool or urine specimen and send to laboratory. Record the type of specimen sent.

Special Considerations
Teaching

• Some patients on complete bed rest have an overhead trapeze frame connected to bed to help lift them on and off bedpan. Teaching this activity helps to maintain strength of patient's arms.
Pediatric

• Constipation in early childhood results from environmental changes such as being hospitalized and reluctance to use a bedpan. Toilet-trained children often regress during hospitalization.
• Repeated withholding of stool leads to stretching or dilating of the rectum and decreases the sensation or "urge" to defecate (Hockenberry and Wilson, 2011).
Gerontologic

• Older adults have some loss of sphincter control and often require a quick response when requesting a bedpan (Kyle, 2009).
• Incidence of constipation is greater because there is impaired rectal sensation to defecate. As a result, the older adult does not perceive the need to defecate.
• With increased age transit time through the bowel increases, causing a normal lengthening of the time between bowel movements (Banning, 2008).

SKILL 34-2   Removing Fecal Impaction Digitally

Fecal impaction is the inability to pass a collection of hard stool. This condition occurs in all age-groups. Physically and mentally incapacitated individuals and institutionalized older adults are at greatest risk. Fecal impaction occurs when there is a history of constipation. However, functional constipation is defined as including two or more of the following factors for at least 3 months: (1) straining with defecation at least one fourth of the time, (2) lumpy or hard stools (or both) one fourth of the time (Fig. 34-3),

Type 1	Separate hard lumps like nuts (difficult to pass)
Type 2	Sausage shaped but lumpy
Type 3	Like a sausage but with cracks on surface
Type 4	Like a sausage or snake, smooth and soft
Type 5	Soft blobs with clear-cut edges (passed easily)
Type 6	Fluffy pieces with ragged edges, a mushy stool
Type 7	Watery, no solid pieces (entirely liquid)

FIG 34-3 Bristol stool form scale. (From O'Donnell LJ, Virjee J, Heaton KW: Detection of pseudodiarrhoea by simple clinical assessment of intestinal transit rate, Br Med J 300:439, ©1990. Reprinted with permission of the BMJ Publishing Group.)

(3) sensation of incomplete evacuation at least one fourth of the time, or (4) two or fewer bowel movements in a week (Kyle, 2009). A variety of interventions successfully relieve constipation and reduce the risk for impaction (e.g., exercise and diet).

Symptoms of fecal impaction include constipation, rectal discomfort, anorexia, nausea, vomiting, abdominal pain, diarrhea (leaking around the impacted stool), and urinary frequency. Prevention is the key to managing fecal impaction. However, once it occurs, digital removal of stool is the only alternative. Digital removal of an impaction is very uncomfortable and embarrassing for a patient. Excessive rectal manipulation causes irritation to the mucosa and subsequent bleeding or vagus nerve stimulation, which can produce a reflex slowing of the heart rate. The skill is performed when the administration of enemas or suppositories is not successful at removing impacted stools.

Delegation and Collaboration
The skill of removing a fecal impaction digitally cannot be delegated to nursing assistive personnel (NAP). The nurse directs the NAP to:
- Help the nurse position a patient for the procedure.
- Observe the stool for color, consistency, rectal bleeding, or bloody mucus and report immediately to the nurse.
- Provide perineal care following each bowel movement.

Equipment
- Clean gloves
- Water-soluble local anesthetic lubricant (NOTE: Some agencies require use of water-soluble lubricant without anesthetic when nurse performs procedure.)
- Waterproof, absorbent pads
- Bedpan
- Bedpan cover (optional)
- Bath blanket
- Basin, washcloths, towels, and soap
- Vital sign equipment

STEP	RATIONALE

ASSESSMENT

1 Assess patient:
  a Ask patient about normal and current bowel elimination pattern, including frequency and characteristics of stool; use of laxatives, enemas, and other medications; level of exercise; urge to defecate but inability to do so; feelings of incomplete emptying; and sensations of bloating, cramping, and excessive gas.

Information provides data in determining contributing factors and preventive measures. Large fecal mass causes rectal distention and increases perception of urge to evacuate rectum (Chien, 2010).

  b Inspect patient's abdomen for distention.

Observation identifies distended or asymmetric areas, which are then investigated on auscultation or palpation. Distention contributes to constipation.

  c Auscultate all four quadrants for presence of bowel sounds.

Hypoactive bowel sounds may result from partial obstruction of the gastrointestinal (GI) tract.

  d Palpate patient's abdomen for distention, discomfort, or masses.

Symptoms are related to accumulation of stool in intestinal tract. Palpable mass may be felt with severe constipation.

  e Measure patient's current vital signs and comfort level on scale of 0 to 10.

Provides baseline measurement. Sacral branch of vagus nerve is stimulated during digital stimulation; this stimulation results in reflex slowing of heart rate (Seidel et al., 2011).

STEP	RATIONALE

Clinical Decision Point *Because of the potential to stimulate the sacral branch of the vagus nerve, patients with a history of dysrhythmias or heart disease have a greater risk for changes in heart rhythm. Be sure to monitor patient's pulse before and during procedure. This procedure is often contraindicated in cardiac patients; if in doubt, verify with the health care provider.*

STEP	RATIONALE
f Perform hand hygiene and apply clean gloves. Observe consistency of stool (see Fig. 34-3), seepage of liquid stool, or continued passage of small amounts of hard stool. Observe anal area for signs of irritation or hemorrhoids. Remove gloves and perform hand hygiene.	Seepage of stool is symptomatic of an impaction high in colon. Patient may be able to pass small pieces of hard stool or have episodes of passing small amounts of liquid stool (Leung and Rao, 2009).
g Determine if patient is receiving anticoagulant therapy.	Procedure may be contraindicated. Manipulation of rectum can cause bleeding, which is prolonged with anticoagulants.
2 Check patient's record for health care provider's order for digital removal of impaction and use of anesthetic lubricant.	Obtain written order before performing procedure because this procedure involves excessive stimulation of vagus nerve.

NURSING DIAGNOSES

• Acute pain	• Constipation	• Diarrhea

Related factors are individualized based on patient's condition or needs.

PLANNING

STEP	RATIONALE
1 Expected outcomes following completion of procedure:	
• Impacted stool is successfully removed.	Indicates that rectum is clear of stool.
• Patient is free of abdominal or rectal discomfort.	Fecal impaction causes direct pain to rectum and indirect abdominal discomfort through abdominal distention.
• Vital signs remain within patient's baseline.	Indicates absence of vagal stimulation.
2 Explain procedure to patient.	Information reduces anxiety and encourages patient participation in therapeutic elimination protocol.

IMPLEMENTATION

STEP	RATIONALE
1 Identify patient using two identifiers (i.e., name and birthday or name and account number) according to agency policy. Compare identifiers with information on patient's identification bracelet.	Ensures correct patient. Complies with The Joint Commission standards and improves patient safety (TJC, 2012).
2 Obtain assistance to help change patient's position if necessary. Raise bed horizontally to comfortable working height.	Promotes patient safety and use of good body mechanics.
3 Pull curtains around bed or close door to room.	Maintains patient's sense of privacy and prevents unnecessary exposure of body parts.
4 Lower side rail on patient's right side. Keeping far side rail raised, help patient to left side-lying position with knees flexed and back.	Promotes patient safety. Provides access to rectum.
5 Drape patient's trunk and lower extremities with bath blanket and place waterproof pad under patient's buttocks.	Maintains patient's sense of privacy and prevents unnecessary exposure of body parts.
6 Place bedpan next to patient.	
7 Perform hand hygiene and apply clean gloves. Lubricate gloved index finger and middle finger of dominant hand with anesthetic lubricant.	Prevents transmission of microorganisms. Reduces discomfort and permits smooth insertion of finger into anus and rectum.
8 Instruct patient to take slow deep breaths during procedure. Gradually and gently insert gloved index finger and feel anus relax around finger. Insert middle finger.	Slow deep breaths help to relax patient. Gradual insertion of index finger helps to dilate anal sphincter.
9 Gradually advance fingers slowly along rectal wall toward umbilicus.	Allows you to reach impacted stool high in rectum.
10 Gently loosen fecal mass by moving fingers in scissors motion to fragment the fecal mass. Work fingers into hardened mass.	Loosening and penetrating mass allows for removal of stool in small pieces, resulting in less discomfort to patient.
11 Work stool downward toward end of rectum. Remove small sections of feces and discard into bedpan.	Prevents need to force finger up into rectum and minimizes trauma to mucosa.
12 Observe patient's response and periodically assess heart rate and look for signs of fatigue.	Vagal stimulation slows heart rate and causes dysrhythmias. Procedure often exhausts patient.

STEP	RATIONALE

Clinical Decision Point *Stop procedure if heart rate drops or rhythm changes from patient's baseline or if patient has dyspnea or complaints of palpitations.*

STEP	RATIONALE
13 Continue to clear rectum of feces and allow patient to rest at intervals.	Rest improves patient's tolerance of procedure, allowing heart rate to return to normal.
14 After removal of impaction perform perineal hygiene.	Promotes patient's sense of comfort and cleanliness.
15 Remove bedpan and inspect feces for color and consistency. Dispose of feces in toilet.	Reduces transmission of microorganisms.
16 If needed, help patient to toilet or clean and store the bedpan. (Procedure may be followed by enema or cathartic.)	Removal of impaction stimulates defecation reflex.
17 Remove gloves by turning them inside out and discarding in proper receptacle. Perform hand hygiene.	Reduces transmission of microorganisms.

EVALUATION

1 Apply clean gloves and perform rectal examination for stool and observe anal and perianal area for irritation or skin breakdown.	Determines if rectum is clear.
2 Reassess vital signs and compare to baseline values. Continue to monitor patient for 1 hour for bradycardia.	Determines extent of vagal stimulation.
3 Auscultate bowel sounds.	Determines presence of peristaltic activity.
4 Palpate abdomen to determine if it is soft and nontender.	Discomfort is relieved.
5 Ask patient to rate comfort level of on scale of 0 to 10.	Procedure can cause discomfort.

Unexpected Outcomes

1 Patient experiences trauma to rectal mucosa as evidenced by rectal bleeding.

2 Patient experiences bradycardia, decrease in blood pressure, and decrease in level of consciousness as result of vagus nerve stimulation.

3 Patient has seepage of liquid stool after procedure complete.

Related Interventions

- Assess anal and perianal region for source of bleeding.
- Stop procedure if bleeding is excessive.

- Stop procedure and measure vital signs.
- Notify health care provider and remain with patient.

- Assess patient for continuing impaction.
- Notify health care provider for possible suppository or enema.
- Increase patient's fluid intake and dietary fiber.

Recording and Reporting

- Record patient's tolerance to procedure, amount and consistency of stool removed, vital signs, and adverse effects.
- Report any changes in vital signs and adverse effects to health care provider.

Special Considerations
Teaching

- If constipation and subsequent impaction are diet related, teach patient about high-fiber nutritional products to increase bulk and the need for adequate fluid intake.
- If necessary, teach family caregivers about the effects of immobility, hydration, and nutrition on normal bowel elimination.

Pediatric

- Do not digitally remove stool in a pediatric patient because of the risk for anal fissures and pain that trigger stool withholding (Hockenberry and Wilson, 2011).

Gerontological

- Many older adults are especially prone to dysrhythmias and other problems related to vagal stimulation; monitor heart rate and rhythm closely (Seidel et al., 2011).
- For older adults, instituting a diet adequate in dietary fiber (6 to 10 g per day) adds bulk, weight, and form to stool and improves defecation.
- Consider developing a regular toileting routine that includes responding to the urge to defecate.

SKILL 34-3 Administering an Enema

[NSO] *Bowel Elimination Module / Lesson 2*

An enema is the instillation of a solution into the rectum and sigmoid colon to promote defecation by stimulating peristalsis. Typically an enema is used to treat constipation or empty the bowel before diagnostic procedures or certain types of abdominal surgery. Preoperative enemas are common for some surgeries.

Cleansing enemas promote complete evacuation of feces from the colon. They act by stimulating peristalsis through infusion of large volumes of solution. Oil-retention enemas act by lubricating the rectum and colon, allowing feces to absorb oil and become softer and easier to pass. Sometimes these enemas are used before digital removal of stool. Medicated enemas contain pharmacologic therapeutic agents. Some are prescribed to reduce dangerously high serum potassium levels (e.g., sodium polystyrene sulfonate [Kayexalate] enema) or to reduce bacteria in the colon before bowel surgery (e.g., neomycin enema).

The volume or type of fluid that breaks up the fecal mass stretches the rectal wall and initiates the defecation reflex. Common types of enemas include:

- *Tap water (hypotonic) enema:* It should not be repeated after first installation because water toxicity or circulatory overload can develop.
- *Physiologic normal saline:* It is the safest enema to administer. Infants and children can tolerate only this type because of their predisposition to fluid imbalance.
- *Hypertonic solution* (e.g., commercially prepared Fleet enema): It is useful for patients who cannot tolerate large volumes of fluid. Only 120 to 180 mL (4 to 6 oz) is usually effective.
- *Harris Flush enema:* It is a return-flow enema in which fluid alternately flows into and out of the large intestine. This stimulates peristalsis in the large intestine and helps to expel intestinal gas.
- *Soapsuds enema (SSE):* It is pure castile soap added to either tap water or normal saline, depending on patient's condition and frequency of administration. Use *only* castile pure soap. Recommended ratio of pure soap to solution is 5 mL (1 teaspoon) to 1000 mL (1 quart) warm water or saline. Add soap to enema bag *after* water is in place to reduce excessive suds.
- *Oil-retention enema:* It uses an oil-based solution. The colon absorbs a small volume, which allows the oil to soften stool for easier evacuation.
- *Carminative solution:* It provides relief from gaseous distention. An example is MGW solution, which contains 30 mL of magnesium, 60 mL of glycerin, and 90 mL of water.

Delegation and Collaboration

The skill of enema administration can be delegated to nursing assistive personnel (NAP). The nurse directs the NAP about:

- How to properly position patients who have mobility restrictions or therapeutic equipment such as drains, intravenous (IV) catheters, or traction.
- Informing the nurse about patient's new abdominal pain (*exception:* a patient reports cramping) or rectal bleeding.
- Informing the nurse immediately about the presence of blood in the stool or around the rectal area or any change in vital signs.

 Video Clip

Equipment
- ❏ Clean gloves
- ❏ Water-soluble lubricant
- ❏ Waterproof, absorbent pads
- ❏ Toilet tissue
- ❏ Bedpan, bedside commode, or access to toilet
- ❏ Basin, washcloths, towel, and soap
- ❏ IV pole
- ❏ Stethoscope

Enema Bag Administration
- ❏ Enema container with tubing and clamp (Fig. 34-4)
- ❏ Appropriate-size rectal tube (adult: 22 to 30 Fr; child: 12 to 18 Fr)
- ❏ Correct volume of warmed (tepid) solution (adult: 750 to 1000 mL; adolescent: 500 to 700 mL; school-age child: 300 to 500 mL; toddler: 250 to 350 mL; infant: 150 to 250 mL)

Prepackaged Enema
- ❏ Prepackaged enema container with lubricated rectal tip (Fig. 34-5)

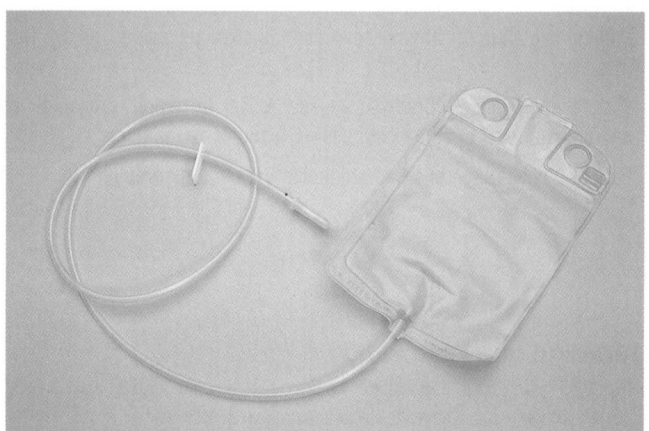

FIG 34-4 Enema bag with tubing.

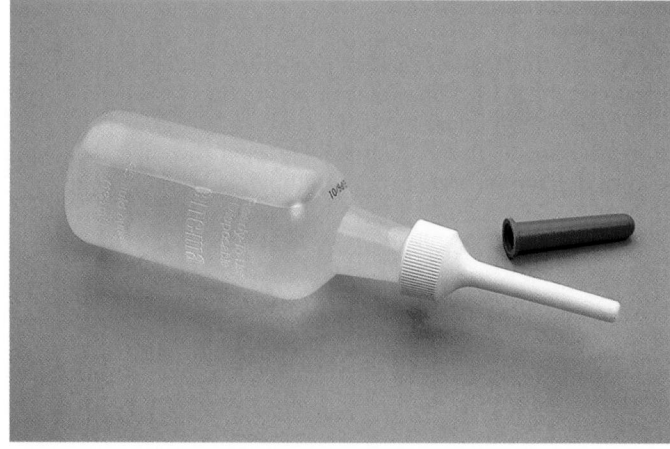

FIG 34-5 Prepackaged enema container with rectal tip and cap.

STEP	RATIONALE

ASSESSMENT

1 Review health care provider's order for enema and clarify reason for administration.

Order by health care provider is usually required for hospitalized patient.

2 Assess last bowel movement, normal versus most recent bowel pattern, presence of hemorrhoids, mobility, and presence of abdominal pain or cramping.

Determines need for enema and type of enema used. Also establishes baseline for bowel function. Hemorrhoids may obscure rectal opening and cause discomfort or bleeding during evacuation.

3 Inspect abdomen for presence of distention and auscultate for bowel sounds.

Establishes baseline for determining effectiveness of enema.

4 Determine patient's level of understanding of purpose of enema.

Allows for planning appropriate teaching measures.

> **Clinical Decision Point** *"Enemas until clear" order means that you repeat enemas until patient passes fluid that is clear of fecal matter. Check agency policy, but usually patient should receive only three consecutive enemas to avoid disruption of fluid and electrolyte balance. It is essential to observe contents of solution passed.*

NURSING DIAGNOSES

- Acute pain
- Constipation
- Risk for constipation

Related factors are individualized based on patient's condition or needs.

PLANNING

1 Expected outcomes following completion of procedure:
  - Stool is evacuated.
  - Enema return is clear.
  - Abdomen is flat, nontender, with no distention.

Solution clears rectum and lower colon of stool.
Indicates that all solid fecal material in colon has passed.
Gas and feces are expelled.

IMPLEMENTATION

1 If enema is medicated, check accuracy and completeness of each medication administration record (MAR) with health care provider's written order. Check patient's name, type of enema, and time for administration. Compare MAR with label of enema solution.

The order is most reliable source and only legal record of drugs or procedure that patient is to receive. Ensures that patient receives correct enema.

2 Identify patient using two identifiers (i.e., name and birthday or name and account number) according to agency policy. Compare identifiers with information on patient's identification bracelet.

Ensures correct patient. Complies with The Joint Commission standards and improves patient safety (TJC, 2012).

3 Provide privacy by closing curtains around bed or closing door.

Reduces embarrassment for patient.

4 Place bedpan or bedside commode in easily accessible position. If patient will be expelling contents in toilet, ensure that toilet is available, and place patient's slippers and bathrobe in easily accessible position.

Bedpan is used if patient is unable to get out of bed.

5 Perform hand hygiene and apply clean gloves.

Reduces transmission of microorganisms.

6 Raise bed to appropriate working height; raise side rail on patient's right side.

Promotes good body mechanics and patient safety.

7 Help patient turn onto left side-lying (Sims') position with right knee flexed. Encourage him or her to remain in position until procedure is complete. Children are placed in dorsal recumbent position.

Allows enema solution to flow downward by gravity along natural curve of sigmoid colon and rectum, thus improving retention of solution.

> **Clinical Decision Point** *Patients with poor sphincter control require placement of a bedpan under the buttocks. Administering enema with patient sitting on toilet is unsafe because curved rectal tubing can abrade rectal wall.*

8 Lower side rail on working side and place waterproof pad, absorbent side up, under hips and buttocks. Cover patient with bath blanket, exposing only rectal area, clearly visualizing anus.

Pad prevents soiling of linen. Blanket provides warmth, reduces exposure of body parts, and allows patient to feel more relaxed and comfortable.

9 Separate buttocks and examine perianal region for abnormalities, including hemorrhoids, anal fissure, and rectal prolapse.

Findings influence approach for inserting enema tip. Prolapse contraindicates enema.

STEP	RATIONALE

10 Administer enema.
  a Administer prepackaged disposable enema:

(1) Remove plastic cap from tip of container. Tip may already be lubricated. Apply more water-soluble lubricant as needed.	Lubrication provides for smooth insertion of rectal tube without causing rectal irritation or trauma. With presence of hemorrhoids, extra lubricant provides added comfort.
(2) Gently separate buttocks and locate anus. Instruct patient to relax by breathing out slowly through mouth.	Breathing out promotes relaxation of external rectal sphincter.
(3) Expel any air from enema container.	Introducing air into colon causes further distention and discomfort.
(4) Insert lubricated tip of container gently into anal canal toward umbilicus (see illustration). *Adult:* 7.5 to 10 cm (3 to 4 inches) *Adolescent:* 7.5 cm to 10 cm (3 to 4 inches) *Child:* 5 to 7.5 cm (2 to 3 inches) *Infant:* 2.5 to 3.75 cm (1 to 1½ inches)	Gentle insertion prevents trauma to rectal mucosa.

Clinical Decision Point *If pain occurs or you feel resistance at any time during procedure, stop and discuss with health care provider. Do not force insertion.*

(5) Roll plastic bottle from bottom to tip until all of solution has entered rectum and colon. Instruct patient to retain solution until urge to defecate occurs, usually 2 to 5 minutes.	Prevents instillation of air into colon and ensures that all content enters rectum. Hypertonic solutions require only small volumes to stimulate defecation.

  b Administer enema in standard enema bag:

(1) Add warmed solution to enema bag: Warm tap water as it flows from faucet, place saline container in basin of warm water before adding saline to enema bag, and check temperature of solution by pouring small amount of solution over inner wrist.	Hot water burns intestinal mucosa. Cold water causes abdominal cramping and is difficult to retain.
(2) If SSE is ordered, add castile soap after water.	Prevents suds in enema bag.
(3) Raise container, release clamp, and allow solution to flow long enough to fill tubing.	Removes air from tubing.
(4) Reclamp tubing.	Prevents further loss of solution.

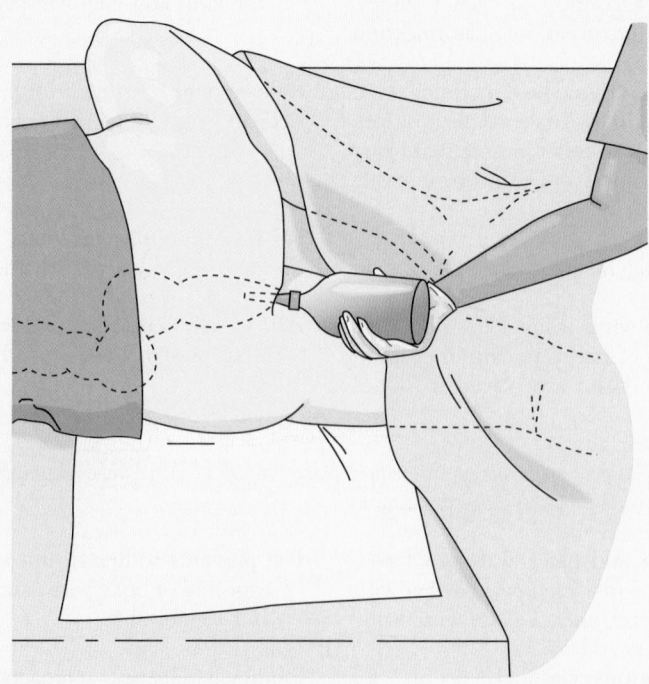

STEP 10a(4)   With patient in left lateral Sims' position, insert tip of commercial enema into rectum. (*From Sorrentino SA:* Mosby's textbook for nursing assistants, *ed 7, St Louis, 2009, Mosby.*)

STEP	RATIONALE
(5) Lubricate 6 to 8 cm (2½ to 3 inches) of tip of rectal tube with lubricant.	Allows smooth insertion of rectal tube without risk for irritation or trauma to mucosa.
(6) Gently separate buttocks and locate anus. Instruct patient to relax by breathing out slowly through mouth. Touch patient's skin next to anus with tip of rectal tube.	Breathing out and touching skin with tube promotes relaxation of external anal sphincter.
(7) Insert tip of rectal tube slowly by pointing it in direction of patient's umbilicus. Length of insertion varies (see Step 10a[4]).	Careful insertion prevents trauma to rectal mucosa from accidental lodging of tube against rectal wall. Insertion beyond proper limit can cause bowel perforation.

Clinical Decision Point *If tube does not pass easily, do not force. Consider allowing a small amount of fluid to infuse and then try to reinsert the tube slowly. The instillation of fluid relaxes the sphincter and provides additional lubrication. Remove an impaction (see Skill 34-2) before administering the enema.*

(8) Hold tubing in rectum constantly until end of fluid instillation.	Prevents expulsion of rectal tube during bowel contractions.
(9) Open regulating clamp and allow solution to enter slowly with container at patient's hip level.	Rapid infusion stimulates evacuation of tubing and can cause cramping.
(10) Raise height of enema container slowly to appropriate level above anus: 30 to 45 cm (12 to 18 inches) for high enema; 30 cm (12 inches) for regular enema (see illustration); 7.5 cm (3 inches) for low enema. Instillation time varies with volume of solution administered (e.g., 1 L may take 10 minutes). You may use an IV pole to hold an enema bag once you get a slow flow of fluid established.	Allows for continuous, slow instillation of solution. Raising container too high causes rapid instillation and possible painful distention of colon. High pressure causes rupture of bowel in infant.

Clinical Decision Point *Temporary cessation of infusion minimizes cramping and promotes ability to retain solution. Lower container or clamp tubing if patient complains of cramping or if fluid escapes around rectal tube.*

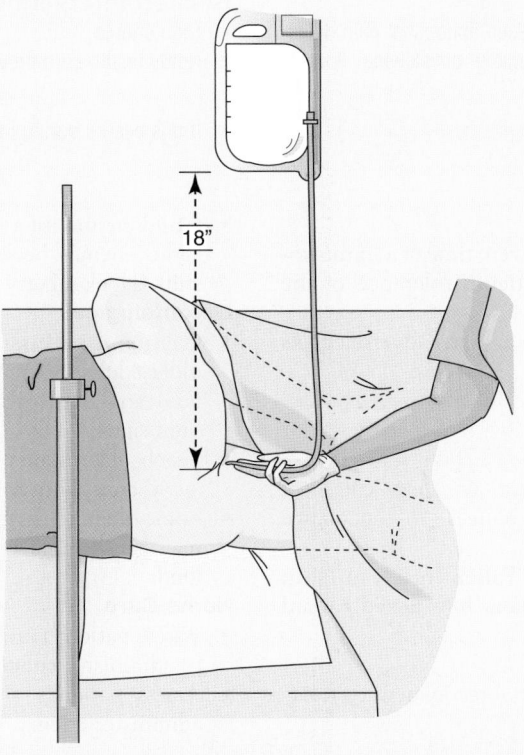

STEP 10b(10)   IV pole is positioned so the bottom of the enema bag is 18 inches above the anus.

STEP	RATIONALE
(11) Instill all solution and clamp tubing. Tell patient that procedure is completed and that you will be removing tubing.	Prevents entrance of air into rectum. Patients may misinterpret sensation of removing tube as loss of control.
11 Place layers of toilet tissue around tube at anus and gently withdraw rectal tube and tip.	Provides for patient's comfort and cleanliness.
12 Explain to patient that some distention and abdominal cramping is normal. Ask him or her to retain solution as long as possible until urge to defecate occurs. This usually takes a few minutes. Stay at bedside. Have patient lie quietly in bed if possible. (For infant or young child gently hold buttocks together for few minutes.)	Solution distends bowel. Length of retention varies with type of enema and patient's ability to contract rectal sphincter. Longer retention promotes stimulation of peristalsis and defecation.
13 Discard enema container and tubing in proper receptacle.	Reduces transmission and growth of microorganisms.
14 Help patient to bathroom or commode if possible. If using bedpan, help to as near normal position for evacuation as possible (see Skill 34-1).	Normal squatting position promotes defecation.
15 Observe character of stool and solution (caution patient against flushing toilet before inspection).	Determines if enema was effective.
16 Help patient as needed to wash anal area with warm soap and water (if nurse administers perineal care, use gloves).	Fecal contents irritate skin. Hygiene promotes patient's comfort.
17 Remove and discard gloves and perform hand hygiene.	Reduces transmission of microorganisms.

EVALUATION

1 Inspect color, consistency, and amount of stool; odor; and fluid passed.	Determines if stool is evacuated or fluid is retained. Note abnormalities such as presence of blood or mucus.
2 Assess for abdominal distention.	Determines if distention is relieved.

Unexpected Outcomes

1 Severe abdominal cramping, bleeding, or sudden abdominal pain develops and is unrelieved by temporarily stopping or slowing flow of solution.

2 Patient is unable to hold enema solution.

Related Interventions

- Stop enema.
- Notify health care provider.

- If this occurs during installation, slow rate of infusion.

Recording and Reporting

- Record the type and volume of enema given, time of administration, characteristics of results, and patient's tolerance of the procedure.
- Report the failure of patient to defecate and any adverse effects to health care provider.

Special Considerations

Teaching

- Instruct patient that enemas are not to treat cause of constipation. Instruct in lifestyle changes to encourage peristalsis.
- Instruct patient in self-administration. Patient needs to lie in dorsal recumbent position with knees and hips flexed toward chest.

Pediatric

- The use of oral stool softeners is the initial recommended treatment of constipation in children.

- Children and infants usually do not receive prepackaged hypertonic enemas because hypertonic solutions cause rapid fluid shift (Hockenberry and Wilson, 2011).

Gerontological

- Caution is necessary when enemas are ordered "until clear" in older adults. Some older adults become fatigued, are at risk for fluid and electrolyte imbalances, and experience changes in vital signs.
- Teach older adults and their caregivers how to modify diet to avoid constipation.
- Some older adults may have difficulty retaining fluid. The nurse may gently hold buttocks together to help with retention of fluid.

Home Care

- Assess patient's and primary caregiver's ability and motivation to administer enema and provide instruction as needed.
- Assess patient's ability to manipulate equipment and self-administer enema.

SKILL 34-4 Insertion, Maintenance, and Removal of a Nasogastric Tube for Gastric Decompression

There are times following major surgery or with conditions affecting the gastrointestinal (GI) tract when normal peristalsis is temporarily altered. Because peristalsis is slowed or absent, a patient cannot eat or drink fluids without causing abdominal distention. The temporary insertion of a nasogastric (NG) tube into the stomach serves to decompress the stomach, keeping it empty until normal peristalsis returns.

An NG tube is a pliable tube inserted through the patient's nasopharynx into the stomach. The tube is hollow, which allows for the removal of gastric secretions and the introduction of solutions into the stomach. There are times when an NG tube is used for enteral feedings, but a softer small-bore feeding tube is preferred for feeding purposes (see Chapter 31). The Levin and Salem sump tubes are the most common for stomach decompression. The Levin tube is a single-lumen tube with holes near the tip (Fig. 34-6). You connect the tube to a drainage bag or an intermittent suction device to drain stomach secretions. The Salem sump tube is preferable for stomach decompression. The tube has two lumens: one for removal of gastric contents and one to provide an air vent, which prevents suctioning of gastric mucosa into eyelets at the distal tip of a tube. A blue "pigtail" is the air vent that connects with the second lumen (Fig. 34-7). When the main lumen of the sump tube is connected to suction, the air vent permits free, continuous drainage of secretions. *Never clamp off the air vent, connect to suction, or use for irrigation.* The health care provider orders the suction setting, which is usually low intermittent.

NG tube insertion uses clean technique. The procedure is uncomfortable, with patients experiencing a burning sensation as the tube passes through the sensitive nasal mucosa. One of the greatest nursing care challenges is keeping a patient comfortable because the tube is a constant irritation to mucosa. Routinely assess the condition of the nares and mucosa for inflammation and excoriation. Supportive care includes changing soiled tape or fixation devices, keeping the nares lubricated and clean, and providing frequent mouth care to minimize the dehydration from mouth breathing.

Delegation and Collaboration

The skill of inserting and maintaining an NG tube cannot be delegated to nursing assistive personnel (NAP). The nurse directs the NAP to:
- Measure and record the drainage from an NG tube.
- Provide oral and nasal hygiene measures.
- Perform selected comfort measures such as positioning or offering ice chips if allowed.
- Anchor the tube to patient's gown during routine care to prevent accidental displacement.

Equipment

- ❏ 14- or 16-Fr NG tube (Smaller-lumen catheters are not used for decompression in adults because they must be able to remove thick secretions.)
- ❏ Water-soluble lubricant
- ❏ pH test strips (measure gastric aspirate acidity); use paper with a range of at least 1.0 to 11.0 or higher
- ❏ Tongue blade
- ❏ Flashlight
- ❏ Emesis basin
- ❏ Asepto bulb or catheter-tipped syringe
- ❏ 2.5-cm (1-inch)–wide hypoallergenic tape or commercial fixation device
- ❏ Safety pin and rubber band
- ❏ Clamp, drainage bag, or suction machine with pressure gauge if wall suction is to be used
- ❏ Towel
- ❏ Glass of water with straw
- ❏ Facial tissues
- ❏ Normal saline
- ❏ Tincture of benzoin (*optional*)
- ❏ Suction equipment
- ❏ Stethoscope
- ❏ Clean gloves

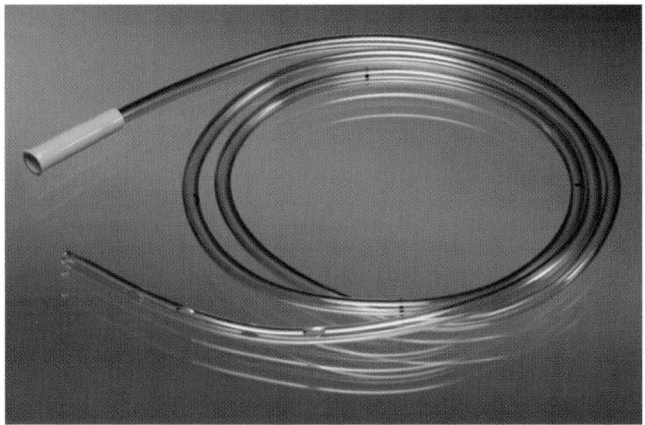

FIG 34-6 Levin tube. (*Courtesy Bard Medical, Covington, Ga.*)

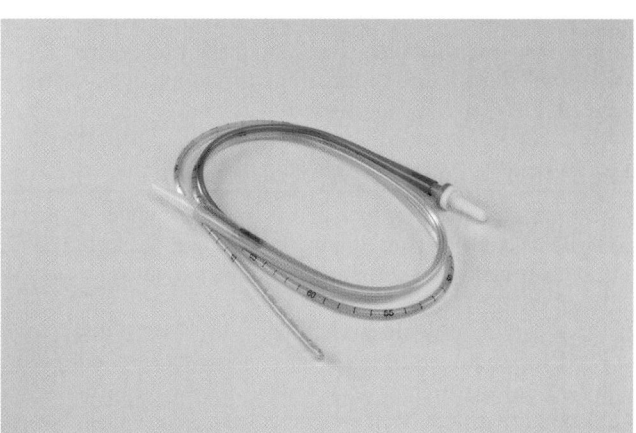

FIG 34-7 Salem sump tube. (*Courtesy Covidien, Mansfield, Mass.*)

STEP	RATIONALE
ASSESSMENT	
1 Inspect condition of patient's nasal and oral cavity.	Determines need for special nursing hygiene measures after tube placement.
2 Ask if patient has had history of nasal surgery or congestion and allergies and note if deviated nasal septum is present.	Alerts nurse to potential obstruction. Insert tube into *uninvolved* nasal passage. Procedure may be contraindicated if surgery is recent.
3 Auscultate for bowel sounds. Palpate patient's abdomen for distention, pain, and rigidity.	In presence of diminished or absent bowel sounds, auscultate abdomen at least 1 minute in each quadrant (Seidel et al., 2011). Documents baseline for any abdominal distention, GI ileus, and general GI function, which later serves as comparison once tube is inserted.
4 Assess patient's level of consciousness and ability to follow instructions.	Determines patient's ability to assist in procedure.

Clinical Decision Point *If patient is confused, disoriented, or unable to follow commands, obtain assistance from another staff member to insert the tube.*

STEP	RATIONALE
5 Determine if patient had previous NG tube and, if so, which naris was used.	Patient's previous experience complements any explanations and prepares patient for NG tube placement.
6 Verify health care provider order for type of NG tube to be placed and whether tube is to be attached to suction or drainage bag.	Requires order from health care provider. Adequate decompression depends on NG suction.

NURSING DIAGNOSES

- Acute pain
- Deficient knowledge regarding purpose of gastric decompression
- Dysfunctional gastrointestinal motility
- Impaired oral mucous membrane
- Risk for impaired skin integrity

Related factors are individualized based on patient's condition or needs.

STEP	RATIONALE
PLANNING	
1 Expected outcomes following completion of procedure:	
• Abdomen is soft, nontender, and without distention.	Correctly positioned NG tube remains patent, drains gastric secretions, and relieves gastric distention.
• Patient's nares and nasal mucosa remain clear, without abrasions or excoriation.	Ensures absence of irritation from NG tube.
• Patient's level of comfort improves or remains the same.	Correctly inserted NG tube prevents abdominal discomfort from progressing.
2 Inform patient that procedure may make him or her gag and there will be a burning sensation in nasopharynx as tube is passed. Develop hand signal with patient.	Increases patient's cooperation and ability to anticipate nurse's action. If patient is unable to tolerate procedure, use of hand signal will alert nurse.

STEP	RATIONALE
IMPLEMENTATION	
1 Identify patient using two identifiers (i.e., name and birthday or name and account number) according to agency policy. Compare identifiers with information on patient's identification bracelet.	Ensures correct patient. Complies with The Joint Commission standards and improves patient safety (TJC, 2012).
2 Place patient in high-Fowler's position. Place pillows behind head and shoulders. Raise bed to horizontal level comfortable for accessing patient.	Promotes patient's ability to swallow during procedure. Good body mechanics prevent injury to you or patient.
3 Place bath towel over patient's chest; give facial tissues to patient. Allow to blow nose if necessary. Place emesis basin within reach.	Prevents soiling of patient's gown. Tube insertion through nasal passages may cause tearing and coughing with increased salivation.
4 Pull curtain around bed or close room door.	Provides privacy.
5 Wash bridge of nose with soap and water or alcohol swab.	Removes oils from nose to allow tape to adhere.
6 Stand on patient's right side if right-handed, left side if left-handed. Lower side rail.	Allows easiest manipulation of tubing.

STEP	RATIONALE
7 Instruct patient to relax and breathe normally while occluding one naris. Then repeat this action for other naris. Select nostril with greater airflow.	Tube passes more easily through naris that is more patent.

8 Measure distance to insert tube:
  a Traditional method:
    Measure distance from tip of nose, to earlobe, and to xiphoid process (see illustration).
  b Hanson method:
    First mark 50-cm (20-inch) point on tube and measure traditionally. Tube insertion should be to midway point between 50 cm (20 inches) and traditional mark.
	Approximates distance from naris to stomach; distance varies with each patient. Tube tip should enter stomach.

9 With small piece of tape placed around tube, mark length that will be inserted.	Indicates length of tube you will insert.
10 Perform hand hygiene and apply clean gloves. Curve 10 to 15 cm (4 to 6 inches) of end of tube tightly around index finger and release.	Aids insertion and decreases stiffness of tube.
11 Lubricate 7.5 to 10 cm (3 to 4 inches) of end of tube with water-soluble lubricant.	Minimizes friction against nasal mucosa and aids insertion of tube. Water-soluble lubricant is less toxic than oil-soluble lubricant if aspirated.
12 Alert patient when procedure will begin.	Decreases patient anxiety and increases patient cooperation.
13 Initially instruct patient to extend neck back against pillow; insert tube gently and slowly through naris with curved end pointing downward.	Facilitates initial passage of tube through naris and maintains clear airway for open naris.
14 Continue to pass tube along floor of nasal passage, aiming down toward patient's ear. If resistance occurs, apply gentle downward pressure to advance tube (do not force past resistance).	Minimizes discomfort of tube rubbing against upper nasal turbinates. Resistance is caused by posterior nasopharynx. Downward pressure helps tube curl around corner of nasopharynx.
15 If there is continued resistance, try to rotate tube and see if it advances. If still resistant, withdraw it, allow patient to rest, lubricate it again, and insert into other naris.	Forcing against resistance causes trauma to mucosa. Allowing patient to rest helps relieve anxiety.

Clinical Decision Point *If unable to insert tube in either naris, stop procedure and notify health care provider.*

STEP	RATIONALE
16 Continue insertion of tube until just past nasopharynx by gently rotating it toward opposite naris. **a** Once past nasopharynx, stop tube advancement, allow patient to relax, and provide tissues.	Relieves patient's anxiety; tearing is natural response to mucosal irritation, and excessive salivation may occur because of oral stimulation.
b Explain to patient that next step requires him or her to swallow. Give patient glass of water unless contraindicated.	Sipping water aids passage of NG tube into esophagus.
17 With tube just above oropharynx, instruct patient to flex head forward, take a small sip of water, and swallow. Advance tube 2.5 to 5 cm (1 to 2 inches) with each swallow of water. If patient is not allowed fluids, instruct to dry swallow or suck air through straw. Advance tube with each swallow.	Flexed position closes off upper airway to trachea and opens esophagus. Swallowing closes epiglottis over trachea and helps move tube into esophagus. Swallowing water reduces gagging or choking. Remove water from stomach by suction after insertion.

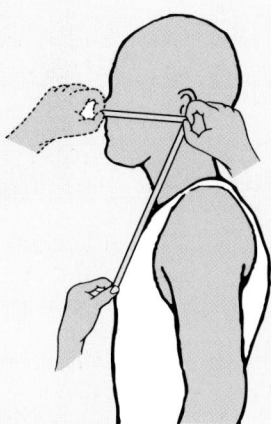

STEP 8a   Technique for measuring distance to insert NG tube.

STEP	RATIONALE
18 If patient begins to cough, gag, or choke, withdraw tube slightly and stop advancement. Instruct patient to breathe easily and take sips of water.	Cough reflex is initiated when tube accidentally enters larynx. Withdrawal of tube reduces risk for laryngeal entry. Small sips of water frequently reduce gagging. Give water cautiously to reduce risk for aspiration.

Clinical Decision Point *If vomiting occurs, help patient clear airway. Perform oral suctioning as needed.*

STEP	RATIONALE
19 If patient continues to cough during insertion, pull tube back slightly.	Tube may enter larynx and obstruct airway.
20 If patient continues to gag and cough or complains that tube feels as though it is coiling behind throat, check back of oropharynx using flashlight and tongue blade. Withdraw tube until tip is back in oropharynx if coiled. Reinsert with patient swallowing.	Tube may coil around itself in back of throat and stimulate gag reflex.
21 After patient relaxes, continue to advance tube with swallowing until you reach tape or mark on tube that signifies that tube is in the desired distance. Temporarily anchor tube to patient's cheek with piece of tape until tube placement is verified.	Tip of tube needs to be within stomach to decompress properly. Anchoring tube prevents accidental displacement while tube placement is verified.
22 Verify tube placement. Check agency policy for preferred methods for checking tube placement.	
a Ask patient to talk.	Patient is unable to talk if NG tube has passed through vocal cords.
b Inspect posterior pharynx for presence of coiled tube.	Tube is pliable and will coil up behind pharynx instead of advancing into esophagus.
c Place towel under end of NG tube and attach Asepto or catheter-tipped syringe to end of tube. Aspirate gently back on syringe to obtain gastric contents, observing color (see illustration).	Gastric contents are usually grassy green, clear, and odorless. Postpyloric tube placement appears golden yellow, yellow-brown, or greenish brown with pH of greater than 6.0 (Hockenberry and Wilson, 2011; Lewis et al., 2011).
d Use gastric (Gastroccult) pH paper to measure aspirate for pH with color-coded pH paper. Be sure that paper range of pH is at least from 1.0 to 11.0 or greater (see illustration).	Gastric aspirates have decidedly acidic pH values typically less than 5.0 (Durai, Venkatraman, and Ng, 2009; Hockenberry and Wilson, 2011). Respiratory secretions are usually greater than 6.0.
e Obtain x-ray film examination of chest and abdomen as ordered.	Radiography is gold standard to verify initial placement of tube (Farrington et al., 2009; Hockenberry and Wilson, 2011; Lewis et al., 2011).
f If tube is not in stomach, advance another 2.5 to 5 cm (1 to 2 inches) and repeat Steps 22a-d to check tube position and verify with radiography.	Tube must be in stomach to provide decompression.

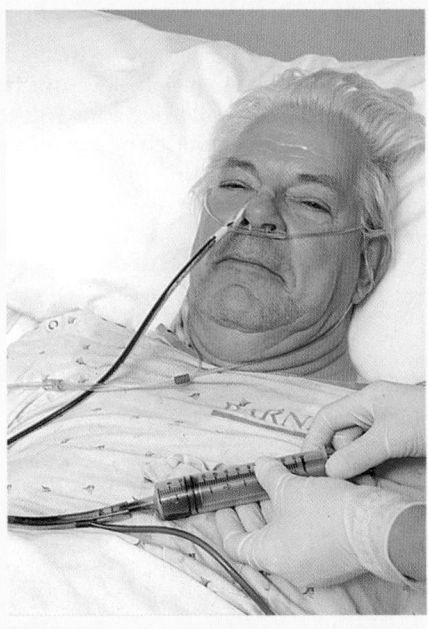

STEP 22c   Aspiration of gastric contents.

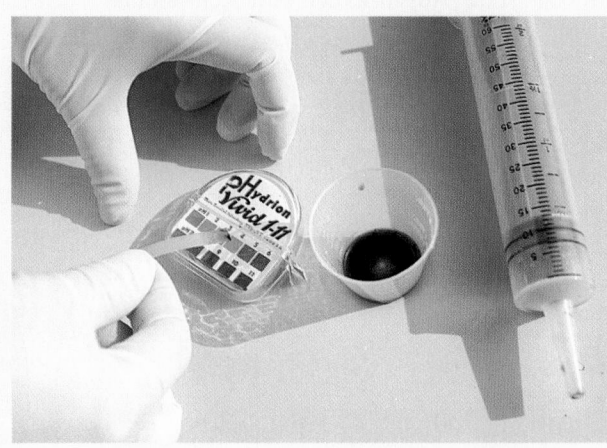

STEP 22d   Checking pH of gastric aspirate.

STEP	RATIONALE
23 Anchor tube.	
a Clamp end of tube or connect tube to drainage bag or suction machine after properly inserted.	Use gravity for drainage bag. Intermittent suction is most effective for decompression. Patient going to operating room often has tube clamped.
b Tape tube to nose; avoid putting pressure on nares.	Prevents tissue necrosis. Tape anchors tube securely.
(1) Cut strip of tape about 10 cm (5 inches) and split down the middle halfway.	
(2) Apply small amount of tincture of benzoin to lower end of nose and allow drying before taping tube to nose *(optional)*. Apply prepared tape to nose, leaving split end free. Be sure that top end of tape over nose is secure.	Benzoin prevents loosening of tape if patient perspires or has oily skin.
(3) Carefully wrap two split ends of tape around tube in opposite directions (see illustrations).	
(4) *Alternative*: Apply tube fixation device using shaped adhesive patch (see illustration).	
c Fasten end of NG tube to patient's gown by looping rubber band around tube in slipknot. Pin rubber band to gown.	Reduces pressure on nares if tube moves. Provides slack for movement without dislodging NG tube.
d When using Salem sump tube, keep pigtail above level of stomach.	Prevents siphoning action that clogs tube.
24 Unless health care provider orders otherwise, elevate head of bed 30 degrees.	Helps prevent esophageal reflux and minimizes irritation of tube against posterior pharynx.
25 Explain to patient that sensation of tube in back of throat decreases somewhat with time.	Helps patient to adapt to continued sensory stimulus.

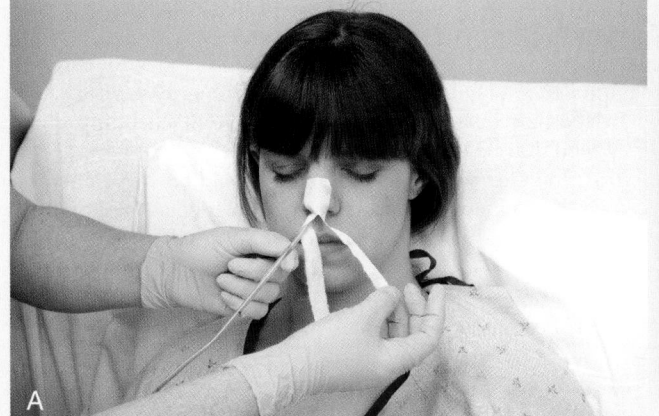 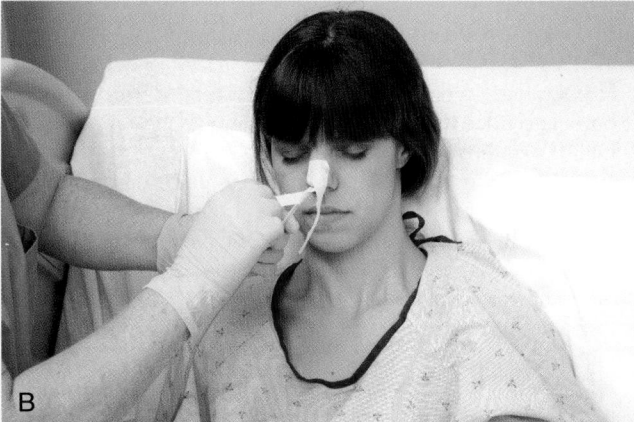

STEP 23b(3)   **A** and **B**, Tape is crossed over and around NG tube.

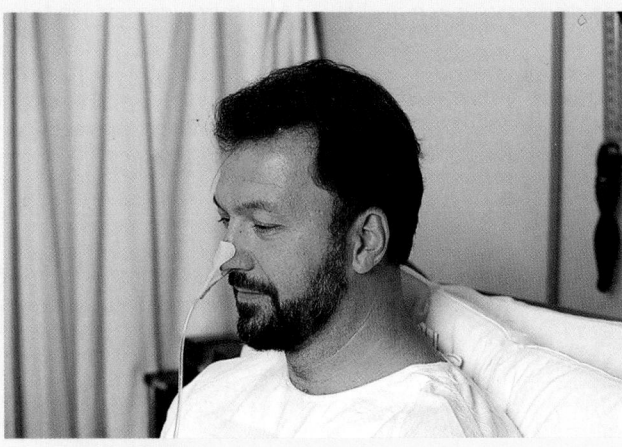

STEP 23b(4)   Patient with tube fixation device.

STEP	RATIONALE

26 Once placement is confirmed:
  a Make either a red mark or use tape on tube to indicate where tube exits nose.
  b *Alternative*: Measure length of tube from nares to connector.
  c Document length of tube in patient's record.
	Mark on tube or tape is guide to indicate continuous correct tube placement.
	
	Information helps to determine tube placement.

Clinical Decision Point *Never reposition an NG tube of a gastric surgical patient, because positioning could rupture the suture line.*

STEP	RATIONALE
27 Attach NG tube to suction as ordered.	Suction setting is usually ordered low intermittent, which decreases gastric irritation from NG tube.

Clinical Decision Point *If lumen of tube is narrow and secretions are thick, NG tube will not drain as desired. Irrigate tube (Step 28). Consult with health care provider for higher suction setting if unable to irrigate tube because of thick secretions.*

STEP	RATIONALE

28 NG tube irrigation:
  a Perform hand hygiene and apply clean gloves.
  b Check for tube placement in stomach (see Step 22). Temporarily clamp tube or reconnect to connecting tube and remove syringe.
  c Draw up 30 mL of normal saline into Asepto or catheter-tip syringe.
  d Clamp NG tube. Disconnect from connecting tubing and lay end of connection tubing on towel.
  e Insert tip of irrigating syringe into end of NG tube. Remove clamp. Hold syringe with tip pointed at floor and inject saline slowly and evenly. Do not force solution.
	Reduces transmission of microorganisms.
	Prevents accidental entrance of irrigating solution into lungs.
	
	Use of saline minimizes loss of electrolytes from stomach fluids.
	
	Reduces soiling of patient's gown and bed linen.
	
	Position of syringe prevents introduction of air into vent tubing, which causes gastric distention. Solution introduced under pressure causes gastric trauma.

Clinical Decision Point *Do not introduce saline through blue "pigtail" air vent of Salem sump tube.*

STEP	RATIONALE

f If resistance occurs, check for kinks in tubing. Turn patient onto left side. Repeated resistance should be reported to health care provider.
  g After instilling saline, immediately aspirate or pull back slowly on syringe to withdraw fluid. If amount aspirated is greater than amount instilled, record difference as output. If amount aspirated is less than amount instilled, record difference as intake.
  h Use an Asepto syringe to place 10 mL of air into blue pigtail.
  i Reconnect NG tube to drainage or suction. (Repeat irrigation if solution does not return.)
29 Removal of NG tube:
  a Verify order to remove NG tube.
  b Auscultate abdomen for presence of bowel sounds.
  c Explain procedure to patient and reassure that removal is less distressing than insertion.
  d Perform hand hygiene and apply clean gloves.
  e Turn off suction and disconnect NG tube from drainage bag or suction. With irrigating syringe, insert 20 mL of air into lumen of NG tube. Remove tape or fixation device from bridge of nose and unpin tube from gown.
  f Stand on patient's right side if right-handed, left side if left-handed.
  g Hand patient facial tissue; place clean towel across chest. Instruct patient to take and hold breath.
	Tip of tube may lie against stomach lining. Repositioning on left side may dislodge tube away from stomach lining. Buildup of secretions causes distention.
	Irrigation clears tubing so stomach should remain empty. Measure and document irrigation inserted in tube as intake.
	
	Ensures patency of air vent.
	
	Reestablishes drainage collection; may repeat irrigation or repositioning of tube until NG tube drains properly.
	
	An order is required for procedure.
	Verifies return of peristalsis.
	Minimizes anxiety and increases cooperation. Tube passes out smoothly.
	Reduces transmission of microorganisms.
	Have tube free of connections before removal. Clears gastric fluids from tube to prevent aspiration of contents or soiling of clothing and bedding.
	
	Allows easiest manipulation of tube.
	
	Some patients wish to blow nose after tube is removed. Towel keeps gown from soiling. Temporary airway obstruction occurs during tube removal.

STEP	RATIONALE
h Clamp or kink tubing securely and pull tube out steadily and smoothly into towel held in other hand while patient holds breath.	Clamping prevents tube contents from draining into oropharynx. Reduces trauma to mucosa and minimizes patient's discomfort. Towel covers tube, which is an unpleasant sight. Holding breath helps to prevent aspiration.
i Inspect intactness of tube.	
j Measure amount of drainage and note character of content. Dispose of tube and drainage equipment into proper container.	Provides accurate measure of fluid output. Reduces transfer of microorganisms.
k Clean nares and provide mouth care.	Promotes comfort.
l Position patient comfortably and explain procedure for drinking fluids if not contraindicated. Instruct patient to notify you if nausea occurs.	Sometimes patients are not allowed anything by mouth (NPO) for up to 24 hours. When fluids are allowed, orders usually begin with small amount of ice chips each hour and increase as patient is able to tolerate more.
30 For all procedures, clean equipment and return to proper place. Place soiled linen in utility room or proper receptacle.	Proper disposal of equipment prevents spread of microorganisms and ensures proper exchange procedures.
31 Remove and discard gloves and perform hand hygiene.	Reduces transmission of microorganisms.

EVALUATION

1 Observe amount and character of contents draining from NG tube. Ask if patient feels nauseated.	Determines if tube is decompressing stomach of contents.
2 Auscultate for presence of bowel sounds. Turn off suction while auscultating.	Sound of suction apparatus is sometimes misinterpreted as bowel sounds.
3 Palpate patient's abdomen periodically. Note any distention, pain, and rigidity.	Determines success of abdominal decompression and return of peristalsis.
4 Inspect condition of nares and nose.	Evaluates onset of skin and tissue irritation.
5 Observe position of tubing.	Prevents tension applied to nasal structures.
6 Ask if patient feels sore throat or irritation in pharynx.	Evaluates level of patient's discomfort.

Unexpected Outcomes

	Related Interventions
1 Patient's abdomen is distended and painful.	• Assess patency of tube. NG tube may not be in stomach. • Irrigate tube. • Verify that suction is on as ordered. • Notify health care provider if distention is unrelieved.
2 Patient complains of sore throat from dry, irritated mucous membranes.	• Perform oral hygiene more frequently. • Ask health care provider whether patient can suck on ice chips, throat lozenges, or local anesthetic medication.
3 Patient develops irritation or erosion of skin around naris.	• Provide frequent skin care to area. • Tape tube on naris to avoid pressure. • Consider switching tube to other naris.
4 Patient develops signs and symptoms of pulmonary aspiration: fever, shortness of breath, or pulmonary congestion.	• Perform complete respiratory assessment. • Notify health care provider. • Obtain chest x-ray film examination as ordered.

Recording and Reporting

- Record length, size, and type of gastric tube inserted and in which naris it was inserted. In addition, record patient's tolerance of procedure, confirmation of tube placement, character of gastric contents, pH value, results of radiography, whether the tube is clamped or connected to drainage bag or to suction, and amount of suction supplied.
- Record difference between amount of normal saline instilled and amount of gastric aspirate removed on intake and output (I&O) sheet. Record the amount and character of contents draining from NG tube every shift.

- Record removal of tube "intact," patient's tolerance of procedure, and final amount and character of drainage.

Special Considerations

Gerontologic

- Check for ill-fitting dentures and remove them for patient's safety and comfort during the insertion.
- Oral and nasal mucosal drying is sometimes present. Adequately lubricate the tube for insertion.

Critical Thinking Exercises

Mr. Simon, a 66-year-old man with a history of severe osteoarthritis, is hospitalized following a total right knee replacement performed 2 days ago. At present he is allowed touch-down weight bearing on his right leg. Mr. Simon's last bowel movement was the day before surgery; thus he has gone 3 days without a bowel movement. Since surgery he received pain medication (an opioid) through his intravenous (IV) line and began taking oral pain medication last night.

His abdomen is nontender, slightly distended, with active bowel sounds in all four quadrants. He attempted a bowel movement with a great deal of straining and expelled small, hard, brown stool. You've talked to the primary care provider and obtained orders for a Fleet enema.

1. You've explained the enema procedure to Mr. Simon and have prepared your supplies. You need to provide a bedpan or commode for Mr. Simon to expel the fecal material following the enema. Make your selection of the type of bedpan or use of commode and provide the rationale.

2. What is the expected outcome of the Fleet enema? Which, if any, instructions will you give to the nursing assistive personnel (NAP)?

3. The NAP just reported to you that Mr. Simon is complaining of stomach pain. Which of the following are correct actions to take? Prioritize your selection.
   a. Notify the health care provider.
   b. Instruct the NAP to palpate Mr. Simon's abdomen.
   c. Give postoperative pain medication as ordered.
   d. Perform an abdominal assessment.
   e. Obtain vital signs (VSs) and instruct the NAP to obtain them every 15 to 30 minutes thereafter.

4. Two days later Mr. Simon has the same symptoms as before receiving the enema. This time he has liquid stool seeping from the rectum. You obtain an order to check for an impaction. You explain the procedure to Mr. Simon and begin the skill as required. As you are removing stool, the NAP who is helping you by monitoring Mr. Simon's vital signs reports that his pulse is 48 beats/min. What does this indicate, and how do you proceed?

REVIEW QUESTIONS

1. One risk associated with digital removal of impacted stool is stimulation of the vagus nerve. The nurse should monitor a patient for which adverse effect?
   1. Urinary incontinence
   2. An elevated pulse rate
   3. Abdominal cramping
   4. A drop in the heart rate

2. During insertion of a nasogastric tube, the nurse has a patient swallow. What is the rationale for swallowing?
   1. It prevents stimulation of the gag reflex.
   2. It closes off the upper airway so the tube enters the esophagus.
   3. It facilitates the tube passing through the nasal passages.
   4. It helps to distract the patient during the procedure.

3. The nurse is placing a bedpan under a frail, immobile female patient. The nurse's actions are appropriate if which method is followed?
   1. Sliding the bedpan under her
   2. Rolling her onto a fracture bedpan
   3. Shove the bedpan under her
   4. Keep her flat after rolling her on the bedpan

4. A patient has an order for enemas "until clear" in preparation for bowel surgery. Which information in a patient's medical record would cause the nurse to question the health care provider's order?
   1. Hemorrhoid surgery 5 weeks ago
   2. Periodic fecal incontinence
   3. Taking medication for an enlarged prostate
   4. A history of glaucoma

5. A patient who had intestinal surgery yesterday has a nasogastric tube for gastric decompression. The patient is nauseated, and his abdomen is distended. The nurse irrigated the tube but met resistance. Which action should the nurse take?
   1. Irrigate the tube again with more normal saline
   2. Turn patient onto left side
   3. Advance the tube several inches
   4. Turn the suction on continuous instead of intermittent

6. The nurse is assessing the abdomen of a patient who is 3 days postoperative from shoulder surgery. The nurse palpates a boggy mass in the transverse colon. In collaborating with the health care provider, which action would the nurse expect to take next?
   1. Administer a Fleet enema
   2. Obtain an x-ray film of the abdomen
   3. Remove the fecal impaction digitally
   4. Wait to see if the patient develops abdominal pain

7. The nurse is assessing a patient's normal bowel elimination habits and anticipating his needs. When should the patient be offered the bedpan?
   1. At bedtime
   2. First thing in the morning
   3. After eating a midday snack
   4. Approximately an hour after breakfast

8. After placing a mobile patient on the bedpan, how high should the nurse place the head of the bed?
   1. 15 to 30 degrees
   2. 30 to 60 degrees
   3. 60 to 90 degrees
   4. Keep the head of the bed flat

9. The nurse is caring for an elderly patient who needs to use a bedpan. Which of the following comfort measures should the nurse use for proper positioning and general comfort? (Select all that apply.)
   1. Keep the head of the bed flat
   2. Place toilet tissue within reach
   3. Stay with patient while using the bedpan
   4. Place a small pillow under lumbar curve in the back
   5. Place the head of the bed at 45-degree angle

10. The nurse has several activities to perform. Which can be delegated to the NAP? (Select all that apply.)
    1. Administering an enema
    2. Removing a fecal impaction
    3. Placing a patient on a bedpan
    4. Inserting a nasogastric (NG) tube
    5. Providing oral care for a patient with a NG tube

REFERENCES

Banning M: Aging and the gut, *Nurs Older People* 20(1):17, 2008.

Chien D: Acquired fecal incontinence in community-dwelling adults, *Nurse Pract* 35(1):15, 2010.

Cohen S: Orthopaedic patient's perceptions of using a bedpan, *J Orthop Nurs* 13(3):784, 2009.

Durai M, Venkatraman R, Ng P: Nasogastric tubes 1: insertion technique and confirming the correct position, *Nurs Times* 105(16):12, 2009.

Farrington M et al: Nasogastric tube placement verification in pediatric and neonatal patients, *Pediatr Nurs* 35(1):17, 2009.

Hockenberry MJ, Wilson D: *Wong's nursing care of infants and children*, ed 9, St Louis, 2011, Mosby.

Kyle G: Constipation, part I: causes and assessment, *Practice Nurs* 20(12):611, 2009.

Leung F, Rao S: Fecal incontinence in the elderly, *Gastroenterol Clin North Am* 38:530, 2009.

Lewis S, et al: *Medical-surgical nursing: assessment and management of clinical problems*, ed 8, St Louis, 2011, Mosby.

Linari L et al: Implementing a bowel program: is a bowel program an effective way of preventing constipation and ileus following elective hip and knee arthroplasty surgery? *Orthopaed Nurs* 30(5):317, 2011.

Ostaszkiewicz J et al: The effects of conservative treatment for constipation on symptom severity and quality of life in community-dwelling adults, *J Wound Ostomy Continence Nurs* 37(2):193, 2010.

Seidel HM et al: *Mosby's guide to physical examination*, ed 7, St Louis, 2011, Mosby.

The Joint Commission (TJC): *National Patient Safety Goals*, Oakbrook Terrace, Ill, 2012, The Commission, available at http://www.jointcommission.org/standards_information/npsgs.aspx.

Touhy T: *Ebersole and Hess's gerontological nursing and healthy aging*, ed 3, St Louis, 2010, Mosby.

Ostomy Care

MEDIA RESOURCES

- ⓔvolve *learning system* http://evolve.elsevier.com/Perry/skills
  - Review Questions
  - ▶ Video Clips
  - Audio Glossary

- NSO Nursing Skills Online

KEY TERMS

Colostomy	Ileal conduit	Ostomy	Stoma
Continent fecal diversion	Ileostomy	Peristomal	Urinary stent
Continent urinary diversion	Orthotopic neobladder	Skin barrier	Urostomy
Effluent			

OBJECTIVES

Mastery of content in this chapter will enable the nurse to:
- Identify the types of fecal and urinary diversions.
- Explain the differences in color and consistency of effluent based on the type of ostomy.

- Pouch a fecal or urinary diversion.
- Describe methods used to maintain integrity of the peristomal skin.
- Catheterize a urinary diversion.

Certain diseases or conditions require surgical intervention to create an opening into the abdominal wall for fecal or urinary elimination. Examples of these conditions include cancer, inflammatory bowel disease, perforation of the colon, or fecal incontinence. The opening is called a *stoma* and is constructed from a section of colon or small intestine. The output from the stoma is called the *effluent*. An opening in the large intestine or colon is a colostomy. A colostomy in the descending or sigmoid colon (Fig. 35-1) generally results in a stool similar to that normally passed through the rectum. If the opening is in the transverse or ascending colon, the effluent varies from thick liquid to semiformed stool. An opening in the ileal portion of the small intestine is an ileostomy (Fig. 35-2), and the fecal effluent will be watery-to-thick liquid and contain some digestive enzymes. Fecal ostomies are either temporary or permanent, depending on the underlying condition and the surgical procedure performed.

A urostomy or ileal conduit (Fig. 35-3) is created from a portion of the intestine that is resected from the ileum. One end of the conduit is sutured closed, and the ureters are implanted through the mucosa. The other end is brought out on the abdominal wall, and a stoma is formed for urine to exit

the body. This ostomy is permanent. A patient with a colostomy, ileostomy, or ileal conduit has no sensation or control over the time or frequency of the output and must wear a pouch to collect the effluent.

Surgical procedures to create continent internal fecal or urinary pouches eliminate the need for an external pouch. The continent ileostomy is a pouch made from a segment of the ileum and placed under the abdominal wall, with a small tract from the pouch opening through the skin. A patient inserts a large catheter through this opening or stoma several times a day to empty fecal effluent in the internal pouch. These procedures are done less frequently now because there are other surgical options available with higher long-term success rates. In the ileal pouch anal anastomosis the surgeon creates an internal reservoir from a segment of the ileum that is then connected to the anal canal above the anal sphincter (Fig. 35-4). The patient will usually have four to six bowel movements per day. Most frequently the surgeon will perform a temporary ileostomy to allow the reservoir to heal.

There are also two types of continent urinary diversions. One is a continent urinary reservoir (Fig. 35-5) created from the intestine. This reservoir into which the ureters are inserted

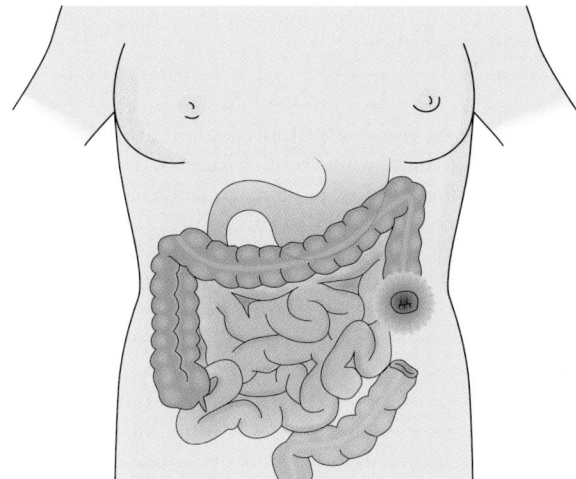

FIG 35-1   Sigmoid colostomy.

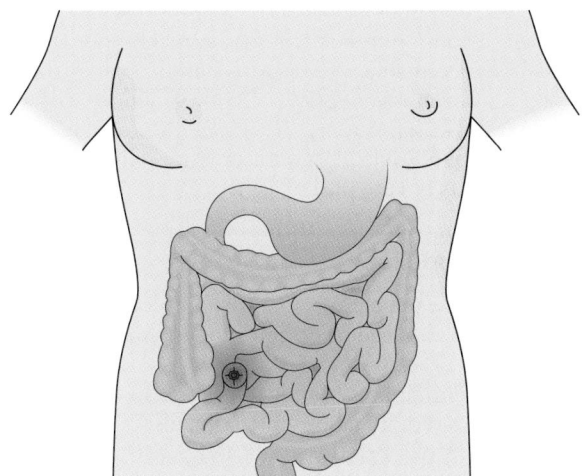

FIG 35-2   Ileostomy.

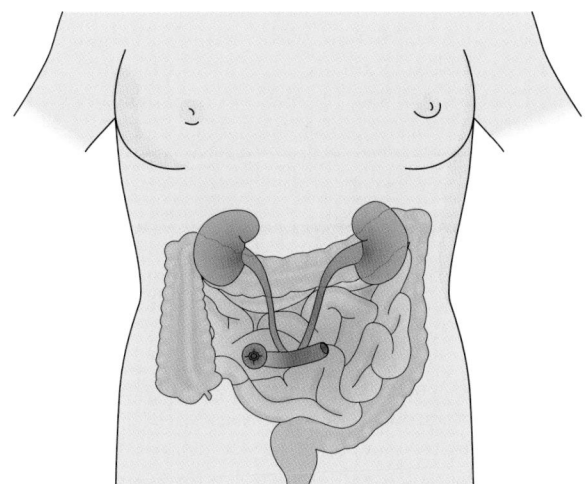

FIG 35-3   Urostomy (ileal conduit).

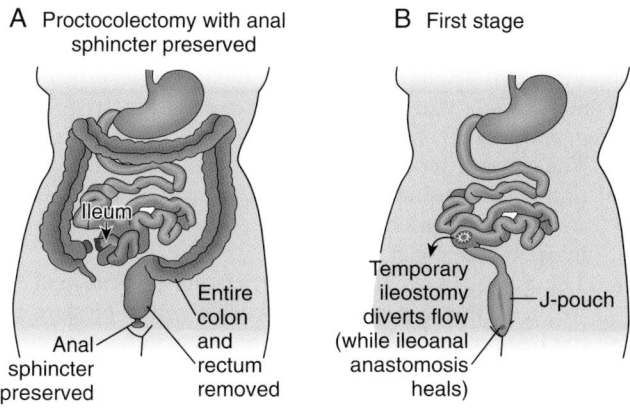

A Proctocolectomy with anal sphincter preserved

B First stage

FIG 35-4   Ileal pouch anal anastomosis.

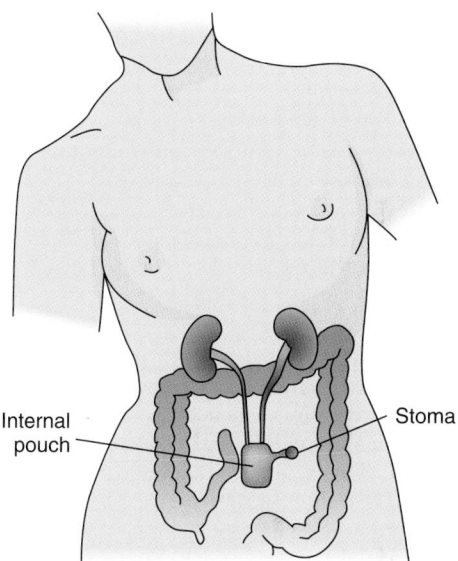

FIG 35-5   Continent urinary diversion.

an orthotopic neobladder, which also uses an intestinal pouch to replace the bladder. Anatomically the pouch is in the same position as the bladder was before removal, allowing the patient to void normally. The patient will have frequent episodes of incontinence of urine after this surgery and will need to follow a bladder-training schedule and perform pelvic muscle exercises until continence is achieved. The postoperative care of patients having continent urinary diversions varies widely with the surgical techniques used, and it is important to learn the surgeon's preferred routine or health care agency procedures before caring for these patients. A recent research study suggests that overall quality of life was rated similarly for both patients with incontinent stomas and those with continent procedures (Gemmill et al., 2010).

EVIDENCE-BASED PRACTICE

Before ostomy surgery, a health care provider or ostomy care nurse should see a patient to mark the stoma site. An ostomy care nurse is a certified wound, ostomy, continence nurse (CWOCN) or an enterostomal therapy (ET) nurse. Evaluating the patient's abdomen while he or she is lying, sitting, and standing allows the nurse and the patient to find an optimal location so it is easy to pouch the new stoma and maintain a reliable seal.

is situated under the abdominal wall, with a narrow tract coming out through the abdominal wall to form a small stoma. A catheter is inserted to empty the urine from the pouch. Patients must be able and willing to catheterize the pouch 4 to 6 times a day for the rest of their lives. The other type of continent urinary diversion is

One of the primary changes in ostomy care is related to stoma care. Pouching systems are more effective, and adhesive technology more advanced. These improvements include a wider variety of sizes and shapes of skin barriers, depths of convexity from shallow to deep, and degrees of flexibility:

- The current trend is to apply a pouch directly to clean dry skin without using skin preparations, paste, or added adhesives unless a patient has a specific problem keeping a pouch intact (Goldberg et al., 2010).
- The adhesives on the skin barriers are pressure and heat sensitive; thus a patient should apply gentle pressure with the hand over the skin barrier for several minutes to adhere the barrier to the skin (Kent, 2008).
- There are new and improved accessory products such as rings or seals for managing abdominal contours that are uneven or peristomal skin that is not intact.
- Some pouches have effective gas filters that allow flatus to escape slowly from the pouch through a charcoal filter. This filter absorbs odor and does not allow leakage of liquid effluent through the filter.
- All of the ostomy companies now have pouches with integrated closures. A Velcro-like closure eliminates the need for a clip to close the bottom of the pouch. It also requires less manual dexterity to empty the pouch (Goldberg et al., 2010).
- A wider selection of products for neonatal and pediatric use has improved the care of that population (Bookout et al., 2011).

PATIENT-CENTERED CARE

With any ostomy requiring a pouching system, a secure seal to prevent leakage of the effluent and protect the skin around the stoma (peristomal skin) is vital to helping patients resume normal activities and accept the changes in their bodies as a result of surgery. It is also a very important factor in facilitating the emotional adjustment to the ostomy (Li, 2009). In addition to the stress of illness and surgical recovery, patients with ostomies face body image changes, fear of social rejection, concern about sexual function and intimacy, and the need for help with personal care.

Use a variety of teaching strategies for patients based on their physical ability, learning style, and emotional readiness to learn. Whenever possible make a referral to an ostomy care nurse (de la Quintana et al., 2010). Ostomy support groups are available to provide support for patients. Information about these groups is available from ostomy care nurses or on the United Ostomy Association of America website, http://www.uoaa.org.

In any culture the presence and care of an ostomy presents unique challenges. New ostomies require monitoring and observation, and patients from some cultures may find this more invasive and embarrassing than those from cultures that are more open about bodily functions. Most patients consider bowel and urinary secretions unfit for public display. Exposure of the lower torso, which is needed for ostomy care, may also be a problem for some patients. Discuss with patients their preferences. For example, it may help to assign gender-congruent caregivers if possible and to encourage the presence of a family member if the patient finds this acceptable.

As you communicate with a patient during ostomy care, be sensitive and avoid communicating anything that the patient may interpret as disrespect or disgust. As always, prepare adequately for the procedure; seek necessary assistance; and maintain a calm, professional demeanor. Do not act offended by the odor or appearance of the effluent in the pouch or the appearance of the stoma. A negative reaction from caregivers only reinforces a patient's feelings that this alteration in bodily function makes them personally and socially unacceptable. A supportive nurse makes the initial period of adjustment easier (Burch, 2011). When a patient comes to the hospital with an ostomy, encourage him or her to resume self-care as soon as possible. Respect a patient's routine of care even if it differs from usual care in the agency.

Safety Guidelines

1 Change ostomy pouches before they become full to avoid leakage, which can lead to chemical or enzymatic injury to the skin.

2 Wear gloves during pouch and stoma care to reduce exposure and transmission of infectious microorganisms.

3 Know the signs of a healthy stoma and peristomal skin.
- *Color/moisture*: Stoma should be red or pink and moist. Report a gray, purple, or black stoma to the charge nurse or health care provider.
- *Size*: In the 4 to 6 weeks after surgery, the stoma will likely decrease in size. Measure with each pouch change.
- Peristomal skin normally is intact with some reddening. Presence of blisters, a rash, or rawlike appearance is abnormal.

SKILL 35-1   Pouching a Colostomy or an Ileostomy

NSO Ostomy Module / Lessons 1, 3, and 4

 Video Clip

Immediately after a fecal surgical diversion, it is necessary to place a pouch over the newly created stoma to contain effluent when the stoma begins to function. The pouch will keep a patient clean and dry, protect the skin from drainage, and provide a barrier against odor. A cut-to-fit, transparent pouching system is preferred because it will cover the peristomal skin without constricting the stoma and allow for visibility of the stoma.

Recognize the difference between a budded stoma (Fig. 35-6) and a flush or retracted stoma (Fig. 35-7). In the immediate postoperative period the stoma may be edematous, and the abdomen distended. These symptoms will resolve over a 4- to 6-week period after surgery, but during this time it will be necessary to revise the pouching system to meet the changing size of the stoma and the changes in body contours (Dietz and Gates, 2010a).

There are many types of pouching systems. All have a protective layer that adheres to the skin, called a skin barrier, and a pouch. A one-piece pouching system (Fig. 35-8) has the two parts integrated together. A two-piece system (Fig. 35-9) has a separate skin barrier and pouch. The flush or retracted stoma may require a convex wafer (Fig. 35-10) for successful placement of a pouch. This type of skin barrier provides gentle pressure on the peristomal skin to push the stoma through the opening in the wafer. You apply the pouch to the skin barrier by attaching it to a flange (a plastic ring) on the barrier. You must use the skin barrier with a flange that fits

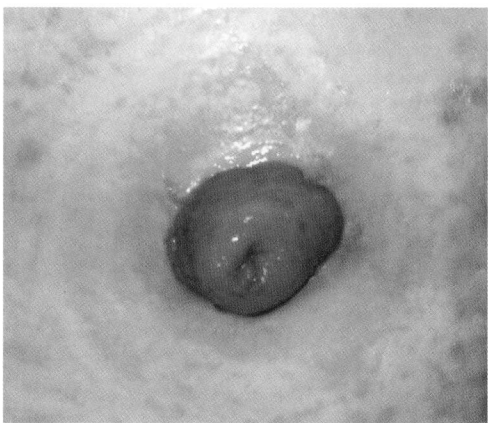

FIG 35-6   Budded stoma. (*Courtesy Jane Fellows.*)

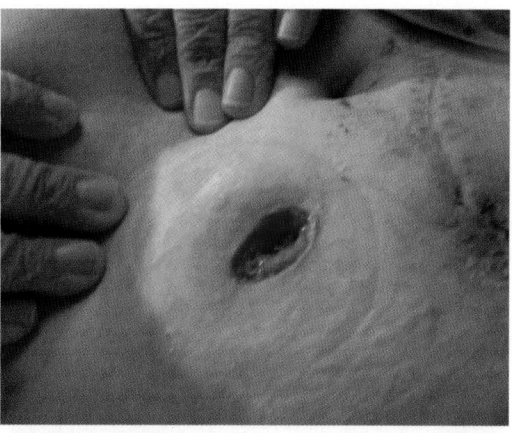

FIG 35-7   Retracted stoma. (*Courtesy Jane Fellows.*)

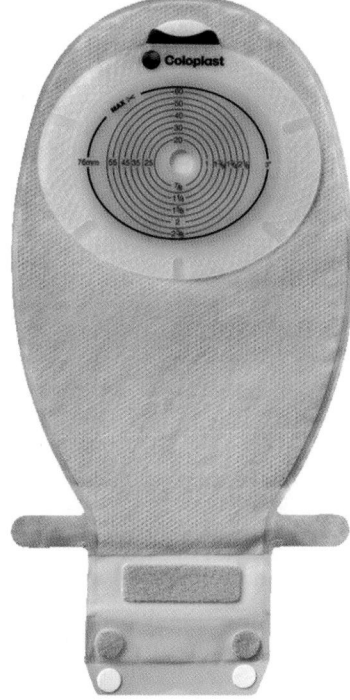

FIG 35-8   One-piece pouch with Velcro closure. (*Courtesy Coloplast, Minneapolis, Minn.*)

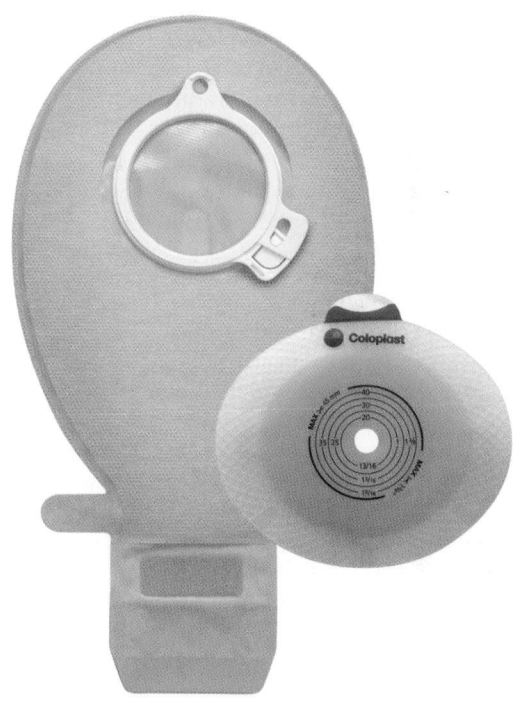

FIG 35-9   Two-piece pouching system with separate skin barrier and attachable pouch. (*Courtesy Coloplast, Minneapolis, Minn.*)

the corresponding size pouch from the same manufacturer to avoid leakage between the skin barrier and the pouch. Some pouching systems have precut openings in the barrier for the stoma, whereas others need to be custom cut to size for the patient's stoma measurement. It is important to understand how to use each of these different pouching systems before applying them on patients (Dietz and Gates, 2010b). The websites for the companies that make ostomy supplies have both patient and health care provider instructions that are helpful in understanding how to use the pouching systems (e.g., http://www.convatec.com; http://www.us.coloplast.com; and http://www.hollister.com).

Delegation and Collaboration
The skill of pouching a new ostomy/ileostomy cannot be delegated to nursing assistive personnel (NAP). In some agencies care of an established ostomy (4 to 6 weeks or more after surgery) can be delegated to NAP. The nurse directs the NAP about:

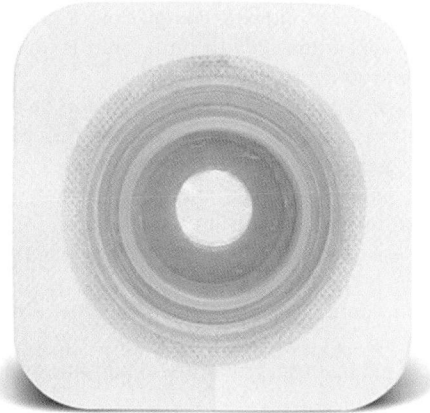

FIG 35-10   Convex skin barrier wafer. (*Used with permission Convatec, Inc. All rights reserved.*)

- The expected amount, color, and consistency of drainage from the ostomy.
- The expected appearance of the stoma.
- Special equipment needed to complete procedure.
- Change in patient's stoma and surrounding skin integrity that should be reported.

Equipment

❑ Skin barrier/pouch—clear, drainable one-piece or two-piece, cut-to-fit or precut size
❑ Pouch closure device such as a clip if needed

❑ Ostomy measuring guide
❑ Adhesive remover (*optional*)
❑ Clean gloves
❑ Washcloth
❑ Towel or disposable waterproof barrier
❑ Basin with warm tap water
❑ Scissors
❑ Waterproof bag for disposal of pouch
❑ Gown and goggles optional if there is risk of splashing when emptying pouch

STEP	RATIONALE

ASSESSMENT

1 Perform hand hygiene and apply clean gloves.	Reduces transmission of microorganisms.
2 Observe existing skin barrier and pouch for leakage and length of time in place. Pouch should be changed every 3 to 7 days for colostomy and 3 to 5 for ileostomy, not daily (Goldberg et al., 2010). In case of an opaque pouch, remove it to fully observe stoma.	Assesses effectiveness of pouching system and detects potential for problems. To minimize skin irritation, avoid unnecessary changing of entire pouching system. When pouch leaks, skin damage from effluent causes more skin trauma than early removal of wafer.

Clinical Decision Point *Repeated leaking may indicate need for different type of pouch. If the pouch is leaking, change it. Taping or patching it to contain effluent leaves the skin exposed to chemical or enzymatic irritation.*

3 Observe amount of effluent in pouch and empty it if it is more than one-third to one-half full by opening clip and draining it into a container for measurement of output. Note consistency of effluent and record intake and output.	Weight of pouch may disrupt seal of adhesive on skin. Monitors fluid balance and bowel function after surgery. Normal colostomy effluent is soft or formed stool, whereas normal ileostomy effluent is liquid.
4 Observe stoma for type, location, color, swelling, presence of sutures, trauma, and healing or irritation of peristomal skin. Remove and dispose of gloves.	Stoma characteristics influence selection of an appropriate pouching system. Convexity in skin barrier is often necessary with flush or retracted stoma.

5 Observe abdomen for best type of pouching system. Consider:
  a Abdominal contour.
  b Presence of scars or incisions.
	Determines pouching system selection.
	Abdominal contours, scars, or incisions affect type of system and adhesion to skin surface.

6 Explore patient's attitude toward learning self-care and identify others who will be helping patient after leaving hospital.	Facilitates teaching plan and timing of care to coincide with availability of caregivers.

NURSING DIAGNOSES

• Alteration in body image	• Readiness for enhanced knowledge	• Risk for impaired skin integrity

Related factors are individualized based on patient's condition or needs.

PLANNING

1 Expected outcomes following completion of procedure: • Stoma is moist and reddish pink. Skin is intact and free of irritation; sutures are intact.	Normal findings in patient with postoperative ostomy that is healing.
• Stoma drains moderate amount of liquid or soft stool, and flatus is in pouch (noted by bulging of pouch). (Flatus may not be observable if pouch has gas filter.)	Stoma is functioning normally. Snug seal around stoma has been attained. Flatus indicates return of peristalsis after surgery.
• Patient, family caregiver, and/or significant others observe stoma and steps of procedure.	Reveals acceptance of alteration in body image and interest in self-care.
• Patient asks questions about procedure and attempts to help with pouch change.	Indicates readiness to learn and begin self-care.
2 Explain procedure to patient; encourage patient's interaction and questions.	Lessens patient's anxiety and promotes patient's participation.
3 Assemble equipment and close room curtains or door.	Optimizes use of time; provides privacy.

STEP	RATIONALE

IMPLEMENTATION

1 Identify patient using two identifiers (i.e., name and birthday or name and account number) according to agency policy. Compare identifiers with information on patient's identification bracelet.

Ensures correct patient. Complies with The Joint Commission standards and improves patient safety (TJC, 2012).

2 Position patient in semireclining or supine during assessment and pouching (**Note:** Some patients with established ostomies prefer to stand). If possible, provide patient with mirror for observation.

When patient is semireclining there are fewer skin wrinkles, which allows for ease of application of pouching system.

3 Perform hand hygiene and apply clean gloves.

Reduces transmission of microorganisms.

4 Place towel or disposable waterproof barrier under patient and across patient's lower abdomen.

Protects bed linen; maintains patient's dignity.

5 If not done during assessment, remove used pouch and skin barrier gently by pushing skin away from barrier. Use an adhesive remover to facilitate removal of skin barrier. Empty pouch and dispose of in an appropriate receptacle. Measure output if needed.

Reduces skin trauma. Improper removal of pouch and barrier can cause peristomal skin irritation or breakdown.

6 Clean peristomal skin gently with warm tap water using washcloth; do not scrub skin. If you touch stoma, minor bleeding is normal. Pat skin dry. When pouching an ileostomy, place disposable washcloth over stoma.

Avoid soap. It leaves residue on skin, which may irritate skin. Pouch does not adhere to wet skin.
Ileostomies leak continuously in some patients.

7 Measure stoma (see illustration). Expect size of stoma to change for first 4 to 6 weeks after surgery.

Allows for proper fit of pouch that will protect peristomal skin.

8 Trace pattern of stoma measurement on pouch backing or skin barrier (see illustration).

Prepares for cutting opening in pouch.

9 Cut opening on backing or skin barrier wafer (see illustration). Be sure that opening is at least $\frac{1}{8}$ inch larger than stoma to avoid pressure on it.

Customizes pouch to provide appropriate fit over stoma.

10 Remove protective backing from adhesive (see illustration).

Prepares skin barrier for placement.

11 Apply pouch over stoma (see illustration). Press firmly into place around stoma and outside edges. Have patient hold hand over pouch to apply heat to secure seal.

Pouch adhesives are heat and pressure sensitive and hold more securely at body temperature.

12 Close end of pouch with clip or integrated closure. Remove drape from patient.

Ensures pouch is secure. Contains effluent.

13 Remove gloves. Perform hand hygiene.

Reduces transmission of microorganisms.

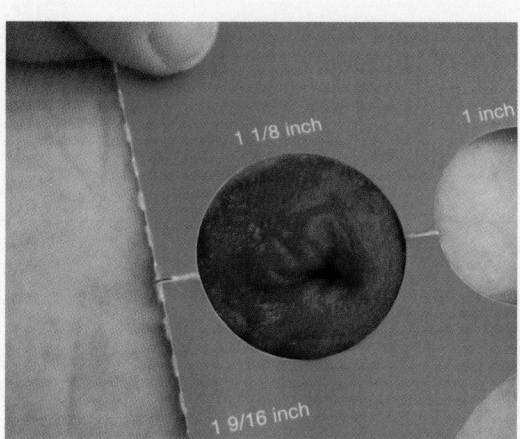

STEP 7   Measure stoma. (*Courtesy Coloplast, Minneapolis, Minn.*)

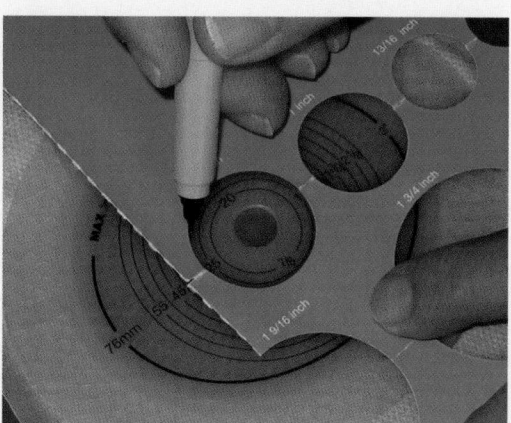

STEP 8   Trace measurement on skin barrier. (*Courtesy Coloplast, Minneapolis, Minn.*)

STEP	RATIONALE

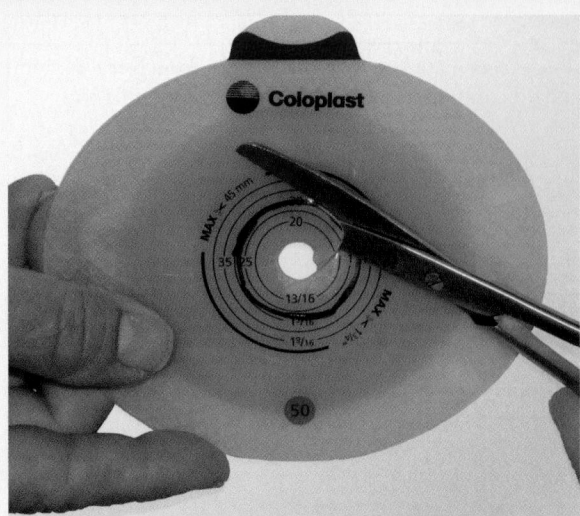

STEP 9   Cut opening in wafer. (*Courtesy Coloplast, Minneapolis, Minn.*)

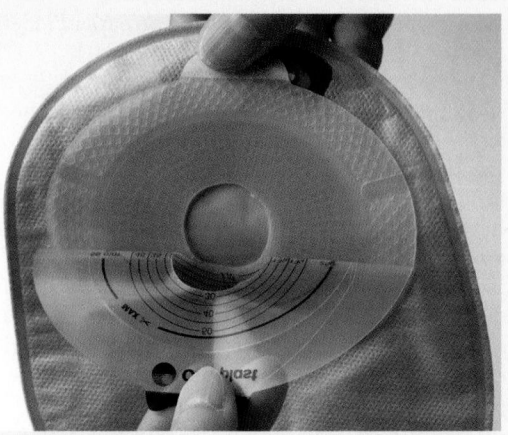

STEP 10   Remove protective backing. (*Courtesy Coloplast, Minneapolis, Minn.*)

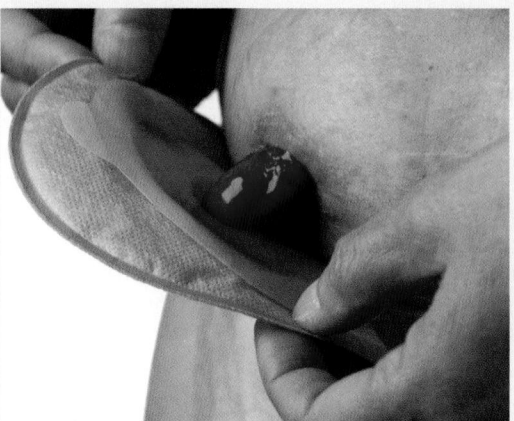

STEP 11   Apply pouch over stoma. (*Courtesy Coloplast, Minneapolis, Minn.*)

EVALUATION

1 Observe condition of skin barrier and adherence to abdominal surface.

Determines presence of leaks.

2 Observe appearance of stoma, peristomal skin, abdominal contours, and suture line during pouch change.

Provides information if another type of pouching system or additional skin care products are needed.

3 Observe patient's and family caregiver's willingness to view stoma and ask questions about procedure.

Determines level of adjustment and understanding of stoma care and pouch application. Allows planning for future education needs and progress toward acceptance of altered body image.

Unexpected Outcomes

1 Skin around stoma is irritated, blistered, or bleeding; or a rash is noted. May be caused by undermining of pouch seal by fecal contents, allergic reaction, or fungal skin eruption.

2 Necrotic stoma is manifested by purple or black color, dry-instead of-moist texture, failure to bleed when washed gently, or tissue sloughing.

3 Patient refuses to view stoma or participate in care.

Related Interventions

- Remove pouch more carefully.
- Change pouch more frequently or use different type of pouching system.
- Consult ostomy care nurse.

- Report to nurse/health care provider.
- Document appearance.

- Obtain referral for ostomy care nurse.
- Allow patient to express feelings.
- Encourage family support.

Recording and Reporting

- Record type of pouch and skin barrier applied, amount and appearance of effluent in pouch, size and appearance of stoma, and condition of peristomal skin.
- Record patient/family level of participation, teaching that was done, and response to teaching.
- Report any of the following to nurse and/or health care provider: abnormal appearance of stoma, suture line, peristomal skin, or character of output.

Special Considerations

Teaching

- Include family caregiver in teaching to facilitate patient's readiness to learn.
- Some patients accept stoma with minimal emotional difficulty; some may never completely adjust to it. Individualize care according to patient's situation and circumstances (Burch, 2011).
- Give patient teaching materials that clearly state each step for a pouch change. Audiotaped or videotaped instructions are also available. For patients with learning disabilities, consider using materials that have illustrations for each step.
- Give patients a list of equipment and name, address, and phone number of a supplier.

Pediatric

- Select pediatric pouches designed especially for neonates, infants, and children; these pouches are smaller and have a more skin-sensitive adhesive on the barrier.
- Because most ostomy surgery done on neonates is for emergencies, often no time is available for preoperative selection of stoma site. The surgery is usually done because the neonate has necrotizing enterocolitis (NEC), Hirschsprung's disease, or congenital disorders (Bookout et al., 2011). The stomas are frequently temporary, with closure of the ostomy when the surgical repair has healed and the neonate is medically ready for surgery. Children and adolescents may have ostomy surgery for conditions such as cancer, inflammatory bowel disease, and trauma.

- Neonates may have multiple stomas on their tiny abdomens following corrective bowel surgeries. Select a cut-to-fit pouch that allows multiple stoma openings in skin barrier yet still fits on neonate's abdomen (Bookout et al., 2011).
- Because infants swallow large amounts of air while sucking, it is normal to expect flatus. Make sure that pouch can accommodate increased amount of flatus after feeding or be prepared to release flatus frequently (Bookout et al., 2011).
- The skin of a preterm infant is not fully developed and is more absorbent than that of a full-term infant. Do not use skin sealants and adhesive removers unless they are approved for preterm-infant use (Bookout et al., 2011).
- As an infant grows in size, so does the stoma. Measure the stoma frequently and make appropriate adjustments in pouching and skin barrier size. Skin barriers for preterm infants must have flexibility to cover the infant's rounded abdominal contour (Bookout et al., 2011).
- Adolescents requiring an ostomy benefit from presurgical contact with other adolescents who have an ostomy (Bookout et al., 2011).

Gerontologic

- Evaluate an older adult's cognitive status for understanding ostomy self-care instructions. Include a family caregiver in the care plan.
- Adapt care approaches for older patients who have impaired manual dexterity or limited vision. If a patient is unable to custom cut the size of the skin barrier, consider having barriers precut by an ostomy equipment supplier or using a precut pouching system.
- Costs of ostomy supplies and reimbursement are an issue for patients on fixed income.

Home Care

- Evaluate home toileting facilities and patients' ability to position to empty pouch directly into a toilet.
- Patient may shower without covering pouch.
- Patients should avoid storing pouches in extremely hot or cold locations. Temperature affects barrier and adhesive materials.

SKILL 35-2 Pouching a Urostomy

Because urine flows continuously from an incontinent urinary diversion, placement of the pouch is more challenging than with the fecal diversion. In the immediate postoperative period urinary stents extend out from the stoma (Fig. 35-11). A surgeon places the stents to prevent stenosis of the ureters at the site where the ureters are attached to the conduit. The stents will be removed during the hospital stay or at the first postoperative visit with the surgeon.

The stoma is normally red and moist. It is made from a portion of the intestinal tract, usually the ileum. It should protrude above the skin. An ileal conduit is usually located in the right lower quadrant. While the patient is in bed, the pouch may be connected to a bedside drainage bag to decrease the need for frequent emptying. When the patient goes home, the bedside drainage bag may be used at night to avoid having to get up to empty the pouch. Each type of urostomy pouch comes with a connector for the

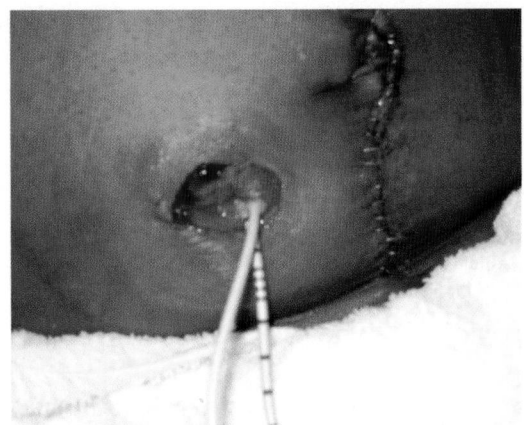

FIG 35-11   Urostomy stoma with stents in place. (*Courtesy Jane Fellows.*)

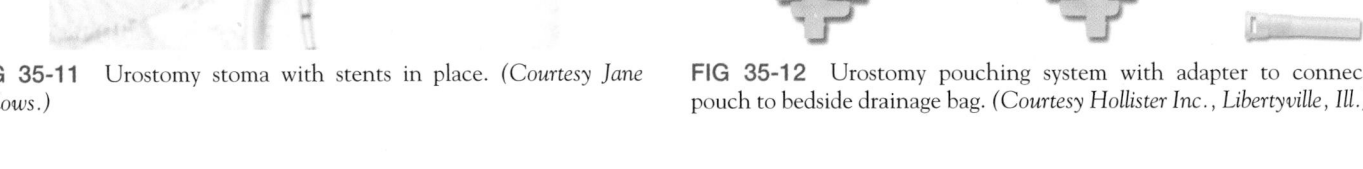

FIG 35-12   Urostomy pouching system with adapter to connect pouch to bedside drainage bag. (*Courtesy Hollister Inc., Libertyville, Ill.*)

bedside drainage bag (Fig. 35-12). Incorrect pouch placement, large volumes of urine in the pouch, or a urinary pouch without an antireflux valve promotes reflux and the risk of infection. You can reduce the risk of reflux by attaching the urinary pouch to straight drainage when high urinary output is expected. A patient must understand the importance of draining the pouch frequently and using clean technique during stomal and skin care.

Delegation and Collaboration

The skill of pouching a new incontinent urinary diversion cannot be delegated to nursing assistive personnel (NAP). In some agencies, care of an established urostomy (4 o 6 weeks or more after surgery) can be delegated to NAP. The nurse directs the NAP about:

- Expected appearance of the stoma.
- Expected amount and character of the output and when to report changes.
- Change in patient's stoma and surrounding skin integrity that should be reported.
  - Special equipment needed to complete procedure.

Equipment

- ❏ Urinary pouch (with antireflux flap and skin barrier;clear, drainable one- or two-piece, cut-to-fit or precut size
- ❏ Appropriate adapter for connection to bedside drainage bag
- ❏ Measuring guide
- ❏ Bedside urinary drainage bag
- ❏ Clean gloves
- ❏ Washcloth
- ❏ Towel or disposable waterproof barrier
- ❏ Basin with warm tap water
- ❏ Scissors
- ❏ Adhesive remover
- ❏ Absorbent wick made from gauze rolled tightly in the shape of a tampon
- ❏ Waterproof bag for disposal of pouch
- ❏ Gown and goggles optional if there is risk of splashing when emptying pouch

STEP	RATIONALE

ASSESSMENT

1 Perform hand hygiene and apply clean gloves.	Reduces transmission of microorganisms.
2 Observe existing skin barrier and pouch for leakage and length of time in place. Pouch should be changed every 3 to 7 days, not daily (Colwell et al., 2004). If urine is leaking under wafer, change pouch.	Assesses effectiveness of pouching system and allows for early detection of potential problems. To minimize skin irritation, avoid changing entire pouching system unnecessarily. Repeated leakage may indicate need for different type of pouch to provide reliable seal.
3 Observe urine in pouch or bedside drainage bag. Empty pouch if it is more than one-third to one-half full by opening valve and draining it into container for measurement.	Urine output provides information about renal status and whether volume is within acceptable limits ($\geq$30 mL/hr). Weight of pouch can disrupt seal. Urine from ileal conduit will contain mucus because of flow through intestinal segment.
4 Observe stoma for color, swelling, presence of sutures, trauma, and healing of peristomal skin. Assess type of stoma. Remove and dispose of gloves.	Consider stoma characteristics in selecting appropriate pouching system. Convexity in skin barrier is often necessary with flush or retracted stoma.
5 Explore patient's attitude toward learning self-care and identify others who will be helping patient after leaving hospital.	Facilitates teaching plan and timing of care to coincide with availability of caregivers.

STEP	RATIONALE

NURSING DIAGNOSES

- Readiness for enhanced knowledge
- Risk for impaired skin integrity

Related factors are individualized based on patient's condition or needs.

PLANNING

STEP	RATIONALE
1 Expected outcomes following completion of procedure:	
• Stoma is moist, reddish-pink with stents protruding from it. Peristomal skin is free of irritation and intact. Sutures are intact.	Normal findings for postoperative urinary diversion.
• Urine drains freely from stents or stoma. Urine is yellow with mucus shreds and is without foul odor. Urine may be pink or contain small blood clots after surgery. Volume of output is within acceptable limits (≥30 mL/hr).	These are normal findings after surgery. Mucus shreds are normal when urine flows through intestinal segment.
• Patient and family caregiver observe stoma and procedural steps.	Shows adjustment to body image change and willingness to learn self-care.
• Patient asks questions about procedure and may help with pouch change.	Indicates readiness to learn and begin self-care.
2 Explain procedure to patient; encourage his or her interaction and questions.	Lessens patient's anxiety and promotes participation.
3 Assemble equipment and close room curtains or door.	Optimizes use of time; provides privacy.

IMPLEMENTATION

STEP	RATIONALE
1 Identify patient using two identifiers (i.e., name and birthday or name and account number) according to agency policy. Compare identifiers with information on patient's identification bracelet.	Ensures correct patient. Complies with The Joint Commission standards and improves patient safety (TJC, 2012).
2 Position patient in semireclining or supine position. If possible provide patient a mirror for observation.	When patient is semireclining, there are fewer skin wrinkles, which allows for ease of pouch application.
3 Perform hand hygiene and apply clean gloves.	Reduces transmission of microorganisms.
4 Place towel or disposable waterproof barrier under patient and across patient's lower abdomen.	Protects bed linen; maintains patient's dignity.
5 Remove used pouch and skin barrier gently by pushing skin away from barrier. If stents are present, pull pouch gently around them and lay towel underneath. Empty pouch and measure output. Dispose of pouch in appropriate receptacle.	Reduces risk for trauma to skin and for dislodging stents. Keeps urine from leaking onto skin.
6 Place rolled gauze at stoma opening. Maintain gauze at the stoma opening continuously during pouch measurement and change.	Using wick at stoma opening prevents peristomal skin from becoming wet with urine during pouch change.
7 While keeping rolled gauze in contact with the stoma, cleanse peristomal skin gently with warm tap water using washcloth; do not scrub skin. If you touch stoma, minor bleeding is normal. Pat skin dry.	Avoid soap. It leaves residue on skin, which can irritate it. Pouch does not adhere to wet skin.
8 Measure stoma (see Skill 35-1, Step 7). Be sure that opening is at least $\frac{1}{8}$ inch larger than stoma to avoid pressure on stoma. Expect size of stoma to change for first 4 to 6 weeks after surgery.	Allows for proper fit of pouch that will protect peristomal skin.
9 Trace pattern on pouch backing or skin barrier (see Skill 35-1, Step 8).	Prepares for cutting opening in pouch.
10 Cut opening in pouch.	Customizes pouch to provide appropriate fit over stoma.
11 Remove protective backing from adhesive surface. Remove rolled gauze from stoma.	Prepares pouch for application to skin.
12 Apply pouch. Press adhesive barrier firmly into place around stoma and outside edges. Have patient hold hand over pouch 1 to 2 minutes to apply heat to secure seal.	Pouch adhesives are heat activated and will hold more securely at body temperature.
13 Use adapter provided with pouches to connect pouch to bedside urinary bag. Keep tubing below level of bag.	Provides for collection and measurement of urine. Allows patient to rest without frequent emptying of pouch.
14 Remove drape from patient. Remove gloves and perform hand hygiene.	Reduces transmission of microorganisms.

STEP	RATIONALE

EVALUATION

1 Observe appearance of stoma, peristomal skin, and suture line during pouch change.	Determines condition of stoma and peristomal skin and progress of wound healing.
2 Evaluate character and volume of urinary drainage.	Determines if stoma and/or stents are patent. Character of urine reveals degree of concentration and alterations in renal function.
3 Observe patient's and family caregiver's willingness to view stoma and ask questions about procedure.	Determines level of adjustment and understanding of stoma care and pouch application.

Unexpected Outcomes

Related Interventions

1 Skin around stoma is irritated, blistered, or bleeding; or a rash is noted as a result of chronic exposure to urine.	• Check stoma size and opening in skin barrier. Resize skin barrier opening if necessary. • Remove pouch more carefully. • Consult ostomy care nurse.
2 No urine output for several hours, or output is less than 30 mL/hr. Urine has foul odor.	• Increase fluid intake. • Notify health care provider. • Obtain urine specimen for culture and sensitivity as ordered.
3 Patient and family caregiver are unable to observe stoma, ask questions, or participate in care.	• Consult ostomy care nurse. • Allow patient to express feelings. • Encourage family support.

Recording and Reporting

- Record type of pouch, time of change, condition and appearance of stoma and peristomal skin, and character of urine.
- Record urinary output on intake and output form.
- Record patient's and family caregiver's reaction to stoma and level of participation.
- Report abnormalities in stoma or peristomal skin and absence of urinary output to nurse in charge or health care provider.

Special Considerations
Teaching

- Teach whenever doing a pouch change even if patient does not appear interested. Do not insist that patient look at stoma; allow time for adjustment.
- Teach patients significance and importance of drinking $1\frac{1}{2}$ to 2 quarts of fluid daily to prevent urinary tract infections (UTIs). Explain that some mucus in urine is expected but patients should report any blood in their urine, excessively cloudy urine, chills, fever (38.3° C [101° F] or higher), and back (flank) pain to their health care provider.
- Give patient teaching materials that state each step clearly. Audiotaped or videotaped instructions are also available. For patients with learning disabilities, consider using material that has illustrations for each step.
- Give patients a list of equipment and name, address, and phone number of a supplier.

Pediatric

- In neonates urinary diversions are less common than fecal ostomies.
- Select pediatric pouches designed especially for neonates, infants, and children; these pouches are smaller and have a more skin-sensitive adhesive on the barrier.

Gerontologic

- Older patients have decreased thirst and may not normally consume adequate fluids. Explain importance of fluid intake to promote healthy renal function and decrease risk for UTIs.
- Evaluate older adult's cognitive status for understanding of ostomy self-care instructions.
- Adapt care approaches for older patients who have impaired manual dexterity or limited vision. For patients who are unable to custom cut the size of their skin barriers, consider having barriers precut by ostomy equipment supplier or using a precut two-piece system.
- Costs of ostomy supplies and reimbursement are an issue for patients on fixed income.

Home Care

- Instruct patient that pouch can be connected to straight drainage at night. Make sure that patient understands that adapter will be needed to connect pouch to the bedside drainage bag.
- Patient may shower without covering pouch.
- Patients should avoid storing pouches in extremely hot or cold locations because temperature will affect barrier and adhesive materials.

SKILL 35-3 Catheterizing a Urinary Diversion

Catheterization of a urinary diversion is the only method to obtain an accurate culture and sensitivity specimen to screen for infection. When it is necessary to obtain a urine specimen from a urinary diversion, the best method is to insert a sterile catheter into the stoma. Obtaining a specimen of urine in a pouch does not provide an accurate finding because of the likely risk for contamination by microorganisms. With the use of strict aseptic technique, catheterization is relatively safe and easy. If a patient uses a two-piece system, remove the pouch from the skin barrier and replace it after catheterization without disturbing the skin barrier. If a patient uses a one-piece system, you have to remove the pouch to obtain the specimen and replace it after the procedure. To prevent trauma to the tissues, you need to understand how the stoma and implanted ureters are constructed for a patient. Reflux of urine into the ureters can cause infection.

Delegation and Collaboration

The skill of catheterizing a urinary diversion cannot be delegated to nursing assistive personnel (NAP). The nurse directs the NAP to:

- Inform nurse if patient complains of peristomal or back pain.
- Inform nurse if there is a change in color, odor, or amount of urine or if there is blood in the urine.

Equipment

- ❏ Urinary catheterization supplies (contained in prepackaged sterile catheter kit or may need to be gathered separately)
  - 14- to 16-Fr sterile catheter
  - Water-soluble lubricant
  - Antiseptic swabs (e.g., povidone-iodine or chlorhexidine)
  - Sterile gloves
  - Sterile specimen container
- ❏ Absorbent gauze wick
- ❏ Bed protection barrier
- ❏ Towels
- ❏ Urinary pouch if needed
- ❏ Clean gloves

STEP	RATIONALE
ASSESSMENT	
1 Observe for signs and symptoms of urinary tract infection (UTI): elevated temperature, chills, foul-smelling urine, and elevated white blood cell (WBC) count.	Determines need to perform catheterization to obtain sterile specimen from urinary diversion. Diversion poses risk for reflux of urine back to kidneys, resulting in infection.
2 Obtain health care provider's order for catheterization.	Invasive procedure requires health care provider's order.
3 Assess patient's understanding of need for procedure and how it is done.	Determines willingness to cooperate and reduces patient's anxiety.
NURSING DIAGNOSES	
• Deficient knowledge regarding catheterization procedure • Risk for infection	
Related factors are individualized based on patient's condition or needs.	
PLANNING	
1 Expected outcomes following completion of procedure:	
• Urine specimen is not contaminated with bacteria during procedure.	Urine obtained correctly. Laboratory results are accurate.
• Patient describes risks for infection and techniques to prevent infection.	Demonstrates patient's learning.
2 Assemble equipment and close room curtain or door.	Optimizes use of time and provides privacy.
3 Explain procedure to patient; if possible, obtain specimen when patient is due to change pouch if using one-piece system.	Lessens anxiety and promotes patient's cooperation. Changing pouch too frequently could result in skin trauma.
IMPLEMENTATION	
1 Identify patient using two identifiers (i.e., name and birthday or name and account number) according to agency policy. Compare identifiers with information on patient's identification bracelet.	Ensures correct patient. Complies with The Joint Commission standards and improves patient safety (TJC, 2012).
2 Position patient sitting if possible and drape towel across lower abdomen.	Gravity facilitates flow of urine. Maintains patient's dignity. Towel absorbs urine.
3 Perform hand hygiene and apply clean gloves.	Reduces transmission of microorganisms.
4 Remove pouch. If patient uses two-piece system, remove pouch but leave barrier attached to skin.	Allows access to stoma.
5 Remove gloves and perform hand hygiene.	Avoids contamination.

STEP	RATIONALE
6 Open sterile catheterization set according to instructions or open needed equipment and place on sterile barrier using aseptic technique (see Chapter 7). If not using catheterization kit, place gauze pad on sterile field and squeeze small amount of lubricant onto gauze. Apply sterile gloves.	Prepares sterile work field.
7 If needed, have patient hold absorbent gauze wick on stoma while you prepare catheterization supplies.	Prevents leakage of urine on peristomal skin, linens, and clothing.
8 Cleanse surface of stoma with antiseptic swabs using circular motion from center outward. Use new swab each time; repeat twice. Wipe off excess antiseptic with dry sterile gauze or cotton ball.	Removes surface bacteria.

Clinical Decision Point *If patient has stents in place, use antiseptic swab to clean the ends of the stents and place the stents in the sterile cup. Allow urine to drip into the cup until you obtain an adequate amount for a specimen. Then go directly to Step 13.*

9 Remove lid from sterile specimen container.	Sterile container collects a small volume of urine.
10 Lubricate tip of catheter with water-soluble lubricant, keeping catheter sterile.	Facilitates passage of catheter through stoma.
11 With dominant hand gently insert catheter tip into stoma. Do not force catheter; redirect course as needed. Place distal end of catheter into specimen container. Use gentle but firm pressure similar to regular catheterization of urethra (see Skill 33-1). Have patient cough or turn slightly.	Use care to avoid trauma to conduit. Movement and coughing may facilitate flow of urine.
12 Hold container below level of stoma. If needed, wait several minutes to get adequate amount of urine.	Culture and sensitivity studies only require 3 to 5 mL of urine (check agency policy).
13 Withdraw catheter slowly; place absorbent pad over stoma.	Keeps skin dry.
14 Apply lid to specimen container.	Prevents accidental spillage.
15 Reapply new pouch or reattach pouch if patient uses two-piece system (see Skill 35-2).	Pouch is necessary to contain urine.
16 Dispose of used pouch and equipment properly.	Avoids unpleasant odor in room.
17 Remove gloves; perform hand hygiene. Label specimen in presence of patient, place in biohazard bag, and send to laboratory at once.	Ensures that laboratory results are assigned to correct patient. Labeling ensures acceptance and processing of specimen by laboratory. Urine that sits for long periods at room temperature will adversely affect laboratory results.

EVALUATION

1 Compare results of culture and sensitivity with expected findings. Mucus is a normal finding if patient has an ileal conduit.	Determines presence of infection. If contamination appears likely, second specimen will be needed.
2 Instruct patient about signs and symptoms of UTI.	Informed patients will seek attention for a problem earlier if aware of signs and symptoms.

Unexpected outcomes

1 Unable to obtain urine specimen.

2 Skin or stoma reveals complications.

Related Interventions

- Reposition patient.
- If there is still no urine, push fluids and try again later.
- Notify nurse and/or health care provider.
- Consult with ostomy care nurse.

Recording and Reporting

- Record time specimen collected; patient's tolerance of procedure; and appearance of urine, skin, and stoma.
- Report results of laboratory test to nurse in charge or health care provider.

Special Considerations
Teaching

- Explain common symptoms of UTI: flank pain, dark or bloody urine, foul-smelling urine, fever (38.3° C [101° F] or higher), confusion.
- Encourage patient to notify health care provider if symptoms of infection develop.
- Reinforce importance of fluid intake (2 L/day).

Critical Thinking Exercises

You are assigned to care for Janeé Bell, a 28-year-old engineer. She has been admitted for elective colon removal secondary to a 10-year history of ulcerative colitis. She is scheduled for an ileal pouch anal anastomosis with J-pouch construction and will have a temporary ileostomy.

1 Which of the following will be part of her preoperative preparation?
   1 A chance to empty a pouch
   2 A nutrition consultation
   3 Stoma site marking with a qualified ostomy care nurse
   4 A barium enema
   Explain your choice.

2 When Janeé returns from surgery, the nurse assesses the stoma. How should the stoma look immediately after surgery? Explain your choice.
   1 Red and moist
   2 Appear just below the skin level
   3 Have stents protruding from it
   4 Pink and dry

3 What information about the ostomy pouch should the nurse include when teaching Janeé about care at home? It must be: Explain your choice.
   1 changed daily.
   2 emptied when it is one-third to one-half full.
   3 emptied every 4 to 6 hours.
   4 changed weekly.

4 Janeé notes that her bowel movement is always liquid. She asks when it will be formed as it was before she got sick. What does the nurse tell her?

REVIEW QUESTIONS

1 The nurse has inserted a catheter into a patient's urinary diversion, but only a few drops of urine have drained. Which action should the nurse perform first to try to obtain an adequate sample? (Select all that apply.)
   1 Remove the catheter and obtain urine from the pouch.
   2 Gently insert the catheter a little more.
   3 Massage the patient's abdomen.
   4 Have the patient turn to side.

2 A patient has a new urostomy secondary to bladder cancer. Which patient behaviors suggest acceptance of his change in bodily function? (Select all that apply.)
   1 He watches you change his pouch.
   2 He asks questions about how the ostomy works.
   3 He empties his pouch.
   4 He says his spouse will be doing the pouch changes.

3 The nurse is caring for a patient with a new permanent sigmoid colostomy and explaining information about care once the patient returns home. Which statement by the patient indicates that he or she requires further instruction on the topic?
   1 "When I wash the stoma, I should just use warm water to clean the skin."
   2 "If I eat a well balanced diet, the stool will be soft and formed."
   3 "I'll need to look at the skin around the stoma each time I change the pouch to be sure that there is no irritation."
   4 "The stoma will stay the shape it is; so it will be easy to buy bags that fit."

4 A patient anticipating an ileostomy because of severe ulcerative colitis asks, "Will I really be able to have a normal life after having this procedure?" What is the most appropriate reply?
   1 "Let's talk about this when you're recovering from the surgery."

2 "I'm going to have a person with an ostomy visit you before the surgery."
3 "Why don't you talk with your surgeon about your concerns?"
4 "Tell me the specific questions you have about life after the surgery."

5 A patient with a urostomy notes a raw, weeping area of the skin in an area under the skin barrier. Which action is most appropriate in this situation?
   1 Cleaning the area with alcohol to help dry it
   2 Consulting an ostomy care nurse
   3 Scheduling the patient for an appointment next week with the health care provider
   4 Having the patient continue his usual skin care regimen of cleaning gently with water

6 The intestinal opening surgically created in the abdomen for a colostomy, ileostomy, or urostomy is called a _____.

7 Place the steps for an ostomy pouch change in the correct order.
   ____ Close the end of the pouch.
   ____ Measure the stoma.
   ____ Cut the hole in the wafer.
   ____ Press the pouch into place over the stoma.
   ____ Remove the old pouch.
   ____ Trace the correct measurement onto the back of the wafer.
   ____ Observe the stoma and the skin around it.
   ____ Clean and dry the peristomal skin.

8 The pathway created for urine to exit the body when the bladder is removed is called an_____.

9 A patient who had colostomy surgery 3 days ago now has air that is filling his pouch, but he has not had any fecal matter from his stoma. Which of the following is the accurate assessment of this situation?
   1 There is infection present causing air to fill the pouch.
   2 The patient has an ileus and should not be allowed to have any oral intake.
   3 This is normal flatus, indicating that bowel function is returning.
   4 The patient should be given a laxative because his bowels are not moving.

10 A patient with a urostomy enters the clinic. Which of the following signs would make you suspect a urinary tract infection (UTI)? (Select all that apply.)
   1 Difficulty recalling name
   2 Pain in the upper abdomen
   3 Dark urine
   4 Foul-smelling urine

REFERENCES

Bookout K, et al: *Pediatric ostomy care: best practice for clinicians*, Mt Laurel, NJ, 2011, WOCN.

Burch J: Stoma management: enhancing patient knowledge, *Br J Commun Nurs* 16(4):162, 2011.

Colwell J, et al: *Fecal and urinary diversions: management principles*, St. Louis, 2004, Mosby.

de la Quintana JP, et al: A prospective, longitudinal, multicenter, cohort quality-of-life evaluation of an intensive follow-up program for patients with a stoma, *Ostomy Wound Management* 56(5):44, 2010.

Dietz D, Gates J: Basic ostomy management, part 1, *Nursing* 40(2):61, 2010a.

Dietz D, Gates J: Basic ostomy management, part 2, *Nursing* 40(5):62, 2010b.

Gemmill R, et al: Going with the flow: quality of life outcomes of cancer survivors with urinary diversion, *J Wound Ostomy Continence Nurs* 37(1):65, 2010.

Goldberg M, et al: *Management of the patient with a fecal ostomy: best practice guidelines for clinicians*, Mt Laurel, NJ, 2010, WOCN.

Kent D: Changing an ostomy pouching system, *Nursing* 38(12):50, 2008.

Li C: Sexuality among patients with a colostomy, *J Wound Ostomy Continence Nurse* 36(3):288, 2009.

The Joint Commission (TJC): *National Patient Safety Goals*, Oakbrook Terrace, Ill, 2012, The Commission, available at http://www.jointcommission.org/standards_information/npsgs.aspx.

MEDIA RESOURCES

- **evolve** http://evolve.elsevier.com/Perry/skills
  - Review Questions
  - ▶ Video Clip
  - Audio Glossary

- Mosby's Nursing Video Skills, 4th edition

KEY TERMS

Analgesia	Hemostasis	Penrose drain	Postural hypotension
Anesthesia	Hemovac drain	Phlebothrombosis	Preoperative
Atelectasis	Hypovolemic shock	Positive expiratory pressure	Preoperative checklist
Coagulopathies	Incentive spirometer	Postanesthesia care unit	Procedural sedation
Decompression	Informed consent	(PACU)	Thrombophlebitis
Dehiscence	Jackson-Pratt drain	PACU phase I	Urinary retention
Ecchymosis	Malignant hyperthermia	PACU phase II	Venous thromboembolism
Evisceration	Obstructive sleep apnea	Postoperative	(VTE)
Extended care	Paralytic ileus		

OBJECTIVES

Mastery of content in this chapter will enable the nurse to:
- Describe the activities needed to prepare a patient for surgery.
- Explain the rationale for preoperative procedures.
- Discuss cultural differences that might affect the implementation of preoperative and postoperative procedures.
- Describe the benefits of structured preoperative teaching.

- Explain the rationale for each of the postoperative exercises.
- Successfully instruct a patient in performing postoperative exercises.
- Discuss the differences in nursing assessment during the immediate postoperative period and the convalescent phase of recovery.
- Conduct an assessment of a postoperative patient.

Surgical care of patients is in a continuous state of technologic advancement. The development of new diagnostic and interventional devices (e.g., endoscopic examination, robotic techniques, and laser surgery) has contributed to a shortened surgical length of stay and changes in roles for health care providers.

Any form of surgery is a stressful event, whether it is a major or a minor surgical procedure occurring in a large medical center or an outpatient center. A patient must frequently make decisions to undergo procedures that are associated with pain, possible disfigurement, dependence, or even the threat of death. Psychologically the experience of surgery can cause considerable fear and anxiety. Physiologically the more complex the surgery, the more likely it is that a patient

will undergo changes in major body systems. Thus it is important that a patient do all preparation for surgery during preadmission testing (PAT) in which a perianesthesia nurse, nurse practitioner, and sometimes the anesthesia provider interview the patient and/or family member, perform pertinent history and physical diagnostic testing, consult if needed, and provide preoperative education to prepare the patient for surgery.

Nurses use a variety of skills to help surgical patients adequately prepare for the physiologic and psychological stressors of surgery. During the preoperative phase the nursing role focuses on physical, psychological, sociocultural, and spiritual preparation and validates existing information, reinforces preoperative teaching, reviews discharge instructions, and provides nursing care to complete preparation for the surgical experience (ASPAN, 2010). A variety of diagnostic tests are coordinated to ensure that the surgeon and anesthesia care providers have the information needed to determine a patient's risks during surgery and the postoperative period. In preparation for surgery, you will instruct the patient and family concerning postoperative care in compliance with The Joint Commission patient and family education standards (TJC, 2012a) (Box 36-1). The instructional topics enable patients and their families to actively participate in the recovery process. Occasionally you will have to perform certain procedures such as surgical skin preparation or inserting an indwelling catheter (see Chapter 33) or nasogastric (NG) tube (see Chapter 34) to protect patients from risks associated with surgery and provide a safe environment.

Although preoperative education improves patient outcomes after surgery, the shift in the provision of surgical services poses special challenges to meet patients' educational needs in a reduced time frame. Because a majority of patients undergo surgery in an ambulatory setting, it is essential that they receive adequate information to ensure that they or their family members can manage postoperative care activities in the home setting. If a patient is to be admitted for same-day surgery, perform the preoperative assessment and teaching of postoperative care instructions several days before surgery. The surgeon's office nurse or, more typically, the preadmission nurse and/or the preoperative nurse in the outpatient department, complete these services. The nurse ensures the completion of operative informed consent permits, blood work, testing (e.g., electrocardiogram [ECG]), and any other ordered procedures based on the American Society of Anesthesiologist (ASA) guidelines before the start of the procedure (ASA, 2012).

During the postoperative phase, when a patient returns from the operating room (OR), you are initially responsible for completing a thorough assessment of physical and mental status and providing continuous monitoring of his or her condition or any changes during the recovery process. The American Society of PeriAnesthesia Nurses (ASPAN) identifies three levels of care provided to the surgical/procedural patient, including postanesthesia phase I, postanesthesia phase II, and extended care. Once a patient's condition stabilizes, focus your efforts on returning the patient to a functional level of wellness as soon as possible within the limitations created by surgery. The speed of a patient's recovery depends on how effectively you anticipate potential complications, initiate necessary supportive and preventive therapies, and actively involve the patient and family in the recovery process.

EVIDENCE-BASED PRACTICE TRENDS

Several evidence-based initiatives target the improvement of surgical care. These initiatives focus on surgical site infections (SSIs), the surgical care improvement project (SCIP), adverse cardiac events, and postoperative venous thromboembolism (VTE). The SCIP program, previously called the *surgical infection prevention project (SIPP)*, is sponsored by the Centers for Medicare and Medicaid Services (CMS) in collaboration with other national partners. The Centers for Disease Control and Prevention (CDC), the Institute for Healthcare Improvement (IHI), The Joint Commission (TJC), CMS, ASPAN, the Association of periOperative Registered Nurses (AORN), and the Council on Surgical and Perioperative Safety (CSPS) have implemented evidence-based initiatives that promote a culture of safety and protect patients from surgical complications.

The CDC's National Nosocomial Infections Surveillance (NNIS) system reports that SSIs account for 4% to 16% of hospital-acquired infections (Drake, 2011). Research indicates that 38% of hospital-acquired infections are SSIs (Drake, 2011). Evidence-based guidelines are identified to reduce SSIs and promote SCIP:

- Do not remove hair unless it will interfere with the operation and remove it using only electric clippers if possible.
- Give the correct antibiotic before surgery and at the appropriate time.
- Maintain blood glucose level after surgery, especially for patients undergoing cardiac surgery.
- Maintain normothermia (core temperature range of 36° C to 38° C [96.8° F to 100.4° F]).
- Receive beta blocker during the perioperative period.
- Remove urinary catheter on postoperative day 1 or 2.

There are also strict guidelines for use of antibiotics. The goal of prophylactic antibiotic therapy is to select the most effective antibiotics for maximum coverage and administer them when they are most beneficial to protect patients from infection with as little risk as possible:

- Overall it is recommended that prophylactic antibiotics be given as close to the time of incision as possible (within 60 minutes) and not be given for longer than 24 hours after surgery.
- However, vancomycin and fluoroquinolones (i.e., ciprofloxacin [Cipro], levofloxacin [Levaquin]) may be given up to 2 hours before incision because of their longer infusion times. Antibiotic use after incision closure does not reduce infection rates; and, when the antibiotics are continued, infections are more likely to be caused by a resistant organism (CDC, 2011; Drake, 2011).

BOX 36-1	The Joint Commission Patient and Family Education Standards

Education provided is appropriate to the patient's needs. The assessment of learning needs addresses cultural and religious beliefs, emotional barriers, desire to learn, physical or cognitive limitations, and barriers to communication as appropriate. When called for by the age of the patient and the length of stay, the hospital assesses and provides for patient's education needs. Patients are educated about:

- The plan for care, treatment, and services (i.e., postoperative monitoring).
- Basic health practices and safety (i.e., out of bed [OOB] only with assistance).
- The safe and effective use of medication (i.e., the patient is only one allowed to self-administer patient-controlled analgesia [PCA]).
- Nutrition interventions, modified diets, or oral health (i.e., progression of diet after surgery).
- Safe and effective use of medical equipment or supplies when provided by the hospital (i.e., incentive spirometer).
- Pain—Understanding pain, the risk for pain, the importance of effective pain management, the pain assessment process, and methods for pain management (i.e., reporting pain, frequency of medications, nonpharmacologic pain-relief techniques).
- Habilitation or rehabilitation techniques to help them reach the maximum independence possible (i.e., early ambulation).

Modified from The Joint Commission: *Accreditation manual for hospitals*, Chicago, 2011, The Commission; and Schick L, Windle P: *PeriAnesthesia nursing core curriculum: preprocedure, phase I and phase II PACU nursing*, ed 2, St Louis, 2010, Saunders.

- Prophylactic antibiotics should be discontinued within 24 hours after the end of surgery in most cases.

Hyperglycemia inhibits the ability of the body to fight infection. Immediate postoperative glucose control is also correlated with a reduction in surgical infection. The presence of hyperglycemia in the immediate postoperative period increases the risk for infection in both patients with diabetes and nondiabetic patients. The higher the serum glucose level, the higher the potential for infection in both patient groups (Drake, 2011).

The prevention of adverse cardiac events calls for the continued use of beta-blocker therapy before and after surgery. Often this medication may be missed because the surgeon is not the patient's primary care provider or the patient continues to be allowed nothing by mouth (NPO) for a period after surgery. This is one of many reasons why The Joint Commission now requires medication reconciliation on admission (or patient encounter with ambulatory care patients) with each transfer and before discharge (Drake, 2011).

It is reported that approximately 15% of all postoperative deaths can be attributed to pulmonary embolus (PE). In addition, it is reported that 15% to 40% of routine surgical patients develop deep vein thrombosis (DVT). This rate is higher for some patients such as those following orthopedic procedures or in critical care units (Ouellette and Patocka, 2012):

- In response to this, the American College of Chest Physicians in 2008 recommends the use of prophylactic pharmacologic and mechanical therapies to prevent venous thromboembolism (VTE). The term *VTE* is now used because it incorporates both DVT and PE.
- Each patient's risk for VTE should be assessed, and patients treated appropriately.
- Mechanical therapies include the use of graduated compression stockings (see Chapter 10) along with intermittent pneumatic compression (IPC) or a venous foot pump. The venous foot pump is primarily limited to when IPC cannot be used such as when surgery or injury occurs to the affected lower extremity.
- Aside from the mechanical device, it is important that pharmacologic regimens such as the administration of low-dose unfractionated heparin, low-molecular-weight heparin, factor Xa inhibitor (fondaparinux [Arixtra]), or warfarin (Coumadin) be included after surgery.

Another trend seen in the United States is the increased prevalence of obesity. Researchers estimate that 68% of adults 20 years of age and older are overweight or obese, with 33.8% of the adult population considered obese (CDC, 2012). Of children and adolescents ages 2 to 19 years, 17% are obese. Being overweight or obese increases the risk for many diseases and health conditions, including hypertension, dyslipidemia, coronary heart disease, type 2 diabetes, stroke, cancers (endometrial, breast, and colon), sleep apnea, and respiratory problems. These conditions increase risks of postoperative complications. Obese patients are at risk for obstructive sleep apnea (OSA), and a majority of patients undergoing surgery are overweight and present signs and symptoms of OSA. After surgery patients with OSA have a greater incidence of airway management problems in postanesthesia care units (PACUs) and postoperative floors and develop postoperative pulmonary complications. Longer lengths of stay and unanticipated postoperative admission to the intensive care unit are common (ASA, 2006; Kaw et al., 2012). The latest trend is to monitor these patients longer in PACU (ASA, 2006; Kaw et al., 2012), admit them to floors with continuous pulse oximetry 24 hours after surgery, encourage deep-breathing exercises, and limit opioid medications.

PATIENT-CENTERED CARE

To provide culturally competent care to a surgical patient, begin by assessing the family hierarchy to determine who needs to be involved in the patient's decisions regarding surgery. When providing preoperative teaching, include family members. The use of professional interpreters for patients who do not speak English is beneficial in providing competent informed patient care.

Before surgery it is important to accommodate a patient's religious and cultural needs and adapt the patient's care to encompass his or her practices and beliefs whenever possible. Identify cultural and religious beliefs and practices that affect patients' and/or family members' reactions to the surgical experience such as who can give consent; blood transfusions; and disposal of body parts, including hair. Preoperative and postoperative time is valued as family time to support a patient by many cultures such as African-Americans. Some Mormons who have received full sacraments request to wear an undergarment. A male Sikh may request to wear a turban or metal bracelet and keep his long hair and beard. An East Indian woman may wish to wear her wedding necklace. For example, allow religious articles (e.g., medals, underclothing) to be worn until just before surgery. It is important to request information from the patient, family, or religious leader about how to remove these articles if absolutely necessary. Similarly, return these articles promptly after surgery.

Before and after surgery it will be helpful to assess patient preferences for pain medication. Some patients believe that pain

TABLE 36-1	Information Needed for Informed Consent
Parameters	**Examples**
Name of procedure/ surgery	Abdominal hysterectomy under general anesthesia
Description of procedure/surgery	Removal of uterus only through an incision in the abdominal wall at the top of the pubic hairline; done while unconscious
Person performing procedure/surgery	Dr. Richard Jones assisted by Dr. William Smith
Benefits of procedure/ surgery	To remove uterus with fibroids and stop excessive bleeding Abdominal route necessary because of anticipated adhesions from prior abdominal surgery
Potential risks and adverse effects of procedure/surgery	Risk of hemorrhage and infection from surgery; risk of excessive sedation and allergic reaction to drugs used with general anesthesia; accidental damage to bladder, intestines, and/or nerves controlling these organs
Approximate length of time for procedure/ surgery	About 1 hour; 1 to 2 hours in postanesthesia care unit (PACU)
Approximate length of time needed for recovery	3 to 4 days on surgical unit; 4 to 6 weeks before resuming physically stressful work
Alternative treatments	Removal of uterus vaginally; radiation to shrink fibroids
Consequences of refusing treatment	Continuation of pain and vaginal bleeding, risk for developing anemia; after menopause fibroids should regress

medication leads to addiction. Buddhists and Hindus prefer to endure the pain without medication. Cultures that value men being in control of their emotions may prevent members from verbalizing pain.

Safety Guidelines

1 Know the type and nature of any previous surgery. Anatomic and physiologic alterations affect a patient's risk for operative problems.
2 Identify the factors and conditions that increase a patient's risks during surgery. Preoperative preparation and postoperative care depend on knowledge of these risk factors.
3 Know the rationale for and extent of impending surgery. Each type of surgical procedure requires a different type of nursing care.

4 Ensure that the patient has signed the informed consent. You are witnessing a patient's signature only and not his or her knowledge. Informed consent is required by law to help protect patient's rights, their autonomy, and their privacy. The surgeon should give the patient information about the extent and type of surgery, alternative therapies, usual risks, benefits, and consequences of not having surgery. See agency policy regarding consent (Table 36-1).
5 Complete the preoperative checklist. Include the global initiative of the World Health Organization (WHO) Surgical Safety Checklist (WHO, 2008).
6 Administer pain-relief therapies according to a patient's perioperative needs. Pain can slow a surgical patient's recovery.
7 Restrict patient activity after administration of preoperative and postoperative sedatives to minimize the risk for patient falls.

SKILL 36-1   Preparing a Patient for Surgery

 Video Clip

Preparing a patient for surgery involves activities and procedures that help to decrease anxiety, ensure patient safety, and decrease the risk for complications. A thorough nursing assessment documents baseline data for future comparisons to determine the effect of instruction and monitor patients at risk for complications during the perioperative experience.

Anxiety interferes with the effectiveness of anesthesia and the ability of patients to actively participate in their care. Provide information to patients about what will occur during the perioperative experience and which sensations a patient can expect to feel. Demonstration of a caring attitude toward a patient, family members, and significant others increases feelings of trust and reduces anxiety (Fig. 36-1). Provide assurance that comfort measures will be implemented to manage pain (see Chapter 15).

Some patients with "do not resuscitate" (DNR) orders require surgery for palliative care. DNR orders should not be upheld or suspended routinely during anesthesia and surgery. A patient's surgeon (attending surgeons and anesthesiologists) are responsible for discussing and documenting issues with a patient and/or family to determine whether to maintain the DNR order or whether it should be partially or completely suspended during surgery. This discussion should describe potential resuscitation efforts that may be required during surgery and whether withholding resuscitation initiatives would alter the patient's goals for having the surgery. Considerations that should be included in the discussion are the goals of the surgical treatment, the possibility of resuscitative measures, a description of what these measures include, and possible outcomes with and without resuscitation. Advance directives must be encouraged and included in a patient's chart. If the patient has opted to alter the DNR order during the intraoperative period, clear documentation should be in the medical record indicating when the DNR order is to be reinstated (AORN, 2010d; ASPAN, 2010).

The risks for postoperative complications are decreased in a number of ways, some of which are specific to the type of procedure. For example, any patient with a surgical incision of the thorax or abdomen will have pain after surgery, and this reduces lung expansion. Before surgery a patient will be encouraged to learn how to use an incentive spirometer to reduce the incidence of atelectasis after surgery. Deep-breathing and coughing exercises are examples of other procedures used to reduce complications.

Food and fluids are withheld routinely for a period of time before surgery. Each patient should have orders written by anesthesia personnel outlining preoperative fasting requirements. Practice guidelines for preoperative fasting in healthy patients undergoing elective procedures allow for the consumption of clear liquids up to 2 hours before surgery, a light breakfast (e.g., tea and toast) 6 hours before the procedure, and a heavier meal 8 hours before the procedure (ASA, 2011). However, in general, to minimize the risk for aspiration, food and fluids are withheld for 8 hours before surgery requiring general anesthesia. The patient may need to be NPO even when spinal or epidural anesthesia is administered. Hypotension caused by autonomic nervous system blockade can induce nausea and vomiting (Lewis et al., 2011). Patients who are dehydrated or are at risk for hypovolemia will have intravenous (IV) fluids ordered. Medications may be given to decrease respiratory and gastrointestinal (GI) secretions, as an adjunct to anesthesia, and to decrease the risk for infection and development of stress ulcers.

The type of surgery determines the preparation required before surgery (e.g., low-residue and clear-liquid diets, enemas, cathartics,

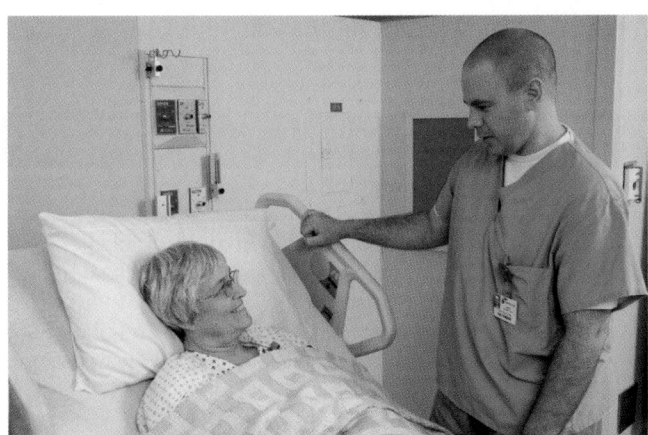

FIG 36-1   Nurse establishes trusting relationship with patient.

and oral antibiotics are for patients who undergo bowel surgery). Encourage patients who smoke to stop the use of all tobacco products for at least 30 days before surgery. Nicotine delays wound healing and increases the risk for wound infection by constricting blood flow (Tonnesen et al., 2009). Patients whose blood work indicates a low hemoglobin level and/or abnormal electrolyte levels or coagulopathies often require inpatient therapy before surgery.

Because many patients are admitted on the day of surgery, much of the preoperative preparation is often the responsibility of the patient or the primary caregiver. Therefore it is important that a preadmission nurse or nurse in the surgeon's practice provide adequate instructions. Patient teaching should include any food and fluid restrictions; which medications, if any, are permitted on the morning of surgery; and the need for surgical site preparation the evening before surgery. It is also important to include action that a patient will need to take if any of these instructions are mistakenly omitted. Written instructions are a useful adjunct to teaching because a patient and/or family can refer to them for any points that are unclear or forgotten. Videos and pamphlets are also useful adjuncts in preparing patients and their families.

The revised Joint Commission standards (2012b) incorporated in the National Patient Safety Goals (NPSGs) implemented the Universal Protocol for Preventing Wrong Site, Wrong Procedure, Wrong Person surgery. This protocol was implemented as an added safety measure to ensure that correct person, procedure, and surgical site are verified at the time of scheduling the procedure, on admission or entry into the agency, and each time the responsibility for care of the patient is transferred to another caregiver. A final verification check involving the entire surgical team occurs immediately before the start of the procedure. If the case involves laterality (right versus left), multiple structures (e.g., fingers, toes, lesions), or multiple levels (e.g., spine), the final verification should include a site marking by the person performing the procedure. The site markings need to be visible after the patient has been prepared and draped. Involve patients in this process when they are awake and aware. Immediately before starting the procedure a "time out" is called. The entire operative team, using active communication, verifies correct patient identity, correct side and site, agreement on the procedure to be done, correct patient position, and availability of correct implants and any special equipment or special requirements. This final verification process should be documented.

Delegation and Collaboration

The skills of preoperative assessment and teaching cannot be delegated to nursing assistive personnel (NAP). Each state has its own delegation rules based on the Board of Nurses. Here are some examples for delegation (ASPAN, 2010).

- Basic infection prevention and control practices
- Care of a patient requiring monitoring and providing comfort measures
- Care of a patient with nausea and vomiting who is receiving IV fluids and oral intake
- Care of a patient with thermoregulatory problems, including hyperthermia and hypothermia
- Care of a patient on continual antiembolism devices who requires assistance with ambulation

Equipment
Equipment for Preanesthesia Phase
- ❏ Stethoscope
- ❏ Blood pressure monitoring equipment
- ❏ Pulse oximetry
- ❏ Thermometer
- ❏ Preoperative checklist

Preadmission
Equipment for preadmission area includes but is not limited to:
- ❏ Method to measure height and weight
- ❏ Blood pressure monitoring equipment
- ❏ Pulse oximeter
- ❏ Access to laboratory, electrocardiogram (ECG), x-ray film and other diagnostic equipment as needed
- ❏ Access to latex-free supplies
- ❏ Emergency cart for adults and pediatrics
- ❏ Stock supplies, including facial tissue; gloves, syringes, and needles (including protective needle devices); emesis basins; alcohol wipes; tongue blades; personal protective equipment; tourniquets; variety of tapes; latex-free supplies

Day of Surgery/Procedure Preparation Area
Each patient bedside unit will have the following:
- ❏ Oxygen equipment, including pulse oximeter
- ❏ Constant and intermittent suction
- ❏ Blood pressure and cardiac monitoring equipment
- ❏ Thermometer
- ❏ Blood glucose monitor
- ❏ Equipment to measure height and weight
- ❏ Surgical preparation supplies
- ❏ Antiembolism stockings and/or intermittent pneumatic compression device (if ordered) (see Chapter 10)
- ❏ Emergency cart for adult and pediatrics

STEP	RATIONALE

ASSESSMENT

1 Determine ability of patient to answer questions regarding health history and pending surgery.

Identifies reliability of patient and need to supplement with information from family members or significant others. Indicates need for further information for informed consent.

2 Collect nursing history and identify surgical risk factors, medications, and history of allergies (see Table 36-2 on p. 888; see Chapter 6).

Allows for anticipation of possible complications and planning for interventions to reduce risks. Allergies, particularly to latex, can be life threatening.

Clinical Decision Point *If patient is having emergency surgery, focus on assessment of primary body system affected.*

STEP	RATIONALE
3 Perform physical examination (see Table 36-2 and Chapter 6). Focus on body systems that surgery will affect, including a comprehensive pain assessment.	Provides baseline data for future assessments and interventions. Also confirms or disputes information from history and may uncover new information.
4 Ask about patient's and family members' knowledge of and expectations of surgery and care. Include questions concerning fears, cultural practices, and religious beliefs if applicable.	Allows you to anticipate patient's/family's priorities and adapt plan so you can give appropriate instruction and support.
5 Review patient's preoperative orders.	Identifies specific procedures, diagnostic tests, and medications that patient will receive.
6 If patient is same-day admit or ambulatory patient, validate that admission preparations were completed as ordered. Specific preparations to review include NPO status, administration of medications, skin preparation, and bowel preparation if applicable.	Failure to complete preparation could lead to perioperative or postoperative complications and may necessitate postponement or cancellation of surgery.
7 Ask if patient has an advance directive. If so, place it in his or her record.	Document conveys patient's wishes if life support measures are necessary.

NURSING DIAGNOSES

- Acute pain
- Anxiety
- Deficient knowledge regarding the surgical experience
- Fear

- Impaired oral mucous membrane
- Impaired physical mobility
- Ineffective airway clearance
- Ineffective breathing pattern
- Ineffective tissue perfusion

- Risk for aspiration
- Risk for impaired skin integrity
- Risk for infection
- Risk for perioperative-positioning injury

Related factors are individualized based on patient's condition or needs.

PLANNING

1 Expected outcomes following completion of procedure:	
• Patient can state which surgical procedure is being performed and risks and benefits of surgery.	Identifies readiness to sign informed consent.
• Patient participates in preoperative and postoperative care.	Preoperative preparations are effective.
• Patient states that anxiety is decreased.	Anxiety interferes with effectiveness of teaching and anesthesia.
2 Explain procedures and allow patient, family members, and significant others to ask questions and express concerns.	Decreases anxiety and increases cooperation.

IMPLEMENTATION

1 Identify patient using two identifiers (i.e., name and birthday or name and account number) according to agency policy. Compare identifiers with information on patient's identification bracelet.	Ensures correct patient. Complies with The Joint Commission standards and improves patient safety (TJC, 2012b).
2 Apply allergy/sensitivity band and other safety bands if applicable.	Alerts surgeons to potential safety issues such as patient's allergies and sensitivities, risk for falls, presence of obstructive sleep apnea, or other conditions.
3 Orient patient to room or presurgical (holding) area. Surgeon obtains informed consent. Act as patient advocate as needed; include considering any culturally sensitive issues. Witness form if allowed by agency.	Decreases anxiety and promotes feelings of control. Surgery cannot be performed legally without informed consent. Patient must receive information about need and extent of surgery, alternatives, risks, and benefits. Patient and/or family may be afraid to ask questions or express concerns regarding diverse practices.

Clinical Decision Point *Patients who are illiterate can sign with a mark if properly witnessed. Minors, unless married or declared emancipated, and individuals considered incompetent cannot legally sign a consent form. Parent or legal guardian must provide consent. Some cultures do not allow female members to give consent. Refer to each state and agency protocol for implementing informed consent.*

4 Check medical record and review or complete preoperative checklist.	Ensures that pertinent laboratory and diagnostic test results are available and that all preoperative preparations are completed (Litwack, 2009).
5 Provide preoperative teaching, including explanation of postoperative exercises (see Skill 36-2), skin preparation, pain-control measures (see Chapter 15), and postoperative care in postanesthesia care unit (PACU) phases I and II and nursing division (see Skill 36-3).	Decreases anxiety and promotes cooperation in care. (Litwack, 2009; Stannard and Krenzischek, 2012)

STEP	RATIONALE
6 Maintain NPO status.	NPO 8 hours after regular meal before surgery in healthy adult patients (ASA, 2011; Litwack, 2009; Stannard and Krenzischek, 2012).

Clinical Decision Point *Patient may brush teeth but should not swallow water. Patient may take oral medications such as beta-blocker medications with sips of water (30 mL). Check with surgeon if they are specifically ordered to be taken before surgery (e.g., antiarrhythmic or seizure medications) and which medications to hold, especially herbals and aspirin. Withhold all other oral medications. You must later check postoperative orders to ensure that scheduled medications unrelated to surgery are not forgotten.*

STEP	RATIONALE
7 Insert intravenous (IV) line and/or indwelling catheter if ordered.	IV line and/or indwelling catheter may be inserted in holding or preanesthesia area to establish route for medication and fluid administration.
8 Provide for hygiene measures, ensuring patient privacy. Instruct patient to remove all clothing, including undergarments, and apply disposable cap and hospital gown with opening in back.	Prevents patient's hair from contaminating sterile surfaces and provides easy access to patient's body in operating room (OR).
9 Instruct patient to remove hairpins; clips; wigs; hairpieces; jewelry, including rings used in body piercing; and makeup (including nail polish and acrylic nails). Religious medals may be pinned to gown if policy permits. Some agencies allow you to remove acrylic nails or nail polish from only one finger if using a pulse oximeter. Check agency policy.	Hair appliances and jewelry anywhere on body may become dislodged and cause injury during positioning and intubation. Rings decrease circulation in fingers. Makeup, nail polish, and false nails impede assessment of skin and oxygenation. In addition, acrylic nails harbor pathogenic organisms (AORN, 2010a).

Clinical Decision Point *Tape wedding rings that cannot be removed. Be careful not to create tourniquet effect with tape around finger.*

STEP	RATIONALE
10 Help patient remove prostheses, including dentures and oral appliances, glasses and contact lenses, artificial limbs and eyes, artificial eyelashes, and hearing aids. Document list of items and their location in preoperative checklist and/or nurses' notes per agency policy.	Prostheses can be lost or damaged during surgery and could cause injury. Oral appliances may occlude airway.

Clinical Decision Point *If patient needs to follow instructions in the OR, leave hearing aid in place. Decision may be made to leave wig or dentures in place until entering OR suite if removal will cause embarrassment. Check agency policy.*

STEP	RATIONALE
11 Inventory all items and give to family member or significant other or have security put valuables in a locked area. Have release form signed if required by agency.	Valuables left in patient's room may be lost or stolen.
12 Apply antiembolism stockings as ordered (see Chapter 10).	Promotes venous return and reduces risk for thrombus formation.
13 Assess vital signs immediately before going to OR.	Abnormal vital signs indicate conditions that increase risk for surgery.

Clinical Decision Point *Report vital signs not within normal range or patient's baseline to anesthesia/surgeon. These results may require surgery to be postponed. Document abnormal vital signs and any action taken in nurses' notes and/or preoperative checklist according to agency policy.*

STEP	RATIONALE
14 If patient does not have an indwelling catheter, help him or her void before receiving preoperative medication.	Prevents incontinence and bladder distention during surgery and urinary retention with overflow after surgery. Preoperative medication causes drowsiness and decreased voiding sensation.
15 Administer preoperative medications as ordered. (These medications may be given in preoperative or holding area. Check preoperative orders.)	Reduces pain, anxiety, respiratory secretions, and amount of anesthesia required. Promotes relaxation. Antibiotics may be ordered prophylactically but are given within 60 minutes of incision.

Clinical Decision Point *Check that informed consent is signed before giving preoperative medications. Times on consent form and medication administration record (MAR) must attest to this. Preoperative medications may alter level of consciousness and make the consent invalid.*

STEP	RATIONALE
16 Place patient on bed rest with call light within reach and inform him or her not to get out of bed without assistance. Allow family members to remain at bedside until patient is transferred to surgical area. Maintain quiet and relaxing environment.	There is an increased chance of injury in attempting to ambulate to void when patient is sedated and unattended. 

EVALUATION

1 Have patient describe surgical procedure and its benefits and risks.

2 Compare all assessment data with patient's baseline and expected normal levels.

3 Have patient repeat preoperative instructions.

4 Monitor patient for signs and symptoms of anxiety and ask how patient and family are feeling.

Confirms level of knowledge needed to sign informed consent.

Evaluates patient's risk for complications and possible need to postpone surgery.

Provides evidence that patient understands instructions.

Increased heart rate and blood pressure, dilated pupils, dry mouth, increased sweating, and muscle rigidity or shaking are responses to stress and anxiety. Asking patient about feelings gives permission to express concerns, which can be further explored.

Unexpected Outcomes

1 Patient is unable to give consent, and family member is unavailable.

2 Vital signs are above or below patient's baseline or expected range.

3 Informed consent has not been signed and witnessed. Surgeon and anesthesiologist did not provide information and/or ensure that consent forms were signed.

4 Patient did not remain NPO, which may indicate that he or she did not understand instructions or forgot.

5 Patient is unable to state instructions.

6 Patient did not void before receiving preoperative medication.

Related Interventions

- In emergency situations obtain telephone consent from next of kin. Two persons must witness oral consent (according to agency policy).
- Document explanation of situation and fact that oral consent was obtained and witnessed.
- At earliest opportunity, person giving oral consent must sign a written consent. Signed telegram or signed fax may also be considered oral consent. Follow agency policy.

- This indicates possible infection; anxiety; pain; or cardiovascular dysfunction, which increases surgical risk.
- Patients who are dehydrated or malnourished may require hydration with IV solutions (see Chapter 28), parenteral nutrition (see Chapter 32), or antibiotic therapy before surgery.

- Patient is not ready for surgery. Patient must sign consent before administration of preoperative medications or any medication that alters central nervous system. Notify physician/surgeon/anesthesiologist.

- Notify surgeon and anesthesiologist. Surgery may be postponed or cancelled.

- Assessment of patient's level of understanding or method of instruction was insufficient. Revision of instruction is necessary.

- Patient did not need to or was unable to void. Assess for renal function and bladder distention. If distended, have patient use urinal or bedpan, or you may need an order for catheterization (see Chapter 33).

Recording and Reporting

- Document all preoperative assessment findings and preparations in nurses' notes and electronic health record (EHR) and/or checklist or flow sheet.
- Document patient's condition on transfer to OR in narrative notes or on flow sheet.
- Document presence of any allergies/sensitivities on armband, in medical record, and in MAR.
- Record disposition of patient valuables/belongings (i.e., whether locked up according to agency policy or sent with family).

- Report lack of signed and witnessed consent form or failure of patient to maintain NPO status and action taken.
- Report and record patient's cultural practices and/or religious beliefs that affect perioperative care and any modification of care planned.

Special Considerations
Teaching

- The Joint Commission patient and family education standards are guidelines to ensure that patient, family member, and/or

TABLE 36-2	Assessment of the Surgical Patient
Assessment Category	**Key Criteria**
Nursing history	Previous personal/family experience with surgery (e.g., complications) and anesthesia (e.g., malignant hyperthermia)
Physical examination	General system review: • Head and neck • Integument • Thorax and lungs • Heart and vascular • Abdomen • Neurologic status • Age • Nutrition • Radiotherapy, chemotherapy, medications that depress immune system • Fluid and electrolyte balance • Preexisting infection • Chronic respiratory disease (emphysema, bronchitis, asthma) • Immunologic disorders (leukemia, acquired immunodeficiency syndrome) • Allergies/sensitivities (including medications, food, latex, and environmental)
Risk factors	• Medication history (prescriptions, including pain-management medications, over-the counter [OTC], and herbal remedies) • Physical or mental impairments • Mobility limitations • Prostheses (including hearing aids) • Smoking habits • Alcohol ingestion • Family support and coping mechanisms • Occupation • Emotional health • Temperature, blood pressure, pulse and respiratory rates • Height and weight • Oxygen saturations • Electrocardiogram • Laboratory values (e.g., Hgb, K^+, glucose, coagulation studies) • Radiology and diagnostic test findings

BOX 36-2	Postanesthesia and Ambulatory Surgery Discharge Criteria

Postanesthesia Discharge Criteria
- Patient awake (or returns to baseline)
- Vital signs stable
- No excess bleeding or drainage
- No respiratory depression
- SaO_2 greater than 90%
- Pain controlled
- Report given

Ambulatory Surgery Discharge Criteria
- All postanesthesia care unit (PACU) discharge criteria met
- No intravenous (IV) narcotics for last 30 minutes
- Minimal nausea and vomiting
- Pain controlled
- Voided (if appropriate to surgical procedure/orders)
- Able to ambulate if age-appropriate and not contraindicated
- Responsible adult present to accompany patient
- Discharge instructions given and understood

children for same-day surgery have been shown to decrease anxiety in both parents and children. Part of preoperative teaching needs to include giving children the opportunity to handle equipment they will see such as an anesthesia mask or drainage tube.
- Take the developmental level of a child into consideration during preoperative preparation. Use toys and games to demonstrate preoperative procedures (Hockenberry and Wilson, 2011).
- Allow parents to accompany their child to the holding area and consider visitation in the PACU after the procedure.

Gerontologic
- Physiologic changes that occur with aging may require admission to hospital before surgery for additional diagnostic tests and stabilization of condition (Table 36-3).
- Teach when patient is alert and rested. Keep teaching sessions short.
- Age-related changes such as decreased vision, hearing, and short-term memory may require presence of family caregiver during preoperative preparation.
- Make sure that a family member or someone will take care of ambulatory patients at home.

Home Care
- Instruct patients admitted on day of surgery about NPO status, skin preparation, and procedures such as enemas and douches before admission. Patients often use enemas or douches at home.
- Patients having surgery performed in ambulatory surgery centers must be accompanied by a family member or friend to allow for discharge after the procedure (Box 36-2).

primary caregiver know about surgical procedure, healing process, sutures, dressing, drains, feeding tubes, pain control, and diet with rationale for each. Adults learn best when they understand the purpose or meaning of what is being taught (Schick and Windle, 2010; TJC, 2012a).

Pediatric
- Involve parents in preoperative preparation to decrease children's anxiety. Preadmission programs to prepare parents and

TABLE 36-3	Physiologic Factors That Place Older Adult Patients at Risk for Surgery	
Alterations	**Surgery Risks**	**Nursing Implications**
Cardiovascular		
Degenerative change in myocardium and valves	Reduced cardiac reserve	Assess baseline vital signs.
Rigidity of arterial walls and reduction in sympathetic and parasympathetic innervation to heart	Predisposes patient to postoperative hemorrhage and rise in systolic and diastolic blood pressure	Maintain adequate fluid balance to minimize stress to heart. Ensure that blood pressure is adequate to meet circulatory demands.
Increase in calcium and cholesterol deposits within small arteries; arterial walls thickened	Predisposes patient to clot formation in lower extremities	Instruct patient in techniques for performing leg exercises and proper turning. Apply antiembolism stockings, sequential compression devices (SCDs) (see Chapter 10).
Integumentary System		
Decreased subcutaneous tissue and increased fragility of skin	Prone to pressure ulcers and skin tears	Assess skin every 4 hours; pad all bony prominences during surgery. Turn or reposition (see Chapter 9).
Pulmonary		
Rib cage stiffens and enlarges	Reduced vital capacity	Instruct patient in proper technique for coughing and deep-breathing exercises and use of spirometer.
Reduced diaphragm excursion	Greater residual capacity or volume of air left in lung after normal breath increases, reducing amount of new air brought into lungs with each inspiration	Encourage deep breathing. Use incentive spirometer to enhance exhalation.
Lung tissue less distensible; alveoli enlarged	Reduced blood oxygenation	Assess oxygen saturation via oximetry (SpO_2).
Renal		
Reduced blood flow to kidneys	Blood loss causes decrease in circulation to the kidney	Monitor urinary output and laboratory data (i.e., blood urea nitrogen [BUN], creatinine).
Reduced glomerular filtration rate and excretory times	Limits ability to remove drugs or toxic substances	Assess for adverse effects of medications.
Reduced bladder capacity	Voiding frequency increases, and larger amount of urine stays in the bladder after voiding	Instruct patient to notify nurse immediately when sensation of bladder fullness develops.
	Sensation of need to void may not occur until bladder is filled	Keep call light or bedpan within easy reach.
Neurologic		
Sensory losses, including reduced tactile sense, increased pain tolerance	Patient less able to respond to early warning signs of surgical complications	Inspect bony prominences for signs of pressure.
Decreased reaction time	Patient becomes confused easily after anesthesia	Orient patient to surrounding environment.
		Observe for nonverbal signs of pain. Maintain safe environment. Institute fall precautions.
Metabolic		
Lower basal metabolic rate	Reduced total oxygen consumption and nutritional needs.	Ensure adequate nutritional intake once diet is resumed.
Reduced number of red blood cells and hemoglobin levels	Reduces ability to carry adequate oxygen to tissues.	Administer necessary blood products. Assess for adequacy of oxygenation, fatigue, and infection.
Change in total amounts of body potassium and water volume	Greater risk for fluid or electrolyte imbalance	Monitor electrolyte levels.

SKILL 36-2 Demonstrating Postoperative Exercises

 Video Clip

Structured preoperative teaching has a positive influence on a surgical patient's recovery (Lewis et al., 2011). You will provide information and teach skills to help patients understand the surgical experience and participate actively in the recovery process. The skills of coughing, deep breathing, turning, and using an incentive spirometer are important in preventing circulatory and respiratory postoperative complications.

In the past teaching occurred the evening before surgery when patients were most anxious. As a result of cost reduction efforts, many patients are admitted to the hospital or ambulatory surgery center the day of surgery. Preoperative teaching is not highly effective at this time because of the patient's high anxiety level (Stannard and Krenzischek, 2012). Many health care agencies have developed comprehensive outpatient education programs to better enable patients to receive the knowledge and skills needed to participate in their own care before coming to the hospital or ambulatory care center. Teaching booklets and videotapes are often available to supplement any instruction a nurse provides.

Postoperative exercises include diaphragmatic breathing and effective coughing, turning, and leg exercises. Patients may use an incentive spirometer, a device that provides visual feedback at a preset inspiratory flow of volume of air that mimics natural sighing or yawning (see Skill 23-3). The surgeon may order incentive spirometry for patients especially at risk for atelectasis or pneumonia (e.g., chronic smokers or patients on prolonged bed rest). Positive expiratory pressure (PEP) therapy is an alternative device to conventional physiotherapy that uses inhalation and exhalation to keep the lungs healthy. When blowing the air out of the lungs, the PEP device provides increased intrathoracic pressure and stenting of the airways that move secretions toward the larger airways, where they can be expelled to prevent the alveoli from collapsing. During the discussion of these exercises, you will explain the relationship between the exercises and the physiologic principles that make them important. Through specific explanations and guided practice you will help develop patient commitment to the recovery process. Demonstrate the exercises and continue to coach the patient through several return practice sessions.

Whenever possible, include family caregivers or other significant people in the practice sessions. Frequently these individuals are with the patient during the postoperative period and can thus serve as coaches. You will also provide patients with information about the sensations typically experienced after surgery such as incisional pain, nausea, tightness of dressings, and which interventions will alleviate them. The information helps patients realistically interpret the events that occur in the postoperative period. As a result, patients are able to decrease anxiety, conserve their energy, and attend to performing the exercises that aid in their recovery.

A potential postoperative complication is venous thromboembolism, including deep vein thrombosis (DVT) and pulmonary embolism. One of the simplest ways to prevent the formation of DVT is to encourage and assist a patient in early ambulation and leg exercises. When this is not possible or the patient's age, past history, or surgical procedure place him or her at an increased risk, use additional devices to help prevent the formation of DVT such as compression stockings and intermittent pneumatic compression devices (see Chapter 10). Another device used to prevent DVT is the venous plexus foot pump (Fig. 36-2). This pump mimics the natural action of walking by intermittently compressing the sole of the foot and then relaxing it so the venous plexus can fill with blood. Neither the intermittent pneumatic compression device nor the venous plexus foot pump should be used on patients with an acute DVT, significant peripheral vascular ischemia, large open wounds or skin grafts, or cancer of the extremity. None of these devices should replace the need for early and frequent ambulation.

Delegation and Collaboration

The skill of teaching postoperative exercises cannot be delegated to nursing assistive personnel (NAP). The NAP can reinforce and help patients perform postoperative exercises. The nurse directs the NAP about:

- Maintaining precautions unique to a particular patient.
- When to report if the patient is unable or unwilling to perform the exercises correctly.

Equipment

- ❏ Pillow (*optional*; used to splint the incision when coughing to reduce discomfort)
- ❏ Incentive spirometer
- ❏ PEP device
- ❏ Stethoscope

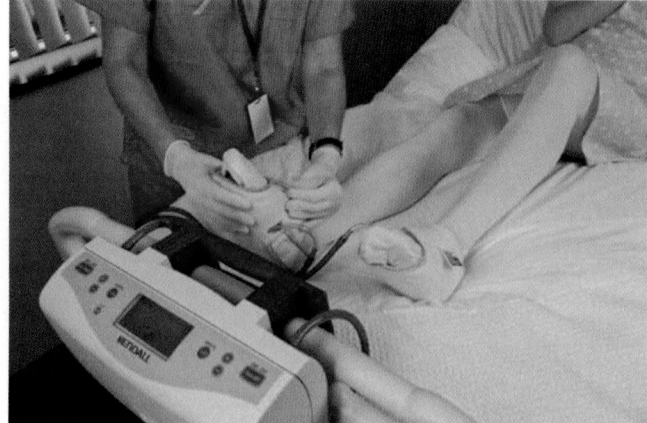

FIG 36-2 Venous plexus foot pump with bedside controls. (*Courtesy Tyco Healthcare Group LP.*)

STEP	RATIONALE

ASSESSMENT

1 Assess patient's risk for postoperative respiratory complications: Identify presence of chronic pulmonary condition (e.g., emphysema, chronic bronchitis, asthma); any condition that affects chest wall movement such as obesity, advanced pregnancy, thoracic or abdominal surgery; history of smoking; and presence of reduced hemoglobin level.	General anesthesia predisposes patient to respiratory problems because lungs are not fully inflated during surgery, cough reflex is suppressed, and mucus collects within airway passages. After surgery inadequate lung expansion can lead to atelectasis and pneumonia. Chronic lung conditions create greater risk for developing respiratory complications. Smoking damages ciliary clearance and increases mucus secretion. A reduced hemoglobin level can lead to reduced oxygen delivery.

Clinical Decision Point *Assess and report to surgeon and/or anesthesiologist if patient has had a cold or upper respiratory infection within past week.*

2 Auscultate lungs.	Establishes baseline for postoperative comparison.
3 Assess patient's ability to deep breathe and cough by placing hand on patient's abdomen; having him or her take a deep breath; and observing movement of shoulders, chest wall, and abdomen. Measure chest excursion during deep breath (see Chapter 6). Ask patient to cough into tissue after taking deep breath.	Reveals maximum potential for chest expansion and ability to cough forcefully; serves as baseline to measure patient's ability to perform exercises after surgery.
4 Assess patient's risk for postoperative thrombus formation (e.g., older adults, immobilized patients, patients with personal or family history of clots, and women over 35 taking birth control pills who smoke). Observe calves for redness, swelling, warmth, tenderness, swollen calf, calf swelling more than 3 cm (1.2 inches) compared with asymptomatic leg. Compare legs for bilateral equality. Palpate pedal pulses. Check for Homans' sign (calf pain on dorsiflexion of foot), which may or may not be present (see Skill 6-4). Calf pain is usually unilateral.	Following general anesthesia, circulation slows, causing a greater tendency for clot formation. Immobilization results in decreased muscular contraction in lower extremities, which promotes venous stasis. The physical stress of surgery creates a hypercoagulable state in most individuals. Manipulation and positioning during surgery may inadvertently cause trauma to leg veins. Symptoms may indicate phlebitis and thrombus formation.

Clinical Decision Point *Homans' sign is not always present when a DVT exists (Schick and Windle, 2010). If you suspect a thrombus, notify surgeon and refrain from manipulating extremity any further. Surgery will usually be postponed. Antiembolism stockings or pneumatic compression cuffs may be ordered for patients at risk for thrombus formation (see Chapter 10).*

5 Assess patient's ability to move independently while in bed.	Patients confined to bed rest, even for limited periods, will need to turn regularly. Determines existence of any mobility restrictions.
6 Assess patient's willingness and capability to learn exercises; note factors such as attention span; anxiety level; level of consciousness; language skills; and level of pain, if any.	Capacity to learn depends on readiness, ability, and learning environment.

Clinical Decision Point *Highly anxious patients or those in severe pain have difficulty learning and performing postoperative exercises.*

7 Assess family's caregiver willingness to learn and to support patient after surgery.	Family's caregiver presence after surgery can be a potential motivating factor for patient's recovery; family member or significant other can coach patient on exercise performance.
8 Assess patient's medical orders before and after surgery.	Requires adaptations in way patient performs exercises.

NURSING DIAGNOSES

• Acute pain	• Impaired physical mobility	• Ineffective tissue perfusion
• Impaired gas exchange	• Ineffective airway clearance	• Risk for impaired skin integrity
• Impaired memory	• Ineffective breathing pattern	• Risk for infection

Related factors are individualized based on patient's condition or needs.

PLANNING

1 Expected outcomes following completion of procedure: • Patient is able to correctly deep breathe, use incentive spirometer, cough, turn, and perform leg exercises throughout postoperative period.	Patient successfully learns exercises. Ability to perform exercises reduces risk for postoperative complications.

STEP	RATIONALE
• After surgery chest excursion meets or exceeds preoperative level.	Helps patient maintain full lung expansion and clear airways after surgery.
• Lungs are clear on auscultation both before and after surgery.	Absence of secretions reduces risk for postoperative pneumonia.
• No redness, warmth, or tenderness in lower extremities; pedal pulses palpable.	Leg exercises prevent occurrence of circulatory and mobility problems after surgery.
• Patient initiates exercises spontaneously.	Patient values importance of exercises to recovery.
2 Prepare equipment as needed.	
3 Prepare room for teaching.	Quiet, private area free from distractions enhances patient's ability to learn.

IMPLEMENTATION

1 Teach diaphragmatic breathing:	
a Help patient to comfortable sitting or standing position. If patient chooses to sit, raise head of bed to semi-Fowler's or Fowler's position and help to side of bed or upright position in chair. If patient is sitting in chair, knees should be at or higher than hips. Use stool if necessary.	Upright position facilitates diaphragmatic excursion by using gravity to keep abdominal contents away from diaphragm. Prevents tension on abdominal muscles, which allows for greater diaphragmatic excursion. Diaphragmatic breathing allows for complete lung expansion and improved ventilation and increases blood oxygenation. Deep breathing also allows air to pass by partially obstructing mucus plugs, thus increasing force with which to expel plug. Coughing loosens secretions and helps to remove them from pulmonary alveoli and bronchi.

Clinical Decision Point *After surgery patient can usually be positioned upright with head of bed elevated. If he or she must remain flat in bed, stress that exercises can still be performed.*

b Stand or sit facing patient.	Patient will be able to observe breathing exercises performed by nurse.
c Instruct patient to place palms of hands across from each other along lower borders of anterior rib cage; place tips of third finger lightly together. Demonstrate for patient.	Position of hands allows patient to feel movement of chest and abdomen as diaphragm descends and lungs expand inside chest wall.
d Have patient take slow, deep breaths, inhaling through nose and pushing abdomen against hands (see illustration). Explain that patient will feel normal downward movement of diaphragm during inspiration. Demonstrate for patient.	Slow, deep breath allows for more complete lung expansion and prevents panting or hyperventilation. Inhaling through nose warms, humidifies, and filters air. Explanation and demonstration focus on normal ventilatory movement of chest. Patient learns to understand how diaphragmatic breathing feels.
e Have patient avoid using chest and shoulder muscles while inhaling.	Using auxiliary chest and shoulder muscles during breathing increases unnecessary energy expenditures and does not promote full lung expansion.

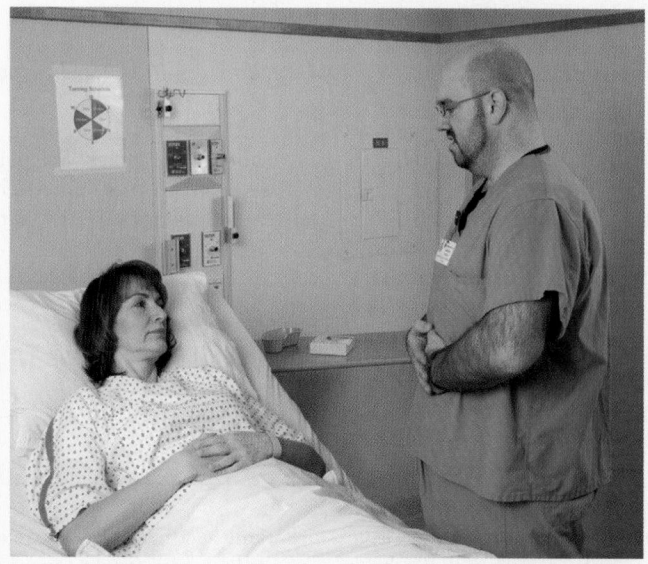

STEP 1d Patient and nurse practice deep breathing.

STEP	RATIONALE
f Take slow, deep breath and hold for count of three; slowly exhale through mouth as if blowing out a candle (pursed lips).	Allows for gradual, controlled expulsion of air.
g Repeat breathing exercise 3 to 5 times.	Allows patient to observe slow, rhythmic breathing pattern.
h Have patient practice exercises. Instruct him or her to take 10 slow, deep breaths every hour while awake during postoperative period until mobile. Another option is to have patient use incentive spirometry (see illustration).	Repetition of exercise reinforces learning. Regular deep breathing prevents or minimizes postoperative respiratory complications. Incentive spirometer gives visual incentive to breathe as deeply as possible.
2 Teach positive expiratory pressure therapy (PEP) and "huff" coughing:	
a Perform hand hygiene. Set PEP device for setting ordered.	Higher settings require more effort.
b Instruct patient to assume semi-Fowler's or high-Fowler's position and place nose clip on patient's nose (see illustration).	Promotes optimum lung expansion and expectoration of mucus.
c Have patient place lips around mouthpiece. Instruct him or her to take a full breath and exhale 2 or 3 times longer than inhalation. Repeat pattern for 10 to 20 breaths.	Ensures that patient does all breathing through mouth. Ensures that patient uses device properly.
d Remove device from mouth and have patient take slow, deep breath and hold for 3 seconds.	Promotes lung expansion before coughing.
e Instruct patient to exhale in quick, short, forced "huffs."	"Huff" coughing, or forced expiratory technique, promotes bronchial hygiene by increasing expectoration of secretions.
3 Teach controlled coughing:	
a Explain importance of maintaining an upright position.	Position facilitates diaphragm excursion and enhances thorax and abdominal expansion.
b Demonstrate coughing. Take two slow, deep breaths, inhaling through nose and exhaling through (pursed lips) mouth.	Deep breaths expand lungs fully so air moves behind mucus and facilitates effective coughing.
c Inhale deeply a third time and hold breath to count of three. Cough fully for two-to-three consecutive coughs without inhaling between coughs (see illustration). (Tell patient to push all air out of lungs.)	Consecutive coughs help remove mucus more effectively and completely than one forceful cough.

Clinical Decision Point *Coughing may be contraindicated after brain, spinal, or eye surgery because of an increase in intracranial pressure.*

d Caution patient against just clearing throat instead of coughing deeply.	Clearing throat does not remove mucus from deeper airways.
e If surgical incision is either thoracic or abdominal, teach patient to place either hands or pillow over incisional area and place hands over pillow to splint incision (see illustration). During breathing and coughing exercises, press gently against incisional area for splinting and support.	Surgical incision cuts through muscles, tissues, and nerve endings. Deep-breathing and coughing exercises place additional stress on suture line and cause discomfort. Splinting incision with hands or pillow provides firm support and reduces incisional pulling and pain.

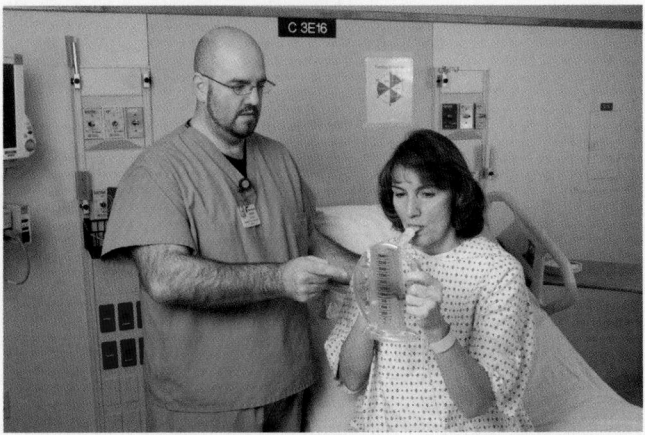

STEP 1h Patient demonstrates incentive spirometry.

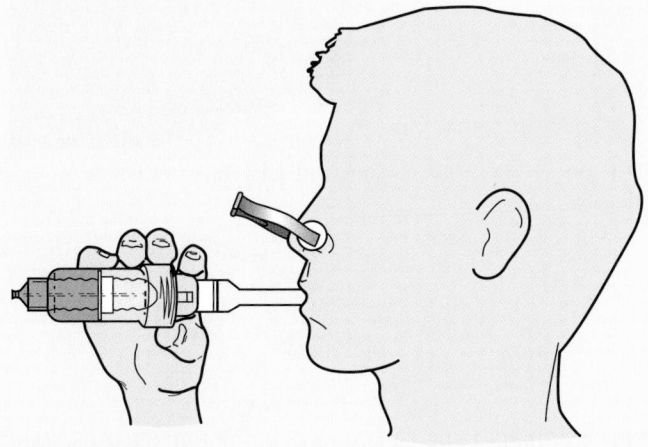

STEP 2b Diagram of use of positive expiratory pressure device.

STEP	RATIONALE
f Patient continues to practice coughing exercises, splinting imaginary incision. Instruct patient to cough 2-to-3 times every hour while awake.	Deep coughing with splinting effectively expectorates mucus with minimal discomfort.
g Instruct patient to examine sputum for consistency, odor, amount, and color changes and notify nurse if any changes are noted.	Sputum consistency, odor, amount, and color changes indicate presence of pulmonary complication such as pneumonia.

Clinical Decision Point *For patients with preexisting pulmonary disease, know usual character of mucus to determine if change has occurred.*

4 Teach turning (example describes turning to right side):	
a Instruct patient to assume supine position and move toward left side of bed. He or she can do this by bending knees and pressing heels against mattress to raise and move buttocks (see illustration).	Positioning begins in this example on left side of bed so turning to right side will not cause patient to roll off edge of bed. Buttocks lift prevents shearing force from body moving against sheets.
b Instruct patient to place right hand or pillow over incisional area to splint it.	Splinting incision supports and minimizes pulling on suture line during turning.
c Instruct patient to keep right leg straight and flex left knee up (see illustration).	Straight leg stabilizes patient's position. Flexed left leg shifts weight for easier turning.

Clinical Decision Point *Some patients such as those who have had back surgery or vascular repair are restricted from flexing their legs after surgery. Some patients are restricted from turning or may need help for positioning (see Chapter 9).*

d Have patient grab right side rail with left hand while pulling toward right and rolling onto right side.	Pulling toward side rail reduces effort needed for turning.
e Instruct patient to turn every 2 hours from side to back to other side while awake. If patient is unable to perform this maneuver, note in chart that staff or primary caregiver must turn patient every 2 hours. You will need to place pillows behind some patients to help maintain side-lying position.	Reduces risk for vascular complications by contraction of leg muscles around veins to improve venous return. Also reduces pulmonary complications by shifting mucus to prevent consolidation.

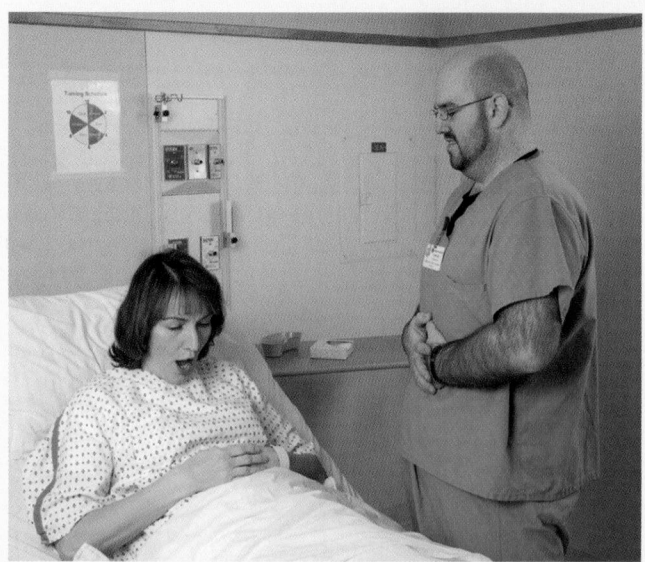

STEP 3c Controlled coughing with placement of hands on upper abdomen.

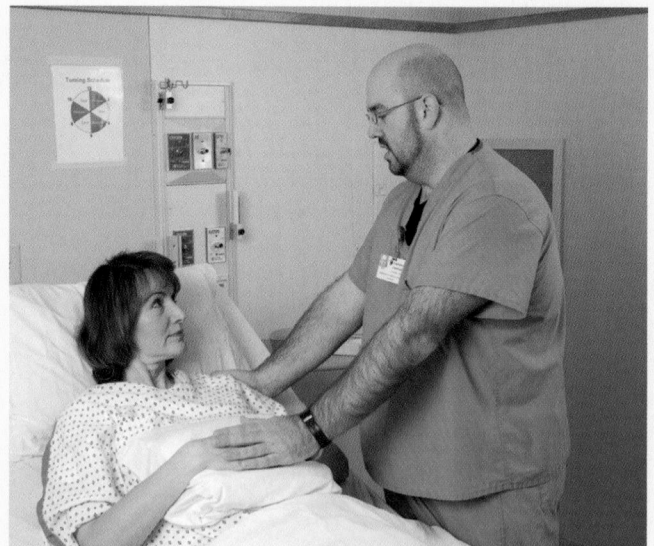

STEP 3e Patient splinting abdomen with pillow.

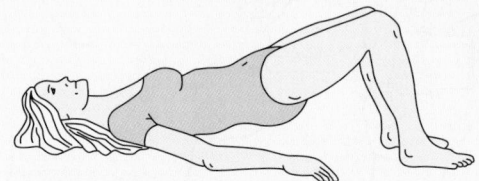

STEP 4a Buttocks lift for moving to side of bed. (*From Lowdermilk D, Perry S: Maternity nursing, ed 7, St Louis, 2006, Mosby.*)

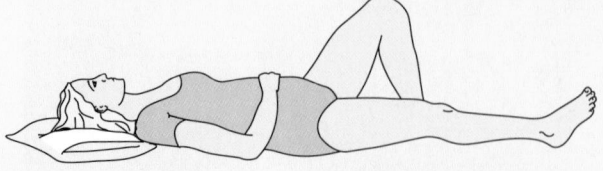

STEP 4c Leg position when turning to the right. (*From Lowdermilk D, Perry S: Maternity nursing, ed 7, St Louis, 2006, Mosby.*)

STEP	RATIONALE
5 Teach leg exercises: **a** Have patient assume supine position in bed. Demonstrate leg exercises by performing passive range-of-motion exercises and simultaneously explaining exercise.	Provides for normal anatomic position of lower extremities and normal joint motion of each joint of lower extremities.

Clinical Decision Point *If patient's surgery involves one or both lower extremities, surgeon must order leg exercises in postoperative period. You can safely exercise leg unaffected by surgery unless patient has preexisting phlebothrombosis (blood clot formation) or thrombophlebitis (inflammation of vein wall).*

STEP	RATIONALE
b Rotate each ankle in one direction and then in other direction. Instruct patient to draw imaginary circles with big toe (see illustration). Repeat 5 times.	Ankle circle exercises maintain joint mobility and promote venous return.
c Alternate dorsiflexion and plantar flexion by moving both feet, pointing toes up toward head and then down toward end of mattress. Direct patient to feel calf muscles contract and relax alternately (see illustration). Repeat 5 times.	Calf pumping stretches and contracts gastrocnemius muscles, which enhances venous return.
d Perform quadriceps setting by tightening thigh and bringing knee down toward mattress and relaxing (see illustration). Repeat 5 times.	Quadriceps-setting exercises contract muscles of upper legs, maintain knee mobility, and improve venous return to heart.
e Patient alternately raises each leg from bed surface; patient begins by keeping leg straight and then bends leg at hip and knee (see illustration). Repeat 5 times.	Leg raise promotes contraction and relaxation of quadriceps muscles and promotes hip and knee movements by keeping leg straight and bending hip and knee joints.

Clinical Decision Point *If patient is unable to perform exercises, note on Kardex or in electronic health record (EHR) that staff or primary caregiver must do passive range of motion to lower extremities every 2 hours while awake. Alternatively notify surgeon and request an order for pneumatic compression cuffs (see Chapter 10).*

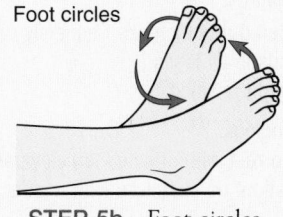

STEP 5b Foot circles.

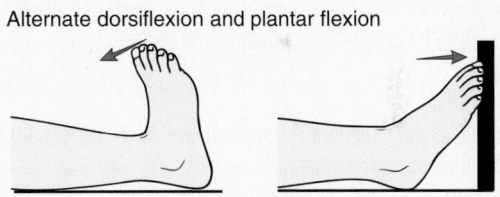

STEP 5c Alternate dorsiflexion and plantar flexion.

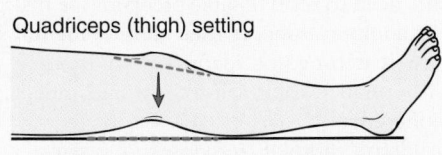

STEP 5d Quadriceps (thigh) setting.

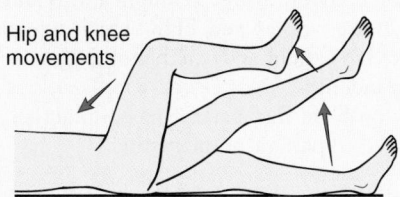

STEP 5e Hip and knee movements. *(From Lewis S et al: Medical-surgical nursing: assessment and management of clinical problems, ed 7, St Louis, 2007, Mosby.)*

STEP	RATIONALE
f Have patient continue to practice exercises at least every 2 hours while awake. Patient is instructed to coordinate turning and leg exercises with diaphragmatic breathing, incentive spirometry, and coughing exercises.	Repetition of exercise sequence reinforces learning. Establishes routine for exercises that develops habit for performance. Sequence of exercises is leg exercises, turning, deep breathing, and coughing. Exercises before coughing enhance ability to move secretions so they may be expectorated.

EVALUATION

1 Observe patient performing all exercises independently.	Provides opportunity for practice and return demonstration of exercises. Ensures that patient has learned correct technique.
2 Observe family caregiver's ability to coach patient.	Family caregiver can help positively or interfere with correct technique.
3 Evaluate patient's chest excursion.	Determines extent of lung expansion.
4 Auscultate patient's lungs.	Breath sounds reveal if airways are clear.
5 Gently palpate calves for redness, warmth, swelling, and tenderness. Assess pedal pulses.	Absent signs and normal pulses usually indicate that no venous thrombosis is present.

Unexpected Outcomes
Related Interventions

1 Patient is unwilling to perform exercises (deep breathing, coughing, and turning) because of incisional pain of thorax or abdomen or surgery in lower abdomen, groin, buttocks, or legs (leg exercises).

- Offer patient pain medication 30 minutes before or have patient use patient-controlled analgesia (PCA) before performing postoperative exercises.

2 Patient is unable to perform exercises correctly. Anxiety and fatigue alter patient's performance.

- Repeat teaching with more demonstrations.
- Patient may benefit from stress-reduction techniques.
- Assess for presence of anxiety, pain, and fatigue.

3 Patient develops pulmonary complications such as atelectasis after surgery. Breaths are shallow; cough is ineffective.

- Notify surgeon of findings.
- Start oxygen as ordered and increase frequency of coughing exercises.
- Assess breath sounds in all lobes.
- Place patient in upright position.

4 Patient develops circulatory complications such as venous stasis or thrombophlebitis after surgery.

- Notify surgeon of findings.
- Place patient on bed rest with affected leg elevated as ordered.
- Continue to have patient do exercises with unaffected leg.

Recording and Reporting

- Record physical assessment findings in narrative notes or flow sheet.
- Report and record any assessed complications and action taken.
- Record in nurses' notes and EHR which exercises you have demonstrated to patient and whether or not patient can perform them independently.
- Report any problem that patient has in practicing exercises to nurse assigned to patient on next shift.

Special Considerations
Teaching

- Health literacy refers to patients' ability to understand their health care issues and effectively care for themselves. It is essential to self-care. Provide instructions in a manner that patients and their families can interpret to improve and minimize errors (Schick and Windle, 2010). Provide education with a combination of procedural explanations, skills teaching, and psychosocial support.
- Explain postoperative exercises to patient and family caregiver, including their importance to recovery and physiologic benefits.

Adults learn best when they understand how they will benefit from activity.

Pediatric

- Have parents encourage and allow children to move within limits posed by surgery.
- Adolescents need to receive same preoperative instructions and teaching as adults to support their developmental stage. Adolescents are searching for identity, and treating them with respect will enhance their self-esteem and independence and increase adherence.
- Young children's normal responses of crying and moving extremities will maintain lung expansion and peripheral circulation. Therefore teaching coughing, deep breathing, and leg exercises is not usually necessary for young children.
- Children need family members and/or nursing staff to assume coach's role of reminding and encouraging.

Gerontologic

- Changes related to aging such as decreased vision, hearing, and short-term memory affect teaching effectiveness. Shorter sessions with frequent reinforcement and use of teaching aids with large print are sometimes necessary. Include family

members or primary caregiver in teaching sessions. Take time to instruct patient properly.
- Aging process decreases ventilatory capacity and increases risk for respiratory complications.
- Aging process decreases muscle mass and decreases venous return, thus increasing the risk for venous stasis.

Home Care
- Review coughing, deep breathing, abdominal splinting, relaxation, pain management, and leg exercises before admission to hospital or surgical clinic and after discharge.

SKILL 36-3 Performing Postoperative Care of a Surgical Patient

Nursing care of a postoperative surgical patient is divided into two phases: immediate recovery and postoperative convalescence. During both phases you will make comprehensive and detailed assessments of a patient's condition. The effects of anesthesia and the physiologic stressors imposed by surgery place patients at risk for a variety of physiologic alterations. It is also important to facilitate communication among all members of the health care team, the patient, and the patient's family or significant other.

The first phase of postoperative care for hospitalized patients is known as the phase I level of care. This extends from the time a patient leaves the operating room (OR) to the time a patient has stabilized in the postanesthesia care unit (PACU), meets the discharge criteria, and has been transferred to the nursing unit or phase II level of care. The first phase is the most critical postoperative phase for assessing aftereffects of anesthesia, including airway clearance, cardiovascular complications, temperature control, and neurologic function. A patient's condition can change rapidly. The perianesthesia nurse must make timely, intelligent, and accurate assessments to select the most appropriate measures of care for a patient.

Each agency has its own policies for directing the process for recovering patients during the immediate postoperative period. For example, frequently patients undergoing cardiac or central vascular repair transfer from the OR to an intensive care unit (ICU). In this situation the patient is not sent to the PACU area. The condition of these patients is potentially unstable and requires further stabilization and monitoring in an ICU setting.

The second phase of recovery is the postoperative convalescent period. ASPAN defines the phase II level of care as when the nursing roles focus on preparation for care in the home or an extended care environment. This period extends from the time a patient is discharged from the PACU to the time he or she is discharged from the inpatient hospital. Outpatient surgical patients undergo convalescence at home. All patients who have undergone surgical procedures have similar postoperative needs. However, nursing care becomes very individualized and depends on the nature of a patient's surgery, preexisting medical conditions, the onset of complications, and the speed of recovery. Not all surgical patients recover at the same rate. During the convalescent period you begin preparation for discharge and actively include the patient, family, and significant others in the process. You promote a patient's independence, educate patient and/or family about any limitations imposed by surgery, and provide resources needed for the patient to assume an improved state of wellness.

Delegation and Collaboration
The skill of initiating and managing postoperative care of a patient cannot be delegated to nursing assistive personnel (NAP). The nurse directs NAPs to:

- Report specific changes in patient's vital signs, behavior, or level of consciousness to the nurse.
- Obtain vital signs at specific intervals.
- Provide comfort and hygiene measures.

Equipment
Phase I Level of Care
- ❏ Equipment for physical assessment
- ❏ Various types and sizes of artificial airways
- ❏ Constant and intermittent suction
- ❏ Oxygen equipment such as mask, oxygen regulator and tubing, and positive-pressure delivery system
- ❏ Pulse oximetry
- ❏ End-tidal CO_2 monitoring
- ❏ Blood pressure monitoring equipment
- ❏ Adjustable lighting
- ❏ Electrocardiogram (ECG) monitor
- ❏ Arterial blood gas supplies
- ❏ Bladder scanner
- ❏ Bedside portable ultrasound to assess pulses
- ❏ Thermoregulation equipment, including thermometers, blanket warmers, and cooling blankets
- ❏ Intravenous supplies (if ordered) (see Chapter 28)
- ❏ Adult and pediatric emergency cart with defibrillator
- ❏ Stock supplies (e.g., facial tissues, dressings, bed pans, urinals, emesis basins)
- ❏ Personal protective equipment
- ❏ Latex free supplies and equipment

Phase II Level of Care
- ❏ Oxygen equipment
- ❏ Constant and intermittent suction
- ❏ Blood pressure monitoring equipment
- ❏ Thermometer
- ❏ Blood glucose testing system
- ❏ Bladder scanner
- ❏ Electrocardiogram (ECG) monitor and pulse oximeter
- ❏ Bag-valve-masks and emergency cart with defibrillator available for adult and children
- ❏ Malignant hyperthermia cart (AORN, 2010b)
- ❏ Latex-free supplies and equipment
- ❏ Transport equipment, including wheelchairs and carts
- ❏ Stock supplies should include: dressings, facial tissues, gloves, bedpans and urinals, syringes, needles and protective needle devices, emesis basins, patient linens, alcohol swabs/wipes, ice bags, tongue blades, and a variety of tapes

STEP	RATIONALE

ASSESSMENT

1 Phase 1: Immediate recovery period

   a Receive hand-off report from circulating nurse and anesthesia provider, including procedure performed, range of vital signs, any complications, estimated blood loss (EBL), other fluid loss, fluid replacement during surgery, type of anesthesia, medications given, type of airway and size, extent of surgical wound, restrictions to movement of position during surgery, and any preoperative medical and/or nursing diagnoses.

Determines patient's general status and allows nurse to anticipate need for special equipment, nursing care, and activities in PACU.

Clinical Decision Point *Patient's usual first complaint is of pain. Know how much sedative and/or analgesic have already been given and how long ago.*

   b On patient's arrival in PACU, review surgeon's orders.

Review provides detailed analysis of patient's physiologic status, allowing nurse to make appropriate observations and interventions. Provides baseline data to determine any change in condition.

   c Consider type of surgical procedure, restrictions to movement, and type of anesthesia used.

Influences type of assessments necessary, type of complications for which to observe, and specific nursing interventions needed.

   d Perform thorough patient assessment, including vital signs; pulse oximetry; pain and systems assessment to include respiratory, cardiac, neurologic, gastrointestinal (GI), genitourinary (GU), metabolic, and fluid status. Assess patient's surgical site and drains, skin integrity, safety, and anxiety level.

Provides baseline for ongoing postoperative evaluations. Identifies priority nursing interventions.

   e Expert opinion states that vital signs should be taken every 5 to 15 minutes during initial stabilization and more frequently if clinically indicated (ASPAN, 2010).

Check agency requirements for vital sign frequency.

   f Discharge from phase I level of care is based on specific criteria, not a time limit. Criteria should address assessment of airway patency, oxygenation, hemodynamic stability, thermoregulation, neurologic stability, intake and output, tube patency, dressings, pain and comfort management, and a postanesthesia scoring system if used. Each agency defines frequency of assessment.

Discharge instructions are developed in consultation with anesthesia department.

Clinical Decision Point *Be sure to turn patient on side (when possible) to observe underlying skin and accumulation of blood or serous drainage not visible otherwise.*

2 Phase II level of care: Convalescent period

   a Obtain phone report from PACU nurse summarizing patient's current status.

Allows you to prepare hospital room with necessary supplies and equipment for patient's special needs.

   b On patient's arrival at division, collect more detailed hand-off report from nurse accompanying patient.

Detailed report helps you plan appropriate assessment and nursing care measures. Data provide baseline to detect any change in patient's condition.

   c Review patient's chart for information pertaining to type of surgery; complications; medications administered; preoperative medical risks; baseline vital signs, including PACU vitals; and patient's usual medications given/not given before surgery.

Nature of surgery, intraoperative complications, and presence of medical risks dictate complications for which to observe. Vital signs provide means to detect postoperative changes. List of patient's usual medications may necessitate a call to surgeon for orders concerning timing and dose of drugs not given before surgery.

   d Review postoperative medical orders.

Offers additional guidelines for type of care to provide.

   e Assess patient's and family's knowledge and expectations of surgical recovery.

Patient will be better prepared to participate in care.

STEP	RATIONALE

NURSING DIAGNOSES

- Acute confusion
- Acute pain
- Deficient fluid volume
- Deficient knowledge regarding postoperative care
- Excess fluid volume
- Impaired gas exchange

- Impaired physical mobility
- Impaired skin integrity
- Impaired spontaneous ventilation
- Impaired swallowing
- Impaired verbal communication
- Ineffective airway clearance

- Ineffective breathing pattern
- Ineffective protection
- Ineffective thermoregulation
- Ineffective tissue perfusion
- Risk for aspiration
- Urinary retention

Related factors are individualized based on patient's condition or needs.

PLANNING

1 Expected outcomes following completion of procedure:

- Patient's vital signs, including oxygen saturation, remain within previous baseline or normal expected range.

  No occurrence of cardiovascular, pulmonary, or thermoregulatory changes except those expected from effects of anesthetic or analgesic.

- Patient reports relief of discomfort after analgesic or other pain-relief measures.

  Pain-relief measures effectively alter patient's reception or perception of pain.

- Surgical wound remains intact without redness, edema, ecchymosis, or discharge. If opaque dressing covers incision, dressing remains dry and intact. Drains, if present, remain patent.

  Indicates wound healing without signs of bleeding or infection.

- Breath sounds remain clear to auscultation; mucus is clear.

  Postoperative exercises and activity promote lung expansion and alveolar stability.

- Return of flatus present within 48 to 72 hours after bowel or abdominal surgery and/or general anesthetic. Normal bowel sounds present within 24 hours in cases of minor surgery.

  You assess the GI system after surgery by noting: (1) return of flatus; (2) first bowel movement; (3) normal vital signs; (4) lack of nausea/vomiting and return of appetite; and (5) absence of signs of ileus such as distention, bloating, and cramps.

- Intake and output (I&O) remain relatively in balance, with urinary output greater than 30 mL/hr.

  Adequate urinary elimination maintained. Fluid intake (intravenous [IV] and/or by mouth [PO]) adequately maintained.

- Legs remain without signs and symptoms of thrombophlebitis.

  Postoperative leg exercises and early ambulation minimize venous stasis and clot formation.

- Patient is able to discuss recovery and discharge plans. Verbalizes no specific physical complaints.

  Patient coping with physical and psychological stress of surgery.

2 Prepare equipment as necessary at bedside and test it for function.

  Ensures proper access of functional equipment.

3 Explain to patient all procedures that you are to perform and rationale for each. On nursing division include family members and/or significant other in explanations. In ambulatory surgery centers families are allowed at bedside during recovery period.

  Involves patient in plan of care and minimizes anxiety. As recovery progresses, patient is able to make more choices regarding how procedures should be performed. Family can serve as coach and help patient remember explanations given.

IMPLEMENTATION

1 Phase 1: Immediate recovery period:

  a Perform hand hygiene.

  Reduces transmission of microorganisms.

  b While receiving hand-off report as patient enters PACU on stretcher/bed, immediately attach oxygen tubing to regulator, hang IV fluids, check IV flow rates, and attach pulse oximeter (see Procedural Guideline 5-3). Connect any drainage tubes to gravity drainage or continuous or intermittent suction as ordered. Attach cardiac monitor. Ensure that indwelling catheter and bag are in drainage position and patent.

  Maintaining oxygenation and circulation are two priorities. Inhaled oxygen improves percentage of oxygen delivered to alveoli. Pulse oximeter provides information on arterial oxygen saturation. IV fluids maintain circulatory volume and provide route for emergency drugs. Drainage tubes must remain patent and in proper position to allow fluid to drain.

  c Conduct ongoing assessment of all vital signs every 5 to 15 minutes until patient stabilizes or per agency protocol. Compare findings with patient's baseline. Provide warm blankets as needed for patient comfort.

  Vital signs reveal onset of postoperative complications from surgery or anesthesia (e.g., respiratory depression, hypo-hyperthermia, pulse irregularity, or hypotension). Acute blood loss may lead to hypovolemic shock with signs of reduced blood pressure, elevated heart and respiratory rates, pale skin, and restlessness. General anesthetic may affect temperature-regulating center, and lower metabolic rate causes hypothermia. Malignant hyperthermia is a rare inherited condition that develops after receiving an anesthetic and is a medical emergency (AORN, 2010b; Schick and Windle, 2010).

STEP	RATIONALE

Clinical Decision Point *If patient underwent a short procedure under procedural sedation, check agency policy for sedation recovery guidelines. The perianesthesia registered nurse (RN) monitoring a patient who receives procedural sedation/analgesia should have no other responsibilities that compromise continuous patient monitoring (AORN 2010c; Schick and Windle, 2010). Monitor oxygenation until patients are no longer at risk for hypoxemia. Monitor ventilation and circulation at regular intervals until patients are suitable for discharge (ASA, 2012).*

d Maintain patent airway:	
(1) Position patient on side with head facing down and neck slightly extended (see illustration). Never position patient with hands over chest (reduces chest expansion).	Extension prevents occlusion of airway at pharynx. Downward position of head moves tongue forward; and mucus or vomitus can drain out of mouth, preventing aspiration.
(2) Place small folded towel or small pillow under patient's head. If patient is restricted to supine position, elevate head of bed approximately 10 to 15 degrees, extend neck, and turn head to side. Have emesis basin available if patient becomes nauseated.	Supports head in extended position. Prevents aspiration if patient should vomit.

Clinical Decision Point *If patient is not able to extend neck, turn head to side if possible; suction oropharynx (see Chapter 25) frequently.*

(3) Encourage patient to cough and deep breathe on awakening and every 15 minutes.	Promotes lung expansion and expectoration of mucus secretions.
(4) Suction artificial airway and oral cavity as secretions accumulate.	Clears airway of secretions.
(5) Once gag reflex returns, have patient spit out oral airway (see illustration). Do not tape oral airway.	Indicates that patient can clear airway independently. If airway is taped, patient will gag and may obstruct airway.
(6) Avoid rapid position changes in patients who had spinal anesthesia, which can cause changes in patient's blood pressure. Good body alignment is needed. Encourage fluid intake.	Rapid movements are avoided so as not to cause spinal headache from loss of cerebrospinal fluid. Increased IV or PO fluids aid body in replacing cerebrospinal fluid.

Critical Decision Point *Because of shorter half-life of drugs used today, many patients have oral airway removed before leaving the OR. PACU nurse must assess that respiratory effort is adequate; otherwise airway may need to be replaced, and patient may need a ventilator.*

e Call patient by name in moderate tone of voice. If there is no response, attempt to arouse patient by touching or gently moving a body part. Explain that patient is in PACU.	Determines patient's level of consciousness and ability to follow commands.
f Assess circulatory perfusion by inspecting color of nail beds, mucous membranes, and skin. Palpate for skin temperature. Test for capillary refill (see Chapter 6).	Pink or normal color of skin, nail beds, and mucous membranes and brisk (3 seconds or less) capillary refill indicate adequate perfusion. Warm extremities reveal adequate circulation.
g Monitor wound drainage:	
(1) Observe condition of dressing and drains for any evidence of bright red blood. Look underneath patient for any pooling of bloody drainage.	Hemorrhage from surgical wound usually occurs within first few hours, indicating that blood vessel was incompletely tied or cauterized during surgery. When dressing becomes saturated, blood oozes down patient's side and collects underneath him or her.

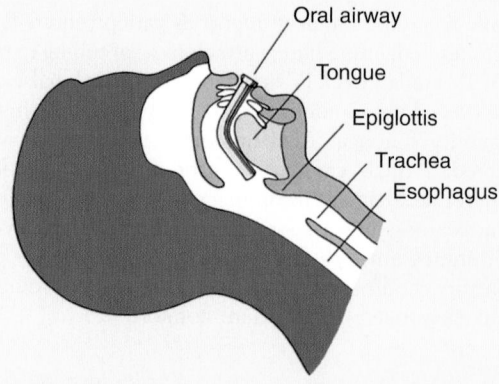

Oral airway
Tongue
Epiglottis
Trachea
Esophagus

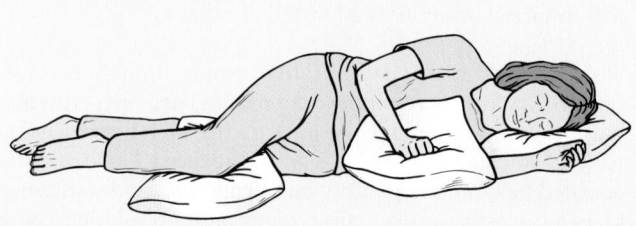

STEP 1d(1) Position of patient during recovery from general anesthesia. (*From Lewis S et al: Medical-surgical nursing: assessment and management of clinical problems, ed 8, St Louis, 2011, Mosby.*)

STEP 1d(5) Oral airway position before removal.

STEP	RATIONALE
(2) Inspect surgical incision for swelling or discoloration. Note condition of surgical dressing, including amount, color, odor, and consistency of drainage. Mark dressing with circle around drainage using black pen. Place time of marking and check area every 10 to 15 minutes, marking any changes and noting vital signs.	Progressive increase or changes in characteristics of drainage warrant call to surgeon because they could indicate hemorrhage (Academy of Medical-Surgical Nurses, 2009; Schick and Windle, 2010). Determines extent of fluid loss and condition of underlying wound. Size, location, and depth of wound influence amount of drainage.
(3) Reinforce pressure dressing or change simple dressing if ordered (see Chapter 39). Continue to monitor condition of incision, surrounding tissue, and amount and color of any drainage if incision is exposed or covered with transparent dressing.	Pressure dressing should not be removed because it helps to maintain hemostasis (termination of bleeding) and absorb drainage. Changing dressings immediately after surgery can disrupt wound edges and aggravate drainage. First dressing changes most often occur 24 hours after surgery and are usually done by surgeon. Minor surgical wounds may not have dressings but simply skin closure; or wounds may be covered with transparent dressing, which allows for observation of incision and surrounding tissue (Academy of Medical-Surgical Nurses, 2009).
(4) Inspect condition and contents of any drainage tubes and collecting devices. Note character and volume of drainage (see illustration) (see Chapter 38).	Determines drainage tube patency and extent and character of wound drainage.
(5) Observe patency and intactness of urinary catheter system (if present). Note volume and character of urine.	Patent drainage system prevents bladder distention. Urine volume monitors renal function and perfusion. Decreased output (less than 30 mL/hour in an adult) is an early sign of hypovolemic shock.
(6) If nasogastric (NG) tube is present, validate correct placement and irrigate per protocol (see Chapter 34) with normal saline if ordered.	Maintains patency of tube to ensure gastric decompression (removal of pressure caused by gas or liquid). Normal saline is isotonic and will not increase loss of fluid and electrolytes from stomach.
(7) Continue monitoring IV fluid rates. Observe IV site for signs of infiltration such as swelling, edema, redness, warmth, discomfort, and leakage of IV fluid (see Chapter 28).	Continuous regular infusion of IV fluids maintains patient's fluid intake to maintain adequate hydration and circulatory function.
h As patient awakens, provide mouth care by placing moistened washcloth to lips, swabbing oral mucosa with toothette dampened in water, or applying petrolatum to lips. Sips of tap water and ice chips may also be ordered.	Patient remains at risk for aspiration and should not receive fluids to rinse mouth. Moist cloth, toothette, or sips of water and/or ice chips can be soothing to dry mucosa.

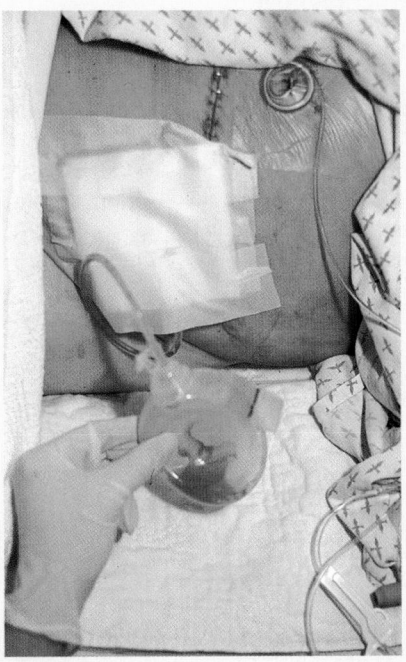

STEP 1g(4)   Note color of drainage in Jackson-Pratt drain.

STEP	RATIONALE
i Continue to monitor and provide pain medication as ordered and when vital signs have stabilized (Schick and Windle, 2010; TJC, 2012a).	Pain increases the stress response and interferes with postoperative exercises. Pain medication can affect vital signs if effect of anesthetic is still present. Patient with spinal anesthesia is unable to feel sensation below level of spinal cord. Patient will need pain medication as regional anesthetic wears off.
j Encourage patient to practice ankle circles and calf-pumping exercises.	These leg exercises encourage venous return. If spinal or epidural anesthetic was used, leg exercises help effects of regional anesthetic to wear off once drug has been substantially metabolized by liver.
k Explain to patient how he or she is progressing and that plans for transfer to a nursing division are being made.	Helps patient remain oriented to surroundings and recovery activities.
l Once all physiologic signs have stabilized, contact surgeon for order to release patient to nursing unit. Measure all I&O before transferring patient to nursing division.	Surgeon is responsible for dictating level of observation and care required by patient. I&O while in PACU is important baseline information to include in report to nurse in nursing division.

Clinical Decision Point *If patient is to be discharged to home, ensure that patient has someone to drive him or her home and observe him or her for signs and symptoms of complications. Review with patient and driver reportable signs and symptoms and emergency care needed.*

2 Phase II level of care: Convalescent period:	
a Make final check of equipment setup in patient's room, including emesis basin and waterproof pads. Be sure that bed is in high position (level with stretcher) and wheels are locked.	During transfer patient's status may change, necessitating quick interventions on arrival. Availability of equipment ensures smooth transfer process. Locked wheels prevent bed from moving during transfer.
b On arrival at patient's room help PACU staff and use three-person carry or slide board to transfer patient to bed (see Chapter 9).	Technique avoids strain on nurses' back muscles and maintains patient's safety.
c Once patient is transferred to bed, immediately attach any existing oxygen tubing, hang IV fluids, check IV flow rate, attach NG tube to suction, and place indwelling catheter in drainage position.	Maintains patient's oxygenation, circulation, and elimination functions. Allows for frequent monitoring of I&O. Provides for patient's comfort. Prevents potentially contaminated urine backflow into sterile bladder, thus decreasing incidence of bladder infections.
d Conduct complete assessment of all vital signs. Compare findings with vital signs in recovery area and patient's baseline values. Depending on agency policy, continue monitoring as ordered and as condition warrants (e.g., a typical order might read: VS q 15 min × 4, q 30 min × 2, q 1 hr × 4). Do not assume that further monitoring is unnecessary if patient appears normal during initial assessment.	Patient should be stabilized once transferred to nursing division. Change in vital signs may reveal onset of postoperative complications.

Clinical Decision Point *Report to anesthesiologist and/or surgeon any findings that differ from previous assessment.*

e Maintain a patent patient airway:	
(1) Position patient on side (if allowed); if patient remains sleepy or lethargic, keep head extended.	Positioning minimizes chances of aspiration.
(2) Encourage deep breathing and coughing, using pillow as an incisional splint every 1 to 2 hours (see illustration).	Promotes lung expansion and expectoration of mucus.

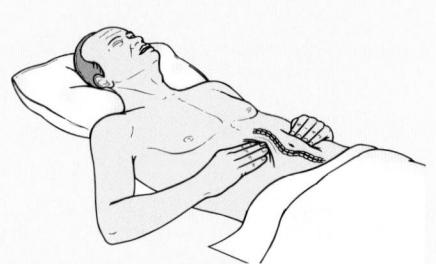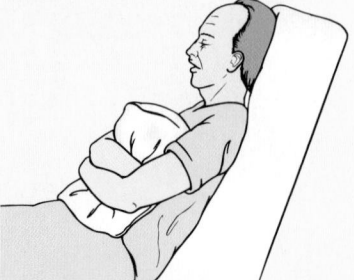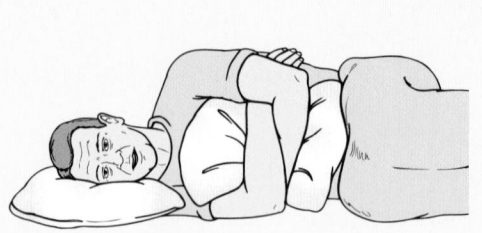

STEP 2e(2) Techniques for splinting incisions. (*From Lewis S et al:* Medical-surgical nursing: assessment and management of clinical problems, *ed 8, St Louis, 2011, Mosby.*)

STEP	RATIONALE
f Be sure that any drainage tubes are connected to proper suction or drainage device. If NG tube is present, validate correct placement, irrigate as ordered, and connect to proper drainage device (see Chapter 34).	Maintains drainage tube patency so wound beds remain dry for healing. Occlusion of NG tube can lead to abdominal distention, vomiting, and aspiration.
g Assess patient's surgical dressing for intactness and presence and character of drainage. Reinforce as ordered. If no dressing present, inspect condition of wound (see Chapter 38).	Wound can hemorrhage quickly during early postoperative period. Observations of wound and dressings provide data to measure progress of wound healing.

Critical Decision Point *If unable to change dressing, mark area of drainage and label with time, date, and initials. Record frequency of reinforcement. Never use felt tip marker to mark dressing because ink can bleed into gauze, contaminating incision site.*

h Assess for bladder distention if patient does not have indwelling catheter. Offer bedpan or urinal if patient senses urge to void.	Anesthetics and analgesics depress sensation of bladder fullness. Patient may still have no sensations below level of spinal or epidural anesthetic.

Critical Decision Point *Initiate measures to stimulate voiding within 4 hours of surgery or removal of indwelling catheter to prevent urinary retention with overflow (see Chapter 33).*

i Measure and record all sources of fluid I&O (see Chapter 6).	Helps in monitoring fluid and electrolyte balance.
j Position patient for comfort; maintain airway and correct body alignment. Avoid positioning on surgical wound site or with pressure on popliteal space.	Good positioning reduces stress on suture line and decreases risks of aspiration and impaired circulation. Comfortable position helps patient relax.
k Encourage patient to continue with leg exercises every 1 to 2 hours. If patient is unable or unwilling to do them, do passive range of motion (see Chapter 10).	Leg exercises increase venous return, which decreases risk for thrombophlebitis. Range-of-motion exercises maintain joint mobility.
l If ordered, apply elastic stockings or pneumatic compression cuffs to lower extremities and attach to compressor (see Chapter 10). Explain to patient that compression cuffs will inflate and deflate intermittently.	Increases venous return. Explanation decreases anxiety and fosters cooperation.
m Explain to patient that you have completed all observations and that you will ask family members or significant other to enter room. Place bed in lowest position with call light within reach and raise side rails as appropriate.	Promotes patient's orientation and sense of well-being. Lowest position minimizes injury if patient becomes confused and tries to get out of bed. Call light and side-rail positioning ensure patient's safety as effects of anesthetic continue to diminish.
n Explain patient's general status to family and/or significant other, describe purpose of any equipment in room, and explain reason for frequent observations and procedures.	Family and significant others normally are anxious to learn about patient's status. Unfamiliar sights (equipment and patient's appearance) also cause anxiety. Family's and significant other's understanding can promote their participation in patient's care.
o Give family simple tasks to perform such as wiping patient's face with washcloth and coaching postoperative exercises.	Give family purpose and reinforces skill in basic care measures.
p Refer to PACU record to determine if pain medication was administered.	Pain relief is essential for patient to be able to perform postoperative exercises. Patient is best judge of their pain. Pain scale provides an objective measure for nurse to interpret patient's progress.
(1) Always ask patient to rate severity of pain on an analog scale or whichever pain scale you use at your agency (TJC, 2012a).	
(2) Administer analgesic if vital signs remain stable or initiate patient-controlled analgesia (PCA) if ordered (see Chapter 15).	
q Provide oral hygiene and repeat as needed.	Maintenance of moist mucous membranes facilitates expectoration of secretions and promotes comfort.
r As patient stabilizes over next hours or days, perform following measures:	Promotes pulmonary and circulatory function to minimize onset of postoperative complications.
(1) Have patient participate in postoperative exercises.	
(2) Encourage use of incentive spirometer if ordered. Watch patient use spirometer first few times to judge efficacy of breathing pattern. Chart level that patient can achieve.	Promotes lung expansion. Helps monitor progress and demonstrates if you need to encourage patient to inhale more deeply.
(3) Begin activity orders. Assess vital signs first time patient sits or stands to judge tolerance.	Early ambulation promotes circulation, lung expansion, and peristalsis. Sudden positional changes cause postural hypotension.
(4) Monitor bowel sounds per protocol and ask if patient has passed flatus.	There is evidence that return of flatus is more accurate than bowel sounds in detecting return of peristalsis after abdominal surgery.
(5) Begin dietary orders slowly according to patient's tolerance. Medicate with antiemetic if patient is nauseated. Give analgesic with antiemetic until patient is eating well.	Promotes normal fluid and electrolyte balance, restores nutritional intake, and promotes normal GI function and wound healing. Analgesics often cause nausea on an empty stomach.

STEP	RATIONALE
(6) Promote normal voiding pattern. Assess bladder volume with bladder scanner. Male patients often need help to stand to void. Female patients need to sit on bedpan in bed or chair so legs can be bent and dangling or helped to bathroom.	Promotes normal urinary elimination and prevents bladder distention and urinary retention with overflow. A more natural voiding position helps patient void.

Clinical Decision Point *If patient does not void within 8 hours after surgery or bladder becomes distended, notify surgeon. You may have to insert urinary catheter.*

(7) Closely monitor progress of wound healing and change dressings as ordered.	Wound infection occurs most often within 3 to 6 days after surgery. Wound dehiscence occurs most often 3 to 11 days after surgery.

Clinical Decision Point *Delayed wound healing may result in wound dehiscence or evisceration. This occurs most frequently after coughing, sneezing, vomiting, or getting up from a sitting position. Remind patient to use caution during these activities and use pillow to splint incision. Evisceration is a medical emergency.*

(8) Monitor and maintain wound drainage devices such as Jackson-Pratt, Hemovac, or Penrose drains. Jackson-Pratt and Hemovac drainage systems must be emptied whenever they are half full of drainage or air and recharged (compressed to discharge air) (see illustration).	Wound drainage devices promote healing from inside to outside and relieve pressure on suture line. Compressing flexible closed container and then plugging drainage hole creates negative suction pressure.
(9) Monitor drainage for color, consistency, and amount every 4 to 8 hours. Compare to previous assessment.	Drainage should progress from sanguineous to serosanguineous to serous in color, become more watery, and decrease in amount as wound heals.
s Gradually increase patient's involvement in decision making and any explanations about surgery and related implications.	Promotes patient's sense of control and independence. Encourages feeling of self-esteem.
t Teach patient and family signs and symptoms of complications such as infection, dehiscence, excessive bleeding; need for nutrition for wound healing; and techniques of wound care if needed.	Early discharge necessitates patient and family involvement because complications often occur after patient goes home.
u Discuss with patient and family or significant other plans for discharge.	Allows nurse to anticipate patient's needs in home setting and discuss any problems that might arise.
v Prepare to make referral for home or convalescent care as patient's condition dictates. Obtain order from surgeon.	If patient continues to need nursing care or rehabilitation after discharge, surgeon's order is necessary. Referral provides continuity of care.

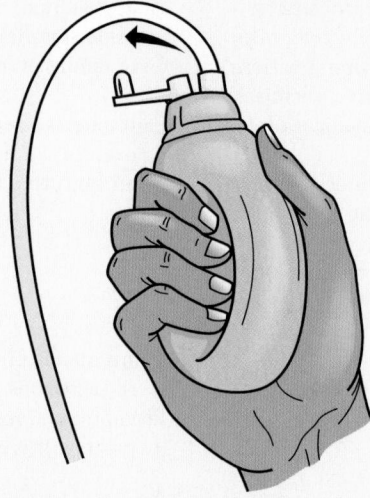

STEP 2r(8)   Charging Jackson-Pratt drainage system.

EVALUATION

1 Compare all vital sign assessment measurements with patient's baseline and expected normal levels.	Evaluates patient's respiratory, cardiovascular, and thermoregulatory status throughout recovery.
2 Measure patient's perception of pain after implementing pain-relief measures such as positioning and use of analgesics.	Determines level of comfort achieved and effectiveness of pain-relief measures.
3 Monitor changes in surgical wound at least every shift.	Provides data to measure progress of wound healing.
4 Monitor lung sounds following postoperative exercises.	Determines status of airways.

STEP	RATIONALE
5 Auscultate bowel sounds at least each shift and ask patient if he or she has passed flatus.	Allows you to evaluate return of peristalsis and diet tolerance.
6 Monitor I&O balance for each shift.	Indicates onset of fluid imbalances.
7 Discuss with patient general level of comfort and progress toward recovery.	Gives patient sense of participation in care. Patient's perceptions are helpful in noting onset of complications. Reveals readiness to learn about discharge.
8 Conduct physical assessments appropriate for patient's unique type of surgery.	Allows nurse to monitor course of recovery.

Unexpected Outcomes

Related Interventions

1 Vital signs are above or below patient's baseline or expected range.

- Ensure that patient is fully awake from anesthesia before giving large doses of opioids.
- Ensure that patient's family does not medicate patient with PCA. Monitor geriatric patient closely for opiate sensitivity—patient may require use of opiate antagonist such as naloxone in presence of bradypnea.
- Medicate for pain as indicated; titrate analgesics to maximize pain relief; assess patient's use and understanding of PCA device.
- Notify surgeon for symptoms of internal bleeding or shock such as hypotension or tachypnea.

2 Patient continues to experience incisional pain. Analgesic dosage may be insufficient.

- Initiate different nonpharmacologic relief measures (positioning, relaxation). Call surgeon for additional analgesic orders.

3 Abnormal or diminished breath sounds are auscultated. This is sometimes caused by bronchial constriction, mucus secretions in large airways, or atelectasis.

- Notify surgeon and request order for incentive spirometer (IS) if not already ordered.
- Change position to promote chest expansion.
- Encourage patient to turn, deep breathe, cough, and use IS more often.
- Assess history of asthma or allergic response to medication when wheezing or stridor is auscultated.

4 Patient exhibits signs of hypovolemia related to hemorrhage.

- Elevate legs but do not lower head past flat position.
- Administer oxygen as ordered.
- Increase rate of IV fluids or administer blood products as ordered.
- Monitor pulse and blood pressure every 5 to 15 minutes.
- Apply pressure dressing to external wound if not contraindicated.

5 Patient complains of calf tenderness and warmth; may exhibit redness and edema in lower extremity (signs and symptoms of venous thrombosis or thrombophlebitis).

- Notify surgeon and anticipate orders for bed rest, leg elevation, and initiation of anticoagulation (e.g., heparin IV drip).
- Do not massage affected leg.
- Continue to have patient do leg exercises with unaffected leg.

6 Bowel sounds are absent or decreased. Postoperative paralytic ileus can develop as a common complication after bowel surgery.

- Intestinal motility may return slowly, depending on anesthetic effects.
- Keep IV line in place.
- Encourage turning and ambulation.
- Continue monitoring bowel sounds and passage of flatus every 4 hours.
- Report findings to surgeon.

7 Patient develops fever, tenderness, and pain at wound site; increased white blood cell count (WBC) or purulent drainage is present. These are signs and symptoms of wound infection.

- Notify surgeon and anticipate orders for culture of wound drainage and IV antibiotics.

8 Patient reports feeling something in wound "give way." Increased serosanguineous drainage occurs. Possibly indicates wound dehiscence or evisceration.

- Report wound dehiscence and/or evisceration to surgeon immediately because it could be life threatening.
- If evisceration has occurred, cover abdominal contents with sterile gauze saturated with sterile normal saline and prepare patient for emergency surgery.

9 I&O measurements and laboratory values reflect fluid volume excess or deficit.

- Continue to monitor strict I&O and check IV rate. Contact surgeon if 24-hour totals continue to reflect imbalance.

10 Patient is unable to discuss discharge plans or has negative view of recovery. Possibly indicates that he or she is coping poorly with stress of surgery.

- Discuss discharge plans and instructions with significant family member or friend.
- Encourage patient to express fears and concerns.
- Refer patient to support group if appropriate.
- Notify surgeon and request referral for counseling if necessary.

Recording and Reporting

- Document patient's arrival in PACU or nursing division; record vital signs, level of consciousness, assessment findings, and all nursing measures initiated in nurses' notes and EHR. Depending on agency policy, continue documentation every 15 minutes until stable, then every 30 minutes ×2, every hour ×4, and every 4 to 8 hours as condition warrants.
- Record vital signs, oxygen saturation, temperature, and I&O on appropriate flow sheets.
- Report any abnormal assessment findings and signs of complications to nurse in charge and/or surgeon.

Special Considerations

Teaching

- If patient had spinal or epidural anesthetic, remind family or significant other that loss of extremity movement is normal for several hours.
- Reinforce preoperative teaching regarding coughing, deep breathing, leg exercises, and information concerning ambulation and pain control.
- Instruct patient and primary caregiver to identify signs and symptoms and appropriate actions to take for infection, respiratory, circulatory, or GI difficulties and wound disruptions.
- Provide important phone numbers to patient and primary caregiver for use in event of emergency and for follow-up care on discharge.
- Teach patient about appropriate wound care, diet recommendations, and activity restrictions.
- Patient teaching for ambulatory surgical patients
  - Surgeon's office and surgery center telephone number (24-hour answer)
  - Follow-up appointment, date, time
  - Review of prescribed medications
  - Guidelines related to specific surgery
  - Dressing and wound care
  - Pain control
  - Activity restrictions
  - Guidelines related to possible effects of anesthesia
  - Dietary restrictions
  - Activity restrictions
  - Signs and symptoms of complications

Pediatric

- Keep parent-child separation to a minimum. When a parent cannot be present, it is important to leave a transitional object (favorite possession) with child.
- Be alert for allergic responses and signs and symptoms of malignant hyperthermia in children who have not been exposed to drugs or anesthetic agents. Family history of allergies makes child at high risk for experiencing similar reactions.
- Vomiting is a major concern in young children because of increased risk for fluid and electrolyte imbalances and risk for aspiration. Vomiting is also more likely because surgery in children is often necessitated by accidental injuries without benefit of NPO status.
- Voiding before discharge from ambulatory surgery is not usually required for young children.
- Undermedicating young children may be based on myth that opiates are more dangerous for infants. The fact is that "by 3 to 6 months of age, healthy infants can metabolize opioids similarly to older children" (Hockenberry and Wilson, 2011). Observing the normalizing of vital signs and behavior after administration of analgesics is a valuable clue that pain really existed before treatment (Hockenberry and Wilson, 2011).

Gerontologic

- The ability of older adults to tolerate surgery depends on extent of physiologic changes that have occurred with aging, presence of any chronic diseases, and duration of surgical procedure.
- Undermedicating older adults is common. Asking patients to rate their pain before and after administration of analgesics and asking which numeric rating is acceptable to them are better methods of individualizing care.

Home Care

- Teach primary caregiver about any postoperative exercises, pain management, home modifications, and diet and activity limitations.
- If patient is discharged with dressing changes, bedroom or bathroom is usually an ideal location for the procedure. Have primary caregiver perform return demonstration of dressing change.

⁇ Critical Thinking Exercises

You are assigned to care for Mrs. Edmonds, a 52-year-old African-American who is 5 feet tall and weighs 113.6 kg (250 lbs). She is married with three adult children and is employed as an attorney. You just received her from the postanesthesia care unit following an abdominal hysterectomy for fibroid tumors and a bladder neck suspension. Her previous medical history includes 30-year, 2-pack-per-day cigarette smoking and type 2 diabetes; and she has been on birth control pills for 20 years. She has an abdominal dressing that has a small amount of shadowing on it, is on oxygen at 2 L via nasal cannula, and has both a Foley catheter and a suprapubic catheter draining pink-tinged urine. She has an intravenous (IV) infusion of $D_5\frac{1}{2}NS$ infusing at 125 mL/hr and a morphine patient-controlled analgesia (PCA) device. She received Ancef IV piggyback approximately 45 minutes before her incision was made and is to receive her second dose 8 hours later.

1 Which risk factors does Mrs. Edmonds have for developing a surgical site infection (SSI), and what is your role in infection prevention at this point in her care?

2 Which topics should be included in Mrs. Edmonds' postoperative teaching, and who should be included?

3 Which other postoperative complications is Mrs. Edmonds at risk for developing, and what are the nursing implications? Provide the rationale.

4 Before performing postoperative exercises, what should the patient be instructed to do?

✓ REVIEW QUESTIONS

1 Prevention of surgical site infections (SSIs) requires numerous actions by both the surgical team and the patient. Select the measures that are used to reduce SSIs. (Select all that apply.)
1 Discharge patient from the hospital as soon as possible.
2 Shampoo hair before neck or back surgery.
3 Give prophylactic antibiotic therapy as close to the time of incision as possible.
4 Shave excess hair with a razor just before the surgery begins.
5 Control hyperglycemia in diabetic and nondiabetic patients.
6 Give a shower or bath after the preoperative enema is evacuated.

2 There are numerous measures to prevent venous thromboembolism during the postoperative period. Which intervention would be most appropriate before the surgery begins?
1 Performing an assessment for Homans' sign
2 Applying compression devices of some type
3 Teaching patient coughing and breathing techniques
4 Instructing patient how to ambulate after surgery

3 A female patient's ethnicity requires that a male member of the family give consent for the scheduled surgery. Which approach by the nurse is the most appropriate?
1 Find out how much the patient understands about the scheduled procedure
2 Have the patient sign the consent first with the male family member observing and then signing afterward
3 Have the male member sign the consent form first and then have the patient sign
4 Refer to agency protocol for implementing this type of informed consent

4 The risk manager is explaining the use of "do not resuscitate" (DNR) orders in the surgical environment during an in-service that is being held for the new surgical team. Which statement is true regarding DNR orders?
1 DNR orders should remain in effect throughout all stages of surgical procedures.
2 DNR orders should automatically be suspended during and immediately following surgical procedures.
3 The surgeon should discuss and document issues with the patient and/or family to determine whether DNR orders are to be maintained or modified during surgical procedures.
4 Patients with DNR orders typically are not generally candidates for surgical procedures.

5 A patient was admitted from the postanesthesia care unit (PACU) to the medical-surgical unit following a colectomy. On initial examination a dime-size amount of drainage is noted on the abdominal dressing. Which intervention should be implemented?
1 Do nothing because this is an expected outcome for the postoperative patient.
2 Mark the dressing with a circle around the drainage.
3 Remove the dressing to assess the exact amount of bleeding.
4 Immediately notify the surgeon.

6 According to the CDC, the recommended goal for use of most prophylactic antibiotic therapy is to give the antibiotic:
1 Within 2 hours of incision time and for no longer than 48 hours after surgery.
2 Within 1 hour of incision time and for no longer than 24 hours after surgery.
3 Within 1 hour of incision time and for no longer than 48 hours after surgery.
4 Within 2 hours of incision time and for no longer than 24 hours after surgery.

7 For patients who are unable to perform exercises, the sequence of exercises to be provided by the patient care provider is:
1 Leg exercises, turn, deep breathe, cough.
2 Deep breathe, cough, leg exercises, turn.
3 Turn, cough, deep breathe, leg exercises.
4 Cough, deep breathe, leg exercises, turn.

8 General anesthesia predisposes patients to the following respiratory problems except:
1 The lungs are not fully inflated during surgery.
2 The cough reflex is suppressed.
3 Mucus collects within airway passages.
4 Spontaneous postoperative pneumothorax.

9 Which assignment would the registered nurse (RN) delegate to the NAP?
1 Manage the postoperative care of the patient
2 Initial assessments on arrival to the PACU
3 Discharge teaching to the ambulatory care patient
4 Care of the patient requiring monitoring and providing comfort measures

10 The three levels of care ASPAN identified during the recovery process are: (Select all that apply.)
1 Preoperative assessment level of care.
2 Postanesthesia phase I level of care.
3 Postanesthesia phase II level of care.
4 Extended care level of care.

REFERENCES

Academy of Medical-Surgical Nurses: *Core curriculum for medical-surgical nursing,* ed 4, Pitman, NJ, 2009, The Academy.

American Society of Anesthesiologists (ASA): Practice guidelines for the perioperative management of patients with obstructive sleep apnea, *Anesthesiology* 104(5):1081, 2006.

American Society of Anesthesiologists (ASA): Practice guidelines for preoperative fasting and the use of pharmacologic agents to reduce the risk of pulmonary aspiration: application to healthy patients undergoing elective procedures, *Anesthesiology* 114(3):495, 2011.

American Society of Anesthesiologists (ASA): *Standards for postanesthesia care,* approved by House of Delegates on October 12, 1988 and last amended on October 21, 2009, found in the Perianesthesia Nursing Standards and Practice Recommendations 2010-2012, 2012, p 137.

American Society of PeriAnesthesia Nurses (ASPAN): *2010-2012 PeriAnesthesia nursing standards and practice recommendations,* Cherry Hill, NJ, 2010, ASPAN.

Association of periOperative Registered Nurses (AORN): *Standards, recommended practices and guidelines,* Denver, 2010a, The Association.

Association of periOperative Registered Nurses (AORN): *Standards and recommended practices for perioperative nursing: malignant hyperthermia guideline,* Denver, 2010b, The Association.

Association of periOperative Registered Nurses (AORN): *Standards and recommended practices for perioperative nursing: managing the patient receiving moderate sedation/analgesia,* Denver, 2010c, The Association.

Association of periOperative Registered Nurses (AORN): *Standards and recommended practices for perioperative nursing: perioperative care of patients with do-not-resuscitate (DNR) orders,* Denver, 2010d, The Association.

Centers for Disease Control and Prevention (CDC): Infection control standards for The Joint Commission, updated 2011, available at www.cdc.gov/ncidod/dhqp/hai.html, accessed March 25, 2012.

Centers for Disease Control and Prevention (CDC), National Center for Health Statistics: Prevalence of overweight and obesity among adults: United States, 1999-2008, last modified February 22, 2012, available at www.cdc.gov/nchs/products/pubs/pubd/hestats/over-weight/overwght_adult_03.htm, accessed March 25, 2012.

Drake K: SCIP core measures: deep impact, *Nurs Manage* 42(5):24, 2011.

Hockenberry M, Wilson D: *Wong's Clinical manual of pediatric nursing,* ed 8, St Louis, 2011, Mosby.

Kaw R, et al: Postoperative complications in patients with obstructive sleep apnea, *Chest* 141(2):438, 2012.

Lewis S, et al: *Medical-surgical nursing, assessment and management of clinical problems,* ed 8, St Louis, 2011, Mosby.

Litwack K: *Clinical coach for effective perioperative nursing care,* Philadelphia, 2009, FA Davis.

Ouellette D, Patocka C: Pulmonary embolism, *Emerg Med Clin North Am* 30(2):329, 2012.

Schick L, Windle P, editors: *PeriAnesthesia nursing core curriculum: preoperative, phase I and phase II PACU nursing,* ed 2, St Louis, 2010, Saunders.

Stannard D, Krenziscek D: *PeriAnesthesia nursing care: a bedside guide for safe recovery,* Sudbury, Mass, 2012, Jones & Bartlett Learning.

The Joint Commission: *Accreditation manual for hospitals,* Chicago, 2012a, TJC, available at http://www.jointcommission.org/accreditation_information.aspx, accessed August 2, 2012.

The Joint Commission (TJC): *National Patient Safety Goals,* Oakbrook Terrace, Ill, 2012b, The Commission, available at http://www.jointcommission.org/standards_information/npsgs.aspx.

Tonnesen H, et al: Smoking and alcohol intervention before surgery: evidence for best practice, *Br J Anaesth* 102(3):297, 2009. ©2009 Oxford University Press.

World Alliance for Patient Safety: WHO surgical safety checklist and implementation manual, Geneva, 2008, World Health Organization.

Intraoperative Care

MEDIA RESOURCES

- **evolve** http://evolve.elsevier.com/Perry/skills
  learning system

  - Review Questions
  - Audio Glossary

KEY TERMS

Asepsis	Perioperative	Scrub nurse	Sterile field
Aseptic technique	Registered nurse first	Sponge	Strike through
Circulating nurse	assistant (RNFA)	Sterile conscience	Surgical scrub
Contamination			

OBJECTIVES

Mastery of content in this chapter will enable the nurse to:
- Describe the meaning of a sterile conscience.
- Describe the roles of a registered nurse in the operating room.
- Identify guidelines for use of sterile technique in the operating room.

- Perform surgical hand antisepsis correctly.
- Describe how to correctly don a sterile surgical gown.
- Apply sterile gloves using the closed technique.

Nurses practicing in the operating room (OR) support patients' surgical experiences from the preoperative phase throughout the intraoperative period and into the various postoperative phases (see Chapter 36). The standards of clinical practice that registered nurses (RNs) follow within the OR provide an optimal level of care that ensures patients' safety and comfort (AORN, 2011a). One should exercise judgment, critical thinking, and interpersonal communication skills and apply the nursing process to ensure that patients receive appropriate nursing care during the perioperative experience.

Members of the surgical team include the surgeon (doctor of medicine [MD] or doctor of osteopathy [DO]), physician's assistant (PA), registered nurse first assistant (RNFA), certified registered nurse anesthetist (CRNA) and/or physician anesthesiologist (MD or DO), circulating nurse (RN), and scrub nurse/technician (RN, licensed practical nurse [LPN], or certified surgical technologist [CST]). The intraoperative phase begins when a patient enters the OR suite and ends with admission to the postanesthesia care unit (PACU). During the intraoperative phase an RN assumes the role of first assistant

to the surgeon, scrub nurse, or circulating nurse. The RNFA is a nurse with advanced education who assists the surgeon with the surgical procedure, performing a combination of nursing and delegated medical functions and/or skills (Box 37-1). The scrub nurse/technician (Box 37-2) is a "sterile" team member who provides the surgeon with instruments and supplies; disposes of soiled sponges; and accounts for sponges, sharps, and instruments on the surgical field. RNs, LPNs, or CSTs may assume the scrub nurse role. The circulating nurse (Box 37-3) is always an RN who is the charge nurse in the room (AORN, 2011b). The circulating nurse is a "nonsterile" member of the surgical team who uses the nursing process and assumes responsibility and accountability for maintaining patient safety and continuity of quality care. This includes supervising the conduct of the scrub technician and delegating tasks to licensed and nursing assistive personnel (NAP) as appropriate. The circulating nurse also assists the first assistant, scrub nurse/technician, and surgeon.

It is essential that perioperative nurses develop a sterile conscience. A sterile conscience requires knowledge of the principles of aseptic technique; self-discipline; good

BOX 37-1 | Role and Responsibilities of a Registered Nurse First Assistant

The registered nurse first assistant (RNFA) role is an expansion of the traditional perioperative nursing role, and areas of responsibility overlap. Responsibilities specific to the practice of first assisting include:

- Participating in "time out" procedure with other surgical team members (safety measure taken to ensure correct patient, correct procedure, correct site and side, correct patient position, and correct implants/equipment present) (TJC, 2011).
- Providing surgical exposure (assisting in retracting tissues and suctioning surgical field).
- Providing hemostasis (control of bleeding).
- Handling and/or cutting tissue.
- Using surgical instruments/medical devices and suturing.
- Performing wound closure.
- Applying human anatomic and physiologic considerations in practice; recognizing structure, function, and location of tissues and organs; manipulating tissues accordingly to avoid injury.
- Ensuring preoperative and postoperative patient management in collaboration with other health care providers.

From Association of periOperative Registered Nurses (AORN): *AORN standards and recommended practices for perioperative nursing—position statement: AORN official statement on RN first assistants*, Denver, 2010a, The Association.

BOX 37-2 | Role of the Scrub Nurse

- Helps circulating nurse prepare OR, open supplies
- Performs surgical hand antisepsis and dons sterile gown and gloves
- Prepares sterile field with procedure-appropriate supplies and instruments, verifying that all are in working order
- Participates in "time out" procedure with other surgical team members (safety measure taken to ensure correct patient, correct procedure, correct site and side, correct patient position, and correct implants/equipment present) (TJC, 2011)
- Performs sponge, sharps, and instrument counts with circulating nurse before incision is made, at the beginning of wound closure, and at the end of the surgical procedure
- Labels all liquids and/or medications on sterile field with sterile marking pen when liquid or medication is out of the original container or package
- Gowns and gloves surgeons and assistants as they enter the OR
- Assists surgeons with sterile draping of patient
- Keeps sterile field orderly and monitors progress of procedure and any breaks in aseptic technique
- Passes sterile instruments and supplies to surgeons and assistants
- Handles surgical specimens per agency policy
- Constantly monitors location of all sponges and sharps in the sterile field

OR, Operating room.

BOX 37-3 | Role of the Circulating Nurse

- Incorporates nursing process in plan of care
- Organizes and prepares OR before start of surgical procedure; checks to see that equipment works properly
- Gathers supplies for surgical procedure and opens sterile supplies for scrub nurse/technician
- Counts sponges, sharps, and instruments with scrub nurse/technician before incision is made, at the beginning of wound closure, and at the end of the surgical procedure
- Ensures that all liquids and/or medications on the sterile field are labeled with sterile marking pen when liquid or medication is out of the original container or package
- Sends for patient at appropriate time
- Conducts preoperative patient assessment, including the following:
  - Explains role and identifies patient
  - Reviews medical record and verifies procedure and consents
  - Confirms dentures and prostheses removed
  - Confirms patient's allergies, nothing by mouth (NPO) status, laboratory values, ECG, x-ray film studies, skin condition, circulatory and pulmonary status
- Safely assists patient to operating table and positions patient according to surgeon preference and procedure type, using safety precautions (e.g., safety belt, securing arms, padding bony prominences)
- Participates in "time out" procedure with other surgical team members (safety measure taken to ensure correct patient, correct procedure, correct site and side, correct patient position, and correct implants/equipment present) (TJC, 2011)
- Applies conductive pad to patient if electrocautery used; may prepare patient's skin; may apply ECG electrodes
- Applies antiembolism stockings and sequential compression device per physician order
- Explains briefly to patient what the circulating nurse and the scrub nurse/technician are doing
- Assists surgical team by tying gowns and arranging equipment
- Assists anesthesia personnel during induction and extubation
- Continuously monitors procedure for any breaks in aseptic technique and anticipates needs of the team; opens additional sterile supplies for scrub nurse/technician
- Handles surgical specimens per agency policy
- Documents on perioperative nurses' notes
- Communicates to family and PACU personnel during the surgical procedure

ECG, Electrocardiogram; *OR*, Operating room; *PACU*, postanesthesia care unit.

communication skills to identify, address, and correct any breaks in sterile technique; and the maturity to overcome personal preferences. If any question exists about sterility of an item, the item is unsterile. For example, if a sterile gown touches the floor while you are putting it on, you discard it and exchange it for a new one.

While the patient is in the OR and the OR team is gowned and gloved, it is recommended that a surgical safety checklist or the World Health Organization (WHO) checklist be completed (WHO, 2008) (Fig. 37-1). The WHO checklist identifies three phases of an operation, each corresponding to a specific period in the normal flow of work: before the induction of anesthesia ("sign in"), before the incision of the skin ("time out"), and before the patient leaves the operating room ("sign out"). In each phase a checklist coordinator must confirm that the surgery team has completed the listed tasks before it proceeds with the operation.

This checklist verifies the patient's identity, ascertains if the patient has any allergies, checks if the surgical site is marked and reverifies the site marking, and asks the patient if he or she has any questions. A time out is conducted immediately before starting any invasive procedure or making an incision (TJC, 2011). Time outs are standardized by each hospital, initiated by a designated member of the team, and involve all the immediate members of the surgical/procedure team who will be participating in the procedure from start to finish. It is during the time out that the team members

---

SURGICAL SAFETY CHECKLIST (FIRST EDITION)

World Health Organization

Before induction of anaesthesia >>>>>>>> Before skin incision >>>>>>>>>>>>>> Before patient leaves operating room

SIGN IN	TIME OUT	SIGN OUT
☐ **Patient has confirmed** • Identity • Site • Procedure • Consent	☐ **Confirm all team members have introduced themselves by name and role**	Nurse verbally confirms with the team:
☐ **Site marked/not applicable**	☐ **Surgeon, anaesthesia professional and nurse verbally confirm** • Patient • Site • Procedure	☐ **The name of the procedure recorded**
☐ **Anaesthesia safety check completed**		☐ **That instrument, sponge and needle counts are correct** (or not applicable)
☐ **Pulse oximeter on patient and functioning**	**Anticipated critical events**	☐ **How the specimen is labelled** (including patient name)
Does patient have a:	☐ **Surgeon reviews:** What are the critical or unexpected steps, operative duration, anticipated blood loss?	☐ **Whether there are any equipment problems to be addressed**
Known allergy? ☐ No ☐ Yes	☐ **Anaesthesia team reviews:** Are there any patient-specific concerns?	☐ **Surgeon, anaesthesia professional and nurse review the key concerns for recovery and management of this patient**
Difficult airway/aspiration risk? ☐ No ☐ Yes, and equipment/assistance available	☐ **Nursing team reviews:** Has sterility (including indicator results) been confirmed? Are there equipment issues or any concerns?	
Risk of >500ml blood loss (7ml/kg in children)? ☐ No ☐ Yes, and adequate intravenous access and fluids planned	**Has antibiotic prophylaxis been given within the last 60 minutes?** ☐ Yes ☐ Not applicable	
	Is essential imaging displayed? ☐ Yes ☐ Not applicable	

This checklist is not intended to be comprehensive. Additions and modifications to fit local practice are encouraged.

FIG 37-1   The WHO surgical safety checklist. (*Used with permission, World Health Organization.*)

---

agree at a minimum that the correct patient has been identified and the correct procedure is scheduled to be done. The time out is documented before the procedure begins (TJC, 2011).

EVIDENCE-BASED PRACTICE TRENDS

Surgical patients are at risk for surgical site infections from the stress of surgery and their procedure. Studies found that surgical staff may transmit pathogens from contact with patients and contaminated items such as tourniquets, linens, or surfaces (e.g., doorknobs, countertops) (Cook, 2011). Avoiding use of any nail enhancements such as artificial nails, acrylics, tips, and gels is another initiative. OR personnel have a responsibility to adhere to specific infection control practices based on individualized agency guidelines.

- Hand hygiene should be performed when OR staff arrive at the health care agency, before and after patient contact, before and after donning gloves and other personal protective equipment, before and after eating, before leaving the health care agency, and when visibly soiled (AORN, 2011c; Cook, 2011).
- Use hand-scrub preparations containing 60% to 90% alcohol combined with chlorhexidine gluconate.
- Artificial fingernail enhancements can increase the risk of colonization and transmission of pathogens to the surgical patient (AORN, 2011c).
- Fingernails should not be longer than ¼ inch in length, and nail polish should not be chipped. There are no recommendations regarding nail polish color (Cook, 2011).

- Rings should not be worn in the surgical area, and watches should be removed before hand hygiene (AORN, 2011c; Cook, 2011).
- Use a brushless, alcohol-based surgical hand product (with added emollients) that limits damage to the user's skin, improves adherence to hand antisepsis protocols, simplifies application technique, and reduces material waste (i.e., water, brushes, and packaging) (Rothrock, 2011).

PATIENT-CENTERED CARE

Often the patient is unsure of what to expect and has concerns about the amount of pain, possible disfigurement, and length of recovery after surgery. Nursing care of the surgical patient requires specialized knowledge that allows you to monitor a patient's intraoperative response to the experience. Patient needs will vary based on their preoperative health and the type of surgical procedure.

Patients should be asked about their cultural preferences and religious beliefs that may affect their acceptance of education, blood administration, and surgical interventions. You need to communicate this information to all health care team members to ensure comprehensive intraoperative care.

Skill Performance Guidelines

1 All items used within a sterile field must be sterile.
2 Gowns used by scrub persons must be sterile before donning. Once in place, gowns are sterile from the front chest and

shoulders to table level and on the sleeves to 5 cm (2 inches) above the elbow.

3 Sterile persons must keep their hands in view, above waist level and below neckline, to avoid contamination.

4 When wearing a sterile gown, do not fold arms with hands tucked in the axillary region. This area is not considered sterile once you have donned the gown. Perspiration can lead to strike through, or contamination that occurs when moisture permeates a sterile barrier.

5 Sterile-draped tables are sterile only at table level. Sides of the drape extending below table level are unsterile.

6 All personnel moving around or within a sterile field must do so in a manner consistent with maintaining the sterility of that field. Scrubbed persons move from sterile areas to other sterile areas, contacting a sterile field only with sterile gowns and gloves. Unscrubbed persons always stay at least 30 cm (12 inches) away from the sterile field while keeping it in constant view; they touch only unsterile areas.

7 Group all sterile supplies and equipment around the sterile-draped patient.

8 Unsterile persons must avoid reaching over the sterile field.

9 Scrubbed persons remain close to the sterile field. When changing position, turn face to face or back to back.

SKILL 37-1 Surgical Hand Antisepsis

In the operating room (OR) setting it is imperative that you achieve surgical hand antisepsis through effective surgical scrub or antiseptic hand rub (AORN, 2011c). To reduce patient risk for acquiring postoperative infections, use of an antimicrobial preparation for hand antisepsis is an integral part of the presurgical scrubbing procedure for OR personnel. Although the skin cannot be sterilized, you can reduce the number of microorganisms greatly by chemical, physical, and mechanical means.

The surgical hand scrub has been the traditional method for surgical asepsis. Through the use of an antimicrobial agent and sterile brushes or sponges, the surgical hand scrub removes debris and transient microorganisms from the nails, hands, and forearms; reduces the resident microbial count to a minimum; and inhibits rapid/rebound growth of microorganisms (AORN, 2011c). Evidence suggests that a brushless technique, with or without water, containing at least 60% alcohol, is an alternative to the traditional hand scrub with a brush with the same microbial efficacy (AORN 2011c; TJC, 2011). Both hand antiseptic methods are currently used in OR settings.

Surgical attire (i.e., scrubs) is worn in the operating room to reduce the chance for contamination between surgical personnel and patients (AORN, 2011d). Keep your fingernails short (¼ inch in length), clean, and healthy. If you wear polish, make sure that it is not chipped or older than 4 days. Never wear artificial nails (AORN, 2011c). Remove watches and bracelets before the surgical scrub. Rings should not be worn in the operating room (Cook, 2011).

The Association of periOperative Registered Nurses (AORN, 2011c) recommends a 3- to 5-minute hand and arm scrub with an approved antimicrobial agent for all surgical procedures. Surgical hand-scrub procedure for all staff using either the anatomic timed scrub or the counted-stroke method should be standardized (AORN, 2011c) (see agency policy). Some procedures, described as clean procedures (e.g., laryngoscopy and proctoscopy), require performing hand hygiene but not necessarily surgical hand antisepsis.

Delegation and Collaboration
The skill of surgical hand antisepsis can be delegated to a surgical technologist or licensed practical nurse. The registered nurse routinely observes surgical hand antisepsis for staff compliance.

Equipment
- Deep sink with foot or knee controls for dispensing water and soap
- Antimicrobial agent approved by agency (dispenser with foot controls)
- Surgical scrub brush with plastic nail file
- Paper face mask, cap or hood, surgical shoe covers
- Protective eyewear/face shield
- Sterile towel
- Sterile pack containing sterile gown

STEP	RATIONALE

ASSESSMENT

1 Determine type and length of time for hand hygiene (see agency policy).

Guidelines vary regarding ideal time needed for surgical scrub.

2 Remove bracelets, rings, and watches.

Jewelry harbors and protects microorganisms from removal. Skin under rings has been shown to harbor more pathogens and should not be worn (Cook, 2011).

3 Inspect fingernails, which must be short (¼ inch), clean, and healthy. Nail polish that is chipped should be removed before entering surgical area. Never wear artificial nails or extenders.

Long nails and chipped or old polish harbor greater numbers of bacteria (AORN, 2011c). Long fingernails can puncture gloves, causing contamination. Artificial nails harbor gram-negative microorganisms and fungus (AORN, 2011c).

4 Inspect condition of cuticles, hands, and forearms for presence of abrasions, cuts, or open lesions.

Cuts, abrasions, exudative lesions, fresh tattoos, or hangnails tend to ooze serum, which may contain pathogens. Individuals with these conditions should not have patient contact until conditions heal (AORN, 2011c).

STEP	RATIONALE

NURSING DIAGNOSIS

- Risk for infection

Related factors are individualized based on patient's condition or needs.

PLANNING

1 Expected outcomes following completion of procedure:

- Patient does not develop signs of surgical site infection.

Indicates that microorganisms are not transferred to patient and sterile field.

IMPLEMENTATION

1 Don surgical shoe covers, cap or hood, face mask, and protective eyewear.

Protective eyewear prevents exposure to blood or body fluids splashing from sterile field, which causes risk for infection (e.g., human immunodeficiency virus [HIV], hepatitis B virus [HBV]).

Clinical Decision Point *Laser surgery requires special protective eyewear to prevent eye damage from stray laser energy.*

2 Perform prescrub wash at beginning of work shift.

Prevents contamination of hands after scrub.

  a Turn water on using foot or knee control and adjust to comfortable temperature.

  b Wet hands thoroughly with water. Follow manufacturer directions for application of soap.

  c Rub hands, covering all surfaces, including backs of hands, fingertips, inner webs, and palms, washing for at least 15 seconds.

A short prescrub wash/rinse at least 15 seconds at beginning of work shift removes gross debris and superficial microorganisms (AORN, 2011c).

  d Rinse well to remove all soap. Dry hands thoroughly with disposable towel and discard towel.

3 Surgical hand scrub (with sponge):

  a Turn on water using foot or knee control. Clean under nails of both hands with disposable nail pick or cleaner (see illustration). Rinse hands and forearms under running water.

Removes dirt and organic materials that harbor microorganisms.

  b Dispense antimicrobial scrub agent according to manufacturer instructions. Apply agent to wet hands and forearms with soft, nonabrasive sponge.

Ensures removal of resident microorganisms on all surfaces of hands and arms (AORN, 2011c).

  c Time a 3- to 5-minute scrub (follow manufacturer instructions). Visualize each finger, hand, and arm as having four sides (see illustrations). Wash all four sides effectively, keeping hand elevated, elbow down. Repeat for other hand, fingers, and arm.

Times vary by product.
Scrubbing all surfaces ensures removal of resident microorganisms on hands and arms (AORN, 2011c).

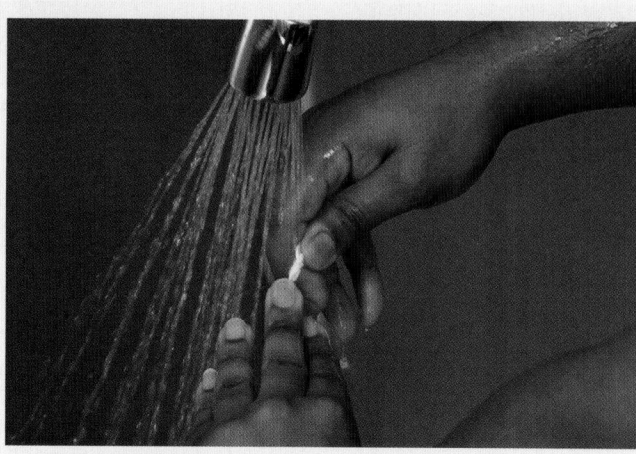

STEP 3a Cleaning under fingernails.

STEP	RATIONALE

d Avoid splashing surgical attire. Discard sponges in appropriate container.

e Rinse hands and arms, running water from fingertips to elbows in one continuous motion, holding hands higher than elbows and away from surgical site (see illustration).

Hands remain cleanest part of upper extremities.

f Turn off water using foot or knee controls and back into OR holding hands higher than elbows and away from surgical attire.

g Approach sterile setup and grasp sterile towel, taking care not to drip water on sterile field (see illustration).

Water contaminates field.

h Keeping hands and arms above waist and outstretched, carefully grasp one end of sterile towel to dry one hand thoroughly, moving from fingers to elbow in rotating motion (see illustration).

Avoids sterile towel contacting unsterile scrub attire and transferring contamination to hands. Dries skin from cleanest (hands) to least clean (elbows).

i Use opposite end of towel to dry other hand.

Avoids transfer of microorganisms from elbow to opposite hand.

j Drop towel into linen hamper or into circulating nurse's hand.

4 Perform spongeless surgical hand scrub with alcohol-based hand-rub product.

a After prescrub wash (Step 2) turn on water using foot or knee control. Clean under nails of both hands with a disposable nail pick or cleaner and rinse hands and forearms under running water. Dry hands thoroughly with paper towel. Turn off water.

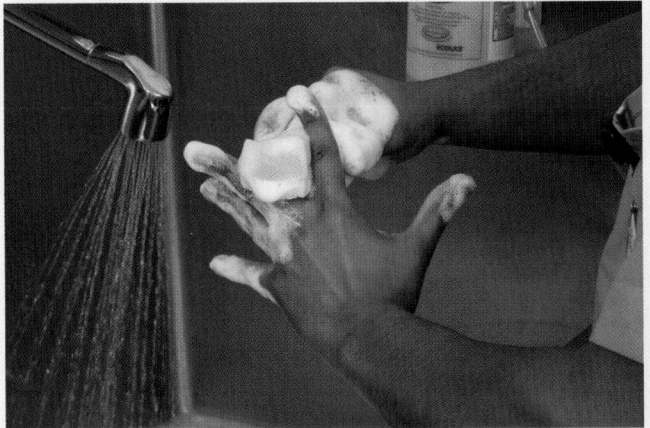 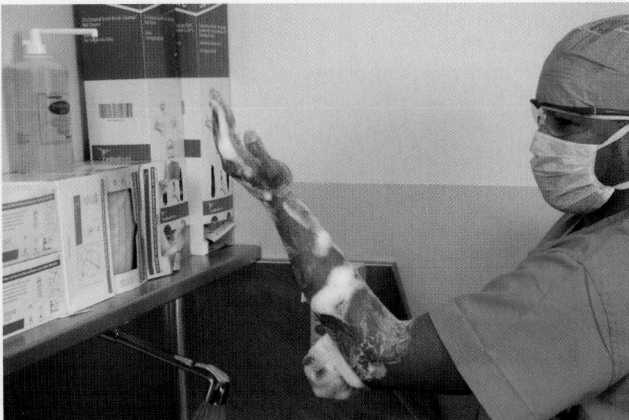

STEP 3c **A,** Scrubbing sides of fingers. **B,** Scrubbing forearms.

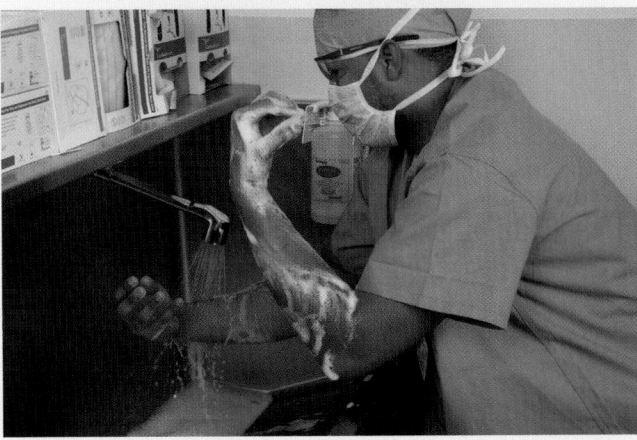 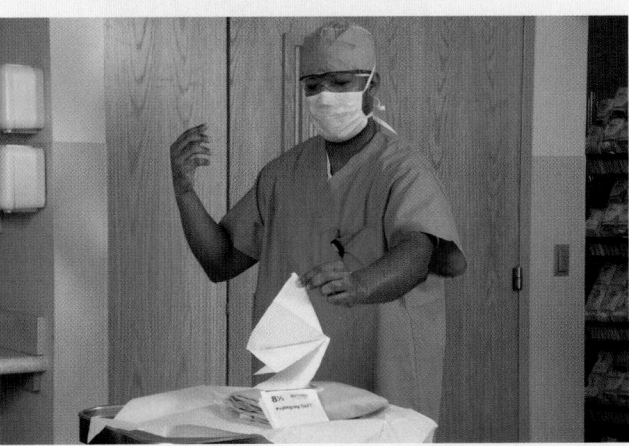

STEP 3e Rinsing arms.

STEP 3g Grasping sterile towel.

STEP	RATIONALE
b Dispense manufacturer-recommended amount of antimicrobial agent hand preparation (see illustration). Apply agent to hands and forearms according to manufacturer instructions for application, recommended volume, and specified time.	Promotes reduction in microorganisms on all surfaces of hands and arms (AORN, 2011c).
c Repeat antimicrobial product application if indicated in manufacturer instructions.	
d Rub thoroughly until completely dry (see illustration). Proceed to OR to don gloves.	

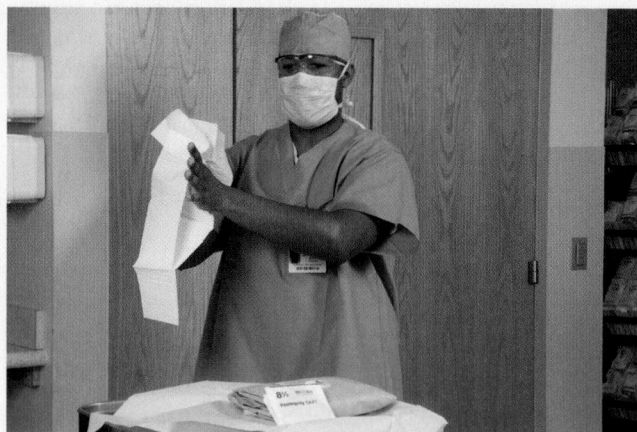

STEP 3h   Drying hands thoroughly.

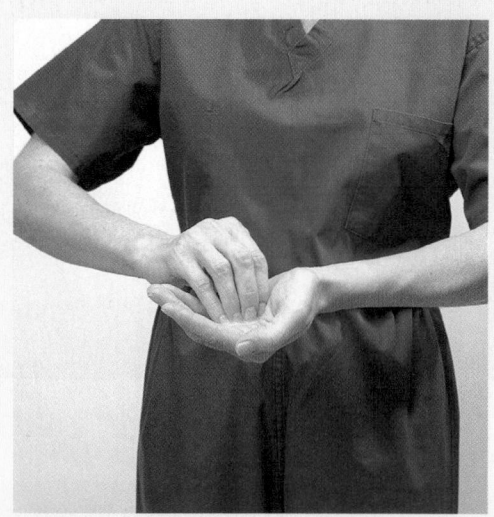

STEP 4b   Dispense antimicrobial agent into hands. (*Photo Courtesy 3M Health Care.*)

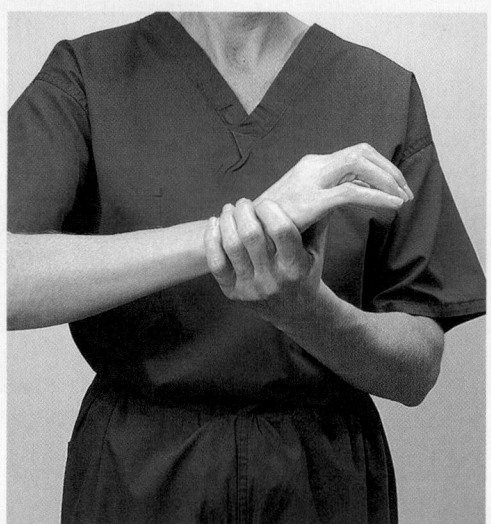

STEP 4d   Rub thoroughly until completely dry. (*Photo Courtesy 3M Health Care.*)

EVALUATION

1 Monitor patient after surgery for signs of surgical site infection (usually occurs 2 to 3 days after surgery).

Signs of infection include redness, heat, swelling, pain, and purulent drainage.

Unexpected Outcomes

1 Redness, heat, swelling, pain, or purulent drainage may develop at surgical site, which often indicates wound infection.

Related Interventions

• Individualize interventions based on patient's situation (e.g., wound care, antibiotic therapy).

Recording and Reporting

- No recording is required for surgical hand antisepsis. Record area and description of surgical site after surgery to provide baseline for monitoring wound.

Special Considerations
Teaching

- Instruct patient and family or significant other how to observe surgical site for signs of infection.

SKILL 37-2 Donning a Sterile Gown and Closed Gloving

Immediately following surgical hand antisepsis, apply a sterile gown and then apply sterile gloves. All members of the surgical team must prepare in this manner before entering the sterile field. Once applied, the surgical gown is considered sterile in the front from chest to waist or table level. The sleeves are considered sterile from 5 cm (2 inches) above the elbow to fingertips. The back of the gown is not considered sterile when worn. Surgical gowns should cover all garments worn underneath. All sterile gowns that are free of tears, punctures, strain, and abrasion provide an effective barrier against microorganisms, particulates, and fluids passing between unsterile and sterile areas (AORN, 2011d).

Use the closed-glove method to apply gloves when you enter the sterile field. If a glove becomes contaminated during the surgery, the circulating nurse, wearing protective unsterile gloves, grasps the outside of the glove and pulls off the glove inside out, leaving the stockinette cuff of the gown in place. Another sterile team member assists in regloving. The open method can be used when only one glove has been contaminated. In some settings the scrub nurse will wear two pairs of sterile gloves. If both of the scrub nurse/technician's gloves become contaminated, the gown is removed first, then the gloves are removed, and then the nurse regowns and regloves using the closed-glove method.

Delegation and Collaboration

The skills of donning a sterile gown and closed gloving can be delegated to a surgical technologist or licensed practical nurse. The registered nurse routinely observes sterile gown application and closed gloving for staff compliance.

Equipment

- ❏ Package of proper-size sterile gloves (latex-free if sensitivity or allergy present)
- ❏ Sterile pack containing sterile gown
- ❏ Clean, flat, dry surface (table or Mayo stand) on which to open gown and gloves
- ❏ Paper face masks, cap or hood, surgical shoe covers
- ❏ Protective eyewear/face shield

STEP	RATIONALE
ASSESSMENT	
1 Select proper size and type of sterile gloves. Select latex-free gloves if you know that patient or any surgical personnel in room are latex sensitive.	Proper fit ensures ease of handling instruments and supplies. Prevents latex allergic response.

Clinical Decision Point *Know your agency policy, because double gloving may be recommended to reduce the risk for glove perforation during a surgical procedure (Fry, 2010; Tanner and Parkinson, 2009; Thomas-Copeland, 2009).*

STEP	RATIONALE
2 Select proper size and type of sterile surgical gown.	Ill-fitting gown impedes movement of extremities.

NURSING DIAGNOSIS

- Risk for infection

Related factors are individualized based on patient's condition or needs.

STEP	RATIONALE
PLANNING	
1 Expected outcomes following completion of procedure: • Patient does not develop signs of surgical site infection.	Nurse maintains aseptic technique and does not contaminate gown or gloves.
IMPLEMENTATION	
1 Donning sterile gown: a Open sterile gown and glove package on clean, dry, flat surface. Scrub nurse (before scrubbing hands) or circulating nurse can do this for you, preferably on small table separate from sterile field containing sterile instruments and supplies.	Provides sterile area for gloving.
b Perform surgical hand antisepsis (see Skill 37-1). Dry hands thoroughly.	
c Pick up gown (folded inside out) from sterile package, grasping inside surface at collar.	Hands are not completely sterile. Inside surface of gown will contact surface of skin and thus is considered contaminated.

STEP	RATIONALE
d Lift folded gown directly upward and step back, away from table.	Prevents gown from touching unsterile object.
e Locate neckband; with both hands grasp inside front of gown just below neckband.	Clean hands may touch inside of gown without contaminating outer surface.
f Keeping gown at arm's length away from body, allow it to unfold with inside of gown toward body. Do not touch outside of gown or allow it to touch floor.	Outside of gown remains sterile.
g With hands at shoulder level, slip both arms into armholes simultaneously (see illustration). Do not allow hands to move through cuff opening. Have circulating nurse pull gown over shoulders by reaching inside arm seams. Pull gown on, leaving sleeves covering hands.	Careful application prevents contamination. Gown covers hands to prepare for closed gloving.
h Have circulating nurse tie gown at neck and waist (see illustration). If gown is wraparound style, do not touch sterile front flap until scrub nurse/technician has gloved (see Step 3b).	Secures gown without contaminating it.
2 Applying gloves using closed-glove method:	
a With hands covered by gown cuffs and sleeves, open inner sterile glove package (see illustration).	Sterile gown cuff will touch sterile glove surface.
b Grasp folded cuff of glove for dominant hand with nondominant hand.	Sterile gown touches sterile glove.

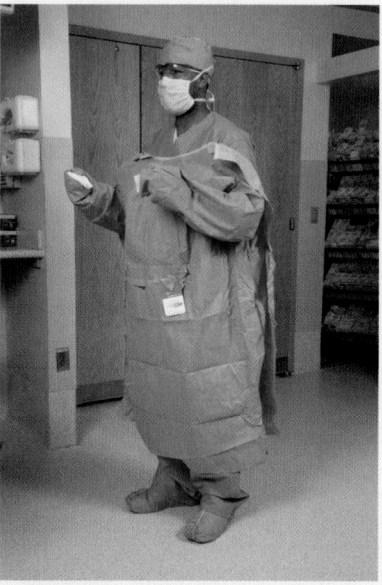

STEP 1g   Placing arms in sleeves.

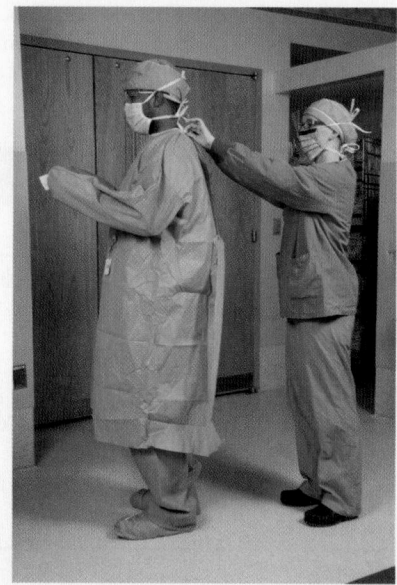

STEP 1h   Circulating nurse ties scrub gown.

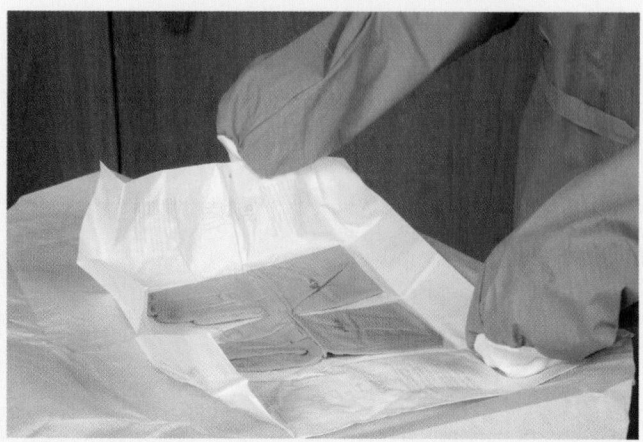

STEP 2a   Scrub nurse opens glove package.

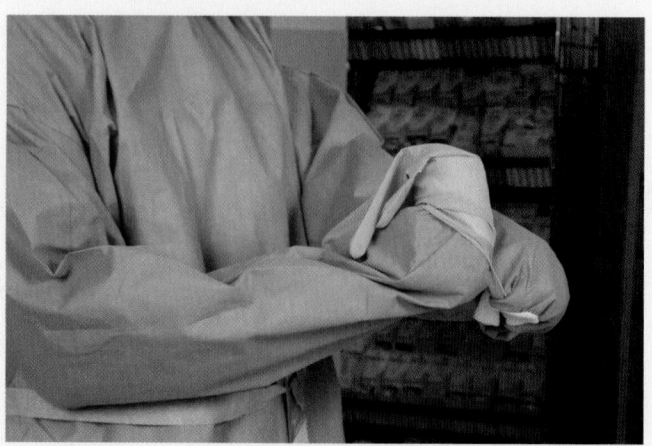

STEP 2d   Glove applied as hands remain inside cuffs.

STEP	RATIONALE
c Extend covered dominant forearm forward with palm up and place palm of glove against palm of dominant hand. Glove fingers point toward elbow.	Positions glove for application over cuffed hand, keeping glove sterile.
d While holding glove cuff through gown with dominant hand on which it was placed, grasp back of glove cuff with nondominant hand and turn glove cuff over end of dominant hand and gown cuff (see illustration).	Positions glove over gown for hand insertion.
e Grasp top of glove and underlying gown sleeve with covered nondominant hand. Carefully extend fingers into glove, being sure that cuff of glove covers cuff of gown.	
f Glove nondominant hand in same manner with gloved, dominant hand (see illustration A). Keep hand inside sleeve. Be sure that fingers are fully extended into both gloves (see illustration B).	Gloves remain sterile.
3 Donning wraparound gown:	
a Grasp sterile front flap/paper tab with gloved hands and untie.	Front of gown is sterile.
b Pass sterile paper tab to member of sterile surgical team or to nonsterile team member (e.g., circulating nurse) (see illustration). Keep gown tie in right hand. Circulating nurse stands still as scrub nurse/technician turns.	Nonsterile team member uses caution not to touch sterile tie when taking sterile paper tab while scrub nurse/technician turns.
c Allowing margin of safety, turn to left one-half turn, covering back with extended gown flap. Retrieve sterile tie only from team member and secure both ties in place.	Maneuver covers entire body with gown. Nonsterile team member pulls off paper tab and discards.

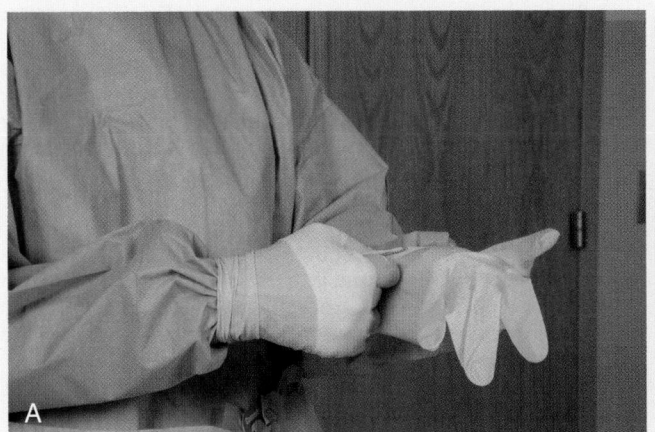 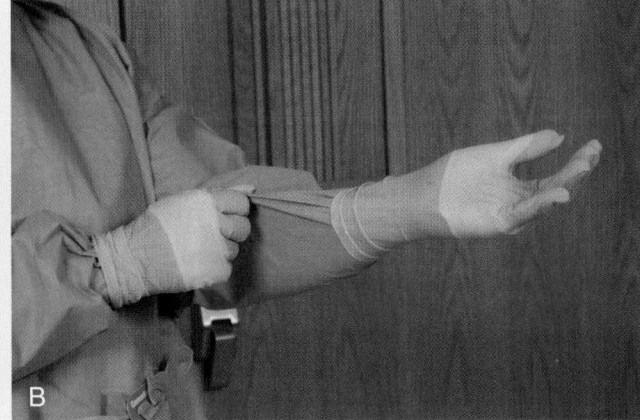

STEP 2f   **A,** Second glove applied. **B,** Gloved fingers extended.

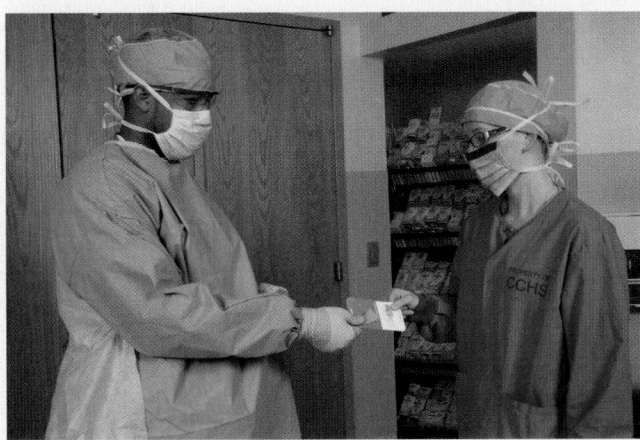

STEP 3b   Paper tab on disposable gown is passed to circulating nurse.

STEP	RATIONALE

EVALUATION

1 Monitor patient after surgery for signs of surgical site infection (usually occurs 2 to 3 days after surgery).

Signs of infection include redness, heat, swelling, pain, and purulent drainage.

Unexpected Outcomes

1 Redness, heat, swelling, pain, or purulent drainage develops at surgical site, which often indicates wound infection.

Related Interventions

• Individualize interventions based on patient's situation (e.g., wound care, antibiotic therapy).

Recording and Reporting

• No recording is required for sterile gowning and gloving. Record area and description of surgical site after surgery to provide baseline for monitoring wound.

Special Considerations
Teaching

• Instruct patient and family to observe surgical site for signs of possible infection. Both staff and patients need to be educated about surgical site infection prevention.

❓ Critical Thinking Exercises

You are assigned to be the circulating nurse for a patient who is having an umbilical hernia repair. She is a 38-year-old Hispanic bookkeeper and mother of five children with no significant medical history except for postpartum hypothyroidism. The surgical team includes Dr. M. Klein; L. Relling, RNFA; Sarah Scott, certified surgical technologist (CST); and Dr. L. Bates, anesthesiologist. Sarah has recently completed an extended orientation but still needs much supervision.

1 Sarah is running late because of the staff meeting this morning. You notice that she omits the prescrub hand wash before performing a brushless antiseptic hand rub. What should you do? Explain your choice.
   1 Tell Sarah to apply extra hand antiseptic to both hands
   2 Tell Sarah that she must start over and perform the prescrub hand wash first
   3 Tell Sarah that she must now perform a surgical hand scrub with a brush
   4 Do nothing because she is going to apply sterile gloves anyway
2 Sarah just had artificial nails applied last night because she is in a wedding tonight. They are polished with no signs of chipping. Is it okay for Sarah to scrub for the hernia repair today? Explain your choice.
   1 Yes because the polish was applied just last night
   2 Yes because the polish is not chipped
   3 No because artificial nails may not be worn
   4 No because artificial nails require a longer scrub
3 While Sarah prepares the sterile field with the appropriate instruments and supplies for the umbilical hernia surgery, you notice that she reaches down to scratch the top of her leg. She continues to set up the sterile field without taking any action. What should she have done?

✅ REVIEW QUESTIONS

1 Many individuals play a vital role as part of the surgical team. What is included in the responsibilities of the circulating nurse?
   1 Performing the surgical hand scrub and donning a sterile gown and gloves
   2 Assisting in retracting tissues and suctioning surgical field
   3 Conducting perioperative assessment and reviewing medical records for accuracy and completeness
   4 Removing liquids and medications from original packages and labels before placing on the sterile back table

2 Many newer methods for the surgical scrub have been researched. Which is the traditional method for surgical asepsis?
   1 Surgical hand scrub
   2 Alcohol foam rub
   3 Brushless scrub
   4 Waterless scrub
3 The scrub nurse is getting ready to do her surgical scrub. What should be done before beginning the scrub?
   1 Remove nail polish even if it is not chipped
   2 Inspect areas from fingertips to elbows for abrasions or open areas
   3 Move rings higher on the knuckles before beginning the scrub
   4 Remove bracelets and artificial nails
4 The closed-glove method is standard in the operating room for many of the participants. The scrub nurse is performing it correctly if which procedure is observed?
   1 Both hands are covered with the cuffs of the gown.
   2 Both hands are exposed through the cuffs of the gown.
   3 The dominant hand is covered with the cuff of the gown.
   4 The nondominant hand is covered with the cuff of the gown.
5 Surgical personnel must have a sterile conscience to provide optimum patient safety. Which situation denotes a breach of sterile conscience?
   1 The scrub nurse accidentally touches the faucet with one hand while scrubbing and rescrubs his hands.
   2 The circulating nurse accidentally touches a sterile item and removes it from the sterile field.
   3 The surgeon thinks he contaminated a sterile glove and has the suspect glove changed.
   4 Before the scrub nurse dries her hands, she drips water on the sterile gown that she is about to put on and applies the gown.
6 If both gloves of a gowned sterile team member become contaminated, one should:
   1 First remove the gloves, then the gown, and regown and reglove using open-glove method.
   2 Remove the gown first, then the gloves, and regown and reglove using closed-glove method.
   3 Remove gown first, then gloves; rescrub and apply new gown and gloves using closed gloving.
   4 Remove gloves and gown, rescrub, and apply new gown and gloves using open gloving.

7 Which of the following statements is true?
1 An unsterile item may be used on the sterile field.
2 Sterile persons must keep their hands in view, above the waist and below the neckline to avoid contamination.
3 When a scrubbed person changes positions at the sterile field with another, turn face to back of the other person.
4 The sides of the drape extending below the table level are considered sterile.

8 The steps for doing a surgical hand scrub include:
1 Inspect hands to ensure that nails are short, no cuts or skin problems. Turn on water; dispense antimicrobial scrub; wash all four sides of fingers, hands, and arms. Do a 3- to 5-minute scrub and rinse off soap. Turn off water using foot or knee controls. Back into operating room (OR) holding hands higher than elbows.
2 Turn on water; dispense antimicrobial scrub; inspect hands to ensure that nails are short, no cuts or skin problems. Wash all four sides of hands, fingers, and arms. Do a 6-minute scrub. Turn off water with paper towel at sink. Back into OR holding hands higher than elbows.
3 Inspect hands to ensure that nails are short, no cuts or skin problems. Turn on water; dispense antimicrobial scrub; wash all four sides of fingers, hands, and arms. Do a 2-minute scrub. Turn off water using foot or knee controls. Back into OR holding hands higher than elbows.
4 Inspect hands to ensure that nails are short, no cuts or skin problems. Use faucet handle to turn on water; dispense antimicrobial scrub; wash all four sides of fingers, hands, and arms. Do a 3-minute scrub. Using a paper towel, turn off faucets. Walk into OR keeping hands higher than elbows.

9 Steps for correctly scrubbing and gowning for a surgical environment include:
1 Applying alcohol-based rub, putting on sterile gloves, putting on sterile gown.
2 Completing 3- to 5-minute hand scrub, putting on sterile gown, putting on sterile gloves.
3 Putting on sterile gown, completing 3- to 5-minute hand scrub, putting on sterile gloves.
4 Completing 3- to 5-minute hand scrub, putting on sterile gloves, putting on sterile gown.

10 Participants in the time out before a procedure or surgery include:
1 Immediate members of the procedure team and others who will be participating in the procedure from the beginning.
2 Only the anesthesiologist, surgeon, scrub nurse, and circulating nurse.
3 Only the surgeon, registered nurse first assistant (RNFA), scrub technician, and circulating nurse.
4 Anesthesiologist, circulating nurse, and scrub technologist.

REFERENCES

Association of periOperative Registered Nurses (AORN): *AORN standards and recommended practices for perioperative nursing—Position statement: AORN official statement on RN first assistants,* Denver, 2011a, The Association.
Association of periOperative Registered Nurses (AORN): *AORN standards, recommended practices, and guidelines—Position statement: statement on one perioperative registered nurse circulator dedicated to every patient undergoing a surgical or other invasive procedure,* Denver, 2011b, The Association.
Association of periOperative Registered Nurses (AORN): *AORN perioperative standards and recommended practices—recommended practices for hand hygiene in the perioperative setting,* Denver, 2011c, The Association.
Association of periOperative Registered Nurses (AORN): *AORN perioperative standards and recommended practices—recommended practices for selection and use of surgical gowns and drapes,* Denver, 2011d, The Association.
Cook K: The hands have it! Hand hygiene in the OR, *OR Nurse* 5(6):14, 2011.
Fry DE et al.: Influence of double-gloving on manual dexterity and tactile sensation of surgeons, *J Am College Surg* (3):325, 2010.
Rothrock J: *Alexander's Care of the patient in surgery,* ed 14, St Louis, 2011, Mosby.
Tanner J, Parkinson H: Double gloving to reduce surgical cross-infection, *Cochrane Database Syst Rev* (10):CD003087, 2009.
The Joint Commission (TJC): Universal protocol for preventing wrong site, wrong procedure, wrong person surgery, 2011, Oakbrook Terrace, Ill, available at http://www.jointcommission.org/standards_information/up.aspx, accessed August 1, 2012.
Thomas-Copeland J: "Do surgical personnel really need to double-glove?" *AORN J* 89(2):322, 2009.
World Health Organization (WHO): *Surgical safety checklist,* 2008, available at http://www.who.int/patientsafety/safesurgery/tools_resources/SSSL_Checklist_finalJun08.pdf, accessed August 1, 2012.

38 Wound Care and Irrigations

MEDIA RESOURCES

- evolve http://evolve.elsevier.com/Perry/skills
  - Review Questions
  - Video Clips
- Mosby's Nursing Video Skills, 4th edition
- NSO Nursing Skills Online

KEY TERMS

Dehiscence
Eschar
Evisceration
Granulation tissue

Healing ridge
Hemostasis
Hemovac drain
Irrigation

Jackson-Pratt (JP) drain
Penrose drain
Primary intention

Secondary intention
Tertiary intention
Staples

OBJECTIVES

Mastery of content in this chapter will enable the nurse to:
- Discuss the response of the body during each stage of the wound-healing process.
- Differentiate between primary- and secondary-intention wound healing.
- Explain factors that impair or promote normal wound healing.

- Perform a wound assessment.
- Perform a wound irrigation.
- Remove sutures or staples.
- Demonstrate care of a wound-drainage system.

Proper wound care is necessary to promote healing that results in an intact skin layer. Intact skin is the first line of defense of the body against invasion by infectious microorganisms. The skin defends the body in other ways by serving as a sensory organ for pain, touch, and temperature; and it has an acid pH, which is often called the *acid mantle*. It also plays a major role in thermoregulation, metabolism, immunity, and fluid balance regulation (Bryant and Nix, 2012).

The skin is the largest external organ. It has two layers: the epidermis and the dermis (Fig. 38-1). The outer layer, the epidermis, has five layers. The outermost layer, the stratum corneum, consists of flattened dead keratinized cells. The thin layer of the stratum corneum prevents dehydration of underlying cells and is a physical barrier to the entry of certain chemicals. The barrier is selective; it allows absorption of topical medications in paste, ointment, and dermal patch forms. The next layers of the epidermis are the stratum lucidum, stratum

granulosum, and stratum spinosum. The innermost layer of the epidermis, the stratum germinativum, is sometimes called the *basal layer*. It is from this single layer of keratinocytes that cells migrate up toward the stratum corneum. Important features of the stratum germinativum are the epidermal protrusions, or "peaks and valleys" that point downward into the dermis. These provide resiliency and integrity to the skin structure. Melanocytes, the cells that give the skin its color, are also in this layer. The area that separates the epidermis from the dermis is called the *dermoepidermal junction* or the *basement membrane zone*.

Beneath the epidermis is the dermis. Collagen (a tough fibrous protein layer), blood vessels, and nerves compose the dermal layer. Collagen composes about 70% of the dermis and is extremely important in wound healing. The dermis restores the physical properties of the skin and its structural integrity. Restoration of both the epidermal and dermal layers is

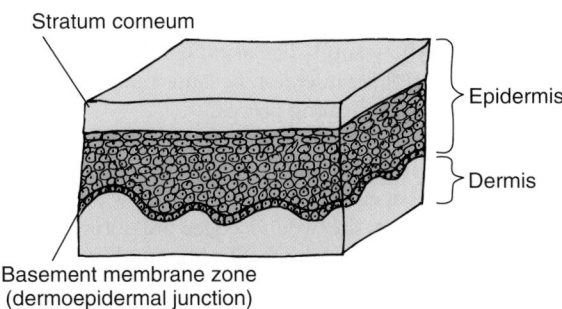

FIG 38-1   Diagram of layers of skin and subcutaneous tissue.

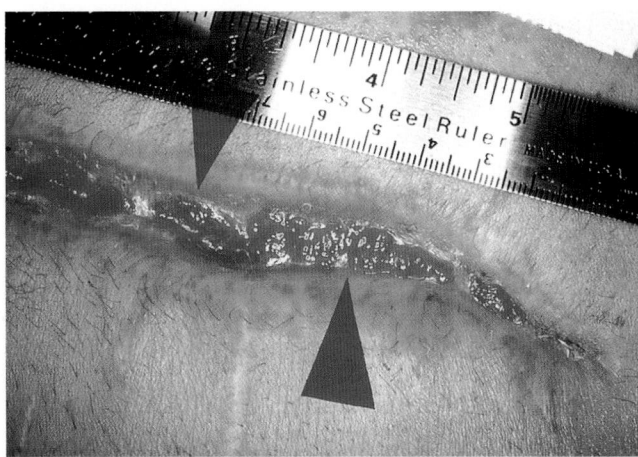

FIG 38-2   Surgical wound with epithelialization occurring: epithelial healing ridge apparent. (*From Bryant RA, Nix DP, editors:* Acute and chronic wounds: current management concepts, *ed 3, St Louis, 2007, Mosby.*)

| BOX 38-1 | Phases of Wound Healing (Full-Thickness Wounds) |

Hemostasis Phase
- Blood vessels constrict; clotting factors activate coagulation pathways to stop bleeding. Clot formation seals the disrupted vessels so blood loss is controlled and acts as a temporary bacterial barrier. Platelets release growth factors, which attract cells needed to begin the repair process.

Inflammatory Phase
- Vasodilation occurs, allowing plasma and blood cells to leak into the wound, noted as edema, erythema, and exudate. Leukocytes (white blood cells) arrive in the wound to begin wound cleanup. Macrophages, a type of white blood cell, appear and begin to regulate the wound repair. The result of the inflammatory phase is a clean wound bed in a patient with a noncomplicated wound.

Proliferative Phase
- Epithelialization (the construction of new epidermis) begins. At the same time new granulation tissue is formed. New capillaries (angiogenesis) are created, restoring the delivery of oxygen and nutrients to the wound bed. Collagen is synthesized and begins to provide strength and structural integrity to the wound. Contraction, which occurs in open wounds, reduces the size of the wound.

Maturation (Remodeling) Phase
- Collagen is remodeled to become stronger and provide tensile strength to the wound. Outer appearance in an uncomplicated wound will be that of a well-healed scar.

Data from Doughty DB, Sparks-Defriese B: Wound healing physiology. In Bryant RA, Nix DP, editors: *Acute and chronic wounds: current management concepts*, ed 4, St Louis, 2012, Mosby.

| BOX 38-2 | Factors That Influence Wound Healing |

- Hypovolemia, hypotension, vasoconstriction, edema, and hypoxia negatively affect wound healing because adequate perfusion and oxygenation are necessary for new vessel development, collagen synthesis, and development of tensile strength.
- An adequate nutritional status is critical for collagen synthesis, tensile strength, and immune function.
- Wound infection prolongs the inflammatory response, and the microorganisms use nutrients and oxygen needed for wound repair.
- A patient with diabetes mellitus may have impaired wound healing because of abnormal and prolonged inflammation, reduced collagen synthesis, and impaired epithelial migration. Hyperglycemia is associated with compromised neutrophil function and impaired migration.
- Corticosteroid therapy or the use of other immunosuppressive agents such as chemotherapy increases the patient's susceptibility to infection.
- Advanced age can contribute to a diminished proliferation of cells critical to repair.

From Doughty DB, Sparks-Defriese B: Wound healing physiology. In Bryant RA, Nix DP, editors: *Acute and chronic wounds: current management concepts*, ed 4, St Louis, 2012, Mosby.

---

necessary to promote healing. Risk for local or systemic infection, impaired circulation, and breakdown of tissue directly impairs the wound-healing ability of the skin layers (Doughty and Sparks-Defriese, 2012).

Physiologically wound healing occurs in the same way for all patients, with skin cells and some tissues (including the vascular tissues) regenerating quickly and others regenerating slowly or not at all. The latter group includes cells of the liver, renal tubules, and central nervous system neurons.

Wound healing is complex and involves a series of physiologic processes among cells and tissues. The location, severity, and extent of the injury and the tissue layer or layers involved all affect the wound-healing process (Doughty and Sparks-Defriese, 2012). A partial-thickness wound (loss of tissue limited to epidermis and possible partial loss of the dermis) heals by the process of regeneration. However, a full-thickness wound (total loss of skin layers and some deeper tissues) heals by scar formation (Box 38-1). In

addition, there are underlying factors that prevent the ability of cells and tissues to regenerate, return to normal structure, or resume normal functioning (Box 38-2).

The healing process proceeds in a series of events, generally described as *phases*. In a full-thickness wound the phases are hemostasis, inflammation, proliferation, and remodeling. During hemostasis a series of overlapping events occur that control blood loss, begin bacterial control, and seal the wound (Doughty and Sparks-Defriese, 2012). The goal of the inflammatory phase is to control infection and clean the wound bed. During the proliferative phase epithelial cells are laid down in the closed incision within 24 to 48 hours, providing a bacterial barrier. During the proliferative stage fibroblasts are at the site of injury. These fibroblasts increase synthesis of collagen, which forms the healing ridge that can be palpated under an intact healing incision by days 5 to 9 (Fig. 38-2) (Doughty and Sparks-Defriese, 2012). Lack of a ridge is cause for concern, and you will need to begin prompt interventions to reduce mechanical strain on the wound.

Types of healing occur by primary, secondary, and tertiary intention (Fig. 38-3, A and B). Healing by primary intention occurs when the edges of a clean surgical incision remain close together. The wound heals quickly, and tissue loss is minimal or absent (Doughty and Sparks-Defriese, 2012). The skin cells regenerate quickly, and capillary walls stretch across under the suture line to form a smooth surface as they join.

Wounds that are left open and allowed to heal by scar formation are classified as healing by secondary intention (Doughty and Sparks-Defriese, 2012). There is tissue loss and open wound edges. Granulation tissue gradually fills in the area of the defect (Fig. 38-4). This process is typical of severe laceration or massive surgical intervention with skin loss. In secondary intention there is a gap between the edges. Connective tissue develops, which supports

new capillaries. This form of healing results in the formation of scar tissue to close the wound. The slowness of this process places a patient at greater risk for infection because there is no epidermal barrier until later in the healing process.

Healing by tertiary intention is sometimes called *delayed primary intention* or *closure*. It occurs when surgical wounds are not closed immediately but left open for 3 to 5 days to allow edema or infection to diminish. Then the wound edges are sutured or stapled closed. Scarring is usually minimal (Doughty and Sparks-Defriese, 2012). During the healing process some type of dressing covers a wound.

The percentage and type of tissue in the wound bed healing by secondary intention provide insight into the severity and duration of the wound, the extent to which it is progressing toward healing, and the effectiveness of current interventions (Nix, 2012). Viable tissue is normally red to pink in color and moist in appearance (Table 38-1). This type of tissue is called *granulation tissue* and indicates a wound moving toward healing. Black, brown, or tan tissue in the wound is slough or eschar and should be removed, or wound healing will be delayed.

Do not remove an initial surgical dressing for direct wound inspection until the health care provider writes an order for removal. Certain situations and some agency policies govern who changes the dressing the first time. Determine if the patient will need pain medication for the dressing change, and plan the best

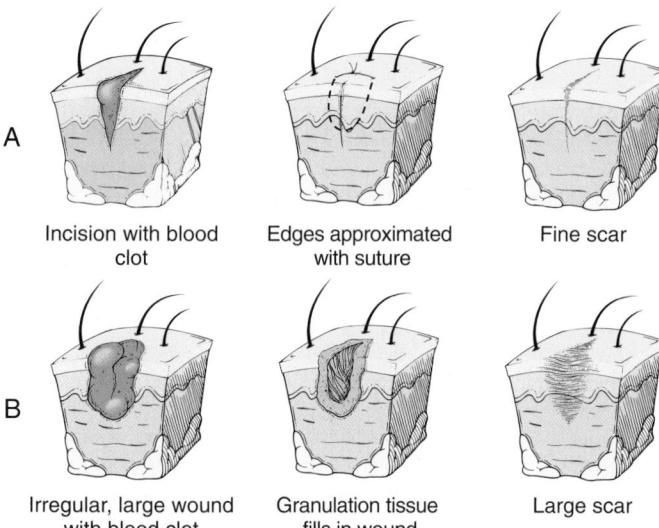

FIG 38-3 Wound healing by primary intention such as with a surgical incision. **A,** Wound healing edges are pulled together and approximated with sutures, staples, or adhesive tapes; and healing occurs by connective tissue deposition. **B,** Wound healing by secondary intention. Wound edges are not approximated, and healing occurs by granulation tissue formation and contraction of the wound edges. (*From Lewis S et al: Medical-surgical nursing: assessment and management of clinical problems, ed 8, St Louis, 2011, Mosby.*)

A — Incision with blood clot — Edges approximated with suture — Fine scar

B — Irregular, large wound with blood clot — Granulation tissue fills in wound — Large scar

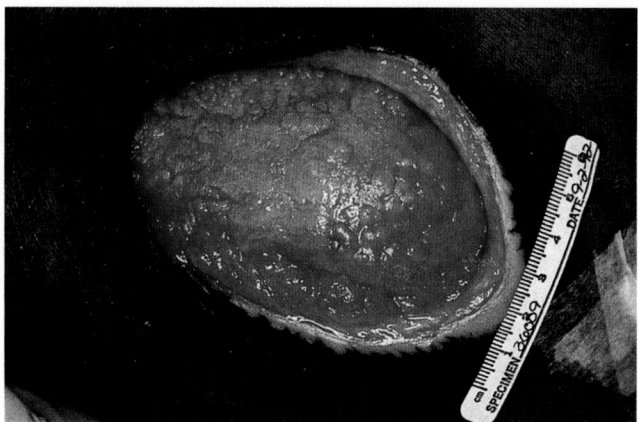

FIG 38-4 Open wound with granulation tissue.

TABLE 38-1	Wound Color/Tissue
Black/brown wounds/eschar	Black or brown tissue is eschar, which represents full-thickness tissue destruction. Black is used to describe necrotic tissue or desiccated tissue such as tendon. It is also related to gangrenous lesions secondary to peripheral vascular disease. If the goal for a wound covered with eschar is debridement, sharp debridement is used to quickly remove the tissue, chemical debridement is used to soften the tissue for removal, or a moist dressing is also considered to loosen the tissue. The method of debridement depends on the overall goal for the patient.
Yellow wounds/ slough	Yellow tissue represents nonviable tissue and in some cases the presence of an infection. It is often yellow, cream colored, or gray slough, which is usually accompanied by purulent drainage. For patients with a low infection risk, the use of moisture-retentive dressings enhances debridement of the yellow tissue. These moisture-retentive dressings may include moist dressings, hydrocolloids, hydrogels, or alginates. If the wound is infected, topical antimicrobials are used.
Red wounds/ granulation	Red tissue represents the presence of granulation tissue. The red color is the result of an increasing amount of new blood vessels in the wound and is considered healthy. The goal in management of a red granulated wound is to select a dressing that maintains a clean and moist wound environment and minimizes damage to healing tissue.

time for analgesic administration to ensure optimal medication effect before wound care. Skin cleaning in the area of the suture line or drain site is indicated when an excessive amount of drainage occurs.

Negative-pressure wound therapy (NPWT) is a wound care treatment that uses the application of subatmospheric (negative) pressure to a wound through suction to facilitate healing and collect wound fluid (Netsch, 2012). NPWT accelerates wound healing by edema and fluid removal, wound contraction, and mechanical stretch perfusion (Netsch, 2012). Several systems are available to provide NPWT; a commonly used brand is called *vacuum-assisted closure (VAC)*. NPWT supports wound healing by optimizing blood flow, removing wound fluid, and maintaining a moist environment. Researchers believe that blood flow increases because of the removal of wound fluid and angiogenesis (development of new blood vessels) and that it stimulates the production of new blood vessels via a mechanical stretch of the tissue (Netsch, 2012). The removal of fluid from the wound decreases tissue edema, which increases dermal perfusion. The dressing placed into the wound maintains a moist environment to facilitate healing. A suction device is placed over the dressing; and the dressing, suction, and wound area are covered with a transparent dressing, which provides the airtight seal necessary for NPWT. The dressing is changed on a scheduled basis, usually no earlier than 48 hours. Chronic wounds such as pressure ulcers, diabetic ulcers, traumatic wounds, and venous stasis ulcers are approved for NPWT (see Chapter 39).

While cleansing a wound, use meticulous hand hygiene and proper infection control procedures before and after removing soiled dressings to limit the risk for health care–acquired infection. Use clean gloves to prevent exposure to body fluids, exudate, or bloody drainage from a wound. During wound cleansing, you deliver fluid or cleansing solution to the wound surface by means of a specific mechanical force. This force helps with the separation and removal of necrotic debris and surface bacteria (Rolstad and others, 2012). To accomplish effective wound cleansing, use an appropriate solution that does not harm the tissue and uses an adequate force to agitate and wash away surface debris and devitalized tissue that contain bacteria (Rolstad and others, 2012).

Irrigation is the most common method of wound cleansing. It uses the mechanical force (either high or low) of a stream of solution to remove debris, bacteria, and necrotic tissue from a wound. The pressure needed to irrigate wounds is between 4 and 15 psi (Table 38-2). Principles of basic wound irrigation include the following:

1 Cleanse in a direction from the least contaminated to the most contaminated area.
2 When irrigating, verify that all the solution flows from the least contaminated to the most contaminated area.

In wound care, the area you are cleansing is considered "clean," and the surrounding skin surfaces are considered "contaminated" even if the wound is not infected. Within the wound the irrigation flow is directed from healthy tissue toward infected tissue, and the flow of irrigation moves from the area being cleansed to an area that is both distal and lower. For postoperative wounds the irrigation solutions should be sterile. For chronic wounds clean solutions can be used. In the event that the irrigant has irritating properties, protect the skin with a skin protectant product and place the collection basin close to the area of the exiting fluid.

The suture line is the "least contaminated" area, and you will always cleanse it first. The center is the most important part of the suture line; therefore, using a sterile swab or gauze, clean the suture line by starting at the center and working toward one end. With

another sterile swab or gauze, start at the center of the incision and work toward the other end. All other cleansing involves moving from one end to the other on each side of the incision. Work in straight lines, moving away from the suture line with each successive stroke.

If a drain is present, clean the drain site using a circular stroke starting with the area immediately next to the drain (Fig. 38-5). Using a new swab, cleanse immediately next to the drain and attempt to clean a little further out from the drain. Continue this process with subsequent swabs until the skin surrounding the drain is cleaned.

TABLE 38-2	Wound Cleansing Considerations	
	Mechanical Force	
	High-Pressure	**Low-Pressure**
Wound base characteristics	Presence of necrotic tissue (eschar, fibrin slough), debris, or other particulate matter Significant bacterial burden Moderate/large amount of exudate	Presence of granulation tissue or new epithelial cells Non/minimum serous or serosanguineous exudate
Clinical outcome(s)	Loosen, soften, and remove devitalized tissue from wound Separate eschar from fibrotic tissue/fibrotic tissue from granulating base	Prevent trauma to viable wound tissue Remove wound care product residue
Solution	Normal saline Volume of solution depends on size of wound	Normal saline Volume of solution depends on size of wound
Delivery systems	35-mL syringe/19-gauge angiocatheter	Pouring saline directly from bottle Bulb syringe Piston syringe

Adapted from Spear M: Wound cleansing: solutions and techniques, *Plast Surg Nurs* 31(1):29, 2011.

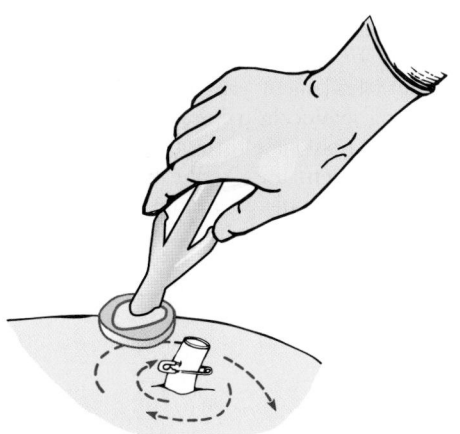

FIG 38-5 Cleansing a drain site.

Infection is present in a wound when microorganisms on the wound surface penetrate into the wound tissues (Stotts, 2012). An infected acute wound usually demonstrates signs of local inflammation; redness and warmth in the area; presence of drainage, pain, or tenderness; and an unusual odor. A surgical site infection (SSI) involves the surgical site and presents within 30 days if there is no implanted device or 1 year if a device is left in place during the procedure. Superficial incision infection involves only skin and subcutaneous tissue at the incision. Deep incision infection involves organs or body cavities in the area of surgery.

Dehiscence is the failure of wound healing in which the surgical wound separates and opens to the fascial level. It occurs fairly early after surgery, by postoperative day 5 to 8 in patients in whom normal healing responses lag (Whitney, 2012). The wound edges open, and serosanguineous drainage is present. These wounds are then allowed to heal by secondary intention. Topical care options include light packing with a moist dressing covered with a dry dressing that is changed on a schedule to prevent the wound bed from drying out (i.e., often every 8 hours). Factors contributing to surgical wound dehiscence include anemia, malnutrition, obesity, and use of steroids.

Evisceration is a failure of wound healing, with total separation of the layers of the wound and protrusion of the internal organs through the wound. This is a surgical emergency, and you need to cover the wound with a moist sterile saline dressing, notify the surgeon immediately, and prepare the patient for emergent surgery.

EVIDENCE-BASED PRACTICE

Nonviable tissue in a wound can delay wound healing and contribute to wound infection. Debridement, the removal of nonviable tissue from the wound, is an essential objective of topical therapy and a critical component of optimal wound management (Ramundo, 2012). Methods of debridement include enzymatic, mechanical, autolytic, or sharp. The type of debridement chosen depends on the goal of wound treatment and the patient's overall condition (EPUAP and NPUAP, 2009). Enzymatic debridement is the topical application of enzymes over the necrotic tissue. The only enzyme available in the United States is collagenase. Collagenase digests the necrotic tissue by dissolving the collagen in the dead tissue (EPUAP and NPUAP, 2009). It is important to follow current guidelines to debride wounds.

- When collagenase is used on a wound, the necrotic tissue is covered with the collagenase, and a moisture-retentive dressing can be used to soften the tissue (Ramundo, 2012).
- Mechanical debridement may include irrigation, which can be done through the use of a 35-mL syringe with a 19-gauge angiocatheter with irrigation pressures delivered between 4 and 15 psi (WOCN, 2010).
- Autolytic debridement can be accomplished by providing moisture via semiocclusive dressing to the wound to begin to loosen the nonviable tissue (Ramundo, 2012).
- Sharp debridement uses sterile instruments to remove the dead tissue and is only performed by a health care provider who is trained, competent, and qualified (EPUAP-NPUAP, 2009).

PATIENT-CENTERED CARE

When caring for patients from other cultures who have acute or chronic wounds, it is important to understand their cultural beliefs and practices and how these might impact wound care. In general, using gender-congruent caregivers and having the family caregiver or a professional translator help with translation and care issues relieves some of the patient's anxiety. In some cultures the meaning of blood and secretions is perceived as dirty; thus it would be advisable to promptly change stained bed lines and gowns. Since some cultures believe that blood is the life force, you should explain the presence of blood-stained secretions and drainage thoroughly.

Be sure to recognize family caregivers when giving explanations about the nursing care regimen. In collectivist cultures presence of family members at the bedside is customary. Among Islamic families it is important to recognize that some Muslims may not be comfortable exposing body parts to a member of the opposite sex (Padela and del Pozo, 2011). Remind patients that traditional home remedies and practices need to be avoided because they may increase the risk for infection in open wounds.

Safety Guidelines

1. Know a patient's age. With age vascular changes occur, collagen tissue is less pliable, and scar tissue is tighter. Because the dermoepidermal junction becomes flatter in older adults, their skin tears more easily from mechanical trauma such as tape removal.
2. Know a patient's nutritional status. Tissue repair and infection resistance are directly related to adequate nutrition, including proteins, carbohydrates, lipids, vitamins, and minerals. Patients who are malnourished are at increased risk for wound infections and wound infection–related sepsis (Stotts, 2012).
3. Understand the risks of obesity. Inadequate vascularization decreases delivery of nutrients and cellular elements required for healing. The patient is at greater risk for wound infection and dehiscence or evisceration (Gallagher-Camden, 2012).
4. Identify factors that decrease oxygenation such as decreased hemoglobin level, smoking, and underlying cardiopulmonary conditions. Adequate oxygenation at the tissue level is essential for white blood cell activity and phagocytosis, for fibroblast proliferation and collagen synthesis, and for reepithelialization (Doughty and Sparks-Defriese, 2012). Tissue repair is negatively influenced by a hematocrit value below 33% and a hemoglobin value below 10 g/100 mL. Hemoglobin level and oxygen release to tissues are reduced in smokers.
5. Know the types of medications prescribed. Steroids reduce the inflammatory response and slow collagen synthesis. Cortisone depresses fibroblast activity and capillary growth. Chemotherapy depresses bone marrow production of white blood cells and impairs immune function.
6. Identify the presence of chronic diseases or chronic trauma such as diabetes mellitus or radiation. Decreased tissue perfusion and failure to release oxygen to tissues result from diabetes mellitus.
7. Skin that has not been wounded is always stronger than healed skin.

PROCEDURAL GUIDELINE 38-1 Performing a Wound Assessment

NSO *Wound Care Module / Lesson 1*

 Video Clip

Wound assessment provides the baseline for planning and evaluating the wound care plan. Normal wound healing occurs in an organized fashion, and evaluating the wound status provides an ongoing assessment of wound healing and helps to determine wound treatments. The frequency of wound assessment depends on the patient's overall condition, policy of the health care setting, type of dressings used, and overall patient goals (Nix, 2012). A variety of wound assessment tools are available, and choice depends on agency policy.

Routine wound assessments provides valuable information regarding the status of the wound. For example, is wound healing progressing as expected, or is it delayed? Is there new drainage? Wound size may increase in a wound with necrotic tissue. Removal of the necrotic tissue may result in a larger wound and is an expected finding. Obtain the health care provider's order as indicated for consultations such as a wound, ostomy, and continence (WOC) nurse or clinical nurse specialist (CNS) to discuss findings. If there is an increase in the amount and consistency of the drainage and if there is new presence of odor, these factors may indicate a wound infection; and a wound culture is often necessary to support appropriate antibiotics.

The following parameters are included in a wound assessment:

- *Location:* Note the anatomic position of the wound on the body.
- *Type of wound:* If possible, note the etiology of the wound (i.e., surgical, pressure, trauma).
- *Extent of tissue involvement:* Full-thickness wound involves both the dermis and epidermis. Partial-thickness wound involves only the epidermal layer. If it is a pressure ulcer, use the staging system of the European Pressure Ulcer Advisory Panel (EPUAP) and the National Pressure Ulcer Advisory Panel (NPUAP) (EPUAP and NPUAP, 2009; see Chapter 18).
- *Type and percentage of tissue in wound base:* Describe the type of tissue (i.e., granulation, slough, eschar) and the approximate amount.
- *Wound size:* Follow agency policy to measure wound dimensions, which includes width, length, and depth.
- *Wound exudate:* Describe the amount, color, and consistency. Serous drainage is clear like plasma; sanguineous or bright red drainage indicates fresh bleeding; serosanguineous drainage is pink; and purulent drainage is thick and yellow, pale green, or white.
- *Presence of odor:* Note the presence or absence of odor, which may indicate infection.
- *Periwound area:* Assess the color, temperature, and integrity of the skin.
- *Pain:* Use a validated pain assessment scale to evaluate pain.

Delegation and Collaboration

The skill of wound assessment cannot be delegated to nursing assistive personnel (NAP). It is the nurse's responsibility to assess and document wound characteristics. The nurse directs the NAP to:

- Report drainage from the wound that is present on sheets or as strike through from the dressing.
- Report the presence of odor in the area of the wound.

Equipment

- ❏ Protective equipment: clean gloves, gown, and goggles if splash/spray risk exists
- ❏ Agency tool to document assessment: measuring guide
- ❏ Cotton-tipped applicator
- ❏ Dressing supplies as ordered
- ❏ Disposable biohazard bag

Procedural Steps

1 Determine agency-approved wound assessment tool and review the frequency of assessment. Examine the last wound assessment to use as comparison for this assessment.
2 Assess comfort level or pain on a scale of 0 to 10 and identify symptoms of anxiety.
3 Explain procedure of wound assessment to patient.
4 Close room door or bed curtains and position patient.
  a Position comfortably to permit observation of wound in well-lighted room.
  b Expose only the wound.
5 Perform hand hygiene and form a cuff on waterproof biohazard bag and place near bed.
6 Apply clean gloves and remove soiled dressings.
7 Examine dressings for quality of drainage (color, consistency), presence or absence of odor, and quantity of drainage (note if dressings were saturated, slightly moist, or had no drainage). Discard dressings in waterproof biohazard bag. Discard gloves.
8 Perform hand hygiene and apply clean gloves.
9 Inspect wound and determine type of wound healing (e.g., primary or secondary intention). A partial-thickness wound heals by reepithelialization, whereas a full-thickness wound heals by the creation of scar tissue and will take longer to heal (Doughty and Sparks-Defriese, 2012).
10 Use agency-approved assessment tool and assess the following:
  a Wound healing by primary intention (surgical wound):
    (1) Assess anatomic location of wound on body.
    (2) Note if incisional wound margins are approximated or closed together. The wound edges should be together with no gaps.
    (3) Observe for presence of drainage. A closed incision should not have any drainage.
    (4) Look for evidence of infection (presence of erythema, odor, or wound drainage).
    (5) Lightly palpate along incision to feel a healing ridge. The ridge will appear as an accumulation of new tissue presenting as firmness beneath the skin, extending to about 1 cm ($\frac{1}{2}$ inch) on each side of the wound between 5 and 9 days after wounding. This is an expected positive sign (Doughty and Sparks-Defriese, 2012).
  b Wound healing by secondary intention (e.g., pressure ulcer or contaminated surgical or traumatic wound):
    (1) Assess anatomic location of wound.
    (2) Assess wound dimensions: Measure size of wound (including length, width, and depth) using a centimeter measuring guide. Measure length by placing a ruler over wound at the point of greatest length (or head to foot). Measure width from side to side (Nix, 2012) (see illustration). Measure depth by inserting cotton-tipped applicator in area of greatest depth and

Continued

PROCEDURAL GUIDELINE 38-1 Performing a Wound Assessment—cont'd

placing a mark on applicator at skin level. Discard measuring guide and cotton-tipped applicator in a biohazard bag.

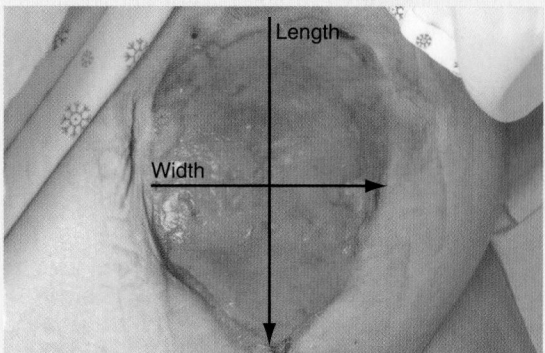

STEP 10b(2)   Measuring wound length and width.

(3) Assess for undermining: Use cotton-tipped applicator to gently probe wound edges. Measure depth and note location using the face of a clock as a guide. The 12 o'clock position (top of wound) would be head of patient, and the 6 o'clock position would be the bottom of the wound toward patient's feet. Document the number of centimeters that area extends from wound edge (e.g., underneath intact skin).

(4) Assess extent of tissue loss: If wound is a pressure ulcer, determine the deepest viable tissue layer in wound bed. If necrotic tissue does not allow visualization of base of wound, the stage cannot be determined.

(5) Notice tissue type, including percentage of tissue intact and presence of granulation, slough, and necrotic tissue.

(6) Note presence of exudate: Amount, color, consistency and odor. Indicate amount of exudate by using part of dressing saturated or in terms of quantity (e.g., scant, moderate, or copious).

(7) Note if any wound edges are rounded toward wound bed; this may be an indication of delayed wound healing. Describe presence of epithelialization at wound edges (if present) because this indicates movement toward healing.

(8) Inspect periwound skin: Include color, texture, temperature, and description of integrity (e.g., open macerated areas). Periwound assessment gives clues about the effectiveness of the wound treatment and possible wound extension (Nix, 2012).

11 Reapply dressings per order. Place time, date, and initials on new dressing.

12 Reassess patient's pain and level of comfort, including pain at wound site, using a scale of 0 to 10, after dressing is applied.

13 Discard biohazard bag, soiled supplies, and gloves per agency policy; perform hand hygiene.

14 Record wound assessment findings and compare assessment with previous wound assessments to monitor wound healing.

Clinical Decision Point *Compare the wound assessment to previous assessment, determine progress toward healing. If there is no movement toward healing or if you notice deterioration, consider a wound care consultation. Lack of wound healing is often related to infection. Notify health care provider and WOC nurse or team.*

SKILL 38-1   Performing a Wound Irrigation

Video Clip

Wound irrigation cleanses and irrigates surgical or chronic wounds such as pressure ulcers. Introduce the cleansing solution directly into the wound with a syringe, syringe and catheter, or pulsed lavage device. When using a syringe, the tip remains 2.5 cm (1 inch) above the wound. If a patient has a deep wound with a narrow opening, attach a soft catheter to the syringe to permit the fluid to enter the wound. Irrigation should not cause tissue injury or discomfort. Avoid fluid retention in the wound by positioning patient on his or her side to encourage the flow of the irrigant away from the wound. It is often helpful to use a 35-mL syringe with a 19-gauge angiocatheter to facilitate optimal pressure for cleansing with minimal risk for tissue injury (Rolstad, Bryant, and Nix, 2012). Ambulatory patients often benefit from the use of a handheld shower for wound cleansing, holding the shower spray approximately 30 cm (12 inches) from the wound.

There are two types of wound irrigation: high-pressure and pulsatile high-pressure lavage. High-pressure irrigation is the cleansing of a debris-filled wound with irrigating fluid delivered at 4 to 15 psi with a 35-mL syringe and a 19-gauge angiocatheter. Use a whirlpool to remove bacteria and debris from the surface of large wounds. Additional benefits include softening and loosening of adherent necrotic tissue and cleansing and removal of wound exudate (Ramundo, 2012).

Wound irrigations promote wound healing by removing debris from a wound surface, decreasing bacterial counts, and loosening and removing eschar. Solutions used for irrigations include normal saline, warm water, and commercially available wound cleansers. Skin cleansers are not the same as wound cleansers, and you never substitute a skin cleanser for a wound cleanser.

Delegation and Collaboration

The skill of sterile wound irrigation cannot be delegated to nursing assistive personnel (NAP). However, you can delegate the cleaning of chronic wounds using clean technique. It is the nurse's responsibility to assess and document wound characteristics. The nurse directs the NAP to:

• Notify the nurse when the wound is exposed so an assessment can be completed.

• Report patient pain.

TABLE 38-3 | Common Wound Dressing Categories

Category	Description/Function	Indications	Side Effects	Examples
Hydrogel	Composed of water or glycerin-based polymers Provides moisture to wound bed Available in sheets or amorphous gel (usually in a tube) Autolytic debridement	Partial- and full-thickness wounds Dry-to-minimal exudate Necrotic wounds	Not indicated for heavily exudating wounds or wounds that are infected	Skintegrity Elasto-Gel Vigilon
Alginate	Highly absorptive products that are retentive gel or fiber-gelling dressings Absorption Available in pads and ropes for packing	Moderate-to-heavy wound exudate Hemostasis	May contribute to wound desiccation if wound exudate is minimal and gel dries	Restore Calcicare SeaSorb Algisite M
Foams	Absorption Available in adhesive and nonadhesive forms	Absorption of moderate-to-heavy exudate	May promote wound dehydration and desiccation if minimal exudate	Biatain Hydrocell PolyMem
Gauze	Absorption Available in woven or nonwoven, cotton or synthetic, sterile and nonsterile	Protection of surgical wounds Absorption of minimal-to-heavy exudate Deliver solution to wound	May adhere to healthy tissue and cause injury on removal	Curity Gauze Sponges KERLIX Super Sponge KLING gauze rolls NU GAUZE packing strips
Hydrocolloids	Made of gelatin, pectin, and carboxymethylcellulose particles suspended in adhesive base Maintain moist environment by forming a gelatinous mass	Autolytic debridement Absorption of minimal to moderate exudate	Some products leave residue in wound on removal; cleanse wound of residue before wound assessment	DuoDERM Exuderm Replicare

Data from Rolstad BS, Byrant RA, Nix DP: Topical management. In Bryant RA, Nix D P, editors: *Acute and chronic wounds: current management concepts*, ed 4, St Louis, 2012, Mosby.

Equipment
- Irrigant/cleansing solution (volume 1.5 to 2 times the estimated wound volume)
- Irrigation delivery system (per order), depending on amount of pressure desired: sterile irrigation 35-mL syringe with sterile soft angiocatheter or 19-gauge needle (WOCN, 2010) or handheld shower
- Protective equipment: sterile gloves, gown, and goggles if splash/spray risk exists
- Waterproof underpad if needed
- Dressing supplies (Table 38-3)
- Disposable waterproof biohazard bag
- Extra towels and padding (to use to protect bed)
- Wound assessment supplies (see Procedural Guideline 38-1)

STEP	RATIONALE
ASSESSMENT	
1 Review order for irrigation of open wound and type of solution to be used.	Open-wound irrigation requires medical order, including type of solution(s) to use.
2 Perform wound assessment and examine recent charted assessment of patient's open wound (see Procedural Guideline 38-1).	
3 Assess patient for history of allergies to antiseptics, medications, tapes, or dressing material.	Known allergies suggest applying a sample of prescribed wound treatment as skin test before flushing wound with large volume of solution or selecting different tape or dressing material.

NURSING DIAGNOSES
- Acute pain
- Chronic pain
- Impaired skin integrity
- Impaired tissue integrity
- Risk for injury

Related factors are individualized based on patient's condition or needs.

STEP	RATIONALE

PLANNING

1 Expected outcomes following completion of procedure:
  - Patient states acceptable level of comfort on pain scale of 0 to 10 after wound irrigation.
  - Wound begins to demonstrate signs of healing; wound is free of excessive drainage, exudate, and inflammation.
  - Skin integrity is maintained; no redness, edema, or inflammation noted in surrounding tissue.

2 If needed, administer analgesic 30 to 45 minutes before starting wound irrigation procedure.

3 Educate patient and family members about procedure.

Premedication, gently administered irrigation, application of clean dressing, and repositioning patient ensure comfort.

Healing progresses in absence of debris and presence of protective coating.

No further skin and tissue damage has resulted from wound irrigation.

Promotes pain control and permits patient to move more easily and be positioned to facilitate wound irrigation (Krasner, 2012).

Promotes cooperation and reduces anxiety.

IMPLEMENTATION

1 Identify patient using two identifiers (i.e., name and birthday or name and account number) according to agency policy. Compare identifiers with information on patient's identification bracelet.

Ensures correct patient. Complies with The Joint Commission standards and improves patient safety (TJC, 2012).

2 Obtain appropriate supplies for wound irrigation and dressing. Form cuff on waterproof biohazard bag and place near bed.

Cuffing helps to maintain large opening, thereby permitting placement of contaminated dressing without touching waste bag itself.

3 Close room door or bed curtains, perform hand hygiene, and position patient.

  a Position comfortably to permit gravitational flow of irrigating solution over wound and into collection receptacle (see illustration).

  b Position patient so wound is vertical to collection basin. Place container of irrigant/cleansing solution in basin of hot water to warm solution to body temperature.

Maintains privacy; frequent hand hygiene reduces microorganisms.

Directing solution from top to bottom of wound and from clean to contaminated area prevents further infection. Position patient during planning stage, keeping in mind bed surfaces needed for later preparation of equipment.

Warmed solution increases comfort and reduces vascular constriction response in tissues.

4 Place padding or extra towel on bed under area where irrigation will take place.

Protects bedding from becoming wet.

5 Expose wound only.

Provides privacy and prevents chilling of patient.

6 Apply gown and goggles. Apply sterile gloves for Steps 7 and 8 and use sterile precautions.

Protects nurse from splashes or sprays of blood and body fluids.

7 Irrigate wound with wide opening:

  a Fill 35-mL syringe with irrigation solution.

  b Attach 19-gauge angiocatheter or 19-gauge needle.

  c Hold syringe tip 2.5 cm (1 inch) above upper end of wound and over area being cleansed.

  d Using continuous pressure, flush wound; repeat Steps 7a to c until solution draining into basin is clear.

Flushing wound helps remove debris and facilitates healing by secondary intention.

Catheter lumen delivers ideal pressure for cleansing and removing debris (Ramundo, 2012).

Prevents syringe contamination. Careful placement of syringe prevents unsafe pressure of flowing solution.

Clear solution indicates removal of debris.

8 Irrigate deep wound with very small opening:

  a Attach soft catheter to filled irrigation syringe.

  b Gently insert tip of catheter into opening about 1.3 cm (0.5 inch).

Catheter permits direct flow of irrigant into wound. Expect wound to take longer to empty when opening is small.

Prevents tip from touching fragile inner wall of wound.

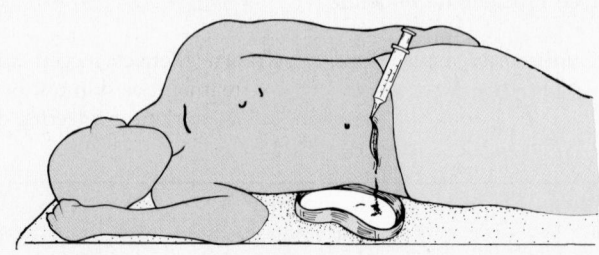

STEP 3a Patient position for wound irrigation.

STEP	RATIONALE

Clinical Decision Point *Do not force catheter into the wound because this will cause tissue damage.*

c Using slow, continuous pressure, flush wound.	Use of slow mechanical force of stream of solution loosens particulate matter on wound surface and promotes healing (Ramundo, 2012).
d While keeping catheter in place, pinch it off just below syringe.	
e Remove and refill syringe. Reconnect to catheter and repeat until solution draining into basin is clear.	
9 Cleanse wound with handheld shower:	
a Perform hand hygiene and apply clean gloves. With patient seated comfortably in shower chair, adjust spray to gentle flow; make sure that water is warm.	Useful for patients able to shower with assistance or independently. May be accomplished at home.
b Shower for 5 to 10 minutes with shower head 30 cm (12 inches) from wound.	Ensures that wound is thoroughly cleansed.
10 When indicated, obtain cultures (see Chapter 43) after cleansing with nonbacteriostatic saline.	WOCN (2010) recommends using quantitative bacterial cultures (tissue biopsy or swab cultures).

Clinical Decision Point *Consider culturing a wound if it has a foul, purulent odor; inflammation surrounds the wound; a nondraining wound begins to drain; or patient is febrile.*

11 Dry wound edges with gauze; dry patient after shower.	Prevents maceration of surrounding tissue from excess moisture.
12 Apply appropriate dressing (see Chapter 39) and label with time, date, and nurse's initials.	Maintains protective barrier and healing environment for wound.
13 Remove mask, goggles, and gown.	Prevents transfer of microorganisms.
14 Dispose of equipment and soiled supplies, remove gloves, and perform hand hygiene.	
15 Help patient to comfortable position.	Reduces transmission of microorganisms.

EVALUATION

1 Have patient rate level of comfort on scale of 0 to 10.	Patient's pain should not increase as result of wound irrigation.
2 Monitor type of tissue in wound bed.	Identifies wound healing progress and determines type of wound cleansing and dressing needed.
3 Inspect dressing periodically (see agency policy).	Determines patient's response to wound irrigation and need to modify plan of care.
4 Evaluate periwound skin integrity.	Determines if extension of wound has occurred or signs of infection are present (warm red periwound skin).
5 Observe for presence of retained irrigant.	Retained irrigant is medium for bacterial growth and subsequent infection.

Unexpected Outcomes	Related Interventions
1 Bleeding or serosanguineous drainage appears.	• Flush wound during next irrigation using less pressure. • Notify health care provider of bleeding.
2 Increased pain or discomfort occurs.	• Decrease force of pressure during wound irrigation. • Assess patient for need for additional analgesia before wound care.
3 Suture line opening extends.	• Notify health care provider. • Reevaluate amount of pressure to use for next wound irrigation.

Recording and Reporting

- Record wound assessment before and after irrigation; amount, color, and odor of drainage on dressing removed; amount and type of solution used; irrigation device used; patient's tolerance of the procedure; type of dressing applied after irrigation.
- Immediately report to the health care provider any evidence of fresh bleeding, sharp increase in pain, retention of irrigant, or signs of shock.

Special Considerations
Teaching

- Instruct patient and primary caregiver regarding wound care technique, observe them doing a return demonstration, and provide written instructions.
- Explain the need for specialized supplies such as irrigating solutions and dressings and the need to maintain asepsis when performing care.
- Instruct patient and primary caregiver in signs of improper wound healing and wound infection.
- Teach patient and caregiver how to make normal saline, especially if cost is an issue. You make normal saline by using 8 teaspoons of salt in 1 gallon of distilled water; keep it refrigerated for 1 month. The saline solution should be allowed to reach room temperature before use.

Pediatric

- Some pediatric patients are very frightened. They might verbally and physically try to prevent nurse from cleaning the wound. Having the child take active part in procedure or working out his or her feelings about wound irrigation with play therapy on a doll with a wound helps the child to be more cooperative with the procedure.
- Neonatal skin is immature and easily damaged from pressure and wound care products. Check that products are approved for use with this population. Remember that in neonates the skin readily absorbs products.

Gerontologic

- Wound irrigations are traumatic, frightening, and painful to some older patients. Assess patient's cooperation before irrigating wound. Be aware of patient's cognitive level of understanding when performing wound irrigation.

Home Care

- Assess patient's home environment to determine adequacy of agencies for performing wound care; check especially for adequate lighting, running water, and storage of supplies.
- Plan wound care in conjunction with patient's total rehabilitation goals. The objective of wound care management in a subacute care setting is to return the patient to his or her home environment.
- Provide support for patient and caregiver during the wound-healing process. Chronic wounds do not heal properly and do not close in a timely manner (Doughty and Sparks-Defriese, 2012).
- Some patients need to receive wound care management in an outpatient wound care clinic. Be sure that patient has directions to clinic and knows where to park and where to obtain dressing supplies.

SKILL 38-2　Removing Sutures and Staples

Agency policy determines whether *only* the health care provider *and* nurse may remove sutures and staples. Always obtain the health care provider's written order before implementing either skill. The time of removal is based on the stage of incision healing and the extent of surgery.

Sutures and staples generally are removed within 7 to 14 days after surgery if healing is adequate (Whitney, 2012). Retention sutures usually remain in place 14 to 21 days. Timing the removal of sutures and staples is important. They must remain in place long enough to ensure initial wound closure with enough strength to support internal tissues and organs. Sutures left in longer than 14 days generally leave suture marks (Whitney, 2012). The health care provider determines and orders removal of all sutures or staples at one time or removal of every other suture or staple as the first phase, with the remainder removed in the second phase.

Sutures are threads of wire or other materials used to sew body tissues together. They come in different sizes and are absorbent or nonabsorbent. They are placed within tissue layers in deep wounds and superficially as the final means for wound closure. The choice of suture technique depends on the type and anatomic location of the wound, thickness of the skin, degree of tension, and desired cosmetic effect (Fig. 38-6) (Whitney, 2012). A patient's history of wound healing, site of wound, tissues involved, and the purpose of the sutures determine the suture material selected. For example, a patient with repeated abdominal surgeries might require wire sutures for greater strength to promote wound closure.

Staples are stainless-steel wire. The location of the incision sometimes restricts their use because there must be adequate distance between the skin and structures that lie below the skin, including bone and vascular structures. The cosmetic result is not always as desirable as that obtained with finer suture material.

Staples do provide ample strength. Removal requires a sterile staple extractor and aseptic technique.

The health care provider and/or nurse judge whether to remove all sutures if any sign of suture line separation is evident during the process of suture or staple removal. It is not uncommon to remove every other suture initially, removing the balance several days to a week later.

Delegation and Collaboration

The skill of staple and/or suture removal cannot be delegated to nursing assistive personnel (NAP). The nurse directs the NAP by:

- Instructing to report to the nurse drainage, bleeding, swelling at the site or an elevation in patient's temperature.
- Instructing to report to the nurse patient's complaints of pain.

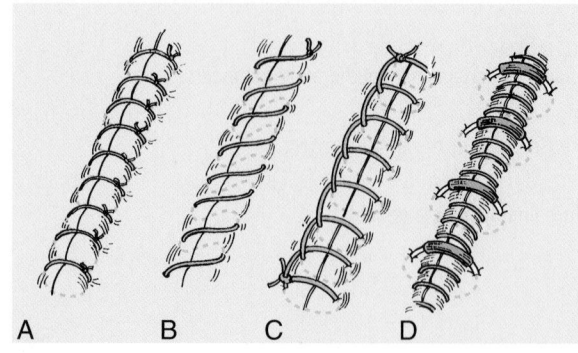

FIG 38-6　Types of sutures. **A,** Intermittent. **B** and **C,** Continuous. **D,** Blanket.

- Providing information about any special hygiene practices following suture removal.

Equipment
❏ Disposable waterproof bag
❏ Sterile suture removal set (forceps and scissors) or sterile staple extractor

❏ Sterile applicators or antiseptic swabs
❏ Steri-Strips or butterfly adhesive strips
❏ Clean gloves
❏ Sterile gloves

STEP	RATIONALE

ASSESSMENT

1 Identify patient with need for suture or staple removal:
  a Check health care provider's order.
  b Review specific directions related to suture or staple removal.

  c Determine history of conditions that may pose risk for impaired wound healing: advanced age, cardiovascular disease, diabetes, immunosuppression, radiation, obesity, smoking, poor cellular nutrition, very deep wounds, and infection.
2 Assess patient for history of allergies.
3 Assess patient's comfort level or pain on scale of 0 to 10.

4 Assess healing ridge and skin integrity of suture line for uniform closure of wound edges, normal color, and absence of drainage and inflammation.

Health care provider's order is required for removal of sutures.
Indicates specifically which sutures are to be removed (e.g., every other suture).

Preexisting health disorders affect speed of healing and sometimes result in dehiscence.

Determines if patient is sensitive to antiseptic or latex.
Provides baseline of patient's comfort level to determine response to therapy.
Indicates adequate wound healing for support of internal structures without continued need for sutures or staples.

Clinical Decision Point *If wound edges are separated or signs of infection are present, the wound has not healed properly. Notify the health care provider because sutures or staples may need to remain in place and/or other wound care initiated.*

NURSING DIAGNOSES

- Impaired skin integrity
- Risk for impaired skin integrity
- Risk for infection

Related factors are individualized based on patient's condition or needs.

PLANNING

1 Expected outcomes following completion of procedure:
  • All suture material or staples are removed.
  • Suture line is intact.
  • Patient states acceptable level of comfort on scale of 0 to 10 following removal of sutures or staples.
2 Explain to patient that suture removal is usually not a painful procedure but patient may feel pulling or tugging of skin.

Removes source of infection or irritation from retained sutures.
Wound is healing and does not require protective dressings.
Some patients require pain medicine before suture or staple removal.
Gains patient cooperation and reduces anxiety.

IMPLEMENTATION

1 Close curtains or room door.
2 Identify patient using two identifiers (i.e., name and birthday or name and account number) according to agency policy. Compare identifiers with information on patient's identification bracelet.

Provides privacy.
Ensures correct patient. Complies with The Joint Commission standards and improves patient safety (TJC, 2012).

Clinical Decision Point *For patient who is highly anxious or who has an extensive wound, consider need to administer analgesic 30 minutes before suture removal.*

3 Position patient comfortably while exposing suture line. Ensure that direct lighting is on suture line.
4 Perform hand hygiene.
5 Place cuffed waterproof disposal bag within easy reach.

Aids visibility and correct placement of forceps or extractor during removal process, ultimately reducing soft tissue injury.
Reduces risk for infection.
Provides for easy disposal of contaminated dressings and prevents passing items over sterile work area.

STEP	RATIONALE

6 Prepare materials needed for suture/staple removal:
  a Open sterile suture removal kit or staple extractor kit.
  b Open sterile antiseptic swabs and place on inside surface of kit.
  c Obtain gloves (sterile gloves if policy indicates).	

7 Perform hand hygiene and apply clean gloves. Carefully remove dressing; discard dressing and gloves in prepared refuse disposal bag.	Reduces transmission of infection.
8 Inspect incision and suture line (see illustration).	Determines adequacy of wound healing.
9 Perform hand hygiene. Apply clean or sterile gloves as required by agency policy.	
10 Clean sutures or staples and healed incision with antiseptic swabs.	Removes surface bacteria from incision and sutures or staples.
11 Remove staples:	
a Place lower tips of staple extractor under first staple. As you close handles, upper tip of extractor depresses center of staple, causing both ends of staple to be bent upward and simultaneously exit their insertion sites in dermal layer (see illustration).	Avoids excess pressure to suture line and secures smooth removal of each staple.
b Carefully control staple extractor.	Avoids suture line pressure and pain.
c As soon as both ends of staple are visible, move it away from skin surface (see illustration) and continue until staple is over refuse bag.	Prevents scratching tender skin surface with sharp pointed ends of staple for comfort and infection control.

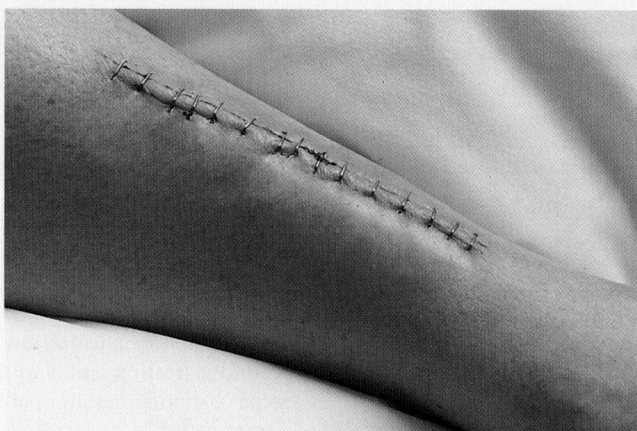

STEP 8   Suture line secured with staples.

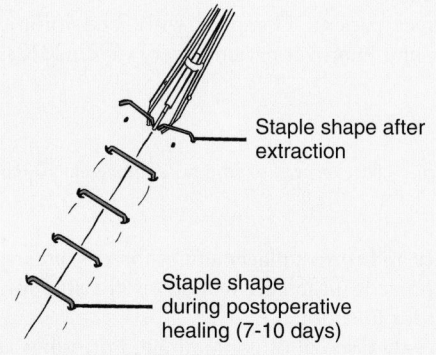

Staple shape after extraction

Staple shape during postoperative healing (7-10 days)

STEP 11a   Staple extractor placed under staple.

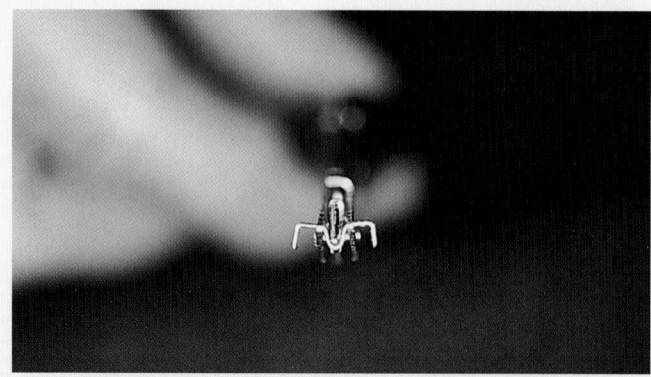

STEP 11c   Metal staple removed by extractor.

STEP	RATIONALE
d Release handles of staple extractor, allowing staple to drop into refuse bag.	Avoids contaminating sterile field with used staples.
e Repeat Steps a to d until all staples are removed.	

12 Remove intermittent sutures:

STEP	RATIONALE
a Place gauze few inches from suture line. Hold scissors in dominant hand and forceps (clamp) in nondominant hand.	Gauze serves as receptacle for removed sutures. Placement of scissors and forceps allows for efficient suture removal.

Clinical Decision Point *Placement of scissors and forceps is very important. Avoid pinching the skin around the wound when lifting up the suture. Likewise avoid cutting the skin around the wound by accident when snipping the suture.*

STEP	RATIONALE
b Grasp knot of suture with forceps and gently pull up knot while slipping tip of scissors under suture near skin (see illustration).	Releases suture.
c Snip suture as close to skin as possible at end distal to knot.	

Clinical Decision Point *Never snip both ends of suture; there will be no way to remove the part of the suture situated below the surface.*

STEP	RATIONALE
d Grasp knotted end with forceps and in one continuous smooth action pull suture through from the other side (see illustration). Place removed suture on gauze.	Smoothly removes suture without additional tension to suture line.

Clinical Decision Point *Never pull exposed surface of any suture into tissue below epidermis. The exposed surface of any suture is considered contaminated.*

STEP	RATIONALE
e Repeat Steps a through d until you have removed every other suture.	
f Observe healing level. Based on observations of wound response to suture removal and health care provider's original order, determine whether remaining sutures will be removed at this time. If so, repeat Steps a to d until you have removed all sutures.	Determines status of wound healing and if suture line will remain closed after all sutures are removed.
g If any doubt, stop and notify the health care provider.	

13 Remove continuous and blanket stitch sutures:

STEP	RATIONALE
a Place sterile gauze a few inches from suture line. Grasp scissors in dominant hand and forceps in nondominant hand.	Gauze serves as receptacle for removed sutures. Placement of scissors and forceps allows for efficient suture removal.
b Snip first suture close to skin surface at end distal to knot.	Releases suture.
c Snip second suture on same side.	Releases interrupted sutures from knot.
d Grasp knotted end and gently pull with continuous smooth action, removing suture from beneath skin. Place suture on gauze compress.	Smoothly removes sutures without additional tension to suture line. Prevents pulling of contaminated portion of suture through skin.

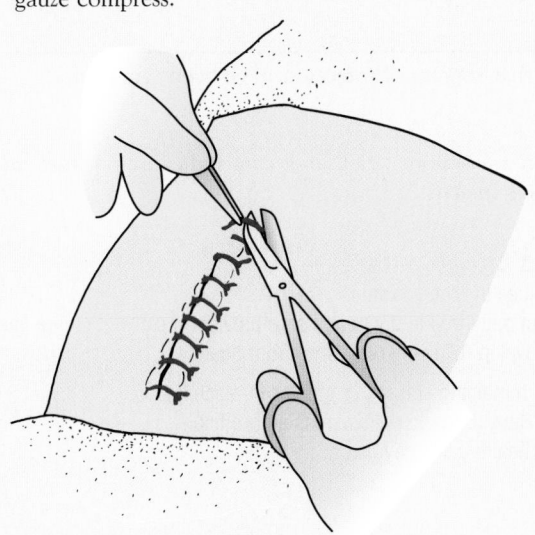

STEP 12b Removal of intermittent suture. Nurse cuts suture as close to skin as possible, away from knot.

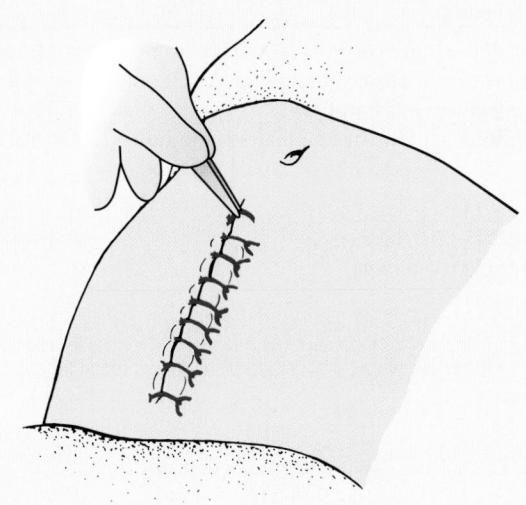

STEP 12d Nurse removes suture and never pulls contaminated stitch through tissues.

STEP	RATIONALE
e Repeat Steps a to d in consecutive order until entire line is removed.	
14 Inspect incision to make sure that all sutures are removed and identify any trouble areas. Gently wipe suture line with antiseptic swab to remove debris and clean incision.	Reduces risk for further incision line separation.

Clinical Decision Point *Make sure that you remove the entire suture and that no part is retained in the patient's wound.*

STEP	RATIONALE
15 Apply Steri-Strips if *any* separation greater than two stitches or two staples in width is apparent to maintain contact between wound edges.	Supports wound by distributing tension across wound and eliminates closure technique scarring.
a Cut Steri-Strips to allow strips to extend 4 to 5 cm (1½ to 2 inches) on each side of incision.	
b Remove from backing and apply across incision (see illustration).	
c Instruct patient to take showers rather than soak in bathtub according to health care provider's preference.	Steri-Strips are not removed and are allowed to fall off gradually.
16 Apply light dressing or expose to air if no clothing will come in contact with suture line. Instruct patient about applying own dressing if needed at home.	Healing by primary intention eliminates need for dressing.
17 Discard all contaminated materials and remove and dispose of gloves.	Reduces transmission of infection.
18 Route reusable items such as staple extractor for resterilization, dispose of sharps (disposable staple extractor and/or scissors) in designated bin, and perform hand hygiene.	Reduces transmission of infection.

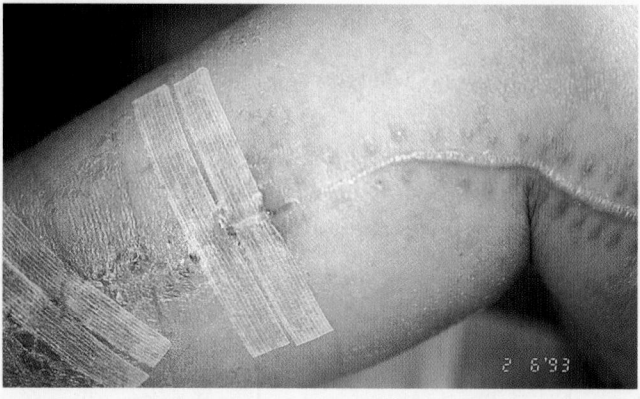

STEP 15b   Steri-Strips over incision.

EVALUATION

1 Assess site where sutures or staples were removed; inspect condition of soft tissues, including skin. Look for any pieces of removed suture left behind.	Ensures that sources of infection have been removed.
2 Determine if patient has pain along incision.	Determines comfort level and can indicate if suture material remains in skin.

Unexpected Outcomes

1 Retained suture is present.

2 Patient experiences wound separation or drainage secondary to healing problems.

Related Interventions

- Notify health care provider.
- Instruct patient to notify health care provider if signs of suture line infection develop following discharge from agency.

- Leave remaining sutures or staples in place.
- Place Steri-Strip closures across suture line.
- Notify health care provider.

Recording and Reporting

- Record the time the sutures or staples were removed and the number of sutures or staples removed. Also document the cleaning of the suture line, appearance of the wound, level of healing of the wound, and type of dressing applied. Document patient's response to suture or staple removal.
- Immediately report to the health care provider if suture line separation, dehiscence, evisceration, bleeding, or purulent drainage occurs.

Special Considerations

Teaching

- Teach patient to observe for any sign of separation of wound edges before removing remaining sutures/staples and inspect incision for continued healing.
- Reinforce instruction about resuming bathing and showering activities, preventing abdominal strain during defecation, and providing adequate nutrition and ambulation.
- Teach patient not to put additional stress on suture line from such activities as lifting or bending. Patients with abdominal surgery or injury need to avoid lifting heavy packages or equipment for several weeks.
- Instruct patient that sometimes there is a small amount of drainage from wound immediately after suture removal.

Pediatric

- Assistance is sometimes necessary to keep infants from moving during the suture removal procedure.
- Topical anesthetic solutions (e.g., lidocaine [Xylocaine], EMLA) applied to intact skin may provide short-term (20 minutes) anesthesia (Krasner, 2012).

Gerontologic

- Some older adults need reassurance about suture/staple removal procedure. Depending on their mental status, they may not understand the procedure.
- Older skin is often at higher risk for dehiscence after sutures/ staples are removed.

SKILL 38-3   Managing Wound Drainage Evacuation

NSO *Wound Care Module / Lesson 2*

If drainage accumulates in the wound bed, wound healing is delayed. Drainage is removed by using either a closed- or open-drain system, even if the amount of drainage is small. The drain is inserted directly through a small stab wound near the suture line into the area of the wound.

An open-drain system (e.g., a Penrose drain [Fig. 38-7]) removes drainage from the wound and deposits it onto the skin surface. Insert a sterile safety pin through this drain, outside the skin, to prevent the tubing from moving into the wound.

To remove the Penrose drain the health care provider may advance the drain in stages since the wound heals from the bottom up. Nursing interventions include caution to prevent accidental removal of the drain during dressing changes and to protect skin surfaces in direct contact with the irritating drainage. Because of the danger of accidental dislodgement and the need to assess the drain placement accurately, do not delegate the care of Penrose drains that are covered with gauze pads to nursing assistive personnel (NAP).

A closed-drain system such as the Jackson-Pratt (JP) drain (Fig. 38-8) or Hemovac drain relies on the presence of a vacuum to withdraw accumulated drainage from around the wound bed into the collection device. A JP drain collects fluid that is in the range of 100 to 200 mL/24 hr; whereas the Hemovac drain accommodates more drainage, usually up to 500 mL/24 hr. The collection device is connected to a clear plastic drain with multiple perforations. Drainage collects in a closed reservoir or a suction bladder (Box 38-3). The closed system collects fluid but operates only if

BOX 38-3	Attaching Wound Suction Devices to Suction

Hemovac
- Connect graduated adapter to emptying port and then to wall suction tubing.
- Set suction level as prescribed or on low if suction level is not specified.

Jackson-Pratt
- Attach tubing to the suction device.
- Squeeze suction device flat to allow all air to be evacuated and close port.

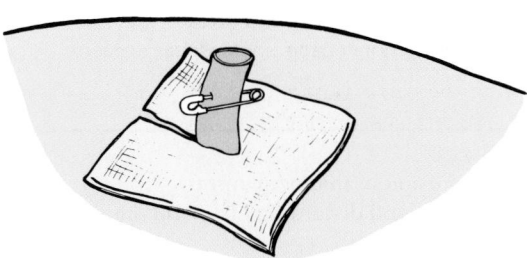

FIG 38-7   Penrose drain with drain-split gauze.

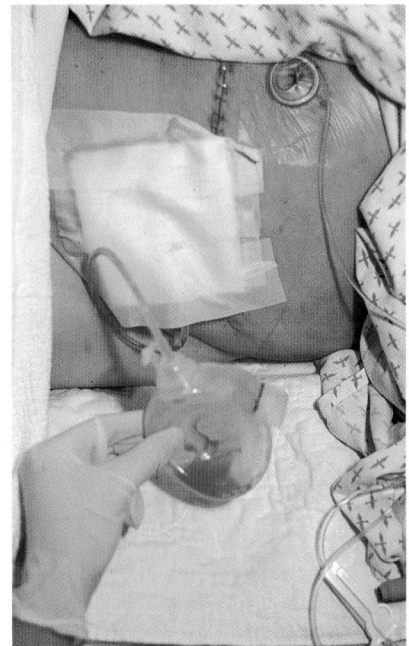

FIG 38-8   Jackson-Pratt wound drainage system.

the tubing is patent and a vacuum exists. You empty the drainage periodically from the reservoir, record the amount, and reestablish the vacuum.

Delegation and Collaboration

The assessment of wound drainage and maintenance of drains and the drainage system cannot be delegated to NAP. However, you may delegate emptying a closed drainage container or pouch, measuring the amount of drainage, and reporting the amount on the patient's intake and output (I&O) record to NAP. The nurse directs the NAP by:

- Discussing any increase in frequency of emptying the drain other than once a shift.

- Instructing to report to the nurse any change in amount, color, or odor of drainage.
- Reviewing the I&O procedure.

Equipment

- ❏ Graduated measuring cylinder
- ❏ Alcohol sponge
- ❏ Gauze sponges
- ❏ Goggles if needed
- ❏ Sterile specimen container if culture is needed
- ❏ Sterile dressings or pouch if drain is needed
- ❏ Clean gloves
- ❏ Safety pin(s)

STEP	RATIONALE
ASSESSMENT	
1 Identify presence, location, and purpose of closed wound drain and drainage system as patient returns from surgery. Assess drainage present on patient's dressing.	Drainage tubing is usually placed near wound through small surgical incision.
2 Identify number of wound drain tubes and what each one will be draining. Label each drain tube with a number or label.	Assigning labeling system to each drain helps with consistent documentation when patient has multiple drainage tubes.
3 Assess if drain tube needs self-suction, wall suction, or no suction by checking health care provider's orders.	Some drain tubes such as Hemovac can be used with self-suction or wall suction.
4 Inspect system to determine presence of one straight tube or Y-tube arrangement with two tube insertion sites.	Allows nurse to plan skin care and identifies quantity of sterile dressing supplies needed.
5 Inspect system to ensure proper functioning. Complete systematic inspection includes insertion site, drainage moving through tubing in direction of reservoir, patency of drainage tubing, airtight connection sites, and presence of any leaks or kinks in system.	Properly functioning system maintains suction until reservoir is filled. Tension on drainage tubing increases injury to skin and underlying muscle.

Clinical Decision Point *Attach tape and a safety pin to drainage tubing with tape and pin to patient's gown so the suction device is below the level of the wound and does not pull on the insertion site.*

STEP	RATIONALE
6 Be sure that Penrose drain has sterile safety pin in place. Penrose drains are sometimes covered with gauze dressing or wound pouch. Use caution and do not accidentally pull on drain while positioning gauze.	Pin prevents drain from being pulled below surface of skin.
7 Identify type of drainage containers that patient has.	Determines frequency for emptying drainage.

NURSING DIAGNOSES

- Impaired skin integrity
- Risk for infection
- Risk for injury

Related factors are individualized based on patient's condition or needs.

PLANNING

STEP	RATIONALE
1 Expected outcomes following completion of procedure:	
• Wound healing continues.	Patient is comfortable, and wound drainage is collected.
• Vacuum is reestablished.	Suction system is intact.
• Tubing is patent.	Fluid is draining away from wound area.
2 Explain procedure to patient.	Promotes patient's cooperation and reduces anxiety.

IMPLEMENTATION

STEP	RATIONALE
1 Close room door or bedside curtains.	Provides privacy.
2 Perform hand hygiene and apply clean gloves.	Reduces transmission of microorganisms.
3 Place open specimen container or measuring graduate on bed between you and patient.	Permits measuring and discarding of wound drainage.
4 Empty Hemovac or ConstaVac:	Avoids entry of pathogens.

STEP	RATIONALE
a Maintain asepsis while opening plug on port indicated for emptying drainage reservoir.	Vacuum will be broken, and reservoir will pull air in until chamber is fully expanded.
(1) Tilt suction container in direction of plug.	Drains fluid toward plug.
(2) Slowly squeeze two flat surfaces together, tilting toward measuring container.	Prevents splashing of contaminated drainage.
b Drain contents into measuring container (see illustration).	Contents counted as fluid output (see Chapter 6).
c Hold uncovered alcohol swab in dominant hand. Place suction device on flat surface with open outlet facing upward; continue pressing downward until bottom and top are in contact (see illustration).	Compression of surface of Hemovac creates vacuum. Cleaning plug reduces transmission of microorganisms into drainage evacuation.
d Holding surfaces together with one hand, and using an alcohol swab, quickly clean opening and plug with other hand and immediately replace plug; secure suction device on patient's bed.	
e Check suction device for reestablishment of vacuum, patency of drainage tubing, and absence of stress on tubing.	Facilitates wound drainage and prevents tension on drainage tubing.
5 Empty Hemovac with wall suction:	
a Turn off suction.	
b Disconnect suction tubing from Hemovac port.	Empties drainage and reestablishes suction to wound bed.
c Empty Hemovac as described in Step 4.	
d Clean port opening and end of suction tubing to open port of Hemovac.	Cleaning plug reduces transmission of microorganisms.
e Set suction level as prescribed or on low if health care provider does not specify suction level.	
6 Empty JP suction drain:	
a Open port on top of bulb-shaped reservoir (see illustration).	Breaks vacuum for drain.
b Tilt bulb in direction of port and drain toward opening. Empty drainage from suction device into measuring container (see illustration). Clean end of emptying port and plug with alcohol wipe.	Reduces transmission of microorganisms.
c Compress bulb over drainage container. While compressing bulb, replace plug immediately.	Reestablishes vacuum.
7 Place and secure drainage system below site with safety pin on patient's gown. Be sure that there is slack in tubing from reservoir to wound.	Pinning drainage tubing to patient's gown prevents tension or pulling on tubing and insertion site.
8 Note characteristics of drainage: measure volume and discard by flushing in commode.	Contents count as fluid output.

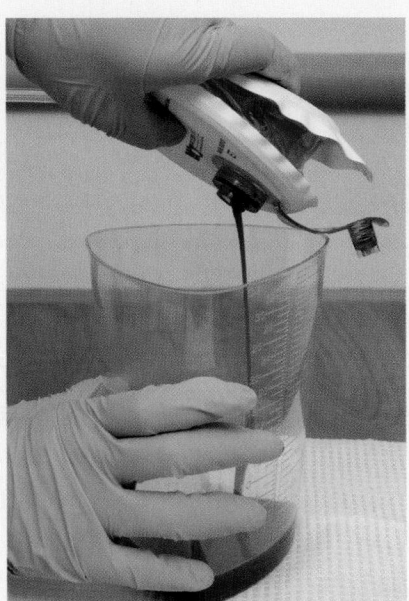

STEP 4b   Hemovac contents drained into measuring container.

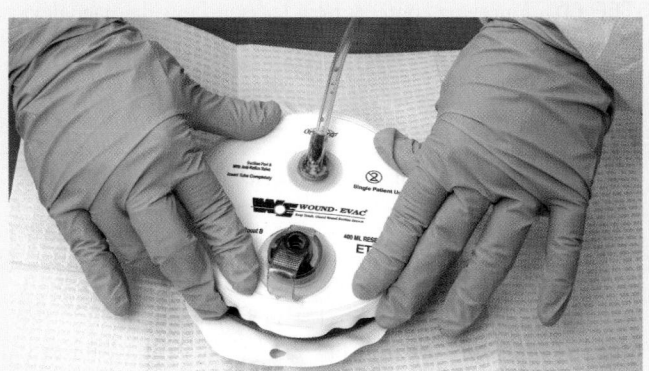

STEP 4c   Hemovac compressed to create suction.

STEP	RATIONALE
9 Discard soiled supplies, remove gloves, and perform hand hygiene.	Reduces transmission of microorganisms.
10 Apply clean gloves. Proceed with dressing change (see Chapter 39) around drain site and inspection of skin if indicated or ordered. Split-drain sponge dressings are often used around drain tubes (see illustration) and taped in place.	Prevents entrance of bacteria into surgical wound.
11 Discard contaminated materials, remove gloves, and perform hand hygiene.	Reduces transmission of microorganisms.

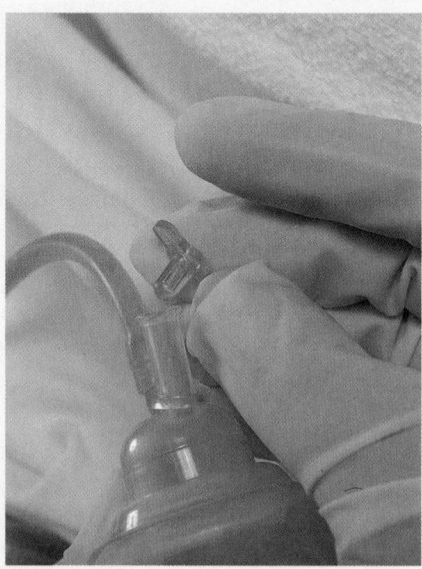

STEP 6a   Opening port of Jackson-Pratt device.

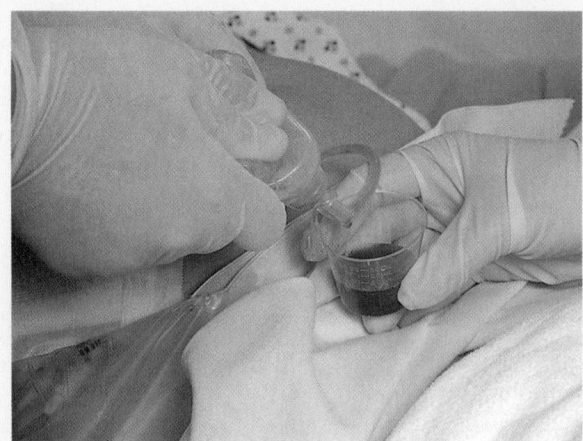

STEP 6b   Emptying contents from Jackson-Pratt drainage device.

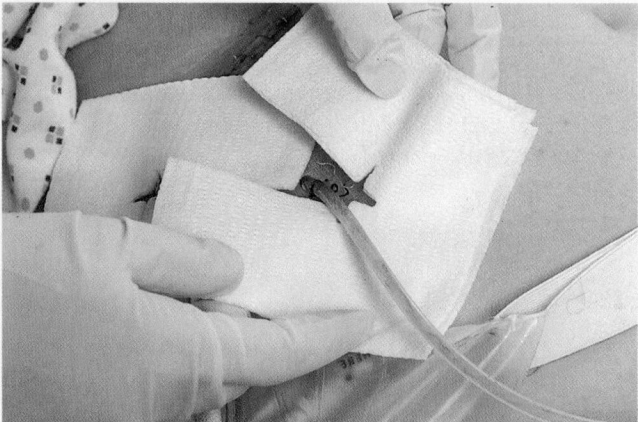

STEP 10   Applying split gauze dressing around Jackson-Pratt drain tube.

EVALUATION

1 Observe for drainage in suction device.	Indicates presence of vacuum, patency of tubing, and functioning of drainage suction device.

Clinical Decision Point *Clots or large collections of debris may block drainage flow. The* **Y***-site in the drainage tubing is especially prone to clogging.*

2 Inspect wound for drainage or collection of drainage fluid under skin, causing seroma.	Drainage should not be significant under suture line. May indicate inadequate functioning of drainage suction device.

STEP	RATIONALE
3 Measure drainage, empty drainage system, record on I&O form.	Empty drainage collection reservoir every 8 to 12 hours and as needed for large drainage volume. Collect diagnostic specimen in presence of unexpected purulence or pungent odor, report findings to health care provider and record in progress note.
4 Assess patient's level of comfort using scale of 0 to 10.	Ensures that procedure does not increase patient's pain.

Unexpected Outcomes	Related Interventions
1 Site where tube exits becomes infected.	• Notify health care provider about presence of signs of infection: purulent drainage, odor, reddened site, increased white blood cell count, and temperature elevation. • Use aseptic technique when changing dressings.
2 Bleeding appears in/or around drainage collector.	• Determine amount of bleeding and notify health care provider if excessive. • Assess for tension on patient's drainage tubing. • Secure tubing to prevent pulling and pain.
3 Patient experiences pain.	• Assess patient's level of pain. • Medicate patient. • Stabilize drainage tubing to reduce tension and pulling against incision. • Notify health care provider if signs of wound infection are present.
4 Drainage suction device is not accumulating drainage.	• Assess drainage tubing for clots. • Assess drainage system for air leaks or kinks. • Notify health care provider.

Recording and Reporting

- Record emptying the drainage suction device; reestablishing vacuum in suction device; amount, color, odor of drainage; dressing change to drain site; and appearance of drain insertion site.
- Record amount of drainage on I&O record.
- Immediately report a sudden change in amount of drainage, either output or absence of drainage flow, to the health care provider. Also report pungent odor of drainage or new evidence of purulence, severe pain, or dislodgement of the drainage tube to the health care provider.

Special Considerations

Teaching

- Instruct patient about anticipated postoperative drainage, expected progress of wound healing and drainage volume, and estimated date of removal of drain as volume diminishes.
- Teach patient or caregiver how to empty and record amount of drainage. If patient is going home with drainage device, ask patient or family caregiver to record amount emptied and bring the recording to the next outpatient visit.

Pediatric

- Have parents help to prevent pediatric patients from dislodging drainage tubes.

Gerontologic

- Be aware that older adults with large amounts of drainage will need additional fluid intake because they are more likely to become dehydrated.
- Take measures to prevent a confused patient from pulling out drain collector.

Home Care

- Provide written instructions in drain care. Include importance of measuring and documenting the amount of drainage. Patient should share the volume of drainage on a daily basis with the health care provider.

Critical Thinking Exercises

The nurse is assigned to care for Mrs. Pereira, who was readmitted to the hospital with wound dehiscence and infection following a colon resection. Her past medical history includes chronic obstructive lung disease and diverticulitis.

1 Which factors from Mrs. Pereira's history contributed to her poor wound healing? (Select all that apply.) Provide a rationale for your answer.
   1 Takes prednisone daily for respiratory disease
   2 Has type 2 diabetes mellitus
   3 Takes aspirin daily because of myocardial infarction (MI) 6 years earlier
   4 Eats six small high-protein meals a day
   5 Is 74 years old
   6 Drinks 2 L of water daily

2 When performing the wound assessment, the nurse notes that the wound base is covered with red, moist granulation tissue. What does the presence of granulation tissue signify in wound healing? Provide a rationale for your answer.

3 Describe why the presence of a healing ridge in a wound healing by secondary intention is important for this patient?

✓ **REVIEW QUESTIONS**

1 A patient has a large abdominal wound, which will require irrigation and packing after discharge from the hospital. Which statement made by the patient indicates a need for further teaching related to her wound irrigation?
   1 "I'll lie so the wound is vertical to the basin during the irrigation."
   2 "I'll use slow, continuous pressure while irrigating my wound."
   3 "I'll warm the irrigation solution to body temperature before I use it."
   4 "I'll irrigate the wound, starting at the bottom and moving to the top."

2 A patient tells the nurse that the health care provider said his sutures are coming out today. Which nursing action is most important before removing the sutures?
   1 Assembling the required equipment
   2 Checking that there is a health care provider's order for the suture removal
   3 Performing hand hygiene in view of the patient
   4 Explaining to the patient what will be happening during the suture removal

3 A patient has an extensive abdominal wound and is to have half of the staples removed and the incision line cleaned. Which actions should the nurse take during the preparation and actual interaction with the patient? (Select all that apply.)
   1 Position the patient in a semi-Fowler's position.
   2 Place upper tip of staple remover under staple to ease removal.
   3 Administer an analgesic 30 minutes before staple removal.
   4 Lift up on the staple when depressing the extractor handles.
   5 Clean the incision before removing the staples, starting at the sides next to the incision.
   6 Remove all of the staples at the top of the incision and leave the rest, beginning at the middle of the incision.

4 The patient is to have sutures removed from his back after surgery. The nurse is performing the procedure correctly by taking which step?
   1 Snipping the suture at the end proximal to the knot
   2 Wiping the area with a disinfectant swab to prevent wound infection
   3 Removing the suture in a smooth, continuous manner
   4 Holding the scissors in the nondominant hand and the pickups in the dominant hand

5 The nurse notes approximately 60 mL of bright red drainage in the Jackson-Pratt drain 6 hours after surgery. Which nursing interventions should be included in the care for this patient? (Select all that apply.)
   1 Emptying the drain 24 hours from now
   2 Pinning the drainage tubing to the patient's gown
   3 Placing Vaseline gauze around the tube insertion site
   4 Securing the drain above the level of the wound
   5 Emptying the drain now
   6 Squeezing the drain flat before putting in the drainage plug

6 A patient had surgery to repair an incisional hernia. His surgical incision was approximated and stapled at the time of the procedure. Which type of wound healing is occurring in the surgical site?
   1 Primary intention
   2 Secondary intention
   3 Tertiary intention

7 In preparing to irrigate a wound, which intervention helps to reduce the risk for infection during wound irrigation? (Select all that apply.)
   1 Using sterile technique
   2 Directing the flow of solution from healthy tissue to infected tissue
   3 Warming irrigation solution to body temperature
   4 Cleaning suture line after doing wound irrigation
   5 Irrigating with a continuous pressure of 3 psi

8 The nurse needs to empty the Jackson-Pratt drain collection device every 8 hours. After draining the fluid from the container, how should he or she reestablish the closed suction system?
   1 Close the port after emptying the drain
   2 Compress the bulb portion of the container and close the port
   3 Pump the container several times before closing
   4 Leave 10 mL of wound fluid in the container to keep the level of suction constant

9 A patient's wound is managed with negative-pressure wound therapy. When you evaluate the negative pressure wound therapy dressing, you note air under the seal of the transparent dressing. What of the following interventions would be appropriate? (Select all that apply.)
   1 Turn up the suction.
   2 Check the seal of the transparent dressing.
   3 Check to be sure that the connections to the suction are intact.
   4 Remove and replace the transparent dressing.
   5 Reevaluate in 30 minutes since this finding may not be significant.

10 The NAP reports to you that the outer dressing from a patient's abdominal wound that is healing by secondary intention has moist, clear, red-tinged drainage. After you verify this finding, how would you describe this type of drainage?
   1 Purulent
   2 Slough
   3 Serous
   4 Blood tinged

REFERENCES

Bryant RA, Nix DP: Principles for practice development. In Bryant RA, Nix DP, editors: *Acute and chronic wounds: current management concepts,* ed 4, St Louis, 2012, Mosby.

Doughty DB, Sparks-Defriese B: Wound-healing physiology. In Bryant RA, Nix DP, editors: *Acute and chronic wounds: current management concepts,* ed 4, St Louis, 2012, Mosby.

European Pressure Ulcer Advisory Panel (EPUAP) and National Pressure Ulcer Advisory Panel (NPUAP): *Treatment of pressure ulcers: quick reference guide,* Washington, DC, 2009, NPUAP.

Gallagher-Camden S: Skin care needs of the obese patient. In Bryant RA, Nix DP, editors: *Acute and chronic wounds: current management concepts,* ed 4, St Louis, 2012, Mosby.

Krasner DL: Wound pain: impact and assessment. In Bryant RA, Nix DP, editors: *Acute and chronic wounds: current management concepts,* ed 4, St Louis, 2012, Mosby.

Nix DP: Skin and wound assessment. In Bryant RA, Nix DP, editors: *Acute and chronic wounds: current management concepts*, ed 4, St Louis, 2012, Mosby.

Netsch DS: Negative pressure wound therapy. In Bryant RA, Nix DP, editors: *Acute and chronic wounds: current management concepts*, ed 4, St Louis, 2012, Mosby.

Padela Al, del Pozo PR: Muslim patients and cross-gender interactions in medicine: an Islamic bioethical perspective, *J Medical Ethics* 37(1):40, 2011.

Ramundo J: Wound debridement. In Bryant RA, Nix DP, editors: *Acute and chronic wounds: current management concepts*, ed 4, St Louis, 2012, Mosby.

Rolstad BS, Byrant RA, Nix DP: Topical management. In Bryant RA, Nix DP, editors: *Acute and chronic wounds: current management concepts*, ed 4, St Louis, 2012, Mosby.

Stotts NA: Nutritional assessment and support. In Bryant RA, Nix DP, editors: *Acute and chronic wounds: current management concepts*, ed 4, St Louis, 2012, Mosby.

The Joint Commission (TJC): *National Patient Safety Goals*, Oakbrook Terrace, Ill, 2012, The Commission, available at http://www.jointcommission.org/standards_information/npsgs.aspx.

Whitney JD: Surgical wounds and incisional care. In Bryant RA, Nix DP, editors: *Acute and chronic wounds: current management concepts*, ed 4, St Louis, 2012, Mosby.

Wound, Ostomy and Continence Nurses Society (WOCN): *Guideline for prevention and management of pressure ulcers*, Mount Laurel, NJ, 2010, WOCN clinical practice guidelines series.

Dressings, Bandages, and Binders

MEDIA RESOURCES

- e**volve** *learning system* http://evolve.elsevier.com/Perry/skills
  - Review Questions
  - ▶ Video Clips

- Mosby's Nursing Video Skills, 4th edition
- NSO Nursing Skills Online

KEY TERMS

Angiogenesis	Evisceration	Macerated	Primary dressing
Dead space	Excoriation	Negative-pressure wound therapy	Secondary dressing
Debridement	Exudate		Stomahesive
Dehiscence	Granulation	Neovascularization	Wound vacuum-assisted closure
Epithelialization	Hydrocolloid	Occlusive dressing	
Erythema	Hydrogel	Pressure dressing	

OBJECTIVES

Mastery of content in this chapter will enable the nurse to:
- Assess a wound correctly.
- Discuss the purposes of dressings, bandages, and an abdominal binder.
- Choose the correct dressing for a wound.
- Understand the technique of a dressing, bandage, or binder application.
- Describe the advantages and disadvantages of the types of dressings.

- Apply dry, moist-to-dry, pressure, transparent, and synthetic dressings correctly.
- Change a negative-pressure wound therapy dressing correctly.
- Demonstrate the technique for applying turned bandages correctly.
- Apply an abdominal binder correctly.

Wound healing is a complex physiologic process. Proper wound management involves manipulating a wound to restore a physiologic wound environment that is characteristic of normal, healthy tissue. Key features of a physiologic wound environment are adequate moisture, temperature control, pH, and control of bacterial burden (Rolstad, Bryant, and Nix, 2011). A wound heals best in a moist environment because this favors epithelial cell migration, promotes extracellular matrix formation, reduces fibrosis, and decreases wound infection (Rolstad, Bryant, and Nix, 2011). Dressings are an important part of wound healing because of their ability to control moisture, debride dead tissue, and protect a wound. They also prevent spread of infection and increase patient comfort. Topical dressings establish and maintain a moist—not wet—wound environment by containing wound fluids, absorbing excess moisture, or donating moisture (Rolstad et al., 2011).

Semiocclusive dressings keep wounds moist, even when no added moisture is supplied.

There are two types of dressings, primary and secondary. A primary dressing is a protective cover that comes in direct contact with a wound bed. Secondary dressings serve a protective or therapeutic function by holding primary dressings in place and increasing the ability to meet wound needs (Rolstad et al., 2011). The ideal dressing is based on its characteristics and outcomes (Box 39-1). For example, a pressure dressing is applied to control bleeding. Use a highly absorbent dressing such as alginate or foam to manage wound drainage. Use a hydrocolloid dressing in a noninfected wound that is draining a moderate amount of exudate.

Most dressings are semiocclusive (also called *moisture retentive*) rather than occlusive. Dressings may contain ingredients such as glycerin, polymers, carboxymethylcellulose, cotton, or rayon. A factor to consider when choosing a dressing is ease of application. A dressing should conform to body contours, be durable yet flexible, and be able to absorb or contain exudate. A dressing should be cost-effective, easy to remove without damaging the healing surface and periwound skin, and acceptable in appearance. Wound care needs can change frequently during the phases of wound healing and often require a variety of wound products (Rolstad et al., 2011).

When changing a dressing, you need to know about wound healing and how to differentiate a normal or expected appearance from abnormal changes in a wound. Assessment of the exudates absorbed by a dressing provides valuable diagnostic information (see Procedural Guideline 38-1).

Primary healing takes place when tissue is cut cleanly and the margins are reapproximated, as in the case of a surgical wound. Repair usually occurs without complication. New capillary circulation bridges the wound quickly in 3 to 4 days, and the wound heals once normal tissue oxygenation is achieved. A wound closed for primary healing is most susceptible to infection during the first 4 days.

Healing by secondary intention occurs when a wound is left open, as in the case of a traumatic wound. Healing results in the formation of granulation tissue from the bottom of the wound and eventual epithelialization from the sides of the wound to close the defect. During epithelialization epithelial cells migrate and proliferate from the wound edges to cover the wound surface. Burns, infected wounds, and deep pressure ulcers heal in this manner (Doughty and Sparks-DeFriese, 2011).

The type of dressing to use depends on the wound characteristics and the goal of wound management, which can be wound debridement or wound healing. Various types of dressings are applied to wounds. Given the many types of available dressings, it may be difficult to decide which dressing is best to use on a particular wound. Numerous dressings and products are available for the management of acute and chronic wounds (Table 39-1). The type of wound care and dressing change required also determines whether to use clean or sterile technique. Clean technique refers to the fact that the nurse maintains medical versus surgical asepsis (e.g., with chronic nonsurgical wounds). A fresh surgical wound requires sterile technique to prevent introducing microorganisms into a healing wound. Current practice recommends using sterile gloves for postoperative dressing changes in the first 24 to 48 hours after surgery.

EVIDENCE-BASED PRACTICE

Negative-pressure wound therapy (NPWT) is designed to create a moist wound healing environment, drain exudate, reduce tissue edema, contract wound edges, and mechanically stimulate a wound bed. An NPWT dressing influences blood perfusion at a wound edge, which may promote angiogenesis and the formation of granulation tissue. No clear evidence shows that NPWT accelerates wound healing compared with other interventions or that one form of NPWT is better than another (Borqquist, Ingemansson, and Malmsiö, 2011). A systematic review of the literature reveals benefits of NPWT:

- Maximal biologic effect of NPWT at the wound edge can be achieved at −80 mm Hg (Borqquist, Ingemansson, and Malmsiö, 2011).
- Foam dressings may be advantageous for large-defect wounds (Borqquist et al., 2011).
- Gauze dressings may be more suitable for smaller wounds or when scar formation is a concern (Borqquist et al., 2011).
- Gauze dressings are a good option for patient comfort (Hurd et al., 2010).
- Intermittent or variable pressure application has a better effect on granulation tissue formation than continuous pressure (Hurd et al., 2010).

PATIENT-CENTERED CARE

An important priority in wound care is patient comfort. Provide patients appropriate analgesic doses 30 minutes before a dressing change to maximize comfort when the dressing and tissues will be manipulated. Consider a patient's cultural view regarding pain. For example, patients from northern European and Asian backgrounds are often more stoic about pain expression, and you will need to offer the pain medication even if the patient does not complain of pain (Galanti, 2008). If a patient's pain is from eroded or denuded skin around the margin of a wound, use skin sealants or barriers. If a patient has ongoing pain from an abdominal wound, consider applying an abdominal binder, which can effectively reduce pain and distress (Cheifetz et al., 2010). It also helps to consistently position patients off of their wounds.

If a patient has a chronic wound, respect the approaches that patient or family caregivers have used to change a dressing at home. Patients might have preferences regarding the time of day to change a dressing or before or after a certain activity. If it is likely

| TABLE 39-1 | Comparison of Wound Care Products | | | | |

Product Category	Indications for Use	Contraindications	Advantages	Disadvantages	Frequency of Change (per Manufacturer Recommendations)
Gauze Dressings Cotton or synthetic material; woven or nonwoven construction	• Protection of surgical incision • Mechanical debridement (moist-to-dry) • Secondary dressing for other wound products • Packing wounds	• Granulating wounds as primary treatment	• Available in many sizes and forms • Sterile and nonsterile	• May adhere to healthy tissue, causing injury when removed • Lint fibers may be left on wound • May interfere with wound healing if gauze dries out in moist-to-dry dressing	• Usually change 2 or 3 times per day as needed.
Transparent Films Adhesive membrane dressings; waterproof, impermeable to fluids and bacteria; allow oxygen and moisture vapor exchange	• Shallow wounds • Dry to minimally exudative wound • Promote autolytic debridement • Stage I or II pressure ulcers	• Infected wounds; wounds that tunnel, undermine, or are full thickness; wounds with moderate to heavy exudate; third-degree burns	• Easy to apply and remove without damage to underlying tissue • Permit viewing of wound • Create second skin; protect from friction • Waterproof • Create moist wound that softens thin slough and eschar • Protective shield to external fluids and bacteria	• May cause skin maceration • May not adhere to moist areas • May cause skin stripping if improperly removed	• Change every 3 or 4 days or as needed. • If using to facilitate autolytic debridement, change every 24 hours.
Hydrocolloids Adhesive dressings that contain gel-forming agents; mold to body contours, considered semiocclusive dressings	• Partial- or full-thickness wound; shallow • Minimal to moderate exudating wounds • Clean stage II and noninfected shallow stage II-IV pressure ulcers • Can be used in combination with absorbent powder or alginate	• Third-degree burns, acutely infected wounds; arterial or diabetic ulcers (use with caution) • Wounds with dry eschar • Use with caution in persons with diabetes or arterial disease	• Available in many sizes • Promote autolytic debridement • Reduce pain • Impermeable to fluids/bacteria • Thermal insulator • Easy to apply and remove	• Potential for periwound maceration if dressing left in place too long • Drainage (gelatinous mass) under dressing often mistaken for pus/infection • Adhesive possibly too aggressive for fragile skin	• Change every 3 to 5 days.
Hydrogel Glycerin-or water-based dressings designed to maintain clean, moist wound; may also absorb small amount of exudate	• Partial- or full-thickness wound; shallow or deep • Dry to minimally exudative wound with or without clean granular wound base • Shallow or deep wounds • Wounds with undermining • Necrotic wounds	• Third-degree burns • Wounds with heavy exudate	• Nonadherent • Cool and soothing • Decrease pain • Facilitates autolysis • Conform to wound	• Potential for maceration or candidiasis of periwound area	• Change daily if adhesive sheets or wound fillers are not used. • Change adhesive covers up to 3 times per week.

TABLE 39-1	Comparison of Wound Care Products—cont'd				
Product Category	**Indications for Use**	**Contraindications**	**Advantages**	**Disadvantages**	**Frequency of Change (per Manufacturer Recommendations)**
Alginates Highly absorbent, nonwoven material that forms gel when exposed to wound drainage; fibrous product derived from brown seaweed	• Moderate to heavily exudating wounds; shallow or deep • Partial- and full-thickness wounds • Leg ulcers, donor sites, traumatic wounds	• Third-degree burns • Nondraining wounds • Dry necrotic wounds	• Nonadhering, nonocclusive • Hemostatic properties • May be packed into tunneled areas • Promote autolytic debridement in exudating wounds • Highly absorbent	• More expensive than gauze or gauze packing strips • Not practical for large wounds • Gelled material may be mistaken for purulence	• Change daily or as often as needed, usually every 24 to 48 hours.
Foam Dressings Absorbent, nonadherent polyurethane or film-coated layer used to protect wounds and maintain moist healing environment	• Moderate to heavily exudating wounds • Partial- and full-thickness wounds; shallow and deep • Stage II to IV pressure ulcers	• Ischemic wound with dry eschar • Third-degree burns • Wounds that tunnel or sinus tracts • Nondraining wounds	• Highly absorbent while maintaining moist wound environment • Often used as secondary dressing along with films and absorbers • Many nonadherent to wound bed	• Nonadhesive foams require secondary dressing • Maceration of periwound may occur if dressing left on too long	• Change every 24 hours or as needed.

Modified from Collins P et al., Wound care literature review 2011, *J WOCN* 39(4S): s*, 2012.; Rolstad BS, Bryant RA, Nix DP: Topical management. In Bryant RA, Nix DP: *Acute and chronic wounds: nursing management*, ed 4, St Louis, 2011, Mosby.

that the patient will continue to have the same type of dressing while at home, be sure to educate him or her and family caregiver on the proper techniques for changing it and disposing of medical waste.

Different cultures and religious practices attribute different meanings to wounds and trauma. It is important to assess and try to understand the different meanings of blood and wounds and how they affect patients and their families. For example, some East Asian cultures interpret loss of blood and secretions as loss of one's spiritual and vital life energy. Some Muslims and Hindus perceive blood as dirty; hence you need to carefully dispose of soiled dressings and linens (Galanti, 2008). Dressing changes always require respect for a patient's privacy. However, sometimes patients from other cultures have additional privacy needs such as the need for gender-congruent caregivers, especially if dressings are located in areas considered private.

Safety Guidelines

1 Know the cause or type of wound. Wounds caused by vascular insufficiency, diabetes mellitus, pressure, trauma, and surgery are all very different and must have an individualized treatment plan. Not knowing the cause of a wound can have serious negative effects if you use treatments that are contraindicated for certain types of wounds.

2 Know the expected amount and type of wound exudate or drainage (Box 39-2). Wounds with large amounts of drainage require more frequent dressing changes or need an absorptive dressing.

3 Determine if wound drainage tubes are present to prevent their accidental dislocation when you remove the old dressing (see Skill 38-3).

BOX 39-2	Types of Wound Drainage

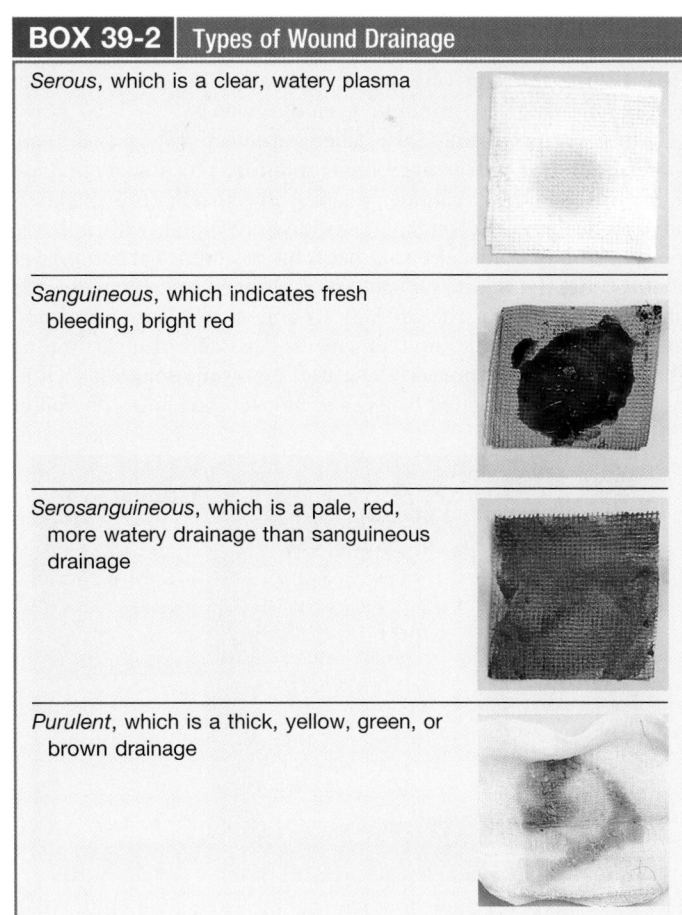

Serous, which is a clear, watery plasma

Sanguineous, which indicates fresh bleeding, bright red

Serosanguineous, which is a pale, red, more watery drainage than sanguineous drainage

Purulent, which is a thick, yellow, green, or brown drainage

4 A wound is a break in skin integrity that increases a patient's risk for infection. Use the appropriate type of gloves when changing a dressing and wash hands thoroughly before and after a dressing change.

5 Be sure that patients in the home setting know infection control principles and how to discard medical waste properly.

SKILL 39-1   Applying a Dressing (Dry and Moist-to-Dry)

NSO *Wound Care Module / Lesson 3*

Dry gauze dressings are for wound healing by primary intention with little drainage (Fig. 39-1). The dressing protects the wound from injury, reduces discomfort, and speeds healing (when used correctly). Dry gauze dressings do not interact with wound tissues and cause little wound irritation. However, gauze does not maintain a moist wound environment unless a wound is highly exudative (Rolstad et al., 2011). In addition, gauze dressings have the disadvantage of moisture evaporating quickly, causing a dressing to dry out. Frequent dressing changes are usually needed, and there are increased infection rates when compared with semiocclusive dressings (Rolstad et al., 2011). Gauze may come impregnated with a variety of substances such as zinc oxide paste, iodinated agents, petrolatum, and crystalline sodium chloride. Impregnated gauze can hydrate a wound and absorbed exudate or deliver antimicrobial agents.

Dry gauze dressings are commonly used for abrasions and nondraining postoperative incisions (see Table 39-1). Telfa gauze dressings contain a shiny, nonadherent surface on one side that does not stick to a wound. Drainage passes through the nonadherent surface to the outer gauze dressing. Dry dressings are not appropriate for debriding wounds. When gauze adheres to drainage on a wound surface, the seal can cause you to pull off healthy tissue when the gauze is removed. When gauze does adhere to a wound, moisten the dressing with sterile normal saline or sterile water before removing it to minimize wound trauma.

Moist-to-dry dressings (also called *wet-to-dry or damp-to-dry*) are gauze moistened with an appropriate solution. The primary purpose is to mechanically debride wounds, specifically full-thickness wounds healing by secondary intention and wounds with necrotic tissue. A moist-to-dry dressing has a moist contact dressing layer that touches the wound surface. The moistened gauze increases the absorptive ability of the dressing to collect exudate and wound debris. This layer dries and adheres to dead cells, thus debriding the wound when removed. Use a sterile isotonic solution such as normal saline or lactated Ringer's to moisten dressings. The outer

absorbent layer is a dry dressing that protects the wound from invasive organisms.

Recent advances in wound care have created a number of new debriding products for use along with moist gauze for debriding necrotic wounds. Autolytic debriding products are applied to wounds to allow enzymes to self-digest dead tissue. Enzymatic debriding agents applied directly to a wound bed act by digesting collagen in necrotic tissue (NPUAP-EPUAP, 2009; Ramundo, 2011). Both autolytic and enzymatic products are used in combination with moist gauze but may also come as prepackaged dressings that do not require any additional gauze.

Dry and moist-to-dry dressings are secured with tape, which may be paper, plastic, woven, or elastic material with adhesive. Frequent removal of tape for dressing changes irritates the skin and causes skin tears. One method to secure a dressing and reduce tape-related injury is a Montgomery tie or strap. A Montgomery tie is a wide strip of tape with holes and laces that is placed on each side of a wound and tied, thus securing gauze dressings during repeated changes. Use strips of a stomahesive or hydrocolloid dressing to create a window on the outer edges of a wound. Then apply tape for the tie over the strips, thereby reducing contact with sensitive periwound tissue.

The purpose of packing a wound is to fill dead space and avoid the potential of abscess formation by a wound closing too soon (Rolstad et al., 2011). Impregnated gauze is useful when there is undermining (i.e., the destruction of tissue under intact skin around the wound perimeter). When there is wound tunneling, a channel has formed that extends from any part of the wound through subcutaneous tissue or muscle. Strip gauze is useful for filling the narrow areas in the channel so the complete dressing can be removed easily during a dressing change (Rolstad et al., 2011). Damp gauze is useful for packing exudative wounds. If a wound is dry, use hydrating packing material such as hydrogel-impregnated or saline-moistened gauze to keep it moist. Box 39-3 summarizes principles for correctly packing a wound.

FIG 39-1   Types of gauze dressings (right to left): 4 × 4, split, ABD, roll, and Telfa.

BOX 39-3 | Principles for Packing a Wound

- Use the wound characteristics to decide which type of packing is appropriate.
- Make sure that the packing material can be safely used to pack a wound.
- Moisten the packing material with a noncytotoxic solution such as normal saline. Never use cytotoxic solutions (e.g., povidone-iodine) to pack a wound.
- If using woven gauze, fluff it before packing it into the wound.
- Loosely pack the wound.
- Do not let the packing material drag or touch the surrounding wound tissue before you put it into the wound.
- Fill all the wound dead space with the packing material.
- Pack the wound until you reach the wound surface; never pack the wound higher than the wound surface.

Every open wound requires cleaning with each dressing change to remove surface bacteria and debris (Rolstad et al., 2011). Usually normal saline is the solution of choice, but commercially prepared wound cleansers are also appropriate. Use an irrigating catheter and syringe for cleaning if a wound is deep (see Chapter 38). Normal saline does not contain a preservative to prevent bacteria from growing in a container; thus any opened saline container must be discarded and replaced in 24 hours. Clearly label all solution bottles with date and time of opening.

Delegation and Collaboration

The skill of applying dry and moist-to-dry dressings may sometimes be delegated to nursing assistive personnel (NAP) if the wound is chronic (see agency policy and Nurse Practice Act). All wound assessments, care of acute new wounds, and wound care requiring sterile technique cannot be delegated. The nurse directs the NAP about:

- Any unique modifications of the dressing change such as the need for use of special tape or taping techniques to secure the dressing.
- Reporting pain, fever, bleeding, or wound drainage to the nurse immediately.

Equipment

- ❏ Clean gloves
- ❏ Sterile gloves
- ❏ Sterile dressing set (scissors, forceps) (*optional*, check agency policy)
- ❏ Sterile drape (*optional*)
- ❏ Sterile dressings: fine mesh gauze, 4 × 4-inch gauze, abdominal (ABD) pads
- ❏ Sterile basin (*optional*)
- ❏ Antiseptic ointment (as prescribed)
- ❏ Wound cleanser (as prescribed)
- ❏ Sterile normal saline or prescribed solution
  - Debriding gel as ordered
- ❏ Tape, Montgomery ties, or bandage as needed (include nonallergenic tape if necessary)
  - Skin barrier (optional if using Montgomery ties)
- ❏ Protective waterproof underpad
- ❏ Waterproof bag
- ❏ Adhesive remover (*optional*)
- ❏ Measurement devices (*optional*): Cotton-tipped applicator, measuring guide, camera
- ❏ Protective gown, goggles, mask (used when splashing from wound is a risk)
- ❏ Additional lighting if needed (e.g., flashlight, treatment light)

STEP	RATIONALE

ASSESSMENT

1 Ask patient to rate his or her level of pain using a pain scale of 0 to 10 and assess character of pain. Administer prescribed analgesic as needed 30 minutes before dressing change.	Superficial wounds with multiple exposed nerves may be intensely painful, whereas deeper wounds with destruction of dermis should be less painful (Krasner, 2011). A comfortable patient will be less likely to move suddenly, causing wound or supply contamination.
	Serves as baseline to measure response to dressing therapy.
2 Assess size, location, and condition of wound. Review previous nurses' notes and electronic health record (EHR).	Helps to plan for proper dressing type, securement and supplies needed, and if assistance is needed during procedure.
3 Assess patient for allergies, especially antiseptics, tape, or latex.	Patients with allergies may have localized or systemic allergic reactions to these supplies.
4 Assess patient's and family caregiver's knowledge of purpose of dressing change.	Determines level of support and explanation required.
5 Assess need, readiness, and willingness for patient or family caregiver to participate in dressing wound.	Prepares patient or family caregiver if dressing must be changed at home.
6 Review medical orders for dressing change procedure.	Indicates type of dressing or applications to use.
7 Identify patients at risk for wound-healing problems, including aging, premature infant, obesity, diabetes mellitus, circulation disorders, nutritional deficit, immunosuppression, radiation therapy, high levels of stress, and use of steroids.	Physiologic changes resulting from aging, chronic illness, poor nutrition, medications that affect wound healing, and cancer treatments have potential to affect wound healing (Doughty, Sparks-DeFriese, 2011).

NURSING DIAGNOSES

• Acute pain	• Deficient knowledge	• Risk for infection
• Chronic pain	• Impaired skin integrity	• Risk for caregiver role strain

Related factors are individualized based on patient's condition or needs.

PLANNING

1 Expected outcomes following completion of procedure:	
• Patient's wound shows evidence of healing by decrease in size and less drainage, redness, or swelling.	Indicates that wound is healing appropriately.

STEP	RATIONALE
• Patient reports pain less than previous assessment after dressing change.	Indicates that dressing procedure and choice are appropriate.
• Dressing remains clean, dry, and intact.	Indicates that proper application and securement are used for dressing.
• Patient or family explains purpose of dressing and method of dressing application.	Indicates that learning has occurred.
2 Explain procedure to patient.	Decreases patient's anxiety.

IMPLEMENTATION

STEP	RATIONALE
1 Identify patient using two identifiers (i.e., name and birthday or name and account number) according to agency policy. Compare identifiers with information on patient's identification bracelet.	Ensures correct patient. Complies with The Joint Commission standards and improves patient safety (TJC, 2012).
2 Close room or cubicle curtains. Perform hand hygiene.	Provides for privacy.
3 Position patient comfortably and drape to expose only wound site. Instruct patient not to touch wound or sterile supplies.	Draping provides access to wound while minimizing exposure. Dressing supplies become contaminated when touched by patient's hand.
4 Place disposable waterproof bag within reach of work area. Fold top of bag to make cuff. Perform hand hygiene and apply clean gloves. Apply gown, goggles, and mask if risk for splashing exists.	Ensures easy disposal of soiled dressings. Prevents contamination of outer surface of bag. Use of personal protective equipment reduces transmission of microorganisms.
5 Gently remove tape, bandages, or ties: use nondominant hand to support dressing and, with your dominant hand, pull tape parallel to skin and toward dressing. If dressing is over hairy area, remove in direction of hair growth. Get patient permission to clip or shave area (check agency policy). Remove any adhesive from skin.	Pulling tape toward dressing reduces stress on suture line or wound edges and reduces irritation and discomfort.
6 With gloved hand or forceps remove dressing one layer at a time, observing appearance and drainage of dressing. Carefully remove outer secondary dressing first; then remove inner primary dressing that is in contact with wound bed. If drains are present, slowly and carefully remove dressings (see illustration) and avoid tension on any drainage devices. Keep soiled undersurface from patient's sight.	Purpose of primary dressing is to remove necrotic tissue and exudate. Appearance of drainage may be upsetting to patient. Avoids accidental removal of drain.
a If moist-to-dry dressing adheres to wound, gently free dressing and alert patient of discomfort.	Moist-to-dry dressing should debride wound. Do not wet dressing; it should be dry.
b If dry dressing adheres to wound that is not to be debrided, moisten with normal saline and remove.	Prevents injury to wound surface and periwound during dressing removal.
7 Inspect wound and periwound for appearance, color, size (length, width, and depth), drainage, edema, presence and condition of drains, approximation (wound edges are together), granulation tissue, or odor (see Chapters 18 and 38). Use measuring guide or ruler to measure size of wound (see Chapter 38). Gently palpate wound edges for bogginess or patient report of increased pain.	Assesses condition of wound and periwound condition. Indicates status of healing.
8 Fold dressings with drainage contained inside and remove gloves inside out. With small dressings remove gloves inside out over dressing (see illustrations). Dispose of gloves and soiled dressing according to agency policy. Cover wound lightly with sterile gauze pad and perform hand hygiene.	Contains soiled dressings, prevents contact of nurse's hands with drainage, and reduces cross-contamination.

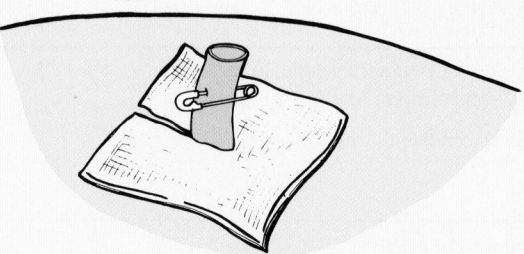

STEP 6   Penrose drain with split gauze.

STEP	RATIONALE
9 Describe appearance of wound and any indicators of wound healing to patient.	Wounds may appear unsettling and frightening to patients; it helps patient to know that wound appearance is as expected and whether healing is taking place.
10 Create sterile field with sterile dressing tray or individually wrapped sterile supplies on over-bed table (see Chapter 8). Pour any prescribed solution into sterile basin.	Sterile dressings remain sterile while on or within sterile surface. Preparation of all supplies prevents break in technique during dressing change.
11 Cleanse wound (see Chapter 38):	
a Perform hand hygiene and apply clean gloves. Use gauze or cotton ball moistened in saline or antiseptic swab (per health care provider order) for each cleansing stroke or spray wound surface with wound cleanser.	Prevents transfer of organisms from previously cleaned area.
b Clean from least to most contaminated area (see Chapter 38) (see illustration).	Cleaning in this direction prevents introduction of organisms into wound.
c Clean around any drain (if present), using circular strokes starting near drain and moving outward and away from insertion site (see illustration) (see Chapter 38).	Correct aseptic technique in cleaning prevents contamination.
12 Use sterile dry gauze to blot in same manner as in Step 11 to dry wound.	Drying reduces excess moisture, which could eventually harbor microorganisms.

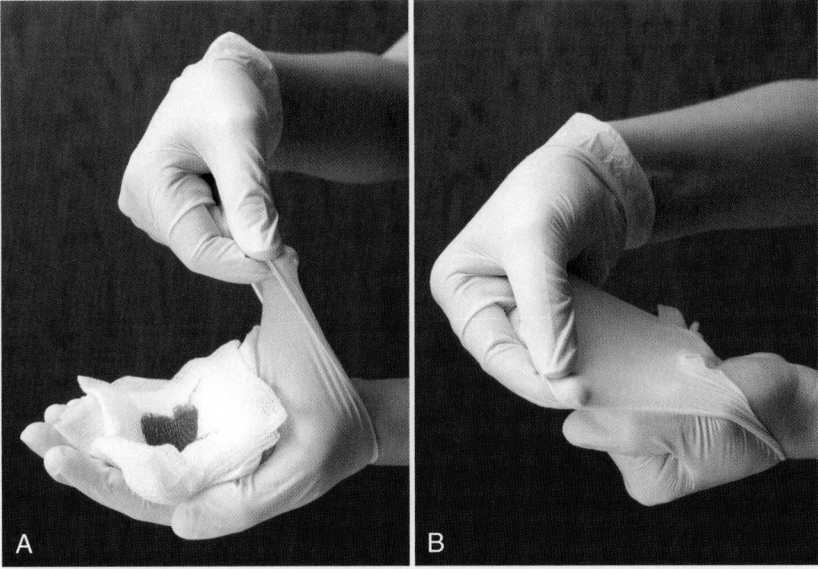

STEP 8 **A** and **B**, Dispose of soiled dressings by placing in gloved hand and pulling glove off over dressing and then off hand.

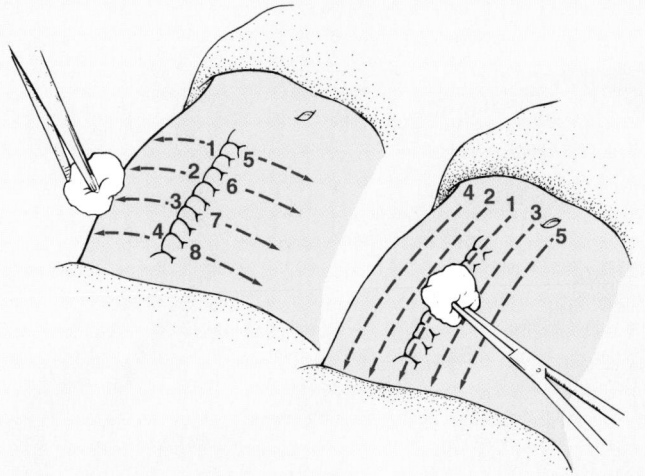

STEP 11b Methods for cleansing a wound, cleansing from least to most contaminated.

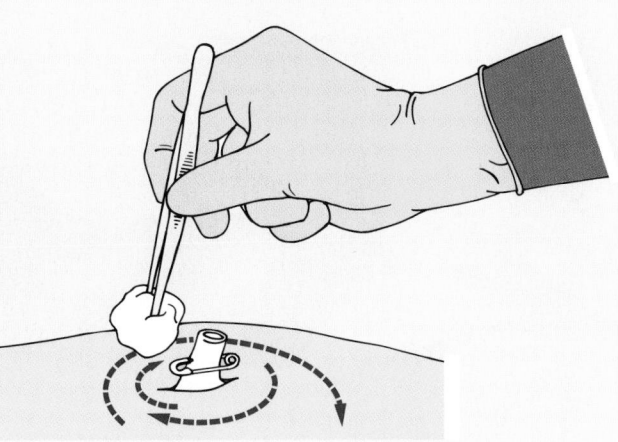

STEP 11c Cleaning around a drain site.

STEP	RATIONALE
13 Apply antiseptic ointment (if ordered) with sterile Q-tip or gauze, using same technique to apply as for cleaning. Dispose of gloves. Perform hand hygiene.	Helps reduce growth of microorganisms.
14 Apply dressing (see agency policy):	
a Dry sterile dressing:	
(1) Apply clean gloves (see agency policy).	Some agencies or condition of wounds may require sterile gloves.
(2) Apply loose woven gauze as contact layer (see illustration).	Promotes proper absorption of drainage.
(3) If drain is present, apply precut, split 4 × 4–inch gauze around drain.	Secures drain and promotes drainage absorption at site.
(4) Apply additional layers of gauze as needed.	Ensures proper coverage and optimal absorption.
(5) Apply thicker woven pad (e.g., Surgipad, abdominal [ABD] pad) (see illustration).	This type of cover dressing is used on postoperative wounds when there is excessive drainage.
b Moist-to-dry dressing:	
(1) Apply sterile gloves (see agency policy).	Reduces transmission of infection.
(2) Place fine-mesh or loose 4 × 4–inch gauze in container of prescribed sterile solution. Wring out excess solution.	Moist gauze absorbs drainage and, when allowed to dry, traps debris.

Clinical Decision Point *If using "packing strips," use sterile scissors to cut the amount of dressing that you will use to pack the wound. Do not let the packing strip touch the side of the bottle. Pour prescribed solution over the packing gauze or strip to moisten it.*

STEP	RATIONALE
(3) Apply moist fine-mesh or open-weave gauze as single layer directly onto wound surface. If wound is deep, gently pack gauze into wound with sterile gloved hand or forceps until all wound surfaces are in contact with moist gauze, including dead spaces from sinus tracts, tunnels, and undermining (see illustration A). Be sure that gauze does not touch periwound skin (see illustration B).	Inner gauze should be moist, not dripping wet, to absorb drainage and adhere to debris. When packing a wound, gauze should conform to base and side of wound (Rolstad et al, 2011). Wound is loosely packed to facilitate wicking of drainage into absorbent outer layer of dressing. Moisture that escapes dressing often macerates the periwound area.

Clinical Decision Point *Do not overpack wound too tightly (Rolstad et al., 2011); it can cause wound trauma when dressing is removed.*

STEP	RATIONALE
(4) Apply dry sterile 4 × 4–inch gauze over moist gauze.	Dry layer pulls moisture from wound.
(5) Cover with ABD pad, Surgipad, or gauze.	Protects wound from entrance of microorganisms.
15 Secure dressing.	
a *Tape:* Apply tape 1 to 2 inches (2.5 to 5 cm) beyond dressing. Use nonallergenic tape when necessary.	Supports wound and ensures placement and stability of dressing.
b Montgomery ties (see illustrations):	Ties allow for repeated dressing changes without removal of tape.

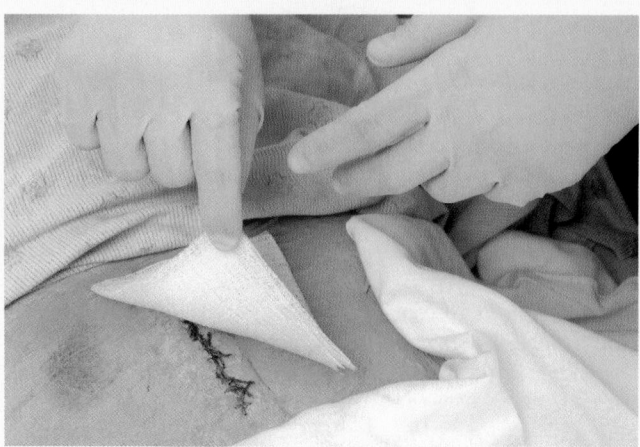

STEP 14a(2)   Placing dry gauze dressing over simple wound.

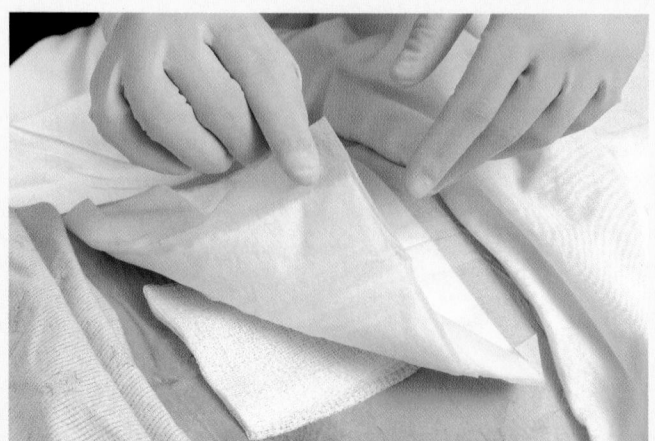

STEP 14a(5)   Placing ABD pad over gauze dressing.

STEP	RATIONALE
(1) Be sure that skin is clean. Application of skin barrier is recommended (see Chapter 18).	Skin barrier (stomahesive) protects intact skin from stretch and tension of adhesive tape.
(2) Expose adhesive surface of tape ends.	
(3) Place ties on opposite sides of dressing over skin or skin barrier.	
(4) Secure dressing by lacing ties across dressing snugly enough to hold it secure but without placing pressure on skin.	
c For dressing an extremity, secure with roller gauze (see illustration) or elastic net.	Roller gauze conforms to contour of foot or hand.
16 Dispose of all dressing supplies. Remove cover gown and goggles and remove gloves inside out; dispose of them according to agency policy.	Reduces transmission of microorganisms. Clean environment enhances patient comfort.
17 Label tape over dressing with your initials and date dressing is changed.	Provides timeline for when next dressing change is to be scheduled.
18 Help patient to comfortable position.	Promotes patient's sense of well-being.
19 Perform hand hygiene.	Reduces transmission of microorganisms.

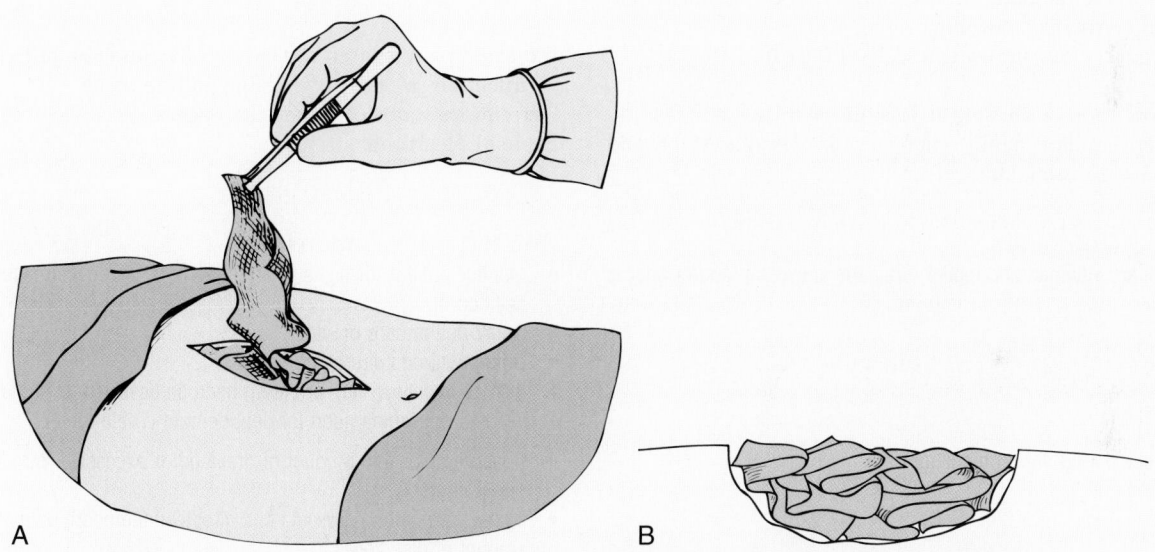

STEP 14b(3) **A,** Packing wound with fine-mesh gauze. **B,** Cross-section of deep wound packed loosely with gauze roll.

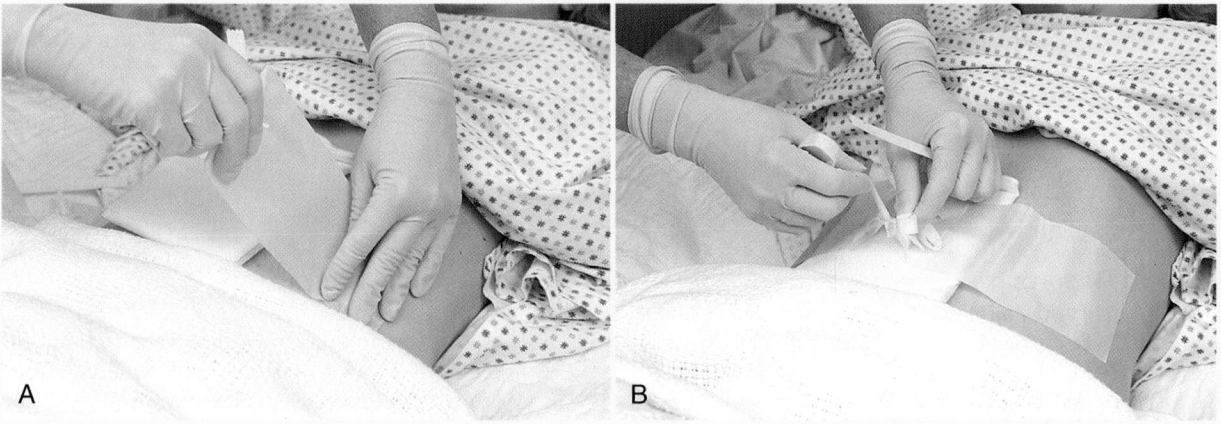

STEP 15b Montgomery ties. **A,** Each tie is placed at side of gauze dressing. **B,** Securing ties encloses dressing.

STEP	RATIONALE

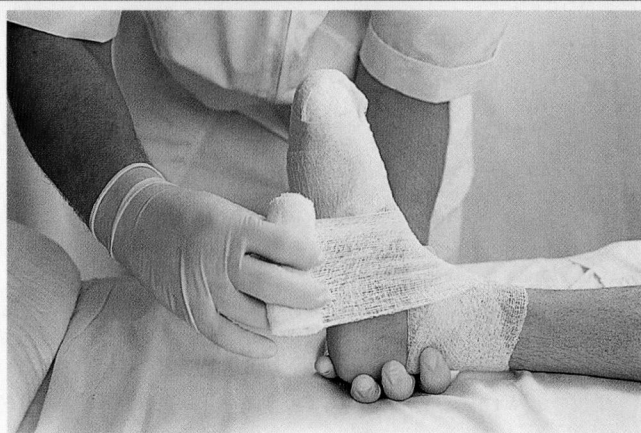

STEP 15c Wrap roller gauze around extremity to secure dressing.

EVALUATION

1 Observe appearance of wound for healing: measure size of wound; observe amount, color, and type of drainage and periwound erythema or swelling.

Determines rate of healing.

2 Ask patient to rate pain using a scale of 0 to 10.

Increased pain is often indication of wound complications such as infection or result of dressing pulling tissue.

3 Inspect condition of dressing at least every shift.

Determines status of wound drainage.

4 Ask patient and/or family caregiver to describe steps and techniques of dressing change.

Evaluates learning.

Unexpected Outcomes

1 Wound appears inflamed and tender, drainage is evident, and/or odor is present.

2 Wound bleeds during dressing change.

3 Patient reports sensation that "something has given way under the dressing."

Related Interventions

- Monitor patient for signs of infection (e.g., fever, increased white blood cell count).
- Notify health care provider.
- Obtain wound cultures as ordered.
- If there is yellow, tan, or brown necrotic tissue, refer to health care provider to determine need for debridement (Table 39-2).

- Observe color and amount of drainage. If excessive, may need to apply direct dressing.
- Inspect area along dressing and directly underneath patient to determine amount of bleeding.
- Obtain vital signs as needed.
- Notify health care provider.

- Observe wound for increased drainage or dehiscence (partial or total separation of wound layers) or evisceration (total separation of wound layers and protrusion of viscera through wound opening).
- Protect wound. Cover with sterile moist dressing.
- Instruct patient to lie still.
- Stay with patient to monitor vital signs.
- Notify health care provider.

Recording and Reporting

- Record appearance and size of wound, characteristics of drainage, presence of necrotic tissue, type of dressing applied, patient's response to dressing change, and level of comfort in nurses' notes and EHR.
- Report any unexpected appearance of wound drainage, accidental removal of drain, bright red bleeding, or evidence of wound dehiscence or evisceration.

Special Considerations
Teaching

- Explain expected wound appearance and risks of improper wound care. Provide patient and family caregiver with a written list of signs to report to the health care provider.
- After demonstrating wound care, allow patient or caregiver to perform dressing change with and without supervision.

TABLE 39-2	Problems Associated with Wounds Requiring Debridement

Problem	Nursing Activities
Solutions used may be irritating to healthy skin around wound.	Protect healthy skin with protective barrier such as stomahesive or apply topical ointments such as zinc oxide. If zinc oxide is used, it should be removed with mineral oil. Avoid scrubbing the skin because scrubbing can cause harm to the epithelial layer.
Wound becomes excessively dry.	A continually moist dressing (with a health care provider's order) might be tried. Eliminate fine-mesh gauze and lightly pack wound with fluffy gauze dampened with prescribed solution.
Wound is deep, and retention of dressing in cavity is suspected.	Irrigate wound copiously with prescribed solution to loosen dressing for removal. Use continuous "ribbon" or strip of gauze to dress deep wounds.
Wound drainage is damaging healthy tissue.	Protect healthy tissue with skin barrier such as a hydrocolloid. Wounds with large amounts of drainage may benefit from occlusive drainage collection device.
Patient's skin is irritated by tape.	Use hydrocolloid under tape, use Montgomery ties as needed, use fabric tape that has multidirectional stretch, secure dressing with binder, or wrap with roll gauze if on extremity.

Pediatric
- Some pediatric patients are fearful of dressing changes. Obtain patient's cooperation and/or have another person available to keep child from moving during dressing change procedure (Hockenberry and Wilson, 2011).
- Older children may need something to do during dressing changes. Listening to music or watching a video helps to relieve some of the boredom or stress during the procedure (Hockenberry and Wilson, 2011).

Gerontologic
- Adhesive tape often irritates older adults' skin and causes skin tears. Use paper tape, nonallergenic tape, or wraps or mesh to prevent tape from contacting patient's skin.
- Another option is to create a stomahesive window. Cut strips of stomahesive into 1-cm ($\frac{1}{2}$-inch) strips. Use a skin barrier to wipe areas of intact skin where you will place strips. Apply the adhesive strips to two or four sides of the wound, framing it. Apply dressing. Apply tape to the stomahesive strips.
- Normal aging changes of skin and tissue and the inflammatory response may delay wound healing (Wysocki, 2011).

Home Care
- Consider resources within the home, ability of a family caregiver, and the amount of time needed to change a particular dressing when selecting a dressing procedure in the home setting. More expensive dressings may be used to decrease frequency of dressing changes.
- Reimbursement for wound care requires a signed health care provider's order, treatment plan, and documentation of the actual care provided.

SKILL 39-2 Applying a Pressure Bandage

A pressure bandage is a temporary treatment to control excessive, sudden, unanticipated bleeding. Hemorrhage may occur during surgical intervention (e.g., cardiac catheterization, arterial puncture, organ biopsy) or after surgery or be a life-threatening occurrence related to accidental trauma (e.g., stabbing, suicide attempt). Pressure dressings are essential to stopping the flow of blood and promoting clotting at the site until definitive action can be taken to stop the source. A number of hemostatic wound products developed for use in trauma settings have shown promise in controlling hemorrhaging wounds (Granville-Chapman, Jacobs, and Midwinter, 2011). One example is HemCon, made from chitosan, a naturally occurring biocompatible polysaccharide that becomes extremely adherent when in contact with blood.

Given the emergent nature of an acute bleeding episode, the aseptic techniques considered essential in most dressing applications are secondary to halting the bleeding. A pressure dressing applied in an emergency is usually temporary; the wound can be cleaned, and dressing changed once the bleeding has been controlled.

Delegation and Collaboration
The skill of applying a pressure dressing in an emergency situation cannot be delegated to nursing assistive personnel (NAP). If application requires more than one person, the NAP can assist. The nurse directs the NAP to:
- Observe the pressure dressing during care activities to make sure that it remains in place and that there is no visible bleeding from the site.
- Observe underneath patient for bleeding after dressing has been applied.

Equipment
- ❏ Necessary dressings: Fine-mesh gauze, abdominal (ABD) pads, hemostatic dressings, roller gauze
- ❏ Adhesive tape; hypoallergenic if necessary
- ❏ Adhesive remover (optional)
- ❏ Clean gloves
- ❏ Protective gown, goggles, mask (used when spray from wound is a risk)
- ❏ Equipment for vital signs

STEP	RATIONALE

ASSESSMENT

1 Anticipate patients at risk for unexpected bleeding, including traumatic injury, arterial puncture, donor graft site, postoperative wound, wounds after surgical debridement, and surgical patient with history of bleeding disorder.

Be familiar with conditions associated with unexpected bleeding to rapidly respond to bleeding.

2 Assess location and circumstance of area where hemorrhage is expected.

Helps to identify proper type and amount of supplies needed.

3 Assess patient for allergies to antiseptics, tape, or latex. If patient is nonresponsive and no history is available, use nonlatex or nonallergenic supplies.

Prevents localized or systemic allergic reaction.

4 Quickly assess patient's anxiety level.

Determines need for education and positive reinforcement during procedure.

5 Consider patient's baseline vital signs before onset of hemorrhage.

If data are available, baseline vital signs indicate status of circulatory function.

NURSING DIAGNOSES

- Decreased cardiac output
- Risk for imbalanced fluid volume
- Impaired skin integrity

Related factors are individualized based on patient's condition or needs.

PLANNING

1 Expected outcomes following completion of procedure:
- Patient shows complete cessation of bleeding and no evidence of hematoma formation.

Hemostasis is achieved.

- Patient maintains stable blood pressure and heart rate.

Hemodynamic stability is achieved with minimal blood loss.

- Distal circulation is maintained with intact pulses (distal to site of injury).

There is no hematoma formation at site of pressure application.

IMPLEMENTATION

Phase I: Immediate action—first nurse

1 Identify external bleeding site. Look underneath patients with large abdominal dressings. NOTE: Wounds to groin area also can result in large amounts of blood loss, which is not always visible.

Quick identification increases response time to stop bleeding. Maintaining asepsis and privacy are considered only if time and severity of blood loss permit.

2 Apply immediate manual pressure to bleeding site.

Hemostasis maintained as supplies are prepared.

3 Seek assistance.

Bandage must be secured quickly.

Phase II: Applying pressure bandage—second nurse

4 Quickly identify source of bleeding.

Determines method of application and supplies to use.

- *Arterial bleeding* is bright red and gushes forth in waves, related to heart rate; if vessel is very deep, flow is steady.
- *Venous bleeding* is dark red and flows smoothly.
- *Capillary bleeding* is oozing of dark red blood; self-sealing controls this bleeding.

5 Elevate affected body part (e.g., extremity) if possible.

Helps slow rate of hemorrhage.

6 First nurse continues to apply direct pressure as second nurse unwraps roller bandage and places within easy reach. Second nurse quickly cuts three to five lengths of adhesive tape and places them within reach; *do not cleanse wound.*

Pressure dressing controls bleeding temporarily. Preparation allows for securing pressure bandage quickly.

7 In simultaneous coordinated actions:

a Rapidly cover bleeding area with multiple thicknesses of gauze compresses. First nurse slips fingers out as other nurse exerts adequate pressure to continue controlling bleeding (see illustrations).

Gauze is absorbent. Layers provide bulk against which local pressure can be applied to bleeding site.

b Place adhesive strips 7 to 10 cm (3 to 4 inches) beyond width of dressing with even pressure on both sides of fingers as close as possible to central bleeding source. Secure tape on distal end, pull tape across dressing, and keep firm pressure as proximate end of tape is secured.

Tape exerts downward pressure, promoting hemostasis. To ensure blood flow to distal tissues and prevent tourniquet effect, adhesive tape must not be continued around entire extremity.

STEP	RATIONALE
c Remove fingers temporarily and quickly cover center of area with third strip of tape.	Provides pressure to source of bleeding.
d Continue reinforcing area with tape as each successive strip is overlapped on alternating sides of center strip. Keep applying pressure.	Prevents tape from loosening.
e When pressure bandage is on extremity, apply roller gauze: apply two circular turns tautly on both sides of fingers that are pressing gauze. Compress over bleeding site. Simultaneously remove finger pressure and apply roller gauze over center. Continue with figure-eight turns. Secure end with two circular turns and strip of adhesive (see Procedural Guideline 39-1).	Roller gauze acts as pressure bandage, exerting more even pressure over extremity.

Clinical Decision Point *Start pressure bandage from distal to proximal, working toward the heart.*

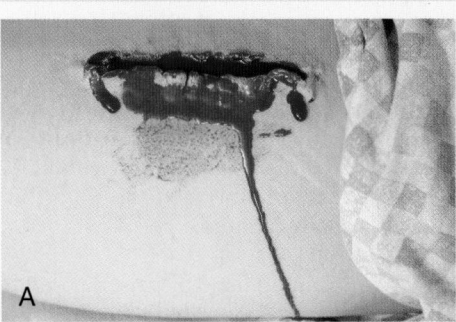 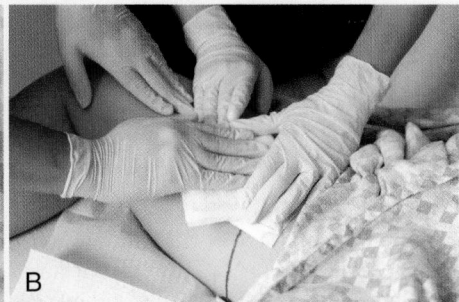

STEP 7a   **A,** Bleeding wound. **B,** Nurses apply pressure dressing.

EVALUATION

1 Observe dressing for control of bleeding.	Effective pressure bandage controls bleeding without blocking distal circulation.
2 Evaluate adequacy of circulation (distal pulse, skin characteristics).	Determines level of perfusion to distal body parts.
3 Estimate volume of blood loss (e.g., count number of dressings used, weigh saturated dressing).	Helps to determine blood and fluid replacement needs.
4 Measure vital signs.	Identifies patient's adaptation to blood loss and early stages of hypovolemic shock.

Unexpected Outcomes

1 There is continued bleeding. Fluid and electrolyte imbalance, tissue hypoxia, confusion, hypovolemic shock, and cardiac arrest develop.

2 Pressure dressing is too tight and occludes circulation.

Related Interventions

- Notify health care provider.
- Reinforce or adjust pressure dressing.
- Initiate intravenous (IV) therapy per order.
- Place patient in Trendelenburg's position; provide covers for warmth.
- Monitor vital signs every 5 to 15 minutes (apical pulse, distal pulses, and blood pressure).
- Inspect areas distal to pressure dressing to ensure that circulation has not been occluded.
- Adjust dressing as needed.
- Notify health care provider.

Recording and Reporting

- Report immediately to health care provider present status of patient's bleeding control, time bleeding was discovered, estimated blood loss, nursing interventions (including effectiveness of applied pressure bandage), apical and distal pulses, blood pressure, mental status, signs of restlessness, and need for health care provider to administer to patient without delay.
- Record interventions taken and patient's response in progress notes and vital sign flow sheet.

Special Considerations
Teaching

- Explain to patient and family (if present) need to monitor vital signs.
- Explain need for patient to remain quiet and stay in position to reduce bleeding.

Pediatric

- Child will calm down if care providers and family remain calm.

Gerontologic
- Because of the normal changes of aging, the older adult has an increased risk for vascular and tissue changes distal to the pressure dressing. Evaluate skin and pulse distal to the pressure bandage frequently.

Home Care
- If patient is at risk for hemorrhage, instruct on the following:
- How family caregiver or patient should apply pressure with clean towels or linen

- Immediate activation of emergency system (9-1-1)
- How to position patient by elevating affected body part (if extremity)
- CAUTION: If a puncture wound occurs from a penetrating object (e.g., knife, toy, building materials), do not remove the object. Removal will cause more rapid blood loss and may damage underlying structures.
- How to position patient to promote elevation of affected body part (if extremity) and promote relaxation

---

SKILL 39-3 Applying a Transparent Dressing

[NSO] *Wound Care Module / Lesson 3*

A transparent film dressing is a clear, adherent, nonabsorptive, polyurethane sheet. Once it is applied, a moist exudate forms over the wound surface, which prevents tissue dehydration and allows for rapid, effective healing by speeding epithelial cell growth. The adhesive is inactivated by moisture and does not adhere to a moist surface. A transparent film has no absorbent capacity, and it is impermeable to fluids and bacteria (Rolstad et al., 2011). The dressings are appropriate for prophylaxis on high-risk intact skin (e.g., high friction areas), superficial wounds with minimal or no exudate, and eschar-covered wounds when autolysis is indicated and safe (NPUAP-EPUAP, 2009). Clinicians commonly use transparent dressings as the dressing of choice over an intravenous (IV) catheter insertion site. The synthetic permeable membrane acts as a temporary second skin, adheres to undamaged skin to contain exudate, minimizes wound contamination, and allows a wound to "breathe." They are also commonly used as secondary dressing to wound products such as alginates and foam.

Transparent dressings come in a variety of sizes. Select one that allows for a 2.5-cm (1 inch) perimeter onto intact skin around the wound (Rolstad et al., 2011). Use a skin barrier on the skin around a wound before dressing application to prevent stripping thin or fragile skin. Because these dressings are clear, you can observe a wound without removing the dressing. For best results these dressings are applied over clean, debrided wounds that are not actively bleeding. The accumulation of fluid with a white, opaque appearance and erythema of the surrounding tissue usually indicate an infectious process; the dressing should be removed, and a wound culture obtained.

Delegation and Collaboration

The skill of applying a transparent dressing for select wounds can be delegated to nursing assistive personnel (NAP) (refer to agency policy). The assessment of the wound and care of sterile or new acute wounds cannot be delegated to NAP. The nurse directs the NAP about:

- Explaining how to adapt the skill for a specific patient.
- Reporting any signs of bleeding, drainage, infection, or poor wound healing immediately to the nurse.

Equipment

- ❏ Sterile gloves (optional)
- ❏ Dressing set (optional)
- ❏ Sterile saline or other cleansing agent (as ordered)
- ❏ Clean gloves
- ❏ Cotton swabs
- ❏ Waterproof bag for disposal
- ❏ Transparent dressing (size as needed)
- ❏ Sterile 4 × 4–inch gauze pads
- ❏ Skin preparation materials (optional)

STEP	RATIONALE

ASSESSMENT

1 Assess location, appearance, and size of wound (see Chapter 38). Determine size of transparent dressing needed. Review previous nurses' notes and electronic health record (EHR).	Determines type of materials needed for dressing change.
2 Review health care provider's orders for frequency and type of dressing change.	Health care provider orders frequency of dressing changes and special instructions.
3 Assess patient for allergies, especially antiseptics, tape, or latex.	Prevents local or systemic allergic reaction.
4 Ask patient to rate level of pain using pain scale of 0 to 10 and assess character of pain. Administer prescribed analgesic as needed 30 minutes before dressing change.	Comfortable patient will be less likely to move suddenly, causing wound or supply contamination. Serves as baseline to measure response to dressing therapy.
5 Assess patient's knowledge of purpose of dressing.	Identifies patient's learning needs.
6 Assess patient's risks for impaired wound healing (e.g., aging, poor nutrition).	Physiologic changes caused by aging, chronic illness, poor nutrition, medications, and cancer treatments have potential to affect wound healing (Doughty and Sparks-DeFriese, 2011).

NURSING DIAGNOSES

• Acute pain	• Impaired skin integrity	• Risk for infection

Related factors are individualized based on patient's condition or needs.

STEP	RATIONALE
PLANNING	
1 Expected outcomes following completion of procedure:	
• Wound heals rapidly with little pain and mobility restriction for patient.	Dressing effective in preventing infection and promoting healing.
• Patient experiences minimal discomfort during dressing change.	Adequate pain control achieved.
2 Explain procedure to patient.	Relieves anxiety and promotes understanding of healing process.
3 Position patient comfortably and to allow for access to dressing site.	Facilitates application of dressing.
IMPLEMENTATION	
1 Identify patient using two identifiers (i.e., name and birthday or name and account number) according to agency policy. Compare identifiers with information on patient's identification bracelet.	Ensures correct patient. Complies with The Joint Commission standards and improves patient safety (TJC, 2012).
2 Close door or cubicle curtains; keep sheet or gown draped over body parts not requiring exposure.	Provides privacy and decreases transfer of microorganisms.
3 Expose wound site, minimizing exposure. Instruct patient not to touch wound or sterile supplies.	Dressing supplies become contaminated when touched by patient's hand.
4 Cuff top of disposable waterproof bag and place within reach of work area.	Cuff prevents accidental contamination of tip of outer bag.
5 Perform hand hygiene and apply clean gloves. Apply personal protective equipment (gown, mask, goggles as needed).	Reduces transmission of infectious organisms from soiled dressings to nurse's hands.
6 Remove old dressing by stretching film in direction parallel to wound rather than pulling.	Stretching action gently breaks dressing seal (Rolstad et al., 2011). Reduces excoriation, tearing, or irritation of skin after dressing removal.
7 Dispose of soiled dressing in waterproof bag, remove gloves by pulling them inside out, dispose of them in waterproof bag, and perform hand hygiene.	Reduces transmission of microorganisms.
8 Prepare dressing supplies. Use sterile supplies for new wounds.	Reduces risk for break in sterile technique.
9 Pour saline or prescribed solution over 4 × 4–inch sterile gauze pads.	Maintains sterility of dressing.
10 Apply clean or sterile gloves (check agency policy).	Allows you to handle dressings.
11 Clean wound and periwound area gently with 4 × 4–inch sterile gauze pads moistened in sterile saline or spray with wound cleanser. Clean from least to most contaminated area (see Skill 39-1).	Reduces introduction of organisms into wound.
12 Pat skin around wound dry thoroughly with dry 4 × 4–inch sterile gauze pads.	Transparent dressing with adhesive backing does not adhere to damp surface (Rolstad et al., 2011).
13 Inspect wound for tissue type, color, odor, and drainage; measure if indicated (see Chapters 18 and 38).	Provides baseline for monitoring wound healing.
14 Remove gloves and perform hand hygiene.	Reduces transmission of microorganisms.

Clinical Decision Point *If wound has a large amount of drainage, choose another dressing that can absorb drainage.*

STEP	RATIONALE
15 Apply transparent dressing according to manufacturer directions. *Do not stretch film during application and avoid wrinkles.* Apply clean gloves.	Wrinkles provide tunnel for exudate drainage.
a Remove paper backing, taking care not to allow adhesive areas to touch each other.	
b Place film smoothly over wound without stretching (see illustrations).	Ensures coverage of wound. Prevents shearing of skin from dressing that is too tight. Stretching can also break wound seal.
c Use your fingers to smooth and adhere dressing.	
d Label dressing with date, your initials, and time of dressing change on outer label of dressing (see illustration).	Provides record for determining when to next change dressing.
16 Discard soiled dressing materials properly. Remove gloves by pulling them inside out and discard in prepared bag. Perform hand hygiene.	Reduces transfer of microorganisms.
17 Help patient to comfortable position.	Enhances patient comfort and relaxation.

STEP	RATIONALE

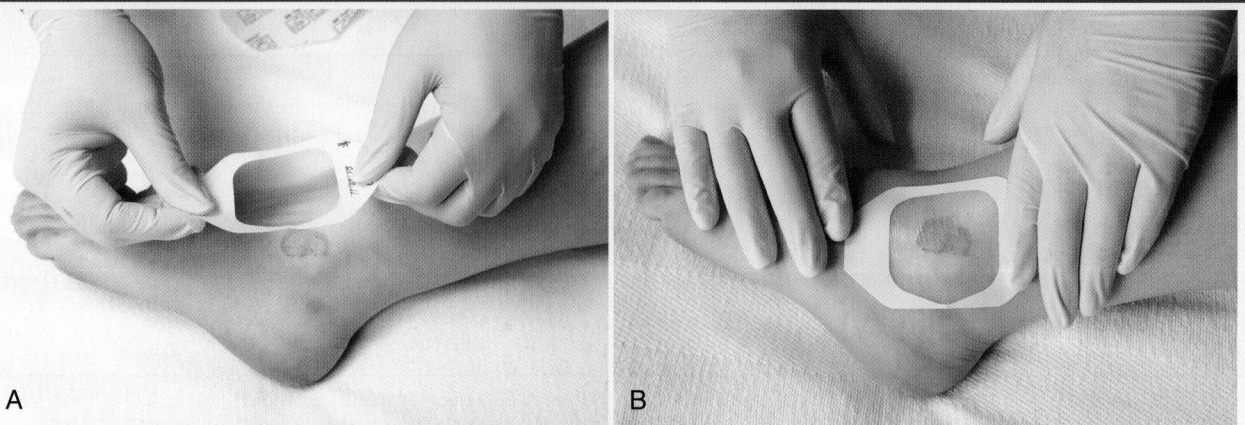

STEP 15b   **A,** Transparent dressing placed over small wound on ankle. **B,** Place film smoothly without stretching.

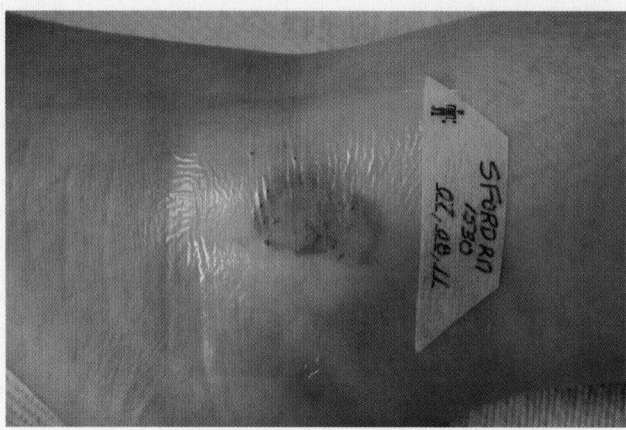

STEP 15d   Transparent dressing correctly labeled.

EVALUATION

1 Inspect appearance of wound and amount of drainage and measure size.
2 Inspect periwound areas.
3 Ask patient to rate pain using scale of 0 to 10.

Determines status of wound healing. Wound is easy to view.

Identifies any injury to surrounding skin.
Determines any change in pain during procedure.

Unexpected Outcomes
1 Wound is inflamed, tender; drainage, necrosis, and/or odor is present.

2 Dressing does not stay in place.

3 Outer layer of patient's skin tears on removal of dressing.

Related Interventions
• Remove dressing and obtain wound culture according to agency policy.
• Different type of dressing may be required.
• Notify health care provider.
• Evaluate size of dressing used for adequate wound margin (2.5 to 3.75 cm [1 to 1½ inches]).
• Dry patient's skin thoroughly before reapplication.
• Adhesive backing may be too strong for fragile skin.
• Consider other nonadhesive-backed transparent dressing.

Recording and Reporting
• Record appearance of wound, presence and characteristics of drainage, and presence of odor. Note patient response to dressing change.
• Report any signs of infection to the health care provider.

Special Considerations
Teaching
• Explain need to change dressing should edges loosen.
• Explain to patient and family that collection of wound fluid under dressing is not "pus" but normal interaction of body fluids with dressing.

Pediatric
- Adhesive backing may cause skin tears on premature babies' immature skin (Hockenberry and Wilson, 2011).
- Children may find this procedure more tolerable if they know that the longer the dressing is left on, the easier it is to remove (Hockenberry and Wilson, 2011).

Gerontologic
- Adhesive backing may be too strong for the skin of older adults. Do not use a film dressing that has an adhesive backing with a

stronger bond to the epidermis than the epidermis has to the dermis.

Home Care
- Wound may be cleaned in shower if approved by health care provider.
- Many types of transparent dressings exist. Explore types with patient and recommend type to which patient has easy access and finds easy to apply.

SKILL 39-4 Applying a Hydrocolloid, Hydrogel, Foam, or Absorption Dressing

NSO *Wound Care Module / Lesson 3*

As management of wound care advances, there are numerous classes of dressings. Match the properties of a dressing with the characteristics of a wound to promote healing. Two classes of dressings include absorbent and hydrating.

Hydrocolloid dressings are a formulation of elastomeric, adhesive, and gelling agents. They promote statistically significant better wound healing outcomes compared with conventional gauze (Rolstad et al., 2011; Baranoski and Ayello, 2012). They are indicated as primary dressings for minimally-to-moderately exudative partial- and full-thickness wounds. Hydrocolloids are used as secondary dressings over fillers such as hydrocolloid powders and pastes (Rolstad et al., 2011). International pressure ulcer guidelines recommend use of hydrocolloids for clean stage II and noninfected shallow stage III pressure ulcers in anatomic locations where the product does not roll or melt (NPUAP-EPUAP, 2009). The dressings have absorptive and hydrating properties. When in contact with wound drainage, the hydrocolloid forms a gel that promotes a moist environment and autolytic and enzymatic debridement. Hydrocolloids come in the form of granules, paste, or wafers. Change dressings when the wound gel appears to have migrated beyond the margins of the wound or the seal is leaking (Rolstad et al., 20011).

Hydrogel dressings are glycerin- or water-based dressings designed to hydrate a wound, thus promoting moist wound healing and autolysis (Rolstad et al., 2011). They are recommended for dry to minimally exudative wounds with or without depth and are a good choice for painful wounds since they do not adhere to a wound base. In addition, international pressure ulcer guidelines recommend hydrogels for dry to minimally exudative pressure ulcers that are noninfected and granulating in anatomic locations that are not at risk for dressing migration (NPUAP-EPUAP, 2009). Hydrogels are nonadherent and have some absorptive properties. The dressings are available as sheets, impregnated gauze, or amorphous gel. They facilitate autolytic debridement of wounds through rehydration. They absorb exudate and encourage healing by maintaining a moist wound healing environment. The gel dressings are nonadherent and must be covered with a secondary dressing to hold them in place. Because of their "cooling" and soothing properties, hydrogel dressings are also used with burns and to soothe radiation burns.

Polyurethane foam dressings are sheets of foamed polymers that contain small open cells capable of holding wound exudate away from a wound bed (Rolstad et al., 2011). Foam dressings are used as primary or secondary dressings to absorb moderate-to-heavy exudates. They are indicated to treat superficial or deep wounds, protect friable periwound skin, pad and protect high-trauma areas (e.g., pretibial area and forearms), and treat infected wounds following appropriate intervention and close monitoring of wound healing. International pressure ulcer guidelines recommend considering foam for use on exudative stage II and shallow stage II pressure ulcers (NPUAP-EPUAP, 2009). Foam dressings are not appropriate when

there is wound tunneling because the dressing expands, which can enlarge the tunnels. The foam dressings protect the wound surface while maintaining a moist, insulated environment. Application directions for the different brands of foam dressings vary.

Alginate dressings include calcium alginate materials, which are manufactured from natural material (seaweed) and known for their absorptive properties, forming a gel over the wound surface to contain exudate. The exudate absorbers are nonadhesive, nonocclusive dressings that conform to the shape of the wound. Alginates create a moist environment and thus promote autolysis, granulation, and epithelialization (Rolstad et al., 2011). These dressings are appropriate for full-thickness wounds with moderate-to-high amounts of drainage. Some alginates become almost amorphous gels in a wound and require irrigation to be removed, whereas others retain a structure that can be lifted out of a wound (Rolstad et al., 2011). You can safely pack deep tracking wounds with calcium-sodium alginate preparation, which allows easy removal with little risk for retained dressing deep in the wound cavity. Alginates and fiber gelling dressings are changed as often as daily; or they are left in place for several days, depending on the amount of exudate and the type of secondary dressing used (Rolstad et al., 2011).

Delegation and Collaboration
The skill of applying a hydrocolloid, hydrogel, foam, or alginate dressing cannot be delegated to nursing assistive personnel (NAP). The nurse directs the NAP about:
- Approach to assist in positioning patient during dressing application.
- What to observe (e.g., leakage of drainage, slippage of dressing) and report back to nurse.

Equipment
- ❏ Sterile gloves *(optional)*
- ❏ Clean gloves
- **Dressing Set** *(optional)*
- ❏ Sterile scissors
- ❏ Sterile drape (optional)
- ❏ Necessary primary dressings: gauze, hydrocolloid, hydrogel, foam, or alginate
- ❏ Secondary dressing of choice
- ❏ Sterile 4 × 4–inch gauze pads
- ❏ Sterile saline or other cleansing solution (as ordered)
- ❏ Skin barrier wipe
- ❏ Tape (nonallergenic paper or adhesive), ties as needed
- ❏ Measuring guide (tape measure, tracing paper, camera as needed)
- ❏ Adhesive remover
- ❏ Waterproof bag
- ❏ Debriding gel (as ordered)
- ❏ Sterile 4 × 4–inch gauze pads
- ❏ Irrigating solution as supplies if indicated (see Skill 38-1)
- ❏ Protective gown, goggles, and mask (used when splashing from wound is a risk)

STEP	RATIONALE

ASSESSMENT

1 Assess for presence of allergies, especially antiseptics, tape, or latex.

Prevents localized or systemic reaction to supplies.

2 Inspect location, size, and condition of wound.

Determines supplies and assistance needed.

3 Ask patient to rate pain using pain scale of 0 to 10 and assess character of pain. Administer prescribed analgesic as needed 30 minutes before dressing change.

Patient may require pain medication before dressing change. Allows for peak effect of drug during procedure.

4 Review health care provider's orders for frequency and type of dressing change. *Do not use alginate or absorptive dressings on nonexudative wounds.*

Health care provider orders mode of therapy.
Dressings are designed to absorb moderate-to-large amounts of wound drainage and should not be used in wounds with minimal or no drainage (Rolstad et al., 2011).

5 Consider using customized shape or size of dressing. Some hydrocolloid dressings are available in custom shapes and sizes to fit difficult body parts (e.g., sacrum, heels, or elbows).

Variety of shapes aids in flexibility of dressing selection and better dressing adherence.

6 Assess patient's knowledge of purpose of dressing and determine need to include family caregiver in dressing wound.

Identifies patient's and family caregiver's learning needs.

NURSING DIAGNOSES

- Acute pain
- Chronic pain
- Deficient knowledge
- Impaired skin integrity
- Risk for infection

Related factors are individualized based on patient's condition or needs.

PLANNING

1 Expected outcomes following completion of procedure:
   - Patient's wound shows evidence of healing as it becomes smaller in size/depth with less drainage, redness, or swelling.

   Dressing effective in promoting healing.

   - Patient reports pain less than previously assessed level (scale of 0 to 10) during and after dressing change.

   Pain control achieved during dressing removal and reapplication.

   - Dressing remains clean, dry, and intact.
   - Patient or family caregiver explains procedure correctly.

   Dressing applied correctly.
   Indicates that learning has occurred.

2 Explain procedure to patient.

Relieves anxiety and promotes understanding of healing process.

3 Position patient comfortably to allow access to dressing site.

Facilitates application of dressing.

IMPLEMENTATION

1 Identify patient using two identifiers (i.e., name and birthday or name and account number) according to agency policy. Compare identifiers with information on patient's identification bracelet.

Ensures correct patient. Complies with The Joint Commission standards and improves patient safety (TJC, 2012).

2 Close room door or cubicle curtains.

Provides for patient privacy.

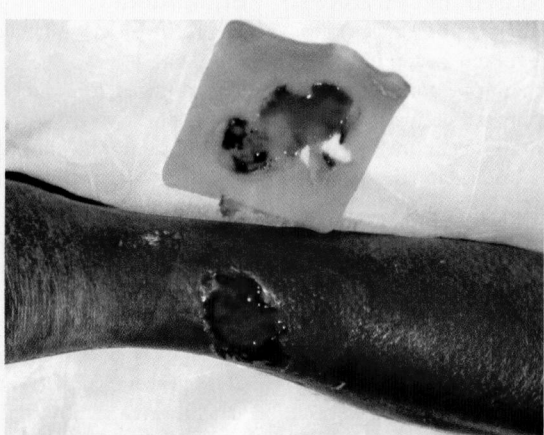

STEP 6 Hydrocolloid dressing after removal from venous ulcer. Purulent-appearing exudate is present on dressing and wound. This is expected with autolysis under the dressing and is not evidence of infection. *(From Bryant R, Nix D: Acute and chronic wounds: current management and concepts, ed 4, St Louis, 2012, Mosby.)*

STEP	RATIONALE
3 Expose wound site and drape patient. Instruct patient not to touch wound or sterile supplies.	Draping provides access to wound while minimizing exposure. Dressing supplies become contaminated when touched by patient's hand.
4 Cuff top of disposable waterproof bag and place within reach of work area.	Prevents accidental contamination of top of outer bag. Nurse should not reach across sterile field.
5 Perform hand hygiene and apply clean gloves. Apply moisture-proof gown, mask, and goggles if there is risk for splashing.	Reduces transmission of infectious organisms.
6 Remove old dressing one layer at a time. Note amount and character of drainage (see illustration). Use caution to avoid tension on any drains.	Reduces irritation and possible injury to skin. Prevents accidental removal of drain.

Clinical Decision Point *Check removal directions for specific brand of dressing used. Some brands need to have old dressing soaked, irrigated, or moistened for removal. With some types of dressings use adhesive remover to ease off dressing but avoid contact of adhesive remover with the wound.*

7 Dispose of soiled dressings in waterproof bag. Remove clean gloves by pulling them inside out and dispose of them in waterproof bag. Cover wound lightly with sterile gauze pad. Perform hand hygiene.	Reduces transmission of microorganisms.

Clinical Decision Point *Hydrocolloid dressings interact with wound fluids and form a soft whitish-yellowish gel, which is sometimes hard to remove and may have a faint odor. A residual gel substance occurs in wound beds with some absorption dressings. This is a normal occurrence; do not confuse these findings with pus or purulent exudate, wound infection, or wound deterioration.*

8 Prepare sterile field with sterile dressing kit or individually wrapped sterile supplies on over-bed table (see Chapter 8).	Creates sterile work area.
9 Pour saline or prescribed solution over 4 × 4–inch sterile gauze pads or open spray wound cleanser. *Option:* For hydrocolloid, alginate. or foam dressings, prepare an irrigation solution if needed (see Skill 38-1).	Hydrocolloid forms viscous, colloidal gel that is easily irrigated out of wound bed (Rolstad et al., 2011).
10 Apply sterile or clean gloves (check agency policy) or use no-touch technique with sterile forceps to clean wound. Remove gauze covering wound.	Allows nurse to handle dressings.

11 Cleanse wound:
  a Cleanse area gently with moist 4 × 4–inch sterile gauze pads, swabbing exudate away from wound. or spray with wound cleanser or irrigate wound bed (see Chapter 38).
  b Clean around any drain, using a circular stroke starting near drain and moving outward away from insertion site (see Skill 39-1).
	Reduces introduction of organisms into wound. Cleaning and irrigating effectively remove residual dressing gel without injuring newly formed delicate granulation tissue in healing wound bed.

12 Use sterile dry 4 × 4–inch gauze pads to blot dry excess saline or cleanser in wound bed and on skin around wound.	Dressing will not adhere to damp surface. Periwound maceration can enlarge wound and impede healing.
13 Inspect appearance and condition of wound (see Chapters 18 and 38). Measure wound size and depth.	Appearance and measurement indicate state of wound healing.
14 Remove gloves and perform hand hygiene,	Reduces transmission of microorganisms.
15 Apply dressing (see manufacturer's directions).	Ensures proper application of dressing. Different brands of dressings require different application techniques.

a Hydrocolloid dressings:
  (1) Select proper size wafer, allowing dressing to extend onto intact periwound skin at least 2.5 cm (1 inch) (Rolstad et al., 2011) (see illustration).
  (2) In the case of a deep wound, apply hydrocolloid granules, impregnated gauze or paste before the wafer.
  (3) Remove paper backing from adhesive side and place over wound. Do not stretch dressing and avoid wrinkles or tenting. Mold wafer to affected body part.
  (4) If cut from larger piece, tape edges with nonallergenic tape to avoid rolling or adherence to clothing (Rolstad, Bryant, and Nix, 2011).
	Hydrocolloid design prevents shear and friction from loosening edges and circumvents need for tape along dressing borders (Rolstad et al., 2011).
	Functions as filler material to ensure contact with all wound surfaces.

STEP	RATIONALE

Clinical Decision Point *Edges may be notched to help mold around wound. Consider using custom shapes to better conform to certain parts of the body such as heels, elbows, and sacrum.*

(5) Hold dressing in place for 30 to 60 seconds. | Hydrocolloids are most effective at body temperature (Rolstad et al., 2011).
(6) Use nonallergenic tape to secure. |

b Hydrogel dressings:

(1) Apply skin barrier wipe to surrounding skin that will come in contact with any adhesive or gel. | Protects periwound skin. Because of high water content of gels, care must be taken to protect periwound skin through use of skin barrier (Rolstad et al., 2011).

(2) Apply gel or gel impregnated gauze directly into wound, spreading evenly over wound bed (see illustration). Fill wound cavity with gel about ½- to ⅓-full or pack gauze loosely, including any undermined or tunneled areas. Cover with moisture retentive dressing or hydrocolloid wafer. *Option:* Hydrogel sheets composed of water should be cut to size of wound *only*. | Hydrogels hydrate and facilitate autolytic debridement of wounds. Filling wound cavity partially full allows for expansion with absorption of exudate.
Avoids overlapping and maceration of periwound (Rolstad et al., 2011).

(3) Cut hydrogel sheet containing glycerin so it extends 2.5 cm (1 inch) out on to intact periwound skin. Cover with secondary moisture-retentive dressing if needed. | Protects skin around wound from maceration

(4) Secure dressing with nonallergenic tape if secondary dressing is not self-adhering.

c Foam dressings:

(1) Know removal and application characteristics of specific brand of foam dressing. | Used with absorptive dressings to accommodate highly draining wounds.
(2) Apply skin barrier wipe to surrounding skin that will come in contact with thin foam dressing adhesive. NOTE: Traditional-thickness nonadhesive may not have adhesive border. | Protects periwound skin from maceration or irritation from adhesive.

(3) Cut foam sheet to extend 2.5 cm (1 inch) out onto intact periwound skin. (Verify which side of foam dressing should be placed toward wound bed and which side should be facing away from wound bed; check product instructions.) | Ensures proper absorption and keeps wound exudate away from wound bed (Rolstad et al., 2011).

(4) Some brands of foam dressings need to be covered with secondary dressing (Rolstad et al., 2011). | Protects wound.
(5) Cut foam to fit around drain or tube.

d Alginate dressings:

(1) Cut sheet or rope to fit size of wound or loosely pack into wound space (see illustration), filling ½ to ⅔ full. | Highly absorptive product expands with absorption of serous fluid or exudate (Rolstad et al., 2011).

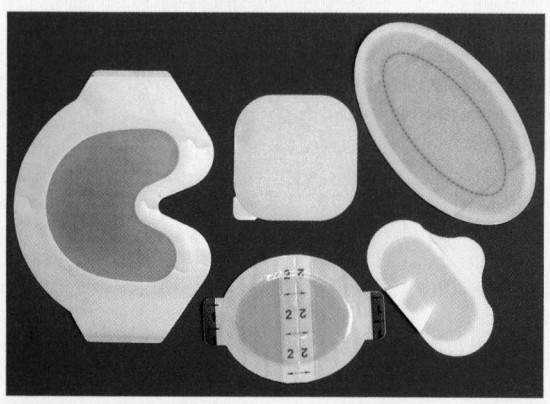

STEP 15a(1) Variety of sizes and shapes of hydrocolloid dressings. (*Courtesy Bonnie Sue Rolstad.*)

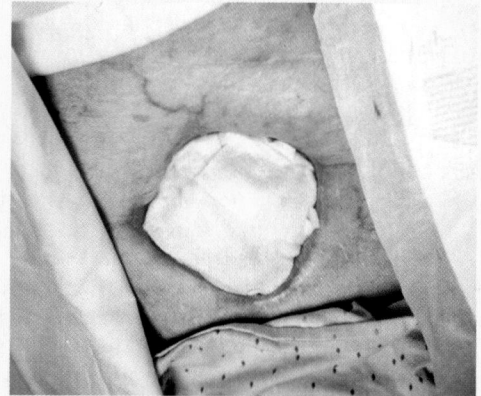

STEP 15b(2) Hydrogel-impregnated gauze used to maintain moist wound bed and fill dead space in this deep abdominal wound with undermining. (*From Bryant R, Nix D: Acute and chronic wounds: current management and concepts, ed 4, St Louis, 2012, Mosby.*)

STEP	RATIONALE
(2) Apply secondary dressing such as transparent film (see illustration) (see Skill 39-3), foam, or hydrocolloid.	Secondary dressing prohibits drainage on bed linens and clothing.
16 Discard soiled dressing materials properly. Remove gloves by pulling them inside out and discard in prepared bag. Perform hand hygiene.	Reduces transfer of microorganisms.
17 Help patient to comfortable position.	Enhances patient comfort and relaxation.

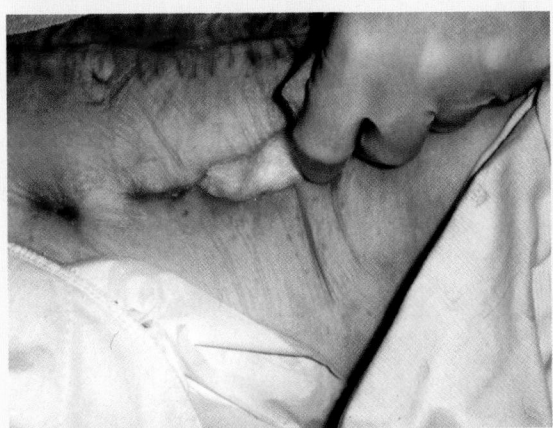

STEP 15d(1) Alginate dressing applied to fill dead space and absorb exudate in full-thickness abdominal wound. *(From Bryant R, Nix D: Acute and chronic wounds: current management and concepts, ed 4, St Louis, 2012, Mosby.)*

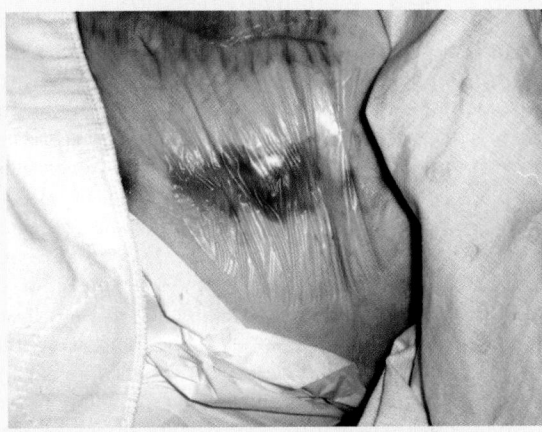

STEP 15d(2) Alginate dressing secured with secondary transparent dressing. *(From Bryant R, Nix D: Acute and chronic wounds: current management and concepts, ed 4, St Louis, 2012, Mosby.)*

EVALUATION

1 Observe condition of wound for healing, including size of wound, color, and character of drainage on ongoing basis.	Determines status of wound healing.
2 Evaluate patient's level of comfort.	Determines if pain resulted from procedure.
3 Ask patient or family caregiver to explain wound care method. *Option:* Have family caregiver demonstrate.	Evaluates level of learning.

Unexpected Outcomes

1 Wound develops more necrotic tissue and increases in size.

2 Dressing does not stay in place.

3 Periwound skin is macerated.

Related Interventions

• In rare instances some wounds do not tolerate hypoxia induced by hydrocolloid dressings. In these patients discontinue use. Notify health care provider.
• Evaluate appropriateness of wound care protocol.
• Evaluate for other factors impairing wound healing.

• Evaluate size of dressing used for adequate margin (2.5 to 3.75 cm [1 to 1½ inches]) or dry skin more thoroughly before reapplication.
• Consider custom shapes for difficult body parts. "Picture frame" edges of hydrocolloid dressing using tape.
• Dressing may be secured with roll gauze, tape, transparent dressing, or dressing sheet.

• Assess moisture control property of dressing or application technique. May need new type of dressing.

Recording and Reporting

• Record appearance of wound, color, size, characteristics of drainage, response to dressing change, condition of periwound skin, and patient's level of comfort in nurses' notes and EHR.
• Graph wound surface area or volume if wound is chronic.
• Write date, time, and nurse's initials in ink (not marker) on the dressing.
• Report signs of infection, necrosis, or deteriorating wound status to health care provider immediately.

Special Considerations
Teaching

• Explain expected wound appearance, fluid or gel accumulation in wound bed, and possible odor with use of specific dressing.
• Because application techniques can vary with different brands, tell patient and family caregiver not to purchase a brand different from the one for which the nurse gave instructions. If a different brand must be used, patient and caregiver should

check with nurse for any additional instructions or modifications in application and removal techniques.

Pediatric

• See Pediatric Considerations for Skills 39-1, 39-2, and 39-3.

Gerontologic

• See Gerontologic Considerations for Skills 39-1, 39-2, and 39-3.
• Avoid early and frequent removal of a hydrocolloid dressing to reduce injury to surrounding intact skin.

SKILL 39-5 Negative-Pressure Wound Therapy (NPWT)

Negative-pressure wound therapy (NPWT) is the application of a vacuum (negative pressure) to a wound through suction to draw edges of a wound together while providing a moist environment to promote healing and collect wound fluid (AHRQ, 2009; Campbell, Smith, and Smith, 2008; Netsch, 2011). The development of NPWT is based on two theories: (1) the removal of excess interstitial fluid decreases edema and concentrations of inhibitory factors and increases local blood flow; and (2) stretching and deformation of the tissue by the negative pressure is believed to disturb the extracellular matrix and introduce biochemical responses that promote wound healing (AHRQ, 2009). The therapy is commonly used for dehisced wounds, diabetic foot ulcers, pressure ulcers, vascular ulcers (includes venous and arterial ulcers), burn wounds, surgical wounds (especially infected sternal wounds), and trauma-induced wounds (AHRQ, 2009; NPUAP-EPUAP, 2009; Petkar et al., 2011). The WOCN (2010) reports increased rates of healing associated with stage III and IV pressure ulcers when using NPWT.

An NPWT system (Fig. 39-2) includes a vacuum pump, drainage tubing, and dressing set. The pump is either stationary or portable, may rely on AC or battery power, allows for regulation of the suction strength, has alarms to indicate loss of suction, and has a replaceable collection canister. The dressing sets contain either foam or gauze dressing to be placed in the wound and an adhesive film drape for sealing the wound. The drainage tubes come in a variety of configurations, depending on the dressings used or wound being treated (AHRQ, 2009).

NPWT generates negative pressure at the wound surface, which removes exudate, contracts the wound bed, prepares a wound for closure, and helps form granulation tissue (Figs. 39-3 and 39-4). Added benefits of NPWT include improved patient comfort and a

reduction in the frequency of dressing changes. Contraindications to NPWT for chronic wounds are exposed vital organs, inadequately debrided wounds, untreated osteomyelitis or sepsis near a wound, untreated coagulopathy, necrotic tissue with eschar, and malignancy within a wound (AHRQ 2009; Netsch, 2011). Patient cooperation and adherence are very important for NPWT to be effective. In addition, it is critical to assess patients routinely for onset of hemorrhage (Netsch, 2011).

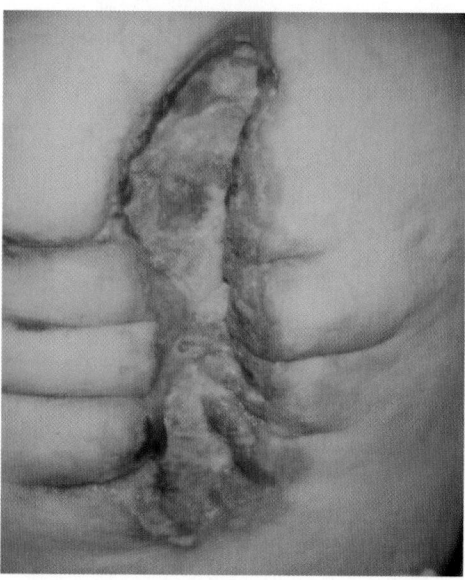

FIG 39-3 Dehisced wound before negative-pressure wound therapy. (*Courtesy KCI Licensing, San Antonio, Tex.*)

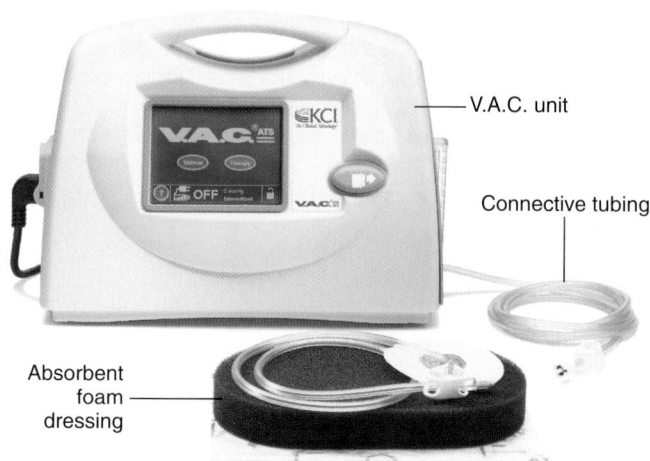

FIG 39-2 The vacuum-assisted closure ATS therapy system. *Top to bottom,* V.A.C. system pump, connective tubing to go between V.A.C. system and dressing, absorbent foam dressing. (*Courtesy KCI Licensing, San Antonio, Tex.*)

V.A.C. unit

Connective tubing

Absorbent foam dressing

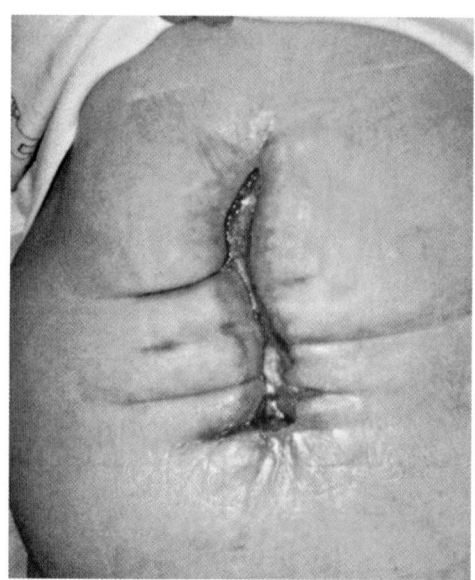

FIG 39-4 Dehisced wound after negative-pressure wound therapy. (*Courtesy KCI Licensing, San Antonio, Tex.*)

NPWT is delivered intermittently or continuously, but most often continuously. A health care provider or wound care specialist orders the cycle and amount of negative pressure to a wound. There are different recommendations for the level of negative pressure to use for wound healing. Check your agency policy. Research has found that the maximal biologic effect of NPWT at the wound edge often can be achieved at −80 mm Hg (Borqquist et al., 2011). There has also been research to show improved microvascular blood flow and granulation tissue formation with intermittent compared to continuous therapy delivered at −125 mm Hg (WOCN, 2010). The target negative pressures for wound healing tend to range from −50 mm Hg to −175 mm Hg, but a setting of −125 mm Hg is most common (Netsch, 2011).

You will typically change an entire NPWT dressing and wound filler every 48 hours or 3 times per week (Netsch, 2011). However, the schedule for changing NPWT dressings varies based on the type and condition of wound. An infected wound may need a dressing change every 24 hours. As a wound heals, the wound base becomes redder; granulation tissue lines the surface of the wound initially, and the wound has a stippled or granulated appearance. Paler areas develop as the wound continues to heal. These changes indicate an increase in fibrous tissue. The example used in this skill is that of the KCI V.A.C. Always refer to manufacturer directions for the type of NPWT used in your agency.

Delegation and Collaboration

The skill of NPWT cannot be delegated to nursing assistive personnel (NAP). The nurse directs the NAP to:
- Use caution in positioning or turning patient to avoid tubing displacement.
- Report any change in integrity of the dressing to the nurse.
- Report any change in patient's temperature or comfort level to the nurse.

Equipment
- ❏ 3 Pairs gloves, clean and sterile
- ❏ Scissors, sterile
- ❏ NPWT unit (requires health care provider's order)
  - NPWT dressing (gauze or foam, see manufacturer recommendations; transparent dressing, adhesive drape)
  - NPWT suction device
  - Tubing for connection between NPWT unit and NPWT dressing
- ❏ Waterproof bag for disposal
- ❏ Skin protectant/stomahesive/hydrocolloid dressing/skin barrier
- ❏ Protective gown, mask, goggles (used when splashing from wound is a risk)

STEP	RATIONALE

ASSESSMENT

1 Assess location, appearance, and size of wound (see Chapter 38).

Provides information about status of wound, presence of complications, and type of supplies and assistance needed.

2 Review health care provider's orders for frequency of dressing change, amount of negative pressure, type of foam or gauze to use, and pressure cycle (intermittent or continuous).

Health care provider's orders list frequency of dressing changes and any special instructions.

3 Ask patient to rate level of pain using pain scale of 0 to 10. Administer prescribed analgesic as needed 30 minutes before dressing change.

Comfortable patient will be less likely to move suddenly, causing wound or supply contamination. Serves as baseline to measure response to dressing therapy.

4 Assess patient's and family caregiver's knowledge of purpose of dressing and whether they will participate in dressing wound.

Identifies patient's learning needs. Prepares patient and family if dressing will need to be changed at home.

NURSING DIAGNOSES

- Acute pain
- Chronic pain
- Deficient knowledge
- Impaired skin integrity
- Risk for infection

Related factors are individualized based on patient's condition or needs.

PLANNING

1 Expected outcomes following completion of procedure:
- Patient's wound shows evidence of healing as wound decreases in size with less drainage, redness, or swelling.

Dressing is effective in promoting healing and preventing infection.

- Patient reports less pain on a scale of 0 to 10 during and after dressing changes.

Analgesic and comfort measures effective in controlling pain.

- Dressing remains intact with airtight seal and prescribed negative pressure.

Dressing is applied correctly and maintains negative pressure.

- Patient or family member demonstrates correct method of dressing changes.

Indicates that patient and family learning has occurred.

2 Explain procedure to patient.

Relieves anxiety and promotes understanding of healing process.

3 When using a KCI V.A.C., put system into "de-V.A.C." mode (see following steps) over period of 45 minutes before removing old dressings.

Found to loosen dressing for easier, less painful removal (Price et al., 2006).

STEP	RATIONALE

IMPLEMENTATION

1 Identify patient using two identifiers (i.e., name and birthday or name and account number) according to agency policy. Compare identifiers with information on patient's identification bracelet.

Ensures correct patient. Complies with The Joint Commission standards and improves patient safety (TJC, 2012).

2 Close room door or cubicle curtains.

Provides for patient privacy and reduces transmission of organisms.

3 Position patient comfortably and drape to expose only wound site. Instruct patient not to touch wound or sterile supplies.

Promotes patient's cooperation and completion of procedure smoothly. Prevents contamination of sterile supplies.

4 Cuff top of disposable waterproof bag and place within reach of work area.

Cuff prevents accidental contamination of top of outer bag.

5 Perform hand hygiene and put on clean gloves. If risk for spray exists, apply protective gown, goggles, and mask.

Reduces transmission of infectious organisms from soiled dressings to nurse's hands.

6 Follow manufacturer directions for removal and replacement because each NPWT unit varies slightly with approach. Turn off NPWT unit by pushing therapy on/off button.

Deactivates therapy and allows for proper drainage of fluid in drainage tubing.

   a Raise tubing above unit and clamp and engage clamp on dressing tubing.

Prevents backflow of any drainage in tubing back into wound.

   b Allow drainage to flow from tubing into drainage collector.

Prevents drainage from exiting tubing when removed.

   c Gently stretch transparent dressing horizontally and remove slowly from dressing and skin.

Protects periwound skin.
Prevents injury to wound tissue.

   d Remove old dressing one layer at a time and discard in bag.
      Keep soiled surfaces away from patient's sight.

7 Perform wound assessment. Observe surface area and tissue type, color, odor, and drainage within wound. Measure length, width, and depth of wound.

Measurement of wound is necessary to assess wound healing progression and justify continuation of NPWT for third-party payers (Netsch, 2011).
Determines condition of wound and need for replacement of dressing.

Clinical Decision Point *This is a time when a wound care nurse or physician might debride the wound. Debridement of eschar or slough, if present, should be performed for removal of deviralized tissue to prepare the wound bed (Netsch, 2011).*

8 Remove and discard gloves in waterproof bag. Avoid having patient see old dressing because sight of wound drainage may be upsetting. Perform hand hygiene.

Reduces transmission of microorganisms. Lessens patient anxiety during procedure.

9 Clean wound.

   a Apply sterile or clean gloves (see agency policy).

   b Clean wound per agency policy. It may be necessary to irrigate with normal saline or other solution ordered by health care provider (see Skill 38-1). Gently blot periwound with gauze to dry thoroughly.

Irrigation removes wound debris and cleans wound bed.
Cleaning periwound is essential for an airtight seal.

Clinical Decision Point *Health care providers may order wound cultures routinely. However, when drainage looks purulent or has a foul odor or if there is a change in amount or color, obtain wound culture. This may be an indication that NPWT may need to be discontinued (Martindell, 2012).*

10 Apply skin protectant, barrier film, stomahesive wafer, or hydrocolloid dressing to periwound skin. It may be necessary to frame periwound with these products.

Maintains airtight seal needed for NPWT wound therapy (Netsch, 2011). Protects periwound skin from moisture-associated skin damage (Martindell, 2012).

11 Fill any uneven skin surfaces (e.g., creases, scars and skinfolds) with skin barrier product (e.g., paste, strip).

Further helps to maintain airtight seal (Netsch, 2011).

12 Remove and discard gloves. Perform hand hygiene.

Prevents transmission of microorganisms.

13 Depending on type of wound, apply sterile or new clean gloves (see agency policy).

Fresh sterile wounds require sterile gloves.
Chronic wounds require clean technique, except when sharp debridement is used at bedside (Wooten and Hawkins, 2005). Do not use same gloves worn to clean wound because cross-contamination may occur.

14 Apply NPWT.

   a Prepare NPWT foam (gauze is an option in other types of NPWT devices).

There are several manufacturers; this skill reviews use of foam in KCI V.A.C.

STEP	RATIONALE
(1) Check wound measurement and select appropriate foam dressing.	Establishes baseline for wound size. Black polyurethane (PU) foam has larger pores and is most effective in stimulating granulation tissue and wound contraction. White soft foam is denser with smaller pores and used when the growth of granulation tissue needs to be restricted (Netsch, 2011; Martindell, 2012).
(2) Using sterile scissors, cut foam to exact wound size, making sure to fit size and shape of wound, including tunnels and undermined areas.	Proper size of foam dressing maintains negative pressure to entire wound.

Clinical Decision Point *Use of black PU foam may cause patients to experience more pain because of excessive wound contraction. You will need to switch patient to the PVA soft foam.*

STEP	RATIONALE
(3) Option: Instill antimicrobial product (e.g., silver impregnated gauze) or topical antibiotic into wound.	Limited research suggests that these products may reduce bioburden of wound (Orgill et al., 2009).
b Gently place foam in wound (see illustration). Be sure that foam is in contact with entire wound base, margins, and tunneled and undermined areas. Count number of foam dressings and document in patient's chart.	Maintains negative pressure to entire wound. Edges of foam dressing must be in direct contact with patient's skin.
c Apply NPWT transparent dressing over foam wound dressing.	
(1) Trim dressing to cover wound so it will extend onto periwound skin approximately 2.5 to 5 cm (1 to 2 inches).	Ensures that wound is properly covered and negative pressure seal can be achieved (Box 39-4). Dressing should be airtight with no tunnels or gaps to ensure a good seal when suction is activated.
(2) Apply transparent dressing, keeping it wrinkle-free (see illustration).	

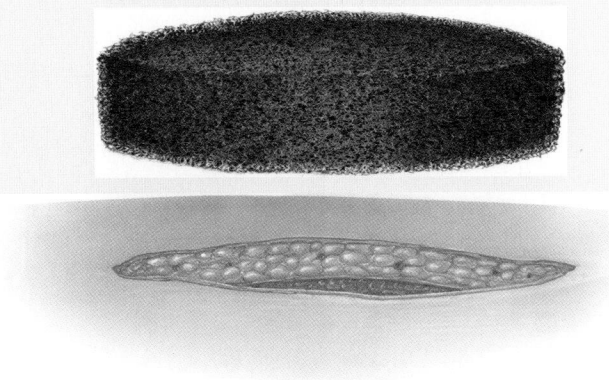

STEP 14b   Place foam in wound. The V.A.C. GranuFoam transparent dressing. *(Courtesy KCI Licensing, San Antonio, Tex.)*

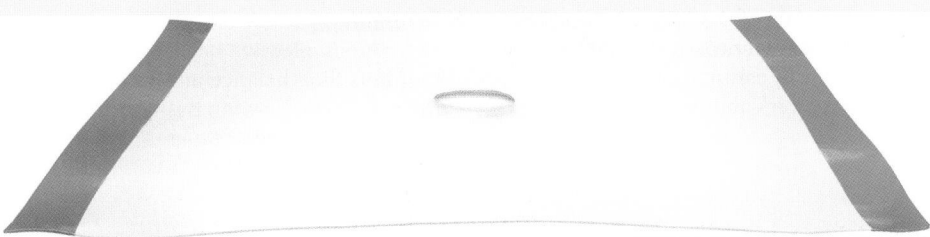

STEP 14c(2)   V.A.C. drape. *(Courtesy KCI Licensing, San Antonio, Tex.)*

BOX 39-4	**Maintaining an Airtight Seal in Negative-Pressure Wound Therapy**

Once negative-pressure wound therapy (NPWT) is initiated, negative pressure must be maintained, and the wound must stay sealed to avoid wound desiccation. Wounds around joints and near the sacrum are problem areas to seal. The following points may help to maintain an airtight seal:

- Choose a wound suitable for therapy.
- Clip hair around wound (check agency policy).
- Cut transparent film to extend 2.5 to 5 cm (1 to 2 inches) beyond wound perimeter.
- Frame the periwound area with skin sealant, skin barrier, hydrocolloid, or transparent film dressing.

- Fill uneven skin surfaces with a skin barrier product.
- Cut or mold transparent dressing to fit wound.
- Avoid wrinkles in transparent film.
- Identify any air leak with a stethoscope and repair with a sealant dressing (e.g., transparent dressing). Only use one or two additional layers for large leaks. Multiple layers reduce moisture vapor transmission and cause maceration of wound.
- Avoid adhesive remover because it leaves a residue that hinders film adherence.

From Netsch DS: Negative-pressure wound therapy. In Bryant RA, Nix DP: *Acute and chronic wounds: nursing management*, ed 4, St Louis, 2011, Mosby; and Thompson G: An overview of negative-pressure wound therapy (NPWT), *Wound Care* 6:523, 2008.

STEP	**RATIONALE**
(3) After wound is completely covered, secure tubing of NPWT unit to transparent film, aligning end of tubing to drainage hole to ensure occlusive seal (see illustration). Do not apply tension to drape and tubing. Set at ordered suction level. Examine system to be sure that seal is intact and therapy is working (see illustration) (this step is different for each type of NPWT).	Excessive tension may compress foam dressing and impede wound healing. It also produces shear force on periwound area (Kinetic Concepts, 2012). Intermittent or continuous negative pressure can be administered at −50 mm Hg to −175 mm Hg, according to health care provider's orders and patient comfort. Average is −125 mm Hg (Netsch, 2011).
15 Record initials and date and time on new dressing.	Provides reference for next dressing change.
16 Help patient to comfortable position. Patients may ambulate with NPWT.	Enhances patient comfort and relaxation.
17 Discard gloves, dispose of any dressing material, and perform hand hygiene.	Prevents transmission of microorganisms.

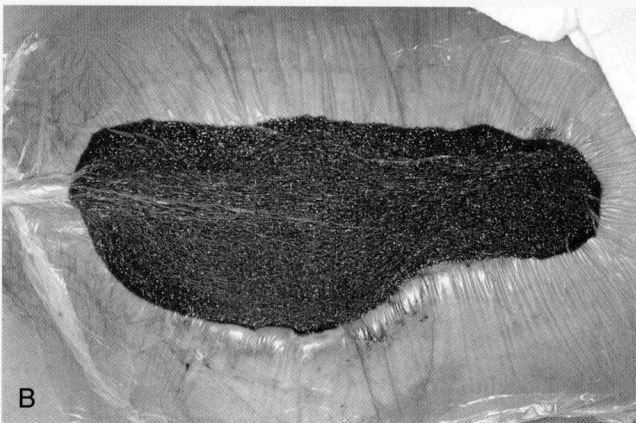

A   B

STEP 14c(3) A, Secure tubing to the foam and transparent dressing unit. (**A** *and* **B** *Courtesy KCI Licensing, San Antonio, Tex.*)

EVALUATION

1 Inspect condition of wound on ongoing basis; note drainage and odor.	Determines status of wound healing.
2 Ask patient to rate pain using scale of 0 to 10.	Determines patient's level of comfort following procedure.
3 Verify airtight dressing seal and correct negative pressure setting.	Determines effective negative pressure being applied.
4 Measure wound drainage output in canister on regular basis.	Monitors fluid balance and wound drainage.
5 Observe patient's or family caregiver's ability to perform dressing change.	Indicates that learning has occurred.

Unexpected Outcomes

1 Wound appears inflamed and tender, drainage has increased, and odor is present.

2 Patient reports increase in pain.

3 Negative pressure seal has broken.

4 Wound hemorrhages.

5 Patient or caregiver is unable to perform dressing change.

Related Interventions

- Notify health care provider.
- Obtain wound culture.
- Increase frequency of dressing changes.

- Patient may need more analgesia.
- Instill normal saline to moisten foam and other filler dressings to allow them to loosen from granulation tissue.
- If using black foam, switch to PVA white soft foam.
- Decrease pressure setting.
- Change from intermittent to continuous cycling.
- Change type of NPWT system.

- Take preventive measures (see Box 39-4).

- Stop NPWT immediately and notify health care provider

- Provide additional teaching and support.
- Obtain services of home care agency.

Recording and Reporting

- Chart in nurses' notes and EHR appearance of wound, characteristics of drainage, placement of NPWT (type of dressing, pressure mode and setting), and patient response to dressing change.
- Report brisk, bright-red bleeding, evidence of poor wound healing, evisceration or dehiscence, and possible wound infection to health care provider immediately.

Special Considerations
Teaching

- Successful NPWT relies on patient's and family caregiver's cooperation with treatment. NPWT can be difficult to use when patient is unable to consciously cooperate (e.g., dementia) (Netsch, 2011).
- Patients and family caregivers need to learn how to administer analgesics appropriately. Patient tolerance of and adherence to NPWT are difficult if dressing changes are painful (Netsch, 2011).
- Educate patients and family caregivers on the signs and symptoms that indicate development of an infection and to report to health care provider immediately.

- Explain expected wound appearance with use of dressing. Instruct patient and caregiver in appearance of foam dressings.
- Instruct patient and family in points to follow to maintain negative pressure seal.
- Explain frequency of dressing changes required. Often the dressing is not changed daily.

Pediatric

- NPWT therapy is not appropriate for fragile neonatal skin.
- Parents need to actively participate in NPWT treatment.

Gerontologic

- Use skin care practices to protect periwound tissue. Transparent film may be irritating to fragile skin. A skin protectant is one method to reduce the risk for tissue injury.
- Therapy may need to start with lower negative pressures such as −75 mm Hg and slowly titrate to more negative pressure.

Home Care

- Patient and family caregiver may benefit from visits from a home care agency to monitor initial treatments.
- Provide information to family and caregiver regarding proper disposal of contaminated products.

PROCEDURE GUIDELINE 39-1   Applying Gauze and Elastic Bandages

NSO *Wound Care Module / Lesson 3*

 Video Clip

Gauze and elastic bandages secure or wrap hard-to-cover areas of the body such as dressings on extremities, amputation stumps, and the hand. Bandages are a secondary dressing, providing protection, pressure, immobilization, and anchoring of underlying dressings or splints. There are numerous types of and applications for bandages. Bandages are available in rolls of various widths and materials, including gauze, elastic, webbing, elasticized knit, and muslin. Gauze bandages are lightweight and inexpensive, mold easily around body contours, and permit air circulation to prevent skin maceration. Elastic bandages apply compression to a body part. Elastic compression to a lower extremity prevents edema by promoting the return of blood from the peripheral to the central circulation. Compression also supports varicosities. Many patients use elastic bandages in the form of stockings to reduce dependent edema in the extremities.

When applying a bandage, select a type of bandage turn (Table 39-3) and width, depending on the size and shape of the body part to be bandaged. For example, 7.5 cm (3-inch)–wide bandages are commonly used for the adult leg. Gauze and elastic bandages are supplied in a roll with an inner and outer surface for easy application. In preparation for bandaging, place the outer surface next to the skin and roll it around the surface to be covered. Apply even tension during application. When applying an elastic bandage to an extremity, start the bandage at the site farthest from the heart (distal) and proceed toward the heart (proximal).

Delegation and Collaboration

The skill of applying an elastic bandage for compression cannot be delegated to nursing assistive personnel (NAP). A nurse assesses the condition of any wound or dressing before applying a bandage. The skill of applying bandages to secure nonsterile dressings can be delegated to NAP (refer to agency policy). The nurse directs the NAP by:

Continued

PROCEDURE GUIDELINE 39-1 Applying Gauze and Elastic Bandages—cont'd

TABLE 39-3 | Types of Bandage Turns

Type	Description	Purpose or Use
Circular turns	Bandage turn overlapping previous turn completely	Anchors bandage at first and final turn; covers small part (finger, toe)
Spiral turns	Bandage ascending body part with each turn overlapping previous one by one-half or two-thirds width of bandage	Covers cylindric body parts such as wrist or upper arm
Spiral-reverse turns	Turn requiring twist (reversal) of bandage halfway through each turn	Covers cone-shaped body parts such as forearm, thigh, or calf; useful with nonstretching bandages such as gauze or flannel
Figure-eight turns	Oblique overlapping turns alternately ascending and descending over bandaged part; each turn crossing previous one to form figure eight	Covers joints, applies low-grade pressure for venous return; snug fit provides excellent immobilization
Recurrent turns	Bandage first secured with two circular turns around proximal end of body part; half turn made perpendicular up from bandage edge; body of bandage brought over distal end of body part to be covered, with each turn folded back over on itself	Covers uneven body parts such as head or stump

- Explaining how to modify the bandage application such as with special taping.
- Reviewing what to observe and report back to the nurse (e.g., patient's complaint of pain, numbness, or tingling after application or changes in patient's skin color or temperature).

Equipment
- ❏ Correct width and number of gauze or elastic bandages
- ❏ Clips or adhesive tape
- ❏ Clean gloves if wound drainage is present
- ❏ *Option:* Pillow

Procedural Steps
1 Review patient's medical record for specific orders related to application of gauze or elastic bandage. Note area to be covered, type of bandage required, frequency of change, and previous response to treatment.
2 Identify patient using two identifiers (i.e., name and birthday or name and account number) according to agency policy. Compare identifiers with information on patient's identification bracelet.
3 Observe adequacy of circulation by palpating temperature of skin and pulses, presence of edema, and sensation (distal to area to be bandaged). Observe skin color and movement of body part to be wrapped. NOTE: Impaired circulation may

result in pain, coolness to touch when compared with the opposite side of the body, cyanosis or pallor of skin, diminished or absent pulses, edema or localized pooling, and numbness and/or tingling of body part.
4 Assess patient's level of comfort (pain scale of 0 to 10). Administer prescribed analgesic as needed before dressing change.
5 Apply clean gloves (if drainage or break in skin is present). Inspect skin of area to be bandaged for alterations in integrity as indicated by presence of abrasion, discoloration, or chafing. Pay close attention to areas over bony prominences.
6 Inspect the condition of any wound for appearance, size, and presence and character of drainage and be sure that it is covered with a proper dressing. If not, reapply dressing (check agency policy for type of gloves to use). Remove clean gloves and perform hand hygiene.
7 Assess for size of bandage:
  a *Gauze or basic elastic bandage to secure a dressing:* Assess size of area to be covered. Each successive roll of gauze/elastic should overlap previous layer. Use smaller widths for upper extremities, larger widths for lower extremities.
  b *Elastic bandage to provide simple compression:* Assess circumference of lower extremity before or shortly after patient gets out of bed in the morning or after patient has been in bed for at least 15 minutes. Select width that will cover and overlap without bulkiness.

PROCEDURE GUIDELINE 39-1 Applying Gauze and Elastic Bandages—cont'd

8 Identify patient's and primary caregiver's present knowledge level and ability to manipulate bandage if bandaging will be continued at home.

9 Close room door or curtains. Position patient comfortably in an anatomically correct supine position in bed.

10 Perform hand hygiene and apply clean gloves if drainage is present.

11 Apply gauze or elastic bandage to secure dressings:

   a Elevate dependent extremity for 15 minutes before applying elastic bandage to promote venous return.

   b Make sure that primary dressing over wound is securely in place.

   c Hold roll of bandage in your dominant hand and use other hand to lightly hold beginning layer of bandage at distal body part.

   d Begin with two circular turns to anchor bandage. Continue transferring roll to dominant hand as you wrap bandage (see illustration).

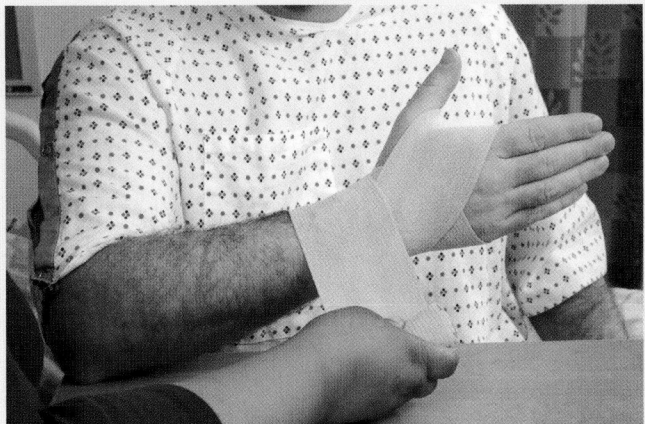

STEP 11d Hold elastic bandage in dominant hand and apply with circular turns.

   e Apply bandage from distal point toward proximal boundary (see illustration), using appropriate turns to cover various shapes of body parts (see Table 39-3). Roll gauze, overlapping each layer by one half to two thirds the width of the bandage.

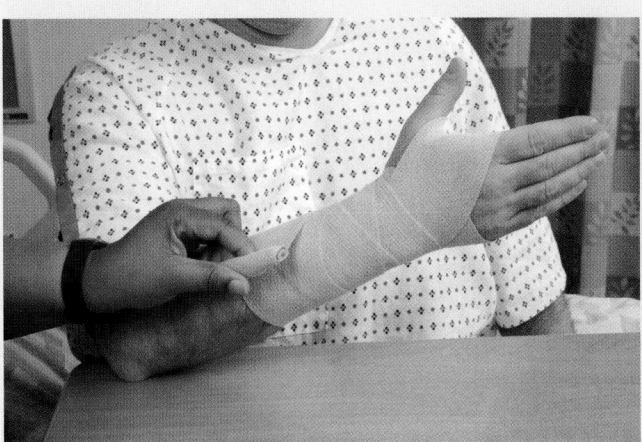

STEP 11e Apply bandage from distal to proximal.

   f Alternate ascending and descending turns (figure-eight pattern) if you are wrapping a joint.

   g Ensure that bandage is snug but not tight and that primary dressing or splint is positioned correctly. A tight bandage may cause numbness and tingling from impaired circulation and/or pressure on peripheral nerves.

   h While unrolling an elastic bandage, stretch bandage slightly. Explain to patient that smooth, even pressure will be applied to improve circulation, reduce swelling, immobilize body part, and provide pressure.

   i End bandage with two circular turns; secure end of gauze or elastic bandage to outside layer of bandage, not skin, with tape or clips (see illustration).

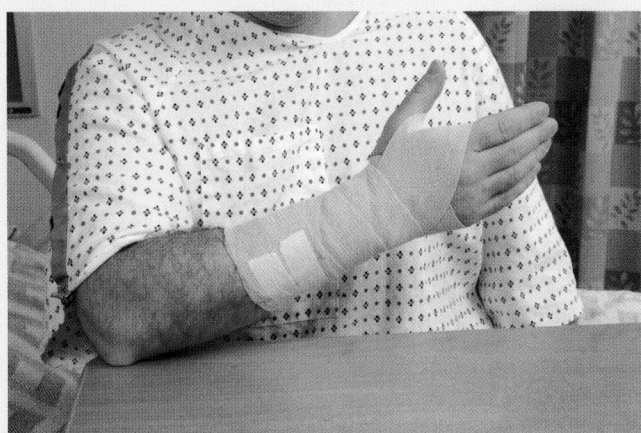

STEP 11i Secure with tape or closure device.

Clinical Decision Point *Keep toes or fingertips uncovered and visible for follow-up circulatory assessment, except in cases in which toes or fingers are treated because of wounds.*

12 Apply elastic bandage over stump (see illustrations):

   a Elevate stump with pillow or support it with the assistance of another person.

   b Secure bandage by wrapping it twice around proximal end of stump or person's waist (depending on size of stump)

   c Make half turn with bandage perpendicular to its edge.

   d Bring body of bandage over distal end of stump.

   e Continue to fold bandage over stump, wrapping from distal to proximal points.

   f Secure with metal clips, Velcro if provided, or tape.

13 Remove gloves if worn and perform hand hygiene.

14 Remove and reapply elastic bandage, securing the dressing once every 8 hours unless otherwise directed by health care provider.

15 Evaluate degree of tightness of bandage.

16 Evaluate distal circulation when bandage application is complete, at least twice during next 8 hours, and then at least every shift.

   a Observe skin color for pallor or cyanosis.

   b Palpate skin for warmth.

   c Palpate distal pulses and compare bilaterally.

   d Ask patient to rate any pain on scale of 0 to 10 and to describe any numbness, tingling, or other discomfort to evaluate for neurologic and vascular changes.

Continued

PROCEDURE GUIDELINE 39-1   Applying Gauze and Elastic Bandages—cont'd

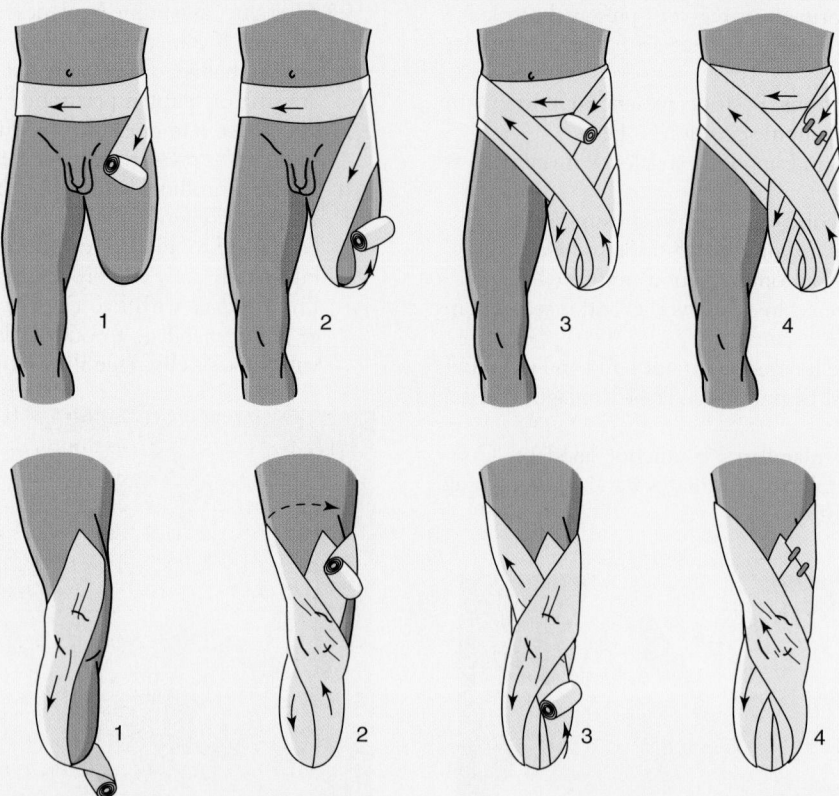

STEP 12   *Top,* Correct method for bandaging midthigh amputation stump. Note that bandage must be anchored around patient's waist. *Bottom,* Correct method for bandaging midcalf amputation stump. Note that bandage need not be anchored around waist. (*From Monahan F et al: Phipps' medical-surgical nursing: health and illness perspectives, ed 8, St Louis, 2006, Mosby.*)

17 Observe mobility of extremity.

18 Evaluate bandage for wrinkles, looseness, and presence of drainage.

19 Have patient or family caregiver demonstrate bandage application.

20 Record patient's baseline and postbandage application, including level of comfort, circulation, type of

bandage applied, presence of any swelling, and range of motion.

21 Record condition of wound or skin integrity if dressing is present and type of bandage applied.

22 Report any changes in neurologic or circulatory status to nurse in charge or health care provider immediately.

PROCEDURAL GUIDELINE 39-2   Applying an Abdominal Binder

Binders are bandages made of large pieces of material specially designed to fit a specific body part. Most binders are made of elastic or cotton. The most common types are the abdominal binder and breast binder. Breast binders are not used as often in current practice. Sports bras are preferred for breast support following certain surgeries (Michaels, Coon, and Rubin, 2011).

An abdominal binder supports large abdominal incisions (e.g., following abdominal laparotomy) that are vulnerable to tension or stress as a patient moves or coughs (Fig. 39-5). The binder also lessens pain in postoperative patients (Larson et al., 2009). In addition, abdominal binders provide a noninvasive intervention for enhancing recovery of walk performance, controlling pain, and improving patient's experience following major abdominal surgery (Cheifetz et al., 2010). Binders support underlying muscles and large incisions, lessening muscle stress when a person moves. The muscles and viscera surrounding an operative site may require support during the postoperative period to reduce trauma and

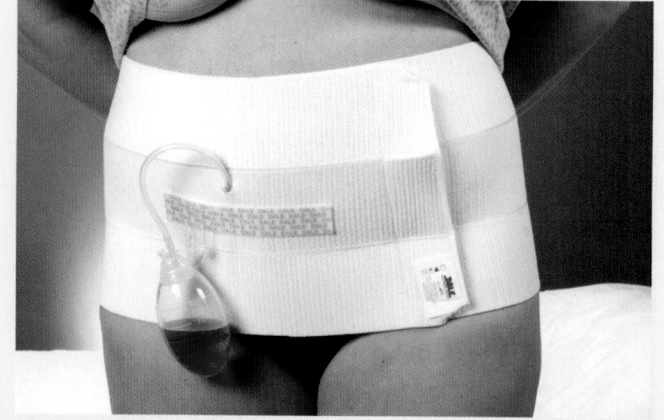

FIG 39-5   Abdominal binder with Velcro closures. (*Courtesy Dale Medical Products, Plainsville, Mass.*)

PROCEDURAL GUIDELINE 39-2 Applying an Abdominal Binder—cont'd

edema. This promotes healing and permits a patient to move more freely without additional discomfort. The basic shape of an abdominal binder is a rectangle that is wide enough to extend from the groin to the waistline and long enough to encircle the abdomen with an overlap for closure.

Delegation and Collaboration

The skill of applying a binder can be delegated to nursing assistive personnel (NAP). A nurse assesses the condition of any incision, the skin, and patient's ability to breathe before binder application. The nurse directs the NAP about:

- How to modify the skill such as special wrapping or manner of securing the binder.
- Reporting patient's complaint of pain, numbness, tingling, or difficulty breathing after applying abdominal binder or any changes in patient's skin color or temperature.

Equipment

- ❑ Clean gloves if wound drainage present
- ❑ Gauze bandage as needed
- ❑ Correct type and size of binder
- ❑ Closures for cloth binder

Procedural Steps

1 Observe patient who needs support of thorax or abdomen; observe ability to breathe deeply, cough effectively, and turn or move independently.
2 Review medical record for order for binder (check agency policy).
3 Identify patient using two identifiers (i.e., name and birthday or name and account number) according to agency policy. Compare identifiers with information on patient's identification bracelet.
4 Inspect skin for actual or potential alterations in integrity. Observe for irritation, abrasion, and skin surfaces that rub against one another.
5 Inspect any surgical dressing for intactness, presence of drainage, and coverage of incision. Change any soiled dressing before applying binder (using clean gloves).
6 Determine patient's level of comfort using scale of 0 to 10. Administer prescribed analgesic 30 minutes before dressing change.
7 Gather necessary data regarding size of patient and appropriate binder to use (see manufacturer guidelines) to ensure proper fit.
8 Determine patient's knowledge of purpose of binder.
9 Close curtains or room door.
10 Perform hand hygiene and apply clean gloves (if likely to contact wound drainage).

11 Apply abdominal binder:
  a Position patient in supine position with head slightly elevated and knees slightly flexed.
  b Help patient roll on side away from you toward raised side rail while firmly supporting abdominal incision and dressing with hands. Fanfold far side of binder toward midline of binder.
  c Place binder flat on bed, right side up. Fanfold far side of binder toward midline of binder so patient can roll over with minimal effort.
  d Place fanfolded ends of binder under patient.
  e Instruct patient or help him or her roll over folded binder. For overweight patients consider asking nurse colleague to assist.
  f Unfold and stretch ends out smoothly on far side of bed. Then stretch out ends on near side of bed.
  g Instruct patient to roll back into supine position.
  h Adjust binder so supine patient is centered over binder, using symphysis pubis and costal margins as lower and upper landmarks.
  i If patient is very thin, pad iliac prominences with gauze bandage.
  j Close binder. Pull one end of binder over center of patient's abdomen. While maintaining tension on that end of binder, pull opposite end of binder over center and secure with Velcro closure tabs or metal fasteners. Provides continuous wound support and comfort.

Clinical Decision Point *At this point recheck patient's ability to breathe deeply and cough effectively. When applied correctly, an abdominal binder over midline abdominal incisions has no significant effect on pulmonary function (Larson et al., 2009).*

12 Assess patient's comfort level and adjust binder as necessary.
13 Remove gloves and perform hand hygiene.
14 Ask patient to rate pain on scale of 0 to 10.
15 Remove binder and surgical dressing to assess skin and wound characteristics at least every 8 hours.
16 Evaluate patient's ability to ventilate properly, including deep breathing and coughing, every 4 hours to determine presence of impaired ventilation and potential pulmonary complications.
17 Record baseline and postbinder condition of skin, circulation, integrity of underlying dressing, and patient's comfort level. Also record type of bandage applied.
18 Report any complications (e.g., pain, skin irritation, impaired ventilation) to nurse in charge.
19 Report reduced ventilation (e.g., pulse oximetry, pulmonary function tests) to health care provider immediately.

Critical Thinking Exercises

Mr. Williams is a 72-year-old patient who has a stage II pressure ulcer over his left heel. The ulcer has required dressing changes for the last 2 weeks. Mr. Williams cares for it at home by applying a hydrocolloid powder on the ulcer and then covering it with a hydrocolloid wafer. His 70-year-old wife is his family caregiver.

1 The patient tells you that he has trouble getting the dressing to stay on the heel during application. Which step is he likely having difficulty performing?

2 While educating Mr. and Mrs. Williams about this dressing, which benefits of the dressing would you describe?

3 Mr. Williams tells you that, when his wife changed the dressing 2 days ago, she noticed that there was a soft whitish gel over the ulcer. He asks you, "Am I getting an infection in there?" What would your response be?

✔ REVIEW QUESTIONS

1 The nurse is removing a moist-to-dry dressing from a packed wound 6 hours after it was placed in the wound. Which observation indicates that the packing technique was incorrect?
   1 The patient experiences some pain when the dressing is removed.
   2 The gauze removed is still wet.
   3 Necrotic tissue is seen in the removed packed gauze.
   4 The wound bed looks pink with some granulation tissue.

2 Place the following steps for application of a hydrocolloid dressing in the correct order:
   1 Hold dressing in place for 30 to 60 seconds.
   2 Secure with nonallergenic tape.
   3 Remove paper backing from adhesive side of wafer and place over wound.
   4 Select proper size so it extends onto periwound skin at least 2.4 cm (1 inch).
   5 Mold wafer to affected body part.

3 A patient has a small surgical wound with necrotic tissue that requires mechanical debridement. Which of the following dressing options is used in this type of wound treatment?
   1 A dry Telfa pad placed between the wound and the outer layer of a gauze abdominal (ABD) dressing
   2 A moist-to-dry dressing placed on the wound bed
   3 A hydrogel gel dressing
   4 Self-adhesive transparent film

4 The nurse is caring for a patient with a painful burn wound. The wound care would be most appropriate if the nurse applied which type of dressing?
   1 Hydrocolloid
   2 Hydrogel
   3 Alginate
   4 Foam

5 A wound care nurse is reviewing the charts of a group of patients to be seen in the clinic. Which patients are most at risk for wound-healing problems? (Select all that apply.)
   1 A 58-year-old woman who is on immunosuppressive drugs for arthritis
   2 A 34-year-old man who has had diabetes mellitus since the age of 12
   3 A 42-year-old woman who has been using steroids for asthma
   4 A 65-year-old African-American man who is 4.5 kg (10 lbs) overweight
   5 An 80-year-old woman with a history of osteoporosis
   6 A 20-year-old man who is receiving radiation near the wound

6 After the nurse applies an abdominal binder to a patient, the patient begins to experience shallow, rapid respirations. What is the first appropriate nursing action?
   1 Notify the health care provider
   2 Elevate the head of the bed
   3 Check the patient's vital signs
   4 Remove and reapply the abdominal binder

7 A patient with a large infected wound needs negative-pressure wound therapy (NPWT) and asks the wound care nurse how the technique works. Which statement by the nurse is most accurate?
   1 Several small foam pieces are packed firmly into the wound bed; solution is poured over the foam, and pressure pushes the fluid into the wound to facilitate healing.
   2 A measured foam pad is placed over the open area along with an occlusive dressing. Negative pressure removes drainage and contracts the wound bed.
   3 The wound bed is flooded with solution, the foam is placed around the edges of the wound bed, and pressure is used to remove the solution and wound drainage.
   4 A skin protectant is coated lightly inside the wound. Several damp gauze pads with the prescribed solution are placed in the wound, and the vacuum device removes the fluid and heals the wound.

8 A patient has an elastic bandage applied to the left leg that holds a large dressing in place over a surgical incision. Which evaluation approach should the nurse use to determine if the patient has neurologic changes?
   1 Palpates distal pulses in left foot
   2 Observes color of skin in left foot
   3 Inspects the surface of the bandage for drainage
   4 Asks the patient to rate his level of pain on a scale of 0 to 10.

9 You are mentoring a student nurse on a surgical floor. You observe the student removing a dry gauze dressing from a patient who had an abdominal laparotomy 24 hours ago. The student applies a pair of clean gloves, uses the dominant hand to remove all of the gauze dressings at one time, and places them in a plastic trash bag. What would be your best reaction to this technique?
   1 "You are using good aseptic technique."
   2 "You should remove one layer of gauze at a time to be sure that you don't pull on any underlying drain."
   3 "Next time, when you remove the dressing, use a pair of sterile gloves."
   4 "When you remove the gauze, you should moisten it first with saline."

10 A patient on the general surgery unit has a 4 inch–long incision that has developed a wound infection. On inspection there is a moderate amount of yellowish drainage that has a distinct odor. The health care provider has ordered a foam dressing. A gauze abdominal (ABD) pad is the secondary dressing for covering the foam. Since the dressing has to be changed every 24 hours, which is the best material to use to secure the ABD pads?
   1 Nonallergenic tape
   2 Transparent film dressing
   3 Montgomery ties
   4 Adhesive tape

REFERENCES

Agency for Healthcare Research and Quality (AHRQ): *Negative-pressure wound therapy devices*, Rockville, Md, 2009, AHRQ, available at http://www.ahrq.gov/clinic/ta/negpresswtd/negpresswtd.pdf, accessed January 8, 2012.

Baranoski S, Ayello E: Wound dressings: An evolving art and science, *Adv Skin Wound Care* 25(2):88, 2012.

Borquist O, Ingemansson R, Malmsiö M: Individualizing the use of negative-pressure wound therapy for optimal wound healing: a focused review of the literature, *Ostomy Wound Manage* 57(4):44, 2011.

Campbell P, Smith G, Smith J: Retrospective clinical evaluation of gauze-based negative-pressure wound therapy, *Int Wound J* 5(2):280, 2008.

Cheifetz O, et al: The effect of abdominal support on functional outcomes in patients following major abdominal surgery: a randomized controlled trial, *Physiother Can* 62(3):242, 2010.

Doughty D, Sparks-DeFriese B: Wound-healing physiology. In Bryant RA, Nix DP: *Acute and chronic wounds: nursing management*, ed 4, St Louis, 2011, Mosby.

Galanti GA: *Caring for patients from different cultures*, ed 4, Philadelphia, 2008, University of Pennsylvania Press.

Granville-Chapman J, Jacobs N, Midwinter MJ: Pre-hospital haemostatic dressings: a systematic review, *Injury* 42(5):447, 2011.

Hockenberry MJ, Wilson D: *Wong's nursing care of infants and children*, ed 9, St Louis, 2011, Mosby.

Hurd T, et al: Impact of gauze-based NPWT on the patient and nursing experience in the treatment of challenging wounds, *Int Wound J* 7(6):448, 2010.

Kinetic Concepts: *The V.A.C. vacuum-assisted closure: V.A.C. therapy clinical guidelines: a reference source for clinicians, product information*, San Antonio, Tex, 2012, Kinetic Concepts, Inc.

Krasner DL: Wound pain: impact and assessment. In Bryant RA, Nix DP: *Acute and chronic wounds: nursing management*, ed 4, St Louis, 2011, Mosby.

Larson CM, et al: The effect of abdominal binders on postoperative pulmonary function, *Am Surg* 75(2):169, 2009.

Martindell D: The safe use of negative-pressure wound therapy, *AJN* 112(6):61, 2012.

Michaels J, Coon D, Rubin P: Complications in postbariatric body contouring: Postoperative management and treatment, *Plastic Reconstr Surg* 127(4):1695, 2011.

National Pressure Ulcer Advisory Panel (NPUAP) and European Pressure Ulcer Advisory Panel (EPUAP): *Prevention and treatment of pressure ulcers*, Washington, DC, 2009, National Pressure Ulcer Advisory Board.

Netsch DSL: *Negative-pressure wound therapy. In Bryant RA, Nix DP: Acute and chronic wounds: nursing management*, ed 4, St Louis, 2011, Mosby.

Orgill D, et al: The mechanisms of action of vacuum-assisted closure: more to learn, *J Surg* 146(1):40, 2009.

Petkar KS, et al: A prospective randomized controlled trial comparing negative-pressure dressing and conventional dressing methods on split-thickness skin grafts in burned patients, *Burns* 37(6):925, 2011.

Price RN, et al: Local anesthetic for change of vacuum-assisted closure in wound care management, *Plast Reconstr Surg* 117(7):2537, 2006.

Ramundo JM: Wound debridement. In Bryant RA, Nix DP, editors: *Acute and chronic wounds: nursing management*, ed 4, St Louis, 2011, Mosby.

Rolstad BS, Bryant RA, Nix DP: Topical management. In Bryant RA, Nix DP: *Acute and chronic wounds: nursing management*, ed 4, St Louis, 2011, Mosby.

The Joint Commission (TJC): *National Patient Safety Goals*, Oakbrook Terrace, Ill, 2012, The Commission, available at http://www.jointcommission.org/standards_information/npsgs.aspx.

Wooten MK, Hawkins K: *WOCN position statement: Clean versus sterile: management of chronic wounds*, Glenview, Ill, 2005, Wound, Ostomy, and Continence Nurses Society.

Wound, Ostomy and Continence Nurses (WOCN) Society: *Guideline for prevention and management of pressure ulcers: WOCN clinical practice guideline series No. 2*, Glenview Ill, 2010, WOCN Society.

Wysocki AB: Anatomy and physiology of skin and soft tissue. In Bryant RA, Nix DP: *Acute and chronic wounds: nursing management*, ed 4, St Louis, 2011, Mosby.

Therapeutic Use of Heat and Cold

MEDIA RESOURCES

- eVolve *learning system* http://evolve.elsevier.com/Perry/skills
  - Review Questions
  - Audio Glossary

KEY TERMS

Compress	Evaporation	Neuropathy	Vasoconstriction
Conduction	Insulator	Piloerection	Vasodilation
Cryotherapy	Maceration	Sitz bath	

OBJECTIVES

Mastery of content in this chapter will enable the nurse to:
- Identify the effects of heat and cold on a patient.
- Differentiate the types of injuries or conditions that benefit from heat and cold applications.
- Identify the risks to patients related to heat and cold applications.
- Explain common guidelines used to protect patients who receive heat and cold applications.
- Correctly apply heat and cold applications.

Local application of moderate heat and cold to body parts provides comfort and pain relief, reduces muscle spasm, improves mobility, and promotes healing. To use heat and cold therapies safely, you need to understand how the body responds to temperature variations normally and the risks connected with these applications.

Exposure to heat or cold causes both systemic and local responses (Table 40-1). The hypothalamus regulates body temperature through a variety of mechanisms that control heat production and loss (Garner and Fendius, 2011). Body temperature is affected by environmental and internal factors. When the skin is exposed to warm or hot temperatures, vasodilation and perspiration occur to promote heat loss. As perspiration evaporates from the skin, cooling occurs. When the skin is exposed to cool or cold temperatures, the systemic response includes vasoconstriction and piloerection to conserve heat. Shivering occurs in response to cooler temperatures, producing heat through skeletal muscle contraction.

Sensory adaptation to local temperature extremes can occur quickly within the body. Although a person may initially feel a temperature extreme, once the sensory receptors adapt, he or she may become unaware of any temperature variation. Eventually excessive heat causes a burning sensation, and excessive cold causes a numbing sensation before pain is sensed. Because of this physiologic phenomenon, there is a high risk for tissue injury from heat and cold applications. Certain patients have a greater risk for injury from warm and cold applications (Table 40-2). You play an important role in maintaining patients' safety in the application of heat and cold. An order for a heat or cold application is always necessary, and it should include the duration of the treatment and the desired temperature to be used when settings can be controlled. In health care agencies materials distribution departments typically set temperature settings on heat and cold devices. Because many of these therapies can be used at home, instruct patients and their families in their proper use.

When using heat or cold therapies, you can use either dry or moist applications. The selection depends on the expected outcome of the therapy. Temperature travels from an external source such as a compress or heating pad to the surface of the skin. A substance that conducts temperatures poorly is a good insulator and thus a protector for skin and tissues. However, there are distinct advantages to using both dry and moist applications (Table 40-3).

EVIDENCE-BASED PRACTICE

The application of ice or cryotherapy is one of the most widely used therapeutic modalities in the management of acute musculoskeletal injuries (Pescasio et al., 2008). The use of cryotherapy has a direct effect on the conduction of pain impulses, which occurs when the skin temperature is lowered (Lane and Latham, 2009). The use of cryotherapy for various injuries has a positive effect on pain relief. First, cold vasoconstricts the vasculature in adjacent tissues and slows bleeding into damaged tissues. Second, cryotherapy decreases the release of inflammatory mediators from the damaged tissues, which hinders protein release from the vasculature and decreases edema. Last, cold has an analgesic effect, which is believed to be caused by slowing of nerve conduction (Gottschalk, 2011). Cold in combination with compression reduces bleeding, edema, and muscle spasm. In addition, it reduces recovery time as part of the rehabilitation program for the treatment of both acute and chronic injuries (Markert, 2011).

Hypothermia and hyperthermia devices are used selectively for specific clinical conditions. They are designed to raise, lower, or maintain temperature through heat or cold transfer between the device and the patient. A systematic review noted that

mild-to-moderate prophylactic hypothermia improves neurologic recovery after brain injury (Fox et al., 2010). In addition, another study, which examined the best method to prevent hypothermia during surgery, tested a variety of warming devices. This study noted that circulating water devices were the most effective in maintaining body temperature control during surgery (Galvao et al., 2010).

- Do not microwave towels or medical products used for heat application.
- Consider patient age, skin and circulation, vital signs, ability to sense temperature, and ability to communicate before applying heat or cold therapies (Ebbinghaus and Kobayashi, 2010).
- A combination of cold and heat therapy is effective in adults and children with musculoskeletal injuries to reduce inflammation and edema and improve joint function (Gottschalk, 2011; Lane and Latham, 2009).

TABLE 40-1	Pathophysiologic Effects of Hot and Cold Applications	
	Cold	**Hot**
Pain	↓	↓
Spasm	↓	↓
Metabolism	↓	↑
Blood flow	↓	↑
Inflammation	↓	↑
Edema	↓	↑
Extensibility	↓	↑

Modified from Garner A, Fendius A: Temperature physiology, assessment and control, *Br J Neurosci Nurs* 6(8): 397, 2011; Physiotherapy Canada: 6. Superficial heat, *Physiother Can* 62(5):47, 2010, DOI:10.3138/ptc2009-09-s6.

TABLE 40-3	Warm Application: Moist versus Dry	
Type	**Advantages**	**Disadvantages**
Moist application	Reduces drying of skin and softens wound exudate	Can cause maceration of skin with prolonged exposure
	Conforms well to body area being treated	Cools rapidly because of moisture evaporation
	Penetrates deeply into tissue layers	Creates greater risk for burns to skin because moisture conducts heat
	Lessens sweating and insensible fluid loss	
Dry application	Less likely to burn skin	Increases insensible fluid loss through sweating
	Does not cause skin maceration	Does not penetrate deep into tissue
	Retains temperature longer because not influenced by evaporation	Causes increased drying of skin

TABLE 40-2	Characteristics of Hot and Cold Application		
	Examples of Conditions	**Precautions**	**Adverse Outcomes**
Cold application	Immediately after direct trauma such as sprain, strains, fractures, muscle spasms; after superficial lacerations or puncture wounds; after minor burns; chronic pain from arthritis, joint trauma; delayed-onset muscle soreness; inflammation	Circulatory insufficiency Cold allergy Diabetes mellitus	Cardiovascular effects (bradycardia) Raynaud's phenomenon Cold urticaria Nerve and tissue damage Slow wound healing Frostbite
Heat application	Inflamed or edematous body part; new surgical wound; infected wound; arthritis; degenerative joint disease; localized joint pain, muscle strains; low back pain; menstrual cramping; hemorrhoidal, perianal, and vaginal inflammation; local abscess	Pregnancy Laminectomy sites Spinal cord Malignancy Vascular insufficiency Eyes, testes, heart	Burns Infections Increased pain Increased inflammation

Modified from Physiotherapy Canada: 6. Superficial heat, *Physiother Can* 62(5):47, 2010, DOI:10.3138/ptc2009-09-s6.

PATIENT-CENTERED CARE

It is important to individualize care to meet a patient's needs and preferences. Remember that patient safety, comfort, and privacy are important when using warm or cold therapies. Burns and skin injuries sustained from hot or cold therapies are serious reportable events and are preventable errors (NQF, 2011). Patients with vascular diseases such as peripheral vascular disease or diabetes are at increased risk for injuries from hot or cold therapies because they have decreased sensation in the hands, feet, and other areas. As a result, a patient may not perceive the sensation of burning or numbness.

Instruct the patient to report any sensations in the affected area such as burning, tingling, pain, excessive redness, or pallor, which may indicate discontinuation of therapy. Involving a patient and family caregivers in these therapeutic modalities helps prepare for discharge and provides an opportunity for a nurse to understand patient or caregiver concerns. When explaining the use of warm and cold therapy to patients, the meaning and significance of the therapy can take on very different interpretations based on a patient's culture. Therefore it is important to assess the culture-specific applications of warm and cold principles for each patient and his or her family members:

- Assess how warm and cold are used normally in the care of the patient in the home.
- Reinforce the purpose of the therapy and identify patient concerns or questions.
- During the application of heat or cold therapy, the patient or his or her extremities may be exposed; maintain comfort and privacy by additional blankets, privacy curtains, and room doors. Some patients refuse being exposed to reduce body temperature.
- Many cultures such as Hispanic, Arab, Asian, African, Caribbean, and Eastern European adhere to the hot-and-cold theory. It is believed that too much exposure to something "hot" or "cold" causes an illness (Giger, 2013).
  - For Asians hot and cold concepts are part of the yin and yang concept that integrates balance and holistic health. The goal of hot and cold principles is to restore balance by providing the opposite of the cause or problem (e.g., pneumonia, cramps, and colic are considered "cold" diseases). For example, wrapping extremities and layering blankets are common treatments for colds.
  - Use cultural brokers such as family members, health care providers, and religious leaders to increase acceptance of critical therapies such as hypothermia or ice packs that contradict a patient's or family's beliefs and practices.

Safety Guidelines

1 Exposed layers of skin are more sensitive to temperature variations than intact skin. Therefore protect damaged skin when applying hot or cold therapy.
2 Know the temperature of the application being used. Many devices such as heating pads or water-flow pads (e.g., Aqua-K pads) have thermostats to regulate temperature. Always check the temperature of a device and of a moist compress applied directly to the skin.
3 Burns and injuries from hot or cold therapies are preventable events (NQF, 2011). If they occur, there are functional implications for patients. In addition, because these are preventable events, there is a potential that the health care costs for these injuries will not be reimbursed to the health care agency.
4 Extremities or perineal areas have decreased fat and underlying tissue and are more sensitive than others to temperature extremes. Modify the intensity of heat and cold when treating sensitive skin areas.
5 Check the patient frequently during a heat or cold application. The condition of the skin indicates whether tissue injury is occurring. Observe for signs of excessive redness, maceration, or blistering.
6 Know your patient's risk for injury from heat or cold. Certain patients are more predisposed to injury than others (see Table 40-2).
7 Do not allow patients to adjust temperature settings. It is common for a patient to adapt to a temperature extreme and then want to adjust the temperature.
8 Never position patients so they cannot move away from the temperature source. This avoids the risk for injuries from temperature exposure. The hospitalized patient should always have a call light within reach.
9 If patients have diabetes mellitus or peripheral vascular diseases, it is important to use caution when applying hot or cold therapies. In addition, these patients require more frequent skin assessment during the treatment.
10 Do not leave a patient unattended if he or she is unable to sense temperature changes or move away from the temperature source. You are responsible for the patient's safety.
11 Discourage a patient from moving an application. This may cause injury to an unprotected area of the body and decrease the effectiveness of therapy.
12 Be aware of the impact that heat application has on a patient's vital signs. In particular, a Sitz bath causes localized vasodilation. If this vasodilation is significant, the patient's blood pressure may decrease, causing dizziness and increasing a patient's risk for falls.

SKILL 40-1   Applying Moist Heat

Application of heat promotes relaxation and healing and relieves muscle spasm and joint stiffness. Factors to consider before application include level of temperature and duration of the heat therapy and the nature of the tissues being treated.

Warm compresses and commercial heat packs (Fig. 40-1) are examples of moist heat applications used for a variety of conditions. A warm compress is a section of sterile or clean gauze moistened with a prescribed heated solution (i.e., normal saline or sterile water) and applied directly to an affected area. Commercially

packaged sterile, premoistened compresses are available in some agencies. They require the use of a special infrared lamp to heat. You heat plain sterile or clean gauze by adding the gauze to a container of warmed solution. A commercial heat pack produces its own moisture by drawing moisture from humidity in the air and retaining it in the hot pack's outer flannel cover.

Moist heat application also includes the use of warm baths, soaks, and sitz baths. A warm bath or soak involves immersion of a body part into a warmed solution. Warm soaks and sitz

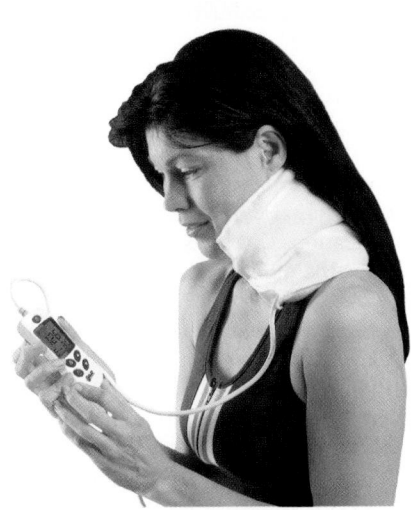

FIG 40-1 Digital moist-heat pack. (*Image used with permission from Theratherm, Chattanooga, a DJO Company. All rights reserved.*)

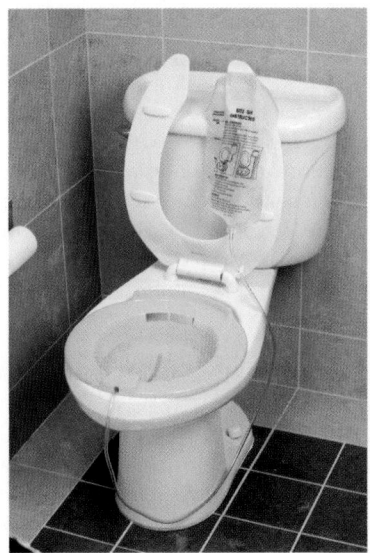

FIG 40-2 Disposable sitz bath. (*Used with permission, Briggs Corporation.*)

baths promote circulation, reduce edema and inflammation, promote muscle relaxation, debride wounds, and apply medicated solutions. If a body part is too large to immerse, you can soak it by wrapping it in a dressing saturated with the prepared, warmed solution.

You give a sitz bath with a special tub or chair basin that allows a patient to sit in water without immersing the legs, feet, and upper trunk (Fig. 40-2). Sitz basins are disposable and especially easy to use in the home. Portable baths fit easily on top of toilets. Patients who have undergone perineal or rectal surgery, who have had an episiotomy during childbirth, or who have painful hemorrhoids or perineal inflammation benefit from a sitz bath.

When preparing a soak or bath, remember that the heated solution is in direct contact with the patient's skin. Be sure to check water temperature frequently to prevent burns. It is desirable to keep the solution temperature constant to enhance the therapeutic effects of the moist heat. Whenever you add heated solution to a soak basin or bath, remove the patient's body part and reimmerse once the solution has mixed.

Delegation and Collaboration

The skill of applying moist heat can be delegated to nursing assistive personnel (NAP). The nurse must assess the condition of the skin and tissues in the area that is treated, evaluate the patient's response, and explain the purpose of the treatment. The nurse instructs the NAP about:

- Proper temperature of the application.
- Skin changes to immediately report to the nurse (e.g., burning or excessive redness).
- Informing the nurse if the patient complains of dizziness or light-headedness.
- Reporting when treatment is complete so an evaluation of the patient's response can be made.

Equipment

All Moist Heat Applications
- ❏ Warmed prescribed solution (i.e., normal saline) or commercially prepared compresses or commercial heat pack
- ❏ Dry bath towel, bath blanket
- ❏ Clean gloves
- ❏ Waterproof pad

Clean Compress
- ❏ Warmed prescribed solution (i.e., normal saline) or commercially prepared compresses
- ❏ Waterproof pad
- ❏ Ties or cloth tape
- ❏ Aquathermia pad (optional)
- ❏ Biohazard waste bag
- ❏ Clean gloves
- ❏ Clean basin
- ❏ Clean gauze or towel

Sterile Compress (see Clean Compress above)
- ❏ Warmed prescribed sterile solution (i.e., normal saline)
- ❏ Sterile gloves
- ❏ Sterile basin
- ❏ Sterile gauze or towel

Soak or Sitz Bath
- ❏ Clean basin, tub, or sitz bath (basin may need to be sterile if body part to be soaked has an open wound)
- ❏ Prescribed solution warmed to appropriate temperature (tap water is commonly used for sitz baths)
- ❏ Prescribed medication (if ordered)

STEP	RATIONALE

ASSESSMENT

1 Refer to health care provider's order for type of moist heat application, location and duration of application, desired temperature, and agency policies regarding temperature.	Ensures safe and correct application.
2 Assess skin around area to be treated. Perform neurovascular assessments for sensitivity to temperature and pain by measuring light touch, pinprick, and temperature sensation (see Chapter 6).	Certain conditions alter conduction of sensory impulses that transmit temperature and pain, predisposing patients to injury from heat applications. Patients with diminished sensation to heat or cold must be monitored closely during treatment.

Clinical Decision Point *Patients with diabetes mellitus, stroke or spinal cord injury, peripheral neuropathy, and rheumatoid arthritis are at greater risk for thermal injury (Physiotherapy Canada, 2010).*

3 Refer to patient's medical record to identify any contraindications to moist heat application: unstable cardiac conditions, active bleeding, nitroglycerin or other therapeutic medicinal patch, acute inflammatory reactions, recent (<72 hours) musculoskeletal injury, and skin conditions such as eczema.	Patients with certain cardiovascular conditions and who exhibit side effects of certain medications may be at risk for sudden changes in blood pressure and blood flow caused by vasodilation (Physiotherapy Canada, 2010). Heat causes vasodilation, which aggravates active bleeding, which can increase hemorrhage or bleeding into the soft tissues adjacent to a musculoskeletal injury (Lane and Latham, 2009). Vasodilation increases the rate of medication absorption when direct heat is applied over a medication patch. Eczema is a heat-sensitive condition, and topical application of heat can worsen condition (Physiotherapy Canada, 2010).

Clinical Decision Point *Reconfirm the health care provider's order when there is an area of active bleeding or inflammation.*

4 Inspect any wound for size, color, drainage, tenderness, and odor (this may be deferred until dressing is removed and heat is applied).	Provides baseline to determine change in a wound following heat application.
5 Assess patient's blood pressure and pulse.	Establishes baseline to determine response to therapy (Physiotherapy Canada, 2010).
6 Assess patient's mobility: ability to position self for soak application, position self in bath, and sit up from bath.	Determines level of assistance needed to position patient for treatment.
7 Assess patient's overall level of comfort using an appropriate pain scale (0 to 10).	Provides baseline for patient's comfort level.
8 Assess patient's and family member's understanding of application and related safety factors.	Determines need for health teaching.

NURSING DIAGNOSES

- Acute pain
- Chronic pain

- Deficient knowledge regarding heat therapy
- Impaired physical mobility

- Impaired skin integrity
- Ineffective peripheral tissue perfusion
- Risk for injury

Related factors are individualized based on patient's condition or needs.

PLANNING

1 Expected outcomes following completion of procedure:	
• Affected area is pink and warm to touch immediately after heat application.	Vasodilation increases blood flow to site.
• After multiple applications, wound shows signs of healing (e.g., tissue granulation; reduced edema, inflammation, drainage).	Moist heat increases blood flow, enhances white blood cell infiltration, and removes waste products from cells (Lane and Latham, 2009).
• Patient denies burning sensation.	Indicates appropriate temperature applied.
• Patient reports measurable decrease in pain.	Heat reduces edema/inflammation and relaxes stiff and strained muscles. Heat applications cause pain signals to be overridden and decrease pain perception in cerebral cortex (Lane and Latham, 2009).
• Blood pressure and pulse are within patient's normal range.	No systemic vascular changes occur. Goal of therapy is to achieve a localized vascular response.
• Patient is able to self-apply therapy safely.	Measures level of learning; necessary for home care.

STEP	RATIONALE
2 Assemble and prepare equipment and supplies.	Organization of supplies prevents unnecessary delays in procedure.
3 Explain steps of procedure and purpose to patient. Describe sensation that patient will feel such as decreasing warmth and wetness. Explain precautions to prevent burning.	Minimizes patient's anxiety and promotes cooperation during procedure.

IMPLEMENTATION

1 Close door if in private room and/or close bedside curtains.	Decreases drafts, thus decreasing transmission of microorganisms. Provides for privacy.
2 Identify patient using two identifiers (i.e., name and birthday or name and account number) according to agency policy. Compare identifiers with information on patient's identification bracelet.	Ensures correct patient. Complies with The Joint Commission Standards and improves patient safety (TJC, 2012).
3 Perform hand hygiene and apply clean gloves.	Reduces transmission of infection.
4 Place waterproof pad under patient (exception: do not do this with sitz bath or a commercial heat pad).	Protects bed linen from moisture and soiling.
5 **Apply moist sterile compress:**	
a Help patient to comfortable position in proper body alignment. Expose body part to be covered with compress and drape patient with bath blanket.	Limited mobility in uncomfortable position causes muscular stress. Prevents cooling.
b Heat prescribed solution to desired temperature by immersing closed bottle of solution in basin of very warm water.	Prevents burns by ensuring proper temperature of solution.
c Remove any present existing dressing covering wound. Dispose of gloves and dressings in biohazard bag.	Reduces transmission of microorganisms.
d Inspect condition of wound and surrounding skin. Inflamed wound appears reddened, but surrounding skin is less red in color.	Provides baseline to measure wound healing.

Clinical Decision Point *If skin surrounding wound is inflamed or reddened or has active drainage, moist heat application may be contraindicated.*

e Perform hand hygiene.	Reduces transmission of microorganisms.
f Prepare compress.	
(1) Open sterile supplies (see Chapter 8). Pour warmed solution into sterile container.	Sterile compress is needed when applied to open wound.
(2) Use sterile technique to add sterile gauze into warmed sterile solution to immerse gauze.	
(3) If using portable heating source, warm solution. NOTE: *If using a commercially prepared compress, follow manufacturer instructions for warming.*	

Clinical Decision Point *To avoid injury to a patient, test temperature of sterile solution by applying drop to your forearm (without contaminating solution). It should feel warm to the skin without burning.*

g Prepare aquathermia pad (option) (see Skill 40-2) or commercial heat pack (if needed).	Aquathermia pad or heat pack is often needed to maintain temperature of a gauze compress.
h Apply sterile gloves if dressing change is sterile; otherwise apply clean gloves.	Allows you to manipulate sterile dressing and touch open wound.
i Pick up one layer of immersed gauze, wring out any excess solution, and apply it lightly to open wound; avoid surrounding skin.	Excess moisture macerates skin and increases risk for burns and infection. Skin is sensitive to sudden change in temperature.
j After a few seconds, lift edge of gauze to assess for redness.	Increased redness indicates burn. Burns and injuries from hot therapies are preventable events (NQF, 2011).
k If patient tolerates compress, pack gauze snugly against wound. Be sure to cover all wound surfaces with warm compress.	Packing compress prevents rapid cooling from underlying air currents.
l Cover moist compress with dry sterile dressing and bath towel. If necessary, pin or tie in place. Remove and dispose of sterile gloves.	Dry sterile dressing prevents transfer of microorganisms to wound via capillary action caused by moist compress. Towel insulates compress to prevent heat loss.

STEP	RATIONALE
m Apply aquathermia, commercial heat pack, or waterproof heating pad (see Skill 40-2) over towel. Keep it in place for desired duration of application.	Provides constant temperature to compress.
n If aquathermia pad or commercial heat pack is *not* used, change warm compress using sterile technique every 5 to 10 minutes or as ordered during duration of therapy.	Prevents cooling and maintains therapeutic benefit of compress.
o After prescribed time, apply clean gloves and remove pad, towel, and compress. Reassess wound and condition of skin and replace dry sterile dressing (using sterile gloves) as ordered.	Continued exposure to moisture macerates skin. Prevents entrance of microorganisms into wound site.
p Help patient to preferred comfortable position.	Maintains patient's comfort.
q Dispose of equipment and soiled compress. Perform hand hygiene.	Reduces transmission of microorganisms.
6 Sitz bath or warm soak to intact skin or wound:	
a Remove any existing dressing covering wound. Dispose of gloves and dressings in proper receptacle and perform hand hygiene.	Reduces transmission of microorganisms.
b Inspect condition of wound and surrounding skin. Pay particular attention to suture line.	Provides baseline to determine response to warm soak.
c When exudate is present, apply clean gloves and clean intact skin around open area with clean cloth and soap and water or sterile gauze, in which case sterile gloves and sterile normal saline or water are needed. Dispose of gloves and perform hand hygiene.	Cleaning prevents transmission of microorganisms.
d Fill sitz bath or bathtub in bathroom with warmed solution. Check temperature (check agency policy).	Ensures proper temperature and reduces risk for burns.
e Help patient to bathroom to immerse body part in sitz bath, bathtub, or basin. Cover patient with bath blanket or towel as needed.	Prevents falls. Covering patient prevents heat loss through evaporation and maintains constant temperature.
f Assess heart rate. Make sure that patient does not feel light-headed or dizzy and that call light is within reach.	Provides baseline to determine if vascular response to vasodilation occurs during treatment.
g Maintain constant temperature throughout 15- to 20-minute soak.	Ensures proper therapeutic effect.
h After 15 to 20 minutes remove patient from soak or bath; dry body parts thoroughly. (Wear clean gloves if drainage is present.)	Avoids chilling. Enhances patient's comfort.
i Drain solution from basin or tub. Clean and place in proper storage area. Dispose of soiled linen and gloves; perform hand hygiene.	Reduces transmission of microorganisms.

EVALUATION

1 Inspect condition of body part or wound treated for evidence of healing. Observe skin color, temperature, edema, and sensitivity to touch.	Evaluates effectiveness of treatment and risk for potential injury.
2 Ask patient to describe level of comfort on scale of 0 to 10. Ask about any sensation of burning following treatment.	Determines if patient was exposed to temperature extreme, resulting in burn. Evaluates patient's subjective response to therapy.
3 Obtain vital signs and compare with baseline.	Determines if systemic vascular response to vasodilation has occurred.
4 Observe patient demonstrate application of therapy and explain its purpose.	Measures level of learning and ability to perform application.

Unexpected Outcomes

1 Patient's skin is reddened and sensitive to touch. Extreme warmth caused burning of skin layer.

2 Patient complains of burning and discomfort.

Related Interventions

- Discontinue moist application immediately.
- Verify proper temperature or check device for proper functioning.
- Notify health care provider and, if there is a burn, complete an incident report (see agency policy).

- Reduce temperature.
- Assess for skin breakdown.
- Notify health care provider.

Recording and Reporting

- Record and report procedure, noting type, location, and duration of application; solution and temperature; condition of body part, wound, and skin before and after treatment; and patient's response to therapy.
- Record preprocedure and postprocedure vital signs (as indicated).
- Record any instructions given and patient's ability to explain and perform procedure.

Special Considerations

Teaching

- If a patient needs to continue heat applications after discharge, have patient or family member give a return demonstration before discharge.
- Teach patient how to gently pack wound to avoid discomfort.
- Caregivers and patients need to learn that careful assessment is needed for patients with reduced sensation to determine if temperature of compress is too hot.

Pediatric

- The skin of infants and children is thin and fragile and therefore easily damaged. Use special caution with application of heat in this population (Hockenberry and Wilson, 2011). Remain with children during procedure for safety and effectiveness.

- It is often helpful to incorporate play into the time a child is required to soak. Placing items with which the child can interact in the basin is helpful. Place boats or other similar water toys in the bath with a child who requires a bath soak. Adult supervision is necessary.

Gerontologic

- An older adult who is receiving long-term steroid therapy or is malnourished can develop thin, fragile skin, which is more easily damaged. Skin becomes less elastic and more prone to tears with aging. An older adult may have impaired circulation to a given skin region or impaired sensation for pain or temperature (Meiner, 2011).
- Older adults who have lost subcutaneous tissue and fat have lost the insulating effect of these tissues and may experience alterations in thermoregulation (Meiner, 2011).
- In some frail older patients with cardiac conditions, it is necessary to monitor vital signs throughout procedure.

Home Care

- When necessary, assess availability of family caregiver to help patient in application of moist heat, family caregiver's understanding of purpose of procedure, and willingness of caregiver to comply with procedure and not leave patient.
- Assess physical environment to determine adequacy of facilities for use by patient. Patient may need assistive devices to get in or out of a tub or a commode chair to set up a sitz bath.

SKILL 40-2 Applying Dry Heat

A water-flow pad such as an aquathermia pad, electric heating pads, and commercial heat packs (Fig. 40-3) are common forms of dry heat therapy. A new product, an air-activated wearable heat wrap, maintains a temperature of 40°C (104°F) and can be worn from 8 to 10 hours (Ebbinghaus and Kobayashi, 2010). Dry heat devices are applied directly to the surface of the skin; for this reason you need to take extra precautions to prevent burns, dry skin, and loss of body fluids. The aquathermia pad (water-flow pad) used in health care settings consists of a waterproof rubber or plastic pad connected by two hoses to an electrical control unit that has a heating element and motor. Distilled water circulates through hollowed channels in the pad to the control unit where water is heated (or cooled). In most health care facilities the central supply department sets the temperature regulators to the recommended temperature. A temperature of 40°C (104°F) is a safe temperature to expose the skin for a long duration (Ebbinghaus and Kobayashi,

2010). Dry-heat treatments penetrate a child's skin superficially about $\frac{1}{5}$ inch (0.5 cm) but maintain temperature changes longer than moist-heat treatments (Ebbinghaus and Kobayashi, 2010).

A conventional heating pad used in the home care setting consists of an electric coil enclosed in a waterproof cover. A cotton or flannel cloth covers the outer pad. The pad connects to an electrical cord that has a temperature-regulating unit for high, medium, or low settings. These pads are not used in health care facilities. Because it is so easy to readjust temperature settings on heating pads, instruct patients not to turn the setting higher once they have adapted to the temperature. Instruct patient and family not to use the highest setting.

Delegation and Collaboration

The skill of applying dry heat can be delegated to nursing assistive personnel (NAP) (see agency policy). The nurse must assess and evaluate the condition of the skin and tissues in the area that is treated and explain the purpose of the treatment. If there are risks or expected complications, this skill cannot be delegated. The nurse directs the NAP about:

- Specific positioning and time requirements to keep the application in place based on health care provider order or agency policy.
- What to observe and report immediately such as excessive redness and pain during application.
- Reporting when treatment is complete so the patient's response can be evaluated.

Equipment

- ❑ Aquathermia or commercial heat pack
- ❑ Distilled water (for aquathermia pad)
- ❑ Bath towel or pillowcase
- ❑ Tape ties or gauze roll

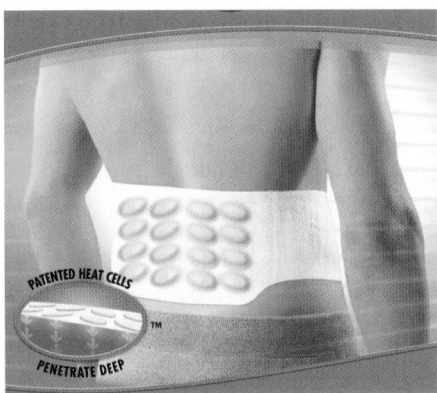

FIG 40-3 Dry heat wrap. (*Image used with permission, ThermaWrap, Pfizer Consumer Healthcare. All rights reserved.*)

STEP	RATIONALE

ASSESSMENT

STEP	RATIONALE
1 Refer to health care provider's order for location of application and duration of therapy. Agency policy usually sets recommended temperature for aquathermia pad.	Order required to help ensure patient's safety. Preset temperature on device reduces risk of skin and tissue injury.
2 Assess condition of skin and underlying tissue in area where you will apply pad for skin integrity, color, temperature, sensitivity to touch, blistering, and excessive dryness (see Chapter 6).	Provides baseline to determine change in skin condition after heat application.
3 Ask patient to describe level of comfort on a scale of 0 to 10. Assess range of motion (ROM) if patient is being treated for muscle sprain.	Provides baseline to determine if pain relief is achieved.
4 Check electrical plugs and cords for obvious fraying or cracking.	Prevents injury from accidental electrical shock.
5 Determine patient's or family member's knowledge of procedure, including steps for application and safety precautions.	Heating pads are frequently used in home. Assessment determines extent of health teaching required.

NURSING DIAGNOSES

- Acute pain
- Chronic pain
- Deficient knowledge regarding heat application
- Impaired physical mobility
- Impaired skin integrity
- Ineffective peripheral tissue perfusion
- Risk for injury

Related factors are individualized based on patient's condition or needs.

PLANNING

STEP	RATIONALE
1 Expected outcomes following completion of procedure:	
• Skin is pink and warm to touch after application.	Vasodilation from heat exposure increases blood flow to affected part.
• Patient reports less pain of inflamed tissues or strained muscles.	Thermoreceptors, special temperature-sensitive nerve endings, are activated by changes in skin temperature. These receptors initiate nerve signals that block pain signal (Gottschalk, 2011).
• Patient's ROM increases.	Heat reduces stiffness and improves ROM (Lane and Latham, 2009).
• Patient correctly applies pad.	Documents learning.
2 Prepare equipment and supplies.	Organization of supplies prevents unnecessary delays in procedure.
3 Explain procedure and precautions.	Improves likelihood of patient's adherence to therapy.

IMPLEMENTATION

STEP	RATIONALE
1 Close door if in private room and/or close bedside curtains.	Provides for patient's privacy.
2 Identify patient using two identifiers (i.e., name and birthday or name and account number) according to agency policy. Compare identifiers with information on patient's identification bracelet.	Ensures correct patient. Complies with The Joint Commission Standards and improves patient safety (TJC, 2012).
3 Perform hand hygiene and position patient to expose area being treated.	Reduces transfer of microorganisms. Patient must be able to assume position for several minutes during application.
4 Apply dry heat device.	
a Aquathermia heating pad	
(1) Cover or wrap area to be treated with a bath towel or enclose pad with pillowcase.	Prevents heated surface from touching patient's skin directly and increasing risk for injury to patient's skin.

Clinical Decision Point *Do not pin wrap to pad because this may cause a leak in device.*

STEP	RATIONALE
(2) Place pad over affected area and secure with tape, tie, or gauze as needed (see illustration).	Pad delivers dry warm heat to injured tissues. Pad should not slip onto different body part.

Clinical Decision Point *Never position patient so he or she is lying directly on pad. This position prevents dissipation of heat and increases risk for burns.*

STEP	RATIONALE
(3) Turn on aquathermia unit and check temperature setting.	Prevents exposure of patient to temperature extremes.
b Apply commercially prepared heat pack: break pouch inside larger pack (follow manufacturer guidelines).	Activates chemicals within pack to warm outer surface.

STEP	RATIONALE
5 Monitor condition of skin over site every 5 minutes and ask patient about sensation of burning.	Determines if heat exposure is causing any burn, blistering, or injury to underlying skin.
6 After 20 to 30 minutes (or time ordered by health care provider), remove pad and store.	Continued exposure results in burns. Muscles located 1 to 2 cm (0.4 to 0.8 inch) below skin surface in children require heat applied for 20 to 30 minutes to be effective (Ebbinghaus and Kobayashi, 2010).
7 Help patient return to preferred comfortable position, dispose of soiled linen, and perform hand hygiene.	Promotes relaxing environment. Reduces transmission of microorganisms.

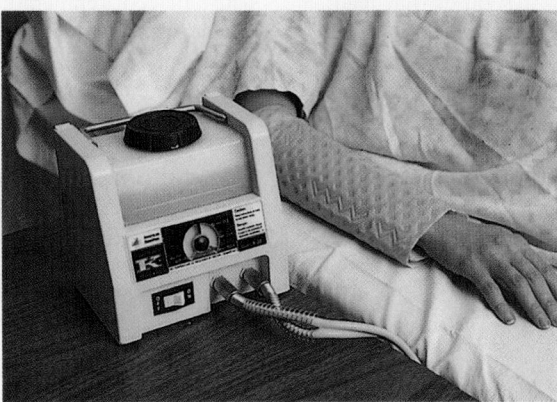

STEP 4a(2) Aquathermia pad.

EVALUATION

1 Inspect condition of skin for integrity, color, temperature, dryness, and blistering. Evaluate again 30 minutes following treatment.	Evaluates response of skin to heat exposure.
2 Assess ROM. Ask patient to rate pain on scale of 0 to 10.	Heat reduces edema and relieves pain from muscle stiffness and spasm (Lane and Latham, 2009). Patient can adequately rate pain relief.

Clinical Decision Point *Do not have patient actively exercise muscle to evaluate results of therapy. Active exercise can aggravate muscle strain.*

3 Observe patient or family caregiver apply pad to be used in home.	Measures level of learning.

Unexpected Outcomes

1 See Skill 40-1, Unexpected Outcomes.

2 Body part is painful to move. Movement stretches burn-sensitive nerve fibers in skin.

3 Patient applies heat incorrectly or is unable to explain precautions.

Related Interventions

- Discontinue aquathermia pad or heat pack use. Wait for swelling to resolve before attempting to reapply.
- Notify nurse in charge or contact health care provider.
- Reinstruct patient or family caregiver as necessary. Consider possible home health referral.

Recording and Reporting

- Record type of application, temperature and duration of therapy, and patient's response.
- Describe any instruction given and patient's/family caregiver's success in demonstrating procedure.
- Report pain level, ROM of body part, skin integrity, color, temperature, sensitivity to touch, blistering and dryness.

Special Considerations
Teaching

- Highlight safety precautions during procedure so they are followed during application.

Pediatric

- The skin of infants and children is thin and fragile and therefore easily damaged. Use special caution in this population. Remain with children during procedure for safety and effectiveness.
- Assess body temperature gain and loss, which occurs more readily in pediatric patients.

Gerontologic

- Older adults are more at risk for burns because of loss of heat sensation. Check site frequently during all treatments.
- Older patients have thin, more fragile skin that is susceptible to burns.

Home Care

- Assess patient and primary caregiver as to their understanding, ability, and motivation to comply with procedure.

- Assess home environment for facilities (e.g., condition of electrical outlets and equipment) to comply with implementation of procedure.

SKILL 40-3   Applying Cold

There are a variety of cold (cryotherapy) modalities such as ice packs, moist cold compresses, chemical cold packs, electromechanical or compression devices, or cold soak immersion of a body part. Cold therapy treats localized inflammatory responses that lead to edema, hemorrhage, muscle spasm, or pain (see Table 40-1). Cold exerts a profound physiologic effect on the body, reducing inflammation caused by injuries to the musculoskeletal system (Markert, 2011). Because reduction of inflammation is the primary goal, cryotherapy is the treatment of choice for the first 24 to 48 hours after an injury (Gottschalk, 2011).

Vasoconstriction resulting from cold application reduces blood flow to the injured part and thus reduces fluid accumulation and slows bleeding and hematoma formation associated with trauma. The lower temperature also suppresses muscle spasm and produces a local anesthetic response, resulting frequently in the reduction of the use of analgesic medications (Lane and Latham, 2009). When used appropriately, cold applications significantly lessen pain and immobility by reducing swelling of injured tissues (Physiotherapy Canada, 2010). This is an important point for nurses to know when deciding on the choice of heat or cold for the treatment of acute injuries. Cold is also indicated as an adjunct analgesic for chronic pain and spasticity control.

A cold compress usually consists of a commercial cold pack or a gauze dressing or washcloth that has been immersed in iced or chilled solution to achieve the desired temperature. The compress may be sterile or clean; however, a clean compress is most common. Any open wounds require sterile applications. There are many sizes or thicknesses of gauze, depending on the site of injury. For example, a cold compress to the eye requires thicker gauze that fits a small area to maintain a cold temperature. Thin gauze works more effectively for larger areas such as the face.

Ice bags and cold packs come in a variety of sizes to fit different body parts (Fig. 40-4). When a commercial ice bag or cold pack is unavailable, use a plastic bag or glove filled halfway with crushed ice. Squeeze the bag or glove to expel air, which hampers cold conduction. In the home a patient can substitute a bag of frozen vegetables (such as peas or corn) for an ice bag. Wrap all of these items in a towel or cloth before application.

There are electrically controlled continuous cold–flow therapy devices that simultaneously provide cold and compression (e.g.,

Cryo/Cuff [Fig. 40-5]). Compression acts with cold to reduce the blood flow and edema formation while providing support to the soft tissues. The cooling pad has the advantage of delivering a constant cool temperature. Elevating the extremity during treatment further augments venous return. A person who undergoes treatment with one of these devices is simultaneously receiving all five components of the *p*rotection, *r*est, *i*ce, *c*ompression, and *e*levation (PRICE) method for managing this type of injury.

Delegation and Collaboration

The skill of applying cold applications can be delegated to nursing assistive personnel (NAP) in special situations (see agency policy). The nurse must assess and evaluate the patient and explain the purpose of the treatment. If there are risks or possible complications, this skill is not delegated. The nurse directs the NAP to:

- Keep the application in place for only the length of time specified in the health care provider's order.
- Immediately report to the nurse any excessive redness on the skin, increase in pain, or decrease in sensation.
- Report when treatment is complete so a nurse can evaluate the patient's response.

Equipment

All Compresses, Bags, and Packs

- ☐ Clean gloves (if blood or body fluids are present)
- ☐ Cloth tape or ties or elastic wrap bandage
- ☐ Soft cloth cover: towel, pillowcase, or stockinette
- ☐ Bath towel or blanket and waterproof pad

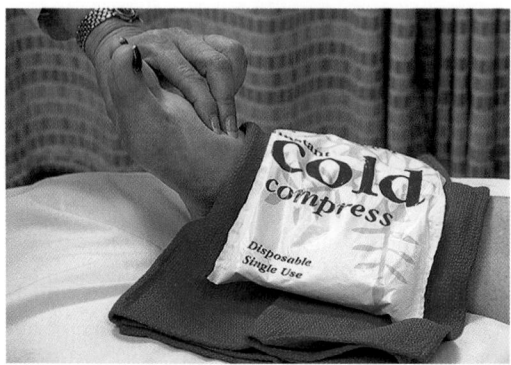

FIG 40-4   Commercial ice pack.

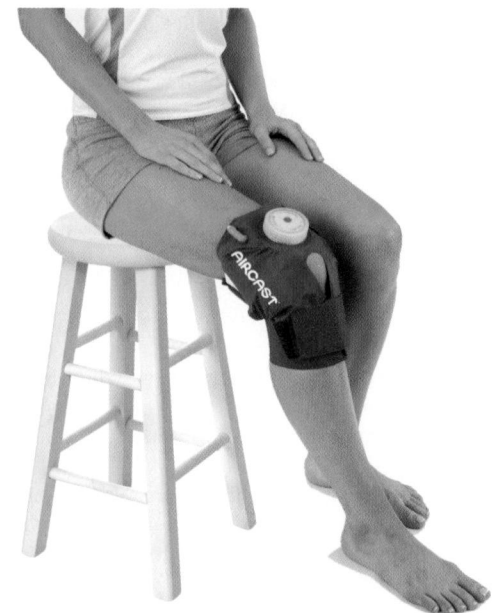

FIG 40-5   Cryo/Cuff includes integrated cooler. (*Image of AirCast Cryo/Cuff used with permission of DJO Global.*)

Cold Compress
- ❑ Absorbent gauze (clean or sterile) folded to desired size
- ❑ Basin
- ❑ Prescribed solution at desired temperature

Ice Bag or Gel Pack
- ❑ Ice bag
- ❑ Ice chips and water

or

- ❑ Reusable commercial gel pack (cold pack)
- ❑ Disposable commercial chemical cold pack

Electrically Controlled Cooling Device
- ❑ Cool water-flow pad or cooling pad and electrical pump
- ❑ Gauze roll or elastic wrap

STEP	RATIONALE
ASSESSMENT	
1 Refer to health care provider's order for type, location, and duration of application. Temperature of a cooling pad will be ordered or preset.	Health care provider's order is required for all cold applications.
2 Inspect condition of injured or affected part. Gently palpate area for edema.	Provides baseline for determining change in condition of injured tissues.

Clinical Decision Point *Keep injured part in alignment and immobilized. Movement can cause further injury to strains, sprains, or fractures.*

STEP	RATIONALE
3 Consider time in which injury occurred.	Apply cold as soon as possible after injury to reduce tissue bleeding and edema (Gottschalk, 2011).
4 Ask patient to describe character of pain and rate severity on a scale of 0 to 10 (or other pain scale when applicable) if able.	Provides baseline for determining pain relief with therapy.
5 Perform neurovascular check and inspect surrounding skin for integrity, circulation, color, temperature, and sensitivity to touch (see Chapter 6).	Determines if patient is insensitive to cold extremes.
6 Assess patient's understanding and/or awareness of procedure.	Patients who are confused or have altered levels of consciousness may not be able to alert nurse that there is decreased sensation or discomfort to underlying skin.

NURSING DIAGNOSES

- Acute pain
- Chronic pain
- Deficient knowledge regarding cold application
- Impaired physical mobility
- Impaired skin integrity
- Ineffective peripheral tissue perfusion
- Risk for injury

Related factors are individualized based on patient's condition or needs.

STEP	RATIONALE
PLANNING	
1 Expected outcomes following completion of procedure:	
• Affected area is slightly pale and cool to touch.	Result of vasoconstriction.
• There is decreased edema and/or bleeding in tissues at site of injury.	Cold reduces blood flow to affected part by reducing protein extravasation from the vasculature and subsequent edema formation (Gottschalk, 2011).
• Patient reports decreased pain as measured on scale of 0 to 10.	Cold decreases local nerve conduction and subsequent pain, creating localized analgesic effect (Gottschalk, 2011).
• Patient correctly states how to apply cold and provides demonstration.	Documents learning.
2 Prepare equipment and supplies.	Organization prevents unnecessary delays.
3 Explain procedure and precautions.	Improves likelihood of patient's adherence to therapy.
IMPLEMENTATION	
1 Close room door and bedside curtain. Perform hand hygiene.	Provides privacy for patient. Reduces spread of microorganisms.
2 Identify patient using two identifiers (i.e., name and birthday or name and account number) according to agency policy. Compare identifiers with information on patient's identification bracelet.	Ensures correct patient. Complies with The Joint Commission Standards and improves patient safety (TJC, 2012).
3 Position patient carefully, keeping body part in proper alignment and only exposing area to be treated, and drape patient with bath blankets.	Prevents further injury to body part. Avoids unnecessary exposure of body parts, maintaining patient's comfort and privacy.
4 Place towel or absorbent pad under area that you will treat.	Prevents soiling of bed linen.

STEP	RATIONALE
5 Apply clean gloves.	Reduces spread of infection.
6 **Apply cold compress:**	
a Place ice and water in basin and test temperature on inner aspect of arm.	Extreme temperature can cause tissue damage.
b Submerge gauze into basin filled with cold solution; wring out excess moisture.	Dripping gauze is uncomfortable to patient.
c Apply compress to affected area, molding it gently over site.	Ensures that cold is directed over site of injury.
d Remove, remoisten, and reapply to maintain temperature as needed.	
7 **Apply ice pack or bag:**	
a Fill bag with water, secure cap, and invert.	Ensures that there are no leaks.
b Empty water and fill bag two-thirds full with small ice chips and water.	Bag is easier to mold over body part when it is not full.
c Express excess air from bag, secure bag closure, and wipe bag dry.	Excess air interferes with cold conduction. Allows bag to conform to area and promotes maximum contact.
d Squeeze or knead commercial ice pack.	Releases alcohol-based solution to create cold temperature.
e Wrap pack or bag with towel, pillowcase, or stockinette. Apply over injury. Secure with tape as needed.	Protects patient's tissue and absorbs condensation. Prevents direct exposure of cold against patient's skin.
8 **Apply commercial gel pack:**	
a Remove from freezer.	
b Wrap pack with towel, pillowcase, or stockinette. Apply pack directly over injury.	Protects patient's tissue and absorbs condensation. Prevents direct exposure of cold against patient's skin.
c Secure with gauze, cloth tape, or ties as needed.	

Clinical Decision Point *Do not reapply ice pack to red or bluish areas; continual use of ice pack makes ischemia worse.*

STEP	RATIONALE
9 **Apply electrically controlled cooling device:**	
a Make sure that all connections are intact and temperature, if adjustable, is set (see agency policy).	Ensures safe temperature application.
b Wrap cool-water flow pad in towel or pillowcase.	Prevents adverse reactions from cold such as burn or frostbite.
c Wrap cool pad around body part.	Ensures even application of cold temperature.
d Turn device on and check correct temperature. (NOTE: Temperature is usually preset in health care settings [check agency policy]).	Ensures effective therapy. Present temperature reduces risk of skin and tissue injury.
e Secure with elastic wrap bandage, gauze roll, or ties.	
10 Remove and dispose of gloves in proper container.	Reduces transmission of microorganisms.
11 Check condition of skin every 5 minutes for duration of application.	Determines if there are adverse reactions to cold (e.g., mottling, redness, burning, blistering, numbness) (Physiotherapy Canada, 2010).
a If area is edematous, sensation may be reduced; use extra caution during cold therapy and assess site more often.	
b Numbness and tingling are common sensations with cold applications and indicate adverse reactions only when severe and coupled with other symptoms. Stop when patient complains of burning sensation or skin begins to feel numb.	When applying cold, skin will initially feel cold, followed by relief of pain. As cryotherapy continues, patient will feel burning sensation, then pain in the skin, and finally numbness (Physiotherapy Canada, 2010).
12 After 15 to 20 minutes (or as ordered by health care provider), apply clean gloves, remove compress or pad, and gently dry off any moisture.	Drying prevents maceration of skin.

Clinical Decision Point *Areas with little body fat (such as knee, ankle, and elbow) do not tolerate cold as well as fatty areas (such as thigh and buttocks). For bony areas decrease time of cold application to lower range.*

STEP	RATIONALE
13 Help patient to comfortable position.	Maintains relaxing environment.
14 Remove and dispose of supplies. Empty basin, if used, and dry. Dispose of soiled linen and gloves. Perform hand hygiene.	Reduces transmission of microorganisms.

STEP	RATIONALE

EVALUATION

1 Inspect affected area for integrity, color, temperature, sensitivity to touch. Reevaluate 30 minutes after procedure.	Determines reaction to cold application.
2 Palpate affected area gently for edema, bruising, and bleeding.	Determines level of edema.
3 Ask patient to report pain level on scale of 0 to 10.	Determines if pain has been relieved.
4 Observe patient, apply cold application, and explain risks of treatment.	Measures level of learning.

Unexpected Outcomes	Related Interventions
1 Skin appears mottled, reddened, or bluish-purple as result of prolonged exposure.	• Stop treatment. • Notify nurse in charge or health care provider. • Different therapy will be needed for injured area.
2 Patient complains of burning type of pain and numbness.	• Stop treatment because these are signs of ischemia. • Notify nurse in charge or health care provider.
3 Patient is unable to describe application or use compress correctly.	• Provide reinstruction and clarification.

Recording and Reporting

- Record procedure, including type, location, and duration of application and patient's response.
- Describe any instruction given and patient's success in demonstrating procedure.
- Report any sensations of burning, numbness, or unrelieved skin color changes to health care provider.

Special Considerations
Teaching

- Injuries requiring this type of therapy usually occur outside of acute care settings. Patients active in sports should know steps to take to minimize extent of injury.

Pediatric

- A greater metabolic rate and larger trunk in relation to the rest of the body make children more prone to hypothermia (Hockenberry and Wilson, 2011). Exercise caution with young patients.
- Infants have an unstable temperature control mechanism; thus mottling of extremities is common and does not always indicate an adverse reaction (Hockenberry and Wilson, 2011).
- Cool soaks also decrease itching with some skin lesions. Use the same precautions and play techniques as with warm soaks.

Gerontologic

- Older adults are more at risk for tissue damage because of altered responses to change in body temperature (Meiner, 2011). Check site frequently during all treatments.

SKILL 40-4   Caring for Patients Requiring Hypothermia or Hyperthermia Blankets

A hypothermia-hyperthermia blanket raises, lowers, or maintains body temperature through conductive heat or cold transfer between the blanket and the patient. When placed on top of a patient, the blanket helps to raise or lower his or her body temperature (Fig. 40-6). When operated manually the unit maintains a set temperature, regardless of the patient's temperature. Because you assess a patient's temperature using conventional thermometers, the temperature of the unit is manually adjusted to reach a different temperature setting. When operating in the automatic setting, the unit continually monitors a patient's temperature with a thermistor probe (rectal, skin, or esophageal). The system increases or decreases the temperature of the circulating water in response to the preset target temperature and actual measured patient temperature.

Patients can have high, prolonged fevers from infectious neurologic diseases and as side effects from anesthesia. Recent research shows that induced hypothermia prevents or moderates neurologic outcomes following neurosurgery or traumatic brain injury and acute stroke (Fox et al., 2010; Linares and Mayer, 2009;

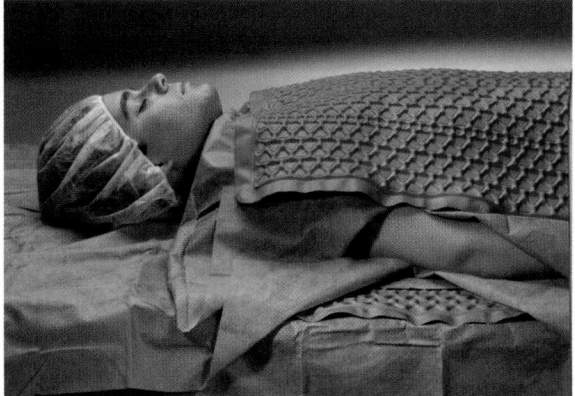

FIG 40-6   Hypothermia cooling blanket is applied over paper sheet before additional top sheet is applied to bed. (*Courtesy Cincinnati SubZero Maxi-Therm Hyper-Hypothermia Blanket.*)

Polderman, 2008; Polderman and Herold, 2009). Mild hypothermia (32° to 34°C [89.6°F to 93.2°F]) in the first hours after an ischemic event and for 72 hours or until stabilization occurs helps prevent permanent damage (Fox et al., 2010).

Delegation and Collaboration

The skill of applying a hypothermia or hyperthermia blanket can be delegated to nursing assistive personnel (NAP) (see agency policy). The nurse is responsible for assessing and evaluating treatment and related patient education. If the patient is unstable and at risk for complications, this skill is not delegated. The nurse directs the NAP to:

- Maintain proper temperature of the application throughout the treatment and discontinue the application as specified in the health care provider's order.

- Inform the nurse of any unexpected patient outcomes (e.g., shivering or redness to the skin).
- Report when treatment is complete so an evaluation of patient's response can be made.

Equipment

- ❏ Hypothermia or hyperthermia blanket with control panel and rectal probe
- ❏ Sheet or thin bath blanket
- ❏ Distilled water to fill the units if necessary
- ❏ Clean gloves
- ❏ Rectal thermometer

STEP	RATIONALE

ASSESSMENT

1 Refer to health care provider's order and check that patient's current body temperature indicates use of hypothermia or hyperthermia blanket.	Instituting therapy requires health care provider's order.
2 Assess vital signs, neurologic status, mental status, and peripheral circulation.	Establishes baseline data to use for comparison during therapy.
3 Verify that other, less intensive measures cannot return patient's body temperature to normal.	Use of hypothermia and hyperthermia blanket is not without risk and should be instituted only when other measures are not effective.

Clinical Decision Point *Antipyretic therapy may be used in combination with a cooling blanket. Temperatures greater than 41°C (105.8°F) have detrimental effects in the neurological patient. As a result some neurological injuries and their sequelae are permanent. A 1°C (1.8°F) rise in body temperature results in a 10% increase in metabolic demands of the body (Kiekkas et al., 2008, 2011).*

4 Assess patient's skin on chest and extremities, paying close attention to bony prominences such as hands and feet.	These areas are more exposed to blanket and consequently are at greater risk for injury. Baseline data enable you to quickly determine if injury to skin or development of pressure ulcer is result of therapy.

NURSING DIAGNOSES

- Hyperthermia
- Impaired skin integrity
- Ineffective peripheral tissue perfusion
- Risk for injury

Related factors are individualized based on patient's condition or needs.

PLANNING

1 Expected outcomes following completion of procedure: • Temperature is within normal range. • Absence of shivering with hypothermia blanket.	Indicates that therapy is effective. Shivering increases metabolic rate and heat production but also increases oxygen consumption. In addition, shivering causes vasoconstriction, which can injure skin of distal body regions (Garner and Fendius, 2011).
• Skin is clear without signs of injury or burns.	Distal regions of patient's skin are at greatest risk for injury from blanket. Indicates that treatment is causing no adverse effects.
2 Explain procedure to patient.	Increases cooperation and reduces anxiety.
3 Position patient comfortably.	
4 Prepare blanket according to agency policy and manufacturer instructions. Manufacturer instructions are usually located on machine.	Agencies have specific policies on maintaining equipment in functional order. Each type of blanket varies from one manufacturer to another.

STEP	RATIONALE
IMPLEMENTATION	
1 Perform hand hygiene and apply clean gloves.	Reduces transmission of microorganisms.
2 Identify patient using two identifiers (i.e., name and birthday or name and account number) according to agency policy. Compare identifiers with information on patient's identification bracelet.	Ensures correct patient. Complies with The joint Commission Standards and improves patient safety (TJC, 2012).
3 Apply lanolin or mixture of lanolin and cold cream to patient's skin where it will touch blanket.	Helps protect skin from heat and cold sensations.
4 Turn on blanket and observe that cool or warm light is on. Precool or prewarm blanket, setting pad temperature to desired level.	Verifies that blanket is correctly set to help reduce (cool) or increase (warm) patient's body temperature. Prepares blanket for prescribed therapy.
5 Verify that pad temperature limits are set at desired safety ranges.	Safety ranges prevent excessive cooling or warming. The blanket automatically shuts off when preset body temperature is achieved.
6 Cover hypothermia or hyperthermia blanket with thin paper or cloth sheet or bath blanket.	Injuries from hot or cold therapies are preventable events (NQF, 2011). Thin sheet protects patient's skin from direct contact with blanket, thus reducing risk for injury to skin. Sheet or blanket covers plastic and provides insulation between patient and appliance.
7 Position hypothermia or hyperthermia blanket on top of patient.	Provides wide distribution of blanket against patient's skin.
a Wrap patient's hands and feet in gauze.	Reduces risk for thermal injury to distal areas of body.
b Wrap scrotum with towels.	Protects sensitive tissue from direct contact with cold.
8 Lubricate rectal probe and insert into patient's rectum.	When using hypothermia or hyperthermia blanket, it is imperative that you continuously monitor patient's core interior (rectal) temperature.
9 Turn and position patient regularly to protect from pressure ulcer development and impaired body alignment (see Chapter 10). Keep linens free of perspiration and condensation.	Patient has increased risk for pressure ulcer development because of skin moisture created by blanket and patient's body temperature.
10 Double-check fluid thermometer on control panel of blanket before leaving room.	Verifies that pad temperature is maintained at desired level.
11 Remove gloves and perform hand hygiene.	Reduces transmission of microorganisms.
EVALUATION	
1 Monitor patient's temperature and vital signs every 15 minutes during first hour and every 30 minutes of therapy thereafter.	Provides continuous evaluation of response of patient's body temperature to therapy during initial and continual therapy.
2 Evaluate automatic temperature control every 30 minutes visually and every 4 hours by taking patient's rectal temperature.	Ensures removal of hypothermia or hyperthermia blanket when patient's temperature returns to desired level. Decreases risk for subnormal body temperature. Verifies accuracy of rectal probe and automatic temperature control device.
3 Observe skin for indications of burns, change in color, and other signs of injury.	Hypothermia and hyperthermia blankets have potential to cause skin injuries.
4 Observe patient for signs of shivering.	Early signs of shivering, which may harm patient, include electrocardiographic changes, facial muscle twitching, or hyperventilation.
5 Determine patient's level of comfort.	Therapy has potential to cause discomfort. Prompt assessment reduces risk for severe injuries.

Unexpected Outcomes

1 Patient's core body temperature decreases or rises rapidly. This indicates that temperature is too extreme and might produce injury to patient.

2 Patient's core temperature remains unchanged.

3 Patient begins to shiver. Shivering increases metabolic rate and heat production, causing patient's core body temperature to rise, and increases oxygen consumption.

4 Skin breaks down, indicating that patient's skin may have received thermal injury (frostbite or burn) from blanket.

Related Interventions

• Adjust blanket temperature no more than 1°F (0.6°C) every 15 minutes to avoid complications.

• Patient may need hypothermic or hyperthermic treatment of additional sites such as axilla, groin, and neck in addition to those covered by blanket.

• Discuss use of antipyretic with health care provider.

• Adjust temperature to more comfortable range and assess if shivering decreases.

• If shivering continues, stop treatment and notify health care provider.

• Stop treatment.

• Notify health care provider.

Recording and Reporting

• Record baseline data: vital signs, neurologic and mental status, status of peripheral circulation, and skin integrity when therapy was initiated.

• Note type of hyperthermia-hypothermia unit used; control settings (manual or automatic, and temperature settings); date, time, duration; and patient's tolerance of treatment.

• Chart on temperature graphic repeated measurements of vital signs to document response to therapy.

• Report any unexpected outcome to health care provider. Further treatment may be needed.

Special Considerations

Teaching

• Instruct patients and their families not to move patient off blanket.

Pediatric

• A greater metabolic rate and larger trunk in relation to the rest of the body make children more prone to hypothermia. Exercise caution with young patients.

• Infants have an unstable temperature control mechanism; thus mottling of extremities is common and does not always indicate an adverse reaction.

Gerontologic

• Some older adults are more at risk for tissue damage because of loss of cold sensation. Check patient frequently during all treatments.

 Critical Thinking Exercises

You are assigned to care for Adam Montgomery, an 82-year-old male patient with diabetes mellitus who is postoperative day 1 for total left knee arthroplasty. The surgeon has ordered an electronically controlled cold compression cuff to be applied to the left knee for 2 to 3 hours, followed by a 1-to 2-hour break with compression loosened. Your patient has been confused off and on since returning to the patient care unit and is receiving hydrocodone 5/500 1 to 2 tablets by mouth every 4 hours for pain.

1 What do you need to do to begin Mr. Montgomery's cold application? (Select all that apply.) Explain your choice(s).
1 Refer to health care provider's order for location and duration of the application
2 Assess current pain level
3 Assess condition of injured or affected body part
4 Explain the procedure and precautions to avoid injury to the skin

2 Mr. Montgomery's risks for cold applications include which of the following? (Select all that apply.)
1 A chronic pain condition
2 A condition causing circulatory insufficiency to extremities
3 An acute injury less than 2 days old
4 An inability to provide feedback about tissue temperature

3 Can you delegate the application of the cold compression cuff to nursing assistive personnel (NAP)? Why or why not?

✓ REVIEW QUESTIONS

1 A patient has been diagnosed with a severe muscle strain of the lower back, and the health care provider has ordered heat applications to the lower back for 48 hours. Which nursing intervention has the greatest priority in this situation?
1 Frequently assessing the setting on the heat delivery system
2 Placing a plastic wrap over the compress for better penetration
3 Frequently assessing the area where the heat is being applied
4 Encouraging the patient to increase his oral fluid intake

2 Which of the following patients would be at risk for injury from heat application? (Select all that apply.)
1 A patient with a lot of body fat
2 A patient being treated for anxiety
3 A patient with peripheral vascular disease
4 A patient with type 1 diabetes
5 A patient with dehydration
6 A malnourished patient
7 A patient who has been on long-term steroid therapy

3 The nurse has just completed a cold application to a patient's knee. Which observation would be expected as a result of the treatment?
1 The affected area is slightly pale and cool to touch.
2 The amount of edema has increased.
3 The patient relates a measurable increase in pain.
4 The affected area is mottled or bluish purple.

4 The nurse is preparing to apply a cold application to a patient's elbow. Which nursing intervention would be indicated?
  1 Decreasing the length of time the cold application would normally be applied
  2 Increasing the length of time the cold application would normally be applied
  3 Keeping the time length of the cold application the same as when the application is over a fatty area
  4 Leaving the cold application in place until it naturally cools to allow for deeper penetration

5 Depending on the application method and duration, the physiologic effects of cold therapy may include which of the following? (Select all that apply.)
  1 Reducing localized pain
  2 Vasodilation
  3 Muscle relaxation
  4 Vasoconstriction

6 A patient placed on a hypothermia blanket begins to shiver. Why should the nurse be concerned about the patient's response to this therapy?
  1 Shivering decreases a patient's metabolic rate and amount of heat loss.
  2 Shivering decreases the amount of oxygen consumption by a patient.
  3 Shivering increases a patient's metabolic rate and heat production.
  4 Shivering causes general vasoconstriction, which is contraindicated for this patient.

7 An alert older patient with limited mobility and strength has a moist heat wrap applied. Which is the most important nursing intervention for this patient?
  1 Checking on patient's response to the therapy in 1 hour
  2 Ensuring that patient's call light is placed within reach
  3 Telling patient to move the heat wrap if it becomes uncomfortable
  4 Securing the device to the affected area with plastic wrap

8 A patient is using a smoking cessation patch and needs a moist heat application. Before the initial application of the heat, which nursing intervention is most important?
  1 Performing a full skin assessment to determine any potential areas of injury
  2 Notifying the health care provider of the patient's use of the medicinal patch
  3 Performing an assessment of the patient's desired comfort level
  4 Ensuring proper body alignment so only the affected area is heated

9 A patient with a strained muscle receives a dry heat application. How does the nurse evaluate the effectiveness of this therapy?
  1 Asks the patient to rate pain using a pain scale
  2 Has the patient gently perform an activity using the affected muscle
  3 Encourages the patient to actively exercise the affected muscle
  4 Watches the patient's face as he uses the affected muscle group

10 A patient just injured his ankle, and a cold pack has been placed on the affected area. What is the appropriate evaluation immediately after injury?
  1 The nurse checks the skin on the patient's ankle 15 to 20 minutes after the cold pack is applied.
  2 The ice pack is wrapped with plastic to ensure even application of the therapy.
  3 The patient sits on a chair while his ankle is placed in a bucket of ice on the floor.
  4 The patient's skin temperature and appearance is checked approximately every 5 minutes.

REFERENCES

Ebbinghaus S, Kobayashi A: Safe heat application for pediatric patients, *J Nurse Care Qual* 25(2):168, 2010.

Fox J, et al: Prophylactic hypothermia for traumatic brain injury: a quantitative systematic review, *CJEM* 12(4):355, 2010.

Galvao CM, et al: Effectiveness of cutaneous warming systems on temperature control: meta-analysis, *J Adv Nurs* 66(4):196, 2010.

Garner A, Fendius A: Temperature physiology, assessment and control, *Br J Neurosci Nurs* 6(8):397, 2011.

Giger J: *Transcultural nursing: assessment and interventions*, ed 6, St Louis, 2013, Mosby.

Gottschalk AW: Ice and cold application for musculoskeletal soft-tissue trauma, *Evidence-Based Practice* 14(5):13, 2011.

Hockenberry MJ, Wilson D: *Wong's nursing care of infants and children*, ed 9, St Louis, 2011, Mosby.

Kiekkas P et al: Physical antipyresis in critically ill adults, *Am J Nurs* 108(7):40, 2008.

Kiekkas P et al: Postoperative hypothermia and mortality in critically ill adults: review and meta-analysis, *Aust J Adv Nurs* 28(4):60, 2011.

Lane E, Latham T: Managing pain using heat and cold therapy, *Pediatr Nurs* 21(6):14, 2009.

Linares G; Mayer SA: Hypothermia for the treatment of ischemic and hemorrhagic stroke, *Crit Care Med* 37(7 suppl):S243, 2009.

Markert S: The use of cryotherapy after a total knee replacement: a literature review, *Orthop Nurs* 30(10):29, 2011.

Meiner SE: *Gerontologic nursing*, ed 4, St Louis, 2011, Mosby.

National Quality Forum (NQF): National voluntary consensus standards for public reporting of patient safety event information, 2011, National Quality Forum, available at http://www.qualityforum.org/Publications/2011/02/National_Voluntary_Consensus_Standards_for_Public_Reporting_of_Patient_Safety_Event_Information.aspx, accessed June 24 2011.

Pescasio M, et al: Clinical management of muscle strains and tears, *J Musculoskeletal Med* 25(11):526, 2008.

Physiotherapy Canada: 6. Superficial Heat, *Physiother Can* 62(5):47, 2010, DOI:10.3138/ptc2009-09-s6.

Polderman KH: Induced hypothermia and fever control for prevention and treatment of neurological injuries, *Lancet* 371:1955, 2008.

Polderman KH, Herold I: Therapeutic hypothermia and controlled normothermia in the intensive care unit: practical considerations, side effects and cooling methods, *Crit Care Med* 37(3):1101, 2009.

The Joint Commission (TJC): *National Patient Safety Goals*, Oakbrook Terrace, Ill, 2012, The Commission, available at http://www.jointcommission.org/standards_information/npsgs.aspx.

41

Home Care Safety

MEDIA RESOURCES

- **evolve** learning system http://evolve.elsevier.com/Perry/skills
  - Review Questions

KEY TERMS

Alzheimer's disease
Dementia
Wandering

OBJECTIVES

Mastery of content in this chapter will enable the nurse to:
- Identify patients at risk for safety problems and possible accidents in the home.
- Promote self-care of patients in the home.
- Describe factors within a home environment that create risks for patient injury.
- Perform a home safety risk assessment.

- Identify interventions that modify the home environment for physical safety.
- Identify interventions to reduce safety risks for patients with sensory, cognitive, and mental status alterations.
- Recommend strategies to ensure safe drug administration within the home.
- Perform a geriatric fall risk assessment.

Home safety is defined as being in an environment and feeling secure in one's surroundings. Home care safety begins before a patient is discharged. Patient Education Management (2009) highlights the need for communication between patient, family caregivers, and home care providers before discharge. Frequently patients deal with problems as they arise rather than preparing and preventing issues. Remember that insurance coverage, including Medicare, can be very limited for home care. Therefore the time spent in the home with a patient must be well planned and used to the fullest.

Healthy People 2020 identifies injury and violence prevention as a topic area, with objectives geared toward preventing unintentional injuries (USDHHS, 2011). *Healthy People 2020* stresses that injuries and violence affect both an individual, the family, and the community. One of the overarching goals of *Healthy People 2020* addresses obtaining a higher quality and longer life through prevention of injury. In accordance with *Healthy People 2020*, home care nurses must assess a patient and home environment for risk. For example, patients with chronic conditions such as diabetes mellitus may be at risk for falls because of neuropathies. Patients living in socioeconomically disadvantaged areas may be at risk for injury as a result of violence or poor living conditions.

Accident prevention begins with making timely and adequate home repairs (e.g., replacing loose floor tile, securing railings on stairwells). However, many patients do not have the resources for maintaining a safe home environment. The nurse plays an important role in improving and maintaining a patient's safety by collaborating with patients, family members, caregivers, and other health care providers in the community in finding the best approaches for meeting a patient's safety needs. The ultimate goal is to create an environment in which patient and family can provide self-care safely and effectively.

Fall prevention is a critical aspect of care for older adults. You can address it by taking a patient history to assess for risks and reasons for recent falls and plan appropriate interventions. Some of the risk factors to consider include previous fall history, older age, incontinence, multiple medications, fewer numbers of activity of daily living limitations, unsteady gait, poor balance, tremors, reduced lower body strength, reduced vision, absence of supervision, cognitive impairments, postural hypotension, and home environmental hazards (Fortinsky et al., 2008; Yamashita et al., 2011). If home care clinicians are given evidence-based interventions related to these risk factors, research suggests that the likelihood of preventing injury increases, which in turn enhances a patient's quality of life and safety.

EVIDENCE-BASED PRACTICE

Older adults can be especially at risk for falls. Often they believe that limiting their activity will help to decrease this risk. Fletcher et al. (2010) conducted a study to understand the fears of falling in older adults. The researchers sought to determine associated risk factors for adults who chose to restrict their activity in the community. The researchers found several risk factors for restriction of activity, including:

- Being female
- The presence of pain
- Previous history of falling

Older adults and their family caregivers may believe that restricting activity will help prevent falls; however, the research findings did not support this belief (Fletcher et al., 2010). Older adults may actually experience a decline in functional abilities and compromised balance as a result of inactivity. Therefore it is important for a nurse to address a patient's fear of falling and to provide education for safe activity in the home and community.

Greene et al. (2009) designed a fall prevention initiative for older adults and conducted a home visit to question patients about their history of falls and awareness of risk factors in their homes. The researchers conducted a brief motor assessment and made recommendations to decrease falls and increase fall risk awareness. In addition, they examined external risk factors such as lighting and the height of a patient's bed, comparing their findings to falls of older adults in nursing homes and assisted-living facilities. The researchers concluded that:

- Characteristics of falls in the home are unique compared to those in other settings. Health care providers must tailor prevention initiatives appropriate to the setting (e.g., home versus nursing home) and patient needs.
- Fall prevention initiatives impact patient behavior, raise caution and awareness, and improve problem solving.

PATIENT-CENTERED CARE

Many factors influence a patient's lifestyle and the manner in which he or she structures and maintains the home environment. Communication is essential in home care and is a continuous process between you and a patient. At the first meeting introduce yourself, explaining how you would like the patient to address you, and ask the patient how you should refer to him or her (Abele, 2011). Recognize that time orientation is different for each culture. For example, Asians, Africans, East Indians, and Native Americans tend to focus on the past and value long-standing traditions. These patients may look to ancestors for guidance in issues of illness and protection. Recognize this and talk with the patient to address safety issues in a culturally congruent manner that respects this time orientation (Abele, 2011).

Collaborate with patients in assessing their home environments. Assess for culture-specific health-related beliefs that may impact his or her willingness to use home care services. For example, Mexican-Americans may prefer to care for their older adult family members in the home without outside assistance (Crist et al., 2011). When assessing the availability of family caregivers in the home, recognize that many collectivist cultures (e.g., Jewish, Hispanic, Arabic, Asian) value an active presence and caring for ill family members. With the patient's permission, include these family members when performing the home safety assessment. Assess and provide support for informal and family caregivers; the presence or absence of these could be the difference between a patient remaining in the home or being readmitted to an acute care facility (Abele and Nies, 2011).

Safety Guidelines

1. When helping a patient change the home environment, retain as much of his or her independence and ability to provide self-care as possible.
2. Ask if patient and/or family caregiver has concerns or questions about safety and if they have any suggestions to improve their safety (Mullin, 2010).
3. Reinforce the importance of preserving patient autonomy as much as possible with family caregivers.
4. Make modifications to the home environment only after consulting with and considering patients' physical strengths, remaining functional abilities, and resources for making change.
5. Be sure that patient and family caregivers know what to do in case of an emergency and how to reach you if needed (Mullin, 2010).

SKILL 41-1 Home Environment Assessment and Safety

The home environment should be a place where individuals feel healthy, comfortable, and safe. People want to be able to move about freely within their homes, regardless of the size of the home, and to have a sense of control over daily living routines. This requires maintaining personal space and a sense of privacy. As the home care nurse you can help a patient maintain independence and reduce risk in the home environment by conducting a safety assessment.

Patients requiring home care often experience physical alterations (e.g., progressive physical changes of aging) that require changes in their home environment. For example, if a patient has poor balance but good upper arm strength, make modifications so he or she can safely walk or move throughout the house, ascend and descend stairs, and enter and exit a bathtub or shower. Teaching a patient to safely use assistive devices (e.g., walker or cane) helps him or her increase mobility and maintain independence (Fig. 41-1).

Respect the concept of personal space. Making changes too rapidly without a patient's consent will cause more problems than benefits. Appreciate the arrangement of a patient's space within the home and do not move things or suggest modifications without permission. Provide a rationale to the patient as to why the changes are beneficial and/or needed. Knowing the rooms that a patient uses most frequently helps in making the adjustments to create a safe environment.

Delegation and Collaboration

The skill of conducting an initial home safety assessment cannot be delegated to nursing assistive personnel (NAP). The nurse directs the NAP to:

- Inform the nurse of suggestions for ways to make the home safer.

Equipment

❑ Home safety checklist

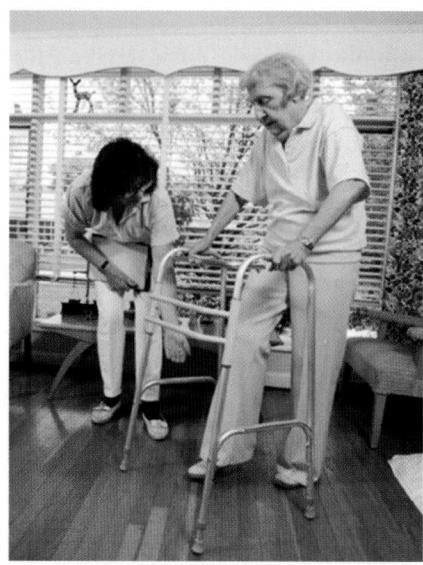

FIG 41-1   Use of walker may help patient remain mobile.

STEP	RATIONALE

ASSESSMENT

1 Review risk factors that predispose patients to accidents within the home:

   a Known visual impairment

Reduced visual function alters patient's balance, depth perception, or adaptation to dark or glaring light (Ebersole et al., 2008).

   b Hearing impairment

Prevents patient from hearing normal environmental sounds clearly as source of orientation. Prevents clear perception of any home-installed alarms (e.g., smoke alarm).

Interferes with communication for patients with co-morbidities to hear and interpret what you are saying (Wallhagen and Pettengill, 2008).

   c Neuromuscular dysfunction (e.g., lower- extremity weakness, unsteady gait, impaired balance, poor ankle dorsiflexion)

Factors predispose patients to fall. Recurrent falls are associated with difficulty standing up from a chair (Touhy, 2010b).

   d Reduced energy or fatigue

Predisposes patients to falls.

   e Incontinence or nocturia

Frequent trips to bathroom often cause patient with other deficits to accidentally trip or fall over barriers.

Dementia does not cause incontinence but it will affect patient's ability to find a bathroom and recognize need to void (Touhy, 2010a).

   f History of stroke, parkinsonism, delirium, seizures, dementia, arrhythmias, gait disturbances, muscle weakness, and syncope

There are usually multiple reasons for falls, including neurologic, sensory, cognitive, medication, and musculoskeletal problems (Touhy, 2010b).

Gait disorders make patients vulnerable to tripping and falling (Ebersole et al., 2008). Age-related changes of neurologic system include slowing of reaction time (Meiner, 2011).

   g Postural hypotension, palpitations, difficulty breathing, or shortness of breath

Dizziness and light-headedness predispose to falls (Touhy, 2010b) and cause patient to be unsteady and compensate for difficulties.

   h Medication usage and history, including polypharmacy and use of sedatives, antihypertensives, antidepressants, and diuretics

Use of multiple medications has been associated with falls. Medications that alter sensorium affect balance and judgment (Muir et al., 2010).

   i History of previous fall

Increases risk for future fall. Recurrent or multiple fallers are more likely to benefit from fall prevention efforts (Fletcher et al., 2009).

2 Determine if patient has had history of falls or other injuries within the home. Be specific in your assessment. Use the mnemonic SPLATT (Meiner, 2011):

Key symptoms are helpful in identifying cause of fall. Onset, location, and activity associated with fall provide further details on causative factors and how to prevent future falls.

SPLATT test allows patient to explain symptoms in own words; it is important to understand circumstances around fall (Meiner, 2011).

STEP	RATIONALE
<ul><li>Symptoms at time of fall</li><li>Previous fall</li><li>Location of fall</li><li>Activity at time of fall</li><li>Time of fall</li><li>Trauma after fall</li></ul>	
3 Have patient who has had a near fall or actual fall maintain a fall diary (Box 41-1).	Information in fall diary is very helpful in determining antecedents and consequences of falling (Meiner, 2011).
4 Conduct a Timed Get Up and Go (TUG) test for basic mobility. Instruct patient to rise from standard chair, walk approximately 3 meters (10 feet), turn around, walk back to chair, and sit in chair again. Time patient while he or she performs activity. Have patient perform test three times and calculate mean score.	Simple screening examination is very useful in detecting difficulties with balance or gait. Normal required time to finish test is less than 20 seconds, with no staggering when turning or need to hold on to something. Helps in diagnosis and treatment of underlying causes; refer to physical therapist for gait and progressive balance training (Ebersole et al., 2008). TUG time performance is associated with a past history of falls, but its predictive ability for future falls remains limited (Beauchet et al., 2011).
5 Determine if patient has fear of falling. Possible indicators include apprehension during ambulation (observed in facial expressions); sweating or trembling while ambulating; clutching people or objects while ambulating; reluctance to change position or ambulate; and new onset of wobbly, reduced mobility after a fall.	Fear of falling occurs variably in older adults. Some patients limit activity because of fear of falling, which is risk factor itself for falling (Muir et al., 2010).

Clinical Decision Point *In addition to patient, include family caregivers as a resource in assessments because they may witness accident trends or patterns.*

STEP	RATIONALE
6 Partner with patient and family caregivers to conduct home safety assessment:	Provides comprehensive review of all areas within home that pose hazardous situations.
a Front and back entrances	
(1) Are walkways to front/back door even and free from holes or cracks?	Entrances pose barriers in surfaces over which patient must walk. Uneven pavement and holes may not be seen by patient, causing tripping and falls.
(2) Are home entrances, including walkways, well lit?	Poorly lit areas prevent individuals from seeing variations in walking surface.
(3) Does patient have nonskid strips/safety treads or bright-colored paint on outdoor steps? Which colors are most easily seen by patient? Are these colors used?	Nonskid surfaces cause fewer slips on stairs. Color on steps permits individual to see edges, accommodating for any reduced depth perception.
(4) Are doormats in good repair with nonskid backing and tapered edge?	Raised edges pose risk for tripping. Doormats without nonskid backing will slide when stepped on, causing patient to lose balance.
(5) Are doors in good repair and do they open and close easily? Can patient open and close all doors easily?	Act of opening and closing door can cause fall. Automatic door openers, level doorknob handles, and hook-and-chain locks may be easier to use (Touhy, 2010b).
(6) Is there sturdy handrail on both sides of stairs leading to entrance?	Handrails provide greater support while ascending and descending stairs. Ideally handrails on both sides of stairwell will provide greatest stability for patient. If entrance space does not allow this, install at least on one side to prevent fall from imbalance (Touhy, 2010b).

BOX 41-1 | **Fall/Near-Fall Diary**

- Keep a notebook and across the longest edge of the paper write the headings: "Date," "Time of Fall," "Activity at Time of Fall," "Symptoms," and "Injury."
- As soon as possible after a fall, have patient or family caregiver complete information under each heading.
- If a family caregiver witnesses the fall, the family member records what happened on a separate piece of paper.

- List emergency contact numbers in the diary for patient to call in case a fall results in serious injury.
- Instruct patient to bring the diary to their health care provider's office at the next scheduled visit or share information with home care nurse on next home visit.

Modified from Meiner SE: *Gerontologic nursing*, ed 4, St Louis, 2011, Mosby.

STEP	RATIONALE
(7) Are steps in good condition with even, flat surfaces?	Uneven surfaces predispose to tripping.
(8) Are doorways and stairs free of clutter?	Reduces risk for tripping and/or falling.
b Kitchen	Kitchen is one of most hazard-oriented rooms in home and poses serious hazards for fire.
(1) Does patient wear clothing with short or close-fitting sleeves when cooking?	Short or close-fitting sleeves are less likely to accidentally catch on fire when person works at stove.
(2) Does patient always stay in kitchen when cooking?	Lack of attention when using fire is risk.
(3) Does patient have loud timer to signal when food is cooked?	Prevents burning food and risk for fire.
(4) Does patient keep stove top and oven clean and grease free?	Grease is highly flammable.
(5) Are stove control dials easy to see and use?	Patient may accidentally use higher flame than is necessary for cooking safely.
(6) Is charged, easy-to-use fire extinguisher close at hand?	Extinguisher should be ready for use at all times.

Clinical Decision Point *Have patient demonstrate steps of how to use extinguisher.*

STEP	RATIONALE
(7) Are emergency numbers for police, fire, and poison control posted on or near telephone?	Emergency phone numbers and extinguisher ensure quick response if fire occurs.
(8) Can items in kitchen cabinets and shelves be reached without climbing on stool or chair?	Climbing on step stools or chairs creates risks for falls.
(9) Is there adequate lighting over sink, stove, and work areas?	Poor lighting makes it difficult to see control knobs or dials and provides inadequate illumination when using sharp knives or utensils.
(10) Are kitchen throw rugs and mats slip resistant?	Rugs or mats that are not slip resistant can easily slide on tile or wood floors.
c Bathrooms	
(1) Can patient unlock bathroom door from both sides of door?	Functional locks prevent person from being trapped in bathroom.
(2) Is tub or shower equipped with nonskid mats, abrasive strips, or surfaces that are not slippery?	Bathrooms are hazardous. Wet floors and tub or shower bottoms can be very slippery, creating risk for falls.
(3) Does bathroom floor have nonslip surface or rug with nonskid backing?	Slippery tile predisposes to falls.
(4) Does patient avoid using slippery bath oils when bathing?	Use of bath oils makes tub surface slippery and increases risk for falls.
(5) Do bathtub and shower have at least one grab bar or handrail placed where patient can reach it?	Grab bars provide extra support while maneuvering into and out of tubs or showers (Home Safety Council, 2011). Grab bars placed in correct place where patient can safely reach them help to steady gait and lessen chance of falls (Meiner, 2011).
(6) Is patient careful not to place towels on grab bars?	Some patients accidentally grab towel instead of bar when needing support. Towel can slip off bar.
(7) Does shower have stable stool or chair and handheld sprayer? Is shower easy to access (walk-in versus step-in to tub area)?	Shower stool allows patient to sit while showering.
(8) Are cold and hot water faucets clearly marked, and is temperature on water heater 120°F (48.8°C) or lower?	Accidental burns can occur from exposure to hot water.
d Bedroom	
(1) Is night-light placed in bedroom and/or bath?	Older adults have altered night vision.
(2) Is working smoke detector just outside bedroom door?	Alarm situated just outside bedroom can awaken person early enough to escape fire.
(3) Can patient turn on light without having to get out of bed in dark? Is flashlight available at bedside?	Getting out of bed without proper lighting or ability to adjust to light changes and reaching for necessary objects put patient at risk for falls.
(4) Is furniture arranged to provide clear path from bed to bathroom?	Obstructed path creates barrier that causes tripping and falls.
(5) Is phone with emergency numbers within easy reach of bed?	If patients develop physical symptoms while in bed, they need to be able to reach phone without having to get out of bed.
(6) Are other alarm systems available? Push buttons that call for help? Nursery listening devices for cognitively impaired or nonambulatory patients?	Alarm systems placed in readily accessible location can alert family caregivers when person requires immediate assistance.

STEP	RATIONALE
e Living room/family room	
(1) Are electrical or extension cords removed from under furniture and carpeting? Kept out of way of traffic?	Patients can easily trip or fall over electrical cords. Hidden cords are trip and fire hazard.
(2) Can patient turn on light without having to walk into dark room?	Darkened room can disorient and prevent patient from seeing uneven surfaces.
(3) Are hallways and walkways free from objects and clutter?	Objects and clutter in common walkway can cause falls.
(4) Are loose area rugs securely attached to floor and not placed over carpeting? (For best safety, consider removing throw rugs.)	Loose edges of rugs are easy for persons to trip over (Touhy, 2010b).
(5) Is furniture arranged in each room so patient can walk around easily?	Furniture creates obstacles to walking in room.
(6) Is all furniture steady and without sharp edges?	Patients often use edge of furniture for support when standing.
f Around the house	
(1) Are all living areas and stairways well lit?	Adequate lighting helps persons see any barriers or uneven walking surfaces.
(2) Is flooring or carpeting throughout house in good repair?	Frayed carpet or irregular surfaces can cause tripping and result in fall.
(3) Are all thresholds level with floor or no more than $\frac{1}{2}$ inch (1.27 cm) in height?	Uneven thresholds can cause tripping.
(4) Is light switch at both top and bottom of stairs?	Prevents individual from having to walk portion of stairs in dark.
(5) Does lighting produce glare or shadows on stairs or floor surfaces?	Older adults are sensitive to glare because their visual pathway becomes distorted.
(6) Do handrails run continuously from top to bottom of flights of stairs?	Handrails provide source of physical support when ascending and descending stairs.
(7) Are handrails securely attached to wall?	
(8) Are step coverings in good condition?	Loosened covering can cause tripping.
(9) Are guns kept in house? Are trigger locks installed on all guns? Are guns stored unloaded? Is ammunition in secure location?	Following gun safety standards decreases risk for injury and death related to gun use (NRA, 2011).
g General fire safety	
(1) Does patient have properly working smoke detectors with fresh batteries?	Smoke alarms properly located, functioning well, and with batteries replaced twice a year can provide timely alert for fire.

Clinical Decision Point *Check to see when smoke-alarm battery was last changed; battery should be changed every 6 months. Instruct patients to change battery each time they change their house clocks for daylight savings.*

STEP	RATIONALE
(2) Does patient have several emergency exit plans in case of fire?	Exit plan helps people anticipate route of escape when fire does occur. Exit should not have locks that are difficult to open or any physical barriers.
(3) Has family determined meeting place in event of emergency such as at mailbox in front of home?	Use of common emergency meeting location is efficient method for determining that all family members are safely out of house.
(4) Does patient use portable space heaters? Are they kept at least 3 feet (1 meter) away from flammable items?	Heaters, furnaces, and chimneys pose risks for fire.
(5) Is furnace area free of things that can catch on fire?	Heating equipment was second-most common cause of home fire fatalities from 2005 through 2009 (National Fire Protection Association [NFPA], 2011).
(6) Does a qualified professional check furnace and chimney annually?	
(7) Does patient who smokes report smoking in bed?	Smoking was leading cause of home fire deaths in 2005 through 2009 (NFPA, 2011). Smoking in bed has added risk of patient falling asleep while cigarette is lit.
h General electrical safety	
(1) Are electrical cords in good condition (i.e., not frayed, spliced, or cracked)?	Damaged cords can short circuit and lead to fire.
(2) Are electrical cords kept away from water?	Use of any appliance or device that is exposed to water creates risk for electrical shock.
(3) Does patient use extension cord/outlet extenders with built-in circuit breaker or fuse?	Prevents overloading of circuit that can lead to fire.
(4) Do all wall outlets and switches have cover plates?	Prevents physical contact with wiring.

STEP	RATIONALE
(5) Does patient use light bulbs of correct wattage for each fixture?	Use of excessive wattage can lead to fire.
(6) Is main electrical fuse box for home easily accessible and clearly labeled?	In event of emergency, fuse box should be easy to access so proper circuit can be cut off.
i Carbon monoxide prevention	
(1) Are furnace flues checked regularly for patency?	Obstructed flues are common cause of carbon monoxide toxicity.
(2) Is there a carbon monoxide detector in home?	
7 Assess patient's financial resources; determine monthly income used for ongoing expenses.	Determines potential for making repairs to home. Reveals need for low-cost community service support.
8 Assess patient's and family caregiver's willingness to make changes. Has patient accepted limitations that pose risk for injury? Determine how important functional independence is for patient.	Some patients perceive attempts to improve safety within home as intrusive. If you show that necessary revisions to home environment will preserve independence, patient will participate more willingly.

NURSING DIAGNOSES

- Anxiety
- Deficient knowledge regarding safety risks
- Ineffective health maintenance
- Impaired home maintenance
- Impaired memory
- Impaired physical mobility
- Risk for falls
- Risk for injury

Related factors are individualized based on patient's condition or needs.

PLANNING

1 Expected outcomes following completion of procedure:	
• Patient and/or family describes potential environmental risks within home that predispose to accidents.	During home safety assessment nurse instructs patient in risks that are of greatest concern.
• Patient and/or family initiate actions to correct environmental risks, making home safer.	Patient sees value in altering living environment.
• Patient remains free of injury.	Environmental barriers are reduced or removed to minimize injuries.
2 Prioritize with patient and family environmental barriers that pose greatest risk.	Patient's own physical and/or cognitive deficits make certain environmental risks more hazardous. Prioritization helps patient make best choices.
3 Recommend calling in reliable contractor if major home repairs are necessary.	Ensures that repairs are made safely and correctly.

IMPLEMENTATION

1 General home safety:	
a Provide direct light source in areas where patient reads, cooks, uses tools, or conducts hobby work. High-intensity light on object or surface that is involved works best.	Visual impairment in older adults usually is a result of cataracts, macular degeneration, glaucoma, or diabetic retinopathy (Touhy, 2010c).

Clinical Decision Point *Avoid fluorescent lighting because it creates excessive glare.*

b Consider satin and nonglossy finishes for walls, cabinets, and countertops in kitchen. Have sheer curtains or adjustable shades in other living areas.	Reduces glare for older adults.
c Apply colored tape or paint to color code controls of stove, oven, dryer, toaster, and other appliances.	Patients with reduced visual acuity may adjust appliance to wrong setting, creating potential risk for fire or burning.
d Consider installing lazy Susans or pull-out drawers with glide mechanisms in kitchen cabinets. Install C-ring handles in lower cabinets.	Makes access to food and kitchen supplies easier.
2 Fall prevention steps:	
a Paint edges of concrete stairs bright yellow, orange, or white.	Patient can see edge of stairs more clearly.
b Install treads with uniform depth of 22.5 cm (9 inches) and 22.5-cm (9-inch) risers (vertical face of steps).	If stairs are of uniform size, patient does not have to continually adjust vision or stride.
c Rearrange furniture to open up space through hallways and major rooms.	Creates unobstructed pathway for ambulation.
d Reduce clutter within living areas (e.g., footstools, flower pots, extension cords, children's toys, stacked newspapers or magazines).	Mobility hazards resulting from clutter are especially a risk at night (Ebersole et al., 2008).

STEP	RATIONALE
e Secure all carpeting, mats, and tile; place nonskid backing under small rugs and doormats. Remove throw rugs/mats in nonessential (dry) areas.	Reduces chance of patient slipping when stepping on rug surface (Touhy, 2010b).
f Pad floor and use specialized tile that absorbs impact of falls.	Cushions person's fall.
g Use low-rise beds, futon beds, or mattress on floor if not contraindicated.	Lowers distance to floor surface.
h Have enough electrical outlets installed to be able to plug light or electronic device (e.g., television, video) into nearby outlet. Secure electrical cords against baseboards.	Prevents need to run extension cords across walkways.
i Install nonskid strips on surface of bathtub and/or shower stall. Be sure that floor is clean and dry (Home Safety Council, 2011).	Reduces chances of slipping on tub/shower stall surface.
j Have grab bar installed in studs at tub, toilet, and/or shower (see illustration). Have patient select vertical or horizontal placement if choice available. Be sure that bar is different color than wall and easy to see.	Bar provides stability for maneuvering in bathroom (Home Safety Council, 2011).
k Have handrails installed along side of any stairway (see illustration). Be sure that stairways are well lit, with switches at top and bottom of steps.	Install at least on one side (Touhy, 2010b). Older adults have difficulty seeing edges of stairs.
l Install appropriate broad-beam lighting for outside walkways.	Provides full illumination.
m Keep lighted phone easily accessible, next to patient's bed.	Prevents patient from having to get up out of bed, often in dark.
n Install motion sensor exterior lighting for walkways/driveway.	Reduces risk for patient falls caused by dark surroundings.
o Have patient use padding or types of clothing that will cushion bony prominences, especially high-risk bony prominences (e.g., hips). Specially designed hip protectors are available.	Helps to absorb impact of falling body.
3 Prevent spread of infection:	
a Teach patient cleaning practices to prevent spread of infection.	Family caregivers need instruction in infection control practices.
b Instruct patient not to share eating and drinking utensils.	Some infections are spread by saliva.
c Instruct patient to clean appliances and surfaces daily.	Regular cleaning prevents risk for contamination and spread of infection.
4 Fire safety:	
a Have smoke detectors installed near each bedroom, in kitchen, and in basement of home. Be sure that detector is on each floor of home.	Fires most frequently start in basement near furnace, dryer, or electrical wiring; kitchen; or in living areas where there is extensive wiring. Alarm should be close to alert patient and family when sleeping.

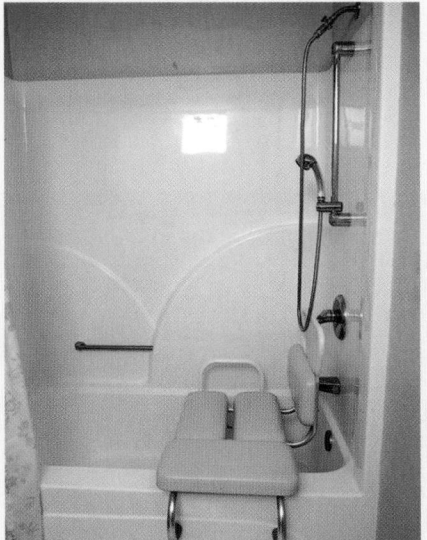

STEP 2j Grab bars and safety seat installed in shower.

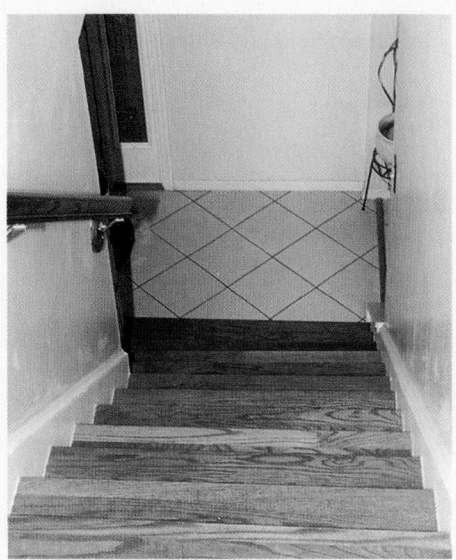

STEP 2k Handrails installed along stairways provide security for patients with visual, balance, and coordination problems.

STEP	RATIONALE
b Have patient select fire extinguisher that is easy to handle and manipulate (see illustration). Ask him or her to read instructions and demonstrate its proper use.	Some older adults or patients with disabilities have difficulty gripping mechanisms on certain extinguishers.
c Have area around furnace cleared of any flammable items.	Reduces risk for fire.
d Instruct patient to be sure that portable space heater has emergency shut off and that equipment housing and electrical cords are intact (Meiner, 2011).	Space heaters can be overturned by accident, which can cause fire; safety mechanism will turn unit off immediately (Meiner, 2011).
e Have patient make appointments for maintenance of furnace and chimney cleaning in appropriate season.	Furnace maintenance prevents short circuits and fires. Accumulation of creosote on chimney walls can lead to fire.
f Have patient check light bulb wattage in all fixtures.	Ensures that proper wattage being used; wattage that exceeds recommendation can cause fire.
g Have patient establish routine during cooking that keeps him or her in kitchen. Be sure that cooking range is clean and items such as potholders and towels are away from burners.	Food cooking on stove can easily boil over or begin to burn when unattended.
h If patient is a smoker, review need to keep ashtrays clean and emptied. Placing small amount of water or sand in bottom of ashtray is useful if patient is visually impaired.	Patient with reduced vision may be unable to tell if cigarette, cigar, or match has extinguished.
i Strongly discourage smoking in bed, smoking in chair when there is possibility of falling asleep, and smoking after taking medication that diminishes alertness. Instruct patient to put cigarette or cigar out at first sign of feeling drowsy (Meiner, 2011).	Risks factors for burns and fire. Patient's reaction time may be slower when tired.
j Recommend that patient install power strips or surge protectors for plugging in multiple appliances/devices.	Prevents risk for electrical short, which can cause fire.
5 Burn safety:	
a Have setting on hot water heater adjusted to 49°C (120°F) or lower.	Prevents scalding burns (Meiner, 2011).
b Instruct patient to always turn cold water on first.	Prevents direct exposure to hot water.
c Install touch pads on lamps.	Light is easy to turn on without risk for touching hot light bulb.
d Use color codes of red for hot and blue for cold on water faucets. (If patient has difficulty distinguishing colors, choose two that are easily distinguished.)	Prevents accidental burning from turning on wrong faucet.
6 Carbon monoxide safety:	
a Have condition of furnace venting checked annually just before turning on furnace.	Improper venting prevents escape of carbon monoxide, a poisonous gas that alters hemoglobin to prevent formation of oxyhemoglobin, and reduces oxygen supply to tissues.
b Caution patients against using gas stove or barbecue grill for heating inside home.	Both are sources of carbon monoxide (Meiner, 2011).
c Have battery-operated carbon monoxide detector installed in home; check or replace battery when you change your clocks in fall and spring (see illustration).	Detector alarms when carbon monoxide reaches unsafe levels. Battery operation will not be affected by power outages (Meiner, 2011).

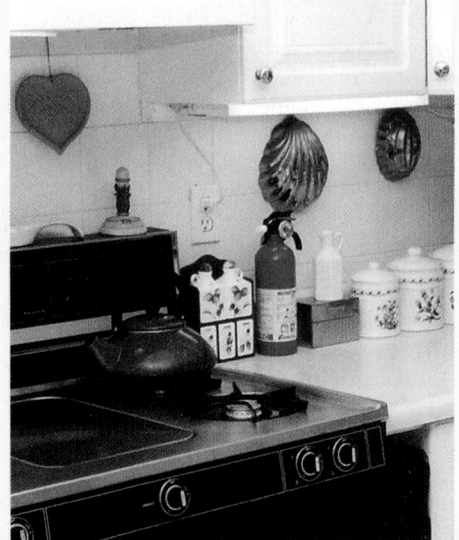

STEP 4b Fire extinguisher accessible in kitchen.

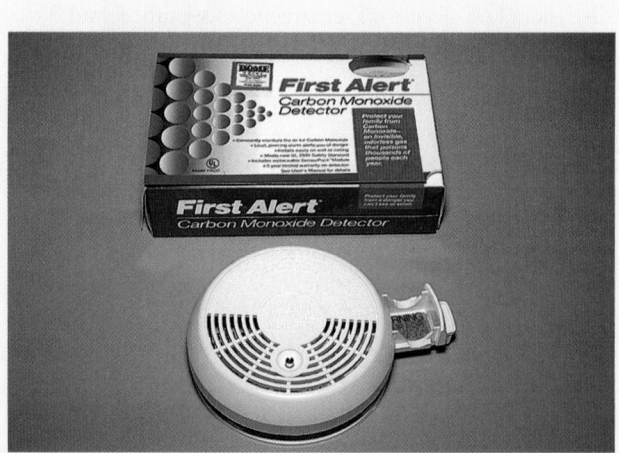

STEP 6c Carbon monoxide detector.

STEP	RATIONALE

7 Firearm safety:
  a Teach patient about dangers associated with keeping guns in home.
  b If guns are in home, teach patient to install trigger locks and store them unloaded in locked cabinet. Teach patient to store ammunition in secured area separate from guns. Store keys in place inaccessible to children.
	Risk of suicide increases in homes with firearms (Edelman and Mandle, 2009).
	Following gun safety standards decreases risk of injury and death related to gun use (Hockenberry and Wilson, 2011).

EVALUATION

1 Have patient and family member(s) identify safety risks revealed in home safety assessment.	Demonstrates what patient recognizes as risk and its relative importance for changing.
2 During follow-up visit or call to home ask patient to discuss plans for making any modification and observe what changes patient has implemented.	Evaluates extent to which patient sees risks as potentially harmful and complies with suggested changes.
3 During follow-up visits or calls ask if patient has experienced any falls or other injuries within home.	Reveals if risks have been eliminated, depending on patient's previous history of injury.
4 Reassess for progression of dementia.	Assesses for potential risk to patient and caregiver.

Unexpected Outcomes

1 Patient and family do not acknowledge risks identified from home safety assessment.

2 Patient fails to make changes agreed on in previous plan.

3 Patient suffers fall or burn within home.

Related Interventions

- Determine if reluctance to make changes is caused by limited resources, disbelief concerning need to make changes, fear of loss of autonomy, or other reasons.
- Review implications of risks to patient's safety and welfare.

- Determine reason for failure to make changes.
- Help prioritize greatest risks.

- Conduct assessment of contributing factors and conditions in environment at time of injury.
- Make revisions based on assessment findings.

Recording and Reporting

- Retain copy of home safety assessment in patient's home care record.
- Record any instruction provided, patient's response, and changes made within environment in progress notes.

Special Considerations

Teaching

- Family and caregivers will benefit from learning how to safely help patient ambulate or transfer from bed to chair or wheelchair to chair, depending on patient's mobility limitations (see Chapter 9).
- Instruct patient and caregiver about what to do in case patient falls, including access to emergency assistance and how to prevent further injury.
- When appropriate, teach caregiver and patient how to use any emergency assistive devices (e.g., devices that are worn around patient's neck and a special monitor connected to patient's telephone). Patients summon help by pressing button on device if phone is inaccessible. Refer the family to local health care agencies and department of aging for options.

Pediatric

- Caution parents when working in the kitchen to never pour hot liquids when an infant or young child is near.

- Remove all crib toys that are strung across crib or playpen when child begins to push up on hands or knees (4 to 7 months) (Hockenberry and Wilson, 2011).
- Keep guns and ammunition in separate, secured places.
- Install safety measures appropriate to developmental level (e.g., cabinet locks and gates).
- Do not let young children use the sink or tub without adult assistance; when child is in tub, stay with him or her (Home Safety Council, 2011).

Gerontologic

- Use "aging in place" resources and designs to accommodate the needs of seniors or disabled individuals without having to completely redesign the home. For example, install grab bars in bathrooms, movable cabinets under the sink so someone in a wheelchair can use the space, and light switches and electrical outlets at heights that can be reached easily (USDHHS Administration on Aging, 2009).
- Place a bedside commode (with bedpan removed) over a conventional toilet seat. Commode level is usually higher than toilet and can also be moved near the bed for nighttime use.

SKILL 41-2 Adapting the Home Setting for Patients with Cognitive Deficits

An important aspect of safety is a person's ability to perform routine activities of daily living (ADLs) and instrumental activities of daily living (IADLs) to make correct decisions about home-management activities. ADLs include a patient's ability to bathe, dress, go to the toilet, transfer, and feed oneself. IADLs include the ability to use a telephone, prepare meals, travel, do housework, take medication, and shop.

Some patients who are unable to perform these activities or who require assistance have physical disabilities and/or cognitive limitations. Cognitive and physical limitations can threaten a person's autonomy. Family members often misunderstand certain behaviors associated with cognitive changes and become concerned about whether the individual can function safely within the home. Be aware that you may face situations in which you have to make decisions about whether a patient is competent to perform self-care.

Common cognitive conditions affecting patients in the home are dementia, delirium, and depression. Delirium can occur in up to 80% of hospitalized patients and continues to manifest symptoms in 30% to 90% of these patients after discharge (Ebersole et al., 2008). Dementia is a chronic generalized impairment of intellectual functioning that leads to a decline in the ability to perform basic ADLs and IADLs. Dementia is characterized by a gradual, progressive, irreversible cerebral dysfunction. Alzheimer's disease is the most common form of dementia and accounts for 50% to 80% of dementia cases (Alzheimer's Association, 2012). As it progresses, older adults become more dependent on family caregivers for assistance. Caregivers will need access to respite programs, which will allow them planned time away from their caregiving role (Mueth, 2011).

Alzheimer's disease is a form of dementia, causing problems with memory, thinking, or behavior; for some individuals with Alzheimer's disease there is a risk for wandering (Alzheimer's Association, 2012). A wandering patient may walk around the house trying repeatedly to carry out a task independently or try to leave his or her place of residence but is stopped by family caregivers. If wandering is an ongoing problem, the family caregiver should provide current photographs of the patient to local police. The patient can also be enrolled in the national MedicAlert + Alzheimer's Association Safe Return program, which provides 24-hour emergency and wandering response services and support services for family and caregivers (Alzheimer's Association, 2011). Local resources can also be explored to ensure safety for the patient inside and outside of the home.

Delegation and Collaboration

The skill of adapting the home environment for patients with cognitive deficits cannot be delegated to nursing assistive personnel (NAP). The nurse is responsible for the assessment of cognitive function. The nurse directs the NAP to:

- Inform the nurse when there is a change in patient's mood, memory, and ability to maintain home.

Equipment

- ❏ Mini-Mental State Examination (MMSE)
- ❏ Short Geriatric Depression Scale (SGDS)
- ❏ Beck Depression Inventory (BDI)
- ❏ Calendar
- ❏ Paper for making lists
- ❏ Medication organizer (*optional*)
- ❏ Bulletin board or poster board (*optional*)
- ❏ Motion detector (*optional*)

STEP	RATIONALE

ASSESSMENT

1 Assess patient over short period of time and be sensitive to his or her sensory needs or disabilities.	Respects human dignity of patient.
2 Be sure that room in which you meet with patient and family is well lit with minimal outside noises or interruptions. Speak clearly and in normal tone of voice.	Optimal environment for assessment of patient's cognitive and mental status provides more valid assessment.
3 Ask patient to describe own level of health and have him or her describe how it affects ability to perform self-care skills (e.g., bathing, dressing, eating, toileting).	Question requires patient to focus on one topic. Allows nurse to assess attention and concentration. Also determines if patient is fully perceptive of physical capabilities.

Clinical Decision Point *Do not create situation in which patient thinks that you are not listening to his or her views. The additional person supplements answers with patient's consent, but patient remains the focus of the interview.*

4 Ask how patient is handling home management responsibilities: "Tell me what bills you pay each month. Can you tell me what each one is for? *Ability to perform ADLs*: Can you tell me about your normal day—when do you get up, eat meals, dress? Do you have problems dressing or bathing?"	Provides good comparison of patient and family perceptions. Interaction will help to measure short-term memory, judgment, and problem solving.

STEP	RATIONALE
5 Assess patient's medications. Review number and type of medications, purpose as prescribed, time of day taken, and dosages. Assess where patient stores medications. Give special attention to pain medications, anticonvulsants, antihypertensives (especially beta-adrenergic blockers), diuretics, digoxin, aspirin, and anticoagulants. Have patient or caregiver keep updated list of medications that can be brought to emergency department if needed. Ask to see medications and/or list used.	Older adults frequently suffer drug interactions from polypharmacy (i.e., concurrent prescribing of multiple medications). Some drugs and/or combinations of drugs place patient at risk for side effects that increase chances of injury as result of physical or cognitive changes. Keeping list of medications allows health care provider easy access to medication history.
6 Determine if patient has a family caregiver who helps with self-care or home-management responsibilities. What level of support is provided by caregiver? How frequently is caregiver available? Does patient perceive satisfaction in caregiver's support? What level of satisfaction does caregiver perceive? Does caregiver have access to and/or take advantage of respite care?	Relationship between family caregiver and patient helps define how difficult it is to provide caregiving support. Role of family caregiver is often stressful, particularly if individual has other responsibilities such as parenting, work, or school. Determines availability of resource to patient and quality of that support.
7 During discussion observe patient's dress, nonverbal expressions, appearance, and cleanliness.	Conditions such as depression and dementia can result in patient's inability to attend to personal appearance.

Clinical Decision Point *Do not confuse behavioral changes with lack of available resources to maintain hygiene. Also be aware of signs and symptoms of abuse or neglect. Report suspected abuse to appropriate social service agency.*

8 Observe immediate home environment.	Behavioral changes associated with cognitive dysfunction are evident in disorderly home and inappropriate placement of objects (e.g., carton of orange juice placed inside kitchen cabinet instead of in refrigerator).

9 If you suspect cognitive or mental status change:
  a Complete Mini-Mental State Examination (e.g., Folstein's examination) for dementia.
  b Complete Short Geriatric Depression Scale (SGDS) for depression. (**NOTE:** Other depression scales are available, such as the Beck Inventory.)
	Test screens orientation, attention and calculation, recall, language, and intelligence (Meiner, 2011).
	SGDS is recommended because it takes 5 minutes to administer and has been tested, validated, and used extensively for depression in older adults (Harvath and McKenzie, 2012).

10 If you suspect that patient is at risk for wandering or is wandering, observe for following behaviors (family caregivers might provide information as well):
  • Repeated shadowing or seeking whereabouts of caregiver
  • Revisiting one destination many times
  • Inability to locate landmarks or getting lost in familiar setting
  • Going into unauthorized or private places
  • Searching for "missing" people or places
  • Walking with no apparent destination or purpose
  • Haphazard or continuous moving, walking, or pacing
  • Walking that cannot easily be redirected
	Alerts family and caregivers of potential safety risks. When wandering extends outside safe environment, patient is at increased risk for injury or death.

11 Assess which current environmental strategies family caregivers are using to deal with wandering (e.g., latches and alarms on doors, visual cues such as STOP signs, constant supervision, and wearing identification band).	Helps to determine level of intervention necessary. Allows for assessment of how family is dealing with issues of wandering and need for additional outside support.
12 Assess caregiver for signs and symptoms of stress.	Helps to determine if caregiver is feeling burdened or overwhelmed and is in need of assistance.

NURSING DIAGNOSES

- Acute confusion
- Caregiver role strain
- Impaired home maintenance
- Impaired memory

- Ineffective health maintenance
- Ineffective role performance
- Risk for injury

- Self-care deficit (feeding, toileting, bathing/hygiene, dressing/grooming)
- Wandering

Related factors are individualized based on patient's condition or needs.

STEP	RATIONALE

PLANNING

1 Expected outcomes following completion of procedure:
- Patient is able to complete home management responsibilities within existing limitations.
- Patient receives appropriate combination of medications for diagnosed conditions.
- Patient is able to perform self-care activities or receives appropriate assistance.
- Family caregivers describe steps to take to minimize wandering.
- Patient experiences fewer episodes of wandering.
- Caregiver identifies community resources for support.

Modifications are made that help patient apply remaining cognitive functions.
Assistive devices enable patient to follow prescribed medication regimen.
Interventions preserve patient's autonomy and maximize patient's functionality.
Instruction prepares caregivers with wandering-management strategies.
Wandering-management strategies are effective.
Services available can include respite care, adult day care programs, and support groups.

2 If patient has difficulty with self-care skills or fine-motor skills, refer family to occupational therapy, homemaker services, or respite care as appropriate.

Occupational therapists provide assistive devices and recommend self-care adaptations. Homemaker services provide added resource for meal preparation and home cleaning. Respite care provides family caregiver temporary rest away from continuous responsibilities.

3 Offer assistive devices to make bathing, dressing, writing, and feeding easier (see illustrations).

Assistive eating devices have larger handles, cup handles. or plate edges to help with meals. Assistive clothing uses Velcro, large zippers, and elastic to facilitate independence when dressing.

4 Consider patient's level of cognitive impairment when making changes in his or her living environment. Some patients may require only minor adaptations, and others will depend more on assistance of caregivers.

Retention of patient's independence and autonomy is ultimate goal.

5 Determine best time of day for approaches that result in desired response.

Some patients are more alert and responsive in morning versus afternoon or vice versa.

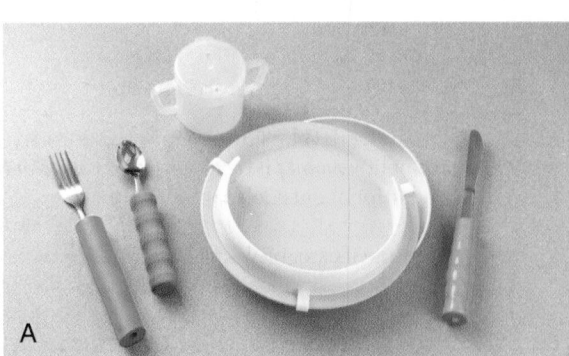
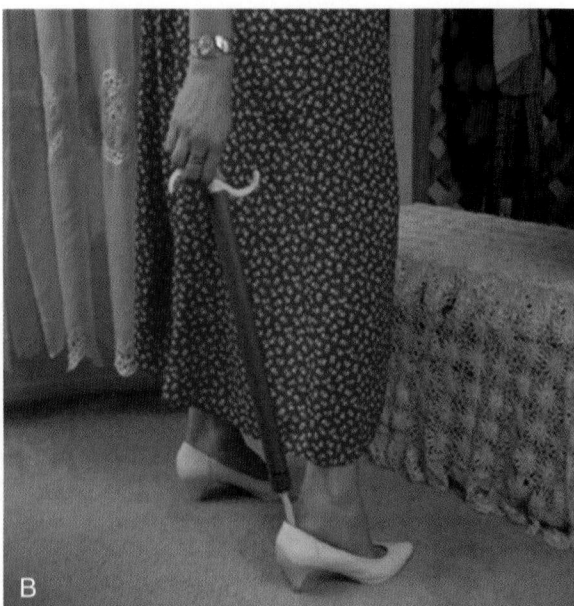

STEP 3 A, Assistive feeding devices. **B,** Assistive device to aid in putting on shoes. (*Image used with permission ArcMate Manufacturing Corporation. All rights reserved.*)

STEP	RATIONALE

IMPLEMENTATION

1 If patient has difficulty remembering when to perform tasks (e.g., paying bills, taking medicines), help to create a list or post reminder notes in conspicuous location (e.g., bulletin board, front of refrigerator), provide medication container organized by days of week, recommend wristwatch with alarm to signal medication administration times.

Memory function in older adults tends to be preserved for relevant, well-learned material (Kazer, 2011). Lists and organizers help patient cope with memory loss and still safely perform activities.

2 When patient has difficulty completing tasks such as writing checks for bills or bringing groceries into home from store, reduce steps it takes to complete task. Consolidate steps or simplify task.

Prevents frustration in completing task and/or forgetting step that leads to task being unfinished.

3 Help patient and caregiver determine routine schedule for ADLs such as eating, bathing, daily exercise, home cleaning, and napping. Have large calendar posted in conspicuous area to write in appointments or special planned events.

Consistency creates sense of security and keeps patient oriented to daily activities. Routines are important in providing security, but patient also needs to have option of making changes as necessary (Kazer, 2011).

4 Instruct family caregiver to focus on patient's abilities rather than disabilities. Use abilities in modifying approaches to perform daily activities. (e.g., if patient has limited use of right hand, try approaches that maximize use of left hand).

Retains patient's autonomy and sense of self-worth.

5 Have caregiver help set up activities so patient can complete task (e.g., chopping vegetables before cooking, placing wash basin on table in bedroom for sponge bath, placing clothes to wear for day on bed, unpacking groceries on countertop for eventual storage, arranging food on plate with items in clockwise orientation [e.g., vegetables at 9, salad at 3, meat at 6]).

Helps patient master task even though unable either physically or cognitively to perform all steps.

6 Discuss with patient, caregiver, and health care provider options for scheduling multiple medications:

Drugs sometimes cause physiologic changes that create risk for injury.

   a Administer medications that are likely to cause confusion at bedtime.

Reduces risk for confusion during waking hours that contribute to disorientation and risk for falling.

Clinical Decision Point *Do not recommend this if patient has nocturia, because patient will be at greater risk for falling.*

---

   b Space antihypertensives and antiarrhythmics at different times to minimize side effects.

These drugs cause blood pressure changes and dizziness, thus increasing risk for falls.

   c When possible reduce number of pain medications used.

Drugs create sedative effects, increasing risk for falls.

   d Have diuretics taken early in day and not at night.

Diuretic effect occurs during day while patient is awake.

   e Discuss with health care provider possibility of taking medications at same time.

If safe and appropriate, taking medications at same time will alleviate problem of patient remembering multiple administration times.

   f Discuss use of medication organizer and dispenser (see illustration).

Organizing medication in daily dispenser helps patient and caregiver avoid medication errors of duplicating or missing medications.

7 Teach family caregiver how to use simple and direct communication:

Relays care and support through therapeutic communication techniques.

   a Sit or stand in front of patient in full view.

Promotes reception of verbal and nonverbal messages.

   b Face patient with hearing impairment while speaking; do not cover mouth.

Patient can see speaker's lips. Prevents voice distortion.

   c Use calm and relaxed approach.

   d Use eye contact and touch.

Helps to reinforce messages.

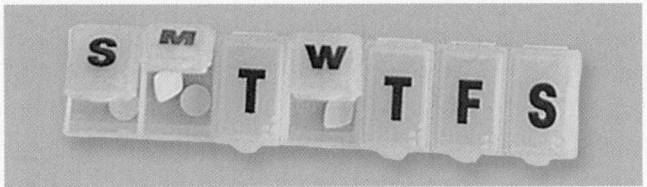

STEP 6f Weekly medication organizer.

STEP	RATIONALE
e Speak slowly, in simple words and short sentences.	Enhances understanding of messages.
f Use nonverbal gestures that complement verbal messages.	
8 Place clocks, calendars, and personal mementos (e.g., pictures, scrapbooks) throughout rooms within home. Enhance environment with addition of tactile boards or three-dimensional art.	Maintaining familiar surroundings maximizes cognitive function.
9 Have family caregiver routinely orient patient to who caregiver is and which activities they are going to complete.	This strategy is useful in patients with progressive dementia. Behavioral symptoms in later stages include delusions, agitation, and hallucinations (Alzheimer's Association, 2012).
10 Be sure that patient has regular naps or rest periods during day.	Fatigue adds to any mental status changes. Provides patient energy to perform planned activities.
11 Have caregiver encourage and support frequent visits by family and friends. Teach caregiver how to use humor and reminiscing about favorite stories to promote social interaction.	Participation in social activities prevents boredom and restlessness.
12 Provide safe place for person to wander (e.g., large family room or fenced yard).	Reduces risk for injury and leaving residence (Kazer, 2011).
13 Use labels to cue or remind person (Alzheimer's Association, 2012).	Helps reorient patient.
14 Recommend that family of wandering patient install door locks or electronic guards.	Reduces chance of patient exiting home unsupervised.
15 Create calm, safe setting that is appropriate for patient's abilities (Alzheimer's Association, 2012).	Prevents falls and minimizes behavioral symptoms.
16 Monitor patient for personal comfort (e.g., hunger, thirst, constipation, full bladder, and comfortable temperature) (Alzheimer's Association, 2012).	Reduces stimuli that prompt wandering.
17 Install motion detector near exit site, with portable alarm that can accompany caregiver.	Alerts caregiver to patient's attempt to exit residence.
18 Consider need for full-time care assistance.	

EVALUATION

1 During follow-up visits ask patient to review home-management activities completed the morning of that day and previous day.	Determines patient's ability to recall events and evaluates if patient completed planned activities.
2 Review with patient and family caregiver revised schedule for medication administration.	Evaluates understanding of regimen.
3 Have caregiver keep track of doses patient takes over a 1-week period.	Tracking doses will confirm if patient is adherent to regimen.
4 Ask caregiver to describe ways that will increase patient's success in completing home-management and self-care activities.	Measures learning.
5 Have caregiver show schedules of daily routines and review specific approaches used. Observe environment for presence of reality orientation cues.	Determines caregiver's success in applying information and making environmental changes.
6 Have family caregivers describe options for minimizing wandering.	Measures learning.
7 Have family caregivers report number of occurrences of wandering.	Determines if reduction in wandering has occurred.

Unexpected Outcomes

1 Patient is unable to complete ADLs as planned.

2 Patient experiences drug interaction from multiple medications.

3 Caregiver is unable to describe/implement techniques that will improve patient's orientation and ability to complete activities.

4 Caregiver is unable to describe/implement strategies to decrease wandering.

5 Patient's wandering increases.

6 Patient misses medication doses or takes a wrong dosage.

Related Interventions

- Further modifications are sometimes necessary.
- Reassess what occurred when task was not completed.

- Have health care provider evaluate patient's medication regimen.
- Recommend feasibility of pharmacy consultation.

- Reinstruction and discussion are necessary.
- Support for caregiver is sometimes necessary before caregiver can learn how to support someone else.

- Consider that caregiver is not able to provide necessary support; need to analyze other options.
- Reinstruction and discussion are necessary.
- Caregiver may not have resources available to adapt environment.

- Reconsider strategies used.
- Reassess factors prompting wandering.

- Review list of medications and method for administering (e.g., medication dispenser). Reconsider strategies to organize and schedule medications.

Recording and Reporting

- Record assessment of patient's cognitive and mental status, recommended interventions, and patient's and caregiver's response in progress notes.
- Report to health care provider any change in patient's behavior that reflects a decline in cognitive or mental status.

Special Considerations

Teaching

- Instruct family caregiver in signs and symptoms of dementia and depression. If patient's functionality continues to decline, caregiver may choose to learn more ADL support skills (e.g., how to help with hygiene, dressing, transfer and turning, toileting).

Pediatric

- Children with cognitive impairment are often not aware of inherent dangers during play and other activities. Parental supervision is critical.

Gerontologic

- Early diagnosis of the cause of dementia is best for the patient and caregiver so prompt treatment can begin, the patient can be included in treatment decisions as much as possible, and the caregiver has an understanding of the behavior (Alzheimer's Association, 2012).
- Consider that a patient may not have a family member who is able or willing to care for him or her. Outside assistance from a professional agency may be required if available; this may also affect patient's ability to stay in his or her home and not be placed in assisted or skilled care.

SKILL 41-3 Medication and Medical Device Safety

At the first home visit, you will review and list all medications and medication bottles that a patient has in their home. It is important to note drug name, dosage, frequency, and route and compare this list with any previous lists, known medications, and discharge instructions. This process is known as medication reconciliation; the goal is to ensure that there are no errors or omissions in a patient's medication regimen, while also assessing if there is any need for change in medications (Institute for Healthcare Improvement, 2012).

Patients in the home frequently manage the administration of medications and the use of medical devices such as syringes, blood glucose monitoring equipment, dressing supplies, and even intravenous (IV) devices. This includes administration, storage, and disposal of medications and medical devices. It is critical that a patient administers medications correctly, uses devices properly, and cleans and removes waste from equipment. Infection control is just one safety principle that a patient and/or family caregiver must learn for the home setting. Make sure that patients know regulations regarding waste disposal and follow the procedures consistent with local and federal laws (e.g., the Environmental Protection Agency recommends placing soiled dressings in securely fastened plastic bags before adding to regular trash).

One of the nurse's responsibilities within the home environment is to help a patient with sensory, mobility, or cognitive deficits. Patients who require special consideration include those with acute sensory or neurologic impairment; those with chronic illness such as diabetes or arthritis; and older adults, who frequently have physical limitations that make manipulating medical devices and dispensing medications difficult. For example, patients with arthritic hands are sometimes unable to open medication containers because of weakness in the hands and the pain created by pressure on the joints.

Delegation and Collaboration

The skill of assessing for and monitoring medication and medical device safety cannot be delegated to nursing assistive personnel (NAP). The nurse directs the NAP to:

- Make suggestions that further ensure patient safety regarding the use of basic infection control practices.
- Make suggestions as to how to dispose of sharps, needles, and contaminated supplies.

Equipment
❑ Colored marking pens
❑ Labels
❑ Puncture-resistant sharps container or 2-L hard plastic bottle with cap

❑ Duct, masking, or adhesive tape
❑ Assistive devices (e.g., syringe magnifier)
❑ Medication organizers

STEP	RATIONALE

ASSESSMENT

1 Assess patient's sensory, musculoskeletal, and neurologic function (see Chapter 6).

2 If family caregiver provides routine assistance, assess his or her function as in Step 1.

3 Assess patient's medication regimen and length of time that patient has been receiving each drug.

Reveals any deficits that will affect preparation and use of medications or medical devices.

Determines level of assistance that caregivers can provide.

Determines complexity of medication regimen and how familiar patient is with regimen.

Clinical Decision Point *Be sure that medication labels are not confusing for a patient. For example, the Spanish word for "eleven" is written as "once." A Spanish patient could confuse a medication direction that requires them to take a medication 1 time a day as 11 times a day.*

4 Ask patient to show you where medications are stored in home. Look at each container.

5 Assess temperature of storage area.

6 Have patient describe daily schedule for drug administration and whether there are any problems in following that schedule.

7 If patient self-administers injections, ask to see where he or she stores supplies and what he or she uses to dispose of used syringes and needles.

8 If patient uses glucose-monitoring device, ask to see where monitor, lancets, and glucose strips are stored. Also ask about how patient disposes of lancets.

Determines condition and labeling of containers.

Medication should not be stored in extreme heat. Insulin should be kept in cool place.

Helps to reveal patient's adherence to or misunderstanding of instructions.

Determines sterility of equipment and whether method of disposal creates risk to patient or family for needlestick injuries.

Allows nurse to examine cleanliness of equipment, sterility of lancets, and condition of glucose strips. Sharps should be disposed of in puncture-proof container.

NURSING DIAGNOSES

- Deficient knowledge regarding medication safety
- Ineffective health maintenance
- Noncompliance
- Risk for infection
- Risk for injury

Related factors are individualized based on patient's condition or needs.

PLANNING

1 Expected outcomes following completion of procedure:
- Patient and family caregiver discuss principles of medication safety.
- Patient and caregiver prepare medications independently.

- Patient and caregiver identify correct conditions for storing medications, medical devices, and supplies.
- Patient and caregiver dispose of used medical equipment and supplies correctly.

Nurse provides knowledge base for safe medication administration.

Adaptations successfully accommodate patient's and/or family caregiver's deficits in handling and manipulating equipment.

Instruction focuses on ensuring infection control measures.

Appropriate receptacles and methods for disposal are made available.

IMPLEMENTATION

1 Educate patient and family caregiver in principles to ensure that medications are safe to use:
  a Never take medicine prescribed for another member of household (Centers for Disease Control and Prevention [CDC], 2012).

  b Do not take any medicine more than a year old or past expiration date on container.

  c Do not place different medicines in same container.
  d Do not place medications in containers different than their original ones.

Medications must be of full strength and used for appropriate pharmacologic reason to have therapeutic benefit.

Expired medication is sometimes toxic or no longer effective.

Prevents accidental "mix-up" of medications and medication error.
Prevents accidental "mix-up" of medications and confusion as to expiration dates.

STEP	RATIONALE
e Always finish prescribed medication; do not save for future illness.	Prevents underdosing or inappropriate dosing.
f Wash hands before and after administering/taking medication.	Contaminated hands are source of infection transmission.
2 Recommend approaches for preparation of medications:	
a For patients with weakened grasp or pain of hands and fingers, have local pharmacist place medications in screw-top container.	Tops of childproof containers are difficult to remove, especially if hand and finger grasp is weakened.

Clinical Decision Point *If patient has children or grandchildren who have easy access to medication storage area or patient's purse, be sure that medications are stored in secure place.*

STEP	RATIONALE
b For patients with visual alterations, have pharmacy type larger labels on all medication containers.	Ensures that patient is able to read drug name and dosage schedule clearly.
c For patients who are legally blind, have Braille labels placed on medication containers.	Labels embossed with drug name, strength, and prescription numbers are easy to read for patient trained in use of Braille.
d For patients taking multiple medications, introduce color-coding system. Use same color for drugs that patient needs to take at same time. Mark tops of bottle caps with colored marking pen.	Technique helps ensure that patient takes correct drugs and doses at correct times of day.
e Provide specially designed syringes with large numerals or syringe magnifier for patients with visual alterations (see illustration).	Ensures that accurate dose of drug is prepared in syringe.
f For patients who have difficulty manipulating syringes, offer a spring-loaded needle insertion aid.	Delivers injection safely without manipulation of plunger.

Clinical Decision Point *Instruct family caregivers in knowing what to do following a needlestick injury: Wash the affected area thoroughly with soap and water and dry. If patient has acquired immunodeficiency syndrome (AIDS), hepatitis, or other communicable disease, caregivers should pursue appropriate laboratory testing.*

STEP	RATIONALE
g Teach caregivers how to properly draw up prescribed volume of medication into syringe. When necessary, have caregiver prepare extra prefilled syringes for patient's use when caregiver is absent.	Ensures that caregiver knows proper preparation techniques. Ensures that patient has access to injections. Watch patient and/or caregiver draw up and dispense medications to determine if more teaching is needed.
3 Recommend approaches for medication and supply storage:	
a Store medications in safe place, preferably in kitchen.	Moisture in bathroom may cause medications to decompose.
b Keep liquid medications and parenteral drugs, especially insulin, in cool place.	Prevents decomposition of drug.

Clinical Decision Point *Although manufacturers recommend storing insulin in the refrigerator, injecting cold insulin can sometimes make the injection more painful. To avoid this, many providers suggest storing the bottle of insulin being used at room temperature. Insulin kept at room temperature will last approximately 1 month. Remember, however, to store extra bottles in the refrigerator if a patient buys more than one bottle at a time to save money (ADA, 2012). If insulin is stored in refrigerator, be sure that drug is in a bin or container, away from food.*

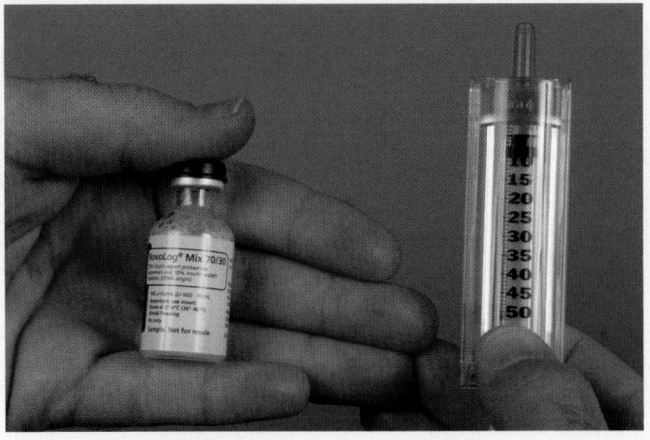

STEP 2e Syringe with magnifier.

STEP	RATIONALE
c Keep medical supplies such as syringes, dressing supplies, and glucose meter in airtight container (e.g., plastic storage bin) and store in cool place such as bedroom closet.	Ensures that supplies are not exposed to moisture or other contaminants.
d Instruct patient and caregiver to use new needle with each medication administration.	Multiple use of same needle puts patient at risk for infection.
4 Review for patient and caregiver proper techniques for disposal of medications, "sharps," and disposable medical supplies:	
a Discard unused portions of drugs or outdated drugs in a bag containing coffee grounds or kitty litter.	Ensures that no one in household uses drug not prescribed for their use or drugs that will be ineffective pharmacologically. Ensures safe disposal to prevent outsider from acquiring medications.
b Obtain sharps container from medical supply store or IV equipment supplier. (If finances are limited, have patient use small-neck plastic bottle such as soda bottle.) Dispose of all needles and lancets in container.	Puncture-proof container prevents exposure to contaminated needlestick. Small-neck container makes it difficult for anyone to easily retrieve used needle or sharp.
c Caution against filling sharps container to point where needles protrude out opening. Discard when three-fourths full, securing top with duct tape or adhesive tape.	Prevents needlesticks.
d Store sharps container in area inaccessible to children.	Prevents injury to child.
e Dispose of soiled dressings, used glucose testing reagent strips, and IV tubing in separate, sealed, plastic garbage bag. Place in second plastic bag (double bagged), and discard appropriately as trash.	Prevents contamination with other items in home. Minimizes chances of caregiver being exposed to infectious waste.
f Consult local public health department or community authorities regarding proper way to dispose of waste, including some medications.	Most communities have strict guidelines for waste and medication disposal.

EVALUATION

1 Have patient and/or caregiver describe steps to take to ensure that medications are safe to use.	Demonstrates learning.
2 Observe patient and/or caregiver prepare and administer medication dose.	Evaluates ability to physically manipulate medications and necessary equipment.
3 Observe home setting for location of medications and supplies.	Evaluates patient's and/or caregiver's adherence to recommendations.
4 Have patient describe how sharps or medical equipment is discarded.	Demonstrates learning.
5 Do pill counts (pills remaining in containers) at successive intervals such as twice a week for 2 weeks.	Helps to verify that patient takes correct number of medications over period of time.

Unexpected Outcomes	**Related Interventions**
1 Patient and/or family caregiver is unable to recall principles for safe use of drugs.	• Reinstruction necessary, or patient and caregiver need chance to ask more questions regarding benefit of precautions. • Offer written, simple, and clear instructions.
2 Patient and/or caregiver has difficulty or is unable to prepare and self-administer medication.	• Offer further assistance in setting up equipment. • Offer assistive aids. • Reinstruct in steps used to prepare medication.
3 Medications and medical devices are not stored in secure or appropriate location.	• Assess whether patient chooses to store items conveniently rather than safely or has limited resources. • Reinstruction and discussion are necessary.
4 Sharps and disposable medical equipment are not disposed of properly.	• Provide reinstruction. • Arrange to provide appropriate containers.
5 Excess or insufficient number of pills found during pill count.	• Review with patient and caregiver daily drug prescribed. Reevaluate use of dosage reminders. • Notify health care provider.

Recording and Reporting
- Record instructions and recommendations to patient and caregiver and results of return demonstrations in progress notes. Notify health care provider of unsafe situation.

Special Considerations
Teaching
- Instruct patients in care of linens. If linens are contaminated with microorganisms, they should be decontaminated by washing with soap/detergent and hot water 140° F (60° C). If patient is using lower temperature washers (<113° F [45° C]), instruct him or her to add hypochlorite bleach to effectively decontaminate linens (Reynolds, 2009).

Pediatric
- It is vital to keep medications and other equipment such as cleaning products out of the reach of children (Home Safety Council, 2011).
- All medicines and cleaning products should have child safety caps (Home Safety Council, 2011).
- If teaching self-management skills, include adult supervision and input. Never refer to medications as candy.

? Critical Thinking Exercises

Mrs. James is a 79-year-old woman who lives with her 84-year-old sister in a split-level four-bedroom home. Mrs. James has a history of metastatic bone cancer and was recently diagnosed with heart failure. In addition to taking multiple oral medications, she undergoes weekly intravenous chemotherapy for progression of her cancer. Mrs. James has no other family closer than a 2-hour drive, and her older sister has advanced glaucoma and diminished hearing. Both women refuse to move from their home, even at the urging of Mrs. James' three children to move closer to one of them. Mrs. James no longer drives, nor does her sister; and she is unable to climb the few steps needed to move beyond the lower living level of the home. Because of this immobility, Mrs. James cannot reach the upstairs bathrooms, which contain showers, and she relies on her older sister to help care for her and maintain the house on a daily basis.

1. Based on her medical history, offer three reasons why Mrs. James is at risk for falls.
2. Mrs. James' children expressed concern that their mother is getting confused about her medication regimen. How would you approach assessing the patient's adherence to the regimen?
   1. Ask her to show you where medications are stored in home.
   2. Have her describe daily schedule for drug administration.
   3. Determine caregiver's knowledge of medication schedule.
   4. Examine the condition of storage area for medications.
3. Mrs. James' children tell you that they are concerned about their mother's and aunt's safety, "We worry that they will get injured. We've tried to convince them to move to a one-level apartment near us, but they refuse." What advice might you give the family?

✓ REVIEW QUESTIONS

1. A woman found wandering in her nightclothes is also dirty, but does not appear to have any injuries. Which topics would a home care nurse include in his discussion with the patient and her family? (Select all that apply.)
   1. The medications she is taking and who supervises her
   2. Any decrease in cognitive function seen within the past few months
   3. Whether she or someone else pays her bills
   4. Any history of wandering
   5. Always have a current photograph available
   6. When she was last seen by her health care provider
2. A 50-year-old teacher with severe rheumatoid arthritis is noting some changes in her mobility. Which simple screening examination could be used to detect difficulties with balance or gait?
   1. The Mini-Mental State Examination (MMSE)
   2. The Timed Get Up and Go (TUG) Test
   3. The SPLATT screening tool
   4. A fall diary

3. A home care patient is changing a dressing daily on a foot ulcer. In what type of container should the nurse teach the patient to place the old dressing for disposal?
   1. A wide-mouth plastic bottle
   2. A small plastic container
   3. The standard garbage can
   4. A plastic garbage bag placed into a second plastic bag
4. A patient has recently noticed that she has near-miss falls more often. Her health care provider recommended that she begin an exercise program. When teaching this patient, the nurse would explain that a program with which focus would be most effective for her?
   1. Endurance exercises
   2. Maintaining range of motion
   3. Incorporating the patient's activity patterns
   4. Strength, gait, and balance
5. An older adult with diabetes mellitus asks the home care nurse how to maintain her diabetic supplies. The nurse knows that teaching was successful when the patient states she should: (Select all that apply.)
   1. Keep the used syringes in a small-neck bottle such as a screw-top soda bottle.
   2. Keep the insulin vials in the refrigerator until shortly before they are needed.
   3. Keep the insulin vials on the kitchen counter until all the insulin has been used.
   4. Keep the glucose meter strips in an airtight bag in the closet until they have been used.
6. While visiting a patient at her home, the patient complains of many trips to the bathroom at night, which "causes her to be light-headed and very tired all day long." Which action should the nurse take first?
   1. Obtain an order for a bedside commode
   2. Suggest the use of night-lights throughout the house
   3. Obtain a complete cultural history of the patient
   4. Determine if she is taking a diuretic
7. A patient with beginning dementia still wants to be independent and cook one meal per day. Which suggestion by the nurse would provide anticipatory guidance regarding safety?
   1. Keep a fire extinguisher in the garage in case of fire.
   2. Make sure that you have enough light in the kitchen.
   3. Use a loud timer to alert you that food is ready.
   4. Keep everything you need in cabinets with a lock.
8. During a home visit the nurse finds one of her patients to be unusually confused and dirty. What is the most appropriate action for the nurse to take initially?
   1. Observe the home environment for cleanliness and availability of supplies
   2. Notify the appropriate state agency that the patient is being abused
   3. Call 9-1-1 and have the patient taken to the hospital for evaluation
   4. Do a brief assessment of the patient's cognitive and mental status

9 An older patient with hearing difficulty lives alone at home. She is taking seven different medications daily at different times of the day and states to the nurse that she is frustrated trying to remember all of her pills and is considering stopping some of the medications. The nurse helps the patient organize the medication by:

   1 Making a visual chart code of the medications so the patient can identify them by color and shape of pill.

   2 Taking the medications away from the patient and returning each day to administer them as ordered.

   3 Bringing the patient a medication pill organizer and helping her fill the organizer for 1 week.

   4 Calling the patient's daughter and instructing the daughter that it is now her responsibility to give her mother daily medication.

10 Both members of an older couple have visual impairments and joint stiffness and pain in their upper extremities. Which activities should the daughter, who lives nearby, suggest to help them maintain appropriate nutrition and some independence?

   1 Cutting up vegetables and fruits and storing in screw-top jars in the refrigerator

   2 Arranging the food on the plate with items in a clockwise orientation

   3 Placing serving-size food items in easy-to-open packages

   4 Taking the parents grocery shopping every week so they can plan their menus

REFERENCES

Abele CL: Cultural diversity and community health nursing. In Nies MA, McEwen M, editors: *Community/public health nursing: promoting the health of populations*, ed 5, St Louis, 2011, Mosby.

Abele CL, Nies MA: Home health and hospice. In Nies MA, McEwen M, editors: *Community/public health nursing: promoting the health of populations*, ed 5, St Louis, 2011, Mosby.

Alzheimer's Association: *Safety center*, 2011, available at http://www.alz.org/safetycenter/we_can_help_safety_medicalert_safereturn.asp, accessed March 27, 2012.

Alzheimer's Association: *Alzheimer's and dementia basics*, 2012, available at http://www.alz.org/alzheimers_disease_what_is_alzheimers.asp, accessed March 27, 2012.

American Diabetes Association: *Living with diabetes: Insulin storage and syringe safety*, 2012, available at http://www.diabetes.org/living-with-diabetes/treatment-and-care/medication/insulin/insulin-storage-and-syringe.html, accessed September 1, 2012.

Beauchet O et al: Timed Up and Go test and risk of falls in older adults: a systematic review, *J Nutr Health Aging* 15(10):933, 2011.

Centers for Disease Control and Prevention: *Prevent unintentional poisoning*, February 2012, available at http://www.cdc.gov/features/poisonprevention/, accessed March 27, 2012.

Crist JD et al: Keeping it in the family: when Mexican-American older adults choose not to use home healthcare services, *Home Healthc Nurse* 29(5):282, 2011.

Ebersole P et al: *Toward health aging: human need & nursing response*, ed 7, St Louis, 2008, Mosby.

Edelman CL, Mandle CL: *Health promotion throughout the lifespan*, ed 6, St Louis, 2009, Mosby.

Fletcher PC et al: Risk factors for falling among community-based seniors, *J Pat Safety* 5(2):61, 2009.

Fletcher PC et al: Risk factors for restriction in activity associated with fear of falling among seniors within the community, *J Patient Safety* 6(3):187, 2010.

Fortinsky RH et al: Extent of implementation of evidence-based fall prevention practices for older patients in home health care, *J Am Geriatr Soc* 56:737, 2008.

Greene D et al: Fall prevention pilot: hazard survey and responses to recommendations, *Occupational Ther Health Care* 23(1):24, 2009.

Harvath T, McKenzie G: Nursing standard of practice protocol: depression in older adults, 2012, available at http://consultgerirn.org/topics/depression/want_to_know_more#ref16, accessed October 1, 2012.

Hockenberry MJ, Wilson DW: *Wong's nursing care of infants and children*, ed 9, St Louis, 2011, Mosby.

Home Safety Council: *Bathroom safety tips*, 2011, available at http://www.homesafetycouncil.org, accessed March 27 2012.

Institute for Healthcare Improvement: *Reconcile medications at all transition points*, 2012, available at http://www.ihi.org/knowledge/Pages/Changes/ReconcileMedicationsatAllTransitionPoints.aspx, accessed March 27, 2012.

Kazer MW: Cognitive and neurological function. In Meiner SE editor: *Gerontologic nursing*, ed 4, St Louis, 2011, Mosby.

Meiner SE: Safety. In Meiner SE editor: *Gerontologic nursing*, ed 4, St Louis, 2011, Mosby.

Mueth EC: Family influences. In Meiner SE, editor: *Gerontologic nursing*, ed 4, St Louis, 2011, Mosby.

Muir SW et al: Modifiable risk factors identify people who transition from non-fallers to fallers in community-dwelling older adults: a prospective study, *Physiother Can* 62(4):358, 2010.

Mullin L: Keeping safety a priority in home care and hospice: one agency's journey, *Home Healthc Nurse* 28(2):63, 2010.

National Fire Protection Association (NFPA): *Home structure fires*, 2011, available at http://www.nfpa.org/assets/files/PDF/OS.Homes.pdf , accessed March 27, 2012.

National Rifle Association (NRA): *NRA gun safety rules*, 2011, available at http://www.nrahq.org/education/guide.asp, accessed March 27, 2012.

Patient Education Management: DP and homecare need improved communication, *Healthc Benchmarks Qual Improve* 16(3):34, 2009.

Reynolds K. Germs in the home environment, *Learn about germs*, 2009, University of Arizona Board of Regents, available at http://learnaboutgerms.arizona.edu/germs_in_the_environment.htm, accessed March 27, 2012.

Touhy TA: Fluids and incontinence. In Touhy TA, Jett KF, editors: *Ebersole and Hess' gerontological nursing and healthy aging*, ed 3, St Louis, 2010a, Mosby.

Touhy TA: Maintaining mobility and environmental safety. In Touhy TA, Jett KF, editors: *Ebersole and Hess' gerontological nursing and healthy aging*, ed 3, St Louis, 2010b, Mosby.

Touhy TA: Communicating with elders. In Touhy TA, Jett KF, editors: *Ebersole and Hess' gerontological nursing and healthy aging*, ed 3, St Louis, 2010c, Mosby.

US Department of Health and Human Services (USDHHS): *Healthy People 2020*, 2011, Injury and Violence Prevention, available at http://www.healthypeople.gov/2020/topicsobjectives2020/overview.aspx?topicid=24, accessed March 27, 2012.

US Department of Health and Human Services (USDHHS) Administration on Aging: *Home modifications*, 2009, available at http://www.aoa.gov/AoARoot/site_utilities/Search.aspx?cx=012624277387271114612:plyugpymdgq&cof=FORID:11&q=home%20modifications%20and%20assistive%20devices#1058, accessed March 27, 2012.

Wallhagen MI, Pettengill E: Hearing impairment: significant but unaddressed in primary care settings, *J Gerontol Nurs* 34(2):36, 2008.

Yamashita T et al: Fall risk factors in community dwelling elderly who receive Medicaid supported home and community-based care services, *J Aging Health* 23(4):682, 2011.

Home Care Teaching

MEDIA RESOURCES

- ℮volve *learning system* http://evolve.elsevier.com/Perry/skills
  - Review Questions
  - Audio Glossary

KEY TERMS

Antipyretic	Gastrostomy feeding tube	Infusion pump	Transtracheal oxygen
Clean technique	High-Fowler's position	Nasogastric feeding tube	catheter
Dementia			

OBJECTIVES

Mastery of content in this chapter will enable the nurse to:

- Identify factors that influence clients' abilities to learn and care for themselves at home.
- Discuss the collaborative nature of home care teaching.
- Assess safety factors that may impair or prohibit a client's ability to perform skills in the home setting.
- Discuss situations and conditions that require a client and/or family to learn skills that support and achieve health maintenance.
- Choose appropriate teaching strategies to use in the home setting.
- Implement and evaluate appropriate learning strategies that support clients' ability to care for themselves in the home.

The health care delivery system has changed, shifting where clients receive care from inpatient facilities to the home. Although acute and long-term care settings continue to provide inpatient services, many clients recover from or are treated for illnesses in their homes. Clients assume greater responsibility for managing their own care, resulting in a greater demand for home care nurses. A home care nurse provides information and resources by collaborating with a client or family caregiver to address the client's health needs, preferences, and values and incorporating their strengths, skills, and capacity (Wolff et al., 2009).

Client teaching is an essential part of nursing practice. All nurses, including home care nurses, have an ethical responsibility to teach their clients. Information needs to be relevant, current, and clearly presented. The Joint Commission's "Speak Up" initiative (TJC, 2011) outlines information for clients related to their rights and role in health care. Included are the rights to be informed about care they will receive, make decisions about their care, refuse care, be listened to, and be treated with courtesy and respect. The home care nurse provides information in a manner appropriate for a client to understand and clarifies information provided to the client by other health care providers, therefore becoming the client's primary source of information.

Home care nurses thoroughly assess factors that affect a client's abilities and willingness to manage self-care. Determine what your clients want to know, how they learn, and what motivates them to learn new information (Meade, 2011). Trust must be established before teaching can begin, and you must remember that you are in their home environment and not an acute care setting. Be respectful of a client's surroundings and time. In addition, make an effort to connect the health message to the client's everyday events and real-life situations and use teach-back methods to ensure client comprehension (Meade, 2011). Teach-back is a way to confirm that you have explained to patients what they need to know in a manner that the patients understand. Patient understanding is confirmed when they explain a topic back to you. For example, after a home health nurse has completed instruction with a patient with diabetes, a teach-back method would include the question, "Now tell me what you do if your blood sugar is lower than 70."

An additional challenge facing home care nurses today is health literacy. Clients who are illiterate often have difficulty reading, writing, and speaking English. *Healthy People 2020* (US Department of Health and Human Services [USDHHS], 2012) has set an objective to improve the health literacy of Americans. To accomplish this, the USDHHS aims to increase the number of clients who report receiving easy-to-understand instructions about managing their illness or health, the rate of providers who ask their clients if they understood the instructions given, and the number of persons reporting that their health care provider always offered assistance in completing forms. It is important for you to remember that many clients have difficulty reading and understanding medical terminology. And no matter what their educational level, the health care system in general is confusing (Brown, 2009). Plan to spend a sufficient amount of time teaching your clients and ensure that they understood your teaching and the information provided. Reinforce verbal instructions with printed, culturally appropriate client education information and use other audiovisual materials when possible.

Home care nurses are creative and adapt teaching to meet each client's unique physical, psychosocial, and cultural needs. It is very important for a client to become an active partner in the plan of care. Refer him or her to community resources to help overcome barriers (e.g., lack of transportation or inadequate funds for medications) and collaborate with the client or caregivers and interdisciplinary teams (e.g., pharmacists, physical therapists, and occupational therapists). Many times a variety of other social services and health-related organizations are involved in making a client's home care plan successful. For collaboration to be successful, identify who is involved in the client's care and establish mutual trust and respect through open and honest communication. When home care nurses successfully implement individualized teaching plans, clients improve their quality of life, need fewer health care provider visits, reduce their health care expenses, and regain health or gain more control over illness.

EVIDENCE-BASED PRACTICE

Clients must understand how to manage their health and illnesses, take discharge medications correctly and safely, and perform related care at home. In discharge planning and home care you will help clients and caregivers make well-informed decisions about their health practices (Meade, 2011). As a teacher and client advocate, you can engage the client or caregiver as participants in care.

With clients discharged sooner and with more health care needs, the home care nurse is challenged to teach them and help them feel secure before and following discharge. A recent study that examined client or caregiver uncertainty surrounding discharge found three main themes: uncertainty through lack of preparation for discharge, uncertainty through lack of information, and uncertainty of "being at home" (Boughton and Halliday, 2009). Another study that examined clients' experiences of living at home on mechanical ventilation provides insight into what clients valued in their home care providers. Clients first wanted an increased quality of life and sense of control; and second, they valued competent health care providers and quality client teaching (Ballangrud et al., 2009). Several effective nursing measures facilitate a client's transition from the health care environment to home.

- Use concise, clear, and consistent information to reduce anxiety in clients and caregivers.
- Use clear written and verbal information to help lessen client or caregiver stress and anxiety and instill a sense of confidence and control when teaching clients and caregivers how to perform specific nursing skills in the home setting (Pittman, 2009).
- Offer clients an opportunity to maintain some control in their lives and health care preferences (Ballangrud et al., 2009).
- Spend quality time with clients and their caregivers and remain organized when providing direct care and client education.
- Provide routine follow-up to determine client or caregiver understanding and/or need for further education about specific home care interventions (Ballangrud et al., 2009).

CLIENT-CENTERED CARE

With appropriate and comprehensive home care teaching, clients can become empowered, resulting in better overall health outcomes. Your client is your primary concern and consideration when teaching. Involve family caregivers as appropriate to ensure their understanding and ability to provide necessary assistance.

Consider principles of cultural diversity when caring for clients in their homes. Know the unique characteristics of the community in which a person lives so you can readily access needed resources. Respect each individual's cultural background and beliefs and his or her ability to understand instructions developed outside of his or her native language. When educating clients of different ethnic groups, be aware of the distinctive aspects of each culture, being careful not to stereotype clients. Collaborate with other nurses and educators to help deal with cultural diversity and ask for help from the people in the cultural group to share values and beliefs.

Respectful communication includes addressing a client in an appropriate manner and using acceptable body language (e.g., avoid direct eye contact) (Jett, 2010). Use an interpreter if you speak a language different from that of the client or if cultural tradition prohibits the client from talking to you directly. The meanings of words can change when translated (e.g., "risk" into Spanish is "riesgo"). This word does not carry the same weight as it does in English; thus you need to explain the *concept* of "danger" for pregnant Mexican women rather than simply translating the word (Scrimshaw, 2009).

Follow ethical principles in your approach to care. Do not limit the information a client can receive, make invalid or unreliable judgments about what a client can learn, or assume that a client should learn to accommodate an unjust treatment (Redman, 2008). Consider alternative teaching methods such as role playing, because often adults do not learn from reading brochures; they may learn by rehearsal, practice, and role playing (McKinney, 2010). Also consider different delivery approaches (e.g., Internet or DVDs) because more adults are accessing the Internet for health information.

Safety Guidelines

1 Assess if a client in the home setting is able to safely perform a skill. If he or she is unable to execute a skill independently,

identify a family caregiver who will help provide it safely in the home setting.

2 Assess and determine if the client has home medical equipment and knows how to use it properly for safe and successful self-care management.

3 Include teaching interventions for other persons in the household who positively or negatively influence the client's self-care management.

4 Provide an opportunity for client or family caregivers to demonstrate skill.

SKILL 42-1 Teaching Clients to Measure Body Temperature

An elevation in body temperature sometimes may be an early warning sign of serious health problems. Clients susceptible to temperature alterations (e.g., immunosuppressed clients) or their family caregivers need to know how to measure temperature correctly so they can seek medical attention earlier. Parents need to know how to measure their children's temperature because children can develop high fevers very quickly; older adults or their caregivers need to know the techniques for temperature measurement because older adults have impaired temperature control mechanisms. Teach clients and family caregivers the skills of measuring body temperature and technique to lower temperature when a fever occurs at home.

A variety of body temperature thermometers are currently available, including mercury, disposable single-use, electronic digital, temporal, and tympanic thermometers. The Environmental Protection Agency (EPA) discourages the use of mercury thermometers. If a mercury thermometer breaks or is not disposed of properly, the mercury vapor gets into the air, posing a major health risk in the home and community (EPA, 2011). Educate clients about the environmental hazards associated with mercury in the home and encourage them to purchase mercury-free thermometers.

Help a client choose the most appropriate thermometer to use in the home based on his or her normal dexterity, vision, and

financial resources. For example, a client with visual impairment from glaucoma or retinopathy is able to read a thermometer with a large digital display more easily. The need for an oral, rectal, or axillary temperature depends on the client's age and health status (see Chapter 5).

Delegation and Collaboration

The skill of teaching clients to measure body temperature cannot be delegated to nursing assistive personnel (NAP). The nurse instructs the NAP to:

- Inform the nurse of client or caregiver concerns about measuring body temperature.

Equipment

- ❏ Thermometer
- ❏ Disposable probe cover (if needed)
- ❏ Water-soluble lubricant (for rectal measurements)
- ❏ Paper or logbook and pencil or pen if frequent measurements are to be taken
- ❏ Disposable clean gloves (for rectal temperature taken by a caregiver)

STEP	RATIONALE

ASSESSMENT

1 Assess client's or family caregiver's ability to manipulate and read thermometer. Have client put on eyeglasses if necessary.

2 Assess client's knowledge of normal temperature range, symptoms of fever and hypothermia, and client's risk for body temperature alterations.

3 Assess client's ability to determine appropriate type of thermometer to be used in varying situations (see Chapter 5).

4 Assess client's or caregiver's previous knowledge and experience in measuring temperature and maintaining thermometer. Have client or caregiver perform return demonstration if they indicate ability to measure temperature.

Physical restrictions in handling or reading thermometer prevent client from being able to read thermometer and often require instructing caregiver instead of client.

Identifies client's ability to initiate preventive health measures and recognize alterations in body temperature.

Determines knowledge of age-related or medical conditions that determine selection of temperature.

Allows assessment of client's or caregiver's knowledge and use of safety precautions, aseptic technique, and time period for insertion.

NURSING DIAGNOSES

- Deficient knowledge regarding temperature measurement skill
- Ineffective thermoregulation
- Risk for infection
- Risk for imbalanced body temperature

Related factors are individualized based on client's condition or needs.

STEP	RATIONALE

PLANNING

1 Expected outcomes following completion of procedure:

- Client or family caregiver is able to correctly measure body temperature.
- Client or caregiver demonstrates proper cleaning and storage of equipment.
- Client or caregiver states normal temperature range and factors that affect temperature, signs and symptoms of fever and hypothermia, and measures to take with abnormal temperatures.

Indicates that skills are learned.

Prevents transfer of microorganisms and maintains integrity of thermometer.
Cognitive learning is achieved.

2 Select setting in home where client is most likely to measure temperature.

3 Discuss and demonstrate with client or caregiver normal temperature ranges; instruct caregiver to remain with client during measurement if age or physical status requires.

Considers client's preferences; is responsive to client's needs (Romano, 2009a).
Learning by doing; active participation is more effective than passive models (Meade, 2011).

IMPLEMENTATION

1 Demonstrate steps of thermometer preparation, insertion, and reading. Provide rationale for steps to client or family caregiver.

The eventual evaluation of psychomotor skill is measured through client's performance and ability to follow directions/instruction (Romano, 2009b). Adults learn best when they understand purpose of procedure.

   a Instruct client to take oral temperature 20 to 30 minutes after smoking or ingesting hot or cold liquids or foods and to wait at least an hour after a hot bath or vigorous exercise. Explain indications for selecting a temperature site other than oral.

Waiting at least 15 minutes after drinking hot or cold liquids or foods improves accuracy of temperature reading (AAP, 2012).

   b Perform hand hygiene. Instruct caregiver to wear clean, disposable gloves.

Client and family caregiver must be knowledgeable of infection prevention techniques.

   c Instruct client or caregiver on proper way to position patient for a temperature measurement (see Chapter 5).

Improves accuracy of readings.

   d Demonstrate temperature measurement technique and have client or caregiver perform each step with guidance. Do not rush him or her.

Allows for correction of errors in technique as they occur and for discussion of potential consequences of errors.

   e Explain any special precautions in using thermometers: oral thermometer must be placed in sublingual pocket; rectal thermometers must be lubricated with water-soluble lubricant; use rectal thermometer only for measuring rectal temperatures; never force a rectal thermometer into rectum.

Ensures accurate reading and avoidance of injury to client.

   f Discuss the typical time frame needed for a temperature to register (based on thermometer type) and how to take a reading.

Ensures accurate reading.

   g Teach proper method for removing, cleaning, and storing thermometer (when applicable) and select suitable storage location.

Prevents transmission of infection. Thermometer is stored properly so it does not break or become inaccurate when not in use.

2 Discuss common symptoms of fever: warm, dry, flushed skin; feeling warm; chills; piloerection; malaise; and restlessness.

Client or caregiver needs to recognize onset of fever in self or family member for early detection and intervention.

3 Discuss common signs and symptoms of hypothermia: cool skin, uncontrolled shivering, loss of memory, and signs of poor judgment. Explain that persons with inadequate home heating, older adults, or those unaware of potential dangers of cold conditions are at risk.

Client or caregiver needs to recognize onset of hypothermia in self or family member for early detection and intervention.

Instruct clients to dress warmly in layers, avoid extreme cold, and ingest warm liquids.

Helps minimize risk of hypothermia by trapping body heat (McLafferty et al., 2009).

Clinical Decision Point *Teach client to take temperature after chills/shivering subsides to obtain an accurate temperature.*

STEP	RATIONALE
4 Discuss importance of notifying health care provider when temperature elevations occur. Review common therapies for temperature reduction that are safe to perform at home, including when to use antipyretics, exposing skin to air, reducing room temperature, increasing air circulation, applying cool moist compresses to skin (e.g., forehead), and drinking fluids (Hockenberry and Wilson, 2011).	Treating fever enhances client comfort. Lowering temperature can reduce risk of febrile seizures in children (Hockenberry and Wilson, 2011).
5 Provide set of written guidelines for client's reference at appropriate level of health literacy.	Clients prefer written materials that are clear and concise; graphics can be used to enhance a point (Pittman, 2009).
6 Give client or caregiver logbook or piece of paper to time and record temperature if frequent monitoring is required. Instruct client to use written record to report temperatures to health care provider.	Keeping organized record of temperatures helps client validate and report temperature fluctuations to health care provider.

EVALUATION

1 Have client or family caregiver independently demonstrate technique for temperature measurement, including body placement and ability to read thermometer three separate times.	When psychomotor skill is performed with confidence and proficiency, it demonstrates mastery of skill (Romano, 2009a).
2 Ask client or caregiver to identify normal temperature range and influence of smoking and hot and cold liquids or foods on oral readings; discuss safety implications for temperature measurement.	Measures cognitive learning and confirms understanding of information.
3 Have client or caregiver describe common signs and symptoms of fever and hypothermia and methods for control.	Measures cognitive learning.
4 Watch client or caregiver clean and store equipment.	Proper cleaning prevents bacterial growth, and proper storage preserves accuracy of thermometer.
5 Watch client record temperature values and times in logbook. Review client's logbook periodically to ensure that temperatures are being recorded correctly.	Health care providers make changes in client care based on information provided by client. To ensure that changes are made appropriately, client needs to record accurate information.

Unexpected Outcomes

1 Client or family caregiver is unable to measure temperature, clean and store thermometer correctly, or verbalize knowledge about fever and temperature measurement.

2 Client reports that mercury glass thermometer has broken.

Related Interventions

- Ask client or caregiver to describe difficulties experienced while performing temperature measurement.
- Use different teaching strategy.
- Plan for client to perform return demonstration during next scheduled home care visit or plan to teach caregiver.
- Instruct client in steps to safely dispose of thermometer (Box 42-1).

BOX 42-1	**Steps to Take in the Event of a Mercury Spill**

- If possible, close the room off from the rest of the house and increase ventilation in the affected room by opening windows or turning on a fan.
- Put on rubber, nitrile, or latex gloves. Do not touch mercury. Do not allow children to help clean up the spill.
- Pick up glass pieces, place them in a folded paper towel, and place glass and towel into plastic zip lock bag.
- Use a squeegee or cardboard to gather mercury beads. Use an eyedropper to collect or draw up visible mercury beads. Slowly and carefully squeeze mercury onto a damp paper towel. Place the paper towel in a zip lock bag and secure. Then put shaving cream on a small brush and "dot" the area or press duct tape in area to pick up smaller beads.

- Place mercury, material used to pick up mercury, and broken glass in a plastic zip lock bag. Triple bag the contaminated objects (place in a total of three sealed bags).
- Place gloves, mercury, and all other wastes into a trash bag. Secure and label the bag.
- Call local health department to determine where to dispose of mercury safely.
- If possible, keep windows open and room well ventilated for at least 24 hours after clean up.
- Instruct client not to use a vacuum cleaner, a broom, or household cleaners when cleaning up mercury spill. Also instruct client not to put mercury down the drain or place contaminated clothing into the washing machine.

Data from EPA: *Mercury releases and spills*, 2011, available at http://www.epa.gov/mercury/spills/index.htm#thermometer; accessed April 5, 2012.

Recording and Reporting

- Record information taught and client's return demonstration in home care record.
- Record temperature in home care record and home documentation system (e.g., logbook).
- Report high and low temperatures to health care provider.

Special Considerations

Teaching

- Instruct client or family caregiver to never force thermometer into rectum or use rectal thermometer after rectal surgery, when the client has a rectal disorder such as tumor or severe hemorrhoids, when the client has a low platelet count, or when it is difficult to position client for proper thermometer placement.
- Use caution in recommending aspirin or any other over-the-counter (OTC) drug or antipyretic medicine in clients whose conditions contraindicate their use (e.g., gastric ulcer, bleeding tendencies, allergic reactions, drug interactions, liver or kidney dysfunction). Encourage client to contact health care provider before using over-the-counter antipyretics.
- Instruct client to never use sponging with isopropyl alcohol to lower fever because of neurotoxic effects (Hockenberry and Wilson, 2011).
- Always leave a phone number and instructions about how to reach home care nurse if needed.

Pediatric

- Stage of growth and development of child will determine site of measurement and type of equipment used (see Chapter 5).
- Different types of thermometers are available for use with children (e.g., temporal artery, tympanic). Reliability of these different thermometers varies; ensure that parents know how to use the equipment correctly and detect the signs and symptoms of a fever (Hockenberry and Wilson, 2011).
- Teach the family to take a child's temperature whenever he or she feels warm to the touch, even if the temperature was recently normal (Hockenberry and Wilson, 2011).

Gerontologic

- Oral temperature for older adults often ranges from 35° to 36.1° C (95° to 97° F); therefore a normal temperature range for adults sometimes reflects a fever in the older adult (Ebersole et al., 2008).
- Older adults are more sensitive to temperature changes and tend to demonstrate symptoms of delirium or dementia with variations of body temperature.
- Altered internal temperature regulation or dehydration occurs frequently in frail, debilitated clients. Temperature measurement becomes very important to prevent severe states of hypothermia or hyperthermia.
- Consider common age-related sensory changes in the older adult and direct teaching strategies to compensate for any alterations (e.g., a magnifying glass to read thermometer).

SKILL 42-2 Teaching Blood Pressure and Pulse Measurement

Clients with a variety of illnesses such as cardiac, kidney, or vascular diseases are susceptible to wide variations in their blood pressure (BP) and pulse. They benefit from knowing how to assess their own BP and pulse because they are able to seek medical attention early when readings vary from their acceptable ranges. In addition, healthy people who exercise learn how their body responds to exercise and are able to determine appropriate exercise plans based on knowing what their pulse and BP are before, during, and after exercise.

Research related to home monitoring of BP has illustrated the importance of regular monitoring outside of acute care settings and medical offices so the provider can treat clients with hypertension appropriately (Powers et al., 2011). If treatment is based on single readings during an office visit, providers do not see an accurate picture of a client's health. To gather this essential information about clients living at home, you will teach them to measure their BP and pulse regularly and interpret readings that are outside of their individualized normal values. For example, teach clients about factors that affect the accuracy of BP readings such as cuff placement, movement of the tubing, speaking during measurement, and position and movement of the extremity or body.

Aneroid sphygmomanometers are available to measure BP in the home (see Chapter 5). Aneroid manometers are safe, lightweight, compact, and portable. In the home many clients choose to use commercial automatic electronic BP devices. These devices may measure pulse rate and produce a BP measurement without needing to use a stethoscope. The devices involve placing a cuff around the arm, the wrist, or a fingertip. A reading is displayed electronically for the client. Electronic BP monitors are often easier to use, but their accuracy compared to manual BP monitoring is still a focus of debate. The level of skill of the person measuring the BP has been cited as a factor that contributes to inaccurate manual readings, thus providing one potential benefit of electronic

monitors (Harvard Health Publications, 2011). It is essential for clients to keep record of all their BP readings and compare those obtained by a health care provider with their electronic monitor to assess the accuracy of readings.

Additional factors that affect the accuracy of BP monitoring are cuff size and placement (Tomlinson, 2010). Have clients learn to place a cuff directly on their skin, not over clothing. Blood pressure cuffs that are too small tend to overestimate BP, whereas cuffs that are too large tend to underestimate it (Tomlinson, 2010). Not all electronic home BP monitors come with interchangeable cuff sizes, which can complicate BP monitoring at home. Help clients and family caregivers determine cuff size, calibration, and accuracy of electronic equipment before they determine which type of BP monitor to purchase.

Delegation and Collaboration

The skill of teaching clients to measure BP and pulse cannot be delegated to nursing assistive personnel (NAP). The nurse instructs the NAP to:

- Report concerns related to BP and measurements to the nurse.

Equipment

For Blood Pressure

❏ Sphygmomanometer or electronic BP reading device (Fig. 42-1) with bladder and cuff: Bladder should completely encircle arm without overlapping; cuff should be secure and fit snugly (Box 42-2).

❏ Stethoscope (two-headed teaching stethoscope is ideal) if using sphygmomanometer

For Pulse

❏ Wristwatch or clock with a second hand

For Both

❏ Pen or pencil and logbook or paper for recording

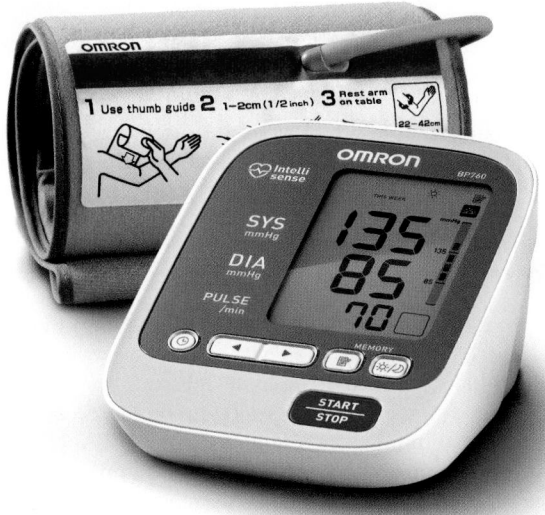

FIG 42-1 Home blood pressure monitoring device. (*Courtesy Omron Healthcare, Bannockburn, Ill.*)

BOX 42-2	Guidelines for Blood Pressure Cuff Size

Adult Sizes
- For "small adult" size: 10 × 24 cm (4 × 9.5 inches)
- For "adult" size: 13 × 30 cm (5 ×11.8 inches)
- For "large adult" size: 16 × 38 cm (6.3 ×15 inches)
- For "adult thigh" size: 20 × 42 cm (7.8 × 16.5 inches)

Pediatric Sizes*
- For newborn or premature infants, use "newborn" size: 4 × 8 cm (1.5 × 3 inches)
- For infants use "infant" size: 6 × 12 cm (2.3 × 4.7 inches)
- For older children use "child" size: 9 × 18 cm (3.5 × 7 inches)
- A standard adult cuff, a large adult cuff, and a thigh cuff for use in children with very large arms may be needed.

*Data from Hockenberry MJ, Wilson D: *Wong's nursing care of infants and children,* ed 9, St Louis, 2011, Mosby.

STEP	RATIONALE

ASSESSMENT

1 Assess client's or family caregiver's psychomotor function: visual (see dial and a clock) and auditory (hear Korotkoff sounds) acuity, ability to manipulate BP monitoring equipment, and ability to feel pulse.

Vision or hearing problems require use of equipment that has been adapted for these conditions (e.g., larger print) (Zaiken and Zeind, 2009). Other deficits may require caregiver to perform skills.

2 Assess client's or caregiver's knowledge of normal BP and pulse range for the client and symptoms and common causes of high or low readings. (Consult with health care provider regarding the normal range desired.)

Identifies client's or caregiver's ability to know when to initiate preventive health measures and recognize alterations in BP and pulse.

3 Assess client's or caregiver's knowledge of what BP and pulse measure, specific medical issues that affect them, and why an awareness of variations is important to client's health.

Identifies client's or caregiver's understanding of potential cause-and-effect relationships between variations in BP and pulse and health status.

4 Assess client's or caregiver's previous knowledge and experience in measuring blood pressure and pulse. Have client or caregiver perform return demonstration if they indicate ability to measure blood pressure or pulse.

Allows nurse to assess client's or caregiver's knowledge and skill performance.

5 Assess home environment for favorable place to measure BP and pulse (e.g., quiet room with comfortable place to sit).

Ensures more accurate measurement.

NURSING DIAGNOSES

- Deficient knowledge regarding pulse/BP measurement
- Ineffective health maintenance

Related factors are individualized based on client's condition or needs.

PLANNING

1 Expected outcomes following completion of procedure:
- Client or family caregiver accurately monitors BP and pulse.
- Blood pressure and pulse are within range expected for client's age and condition (see Chapter 5).
- Client or caregiver explains importance of measuring BP and pulse, best time for measurement, and when to communicate with health care provider to evaluate changes in treatment regimen.

Learning has occurred.

Cardiovascular status is stable at a level that is determined for client by his or her health care provider.

Measures cognitive learning.

2 Encourage client or caregiver to perform measurements on routine schedule for long-term monitoring plan.

Daily activities and many extrinsic and intrinsic factors affect measurement fluctuations. A routine schedule allows for daily comparisons.

STEP	RATIONALE
3 Encourage client to avoid exercise, caffeine, and smoking for 30 minutes before assessment to avoid inaccuracy.	These factors cause elevations in BP and pulse (Vidt et al., 2010).
4 Have client or caregiver perform measurement in comfortable position, with arm supported and feet flat on floor, and in warm and quiet environment.	Maintains client's comfort during measurement. Systolic and diastolic BP increases with crossed-leg position (Frese et al., 2011).

IMPLEMENTATION

1 Blood pressure measurement:	
a Explain importance of having client sit quietly for 5 minutes with back supported and feet on floor before measurement.	Reduces anxiety that can falsely elevate BP readings (Vidt et al., 2010).

b Discuss with client best sites for assessing BP. For self-measurement brachial artery is almost always used. Explain to avoid applying cuff to arm with:
    • Intravenous (IV) catheter with or without fluids infusing
    • Arteriovenous shunt
    • Breast or axillary surgery
    • Trauma, inflammation, or disease
	Most accessible sites are easiest to measure for accuracy of assessment. Appropriate site selection promotes accuracy in reading and minimizes potential for trauma. Application of pressure from inflated bladder temporarily impairs blood flow and compromises circulation in extremity that already has impaired circulation.

c Demonstrate steps for measuring BP (see Chapter 5):	The eventual evaluation of a psychomotor skill is measured through client's performance and ability to follow directions/instructions (Romano, 2009b).
(1) Use of sphygmomanometer and stethoscope:	
(a) Teach palpating artery, positioning cuff, wrapping cuff, placing stethoscope, inflating and releasing cuff, listening for Korotkoff sounds.	Prepares client or family caregiver for measuring blood pressure.
(b) Describe sounds of measurement and relationship to observation of gauge during BP reading. Caution client about level and length of time appropriate for cuff inflation.	Ensures accurate reading. Prolonged inflation of cuff impairs circulation to extremity.
(c) Teach client or caregiver to routinely clean diaphragm and earpieces of stethoscope with rubbing alcohol or damp cloth.	Stethoscopes are frequently contaminated with microorganisms. Cleaning stethoscope routinely prevents transmission of microorganisms.

Clinical Decision Point *If client or caregiver needs to use stethoscope to take blood pressure, use double-headed teaching stethoscope to verify accuracy of reading or read BP 1 to 2 minutes after client's attempt to verify accuracy. If client is having difficulty hearing Korotkoff sounds, ensure that he or she is applying cuff appropriately and using the correct size cuff. Also determine correct use of equipment (e.g., cuff may have been deflated too quickly or too slowly; cuff may not have been pumped high enough for systolic readings).*

(2) Use of electronic blood pressure monitor:	
(a) Teach correct placement of cuff and use of electronic equipment for proper cuff inflation.	Using electronic equipment correctly helps ensure accurate BP readings.
2 Pulse measurement:	
a Discuss with client or caregiver best sites for assessing pulse: radial and carotid.	Radial and carotid sites are accessible and usually easiest to palpate.

Clinical Decision Point *If carotid site is chosen, caution client against vigorously massaging neck while attempting to locate pulse or attempting to locate both arteries at the same time. Stimulation of carotid sinus leads to reflex slowing of heart rate from vagal stimulation. In addition, simultaneous occlusion of both carotid arteries decreases blood to brain, resulting in fainting.*

b Demonstrate steps for palpating pulse (see Chapter 5): position of artery on wrist or neck, how to locate artery, using fingertips for palpation, compressing artery, palpating pulse before counting, counting pulse, and calculating pulse rate (see illustration).	The eventual evaluation of psychomotor skill is measured through client's performance and ability to follow directions/instructions (Romano, 2009b).

STEP	RATIONALE
(1) Instruct in use of gentle pressure; reinforce not to press hard over pulse site.	Pressing too hard may occlude artery.
(2) Instruct in use of watch or clock with second hand to count pulse.	Ensures correct timing of pulse.
(3) Instruct to count for full 60 seconds, starting with second hand at 12:00 position.	Consistent timing of procedure reduces confusion or forgetfulness about time period or starting point used for pulse measurement. A full 60-second count increases accuracy of measure.
3 Educate client about normal desired BP and pulse ranges, purposes for monitoring, and when to take measurements (e.g., before and after taking cardiac or antihypertensive medications; before, during, and after exercise).	Client needs to be able to determine when values are not in desired ranges and when measurements need to be taken.
4 Describe symptoms that indicate need to perform BP and/or pulse measurement.	Promotes understanding of health status alterations that need medical intervention.

Clinical Decision Point *Discuss importance of notifying health care provider and withholding medications when abnormal values in BP or pulse occur (e.g., hypotension or bradycardia). Client needs to understand preventive measures to take and to follow health care provider's directions if alterations develop.*

5 Have client or caregiver attempt each step of skill on you or family member.	You can correct any errors in technique as they occur.
6 Observe client demonstrate techniques on self. When measuring BP, do not allow multiple repetitive BP attempts on any one limb.	After developing confidence in measuring values in others, client is ready to measure own values. Making repeated BP attempts restricts circulation and alters measurement.
7 Teach client to monitor BP and pulse even if they remain in normal range.	Continuous monitoring provides important information that evaluates effectiveness of medications or other treatments.
8 Provide client with printed instructions with written or pictorial guide or with videotape/DVD demonstration of procedure if possible.	Printed and audiovisual teaching materials help stimulate client's visual and auditory senses, which enhances teaching (Pittman, 2009).
9 Give client logbook or piece of paper to record BP and pulse and time they were taken. In addition, client records whether or not medications that affect BP or pulse were taken. Instruct client to use written record to report readings to health care provider.	Keeping organized record of BP and pulse readings and medications empowers client and provides accurate information to health care providers.
10 Instruct client in proper care of equipment (e.g., storage, cleaning, and battery care).	Improper care and storage of equipment affects accuracy of measurement.

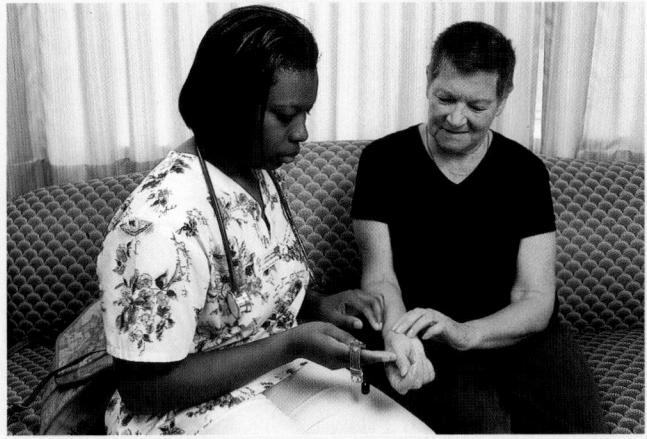

STEP 2b   Nurse observing client checking radial pulse.

EVALUATION

1 Observe client or family caregiver demonstrate technique for BP and/or pulse measurement on at least three different occasions and verify that client adds information to logbook correctly.	Feedback through return demonstration of psychomotor learning is best means to evaluate learning.
2 Ask client if readings are within desired range and when to report abnormal readings to health care provider.	Determines client's ability to know when readings are within proper range and what to do when abnormal readings are obtained.

STEP	RATIONALE
3 Ask client to describe reason for BP and pulse monitoring and any related medications (e.g., antihypertensives, anti-dysrhythmics) or treatment (e.g., diet and exercise).	Determines if client understands monitoring and related therapies.
4 Have client or caregiver demonstrate proper care of equipment.	Demonstrates learning.

Unexpected Outcomes	Related Interventions
1 Client or family caregiver is unable to measure BP or pulse (e.g., inability to manipulate equipment, visualize numbers on equipment or clock, hear BP sounds).	• Alter teaching plan to accommodate client's problems (e.g., use other types of equipment that are easier to manipulate, see, or hear). • Reinforce information taught and continue return demonstrations until client is able to perform skill. • Teach skill to a different family caregiver.
2 Client or caregiver has difficulty explaining purposes of measurement or implications of therapy.	• Review and reinforce information that client or caregiver does not understand.

Recording and Reporting

- Record teaching, client responses, and demonstration in home care record.
- Record BP and pulse in home care record and home documentation system (e.g., logbook).
- Report changes in readings of BP and/or pulse.

Special Considerations

Teaching

- Educate client about risks for hypertension (see Chapter 5).
- Ensure that client understands health care provider's recommendations for treatment regimen, including potential side effects and interactions of any medication therapies (e.g., clients taking thyroid medications might need to withhold them when BP is above normal range or pulse is above 100 beats/min). Confirm specific guidelines for BP and pulse with health care provider; document information in home care record; and provide clear, written instructions for the client.
- Always leave a phone number and instructions about how to reach home care nurse if needed.

Pediatric

- Readings (BP or pulse) are often inaccurate if an infant or child is anxious and uncooperative. Blood pressure is also inaccurate when the cuff size is inappropriate. Having others divert the child's attention or taking his or her BP or pulse while he or is seated on the parent's lap usually helps calm the child (Hockenberry and Wilson, 2011).

- Young children will be more likely to cooperate if allowed to touch and/or play with equipment before procedure. Consider performing the procedure first on the parent or another person significant to child. This allows the child to observe that the procedure is safe.
- Use the radial pulse in children over 2 years of age. Femoral or brachial pulse is the best site for palpation of pulse for children under 2 years of age (Hockenberry and Wilson, 2011).
- In infants teach parents to observe and count the pulse on anterior fontanel. Remind parents *not* to palpate the pulse.

Gerontologic

- Musculoskeletal changes such as arthritis or other joint conditions may impair a client's ability to position limb comfortably and/or perform fine-motor skills required to measure BP and pulse (Upadhyaya, 2011).
- Older adults, especially those who are frail or who have lost upper arm mass, require a smaller BP cuff.
- Home BP monitoring is not a replacement for BP monitoring by health care professionals in older adults, but it can serve to provide more information to ensure the best treatment.

SKILL 42-3 Teaching Intermittent Self-Catheterization

Most clients urinate and empty their bladder 4 or 5 times a day (SUNA, 2010). However, some clients are not able to empty their bladder. Infections in the bladder or kidneys and damage to the kidneys sometimes result from incomplete emptying of the bladder. Clean intermittent self-catheterization (CISC) is a safe and effective way to empty the bladder. The client performs self-catheterization with clean technique, eliminating the need to wear gloves. Clients who use CISC have a variety of health problems that affect the neuromuscular control of the bladder (e.g., spinal cord injury, multiple sclerosis, spina bifida, bladder outlet obstruction, continent urinary diversion) (SUNA, 2010). Current practice supports CISC for use in the home to provide a means to completely empty the bladder, prevent urinary tract infections (UTIs), and prevent further bladder and kidney damage (NIH, 2010). Inadequate or excessive fluid intake, poor catheterization technique and catheter care, and traumatic catheterization can cause UTIs. Teaching proper self-catheterization technique is crucial in preventing infections (Newman and Willson, 2011).

Using CISC helps clients believe that they are more in control of their daily needs, which enhances their quality of life. It also helps some clients become continent, maintain a positive body image, and experience less anxiety and embarrassment. In addition, CISC allows clients to express their sexuality and sustain satisfying relationships with significant others. However, the skill requires physical and manual dexterity, and clients must adhere to a regular schedule for it to be successful (SUNA, 2010). When the client is unable to perform CISC independently, teach his or her family caregiver how to perform the skill. For clients with certain medical conditions (e.g., immunosuppressed clients) sterile or aseptic technique is the recommended method of self-catheterization rather than CISC (Newman and Willson, 2011).

Delegation and Collaboration

The skill of teaching intermittent self-catheterization cannot be delegated to nursing assistive personnel (NAP).

Equipment

- ❏ Soap, water, and clean washcloth
- ❏ Mirror (optional)
- ❏ Urethral catheter (smallest size that is able to pass easily into the bladder and completely drain client's urine)
- ❏ Lubricant (e.g., water-soluble jelly)
- ❏ Container for collection of urine (e.g., urinal)—not needed for clients emptying urine directly into toilet
- ❏ Mild soap (e.g., Ivory)
- ❏ Catheter storage item or container (e.g., brown paper bag, clean towel)
- ❏ Disposable clean gloves (for family caregiver)
- ❏ Paper or logbook and pencil or pen (optional)

STEP	RATIONALE

ASSESSMENT

1 Review client's medical record, including order for CISC and nurses' notes. Gather information about voiding history, existing medical and surgical history, client's usual daily fluid intake, postvoid residual amounts, and daily voiding routine.	Determines reason for CISC, frequency of catheterization, and previous responses to client education.
2 Assess client's ability to perform CISC, including developmental level, level of consciousness, motor function, and psychosocial status.	Client must be physically able to reach urethra and move equipment as needed. Client who cannot see urethra can be taught to feel for proper location of urethral opening (NIH, 2010).
3 Assess client's or family caregiver's knowledge about CISC and observe performance of CISC if patient has performed previously.	Effective client or caregiver education builds on previous knowledge; observation is effective way to evaluate performance of psychomotor skills (Romano, 2009b).

NURSING DIAGNOSES

- Impaired urinary elimination
- Urinary retention
- Readiness for enhanced urinary elimination
- Reflex urinary incontinence
- Deficient knowledge regarding self-catheterization

Related factors are individualized based on client's condition or needs.

PLANNING

1 Expected outcomes following completion of procedure:	
• Client or family caregiver states signs and symptoms that indicate need for CISC.	Indicates ability to identify appropriate times to use CISC.
• Client or caregiver correctly demonstrates how to perform CISC and clean and store equipment.	Return demonstration of skill indicates learning (Romano, 2009b).
• Client or caregiver verbalizes signs and symptoms of complications of CISC (e.g., UTI, urethral bleeding, urethritis, stricture, creation of a false passage) and when to contact health care provider (Newman and Willson, 2011).	Urinary complications are common in clients who use CISC; urethral, scrotal, and/or bladder complications can occur (Newman and Willson, 2011). Verbalization of signs and symptoms of complications helps clients or caregivers identify potential problems early and seek appropriate care.
2 Select setting in home that client or caregiver will most likely use when performing CISC.	Respecting client's needs, values, and choices is key in client-centered care (Romano, 2009a).
3 Help client or caregiver select catheter that is easiest to use, causes least amount of trauma, and is most comfortable.	Variety of single-use and reusable catheters is currently available.

IMPLEMENTATION

1 Teach client or family caregiver how to perform appropriate hand hygiene using soap and water. If caregiver is performing skill, have him or her apply a pair of disposable clean gloves.	Prevents risk for UTI and trauma, which can lead to urethral strictures (SUNA, 2010). Prevents transmission of infection.
2 Help client get into comfortable position: Some men prefer to stand, whereas others prefer to sit. Female clients often need to try different positions to decide which position is most comfortable (SUNA, 2010). Position client in place that has adequate lighting.	Client needs adequate lighting to see meatus and equipment.
3 Teach client how to clean urethral meatus:	
a *For women:* Have client spread labia with one hand and clean urethral opening with warm soapy water and clean washcloth with other hand. Have female clean in direction from urethral meatus toward rectum.	Retraction of labia allows for female urethral meatus to be cleaned, reducing risk for infection (NIH, 2010; SUNA, 2010). Reduces transmission of infection from rectal area to meatus.

STEP	RATIONALE
b *For men:* If client has not been circumcised, teach him to retract foreskin to expose urethral meatus. Teach client to hold penis perpendicular to body with one hand and clean urethral opening with warm soapy water and clean washcloth with other hand. Have male clean in a circular motion from meatus outward.	Ensures cleaning of meatus and reduces risk for infection (NIH 2010; SUNA 2010).
4 Teach female client how to insert catheter:	
a Using mirror, help client locate meatus. Explain that it is just below clitoris and just above vaginal opening.	Mirror helps female client visualize anatomy (NIH 2010; SUNA 2010).

Clinical Decision Point *If female client is unable to visualize anatomy or wants to learn how to find meatus while in a sitting position, teach touch technique by helping client use fingers to find her urethral opening (NIH, 2010). Teach client to put one finger over the clitoris and another finger over the vaginal opening. Then help her use these two fingers to find the urethral opening. Another method is the tunnel technique. When women sit with their hips flexed forward, the labia create a "tunnel" that leads to the urethral opening. Teach the woman to slightly separate labia near the clitoris and angle the catheter backward into the urethral opening while placing a finger over the vaginal opening.*

STEP	RATIONALE
b Have client lubricate tip of catheter with water-soluble jelly by rotating tip to spread lubricant around bottom 2.5 to 5 cm (1 to 2 inches) of catheter.	Lubrication reduces urethral trauma (NIH, 2010; SUNA 2010).
c Place outflow end of catheter into urine collection container or let hang over toilet bowl. Slowly and gently insert tip of catheter 5 to 10 cm (2 to 4 inches) into meatus until urine begins to flow.	Appearance of urine indicates that catheter tip is in bladder.

Clinical Decision Point *If client feels resistance at the internal sphincter, teach her to apply firm, gentle, steady pressure until muscles relax and allow catheter to pass (SUNA, 2010).*

STEP	RATIONALE
5 Teach male client how to insert catheter:	
a Have client lubricate tip of catheter with water-soluble jelly by rotating tip to spread lubricant around bottom 13 to 18 cm (5 to 7 inches) of catheter.	Lubrication reduces urethral trauma. Dry catheters may cause excoriations in urethra, which can lead to an entry point for bacteria contamination (Newman and Willson, 2011).
b Place outflow end of catheter into urine collection container or let hang over toilet bowl. Slowly and gently insert tip of catheter 15 to 20 cm (6 to 8 inches) into meatus until urine begins to flow. Tell client that catheter often needs to be inserted all the way for urine to begin to flow.	Male urethra is longer than female urethra. Flow of urine indicates that catheter tip is in bladder.

Clinical Decision Point *Men may experience some resistance when the catheter reaches the prostatic urethra or the neck of the bladder. If client feels resistance, teach him to apply firm, gentle, steady pressure to fatigue the external sphincter and cause muscle relaxation (SUNA, 2010).*

STEP	RATIONALE
6 Instruct client to hold catheter in place while urine flows into container or toilet.	Release of catheter during procedure often causes catheter to accidentally come out before bladder is completely emptied.
7 When urine flow stops, teach client to slowly and gently remove catheter. Then have client perform hand hygiene.	Removing catheter slowly allows pockets of urine that can accumulate at base of bladder to drain (SUNA, 2010).
8 Give client logbook to record amount of urine if needed.	Some clients need to keep track of their urinary output.
9 Instruct client to clean catheter with mild soap (e.g., Ivory) and water immediately after use. Rinse catheter completely, allow to air dry, and store in clean dry towel or brown paper bag.	Prevents UTIs.
10 Teach client to replace catheter every 2 to 4 weeks (NIH, 2010) or when it becomes cracked or brittle, has any buildup of sediment, or loses its form.	Appropriate disposal and replacement of equipment prevents complications of CISC (SUNA, 2010).

EVALUATION

STEP	RATIONALE
1 Observe client or family caregiver independently demonstrate technique for CISC.	Feedback through return demonstration of psychomotor skill is best means of evaluating learning of skill.
2 Ask client to identify plan for timing of CISC and steps to take when problems arise.	Measures client's cognitive learning and ability to problem solve.
3 Review client's logbook and observe client enter information about urine output if indicated.	Confirms that client understands record keeping and importance of tracking urine output.

Unexpected Outcomes

1 Client is unable to easily pass catheter into bladder.

2 Client states he or she is having symptoms of UTI (e.g., flank or abdominal pain, malaise, fever, chills).

Related Interventions

- Teach client not to force catheter into bladder.
- Tell client to go to nearest urgent care center or emergency department if bladder is full and client is unable to insert catheter.
- Consider initiating consultation with urologist.

- Inform client's health care provider of symptoms and anticipate treatment with antibiotic.

Recording and Reporting

- Record teaching, client responses, and demonstration in home care record.
- Record urine output in home care record and home documentation system (e.g., logbook).
- Report signs and symptoms of UTIs and difficulty performing CISC.

Special Considerations
Teaching

- It is common for clients who perform CISC routinely to have an abnormal urinalysis. Clients should only be treated for UTIs if they have symptoms of an infection (e.g., back pain, pelvic tenderness, malaise, confusion, foul-smelling urine, urgency) (SUNA, 2010).
- Always leave a phone number and instructions about how to reach home care nurse if needed.

Pediatric

- Children who are motivated and physiologically and developmentally ready need to learn how to catheterize themselves.

- Consult a pediatric urologist; children need special assessment and teaching (SUNA, 2010).
- When teaching children to perform CISC, use developmentally appropriate teaching strategies.
- Concerns of children and adolescents who use CISC include leakage and being wet. They also are often concerned about what their peers know. Allow children to voice their concerns and help them problem solve what they will do in a variety of situations.

Gerontologic

- CISC is very effective in older adults because it helps restore continence, decreases urinary urge and nocturia, and improves quality of life.
- Older adults may have difficulty performing CISC because of limited manual dexterity. Individualize care for a client's needs and functional abilities. Educate the client or caregivers (Ebersole et al., 2008).

SKILL 42-4   Using Home Oxygen Equipment

Medical oxygen is classified by the Food and Drug Administration (FDA) as a drug; therefore a prescription from a health care provider is required for home use (Brinkerhoff, 2009; CMS, 2008). The prescription includes the following components: drug/apparatus, dose, route of administration, and duration. The most common route of administration of oxygen in the home is by nasal cannula; however a face mask, tracheal mask, or tracheal catheter can also be used (Brinkerhoff, 2009).

Oxygen-conserving devices (OCDs) were introduced to reduce the weight of portable oxygen systems and extend operating time by not wasting oxygen through continuous flow (McCoy, 2010). There are three types of OCDs:

1 *Reservoir nasal cannula*: Stores oxygen in a small chamber during exhalation for subsequent delivery during early phase inhalation.
2 *Demand pulsing oxygen delivery systems*: Deliver a burst of oxygen at the onset of inspiration; small oxygen pulses are very effective in oxygenating the client.
3 *Transtracheal oxygen catheter*: Delivers oxygen directly through a catheter placed between the second and third tracheal rings (American Thoracic Society, 2011) (Table 42-1).

Oxygen sources in the home include liquid oxygen systems, compressed oxygen in tanks, or oxygen concentrators (Fig. 42-2, A) (Lewis et al., 2011). Some oxygen tanks (e.g., compressed) are large and stationary. Portable tanks are easy to move, weigh more than 10 lbs, are not designed to be carried, and deliver oxygen for about 5 hours at 2 L/min. Ambulatory tanks weigh less than 10 lb, are designed to be carried (Fig. 42-2, B), and deliver oxygen for at

least 4 hours at 2 L/min. Table 42-2 compares the different types of home oxygen delivery systems.

Compressed oxygen requires a regulator and flowmeter. The client receives delivery of several large oxygen tanks to the home. The size of the tank and flow rate determine how long compressed oxygen tanks will last (Table 42-3). Liquid systems take up less

TABLE 42-1	Oxygen Flow and Appropriate Uses for Oxygen Delivery Devices		
Device	**Flow (L/min)**	**FiO₂ Range (%)**	**Uses**
Nasal cannula	1-6	24-44	Clients requiring low concentrations of oxygen therapy
Simple face mask	6-12	35-50	Clients who require short-term oxygen therapy with moderate FiO₂ needs
Oxygen-conserving cannula	Up to 8	30-50	Clients in need of long-term home therapy
Partial and nonrebreather mask	10-15	60-90	Clients in acute respiratory failure or in emergency situations

Data from Lewis et al: *Medical surgical nursing: assessment and management of clinical problems*, ed 8, St Louis, 2011, Mosby.

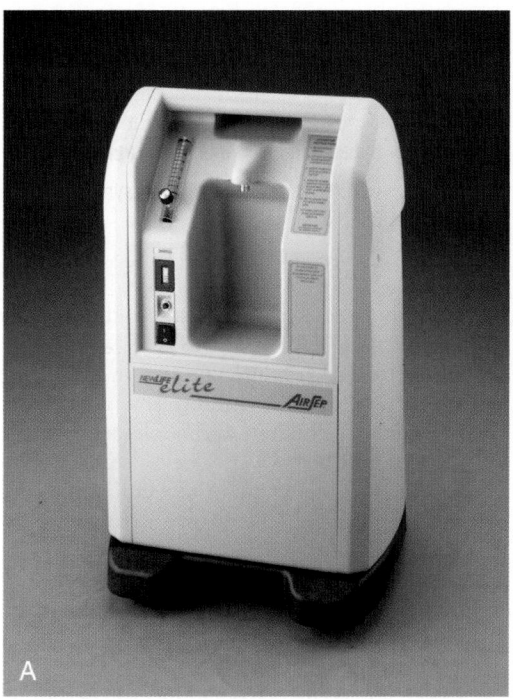
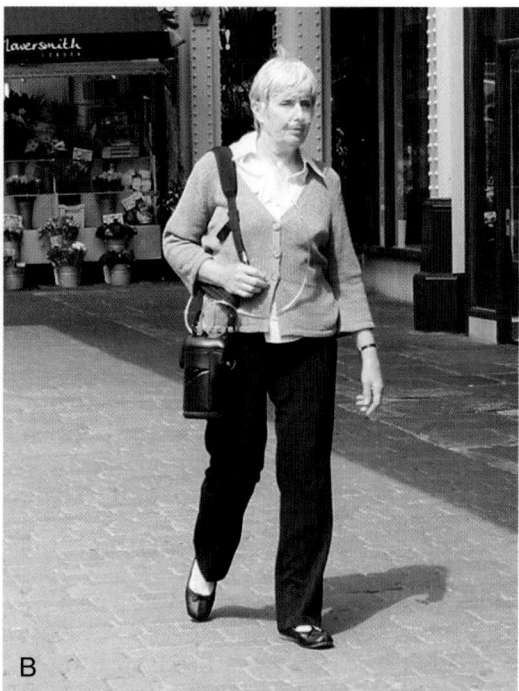

FIG 42-2 **A,** Portable oxygen concentrator for home use. **B,** Ambulatory tank is small enough to be carried easily. *(Courtesy AirSep Corporation.)*

TABLE 42-2	Home Oxygen Delivery Systems	
	Advantages	**Disadvantages**
Compressed Oxygen		
Oxygen is stored under pressure in a cylinder equipped with a regulator that controls the flow rate.	An oxygen-conserving device may be attached to the system to avoid waste; device releases gas only on inhalation and cuts it off with exhalation; does not require an electrical source; smaller tanks are available.	Large tanks are heavy and only suitable for stationary use. Client must know how to read regulator and understand when to call medical supplier for replacement cylinder.
Liquid Oxygen Systems		
Oxygen is stored as a very cold liquid in a vessel very similar to a thermos. When released, the liquid converts to a gas and is breathed in just like compressed gas.	Storage method takes up less space than the compressed gas cylinder; it can transfer the liquid to a small, portable vessel at home.	It is more expensive than compressed gas, and the vessel vents when it is not in use. An oxygen-conserving device may be built into the vessel to conserve the oxygen.
Oxygen Concentrator		
It separates the oxygen out of the air, concentrates it, and stores it.	It does not have to be resupplied and it is not as costly as liquid oxygen. Extra tubing permits the user to move around with minimal difficulty. Small, portable systems have been developed that afford even greater mobility.	It must have a cylinder of oxygen as a backup in the event of a power failure.

space because oxygen is stored in a liquid state. Liquid oxygen is stored at or below −297° F (−183° C) and requires the use of a small ambulatory tank that is filled from a reservoir in the home (Fig. 42-3). Table 42-4 shows how long a liquid oxygen system will last, depending on the prescribed flow rate. The oxygen concentrator method extracts oxygen from room air and supplies oxygen to the client at prescribed flow rates. Oxygen concentrators deliver a lower percentage of oxygen to the flowmeter. Therefore, if a client is switched to a concentrator, the flow rate usually needs to be adjusted. The client who uses a concentrator needs to have a backup system such as a portable oxygen tank in case of power failure.

Home oxygen equipment and supplies are designated as durable medical equipment (DME) by Medicare; a certificate of medical necessity (CMN) is required for clients who receive Medicare (CMS, 2008). Governmental or private insurance often pays for home oxygen therapy if there are written orders from the health care provider.

Clients and their family caregivers need extensive teaching to use oxygen therapy correctly and safely. Instruct a client to have an all-purpose fire extinguisher close by and learn how to use it and to keep the oxygen supplier's number handy. In addition, provide client education about the safe use of oxygen in the home (Box 42-3). When initiating and managing ongoing oxygen

TABLE 42-3 | Oxygen Cylinder Timetable*

	Large (H-K) Tank		Small (E) Tank	
L/min	2200 lbs Full	1000 lbs ½ Full	625 L Full	284 L ½ Full
1	115 hr	52 hr	10 hr	5 hr
2	56 hr	26 hr	5 hr	2 hr
3	37 hr	17 hr	3 hr	1 hr
4	28 hr	13 hr	3 hr	1 hr
5	22 hr	10 hr	2 hr	54 min
6	18 hr	8 hr	<2 hr	47 min

The following formulas can also be used to determine the length of time a tank will last:

For E Cylinders
Pressure on cylinder gauge (psi): 500 psi (safety factor) × 0.3 (E cylinder factor) ÷ L/min = minutes

For H Cylinders
Pressure on cylinder gauge (psi): 500 psi (safety factor) × 3.1 (H cylinder factor) ÷ L/min = minutes

EXAMPLE: If E cylinder reads 1500 psi and liter flow rate is 4 L/min:
Time left: 1500 − 500 × 0.3 ÷ 4 = 1000 × 0.3 ÷ 4 = 300 ÷ 4 = 75 minutes (1 hr 15 min)

NOTE: Do not allow oxygen cylinder pressure to fall below 500 psi, or the client may run out of oxygen.
*All times are approximate.

TABLE 42-4 | Liquid Oxygen Timetable

	Stationary Reservoirs		Portable Units	
L/min	41 L	31 L	1/2 L	1 L
0.25	1400 hr	1060 hr	28 hr	44 hr
0.50	1125 hr	850 hr	18 hr	27 hr
1	560 hr	425 hr	9 hr	15½ hr
1.5	375 hr	283½ hr	6 hr	11½ hr
2	281 hr	213 hr	4½ hr	8½ hr
3	187½ hr	142 hr	3 hr	6 hr

BOX 42-3 | Safe Home Oxygen Therapy

Fire Safety
Although oxygen is not flammable, it needs fire to burn, therefore:
- Use and store oxygen in a well-ventilated area.
- Keep cylinders and vessels at least 8 feet (2.4 meters) away from heaters.
- Do not use open flames (e.g., matches, fireplaces, stoves, space heaters, candles) when oxygen is in use.
- Do not allow smoking in the house. Post "No Smoking" signs inside and outside the house.
- Avoid using electrical appliances that produce sparks (e.g., electric razors).
- Install smoke detectors and have a fire extinguisher available in the home. Test smoke detectors twice a month.
- Help client or family caregiver plan a fire evacuation route. Have two routes out of every room and an outside meeting place.

Oxygen Storage and Handling
- Store oxygen tanks upright in carts or stands to prevent tipping or falling or place tanks flat on the floor when not in use.
- Do not store oxygen tanks in the trunk of a car.
- When transporting oxygen in a vehicle, ensure that tanks are secured properly in the passenger area with the windows opened 2 to 3 inches (5 to 7.5 cm) to allow adequate ventilation.

Concentrator Safety
- Plug concentrators into properly grounded outlets.
- Do not use extension cords, power strips, or multioutlet adapters with concentrators.
- Ensure that power supply or circuit meets or exceeds the amperage requirements of the concentrator.

Liquid Oxygen Safety
- Avoid direct contact with liquid oxygen because it can cause frostbite. The vapors are also extremely cold; can damage delicate tissues such as eyes.
- Do not touch connectors that are frosted or icy.
- Keep ambulatory tanks upright; do not lay them down or place on their side.

Adapted from Lewis et al: *Medical surgical nursing: assessment and management of clinical problems*, ed 8, St Louis, 2011, Mosby; National Fire Protection Association, 2008, available at http://www.nfpa.org/assets/files//pdf/os.oxygen.pdf, accessed April 5, 2012.

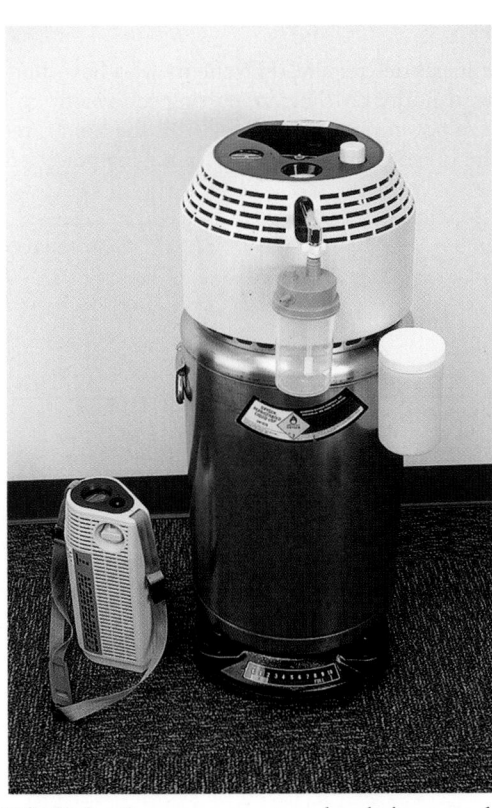

FIG 42-3 Oxygen reservoir and ambulatory tank.

therapy, collaborate with the client, health care provider, family caregivers, DME provider, and payer.

Delegation and Collaboration

The skill of teaching clients how to use home oxygen equipment cannot be delegated to nursing assistive personnel (NAP).

Equipment

- ❏ Nasal cannula, oxygen mask (see Chapter 23), OCD, or other prescribed delivery device
- ❏ Oxygen tubing
- ❏ Home oxygen delivery system (compressed oxygen, oxygen concentrator, or liquid oxygen) with all required equipment (varies with supplier and system used)
- ❏ "No Smoking/Oxygen in Use" sign for each entrance to the home

STEP	RATIONALE

ASSESSMENT

1 While client is still in hospital, determine client's or family caregiver's ability to use oxygen equipment correctly. In home setting reassess for appropriate use of equipment.

Physical or cognitive impairments indicate need to teach caregiver how to operate home oxygen equipment. Determines specific components of skill that client and family caregiver are able to complete easily.

2 Assess home environment for adequate electrical service if oxygen concentrator is used.

Oxygen concentrators require electricity to work (American Thoracic Society, 2011). Continuous oxygen therapy must not be interrupted.

3 Assess client's or family caregiver's knowledge of purpose of oxygen and ability to observe for signs and symptoms of hypoxia, including apprehension, anxiety, decreased ability to concentrate, decreased levels of consciousness, increased fatigue, dizziness, behavioral changes, increased pulse, increased respiratory rate, pallor, and cyanosis.

Hypoxia sometimes occurs at home when client uses oxygen. Possible causes of hypoxia include poor tubing connections; use of long oxygen tubing; or worsening of client's physical problem, with change in respiratory status.

4 Determine appropriate resources in community for equipment and assistance, including maintenance and repair services and medical equipment supplier.

Ensures readily available assistance for clients with home oxygen systems.

5 Determine appropriate backup systems for compressor in event of power failure (e.g., notify local emergency medical services [EMS]). Have spare oxygen tank available for emergency use.

Many municipalities require that clients who have home oxygen equipment notify EMS before putting equipment in the home. In case of power outage, EMS will call the home, and in some cases the home is on priority list for having power restored.

NURSING DIAGNOSES

- Anxiety
- Deficient knowledge regarding oxygen therapy
- Ineffective health maintenance

Related factors are individualized based on client's condition or needs.

PLANNING

1 Expected outcomes following completion of procedure:
- Client receives oxygen at prescribed rate.

Oxygen system set up correctly.

- Client or family caregiver verbalizes purpose and correct use of home oxygen.

Provides measurable criteria to determine level of understanding.

- Client or caregiver demonstrates how to maintain oxygen system.

Indicates learning has occurred.

- Client or caregiver states indications for calling DME provider to replenish oxygen supply and reorder oxygen delivery supplies.

Client needs constant supply of oxygen at home.

- Client or caregiver verbalizes safety guidelines for oxygen use (e.g., place "No Smoking/Oxygen in Use" signs at entrances to home) (Lewis et al., 2011).

Provides measure of understanding of oxygen use.

- Client or caregiver verbalizes emergency plan of care (Lewis et al., 2011).

Ensures safe, continuous delivery of home oxygen.

2 Select setting in home where client is most likely to use oxygen equipment.

Practicing in same environment where skill is routinely performed facilitates comprehension and learning.

STEP	RATIONALE

IMPLEMENTATION

1 Instruct client or family caregiver on how to perform hand hygiene before handling oxygen equipment.

Reduces transmission of microorganisms.

2 Place oxygen delivery system in clutter-free environment that is well ventilated; away from walls, drapes, curtains, bedding, and combustible materials; and at least 8 feet (2.4 meters) from heat sources.

Keeps system balanced and prevents injury.

Clinical Decision Point *Do not place oxygen delivery system in a closet.*

3 Demonstrate steps for preparation and maintenance of oxygen therapy:

Demonstration is reliable technique for teaching psychomotor skill and enables client to ask questions.

  a Compressed oxygen system:

    (1) Turn cylinder valve counterclockwise two to three turns with wrench.

Turns on oxygen.

    (2) Check cylinders by reading amount on pressure gauge.

Verifies adequate oxygen supply for client use.

    (3) Store wrench with oxygen tank or in other safe place.

Storing wrench in safe place ensures that it is available whenever needed.

  b Oxygen concentrator system:

    (1) Plug concentrator into appropriate outlet.

Provides power safely to concentrator.

    (2) Turn on power switch.

Starts concentrator motor.

    (3) Alarm will sound for few seconds.

Alarm turns off when desired pressure inside concentrator is reached.

  c Liquid oxygen system:

    (1) Check liquid system by depressing button at lower right corner and reading dial on stationary oxygen reservoir or ambulatory tank.

Verifies adequate oxygen supply for client use.

    (2) Collaborate with DME provider to provide instruction in refilling ambulatory tank when it becomes empty.

Ensures continuous oxygen therapy is not interrupted.

Clinical Decision Point *Only fill ambulatory tanks when they are empty. Liquid oxygen is stored at or below −297° F (−183° C) inside reservoir, and the temperature inside the ambulatory tank is warmer. If cold oxygen from the reservoir mixes with warmer oxygen left in the ambulatory tank, the ambulatory tank malfunctions.*

    (3) To refill liquid oxygen tank:

      (a) Wipe both filling connectors with clean, dry, lint-free cloth.

Removes dust and moisture from system.

      (b) Turn off flow selector of ambulatory unit.

      (c) Attach ambulatory unit to stationary reservoir by inserting female adapter from ambulatory tank into male adapter of stationary reservoir (see illustration).

Secures connection between oxygen reservoir and ambulatory tank.

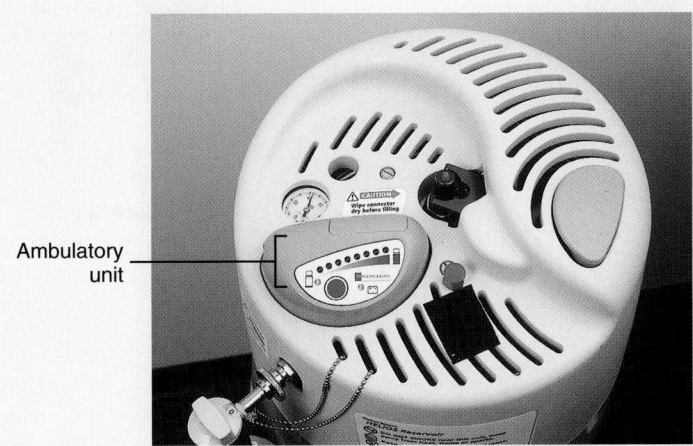

Ambulatory unit

STEP 3c(3)(c)   Top view of stationary reservoir.

STEP	RATIONALE
(d) Open fill valve on ambulatory tank (e.g., lever, button, key) and apply firm pressure to top of stationary reservoir (see illustration). Stay with unit while it is filling. You will hear loud hissing noise. Tank should be filled in about 2 minutes.	Prevents leakage of oxygen during filling process. If oxygen leaks during filling process, connection between ambulatory tank and reservoir potentially ices up, and ambulatory and reservoir tanks stick together.
(e) Disconnect ambulatory unit from stationary reservoir when hissing noise changes and vapor cloud begins to form from stationary unit.	Overfilling causes ambulatory unit to malfunction as result of high pressure in tank.

Clinical Decision Point *If ambulatory unit does not separate easily, valves from reservoir and ambulatory unit are frozen together. Wait until valves warm to disengage (about 5 to 10 minutes). Do not touch any frosted areas because contact with skin causes skin damage from frostbite.*

STEP	RATIONALE
(f) Wipe both filling connectors with clean, dry, lint-free cloth.	Ice often forms during filling process. Removes moisture from oxygen system.
4 Connect oxygen delivery device (e.g., nasal cannula) to oxygen delivery system (see Chapter 23) (see illustration).	Connects oxygen source to delivery method.
5 Adjust oxygen flow rate (L/min).	Ensures ordered oxygen dose is delivered.
6 Have client or caregiver apply oxygen delivery device (e.g., nasal cannula) correctly (see Chapter 23). Ensure that client has two sets of oxygen delivery devices and tubing.	Delivers oxygen to client. Extra set of equipment is used when equipment is cleaned or in case of equipment malfunction.
7 Instruct client not to change oxygen flow rate.	Provides prescribed amount of oxygen. Exceeding prescribed amount of oxygen is sometimes harmful (e.g., client with chronic obstructive pulmonary disease [COPD]).
8 Have client or caregiver perform each step with guidance. Provide written material for reinforcement and review.	Allows for correction of any errors in technique and discussion of their implications.
9 Instruct client or caregiver to notify health care provider if signs or symptoms of hypoxia or respiratory tract infection occur (e.g., fever, increased sputum, change in color of sputum, foul sputum odor).	Respiratory tract infections increase oxygen demand and often affect oxygen transfer from lungs to blood, creating exacerbation of client's pulmonary disease.
10 Discuss emergency plans for power loss, natural disaster, and acute respiratory distress. Have client or caregiver call 9-1-1 and notify health care provider and home care agency.	Ensures appropriate response and can prevent worsening of client's condition.

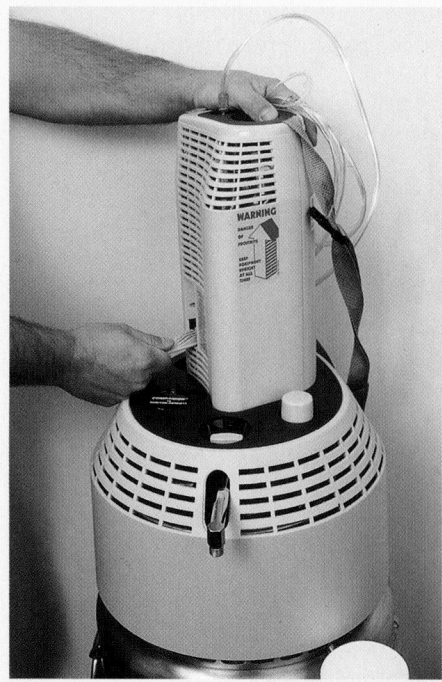

STEP 3c(3)(d)   Fill valve on ambulatory tank is opened while applying firm pressure to top of ambulatory tank.

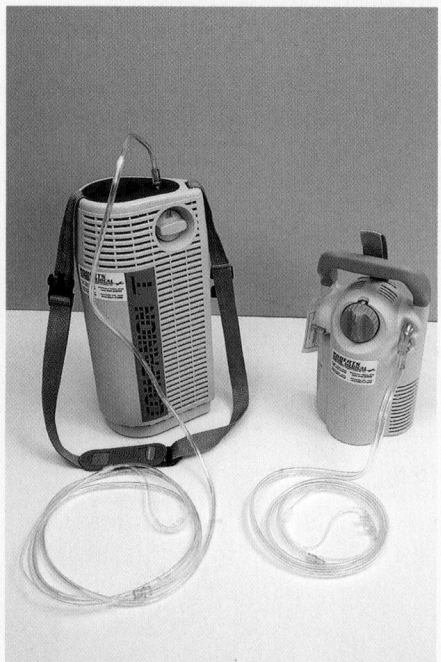

STEP 4   Oxygen delivery device (nasal cannulas) and tubing attached to ambulatory oxygen tanks.

STEP	RATIONALE
11 Instruct client in safe home oxygen practices, including placing "No Smoking/Oxygen in Use" signs at each entrance to home, not allowing smoking in house, keeping oxygen tanks 8 feet (2.4 meters) away from open flames, and storing oxygen tanks upright.	Ensures safe use of oxygen in home and prevents injury to client and family (Lewis et al., 2011).

EVALUATION

1 Monitor rate at which oxygen is being delivered during each home visit.	Determines if client or caregiver is regulating oxygen at prescribed rate.
2 Ask client or family caregiver about ease or problems associated with home oxygen.	Determines ability of client or caregiver to deal with stressors associated with home oxygen use. Also indicates client's risk for inappropriate oxygen use.
3 Ask client or caregiver to state safety guidelines, emergency precautions, and emergency plan.	Determines client's or caregiver's knowledge of what to do if power fails, there is a failure in equipment, or client's status worsens.

Unexpected Outcomes	Related Interventions
1 Client has signs and symptoms associated with hypoxia (see Assessment, Step 3).	• Determine if oxygen delivery device and oxygen source are delivering oxygen properly. • Determine if prescribed oxygen flow rate is set properly. • Assess client for change in respiratory status such as airway plugging, respiratory tract infection, or bronchospasm. • Instruct client or family caregiver when to notify health care provider or activate EMS because of signs of hypoxia.
2 Client uses unsafe practices with oxygen therapy, uses oxygen around fire or cigarette smoking, or sets incorrect flow rate.	• Reinforce client education and perform follow-up reassessment (see Box 42-3). • Include caregiver in instruction and set up problem-solving exercises with client.
3 Client is unable to fill ambulatory system.	• Identify and instruct family caregiver who can help client fill tank.

Recording and Reporting

- Record teaching plan, information provided to client, and client's or family caregiver's ability to discuss information in home care record.
- Communicate client's or caregiver's learning progress to other health care providers involved in client's care.
- Record oxygen delivery system, related supplies, and prescribed oxygen flow rate in home care record.
- Report respiratory complications/concerns to health care provider.

Special Considerations
Teaching

- Potential for oxygen desaturation and decreased oxygen delivery to brain impairs client's ability to remember previous learning. Provide frequent teaching sessions and written or pictorial instructions to reinforce previous learning of teaching plan.
- Instruct client or caregiver in appropriate cleaning, disinfecting, and maintaining all oxygen delivery systems and supplies. Verify instructions with manufacturer guidelines and DME provider's instructions.
- Instruct client or caregiver to check mask and tubing by placing hands or face over mask or cannula to feel airflow and check

that mask is not too tight; tight mask often leaves marks on skin. Apply cotton or gauze sponge at pressure points.
- Always leave a phone number and instructions about how to reach home care nurse if needed.

Pediatric

- Keep equipment out of reach of any children in home. Do not allow children to handle or operate home oxygen equipment.
- Oxygen is not flammable, but fire needs it to burn. Keep children away from fire and flames at all times; as appropriate, educate about dangers of oxygen coming into contact with fire (National Fire Protection Association, 2008).

Gerontologic

- Older adults have less efficient respiratory systems and less surface area for gas exchange; thus they are at greater risk for cerebral anoxia and confusion when they experience decreased oxygen levels. They may be unable to recognize respiratory problems or problems with their oxygen delivery system; therefore they need frequent contact with a designated caregiver.

SKILL 42-5   Teaching Home Tracheostomy Care and Suctioning

Performing tracheostomy care and suctioning in the home is similar to performing them in the hospital except for one key variable: the use of *medical asepsis* or *clean technique*. The home environment has fewer germs than hospitals; therefore clean technique can be used. Aseptic technique is used in the hospital because the client is more susceptible to infection and more virulent or pathogenic microorganisms are usually present. In the home setting the majority of clients use clean technique. Use judgment in choosing the correct technique for each client (e.g., use aseptic technique with clients who are immunocompromised; are infected [not colonized]; or have family caregivers infected with viral, bacterial, or fungal microorganisms). Clients living in unclean conditions also need to be suctioned using aseptic technique whenever possible to try to prevent infection. All caregivers need to use standard precautions when suctioning with either clean or aseptic technique.

Caring for a tracheostomy at home begins in the hospital (see Chapter 25) with teaching and return demonstration. The client or family caregiver usually learns better when instruction in less invasive techniques such as tracheal stoma care precedes more invasive techniques such as inner cannula care and suctioning. Continually develop, implement, and evaluate the teaching plan based on client performance. It is imperative that clients and their caregivers have the ability to practice suctioning frequently before discharge to develop confidence with skill performance; otherwise arrangements to provide 24-hour care are necessary before discharge.

Delegation and Collaboration

The skill of teaching home tracheostomy care and suctioning cannot be delegated to nursing assistive personnel (NAP).

Equipment

❑ Suction machine with connecting tube
❑ Clean or sterile gloves
❑ Three small basins
❑ Mild, soapy water or solution of 3% hydrogen peroxide
❑ Normal saline
❑ Appropriate-size sterile or clean and disinfected suction catheter (diameter no greater than half the diameter of the tracheostomy tube [e.g., if tracheostomy tube is 8 mm (0.3 inches), then use 16-Fr or smaller suction catheter])
❑ Tracheostomy care kit or clean 4 × 4–inch gauze pads (nonshredding)
❑ Small nylon bottle brush or pipe cleaners or disposable inner cannula
❑ Cotton-tipped applicators
❑ Tracheostomy ties (twill tape [⅜-inch preferably] or Velcro-type tie holders)
❑ Mirror
❑ Wet washcloth or paper towel (*optional*)
❑ Dry cloth, towel, or paper towel (*optional*)
❑ Protective eyewear (*optional*)
❑ Trash bag (plastic, leakproof preferred)
❑ Disposable apron (*optional*)
❑ Bag-valve-mask (BVM) with oxygen supply (*optional*)

STEP	RATIONALE

ASSESSMENT

1 Assess client's or family caregiver's ability to measure a pulse and to perform tracheostomy care and suctioning properly. Also assess client's level of consciousness, ability to attend and problem solve, and fine-motor function.

Instructing caregiver is essential if client's physical and cognitive impairment prevents ability to perform tracheostomy care and suctioning. Emergency situations usually require family caregiver or significant other to suction.

2 Assess client's or caregiver's knowledge of indications for the need to perform:

a Tracheostomy care, including presence of excess peristomal secretions, excess intratracheal secretions, soiled or damp tracheostomy dressing/ties, and diminished airway through tracheostomy tube.

b Suctioning, including presence of gurgling, wheezes on inspiration or expiration, restlessness, ineffective coughing, tachypnea, cyanosis, acutely decreased level of consciousness, tachycardia or bradycardia, acutely shallow respirations, or acute dyspnea.

Knowledge needed for client or caregiver to accurately assess need to provide tracheostomy care. Signs and symptoms are related to presence of secretions at stoma site or within tracheostomy tube.

Knowledge allows client or caregiver to accurately determine need to perform tracheostomy tube suctioning. Physical signs and symptoms result from lower airway obstruction and tissue hypoxia.

3 Observe client or caregiver perform complete tracheostomy tube care and suctioning.

Determines which specific components of skill that client or caregiver can complete easily and which are more difficult and require reinforcement.

NURSING DIAGNOSES

- Deficient knowledge regarding tracheostomy care
- Ineffective breathing pattern
- Ineffective health maintenance
- Risk for caregiver role strain
- Risk for infection

Related factors are individualized based on client's condition or needs.

STEP	RATIONALE

PLANNING

1 Expected outcomes following completion of procedure:

- Client or family caregiver identifies signs and symptoms indicating need for tracheostomy care and suctioning.

  Client or caregiver is able to institute preventive means to maintain airway.

- Client or caregiver states factors that influence tracheostomy airway functioning.

  Tracheostomy often impairs normal airway clearance, humidification, and gas exchange.

- Client or caregiver correctly demonstrates complete tracheostomy tube care and suctioning in controlled setting.

  Provides validation of ability to perform procedure.

- Client or caregiver identifies signs of stoma inflammation or respiratory tract infection and when to notify health care provider.

  Measures cognitive learning.

- Lower and upper airways are cleared of secretions, as evidenced by absent or diminished wheezes and gurgles in large airways, normalization of pulse and respiratory rate, increased depth of respirations, absence of cyanosis, improved color, and decreased dyspnea.

  Suctioning by client or caregiver is successful.

- Stoma site is clean and free of infection and transesophageal fistula; inner cannula is free of secretions.

  Tracheostomy care is successful.

2 Select setting in home that client or caregiver is most likely to use when completing tracheostomy tube care.

Practicing skill in same setting where skill will be routinely performed facilitates comprehension and learning.

3 Discuss and demonstrate with client or caregiver proper position for procedure (high-Fowler's position in front of mirror).

Promotes understanding of comfort and safety principles and facilitates visibility.

IMPLEMENTATION

1 Suctioning:

a Verify health care provider's orders for suctioning.

Invasive procedure requires an order.

b Instruct client or caregiver on techniques for hand hygiene and application of clean gloves.

Reduces transmission of microorganisms.

c Explain and demonstrate step-by-step preparation and completion of tracheostomy tube suctioning using either open or closed suctioning (see Chapter 25) (see illustration).

Demonstration is reliable technique for teaching psychomotor skill and enables client or caregiver to ask questions throughout procedure. Steps used to suction clients in hospital are also used in home.

Clinical Decision Point *Instillation of normal saline before suctioning, once a common practice, is no longer recommended. Use of normal saline adversely affects arterial and global tissue oxygenation and dislodges bacterial colonies; therefore this can contribute to lower airway contamination (Halm and Krisko-Hagel, 2008).*

d After client or caregiver suctions tracheostomy, teach how to suction nasal and oral pharynx and perform mouth care. Encourage client or caregiver to brush teeth with small soft toothbrush 2 times a day and use mouth moisturizer and moisturize lips every 2 to 4 hours.

Dental plaque harbors microorganisms.
Suctioning removes secretions from trachea and lower airway that clients are not able to clear by coughing (Cleveland Clinic, 2009).

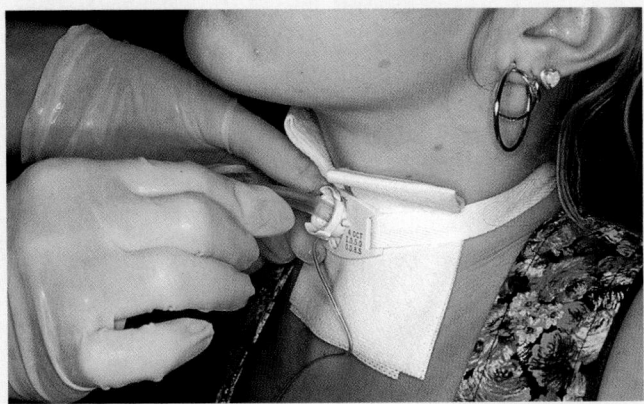

STEP 1c Insertion of suction catheter into tracheostomy tube.

STEP	RATIONALE
e At conclusion of procedure, have client take two to three deep breaths; reassess status of breathing.	Deep breathing reduces oxygen loss and prevents hypoxia. Expect client's respiratory status to improve following suctioning.
f Demonstrate how to disconnect suction catheter; coil and discard catheter in appropriate receptacle. If catheter is to be cleaned and disinfected, set aside. Have client or caregiver remove soiled gloves and dispose in appropriate container; perform hand hygiene.	Prevents transmission of microorganisms.
2 Tracheostomy care:	
a Have client sit at a table with mirror. Teach skills of tracheostomy care, including cleaning stoma and tracheostomy tube and changing tracheostomy ties and dressing (see illustrations and Chapter 25).	Steps used to provide tracheostomy care in hospital are also used in home. *Exception:* Mild soap and water can be used to clean a tracheostomy tube (Cleveland Clinic, 2009). Use hydrogen peroxide solution only to remove heavy secretions.

Clinical Decision Point *During tracheostomy care a client is at risk for the tracheostomy tube coming out. Instruct client or caregiver to never remove the old tracheostomy tube ties until the new ties are secured properly. Keep two tracheostomy tubes, one the same size as the client's and one a size smaller, at the client's bedside so he or she can insert a new tube if the tube comes out.*

STEP	RATIONALE
b Instruct client or caregiver to apply clean gloves. Demonstrate technique for cleaning reusable supplies in warm soapy water. Rinse thoroughly and dry between two layers of clean paper towels. Store supplies in loosely closed clear plastic bag; label bag.	Prevents transmission of microorganisms. Air must circulate, or humidity in bag can promote microorganism growth.
c Have client or caregiver remove and discard gloves. Perform hand hygiene.	Reduces transmission of microorganisms.
d Explain the procedure for disinfecting reusable supplies. This needs to be done at least weekly. To disinfect supplies use one of the following methods:	Removes organisms and reduces risk for infection.
(1) *Method 1*: Boil reusable (boilable) supplies for 15 minutes. Allow to cool and dry.	
(2) *Method 2*: Soak reusable supplies in equal parts of vinegar and water for 30 minutes. Remove, rinse thoroughly, and dry.	
(3) *Method 3*: Soak reusable supplies in prepared solutions of quaternary ammonium chloride compounds according to manufacturer instructions. Rinse and dry.	
3 Have client or caregiver perform each step with guidance from you.	Adults learn psychomotor skills best by active participation, and you can correct any errors in technique as they occur and discuss their implications.

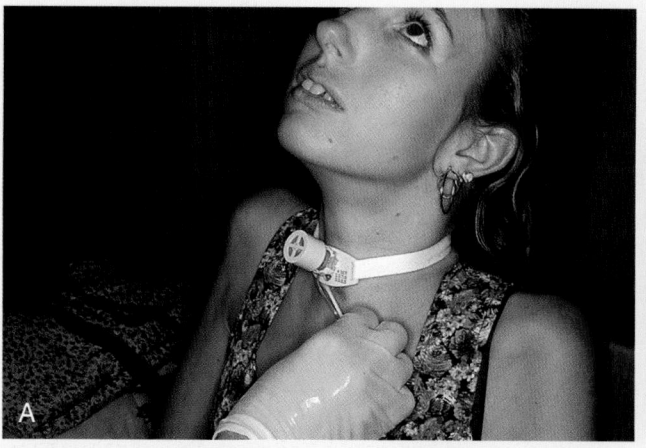 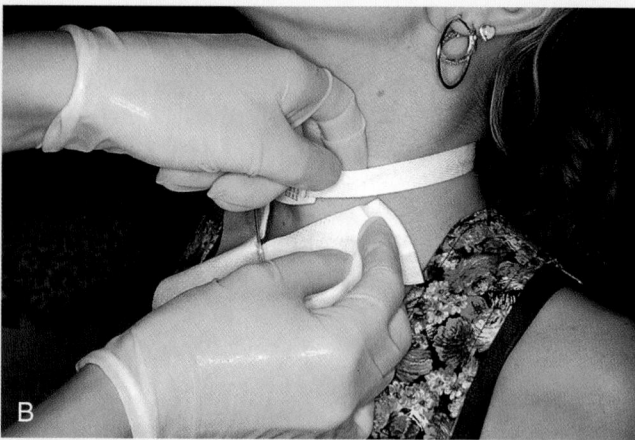

STEP 2a   A, Cleaning area around tracheal stoma. **B,** Applying clean tracheostomy dressing.

STEP	RATIONALE
4 Teach client or caregiver signs and symptoms of the following: **a** Stoma infection (redness, tenderness, drainage) **b** Respiratory tract infection (fever, increased sputum, change in color of sputum, foul sputum odor, increased cough, chills, night sweats) **c** Transesophageal fistula (air leaking through stoma, nose, or mouth with cuff properly inflated; more air needed to inflate cuff; aspiration of food or liquid during suctioning; excessive belching; coughing when swallowing)	Client or caregiver must be able to recognize onset of complications associated with long-term tracheostomy use early so medical treatment can begin, reducing risk for more serious negative outcomes. Emphasize importance of notifying health care provider when signs and symptoms of complications occur.

EVALUATION

1 Ask client or family caregiver to state signs of stoma or respiratory tract complications.	Prompt identification of symptoms results in early treatment and decreases risk for complications that may lead to hospital readmission.
2 Observe client or caregiver demonstrate technique for tracheostomy tube care and suctioning.	Feedback through independent demonstration of psychomotor skill is reliable method to evaluate learning.

Unexpected Outcomes	Related Interventions
1 Stoma site is reddened or hard, with or without drainage.	• Evaluate client's or family caregiver's technique. • Increase frequency of tracheostomy care.
2 Copious colored secretions are present around stoma or when client or caregiver suctions tracheostomy.	• Have client use sterile technique for suctioning and tracheostomy care. • Secretions may be pink, rust colored, or blood tinged, depending on problem; documenting color helps health care provider diagnose problem. • Evaluate for adequate humidity (use room humidifier or tracheostomy collar humidity, if needed) (see Chapter 25). • Notify health care provider.
3 Bloody secretions are suctioned.	• Evaluate suctioning technique, suctioning frequency, and size of catheter used. • Usual length to insert catheter is length of tracheostomy tube plus $\frac{1}{4}$ inch. • Assess for signs of infection.
4 No secretions are suctioned.	• Evaluate client's fluid status, need for increased humidity. • Determine if appropriate size of suction catheter is used. • Reassess need to suction.
5 Tracheostomy tube comes out during a home visit.	• Replace tracheostomy tube to maintain an airway. • Activate emergency medical system (EMS) if needed.
6 Skin breakdown is present at stoma site.	• Assess site for pressure areas or site infection. • Remove pressure source.

Recording and Reporting
• Record client instruction and client's or family caregiver's ability to demonstrate tracheostomy care and suctioning in home health record.
• Develop a system of recording home care for client or caregiver to document and keep track of tracheostomy care provided.

Special Considerations
Teaching
• Some clients benefit by using a mirror to visualize stoma area.
• Tracheostomy tubes are changed every 3 to 4 weeks in adults and every 1 to 2 weeks in children. Two people are required to change the tracheostomy tube. Procedural Guideline 42-1 provides guidelines for changing a tracheostomy tube at home.
• Always leave a phone number and instructions about how to reach home care nurse if needed.

Pediatric
• Encourage parents to give tracheostomy care as soon as child is stable in the hospital. The more time they have to practice these skills, the more comfortable they become in caring for the child at home.
• Children with tracheostomies need to socialize and play with other children who are close to their own age. Encourage parents to take children out of the home. However, an additional adult needs to travel in the car with the child to help if problems arise while in the car (Hockenberry and Wilson, 2011).
• To prevent hypoxia, teach parents that suctioning needs to last no more than 5 seconds. Allow the child to rest for at least 30 to 60 seconds between suctioning passes and do not suction more than 3 times (Hockenberry and Wilson, 2011).
• Teach families and caregivers pediatric cardiopulmonary resuscitation, including use of BVM or mouth-to-tracheostomy technique. They also need to notify the local EMS of the child's

condition and the presence of a tracheostomy and provide EMS with a list of equipment in the home (Hockenberry and Wilson, 2011).

- Encourage parents to have a cool-mist humidifier in same room as child; humidity helps keep secretions thin and decreases the likelihood of mucus plugging (Hockenberry and Wilson, 2011).
- Caring for a child with a tracheostomy often disrupts parents' ability to socialize and can cause sleep deprivation. Develop a plan that includes respite care to allow parents time to meet their own needs (Zia et al., 2010).
- Teach families and caregivers to avoid dressing the child in clothes that could cover the tracheostomy opening such as turtlenecks and clothes that have a tight-fitting collar. Avoid

clothing, toys, and pets that shed fine hair or lint because they could get into the tracheostomy and cause breathing problems (Hockenberry and Wilson, 2011).

Gerontologic
- Older adults lose some properties of elastic recoil and often have greater difficulty in clearing airway secretions through cough. As a result they require more suctioning and airway care and have increased risk for infection (Ebersole et al., 2008).
- Assess for cognitive, mobility, or sensory impairments that impair ability to manage artificial airway at home and teach caregiver if client is unable to manage airway independently.
- Anxiety accompanies decreased ability to breathe and may cause the older adult to become too nervous to perform suctioning independently.

PROCEDURAL GUIDELINE 42-1 Changing a Tracheostomy Tube at Home

To change a tracheostomy tube in the home, it is best to have two people present in case of emergency. Before beginning, ensure that all necessary supplies have been gathered and the client and family caregiver are in a place in the home that is comfortable for the procedure. The client or family caregiver is observed by a home care health professional the first time the caregiver changes a tracheostomy in the home setting.

Delegation and Collaboration
The skill of changing a tracheostomy tube cannot be delegated to nursing assistive personnel (NAP).

Equipment
❑ Clean gloves
❑ Suction catheter
❑ Suction machine
❑ Bag-valve-mask
❑ Face mask
❑ New sterile tracheostomy tube (Fig. 42-4)
❑ Gauze tracheostomy dressing

Procedural Steps
1 Do not allow client to have anything by mouth (NPO) or hold tube feedings for at least 1 hour before procedure.
2 Explain procedure to client before tracheostomy is changed to alleviate anxiety. Have family caregiver assist.
3 Have caregiver perform hand hygiene and apply clean gloves.
4 Remove new tracheostomy tube from sterile container. If the tube has a cuff, be sure it is deflated. Remove inner cannula and insert obturator into outer cannula. Attach clean tracheostomy ties or tracheostomy tube holder to neck plate, checking integrity of cuff.
5 Suction existing tracheostomy tube and have bag-valve-mask and face mask available.

6 Have family caregiver use fingers to hold tracheostomy faceplate in place. Loosen tracheostomy ties and deflate tracheostomy tube cuff (if tracheostomy has one).
7 Have patient take a deep breath, relax, and then direct caregiver to pull out old tracheostomy tube with a gentle, steady pressure in same direction as an inner cannula would be removed. Be sure patient is breathing without distress. Remove gloves and perform hand hygiene.
8 Apply sterile gloves. Insert new tracheostomy through stoma with gentle force, then push back and then down, following direction of the airway. Remove obturator. Allow air to flow in; insert inner cannula and lock in place.
9 Secure new tracheostomy ties or tube holder, inflate cuff (if present), and place new gauze dressing around stoma if necessary.
10 Evaluate patient's ease of breathing, respiratory rate.

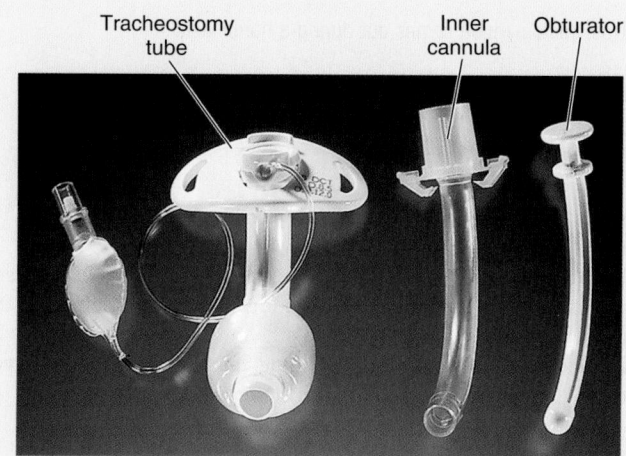

FIG 42-4 Tracheostomy tube. (*Courtesy Mallinckrodt, Inc. Shiley Tracheostomy Products, St. Louis, MO.*)

SKILL 42-6 Teaching Medication Self-Administration

The National Institute for Health and Clinical Excellence (NICE, 2009) found that approximately 50% of prescribed medications are used incorrectly and that some clients do not choose to take their prescribed medication. The goals of NICE include identifying and addressing issues that can influence clients' adherence to their medication regimen. You will be involved in teaching clients how to correctly administer medications, but first you must seek to identify and address any issues that are of concern to your clients.

Compliance was used in the past to describe if clients' behaviors matched that of health care providers' recommendations when it came to taking prescribed medications or adhering to prescribed treatments (Kaufman and Birks, 2009). Recent literature supports the term *adherence* since this emphasizes a client's role in decision making, taking into account freedom of choice (Kaufman and Birks, 2009). One method that has been identified to increase adherence is to support clients' decisions in how to take their medications. Use teaching methods that incorporate active listening so you can adapt clients' needs and concerns into their medication regimen.

Some barriers to medication adherence include fear of adverse reactions from medications, belief that a medication does not help, inconvenience of taking medication, cost of medication, inadequate knowledge, forgetfulness, and lack of social support (Santhosh and Naveen, 2011). Considering these potential barriers, you can provide information and support to ensure that a client or family caregiver is making a well-informed decision when it comes to whether or not to take a medication. Once a client has mastered the skill of administering medications, you must continue to validate that the skill is being performed correctly and assess for new issues and concerns.

Delegation and Collaboration

The skill of teaching clients medication self-administration cannot be delegated to nursing assistive personnel (NAP). The nurse directs the NAP to:

- Communicate to the nurse problems that clients report having with medication self-administration.

Equipment

- ❏ Medication
- ❏ Liquid to take with medication
- ❏ Medication administration record or other up-to-date list of current medications from health care provider
- ❏ Diary or medication log
- ❏ Container for daily or weekly preparation
- ❏ Measuring devices as needed (e.g., medicine cup, teaspoon)
- ❏ Teaching tools (e.g., charts, written instructions, color codes for medicine containers)

STEP	RATIONALE

ASSESSMENT

STEP	RATIONALE
1 Assess client's cognitive, sensory, and motor function; level of consciousness, sight, hearing, touch, health literacy level, swallowing ability, mobility, activity tolerance, social support, and willingness to cooperate.	Cognitive, sensory, and motor deficits frequently influence client's ability to take or prepare prescribed medication correctly and participate in instruction.
2 Assess resources client has to obtain medications when needed (e.g., finances, social support, and transportation).	Lack of resources is a major factor that will negatively affect adherence with medication self-administration regimen (Santhosh and Naveen, 2011).
3 Assess client's learning readiness and ability to concentrate; consider presence of pain, nausea, or fatigue and client interest in instruction.	Presence of significant illness, frailty, or confusion affects person's ability to attend to teaching plan. Indicates need to rely on family caregiver for learning and implementation (if available) on short- or long-term basis.
4 Assess client's and family caregiver's knowledge regarding medication therapy: names of drugs, how to administer, purpose or action, daily doses and times to be taken, side effects to expect, and what to do if problems occur.	Clients need to be able to understand information about their medications and remember it (Kaufman and Birks, 2009). Caregivers' self-confidence in administering medication influences their ability to manage medication for client (Lau et al., 2010).
5 Assess client's belief in need for medication therapy. Consider prior experiences, ethnic values, religious beliefs, personal experiences with medications, and significant others' values about medications.	Many factors influence client's willingness to follow drug regimen.
6 Assess client's prescribed and over-the-counter (OTC) medications, including use of herbal supplements: Has more than one health care provider prescribed medications? Are labels clearly marked? Are time schedules confusing? Do different drugs look alike? Does client store medications together or out of original containers? Are expiration dates on bottles still current?	Determines sources of confusion affecting client's adherence. Adherence with medication therapy (especially in older adults) is often complicated by polypharmacy (multiple chronic conditions are often treated with multiple medications sometimes prescribed by more than one health care provider). Adherence is more complicated when medication regimens are complex.
7 Assess client's understanding of effects and interactions between prescribed medications and ingestion of certain foods, OTC drugs, and herbal supplements.	Medication interactions, including those with OTC drugs, herbals, and certain foods, can seriously affect medication effectiveness and/or create negative side effects (Santhosh and Naveen, 2011).
8 Be sure family caregiver knows client's drug allergies.	As new drugs are prescribed, the family caregiver often becomes the one to monitor for inappropriate drug prescription.

STEP	RATIONALE

NURSING DIAGNOSES

- Anxiety
- Deficient knowledge regarding medication self-administration
- Readiness for enhanced knowledge
- Ineffective health maintenance
- Ineffective individual or family therapeutic regimen management

Related factors are individualized based on client's condition or needs.

PLANNING

1 Expected outcomes following completion of procedure:
- Client or family caregiver is able to state purpose of each medication and why it is beneficial.
- Client identifies common adverse effects and relief measures.
- Client or caregiver is able to state when to notify health care provider about medication problems.
- Client reads each label and explains when each medication should be taken.
- Client or caregiver demonstrates self-administration of medication by prescribed route.

Demonstrates cognitive learning.

Enhances adherence to medication therapy.
Empowers client to participate in care.

Prevents medication administration errors.

Demonstrates skill achieved.

2 Prepare environment for teaching session:
  a Select room that is well lit.
  b Provide comfortable seating.
  c Be sure that client is close and can see nurse clearly.
  d Control sources of noise and distractions.

Room environment needs to minimize existing sensory alterations. Comfortable environment free of distractions promotes client's attention.

3 Prepare teaching materials:
  a Use an approach that matches client's learning preference:
    (1) Written materials printed in large bold letters (set in 14-point or larger type).
    (2) DVD or Internet instructional programs.
    (3) Illustrations of medication safety guidelines.
  b Give written schedules or individualized instruction sheets.

Client-centered care focuses on working in partnership with clients to provide high-quality, appropriate, and cost-effective health care (Kaufman and Birks, 2009).

Makes teaching patient-centered.

4 Ensure that client is wearing glasses or hearing aids if needed during teaching session.

Use of glasses or hearing aids increases client's sensory perception and likelihood of attending to teaching session and understanding content.

5 Consult with health care provider to review medications that client is receiving and simplify regimen if possible.

Review of medications helps minimize risk for drug interactions from multiple medications and ensures accuracy of medication regimen. Simplification of regimen improves adherence, particularly related to daily frequency of prescribed doses.

6 Arrange teaching time to allow participation of family members (see illustration).

Caregiver can serve as positive resource to client and often reinforce information provided (Lau et al., 2010).

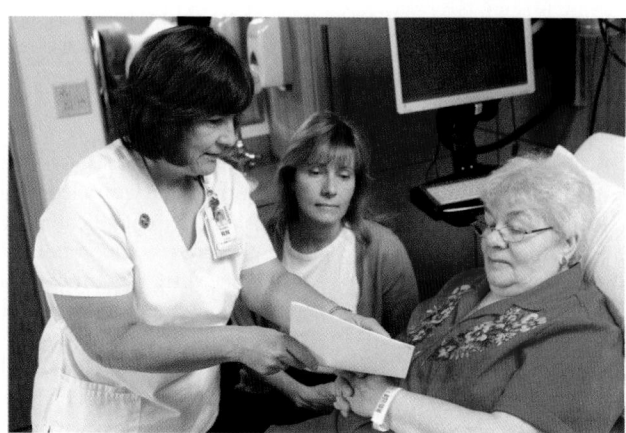

STEP 6 Client and family member participate in medication self-administration teaching program.

STEP	RATIONALE

IMPLEMENTATION

1 Instruct client or family caregiver on importance of performing hand hygiene before medication self-administration.

Reduces transmission of microorganisms.

2 Present information clearly and concisely:

Improves client's ability to attend and understand (Kaufman and Birks, 2009).

a Face learner in well-lit room.

Allows visualization of client's nonverbal responses to education. Client with hearing loss or visual problem is able to see your expressions, read written information, and hear your voice more clearly.

b Use short sentences and speak in slow, low-pitched voice.

Enhances understanding of information.

c Provide descriptions in understandable terms.

Prevents confusion of terminology. Clients learn more quickly when you present information at level of learner (Kaufman and Birks, 2009).

3 Provide frequent pauses so client or caregiver can ask questions and express understanding of content.

Increases learner participation. Ongoing feedback ensures that client is acquiring information.

4 Instruct client or caregiver on the following content: purpose of regularly scheduled and prn (as needed) medications and their desired effects, how medication works and why it helps, dosage schedules and rationale, common side effects, what to do to relieve side effects, what to do if dose is missed, when to call health care provider with problems, who to call with problems, medication safety guidelines, and implications when medications are not taken.

Provides client or caregiver with sufficient information to understand and take medications safely at home.

5 Instruct client in appropriate route of medication delivery, including oral, subcutaneous, intramuscular, inhalation, and topical.

Client needs to be proficient in all routes of medication administration. Adverse effects often occur if medications are administered incorrectly.

6 Provide frequent, short teaching sessions. Plan to have several teaching sessions, especially if client needs to take multiple medications. Leave instruction aids in home for client to review if possible.

Frequent sessions improve client's attention and retention of information discussed. Reference to charts, written information, and other teaching tools as resources enhances learning (Kaufman and Birks, 2009).

7 Provide teaching about OTC medications and herbal supplements.

Clients may not understand effects of OTC and herbal supplements (Santhosh and Naveen, 2011).

8 Provide client with special charts, diagrams, learning aids, written information, and Internet/Intranet resources (see illustration).

Clear written information, charts, and other resources such as the Internet/Intranet enhance client learning and allow for reinforcement of information.

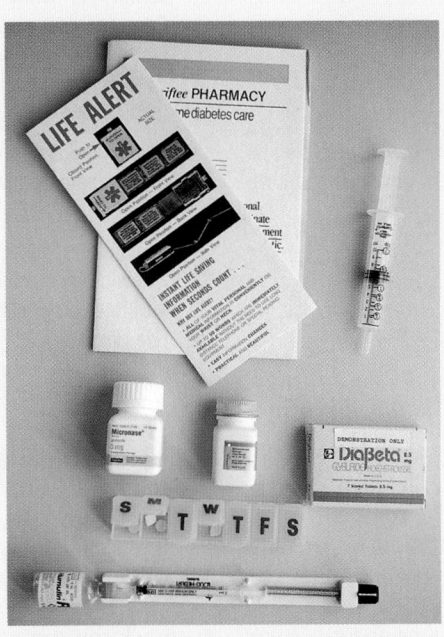

STEP 8 Examples of aids for client medication self-administration.

STEP	RATIONALE
9 Offer assistance as client practices preparing medication (e.g., "Let's prepare the medications you will take with your meals or the medicines you take first in the morning").	Allows for observation of client's ability to read labels correctly and prepare all medications for prescribed times.
10 Have pharmacy provide clear, large-print labels for medication bottles and medication teaching handouts if appropriate.	Improves client's ability to read and follow directions.
11 Have pharmacy provide containers that client can open independently if manual dexterity is limited.	Most pharmacies dispense pills in "childproof" containers, which client with limited mobility of fingers/hands often finds difficult to manipulate or open.

Clinical Decision Point *If there are pets or small children in the home or children who frequently visit the home, help client establish a "safe place" for medication storage to reduce risk for accidental ingestion by pets or children.*

STEP	RATIONALE
12 Facilitate arrangements for pharmacy to receive written prescriptions in timely fashion if required for dispensing. Arrange for pharmacy to deliver medications to home if client is unable to arrange for transportation to pharmacy.	Availability of drugs influences adherence.

EVALUATION

1 Ask client or family caregiver to explain information about each drug: purpose; actions; routes; timing of medications and maximum frequency of use of either prescribed or OTC medications; side effects and interactions; and foods, herbals, or OTC medications to avoid.	Clients and caregivers need to be able to understand medication information they are given and remember this information (Kaufman and Birks, 2009).
2 Identify client's problem-solving abilities (e.g., when to call health care provider or refer to printed information for resources).	Developing techniques to gain information and solve problems assists in client adherence and reduces potential problems from medication regimen (Kaufman and Birks, 2009).
3 Have client or caregiver prepare doses for all prescribed medications.	Indicates understanding of medication dosages and schedules.
4 Ask client to verbalize any remaining questions regarding medication management.	Offers opportunity for clarification and minimizes any remaining confusion or misunderstanding.

Unexpected Outcomes

1 Client or family caregiver makes errors in preparing medications or is unable to recall and/or explain information discussed in teaching sessions.

2 Medication self-administration plan is not possible because of client's self-care deficits. This is very common when client develops cognitive changes.

3 Client refuses to take medications as prescribed.

Related Interventions

- Provide additional instruction and/or teaching materials for consultation when information is forgotten or unclear.
- Ensure that written instructions are at client's level of understanding. Some commercially prepared booklets contain instructions that are too complex or contain medical jargon that is difficult to understand.
- Consider use of pictures, color coding, diagrams, and tape-recorded instructions for reading or sight impaired.
- Periodically observe client or caregiver prepare and administer medications.
- Develop alternative plan, which often relies on family caregivers to provide safe administration of home medication regimen.

- Explore and identify reasons for noncompliance, which often include the following: cost, side effects, complexity of regimen, problems with swallowing or other side effects, and cultural preferences.
- See Box 42-4.

Recording and Reporting

- Document instruction provided and learning outcomes achieved by client in home care record.
- Develop a system of recording (patient diary) for client or family caregiver to use to document adherence to dosage schedules and self-monitoring of any problems.
- Always leave a phone number and instructions about how to reach home care nurse if needed.

Special Considerations
Teaching

- See Chapter 41 for guidelines for medication safety.
- If it is difficult to plan a separate teaching session, instruct client while administering medications.
- Examples of learning aids include homemade calendars for each week that contain plastic bags containing medications to take at specific times, egg cartons divided into color-coded sections

BOX 42-4	Evidence-Based Nursing Interventions to Enhance Adherence to Medication Therapy

- Involve clients as partners in collaboration. Encourage them to express their views and share in the decision making with you.
- Urge clients to take medications.
- Be empathetic regarding clients' feelings.
- Encourage a sense of control for the client by providing information about diagnosis and treatment.
- Recognize caregiver needs and provide information and support. Understand that caregiver may have competing responsibilities (e.g., employment, other dependents).
- Client's attitude will affect his or her willingness to work with health care providers and be compliant with treatments.

Modified from Kaufman G, Birks Y: Strategies to improve clients' adherence to medication, *Nurs Stand* 23(49):51, 2009; Lau DT et al.: Exploring factors that influence informal caregiving in medication management for home hospice clients, *J Palliat Med* 13(9):1085, 2010; Santhosh YL, Naveen MR: Medication adherence behavior in chronic diseases like asthma and diabetes mellitus, *Int J Pharm Pharm Sci* 3(3):238, 2011.

with medications for the day, clock faces for clients who cannot read or see clearly, color coding for drug types (e.g., blue for sedative, red for pain pill), and pillboxes that identify days of the week and times of day.

Pediatric

- Instruct adults to keep all medications locked and securely out of reach of children.
- Encourage caregivers not to tell children that medications are treats because this increases the risk for child overdosing by mistaking medicine for candy.

- Successful medication teaching involves the child's parents or other caregivers and the child and siblings whenever possible. To provide effective medication teaching to children, take the child's developmental and cognitive abilities into consideration when planning teaching sessions (Hockenberry and Wilson, 2011).
- Parents need to supervise older children as they begin taking responsibility for their own treatment.

Gerontologic

- Capacity for learning new information remains as people age (in the absence of dementia); however, older clients often need additional time to accomplish learning. Allow adequate time and number of teaching sessions to support successful learning. Effective teaching strategies for older adults include memory aids, information written in large letters (14 point is recommended), involvement of caregiver, follow-up teaching sessions either over the telephone or in person, and computer-assisted teaching guides (Ebersole et al., 2008).
- Cognition problems coupled with complexity of medication regimens have a negative effect on safe medication self-administration in older adults. Attempt to decrease the complexity of medication regimens in clients with cognitive deficits whenever possible to promote safe medication self-administration practices.
- Older adults often have to take medications in multiple routes (e.g., oral, inhaled, injections). Many times problems with physical dexterity, eyesight, cognitive skills, and memory negatively affect adherence to medication schedules. Establish a therapeutic nurse-client relationship to help clients overcome these barriers to adherence.

SKILL 42-7   Managing Feeding Tubes in the Home

Enteral nutrition therapy in the home setting is usually effective when a client tolerates at least 70% of feeding intake without complications and is medically stable, the client or family caregiver is able to administer feedings, and there is sufficient time in a controlled environment to learn the skill. A recent study revealed that the majority of clients requiring home enteral nutrition are adults over the age of 60 years (Hitchings et al., 2010). Clients benefit when they are able to see tube feeding equipment and devices when learning how to administer home enteral nutrition. Provide hands-on experience and client involvement with decision making about home enteral nutrition whenever possible.

This procedure in the home setting follows the guidelines and skills described in Chapter 31 (see Skills 31-1, 31-2, 31-3, and 31-4 and Procedural Guideline 31-1). Most patients who receive enteral nutrition in the home have either gastrostomy or jejunostomy tubes. This skill focuses on teaching the client or caregiver in the home. Frequently in this setting the nurse is responsible for

reinsertion of gastrostomy feeding tubes, and the health care provider is responsible for reinsertion of jejunostomy tubes.

Delegation and Collaboration

The skill of management of feeding tubes in the home cannot be delegated to nursing assistive personnel (NAP). The nurse inserts feeding tubes, verifies tube placement, assesses for residual volume, and administers medications through feeding tubes. Administration of enteral tube feeding via syringe is sometimes delegated to NAP (verify agency policy). The nurse directs the NAP to:

- Report when client has difficulty with feeding, coughing, gagging, respiratory distress, discomfort, or vomiting.

Equipment

See Skills 31-1, 31-2, 31-3, and 31-4 and Procedural Guideline 31-1 for list of equipment

❑ Paper or log book to record daily weights, intake and output (I&O), temperature, feeding residuals

---

STEP	RATIONALE

ASSESSMENT

| 1 Assess client's health status, including presence of discomfort and fatigue and ability to successfully manage enteral feedings in home. | Increases successful home management with fewer complications. |
| 2 Assess client's and family caregiver's physical, emotional, financial, and community resources. | Availability of resources increases ability for self-care home management. |

STEP	RATIONALE
3 Assess environmental conditions of home (sanitation, storage of equipment, work area, supplies, and power source).	Ensures safe environment and decreases risks of infection and complications.
4 Assess client's and caregiver's understanding of purpose of enteral feedings and positive expected outcomes.	Understanding rationale of treatment is critical to enhancing participation and cooperation in care.
5 Assess client's and caregiver's understanding of storage and management of equipment and supplies and where and how to obtain supplies.	Ensures safe home management and decreases risk for complications. Home care delivery companies usually deliver a month's supply at a time. If client stores feeding containers in garage, it must be brought into the house a couple hours before using in colder months to warm to room temperature (Best and Hitchings, 2010). The garage is not a good storage place during hot weather; use a basement if possible.
6 Assess client's and caregiver's ability to manipulate feeding equipment.	Sometimes caregiver needs to administer enteral feedings.

NURSING DIAGNOSES

- Anxiety
- Deficient knowledge regarding tube feeding self-administration
- Feeding self-care deficit
- Imbalanced nutrition: less than body requirements
- Risk for aspiration
- Ineffective health maintenance

Related factors are individualized based on client's condition or needs.

PLANNING

1 Expected outcomes following completion of procedure:	
• Client or family caregiver verbalizes purpose of enteral feedings and enhanced nutritional health.	Provides measurable criteria to determine level of cognitive understanding.
• Client or caregiver demonstrates proper use of equipment and handling of formulas.	Provides demonstration of skills needed to manage home enteral nutrition.
• Client or caregiver demonstrates accurate administration of enteral feedings and medications.	Provides demonstration of skills needed to administer home enteral nutrition.
• Client or caregiver verbalizes understanding of signs and symptoms and management of complications of feeding.	Confirms that client or caregiver has knowledge needed to respond when problems with feedings develop.

IMPLEMENTATION

1 Have client or family caregiver perform hand hygiene.	Reduces transmission of microorganisms.
2 Discuss with client or family caregiver purpose of enteral feeding and enhanced nutritional health.	Reinforces importance of regular feedings.
3 Help client or caregiver determine a feeding schedule that will maintain nutritional requirements and fit within client's or family's schedule.	Promotes adherence to enteral nutrition therapy. A patient-centered approach increases client confidence in managing his or her own feedings (Best and Hitchings, 2010).

Clinical Decision Point *Explain that caregiver needs to communicate to home health or health care provider any changes in feeding schedules made to fit daily routine.*

4 Have client or caregiver apply clean gloves. Demonstrate how to identify placement of feeding tube: aspiration of gastric fluid, checking pH of gastric fluid, and acceptable pH range (see Skill 31-2).	Some nasally placed tubes are inadvertently placed in respiratory system and migrate to esophagus or into respiratory tract. Check pH periodically (Best and Hitchings, 2010). Aspirated secretions with low pH are strong indicator of gastric placement. However, high pH cannot differentiate between aspirated secretions obtained from respiratory and intestinal tube placements.

Clinical Decision Point *Instruct client to avoid administration of all feedings, flushes, or medications if there is any doubt as to placement of enteral feeding tube.*

5 Observe client or caregiver determine placement of nasally placed tube.	Identifies if there are areas for further teaching.
6 Observe client or caregiver check for gastric residual volume by aspirating gastric contents. Instruct to return aspirated contents to stomach unless volume exceeds 250 mL (Bankhead et al., 2009).	Aspirates more than 250 mL indicate need to initiate interventions such as changing from intermittent to continuous feedings, evaluating possibility of decreasing opioid analgesics, and starting medication that enhances gastric motility (e.g., metoclopramide [Reglan]) to reduce aspiration risk.

STEP	RATIONALE

Clinical Decision Point *If gastric aspirates are more than 250 mL and there is no abdominal pain, instruct client or caregiver to return gastric contents and recheck in 1 hour. If aspirates remain more than 250 mL after an hour, instruct the client or caregiver not to stop the infusion for 4 hours and recheck (Bankhead et al., 2009). If the residual is still more than 250 mL, instruct client or caregiver to contact home care nurse or health care provider (Kenny and Goodman, 2010).*

STEP	RATIONALE
7 Discuss use of medical asepsis in setting up and changing administration sets, mixing formulas (do not add formula to hanging bag), refrigerating unused formula, limiting amount of formula "hung" at one time to amount that can be infused in 4- to 6-hour period (less time in warmer weather), and maintaining and caring for bag.	Medical aseptic technique minimizes risk for microorganism contamination. Refrigeration and limiting "hang" time reduce microorganisms. Changing administration sets every 24 hours reduces microorganism growth.
8 Instruct client or caregiver that client needs to sit up in chair or have head of bed elevated at least 30 to 45 degrees while receiving feedings or medications or when tube is flushed. If this is not possible, place client in reverse Trendelenburg's position.	Decreases risk for aspiration. Aspiration is indicated by increased coughing, difficulty in breathing, or increased sputum (Hitchings et al., 2010).
9 Observe client or caregiver mixing, administering, and storing formulas. Discuss flushing of tube after administration of feedings or medications.	Identifies competence and need for further teaching. Regular flushing of tube prevents clogging.
10 Observe client or caregiver changing administration sets; and cleaning bags. Then have them dispose of supplies, remove gloves and perform hand hygiene.	Reduces transmission of infection.
11 Observe client or caregiver administering medications and flushing tube (see Skill 21-2).	Ensures that medications are given correctly.

Clinical Decision Point *Verify that medications do not include any sublingual, enteric-coated, or sustained-release medications.*

STEP	RATIONALE
12 Discuss and observe use of infusion pump if client is receiving continuous feeding (see Chapter 31).	Use of tube-feeding infusion pumps is complex and requires reinforcement.
13 Discuss measures to stabilize feeding tube in clients with abdominal tubes and to cleanse and protect skin insertion site.	Prevents tube from dislodging and prevents skin breakdown.
14 Provide contact information for ordering equipment and supplies or who to call in case of equipment failure.	Ensures that caregiver is able to respond in an emergency.
15 Discuss emergency plan and actions to take for signs and symptoms of aspiration such as elevating head of bed, oral suctioning, and calling health care provider.	Ensures understanding of management of equipment, supplies, emergency plan, and collaboration.
16 Discuss who to contact and when for signs of diarrhea, constipation, or weight loss.	Provides support to client or caregiver.

EVALUATION

1 Ask client or family caregiver to state purpose of home enteral nutrition therapy.	Demonstrates cognitive learning.
2 Observe client or caregiver performing medical asepsis techniques, checking tube placement, aspirating residuals, administering medications and solutions, and using/cleaning equipment.	Demonstrates psychomotor learning.
3 Ask client or caregiver to state measures used to prevent complications (e.g., verification of tube position before each feeding, elevation of client's head during feeding, stabilization and flushing of tubing).	Ensures safe home management and identification of areas for teaching.
4 Ask client or caregiver how to care for open formula cans.	Ensures safe home management for preventing foodborne illness.
5 Ask client or caregiver about ways to manage complications (e.g., signs of intolerance: nausea, abdominal distention, diarrhea, skin problems, and fluid deficit).	Ensures safe home management and identification of areas of teaching (Hitchings et al., 2010).

Unexpected Outcomes	Related Interventions
1 Feeding tube becomes displaced.	• Instruct family caregiver to notify home care nurse whenever this happens and stop feeding. • Nurse will reposition feeding tube and verify placement before initiating any enteral feeding.
2 Signs and symptoms of aspiration are present.	• Stop feeding. Raise head of bed. • Verify tube position. • Notify health care provider.
3 Client develops diarrhea.	• Notify health care provider. • Consider change in strength, type, or rate of enteral feeding or administration of antidiarrheal agents (Hitchings et al., 2010).
4 Skin surrounding stoma breaks down, or drainage around insertion site develops.	• Clean stoma area more frequently. • Apply antibiotic ointment around stoma as ordered. • Contact health care provider.

Recording and Reporting

• Record instructions given to client or family caregivers and their response in home care record.
• Record specifics of enteral feeding plan, including type and size of tube in home, formula, and amounts to be administered in specific time frames.
• Client or caregivers need to document I&O, daily weights, amount of gastric fluid aspirated before each feeding (or every 4 hours if receiving continuous feeding), date and time of feedings, amount and type of formula, any additives, and date and time that administration sets are changed.

Special Considerations

Teaching

• Performing skill without nurse in attendance provokes anxiety. Always leave a phone number and instructions about how to reach home care nurse if needed.

Pediatric

• Children are at risk for aspiration and fluid and electrolyte imbalance; thus teach parent to monitor child carefully (Hockenberry and Wilson, 2011).
• Children who receive long-term home enteral feedings often experience developmental and growth delays. Other common problems include sleep disturbance, tube blockages, problems with delivery of equipment, and equipment malfunction. Therefore these children require close follow-up and frequent nutritional monitoring.
• Teach parents or caregiver to position children who cannot sit up during or after a tube feeding on their right side during the tube feeding and for approximately 1 hour after the feeding (Hockenberry and Wilson, 2011).

Gerontologic

• Assess for changes and limitations in sensory function, mobility, or dexterity that indicate a need to teach a caregiver how to administer feedings.
• Day enteral tube feeding is best choice because overnight feeding has an increased risk of aspiration in clients with an incompetent swallow. Feeding increases the need for urination; client may forget to disconnect before getting out of bed, get tangled in the tubing, and/or experience urinary/fecal incontinence because he or she cannot get to the toilet quickly enough (Hitchings et al., 2010).
• Elderly are especially at risk for drug interactions with nutrients because of increased number of different medications (polypharmacy) (Hitchings et al., 2010).

SKILL 42-8   Managing Parenteral Nutrition in the Home

Parenteral nutrition (PN) in the home is indicated for clients who cannot take adequate nutrition by mouth and when enteral feedings are contraindicated (e.g., cancer, renal failure, motor neuron disorders, cardiac disease, chronic respiratory or gastrointestinal disorders) (Holmes, 2011). In the home PN is often called *total nutrient admixture (TNA)*. Nurses who manage PN in the home collaborate frequently with registered dietitians and other health care providers to ensure that clients receive sufficient calories, protein, and fluid. PN is administered through a long-term central venous catheter (CVC) such as a tunneled CVC (e.g., Groshong or Hickman catheter), an implantable port, or a peripherally inserted central catheter (PICC) (see Chapter 28). There are risks of complications for infusion, including intravenous (IV)–related blood clots and blood stream infection.

PN is an individually formulated and complete supplement that includes a mixture of amino acids, dextrose, fat emulsions, vitamins, electrolytes, minerals, and trace elements. Administering PN in the home is time consuming, placing a burden on the family caregiver (Smith and Ross, 2010).

Usually administration of PN in the home takes about 12 hours; thus many clients choose to receive their PN during the night. Because of the risks involved with PN and because management in the home is very complex, clients receive their first infusion of PN in an acute care setting. After discharge a home care nurse visits frequently. Carefully assess the reaction of the client or caregiver to the use of the technology needed to administer PN at home and provide emotional support. Although administering PN in the home increases clients' autonomy, it often interferes with their ability to maintain their normal routines. Work with the client or caregiver to stress the benefits and offer support in dealing with related issues.

Delegation and Collaboration

The skill of managing parenteral nutrition in the home cannot be delegated to nursing assistive personnel (NAP).

Equipment

- ❏ IV solution of PN or TNA
- ❏ IV tubing with optional filter (0.2 μm for dextrose/amino acids, 1.2 μm for TNA)
- ❏ Electronic IV infusion pump with alarms and protection from free flow
- ❏ Home blood glucose monitoring equipment
- ❏ Alcohol swabs
- ❏ Clean gloves
- ❏ Paper or logbook and pencil or pen

STEP	RATIONALE

ASSESSMENT

1 Assess client's nutritional status and risk for malnutrition by using a nutrition screening tool (see Chapter 30) and performing a physical examination. Identify signs and symptoms of malnutrition (e.g., weight loss or weight below ideal level; muscle atrophy, wasting, or weakness; lethargy; unable to eat for more than 6 days). Include measurement of vital signs.

Nutritional assessment helps to identify clients who are malnourished or vulnerable to nutritional decline (Holmes, 2011).

2 Assess client's fluid and electrolyte levels, serum albumin, total protein, transferrin, prealbumin, triglycerides, and glucose levels.

Provides baseline assessment data (Holmes, 2011).

3 Assess client's venous access device for edema, drainage, tenderness, and signs of inflammation (see Chapter 28). Measure circumference of upper arm if client has PICC; mark place on arm where measurement was taken.

Infection is a common complication when client has venous access device. Measurement of arm helps detect infiltration of PICC. Mark on arm ensures consistent measurements over time.

4 Verify health care provider's order for nutrients, vitamins, minerals, trace elements, electrolytes, and flow rate.

Ensures safe and accurate PN administration.

5 Assess client's or family caregiver's anxiety level and readiness to learn.

Anxiety prevents learning. Skill is highly complex, and client needs to be ready to learn.

6 Assess client's or caregiver's previous knowledge and experience in managing PN in the home. Have client or caregiver perform return demonstration if able to perform skill.

Determines level of understanding before beginning teaching session.

NURSING DIAGNOSES

- Adult failure to thrive
- Anxiety
- Caregiver role strain
- Fatigue
- Imbalanced nutrition: less than body requirements
- Deficient knowledge regarding TPN
- Readiness for enhanced nutrition
- Risk for infection
- Social isolation

Related factors are individualized based on client's condition or needs.

PLANNING

1 Expected outcomes following completion of procedure:
- Client or family caregiver is able to administer PN correctly.
- Client or caregiver demonstrates proper care of CVC.
- Client or caregiver states signs and symptoms that need to be reported to health care provider.

Indicates that skills are effectively learned.
Prevents infection and ensures patency of venous access device.
Ensures safe administration of PN in home.

2 Select setting in home where client is most likely to administer PN.

Practicing in same environment where skill is routinely performed facilitates comprehension and learning.

IMPLEMENTATION

1 Provide name and phone number of persons or resources available 24 hours a day, 7 days a week in case problems arise.

Provides assurance and allows client or family caregiver to troubleshoot problems and answer questions.

2 Explain type/name of infusion, dosage, expected outcomes, and components of PN. Explain that PN needs to be stored in refrigerator.

Allows client or caregiver to verify that correct PN is infused and client or caregiver understands expected outcomes of care. Refrigeration maintains integrity of PN.

3 Have client or caregiver perform each step with guidance from nurse. Do not rush client.

Allows you to correct errors in technique as they occur and discuss implications.

4 Instruct client or caregiver to inspect bag label, ensure that client's name is on label, ensure that bag has not expired, and check bag for leaks.

Ensures that right client receives right PN. Bag needs to be intact to maintain closed system and ensure that client receives all prescribed nutrients.

5 Suggest taking PN solution out of refrigerator for 30 to 60 minutes before scheduled infusion time.

Chilled solution often causes discomfort; allowing solution to warm enhances comfort during infusion.

6 Explain need to inspect fluid in bag for color and precipitates.

Changes in color or precipitates in bag indicate disruption in PN.

STEP	RATIONALE

Clinical Decision Point *If precipitate appears, components of mixture are separated, or color changes, explain that solution needs to be discarded.*

STEP	RATIONALE
7 Perform hand hygiene and apply clean gloves. Demonstrate how to attach IV tubing to bag, how to attach filter to IV tubing (*optional*), how to prime IV tubing, and how to load IV tubing into electronic infusion pump (see Chapter 28).	Prepares PN solution for IV administration.
8 Wipe CVC port with alcohol and show how to flush CVC and connect IV tubing to port (see Chapter 28). Use needleless system whenever possible.	CVC needs to be patent, and IV tubing needs to connect to CVC to allow PN to be administered. Needleless systems prevent needlestick injuries.
9 Explain how to determine appropriate rate of infusion and program infusion pump (see Skill 28-2). Caution patient and caregiver against changing rate to "catch up."	Ensures that PN is administered at appropriate rate.
10 Remove and dispose of gloves; perform hand hygiene.	Prevents spread of microorganisms.
11 When infusion is completed, explain how to disconnect IV tubing and flush CVC (see Chapter 28). Ensure that client or caregiver performs hand hygiene before and after disconnecting line.	Flushing CVC following infusion maintains patency of vascular access device. Meticulous hand hygiene prevents infection.
12 Describe appropriate use and storage of infusion pump and supplies. Explain appropriate tubing replacement schedules (e.g., every 24 hours for TNA, 72 hours for three-in-one solutions).	Maintains integrity of equipment; appropriate timing of tubing changes prevents infection.
13 Help to develop plan for appropriate disposal of supplies, including needles, syringes, and unused medications or solutions, using principles of standard precautions.	Implementation of standard precautions is necessary to prevent transmission of communicable diseases and needlestick injuries.
14 Demonstrate appropriate care of CVC site; discuss how to change dressings, frequency of dressing changes, and signs of infection (see Skill 28-6).	Prevents infection at CVC insertion site.
15 Teach client and/or caregiver about signs and symptoms that indicate potential complications from PN therapy (e.g., infection and phlebitis at CVC site, refeeding syndrome, hyperglycemia, hypernatremia, hypophosphatemia, hypokalemia, hypomagnesemia) and when to call for help.	Knowledge of complications of PN therapy allows for early detection and appropriate action.
16 Demonstrate use of self–blood glucose monitor. Explain frequency of testing, normal glucose values, and what to do if values fall outside of expected range (see Chapter 43).	PN increases blood glucose levels, which negatively affects client outcomes. Frequent monitoring of glucose level helps detect problems early. Expect testing frequency to decrease as client's condition and response to PN stabilizes.
17 Provide client with logbook to record administration of PN, weights, intake and output, and blood glucose levels.	Allows health care providers and clients to evaluate outcomes and detect adverse effects of nutritional therapy.
18 Help client develop a plan to reorder supplies, PN fluid, and prescribed additives; for emergencies (e.g., what to do if electricity goes out); and for a home safety plan (e.g., how to get to bathroom without tripping over IV tubing).	Plans allow for continuous, safe, and effective administration of PN.

EVALUATION

1 Have client or family caregiver independently demonstrate initiation, infusion, and discontinuation of PN infusion and CVC site care.	Feedback through return demonstration of psychomotor skill is best means of evaluating mastery of skill.
2 Watch client clean and store PN, equipment, and supplies.	Proper cleaning and storage prevents bacterial growth.
3 Ask client or caregiver to identify expected outcomes of nutritional therapy.	Measures client cognitive learning and confirms understanding of information.
4 Have client or caregiver describe common signs and symptoms of infection and other complications of PN.	Measures cognitive learning.
5 Watch client record information in logbook. Review client's or caregiver's log book periodically to ensure that information is being recorded correctly.	Health care providers make changes in client care based on information provided by client. To ensure that changes are made appropriately, client needs to record accurate information.

Unexpected Outcomes

1 Client or family caregiver is unable to manage home PN therapy or verbalize information that was taught.

2 Client or caregiver reports signs and symptoms of complications from PN or CVC.

Related Interventions

- Ask client or caregiver to describe difficulties experienced while performing skill.
- Use different teaching strategy.
- Teach caregiver further and evaluate need to increase frequency of home visits to ensure safe administration of PN at home.
- Inform health care provider.
- Tell client or caregiver to call EMS if signs and symptoms are severe.

Recording and Reporting

- Record information taught, client's response, and outcomes of PN therapy (e.g., weight, electrolyte and glucose levels, physical assessment findings) in home care record.
- Record appearance of CVC site, infusions, glucose monitoring results, client's weight in home documentation system (e.g., logbook).

Special Considerations

Teaching

- Assess client's psychosocial status while providing information. Many clients experience a decrease in the quality of life when PN feedings are started in the home, which often increases anxiety and decreases comprehension of information.
- Eating is often a social event. When clients do not eat, they tend to feel socially isolated. Teach clients and family caregivers the importance of maintaining social relationships and enhancing social support during PN therapy. Refer client to support groups and other resources such as the Oley Foundation (http://oley.org/index.html) (Hockenberry and Wilson, 2011).
- Always leave a phone number and instructions about how to reach home care nurse if needed.

Pediatric

- The risk for displacement of the CVC increases as the child grows. Ensure that the placement of the venous access device is confirmed with x-ray film examination as the child grows.
- Teach the caregiver to socialize child with other children to enhance development (Hockenberry and Wilson, 2011).

Gerontologic

- Frail older adults are at high risk for electrolyte disturbances. Frequently assess and monitor their response to PN and their laboratory values.
- Carefully assess client's ability to perform skill. Management of PN at home is complex and requires manual dexterity, visual acuity, and high-level critical thinking and decision-making skills. Include caregiver or other family members in teaching plan to help with management of home PN.

Critical Thinking Exercises

You are scheduled to visit an 80-year-old retired banker who lives in a private home with his 77-year-old wife. The client was recently hospitalized for atrial fibrillation, an abnormal heart rhythm, and was sent home on digoxin, a cardiac glycoside, to control his arrhythmia. The client has impaired visual acuity and is hard of hearing. When you call him to set up the home visit, you find that, in addition to his recent arrhythmia, he has an elevated temperature. This is your first home visit.

1 What information would you like to have about the client before you go to his home to help him with safely managing his new medical condition and medication and address the temperature?

2 You teach the client how to take his pulse before he takes his digoxin. For how long do you tell him to take his pulse? Explain your choice.
1 For 15 seconds and then multiply by 4
2 For 30 seconds and then multiply by 2
3 For a full minute
4 For 2 minutes

3 The client tells you that he cannot feel his radial pulse after repeated attempts. What is your next step?

4 Describe three teaching strategies you could use to enhance client's ability to learn how to take medications correctly.

5 The client informs you that his temperature has been 100° F (37.7° C) for the past 2 days. However, his wife is concerned that he is not checking his temperature accurately and that it is actually much higher. What will you do to assess if the client is checking his temperature correctly?

REVIEW QUESTIONS

1 A client has purchased a new electronic blood pressure monitoring device. Which nursing action will verify the accuracy of her blood pressure monitor?
1 Calling the client after 2 weeks of monitoring and asking for the readings obtained
2 Having her check her neighbor's blood pressure with the new monitor
3 Checking her blood pressure with a manual aneroid sphygmomanometer 1 to 2 minutes after she checks it with her monitor
4 Asking her to describe when and how she should take her blood pressure with her new monitor

2 A client is being discharged from the hospital with home oxygen therapy. What should be included in the nurse's teaching session with him and his family? (Select all that apply.)
1 He should not allow people in the home to smoke.
2 He should be able to attend his son's Boy Scout campfire.
3 He should use an electric razor when shaving.
4 He should have two complete sets of oxygen delivery devices.
5 The oxygenation delivery systems can be placed behind the bedroom curtains so the room looks neat and uncluttered.
6 When filling an ambulatory liquid tank from the stationary reservoir, the first thing to do is to wipe the connectors of both tanks with a lint-free cloth.

3   A client's family is being taught how to suction the client's tracheostomy in preparation for her discharge home. What information should be included in the teaching session?
1   Instill normal saline to help prevent hypoxia during suctioning.
2   Set the suction pressure on the suction machine between 160 and 180 mm Hg.
3   Teach how to perform oral suction after tracheostomy suction.
4   Place client in a supine position.
5   Grasp the suction catheter with the nondominant hand.

4   An 83-year-old client cares for himself at home. Which nursing intervention will enhance adherence to his medication regimen?
1   Teach him everything he needs to know in 1 day and return in 2 weeks.
2   Include him in deciding the system used to help him remember to take his medications.
3   Provide large-print instructions that are written in dark blue ink.
4   Provide medication information when his daughter and infant grandchild are visiting him.

5   An older adult had a recent stroke and is receiving home enteral nutrition. Which action(s) should the nurse have instructed the family caregiver to take if the client begins to have difficulty breathing and coughing? (Select all that apply.)
1   Call the health care provider.
2   Raise the head of the bed.
3   Verify tube placement.
4   Stop the feeding.

6   The home care nurse receives a call from the wife of an elderly couple, who says that her frail husband doesn't feel well at all and his temperature is 99.2° F (37.3° C) orally. Which response by the nurse would be most appropriate?
1   "How much liquid has he had to drink since yesterday?"
2   "Take him to the emergency department because he needs care."
3   "Which specific symptoms is your husband experiencing?"
4   "When did he beginning noticing a change in his health?"

7   A client who is monitoring his blood pressure at home is consistently getting much higher readings than the readings taken when he visits his health care provider's office. Which question is most important for the home health nurse to ask?
1   "What time of day are you checking your blood pressure?"
2   "How tight is the blood pressure cuff before you inflate it?"
3   "Are you concerned about the difference in the readings?"
4   "How long ago did the difference in the readings begin?"

8   The nurse is teaching a client how to perform clean, intermittent catheterization. Which statement by the client reflects accurate teaching by the nurse?
1   "I need to clean the urethral opening with three betadine wipes."
2   "I should use a sterile catheter each time I catheterize myself."
3   "I should have an extra catheter washed and ready to use."
4   "I should use sterile gloves to prevent contamination of the urine."

9   The daughter of an older client asks why her mother periodically becomes more confused when she is trying to cough up thick mucus than she did several years ago. Which response by the nurse is most accurate?
1   "Your mother is becoming weaker, which is causing the problem."
2   "As your mother ages, she is losing some of the elastic recoil."
3   "Oxygen levels decrease with forceful coughing more as aging occurs."
4   "Her anxiety is causing her to not to cough as effectively as before."

10   A mother of a school-age child with a newly diagnosed chronic illness is receiving education about the new medication regimen from the nurse. Which statement by the mother requires that the nurse provide additional information?
1   "I'm not sure why my child needs all these medications."
2   "Medications need to be stored in a locked area so my 3-year-old can't get them."
3   "I need to make a chart outlining when to give the medications."
4   "I need to call the pharmacy when I notice that only a few doses of medication are left."

REFERENCES

American Academy of Pediatricians (AAP): *How to take a child's temperature*, 2012, available at http://www.healthychildren.org/English/health-issues/conditions/fever/pages/How-to-Take-a-Childs-Temperature.aspx?nfstatus=401&nftoken=00000000-0000-0000-0000-000000000000&nfstatusdescription=ERROR%3a+No+local+token, accessed April 5, 2012.

American Thoracic Society: *Oxygen sources and delivery devices*, 2011, available at http://www.thoracic.org/clinical/copd-guidelines/for-health-professionals/management-of-stable-copd/long-term-oxygen-therapy/oxygen-sources-and-delivery-devices.php, accessed April 5, 2012.

Ballangrud R, et al: Clients' experience of living at home with a mechanical ventilator, *J Adv Nurs* 65(2):425, 2009.

Bankhead R, et al: Enteral nutrition practice recommendations, *JPEN J Parenter Enteral Nutr* 33:122, 2009.

Best C, Hitchings H: Enteral tube feeding-from hospital to home, *Br J Nurs* 19(3):174, 2010.

Boughton M, Halliday L: Home alone: client and career uncertainty surrounding discharge with continuing clinical care needs, *Contemp Nurse* 33(1):33, 2009.

Brinkerhoff S: Oxygen therapy in the home: safety precautions and implications for home healthcare clinicians, *Home Healthcare Nurse* 27(7):417, 2009.

Brown T: Literacy and healthcare: the challenge of communication in home healthcare and hospice, *Home Healthc Nurse* 27(1):63, 2009.

Centers for Medicare and Medicaid Services (CMS): *Medicare coverage of durable medical equipment and other devices*, 2008, available at http://www.medicare.gov/Publications/Pubs/pdf/11045.pdf, accessed April 5, 2012.

Cleveland Clinic: *Tracheal suction guidelines*, 2009, available at http://my.clevelandclinic.org/services/tracheostomy/hic_tracheal_suction_guidelines.aspx, accessed April 5, 2012.

Ebersole P, et al: *Toward healthy aging: human needs and nursing response*, ed 7, St Louis, 2008, Mosby.

Environmental Protection Agency (EPA): *Thermometers*, 2011, available at http://www.epa.gov/mercury/thermometer-main.html, accessed April 5, 2012.

Frese E, et al: Blood pressure measurement guidelines for physical therapists, *Cardiopulm Phys Ther J* 22(2):5, 2011.

Halm MA, Krisko-Hagel K: Instilling normal saline with suctioning: beneficial technique or potentially harmful sacred cow? *Am J Crit Care* 17(5):469, 2008.

Harvard Health Publications: The hidden burden of high blood pressure, *Harv Health Lett* 21(11):3, 2011.

Hitchings H, et al: Home enteral tube feeding in older people: consideration of the issues, *Br J Nurs* 19(18):1150, 2010.

Hockenberry MJ, Wilson D: *Wong's nursing care of infants and children*, ed 9, St Louis, 2011, Mosby.

Holmes S: Importance of nutrition in palliative care of clients with chronic disease, *Primary Health Care* 21(6):31, 2011.

Jett KF: Culture and aging. In Touhy TT, Jett KF, editors: *Ebersole and Hess' gerontological nursing and healthy aging*, ed 3, St Louis, 2010, Mosby.

Kaufman G, Birks Y: Strategies to improve clients' adherence to medication, *Nurs Stand* 23(49):51, 2009.

Kenny DJ, Goodman P: Care of the patient with enteral tube feeding: an evidence-based practice protocol, *Nurs Res* 59(15):522, 2010.

Lau DT, et al: Exploring factors that influence informal caregiving in medication management for home hospice clients, *J Palliat Med* 13(9):1085, 2010.

Lewis SL, et al: *Medical-surgical nursing: assessment and management of clinical problems*, ed 8, St Louis, 2011, Mosby.

McCoy R: What's new with home oxygen therapy? *J Respir Care Practitioners* 23(1):14, 2010.

McKinney M: Coaching with care: client advocates help guide post-hospital care in an effort to improve outcomes, reduce readmissions, *Mod Healthc* 40(33):30, 2010.

McLafferty E, et al: Prevention of hypothermia, *Nurs Older People* 21(4):34, 2009.

Meade CD: Community health education. In Nies MA, McEwen M, editors: *Community/public health nursing: promoting the health of populations*, ed 5, St Louis, 2011, Mosby.

National Fire Protection Association: *Fires and burns involving home medical oxygen*, 2008, available at http://www.nfpa.org/assets/files//pdf/os.oxygen.pdf, accessed April 5, 2012.

National Institute for Health and Clinical Excellence (NICE): *NICE supports clients to get more involved in the decision-making process regarding their prescribed medicines,* 2009, The Institute.

National Institutes of Health (NIH): *Clean intermittent self-catheterization,* 2010, available at http://www.nlm.nih.gov/medlineplus/ency/patientinstructions/000144.htm, accessed April 5, 2012.

Newman DK, Willson MM: Review of intermittent catheterization and current best practices, *Urologic Nurs* 31(1):12, 2011.

Pittman TJ: Teaching tools. In Lowenstein AJ, et al, editors: *Teaching strategies for health education and health promotion: working with clients, families, and communities,* Sudbury, Mass, 2009, Jones and Bartlett.

Powers BJ, et al: Measuring blood pressure for decision making and quality reporting: where and how many measures? *Ann Intern Med* 154(12):781, 2011.

Redman BK: When is client education unethical? *Nurs Ethics* 15(6):813, 2008.

Romano JC: Teaching on the fly. In Lowenstein AJ, et al, editors: *Teaching strategies for health education and health promotion: working with clients, families, and communities,* Sudbury, Mass, 2009a, Jones and Bartlett.

Romano JC: Getting started. In Lowenstein AJ, et al, editors: *Teaching strategies for health education and health promotion: working with clients, families, and communities,* Sudbury, Mass, 2009b, Jones and Bartlett.

Santhosh YL, Naveen MR: Medication adherence behavior in chronic diseases like asthma and diabetes mellitus, *Int J Pharm Pharm Sci* 3(3):238, 2011.

Scrimshaw SC: Methods for working with cultural diversity. In Lowenstein AJ, et al, editors: *Teaching strategies for health education and health promotion: working with clients, families, and communities,* Sudbury, Mass, 2009, Jones and Bartlett.

Smith CE, Ross VM: Complex home care. Part III. Economic impact on family caregiver quality of life and clients' clinical outcomes, *Nurs Econ* 28(6):393, 2010.

Society of Urologic Nurses and Associates (SUNA): *Adult intermittent self-catheterization: client fact sheet,* 2010, available at http://www.suna.org/members/selfCatheterization.pdf, accessed April 5, 2012.

The Joint Commission (TJC): *Speak up: know your rights,* 2011, available at http://www.jointcommission.org/assets/1/18/Speakup_Rights.pdf, 2011, accessed April 5, 2012.

Tomlinson BU: Accurately measuring blood pressure: factors that contribute to false measurements, *MEDSURG Nurs* 19(2):90, 2010.

US Department of Health and Human Services (USDHHS): *Healthy people 2020,* 2012, available at http://healthypeople.gov/2020/topicsobjectives2020/objectiveslist.aspx?topicId=18, accessed April 5, 2012.

Upadhyaya RC: Musculoskeletal function. In Meiner SE, editor: *Gerontologic nursing,* ed 4, St Louis, 2011, Mosby.

Vidt DG, et al: Taking blood pressure: too important to trust to humans? *Cleveland Clinic J Med* 77(10):683, 2010.

Wolff JL, et al: Optimizing client and family involvement in geriatric home care, *J Healthhc Qual* 31(2):24, 2009.

Zaiken K, Zeind CS: Teaching clients about medications. In Lowenstein AJ, et al, editors: *Teaching strategies for health education and health promotion: working with clients, families, and communities,* Sudbury, Mass, 2009, Jones and Bartlett.

Zia S, et al: Pediatric tracheostomy: complications and role of home care in developing country, *Pediatr Surg Int* 26:269, 2010.

Specimen Collection

MEDIA RESOURCES

- **evolve** *learning system* http://evolve.elsevier.com/Perry/skills
- **NSO** Nursing Skills Online
  - Review Questions
  - ▶ Video Clips
  - Audio Glossary

KEY TERMS

Aspirate	Expectorate	Melena	Sensitivity
Blood culture	Glucose monitoring	Midstream collection	Timed urine collection
Clean-voided specimen	Guaiac test	Occult blood	Urgency
Culture	Hematuria	Point-of-care test	Vacutainer tube
Double-voided specimen	Ketones	Reagent	Void
Dysuria			

OBJECTIVES

Mastery of content in this chapter will enable the nurse to:

- Explain the rationale for the collection of each specimen.
- Identify special conditions necessary for collection of each specimen.
- Explain instructions to encourage patient cooperation for successful collection of each specimen.
- Recognize the impact of patient-centered issues on patient's cooperation with collection of specimens.
- Identify measures to minimize anxiety and promote safety during specimen collection.
- Discuss nursing responsibilities for processing a specimen after collection.

- Chart appropriate information in a patient's electronic health record (EHR) or written record after collection of a specimen.
- Use correct technique for collecting clean-voided, timed, and catheterized urine specimens.
- Use correct technique for collecting specimens and cultures for blood and other body fluids.
- Use correct technique to perform venipuncture.
- Use infection control practices during specimen collection techniques.
- Use correct technique to perform arterial puncture for blood gas measurement.

Laboratory test results aid in the diagnosis of health care problems, provide information about the stage and activity of a disease process, and measure a patient's response to therapy. Proficiency in performing point-of-care (POC) tests, assistance with diagnostic testing, and specimen collection and analysis are nursing responsibilities. Skill and judgment in obtaining specimens affect patient comfort and safety and ensure accuracy and quality of diagnostic procedures. Accountability, attention to monitoring patient outcomes, and current health care economics increase the demand for accurate and timely laboratory tests.

When there are questions about laboratory tests, consult reference books or the agency procedure manual or laboratory. Each agency may establish its own values for each test, which are printed on the agency laboratory slips. It is important that you know the significance of any abnormal finding. Discuss any major deviations immediately with the health care provider.

EVIDENCE-BASED PRACTICE

Evidence-based research specific to nursing practices of specimen collection techniques needs further exploration to provide and ensure safety, quality care, and best practices. Blood cultures are one type of specimen collection obtained by venipuncture to confirm the diagnosis of infection. Blood cultures are usually incubated to examine for bacterial growth, but early test results are available within 48 hours. If results are negative, antibiotics are unnecessary, and the health care provider can seek alternative diagnoses. When results are positive and bacteria grow in the blood culture, the health care provider needs to ensure that the growth was not caused by contamination from the skin but by a true bacterium. During this time unnecessary testing may occur, hospital stays are extended, and unneeded antibiotics may be administered. Studies have indicated that in the adult population blood cultures are contaminated 1% to 6% of the time (Weddle et al., 2010). In the pediatric population these contamination rates can be 9% or higher. There are interventions that can reduce the contamination of blood cultures during venipuncture.

- Use skin preparations such as iodine, chlorhexidine, or alcohol before venipuncture.
- Obtain culture only through percutaneous venipuncture.
- Obtain two different culture specimens at the same time.
- Developing a dedicated phlebotomy team has been shown to reduce contamination rates.

PATIENT-CENTERED CARE

Nurses and other health care providers support patient-centered care by assessing and adapting for patient's psychosocial and physiologic factors before, during, and after specimen collection. During phlebotomy physiologic factors such as discomfort, pain, or dehydration may affect your ability to collect a specimen. Psychosocial factors to consider include age, gender, anxiety, embarrassment, fear, ethnicity, and patients' values and beliefs (Pagana and Pagana, 2011).

Patients often experience embarrassment or discomfort when giving a sample of body excretions or secretions. It is important to handle excretions or secretions discretely and provide a patient with as much privacy as possible. Given clear instructions, patients are able to obtain their own specimens of urine, stool, and sputum without unnecessary exposure. Choose words that are clearly understood; many patients, especially children, do not understand the terms *void*, *urine*, or *stool*.

Cultural considerations are important when collecting specimens and performing diagnostic procedures. Culture and beliefs may affect a patient's response and willingness to participate in specimen collection. Southeast Asians consider blood to be a vital life force that is irreplaceable. They may become anxious about a needle penetrating the skin, allowing blood to seep out. The insertion of a foreign object into the mouth (e.g., swab, tongue blade) to collect specimens may be threatening to Southeast Asians who believe that diseases can be introduced through the mouth and the head is the seat of one's life force (Stuart, Stuart, and Cherry, 2011).

Consider both cultural and language barriers when delegating specimen collection to patients and family members. For example, Muslims and Hindus designate which hand is to be used for clean and dirty tasks. Collecting their own stool and urine specimens may be difficult because only the left hand can be used for "dirty" activities. Language barriers make it difficult to explain the purpose of tests and collection techniques. Be sure to provide repeated return demonstrations to ensure that patient or family member understands how to perform a procedure.

Whenever possible, use gender-congruent caregivers when collecting vaginal, rectal, and urinary specimens from patients whose cultural values demand modesty and distinct separation of gender roles. Provide privacy when giving instructions and during specimen collection.

Safety Guidelines

1. Adapt to a patient's need and ability to safely perform and/or participate in specimen collection procedures.
2. Verify the type of procedure scheduled and the procedure site with the patient.
3. Follow standard precautions (see Chapter 7) when collecting specimens of blood or body fluids.
4. Properly label all specimens with patient's identification, date and time the specimen is obtained, name of the test, and source of the specimen/culture for each container (TJC, 2012).
5. Deliver specimens to the laboratory within the recommended time or ensure that they are stored properly for later transport.
6. Follow procedures for special conditions (e.g., iced specimens, special containers with preservatives) required for transport of specimens. Specific required prerequisite conditions include fasting and nothing by mouth (NPO) and may need to be completed before the collection of a specimen (Pagana and Pagana, 2011).
7. Know agency policy regarding infection control practices for transportation of all specimen containers of body substances.
8. Follow procedures for medications or dietary intake that may result in some deviations from normal values.
9. Follow precautions for collecting specimens from patients who are in protective isolation.

SKILL 43-1 Urine Specimen Collection: Midstream (Clean-Voided) Urine; Sterile Urinary Catheter

NSO *Specimen Collection Module / Lessons 1 and 2*

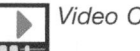 *Video Clip*

A urinalysis provides information about kidney or metabolic function, nutrition, and systemic diseases. Urine collection uses a variety of methods, depending on the purpose of the urinalysis and the presence or absence of a urinary catheter. Guidelines for assessment, planning, and evaluation are similar, regardless of the method of collection. Routine urinalysis includes measurement of nine or more elements, including urine pH, protein and glucose levels, ketones, specific gravity, white blood cell (WBC) count, and presence of bacteria and/or blood (Pagana and Pagana, 2011).

Types of Urine Tests and Specimens

A *random urine specimen for routine urinalysis* is collected using a specimen "hat" (Fig. 43-1), which you place under a toilet seat to collect voided urine. You then place approximately 120 mL of urine in a specimen container, properly labeled, and send to the laboratory.

A *culture and sensitivity (C&S) of urine* is performed to identify if bacteria are present (culture) and determine the most effective antibiotic for treatment (sensitivity). Use sterile technique to ensure that any microorganisms present originate in the urine and not from the patient's skin, the hands, or the environment. You collect specimens for C&S either as a clean-voided midstream specimen or under sterile technique from a urinary catheter. Urine collected by this method may also be analyzed for the same components as a routine urinalysis.

A *timed urine specimen for quantitative analysis* requires urine to be collected over 2 to 72 hours. The 24-hour timed collection (see Procedural Guideline 43-1) is most common and allows for measurement and quantitative analysis of elements such as amino acids, creatinine, hormones, glucose, and adrenocorticosteroid excretion.

Chemical properties of urine are tested by immersing a specially prepared test strip of paper (Chemostrip) into a clean urine specimen. The test detects the presence of glucose, ketones, protein, or blood not normally present in the urine (see Procedural Guideline 43-2). When the screening test for the presence of substances in the urine is positive, additional laboratory tests are used to determine a patient's diagnosis or measure the effectiveness of treatment.

Delegation and Collaboration

The skill of collecting urine specimens can be delegated to nursing assistive personnel (NAP). The nurse informs the NAP about:

- When to obtain the specimens.
- Patient mobility restrictions that will affect collection technique.
- Reporting to the nurse if the urine is not clear (e.g., contains blood, cloudiness, or excess sediment).
- Reporting when a patient is unable to initiate a stream or has pain or burning on urination.

Equipment

❏ Completed identification labels with appropriate patient identifiers
❏ Completed laboratory requisition, including patient identification, date, time, name of test, and source of culture
❏ Small plastic biohazard bag for delivery of specimen to laboratory (or container specified by agency)

Clean-Voided Urine Specimen

❏ Commercial kit for clean-voided urine (Fig. 43-2) containing:
- Sterile cotton balls or antiseptic towelettes
- Antiseptic solution (chlorhexidine or povidone-iodine solution)
- Sterile water or normal saline
- Sterile specimen container
- Urine cup
❏ Clean gloves
❏ Soap, water, washcloth, and towel
❏ Bedpan (for nonambulatory patient), specimen hat (see Fig. 43-1) (for ambulatory patient)

Sterile Urine Specimen from Urinary Catheter

❏ 20-mL Luer-Lok for routine urinalysis or 3-mL safety Luer-Lok syringe for culture
❏ Alcohol, chlorhexidine, or other disinfectant swab
❏ Clamp or rubber band
❏ Specimen container (nonsterile for routine urinalysis; sterile for culture)
❏ Clean gloves

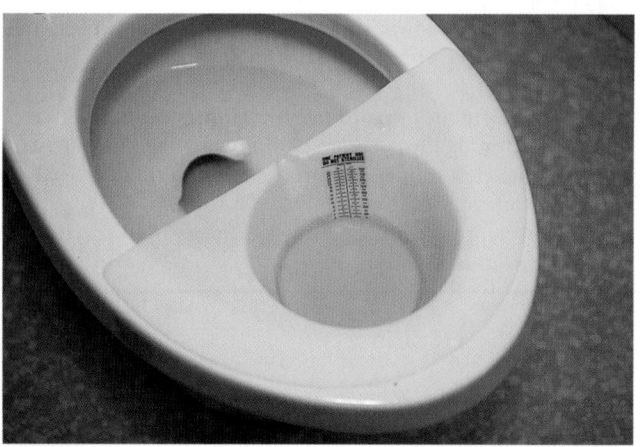

FIG 43-1 Specimen hat.

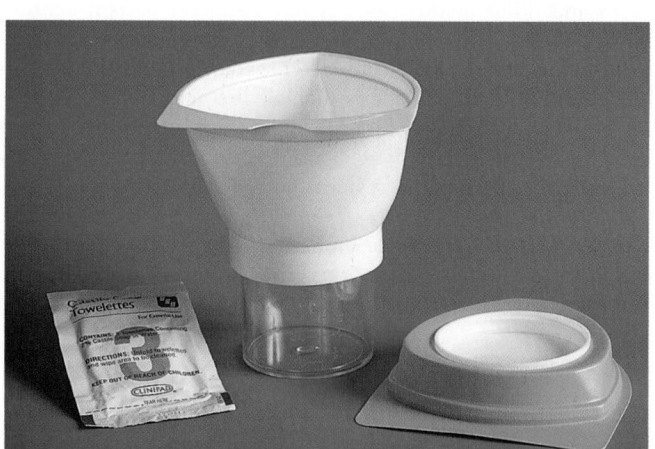

FIG 43-2 Clean-voided specimen collection kit.

STEP	RATIONALE

ASSESSMENT

1 Assess patient's or family members' understanding of purpose of test and method of collection.	Information allows you to clarify misunderstanding; promotes patient cooperation.
2 Assess patient's ability to help with urine specimen collection; able to position self and hold container.	This determines degree of assistance patient requires.
3 Assess for signs and symptoms of urinary tract infection (UTI) (frequency, urgency, dysuria, hematuria, flank pain, fever; cloudy, malodorous urine).	These are indicators of UTI.
4 Refer to agency procedures for specimen collection methods.	Agency policies may vary regarding collection and/or handling of specimens.

NURSING DIAGNOSES

- Acute pain
- Anxiety

- Deficient knowledge regarding specimen collection

- Risk for infection

Related factors are individualized based on patient's condition or needs.

PLANNING

1 Expected outcomes following completion of procedure:	
• Specimen free of contaminants is collected.	Proper collection technique prevents substances from changing normal characteristics of urine.
• Patient discusses procedure for specimen collection.	Procedure is safely performed.
• Patient discusses purpose and benefits of specimen collection.	Evaluates patient's learning.

IMPLEMENTATION

1 Perform hand hygiene, check labels, and complete laboratory requisition for specimen container.	Reduces transfer of microorganisms. Organizes procedure.
2 Identify patient using two identifiers (i.e., name and birthday or name and account number) according to agency policy. Compare identifiers in MAR/medical record with information on patient's identification bracelet and/or ask patient to state name.	Ensures correct patient. Complies with The Joint Commission standards and improves patient safety (TJC, 2012).
3 Provide privacy for patient; close curtains around bed or close room door. Allow mobile patients to collect specimen in bathroom.	Privacy allows patient to relax and produce specimen more easily.
4 Collect clean-voided urine specimen.	
a Apply clean gloves. Give patient cleaning towelette or towel, washcloth, and soap to clean perineum or help with cleaning perineum. Help bedridden patient onto bedpan to facilitate access to perineum. Remove and dispose of gloves.	Patients prefer to wash their own perineal areas when possible. Cleaning prevents contamination of specimen after urine passes from urethra.
b Using surgical asepsis, open outer package of commercial specimen kit.	Maintains sterility of equipment.
c Apply clean gloves.	Prevents contact of microorganisms on your hands.
d Pour antiseptic solution over cotton balls (unless kit contains prepared antiseptic towelettes).	Cotton ball or towelette is used to clean perineum.
e Open specimen container, maintaining sterility of inside specimen container, and place cap with sterile inside up. Do not touch inside of cap or container.	Contaminated specimen is most frequent reason for inaccurate reporting of urine C&S.
f Use aseptic technique to help patient or allow patient to independently clean perineum and collect specimen. Amount of assistance needed varies with each patient. Inform patient that antiseptic solution will feel cold.	Maintains patient's dignity and comfort.

STEP	RATIONALE
(1) *Male:*	
(a) Hold penis with one hand; using circular motion and antiseptic towelette, clean meatus, moving from center to outside 3 times with different towelettes (see illustration). Have uncircumcised male patient retract foreskin for effective cleaning of urinary meatus and keep retracted during voiding. Return foreskin when done.	Reduces number of microorganisms at urethral meatus and moves from areas of least to most contamination. Return of foreskin prevents stricture of penis.
(b) If agency procedure indicates, rinse area with sterile water and dry with cotton balls or gauze pad.	Prevents contamination of specimen with antiseptic solution.
(c) After patient initiates urine stream into toilet or bedpan, have him pass urine specimen container into stream and collect 90 to 120 mL of urine (Pagana and Pagana, 2011) (see illustration).	Initial urine flushes out microorganisms that normally accumulate at urinary meatus and prevents transfer into specimen.
(2) *Female:*	
(a) Either nurse or patient spreads labia minora with fingers of nondominant hand.	Provides access to urethral meatus.
(b) With dominant hand clean urethral area with antiseptic swab (cotton ball or gauze). Move from front (above urethral orifice) to back (toward anus). Use fresh swab each time; clean 3 *times;* begin with labial fold farthest from you, then labial fold closest, and then down center (see illustration).	Prevents contamination of urinary meatus with fecal material. Cleaning down center last decreases contamination from labia.
(c) If agency procedure indicates, rinse area with sterile water and dry with cotton ball.	Prevents contamination of specimen with antiseptic solution.
(d) While continuing to hold labia apart, patient initiates urine stream into toilet or bedpan; after stream is achieved, pass specimen container into stream and collect 90 to 120 mL of urine (Pagana and Pagana, 2011) (see illustration).	Initial stream flushes out resident microorganisms that accumulate at urethral meatus and prevents transfer into specimen.

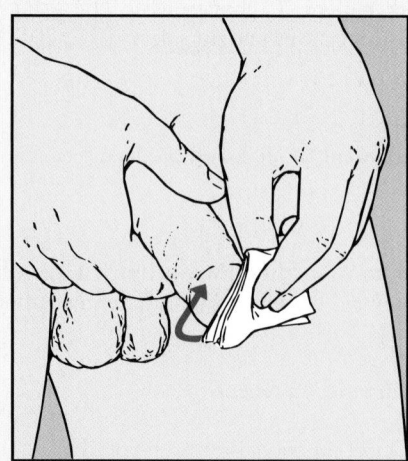

STEP 4f(1)(a)   Cleaning technique (male).

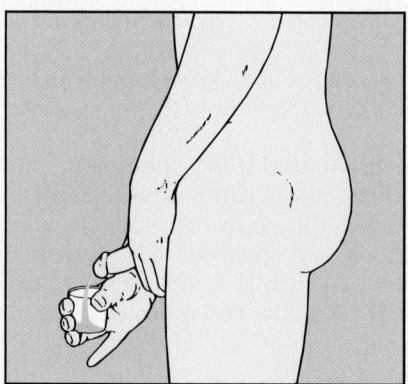

STEP 4f(1)(c)   Collecting midstream urine specimen (male).

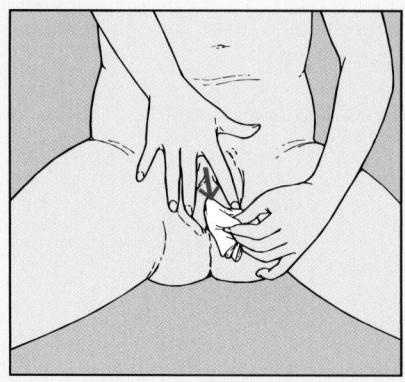

STEP 4f(2)(b)   Clean from front to back, holding labia apart.

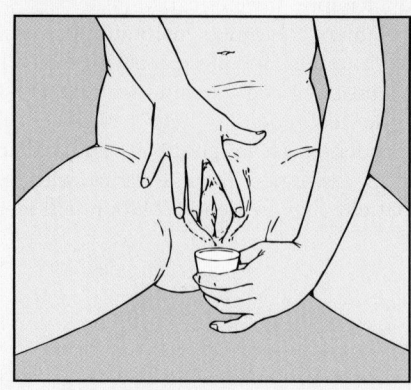

STEP 4f(2)(d)   Collection of midstream urine specimen (female).

STEP	RATIONALE
g Remove specimen container before flow of urine stops and before releasing labia or penis. Patient finishes voiding into bedpan or toilet. Offer to help with personal hygiene as appropriate.	Prevents contamination of specimen with skin flora. Prevents sediment from bladder getting into specimen.
h Replace cap securely on specimen container, touching only outside.	Retains sterility of inside of container and prevents spillage of urine.
i Clean urine from exterior surface of container.	Prevents transfer of microorganisms to others.
5 Collect urine from indwelling urinary catheter.	
a Explain that you will use syringe without need to remove urine through catheter port and that patient will not experience any discomfort.	Minimizes anxiety when you manipulate catheter and aspirate urine with syringe from catheter port.
b Explain that you will need to clamp catheter for 10 to 15 minutes before obtaining urine specimen and that urine cannot be obtained from drainage bag.	Allows urine to accumulate in catheter. Urine in drainage bag is not considered sterile.
c Apply clean gloves. Clamp drainage tubing with clamp or rubber band for as long as 15 minutes below site chosen for withdrawal (see illustration).	Permits collection of fresh sterile urine in catheter tubing rather than draining into bag.
d After 15 minutes position patient so catheter sampling port is easily accessible. Location of port is where catheter attaches to drainage bag tube (see illustration). Clean port for 15 seconds with disinfectant swab and allow to dry.	Prevents entry of microorganisms into catheter.
e Attach needleless Luer-Lok syringe to built-in catheter sampling port (see illustration). Some needleless ports use blunt plastic valve or slip-tip syringe inserted into port diaphragm.	Guideline recommends use of Luer-Lok needleless system. Needleless system prevents injury by needlestick.

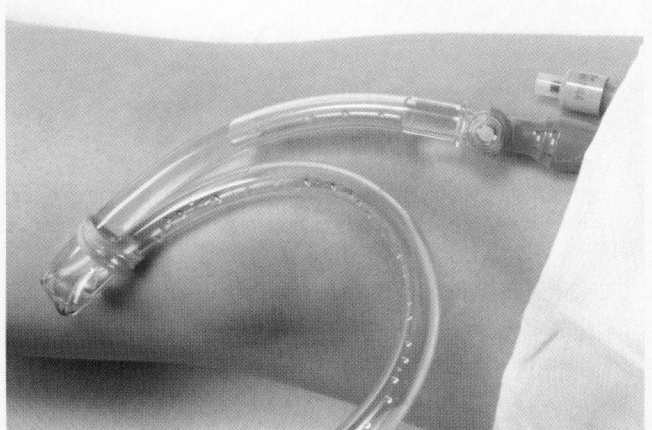

STEP 5c   Rubber band used to clamp catheter drainage tube.

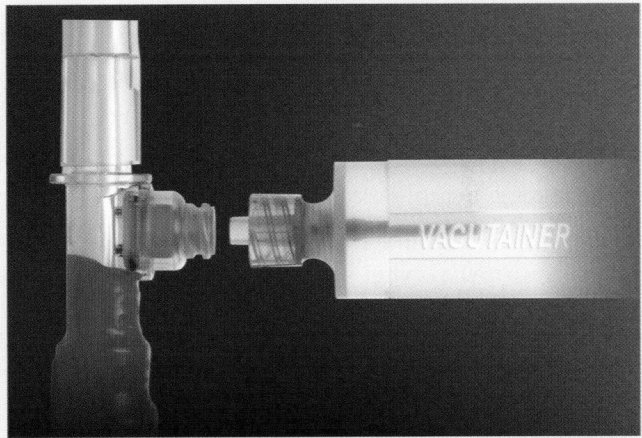

STEP 5d   Port with syringe attached.

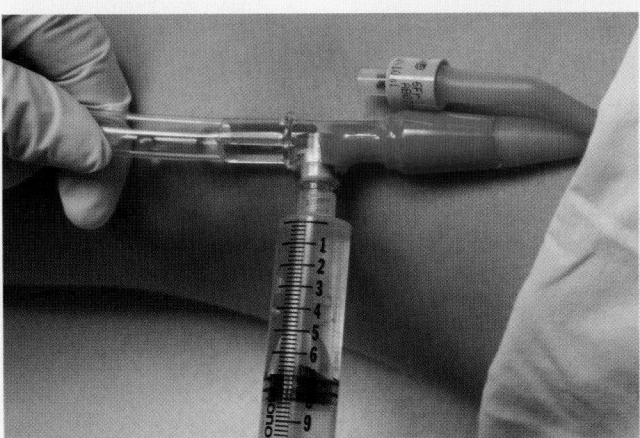

STEP 5e   Access urinary catheter port with Luer-Lok syringe or syringe with blunt plastic valve.

STEP	RATIONALE
f Withdraw 3 mL for culture or 20 mL for routine urinalysis.	Allows collection of urine without contamination. Proper volume is needed to perform test.
g Transfer urine from syringe into clean urine container for routine urinalysis or into sterile urine container for culture.	Prevents contamination of urine during transfer procedure.
h Place lid tightly on container.	Prevents contamination of specimen by air and loss by spillage.
i Unclamp catheter and allow urine to flow into drainage bag. Ensure that urine flows freely.	Allows urine to drain by gravity and prevents stasis of urine in bladder.
6 Securely attach label to container (not lid). In patient's presence, confirm label identifiers (two identifiers, specimen source, and collection date and time). If patient is female, indicate if she is menstruating.	Ensures that specimen is identified correctly for proper diagnosis (TJC, 2012).
7 Dispose of soiled supplies. Remove and dispose of gloves and perform hand hygiene.	Prevents transmission of microorganisms.
8 Send specimen and completed requisition to laboratory within 20 minutes. Refrigerate specimen if delay cannot be avoided.	Delay of analysis may significantly alter test results (Pagana and Pagana, 2011).

EVALUATION

1 Inspect clean-voided specimen for contamination with toilet paper or stool.	Contaminants prevent specimen from being used.
2 Evaluate patient's urine C&S report for bacterial growth.	Routine cultures identify organism(s), and sensitivity study identifies antimicrobial medications that may be effective against pathogen.
3 Observe urinary drainage system in catheterized patient to ensure that it is intact and patent.	System must remain closed to remain sterile.
4 Ask patient to describe midstream urine collection procedure.	Validates patient's understanding.

Unexpected Outcomes

1 Urine specimen is contaminated with stool or toilet paper.

2 Patient is unable to void, or urine does not collect in drainage tube.

3 Urine culture reveals bacterial growth (determined by colony count of more than 10,000 organisms per milliliter).

4 Lumen leading to balloon that holds catheter in bladder is punctured.

Related Interventions

- Repeat patient instruction and specimen collection. If unable to obtain specimen through clean voiding, patient may need catheterization (see Skill 33-1).
- Offer fluids if permitted to enhance urine production.
- Report findings to health care provider.
- Administer medications as ordered.
- Monitor patient for fever and dysuria.
- Notify health care provider.
- Prepare for removal and insertion of new catheter.
- Collect specimen.

Recording and Reporting

- Record collection of specimen in nurses' notes and electronic health record (EHR) or per agency policy; note method used to obtain specimen, date and time collected, type of test ordered, appearance, odor and color of urine, and disposition to laboratory.
- Report any abnormal findings to health care provider.

Special Considerations
Teaching

- Discuss signs and symptoms of UTI with patient and family member.
- Explain significance of cleaning genital area before collecting specimen.

Pediatric

- Use a sterile plastic urine-collecting bag (Fig. 43-3) that adheres to the perineum of an infant or a non–toilet-trained child (Hockenberry and Wilson, 2011).

Gerontologic

- Older adults may need assistance in positioning to obtain specimen.

Home Care

- Specimens for culture should not be collected at home because time delay before laboratory culture could greatly enhance bacterial growth. If patient collects the urine specimen, he or she should keep it on ice until it reaches the laboratory for testing.

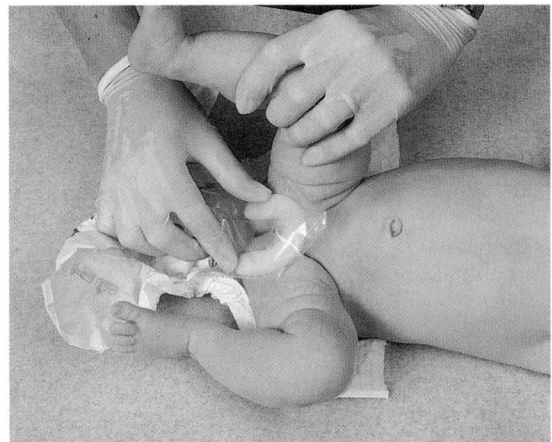

FIG 43-3 Application of urine collection bag. (*From Warekois RS, Robinson R:* Phlebotomy worktext and procedures manual, *ed 3, St Louis, 2012, Mosby.*)

PROCEDURAL GUIDELINE 43-1 Collecting a Timed Urine Specimen

Some tests of renal function and urine composition require urine to be collected over 2 to 72 hours. The 24-hour timed collection is used most often and measures elements such as amino acids, creatinine, hormones, glucose, and adrenocorticosteroids, the levels of which fluctuate throughout the day. A timed urine collection provides a means to measure the concentration or dilution of urine.

Timed urine collections begin after a patient urinates. Discard the first specimen and then collect every successive specimen until the time period has ended. Transfer each specimen immediately to a large collection bottle with or without preservative, kept in the patient's bathroom. Any missed specimens make test results inaccurate. The patient should always provide the last specimen as close as possible to the end of the collection period. The specimen may be placed on ice to prevent deterioration.

Delegation and Collaboration

The skill of collecting a timed urine specimen can be delegated to nursing assistive personnel (NAP). The nurse informs the NAP about:

- When timed collection begins, proper method to store the collected urine, where to place signs that a timed urine collection is in progress, and saving all urine.
- Reporting when blood, mucus, or foul odors are present in the urine specimen or if there is a break in the collection procedure.

Equipment

- ❑ Large collection bottle with cap that usually contains a chemical preservative
- ❑ Bedpan, urinal, specimen hat, bedside commode, or pediatric potty-chair
- ❑ Graduated measuring container for intake and output (I&O) measurement
- ❑ Large basin to hold collection bottle surrounded by ice if immediate refrigeration is required
- ❑ Specimen identification label and completed laboratory requisition (with appropriate patient identifiers and specimen information)
- ❑ Instructional signs that remind patient and staff of timed urine collection

- ❑ Clean gloves
- ❑ Plastic biohazard plastic bag or container (see agency policy)

Procedural Steps

1 Identify patient using two identifiers (i.e., name and birthday or name and account number) according to agency policy. Compare identifiers on MAR/medical record with information on patient's identification bracelet and/or ask patient to state name.

2 Explain the reason for specimen collection, how patient can help, and that urine must be free of feces and toilet tissue.

3 Place specimen collection container in the bathroom and, if indicated, in a pan of ice. Post signs to remind staff, family and visitors, and patient of timed urine collection on patient's door and toileting area. If patient leaves unit, be sure that personnel in receiving area collect and save all urine.

4 If possible, have patient drink two to four glasses of water about 30 minutes before times of collection to facilitate ability to void at the appropriate time for test to begin.

5 Perform hand hygiene and apply clean gloves. Discard the first voided specimen as the test begins. Indicate time test began on laboratory requisition. For accurate results the patient must begin the test with an empty bladder. Begin collecting all urine for designated time.

6 Measure volume of each voiding if I&O are to be recorded. Place all voided urine in labeled specimen bottle with appropriate additives.

7 Unless instructed otherwise, keep specimen bottle in specimen refrigerator or container of ice in bathroom to prevent decomposition of urine.

8 Encourage patient to drink two glasses of water 1 hour before timed urine collection ends. Encourage patient to empty bladder during last 15 minutes of urine collection period.

9 Perform hand hygiene and apply clean gloves. Collect final specimen at end of collection period. Label specimen (two identifiers, specimen source, collection date and time, number of bottle) in patient's presence, attach appropriate requisition, and send to laboratory. Remove gloves and perform hand hygiene.

10 Remove signs. Tell patient that specimen collection period is completed.

PROCEDURAL GUIDELINE 43-2 Urine Screening for Glucose, Ketones, Protein, Blood, and pH

Video Clip

Tests for chemical properties of urine are part of the routine urinalysis completed in the laboratory or as a point-of-care test performed at the bedside or in the home. The use of a Multistix reagent test strip may simultaneously assess for up to nine chemical properties, specific gravity, pH, protein, glucose, ketones, blood bilirubin, urobilinogen, leukocytes, and nitrates. The test is easy to perform and causes no pain. This type of screening is used when more detailed laboratory testing is not available (e.g., health care provider's office, clinic, or long-term care setting). The use of urine testing for managing blood glucose is no longer recommended. Capillary blood monitoring is an accurate assessment of serum glucose levels (Pagana and Pagana, 2011).

Delegation and Collaboration

The skill of urine screening for chemical properties can be delegated to nursing assistive personnel (NAP). The nurse informs the NAP to:

- Obtain the specimen correctly (e.g., before meals, following a "double-voided" specimen).
- Report the results of the test or any odor, blood, or mucus in the urine specimen.

Equipment

- ❏ Bedpan, urinal, specimen hat, bedside commode, or pediatric potty-chair
- ❏ Container for urine from catheter
- ❏ Watch with second hand or digital counter
- ❏ Reagent test strip (check expiration date on container)
- ❏ Test strip color chart
- ❏ Paper towel
- ❏ Clean gloves
- ❏ Small biohazard plastic bag for delivery of specimen to laboratory (or container specified by agency)

Procedural Steps

1. Identify patient using two identifiers (i.e., name and birthday or name and account number) according to agency policy. Compare identifiers on MAR/medical record with information on patient's identification bracelet and/or ask patient to state name.
2. Determine if double-voided specimen is needed for glucose testing. If required, ask patient to void, discard, and then drink a glass of water.
3. Perform hand hygiene and apply clean gloves. Ask patient to collect a fresh, random urine specimen. If patient is catheterized, remove a 5-mL specimen from the catheter port (see Skill 43-1).

4. Immerse end of reagent strip into urine container. Remove the strip immediately and tap it gently against the side of the container to remove excess urine.
5. Hold strip in horizontal position to prevent mixing of chemical reagents (see illustration).

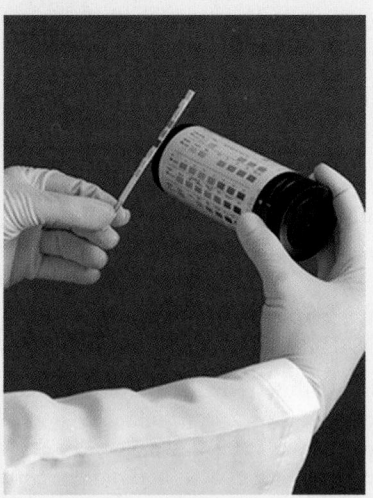

STEP 5 Testing urine using reagent strip.

6. Precisely time the number of seconds specified on container and compare color of strip with color chart on container (Table 43-1).
7. When appropriate, discuss test results with patient. Discard urine. Remove and discard gloves; perform hand hygiene.
8. Record results immediately on appropriate testing flow sheet. Report reading to health care provider.

TABLE 43-1	Color Chart for Reagent Strip	
Test	**When to Read**	**Range of Results**
pH	Anytime	4.6-8.0
Protein	Anytime	None or up to 8 mg/100 mL
Glucose	10 seconds (qualitative)	(−) to +4
	30 seconds (quantitative)	(−) to +4 (270)
Ketones	15 seconds	(−) to +3 (large)
Blood	25 seconds	(−) to +3 (large)

SKILL 43-2 Measuring Occult Blood in Stool

NSO Specimen Collection Module / Lesson 4

 Video Clip

Hemoccult testing is useful for screening for the presence of occult (invisible) blood in the stool for conditions such as colon cancer, bleeding gastrointestinal (GI) ulcers, and localized gastric or intestinal irritation. Use caution; a false-positive result may occur if a patient has ingested red meat within 3 days of testing or is taking certain medications (e.g., iron). A false-negative may result if that patient is taking vitamin C (Pagana and Pagana, 2011). The test measures microscopic amounts of blood in the stool. Normally a person loses small amounts of blood daily in the feces as a result of minor abrasions of the nasopharyngeal or oral mucosa. If greater than 50 mL of blood enters the feces from the upper GI tract, the blood causes melena (darkening of feces). When blood is present, further testing is indicated to determine the source of the bleeding.

Patients are often instructed on how to collect stool specimens for the test in the home. Only a small amount of stool is needed to perform the test successfully. The most common guaiac tests are the Hemoccult slides and the Hematest tablets. A new deoxyribonucleic acid (DNA) stool sample test promises to be twice as sensitive as the current guaiac testing for precancerous benign and malignant tumors. The DNA stool sample test identifies nonbleeding polyps with abnormal DNA (Pagana and Pagana, 2011).

Delegation and Collaboration
The skill of testing stool for occult blood can be delegated to nursing assistive personnel (NAP). The nurse informs the NAP to:
- Report immediately if blood is detected and not to discard stool from a positive test so the nurse may repeat the testing.

Equipment
- Soap, water, washcloth, and towel
- Paper towel
- Clean gloves
- Wooden applicators

Hemoccult Test
- Cardboard Hemoccult slide (Fig. 43-4)
- Hemoccult developing solution

Hematest
- Hematest tablets (must be protected from moisture, heat, and light)
- Guaiac paper
- Clean container of tap water

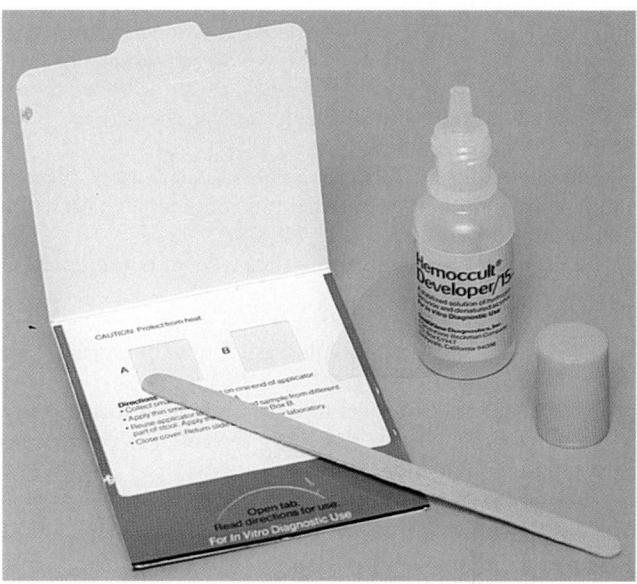

FIG 43-4 Hemoccult testing kit for measuring occult blood.

STEP	RATIONALE

ASSESSMENT

1 Assess patient's or family member's understanding of need for stool test.	Provides information on which to base necessary health teaching.
2 Assess patient's ability to cooperate with procedure and collect specimen.	To avoid embarrassment, patients often prefer to collect own stool specimen. Some patients require assistance.
3 Assess patient's medical history for GI disorders (e.g., history of bleeding, colitis, or hemorrhoids).	You can institute routine screening. Hemorrhoids can cause bleeding that may be misinterpreted as upper GI bleeding.
4 Review patient's medications for drugs that contribute to GI bleeding.	Anticoagulants increase risk for bleeding in GI tract, even from minor trauma to mucosa. Long-term use of steroids, nonsteroidal antiinflammatory drugs (NSAIDs), and acetylsalicylic acid (aspirin) can irritate mucosa and result in bleeding (Pagana and Pagana, 2011).
5 Refer to health care provider's orders for medication or dietary modifications or restrictions before test.	Specimens will be positive if contaminated by menstrual blood, hemorrhoid blood, or povidone-iodine. Diets rich in meats, green leafy vegetables, poultry, and fish may produce false-positive results.

NURSING DIAGNOSES

- Anxiety
- Bowel incontinence
- Constipation
- Deficient knowledge regarding collection and testing of stool specimen
- Diarrhea

Related factors are individualized based on patient's condition or needs.

STEP	RATIONALE

PLANNING

1 Expected outcomes following completion of procedure:

• Test for occult blood is negative.

Patient has only small amount of blood in feces because of normal nasopharyngeal and oral mucosa abrasions.

• Patient discusses purpose and benefits of testing stool for blood.

Validates learning.

2 Explain procedure to patient and/or family member. Discuss reason for specimen collection and how patient can help. Explain that feces must be free of urine and toilet tissue.

Patient who understands procedure is more likely to cooperate and may be able to obtain specimen independently. Also prevents accidental disposal of specimen.

3 Arrange for any needed dietary or medication restrictions.

Ensures accuracy of test results.

IMPLEMENTATION

1 Perform hand hygiene

Reduces transmission of microorganisms.

2 Identify patient using two identifiers (i.e., name and birthday or name and account number) according to agency policy. Compare identifiers on MAR/medical record with information on patient's identification bracelet and/or ask patient to state name.

Ensures correct patient. Complies with The Joint Commission standards and improves patient safety (TJC, 2012).

3 Apply clean gloves. Obtain uncontaminated stool specimen and place in clean, dry container not contaminated with urine, water, or toilet tissue.

Prevents transmission of microorganisms. Allows for accurate testing when specimen is not contaminated with other products.

4 Use tip of wooden applicator to obtain small portion of feces.

Small specimen is sufficient for measuring blood content.

5 Measure for occult blood.

  a Perform Hemoccult slide test:

    (1) Open flap of Hemoccult slide. Apply thin smear of stool on paper in first box.

Guaiac paper inside box is sensitive to fecal blood content.

    (2) Obtain second fecal specimen from different portion of stool and apply thinly to second box of slide (see illustration).

Occult blood from upper GI tract is not always equally dispersed throughout stool. Findings of occult blood are more conclusive for GI bleeding when entire specimen is found to contain blood.

    (3) Close slide cover and turn slide over to reverse side. Open cardboard flap and apply 2 drops of Hemoccult developing solution on each box of guaiac paper (see illustration).

Developing solution penetrates underlying fecal specimen. Change in color of guaiac paper indicates blood.

    (4) Read results of test after 30 to 60 seconds. Note color changes.

Ensures correct results. Bluish discoloration indicates occult blood (guaiac positive). No change in color of guaiac paper indicates negative results.

    (5) Dispose of test slide in proper receptacle.

Reduces transfer of microorganisms.

  b Perform test using Hematest tablets:

Tablet contains solid form of developing solution.

    (1) Place stool on guaiac paper. Then place Hematest tablet on top of stool specimen. Apply 2 to 3 drops of tap water to tablet, allowing water to flow onto guaiac paper.

Tap water dissolves Hematest tablet and thus dispenses developing solution over specimen and guaiac paper.

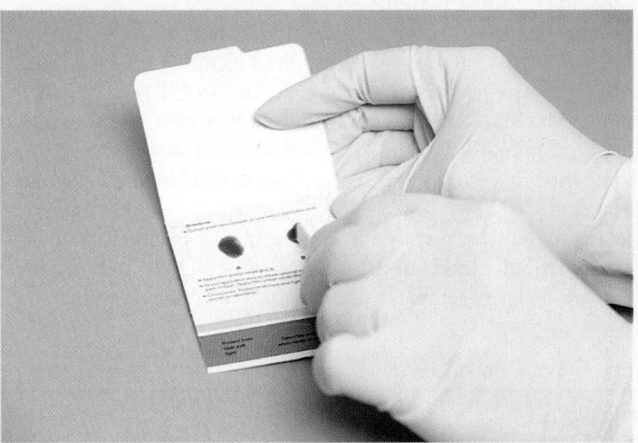

STEP 5a(2)   Application of stool specimen to both spots on Hemoccult slide.

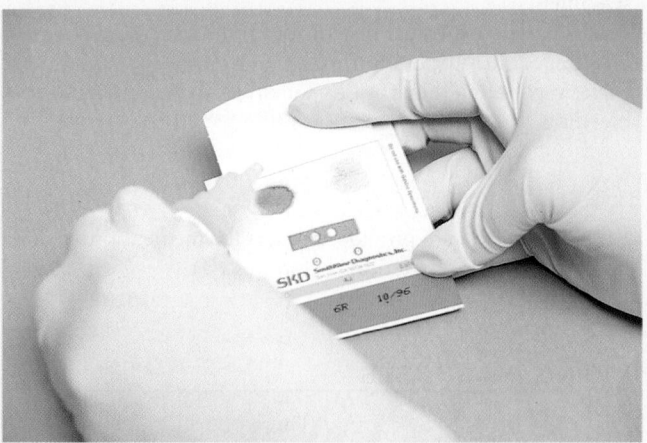

STEP 5a(3)   Application of developing solution.

STEP	RATIONALE
(2) Observe color of guaiac paper within 2 minutes.	Bluish discoloration is guaiac positive. Do not read color after 2 minutes. False findings may occur.
(3) Dispose of tablet and paper in proper receptacle.	Reduces transfer of microorganisms.
6 Wrap wooden applicator in paper towel, grasp in nondominant hand, remove gloves over wrapped applicator. Discard in proper receptacle. Perform hand hygiene.	Reduces transfer of microorganisms.

EVALUATION

1 Ask patient to explain collection procedure.	Documents level of learning.
2 Note color changes in guaiac paper.	Reveals blood in feces.

> **Clinical Decision Point** *Single positive test result does not confirm bleeding or indicate colorectal cancer. To confirm positive results, test must be repeated while patient is on meat-free, high-residue diet with more in-depth diagnosis (Van Leeuwen et al., 2011).*

3 Note character of stool specimen.	Certain abnormal constituents of stool may be visible.

Unexpected Outcomes
1 Test for occult blood is positive.

Related Interventions
• Continue to monitor patient.
• Notify health care provider.

Recording and Reporting
• Record results of test and include stool characteristics in nurses' notes.
• Report positive test results to health care provider.

Special Considerations
Teaching
• Explain rationale regarding why patient needs to obtain specimens from two different areas of stool specimen.
• If patient has been on long-term steroid or anticoagulant drug therapy, explain how these drugs may result in occult blood in stools.
• If health care provider orders meat-free diet before test, explain its significance to test results (red meats can cause false-positive results).
• Discuss reason for multiple testing of stool for occult blood. Patients are usually requested to obtain specimen every day for 3 days.

Pediatric
• Children of school age and older are concrete thinkers and often very curious. They may ask many questions about the test. Answer questions honestly and at child's level of understanding. Allow child to watch, if desired, while performing test.
• Testing reagent is often poisonous; thus keep it out of reach of the small child.

Home Care
• Many patients or family caregivers are instructed to collect specimens at home and return them to clinic or health care provider's office. Be sure they know infection control principles.
• Alert patient that presence of chemical home products such as toilet bowl cleaner in the stool specimen will interfere with the results (Fischbach and Dunning, 2009).

SKILL 43-3   Measuring Occult Blood in Gastric Secretions (Gastroccult)

[NSO] *Specimen Collection Module / Lesson 3*

Analysis of gastric secretions or emesis can detect blood that is not always visible. Gastroccult testing helps to reveal bleeding in the esophagus or stomach. The test can verify the presence of blood when red or black coloration of the gastric contents is noted or when the gastric contents or emesis has the appearance of coffee grounds. The test measures microscopic amounts of blood in the gastric secretions. It is a useful diagnostic tool for conditions such as upper gastrointestinal (GI) ulcers or bleeding. Because the test is easy to perform, patients are often instructed in how to test emesis in the home.

Delegation and Collaboration
The skill of Gastroccult testing can be delegated to nursing assistive personnel (NAP) for test on emesis. You cannot delegate the skill of Gastroccult testing to NAP if the specimen is collected from a nasogastric (NG) or nasoenteral tube. The nurse informs the NAP to:
• Report immediately if blood or coffee-ground emesis is visible in NG or NI tube secretions.
• Save specimen for repeat testing.

Equipment
❑ Facial tissues
❑ Emesis basin
❑ Wooden applicator or 3-mL syringe

❑ Bulb or catheter tip syringe
❑ Cardboard Gastroccult test slide
❑ Gastroccult developing solution
❑ Clean gloves

STEP	RATIONALE

ASSESSMENT

1 Assess patient's or family members' understanding of need for test.	Provides nurse with information on which to base necessary health teaching.
2 Assess patient's medical history for bleeding or GI disorders.	You can institute routine screening.
3 Assess patient's medical history for GI disorders (e.g., history of bleeding, colitis).	Anticoagulants increase risk for bleeding in GI tract, even from minor trauma to mucosa. Long-term use of steroids, nonsteroidal antiinflammatory drugs (NSAIDs), and acetylsalicylic acid (aspirin) can irritate mucosa.

NURSING DIAGNOSES

- Anxiety
- Deficient knowledge regarding occult blood testing
- Fear

Related factors are individualized based on patient's condition or needs.

PLANNING

1 Expected outcomes following completion of procedure:	
• Test for occult blood is negative.	Patient has only small or no amount of blood in gastric secretions.
• Patient discusses purpose and benefits of testing gastric contents for blood.	Validates learning.
2 Explain procedure to patient and/or family member. Discuss why specimen collection is necessary.	Patient who understands procedure is more likely to be less anxious and more cooperative.

IMPLEMENTATION

1 Perform hand hygiene.	Reduces transmission of microorganisms.
2 Identify patient using two identifiers (i.e., name and birthday or name and account number) according to agency policy. Compare identifiers in MAR/medical record with information on patient's identification bracelet and/or ask patient to state name.	Ensures correct patient. Complies with The Joint Commission standards and improves patient safety (TJC, 2012).
3 Verify NG tube placement (see Chapter 34).	Ensures aspiration of gastric contents.
4 Obtain specimen by disconnecting suction or gravity drainage tube from NG or nasoenteral tube. Using a bulb or catheter tip syringe, aspirate 5 to 10 mL of fluid from NG or nasoenteral tube.	Only small amount of specimen is needed for testing.

Clinical Decision Point *Observe specimen. If you find red blood or coffee-ground material, report these findings immediately to health care provider.*

5 To obtain sample of emesis, use 3-mL syringe or wooden applicator to obtain sample from emesis basin.	Small specimen is sufficient for measuring blood content.
6 *Perform Gastroccult test:*	
a Using wooden applicator or syringe, apply 1 drop of gastric sample to Gastroccult blood test slide.	Sample must cover test paper for test reaction to occur.
b Apply 2 drops of commercial developer solution over sample and 1 drop between positive and negative performance monitors (see illustration).	
c Verify that performance monitor turns blue in 30 seconds.	Indicates proper function of testing paper.
d After 60 seconds compare color of gastric sample with that of performance monitor.	If sample turns blue, test is positive for occult blood. If sample turns green, it is negative for occult blood.
e Dispose of test slide, wooden applicator, and syringe in proper receptacle. If needed, reconnect enteral tube to drainage system or suction. Remove gloves. Perform hand hygiene.	Reduces transmission of microorganisms.

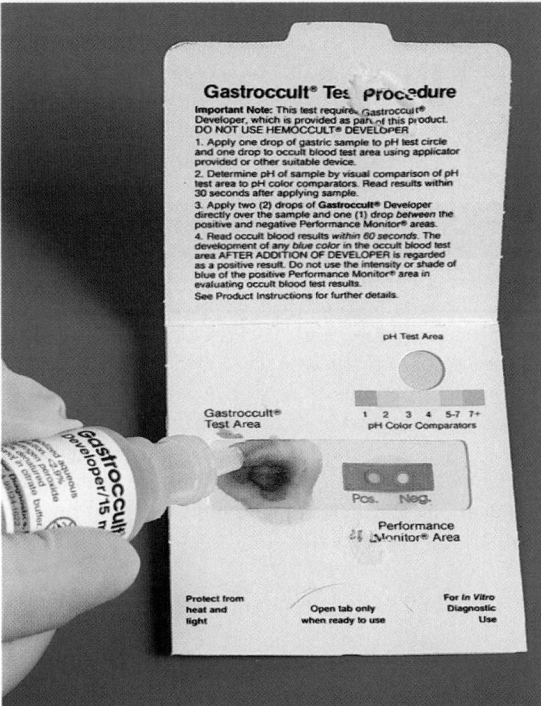

STEP 6b   Applying developing solution to Gastroccult test area.

EVALUATION

1 Ask patient to explain reason for procedure.	Validates level of understanding.
2 Note color changes in guaiac paper.	Reveals blood in gastric secretions.
3 Note character of gastric secretions.	Blood may be visible, or coffee-ground material denoting blood may be observed.

Unexpected Outcomes	**Related Interventions**
1 Test for occult blood is positive.	• Continue to monitor patient.
	• Notify health care provider.

Recording and Reporting
• Record results of test and presence of any unusual characteristics of gastric contents in nurses' notes.
• Report positive test results to health care provider.

Special Considerations
Teaching
• Explain that long-term steroids cause increase risk for bruising, skin is more fragile, and anticoagulants increase risk for bleeding.

Pediatric
• Children of school age and older are concrete thinkers, are often very curious, and may ask many questions about test. Answer questions honestly and at child's level of understanding. Allow child to watch, if desired, while test is performed.

Home Care
• Many patients or family caregivers can perform the Gastroccult test on emesis. Be sure they know infection control principles.

SKILL 43-4   Collecting Nose and Throat Specimens for Culture

When patients have signs and symptoms of upper respiratory or sinus infection, a nose or throat culture is a simple diagnostic tool to identify the presence and type of microorganisms. You should obtain cultures before antibiotic therapy is initiated because antibiotics may interrupt the growth of the organisms in the laboratory. If a patient is receiving antibiotics, notify the laboratory and identify which specific antibiotics he or she is receiving (Pagana and Pagana, 2011).

Collection of a specimen from the nose and throat can cause discomfort and gagging because of sensitive mucosal membranes.

It is important to collect a throat culture before mealtime or at least 1 hour after eating or drinking to decrease the chance of inducing vomiting. A patient's clear understanding of the specimen collection technique minimizes anxiety or discomfort.

Delegation and Collaboration
The skill of obtaining specimens from the nose and throat cannot be delegated to nursing assistive personnel (NAP). The nurse informs the NAP to:

- Report any complaint of shortness of breath, difficulty breathing, and other signs of respiratory distress.

Equipment
- ❑ Two sterile swabs in sterile culture tubes (flexible wire swab with cotton tip may be used for nose cultures)
- ❑ Nasal speculum (*optional*)
- ❑ Emesis basin or clean container (*optional*)
- ❑ Tongue blades and penlight
- ❑ Facial tissues/gauze
- ❑ Clean gloves
- ❑ Completed identification labels with proper patient identifiers
- ❑ Completed laboratory requisition (date, time, name of test, patient identification, source of culture)
- ❑ Small biohazard plastic bag for delivery of specimen to laboratory (or container specified by agency)

STEP	RATIONALE

ASSESSMENT

1 Assess patient's understanding of purpose for procedure and ability to cooperate. You may need assistance to obtain throat cultures from confused, combative, or unconscious patients.

Provides basis to determine need for health teaching and assistance.

2 Inspect condition of nares and drainage from nasal mucosa and sinuses.

Reveals physical signs that indicate infection or allergic irritation. Clear drainage usually indicates allergy. Yellow, green, or brown drainage usually indicates infection.

3 Determine if patient experiences postnasal drip, sinus headache or tenderness, nasal congestion, sore throat, or exposure to others with similar symptoms.

Symptoms help reveal nature of problem.

4 Apply clean gloves. Assess condition of posterior pharynx (see Chapter 6).

Reveals local inflammation or lesions of pharynx.

5 Assess patient for signs of infection, including fever, chills, and/or fatigue.

Infection originating within nasopharynx can become systemic, requiring antibiotic therapy.

6 Review health care provider's orders to determine if nose, throat, or both cultures are needed.

Prevents exposing patient to unnecessary discomfort of repeated cultures.

NURSING DIAGNOSES
- Acute pain
- Chronic pain
- Deficient knowledge regarding specimen collection
- Risk for infection

Related factors are individualized based on patient's condition or needs.

PLANNING

1 Expected outcomes following completion of procedure:
   - There is no bacterial growth in specimens.
   - Patient does not experience bleeding of nasal mucosa.
   - Specimen is not contaminated.
   - Patient discusses purpose of nose and throat cultures.

Absence of bacterial infection.
Procedure is atraumatic.
Evidenced by results of laboratory analysis.
Validates learning.

2 Plan to do culture before mealtime or at least 1 hour after eating.

Procedure often induces gagging; timing decreases patient's chances of vomiting.

3 Explain procedure to patient and/or family member. Discuss reason for specimen collection and how patient can help.

Understanding procedure usually decreases anxiety and promotes cooperation.

4 Explain that patient may have tickling sensation or gagging during swabbing of throat. Nasal swab may create urge to sneeze. Each procedure only takes a few seconds to complete.

Helps patient relax.

IMPLEMENTATION

1 Identify patient using two identifiers (i.e., name and birthday or name and account number) according to agency policy. Compare identifiers in MAR/medical record with information on patient's identification bracelet and/or ask patient to state name.

Ensures correct patient. Complies with The Joint Commission standards and improves patient safety (TJC, 2012).

2 Ask patient to sit erect in bed or chair facing you. Acutely ill patient or young child may lie back against bed with head of bed raised to 45-degree angle in semi-Fowler's position.

Provides easy access to nasal or oral structures.

3 Perform hand hygiene. Have swab in tube ready for use. Loosen top so swab can be removed easily.

Reduces transmission of microorganisms. Allows you to grasp swab easily without danger of contamination. Most commercial tubes have tops that fit securely over end of swab. Allows touching outer tops without contaminating swab stick.

STEP	RATIONALE
4 Collect throat culture.	
a Apply clean gloves.	Reduces transmission of microorganisms.
b Instruct patient to tilt head backward. For patients in bed, place pillow behind shoulders.	Facilitates visualization of pharynx.
c Ask patient to open mouth and say "ah." To visualize pharynx, depress tongue with tongue blade and note inflamed areas of pharynx or tonsils. Depress anterior third of tongue only and illuminate with penlight as needed.	Permits exposure of pharynx, relaxes throat muscles, and minimizes gag reflex. Area to be swabbed should be visualized clearly.

Clinical Decision Point *Placement of tongue blade along back of tongue more likely initiates gag reflex. If patient gags, remove tongue blade and allow him or her to relax before reinserting.*

STEP	RATIONALE
d Insert swab without touching lips, teeth, tongue, cheeks, or uvula.	Prevents contamination with organisms from oral cavity (Pagana and Pagana, 2011).
e Gently but quickly swab tonsillar area side to side, making contact with inflamed or purulent sites (see illustration).	These areas contain most microorganisms.
f Carefully withdraw swab without touching oral structures.	Collects microorganisms from throat tissues without contamination from mouth and tongue.
5 Collect nasal culture.	
a Apply clean gloves.	Reduces transmission of microorganisms.
b Encourage patient to blow nose and then check nostrils for patency with penlight. Select nostril with greatest patency.	Clears nasal passages of mucus containing resident bacteria.
c In sitting position have patient tilt head backward. Patients in bed should have small pillow behind shoulders.	Provides access to nasal passages and facilitates visualization of nasal septum and sinuses.
d Gently insert nasal speculum in one nostril (*optional*).	Allows retraction of mucosa for easier swab insertion.
e Carefully pass swab into nostril until it reaches that portion of mucosa that is inflamed or containing exudate. Rotate swab quickly. NOTE: If you need to obtain nasopharyngeal culture, use special swab on flexible wire that can be flexed downward to reach nasopharynx.	Swab should remain sterile until it reaches area to be cultured. Rotating swab covers all surfaces where exudate is present.
f Remove swab without touching sides of speculum or nasal canal.	Prevents contamination of swab by resident bacteria.
g Carefully remove nasal speculum (if used) and place in basin. Offer patient facial tissue.	Minimizes period of time that patient experiences discomfort.
6 Insert swab into culture tube. Use gauze to protect your fingers while crushing ampule at bottom of tube to release culture medium (see illustrations).	Placing tip within culture medium maintains life of bacteria for testing.
7 Place tip of swab into liquid medium and place top securely on top of tube.	Preserves specimen for testing.
8 Securely attach completed identification label and laboratory requisition to culture tube and confirm identifiers, specimen source, and collection date and time in front of patient (see agency policy). Note on laboratory requisition if patient is taking antibiotic or if specific organism is suspected (e.g., *Bordetella pertussis*).	Incorrect identification of specimen could result in diagnostic or therapeutic errors.

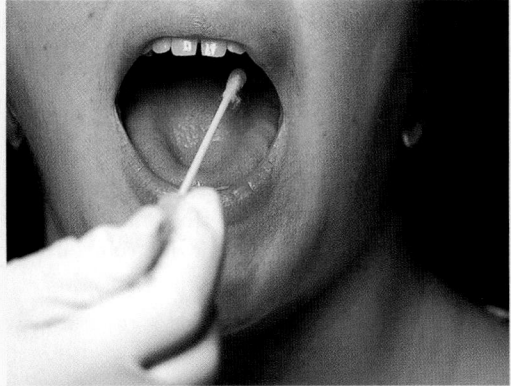

STEP 4e Collection of specimen from posterior pharynx.

STEP	RATIONALE
9 Enclose specimen in plastic biohazard bag (according to agency policy) and send immediately to laboratory.	Specimen not sent to laboratory immediately or refrigerated allows growth of organisms and inaccurate results.
10 Return patient to position of comfort. Remove and dispose of gloves and perform hand hygiene.	Provides for patient comfort. Reduces transmission of microorganisms.

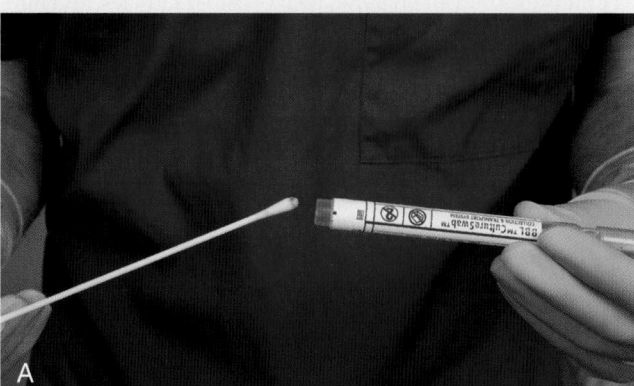 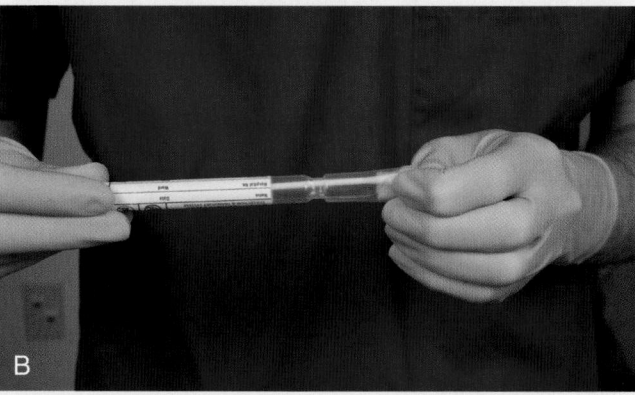

STEP 6   Activating culture tube. **A,** Place swab into tube. **B,** Crush end of tube to release liquid medium.

EVALUATION

1 Check laboratory record for results of culture test.	Results reveal type of organisms in nose or pharynx and antibiotics most likely to be effective.
2 Ask patient to explain purpose of culture.	Demonstrates learning.

Unexpected Outcomes	Related Interventions
1 Nose and throat cultures reveal bacterial growth.	• Notify health care provider of findings. • Administer medications as ordered.
2 Patient experiences minor nasal bleeding.	• Apply mild pressure and ice pack over bridge of nose. • Notify health care provider of patient's condition.
3 Specimen is contaminated.	• Repeat specimen collection.

Recording and Reporting

• Describe appearance of nasal and oral mucosal structure and record specimen collection, date, time, and disposition in nurses' notes.
• Report unusual test results to health care provider.

Special Considerations

Teaching

• Instruct patient that procedure may cause slight discomfort and gagging is common.
• Discuss patient's role in collecting specimen.
• Discuss reason for time delay in receiving culture results.

Pediatric

• Allowing young children to visualize and examine speculum decreases their fear.
• Immobilization of child's head and arms is important when obtaining specimen. You should do this in a firm, gentle, kind manner. Ask another nurse to help if necessary.
• Ask parents to act as coach and suggest that they hold their child on their lap. Do not ask parents to restrain child.

• Showing tongue blade and penlight to child and demonstrating how to say "ah" helps to decrease anxiety.
• School-age child will be more cooperative if given opportunity to ask questions about procedure and results.
• Nasal and nasopharyngeal specimen screening may be done for actual infection or nonsymptomatic carriers in respiratory infections, including respiratory syncytial virus (RSV) (Pagana and Pagana, 2011).
• Do not attempt throat culture if you suspect acute epiglottitis because trauma from swab might cause increase in edema, resulting in occlusion of airway (Hockenberry and Wilson, 2011).

Gerontologic

• Some older adults need help in keeping mouth open to obtain specimen.
• Some older adults have poor dentition. Take care not to break a tooth and consider removal of dentures.
• In confused patients someone may need to hold patient's hands while you collect the sample.

SKILL 43-5 Obtaining Vaginal or Urethral Discharge Specimens

Normally drainage from the vagina or urethra is thin, nonpurulent, whitish or clear, and small in amount. Factors such as poor hygiene practices can cause an accumulation of discharge. If a patient develops an increased amount of discharge or if there is a change in the character of discharge from the vagina or urethra, medical follow-up is necessary.

Patients most commonly requiring cultures of vaginal or urethral discharge have signs and symptoms of sexually transmitted disease (STD) or urinary tract infection. Patients suspected of having an STD may be embarrassed by their condition. Show respect and understanding toward a patient. When collecting vaginal or urethral specimens, work quickly and calmly, maintaining the patient's privacy at all times.

Delegation and Collaboration
The skill of obtaining vaginal or urethral discharge specimens cannot be delegated to nursing assistive personnel (NAP).

Equipment
- ❏ Sterile swab in sterile culture tube (commercially available culture tubes have swab and tube with ampule containing special transport medium)
- ❏ Sheet, blanket, or paper drape
- ❏ Clean gloves
- ❏ Penlight or gooseneck lamp
- ❏ Completed identification labels with proper patient identifiers
- ❏ Completed laboratory requisition (date, time, name of test, patient identification, source of culture)
- ❏ Small biohazard plastic bag for delivery of specimen to laboratory (or container specified by agency)

STEP	RATIONALE

ASSESSMENT

1 Assess patient's understanding of need for culture and ability to cooperate with procedure.

Provides you with information on which to base necessary health teaching.

2 Perform hand hygiene and apply clean gloves. Assess condition of external genitalia and urethra, meatus, and vaginal orifice. Observe for redness; swelling; complaint of tenderness; and discharge that is whitish, mucoid, or purulent or a whitish discharge like cottage cheese. Remove and discard gloves and perform hand hygiene. NOTE: This step may be done during collection.

Reduces transmission of microorganisms. Assessment findings and specimen test results reveal nature of problem.

3 Ask patient about dysuria, localized pruritus of genitalia, or lower abdominal pain.

Symptoms of urinary tract or vaginal infection.

4 If symptoms suggest STD, gather and record patient's sexual history.

Determines sexual activity and if there has been sexual contact with a person known to have an STD. If culture results are positive, tell patient to receive treatment and have sexual partners evaluated (Pagana and Pagana, 2011).

5 Refer to health care provider's order to determine if culture is to be vaginal or urethral.

Patient may require one or both types of cultures.

NURSING DIAGNOSES

- Acute pain
- Anxiety
- Deficient knowledge regarding specimen collection
- Risk for infection

Related factors are individualized based on patient's condition or needs.

PLANNING

1 Expected outcomes following completion of procedure:
- Specimen is not contaminated.

Results on laboratory test will reveal whether skin cells or mucosal cells have contaminated specimen.

- Vaginal or urethral cultures do not reveal growth of microorganisms.

Evidence of absence of infection.

2 Explain procedure to patient and/or family member. Discuss reason for specimen collection and how patient can help. Instruct female patient not to douche 24 hours before culture is obtained. Male is not to urinate 1 hour before urethral culture is obtained.

Patient who understands procedure is less anxious and more likely to cooperate. Douching of vaginal canal would remove discharge containing pathogens. Urinating by male washes secretions out of urethra (Pagana and Pagana, 2011).

STEP	RATIONALE

IMPLEMENTATION

STEP	RATIONALE
1 Perform hand hygiene. Apply clean gloves.	Reduces transmission of microorganisms.
2 Draw bedside curtains or close room door. Place "Do Not Enter" sign on door (if available).	Provides privacy for patient and demonstrates respect for patient's well-being.
3 Identify patient using two identifiers (i.e., name and birthday or name and account number) according to agency policy. Compare identifiers in MAR/medical record with information on patient's identification bracelet and/or ask patient to state name.	Ensures correct patient. Complies with The Joint Commission standards and improves patient safety (TJC, 2012).
4 Help patient to proper position, raise gown, and drape body parts to be exposed: **a** *Female*: Dorsal recumbent position with sheet draped over each leg and genitalia. **b** *Male*: Sitting on chair or bed or lying supine with sheet draped across lower trunk and genitalia.	Provides easy access to perineal area. Draping minimizes exposure of body parts, minimizing anxiety.
5 Direct light source onto perineum (may not be needed for male patient).	Allows better visualization of external urethral or vaginal structures.
6 Open culture tube and hold swab in dominant hand.	Provides for easier manipulation of swab during culture collection.
7 Instruct patient to deep breathe slowly.	Helps patient to relax. Tensing of muscles around pelvic floor may cause discomfort during swabbing.
8 Obtain specimens. **a** *Female*: (1) With nondominant hand fully separate labia to expose vaginal orifice.	Exposes perineum and ensures that specimen is of vaginal discharge.
(2) Touch tip of swab into discharge pool, being careful not to touch skin or mucosa along perineum or vaginal canal. If no discharge is visible, gently insert swab 1 to 2.5 cm ($\frac{1}{3}$ to 1 inch) into vaginal orifice and rotate before removal.	Discharge contains greatest concentration of microorganisms.
(3) To expose urethral meatus use nondominant hand to pull gently on labia minora upward and back to separate.	Allows better visualization of urethral orifice.
(4) Use clean swab; gently apply to tip of meatus where discharge is visible. Avoid touching labia.	Discharge contains greatest concentration of microorganisms.

Clinical Decision Point *If discharge near vagina appears different from discharge along perineum, collect separate specimens from each area because, if two organisms are present, they could be cross-contaminated on a single swab. Label specimen with area of patient's body that you swabbed.*

STEP	RATIONALE
b *Male*: (1) Grasp patient's penis proximal to glans with nondominant hand; if male is uncircumcised, gently retract foreskin.	Provides clear exposure of urethral meatus.
(2) Use dominant hand to hold swab. Apply gently to area of discharge at urinary meatus.	Discharge contains greatest number of microorganisms.
(3) If no discharge is apparent, health care provider may order swab to be introduced into urinary meatus. Hold male genitalia firmly but gently.	Excess manipulation can cause erection.
(4) Return foreskin to natural position.	Tightening of foreskin around shaft of penis can cause localized discomfort, edema, and potential necrosis.
9 Return each swab to culture tube and secure top.	Retains microorganisms within tube.
10 If using commercial culture tube, wrap ampule with gauze to prevent injury to your fingers while crushing. Immediately squeeze end of tube to crush ampule (see Skill 43-4). Push tip of swab into fluid medium.	Medium supports life of microorganisms until culture is analyzed.
11 Remove and discard gloves. Perform hand hygiene.	Reduces transmission of microorganisms.
12 Label each culture tube with identification label, affix completed requisition, and confirm identifiers in front of patient (TJC, 2012).	Incorrect specimen identification could lead to diagnostic or therapeutic error.

STEP	RATIONALE
13 Send specimen to laboratory immediately or refrigerate.	Bacteria multiply quickly. Prompt analysis ensures accurate results.
14 Help patient to comfortable position, assist with personal hygiene, and remove and discard drape.	Reinforces patient's sense of self-esteem. Reduces transmission of microorganisms.

EVALUATION

1 Review laboratory results for evidence of pathogens.	Results will reveal type of organisms present. Certain organisms are common to vaginal tract. Urethra should be free of microorganisms.
2 Continue to monitor whether discharge is present; if so, observe color and amount.	Characteristics of discharge indicate specific type of infection.
3 Observe specimen for presence of feces.	Need to obtain another specimen if it contains feces.

Unexpected Outcomes	Related Interventions
1 Vaginal or urethral cultures reveal growth of pathogenic microorganisms.	• Notify health care provider of findings and follow new orders. • Continue to monitor patient.
2 Specimen is contaminated with epidermal cells.	• Repeat specimen collection.

Recording and Reporting
- Record types of cultures obtained and date and time sent to laboratory in nurses' notes and EHR.
- Report laboratory results to nurse in charge or health care provider.

Special Considerations
Teaching
- Discuss sexuality and safe sex practices with patient if appropriate.
- Patients with urethral or vaginal discharge often require instruction about perineal hygiene measures.
- If topical treatments (e.g., suppositories) are ordered, instruct patient in proper administration of medication (see Chapter 21).

Pediatric
- A second nurse can help with specimen collection from an infant or young child by gently holding child's legs apart

in froglike position. Have parent present to encourage cooperation.
- Parents should understand that obtaining vaginal specimen will not affect virginity of child.
- Be sensitive to cultural variations and beliefs pertaining to genitalia (i.e., female circumcisions).
- In addition to collecting the specimen on adolescent patients, this may also open up the possibility of discussions related to sexuality during which they may have questions but are not comfortable initiating on their own.

Gerontologic
- Clear explanation regarding importance of obtaining sample is extremely helpful to alleviate or diminish anxiety and gain cooperation.

PROCEDURAL GUIDELINE 43-3 Collecting a Sputum Specimen by Expectoration

Sputum is mucus secretions produced by cells of the lungs, bronchi, and trachea. You collect a specimen either by having a patient cough and expectorate into a sterile specimen container or by suctioning into a sterile sputum trap (see Skill 43-6). In a healthy state sputum production is minimal; a disease state can increase the amount and character of sputum. Sputum specimens are collected to identify cancer cells, for culture and sensitivity (C&S) to identify pathogens and determine the antibiotics to which they are sensitive, and for acid-fast bacillus to diagnose pulmonary tuberculosis.

Delegation and Collaboration
The skill of collecting a sputum specimen by expectoration can be delegated to nursing assistive personnel (NAP). The nurse instructs the NAP to:
- Immediately report the presence of blood in the sputum or changes in the patient's vital signs.

Equipment
- ❑ Completed identification labels with appropriate patient identifiers
- ❑ Completed laboratory requisition, including appropriate patient identification, date, time, name of test, and source of culture
- ❑ Small biohazard plastic bag for delivery of specimen to laboratory (or container as specified by agency)
- ❑ Sterile specimen container with cover
- ❑ Clean gloves
- ❑ Facial tissues
- ❑ Emesis basin (*optional*)
- ❑ Toothbrush (*optional*)
- ❑ Disinfectant swab (optional)

Procedural Steps
1 Identify patient using two identifiers (i.e., name and birthday or name and account number) according to agency policy.

Continued

PROCEDURAL GUIDELINE 43-3   Collecting a Sputum Specimen by Expectoration—cont'd

Compare identifiers in MAR/medical record with information on patient's identification bracelet and/or ask patient to state name.

2 Provide opportunity to clean or rinse mouth with water. Patient should not use mouthwash or toothpaste because the products may alter culture results.

3 Perform hand hygiene and apply clean gloves. Provide sputum cup and instruct patient not to touch the inside of the container.

4 Have the patient take three-to-four deep slow breaths with full exhalation. Then take full inhalation followed immediately by a forceful cough, expectorating sputum directly into specimen container.

5 Repeat until 5 to 10 mL of sputum (not saliva) has been collected.

6 Secure lid on container tightly. If any sputum is present on outside of container, wipe it off with disinfectant.

7 Offer patient tissues after patient expectorates, dispose of tissues, and offer mouth care.

8 Remove and dispose of gloves. Perform hand hygiene.

9 Securely attach properly completed identification label and laboratory requisition to side of specimen container (not lid). Confirm identifiers in patient's presence.

10 Enclose specimen in a plastic biohazard bag.

11 Send specimen to laboratory immediately.

SKILL 43-6   Collecting a Sputum Specimen by Suction

Video Clip

Sputum is produced by cells lining the respiratory tract. Although production is minimal in the healthy state, disease states can increase the amount or change the character of sputum. Examination of sputum aids in the diagnosis and treatment of several conditions, ranging from simple bronchitis to lung cancer.

Suctioning is often indicated to collect sputum from patients unable to spontaneously expectorate a sample for laboratory analysis. Sometimes suctioning provokes violent coughing, which can induce vomiting and constriction of pharyngeal, laryngeal, and bronchial muscles. In addition, it may cause hypoxemia or vagal overload, causing cardiopulmonary compromise and increased intracranial pressure.

Delegation and Collaboration

The skill of collecting sputum specimens by suction cannot be delegated to nursing assistive personnel (NAP). The nurse instructs the NAP to:

- Notify the nurse if the patient expectorates bloody sputum.

Equipment

Suctioned Specimen

❏ Completed identification labels with proper patient identifiers
❏ Completed laboratory requisition, including patient identification, date, time, name of test, and source of culture
❏ Suction device (wall or portable)
❏ Sterile suction catheter (size 14, 16, or 18 Fr [not large enough to cause trauma to nasal mucosa]) or suction catheter with sleeve
❏ Sterile gloves and clean gloves
❏ Sterile water in container
❏ In-line specimen container or sputum trap
❏ Small plastic bag for delivery of specimen to laboratory (or a container as specified by agency)
❏ Oxygen therapy equipment if indicated
❏ Protective eyewear
❏ Disinfectant wipe

STEP	RATIONALE

ASSESSMENT

1 Check health care provider's orders for type of sputum analysis and specifications (e.g., amount of sputum, number of specimens, time of collection, method to obtain). Specimens for acid-fast bacillus (AFB) require three consecutive morning samples.

Specific test dictates when or how frequently specimens are collected. Ideal time to collect sputum is early morning because bronchial secretions tend to accumulate during the night. Bacteria also accumulate as secretions pool.

2 Assess patient's level of understanding of procedure and its purpose.

Provides baseline to establish teaching plan.

3 Assess when patient last ate meal (or had tube feeding).

It is best to obtain specimen 1 to 2 hours after or 1 hour before meal to minimize gagging, which can cause vomiting and aspiration.

4 Determine type of assistance needed by patient to obtain specimen.

Positioning, postural drainage, and deep breathing and coughing exercises may improve ability to cough productively. Suctioning is often indicated when patient is unable to cough and expectorate.

5 Assess patient's respiratory status, including respiratory rate, depth, pattern, and color of mucous membranes.

Active coughing may alter respiratory status.

Respiratory status can depend on amount of sputum in tracheobronchial tree.

STEP	RATIONALE

NURSING DIAGNOSES

- Deficient knowledge regarding specimen collection procedures
- Ineffective airway clearance
- Ineffective breathing pattern
- Risk for aspiration
- Risk for infection

Related factors are individualized based on patient's condition or needs.

PLANNING

STEP	RATIONALE
1 Expected outcomes following completion of procedure:	
• Patient's respirations are same rate and character before and after procedure.	Specimen collection did not alter respiratory status.
• Patient maintains comfort level and experiences minimal anxiety.	Suctioning tends to cause anxiety.
• Sputum is not contaminated by saliva or oropharyngeal flora.	Sputum must originate from tracheobronchial tree for accurate results.
• Laboratory tests do not reveal abnormal cells or microorganisms.	Absence of infection or abnormal cells.
• Patient discusses purpose and benefit of sputum collection.	Validates learning.
2 Explain steps of procedure and purpose. Instruct patient to breathe normally during suctioning to prevent hyperventilation.	Promotes understanding and cooperation.

IMPLEMENTATION

STEP	RATIONALE
1 Close curtains or room door.	Provides privacy.
2 Identify patient using two identifiers (i.e., name and birthday or name and account number) according to agency policy. Compare identifiers in MAR/medical record with information on patient's identification bracelet and/or ask patient to state name.	Ensures correct patient. Complies with The Joint Commission standards and improves patient safety (TJC, 2012).
3 Position patient in high- or semi-Fowler's position for suctioning.	Promotes full lung expansion and facilitates ability to cough.

Clinical Decision Point *If patient has surgical incision or localized area of discomfort, have him or her place pillow or hands firmly over affected area. Splinting of painful area minimizes muscular stretching and discomfort during coughing and thus makes cough more productive.*

STEP	RATIONALE
4 Perform hand hygiene and apply clean glove to nondominant hand. Prepare suction machine or device and determine if it functions properly.	Adequate amount of suction is necessary to aspirate sputum.
5 Connect suction tube to adapter on sputum trap. Open sterile water.	Establishes suction that passes through sputum trap to aspirate specimen.
6 Using sterile technique, apply sterile glove to dominant hand or use clean glove if suction catheter has plastic sleeve.	Tracheobronchial tree is sterile body cavity. Allows you to manipulate suction catheter without contamination.
7 With gloved hand connect sterile suction catheter to rubber tubing on sputum trap.	Aspirated sputum will go directly to trap instead of to suction tubing.
8 Lubricate suction catheter tip with sterile water (*with suction off*).	Lubrication allows for easier insertion of catheter.
9 Gently insert tip of suction catheter through nasopharynx, endotracheal tube, or tracheostomy tube without applying suction (see Chapter 25).	Minimizes trauma to airway as catheter is inserted.
10 Gently and quickly advance catheter into trachea. Warn patient to expect to cough.	Entrance of catheter into larynx and trachea triggers cough reflex.
11 As patient coughs, apply suction for 5 to 10 seconds, collecting 2 to 10 mL of sputum.	Ensures collection of sputum from deep within tracheobronchial tree. Suctioning longer than 10 seconds can cause hypoxia and mucosal damage.
12 Release suction and remove catheter; turn off suction.	Suction can damage mucosa if applied during withdrawal.
13 Detach catheter from specimen trap and dispose of catheter in appropriate receptacle.	Decreases risk for spreading microorganisms.
14 Secure top on specimen container tightly. For sputum trap, detach suction tubing and connect rubber tubing on sputum trap to plastic adapter (see illustration).	Contains microorganisms within container, preventing exposure to personnel handling specimen.

STEP	RATIONALE
15 If any sputum is present on outside of container, wipe it off with disinfectant.	Prevents spread of infection to people handling specimen.
16 Offer patient tissues after suctioning. Dispose of tissues in emesis basin or appropriate container.	Maintains cleanliness and comfort.
17 Remove and dispose of gloves. Perform hand hygiene.	Reduces transmission of microorganisms.
18 Label specimen with identification label on side of specimen container (not lid). Confirm identifiers in front of patient (TJC, 2012). Place specimen in small plastic bag (or container specified by agency) and attach requisition.	Incorrect identification could lead to diagnostic or therapeutic error. Plastic bag or container reduces risk for health care worker's exposure to sputum.
19 Send specimen immediately to laboratory or refrigerate.	Bacteria multiply quickly. Prompt analysis ensures accurate results.
20 Offer patient mouth care if desired.	Promotes comfort.

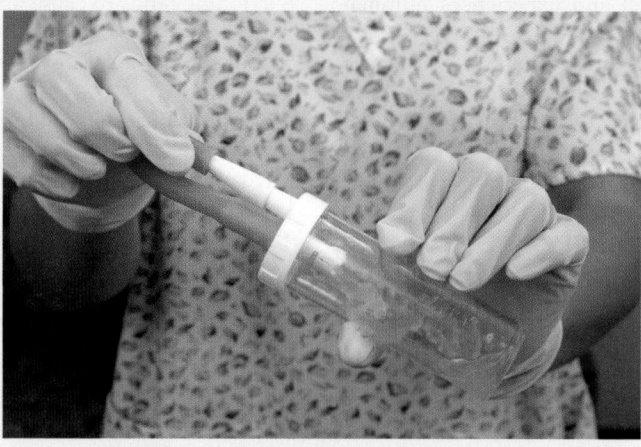

STEP 14   Closing sputum specimen trap.

EVALUATION

1 Observe patient's respiratory status throughout procedure, especially during suctioning. If under distress, measure oxygen saturation with pulse oximeter.	Excessive coughing or prolonged suctioning can alter respiratory pattern and cause hypoxia. Determines oxygenation status.
2 Note anxiety or discomfort in patient.	Procedure can be uncomfortable. If patient becomes short of breath, anxiety will develop.
3 Observe character of sputum: color, consistency, odor, volume, viscosity, and/or presence of blood.	Characteristics may indicate disease entities.
4 Refer to laboratory reports for test results.	Indicates if abnormal cells or microorganisms are present in sputum.
5 Evaluate patient's ability to describe/demonstrate sputum collection process.	Reinforces patient's ability to collect future expectorated specimens.

Unexpected Outcomes

1 Patient becomes hypoxic with increased respiratory rate and effort and shortness of breath.

2 Patient remains anxious or complains of discomfort from suction catheter.

3 Inadequate amount of sputum collected.

4 Patient complains of pain when coughing to produce sputum.

Related Interventions

- Discontinue suctioning immediately.
- Administer oxygen (if ordered).
- Notify health care provider of patient's condition.
- Continue to monitor patient's vital signs and pulse oximetry.

- Discontinue procedure until stable.
- Administer oxygen (if ordered).
- Notify health care provider of patient's change in condition.
- Continue to monitor patient's vital signs and pulse oximetry.

- Repeat specimen collection after patient takes several deep breaths.

- Encourage patient who is recovering from surgical procedure to splint incision before coughing.
- Obtain order for pain medication as needed (prn).
- Inform health care provider of changes in patient's condition.

Recording and Reporting

- Record method used to obtain specimen, date and time collected, type of test ordered, and transport to laboratory in nurses' notes. Describe characteristics of sputum specimen. Describe patient's tolerance of procedure.
- Report unusual sputum characteristics to nurse in charge or health care provider.
- When laboratory reports are available, report abnormal findings to health care provider. If AFB sputum culture is positive, initiate appropriate isolation techniques.
- Most agencies require nurses to note on specimen requisition if patient is receiving antibiotics.

Special Considerations
Teaching
- Demonstrate proper splinting technique for postoperative patients.

- If aerosol treatment is indicated, teach patient purpose of procedure, explaining that it will stimulate coughing and sputum expectoration.

Pediatric
- Children need very clear instructions or demonstration for deep breathing. Infants and young children will be unable to cooperate; aerosol treatment may be indicated.
- You may need help to restrain a young child's head and arms during suctioning; parent may help by providing support.
- Use smaller catheter size for young children. It may be possible to elicit a cough by tickling the back of the throat with the suction catheter.

SKILL 43-7 Obtaining Wound Drainage Specimens

[NSO] *Specimen Collection Module / Lesson 5*

When caring for a patient with a wound, assess the condition of the wound and observe for the development of infection. Localized inflammation, tenderness, and warmth at the wound site and purulent drainage are signs and symptoms of wound infection. Identification of the causative organism confirms an infection and provides guidelines for accurate treatment. A specimen of wound drainage is analyzed to determine the type and number of pathogenic microorganisms.

Always collect a wound culture sample from fresh exudate from the center of a wound after removing old drainage. Resident colonies of bacteria on the skin grow in wound exudate and may not be the true causative organisms of infection. Use separate techniques to collect specimens for measuring aerobic versus anaerobic microorganisms. Aerobic organisms grow in superficial wounds exposed to the air. Anaerobic organisms grow deep within body cavities, where oxygen is not normally present.

Delegation and Collaboration
The skill of obtaining wound drainage specimens cannot be delegated to nursing assistive personnel (NAP). The nurse instructs the NAP to:

- Report foul odor, increase in drainage, and increase in temperature or patient complaint of discomfort.

Equipment
- ❏ Culture tube with swab and transport medium for aerobic culture
- ❏ Anaerobic culture tube with swab (tubes contain carbon dioxide or nitrogen gas)
- ❏ 5- to 10-mL syringe and 19-gauge needle
- ❏ Two pairs of clean gloves and sterile gloves
- ❏ Protective eyewear
- ❏ Antiseptic swab
- ❏ Sterile dressing materials (determined by type of dressing)
- ❏ Paper or plastic disposable bag
- ❏ Completed specimen identification label with proper patient identifiers
- ❏ Completed laboratory requisition (date, time, name of test, patient identification, and source of culture)
- ❏ Small plastic biohazard bag for delivery of specimen to laboratory (or container specified by agency)

STEP	RATIONALE

ASSESSMENT

1 Assess patient's understanding of need for wound culture and ability to cooperate with procedure.	Use data to develop teaching plan. Wound is painful site. Collection of specimen may cause anxiety or fear.
2 Assess patient for signs of fever, chills, or excessive thirst. Note in medical record laboratory results if white blood cell (WBC) count is elevated.	Signs and symptoms indicate systemic infection.
3 Ask patient about extent and type of pain at wound site using a scale of 0 to 10. If patient requires analgesic before dressing changes, give medication 30 minutes before beginning procedure to reach peak effect.	Pain at wound site often increases with infection.
4 Determine when dressing change is scheduled (see Chapter 39). Perform wound assessment as part of actual procedure.	
5 Review health care provider's orders for aerobic or anaerobic culture.	Specimens are taken from different sites and placed in different containers, depending on type of culture.

STEP	RATIONALE
6 Perform hand hygiene and apply clean gloves. Remove old dressings covering wound. Fold soiled sides of dressing together and dispose properly. Remove gloves. Apply sterile gloves to palpate wound. Observe for swelling, separation of wound edges, inflammation, and drainage. Palpate gently along wound edges and note tenderness or drainage. Remove and discard gloves.	Gloves minimize exposure to microorganisms Signs indicate wound infection.

NURSING DIAGNOSES

• Acute pain	• Deficient knowledge regarding wound drainage culture procedure	• Risk for infection
• Anxiety		• Risk for injury
• Chronic pain	• Impaired tissue integrity	

Related factors are individualized based on patient's condition or needs.

PLANNING

1 Expected outcomes following completion of procedure:	
• Wound culture does not reveal bacterial growth.	Wound remains free of pathogenic microorganisms.
• Culture swab is not contaminated by bacteria from skin.	Test results indicate type of cells present.
• Patient discusses purpose and procedure for specimen collection.	Validates learning.
2 Determine if analgesia is necessary. Administer analgesic 30 minutes before dressing change and/or specimen collection.	Minimizes discomfort during procedure. Provides patient-centered care.
3 Explain reason for wound culture and how it will be collected.	Promotes understanding and cooperation and eases anxiety.
4 Explain that patient may feel tickling sensation when wound is swabbed.	Anticipation of expected sensations minimizes anxiety.

IMPLEMENTATION

1 Close bedside curtains or door to room.	Provides privacy.
2 Identify patient using two identifiers (i.e., name and birthday or name and account number) according to agency policy. Compare identifiers in MAR/medical record with information on patient's identification bracelet and/or ask patient to state name.	Ensures correct patient. Complies with The Joint Commission standards and improves patient safety (TJC, 2012).
3 Perform hand hygiene and apply clean gloves.	Provides baseline for condition of wound.
4 Clean area around wound edges with antiseptic swab. Wipe from edges outward. Remove old exudate.	Removes skin flora, preventing possible contamination of specimen.
5 Discard swab and remove and dispose of soiled gloves in appropriate receptacle. Perform hand hygiene.	Reduces spread of infection.
6 Open packages containing sterile culture tube and dressing supplies. *Apply sterile gloves.*	Provides sterile field for picking up and handling sterile supplies.
7 Obtain cultures.	
a Aerobic culture:	
(1) Take swab from culture tube, insert tip into wound in area of drainage, and rotate swab gently. Remove swab and return to culture tube (wrap outside of ampule with gauze to prevent injury to your fingers). Crush ampule of medium and push swab into fluid.	Swab should be coated with fresh secretions from within wound. Medium keeps bacteria alive until analysis is complete.
b Anaerobic culture:	
(1) Take swab from special anaerobic culture tube, swab deeply into draining body cavity, and rotate gently. Remove swab and return to culture tube.	Specimen is taken from deep cavity where oxygen is not present. Carbon dioxide or nitrogen gas keeps organisms alive until analysis is complete. Air injected into tube would cause organisms to die.
Or	
(2) Insert tip of syringe (without needle) into wound and aspirate 5 to 10 mL of exudate. Attach 19-gauge needle, expel all air, and inject drainage into special culture tube.	Sterile large-bore needle (19-gauge) allows exudate to be transferred from sterile syringe into special culture tube without contamination.
8 Remove and dispose of gloves. Perform hand hygiene.	Reduces transfer of microorganisms.

STEP	RATIONALE
9 Place correct specimen label on each culture tube. Verify identifiers in front of patient (TJC, 2012). NOTE: Indicate on specimen if patient is receiving antibiotics.	Ensures correct results for correct patient.
10 Send specimens to laboratory immediately.	Bacteria multiple rapidly. Prompt analysis ensures accurate results.
11 Clean wound per health care provider's order. Apply new sterile dressing (see Chapter 39) using aseptic technique. Secure dressing with tape or ties.	Protects wound from further contamination; aids in absorbing drainage and debridement of wound.
12 Remove and dispose of gloves and soiled supplies in appropriate receptacle according to agency policy. Perform hand hygiene.	Reduces transmission of microorganisms.
13 Help patient to comfortable position.	Promotes patient's ability to relax.

EVALUATION

1 Obtain laboratory report for results of cultures.	Report indicates if pathogenic organisms are identified.
2 Observe character of wound drainage.	Characteristics can reveal abnormal status and infection.
3 Observe edges of wound for redness and bleeding.	Indicates trauma to healing tissue.
4 Ask patient about purpose of wound culture.	Validates learning.

Unexpected Outcomes	Related Interventions
1 Wound cultures reveal heavy bacterial growth.	• Monitor patient for fever, chills, or excessive thirst, which indicate systemic infection. • Inform health care provider of findings.
2 Wound culture is contaminated from superficial skin cells.	• Monitor patient for fever and pain. • Inform health care provider of findings. • Repeat collection of specimen as ordered.
3 Patient describes increased pain.	• Provide analgesia. • Notify health care provider.

Recording and Reporting

- Record types of specimens obtained, source, and time and date sent to laboratory and describe appearance of wound and characteristics of drainage in nurses' notes.
- Report any evidence of infection to charge nurse and health care provider.
- Record patient's tolerance of procedure and response to analgesics.

Special Considerations
Teaching

- Instruct patient to inform you if procedure causes pain or if you need to stop because unable to tolerate pain.

- Teach patient to assess status of wound for changes and signs and symptoms of infection.

Pediatric

- If procedure is to be performed on a child and is anticipated to be painful, some agencies prefer performing it in area other than child's room, thus maintaining feeling that child's room is safe place (Hockenberry and Wilson, 2011).
- It is often helpful to have an additional nurse or other adult available to help with a specimen collection in a young child or infant.

Home Care

- Teach patient antiseptic practices (e.g., handwashing, disposal of dressings, and clean technique for applying dressing).

SKILL 43-8 Collecting Blood Specimens and Culture by Venipuncture (Syringe and Vacutainer Method)

NSO *Vascular Access / Drawing Blood and Administering Fluid Module*

Blood tests are one of the most commonly used diagnostic aids in the care and evaluation of patients. In any health care setting they can yield valuable information about a patient's nutritional, hematologic, metabolic, immune, and biochemical status. Tests allow health care providers to screen patients for early signs of physical illness, monitor changes in acute or chronic diseases, and evaluate responses to therapies.

You are often responsible for collecting blood specimens; however, many agencies have specially trained phlebotomists who are responsible for drawing venous blood. Be familiar with your agency policies and procedures and your state Nurse Practice Act regarding guidelines for drawing blood samples.

The three methods of obtaining blood specimens are (1) skin puncture, (2) venipuncture, and (3) arterial puncture. All procedures require sterile technique. Anticipate a patient's anxiety because the procedures are painful; and often just the appearance of a needle is frightening, especially to children. A calm approach and skilled technique help to limit anxiety.

Venipuncture is the most common method of obtaining blood specimens. This method involves inserting a hollow-bore needle into the lumen of a large vein to obtain a specimen using either a needle and syringe or a Vacutainer device that allows the drawing of multiple samples. Because veins are major sources of blood for laboratory testing and routes for intravenous (IV) fluid or blood replacement, maintaining their integrity is essential. You need to be skilled in venipuncture to avoid unnecessary injury to veins.

Skin puncture, also called *capillary puncture,* is the least traumatic method of obtaining a blood specimen. A sterile lancet or needle is used to puncture a vascular area on a finger or earlobe in an adult or child. You place a drop of blood on a test slide, wick a drop of blood to a test slide, or collect it within a thin glass capillary tube for laboratory analysis. Changes in health care economics and delivery result in the increased use of skin puncture. Point-of-care (POC) clinical laboratory tests at the bedside most frequently use skin puncture (Pagana and Pagana, 2011).

Blood cultures aid in detection of bacteria in the blood. It is important that at least two culture specimens be drawn from two different sites. Because bacteremia may be accompanied by fever and chills, blood cultures should be drawn when these symptoms are present (Pagana and Pagana, 2011). Bacteremia exists when both cultures grow the infectious agent. Only one culture growing bacteria is considered contamination. Draw all cultures before antibiotic therapy begins because the antibiotic may interrupt the growth of an organism in the laboratory. If the patient is receiving antibiotics, notify the laboratory and inform them of specific antibiotics the patient is receiving (Pagana and Pagana, 2011).

Delegation and Collaboration

The skill of collecting blood specimens by venipuncture can be delegated to specially trained nursing assistive personnel (NAP). In some agencies, phlebotomists obtain the venipuncture samples. Agency and government regulations and policies differ regarding personnel who may draw blood specimens. The nurse informs the NAP to:
- Report any patient discomfort or signs of excessive bleeding from the puncture site to the nurse.

Equipment

All Procedures
- ❏ Chlorhexidine or antiseptic swab (check agency policy for use of 70% alcohol)
- ❏ Clean gloves
- ❏ Small pillow or folded towel
- ❏ Sterile 2 × 2–inch gauze pads
- ❏ Tourniquet
- ❏ Adhesive bandage or adhesive tape
- ❏ Completed identification labels with proper patient identifiers
- ❏ Completed laboratory requisition (appropriate patient identification, date, time, name of test, and source of culture)
- ❏ Small plastic biohazard bag for delivery of specimen to laboratory (or container specified by agency)
- ❏ Sharps container

Venipuncture with Syringe
- ❏ Sterile safety needles (20- to 21-gauge for adults; 23- to 25-gauge for children)
- ❏ Sterile 10- to 20-mL Luer-Lok safety syringes
- ❏ Needle-free blood transfer device
- ❏ Appropriate blood specimen tubes

Venipuncture with Vacutainer
- ❏ Vacutainer and safety access device with Luer-Lok adapter
- ❏ Sterile double-ended needles (20- to 21-gauge for adults; 23- to 25-gauge for children)
- ❏ Appropriate blood specimen tubes

Blood Cultures
- ❏ Sterile double needles (20- to 21-gauge for adults; 23- to 25-gauge for children)
- ❏ Two 20-mL sterile syringes
- ❏ Anaerobic and aerobic culture bottles (check agency policy)

Central Venous Catheter Collection
- ❏ Two empty 10-mL sterile syringes
- ❏ Sterile 10-mL normal saline flushes
- ❏ Vacutainer and safety access device Luer-Lok adapter
- ❏ Appropriate blood specimen tubes

STEP	RATIONALE

ASSESSMENT

1 Determine whether patient understands purpose of procedure and ability to cooperate.

2 Determine if special conditions need to be met before specimen collection (e.g., patient allowed nothing by mouth [NPO], specific time for collection in relation to medication given, need to ice specimen).

3 Assess patient for possible risks associated with venipuncture: anticoagulant therapy, low platelet count, bleeding disorders (history of hemophilia). Review medication history.

4 Assess patient for contraindicated sites for venipuncture: presence of IV infusion, hematoma at potential site, arm on side of mastectomy, or hemodialysis shunt.

5 Review health care provider's orders for type of tests.

Provides data for you to establish teaching plan and provides emotional support. Some patients' past experiences increase anxiety.

Some tests require meeting specific conditions to obtain accurate measurement of blood elements (e.g., fasting blood sugar, drug peak and trough level, timed endocrine hormone levels).

Patient history may include abnormal clotting abilities caused by low platelet count, hemophilia, or medications that increase risk for bleeding and hematoma formation.

Drawing specimens from such sites can result in false test results or may injure patient. Samples taken from vein near IV infusion may be diluted or contain concentrations of IV fluids. Postmastectomy patient may have reduced lymphatic drainage in arm on operative side, increasing risk for infection from needlesticks. Never use arteriovenous shunt to obtain specimens because of risks for clotting and bleeding. Hematoma indicates existing injury to vessel wall.

Multiple samples are often needed. Health care provider's order is required.

STEP	RATIONALE

Clinical Decision Point *Some specimens have special collection requirements before or after specimen collection; examples follow:*
- *Cryoglobulin levels: Use prewarmed test tubes.*
- *Ammonia and ionized calcium levels: Place tube in ice for delivery to laboratory.*
- *Lactic acid levels: Do not use tourniquet.*
- *Vitamin levels: Avoid exposure of test tube to light.*

NURSING DIAGNOSES

• Anxiety	• Fear	• Risk for injury
• Deficient knowledge regarding blood specimen collection process	• Risk for infection	

Related factors are individualized based on patient's condition or needs.

PLANNING

1 Expected outcomes following completion of procedure:	
• Venipuncture site shows no evidence of continued bleeding or hematoma at venipuncture site after specimen collection.	Indicates that hemostasis is achieved.
• Patient denies anxiety or discomfort.	Explanation relieves anxiety; procedure is performed quickly. Removal of painful stimulus lessens anxiety.
• An adequate sample is collected for testing (see agency policy or laboratory manual).	Appropriate laboratory analysis can be conducted.
• Patient discusses purpose, procedure, and benefits of venipuncture.	Validates learning.
2 Explain procedure to patient: describe purpose of tests; explain how sensation of tourniquet, alcohol swab, and needlestick will feel.	Anticipatory guidance helps to reduce anxiety.

IMPLEMENTATION

1 Bring equipment to bedside and organize.	Facilitates procedure.
2 Identify patient using two identifiers (i.e., name and birthday or name and account number) according to agency policy. Compare identifiers in MAR/medical record with information on patient's identification bracelet and/or ask patient to state name.	Ensures correct patient. Complies with The Joint Commission standards and improves patient safety (TJC, 2012).
3 Close bedside curtain or room door. Perform hand hygiene.	Provides for privacy. Reduces transmission of infection.
4 Raise or lower bed to comfortable working height.	Reduces strain on your back muscles and improves access to venipuncture site.
5 Help patient to supine or semi-Fowler's position with arms extended to form straight line from shoulders to wrists. Place small pillow or towel under upper arm. (*Option:* Lower arm briefly so it fills veins in hand and lower arm with blood.)	Helps to stabilize extremity because arms are most common sites of venipuncture. Supported position in bed reduces chance of injury to patient if fainting occurs.
6 Apply tourniquet so it can be removed by pulling an end with single motion.	Tourniquet blocks venous return to heart from extremity, causing veins to dilate for easier visibility.
a Position tourniquet 5 to 10 cm (2 to 4 inches) above venipuncture site selected (antecubital fossa site is most often used).	
b Cross tourniquet over patient's arm (see illustration). May place tourniquet over gown sleeve to protect skin.	Older adult's skin is very fragile.
c Hold tourniquet between your fingers close to arm. Tuck loop between patient's arm and tourniquet so you can grasp free end easily (see illustration).	Pull free end to release tourniquet after venipuncture.

Clinical Decision Point *Palpate distal pulse (e.g., radial) below tourniquet. If pulse is not palpable, remove tourniquet, wait 60 seconds, and reapply it more loosely. If tourniquet is too tight, pressure will impede arterial blood flow.*

7 Do not keep tourniquet on patient longer than 1 minute.	Prolonged tourniquet application causes stasis, localized acidemia, and hemoconcentration (Pagana and Pagana, 2011).
8 Ask patient to *gently* open and close fist several times, finally leaving fist clenched.	Facilitates distention of veins by forcing blood up from distal veins. Vigorous open and close may cause erroneous laboratory results from hemoconcentration (Pagana and Pagana, 2011).

STEP	RATIONALE
9 Quickly inspect extremity for best venipuncture site, looking for straight, prominent vein without swelling or hematoma. Of three veins located in antecubital area, median cubital vein is preferred (see illustration).	Straight and intact veins are easiest to puncture.
10 Apply clean gloves. Palpate selected vein with finger (see illustration). Note if vein is firm and rebounds when palpated or if it feels rigid or cordlike and rolls when palpated. Avoid vigorously slapping vein, which can cause vasospasm.	Patent, healthy vein is elastic and rebounds on palpation. Thrombosed vein is rigid, rolls easily, and is difficult to puncture.
11 Obtain blood specimen.	
a Syringe method:	
(1) Have syringe with appropriate needle securely attached.	Needle must not dislodge from syringe during venipuncture.
(2) Clean venipuncture site with antiseptic swab, with first swab moving back and forth on horizontal plane, another swab on vertical plane, and last in circular motion from site outward for about 5 cm (2 inches) for 30 seconds. Allow to dry.	Antimicrobial agent cleans skin surface of resident bacteria so organisms do not enter puncture site. Allowing antiseptic to dry completes its antimicrobial task and reduces "sting" of venipuncture. Alcohol left on skin can cause hemolysis of sample and retraction of tissue away from puncture site.
(a) If drawing sample for blood alcohol level or blood cultures, use only antiseptic swab, not alcohol swab.	Ensures accurate test results.
(3) Remove needle cover and inform patient that "stick" lasts only a few seconds.	Patient has better control over anxiety when prepared for what to expect.

Clinical Decision Point *Observe needle for defects such as burrs, which can cause increased discomfort and damage to patient's vein (McCall and Tankersley, 2012).*

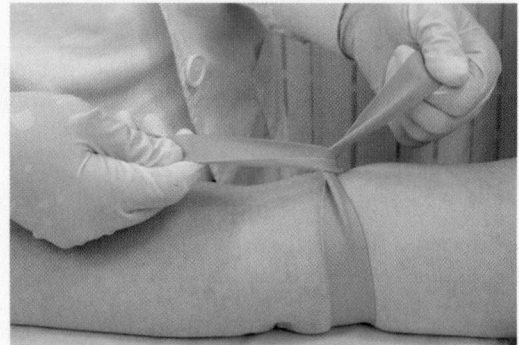

STEP 6b   Cross tourniquet over arm.

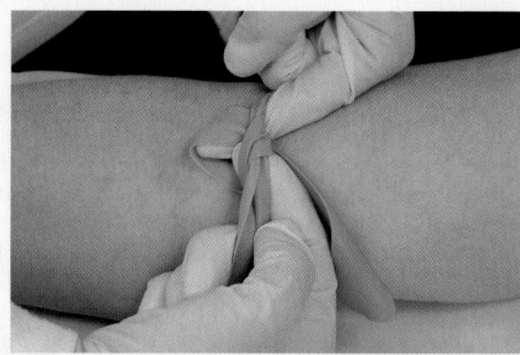

STEP 6c   Tuck loop between patient's arm and tourniquet.

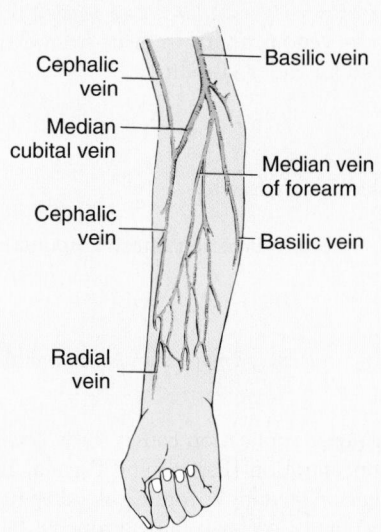

STEP 9   Location of antecubital veins.

Cephalic vein
Basilic vein
Median cubital vein
Median vein of forearm
Cephalic vein
Basilic vein
Radial vein

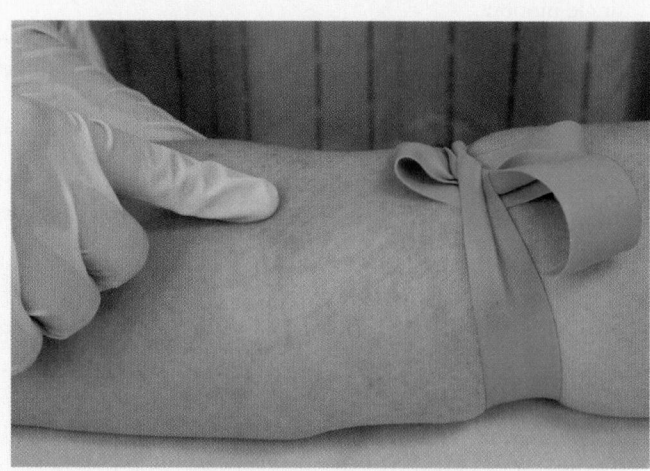

STEP 10   Palpate vein.

STEP	RATIONALE
(4) Place thumb or forefinger of nondominant hand 2.5 cm (1 inch) below site and gently pull skin taut. Stretch skin steadily until vein is stabilized.	Stabilizes vein and prevents rolling during needle insertion.
(5) Hold syringe and needle at 15- to 30-degree angle from patient's arm with bevel up.	Reduces chance of penetrating both sides of vein during insertion. Bevel up decreases chance of contamination by not dragging bevel opening over skin and allows point of needle to first puncture skin, reducing trauma.
(6) Slowly insert needle into vein, stopping when "pop" is felt as needle enters vein (see illustration).	Prevents puncture through vein to opposite side.
(7) Hold syringe securely and pull back gently on plunger.	Syringe held securely prevents needle from advancing. Pulling on plunger creates vacuum needed to draw blood into syringe. If plunger is pulled back too quickly, pressure may collapse vein.
(8) Observe for blood return (see illustration).	If blood flow fails to appear, needle may not be in vein.
(9) Obtain desired amount of blood, keeping needle stabilized.	Test results are more accurate when required amount of blood is obtained. You cannot perform some tests without minimal blood requirement. Movement of needle increases discomfort.
(10) After obtaining specimen, release tourniquet.	Reduces bleeding at site when needle is withdrawn.
(11) Apply 2 × 2–inch gauze pad without applying pressure. Quickly but carefully withdraw needle from vein and apply pressure following removal of needle (see illustration). Check for hematoma.	Pressure over needle can cause discomfort. Careful removal of needle minimizes discomfort and vein trauma. Hematoma may cause compression injury (McCall and Tankersley, 2012).
(12) Activate safety cover and immediately discard needle in appropriate container.	Prevents needlestick injury.

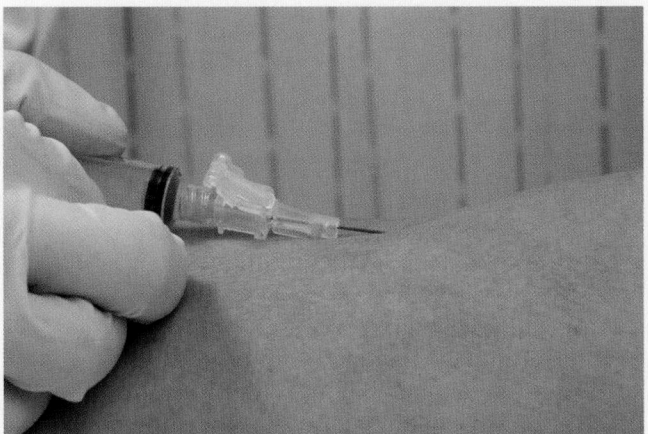

STEP 11a(6)   Inserting needle into vein.

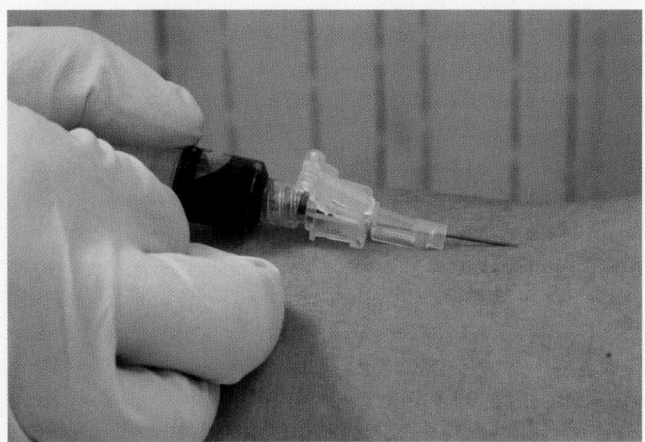

STEP 11a(8)   Observe for blood return.

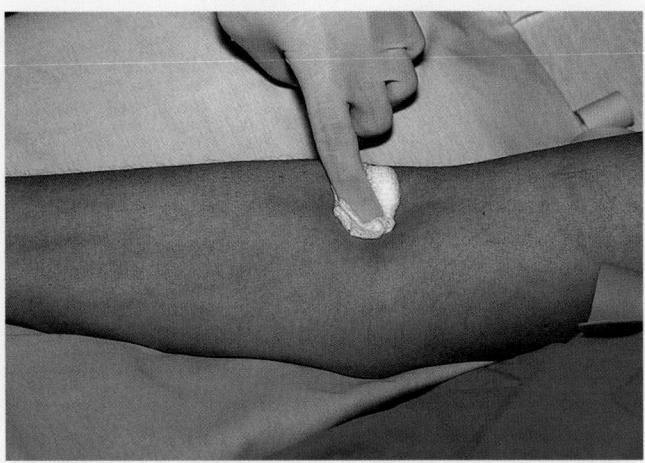

STEP 11a(11)   Application of gauze to puncture site.

STEP	RATIONALE
(13) Attach blood-filled syringe to needle-free blood transfer device. Attach tube and allow vacuum to fill tube to specified level. Remove and fill other tubes as appropriate (see illustration). Gently rotate each tube back and forth 8 to 10 times.	Additives prevent clotting. Shaking can cause hemolysis of red blood cells (RBCs).
b Vacutainer system method:	
(1) Attach double-ended needle to Vacutainer tube (see illustration).	Long end of needle is used to puncture vein. Short end fits into blood tubes.
(2) Have proper blood specimen tube resting inside Vacutainer device but do not puncture rubber stopper.	Puncturing causes loss of tube vacuum.
(3) Clean venipuncture site by following Steps 11a(2) and 11a(2)(a) for antiseptic swab. Allow to dry.	Cleans skin surface of resident bacteria so organisms do not enter puncture site. Drying maximizes effect of antiseptic.
(4) Remove needle cover and inform patient that "stick" will occur, lasting only a few seconds.	Patient has better control over anxiety when prepared about what to expect.
(5) Place thumb or forefinger of nondominant hand 2.5 cm (1 inch) *below* site and gently pull skin taut. Stretch skin down until vein stabilizes.	Helps to stabilize vein and prevent rolling during needle insertion.
(6) Hold Vacutainer needle at 15- to 30-degree angle from arm with bevel up.	Smallest and sharpest point of needle will puncture skin first. Reduces chance of penetrating sides of vein during insertion. Keeping bevel up causes less trauma to vein.
(7) Slowly insert needle into vein (see illustration).	Prevents puncture on opposite side.
(8) Grasp Vacutainer securely and advance specimen tube into needle of holder (do not advance needle in vein).	Pushing needle through stopper breaks vacuum and causes flow of blood into tube. If needle in vein advances, vein may become punctured on other side.
(9) Note flow of blood into tube, which should be fairly rapid (see illustration).	Failure of blood to appear indicates that vacuum in tube is lost or needle is not in vein.

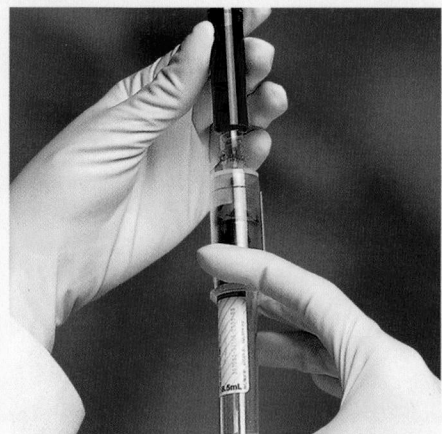

STEP 11a(13) Attach blood filled syringe to needle-free blood transfer device.

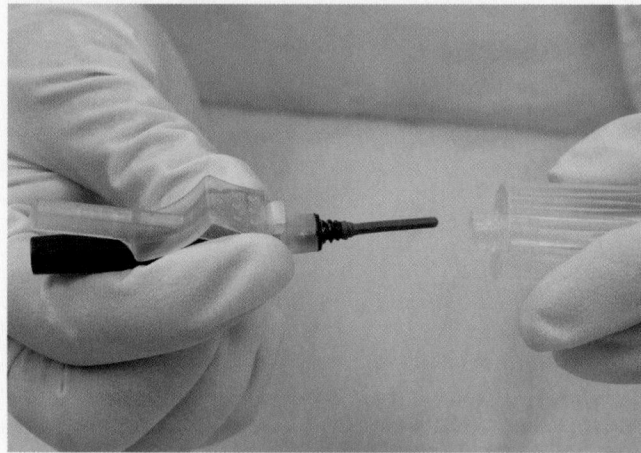

STEP 11b(1) Attaching double-ended needle to Vacutainer tube.

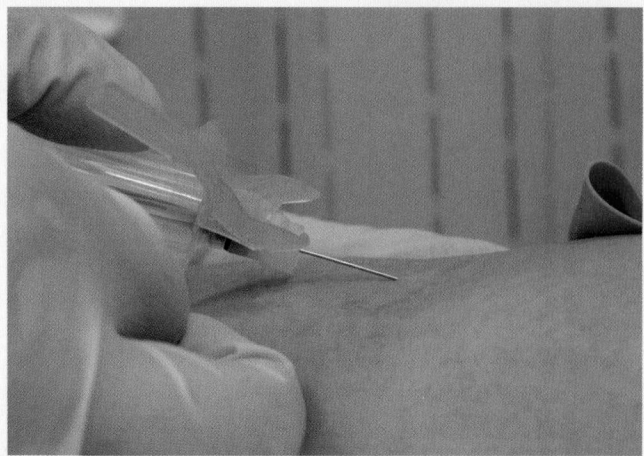

STEP 11b(7) Inserting Vacutainer needle into vein.

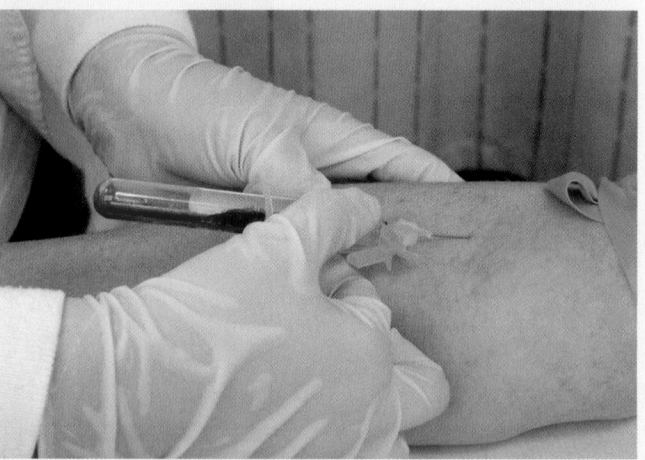

STEP 11b(9) Blood flowing into tube.

STEP	RATIONALE
(10) After filling specimen tube, grasp Vacutainer firmly and remove tube. Insert additional specimen tubes as needed. Gently rotate each tube back and forth 8 to 10 times.	Vacuum in tube stops flow at amount to be collected. Grasping prevents needle from advancing or dislodging. Tube should fill completely because additives in certain tubes are measured in proportion to filled tube. Ensures proper mixing with additive to prevent clotting.
(11) After last tube is filled and removed from Vacutainer, release tourniquet.	Reduces bleeding at site when needle is withdrawn.
(12) Apply 2 × 2–inch gauze pad over puncture site without applying pressure and quickly but carefully withdraw needle with Vacutainer from vein.	Pressure over needle can cause discomfort. Careful removal of needle minimizes discomfort and vein trauma.
(13) Immediately apply pressure over venipuncture site with gauze or antiseptic pad for 2 to 3 minutes or until bleeding stops. Observe for hematoma. Tape gauze dressing securely.	Direct pressure minimizes bleeding and prevents hematoma formation. Hematoma may cause compression and nerve injury. Pressure dressing controls bleeding.
(14) Dispose of syringe, needle, gauze, and other supplies in appropriate containers.	Safe disposal of supplies exposed to body fluids prevents transfer of microorganisms.

c Blood culture:

STEP	RATIONALE
(1) Clean venipuncture site as in Step 11a(2) with antiseptic swab or follow agency policy. Allow to dry.	Antimicrobial agent cleans skin surface so organisms do not enter puncture site or contaminate culture. Drying ensures complete antimicrobial action and decreases stinging.
(2) Clean bottle tops of culture bottles for 15 seconds with agency-approved cleaning solution. Allow to dry.	Ensures that bottle top is sterile.
(3) Collect 10 to 15 mL of venous blood using syringe method (see Step 11a) in 20-mL syringe from two different venipuncture sites.	Two blood cultures must be collected from two different sites to confirm culture growth (Pagana and Pagana, 2011).
(4) With each specimen activate safety guard and discard needle. Replace with new sterile needle before injecting each blood sample into culture bottle.	Maintains sterile technique and prevents contamination of specimen.
(5) If both aerobic and anaerobic cultures are needed, fill anaerobic bottle first.	Anaerobic organisms may take longer to grow (Pagana and Pagana, 2011).
(6) Gently mix blood in each culture bottle.	Mixes medium and blood.

d Central venous catheter (CVC) collection:

STEP	RATIONALE
(1) Select appropriate port on IV catheter (see illustration). Turn off all IV pumps and clamp lumens.	If more than one lumen, select distal lumen if possible (Alexander et al., 2010). Prevents dilution of sample with medication or total parenteral nutrition (TPN).
(2) Wipe all Luer-Lok caps with alcohol-wipe antiseptic solution or remove Luer-Lok alcohol-impregnated cap (DualCap System) (see illustration). Attach 10-mL saline prefilled syringe to selected port. Release clamp. Aspirate gently for blood return. Flush with 5 to 10 mL normal saline (NS) (check agency policy). Do not use syringe smaller than 10 mL. Remove syringe.	Luer-Lok–impregnated caps recommended by INS (2011). 70% isopropyl alcohol impregnated Luer-Lok cap (DualCap System) eliminates issue of wiping CVC ports adequately (Buchman et al., 2009). Aspirating and flushing ensures patency of selected lumen and catheter in vein. Pressure from small syringe may damage catheter.

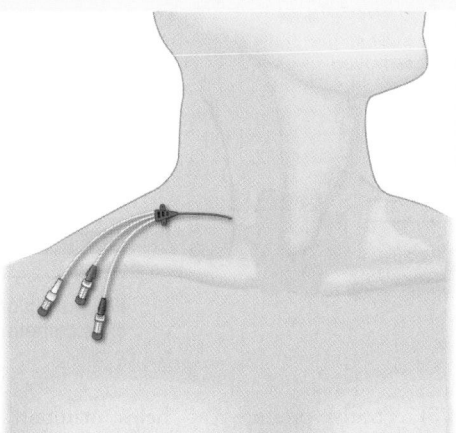

STEP 11d(1) Triple-lumen central venous catheter; select appropriate distal lumen port.

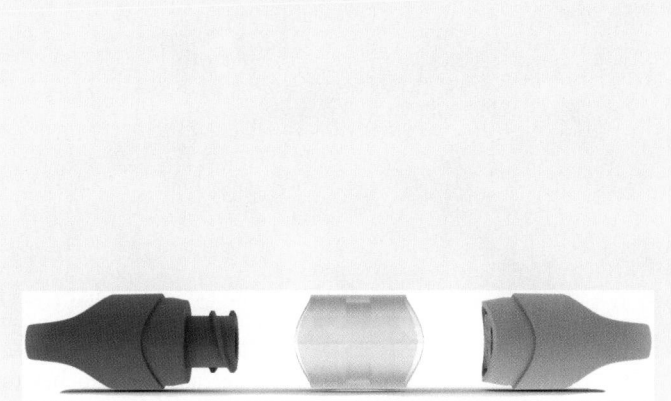

STEP 11d(2) DualCap System. Disinfects and protects both IV catheter needleless Luer access and end of IV tubing.

STEP	RATIONALE
(3) Wipe port with alcohol wipe. For **syringe method** attach syringe to selected port, aspirate 5 mL of blood, and discard. Reclamp catheter. Wipe port, attach 10- to 20-mL Luer-Lok syringe, unclamp catheter, and aspirate desired amount of blood. Reclamp catheter and remove syringe. Clean catheter port with alcohol. To transfer blood from syringe to specimen tube, use a Vacutainer holder with Luer-Lok attachment. Insert appropriate specimen tube into Vacutainer holder. Attach syringe to Luer-Lok attachment and fill desired tubes.	Discard ensures that blood sample is not contaminated with IV fluids, medication, or other products. Tubes have vacuum and automatically fill to necessary amount.
(4) For **Vacutainer method**, clamp catheter and attach needleless connecter to Vacutainer holder. Place blood tube into Vacutainer holder. Disinfect injection or access cap with alcohol. Insert Vacutainer needleless connection into injection or access cap, unclamp catheter, and advance blood tube into holder to activate blood flow. Allow blood to fill tube, clamp catheter, and discard first tube in appropriate biohazard container. Attach specimen tubes to Vacutainer with Luer-Lok adapter, unclamp catheter, and obtain blood specimens (see illustration).	Tubes have vacuum and automatically fill to necessary amount.
(5) After all specimens are collected, clamp catheter. Remove Vacutainer holder and needleless connection from injection or access cap and disinfect with alcohol.	Reduces risk for contamination by bloodborne pathogens.
(6) Attach 10-mL prefilled NS syringe and flush with 5 to 10 mL NS using push, pause method. Ensure positive pressure for lumen. Cap with spring automatically has positive pressure; thus syringe can be removed, and lumen locked (see illustration). For caps without positive pressure, hold syringe plunger steady at completion of flush, lock off lumen with slide clamp, and remove syringe. Reattach alcohol-impregnated cap.	Push, pause creates turbulence that helps to clear lumen. Positive pressure prevents blood from flowing into tip of catheter and forming clot.
(7) Blood tubes contain additives; gently rotate back and forth 8 to 10 times.	Additives mix with blood to prevent clotting. Shaking can cause hemolysis of RBCs producing inaccurate test results.
12 Check tubes for any sign of external contamination with blood. Decontaminate with 70% alcohol if necessary.	Prevents cross-contamination. Reduces risk for exposure to pathogens present in blood.
13 Remove gloves and perform hand hygiene after specimen is obtained and any spillage is cleaned.	Reduces risk for exposure to bloodborne pathogens.
14 Help patient to comfortable position.	

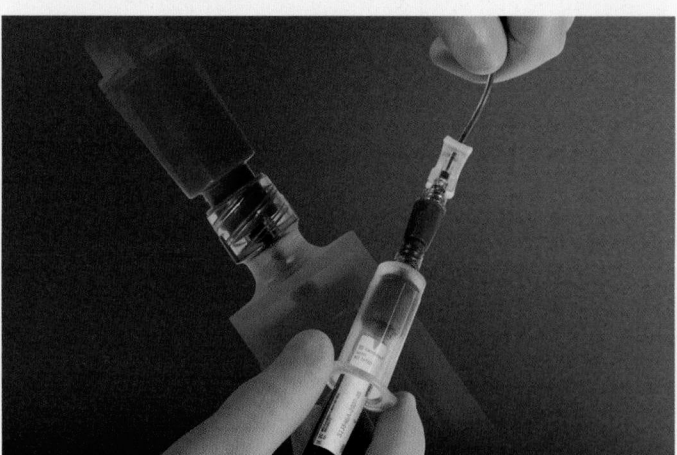

STEP 11d(4)　Male Luer-Lok Vacutainer adapter attaches to port; blood draws directly into specimen tubes. (*Courtesy and copyright* © *Becton Dickinson.*)

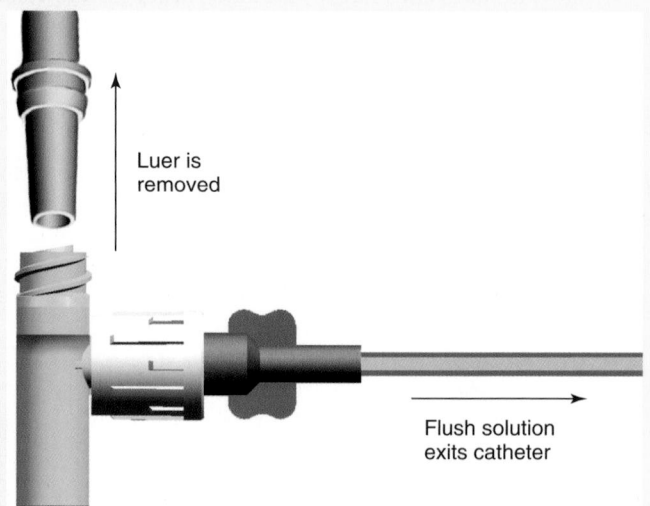

Luer is removed

Flush solution exits catheter

STEP 11d(6)　Positive-pressure cap helps maintain patency of vascular access device. (*With permission, courtesy ICU Medical, San Clemente, Calif.*)

STEP	RATIONALE
15 Securely attach properly completed identification label to each tube and affix proper requisition. Verify identifiers in front of patient (TJC, 2012).	Incorrect identification of specimen could result in diagnostic or therapeutic errors.
16 Place specimens in plastic biohazard bag and send to laboratory. Cultures must be sent to laboratory within 30 minutes (Pagana and Pagana, 2011).	Minimizes spread of microorganisms.
17 Perform hand hygiene.	Reduces transfer of microorganisms.

EVALUATION

1 Reinspect venipuncture site for homeostasis.	Determines if bleeding has stopped or hematoma has formed.
2 Determine if patient remains anxious or fearful.	Some patients require more blood tests in future. Address concerns and let patient express anxiety.
3 Check laboratory report for test results.	Reveals constituents of blood specimen.
4 Ask patient to explain purposes of tests.	Validates learning.

Unexpected Outcomes	Related Interventions
1 Hematoma forms at venipuncture site.	• Apply pressure using 2 × 2–inch gauze dressing. • Continue to monitor patient for pain and discomfort.
2 Bleeding at site continues.	• Apply pressure to site; patient may also apply pressure. • Monitor patient. • Notify health care provider.
3 Signs and symptoms of infection at venipuncture site occur.	• Notify health care provider. • Apply moist heat to site (see Chapter 40).
4 Laboratory tests reveal abnormal blood results.	• Notify health care provider.

Recording and Reporting

• Record method used to obtain blood specimen, date and time collected, type of test ordered, disposition of specimen, and description of venipuncture site.
• Report any STAT or abnormal test results to health care provider.

Special Considerations

Teaching

• Instruct patient to briefly apply pressure to venipuncture site. Patients with bleeding disorders or those undergoing anticoagulant therapy should apply pressure for at least 5 minutes.
• Instruct patient to notify nurse or health care provider if persistent or recurrent bleeding or expanding hematoma develops at venipuncture site.

Pediatric

• Explain procedure to child at developmentally appropriate age and provide atraumatic care (Hockenberry and Wilson, 2011).
• Because children often fear that loss of their blood is a threat to their lives, explain to them that their blood is continually being produced. An adhesive bandage gives them assurance that

their blood will not leak out through puncture site (Hockenberry and Wilson, 2011).
• At times it is advantageous to draw children's blood specimens in a treatment room instead of in bed or room to maintain feeling that their room is a safe place (Hockenberry and Wilson, 2011).
• When performing venipuncture on children, explore sources for vein access: scalp, antecubital fossa, saphenous, and hand veins.
• Application of EMLA cream to the venipuncture site may be ordered before the stick to reduce pain in infants and young children (Hockenberry and Wilson, 2011).
• Vacutainers are not recommended in children under 2 years of age because of possible vein collapse with their use.

Gerontologic

• Older adults have fragile veins that are easily traumatized during venipuncture. Sometimes application of warm compresses may help to obtain samples. Using small-bore catheter may be beneficial.

Home Care

• In home care setting a blood pressure cuff rather than a tourniquet can be used for venipuncture.

SKILL 43-9 Blood Glucose Monitoring

Blood glucose monitoring allows patients with diabetes mellitus to self-manage their disease. Obtaining capillary blood by skin puncture is an alternative to reduce the frequency of needlesticks when you cannot perform venipuncture. The procedure is less painful than venipuncture, and the ease of the skin puncture method makes it possible for patients to

perform this procedure. The development of reagent strips, home glucose monitors, and the skin puncture method has revolutionized home management care of patients with diabetes mellitus.

Glucose levels can be evaluated by performing a skin puncture and using either a visually read test (e.g., Chemstrip bG, Glucostix) or a reflectance meter. The visually read test does not require an expensive machine, but the patient must be able to visually interpret the results. A single drop of blood is applied to a specifically prepared reagent strip; the strip is read, and the results are compared to the color chart on the container. Measurement by a visually read test may not be accurate but can be useful for screening.

Blood glucose reflectance meters are lightweight and run on batteries (e.g., AccuChek III, OneTouch) (Fig. 43-5). After a drop of blood from the skin puncture is dropped or wicked onto a reagent strip, the meter provides an accurate measurement of blood glucose level in 5 to 50 seconds. Point-of-care (POC) blood glucose testing meters should be dedicated for single-patient use. If single-patient use is not possible, meters must be cleaned and disinfected (US FDA, 2011).

Reflectance meters use a wet-wash or dry-wipe method of testing. To perform a wet wash, the user flushes the blood-coated reagent strip with water before inserting the strip into the glucose meter. The dry-wipe method requires the user to wipe off the blood-coated reagent strip with a dry cotton ball before making a reading. Some products do not require blood to be flushed or wiped before a reading. The various methods allow measurement of blood glucose between 20 and 800 mg/dL, thus providing a sensitive measurement of blood glucose level.

The meters differ in several ways, including amount of blood needed for each test, testing speed, overall size, ability to store test results in memory, cost of the meter, and cost of test strips (ADA, 2011). Some larger meters are voice activated, which provides support for the older adult or patient with visual impairments. The amount of time to complete the glucose testing with the current glucose meters varies from 5 to 50 seconds. You can program some meters to monitor the glucose levels for a continuous 72 hours.

Improved technology introduced two methods for glucose measurement now available on the market. A minimally invasive glucose meter uses a very small, fine plastic sensor inserted through the abdomen and provides continuous readings of blood glucose levels (Fig. 43-6, A). A biosensor is taped on the external abdomen. Using a handheld wireless meter, a patient activates the biosensor to transmit the blood glucose level at any time without puncturing the skin (Fig. 43-6, B). Another model, considered a noninvasive glucose meter, does not prick the skin with a needle but uses precise laser technology or light beam to puncture the skin, resulting in less damage to tissue. For the patient with diabetes mellitus who requires assessment of trends and patterns, these systems are ideal.

Testing of glycosylated hemoglobin (HbA_{1c}) evaluates the amount of glucose available in the bloodstream over the 120-day life span of a red blood cell. HbA_{1c} provides an accurate long-term index of a patient's average blood glucose level drawn by venous puncture (Pagana and Pagana, 2011).

Delegation and Collaboration

Assessment of a patient's condition cannot be delegated to nursing assistive personnel (NAP). When the patient's condition is stable, the skill of obtaining and testing a sample of blood for blood glucose level can be delegated to NAP. The nurse informs the NAP by:

- Explaining appropriate sites to use for puncture and when to obtain glucose levels.
- Reviewing expected blood glucose levels and when to report unexpected glucose levels to the nurse.

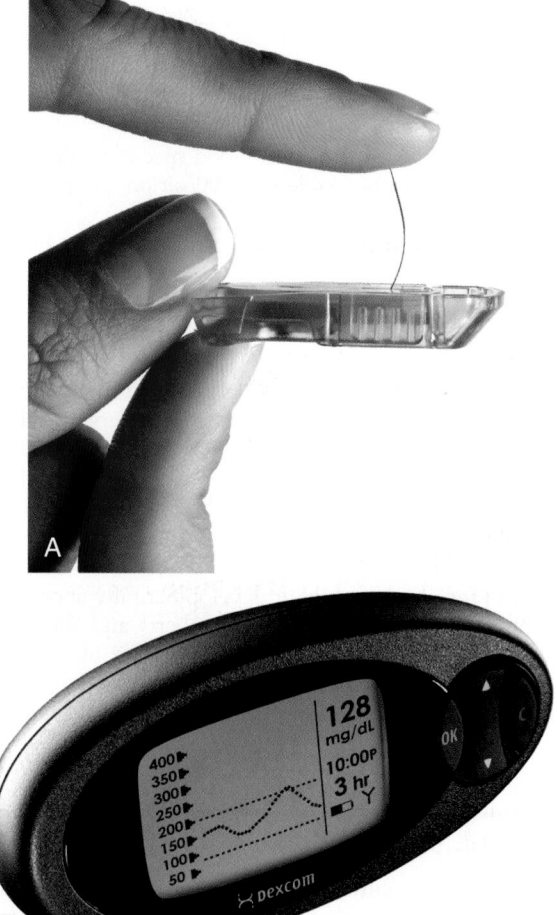

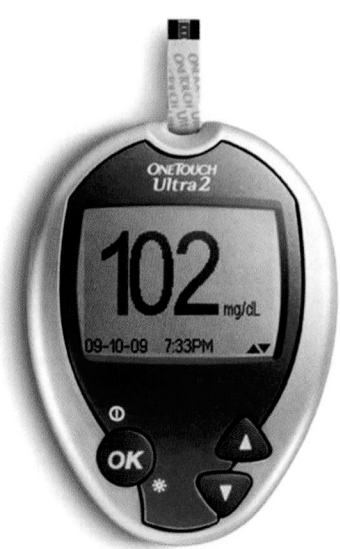

FIG 43-5   Blood glucose monitor. (*Courtesy LifeScan, Milpitas, Calif.*)

FIG 43-6   **A,** Tiny sensor implanted under skin transmits continuous reading to receiver. **B,** Monitor displays and stores readings. (*Courtesy DexCom.*)

Equipment

- ❑ Antiseptic swab
- ❑ Cotton ball
- ❑ Lancet device, either self-activating or button activated
- ❑ Blood glucose meter (e.g., Accucheck III, OneTouch)
- ❑ Blood glucose test strips appropriate for meter brand used
- ❑ Clean gloves
- ❑ Paper towel

STEP	RATIONALE

ASSESSMENT

1 Assess patient's understanding of procedure and purpose of blood glucose monitoring. Determine if patient understands how to perform test and its importance in glucose control.	Provides baseline for developing teaching plan.
2 Determine if specific conditions need to be met before or after sample collection (e.g., fasting, postprandial, after certain medications, before insulin doses).	Dietary intake of carbohydrates and ingestion of concentrated glucose preparations alter blood glucose levels.
3 Determine if risks exist for performing skin puncture (e.g., low platelet count, anticoagulant therapy, bleeding disorders).	Abnormal clotting mechanisms increase risk for local ecchymosis and bleeding.
4 Assess area of skin to be used as puncture site. Inspect fingers or forearms for edema, inflammation, cuts, or sores. Avoid areas of bruising and open lesions. Avoid using the hand on the side of a mastectomy.	Sides of fingers are commonly selected because they have fewer nerve endings. Measurements from alternative sites are meter specific and may be different from those at traditional sites (Corbett, 2008). The puncture site should not be edematous, inflamed, or recently punctured because these factors cause increased interstitial fluid and blood to mix and also increase risk for infection.
5 Review health care provider's order for time or frequency of measurement.	Health care provider determines test schedule on basis of patient's physiologic status and risk for glucose imbalance.
6 For patient with diabetes who performs test at home, assess ability to handle skin-puncturing device. Patient may choose to continue self-testing while in hospital.	Patient's physical health may change (e.g., vision disturbance, fatigue, pain, disease process), preventing him or her from performing test.

NURSING DIAGNOSES

- Anxiety
- Deficient knowledge regarding blood glucose monitoring
- Ineffective health maintenance
- Ineffective therapeutic regimen management

Related factors are individualized based on patient's condition or needs.

PLANNING

1 Expected outcomes following completion of procedure:	
• Puncture site shows no evidence of bleeding or tissue damage.	Hemostasis is achieved. Lancet or needle did not puncture skin too deeply.
• Blood glucose measurements are accurate.	Normal fasting glucose is 70 to 110 mg/dL, indicating good metabolic control (Pagana and Pagana, 2011).
• Patient can verbalize procedure for self-monitoring blood glucose.	Demonstrates psychomotor learning.
• Patient explains test results.	Validates knowledge.
2 Explain procedure and purpose to patient and/or family. Offer patient and family opportunity to practice testing procedures. Provide resources/teaching aids for patient and family caregiver.	Promotes understanding and cooperation.

IMPLEMENTATION

1 Identify patient using two identifiers (i.e., name and birthday or name and account number) according to agency policy. Compare identifiers in MAR/medical record with information on patient's identification bracelet and/or have patient state name.	Ensures correct patient. Complies with The Joint Commission standards and improves patient safety (TJC, 2012).
2 Perform hand hygiene. Instruct adult to perform hand hygiene, including forearm (if applicable) with soap and water. Rinse and dry.	Promotes skin cleansing and vasodilation at selected puncture site. Reduces transmission of microorganisms.
3 Position patient comfortably in chair or in semi-Fowler's position in bed.	Ensures easy accessibility to puncture site. Patient will assume position when self-testing.

STEP	RATIONALE
4 Remove reagent strip from vial and tightly seal cap. Check code on test strip vial. Use only test strips recommended for glucose meter. Some newer meters do not require code and/or have disk or drum with 10 or more test strips.	Protects strips from accidental discoloration caused by exposure to air or light. Code on test strip vial must match code entered into glucose meter.
5 Insert strip into meter (refer to manufacturer directions (see illustration). Do not bend strip. Meter turns on automatically.	Some machines must be calibrated; others require zeroing of timer. Each meter is adjusted differently.
6 Remove unused reagent strip from meter and place on paper towel or clean, dry surface with test pad facing up (see manufacturer directions).	Moisture on strip can alter accuracy of final test results.
7 Meter displays code on screen that must match code from test strip vial. Press proper button on meter to confirm matching codes. Meter is ready for use.	Codes must match for meter to operate. Meters have different messages that confirm that meter is ready for testing and blood can be applied.
8 Perform hand hygiene and apply clean gloves. Prepare single-use lancet or multiple-use lancet device. NOTE: Some meters recommend that this step be completed before preparing test strip. Remove cap from lancet device; insert new lancet. Some lancet devices have disk or cylinder that rotates to new lancet.	Reduces transmission of microorganisms. Never reuse a lancet because of risk of infection.
a Twist off protective cover on tip of lancet. Replace cap of lancet device.	
b Cock lancet device, adjusting for proper puncture depth.	Each patient varies as to depth of insertion needed for lancet to produce blood drop.
9 Obtain blood sample.	
a Wipe patient's finger or forearm lightly with antiseptic swab. Choose vascular area for puncture site. In stable adults select lateral side of finger. Avoid central tip of finger, which has denser nerve supply (Pagana and Pagana, 2011).	Removes microorganisms from skin surface. Side of finger is less sensitive to pain.
b Hold area to be punctured in dependent position. Do not milk or massage finger site.	Increases blood flow to area before puncture. Milking may hemolyze specimen and introduce excess tissue fluid (Pagana and Pagana, 2011).
c Hold tip of lancet device against area of skin chosen for test site (see illustration). Press release button on device. Some devices allow you to see blood sample forming. Remove device.	Placement ensures that lancet enters skin properly.
d With some devices a blood sample begins to appear. Otherwise gently squeeze or massage fingertip until round drop of blood forms (see illustration).	Adequate-size blood sample is needed to test glucose.
10 Obtain test results.	Exposure of blood to test strip for prescribed time ensures proper results.

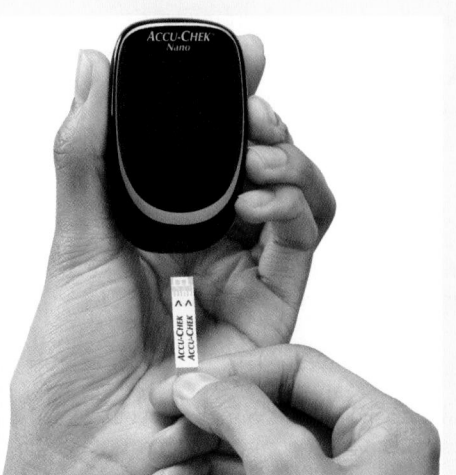

STEP 5 Load test strip into meter. (*Courtesy Accucheck Glucometer.*)

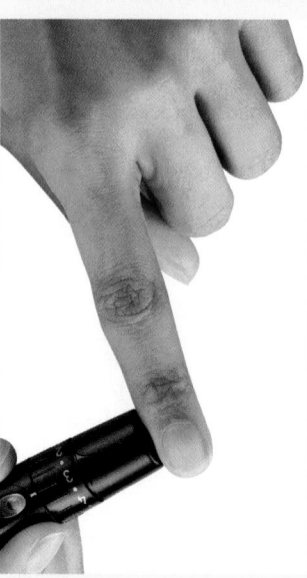

STEP 9c Prick side of finger with lancet. (*Courtesy Accucheck Glucometer.*)

STEP	RATIONALE

Clinical Decision Point *Some meters (e.g., OneTouch [LifeScan]) require blood sample to be applied to test strip already in the meter. Once the drop of blood is applied, the meter automatically calculates the reading.*

a Be sure that meter is still on. Bring test strip in meter to drop of blood. Blood will be wicked onto test strip (see illustration). Follow specific meter instructions to be sure that you obtain adequate sample.

Blood enters strip, and glucose device shows message on screen to signal that enough blood is obtained.

Clinical Decision Point *Do not scrape blood onto the test strips or apply it to wrong side of test strip. This prevents accurate glucose measurement.*

b Blood glucose test result will appear on screen (see illustration). Some devices "beep" when completed.

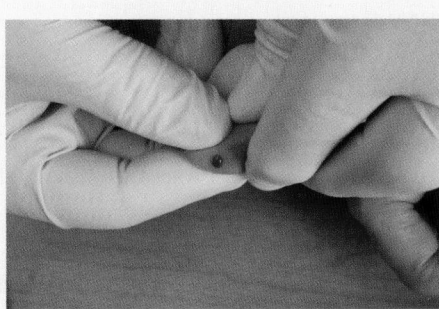

STEP 9d Gently squeeze puncture site until drop of blood forms.

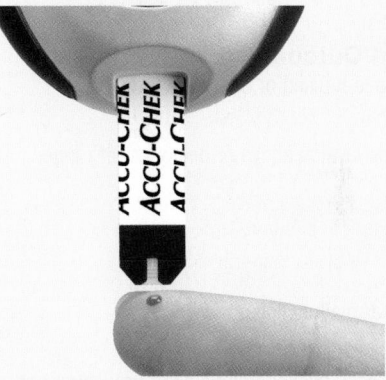

STEP 10a Touch test strip to blood drop. Blood wicks into test strip. (*Courtesy Accucheck Glucometer.*)

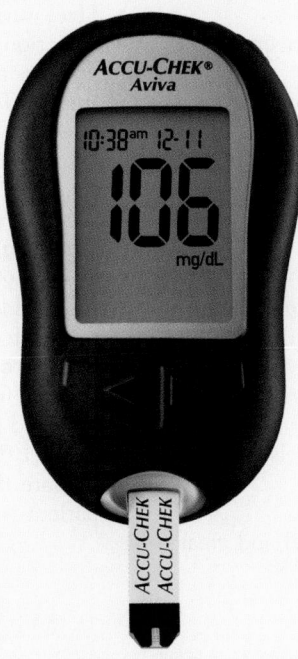

STEP 10b Results appear on meter screen. (*Courtesy Accucheck Glucometer.*)

STEP	RATIONALE
11 Turn meter off. Some meters turn off automatically. Dispose of test strip, lancet, and gloves in proper receptacles.	Meter is battery powered. Proper disposal reduces risk for needlestick injury and spread of infection.
12 Perform hand hygiene.	Reduces transmission of microorganisms.
13 Discuss test results with patient and encourage questions and eventual participation in care if this is a new diabetes mellitus diagnosis.	Promotes participation and compliance with therapy.

EVALUATION

1 Reinspect puncture site for bleeding or tissue injury.	Site can be source of discomfort and infection.
2 Compare glucose meter reading with normal blood glucose levels and previous test results.	Determines if glucose level is normal.
3 Ask patient to discuss procedure.	Validates level of learning.
4 Ask patient to explain test results and perform next reading.	Results of test may cause anxiety. Patient may misunderstand specific step of procedure. Return demonstration reinforces learning.

Unexpected Outcomes	Related Interventions
1 Puncture site is bruised or continues to bleed.	• Apply pressure. • Notify health care provider if bleeding continues.
2 Blood glucose level is above or below target range.	• Continue to monitor patient. • Check if there are medication orders for deviations in glucose level. • Notify health care provider. • Administer insulin or carbohydrate source as ordered, depending on glucose level.
3 Glucose meter malfunctions.	• Review instructions for troubleshooting glucose meter. • Repeat test.
4 Patient expresses misunderstanding of procedure and results.	• Repeat instructions to patient. • Have patient demonstrate procedure.

Recording and Reporting

- Record procedure and glucose level in nurses' notes or special flow sheet and action taken for abnormal range.
- Describe patient response, including appearance of puncture site, in nurses' notes.
- Describe explanations or teaching provided in nurses' notes.
- Record and report abnormal blood glucose levels.

Special Considerations

Teaching

- Provide information on where patient with diabetes mellitus can obtain testing supplies. When possible, teach with the same meter that patient will use at home.
- Provide patient with information on where to obtain assistance if glucose meter has malfunctioned.
- Stress importance of the timing of blood glucose levels, particularly in patients with diabetes mellitus.

Pediatric

- Allow young children to choose puncture site; heel and great toe are common puncture sites in infants.

- Heel warming helps to obtain specimen from a neonate.
- Infection or abscess of the heel and necrotizing osteochondritis are the most serious complications of heelstick puncture in infants. To avoid osteochondritis make sure that puncture is not deeper than 2 mm and is made at the outer aspect of the heel (Hockenberry and Wilson, 2011).
- Allow young child with parent to demonstrate technique; incorporate a play activity for further understanding.

Gerontologic

- Warming fingertips may facilitate obtaining specimen.
- Some older adults have vision or dexterity problems that interfere with performing self-fingersticks.

Home Care

- Provide information on correct disposal of sharps in nonpermeable and puncture-resistant container.
- Suggest that patient attend diabetic support group if needed.
- Be sure that patient's family caregiver can perform test when patient is ill or is unable to manipulate devices.

SKILL 43-10   Obtaining an Arterial Specimen for Blood Gas Measurement

You assess effectiveness of oxygenation and ventilation by measuring arterial blood gases (ABGs). Measurement of ABGs provides valuable information in assessing and managing a patient's respiratory and metabolic disturbances (Pagana and Pagana, 2011). The parameters measured in an ABG include arterial blood pH, partial pressure of oxygen (PaO_2), partial pressure of carbon dioxide ($PaCO_2$), and arterial oxygen saturation (SaO_2). The ABG sample is easy to obtain and analyze to provide a clear picture of acid-base balance, oxygenation, and ventilation.

Each agency has a policy regarding who is allowed to obtain ABG samples. Many agencies allow nurses in specialty areas (e.g., critical care) to obtain them; others specify a certified respiratory therapist, and some require institutional certification of this skill. A decision to draw ABG samples may be a direct result of your physical assessment (see Chapter 6).

Delegation and Collaboration

The skill of obtaining an arterial blood gas sample cannot be delegated to nursing assistive personnel (NAP). The nurse informs the NAP to:

- Report any bleeding from arterial puncture site.
- Report any changes in patient vital signs, level of consciousness, or restlessness.

Equipment

- ❑ Commercial blood gas kit or individual supplies, including:
- ❑ 3-mL heparinized syringe
- ❑ 23- or 25-gauge needle with safety guard
- ❑ Filter cap (allows expelling of air and retains blood)
- ❑ Alcohol swabs (2)
- ❑ 2 × 2–inch gauze pad
- ❑ Tape
- ❑ Heparin (1 : 1000 solution)
- ❑ Cup or plastic bag with crushed ice
- ❑ Clean gloves
- ❑ Protective eyewear
- ❑ Completed identification labels with proper patient identifiers
- ❑ Completed laboratory requisition with date, time, name of test, patient identification, and source of specimen
- ❑ Small plastic biohazard bag for delivery of specimen to laboratory (or container specified by agency)

STEP	RATIONALE

ASSESSMENT

1 Assess for factors that influence ABG measurements:	Allows you to eliminate factors that interfere with accurate measurement.
a Hypoventilation or hyperventilation	Hypoventilation can cause retention of CO_2, and hyperventilation can cause decreased CO_2 levels (Hockenberry and Wilson, 2011).
b Body temperature	Change in body temperature as little as 1° F can alter blood gas values (Hockenberry and Wilson, 2011).
2 Identify medications that may influence ABG measurement (e.g., anticoagulants, diuretics).	Certain medications increase risk for bleeding at puncture site or may cause hemoconcentration.
3 Assess respiratory status, including rate, depth, rhythm, adventitious sounds, use of accessory muscles.	Physical signs and symptoms may indicate need for ABG sample.
4 Review criteria for choosing site for ABG sample.	Prevents causing compromised circulation from puncture.

Clinical Decision Point *Factors that contraindicate use of arterial site include amputation, contractures, localized infection, dressing or cast, mastectomy, or arteriovenous shunts.*

a Assess collateral blood flow. *Perform Allen test.*	Allen test assesses collateral circulation before performing arterial puncture on radial artery. Positive Allen test ensures that there is collateral circulation to hand in case thrombosis of radial artery occurs following puncture (Pagana and Pagana, 2011).
(1) Have patient make tight fist and raise hand above heart.	Removes as much blood from hand as possible.
(2) Apply direct pressure to both radial and ulnar arteries (see illustration).	Obstructs arterial blood flow to hand.
(3) Have patient lower and open hand (see illustration).	Fingers and hand should be pale and blanched, indicating lack of arterial blood flow.
(4) Release pressure over ulnar artery; observe color of fingers, thumbs, and hand (see illustration).	Flushing identifies that circulation through ulnar artery is good and that ulnar artery alone is capable of providing blood supply to entire hand. Therefore you can use radial artery for puncture.

Clinical Decision Point *If there is no flushing in 15 seconds, Allen test is negative and should be repeated on the other arm or choose another artery for puncture (Pagana and Pagana, 2011).*

STEP	RATIONALE
b Assess accessibility of vessel.	Palpating, stabilizing, and performing venipuncture of superficial artery is easier. Superficial arteries are located at distal ends of extremities.
c Assess tissue surrounding artery.	Muscle, tendon, and fat have decreased sensation to pain. Bony periosteum and nerves are highly sensitive to pain.
d Assess that arteries are not directly adjacent to veins.	Helps reduce chance of venous puncture and possibility of inaccurate samples.
5 Assess arterial sites for use in obtaining specimen.	Arterial blood may be obtained from areas where strong pulses are palpable (i.e., radial, brachial, or femoral artery) (Pagana and Pagana, 2011).

Clinical Decision Point *Previous puncture sites or preexisting conditions may eliminate potential sites (see agency policy). Artery should be easily accessible.*

a Radial artery	Safest, most accessible site for puncture; is superficial, is not adjacent to large veins, usually has adequate collateral circulation by ulnar artery, and is relatively painless if periosteum is avoided. Used when Allen's test is positive.
b Brachial artery	Has reasonable collateral blood flow, is less superficial, is more difficult to palpate and stabilize, carries increased risk for venous puncture, and results in increased discomfort for patient if brachial nerve is punctured. Used when radial artery is inaccessible or Allen's test is negative.
c Femoral artery	Nurses without specialized training should not use this artery. Has no adequate collateral flow if obstructed below inguinal ligament, is difficult to stabilize, is deep, and is directly adjacent to femoral vein. Is best artery to use in emergency (e.g., cardiac arrest or hypovolemic shock when pulses are difficult to palpate).

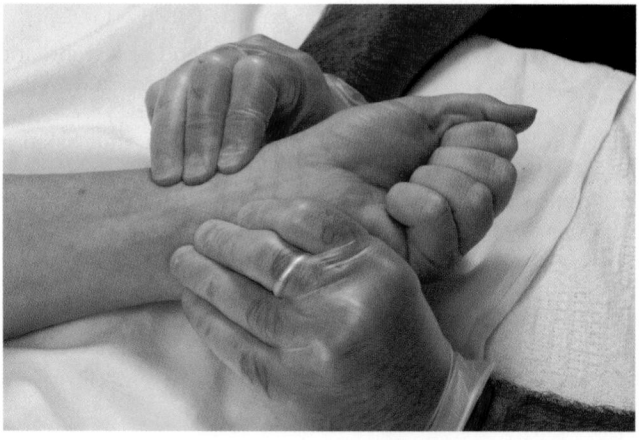

STEP 4a(2) Applying pressure to radial and ulnar arteries.

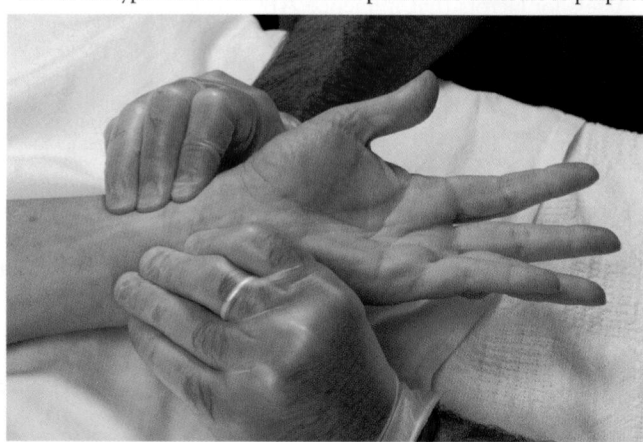

STEP 4a(3) Patient opening hand; note color.

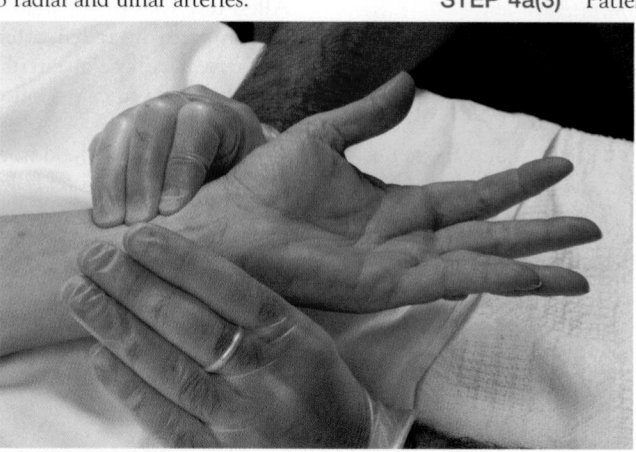

STEP 4a(4) Releasing pressure over ulnar artery, and noting color of hand.

STEP	RATIONALE
6 Review baseline ABG values for patient.	Provides baseline for comparison and evaluation of therapies.
7 Determine patient's knowledge about ABG procedure.	Obtaining blood specimen is painful. Patient who is knowledgeable will be more cooperative.

NURSING DIAGNOSES

- Anxiety
- Deficient knowledge regarding arterial blood gases
- Impaired gas exchange
- Ineffective airway clearance
- Ineffective breathing pattern
- Ineffective peripheral tissue perfusion
- Risk for injury

Related factors are individualized based on patient's condition or needs.

PLANNING

1 Expected outcomes following completion of procedure:	
• Patient's ABG values are within normal range.	Indicates adequate oxygenation.
• Patient's extremity distal to puncture remains warm and pink, has adequate capillary refill, and is free of pain.	Indicates adequate arterial circulation to extremity.
• Patient denies anxiety, and respiratory rate remains within baseline.	Anxiety increase respiratory rate, which can alter ABG results.
• Patient correctly discusses ABG procedure.	Indicates learning.
2 Prepare heparinized syringe (if not in commercial kit).	Heparin mixes with specimen to prevent clotting.
a Aspirate 0.5 mL sodium heparin (1000 units/mL) into syringe from vial or ampule.	Prevents blood sample from clotting before reaching laboratory. Excessive heparin can affect pH of arterial sample.
b Withdraw plunger entire length of syringe. Maintain asepsis.	Coats inside of barrel of syringe with heparin.
c Eject all heparin in barrel out of syringe.	In hub of syringe 0.15 to 0.25 mL of sodium heparin remains; 0.05 mL of sodium heparin adequately anticoagulates 1 mL of blood; 0.15 mL adequately anticoagulates 3 mL without affecting pH level.
3 Explain steps and purpose of procedure to patient.	Reduces anxiety and promotes understanding and cooperation.

IMPLEMENTATION

1 Identify patient using two identifiers (i.e., name and birthday or name and account number) according to agency policy. Compare identifiers in MAR/medical record with information on patient's identification bracelet and/or ask patient to state name.	Ensures correct patient. Complies with The Joint Commission standards and improves patient safety (TJC, 2012).
2 Perform hand hygiene.	Reduces transmission of infection.
3 Palpate selected radial, femoral, or brachial site with fingertips.	Determines area of maximal impulse for puncture site.
4 Using radial artery, elevate patient's wrist with small pillow and ask him or her to extend fingers downward. Stabilize artery by slight hyperextension of wrist.	This flexes wrist and positions radial artery closer to surface (Fischbach and Dunning, 2009). Reduces mobility of artery and makes insertion of needle easier.
5 Apply clean gloves. Clean area of maximal impulse with alcohol swab or antiseptic swab (check agency or manufacturer recommendation). Wipe in circular motion away from site or use back-and-forth strokes. Allow to dry.	Reduces number of resident bacteria on surface of skin. Drying maximizes antibacterial effects.
6 Hold 2 × 2 inch–gauze pad with same fingers used to palpate artery.	Keeps gauze pad accessible for covering puncture site when necessary.
7 Use corner of sterile gauze pad or alcohol wipe to point to chosen site.	Maintaining location of artery improves likelihood of successful puncture.
8 Hold needle bevel up and insert at 45-degree angle into artery. Prepare patient for needlestick because radial sticks are painful.	Angle allows for better arterial flow into needle. Prepared patient will be less likely to withdraw arm.
9 Stop advancing needle when blood is noted returning into hub of needle or syringe.	Quick return of blood indicates that arterial flow is obtained. Prevents puncturing through both sides of artery.
10 Allow arterial pulsations to pump 2 to 3 mL of blood into heparinized syringe slowly (see illustration).	Allowing pulsations to assist in filling syringe reduces presence of air bubbles in sample. Bubbles alter ABG results.
11 When sampling is complete, hold 2 × 2–inch gauze pad over puncture site, withdraw syringe and needle, and activate safety guard over needle.	Pad minimizes pulling of skin as needle is withdrawn. Decreases contamination from blood and accidental needlestick.
12 Apply pressure over and just proximal to puncture site with pad (see illustration).	Insertion of needle into artery is just proximal to insertion site through skin. Gauze absorbs any blood that might ooze from site.

STEP	RATIONALE
13 Maintain continuous pressure on and proximal to site for 3 to 5 minutes (approximately 15 minutes if patient is undergoing anticoagulant therapy or has bleeding disorder) (Pagana and Pagana, 2011). Have another nurse perform Step 16 if prolonged pressure is needed.	To avoid hematoma formation, apply and hold pressure or apply a pressure dressing to arterial puncture site for 3 to 5 minutes (Pagana and Pagana, 2011). Prevents delay in preparing syringe in ice.
14 Visually inspect site for signs of bleeding or hematoma formation.	Determines if continued need exists to exert pressure. Because artery rather than vein has been accessed, monitor puncture site for bleeding.
15 Palpate artery below or distal to puncture site.	Determines if pulse quality has changed, indicating alteration in arterial flow.
16 Take syringe, remove safety needle, and discard needle in appropriate biohazard container. Attach filter cap to syringe (available in kit) to expel air or cover tip of syringe with 2 × 2–inch sterile gauze to expel air (see agency procedure). Some kits may have all supplies, including syringe with heparin, needle with safety needle cap, and filter cap that allows air to vent and not blood (see illustration).	Decreases chance of contamination from room air. Air bubbles in specimen can falsely elevate or decrease results, depending on patient's blood gas concentration (Hockenberry and Wilson 2009; Van Leeuwen et al., 2011).
17 Prepare syringe for laboratory analysis (according to agency policy). Common principles include:	
• Place patient identification label on syringe in front of patient (TJC, 2012), confirming identifiers.	Permits proper identification of sample for laboratory.
• Place syringe in cup of crushed ice.	Failure to place ABG sample in ice bath may affect results of pH, PaO_2, and $PaCO_2$ (Van Leeuwen et al., 2011).

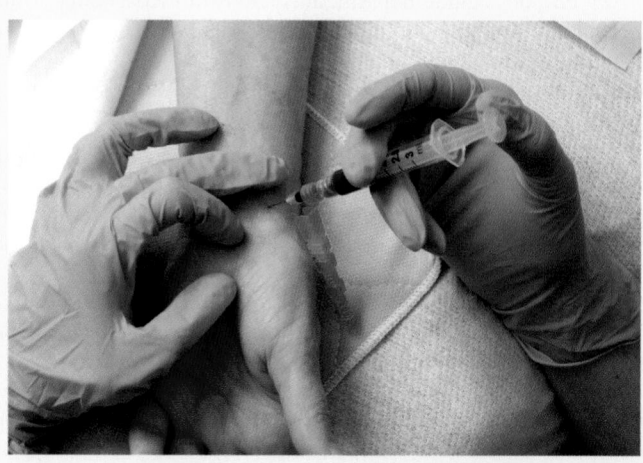

STEP 10 Blood flowing into syringe.

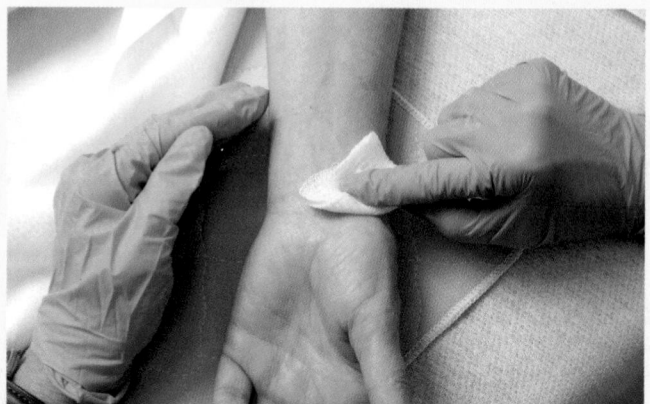

STEP 12 Applying firm pressure to arterial puncture site.

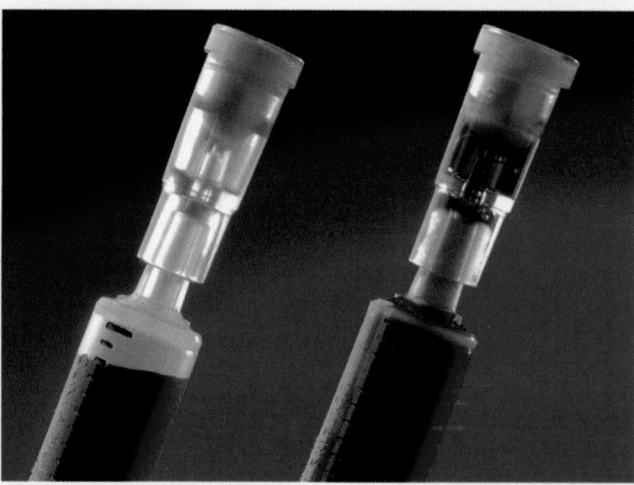

STEP 16 Filter-Pro Air Bubble Removal Device expels air safely from syringe without accidentally expelling blood and aerosolizing sample. (*With permission from Smiths Medical, Carlsbad, Calif.*)

STEP	RATIONALE
• Attach properly labeled requisition to blood gas sample, including most recent hemoglobin, mode and flow of oxygen, and patient's temperature.	Prevents mislabeled specimens in laboratory. Ensures that correct results are received for correct patient. Hyperthermia and hypothermia influence oxygen release from hemoglobin at tissue level (Fischbach and Dunning, 2009). Temperature affects amount of gas in solution. Fever increases actual PaO_2 and $PaCO_2$ (Van Leeuwen et al., 2011).
18 Place cup and sample in biohazard bag. Send sample to laboratory immediately.	Prevents alteration in gas tensions resulting from metabolic processes that continue after blood is drawn (Fischbach and Dunning, 2009).
19 Remove gloves and perform hand hygiene.	Reduces transmission of microorganisms.

EVALUATION

1 Inspect puncture site and area distal to puncture site for complications.	An artery can be obstructed, or important structures anatomically juxtaposed to an artery can be penetrated (Pagana and Pagana, 2011).
2 Review results of sample as soon as possible.	Identifies any abnormality and expedites initiation of treatment.

Unexpected Outcomes

1 Patient has abnormal ABG values.

2 Patient has hematoma formation at puncture site.

3 Puncture site is bruised or continues to bleed.

Related Interventions

• Continue to monitor patient.
• Notify health care provider of findings and obtain further orders.

• Apply warm compresses to enhance absorption of blood (see Chapter 40).
• Continue to monitor patient.
• Notify health care provider.

• Apply pressure.
• Notify health care provider if bleeding continues.

Recording and Reporting

• Record results of Allen test, location and condition of puncture site, patient's tolerance of procedure, and disposition of specimen to laboratory in nurses' notes.
• Report ABG results to health care provider as soon as available.
• Report patient's FiO_2 and any ventilator settings (e.g., tidal volume [V_T], respiratory frequency [RF], mode of ventilation).
• Record results of test in nurses notes.

Special Considerations
Teaching
• Teach patient to report numbness, burning, and/or tingling during and after in hand that had radial artery puncture.

Pediatric
• In neonatal and pediatric patients you can use capillary blood gas. Procedures are similar to those for obtaining heelsticks.
• When dealing with neonatal patients, especially premature infants, normal values for ABGs often differ from those of adults.
• Arterial blood samples from punctures are painful and cause crying and breath holding that affect the accuracy of blood gas values (decreases PaO_2) (Hockenberry and Wilson, 2011).

Gerontologic
• Pay special attention during interpretation of ABGs for patients with chronic pulmonary conditions. In these patients compensatory mechanisms may allow normal pH in face of markedly elevated $PaCO_2$.

Critical Thinking Exercises

Mrs. Yamamoto is a 76-year-old who was admitted with pneumonia today. She has a productive cough. She also has a history of diabetes mellitus. Her blood glucose level on admission is 208 mg/dL. She speaks and understands minimal English. Her daughter translates for her and states that her blood glucose level is normally well controlled with oral hypoglycemic medication.

1 Which test(s) would you expect to be ordered? (Select all that apply.)
 1 Sputum specimen today
 2 Throat culture in morning
 3 Midstream urine culture at noon
 4 Fingerstick for blood glucose levels before meals and at bedtime
2 Immediate results will be available for which of the tests?
3 Briefly describe how you would teach Mrs. Yamamoto about providing a sputum specimen.
4 What do you need to assess to determine Mrs. Yamamoto's ability to test her own blood glucose levels at home?

REVIEW QUESTIONS

1 A urine specimen for culture and sensitivity is being collected from a male patient. Which steps would be used to obtain an accurate specimen? (Select all that apply.)
 1 Two patient identifiers are checked.
 2 Help patient to perform pericare before the sterile part of the procedure.
 3 Wipe the head of the penis back and forth 3 times with each swab.
 4 Collect 10 to 20 mL for the sample.
 5 Have the patient initially void into a bedpan or clean container.
 6 Have patient hold penis above the sterile specimen cup without touching the container.
2 A 24-hour urine (timed urine collection) is being started. Which step is essential to have an accurate collection?
 1 Discarding the first urine specimen
 2 Including the first specimen for the test
 3 Discarding both the first and last specimen
 4 Discarding the last specimen

3 A patient is scheduled to obtain a stool sample for occult blood several days from now. Which food should be avoided before the stool sample is obtained because it can alter the results of the test?
  1 Potatoes
  2 Tomatoes
  3 Bananas
  4 Apples

4 The nurse is preparing to obtain a throat culture. Which step(s) would facilitate obtaining an accurate specimen? (Select all that apply.)
  1 Placing patient in a sitting position or with head elevated at a 45-degree angle
  2 Having patient lean her head forward
  3 Having patient swallow a small amount of water to rinse away food from the culture site before swabbing the area
  4 Swabbing the tonsillar area
  5 Swabbing the uvula
  6 Having patient blow her nose

5 The nurse is preparing to obtain a culture from a male patient with a urethral discharge. Which objective data should the nurse observe for in the genital area before obtaining the culture?
  1 Redness
  2 Lower abdominal discomfort
  3 Urethral stinging
  4 Itching

6 Place the steps for collecting a wound culture specimen in the correct order.
  1 Open packages containing sterile culture tubes and dressing supplies.
  2 Identify patient using two identifiers.
  3 Clean area around wound edges.
  4 Apply clean gloves. Remove old dressings and dispose of in appropriate receptacle.
  5 Apply sterile gloves. Obtain culture.

7 Place the following steps for collecting a sterile urine specimen from a Luer-Lok catheter port in the correct order.
  1 Attach a Luer-Lok syringe to the Luer-Lok port.
  2 Clamp the drainage tube with a clamp or rubber band for 15 minutes.
  3 Clean catheter entry port and wait for disinfectant to dry.
  4 Unclamp catheter and allow urine to flow into drainage bag.
  5 Aspirate 3 mL of urine into the syringe attached to the Luer-Lok.

8 Place in order the steps for performing a skin puncture for blood glucose monitoring.
  1 Instruct adult patient to perform hand hygiene.
  2 Apply clean gloves.
  3 Compare code on glucose meter screen to code on test strip vial.
  4 Drop or wick blood on to reagent strip.
  5 Clean site with an antiseptic swab or wipe.

9 A nursing assistive personnel (NAP) received instructions from the nurse to collect a sterile urine specimen from the Luer-Lok port of an indwelling catheter. The nurse identifies that the NAP needs further instruction when he or she states:
  1 "It's not my role to collect a specimen from the port of an indwelling catheter."
  2 "I'll use an 18-gauge needle to draw out the urine for the specimen."
  3 "I'll use a 20-mL Luer-Lok syringe to collect urine for a routine urinalysis."
  4 "I'll use a Luer-Lok syringe to draw the urine specimen."

10 Which sites are most often used for the Allen test before the collection of an arterial blood gas?
  1 Radial and ulnar pulses
  2 Radial and brachial pulses
  3 Radial and carotid pulses
  4 Popliteal and posterior tidal pulses

REFERENCES

Alexander M, et al: *Infusion nursing: an evidence-based approach*, ed 3, St Louis, 2010, Saunders.

American Diabetic Association (ADA): *Diabetes forecast: the healthy living magazine*, 2011.

Buchman A, et al: A new central venous catheter cap: decreased microbial growth and risk for catheter-related bloodstream infection, *J Vasc Access* 10(1):11, 2009.

Corbett JV: *Laboratory tests and diagnostic procedures with nursing diagnoses*, ed 7, Upper Saddle River, NJ, 2008, Prentice-Hall.

Fischbach F, Dunning MB.: *A manual of laboratory and diagnostic tests*, ed 8, Philadelphia, 2009, Lippincott Williams & Wilkins.

Hockenberry MJ, Wilson D: *Nursing care of infants and children*, ed 9, St Louis, 2011, Mosby.

Infusion Nurses Society (INS): *Infusion nursing: Standards of practice*, Norwood, Mass, 2011, Lippincott, Williams, & Wilkins.

McCall R, Tankersley C: *Phlebotomy essentials*, ed 5, Philadelphia, 2012, Lippincott Williams & Wilkins.

Pagana K, Pagana T: *Mosby's diagnostic and laboratory test reference*, ed 10, St Louis, 2011, Mosby.

Stuart B, Stuart J, Cherry C: *Pocket guide to culturally sensitive health care*, Philadelphia, 2011, Davis.

The Joint Commission (TJC): *National Patient Safety Goals*, Oakbrook Terrace, Ill, 2012, The Commission, available at http://www.jointcommission.org/standards_information/npsgs.aspx.

US Food and Drug Administration (FDA): How to report problems with glucose meters and continuous glucose monitoring systems, 2011, http://www.fda.gov/MedicalDevices/ProductsandMedicalProcedures/InVitroDiagnostics/GlucoseTestingDevices/ucm162002.htm/standards_information/npsgs.aspx.

Van Leeuwen A, et al: *Davis's comprehensive handbook of laboratory and diagnostic tests with nursing implications*, ed 4, Philadelphia, 2011, Davis.

Weddle G, et al: Role of nursing unit factors on performance of phlebotomy and subsequent blood culture contamination rates, *J Nurs Care Qual* 25(2):176, 2010.

Diagnostic Procedures

MEDIA RESOURCES

- evolve http://evolve.elsevier.com/Perry/skills
  learning system

  - Review Questions
  - Audio Glossary

KEY TERMS

Abdominal girth	Deep sedation	Lavage	Percutaneous coronary intervention (PCI)
Aldrete score	Epidural blood patch	Lumens	
Aspiration	Fiber optic	Manometer	Precordial
Biopsy	Glabellar tap	Medullary	Radiopaque
Bone marrow	Herniation	Minimal sedation	Stopcock
Capnography	Intestinal obstruction	Moderate sedation	Thrombocytopenia
Cerebrospinal fluid (CSF)	Intravenous conscious sedation (IV sedation)	Modified Ramsay sedation scale	Trocar
Cytology			

OBJECTIVES

Mastery of content in this chapter will enable the nurse to:
- Identify the physiologic indications for diagnostic procedures.
- Describe the health care team collaboration and teamwork required before, during, and after procedures, including delegation to nursing assistive personnel.
- Perform appropriate physical and psychosocial assessments before, during, and after diagnostic procedures.

- Effectively assist health care providers with angiogram, cardiac catheterization, intravenous (IV) pyelogram, bone marrow aspiration/biopsy, lumbar puncture, paracentesis, thoracentesis, bronchoscopy, and endoscopy.
- Demonstrate understanding of nursing responsibilities related to the use of intravenous sedation during diagnostic/surgical procedures.

Diagnostic procedures are performed at patients' bedsides or in specially equipped rooms within a hospital or outpatient care setting. As a nurse you are responsible for assessing a patient's knowledge of a procedure; preparing the patient; providing a safe environment and emotional support throughout the procedure; providing preprocedure and postprocedure assessment, care, and documentation; and providing discharge teaching. In addition, you are responsible for the oversight of any nursing care delegated to nursing assistive personnel (NAP). When procedures are completed in outpatient settings, it is the discharge nurse's responsibility to provide detailed printed home care instructions for postprocedure care, provide a complete reconciliation and instructions for all medications taken by a patient before the procedure and after discharge, and teach postprocedure care to the patient or caregiver. The health care provider is responsible for providing the patient with an explanation of the test/procedure, risks, benefits, treatment options, and outcomes before the procedure as part of the *informed consent* process.

EVIDENCE-BASED PRACTICE

Patients have diagnostic procedures in a variety of settings: inpatient, outpatient, and specialty diagnostic imaging centers. It is a challenge for nurses working in these settings to ensure that patients requiring diagnostic testing understand their testing and postprocedural care requirements. Some tests require intravenous (IV) sedation along with the diagnostic procedure, such as a gastrointestinal endoscopy; others require contrast media or aspirations; and some diagnostic tests that are noninvasive. Diagnostic procedures are not without risk. It is important that you understand your patients' diagnostic procedures, including why the procedure is needed, which preprocedural assessments are needed, expected outcomes, your role during the procedure, and appropriate postprocedural nursing care, to help ensure patient safety.

IV sedation is used for diagnostic or surgical procedures that do not require complete or general anesthesia. It is performed in acute care, surgical care, and outpatient care settings. Sedation classifications include "minimal," "moderate," or "deep" sedation/analgesia, depending on the depth of sedation (ASA, 2009). Based on current evidence-based practice, health care agencies maintain standards for preassessment, preparation, and monitoring of patients who will receive IV procedural sedation. Objective scales such as the American Society of Anesthesiologists (ASA) physical status classification system are used to determine if patients are at risk for undesirable outcomes. Use of an objective scale helps to reduce the risk for complications by determining when it is prudent to involve an anesthesiologist to help manage the care of a complicated patient condition (ASA, 2009). These objective scales incorporate evidence-based guidelines to reduce the risk for sedation-induced complications such as cardiac arrhythmias, respiratory failure, renal failure, neurologic disorders related to the use of paralytic agents, or bleeding disorders resulting from hepatic failure.

The use of vascular closure devices (VCDs) is common after procedures involving an arteriotomy or opening in an artery. VCDs are designed to reduce the time to hemostasis at the access (puncture) site and allow for earlier sheath removal. The use of VCDs contributes to earlier postprocedural resumption of normal activities and decreased treatment costs. A recent meta-analysis noted the effectiveness of the VCDs in obtaining prompt hemostasis over manual compression in the adult (Biancari et al., 2010). However, the researchers also noted an increased risk for lower limb ischemia, arterial stenosis, and other arterial complications (Biancari et al., 2010). They also leave behind foreign material, resulting in an increased risk for site infection (Hermanides et al., 2011; Hon et al., 2009).

- Timely and complete neurovascular checks are critical to identify postprocedure limb ischemia or other arterial complications.
- Instruct patient and caregiver to notify the nurse if the extremity feels moist, cold, tingling, or burning.

Patients undergoing lumbar puncture (LP) are at risk for experiencing postpuncture headaches as a side effect of the procedure. The symptoms range from a dull ache with a stiff neck to nausea. These symptoms can last several days and are incapacitating at times. Although an epidural blood patch may be effective in treating postpuncture headaches in some patients, it is not effective in preventing these headaches (Boonmak and Boonmak, 2010).

- In children the early use of a topical anesthetic EMLA before the puncture is showing some clinical effects in preventing postpuncture headaches but needs further testing (Fein et al., 2010).
- Rest, fluids (including caffeinated beverages), and analgesics are effective measures for managing this headache pain (Stannard, 2011).

PATIENT-CENTERED CARE

Any diagnostic procedure can create a sense of powerlessness for patients. The unknown (i.e., not knowing what a test may reveal or not completely understanding what a test involves or feels like) can also create fear and anxiety. It is important to involve patients in a discussion of what a test involves and giving them opportunity to ask questions. Learn what their fears are because you may have the opportunity to alleviate them. For example, if a patient worries about being physically exposed during a procedure, communicate with procedure staff to see if there is a way to minimize exposure and use more draping.

When a patient is chronically ill or fatigued or has decreased functional status, plan the diagnostic testing schedule to provide rest periods between multiple tests performed on the same day. Provide reassurance to a patient throughout a procedure. Most of these procedures cause moderate discomfort, and the patient tolerates them better if you remain at the side and explain each step.

 Safety Guidelines

Before a procedure:

1 It is essential to patient safety to be sure that patient undergoes the correct procedure. Ensure proper identification of a patient by using a minimum of two identifiers, verifying the correct procedure (and site, when applicable). This includes verbal verification and written/computerized documentation of the preceding information on patient arrival, again in the procedure room, and just before starting a procedure (TJC, 2012) (see agency policy).

2 Assess for completion of relevant documentation (e.g., history and physical, signed procedure consent form, nursing assessment, and preanesthesia assessment) necessary for performing a safe procedure.

3 Identify any medications for which uninterrupted dosing is required (e.g., anticonvulsants, antibiotics, and certain cardiac medications). If the procedure requires a patient to have nothing by mouth (NPO), discuss medications with the health care provider to decide if the patient should take any medications before the procedure. When insulin or oral hypoglycemic medications are given to patients before procedures, arrange to have either the patient's meal or other nutritional support available on completion of the procedure.

4 Verify that informed consent was obtained before administering any sedatives. The health care provider performing the procedure is responsible for obtaining informed consent from a patient. In some agencies after the health care provider discusses the procedure and obtains verbal consent, the registered nurse obtains the patient's signature on the consent form. (Check agency policy to determine if a consent form is required and the expectations of the nurse in this process.) *When there is no evidence of informed consent in the patient medical record, hold any preprocedure medications that may alter the patient's level of consciousness and notify the health care provider performing the procedure and staff in any receiving area.*

During a procedure:

1 If a procedure involves the use of radiation:
   a Minimize the amount of radiation exposure by using protective shielding devices such as a lead apron and goggles, radioprotective gloves, and/or thyroid shield.
   b Monitoring staff radiation exposure may require the use of a dosimeter (see agency policy).
   c Remain positioned as far away from the radiographic equipment as possible while still performing required patient care.
2 Monitor physiologic parameters indicated by the procedure.
3 Position patients carefully to avoid musculoskeletal or neurologic injury.
4 Label any specimens obtained during a procedure properly.

After the procedure:

1 Know possible procedural complications and conduct appropriate assessments for early detection.
2 Monitor oxygen saturation and vital signs to detect sedation failure and adverse effects (e.g., vomiting, hypoxic events) (AHRQ, 2010).
3 Know the use, side effects, and complications of the sedative agent(s) and reversal agents to be administered.
4 Be able to recognize cardiac dysrhythmias.
5 Institute fall precautions until patient has recovered from effects of sedatives.

SKILL 44-1 Intravenous Moderate Sedation During a Diagnostic Procedure

Certain diagnostic or therapeutic procedures require patients to receive intravenous (IV) moderate sedation. Moderate sedation/analgesia produces a minimally depressed level of consciousness induced by the administration of pharmacologic agents in which a patient retains a continuous and independent ability to maintain protective reflexes and a patent airway and is aroused by physical or verbal stimulation. Moderate sedation improves a patient's cooperation with a procedure, allows a rapid return to his or her preprocedure status, and minimizes the risk for injury. It often raises a patient's pain threshold and provides amnesia concerning the actual procedural events. In addition, no interventions are required during a procedure to maintain a patent airway, and spontaneous ventilation is adequate (ASA, 2009).

Deep sedation is one risk associated with moderate sedation when a patient's level of consciousness depresses past the point at which he or she cannot maintain a patent airway. Because of this risk, the use of IV moderate sedation is closely controlled and normally restricted to physicians and registered nurses (RNs) who receive specialized training or credentialing (AORN, 2011). Know the agency policy for recommended and maximum doses of medications and monitoring and documentation requirements when using IV sedation.

The most common types of medications used to achieve moderate sedation include benzodiazepines and opiates. Benzodiazepines reduce anxiety and promote muscle relaxation. Midazolam (Versed) also produces an amnesic effect. Opiates such as morphine sulphate or fentanyl (Sublimaze, Duragesic) help control pain while achieving sedation. Propofol (Diprivan), a safe, rapid-acting hypnotic, is also commonly used and may offer a faster recovery time than the combination of benzodiazepines and opiates (Ellett, 2010; Muller and Wehrmann, 2011).

Patient risks during IV sedation include hypoventilation, airway compromise, hemodynamic instability, and/or altered levels of consciousness that include an overly depressed level of consciousness or agitation and combativeness. Emergency equipment appropriate for the patient's age and size (see Chapter 27) and a staff competent in airway management, oxygen delivery, and use of resuscitation equipment are essential. During a procedure patients need continuous monitoring (recorded at least every 5 minutes) of heart and respiratory rate and rhythm, blood pressure, oxygen saturation, and level of consciousness (see agency policy) (AHRQ, 2010). End-tidal CO_2 is also becoming a common parameter for monitoring sedation tolerance. Monitoring continues after the procedure (see agency policy).

Delegation and Collaboration

The skill of assisting with IV moderate sedation, including the preprocedure assessment, cannot be delegated to nursing assistive personnel (NAP). In most agencies an RN or health care provider assesses and monitors a patient's level of sedation, airway patency, and level of consciousness. Roles in monitoring depend on scope-of-practice guidelines as determined by state regulations (see agency policy).

Equipment

❑ Personal protective equipment (PPE): Gloves, mask, gown, eye protection
❑ Sedation as prescribed: Benzodiazepines (e.g., midazolam [Versed], opiates, and propofol [Diprivan], fentanyl [Sublimaze])
❑ Emergency equipment: Crash cart, cardiac monitor/defibrillator, and endotracheal intubation/airway management equipment in various sizes and appropriate for patient's age
❑ Equipment for insertion of a peripheral IV catheter (CDC, 2011) (see Chapter 28)
❑ Oxygen and airway supplies: Bag and mask device, oral/nasopharyngeal airways
❑ Suction equipment (see Chapter 25)
❑ Sphygmomanometer or noninvasive blood pressure monitor
❑ Pulse oximeter or end-tidal CO_2 monitor
❑ Electrocardiogram (ECG) monitor
❑ Appropriate reversal drugs (e.g., flumazenil [Romazicon] for reversal of benzodiazepines, naloxone [Narcan] for reversal of opiates) and labels for each
❑ Pain medication (opioids) for procedures anticipated to cause discomfort

STEP	RATIONALE

ASSESSMENT

1 Verify type of procedure scheduled and procedure site with patient.

Ensures correct patient. Complies with The Joint Commission standards and improves patient safety (TJC, 2012).

2 Verify that a preprocedure medication reconciliation and history and physical (H&P) examination were completed.

Accrediting agencies such as The Joint Commission require a documented preprocedure medication history and H&P before administration of procedural IV sedation.

3 Verify that informed consent was obtained before administering any sedatives.

Federal regulations, many state laws, and accreditation agencies require informed consent for procedure.

4 Assess patient's past history of adverse reaction to IV sedation (e.g., hemodynamic instability, nausea or vomiting, airway compromise, altered level of consciousness).

Patients with history of these reactions are at higher risk for procedural complications if IV sedation is used.

5 Verify patient's ASA Physical Status Classification (Box 44-1).

ASA recommends that patients receiving classification of 3 or higher have anesthesia consultation before receiving IV sedation (ASA, 2009).

Critical Decision Point *Consultation with an anesthesiologist is often required by the agency if a patient has an ASA classification of 3 to 6 or history of or evidence for difficult intubation, sleep apnea, or complications related to sedation/anesthesia.*

---

6 Assess patient for history of airway abnormalities, liver failure, lung disease, heart failure, hypotonia, morbid obesity, severe gastroesophageal reflux, and history of adverse reaction to sedatives (AHRQ, 2010).

Risk factors that increase likelihood of adverse event (AHRQ, 2010).

7 Assess patient's current or past history for substance abuse or liver/kidney disease.

A history of substance abuse and/or liver/kidney disease usually requires dose adjustment of sedative agents.

8 Verify that patient has not ingested food or fluids, except for oral medications, for at least 4 hours (check specific agency requirements).

Because risk of moderate sedation is loss of airway protection, empty stomach reduces risk for aspiration.

9 Determine if patient is allergic to latex, antiseptic, tape, or anesthetic solutions.

Allergic reactions to latex or tape range from mild skin reaction to anaphylaxis. Common allergic reactions to local anesthetic agents include central nervous system (CNS) depression, respiratory difficulty, and hypotension.

10 Assess patient's level of understanding of procedure, including any concerns.

Determines extent of instruction or level of support required.

11 Assess baseline heart rate, breath sounds, respiratory rate, blood pressure, level of consciousness, pain level, and oxygen saturation (SpO_2).

Establishes baseline for comparison during and after procedure.

12 Determine patient's height and weight.

Needed to calculate drug dosages.

13 Assess patient's baseline status via agency's designated scoring system. Many agencies use an "Aldrete score" (Aldrete, 2007; Table 44-1).

Establishes baseline for comparison after procedure.

NURSING DIAGNOSES

- Acute pain
- Anxiety
- Deficient knowledge regarding procedure
- Risk for aspiration
- Risk for injury

Related factors are individualized based on patient's condition or needs.

BOX 44-1	ASA Physical Status Classification System

ASA 1 = Normal healthy patient
ASA 2 = Patient with mild systemic disease
ASA 3 = Patient with severe systemic disease
ASA 4 = Patient with severe systemic disease that is a constant threat to life
ASA 5 = Moribund patient who is not expected to survive without the operation
ASA 6 = Declared brain-dead patient whose organs are being removed for donor purposes
"E" is added if the procedure is performed as an emergency.

From American Society of Anesthesiologists: *Relative value guide*, 2012, available at http://www.asahq.org/clinical/physicalstatus.htm, accessed September 11, 2011/.

STEP	RATIONALE

PLANNING

1 Expected outcomes following completion of procedures:
- Adhere to Universal Protocol (Box 44-2)
- Patient's airway remains patent.

- Patient's level of comfort is equivalent to score of 4 or less on pain scale of 0 to 10.

2 Explain to patient that IV sedation will cause relaxation and amnesia but that he or she will be awake during procedure. If patient will not be able to verbalize because of nature of procedure, teach him or her agreed-on nonverbal signals such as "yes," "no," and "pain."

3 Explain that close monitoring of vital signs and frequent checks to determine that patient is awake are normal and do not mean that there are problems.

4 Explain to patient major steps of procedure.

5 Position patient as needed for procedure.

Rationale column:

Maintains patient safety (TJC, 2012).
Moderate sedation is monitored successfully without progression to deep sedation.
Procedure managed to minimize patient's pain.

Encourages cooperation and minimizes risks and anxiety about procedure.

Reduces patient anxiety during procedure.

Reduces patient anxiety during procedure.

IMPLEMENTATION

1 Identify patient using two identifiers (i.e., name and birthday or name and account number) according to agency policy. Compare identifiers in MAR/medical record with information on patient's identification bracelet and/or ask patient to state name.

2 Establish peripheral IV access (CDC, 2011) (see also Chapter 28).

3 Implement Universal Protocol in presence of appropriate health care team members (as applicable) and in accordance with agency policy (see Box 44-2).

Rationale column:

Ensures correct patient. Complies with The Joint Commission standards and improves patient safety (TJC, 2012).

Provides access for administration of sedation and any emergency medications (as needed).
Ensures patient safety by correctly identifying correct patient to correct procedure.

TABLE 44-1 | **Aldrete Scoring System**

		Score
Activity (moving voluntarily on command)	4 extremities	2
	2 extremities	1
	0 extremities	0
Respiration	Able to deep breathe and cough freely	2
	Dyspnea, shallow or limited breathing	1
	Apneic	0
Circulation	BP ± 20 mm Hg of presedation level	2
	BP ± 20-50 mm Hg of presedation level	1
	BP ± 50 mm Hg of presedation level	0
Consciousness	Fully awake	2
	Arousable on having name called	1
	Not responding	0
Color	Normal	2
	Pale, dusky, blotchy, jaundiced, or other change	1
	Cyanotic	0

From Aldrete JA: The post-anesthesia recovery score revisited, *J Clin Anesth* 7:89, 1995; Aldrete JA: Post-anesthetic recovery score, *J Am Coll Surg* 205(5):3, 2007.
BP, Blood pressure.

BOX 44-2 | **The Joint Commission Universal Protocol**

- Verification of correct person, correct site, and correct procedure occurs.
- Procedure site is marked before moving to procedure area.
- A "Time-Out" is performed immediately before starting procedures.
- When patient is in preprocedure area (immediately before moving him or her to procedure room), a checklist (e.g., paper, electronic, or other medium such as a wall-mounted white board) is used to review and verify that required items are available and are accurately matched to the patient.

From The Joint Commission: *National Patient Safety Goals*, 2012, TJC, http://www.jointcommission.org/assets/1/18/UP_Poster1.PDF, accessed August 23, 2012.

STEP	RATIONALE
4 During the diagnostic procedure, monitor heart rate and oxygen saturation (SpO$_2$) continuously via pulse oximetry equipment. Some agencies also use end-tidal CO$_2$ monitoring (capnography). Monitor patient's airway patency, respiratory rate and depth, blood pressure, and level of consciousness and responsiveness every 5 minutes (AHRQ, 2010). Keep oxygen and suction equipment nearby.	Vital signs, oximetry, and capnography provide comparison with patient's baseline status. Oxygen and suction equipment may be required in an emergent situation.
5 Observe for verbal or nonverbal evidence of pain, facial grimacing, and eye opening.	Physical responses indicate level of sedation.
6 Assess level of sedation using Modified Ramsay Sedation Scale (Table 44-2) or other criteria adopted by agency.	Determines patient's level of sedation. Numeric rating scale offers consistent assessment and accurate judgment of patient's changing status and verbal/physical stimulation.

Critical Decision Point *Report a Ramsay sedation score higher than 3 (responsive to commands only) to the health care provider.*

7 Reposition patient as needed without interrupting diagnostic procedure.	Prevents pressure- and position-related injuries (AHRQ, 2010).

EVALUATION

1 Monitor patient throughout procedure using the Modified Ramsay Sedation Scale (or other criteria adopted by the agency).	Provides data to verify patient's expected return to baseline status.
2 *After procedure*: Use Aldrete score (see Table 44-1) and monitor level of consciousness, respiratory rate, SpO$_2$, blood pressure, heart rate and rhythm, and pain score according to agency policy (AHRQ, 2010) (e.g., every 5 minutes for at least 30 minutes, then every 15 minutes for an hour, and then every 30 minutes until patient meets discharge criteria).	Enables prompt detection of any airway compromise or protective reflexes caused by delayed action of medications.
3 Ask patient to repeat back what he or she understands regarding procedure or any postprocedure patient instructions, including medication orders and instructions.	Verifies patient understanding of procedure or discharge education.
4 Have patient's "designated driver" explain any postprocedure education and sign appropriate documents.	Patients who receive conscious sedation are restricted from driving for 24 to 48 hours, depending on procedure, type of sedation, and postprocedure restrictions.

Unexpected Outcomes	Related Interventions
1 Oversedation, evidenced by decreasing SpO$_2$ (cyanosis, slow shallow respirations with periods of apnea), tachycardia, sedation score of 4 (exhibiting brisk response to light glabellar tap or loud auditory stimulus) or higher on Modified Ramsay Sedation Scale or less than 8 on Aldrete scale.	• Support patient's breathing via positioning and manual bagging. • Immediately notify health care provider. • Be prepared to administer reversal agents. Naloxone (Narcan) is for reversal of opioids, and flumazenil (Romazicon) is for reversal of benzodiazepines.

Clinical Decision Point *If reversal agents are used, level of consciousness and vital signs should return to acceptable levels for a period of 2 hours from time of administration of reversal agent before monitoring ends (AHRQ, 2010).*

2 Patient develops cardiac instability evidenced by irregular heart rate, change in pulse rate, or change in blood pressure.	• Initiate oxygen therapy, ensure IV access, and obtain ECG as ordered. • Immediately notify health care provider.

TABLE 44-2	Modified Ramsay Sedation Scale		
Minimal sedation (anxiolysis)		1	Anxious and agitated or restless or both
		2	Cooperative, oriented, and tranquil
Moderate sedation/analgesia (conscious sedation)		3	Responds to commands spoken in a normal voice
Deep sedation/analgesia		4	Brisk response to a light forehead tap or loud auditory stimulus
		5	Sluggish response to a light forehead tap or loud auditory stimulus
		6	No response to a light forehead tap or loud auditory stimulus

Data from American Society of Anesthesiologists: *Continuum of depth of sedation: definition of general anesthesia and levels of sedation/analgesia*, The Society, October 2009, available at http://www.asahq.org/For-Members/Standards-Guidelines-and-Statements.aspx, accessed August 23, 2012; and Sessler C et al: Evaluating and monitoring analgesia and sedation in the critical care unity, *Crit Care* 12(suppl 3):S2, 2008.

Recording and Reporting

- Document vital signs, SpO_2, end-tidal CO_2, and sedation level at baseline, then every 5 minutes during the procedure, and every 15 minutes for at least 30 minutes after the procedure according to agency policy.
- Record dosage, route, and time of administration for drugs given during and after the procedure, including reversal agents. Record significant patient reactions during the procedure. Include IV fluids and blood products if administered.
- Immediately report to patient's health care provider any respiratory distress, cardiac compromise, or unexpected altered mental status.
- Document discharge teaching, medication reconciliation, discontinuation of IV access, final/discharge assessment, and to whom/how discharged (e.g., designated driver, ambulance/transporter, nursing home).

Special Considerations
Teaching

- Explain that it is unlikely for patients to remember the procedure because of the amnesic effect of the sedative(s).
- Before the procedure, instruct patient to arrange for transportation home after the procedure because (at most agencies) patient will not be permitted to drive for 24 hours after receiving sedation.
- Provide patients and family caregivers with discharge instructions that include complications that may occur; how to manage complications; and physical signs and symptoms to report to the health care provider, including contact information and postprocedure medication reconciliation and instructions.

Pediatric

- Children are more likely than adults to sustain a serious complication resulting from anesthesia. Such complications are often linked to either the cardiovascular or respiratory system. For this reason the American Academy of Pediatrics recommend that personnel who are able to manage a child's airway be present for the procedure (AAP, 2012).
- A preprocedure medical evaluation is required. To safely administer sedation to a pediatric patient, consider anatomic and physiologic variations, preprocedure assessments, and pharmacologic techniques (AAP, 2012).
- During the preprocedure assessment answer the parent's questions in a relaxed and confident manner. When communicating with children, take into account the child's developmental stage.

Gerontologic

- Closely monitor the effects of medications on patient's respiratory status and pulse. These drugs interfere with breathing or increase or decrease heart rate as a result of reduced drug clearance through the kidneys or liver (Lewis et al., 2011).
- Physical limitations of the patient, including hearing and vision loss, contribute to frustration and confusion, compounding the sense of loss of control.

Home Care

- Instruct the patient to avoid making any legally binding decisions until at least 24 hours after the procedure.

SKILL 44-2   Contrast Media Studies: Arteriogram (Angiogram), Cardiac Catheterization, and Intravenous Pyelogram

Contrast media studies involve visualization of blood vessels and internal organs by intravascular injection of a radiopaque medium. An arteriogram (angiogram) permits visualization of the vasculature and arterial system of an organ (Fig. 44-1). Arteriography is usually performed by an interventional radiologist to diagnose arterial or venous occlusions; stenosis; emboli; thromboses; aneurysms; tumors; congenital malformations; or trauma to the brain, heart, lung, kidneys, or lower extremities.

Cardiac catheterization is a specialized form of angiography performed by an interventional cardiologist. An intravenous or intraarterial catheter introducer is inserted into the left or right side of the heart via a major peripheral vessel, usually the femoral artery and/or vein. The test studies pressures within the heart, cardiac volumes, valvular function, and patency of coronary arteries. Cardiac catheterizations are performed in specially equipped laboratories (Fig. 44-2). A contrast medium is injected, and the structures and functions of the heart and lungs are assessed.

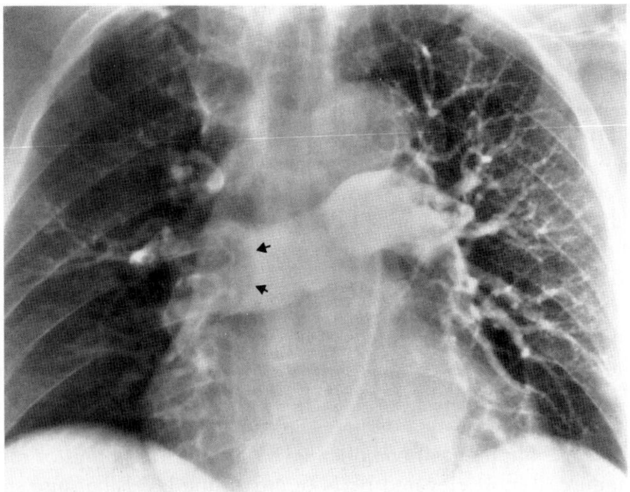

FIG 44-1   Pulmonary arteriogram shows obstruction (*arrows*) of right pulmonary artery. (*From Eisenberg R, Johnson N: Comprehensive radiographic pathology, ed 4, St Louis, 2007, Mosby.*)

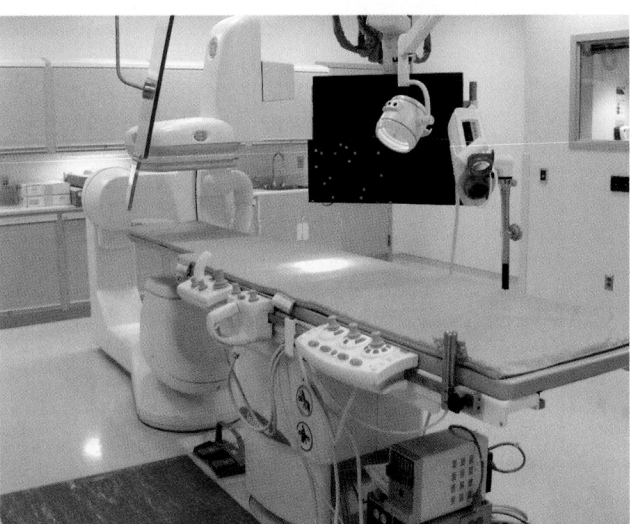

FIG 44-2   Cardiac catheterization laboratory. (*Image used with permission, Flagstaff Medical Center, Northern Arizona Healthcare. All rights reserved.*)

Cardiac catheterizations are contraindicated in patients who would refuse needed surgery, are allergic to iodine contrast media, are uncooperative or cannot lie still during the entire procedure, or are susceptible to dye-induced renal failure. Precautions to help prevent dye-induced renal failure are controversial and include ensuring that the patient is well-hydrated using bicarbonate solution or sodium chloride with or without prophylactic N-acetylcysteine (Mucomyst) (Lewis et al., 2011). Intravenous pyelography (IVP) is a venographic examination of the flow of radiopaque contrast medium through the kidneys, ureters, and bladder to identify obstruction, hematuria, stones, bladder injury, or renal artery occlusion. Dye is injected into a peripheral vein, and serial radiographs are taken over the subsequent 30 minutes.

Delegation and Collaboration

The skill of assisting with angiography and IVP can be delegated to nursing assistive personnel (NAP) if the patient is stable and no intravenous (IV) sedation is used. The registered nurse (RN) directs the NAP about:

- When to obtain and report vital signs, urinary output, and weight.
- Which signs and symptoms to report to the nurse.

- Accompanying the patient to the procedure room and assisting specially trained and licensed radiology personnel with the specific angiography procedure.

The skill of assisting with cardiac catheterization can be delegated to specially trained NAP with a nurse continuously present. The nurse provides continuous patient assessment and monitoring for serious complications. The NAP helps with patient transport, positioning, and obtaining supplies.

Equipment

- ❑ Protective supplies: Mask, goggles, sterile gown, and sterile gloves
- ❑ Sterile packs containing catheters/equipment for performing procedures
- ❑ Equipment for peripheral IV access
- ❑ Medications such as sedatives (e.g., diazepam [Valium], midazolam [Versed], propofol [Diprivan]) for IV sedation or analgesics for relaxation and pain control
- ❑ Emergency equipment: Oxygen, endotracheal intubation/airway management equipment, emergency cart, cardiac monitor/defibrillator, sedative reversal agents
- ❑ Pulse oximeter, end-tidal CO_2 monitor, blood pressure (BP) equipment

STEP	RATIONALE

ASSESSMENT

1 Verify type of procedure scheduled and procedure site with patient.

Ensures correct patient. Complies with The Joint Commission standards and improves patient safety (TJC, 2012).

2 Verify that informed consent was obtained before administering any sedatives.

Federal regulations, many state laws, and accreditation agencies require informed consent for procedure.

3 Determine if patient is taking anticoagulants, aspirin, or any nonsteroidal medication.

Medication increases risk for bleeding and is often stopped before procedure.

4 Assess patient for history of any allergies to iodine dye, shellfish, or latex and whether patient has had previous reaction to contrast agent (Schabelman and Witting, 2010). If so, notify cardiologist or radiologist.

Allergic individuals in general are at mildly increased risk for developing adverse reactions to radiocontrast media (Beaty et al., 2008). Hypoallergenic contrast medium is sometimes used.

5 Review medical record for contraindications:

a *All contrast media:* Pregnancy unless benefits of test outweigh risks to fetus.

Radioactive iodinated contrast media crosses blood-placental barrier.

b *Angiography:* Anticoagulant therapy, bleeding disorders, thrombocytopenia, dehydration, uncontrolled hypertension, renal insufficiency, and pregnancy.

Anticoagulants and bleeding disorders interfere with patient's blood clotting abilities and may cause blood loss.

Dehydration and renal insufficiency are contraindications to use of ionic radiographic contrast media because patient has impaired ability to excrete contrast media via kidneys.

c *Cardiac catheterization:* History of severe cardiomyopathy, severe dysrhythmias, uncontrolled heart failure (HF).

Introduction of catheter into myocardium increases risk for dysrhythmias (Pagana and Pagana, 2010).

d *IVP:* History of dehydration, known renal insufficiency (with blood urea nitrogen [BUN] level >40 mg/100 mL, or creatinine >2 mg/dl) (Pagana and Pagana, 2010).

Iodinated dye is sometimes nephrotoxic and worsens existing renal disease.

e Determine whether patient took metformin hydrochloride (Glucophage) within previous 48 hours. If so, notify health care provider immediately.

Taking metformin hydrochloride 48 hours before receiving iodinated contrast media can lead to acute renal failure and lactic acidosis (Ott, 2008).

6 Assess patient's bleeding and coagulation status (e.g., complete blood count [CBC], platelets, prothrombin time [PT], activated partial thromboplastin time [aPTT], and international normalized ratio [INR]) and assess patient's renal function (e.g., BUN, creatinine levels) before procedure. Assess electrolytes (sodium and potassium).

Abnormal laboratory findings may contraindicate procedure because of potential complications of hemorrhage and/or renal failure. Report elevated BUN or creatinine levels because such patients are at risk for renal failure induced by contrast media (Pagana and Pagana, 2010). Abnormal electrolytes may reveal possible electromechanical problems.

STEP	RATIONALE
7 Obtain vital signs and peripheral pulses. For arterial procedures mark patient's peripheral pulses before procedure. For cardiac catheterization also auscultate heart and lungs and obtain weight.	Provides baseline data and locations for comparison with findings during and after procedure.
8 Assess patient's hydration status, including condition of mucous membranes, and recent 24-hour intake.	Severe dehydration can lead to renal failure (Pagana and Pagana, 2010).
9 Assess patient's level of understanding of procedure, including any concerns.	Determines extent of instruction or level of support required.
10 Determine type of arteriogram scheduled (e.g., carotid, femoral, brachial). If cardiac catheterization, verify if test is for right or left heart or both. For IVP ask if study is for one or both kidneys.	Enables you to anticipate patient teaching needs and postprocedure interventions.
11 Determine and document last time of ingested food, drink, or medications.	Prevents possible aspiration because patient is sedated. Excessive hydration causes dilution of contrast medium, making structures more difficult to visualize. Patients should be NPO for 6 to 8 hours before procedure.

Clinical Decision Point *Exceptions occur for patients at risk for contrast media–induced renal impairment who are specifically instructed to drink increased fluids in the hours before the procedure or those instructed by the health care provider to take medications before the procedure. Good preprocedure hydration reduces the risk for renal impairment caused by contrast media (Pagana and Pagana, 2010).*

STEP	RATIONALE
12 Review health care provider's orders for preprocedure medications, hydration, antihistamines, and IV sedation:	Increased sedation is necessary in anxious or confused patients. Increased hydration is often required for renal insufficiency, and antihistamines for possible allergic reaction.
a Atropine	Decreases salivary secretions and increases heart rate when bradycardia is present.
b Diphenhydramine (Benadryl)	Used prophylactically to block histamine and decrease allergic response.
c Preprocedural sedative	Decreases anxiety and promotes relaxation.

NURSING DIAGNOSES

- Acute pain
- Anxiety
- Decreased cardiac output
- Deficient knowledge regarding procedure
- Fear
- Risk for infection
- Risk for injury

Related factors are individualized based on patient's condition or needs.

PLANNING

1 Expected outcomes following completion of procedure:	
• Patient does not experience any procedure or postprocedure complications such as significant changes in vital signs, diminished or absent peripheral pulses, allergic response, or decreased or absent urine output.	Procedure performed without complication.
• Patient's level of comfort is equal to score of 4 or less on pain scale of 0 to 10. Expected discomfort includes soreness at catheter insertion site and possible backache.	Patient tolerates procedure.
• Patient tolerates increased fluid intake and urinates sufficiently (at least 30 mL/hr or 0.5 mL/kg/hr) to excrete radiographic dye.	Adequate renal function.
• Patient recovers from IV sedation without respiratory complications or change in level of consciousness.	Appropriate level of sedation.
2 Explain to patient purpose of procedure and what will happen during it.	Helps to minimize patient's anxiety.
3 Remove all of patient's jewelry, metal objects, and body piercings.	Eliminates objects that interfere with radiography visualization of vessels and could be conductive material during electrocautery.
4 Preprocedure preparation:	
a *For IVP:* Verify that patient has completed necessary bowel preparation of orally administered evacuation preparation 24 hours before test and evacuation enema 8 hours before test (check agency policy).	An evacuated lower intestine and bowel improves visualization of urinary structures.

STEP	RATIONALE
b *For cardiac catheterization:* Determine whether hair at site of catheter insertion needs clipping or preparation with antiseptic just before procedure. Allow antiseptic to dry. Do not shave site.	Reduces risk for site-related infection. Drying promotes maximal antibacterial activity. Shaving results in increased chance for infection.
5 For cardiac catheterization it is common to verify availability of emergent cardiac surgery because of risk for complete coronary artery occlusion from dislodged plaque or inadvertent perforation of vasculature (check agency policy). Also verify patient's ASA classification before procedure.	Prepares backup plan for possible procedural outcomes that would require emergency surgery.

IMPLEMENTATION

1 Identify patient using two identifiers (i.e., name and birthday or name and account number) according to agency policy. Compare identifiers with information on patient's identification bracelet. Verify type of procedure scheduled and procedure site with patient.	Ensures correct patient. Complies with The Joint Commission standards and improves patient safety (TJC, 2012).
2 Have patient empty bladder or bowels before procedure.	Ensures that patient will not need to void during procedure.
3 Prepare cardiac monitor, pulse oximeter, and/or end-tidal CO_2 monitor.	Provides easy access to equipment for monitoring patient status during and after procedure.
4 Perform hand hygiene and apply appropriate protective equipment.	Reduces transmission of microorganisms.
5 Provide IV access using large-bore cannula. Remove gloves.	Provides access for delivery of IV fluids and/or drugs.
6 Assist patient in assuming a comfortable supine position on x-ray table. Some patients undergoing IVP may be in supine or in a slight Trendelenburg's position. Immobilize extremity that will be injected. Pad any bony prominences.	For arterial procedures, patient may need to maintain position for 1 to 3 hours. Padding the bony prominences reduces the risk for impaired skin integrity.
7 Take "Time-Out" to verify patient's name, type of procedure to be performed, and procedure site with patient.	"Time-Out" verification just before starting an invasive procedure includes health care provider and all involved personnel and is a safety precaution to prevent wrong patient, wrong site, and wrong procedure errors (TJC, 2012).
8 Monitor vital signs, pulse oximetry (SpO_2), end-tidal CO_2 and, for arterial procedures, palpate peripheral pulses.	Data provides comparison with baseline to determine patient's response to procedure.
9 Inform patient that during injection of dye it is common to experience some chest pain and severe hot flash that is quite uncomfortable but lasts only a few seconds.	Dye causes feeling of warmth, flushing, or metallic taste shortly after injection.
10 Physician cleanses arterial puncture site for catheter insertion (femoral, radial, carotid, or brachial) with antiseptic.	Reduces transmission of microorganisms.
11 All members of the team apply mask and goggles, sterile gown, head cover, and sterile gloves. Drape patient with sterile drapes, leaving puncture site exposed.	Maintains surgical asepsis.
12 Physician anesthetizes skin overlying arterial puncture site.	Provides local anesthetic to area of incision or puncture.
13 For arterial procedures, the physician does the following:	
a Punctures artery; inserts introducer (think plastic tube) into artery. Guidewire is inserted through introducer and advanced; flexible catheter is inserted over guidewire and advanced into heart. Introducers allow for use of various procedure catheters, depending on need (e.g., balloon angioplasty, stent placement, ablation).	Permits access to artery and coiling of catheter in artery.
b Advances catheter to desired artery or cardiac chamber, removes guidewire, and injects contrast medium through catheter.	Permits radiographic visualization of structures, aneurysms, occlusions, or anomalies.
14 During dye injection, specialized machinery takes rapid sequence of x-ray films.	Permits radiographic records of visualization of dye through artery and any abnormalities present.
15 If iodinated dye is used, observe patient for signs of anaphylaxis, including respiratory distress, palpitation, itching, and diaphoresis.	Allergic reactions can be life threatening.
16 During cardiac catheterization the nurse assists with measuring cardiac volumes and pressure.	Provides data related to cardiac output, central venous pressure (CVP), ventricular pressures, and pulmonary artery pressure.

STEP	RATIONALE

Clinical Decision Point *Be prepared to end the cardiac catheterization procedure early in the event of severe unrelieved chest pain, neurologic symptoms of a cerebrovascular accident, cardiac dysrhythmias, or hemodynamic changes (Pagana and Pagana, 2010).*

17 Nurse administering IV sedation monitors levels of sedation, level of consciousness, and vital signs (see Skill 44-1).	Proper IV sedation does not cause loss of consciousness.
18 Physician withdraws catheter and applies manual pressure to puncture site until homeostasis occurs (5 to 15 minutes or longer).	Five to fifteen minutes of manual pressure is often enough to stop active site bleeding. However, certain amount of bed rest is needed to achieve reliable hemostasis. Check agency policy for postprocedure bed rest requirements. This may vary from 2 to 6 hours when no arteriotomy closure device is used.
a *Option:* Physician may choose to use an arteriotomy closure device (ACD), which can be categorized as either passive-closure device (helps with compression such as clamps/tamping devices, assisted or enhanced coagulation, and sealants) or active-closure devices (immediate closure with suture devices, clips, and collagen plug devices).	Use of ACDs is reasonable after invasive cardiovascular procedures performed via femoral artery to achieve faster hemostasis, shorter duration of bed rest, and possibly improved patient comfort. Use of devices should be weighed against risk of complications (Patel et al., 2010).

Clinical Decision Point *Before removing catheter sheath, check for health care provider's orders for instructions for treating a vasovagal reaction. Manual pressure applied to the groin/femoral area can stimulate the baroreceptors and cause a vasovagal reaction in which the patient becomes bradycardic and hypotensive. Vasovagal reactions are usually brief and self-limiting. When applying pressure to the groin after sheath removal, be alert for a vasovagal reaction and prepared to treat it by lowering the head of the bed to the flat position and giving a bolus of IV fluids.*

19 If a percutaneous coronary intervention (PCI) such as a percutaneous transluminal coronary angioplasty (PTCA) or directional coronary atherectomy (DCA) was performed during cardiac catheterization, a femoral introducer/sheath is often left in place and removed in several hours.	Postinterventional sheaths provide emergency access to vasculature in event that coronary artery becomes occluded, allowing time for anticoagulants to wear off.
20 Remove and discard gloves. Perform hand hygiene.	Reduces transmission of microorganisms.
21 Postprocedure:	
a For arterial procedures:	
(1) Keep affected extremity immobilized for 2 to 6 hours after removal of sheath (see agency policy). Use orthopedic bedpan for female patient as needed for bowel or bladder evacuation while on bed rest.	There is evidence of no benefit relating to bleeding and hematoma formation in patients who have more than 3 hours of bed rest following transfemoral diagnostic cardiac catheterization. There is evidence of benefit relating to decreased incidence and severity of back pain after 3 hours of bed rest. Inconclusive evidence suggests that bed rest for 2 hours following transfemoral cardiac catheterization may be sufficient (Chair and Fernandez, 2008).
(2) Emphasize need to lay flat for 6 to 12 hours (and possibly overnight if sheath is left in groin).	Helps to prevent disruption of hemostasis.
b Encourage patient to drink 1 to 2 L of fluid after procedure.	Facilitates elimination of contrast material and prevents renal damage (Pagana and Pagana, 2010).

EVALUATION

1 Evaluate patient's body position and comfort during procedure.	Position can cause stress on insertion site and patient's musculoskeletal structures.
2 Monitor vital signs and oxygen saturation and assess for signs of cardiac complications every 15 minutes for 1 hour, every 30 minutes for 2 hours, or until vital signs are stable.	Verifies patient's physiologic status and evaluates effect of procedure. Signs of cardiac complications include chest pain or pressure, new dysrhythmias, and/or shortness of breath.
3 Monitor for complications:	
a Perform neurovascular checks by palpating peripheral pulses on affected extremity and comparing right and left extremities for skin color, temperature, and sensation. Use Doppler ultrasonic stethoscope to locate pulses that are not palpable (see Chapter 6).	Enables prompt detection of circulatory impairment caused by intravascular clotting or bleeding at procedure site. Signs of reduced circulation include diminishing distal pulses and/or coolness, mottling, pallor, pain, numbness, and tingling in affected extremity.
b With vital signs assess vascular access site for bleeding and hematoma.	Verifies expected sealing of puncture.
c Auscultate heart and lungs and compare with preprocedure findings.	Evaluates patient response to procedure.

STEP	RATIONALE
d Observe patient for possible delayed reaction to iodine dye (if used)—dyspnea, hives, tachycardia, and rash (Pagana and Pagana, 2010).	Reaction may occur up to 6 hours after injection of dye.
4 Evaluate level of sedation, level of consciousness, and SpO_2. Use Aldrete scale (see Skill 44-1).	Determines patient's response to IV sedation.
5 Assess postprocedure laboratory values—CBC, prothrombin time, aPTT, INR, electrolytes, BUN/creatinine.	Detects changes in laboratory values that indicate onset of complications such as bleeding.
6 Have patient rate discomfort on pain scale of 0 to 10.	Pain is early sign of complications.

Unexpected Outcomes

1 Vasovagal response occurs (at time of femoral puncture or after procedure with femoral pressure). Symptoms include feeling faint, dizzy, and light-headed and possible momentary loss of consciousness. Bradycardia is caused by stimulation of vagus nerve via baroreceptors.

2 Evidence of oversedation:
  • Prolonged reduced level of consciousness.

3 Pedal pulses are nonpalpable bilaterally 2 hours after arteriogram with change in skill color and temperature.

4 Hematoma or hemorrhage is present at catheter insertion site.

5 Patient has allergic reaction to contrast medium with symptoms of flushing, itching, and urticaria.

6 Renal toxicity from contrast medium occurs:
  • Urine output less than 30 mL/hr or 0.5 mL/kg/hr.

7 Patient experiences retroperitoneal bleeding (when femoral access site is used):
  • Low back pain radiating to both sides of body (hallmark sign).
  • Tachycardia.

Related Interventions

• Support airway (through positioning).
• Lower table or head of bed to flat position or to Trendelenburg's position if ordered.
• Be prepared to administer bolus of IV fluid (normal saline).

• See Skill 44-1.

• Assess pulse with Doppler.
• Immediately notify health care provider.

• Apply pressure over insertion site.
• Monitor catheter site every 15 to 30 minutes for 2 to 3 hours; follow agency protocol.
• Notify health care provider if interventions do not stop bleeding or if patient has symptoms of acute blood loss (hypotension, tachycardia, decreased level of consciousness).

• Monitor vital signs and observe for symptoms of anaphylaxis.
• Notify health care provider.
• Follow specific postprocedure orders related to findings.
• Prepare to administer antihistamine or epinephrine if ordered.

• Place on strict intake and output (I&O) monitoring.
• Monitor closely for signs of fluid overload.
• Review electrolyte, urea nitrogen, and creatinine levels.

• Prepare patient for emergency surgery.
• Monitor vital signs every 5 to 15 minutes.
• Monitor distal pulses hourly.

Recording and Reporting

• Record patient's status: vital signs, SpO_2/end-tidal CO_2, status of peripheral pulses for equality and symmetry, blood pressure for hypotension, temperature and color of catheterized extremity, condition of IV site, and level of patient responsiveness. Record any drainage from puncture site, appearance of dressing, and condition of puncture site.

• Report to health care provider any vital sign change, excessive bleeding or increasing hematoma at puncture site, decreased or absent peripheral pulses, persistent pain, altered neurologic status, dysrhythmias, decreased SpO_2 or increased end-tidal CO_2, or decreased responsiveness after sedation.

Special Considerations

Teaching

• See Skill 44-1, Teaching Considerations.
• Prepare patient to stay in the hospital if complications occur or if an intervention necessitates prolonged postprocedure vascular checks.
• Because the dye can transfer to breast milk, teach women who are breast-feeding to substitute formula or previously pumped

breast milk for infant feedings, disposing of any pumped breast milk for 24 hours after the procedure (Pagana and Pagana, 2010).

Pediatric

• Infants and children are particularly susceptible to the diuretic effects of radiocontrast dyes because of their small body size and immature renal/hepatic systems. In addition, those with congenital cardiac anomalies develop compensatory erythrocytosis and thus experience complications from dehydration very quickly. Emphasize to the parent(s) or caregiver the importance of fluid intake with the child after the procedure. Urinary output should exceed 1 mL/kg/hr (Hockenberry and Wilson, 2011).

Gerontologic

• Physical exposure and low room temperature contribute to hypothermia in frail older adults who are unable to communicate that they are cold. Use heated blankets or forced-air heat to maintain core temperature at comfortable, safe levels (Lewis et al., 2011).

• In older adults slight alterations in vital signs or behavior are signs for impending problems; therefore close monitoring is important.

Home Care

- On discharge, provide patient with written instructions to contact the health care provider (or affiliated emergency department) if the following occur after arteriogram or cardiac catheterization:
  - Bleeding from the catheterization puncture site; apply gentle pressure with a clean gauze or cloth
  - Formation of a knot or lump under the skin that increases in size
  - Worsening of a bruise or its movement down the extremity rather than disappearing
  - Pain at puncture site or in the extremity used for the catheterization
  - Extremity is pale and cool to the touch where arterial puncture is made

- Appearance of redness, swelling, or warmth of the affected extremity
- After arteriogram or cardiac catheterization, instruct patient not to drive or climb stairs for 24 hours; to avoid sports, strenuous activity/housework, and lifting (e.g., groceries, children) for 3 days; and to avoid taking baths until wound is healed.
- On discharge after an IVP, instruct patient to:
  - Drink at least 64 ounces (1 to 2 liters) of water to help flush the contrast media through the kidneys.
  - Watch for signs of a delayed reaction to the contrast medium for 24 hours after the procedure and call the health care provider or go to the nearest emergency department.

> **SKILL 44-3** Assisting with Aspirations: Bone Marrow Aspiration/Biopsy, Lumbar Puncture, Paracentesis, and Thoracentesis

Aspirations are sterile invasive procedures involving the removal of body fluids or tissue for diagnostic procedures (Table 44-3). The nurse assists the health care provider during an aspiration procedure. Informed consent is required for these invasive procedures.

Bone marrow aspiration is the removal of a small amount of the liquid organic material in the medullary canals of selected bones. The sternum and the posterior superior iliac crests are the most common in adults. In children the anterior or posterior iliac crests are used, and in infants the proximal tibia is used (Hockenberry and Wilson, 2011; Pagana and Pagana, 2010). A biopsy is the removal of a core of marrow cells for laboratory analysis. Both aspiration and biopsy diagnose and differentiate leukemia, certain malignancies, anemia, and thrombocytopenia. The marrow is examined in a laboratory to reveal the number, size, shape, and development of red blood cells (RBCs) and megakaryocytes (platelet precursors). Bone marrow cultures help differentiate infectious diseases such as tuberculosis (TB) or histoplasmosis. This procedure takes approximately 20 minutes to perform. Potential complications of bone marrow aspiration or biopsy include bleeding, especially if coagulopathy is present; infection; and, less commonly, organ puncture.

A lumbar puncture (LP), called a *spinal puncture or tap*, involves the introduction of a needle into the subarachnoid space of the spinal column. The purpose of the test is to measure pressure in the subarachnoid space; obtain cerebrospinal fluid (CSF) for visualization and laboratory examination; and inject anesthetic, diagnostic, or therapeutic agents. CSF is examined in a laboratory to help diagnose spinal cord tumors, central nervous system (CNS) infections, hemorrhage, and degenerative brain disease. The procedure takes approximately 30 minutes to perform.

The major contraindication for LP is evidence of increased intracranial pressure (ICP). The LP causes a sudden release of pressure and possible herniation of the brain structures through the foramen magnum. This herniation compresses the brainstem, which contains the vital cardiac, respiratory, and vasomotor centers; and sudden death results. In elective LP preprocedure computed tomography results are reviewed for evidence of brain shift to rule out ICP.

Abdominal paracentesis involves aspiration of peritoneal fluid from the abdomen. Cytologic analysis of the aspirate determines presence of bacteria, blood, glucose, and protein to help diagnose the causes of an abdominal effusion. Paracentesis may also be a

TABLE 44-3	**Summary of Aspiration Procedures**			
Aspiration Procedure	**Preparation/Assessment Specific to Test**	**Position and Site**		**Special Considerations**
Bone marrow aspiration	Assess complete blood count for abnormalities.			Patients with arthritis or orthopnea may have difficulty assuming the positions. Pressure is applied to the site following procedure.

"X" marks site of aspiration. (*From Ignatavicius DD, Workman ML*: Medical-surgical nursing: Patient-centered collaborative care, *St Louis, ed 6, 2010, Saunders.*)

Continued

TABLE 44-3 | Summary of Aspiration Procedures—cont'd

Aspiration Procedure	Preparation/Assessment Specific to Test	Position and Site	Special Considerations
Lumbar puncture	Assess neurologic status, including movement, sensation, and muscle strength of legs to provide a baseline for comparison.	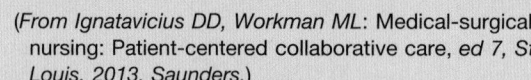 Lateral decubitus position L1 L3 L5 L2 L4 Subarachnoid space *(From Ignatavicius DD, Workman ML: Medical-surgical nursing: Patient-centered collaborative care, ed 7, St Louis, 2013, Saunders.)*	*Risk for spinal headache*: Instruct patient to remain flat and logroll according to health care provider's orders. Observe for excessive drainage at site. Fluid loss at site can predispose patient to headache and infection.
Paracentesis	Assess bladder for distention and determine last voiding. Weigh patient, inspect and palpate abdomen, and measure abdominal girth at largest point. Mark location.	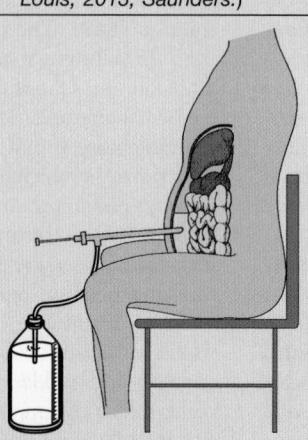 *(From Pagana KD, Pagana TJ: Mosby's manual of diagnostic and laboratory tests, ed 4, St Louis, 2010, Mosby.)*	After fluid is removed, pressure on diaphragm is released, and breathing becomes much easier. *Risk for trauma*: Have patient empty urinary bladder before procedure.
Thoracentesis	Assess respiratory rate and depth, symmetry of chest on inspiration and expiration, cough, and sputum. Help patient remain still during procedure to prevent trauma to visceral pleura. Patient will need to hold breath and avoid coughing during procedure.	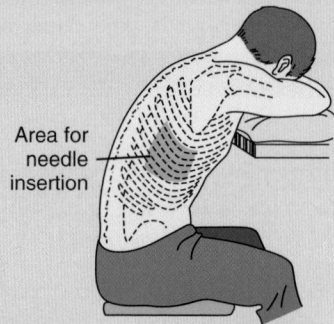 Area for needle insertion Ribs Parietal pleura Visceral pleura Lung tissue (parenchyma) Pleural effusion Syringe Diaphragm	Monitor blood pressure for hypotension if large quantity of fluid is removed. *Risk for pneumothorax*: Observe for sudden shortness of breath, tracheal deviation, anxiety, altered vital signs, and decreased oxygen saturation.

palliative measure to provide temporary relief of abdominal and respiratory discomfort caused by severe ascites. Lavage paracentesis, in which a lavage of solution is instilled and then withdrawn, is done to detect the presence of bleeding, as in cases of blunt abdominal trauma or tumor cells when cancer is suspected. Although not contraindicated, paracentesis is performed with caution in patients with coagulopathies, with portal hypertension accompanied with abdominal collateral circulation, and in those who are pregnant. The procedure takes approximately 30 minutes to perform.

Thoracentesis is performed to analyze or remove pleural fluid or instill medications intrapleurally. Cytologic studies of specimens reveal presence of blood, glucose, amylase, lactate dehydrogenase (LD), and cellular composition. Cytologic specimens are also examined for malignancy, differentiated between transudative and exudative characteristics, and cultured for pathogens. The following cause transudate in the pleural space: ascites, cirrhosis (hepatic), heart failure, hypertension (pulmonary, systemic), nephritis, and nephrosis. Therapeutic thoracentesis relieves pain, dyspnea, and signs of pleural pressure. The test takes approximately 30 minutes to perform.

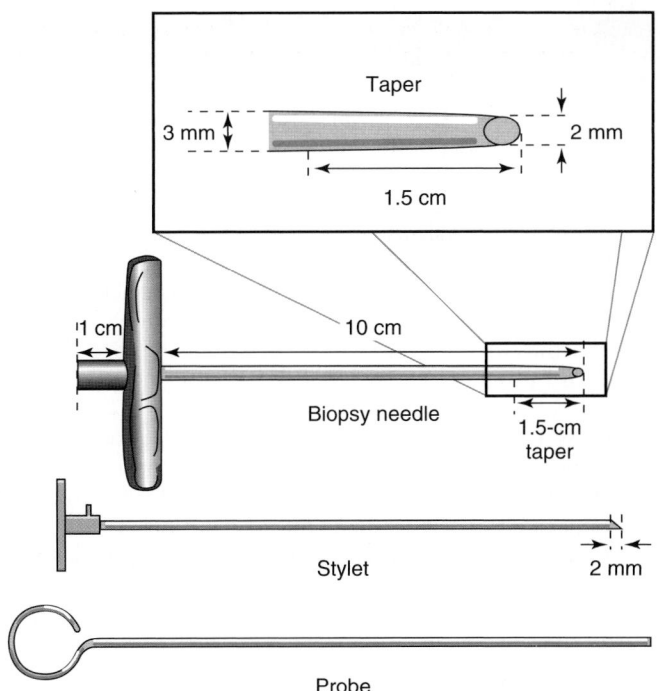

FIG 44-3 Bone marrow biopsy needle showing shape and size. (*From Monahan F et al: Phipps' medical-surgical nursing: health and illness perspectives, ed 8, St Louis, 2007, Mosby.*)

Delegation and Collaboration

The skill of assisting with aspirations can be delegated to nursing assistive personnel (NAP) if the patient is stable (check agency policy). However, assessment of the patient's condition must be completed by the nurse and cannot be delegated. The nurse directs the NAP about:

- How to properly position the patient during the procedure.
- When to take and report vital signs.
- Which signs and symptoms experienced by the patient to immediately report to the RN.

Equipment

- ❏ Protective equipment: Masks, goggles, gowns, head cover, sterile gloves for all health care personnel performing the procedure
- ❏ Test tubes, sterile specimen containers, laboratory requisitions, and labels
- ❏ Analgesia (if ordered)
- ❏ Antiseptic solution
- ❏ 4 × 4–inch sterile gauze pads, tape, Band-Aid
- ❏ Sphygmomanometer, pulse oximeter/end-tidal CO_2 monitor
- ❏ Aspiration tray: Most agencies provide trays specific to the aspiration procedure. Standard tray includes antiseptic solution

(e.g., povidone-iodine; chlorhexidine); gauze sponges (4 × 4 inch); sterile towels; local anesthetic solution (e.g., lidocaine 1%); two 3-mL sterile syringes with 16- to 27-gauge needles. Additional equipment for specific aspirations includes:

- Bone marrow aspiration: Two bone marrow needles with inner stylet (Fig. 44-3)
- LP: Manometer to measure spinal pressure and at least four test tubes
- Paracentesis: Intravenous (IV) fluids as ordered, vacuum bottles to collect fluid, stopcock with extension tubing, sterile collection containers, measuring tape
- Thoracentesis: Vacuum bottles to collect fluid, stopcock with extension tubing

STEP	RATIONALE

ASSESSMENT

1 Verify type of procedure scheduled, purpose, and procedure site with patient and medical record.

2 Verify that informed consent was obtained before administering any analgesia or antianxiety agents.

3 Review medical record for contraindications.

  a *LP:* Increased intracranial pressure (IICP), spinal deformities, and clotting disorders

  b *Paracentesis:* Clotting disorders, intestinal obstructions, and pregnancy

  c *Bone marrow biopsy:* Patient cannot maintain position during procedure.

  d *Thoracentesis:* Patient cannot maintain position during procedure.

Ensures correct patient. Complies with The Joint Commission (2012) requirements and improves procedure safety.

Federal regulations, many state laws, and accreditation agencies require informed consent for procedures.

Factors can cause hemorrhage, and ICP may cause brainstem herniation.

Paracentesis in pregnant woman may injure fetus.

STEP	RATIONALE
4 Determine patient's ability to assume position required for procedure and ability to remain still (see Table 44-3). Discuss with health care provider need for premedication for anxious patients.	Movement during procedure can cause complications such as bleeding and injury to nerves or tissue. Required position depends on site used for aspiration.
5 Before procedure: Obtain vital signs, oxygen saturation (SpO_2)/ end-tidal CO_2 value, and weight. For paracentesis obtain abdominal girth measurement. (Use ink pen to mark measurement location for abdominal girth measurement.) For LP assess lower extremity movement, sensation, and muscle strength.	Provides baseline for comparison with vital signs during and after procedure. Patients will have decreased abdominal girth and lose weight after paracentesis.
6 Instruct patient to empty bladder.	Reduces risk for bladder trauma during paracentesis. Promotes patient comfort.
7 Assess patient's coagulation status: use of anticoagulants, complete blood count (CBC), platelet count, clotting factors, activated partial thromboplastin time (aPTT), international normalized ratio (INR), and prothrombin time (PT).	Invasive procedures are contraindicated in patients with coagulation disorders because of risk for bleeding (Pagana and Pagana, 2010).
8 Determine whether patient is allergic to antiseptic, latex, or anesthetic solutions.	Precautions can be taken to decrease chance of allergic reactions.
9 Assess patient's level of understanding of procedure, including any concerns.	Determines extent of instruction and level of support required.
10 Assess baseline pain level, using scale of 0 to 10.	Determines need for preprocedure analgesia. Pain control helps patients maintain proper position and tolerate aspiration procedure.

NURSING DIAGNOSES

- Acute pain
- Anxiety
- Deficient knowledge regarding procedure

- Fear
- Impaired gas exchange
- Impaired mobility

- Ineffective breathing pattern
- Risk for infection
- Risk for injury

Related factors are individualized based on patient's condition or needs.

PLANNING

1 Expected outcomes following completion of procedure:	
• Patient describes purpose of procedure.	Demonstrates understanding and improves likelihood of cooperation.
• Patient assumes and maintains required position and remains still throughout procedure.	Correct position facilitates safe and timely completion of the procedure.
• There is no bleeding at needle insertion site.	Precautions during procedure prevent bleeding.
• Amount of aspirate is sufficient to perform laboratory testing.	
• Patient's level of comfort equals score of 4 or less on pain scale of 0 to 10.	Procedure performed with minimal discomfort to patient.
• Vital signs, SpO_2, and end-tidal CO_2 remain within normal limits during and after aspiration procedure.	Removal of abdominal (ascites) or pleural fluid increases lung expansion and improves gas exchange.
• Patient undergoing paracentesis has reduced abdominal girth and improved respirations.	Fluid successfully removed from peritoneal space.
2 Explain steps of skin preparation, anesthetic injection, needle insertion, position required.	Anticipation of expected sensations and procedural activities reduces anxiety.
3 If ordered, premedicate for pain 30 minutes before procedure. *Option:* In some cases patients will receive anti-anxiety medications.	Pain and anxiety control helps patient to remain in position, minimizes discomfort from needle insertion, and decreases anxiety.
4 Before thoracentesis verify recent chest x-ray film examination.	Provides preprocedure baseline to determine location of pleural fluid.

IMPLEMENTATION

1 Identify patient using two identifiers (i.e., name and birthday or name and account number) according to agency policy. Compare identifiers with information on patient's identification bracelet.	Ensures correct patient. Complies with The Joint Commission standards and improves patient safety (2012).
2 Perform hand hygiene.	Reduces transmission of microorganisms.

STEP	RATIONALE
3 Set up sterile tray or open supplies to make accessible for health care provider.	Maintains integrity of sterile field and promotes prompt completion of procedure.
4 Take "Time-Out" to verify patient's name, type of procedure scheduled, and procedure site with patient and health care team.	"Time-Out" verification just before starting procedure includes physician and all personnel and is safety precaution to prevent wrong patient, wrong site, and wrong procedure errors (TJC, 2012).
5 Help patient maintain correct position. Reassure patient while explaining procedure.	Decreases chance of complications occurring during procedure. Explanations increase patient comfort and relaxation.
a Bone marrow:	
• *Adults:* For sternal biopsy place in supine position. For iliac crest biopsy place in prone or lateral recumbent position.	Provides best access to bone containing marrow.
• *Children:* For iliac crest biopsy place in prone or lateral recumbent position.	
b LP:	
Position in lateral recumbent (fetal) position with head and neck flexed (see Table 44-3).	Provides full curvature and flexion of spinal column to allow maximal space between vertebrae.
c Paracentesis:	
Position in bed in semi-Fowler's position or sitting upright on side of bed or in chair with feet supported (see Table 44-3).	Position uses gravity to cause fluid to accumulate in lower abdominal cavity, where it is drained more easily.
d Thoracentesis:	
Place in orthopneic position (upright position with arms and shoulders raised and supported on padded over-bed table) (see Table 44-3). If patient is unable to tolerate, help to side-lying position with affected lung positioned upward.	Expands intercostal space for needle insertions.

Clinical Decision Point *Emphasize the importance of remaining immobile during procedure to prevent trauma, especially with the LP. Sudden movement is a risk for spinal cord nerve root damage. Sudden movement during paracentesis or thoracentesis risks damage of the abdominal or pulmonary structures. Also instruct patient not to cough, sneeze, or breathe deeply during the procedures because these actions increase the risk for needle displacement and damage of other structures.*

6 Explain to patient that pain may occur when lidocaine (local anesthetic) is injected into tissues. Pressure may also occur when tissue or fluid is aspirated.	Aspiration is painful but lasts for only a few moments. If patient is having bone marrow aspirate, deep pressure feeling is frequently experienced as bone marrow is withdrawn (Pagana and Pagana, 2010).
7 Physician applies sterile gloves, mask, gown, and goggles; cleans patient's skin with antiseptic solution; and drapes site with sterile drape.	Removes surface bacteria from skin at area of puncture site. Creates sterile field.
8 Physician injects local anesthetic and allows time for anesthesia to occur.	Provides optimal effect of local anesthesia.
9 Physician inserts needle or trocar into spinal space or body cavity involved (see Table 44-3). To aspirate tissue or body fluids for specimen analysis, syringe is attached to trocar or needle, and aspirate is placed into specimen container.	Success depends on positioning, accurate insertion site, and patient remaining still.
10 Nurse assesses patient's condition during procedure, including respiratory status, vital signs if indicated, and any complaints of pain.	Identifies any changes that indicate complication.

Clinical Decision Point *Increased or worsening abdominal or thoracic pain is significant in paracentesis and thoracentesis. Severe abdominal pain indicates a possible bowel perforation following a paracentesis. Following a thoracentesis abdominal pain results from diaphragmatic, liver, or spleen perforation. Inspiratory chest pain results from perforation of the lung.*

11 Note characteristics of aspirate:	
a *Bone marrow aspirate:* Marrow may appear red or yellow.	Normal marrow.
b *LP:* Record opening pressure; observe fluid for color, cloudiness, or blood.	Normal CSF is clear and colorless. Cloudiness is result of protein, which indicates an infection.
c *Paracentesis:* Fluid may appear yellow, cloudy, bile-stained green, or blood tinged. Peritoneal lavage fluid may appear bright red.	Blood-tinged fluid is caused by traumatic tap. In patient with abdominal trauma bloody lavage identifies active bleeding.

STEP	RATIONALE
d *Thoracentesis:* Pleural fluid may appear clear yellow, puslike, or cloudy.	Clear yellow is normal. Transudate and exudates are typically yellow, straw color.
	Blood-tinged fluid indicates malignancy, pulmonary infarction, or severe inflammation. Puslike fluid indicates infection (empyema); milky fluid indicates chylothorax (i.e., leak from thoracic duct resulting in lymphatic drainage in pleural cavity).
12 Properly label specimens in presence of patient and transport to laboratory in proper containers. Label specimens in order of collection.	Ensures that correct laboratory results are assigned to right patient. Test tubes are numbered in sequence of collection (e.g., 1 through 4).
13 Physician removes needle/trocar and applies pressure over insertion site until drainage ceases. If necessary, help with direct pressure and application of gauze dressing.	Assists in homeostasis and secures insertion site.
14 All team members in procedure remove protective equipment, discard in appropriate receptacle, and perform hand hygiene.	Reduces transmission of infection.

EVALUATION

1 Monitor level of consciousness, vital signs, and SpO_2/end-tidal CO_2. Check agency policy; sometimes vital signs are obtained every 15 minutes for 2 hours.	Verifies patient's physiologic status in response to procedure or any potential complications.
2 Inspect dressing over puncture site for bleeding, swelling, tenderness, and erythema. Inspect area under patient for bleeding. Avoid disrupting healing clot at site if pressure dressing is present.	Determines further blood loss from puncture site. Infection is potential complication, especially if patient is leukopenic (Pagana and Pagana, 2010).
3 Evaluate pain score to determine if patient's level of comfort is equivalent to a score of 4 or less on pain scale of 0 to 10.	Determines if patient is having increased pain to warrant postprocedure analgesia.
4 Following paracentesis, measure abdominal girth and respirations and compare to preprocedure measurements.	Determines amount of change in abdominal size and ability to ventilate.

Unexpected Outcomes

1 Oversedation occurs.

2 Site complications occur:

  a *Bone marrow:* Tenderness or erythema at site.

  b *LP:*

    (1) Postprocedure headache (PPHD) is evidenced by headache, blurred vision, and tinnitus.

    (2) Excess loss of CSF is indicated by decreased level of consciousness, hearing loss, dilated pupils, and decreased ICP.

  c *Paracentesis:* Leakage of fluid from site and acute abdominal pain occur.

  d *Thoracentesis:* Pneumothorax is evidenced by sudden dyspnea, tachypnea, and asymmetric chest excursion.

Related Interventions

• See Skill 44-1.

• Notify health care provider and obtain further orders.
• Administer analgesic as ordered.
• Continue to monitor site.

• Monitor fluid loss.
• Physician may inject blood patch into epidural space.
• Medicate for pain as ordered.

• Maintain airway.
• Transfer to intensive care unit (ICU) per physician order.

• Reinforce dressing; may also be instructed to place sterile collection bag over site.
• Monitor vital signs and SpO_2.
• Assess abdomen for bowel sounds.

• Administer oxygen.
• Monitor vital signs and SpO_2.
• Anticipate chest x-ray film examination and possible chest tube insertion.

Recording and Reporting

• Record in patient's chart name of procedure; preprocedure preparation; location of puncture site; amount, consistency, and color of fluid drained or specimen obtained; duration of procedure; patient's tolerance (e.g., vital signs, SpO_2) and comfort level; laboratory tests ordered and specimen sent; type of dressing; postprocedure activities (e.g., chest x-ray film examination); and other procedure-specific assessments (e.g., extremity assessment, abdominal girth, level of consciousness).

• Immediately report to health care provider any change in vital signs and SpO_2, unexpected pain/discomfort, and any excessive drainage from dressing over puncture site.

Special Considerations
Teaching
- Instruct patient that some people experience tenderness at the puncture site for several days after the study and that mild analgesia often helps to relieve some of the discomfort.

Pediatric
- Conscious or unconscious sedation is commonly used. If using unconscious sedation, an anesthesiologist or nurse anesthetist will be needed for the procedure.
- Prepare preschool children before the procedure; make a game out of having child recall the next procedural step, which can serve as a distraction (Hockenberry and Wilson, 2011).

Gerontologic
- Older adults with arthritis need help to stay in the required position.

- Older adults have reduced elastic lung recoil, weaker cough efficiency, and decreased chest expansion. Restlessness may indicate hypoxia following thoracentesis.
- Be aware that older adults may have specific fears and anxiety related to postprocedure falling and fatigue.

Home Care
- Teach patients and family caregivers about specific postprocedure complications and when to report them to the health care provider.
- If patient is transferred to long-term care facility, ensure thorough communication between agencies regarding results of procedure and patient condition.

SKILL 44-4 Assisting with Bronchoscopy

Bronchoscopy is the examination of the tracheobronchial tree through a lighted tube containing mirrors. A flexible fiberoptic bronchoscope has lumens that allow both visualization and simultaneous administration of oxygen (Fig. 44-4). The fiberoptic bronchoscope is used for obtaining sputum, foreign bodies, and biopsy specimens. Laser ablation of endotracheal lesions may also be performed through the bronchoscope.

Bronchoscopy may be an emergency or elective procedure and may be performed for diagnostic or therapeutic reasons. The main purposes of this procedure include aspirating excessive sputum or mucus plugs that airway suctioning cannot remove; visualizing the tracheobronchial tree for assessment of abnormalities of the mucosa, abscesses, aspiration pneumonia, strictures, and tumors; obtaining deep tissue biopsy and sputum specimens; and/or removing foreign bodies. This procedure is contraindicated in patients who cannot tolerate interruption of high-flow oxygen unless intubated. Potential complications of bronchoscopy include fever, infection, hypoxemia, bronchospasm and/or laryngospasm, pneumothorax, aspiration, dysrhythmias and hypotension, hemorrhage (after biopsy), and cardiac arrest.

The procedure is performed at the bedside or in a specially equipped endoscopy room. Usually a pulmonary specialist or surgeon performs the procedure in approximately 30 to 45 minutes.

Delegation and Collaboration
The skill of assisting with bronchoscopy cannot be delegated to nursing assistive personnel (NAP). The nurse directs the NAP to:
- Measure follow-up postprocedure vital signs (after RN's initial assessment).
- Position the patient appropriately (based on procedure and patient limitations).
- Immediately report to the nurse if the patient has possible respiratory distress or is coughing up blood.

Equipment
- ❏ Bronchoscopy tray, if available from central supply, which includes flexible fiberoptic bronchoscope (see Fig. 44-4); 4 × 4–inch gauze sponges; local anesthetic spray (lidocaine); sterile tracheal suction catheters; diazepam (Valium), midazolam (Versed), or other sedative for intravenous (IV) sedation
- ❏ Oxygen, resuscitative equipment
- ❏ Pulse oximeter/end-tidal CO_2 monitor, cardiac monitor
- ❏ Sterile gloves
- ❏ Sterile water-soluble lubricating jelly (NOTE: Petroleum-based lubricants are not used because of the hazard of aspiration and subsequent pneumonia.)
- ❏ Protective equipment: Mask, gown, gloves, head cover, and goggles for all health care providers
- ❏ Emesis basin
- ❏ Suction machine and connecting tube
- ❏ Blood pressure equipment

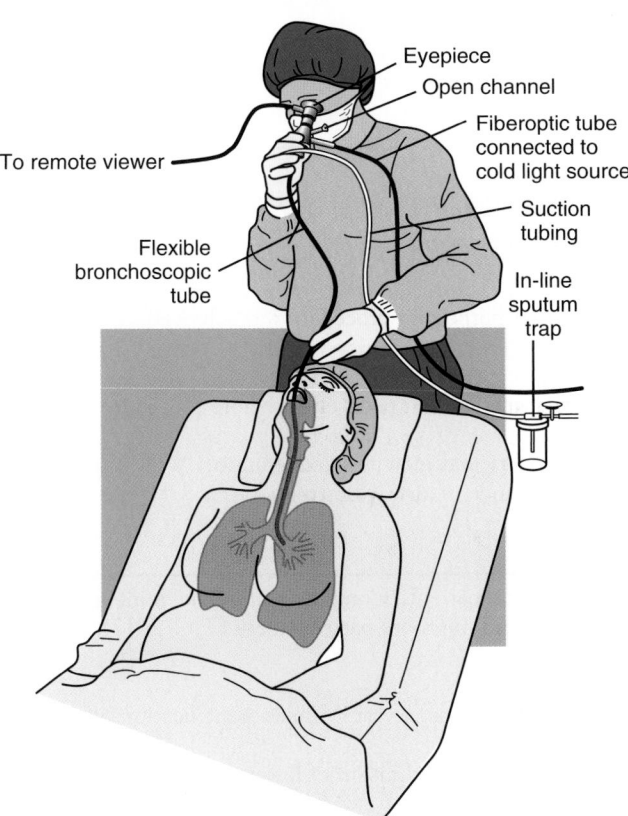

FIG 44-4 Flexible fiberoptic bronchoscopy.

STEP	RATIONALE

ASSESSMENT

1 Verify type of procedure scheduled and procedure site with patient.	Ensures correct patient. Complies with The Joint Commission standards and improves patient safety (TJC, 2012).
2 Verify that informed consent was obtained before administration of any sedatives.	Federal regulations, many state laws, and accreditation agencies such as The Joint Commission require informed consent for procedure.
3 Assess patient's history for inability to tolerate interruption of high-flow oxygen unless intubated.	Determines need for oxygen administration during procedure.
4 Obtain baseline vital signs, pulse oximetry (SpO$_2$) and end-tidal CO$_2$ values.	Baseline data provide for comparison with findings during and after procedure.
5 Assess type of cough, sputum produced, heart and lung sounds.	Provides for comparison with respiratory status during and after procedure.
6 Determine purpose of procedure: for sputum aspiration, assessment, tissue biopsy, or removal of foreign body.	Anticipates equipment needs of physician and type of information to convey to patient during teaching.
7 Determine whether patient is allergic to local anesthetic used for spraying throat (usually lidocaine).	Allergy causes laryngeal edema or laryngospasm.
8 Assess need for preprocedure medication (usually atropine and opioid or sedative).	Atropine decreases secretions and inhibits vagally stimulated bradycardia; opioids or sedatives relieve anxiety and decrease discomfort.
9 Assess time patient last ingested food/fluids or medications. Patient must be NPO for at least 8 hours before a bronchoscopy; however, some medications may be taken before procedure by physician order.	Reduces risk for aspiration.
10 Assess patient's level of understanding of procedure, including any concerns.	Determines extent of instruction and level of support required.

NURSING DIAGNOSIS

• Anxiety	• Impaired gas exchange	• Risk for aspiration
• Deficient knowledge regarding procedure	• Ineffective airway clearance	• Risk for infection
• Fear	• Ineffective breathing pattern	• Risk for injury

Related factors are individualized based on patient's condition or needs.

PLANNING

1 Expected outcomes following completion of procedure:	
• Patient recovers from sedation without respiratory complications or change in level of consciousness.	Sedation adequate, and patient tolerates procedure.
• Patient's level of comfort is equivalent to score of 4 or less on pain scale of 0 to 10.	Minimal trauma caused by bronchoscope.
• Physician is able to observe, suction, and obtain specimens from tracheobronchial tree.	Indicates that purpose of procedure was achieved.
• Patient explains procedure and assumes appropriate position.	Demonstrates patient's understanding.
2 Administer atropine, opioid, or antianxiety agent 30 minutes before procedure.	Ensures that medication takes effect before procedure.
3 Explain procedure to patient.	Reduces anxiety and increases cooperation.
4 Remove and safely store patient's dentures and/or eyeglasses.	Minimizes chance of airway obstruction.

IMPLEMENTATION

1 Identify patient using two identifiers (i.e., name and birthday or name and account number) according to agency policy. Compare identifiers with information on patient's identification bracelet.	Ensures correct patient. Complies with The Joint Commission standards and improves patient safety (TJC, 2012).
2 Assess current IV access or establish new IV access with large-bore cannula (see Chapter 28).	Provides immediate access for IV fluids or medications if emergency occurs.
3 Help patient assume position desired by physician: usually semi-Fowler's.	Provides maximal visualization of lower airway and adequate lung expansion.

STEP	RATIONALE
4 Take "Time-Out" to verify patient's name, type of procedure scheduled, and procedure site with patient and health care team.	"Time-Out" verification just before starting procedure includes physician and all personnel and is safety precaution to prevent wrong patient, wrong site, and wrong procedure errors (TJC, 2012).
5 Perform hand hygiene and apply protective equipment. Position tip of suction catheter for easy access to patient's mouth.	Reduces transmission of microorganisms. Removes secretions to reduce risk for aspiration.
6 Physician usually sprays nasopharynx and oropharynx with topical anesthetic. Lidocaine is commonly used 10 to 15 minutes before procedure. When a patient is intubated or has tracheostomy, anesthetic spray is usually not needed.	Provides swift anesthesia of oropharynx.
7 Instruct patient not to swallow local anesthetic; provide emesis basin for expectorating it.	Reduces unintended anesthesia of esophagus.
8 Another physician or staff member attaches bronchoscope to machine light source.	Enhances visualization during procedure.
9 Physician applies goggles, mask, and sterile gloves; introduces bronchoscope into mouth to pharynx; passes through glottis and into trachea and bronchi (see Fig. 44-4). More anesthetic spray may be used at glottis to prevent cough reflex. For intubated patients the flexible bronchoscope is introduced through their endotracheal tube.	Bronchoscope must be passed through upper airway structures to promote visualization of lower airways. Trachea and bronchi are observed for lesions and obstructions. Adaptor accompanies bronchoscope and is used for bag-valve-mask or ventilator use.
10 Physician suctions mucus and performs bronchial washing with cytologic specimens taken with wire brush or curette. Biopsy specimens may also be obtained.	Cytologic specimens are obtained to diagnose carcinoma.
11 Help patient through procedure by providing explanations, verbal reassurance, and support.	Although premedicated and drowsy, remind patient not to change position and to cooperate. Reinforce that patient will be able to breathe during procedure.
12 Assess patient's pulse, blood pressure, respirations, SpO$_2$, end-tidal CO$_2$, and breathing capacity during procedure: observe degree of restlessness, capillary refill, and color of nail beds.	Bronchoscope can cause feelings of suffocation and vasovagal response and laryngospasm. Because airway is partially occluded, patient can develop hypoxia during procedure.
13 Note characteristics of suctioned material. Expect small amount of blood mixed with aspirate because of tissue trauma.	Information used to record and report and make further patient observations.
14 Using gloved hand, wipe patient's mouth and nose to remove lubricant after bronchoscope is removed.	Promotes hygiene and comfort.
15 Instruct patient not to eat or drink until tracheobronchial anesthesia has worn off and gag reflex has returned, usually 2 hours. Use tongue depressor to touch pharynx to test for presence of gag reflex.	Prevents aspiration.
16 Remove protective equipment, discard, and perform hand hygiene.	Reduces transmission of microorganisms.

EVALUATION

1 Monitor vital signs, SpO$_2$, and end-tidal CO$_2$.	Verifies physiologic response to procedure.
2 Observe character and amount of sputum. Physician may order serial sputum collection for 24 hours for cytologic examination.	Evaluates for complication of bronchial perforation, indicated by severe hemoptysis. Slight blood-tinged sputum is normal after this procedure.
3 Observe respiratory status closely; palpate for facial or neck crepitus.	Detects early sign of bronchial perforation (Chernecky and Berger, 2008).
4 Assess for return of gag reflex. It usually returns in approximately 2 hours.	Helps prevent aspiration pneumonia, which is risk until gag reflex returns.
5 Ask patient to describe postprocedure normal and abnormal symptoms.	Evaluates patient's understanding.

Unexpected Outcomes	Related Interventions
1 Vasovagal response caused by stimulation of baroreceptors during bronchoscope insertion, causing symptoms of: • Feeling nauseous, faint, dizzy, and/or light-headed. • Diaphoresis with slow, steady pulse. • Unconsciousness for few seconds.	• Lower head of table. • Continue vital signs monitoring. • Lower head of table. • Support airway (positioning/suctioning).
2 Laryngospasm and bronchospasm as evidenced by: • Sudden, severe shortness of breath.	• Call physician immediately. • Support airway (positioning). • Prepare emergency resuscitation equipment. • Anticipate possible cricothyrotomy.
3 Hypoxemia as evidenced by: • Gradual shortness of breath. • Decreasing level of consciousness.	• Monitor SpO_2. • Maintain airway and breathing. • Notify physician immediately.
4 Hemorrhage as evidenced by: • Acute blood loss • Hypotension and tachycardia • Decreasing level of consciousness	• Notify physician immediately. • Monitor vital signs. • Be prepared to administer IV fluids.
5 Oversedation (see Skill 44-1)	

Recording and Reporting

• Record procedure(s) performed (e.g., biopsy), character of sputum, duration of procedure, patient's tolerance and if any complications, and the collection and disposition of specimen(s). Document time of gag reflex return.

• Report bleeding or respiratory distress following the procedure or any changes in vital signs beyond patient's normal limits to physician immediately. Report results of procedure to appropriate health care personnel.

Special Considerations

Teaching

• Before the procedure instruct patient to perform good mouth care to decrease risk for introducing bacteria into lungs during the procedure.

• In some cases patients may receive IV sedation (refer to Skill 44-1, Teaching Considerations).

• If ordered, teach patient how to perform controlled coughing techniques for obtaining serial sputum samples (see Chapter 43).

Pediatric

• In children the procedure is most frequently performed under general anesthesia to remove foreign bodies from the larynx or trachea. Follow-up care after the foreign body is removed includes chest physiotherapy, monitoring for respiratory distress, and education of parents.

• Children are at higher risk for hypoxemia than adults because their bronchus is smaller and the bronchoscope decreases the available breathing space (Pagana and Pagana, 2010).

Gerontologic

• Physical exposure and room temperature contribute to hypothermia in frail older adults who are unable to communicate that they are cold. Use warmed blankets or forced-air heat to maintain core temperature at comfortable, safe levels (Lewis et al., 2011).

• Postprocedure restlessness often indicates hypoxemia or pain. Thoroughly assess pulmonary capacity before administering opioids, which may depress the respiratory centers.

Home Care

• Instruct ambulatory care patients to notify the physician if the following symptoms develop: fever, chest pain or discomfort, dyspnea, wheezing, or hemoptysis.

• Throat discomfort is managed with throat lozenges or warm saline gargles.

SKILL 44-5 Assisting with Gastrointestinal Endoscopy

Endoscopy allows direct visualization of an internal organ or structure by means of a long, flexible fiberoptic scope. The tip of the scope has a light source and camera lens that allows visualization of the lining of the gastrointestinal (GI) structures on a large display screen (Fig. 44-5). For visualization of the upper GI tract, esophagoscopy, gastroscopy, gastroduodenojejunoscopy (GDJ), or duodenoscopy is performed; or more frequently esophagogastroduodenoscopy (EGD), which permits visualization of the esophagus, stomach (Fig. 44-6), and duodenum in one examination. Besides direct observation, endoscopy enables biopsy of suspicious tissue, polyp removal, and performance of many other procedures such as direct visual guidance for fine-needle aspiration biopsies and dilation and stenting of strictures. For visualization of the hepatobiliary tree and pancreatic ducts, an endoscopic retrograde cholangiopancreatography (ERCP) is performed. For visual examination of the lower GI tract, proctoscopy, sigmoidoscopy, or colonoscopy is performed. Typically these patients receive intravenous (IV) moderate sedation.

Risks of endoscopic procedures include intestinal perforation, hemorrhage, peritonitis, aspiration, respiratory depression, and/or myocardial infarction secondary to vasovagal response. Both upper and lower GI endoscopic examinations may be performed in a specially equipped endoscopic unit or at the patient's bedside.

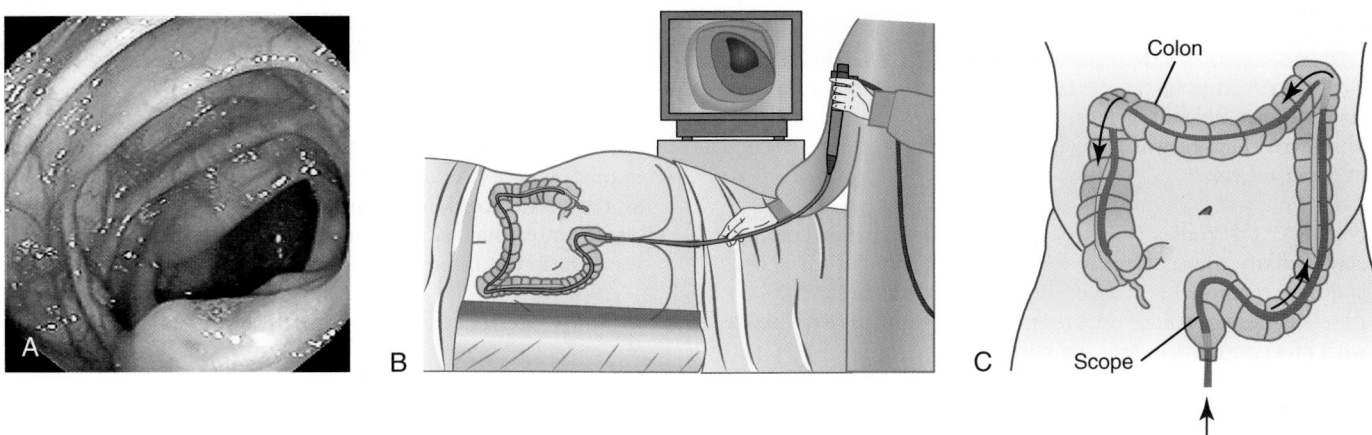

FIG 44-5 **A,** Scope view of healthy colon. **B,** Overview of colonoscopy process. **C,** Path of scope through colon.

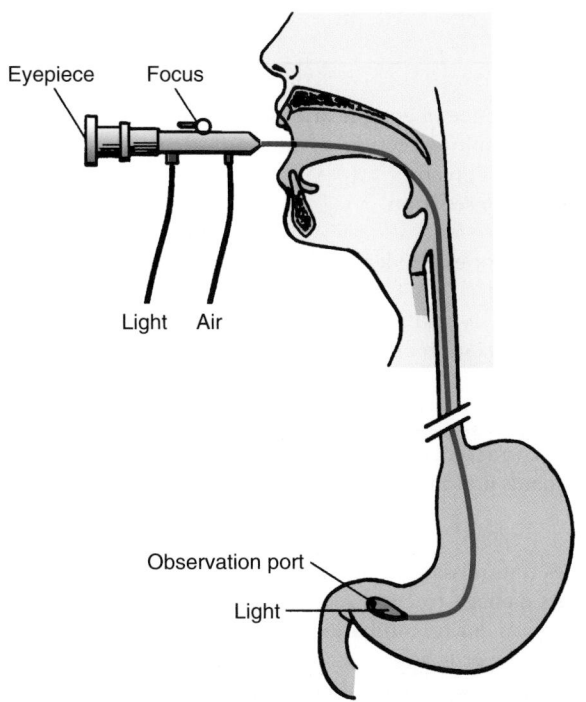

FIG 44-6 Stomach may be visualized by means of a fiberscope.

Delegation and Collaboration

The skill of assisting with endoscopy cannot be delegated to nursing assistive personnel (NAP). The nurse directs the NAP about:

- How to assist with patient positioning.

Equipment

- ❏ Protective equipment: Mask, gown, gloves, head cover, goggles for all health care personnel
- ❏ Endoscopy tray
- ❏ Fiberoptic endoscope and camera (see Fig. 44-5)
- ❏ Solutions for biopsy specimens
- ❏ Local anesthetic spray
- ❏ Tracheal suction equipment (see Chapter 25)
- ❏ Blood pressure equipment
- ❏ Sterile water-soluble jelly
- ❏ Sterile gloves for physician
- ❏ Emesis basin
- ❏ IV fluid and equipment for IV start (*optional*)
- ❏ Diazepam (Valium), midazolam (Versed), or other sedative for IV sedation (*optional*)
- ❏ Sedative reversal agents
- ❏ Carbon dioxide source to inflate colon (for lower GI procedures)
- ❏ Oxygen, resuscitative equipment, pulse oximeter/end-tidal CO_2 monitor

STEP	RATIONALE

ASSESSMENT

1 Verify type of procedure scheduled and procedure site with patient.	Ensures correct patient. Complies with The Joint Commission standards and improves patient safety (TJC, 2012).
2 Verify that informed consent was obtained before administering sedation.	Federal regulations, many state laws, and accreditation agencies such as The Joint Commission require informed consent for procedure.
3 Determine if GI bleeding is present. Observe character of emesis, stool, and nasogastric (NG) tube drainage for frank blood or material that looks like coffee grounds.	Test is contraindicated in patients with severe upper GI bleeding because viewing lens becomes covered with blood clots, preventing visualization (Pagana and Pagana, 2010).
4 Obtain vital signs and oxygen saturation/end-tidal CO_2 values.	Baseline data provide for comparison with findings during and after procedure.

Clinical Decision Point *If patient is bleeding actively, physician may order lavage of the stomach and aspiration to clear clots before procedure is attempted.*

STEP	RATIONALE
5 Determine purpose of procedure: biopsy, examination, or coagulation of bleeding sites.	Anticipates appropriate equipment needs.
6 Verify that patient was NPO for at least 8 hours for endoscopy of upper GI tract.	Introduction of endoscope increases risk for vomiting resulting from stimulation of gag reflex. Empty stomach reduces risk for aspiration of stomach contents.
7 For lower GI studies (proctoscopy, sigmoidoscopy, or colonoscopy), verify that patient followed clear liquid diet for 2 days and has completed any ordered bowel-cleansing regimen.	An empty intestinal tract promotes endoscopic insertion and good visualization of interior walls.
8 Assess patient's level of understanding and previous experience with procedure, including any concerns.	Determines extent of instruction and level of support required.

NURSING DIAGNOSES

- Anxiety
- Deficient knowledge regarding procedure
- Fear
- Impaired gas exchange
- Ineffective breathing pattern
- Risk for aspiration
- Risk for infection
- Risk for injury

Related factors are individualized based on patient's condition or needs.

PLANNING

1 Expected outcomes following completion of procedure:	
• Patient does not aspirate and has no postprocedure bleeding.	Indicates absence of complications and tolerance of procedure.
• Patient's level of comfort is equivalent to score of 4 or less on pain scale of 0 to 10.	Provides reliable detection of increasing pain so postprocedure analgesia is given.
• Patient is without respiratory complications or change in level of consciousness.	Recovers from sedation.
• Patient describes purposes and steps of procedure.	Documents patient understanding.
2 Prepare patient:	
a Explain steps of procedure, including sensations to expect.	Relieves anxiety and answers patient's questions.
b Administer pain medication or preprocedure medication.	Promotes relaxation and reduces anxiety.

IMPLEMENTATION

1 Identify patient using two identifiers (i.e., name and birthday or name and account number) according to agency policy. Compare identifiers with information in patient's identification bracelet.	Ensures correct patient. Complies with The Joint Commission standards and improves patient safety (TJC, 2012).
2 Perform hand hygiene and apply protective equipment.	Reduces transmission of microorganisms.
3 Remove patient's eyeglasses, dentures, or other dental appliances.	Prevents damage to eyeglasses or damage/dislodgement of dental structures during intubation phase.
4 Take "Time-Out" to verify patient's name, type of procedure scheduled, and procedure site with patient and health care team.	"Time-Out" verification just before starting procedure includes physician and all personnel and is safety precaution to prevent wrong patient, wrong site, and wrong procedure errors (TJC, 2012).
5 Ensure that IV line is patent and administer IV sedation as ordered (see Skill 44-1).	Provides route for emergency medications and creates immediate conscious sedation.
6 Help patient assume proper position for procedure and apply appropriate drape.	Improves efficiency of procedure and ability of physician to visualize site. Drape provides comfort and minimizes exposure.
a *Upper GI procedures:* Assist patient in maintaining left lateral Sims' position.	Sims' position allows easy passage of upper or lower endoscope. Provides airway clearance if patient gags and vomits gastric contents.
b *Lower GI procedures:* Assist patient in maintaining left lateral decubitus position. Drape patient for privacy.	Left lateral decubitus position provides access to lower GI tract.
7 Physician performs hand hygiene and puts on protective equipment.	Reduces transmission of microorganisms.
8 **Upper GI procedures:**	
a Help physician spray nasopharynx and oropharynx with local anesthetic.	Topical anesthetic decreases gag reflex caused by passage of endoscope, thus improving safety and comfort.
b Administer atropine if ordered.	Reduces quantity of secretions, therefore reducing risk for aspiration.
c Position tip of suction cannula for easy access in patient's mouth.	Drains oral secretions to reduce risk for aspiration.

STEP	RATIONALE
9 Lower GI procedures:	
a Prepare lubricant for fiberoptic endoscope.	Facilitates passage of tubing.
10 Physician slowly passes endoscope into mouth or through anus to view esophagus, stomach, colon, or rectum and advances to desired depth while visualizing lining of structures.	Provides visualization of all structures to detect polyps, cancerous lesions, or areas of inflammation and stricture.
11 Physician insufflates air through endoscope into upper GI tract or carbon dioxide into lower GI tract in case of colonoscopy.	Distends GI structures for better visualization. Carbon dioxide insufflation produces less postprocedure abdominal cramping than air insufflation because it is more readily absorbed (Chernecky and Berger, 2008).
12 Help patient throughout procedure:	
a Anticipate needs and promote comfort.	Patient is unable to speak after tube is passed into throat.
b Tell patient what is happening as each portion of procedure is carried out (e.g., abdominal cramping).	Reassures patient about procedure and how long it will last.
c For upper GI procedures, suction if there are excessive oral secretions or vomitus.	Prevents aspiration of oral secretions or gastric contents.
13 Place tissue specimens in proper laboratory containers or on proper slides. Seal as needed. Date, time, and initial all specimen containers before sending to laboratory.	Ensures proper specimen preservation and labeling and preparation of specimens for microscopic examination.
14 Help patient return to comfortable position.	Promotes relaxation.
15 Help to dispose of equipment and perform hand hygiene.	Reduces transmission of infection.
16 In recovery, after sedation resolves, inform patient not to eat or drink until gag reflex returns.	Reduces risk for aspiration.

EVALUATION

1 Monitor vital signs and oxygen saturation according to agency policy, which can be every 15 minutes for 2 hours.	Change in vital signs may indicate new bleeding in GI tract or oversedation.
2 Assess for levels of sedation and consciousness (see Skill 44-1).	Determines patient's response to IV sedation.
3 Ask patient to describe level of comfort using pain scale of 0 to 10. Observe for pain.	Monitors for sudden abdominal pain, which can indicate rupture of abdominal organs.
4 Evaluate emesis or aspirate for frank or occult blood (see Chapter 43).	Monitors for GI bleeding.
5 Assess for return of gag reflex, usually in 2 to 4 hours. Provide oral hygiene when gag reflex returns.	Determines when effects of anesthetic have disappeared. Gag reflex prevents aspiration.
6 Ask patient to state postprocedure dietary and activity limitations.	Evaluates patient understanding.

Unexpected Outcomes	Related Interventions
1 Vasovagal response caused by stimulation of baroreceptors during endoscope insertion as evidenced by:	
• Feeling nauseous, faint, dizzy, and/or light-headed.	• Lower head of table.
• Diaphoresis with slow, steady pulse.	• Support airway.
• Few seconds of unconsciousness.	
2 For upper GI procedures: Laryngospasm and bronchospasm as evidenced by:	
• Sudden, severe shortness of breath	• Call physician immediately.
	• Support airway (positioning).
	• Prepare emergency resuscitation equipment.
	• Anticipate possible cricothyrotomy.
3 For upper GI procedures: Hypoxemia as evidenced by:	
• Gradual shortness of breath	• Monitor SpO$_2$.
• Decreasing level of consciousness	• Maintain airway and breathing.
	• Notify physician immediately.
4 Pulmonary aspiration as evidenced by:	
• Dyspnea, tachypnea, decreasing levels of oxygen saturation.	• Support airway.
	• Follow specific postprocedural orders related to findings.
	• Monitor oxygen saturation.
5 Abdominal pain, fever, or bleeding, indicating damage to intestinal wall.	• Continue to monitor vital signs.
	• Notify physician of findings.
6 Oversedation with decreasing level of consciousness.	• See Skill 44-1.

Recording and Reporting

- Record the procedure, duration, patient's tolerance, complications and interventions, and collection and disposition of specimen.
- Report onset of bleeding, abdominal pain, dyspnea, and vital sign changes to physician.

Special Considerations
Teaching

- Upper GI endoscopy:
  - Explain method for endoscope insertion. Prepare patient for a slight feeling of not being able to breathe. Assure him or her that this feeling is common but that air is delivered through the endoscope and suffocation will not occur.
  - Teach patient simple hand signals for pain or discomfort because he or she will not be able to speak after the endoscope is positioned in the esophagus.
- Lower GI procedures (colonoscopy, sigmoidoscopy, proctoscopy):
  - Explain that it is normal to experience increased flatus and abdominal cramping.
  - Small amounts of blood in the stool are common if a biopsy was taken.

Pediatric

- Introduction of the endoscope in infants and small children who have a narrow and collapsible airway may result in respiratory distress.

Gerontologic

- Older adults frequently have reduced drug clearance from decreased glomerular filtration rate (GFR) and nephron activity or decreased hepatic function. It is important to monitor the effects of medications given to older adults (Meiner, 2011).
- Because of age-related changes in older adults, the gastric mucosa is thinner, which increases the incidence of irritation and ulceration (Meiner, 2011).
- Physical exposure and room temperature contribute to hypothermia in frail older adults who are unable to communicate that they are cold. Use warmed blankets or forced-air heat to maintain core temperature at comfortable, safe levels (Lewis et al., 2011).
- Some older adults experience dehydration, electrolyte imbalance, and exhaustion from pretest preparation. If the procedure is done on an ambulatory care basis, it is helpful to have someone stay with the patient for at least 24 hours afterwards.

Home Care

- Explain that patient might have hoarseness or a sore throat after an upper GI procedure. Patient can have ice chips or anesthetic lozenges after gag reflex returns.
- Instruct patient or family to notify physician if patient has a fever, abdominal pain, rigid abdomen, and rectal bleeding or stool in blood.

SKILL 44-6 Obtaining an Electrocardiogram

A 12-lead electrocardiogram (ECG) is a graphic representation of the electrical activities, or conduction system, of the heart. The electrical impulse for each heartbeat originates within the sinoatrial (SA) node, the "pacemaker" of the heart. The rate of impulses initiated at the SA node for an adult at rest is about 60 to 100 beats/min. The electrical impulses are then transmitted through the atria to the atrioventricular (AV) node. The AV node assists with atrial emptying by delaying the impulse before transmitting it through the bundle of His and the ventricular Purkinje network. The normal sequence on the ECG records the path of these electrical impulses, called *normal sinus rhythm (NSR)*, which contains PQRST waves (Fig. 44-7). The PR interval represents atrial depolarization during which the atria empty their blood supply into the ventricles. The QRS interval represents ventricular depolarization, during which ventricular contraction occurs. The remainder of the waveform through the end of the T wave signifies ventricular repolarization.

The electrical activity of the conduction system is recorded on a 12-lead ECG to determine baseline cardiac function (e.g., preoperative, prediagnostic testing), to evaluate response to cardiac medications, to monitor recovery after a myocardial infarction (MI), or when a patient experiences chest discomfort (Chernecky and Berger, 2008). An ECG monitors the regularity and path of the electrical impulse through the conduction system; however, it does not reflect muscular work of the heart.

Disturbances in conduction result when impulses cannot travel through the normal pathways. These rhythm disturbances are called *dysrhythmias*, meaning a deviation from the NSR (Table 44-4). Dysrhythmias occur as a response to ischemia, valvular abnormality, anxiety, drug toxicity, or acid-base or electrolyte imbalance. Some common dysrhythmias include tachycardia (greater than 100 beats/ min), bradycardia (less than 60 beats/ min), premature ventricular or atrial contractions (premature ventricular contractions [PVCs], premature atrial contractions [PACs]), atrial fibrillation, or heart block (delayed or absent beat).

The electrical impulses are conducted to the surface of the body and detected by electrodes placed on the limbs and torso. The electrodes carry these impulses to a continuously running graph that plots the ECG wave pattern. The appearance of the ECG pattern helps diagnose whether there are any abnormalities in the electrical conduction through the heart. A 12-lead ECG machine includes 10 leads and electrodes. One electrode is placed on each of the four extremities, and six electrodes are placed at specific sites on the chest (precordial). The 12 "leads" that are produced are 12 different graphic pictures, based on how the electricity flows between specific electrodes. They are the bipolar limb leads I, II, III; augmented limb leads aV_R, aV_L, aV_F; and precordial chest leads

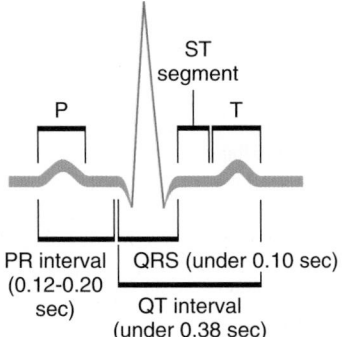

FIG 44-7 Normal ECG waveform. (*From Pagana KD, Pagana TJ: Mosby's manual of diagnostic and laboratory tests, ed 4, St Louis, 2010, Mosby.*)

TABLE 44-4 | Common Basic Cardiac Dysrhythmias

Rhythm Characteristics	Appearance	Clinical Significance
Sinus tachycardia: Regular rhythm, rate 100-180 beats/ min, normal PQRS complex	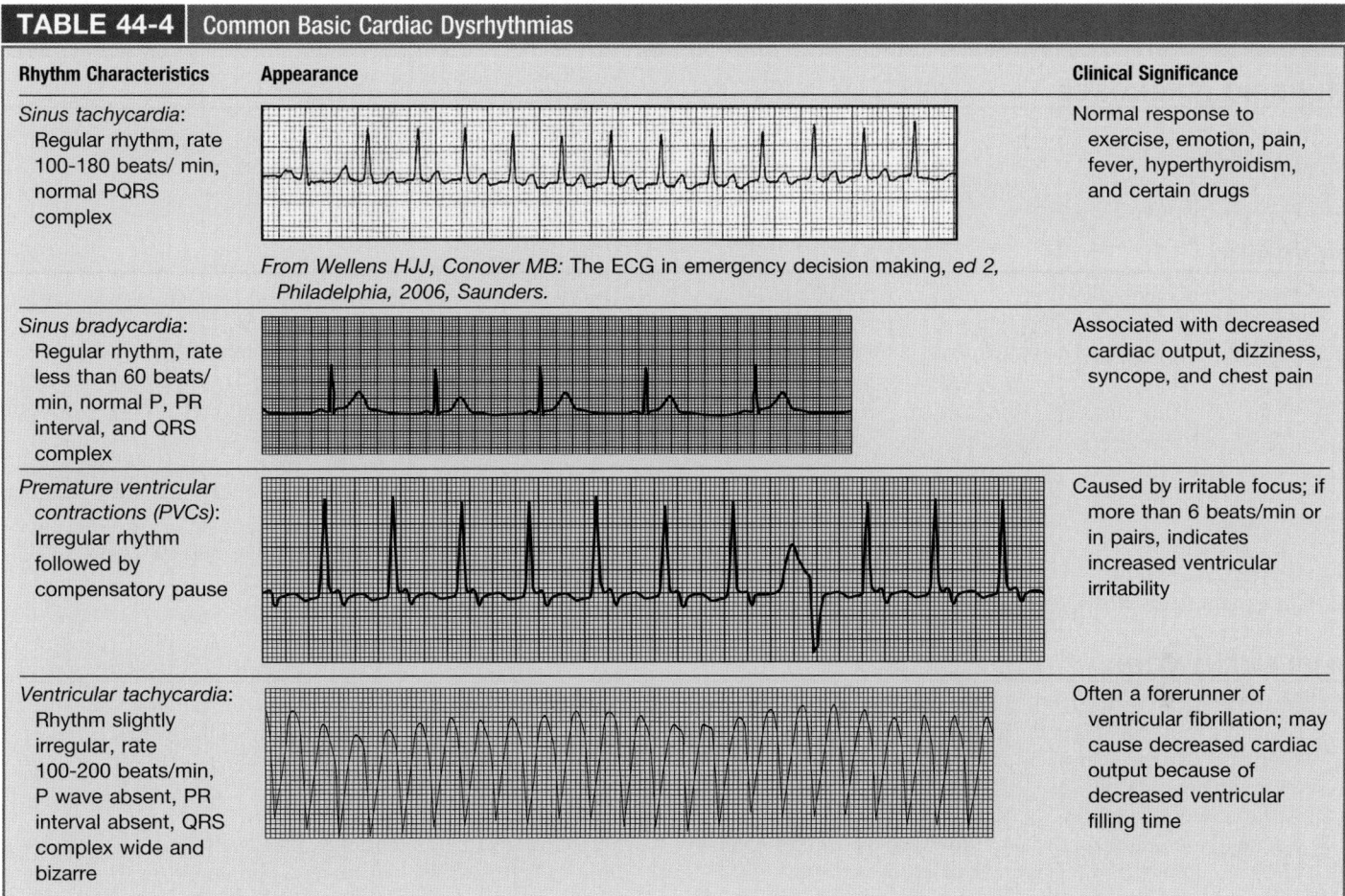 *From Wellens HJJ, Conover MB:* The ECG in emergency decision making, *ed 2, Philadelphia, 2006, Saunders.*	Normal response to exercise, emotion, pain, fever, hyperthyroidism, and certain drugs
Sinus bradycardia: Regular rhythm, rate less than 60 beats/ min, normal P, PR interval, and QRS complex		Associated with decreased cardiac output, dizziness, syncope, and chest pain
Premature ventricular contractions (PVCs): Irregular rhythm followed by compensatory pause		Caused by irritable focus; if more than 6 beats/min or in pairs, indicates increased ventricular irritability
Ventricular tachycardia: Rhythm slightly irregular, rate 100-200 beats/min, P wave absent, PR interval absent, QRS complex wide and bizarre		Often a forerunner of ventricular fibrillation; may cause decreased cardiac output because of decreased ventricular filling time

V_1 to V_6. Because the leads are specific to portions of the anatomy of the heart, abnormalities in conduction help determine which part of the heart has sustained damage. Although a 12-lead ECG is considered diagnostic, a 3- or 5-lead ECG is considered interpretive (see Fig. 44-7).

Three- or five-lead ECG tracings are used during emergencies and pacemaker insertion. In a three- or five-lead procedure, one electrode is substituted sequentially for the six chest electrodes. For diagnostic procedures requiring a continuous ECG recording over an extended period of time, use a Holter monitor. A Holter monitor is a small, portable device that records electrical activity of the heart for up to 24 hours. The ECG is recorded on magnetic tape or in a digital record and monitors cardiac rhythm during activity, rest, and sleep.

Delegation and Collaboration

The skill of obtaining an ECG reading can be delegated to nursing assistive personnel (NAP). The nurse directs the NAP to:

- Immediately notify the nurse if the patient states any chest pain or appears anxious.

Equipment

- ❑ 12-lead ECG machine
- ❑ ECG leads and electrodes (self-stick adhesive)
- ❑ Electrode gel *(optional)*
- ❑ Alcohol wipes
- ❑ Hair clippers *(optional)*

STEP	RATIONALE

ASSESSMENT

1 Verify type of ECG ordered.	Ensures correct patient. Complies with The Joint Commission standards and improves patient safety (TJC, 2012).
2 Determine rationale for obtaining ECG (e.g., baseline assessment or diagnostic [chest pain]).	If ECG is ordered for active chest pain, test must be performed immediately.
3 Assess patient's level of understanding of procedure, including any concerns.	Determines extent of instruction and level of support required.
4 Assess patient's ability to follow directions and remain still in supine position.	Provides clear, accurate recording without electrical artifacts, which distort wave form.

STEP	RATIONALE

NURSING DIAGNOSES

- Acute pain
- Anxiety
- Deficient knowledge regarding procedure
- Fear

Related factors are individualized based on patient's condition or needs.

PLANNING

1 Expected outcomes following completion of procedure:
- Patient tolerates procedure without anxiety or discomfort.
- Clear recording of ECG waveform is obtained.

Appropriate preparation decreases anxiety.

Normal ECG waveform (see Fig. 44-7) consists of P, Q, R, S, and T waves plotted on graph paper. Each small block on graph paper measures 0.04 second. A "normal" ECG waveform demonstrates the following:

PR interval = 0.12 to 0.20 second

QRS width = less than 0.10-second QT interval = less than 0.38 second

ST segment is isoelectric (on same horizontal level as PR interval)

2 Close room door or bedside curtains.

Provides privacy.

IMPLEMENTATION

1 Identify patient using two identifiers (i.e., name and birthday or name and account number) according to agency policy. Compare patient identifiers with information on patient's identification bracelet.

Ensures correct patient. Complies with The Joint Commission standards and improves patient safety (TJC, 2012).

2 Perform hand hygiene.

Reduces transmission of microorganisms.

3 Remove or reposition patient's clothing to expose only patient's chest and arms. Keep pelvis and thighs covered.

Facilitates correct placement of cardiac leads.

Minimizes patient's embarrassment. Improper lead placement produces electrical artifact, which requires repeating test (Chernecky and Berger, 2008).

4 Place patient in supine position.

Exposes patient for lead placement.

5 Instruct patient to lie still without talking (12-lead ECG only) and to not cross legs.

Body movement produces artifact, which necessitates repeating test (Chernecky and Berger, 2008).

6 Clean and prepare skin; wipe sites with alcohol. It is often necessary to clip hair from chest if large amounts are present. In patients who are very thin and emaciated, it is difficult to secure electrodes because of bony structure and decreased amount of subcutaneous tissue.

Skin preparation helps remove oils that prevent adherence of electrodes.

7 Apply self-sticking electrode, being careful to use pressure on perimeter only, and attach leads. (If self-sticking leads are not available, apply electrode paste to skin before attaching leads.)

Position of leads promotes proper display of ECG on paper. Pressure on center of lead displaces electroconductive gel and results in poor tracing.

a For 12-lead ECG:

(1) Chest (precordial leads) (Fig. 44-8):

Proper position of leads promotes accurate display of ECG on paper.

(a) V_1—Fourth intercostal space (ICS) at right sternal border

(b) V_2—Fourth ICS at left sternal border

(c) V_3—Midway between V_2 and V_4

(d) V_4—Fifth ICS at midclavicular line

(e) V_5—Left anterior axillary line at level of V_4 horizontally

(f) V_6—Left midaxillary line at level of V_4 horizontally

(2) Extremities: one lead on each extremity. Place on lower portion of each extremity, avoiding any bone prominences.

Positioning of leads in this manner produces fewer artifacts.

(a) aV_r—Right wrist

(b) aV_l—Left wrist

(c) aV_f—Left ankle

(d) aV_7—Right ankle

STEP	RATIONALE
8 Turn on ECG machine, enter required demographic information into computer, and obtain tracing.	Transfers electrocardiac conduction to ECG tracing paper for subsequent analysis by cardiologist.
a Simultaneous 12-channel recording: Enter patient's name and medical record number into ECG machine menu. Obtain test tracing.	
• Reposition leads as needed. Activate machine to obtain simultaneous tracing of all 12 leads. If patient experiences chest pain, document occurrence on ECG printout.	Chest pain experienced during study is often correlated to arrhythmia on ECG (Pagana and Pagana, 2010).
b Three or five-lead recording:	
(1) After placing limb electrodes, apply electroconductive gel over V_1 to V_6 locations (described previously).	
(2) Turn lead selector to lead "1," turn on machine, and begin recording. If tracing is clear, run sequential 6-second tracings for leads I, II, III, aV_R, aV_L, and aV_F by turning lead selector to corresponding settings.	
(3) Stop machine, position V electrode over V_1 position, and run a 6-second tracing. Repeat sequentially by moving V electrode over V_2, V_3, V_4, V_5, and V_6 positions.	
c For continuous interpretation/monitoring:	
(1) Apply limb electrodes. Apply electroconductive gel over location for single chest lead where designated by agency policy or as ordered.	
(2) Maintain either two upper limb electrodes (3-lead), or four limb electrodes (5-lead).	
9 Disconnect leads and wipe off excess electrode paste from chest. If serial tracings are expected, some cardiologists will have you mark where leads were placed to ensure subsequent tracings from same electrode sites.	Promotes comfort and hygiene.
10 Deliver ECG tracing to appropriate laboratory or health care provider. Provide any previous ECG tracings.	Provides for review of ECG by cardiologist. Comparison with previous readings helps to detect abnormalities.

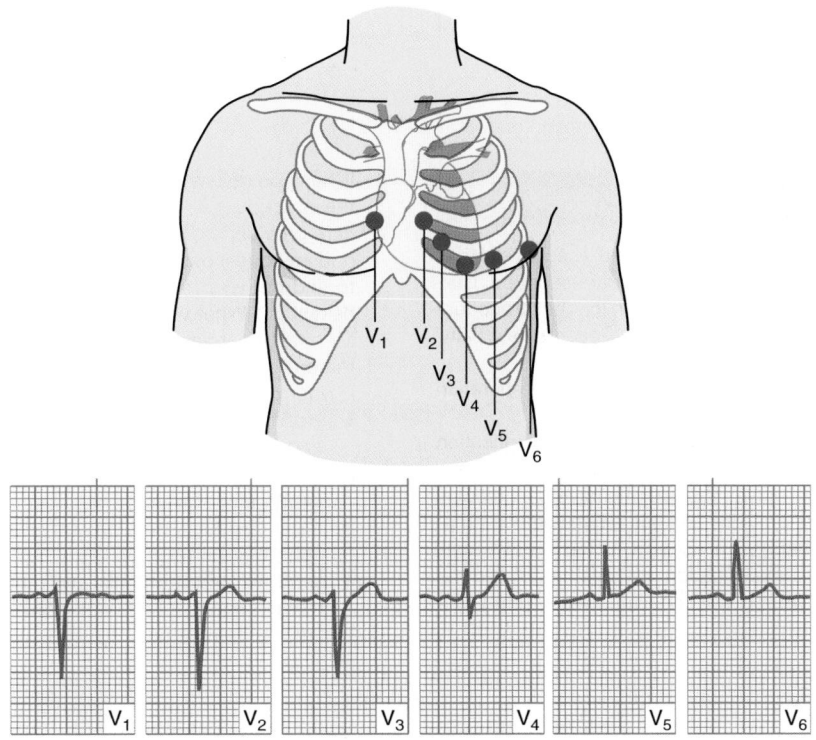

FIG 44-8 Anatomic placement of precordial leads. (*From Monahan F et al:* Phipps' medical-surgical nursing: health and illness perspectives, *ed 8, St Louis, 2006, Mosby.*)

STEP	RATIONALE

EVALUATION

1 Although procedure is painless, it is important to note and document if patient is experiencing any chest discomfort during ECG recording.

Helps correlate ECG changes to symptoms of chest pain.

Unexpected Outcomes

1 ECG cannot be interpreted because of absence of tracing in one or more leads; presence of electrical artifact in tracing.

Related Interventions

- Inspect electrodes for secure placement.
- Reposition any leads that move as result of patient breathing or movement or vibrations in environment and repeat tracing.
- Remind patient who moves that it is necessary to lie still to obtain an accurate tracing.
- If artifact looks like 60-cycle interference (looks like very thick-lined waveform), unplug battery-operated equipment in room one item at a time to see if interference disappears. NOTE: 60-cycle interference is rare.

2 Patient has chest pain or anxiety.

- Continue to monitor.
- Reassess factors contributing to anxiety.
- Follow specific postprocedure orders related to findings.
- Notify health care provider.

Recording and Reporting

- Record when ECG was obtained (date and time) and where tracing was sent, rationale for obtaining ECG (e.g., pain, discomfort, before surgery, after surgery), and baseline vital signs. Include rhythm strip in patient's chart (check agency policy).
- Report any arrhythmias or patient chest pain to health care provider immediately.

Special Considerations

Teaching

- If Holter monitoring is being used, instruct patient to maintain an accurate diary of activities (detailed documentation of

activities and occurrence of chest pain help to diagnose condition). Also inform patient that the Holter monitoring interpretation will be available in a few days.

Gerontologic

- Be aware that medications such as antiarrhythmics can affect results.

? Critical Thinking Exercises

Mr. Hall, a 67-year-old African-American, is a retired executive. He is scheduled for a cardiac catheterization under moderate sedation. Currently he is taking warfarin (Coumadin). The order for the procedure faxed from the health care provider's office lists "new-onset chest pain" as the clinical indication for the procedure.

1 Which laboratory data would you review as part of your preparation of Mr. Hall for his procedure?
2 Describe the steps you would take to perform patient verification safety procedures for Mr. Hall.
3 Cardiac catheterization often involves the use of intravenous moderate sedation. The health care provider has not requested the presence of an anesthesiologist during the procedure. You are responsible for verifying Mr. Hall's ASA classification before the procedure. Which ASA classification would you consider appropriate for Mr. Hall?
  1 ASA 1
  2 ASA 2
  3 ASA 3E
  4 ASA 4
  5 ASA 5E
  6 ASA 6

4 When you review Mr. Hall's chart, you see that the consent form for the procedure is unsigned. When you ask him whether the health care provider explained the procedure and the risks and asked if he had any questions, he replies, "My doctor told me that I needed this to find out why my chest pain is happening. But I don't know how risky it is." What would you do?
5 Mr. Hall's cardiac catheterization procedure is finished. The right femoral site was used for catheter insertion. Which items take priority in your postprocedure assessments of Mr. Hall?
  1 Heart rate and rhythm, respiratory effort, oxygen saturation/end-tidal CO_2, procedure site for bleeding control, pedal pulses
  2 Blood pressure, pain level, neurologic checks, complete blood count, electrolytes
  3 Pupil checks, level of consciousness, breath sounds, bowel sounds
  4 Level of consciousness, pain level, neurologic checks, and oxygen saturation/end-tidal CO_2 levels

REVIEW QUESTIONS

1 The registered nurse is reassessing a patient who is recovering after a cardiac catheterization via a femoral artery approach. Which set of postprocedure assessment data should be reported immediately to the physician?
1 Increase in heart rate from 92 to 116 beats/min and low back pain radiating to the sides
2 Occasional premature ventricular contractions (PVCs) and mild tenderness at catheter insertion site
3 Urine output of 40 mL in the first hour after catheterization and decrease in oxygen saturation from 99% to 96%
4 Bloody drainage visible at the edge of the dressing

2 On the urologic unit each of the registered nurse's patients is scheduled for an intravenous pyelogram. For which patient is this procedure contraindicated?
1 The patient with renal insufficiency
2 The patient with a urinary tract infection
3 The patient with possible kidney stones
4 The patient with only one kidney

3 The nurse is helping a patient who has just had a paracentesis performed. Which assessment data indicate that the desired results from the procedure have occurred?
1 Increased abdominal girth, decreased respiratory effort, increased respiratory rate
2 Increased abdominal girth, increased respiratory effort, decreased respiratory rate
3 Decreased abdominal girth, decreased respiratory effort, decreased respiratory rate
4 Decreased abdominal girth, increased respiratory effort, increased respiratory rate

4 The nurse is providing a 77-year-old male instructions about how to prepare for his colonoscopy next week. Which information should be included in his instructions?
1 Eat only soft foods for 3 days before the day of the procedure. Administer a cleansing enema in the morning before the test. Consume no food or fluids for 4 hours before the procedure.
2 Have a full-liquid diet the day before the procedure. Drink a bowel-cleansing preparation the night before the procedure. Take the prescribed antibiotic the morning of the procedure.
3 No diet modifications are needed in the days before the procedure. Fast from food and fluids, except for medications, the night before the procedure. Have a bowel movement the morning before the procedure.
4 Consume clear liquids the day before the procedure. Complete the bowel preparation the afternoon and evening before the procedure. Fast from food and fluids for 8 hours before the procedure. Take only medications that are ordered by the physician the morning of the procedure.

5 Place the steps listed here in the correct order for helping a patient who is undergoing a lumbar puncture.
1 Help patient maintain lateral recumbent position with head and neck flexed.
2 Properly label specimen in presence of patient.
3 Assess patient's condition during procedure.
4 Take "Time-Out" to verify patient's name, type of procedure scheduled, and procedure site.
5 Explain to patient that pain may occur when lidocaine (local anesthetic) is injected into the site.
6 Record the opening intracranial pressure; observe fluid for color.

6 You are caring for a patient before a colonoscopy. The patient asks if he can ask you questions during the procedure. Your best response would be which of the following?
1 "You'll be receiving a sedative that will make you sleep throughout the procedure."
2 "You'll actually be awake throughout the procedure and can ask questions at any time."
3 "You'll be awake during the procedure but not able to talk; so let me go over some nonverbal signs you can use to communicate with us."
4 "You'll be relaxed and able to talk with us, but you won't remember the discussion."

7 A patient underwent a bronchoscopy and is now entering the recovery area. The patient develops sudden, severe shortness of breath. You should take which of the following set of actions?
1 Monitor SpO_2 and lower head of procedure table.
2 Support patient's airway, call physician immediately, and prepare for possible resuscitation.
3 Measure vital signs and prepare for administration of intravenous (IV) fluids.
4 Observe for blood-tinged mucus, suction airway, and lower head of procedure table.

8 You are caring for a patient who has undergone conscious sedation for a cardiac catheterization. Which criteria below best represent what you measure to determine the patient's response to sedation?
1 Complete blood count (CBC) level, hydration status, and respiratory rate
2 Femoral pulse, end-tidal carbon dioxide (CO_2), and gag reflex
3 Heart rate, arterial oxygen saturation (SpO_2), and level of consciousness
4 Prothrombin time, SpO_2, and respiratory rate

9 When preparing a patient for a 12-lead electrocardiogram (ECG), it is necessary to apply six precordial chest leads. Match the lead on the left with the correct position on the right.
1 V_1 ___ a Fifth intercostal space (ICS) at midclavicular line
2 V_2 ___ b Left midaxillary line at level of V4 horizontally
3 V_3 ___ c Left anterior axillary line at level of V4 horizontally
4 V_4 ___ d Fourth ICS at right sternal border
5 V_5 ___ e Midway between V2 and V4
6 V_6 ___ f Fourth ICS at left sternal border

10 Which of the following patients would be unable to undergo an angiogram? (Select all that apply.)
1 44-year-old female who is taking warfarin (Coumadin)
2 52-year-old male suspected of having an abdominal aneurysm
3 77-year-old female who is suspected of having an arterial occlusion of the renal artery
4 65-year-old female who is 30 weeks' pregnant

REFERENCES

Agency for Healthcare Research and Quality (AHRQ): *National Guideline Clearing House, ACR-SIR practice guideline for sedation/analgesia*, Rockville Md, 2010, AHRQ, http://www.guideline.gov/content.aspx?id=32523&search=conscious+sedation#Section396 accessed April 6, 2012.

Aldrete JA: Post-anesthetic recovery score, *J Am Coll Surg* 205(5):3, 2007.

American Academy of Pediatrics (AAP): Guidelines and management of pediatric patients during and after sedation for diagnostic and therapeutic procedures, *Pediatrics* 129(4): e1103, 2012.

American Society of Anesthesiologists (ASA): *Continuum of depth of sedation: definition of general anesthesia and levels of sedation/analgesia*, Committee of Origin: Quality Management and Departmental Administration, The Society, October, 2009, available at http://www.asahq.org/For-Members/Standards-Guidelines-and-Statements.aspx, accessed August 23, 2012.

Association of periOperative Registered Nurses (AORN): *Standards, recommended practices, and guidelines*, Denver, 2011, The Association.

Beaty AD, et al: Seafood allergy and radiocontrast media: are physicians propagating a myth? *Am J Med* 121(2):158, 2008.

Biancari F, et al: Meta-analysis of randomized trials on the efficacy of vascular closure devices after diagnostic angiography and angioplasty, *Am Heart J* 159(4):518, 2010.

Boonmak P, Boonmak S: Epidural patching for preventing and treating post-dural puncture headache, *Cochrane Database Rev* (1):CD001791, 2010.

Centers for Disease Control and Prevention (CDC): *2011 Guidelines for the prevention of intravascular catheter-related infections,* Atlanta, 2011, CDC, available at http://www.cdc.gov/hicpac/bsi/bsi-guidelines-2011.html, accessed August 23, 2012.

Chair SY, Fernandez R: The clinical effectiveness of length of bed rest for patients recovering from trans-femoral diagnostic cardiac catheterization, *Int J Evidence Based Healthc* 6(4):352, 2008.

Chernecky CC, Berger BJ: *Laboratory tests and diagnostic procedures,* ed 5, Philadelphia, 2008, Mosby.

Ellett ML: A literature review of the safety and efficacy of using propofol for sedation in endoscopy, *Gastroenterol Nurs* 33(2):111, 2010.

Fein D, et al: Pattern of pain management during lumbar puncture in children, *Pediatr Emerg Care* 26:357, 2010.

Hockenberry MJ, Wilson D: *Wong's nursing care of infants and children,* ed 9, St Louis, 2011, Mosby.

Hon L-Q, et al: Vascular closure devices: a comparative overview, *Curr Probl Diagn Radiol* 38(1):33, 2009.

Lewis S, et al: *Medical-surgical nursing,* ed 8, St Louis, 2011, Mosby.

Meiner SE: *Gerontologic nursing,* ed 4, St Louis, 2011, Mosby.

Muller M, Wehrmann T: How best to approach endoscopic sedation? *Nat Rev Gastroenterol Hepatol* 12:8(9):481, 2011.

Ott L: Assessing blood flow with CT angiography, *Nursing* 28(1):26, 2008.

Pagana KD, Pagana TJ: *Mosby's manual of diagnostic and laboratory tests,* ed 4, St Louis, 2010, Mosby.

Patel MR, et al: Arteriotomy closure devices for cardiovascular procedures: a scientific statement from the American Heart Association, *Circulation* 122:1882, 2010.

Schabelman E, Witting M: The relationship of radiocontrast, iodine, and seafood allergies: a medical myth exposed, *J Emerg Med* 39(5):701, 2010.

Stannard D: Epidural blood patching for preventing and treating post-dural puncture headache, *J Perianesthesia Nurs* 26(6):411, 2011.

The Joint Commission (TJC): *National Patient Safety Goals,* Oakbrook Terrace, Ill, 2012, The Commission, available at http://www.jointcommission.org/standards_information/npsgs.aspx, accessed November 2011.

Answer Key

CHAPTER 1

Answers to Critical Thinking Questions

1 Does a (I) low carbohydrate diet compared with a (C) high carbohydrate diet affect (O) gastrointestinal symptoms of (P) adult patients with inflammatory bowel disease (T) within 3 months?

2 A systematic review is a summary of all evidence that exists regarding a particular clinical problem or issue in the literature. Basically a researcher has asked a PICOT question and then examined all of the well-designed relevant randomized controlled trials (RCTs) that ask the same question. A systematic review explains if the evidence exists for a practice change.

3 A case control study

Answers to Review Questions

1 **The correct order is 5, 1, 6, 4, 2, 3.**

2 **2 Rationale:** In this case the knowledge that there is new information about wound care triggers a question about antiinfection solutions. The trigger was not a result of a problem or trend on the nurse's unit. Peer focused and PICOT focused are not triggers for questions.

3 **4 Rationale:** Question four has the primary components of an identified patient population (P), the intervention thought to be worthwhile (I), and a desired outcome (O). The question also has a comparison intervention. Questions 1 and 2 have no outcome. Question 3 has no population or area of interest.

4 **3 Rationale:** This is an example of a problem (i.e., lower patient satisfaction scores), triggering interest in a question for EBP.

5 **P**—female obstetric patients, **I**—hourly rounding, **C**—none, **O**—perception of nursing care or patient satisfaction, **T**—none.

6 **4 Rationale:** Qualitative studies examine individuals' experiences with health problems or life experiences and the contexts in which the experiences occur. These studies would be helpful in the nurse's review.

7 **2 Rationale:** The best outcome measure to detect a change in pain acuity is the patient's report of pain severity. Ability of patients to follow coaching or the time it takes to perform guided imagery is not an outcome that determines if guided imagery was effective. Frequency of using pain medication can be an outcome to measure a patient's pain experience, but it is not the best measure of pain acuity.

8 **1 Rationale:** A background question is broad and general. When the question is answered, it provides general knowledge. In contrast, a foreground question such as the other three examples is relevant to a specific practice issue.

9 **2, 3 Rationale:** It is important to build staff support for the EBP process by educating all involved and keeping staff informed. It is best to involve all staff, using an interdisciplinary approach when possible. Do not involve all staff in data collection. Involve only a few who can collect data consistently in the same way.

10 **2, 3 Rationale:** Resources for implementation of an EBP change include staff from all disciplines (as appropriate) and administrative support and costs of the implementation. Accuracy of the device is not a resource but a clinical factor that should be addressed in your literature review supporting use of the device. Patient satisfaction could be an outcome measure that you choose to include in the pilot.

CHAPTER 2

Answers to Critical Thinking Exercises

1 Additional information that would be helpful as you assume care for Mrs. Hampton includes:

- Level of consciousness and findings from neurologic assessment.
- Patient's medical history, including medications; information regarding any recent changes in medication or treatment plan.
- Blood glucose level, home insulin schedule and dosages, whether home insulin was administered before presenting to hospital.
- Results of any testing completed such as computed tomography (CT) scan of head or magnetic resonance imaging (MRI).
- Patient's plans or expectations for discharge (e.g., plans to return home with assistance of husband).
- Referrals that have been made for physical therapy and speech therapy.
- Discharge planning that has been started by the discharge planner or case manager.

2 You introduce yourself to Mr. and Mrs. Hampton, explain that you are the nurse who will be caring for Mrs. Hampton during the day shift, and accompany them to the assigned room. Orient them to the room and help put Mrs. Hampton's belongings away after making sure that all of her personal belongings were brought with her. Show the Hamptons the call light system and how to get help if needed. Provide Mr. Hampton with a comfortable chair and support his interactions with his wife. Allow Mr. Hampton to participate in Mrs. Hampton's care to the extent that he is comfortable. Reinforce the reasons for the transfer and answer any questions that the Hamptons have about it. Allow them the opportunity to express their anxiety about the move from the intensive care unit.

3 Ask Mr. Hampton to bring a copy of the advance directive to the hospital. Notify the health care provider that Mrs. Hampton has an advance directive. Document in the medical record the presence of an advance directive and the request made for Mr. Hampton to bring the document to the hospital. Ask Mrs. Hampton to explain the substance of the advance directive to determine her understanding of it. Place a copy of the advance directive in the medical record.

4 Recognize that Mr. Hampton's anxiety is normal and allow him to express his concerns related to taking his wife home. Ask Mr. Hampton about family or other help that is available. Have him describe the home and identify which problems may be related to Mrs. Hampton's mobility and risk for falls. Discuss with Mr. Hampton changes that can be made in the home to improve safety (e.g., removal of throw rugs, having grab bars installed in the bathroom at the toilet and tub (see Chapter 41). Have the discharge planner or case manager work with Mr. Hampton to get the home equipment that is needed to help Mrs. Hampton bathe and navigate through her home. Get confirmation from physical therapy that Mrs. Hampton uses her walker correctly.

Answers to Review Questions

1 **1, 2, 4, 6 Rationale:** The nurse is responsible for identifying allergies and, if present, places an allergy band on the patient. It is also the nurse's role to clarify the specific details pertaining to the patient's advance directive. All the other activities may be done by the admission clerk.

2 **4 Rationale:** The discharge planning process is comprehensive and multidisciplinary, including representatives from all the services who provided care.

3 **2 Rationale:** The patient's current status must be accurate to anticipate the needs that may occur during the transfer or discharge.

4 **2 Rationale:** Toddlers do better in unfamiliar settings when they have items that they are used to having to comfort them. They also think in the present; thus having something they can hold onto is most important. The other information from the parents regarding the child's rituals and preferences is important but might not be used, depending on the child's medical needs.

5 **3 Rationale:** Matching the services provided at the skilled care facility provides the best referral for the individualized needs of the patient. This assists with promoting positive patient outcomes.

6 **2 Rationale:** Respecting and understanding the patient's health beliefs and customs leads to the development of an individualized plan of care for patients with different cultures, religions, and beliefs.

7 **2 Rationale:** Introducing yourself as the nurse and other staff and orienting the patient should be completed to ensure some reduction in patient anxiety with his or her new surroundings. Other components of the admission process are completed as appropriate to the patient's needs and condition.

8 **1 Rationale:** When a patient in any type of unit or facility leaves without a written order from his or her health care provider, it is defined as *against medical advice.*

9 Transitional care is defined as nursing actions implemented to ensure coordination and continuity of care for patients who are transferring between different care settings or care levels.

10 **3 Rationale:** The Joint Commission suggests a reading level of fifth grade or below for all written documents used for patient teaching and information.

CHAPTER 3

Answers to Critical Thinking Exercises

1 Ensure that the environment is quiet and free from disturbance. Show empathy and respect, speak slowly and clearly, and face the patient when speaking to her. Give the patient time to process and respond to the information. Obtain an accurate health history; use collateral sources to obtain health information. Perform a mini-mental examination or tool used by your institution to establish a baseline of the patient's cognitive status. Repeat information as needed. Encourage patient to use any form of communication that she feels comfortable using. Avoid arguing with her.

2 Pause and consider your feelings and thoughts that are interacting with the cognitively impaired patient. Assess orientation status of patient. Try a calm, firm approach using a comfortable voice. Use simple language. Make sure that patient has hearing aid and/or glasses.

3 Strategies useful to communicate effectively with a cognitively impaired patient include use of touch to aid concentration and offer encouragement, pictorial drawings, gestures, and yes-or-no questions.

Answers to Review Questions

1 **4 Rationale:** A therapeutic nurse-patient relationship is goal directed. It can also include the need to help a patient discuss any pertinent topics, whether comfortable or uncomfortable.

2 **1 Rationale:** Therapeutic communication is goal directed, which in this situation is better pain management for the patient.

3 **3 Rationale:** The use of "why" questions may cause defensiveness in the patient and hinder communication. The other options promote communication by encouraging the patient to communicate.

4 **3 Rationale:** The nurse needs to first assess the level of anxiety so appropriate communication techniques and strategies can be used. The patient may not have the insight to understand what is currently causing his or her behavior.

5 **2 Rationale:** Speaking louder and bringing in other team members may be perceived as threatening and may cause the patient's behavior to become out of control faster. The patient may not be aware of his or her behavior; therefore asking about comfort measures to relieve the threatening behavior may also cause him or her to escalate. The nurse may need to leave the room quickly. By positioning himself or herself near the door, he or she should not be trapped by the patient.

6 **3 Rationale:** Direct eye contact and excessive touch can be offensive to persons from certain cultures. The patient's right to privacy must be guarded; therefore the use of a medical interpreter provides for correct, confidential communication.

7 **4 Rationale:** Patients with anxiety need assistance in clarifying factors that cause the anxiety and coping more effectively. Active

listening helps to identify the source of the anxiety. Meeting basic needs and being nonjudgmental and accepting of feelings is important but not your first step. Ultimately once a cause for anxiety is known, you can help the patient by letting him or her make as many choices about care as possible.

8 **2 Rationale:** Distraction is often effective for this type of patient. Strategies that may have worked before may not be as effective now. There is no time to call the family when the patient is already hostile. A show of force could make the patient agitated.

9 **4 Rationale:** Even though being positive about the situation is a strategy, this patient is grieving for the loss of his extremity and is depressed. Antidepressant medications are not given initially. The patient needs the opportunity to express feelings, especially anger, which is normal behavior. The health care provider, not the physical therapist, would be consulted about when he would be evaluated for a prosthesis.

10 **4 Rationale:** The method of instruction should be based on the patient's preferred method of learning. It can incorporate a variety of methods that would be appropriate for the information being conveyed and how the patient learns best. The other options are either demeaning (option 1), too narrow in scope and closed ended (option 2) or family-centered instead of patient-centered (option 3).

CHAPTER 4

Answers to Critical Thinking Exercises

1 Vital signs and glucose testing can be recorded by nursing assistive personnel (NAP) on flow sheets. It is appropriate for the NAP to document repetitive care aspects. As a nurse you must give the NAP specific information as to when you want to be notified about vital sign data (e.g., temperature above 99° F [37.2 C] orally, heart rate greater than 100 beats/min, blood pressure less than 100/70 mm Hg or greater than 130/85 mm Hg, and glucose measurement less than 60 mg/dL or greater than 120 mg/dL). Pain assessment and preoperative teaching must be done and recorded by the nurse.

2 You specify in your report to the NAP that he or she is to notify you if there is any change in the pain; if there are any symptoms of hypoglycemia, such as dizziness, pallor, or confusion; and if the patient expresses any lack of understanding about the preoperative teaching.

3 Include the following elements: location of pain, description of type of pain, duration, information obtained from palpation of area, pain intensity on a scale of 0 to 10, patient comments, results of pain relief measures.

4 Notify the physician using SBAR.

S (Situation): Give patient's name and room number. Give vital signs of 90/50, pulse 110, and respirations 24. Patient is complaining of dizziness and feeling sweaty.

B (Background): Patient history, events leading up to the change in vital signs.

A (Actions taken): Placed patient back in bed.

R (Recommendation): Start IV fluids, apply oxygen, check intake and output.

5 Document fully the patient's current understanding of the preoperative teaching. Document return verbalization of understanding or demonstration of teaching to validate that learning has taken place.

Answers to Review Questions

1 **1, 3, 4 Rationale:** Documentation is to be entered by the nurse who provided the care or made the observation, not by anyone else.

2 **3 Rationale:** Military time is one 24-hour time cycle; thus for this example you would begin with 1200 (noon) and add 4 (four) hours, which adds up to 1600 hours in military time.

3 **1 Rationale:** Focus charting begins with the concern or problem being experienced (data), what was done about the problem (action), and the patient's outcome (response).

4 **3 Rationale:** The purpose is identification of trends in clinical care.

5 **3 Rationale:** SBAR is a standardized approach for transferring information during shift report.

6 1 **Rationale:** Because of the complexity of the patient's medical condition and family situation, SBAR documentation provides a framework for cross-discipline communication in an efficient, timely format.

7 4 **Rationale:** All nursing care is based on the patient's needs, which are identified during the assessment process. Both objective and subjective data are included but not the nurse's hunches or personal thoughts.

8 2 **Rationale:** The information must be focused only on the patient and would show an improvement in the patient's condition. The other options either show a negative situation or are not focused on the patient.

9 2 **Rationale:** Whenever unexpected adverse events resulting in injury either to caregivers or the recipients of care occur, an incident report needs to be completed.

10 3 **Rationale:** Data should be objective, reflecting the patient's status. Never document in the record that an incident report was completed.

CHAPTER 5

Answers to Critical Thinking Exercises

1 The nurse must obtain all admission vital signs. All of the routine vital signs can be delegated. Temperature should be tympanic or temporal because patient is sedated and may not be able to hold an oral thermometer. Blood pressure can be taken on the right arm or leg.

2 The NAP reported a change in BP; the priority nursing intervention is for the nurse to immediately obtain a new blood pressure reading and further assess the patient. Once the nurse determines that the patient is indeed stable, other explanations for the differences can be explored. Possible explanations for differences are technique, equipment, and patient-related findings. Technique includes site of blood pressure measurement and whether the nursing assistive personnel (NAP) used the proper method. The nurse may want to observe the NAP's technique in blood pressure measurement. Equipment differences include using a cuff that is too small or an electronic blood pressure machine. An example of a patient-related finding is that the patient was in pain in the emergency department, thus raising blood pressure. After receiving pain medication the blood pressure decreases.

3 The NAP was instructed to report any respiratory rate less than 16 immediately. The nurse needs to reinforce that instruction and determine why this directive was not followed. The respiratory rate has likely been affected by the pain medication, which can depress the respiratory center of the brain.

4 The NAP should be told to obtain the respiratory rate before waking the patient and taking the blood pressure. A sleepy patient is unlikely to have a respiratory rate of 20. The blood pressure was obtained in the right arm, which had a IV present. The nurse should instruct the NAP to retake the BP and should observe the NAP during this measurement. Therefore the nurse can identify and correct any problems with obtaining the BP.

Answers to Review Questions

1 1, 2 **Rationale:** It is common to find sweat in the axilla of a patient with fever. Drying the axilla helps the probe make better contact with the skin. The axillary route would be best because of the patient's confusion. As with other sites for measuring body temperature, the probe must be held in the appropriate position for maximum contact.

2 2 **Rationale:** With aging cerumen (earwax) tends to be drier and can interfere with an accurate tympanic temperature measurement. The cerumen acts as a barrier; therefore the temperature reading would not be reliable.

3 2 **Rationale:** With increased fluid in the abdomen, the patient's respiratory status can be compromised. For patient comfort and accuracy of assessment, his or her head should be elevated.

4 4 **Rationale:** Crossing the legs can falsely increase the systolic and diastolic blood pressure. The cuff should be on the bare arm, but uncrossing the legs is more important. The other two statements are true but would not necessarily promote an accurate reading.

5 3 is the correct sequencing for obtaining a two-step blood pressure measurement using the brachial artery.

6 2 **Rationale:** Electronic blood pressure measurement devices can be used for the patient with diabetes mellitus. Patients with constant body movement, irregular heart rates, peripheral vascular disease, and seizures are not candidates for use of the electronic blood pressure devices.

7 4 **Rationale:** Older adults are less like to demonstrate a high fever. Heart rate increases with fever, not infection.

8 3 **Rationale:** Abnormal radial pulse should be rechecked with apical heart rate assessment. The radial pulse may be too weak to count.

9 3, 4 **Rationale:** Pulse deficit should be determined with a 60-second count starting with zero, and any peripheral artery can be used. Both health care providers must count simultaneously.

10 2, 3 **Rationale:** These are American Heart Association definitions of prehypertension, which are systolic values greater than 120 or diastolic values greater than 80.

CHAPTER 6

Answers to Critical Thinking Exercises

1 Focused systems assessments would include musculoskeletal (focused on R hip), skin (IV site and surgical wound), cardiovascular and respiratory (postoperative status), abdomen (screening for return of peristalsis), peripheral neurovascular (circulation to affected leg), perineal (catheter insertion site), and intake and output.

  a Key elements of each system:

    (1) *Cardiovascular:* Blood pressure (BP); heart rate (HR); inspection, palpation, and auscultation of the heart

    (2) *Musculoskeletal:* Range of motion and position of affected extremity. ROM will be limited until physician orders activity

    (3) *Peripheral neurovascular:* Inspecting and palpating extremities; checking peripheral pulses, edema, skin color and temperature, capillary refill of nail beds; sensation, movement

    (4) *Respiratory:* Checking rate and depth of respirations, chest excursion, lung sounds

    (5) *Skin:* Condition of skin around IV site. Condition of skin around surgical incision. Presence of pressure areas in dependent body parts

    (6) *Abdominal:* Checking size and shape of abdomen, palpating bladder, assessing bowel sounds

    (7) *Intake and output:* Intake, output (Foley, Jackson-Pratt drain), intravenous site patency

2 A crackling noise on inspiration indicates crackles. Crackles indicate fluid in the alveoli and small airways. Priority nursing diagnosis is ineffective airway clearance.

3 This indicates a normal heart rate, which is between 60 and 100 beats/min, regular rate and rhythm.

4 The nurse must listen for 5 minutes over each quadrant before deciding that bowel sounds are absent. It is common for bowel sounds to be hypoactive for 24 hours or more after surgery.

5 See Skill 6-4 for specifics. Unilateral leg edema is one of the most reliable findings of deep vein thrombosis. Other symptoms include pain or tenderness, erythema, increased warmth, and firmness of affected area.

Answers to Review Questions

1 4 **Rationale:** Palpation or percussion of the abdomen can cause bowel sounds to be heard, although peristalsis can be absent. All the other responses are correct.

2 3 **Rationale:** Comparison of areas side to side is extremely important in evaluating a patient's neurologic system. This prevents omissions between the affected and unaffected areas.

3 2 **Rationale:** Diarrhea would be accompanied by hyperactive bowel sounds, and because so much fluid had already been lost, the urine would be darker, therefore concentrated.

4 3 **Rationale:** Having the patient breathe deeper enables the nurse to fully assess lung sounds in the bases of his or her lungs.

5 **780 mL** **Rationale**: 3 ounces = 90 mL (orange juice) + 120 mL (milk) + 90 mL (popsicle) + 360 mL (cola) + 120 mL ice (ice is calculated as half its volume).

6 **1, 5** **Rationale**: The general survey includes assessment of vital signs, height and weight, general behavior, and appearance.

7 **3** **Rationale**: A lesion colored blue/black or with variegated, nonuniform pigmentation or variations/multiple colors (tan, black) with areas of pink, white, gray, blue or red may indicate melanoma.

8 **4** **Rationale**: The sounds are abnormal. Crackles sound like crushing cellophane; rhonchi sound like blowing air through fluid with a straw. Wheezes are musical.

9 **4** **Rationale**: S_1 and S_2 are normal components of the cardiac cycle and an expected physical assessment finding.

10 **2, 3, 4, 1** **Rationale**: Percussion and palpation are completed after inspection and auscultation because of the risk for causing increased bowel sounds that could be interpreted as an abnormal finding.

CHAPTER 7

Answers to Critical Thinking Exercises

1 Joe should wash his hands with soap and water and put on gloves to continue his assessment, explaining the rationale for this to Mr. Nesbitt. He should put Mr. Nesbitt on contact precautions because the drainage from his sacral wound may contain pathogens. His gloves should be changed if they become soiled.

2 After assessing the wound, if his gloved hand contacted it, it would be necessary to remove the gloves, perform hand hygiene, and reglove before checking the Foley catheter, especially if he touched the catheter. However, gloves would not be necessary to visually inspect the position and condition of the tubing. Hand hygiene should be performed when Joe leaves the patient's room.

3 Contact precautions do not require use of a mask. However, if the nurse has a respiratory infection, he or she might choose to wear a mask to protect the patient from exposure.

Answers to Review Questions

1 **4** **Rationale**: Soap and water are essential for visibly dirty hands according to the Centers for Disease Control and Prevention.

2 **2** **Rationale**: Lathering the hands with the cleaning agent using friction is the best method to remove dirt and transient bacteria.

3 **1, 2, 3, 4, 5** **Rationale**: All of the first five factors relate to patient/family needs, the type of isolation devices needed, and organizing nursing care. Item 6 does not impact the delivery of nursing while on isolation precautions.

4 **2** **Rationale**: A mask provides a barrier when the patient has droplet precautions.

5 **3, 4** **Rationale**: Gowns are used once and discarded because of the chance of being contaminated. Hand hygiene should always be performed before and after going into a room.

6 **1** **Rationale**: Microorganisms causing pneumonia exist in droplets of mucus and do not remain suspended in air; therefore they can be spread by direct contact with secretions, especially by unclean hands.

7 **1, 2** **Rationale**: Gloves form a barrier that prevents entrance of microorganisms on the nurse's hands into the urinary device and protects the nurse from exit of microorganisms in the urine.

8 **2** **Rationale**: Soap and water flush spores from hands more efficiently.

9 **4** **Rationale**: Health care worker's hands are the greatest source of microorganisms.

10 **3** **Rationale**: Explaining the reason for isolation and answering questions relieve patient's anxiety.

CHAPTER 8

Answers to Critical Thinking Exercises

1 Insertion of an indwelling urinary catheter requires wearing sterile gloves. Clean gloves are used for nasogastric tube and oral cavity suction. No gloves are necessary to measure blood pressure.

2 Ask Mrs. Lorenzo if she has an allergy to latex or if she has ever had a previous reaction to the following items within hours of exposure: adhesive tape, dental or face mask, golf club grip, ostomy bag, rubber band, balloon, bandage, elastic underwear, IV tubing, rubber gloves, condom. Use latex-free products when caring for Mrs. Lorenzo.

3 Nothing. Only 2.5 cm (1 inch) from the border of the drape to the edge is considered contaminated.

Answers to Review Questions

1 **2** **Rationale**: The pair of synthetic gloves affords some protection from the latex. All other options offer no protection.

2 **2** **Rationale**: The area below the waist is more likely out of direct vision and can become contaminated easier by contact with a nonsterile surface.

3 **1** **Rationale**: The inside of the glove becomes unsterile when it comes in contact with the ungloved hand.

4 **4** **Rationale**: Individuals with spina bifida are at risk for latex allergy; thus the nurse should use a nonlatex catheter and nonlatex gloves. Individuals with spina bifida who have a latex sensitivity may also be allergic to bananas, avocados, kiwi fruit, and tomatoes, but not eggs.

5 **3** **Rationale**: The label of the bottle should be facing the student's palm so it does not become distorted or ruined if fluid runs down the bottle.

6 **1** **Rationale**: Provides steam under pressure, the most effective means of sterilizing instruments and packaged dressings.

7 **1** **Rationale**: When a nurse is sick and needs to get close to an open wound of a patient whose immune system is not functioning well, it is appropriate to ask someone else to change the dressing rather than put the patient at risk. This is the best answer and the only one that keeps the sick nurse away from the patient.

8 **3** **Rationale**: Opening the first flap toward the nurse would require the nurse to reach over the sterile field to completely open the pack. The flap should open away from the nurse.

9 **"position"** **Rationale**: The NAP can be most effective by helping the patient assume and maintain the position that the nurse needs to perform the procedure.

10 **1, 3, 4** **Rationale**: Procedures listed invade sterile body cavities.

CHAPTER 9

Answers to Critical Thinking Questions

1 Additional information may include the following: vital signs, transfer restrictions until CT scan performed, ability to move hands and arms, presence of paralysis, level of orientation and alertness (cognitive status), and patient's level of comfort.

2 1, 2, and 3 are correct answers. Mr. Clark is in pain most likely related to his lacerations and fractures. Pain management is a priority at this time. In addition to pain management, explaining to Mr. Clark the purpose of the CT scan helps elicit his cooperation. He is most likely fearful of movement because of his pain and uncertainty of his condition. Describing the method of transfer and showing him that there will be additional personnel to help transfer him to the stretcher increases his trust and cooperation. Option 4 is incorrect. You may inform Mr. Clark that it is a health care provider's order, but the patient has the right to refuse treatment. You are more likely to elicit Mr. Clark's cooperation by determining the underlying reasons for his refusal to transfer.

3 Mr. Clark should be logrolled until the results of the CT scan have been determined. A nurse must supervise and aid NAP and all personnel when log rolling a patient with a spinal cord injury to keep the spinal column in straight alignment to prevent further injury.

4 Considering his weight and injuries, a slide board with the assistance of three caregivers should be used. Appropriate transfer equipment (such as a slide board) in combination with proper body mechanics reduces the risk of injuries to health care providers.

Answers to Review Questions

1 **3** **Rationale**: The three-person lift for horizontal transfer from the bed to the stretcher is no longer recommended. Physical stress can be decreased significantly by using a slide board.

2 3 **Rationale:** Keeping the knees bent allows for better balance and leverage; keeping the trunk erect helps prevent muscle fatigue because the muscles are working together.

3 3 **Rationale:** A transfer belt is contraindicated around the patient's waist after abdominal surgery. It is far better to have the patient sit on the side of the bed dangling for a few minutes with the nurse there to allow for a smoother transition from supine to upright position for the first time. This also allows the nurse to assess for orthostatic hypotension.

4 2 **Rationale:** The patient's pain may be at a level at which he does not want to move. There are no data to support any of the other options.

5 2 **Rationale:** The patient's skeleton must be kept in alignment, which requires the patient to be turned as a total unit, using enough staff for the turning and positioning. The patient should not participate in the activity because of the instability of the spinal cord.

6 2 **Rationale:** Rebound hypertension would result after prolonged bed rest. There is no indication that the patient is experiencing difficulty with proprioception. There is no indication that the patient has pathology related to the central nervous system.

7 4 **Rationale:** Because of the patient's weight and limited ability to bear weight, a ceiling lift provides the best and safest technique to transfer this patient. A transfer board is used when transferring a patient from a bed to stretcher. A stand-assist device requires the patient to possess full weight-bearing capacity. A three-person carry is inappropriate and no longer recommended.

8 2 **Rationale:** By logrolling and moving the patient as a unit, the nurse prevents twisting and damage to the unstable spinal cord. The step-by-step method causes twisting and bending of the spine, causing further damage. The patient should remain nonweight bearing to prevent further damage to the injured spine. The use of a mechanical lift poses the risk of twisting and bending the spine during transfer.

9 4 **Rationale:** Spacing your feet farther apart allows you to widen your base of support. Leaning back shifts your center of gravity and causes a decrease in stability. Tensing and tightening back muscles could cause back strain. Keeping your knees in a locked position is not correct body mechanics—maintain trunk erect and knees bent so multiple muscle groups work together.

10 4 **Rationale:** A slide board is the most appropriate method to transfer this patient. Carefully assessing the need for additional assistance and the patient's ability to help provides better protection from injury than body mechanics alone.

CHAPTER 10

Answers to Critical Thinking Questions

1 Mr. Timber reports a pain level of 8 on a scale of 0 to 10. A nursing priority is to provide pain management strategies and lower his level to an agreed-on range. In addition, Mr. Timber may have concerns about his ability to safely ambulate without falling or injuring himself. Spending time with him and explaining about and demonstrating the use of crutches will help to minimize his anxiety and concerns.

2 To minimize the effects of orthostatic hypotension allow Mr. Timber to sit with the head of the bed elevated for several minutes before dangling him on the side of the bed. During dangling instruct him to take several deep breaths and move his feet up and down and in a circular motion to promote venous return via intermittent contraction and relaxation of the skeletal leg muscles.

3 Assess the safety of the CPM machine by inspecting the electrical cord for fraying and damage. In addition, put the CPM machine through one full cycle before applying to patient to ensure that the machine is functioning properly. Assess the setup of the machine before placing on the patient's bed: check the stability of the frame, the flexion/extension controls, the padding to exposed metal parts or hard surfaces, and the on/off switch.

4 The appropriate crutch gait for Mr. Timber is the three-point alternating, or three-point gait, which requires the patient to bear all of his weight on one foot. Several teaching considerations are needed for

Mr. Timber. It is important that these considerations are individualized to meet his learning needs. Some examples of teaching considerations for Mr. Timber are the following:

- Instruct patient with axillary crutches about the dangers of pressure on the axillae, which occurs when leaning on the crutches to support body weight.
- Explain why patient must use crutches measured for him or her.
- Demonstrate how to routinely inspect crutch tips. Rubber tips should be securely attached to the crutches. When tips are worn, they should be replaced. Rubber crutch tips increase surface friction and help prevent slipping.

Answers to Review Questions

1 2 **Rationale:** Range-of-motion exercises are done only until resistance is met, not until pain is felt by the patient.

2 4 **Rationale:** Risk for activity intolerance is common for patients who have been immobile for a period of time and are beginning to exert more energy. This diagnosis places the patient initially at risk when exercise begins to increase.

3 3 **Rationale:** If a blood clot is suspected in a leg, the patient should be kept calm and quiet in bed, and the nurse should inform the physician. There should be no rubbing or movement of the leg. The elastic stockings and sequential compression devices are for prevention and, if a DVT is suspected, the health care provider should be notified immediately.

4 3 **Rationale:** NAP can make sure that the patient's environment is free from potential threats to patient safety such as spills or clutter.

5 4 **Rationale:** The nurse stands on the patient's right side or strong side for support.

6 3 **Rationale:** By changing the heel size, the patient's height will be either higher or lower than when the height of the crutches was adjusted initially. Two-to-three fingers should fit between the axilla and the crutch, and the elbow should be slightly bent for proper fit.

7 1 **Rationale:** When a patient is using a supportive device such as a cane, the nurse stands on the weak side. The patient's cane would be in the right hand since the weakness is on the left.

8 4 **Rationale:** The arms of the chair are more stable to use when standing. The walker could tip over. Rocking the patient works when another person is helping to stand a patient. Moving toward front or edge of chair helps make it easier to stand.

9 4 **Rationale:** The patient should always be checked first, before equipment or implementing any treatment.

10 1, 3, 4 **Rationale:** Pallor, nausea, and dizziness are all signs of orthostatic hypotension. Bradycardia is incorrect; tachycardia is actually a symptom. Irritability is not a classic sign of the condition.

CHAPTER 11

Answers to Critical Thinking Exercises

1 The correct answer is C. A fiberglass cast sets up and is dry in 15 to 20 minutes, so it is not necessary to prevent indentation nor does the cast remain damp after that time period. A plaster of Paris cast will take much longer and is susceptible to indentation and dampness and the need to assist in the drying process.

2 The correct answer is B. The patient is receiving pain medication, and the assessment data indicate muscles spasms. You do not release the traction because the traction is in place to reduce the muscle spasms.

3 The correct answer is D. A heating pad would increase the swelling at this point. The key data are increased swelling and pain that is out of proportion to what is expected, given that she is being medicated and the extremity is elevated. The concern is compartment syndrome and altered neurovascular status. To bivalve the cast, cut it in two lengthwise along each side. In addition, the wadding underneath is cut to relieve the pressure. Although a window may be cut in a cast to visualize a wound underneath, it does not relieve pressure. Typically, wrist fractures are initially placed in an ace and splint configuration to accommodate initial swelling.

Answers to Review Questions

1 **2** **Rationale:** A plaster cast needs to breathe and should not be covered. Exposure to water causes the cast to crumble. Sharp edges should be covered with tape or moleskin to prevent skin damage.

2 **2** **Rationale:** The first step involves positioning. Then explaining before using the saw will decrease anxiety. The skin must be inspected for integrity before using an enzyme wash.

3 **2, 4** **Rationale:** Shaving can create micro nicks that can become inflamed under traction. The boot should fit snugly to prevent slipping. The heel should sit properly in the boot without the need for padding, which can increase pressure. Weight is added slowly and gently to prevent muscle spasm and pain. Neurovascular status is assessed distal to the traction.

4 **Every 2 hours** **Rationale:** Permanent neurovascular deficits can occur in as little as 6 hours.

5 **A, B, C, E, G** **Rationale:** Symptoms indicate swelling under the cast. Elevation promotes venous return and decreases edema. Heat and lowering the cast increase edema. More frequent neurovascular checks are needed because swelling could increase. Checking for the degree of tightness will reflect any change. The health care provider must be notified. Analgesics do not relieve edema and could mask increasing symptoms.

6 **2** **Rationale:** A cotton T-shirt should be worn under the brace to protect the skin. The brace should be examined for anything that might damage the skin. Joints are cleaned with pipe cleaners and oiled weekly. Ammonia damages any plastic parts.

7 **4** **Rationale:** Crusting and clear drainage are expected from pin sites. Ashen color indicates possible circulatory problems but not infection. Erythema (redness), warmth, or purulent drainage from the pin sites indicates infection.

8 **2** **Rationale:** Nursing does not determine the amount of weight to be applied or manipulate the traction pins. If a pin moved, the nurse should notify the health care provider. The pull of the traction should be in a straight line, with the rope going over the pulley in a 90-degree angle.

9 **3** **Rationale:** Patients should use the overhead trapeze to move in bed. Weights are never removed from skeletal traction because the callus formation may be damaged and delay healing. If weights do not hang freely at the end of the bed, the pull of the traction is affected. Proper limb alignment ensures proper pull of the traction.

10 **1** **Rationale:** Itching is expected but can be managed with medication.

CHAPTER 12

Answers to Critical Thinking Exercises

1 Complete assessment with emphasis on pressure ulcer risk, current mobility status, and skin integrity.

2 Determine patient's level of pressure ulcer risk and then determine whether pressure reduction or relief is needed. Mr. Hoji is at high risk for pressure ulcers. He has decreased mobility and sensation. He needs pressure relief. The rationale is that he has no ability to independently change position. In addition, because of impaired sensation, he cannot perceive pressure on his skin and tissues.

3 Anxiety and nausea are common with air-suspension beds; the patient's comfort can be improved with pharmacologic agents to reduce anxiety and nausea, but the nurse should also provide reassurance to the patient about the safety of the bed and that his needs will be addressed. In addition, when lateral rotation is also used, the patient's nausea increases. When patients are prescribed an antiemetic such as prochlorperazine (Compazine) be sure that this medication is given routinely as opposed to an "as needed" (prn) order. Explaining to the patient that these sensations are temporary and will gradually improve is important. However, the patient cannot really process this information unless he is comfortable. For these reasons pharmacologic agents to control anxiety, nausea, and any pain are beneficial to patients on support surfaces.

Answers to Review Questions

1 **3** **Rationale:** Patients tend to perspire on this bed. The surface of the bed quickly removes fluids from contact with the patient's skin; thus the evidence of perspiration may be minimized. The perspiration and/or diaphoresis can go undetected, and the increase in insensible fluid loss may not be noticed until the patient develops dehydration or electrolyte changes.

2 **2** **Rationale:** Stop the rotation of the bed and assess the patient further. He or she may experience orthostatic hypotension when the bed rotates. Stopping rotation while remaining with the patient and conducting further blood pressure assessments will indicate if the problem diminishes. The rotation can begin again, perhaps at a decreased angle and at a slower cycle.

3 **4** **Rationale:** Consider changing to a pressure-relief device because this patient is not responding to pressure reduction. The patient needs to move to a pressure-relief system because of the development of pressure ulcers on more than one position area (e.g., supine and left lateral positions).

4 **1** **Rationale:** A patient's ability to assist with transfer to the bed is the least factor to be considered. A severely overweight patient has problems with mobility and therefore needs a bed that will enable the caregiving staff to reposition and provide care while relieving pressure on the skin.

5 **1** **Rationale:** A patient should never be placed in prone position on an air-fluidized bed because of the chance of suffocation. All of the other options are appropriate.

6 **1** **Rationale:** A person with paraplegia does not have normal sensation below the waist. Thus he should not rely on his own "feeling" to adjust the inflation of his seat cushion. Continued redness indicates that a stage I pressure ulcer is developing and should be reported immediately to the nurse or case manager.

7 **3** **Rationale:** The nurse should check with a hand placed under the seat cushion after proper inflation to be sure that the cushion is providing pressure relief. The nurse's hand should not feel a patient's ischia, but the nurse should also note that overinflation of the cushion can damage tissue and cause pressure areas. A general rule of thumb is about 1 inch of support between the patient's ischia and the bottom of the chair.

8 **3** **Rationale:** Current best practice shows a decrease in nurse injury associated with the use of mechanical lifts in the hospital and long-term care. Safe lifting protocols and practices are being integrated into nursing curricula and include the use of mechanical lifts as routine practice.

9 **1** **Rationale:** Best practice suggests that assessing the person's risk factors provides the best basis for choosing a pressure-relieving device.

10 **The correct order is 3, 2, 5, 4, 1** **Rationale:** Proper application of an air mattress overlay is essential to reduce the risk of pressure on a patient's skin or tissues. Ensuring that the sheet is free of wrinkles also reduces the risk for impaired skin integrity. Inflating the mattress before patient transfer verifies that the mattress inflates properly and to the manufacturer's recommended pressure. The intermittent cycling of the air mattress continually alternates pressure against the skin and soft tissue.

CHAPTER 13

Answers to Critical Thinking Exercises

1 Diarrhea may cause Mr. Werneck to have to get out of bed often to use toilet facilities. The diarrhea can cause electrolyte and fluid imbalances that increase risk for dizziness or orthostatic hypotension. The weakness in his leg and his sense of fatigue also add to his risk. Antihypertensive medications increase risk for orthostatic hypotension, which increases fall risk. Being in his room alone after visiting hours might prompt him to walk more on his own. Finally, his age is also a risk factor.

2 Provide a bedside commode to eliminate the need to walk to the bathroom. Inform his wife of her husband's risk for falls and involve her in reminding the patient to sit up and dangle his feet before he

attempts to get up to sit on the commode. Keep the call light close by and respond promptly if patient complains of discomfort or needs assistance to get up. Place a nonskid pad alongside the bed. Place Mr. Werneck in a room close to the nurses' station.

3 Call for help, assess the patient for injury, and stay with him until assistance arrives.

Answers to Review Questions

1 **4 Rationale:** Never leave a seizing patient alone and observe his breathing status. Loss of the airway and protection from injury are primary issues when a patient has a seizure. It is appropriate to turn a patient on his or her side, but airways are not placed by NAP. The patient needs to be watched so he doesn't bump his head, but he shouldn't be held firmly during a seizure. Side rails should be raised, not lowered, if a patient has a seizure.

2 **4 Rationale:** If dentures are loose, they can be removed after the postictal phase of the seizure. Never try to remove anything from the mouth when a patient is showing warning signs of a seizure or during a seizure. Immediately after a seizure the patient may still be unconscious, and there is still a risk that he or she will bite down on your hands. If the dentures are firmly in place, leave them alone.

3 **2 Rationale:** If a head or neck injury is suspected, a cervical collar should be placed on the patient to prevent additional injury. It is the only answer that protects the patient from further injury. Using three people would protect the caregivers from injury.

4 **3 Rationale:** According to The Joint Commission standards, a patient must be seen by a health care provider within 1 hour to perform an assessment after restraints are applied. The assessment will either support the use of continued restraints or their removal. The other actions are not mandated by standards.

5 **3 Rationale:** For safety sake, one restraint should be removed at a time with an additional staff member present because of the erratic patient behavior.

6 **3, 4 Rationale:** QSEN skills for safety competency include demonstrating effective use of strategies such as evidence-based assessment guidelines to reduce risk of harm to patients. In addition, communication to staff members of any observations related to errors such as a fall occurrence is essential. Reliance on memory is not a safety competency, nor is the use of a new technology without having received proper training.

7 **2 Rationale:** The one evidence-based intervention among the choices is a standard vision assessment. Restraints do not prevent falls. Diversional activities and the RAWS are designed to reduce the use of restraints, not prevent falls.

8 **3 Rationale:** The patient should not be involved in securing the fire. He or she should be evacuated as quickly and safely as possible.

9 **2, 3, 4, 1 Rationale:** Follow the acronym RACE—**R**escue, **A**ctivate alarm, **C**ontain fire, **E**vacuate patient.

10 **1, 3, 4 Rationale:** A patient-centered approach involves considering the patient's and family member's cultural perspectives and the meaning that restraints have for them. A restraint can be perceived as a form of punishment. In addition, when possible, always consider a patient's or family member's preference for type of restraint to use. It is important to apply evidence in an assessment, but a patient-centered approach includes the views and opinions of the patient and family.

CHAPTER 14

Answers to Critical Thinking Exercises

1 Rescue workers should wear respiratory and skin personal protective equipment (PPE) and locate selves upwind and uphill unless cyanide is suspected.

2 A 22-year-old with cyanosis, a respiratory rate of 35 breaths/min, and confusion would be color coded immediate, red. A 14-year-old with a diffuse red rash on the extremities would be color coded minimal, green. A 56-year-old with controlled bleeding of deep lacerations received from falling debris would be color coded delayed, yellow. A 41-year-old with burns on 50% of the body would be color coded immediate, red. Those coded red would receive highest priority.

3 The primary objective for initial care is decontamination. Decontamination is the process used to remove harmful contaminants from the surface of the skin. It is achieved by removing clothing and scrubbing the skin and by hydrolysis, a process of chemical dilution using large volumes of water.

4 Clothing should be cut off rather than pulled over the head to prevent contamination of the head and hair. Clothing should then be placed in a biohazard bag, labeled, and sealed to reduce the likelihood of secondary chemical contamination.

5 Children may be frightened by separation from their parents, the appearance of rescue workers in PPE, and decontamination procedures. To avoid secondary contamination do not immediately pick up a child. Offer verbal encouragement and praise to facilitate treatment. Observe children closely for symptoms of exposure because they are more prone to the effects of chemical toxins (being closer to the ground and having a higher respiratory rate than adults). Children are also more susceptible to hypothermia with decontamination procedures.

Answers to Review Questions

1 **1 Rationale:** Practice makes staff more familiar with disaster protocols in the event of a true disaster.

2 **4 Rationale:** A nurse who must inform a mother that her three children did not survive would have the most difficult job.

3 **2 Rationale:** A disaster victim who arrives at the ED with labored respirations, cool skin, a pulse of 120 beats/min, and a blood pressure of 90/60 mm Hg should receive the highest level of priority of care because of the presenting signs. This victim stands a good chance of survival with appropriate care.

4 **2 Rationale:** Contact isolation is needed because of the mechanism of transmission.

5 **1 Rationale:** The health care workers must be protected first because of the chance of spreading whatever contamination may be present. If the health care workers become infected, no one will be available to care for the victims.

6 **4 Rationale:** Assessment cannot be delegated to NAP at any time. The nurse may direct the NAP to gather supplies and use appropriate PPE to prevent contamination.

7 **2 Rationale:** Rapid decontamination of the patient is more important than determining the exact agent and decreases the risk of secondary exposure to health care providers.

8 **3 Rationale:** Level A protection is used in highly contaminated areas. Level B is used by first responders and includes a self-contained breathing apparatus. Level C first responders (emergency personnel first on the scene) and hospital personnel are trained and fitted to use level C protection. Level D consists of the standard work uniform and the implementation of standard precautions.

9 **1 Rationale:** Potassium iodide is the treatment of choice for radioactive exposure.

10 **4 Rationale:** Vaccination within 3 days of exposure completely prevents the disease or significantly reduces its effect. Vaccination 4 to 7 days after exposure offers some protection from disease or decreases its severity.

CHAPTER 15

Answers for Critical Thinking Questions

1 Every 4 hours for assessment is appropriate for someone in her condition; and, as with many elderly patients, the verbal scale is easier to use than the numeric scale. You may have to explain it each time because Mrs. Silver is legally blind. The FACES scale could not be used correctly by Mrs. S. because she is unable to see it.

2 Guided imagery and massage are good options. Repositioning off of her right side would likely be helpful as well. .

3 The nurse should explain that the pain could be contributing to the constipation. The patient's immobility also adds to the problem. However, morphine also can lead to constipation. The nurse should assess the patient's diet and confer with the health care provider about an alternative pain medication and possibly a stool softener.

Answers for Review Questions

1 **3** **Rationale:** Frequent button pushing indicates an increase in pain; thus a pain assessment is needed. Assessment alone does nothing to help the patient; action must be taken right away to make him or her comfortable again. Pain is not "normal" and should never be ignored. It may be expected after surgery but should still be treated appropriately. A patient is limited to the amount of medication ordered until the prescriber is notified and orders received, but patients are never told that they can only push so many times an hour.

2 **3** **Rationale:** Teenagers usually are comfortable with technology; at this developmental stage the autonomy of being able to determine when to take their pain medication is very satisfying and reassuring.

3 **2** **Rationale:** A person with sleep apnea already has periods of decreased oxygenation as a result of episodes in which they briefly stop breathing while asleep (apnea). Obesity often causes partial obstruction of the trachea, especially when the pharynx is relaxed during sleep. These patients need frequent pain and sedation assessment. When they receive prn medications, the nurse assesses pain and sedation with each injection of analgesia.

4 **4** **Rationale:** The orders should always be checked independently by two registered nurses; the pump is programmed to the checked and double-checked dosage. If the two nurses do not agree, they need to recheck their calculations.

5 **2** **Rationale:** Monitoring frequency should be based on patient factors (e.g., whether they are opioid naïve, type of surgery or illness, previous sleep apnea). Using a standard scale (individual institutional policy) ensures that each caregiver bases the assessment on the same patient factors. Detecting and treating oversedation helps to prevent respiratory depression, a life-threatening situation if not corrected quickly; oversedation proceeds respiratory depression. Simply awakening a patient does not mean that consistent assessment is used. Once a shift is not enough to observe for oversedation. Medications may need to be adjusted if oversedation is present.

6 **From top to bottom, four, one, two, three.** **Rationale:** Treating patient's pain is the number one priority. Using a pain scale is important to assess and document actual pain at the time of occurrence. Positioning patients helps with pain management. Assessing and treating the patient's pain are priorities over searching through the chart to see if patient was ever nonverbal.

7 **2** **Rationale:** Vital signs are not a reliable indicator for persistent/chronic pain as the body adapts to the changes caused by pain. Patients are not used to determining pain intensity. With acute/transient pain, changes in the vital signs may be seen initially; but one person's blood pressure may rise dramatically with severe pain, whereas another's may drop significantly.

8 **2** **Rationale:** Elderly patients do very well on opioids; but, because of age-related decline in liver and kidney function, the opioids need to be started at very low doses, and dosage increases should be slower.

9 **1** **Rationale:** ATC dosing is the most effective by stabilizing the blood level of the drug, which helps provide reliable pain control.

10 **3** **Rationale:** Rather than looking for hidden meanings, believe a patient's self-report of pain. Although a patient might think that anxiety may be relieved by pain medication, teaching is needed. If the symptoms are anxiety based with no underlying pain, try some complementary methods. If a patient is unable to relax, contact the health care provider or nurse practitioner for orders for medication for relaxation. It is extremely rare that a patient will say that she is having pain to gain attention, although some patients have learned that it is one way to get someone to come to their room. Try to spend time with the patient and help her with other needs and then do a pain assessment. Requesting additional pain relief is not a symptom of addiction.

CHAPTER 16

Answers to Critical Thinking Exercises

1 Because you do not know what Mr. Corbin has been told about his situation, begin by exploring his perceptions of his health status and validate his feelings. "Tell me what you were told about your illness. I would like to understand better." Discussion helps reveal misperceptions or the need for factual information to help Mr. Corbin gain a sense of control. Mr. Corbin has also opened the door for a conversation about his emotional state. Paraphrase by saying, "It sounds like you are feeling all alone and don't know where to go for help. Is that right?" Sit down while speaking and ensure privacy by closing the door.

2 The correct answer is 2. The nurse should gather more assessment data before selecting an intervention (choices 1 and 4). Perform a physical assessment of the patient's abdomen and ask about normal bowel patterns, current pain medications, and recent diet and fluid intake. Assess the type, timing, location, precipitating and relieving factors, and intensity of Mr. Corbin's abdominal pain. Allow him to describe his own symptoms instead of asking his wife (choice 3). Ask him about other symptoms he may be experiencing.

3 Assess what Mr. Corbin and his wife already know about hospice care and what it means to them. People face many changes when opting to receive home hospice care. Their familiar health care patterns and relationships will change, and caregivers will come into their home. To accept hospice care admits that death is presumed likely within the next few months or sooner. Symptom management becomes the primary focus of care. Assess the Corbin family's degree of openness and awareness concerning death. The family must provide the care for all daily activities, necessitating some temporary changes in roles and schedules. However, families do have access to professional and volunteer hospice team members throughout their experience. Hospice professionals provide teaching, support, counseling, home visits as needed, and 24-hour contact for medical emergencies or questions. Family members need a support system to meet the challenges of helping their loved one die at home.

Answers to Review Questions

1 **3** **Rationale:** Palliative care prioritizes care based on patient needs and preferences. Nurses help patients identify their own goals of care. An open-ended question always elicits more information than a closed-ended one.

2 **3** **Rationale:** It is normal after a significant loss to experience the presence of the lost person and have difficulty resuming life activities.

3 **4** **Rationale:** Others do not consider the woman's loss to be significant enough for her grief expression; thus she feels disenfranchised.

4 **1** **Rationale:** When patient and family members are ready to discuss goals of care, it is best to include the patient, family members, and members of the care team so patient preferences can be expressed and health care team can provide needed information.

5 **4** **Rationale:** Options 1, 2, and 3 offer solutions to fix the problem. Disease process, medications, social withdrawal, and a slowing of bodily functions cause persons nearing the end of life to lose their interest in food.

6 **2** **Rationale:** When a loss has been long anticipated, some people experience relief that the experience has come to an end. They have been grieving for some time before the actual loss happens.

7 **6** **Rationale:** Palliative care interventions are available to patients who wish to have good symptom management and also continue their disease-modifying treatments.

8 **2** **Rationale:** People from some cultures do not want full disclosure ("honesty") related to their prognosis, nor do all people value self-determination as practiced in Western medical culture.

9 **1** **Rationale:** Persons specially educated are best for making for organ donation requests. Many times family members give consent based on their knowledge of the deceased's values (options 2 and 3). Because the options for donating organs and tissue are numerous, request for organ or tissue donation is routinely made (option 4) of most patients.

10 **The correct order is 9, 6, 5, 7, 2, 3, 1, 4, 8 Rationale:** Perform all preliminary activities, including elevating patient head (completed first in case of delays in other activities), confirming organ donation, talking to family, and requesting support persons for the family. Perform activities that could lead to resoiling the body (specimens and tube removal) before bathing and positioning the patient. Tag the body before transport to the morgue but after patient family has viewed the body.

CHAPTER 17

Answers to Critical Thinking Exercises

1 The correct answers are 1, 3, and 4. Patients with diabetes should wear socks made of natural fibers to aid in absorption of perspiration. Cotton socks are most commonly recommended. A professional should trim nails to minimize chance of injury and infection. It is recommended that patients with diabetes mellitus should not soak feet for two reasons: (1) decreased sensation in lower extremities caused by peripheral neuropathy makes it difficult to determine temperature; and (2) soaking the feet causes maceration of the skin around the nails and feet, which can cause infection.

2 The correct answer is 2. Patients with diabetes should have a podiatrist who performs foot and nail care at least annually. Patients should be taught signs and symptoms that warrant the need to seek medical attention.

Answers to Review Questions

1 **3 Rationale:** Moving a cloth on the skin during bathing not only cleans but also removes dead skin cells.

2 **4 Rationale:** A patient with arthritis in her neck may have pain and limited movement. This could cause a problem when her head is turned and repositioned while her hair is washed.

3 **4 Rationale:** A patient who becomes aggressive or uncooperative would do best with a warm, disposable bath in bed. It provides a more thorough bath in the safest environment for both patient and caregiver.

4 **3 Rationale:** Muslims use the left hand for cleaning the genital area. The right hand is reserved for eating and praying. As long as the caregiver is a woman, it is not necessary to have another woman present. If the nurse is right-handed, she should switch and perform the perineal care using her left hand to show respect for her patient's beliefs. Gloves should be used for all patients when doing perineal care.

5 **4 Rationale:** Before administering oral care to an unconscious patient, check the gag reflex to determine risk for aspiration. A pupil check indicates if intracranial pressure is developing. The Glasgow Coma Scale measures level of consciousness. It is important to inspect the oral cavity, but this will not reveal any risk for aspiration.

6 **1, 3, 4 Rationale:** A bed bath, tub bath, and shower are all considered cleaning baths. An herbal bath is a therapeutic bath because it is ordered for a specific effect.

7 **3 Rationale:** Oral care with peroxide is not recommended with mechanically ventilated patients. Normal saline can be used to moisten the mucosa; however, it is not associated with prevention of VAP. Oral care using chlorhexidine has proved to reduce VAP in mechanically ventilated cardiac surgery patients. It has also shown benefit with patients who do not have a pneumonia diagnosis before intubation.

8 **2** In the absence of a blink reflex, the eyelids should be kept closed with an eye patch or shield after gently closing the eye with the back of your fingertip. Taping the eyelids closed is not accepted practice; and leaving the eyes open causes excessive dryness of the eye, leading to corneal drying, abrasions, and eye infection.

9 **The correct order is 1, 4, 3, 2, 5 Rationale:** Assessing the environment for safety should always precede care. Making sure that you have your supplies arranged nearby eliminates leaving the bedside and interrupting care. Raising the bed to working height is a necessary part of safe body mechanics to avoid injury to the caregiver. Lowering the side rail allows easy access to the patient for positioning and performing the procedure.

10 **Mucositis.** Mucositis is inflammation of the mucous membrane of the mouth.

CHAPTER 18

Answers to Critical Thinking Exercises

1 Ms. Willett is unable to move well in bed or change position because of the immobilizer and the pain that she is experiencing. She is also on bed rest. She is a high risk under the activity subscale on the Braden Scale because of her bed rest.

2 The correct answer is 2, eschar, nonstageable. Granulation tissue is red and moist and is found in wounds that are moving toward healing; this wound can be stage II or III, depending on the depth of the tissue loss. Slough tissue can be tan, yellow, brown, or gray; is moist; and is found in wounds that require interventions to clean this tissue from the wound. Staging may be difficult if the base of the wound is not clearly defined. Erythema stage I is intact red skin that is warm to the touch. Eschar, nonstageable, the correct answer, is dead devitalized tissue that may need to be removed to allow the area to heal. As long as the eschar covers the ulcer, it cannot be staged; staging is done when the base of the wound is visible. An eschar-covered wound does not allow the wound base assessment.

3 The correct answer is 1. A sheet burn opens the top layer of skin, and the area is slightly moist. Blistering is caused when the two layers of skin, dermis and epidermis, separate and allow fluid to accumulate. A blistered area is intact. Bruising results in breakage of the local capillaries and discoloration of the tissues. The correct answer is erythema.

4 It is likely that the erythema has occurred because of unrelieved pressure over Ms. Willet's sacrum. She is on bed rest and not moving well because of her pain and the immobilizer. This area is at risk for pressure ulcer development. The nurse should palpate the reddened area. If it does not blanch, the nurse can suspect tissue damage.

Answers to Review Questions

1 **1, 2 Rationale:** The patient with the surgical wound most likely has an infection that delays wound healing because the inflammatory phase of wound healing is prolonged. A steroid such as cortisol also delays the inflammatory phase of wound healing. Vitamin C and a moist dressing are factors that promote wound healing.

2 **2 Rationale:** This provides an early baseline assessment and periodic reassessment throughout the confinement.

3 **2 Rationale:** The patient has numerous risk factors that necessitate the consultation with the wound clinical nurse specialist about the most appropriate bed surface to reduce pressure.

4 **2, 3, 4 Rationale:** The use of an incentive spirometer does not cause prolonged pressure; thus a pressure injury to the lips is unlikely. The patient is at risk for a pressure injury from the nasogastric tube (nares), IV tubing (skin along arm or wherever patient lies on tubing), and the drainage tube (wherever patient lies over tubing).

5 **2 Rationale:** This type of dressing protects the wound base and provides a moist environment, which in this case is essential to support the growth of new tissue.

6 **2 Rationale:** The head is the most common site of pressure ulcers in neonates and very young children because the skin is thin, little hair is present to absorb pressure, and they are often unable to reposition themselves adequately to reduce pressure.

7 **2 Rationale:** A moist saline gauze dressing provides a moist environment to the wound and wicks away excessive drainage, facilitating healing.

8 **2 Rationale:** A hydrocolloid dressing interacts with the moist wound base and forms a gel over the wound to support moist wound healing.

9 **3 Rationale:** All four patients have some risk factors for developing a pressure ulcer. However, the 50-year-old patient has more factors (3) placing him at risk: poor circulation from diabetes, limited mobility from his postoperative status, and presence of diaphoresis.

10 **3 Rationale:** The correct sequence of steps is to explain the purpose of the dressing change to the patient; position the patient to provide easy access for cleaning the wound; once cleaned, assess the wound and measure to determine correct size of dressing; and

apply the dressing so it extends at least 2.5 cm (1 inch) beyond the wound edge and press gently to adhere.

CHAPTER 19

Answers to Critical Thinking Exercises

1 The correct answer is 3. Apply gloves when drainage is present. It is important to turn off the aid volume to prevent feedback (whistling) during removal. Grasping the device prevents accidentally dropping the aid. Wash the ear canal to remove any drainage or wax. The brush supplied with the aid is used to dislodge any wax that is transferred from the ear canal to the aid. Storing the aid in its storing case further reduces the risk of damage to the aid.

2 The correct choices are 1 and 3. The batteries are very toxic to children and pets when swallowed, and a child would need to be seen by a health care professional should this occur. The aids are small and present a choking hazard to a child. Teaching Mr. Kupec to have his grandchildren face him (option 2) increases his hearing clarity when the children are speaking, but it is not related to child safety. Offering to show the children the hearing aid (option 4) addresses some of their curiosity but is not a safety measure.

3 Of key importance to teach Mr. Kupec and his wife are: (1) how to clean the aids; (2) when to see an audiologist to evaluate the efficacy of the aids; (3) safety factors; and (4) any insurance or financial data regarding care, insurance, and replacement of the aids.

Answers to Review Questions

1 **2 Rationale:** The patient will be unable to care for her contact lenses immediately after surgery. No signs or symptoms have been presented to justify any of the other choices.

2 **4 Rationale:** Some disposable contact lenses are intended to be cleaned and reused. Furthermore, there is increased risk for infection with any contact lens use.

3 **4 Rationale:** The chemical should be removed as soon as possible to minimize the risk for permanent damage to the eye. Although a basin may be positioned to catch a dislodged contact lens, taking time to remove the lens delays removing the chemical from the eye and increases the risk for permanent damage. Testing the pH of secretions may be performed after an initial period of irrigation to determine the need to continue.

4 **1 Rationale:** The artificial eye should be cleaned only as often as necessary to prevent discomfort. The other statements are correct and indicate adequate teaching.

5 **2, 3 Rationale:** Make sure that a patient can see your face to facilitate comprehension. Speaking more slowly while using the same appropriate tone causes less frustration for a patient and allows you to assess whether other approaches need to be used. Raising voice volume distorts the voice and may make understanding more difficult. If a patient appears not to understand, a different choice of words may help; but a rapid series of statements or questions deprives him or her of the longer processing time needed to compensate for a hearing impairment. Gestures may not be helpful in many circumstances.

6 **4 Rationale:** Only the natural eye can react to stimuli such as when accommodation is done. Both eyes would produce tears and lubrication. Movement is present if the eye muscles have been attached to the ocular implant beneath the artificial eye, but the artificial eye would not have more natural movement than the natural eye.

7 **3 Rationale:** Heat from the blow dryer can damage hearing aids. Other substances such as hair spray or cologne also need to be kept away from the aids. The hearing aids need to be stored away from children and dogs and cats. Dogs in particular and cats are attracted to the scent of used hearing aids. Use of a desiccant prolongs the life of batteries and the hearing aid.

8 **2 Rationale:** Before any interventions are taken, the nurse must first assess a patient's ear for signs of irritation, including any presence of infection. From there the nurse can determine what needs to be done. This follows the sequence of the nursing process to first assess before implementing. Teaching a patient how to reposition his hearing aids if they are uncomfortable would be appropriate

based on the assessment findings. Reducing the volume of the hearing aid in the ear not causing a problem is inappropriate.

9 **4 Rationale:** The patient's corneas are susceptible to dryness and injury because of his or her condition since the patient does not have voluntary control to keep the eyes closed. It is essential that the corneas be kept moist by instillation of an eye lubricant, but eye irrigations would not be performed. The eyes should not be taped closed. Checking for the papillary response has nothing to do with a patient's eyes care.

10 **4 Rationale:** The nurse needs to have more information about the pain and any signs or symptoms that a patient is having such as ear drainage, any odor, and quality and quantity of pain. This assessment must be done first. Based on the information, the nurse makes the appropriate recommendations. Although the use of soap and water is appropriate, it has nothing to do with the problem expressed. Earwax helps to protect the ears, although too much can interfere with hearing. Nothing should be put into the ear until perforation of the eardrum has been ruled out.

CHAPTER 20

Answers to Critical Thinking Exercises

1 The antidepressant, hormone, cardiac drug (beta-blocker), and antihypertensive medications can all potentially create adverse effects in older adults. The weakness and dizziness are likely side effects of the metoprolol and the antihypertensive. Because he takes multiple medications, there should be concern that there is possible drug interaction, with either summation or synergism occurring.

2 The health care provider has the option of lowering the dose in the older adult to determine if therapeutic effects can still be achieved.

3 You would need to evaluate if the patient has the motor dexterity or visual acuity to split tablets.

Answers to Review Questions

1 **1 Rationale:** Many medications bind to albumin (protein). If a patient is malnourished, the level of protein can be lowered; and toxicity can be a problem, especially if the medication would normally bind to the protein. The patient should always be watched for the other problems.

2 **1 Rationale:** The trough is drawn when the level of the medication is the lowest, which occurs right before the next dose is due.

3 **1 Rationale:** The patient is nauseated; therefore it is important to judge which route is best for her because of the chance of vomiting the medication.

4 **4 Rationale:** 0.5 g = 500 mg. If each tablet is 250 mg, two tablets are needed.

5 **4 Rationale:** The nurse must know how the medication is metabolized and excreted (i.e., through the liver, kidneys, or intestines). Whichever system is affected can affect the manner and amount of drug absorbed or excreted.

6 **3 Rationale:** If sediment is seen at the bottom of the container of a clear liquid medication, the medication should be discarded or sent back to the pharmacy with an explanation according to institutional policy. The medication components may have gone through a change during transport or storage, or the medication may have expired.

7 **4 Rationale:** The nurse needs to check if the mouthwash contains anything that might interact with the patient's medications for possible interactions. The pharmacist or health care provider could also be contacted. The nurse could also recommend switching to a safer mouthwash unless it is contraindicated. None of the other answers is a priority or relevant.

8 **3 Rationale:** The Joint Commission has prohibited the use of MSO4 as an abbreviation for morphine sulfate. The nurse needs to call the health care provider who prescribed the order for clarification and to read back the order to the health care provider. This would then be transcribed as a verbal order and noted per institutional policy.

9 **3 Rationale:** The patient needs to be assessed and not left alone since this response to the medication was unpredicted and the

patient outcome is not known. The health care provider needs to be notified, and orders may be given for medical intervention. This type of medication can cause difficulty in the elderly population. Naloxone is used for opioid toxicity and is not appropriate.

10 1 **Rationale:** These medications may be appropriate or inappropriate for this patient, but it won't be known until they are identified. The nurse is attempting to assess and obtain a medication history. Since the patient doesn't know the name of the medication, the nurse should check to see if the patient brought the medications with him. Identification of medications is done by the pharmacist, not the nurse. The older adult has alterations in the absorption, distribution, metabolism and excretion of medications and needs to be monitored. Option 2 has nothing to do with the question.

CHAPTER 21

Answers to Clinical Thinking Exercises

1 A spacer device would be helpful for Mrs. Martin. She would just need to breathe in and out of the spacer device to receive the medication after pressing the metered-dose inhaler (MDI) canister.

2 The nurse should explain to Mrs. Martin that the old medication should be removed before applying new medication. The layer of old medication reduces the antibacterial action of the ointment. The nurse should demonstrate to Mrs. Martin how to care for the wound and watch as she performs it herself.

3 The nurse needs to review the correct technique for transdermal patch application and removal with Mrs. Martin. The old patches should be removed, folded with sticky sides together, wrapped in paper, and discarded. The new patch should be applied to a new area of skin, and the old site washed with soap and water to remove residue. Mrs. Martin may need to check to see if her health care provider would like her to have a nitrate-free period overnight. If so, the patch would be removed at bedtime, with a new patch applied in the morning.

Answers to Review Questions

1 4 **Rationale:** An oral-dosing syringe has the appropriate markings for accuracy and usually has a protective colored tip to prevent it from being lost in the infant's environment.

2 3 **Rationale:** Explain that the tablet is formulated to release slowly over time and should not be crushed, broken, or chewed.

3 4, 5, 6 **Rationale:** The tube should be adequately flushed after the last dose of medication to decrease the chance of crusting inside the tube and to ensure that all the medication has left it. Gastric residual should be checked before giving the medications. If too much gastric content is still left in the stomach, there may be a problem with the patient's rate of absorption, which can affect the medication absorption as well. The head of the bed should be left elevated to prevent aspiration.

4 2 **Rationale:** Because the patient is immunocompromised and has a large wound, sterile gloves should be used when applying medication because of the risk for infection.

5 1 **Rationale:** Applying the patch to a different area each time prevents skin irritation, which would affect the absorption rate.

6 2 **Rationale:** Wearing gloves minimizes the likelihood of the nurse being exposed to the medication.

7 1 **Rationale:** Steroid use can cause oral candidiasis, and therefore the mouth should be rinsed to avoid complications.

8 4 **Rationale:** Warming the medication is less irritating to the nerves in the ear and will reduce vertigo.

9 1 **Rationale:** This is the correct position for administering medication to the maxillary sinus.

10 2, 1, 5, 3, 4 **Rationale:** This is the correct order of action for administering ophthalmic ointment to a patient.

11 2 **Rationale:** Keeping the head of the bed elevated prevents aspiration and maintains an open airway.

12 3 **Rationale:** NAP have a limited scope of practice; the most appropriate delegation is to have them report changes in a patient's status.

CHAPTER 22

Answers to Critical Thinking Exercises

1 The nurse needs to know:
The drug classification, desired effect, and nursing implications related to heparin therapy; and the safe medication dose, which must be compared to the order before administration. The nurse needs to calculate how many milliliters to draw from the vial and if a filter needle is required.

2 The nurse needs to know:
Current diet.
Use of over-the-counter supplements and other prescribed medications.
If anything is affecting the blood flow to subcutaneous tissues of the abdomen.
Nutritional and fluid status and skin turgor.
Partial thromboplastin time to evaluate the desired effect.

3 The nurse should always use the smallest syringe possible when preparing medication. Usually a 25-gauge, $\frac{3}{8}$- to $\frac{5}{8}$-inch needle deposits medication into the subcutaneous tissue of a normal-size patient; however, this patient is overweight and may need a different-size needle. Use the abdomen, staying 5 cm (2 inches) away from the umbilicus.

4 The nurse needs to assess:
If the medication needs to be diluted before administering it by IV push.
The rate per minute of administration.
The compatibility of IV medications with IV fluids.
The condition of the IV site.
The level of the patient's pain.

Answers to Review Questions

1 2 **Rationale:** The nurse should calculate and determine how much medication needs to be injected into the patient while considering which route is being used. This needs to be done before the diluent and powder are mixed.

2 1 **Rationale:** The medication from the vial is withdrawn first to prevent any contamination of the vial with medication from the ampule.

3 4 **Rationale:** A 22-gauge, $1\frac{1}{2}$-inch needle will penetrate the ventrogluteal area and disperse the aqueous-based medication easily. The other needle sizes are either too small or too large.

4 1 **Rationale:** The patient is experiencing infiltration of the IV infusion, and the site needs to be changed.

5 3 **Rationale:** Assessment of the condition of the IV insertion site is the priority. If there is a problem with the site, the medication cannot be given.

6 2 **Rationale:** An induration of greater than 10 mm in a healthy individual indicates tuberculosis exposure and requires follow-up.

7 1 **Rationale:** Symptoms indicate paresthesia and should not be present after an IM injection.

8 **Match:** 1, b; 2, c; 3, a

9 4 **Rationale:** Management of hypoglycemia includes drinking 4 ounces of fruit juice or regular soda or 8 ounces of skim milk or eating 6 to 10 hard candies.

10 **Fill in:** Dyspnea, wheezing, and circulatory collapse are symptoms of anaphylactic reactions.

CHAPTER 23

Answers to Critical Thinking Exercises

1 Additional information may include the following:
a Pulmonary system
(1) Measure pulse oximetry.
(2) Observe breathing pattern.
(3) Observe for use of accessory muscles and nasal flaring.
(4) Auscultate lungs for adventitious sounds and note if lung sounds clear with coughing.
(5) Observe sputum for color, thickness, amount, and patient ability to clear airway.

b Cardiac system
   (1) Vital signs
   (2) Heart rate and rhythm
c Neurologic system
   (1) Level of consciousness (LOC)
   (2) Orientation
   (3) Ability to follow instructions
      Mr Landon is very fatigued and short of breath, which makes taking a history difficult. Obtaining cardiopulmonary data through a focused assessment enables the nurse to identify pertinent data about the patient's status before treatment. In addition, a brief neurologic examination obtains baseline LOC and orientation and helps to determine the patient's ability to follow instructions. These baseline data help to determine the patient's present cardiopulmonary and oxygenation status without increasing his level of fatigue. Remember, in patients without underlying cardiac disease, the body adapts to decreased oxygenation or increased oxygen demands by increasing heart rate and blood pressure. In addition, the nurse has a sense of the patient's understanding of care and ability to participate in it (e.g., coughing and deep breathing, anticipated oxygen therapy).

2 Administration of oxygen therapy
   a The FiO_2 level is between 24% and 28%.
   b Hypercarbia is a risk for patients with COPD because the oxygen therapy may override the adapted respiratory drive. As a result, CO_2 is retained, and there is an increased risk for respiratory failure in this patient.

3 The strap on the cannula may be too tight or placed incorrectly. Inspect the external ears where the cannula strap rests to observe for any skin irritation. Adjust the fit of the cannula and place pressure-relieving devices (e.g., ear protectors or folded 4 × 4) under the elastic strap of the cannula.
   • The oxygen may dry out the nasal mucosa, and the cannula itself can irritate the patient's nares. Inspect nares for skin irritation. Evaluate the humidification level of the oxygen therapy; perhaps more humidification is needed.

4 d Partial rebreather mask mixes exhaled carbon dioxide with oxygen and causes an increase in carbon dioxide. Because Mr. Landon has underlying COPD and pneumonia, he is at risk for carbon dioxide retention, and this risk is further increased by the partial rebreather mask.

Answers to Review Questions

1 1 **Rationale:** A respiratory rate of 24 breaths/min could be seen in a dyspneic patient. All of the other options would be seen when hypoxia has been present for a long period of time.

2 2 **Rationale:** If the reservoir is deflated, the patient can breathe large amounts of carbon dioxide.

3 2 **Rationale:** A patient with COPD often has difficulty holding the breath at the end of inhalation. There is no reason the patient would not be able to hold the mouthpiece. Patients do not blow into an incentive spirometer. Three readings are made with a peak flow meter.

4 4 **Rationale:** When the oxygen rate is 4 L/min or greater, humidification is needed to prevent drying of the nasal mucous membrane. Under 4 L the moisture can be provided by the nasal passages.

5 2 **Rationale:** A Venturi mask is the only method of delivering an FiO_2 of 80% with the stated liters per minute. The nasal cannula delivers 44% at most, the partial rebreather must be set at a minimum of 8 liters, and the nonrebreather must be set at a minimum of 6 liters.

6 3 **Rationale:** Pulse oximetry measures arterial saturation immediately. Options 1 and 2 do not address the adequacy of oxygenation. Option 4 provides information about the presence of secretions or airway narrowing but not about the adequacy of oxygen therapy.

7 2 **Rationale:** Petroleum jelly products should not be used around oxygen because of the possibility of friction, which can cause a fire. Options 1, 3, and 4 demonstrate that the patient needs education.

8 2 **Rationale:** Noninvasive positive-pressure ventilation (NIPPV) *maintains positive airway pressure* and *improves alveolar ventilation* without the need for an artificial airway.

9 2, 3 **Rationale:** When caring for an intubated patient, nurses are encouraged to use verbal and nonverbal communication. Alphabet charts, pen and paper, slates or chalkboards, and computers are some common communication tools. Intubated patients do not have a hearing loss; thus speaking loudly may frustrate them and does not promote communication. Families can speak to the patient, but the patient still needs a mechanism of communication.

10 3 **Rationale:** When a patient is on humidified oxygen via tracheostomy, water can accumulate in the tubing. It is important to empty this water from the tubing so the patient may receive adequate oxygenation. This sound may be disturbing to the patient. Options 1, 2, and 4 do not address the problem of water in the tubing.

CHAPTER 24

Answers to Critical Thinking Exercises

1 Place bed in Trendelenburg's and use three positions: left side-lying to drain right lower lobe bronchus, right side-lying to drain left lower lobe bronchus, and left side-lying with one-quarter turn back onto pillow to drain right middle lobe.

2 Chest examination would reveal decreased breath sounds at bases posteriorly and over right lateral chest wall. A decreased chest wall excursion is expected, more pronounced on the right side. It is also important to assess patient's cough and sputum production. In this case you might expect patient to complain of increased dyspnea, and the respiratory rate and oxygen saturation may change.

3 Improvement of lobar collapse on chest x-ray film is a common clinical finding after the successful application of CPT. In addition, you would expect oxygen saturation oxygenation to improve and dyspnea, tachypnea, and fever begin to resolve.

4 Documentation includes the following: (a) tolerated CPT to bilateral lower lobes and right middle lobe using Trendelenburg's position; (b) breath sounds increased at both bases and right middle lobe area after treatment with decreases in rhonchi and palpable fremitus; (c) coughed up 30 mL of thick yellow secretions and drank two 8-ounce glasses of water during therapy session; (d) instructed family in how to position patient at home and how to do percussion and vibration; they performed an excellent return demonstration; and (e) repeat chest x-ray film showed reexpansion of right middle lobe and increased aeration of bilateral lower lobes.

Answer to Review Questions

1 2 **Rationale:** Steroids are a classification of medications that increase the risk for pathologic rib fractures.

2 1 **Rationale:** To help liquefy secretions, patients need a minimum of 1500 mL daily unless contraindicated by other physiologic problems. Setting up a fluid intake schedule would best help alleviate this problem.

3 3 **Rationale:** The oxygen saturation levels are reasonable considering what is being done to the patient. If the patient says he feels all right, continue with the therapy while continuing to monitor him. If the patient doesn't feel well, stop the session and assess further.

4 2 **Rationale:** Because the residual amount from the stomach is greater than 100 mL, the treatment should be held. Positioning could lead to regurgitation of gastric contents. Normally when a patient is receiving tube feedings and has a residual volume, be sure that the head of the bed is up.

5 1 **Rationale:** A patient with congestive heart failure is often short of breath during any exercise. Chest physiotherapy causes exertion and can worsen shortness of breath; as a result the patient needs short rest periods between the different positions. Maintaining normal hydration and oral hygiene are important for every patient.

6 1 **Rationale:** Right side-lying Trendelenburg's position aids in the drainage from the left lower lobe.

7 1 **Rationale:** Sitting up in a chair and leaning backward onto a pillow promotes drainage from the area. The upright position especially helps with the air-filled abscesses.

8 2 **Rationale:** Postural drainage should be avoided for 1 to 2 hours after meals. If he finished his lunch at 1 PM, the soonest that postural drainage can be done is at 2 PM.

9 2 **Rationale:** Forceful cough is the best option given for this type of patient to clear his secretions. Increasing fluids helps thin the secretions but does not help him to cough. Postural drainage and vibration and shaking are contraindicated because of the chance of fracturing a rib or causing injury to this frail patient.

10 3 **Rationale:** A current assessment of the patient is needed before decisions regarding treatment can be made. There can be a number of causes for the dyspnea and the bleeding. The health care provider will be notified but will expect current patient information to be available.

CHAPTER 25

Answers to Critical Thinking Exercises

1 1 **Rationale:** Yankauer suctioning is the method of choice for the upper airways; this enables the patient to clear oral secretions as needed; and it is a clean, nonsterile procedure.

2 1, 2, 3 **Rationale:** Hand hygiene has a direct benefit in reducing nosocomial infections and the transfer of microorganisms to health care professionals. Sterile suction technique reduces nosocomial infection in patients with new artificial airways or new tracheostomies or patients with acute illnesses/trauma. Clean suction technique can be used in patients who have permanent airways, usually a tracheostomy, and are free of any pulmonary infections. Frequently clean technique is used in the home environment.

3 1, 3, 5 **Rationale:** It is important to notify the health care provider because new care orders may be necessary for this patient; these orders may include antibiotics, chest physiotherapy, or diagnostic tests such as bronchoscopy. In some patients increasing fluids may help to liquefy pulmonary secretions. Before increasing fluids, be sure to determine that it is not contraindicated for this patient. For example, patients with cardiac or renal diseases may not be able to tolerate an increase in fluids. A sputum specimen for culture and sensitivity is needed because a change in thickness and/or sputum color frequently indicates an infectious process. An order is needed for a specimen. Antibiotics may be started before results of the test are available.

Answers to Review Questions

1 1 **Rationale:** Oropharyngeal suction uses a Yankauer or tonsillar tip suction device to remove large amounts of thick mucus. This would be most appropriate for a patient who cannot clear her airway by herself and does not have an artificial airway.

2 1, 3 **Rationale:** There are usually fewer infectious microorganisms in the trachea compared with the mouth. Suction from the least contaminated to the most contaminated.

3 4 **Rationale:** The common symptom of hypoxia is lethargy. Patients exhibit anxiety and restlessness, not a feeling of calmness, with hypoxia. In addition, patients will have tachycardia and potential dysrhythmias secondary to hypoxia. Hypoxia can cause all patients to be confused with a diminished level of consciousness.

4 3 **Rationale:** Whenever there is a drop in the patient's oxygen saturation, the patency of the patient's airway should be assessed for an open airway. This follows the ABCs of cardiopulmonary assessment.

5 1 **Rationale:** This is one of the times that notifying the health care provider is indicated. The patient has already been repositioned and suctioned, and there are no data to support that the nurse is allowed to reposition the endotracheal tube. The health care provider may need to order an x-ray film to check the placement of the endotracheal tube.

6 **The correct order for this situation is 2, 4, 5, 1, 3, 6.**

7 3 **Rationale:** To prevent oxygen desaturation, quickly clean the inner cannula. It should not be cleaned with hydrogen peroxide; use normal saline. Be sure to "lock it down" when appropriate after cleaning it. Leaving it unlocked increases its risk of becoming dislodged.

8 **The correct order is 2, 5, 1, 4, 3.**

9 3, 4 **Rationale:** Based on research, the following statements are true: Elevate the head of the bed 30 to 45 degrees to prevent aspiration. Change patient position every 2 hours to decrease risk for atelectasis, pulmonary infections, decubiti, discomfort, and urinary stasis. Provide oral care with chlorhexidine by swab every 8 hours. If chlorhexidine is contraindicated, a toothbrush can be used to remove dental plaque organisms. Maintaining the endotracheal cuff pressures at 20 cm H_2O is necessary to decrease movement of secretions to the lower airways.

10 2, 3 **Rationale:** Know patient's normal range of vital signs and oxygen saturation levels. Baseline vital signs compared with current measures identifies individual abnormalities and the onset of worsening of an illness. Identify conditions that increase patient's risk for aspiration of gastric contents into the lung, resulting in airway obstruction. These include the presence of enteral feeding tubes or other nasal or oral gastric tubes, a decreased level of consciousness, and a decreased swallowing ability. Review patient's condition from the past 12 or 24 hours. These are relative baseline measurements that help to distinguish between gradual and acute changes in his or her status. Perform a systematic respiratory assessment of upper and lower airways, including identifying respiratory rate, respiratory pattern, respiratory muscles used, breath sounds, ability to cough effectively, integrity of the rib cage, and the characteristics of sputum production. Identify and become familiar with the use of equipment available at the institution. Knowing how to operate the equipment before using it will benefit both you and the patient. Test all equipment before use. Have adequate supplies on hand at the bedside. Equipment must work properly to provide safe nursing care.

CHAPTER 26

Answers to Critical Thinking Exercises

1 Vital signs document patient's cardiopulmonary status and identify any early changes. Prompt detection and correction of air leaks related to the chest tube decrease the risks for chest tube complications and duration of chest tube placement. The hourly monitoring of chest tube drainage is to provide timely observations on the amount and type of drainage. During the first 3 hours 100 mL/hr is expected, and patient coughing and position changes can result in a temporary increase in drainage.

2 Avoid dependent chest tube loops; change position of patient and drainage tubes to prevent drained blood from pooling in the chest or tube.

3 This drainage is dark red, not bright red; it is not a large volume; and it is probably caused by the rapid discharge of accumulated drainage from the chest. This discharge of fluid was probably stimulated by the patient's activity from bed to chair. However, because this is a fresh postoperative patient, you would take his vital signs to determine his tolerance to activity and monitor cardiopulmonary status. You would also continue to monitor chest tube drainage to be sure that the volume did not increase excessively, and you would implement measures to assist in maintaining chest tube patency (see Answer 2).

Answers to Review Questions

1 2 **Rationale:** Explaining that by controlling pain he will be able to be active and cough well is a true statement. However, there is no guarantee that the medication will not make him sleepy.

2 3 **Rationale:** The pneumothorax is getting worse, possibly leading to a tension pneumothorax. The signs and symptoms indicate respiratory distress. If these symptoms are present, notify the health care provider immediately.

3 1 **Rationale:** Monitoring chest tube drainage and maintaining chest tube patency are the key priorities when a patient has a chest tube.

4 1 **Rationale:** Apical (second or third intercostal space) and anterior chest tube placement promotes removal of air.

5 3 **Rationale:** Placing an occlusive dressing over the chest tube site helps prevent the air leak from getting worse and prevents bacteria from entering the site. It is essential to check vital signs to assess the status of the patient.

6 **4** **Rationale:** As noted in the skills, none of these activities can be delegated to NAP.

7 **4** **Rationale:** The patient has a chest tube that is smaller in diameter than what one should be to drain blood. The tube should be a 24 to 32 Fr size. The nurse's priority is to be sure the tube does not become occluded. Vital sign monitoring is important, but the patient at this time is stable. The appearance of the drainage is not unusual at this time.

8 **1** **Rationale:** The patient must not be in a prone position to complete the chest tube removal. The skill reads to help patient sit on edge of bed or lie supine or on the side without chest tubes. The following statements are true related to chest tube removal: The nurse administers the ordered analgesia 30 minutes before the procedure. The nurse offers emotional support during tube insertion. The nurse has suction available.

9 **3** **Rationale:** You should notify the health care provider immediately since these symptoms indicate a change in chest tube drainage appearance to bright red blood and an unexpected amount of drainage. This information, along with the vital signs and complaint of dyspnea, indicates respiratory distress.

10 **Intrathoracic pressure** **Rationale:** There continues to be controversy as to whether to "strip" or "milk" a chest tube. Stripping or milking a chest tube is a process used to clear a tube of clots. Milking or stripping is the manual compression of a chest tube in an attempt to move chest tube drainage toward the collection device. Stripping causes a dangerous increase in intrathoracic pressure, which causes damage to the lung tissue.

CHAPTER 27

Answers to Critical Thinking Exercises

1 2 Rationale: On finding an unconscious patient, you must call for help immediately to mobilize necessary equipment for defibrillation.

2 1 Rationale: You must verify that the victim is pulseless before initiating AED use and/or chest compressions.

3 2 Rationale: Cardiopulmonary resuscitation (CPR) interruptions should be minimized. Only very brief interruptions should be allowed for changing CPR personnel during pulse checks, AED analysis, or defibrillation.

4 2 Rationale: Assessment of the return of patient's spontaneous pulse and respirations and cardiac rhythm analysis need to occur every 2 minutes during a chest compression interruption.

5 Reassessment of the primary survey will continue even after the code team has arrived. Helping the code team perform the secondary survey may include handing off the requested supplies from the crash cart, setting up suction, establishing peripheral or central IV access, chest auscultation on intubation, connecting to a monitor/defibrillator, relaying significant patient information to the code team, or administering or handing off medications. Delegation of other actions may include having someone help the victim's roommate or visitors away from the code scene, assigning pastoral care or other nurses to communicate with family members, delegating someone to remove excess furniture or equipment from the room, having someone bring the patient's chart to the bedside, assigning a fresh person to perform chest compressions, or assigning another nurse to record/document the events of the code.

Answers to Review Questions

1 **3** **Rationale:** Goals of resuscitation are aimed at restoring cardiopulmonary and neurologic function.

2 **1, 2, 3** **Rationale:** Rapid-response teams are created with the intention of intervening early to avoid cardiac arrest; transfer to ICU if needed and reduce hospital mortality rate.

3 **1** **Rationale:** Family and patient's religious and cultural practices need to be considered, especially regarding resuscitation and/or end-of-life care.

4 **4** **Rationale:** It may stimulate vomiting or laryngospasm if inserted in the semiconscious patient.

5 **1** **Rationale:** Follow the C (circulation) D (defibrillation) A (airway) B (breathing) sequence of steps. It is essential to continue

compressions if no pulse is present until the AED prompt says not to touch the patient.

6 **3** **Rationale:** The jaw-thrust technique prevents head extension and neck movement, which is crucial to prevention of paralysis or spinal cord injury.

7 **2** **Rationale:** Basic life support certification provides hands-on training with an AED for laypersons, nursing assistive personnel (NAP), and licensed health care professionals.

8 **4** **Rationale:** Chest compressions at 100/min are essential for perfusing vital organs, including the heart and brain.

9 **4** **Rationale:** Immediately after a shock, chest compressions should be continued for 2 minutes to provide minimal interruption in organ perfusion.

10 **4** **Rationale:** If enough air fills the lung on artificial breaths, the chest will rise, indicating effectiveness.

CHAPTER 28

Answers to Critical Thinking Exercises

1 The correct microdrip rate would be 100 gtt/min. The correct macrodrip rate would be 25 gtt/min.

2 The following steps are necessary before starting a new bag of IV solution:
- You should first check the health care provider's order to ensure that there is a written order for the solution, rate of administration, additives, and medications.
- Check the IV solution for integrity, including but not limited to discoloration, cloudiness, leakage, and expiration date.
- Check references for information on IV fluids composition, purpose, potential incompatibilities, and side effects.
- Provide explanation of the procedure to the patient. Allay any anxieties and answer any questions the patient may have.
- Check laboratory data to evaluate any abnormalities before changing the IV solution.
- Assess patency of current venous access device (VAD) site, observing for any signs or symptoms of complications such as redness, swelling, or complaints of discomfort.

3 The presence of discomfort at the site warrants closer inspection for signs of phlebitis or infiltration. The nurse should also check to be sure that the slower rate is not positional or that the IV tubing is not kinked. If the patient has early signs of phlebitis or infiltration, stop the infusion and restart IV in area above the affected area or in other extremity if appropriate.

4 Document the following:
- All signs and symptoms of complications of the IV catheter, such as tenderness and pain at site, redness, swelling
- Discontinuation of the IV size and length of catheter, amount of fluid infused, medication administered
- Interventions initiated, such as warm compresses
- Patient response to procedure

Answers to Review Questions

1 **2** **Rationale:** The formula is

$$\frac{1000 \text{ mL} \times 15 \text{ gtt/mL}}{12 \text{ hours} \times 60 \text{ min/hr}} = 21 \text{ gtt/min}$$

2 **3** **Rationale:** Phlebitis is evidenced by what the patient is experiencing. Coolness and swelling would be seen with infiltration. There are no data to support the other two options.

3 **3** **Rationale:** The smallest device possible with the smallest gauge is recommended to prevent complications to inner layers of the veins.

4 **The correct order is 2, 4, 1, 3** **Rationale:** After the tape is removed, the old or current dressing (TSM) is removed; once the dressing is removed, the site is observed for signs and symptoms of IV-related complications; site is cleaned with antiseptic swab to remove any surface microorganisms before new dressing is applied; new dressing (TSM) is applied to protect site and prevent any microorganisms from entering the insertion site.

5 **False** **Rationale**: A midline catheter is considered a peripheral device because of the location of the final tip placement, which is not in the superior vena cava (SVC); it terminates below the axilla.

6 **2** **Rationale**: Although it is desirable to place an IV infusion in the patient's nondominant hand, this patient has a medical condition that dictates that the IV catheter be placed in her dominant hand or arm.

7 **1** **Rationale**: The patient is susceptible to bleeding; thus pressure should be applied whenever a device such as a catheter is removed from his body while he still has prolonged bleeding times. You or the patient (if capable) can apply the pressure for the required period of time.

8 **4** **Rationale**: The tip of the catheter should be in the superior vena cava above the right atrium of the heart.

9 **1** **Rationale**: Current evidence states that chlorhexidine skin antisepsis has been shown to reduce the risk of catheter-associated infections when used as a skin prep.

10 **4** **Rationale**: Solution with an osmolarity of greater than 600 mOsm/L needs to be administered by a catheter placed in the SVC. The only correct option is the implanted venous port. Although the PICC is a central device, the tip placement is not in the SVC.

CHAPTER 29

Answers to Critical Thinking Questions

1 You should review the potential benefits and risks associated with blood transfusions. Describe and discuss options such as autologous transfusion and blood alternatives. Ms. Cooper needs to know if bleeding and blood loss may occur during her surgery. Blood transfusion may be a therapeutic regimen in her recovery. Also explain that comprehensive testing and screening of blood products now reduces incidence of infection and disease transmission. Patient's blood sample is mixed with donor's blood sample to determine the compatibility of the two. This will ensure that she gets the correct blood type. Explain the process for verification of the patient identification and blood unit label information to prevent transfusion errors.

As with any invasive procedure, the risk for infectious transmission may occur. Because transfusions are administered directly in the vascular system, nurses perform hand hygiene to prevent infection.

If transfusions are not used when clinically indicated, recovery may be impaired. Ms. Cooper has the right to refuse blood transfusions. Because Ms. Cooper's surgery is elective, she has the option of providing autologous blood, which is her own blood donated in advance, to be used in the event that she requires postoperative blood products.

2 Ms. Cooper needs to schedule an appointment with the blood bank to donate her own blood for personal use. Her blood cell counts, including hemoglobin and hematocrit, must be within the normal range. No donations may be made within 72 hours of surgery.

3 Ms. Cooper can receive all blood types in a transfusion. Her blood cells carry A and B antigens.

4 You should verify the health care provider's orders for the transfusion of the blood product. A signed consent form should be in the medical record. A vascular access device that is patent without complications must be assessed before initiation. You should have a 0.9% NaCl infusion setup with Y-tubing for the blood product. Obtaining baseline vital signs is necessary.

The patient's name and identification number on an arm identification bracelet should match the transfusion form information. The unit number, component, ABO, and Rh on blood product and transfusion record should match. You must verify this information with another staff member as required by facility policy. Most facilities have a transfusion form that should be completed to record the name of the blood product; identification number and expiration date; patient's and donor's blood type; and patient identification, including name and date of birth.

The blood product should not be at room temperature for more than 30 minutes before the initiation of transfusion. When there is a delay in initiating the blood transfusion, the blood product should be returned to the blood bank. Once the product is initiated, it should be infused within 4 hours to decrease the risk for pathogen growth.

You should remain with a patient for the first 15 minutes of transfusion and monitor him or her throughout the transfusion. You may direct the nursing assistive personnel (NAP) to take frequent vital signs and inquire about the patient's comfort. However, you maintain responsibility for assessing and monitoring him or her. If any adverse signs and symptoms are present, you should implement appropriate actions and notify the health care provider.

5 If patient symptoms suggest a mild allergic reaction, **stop transfusion** and administer antihistamine per health care provider's order. Restart transfusion per health care provider's order. If symptoms are unclear, slow the transfusion and assess patient for rash or hives and respiratory symptoms such as coughing, wheezing, or throat or oral mucous membrane itching. You should ask patient to describe when and where the signs and symptoms occurred. The assessment should include the back and trunk because this is a common area of occurrence. Take a set of vital signs. Notify the health care provider for orders, which usually include administration of antihistamine and continuing the transfusion. You should continue monitoring the signs and symptoms, noting whether they dissipate or get worse. If they continue to worsen, the physician should again be notified. Record the response on the medical record.

Answers to Review Questions

1 **3** **Rationale**: Normal saline is the only intravenous solution that should be used with blood because of its isotonic quality. Dextrose solutions cause hemolysis of the red blood cells.

2 **3** **Rationale**: Only negative blood types can be given to a patient with a negative blood type.

3 **4** **Rationale**: When blood is stored, there is continual destruction of red blood cells, which release potassium from the cells into the plasma. If blood is transfused rapidly, there may be transient hyperkalemia before the potassium is reabsorbed. The hematocrit and hemoglobin values would indicate whether a patient needs a blood transfusion. The sodium level is not relevant to this situation.

4 **2** **Rationale**: Comparing a patient's identification bracelet with the blood bag label number is the most important step to take.

5 **4** **Rationale**: It is essential to maintain an IV access, but you do not want the patient to receive any more of the current blood. Another blood administration set should be primed with a new bag of normal saline in case more blood needs to be given. Remember to keep the old blood bag and saline and the administration set and send them to the appropriate department per protocol for analysis.

6 **4, 2, 1, 3 is the correct order of steps.**

7 **3** **Rationale**: The addition of adenine adds 35 days to the shelf life of the blood.

8 **2** **Rationale**: HLAs are immunogenic antigens, which cause serious transfusion reactions such as TRALI. Fetal hemolysis and Rh incompatibility are not a direct result of HLAs.

9 **4** **Rationale**: No medications or solutions (other than 0.9% normal saline solution [NS]) are to be administered with blood. Blood should never be stopped to administer another medication or solution; therefore starting a new IV is the most appropriate action.

10 **2** **Rationale**: Only a registered nurse (RN) (or in some states a licensed practical nurse [LPN]) may administer blood or blood products; the task may not be delegated.

CHAPTER 30

Answers to Critical Thinking Exercise

1 Mr. Jasper's BMI is 18.7; he is at the lower limit of "normal weight." With his condition he is at risk for being underweight unless his nutritional status improves.

2 Several actions should be considered: (a) Include the daughter in the teaching plan. The patient and significant others might have misconceptions about which foods are safe and nutritional. (b) Explain that the purpose of dietary modifications is to prevent him from aspirating (i.e., having fluid/food enter his lung) and having pneumonia. Teach

the signs and symptoms of aspiration. (c) Explain that thin liquids create safety risks in swallowing because of the speed with which they move. Increasing the viscosity or thickness of the liquid slows movement through the mouth and pharynx and promotes protection of the airway. (d) Explain the reason for not giving him bites of the cookie. His dry mouth will prevent him from forming a food bolus; thus he will experience dysphagia, potentially leading to aspiration. (e) Teach the daughter to provide verbal cueing while feeding. Remind patient to chew and think about swallowing. This will result in a more normal swallow to help prevent aspiration. (f) Suggest that patient's meals be eaten in a quiet area in the dining room to minimize distractions so he will be able to more easily focus on chewing and swallowing. (g) Teach the risk of backward head tilts. Food and fluids are more likely to be misdirected into the airway in this position. An alternative is a chin-tuck maneuver, which helps in airway protection.

3 A soft, low-residue diet includes pastas; casseroles; moist, tender meats; and canned, cooked fruits and vegetables.

Answers to Review Questions

1 **4** **Rationale:** The patient is classified at risk for malnutrition. Although gaining weight is important, determining knowledge base related to nutrition is the priority and serves as the baseline for teaching.

2 **93% or below. 95 × 0.02 = 1.9; 95 − 1.9 = 93** **Rationale:** Bedside assessment is not sufficient for evaluating the frequency of silent aspiration, because a silent aspiration does not have specific symptoms. Recommendations include accompanying fluid administration with measurement of pulse oximetry. A drop in oxygen greater than or equal to 2% saturation indicates silent aspiration.

3 **1** **Rationale:** The nurse screens for actual and potential nutritional alterations. Nurses focus on the effects of an illness or a disease on a patient's nutritional status such as recent weight loss and decreased oral intake.

4 **1** **Rationale:** In adults weight is usually stable, A loss of 10 lbs (4.5 kg) during a 6-month period whether intentional or unintentional is a critical indicator for further assessment, especially in the older adult.

5 **4** **Rationale:** Provides comfort. If a patient has nausea or pain, offer appropriate antiemetics or analgesics at least 30 minutes before mealtime.

6 **1** **Rationale:** The single most important measure to prevent aspiration is to place the patient on NPO until a swallowing evaluation determines that dysphagia poses no substantial risk.

7 **1** **Rationale:** Single textures are easier to swallow than multiple textures or thin liquids (low viscosity) such as water, coffee, tea, and anything that liquefies in the mouth at room temperature. Swallowing thin liquids requires the most coordination and control and creates safety risks in swallowing for patients with impaired oral motor control because of their speed and decreased texture. Jell-O and orange sherbet are thin liquids. Shredded wheat and milk are multiple textures.

8 **4** **Rationale:** Glossitis and smooth tongue may be indicators of malnutrition.

9 **2** **Rationale:** Cream is not a clear liquid.

10 **2** **Rationale:** Orthodox Jews do not eat shell fish.

CHAPTER 31

Answers to Critical Thinking Questions

1 Assessment of the risk for placement error during feeding tube insertion centers on the patient's mental status, ability to cooperate with the procedure, presence of cough and gag reflexes, and clinical factors such as the presence of an artificial airway. When numerous risk factors for inadvertent pulmonary intubation are present, additional safety measures such as a CO_2 sensor or an electromagnetic tracking device can enhance the safety of the procedure if these devices are available.

2 The patient may have difficulty understanding the explanation for the procedure. Use simple phrases and take time to explain it. Show him what the feeding tube looks like. He will have trouble communicating,

depending on his level of alertness. If he can communicate, have him use his right hand to make signals. You may need assistance to position him for the insertion. If he has a reduced gag reflex, you might not offer him water or ice chips for swallowing. Plan to have to coach him to successfully swallow during tube insertion.

3 Aspiration of stomach contents to test pH or measure gastric residual volume (GRV) can lead to clogging of the tube. Another common cause of feeding tube occlusion is fragments from improperly crushed medications. Irrigation of the tube with water at scheduled intervals and before and after aspiration of gastric contents and medication administration is the most effective way to prevent this complication.

4 Because no single method for checking position of feeding tubes is completely reliable, a variety of techniques are used in combination. They include marking and monitoring the external length of the tube, noting the color, pH, and appearance of fluid withdrawn through the tube, and observing for changes in gastric residual volume. A repeat abdominal radiograph should be obtained (requires health care provider's order) if bedside checks raise any doubt regarding the location of the tube.

Answers to Review Questions

1 **3** **Rationale:** Continue tube feeding as ordered. A gastric residual volume of 150 mL falls below recommended limits for stopping feeding (250 to 500 mL). Slowing the rate or stopping the feeding for a residual volume of 150 mL will result in inadequate nutrition. Return to the stomach residual volumes of 250 mL or less to avoid loss of nutrients, fluid, and electrolytes.

2 **3, 4, 5, 6** **Rationale:** Both 1 and 2 are incorrect. Room number is not a valid patient identifier, and head of bed must be elevated to a minimum of 30 degrees.

3 **1** **Rationale:** The feeding must be stopped while patient's status is being evaluated. If the tube has become misplaced, this action prevents additional fluid from being instilled. The nurse would perform all of the actions listed and in the order they appear in the options listed.

4 **2** **Rationale:** Sorbitol can cause diarrhea. None of the other options is correct.

5 **2** **Rationale:** Slow weight gain is expected. A gain of more than 2 lbs (0.9 kg) in 24 hours usually indicates fluid retention. This patient has gained 4 lbs in 48 hours and is probably retaining fluid. Asking the patient how he feels would provide subjective data; objective data are needed to determine why the patient is gaining weight rapidly.

6 **4** **Rationale:** X-ray film confirmation of a blindly inserted tube is the only reliable method for verifying correct placement and is mandatory before the tube is used for administration of fluids or medication.

7 **3** **Rationale:** A jejunostomy tube would be the safest route because it bypasses the face and is farthest from the lungs, decreasing the chance of aspiration the most, which is essential when facial injuries are present.

8 **3** **Rationale:** Although the gastrointestinal tract is not sterile, enteral formulas provide an ideal medium for bacterial growth. All components of the system must be handled aseptically to prevent transmission of organisms and development of diarrhea.

9 **3** **Rationale:** The nurse needs to wait at least an hour after medications are given to allow for absorption. The syringe used should be 60 mL to allow for ample room for both aspiration and irrigation. The patient should be kept with the head of the bed at least 30 degrees (preferably 45 degrees). A small amount of gastric fluid aspirated slowly can be tested for the appropriate pH level, which would indicate proper technique and proper tube placement.

10 **1** **Rationale:** Absent bowel sounds are not a contraindication to feeding; but a change from baseline in the abdominal examination, particularly if tenderness or distention is present, should be conveyed to the ordering health care provider to determine if tube feeding can safely proceed. Administration of enteral nutrition is often unnecessarily delayed until bowel sounds are heard.

CHAPTER 32

Answers to Critical Thinking Exercises

1 Vital signs, electrolyte levels, weight, and fluid status (auscultating lung sounds, checking for edema).

2 Provides baseline for measuring tolerance to high concentration of glucose infusion.

3 The fever is a likely indication of an infection, which could be the result of a catheter site or bloodstream infection. You should notify the health care provider immediately.

4 You would caution Mr. Giles about his enthusiasm and explain that it is unlikely that he has gained all of the weight from a restoration in nutritional status. It is likely that most of the weight gain is from fluid retention. Your assessment would include auscultating lung sounds, checking for edema in the extremities, and comparing heart rate with baseline.

Answers to Review Questions

1 **1, 3 Rationale:** The fluid for the total PN is hyperosmolar. However, you should avoid complex terms in the explanation. Explaining that the smaller veins cannot tolerate the concentration of the nutrients very well and become irritated more easily is more easily understood by the patient.

2 **1 Rationale:** Elevated temperature, chills, nausea and vomiting, and chest pain indicate lipid infusion intolerance. Option 2 could indicate a problem with the catheter placement. Option 3 could indicate infection, and option 4 is nonspecific.

3 **2 Rationale:** The Infusion Nurses Society recommends changing IV administration sets for 3 : 1 PN every 24 hours and immediately on suspected contamination.

4 **1 Rationale:** PN is a nutritional support measure to ensure adequate intake while patient is NPO. Option 2 is not correct because enteral feedings may be given in some cases concurrently with PN. Option 3 is not correct because PN is a nutritional measure, not an effective treatment for cancer. Option 4 is not correct because the risks and costs associated with PN are too high for its use as a supplement.

5 **4 Rationale:** PN is a complete mixture of each of these components.

6 **3 Rationale:** This filter is used to prevent particulate matter and large lipid droplets from reaching a patient and risking pulmonary embolism. Option 1 is not correct, because without a filter the risk of pulmonary embolism is great. Option 2 is not correct because lipid will not flow through such a small filter. This filter is used for PN that does not contain lipid. Option 4 is not correct because such filters are not used.

7 **4 Rationale:** Bloodstream infections are a risk both in hospitalized and home PN patients. Option 1 is not correct because PN does not cause gastrointestinal distress since it is infused intravenously. However, bowel obstruction may be a reason to infuse PN. Option 2 is not correct because PN is administered intravenously and not associated with pneumonia. Option 3 is not correct, because PN may be given in a clinical setting in which albumin levels are more likely to be low.

8 **3 Rationale:** Liver disease is associated with multiple bloodstream infections, severe gastrointestinal disease, and longer PN duration. Option 1 is not correct, although it may be associated with short-term PN infusion. Option 2 is not correct because PN lipid contains no cholesterol and long-term PN patients with severe GI disease more often have low cholesterol. Option 4 is not correct.

9 **5 Rationale:** All of the above conditions are clinical situations in which PN is indicated.

10 **1 Rationale:** Patients with short-bowel syndrome or severe dysmotility have permanent and severe malabsorption and require the nutrients that PN provides, even with oral food intake. Option 2 is not correct because the risks and costs associated with long-term PN outweigh the benefits as a diet supplement. Option 3 is not correct because PN is an expensive therapy that carries the risk of catheter-related bloodstream infection (CRBSI); thus it would not be justifiable based only on preference. Option 4 is not correct

because such a patient will be unable to add vitamins to the infusion bag and control the home infusion pump safely.

CHAPTER 33

Critical Thinking Exercises

1 The following assessments would be pertinent for this patient:
- Determine cultural considerations that would be appropriate as you care for this patient.
- Assess understanding and knowledge of her condition and treatment plan.
- Assess the intake and output (I&O) record. Identify any trends, voiding patterns (e.g., increased incontinence, frequency), and the last time the patient voided.
- Assess the ability of the patient to participate in the plan of care, which includes language, sensory, cognitive, and mobility.
- Assess the lower one third of the abdomen for distention and/or tenderness.
- Assess for signs and symptoms of a UTI.

2 An assessment of the PVR urine is very important for this patient. An abnormal PVR urine would indicate inadequate bladder emptying. She has a history of urinary retention plus a number of other conditions that increase her risk for bladder dysfunction and urinary retention such as stroke, history of UTIs, and type 2 diabetes. Her incontinence needs to be further evaluated, and PVR will determine if this incontinence is caused by an overflow of urine as a result of urinary retention. In addition, if the patient's bladder is emptying, a PVR would help rule out the use of catheterization.

3 The health care provider has ordered the option to use a bladder scanner or to catheterize the patient. Whenever possible, you should avoid catheterization because of the increased risk for UTI; thus the use of the bladder scanner would be appropriate. The initial assessment with the bladder scanner will dictate if you need to insert an indwelling catheter (e.g., if the bladder scanner shows a volume greater than 400 mL).

4 The following teaching would be appropriate when assessing PVR:
- Explain rationale for the procedure in simple, easy terminology.
- Explain the procedure, including that the measurement needs to be made within 10 minutes of voiding.
- Instruct the patient to void in a measurement container.
- Explain that the bladder scanner looks inside the body and measures the volume of urine left in the bladder after voiding. It does not hurt.

Answers to Review Questions

1 **3 Rationale:** Hygiene minimizes skin irritation and infection from continued exposure to urine. There needs to be 2.5 to 5 cm (1 to 2 inches) of space between tip of the glans penis and the end of the catheter. Excess space may cause pooling of urine, causing excessive exposure to urine. Shaving the pubic area increases the risk for skin irritation. The condom should be secure but not tight. Application of tape is contraindicated because it could interfere with circulation, increasing risk for necrosis of the penis.

2 **2 Rationale:** This is the correct order in which to insert an indwelling urinary catheter.

3 **3 Rationale:** Advancing the catheter to the bifurcation avoids inflating the catheter balloon in the prostatic urethra, causing trauma and pain. Catheter balloons are never inflated with saline. Securing the catheter drainage tubing to the bed sheets increases the risk for accidental pulling or tension on the catheter. Advancing the catheter until urine flows and then inserting 1/4 inch (0.6 cm) more is not unique to the male patient.

4 **2, 3 Rationale:** By allowing the balloon to drain by gravity, the development of creases or ridges in the balloon may be avoided, minimizing trauma to the urethra during withdrawal. All patients who have a catheter removed should have their voiding monitored with a voiding record or bladder diary. The size syringe used to deflate the balloon is dictated by the size of the balloon. Catheters should be pulled out slowly and smoothly. Pulling fluid out of the

balloon with force can cause the formation of creases or ridges in the balloon.

5 **3, 4** **Rationale:** An established suprapubic catheter insertion site can be cleaned with medical aseptic technique. Always inspect a site for signs of infection. Anchor the catheter to the abdomen to minimize trauma and increase comfort. Wiping the catheter toward the insertion site violates principals of asepsis. Avoid applying tension to the catheter in all circumstances to minimize discomfort and potential for damage to the bladder wall.

6 **2** **Rationale:** The most appropriate action would be to ensure that the catheter is not occluded. Fluids should not be encouraged if the catheter is blocked. Irrigation and catheter removal are more invasive interventions that may be appropriate, depending on the cause of the decreased urine flow.

7 **3** **Rationale:** Adequately assess bladder function after a catheter is removed; voiding frequency and amount should be monitored. Unless contraindicated, fluids should be encouraged. To promote normal micturition, patients should be placed in as normal a posture for voiding as possible. Suprapubic tenderness and pain are possible indicators of urinary retention and/or a urinary tract infection.

8 **3** **Rationale:** Evidence-based guidelines support the use of indwelling catheters in the presence of urinary retention. Another indication for catheterization is healing of open sacral or perineal wounds in incontinent patients. A stage I ulcer is not an open wound but would require close observation. All other patient conditions are not appropriate for an indwelling catheter because of the increased risk for catheter-associated urinary tract infection (CAUTI).

9 **3** **Rationale:** Evidenced-based guidelines for the prevention of CAUTI support the use of the smallest size catheter and balloon possible, which in an adult is a size 14 Fr, 5 mL balloon.

10 **2** **Rationale:** An appropriate first action would be to assess the patency of the drainage system. Urine output in the drainage bag should be more than the volume of the irrigant solution infused. If the system is not draining urine and irrigant, the irrigant should be stopped immediately. The catheter may be occluded, and the bladder distended.

CHAPTER 34

Answers to Critical Thinking Questions

1 A fracture bedpan is best; it is easier to place in patients with restricted mobility. Mr. Simon can help with placement by using a side rail or trapeze bar. A commode is contraindicated because Mr. Simon is only able to use touch-down weight bearing and therefore may not transfer from bed to commode easily or timely.

2 It is expected that the Fleet enema would stimulate a bowel movement, and the fecal material expelled may be hard or range from hard-to-soft stool. In addition, Mr. Simon may have subsequent bowel movements throughout the day. You must instruct the nursing assistive personnel (NAP) about the expected outcome of the enema. In addition, you must instruct the NAP to immediately report to you any complaints of abdominal pain or discomfort, rectal bleeding, blood in the stool, enlarged abdomen, or changes in vital signs.

3 **d, e, a** **Rationale:** First you must perform an abdominal assessment. Mr. Simon's pain could be caused by many factors ranging from benign gas to perforation. You need to collect data as baseline to monitor progression of pain and other abdominal signs and symptoms. In addition, you need data when you call his health care provider. Next obtain VSs and instruct the NAP to obtain them every 15 to 30 minutes thereafter. You need to obtain the first set of VSs as a baseline and compare with the patient's range. The NAP then monitors these VSs at your direction for frequency. This obtains valuable information while you are contacting the health care provider. Finally you should notify the health care provider. You should now have abdominal assessment and your VSs measurement data to report.

You do not do the following: Instruct the NAP to palpate Mr. Simon's abdomen. Assessment is a nursing responsibility. However, you may instruct the NAP to notify you if it appears that Mr. Simon's abdomen is getting bigger or his level of pain changes.

Nor do you give postoperative pain medication as ordered. Although Mr. Simon indeed has pain medication, that medication is to control postoperative knee pain. It will take away or diminish his abdominal pain. Until the cause of Mr. Simon's abdominal pain is identified, the presence of pain and changes in quality and intensity are important clinical assessment findings that should not be masked by analgesia.

4 The patient may be experiencing a slowed heart rate as a result of vagal stimulation. Immediately stop the procedure and retake the vital signs. Notify the prescriber if the vital signs remain low.

Answers to Review Questions

1 **4** **Rationale:** This may be the result of vagus stimulation, and you should stop the procedure.

2 **2** **Rationale:** Swallowing closes off the upper airway and prevents the tube from entering the lungs.

3 **2** **Rationale:** Rolling patient onto a fracture pan prevents friction or injury to underlying skin and tissue. A frail patient is likely to have fragile skin.

4 **1** **Rationale:** Surgery just 5 weeks ago would require particular precaution not to disturb the surgical site and prevent trauma to the rectum. An enema would appear to be contraindicated; thus verifying the order would be appropriate.

5 **2** **Rationale:** Turning a patient to the left side will release the tube from the stomach lining. It is not within a nurse's scope of practice to advance a nasogastric tube after a patient has abdominal surgery or increase the suction.

6 **1** **Rationale:** Postoperative patients generally receive opioids, which have a common side effect of constipation, for pain. Therefore the best answer is to administer an enema. An x-ray film would not be necessary at this time. The stool is too high in the colon to remove digitally. Waiting for pain is not an appropriate action.

7 **4** **Rationale:** The bedpan should be offered an hour after breakfast. Peristalsis is strongest after the first meal of the day.

8 **2** **Rationale:** Elevating the head of the bed to 30 to 60 degrees prevents hyperextension of the back and supports the upper torso.

9 **2, 4, 5** **Rationale:** Toilet paper should be within easy reach, the head of the bed should be 30 to 60 degrees, and a small pillow under the lumbar curve will reduce stress on back. You should allow the patient to be alone for privacy. A flat bed places more stress on the back.

10 **1, 3, 5** **Rationale:** Administering an enema, placing a patient on a bedpan, and providing oral care for a patient with an NG tube may all be delegated to NAP. Removing a fecal impaction and inserting an NG tube require the training and skill of a nurse.

CHAPTER 35

Answers for Critical Thinking Questions

1 **3** **Rationale:** Stoma site should be marked before surgery to avoid having a stoma in a location that would make pouching difficult such as in a fold or crease or a location that the patient cannot see. It is not feasible for a patient to empty a pouch until after surgery. A nutrition consultation may be needed after surgery, but often there are few dietary restrictions with an ileostomy. The diagnosis of ulcerative colitis has already been made; thus this diagnostic test for colon disease would be unnecessary before surgery.

2 **1** **Rationale:** The stoma should be red and moist. Retraction of the stoma below skin level is usually secondary to necrosis and does not occur until about 2 weeks after surgery. Stents protruding from a stoma are seen with a urostomy, not an ileostomy. The stoma may be pink after surgery, but it would be moist and producing mucus.

3 **2** **Rationale:** To avoid having the pouch get too heavy and loosen from the skin, it should be emptied when it is one-third to one-half full. The pouch should not be changed daily because this could cause skin breakdown. Pouch emptying cannot be done on a

prescribed schedule. The frequency varies with food and fluid intake. An expected wear time for an ileostomy pouch is 3 to 5 days.

4   You will explain that the effluent from an ileostomy is always liquid, although it may be thick or thin. This is a normal finding with an ileostomy. The patient should not expect a formed bowel movement.

Answers for Review Questions

1   **2, 3, 4   Rationale:** All of these actions may facilitate additional drainage through the catheter. You cannot use urine from the pouch because it may be contaminated.

2   **1, 2, 3   Rationale:** Being receptive to teaching and active participation in care shows the patient's acceptance of his bodily function changes. Assigning care to his spouse is delaying or denying the return to self-care.

3   **4   Rationale:** The stoma will initially be edematous. The swelling will decrease normally over 4 to 6 weeks, and the size may change during that time.

4   **4   Rationale:** Assessment is the first step of the nursing process; and, by using an open-ended question, you can determine a patient's specific concerns. Shifting responsibility to the health care provider is inappropriate, and waiting until after the surgery to address the issue only increases a patient's anxiety. Having a person with an ostomy visit the patient before surgery may be helpful, but assessment needs to be done first.

5   **2   Rationale:** The patient needs assistance immediately before the enzymes from the urinary drainage break down the skin any further. The ostomy care nurse is the best resource person to contact.

6   The intestinal opening surgically created in the abdomen for a colostomy, ileostomy, or urostomy is called a *stoma.*

7   The correct order for the steps in changing an ostomy pouch is:
1   Observe the stoma and the skin around it.
2   Remove the old pouch.
3   Clean and dry the peristomal skin.
4   Measure the stoma.
5   Trace the correct measurement onto the back of the wafer.
6   Cut the hole in the wafer.
7   Press the pouch into place over the stoma.
8   Close the end of the pouch.

8   The pathway created for urine to exit the body when the bladder is removed is called an *ileal conduit.*

9   **3   Rationale:** Air in the pouch is a normal and expected sign following ostomy surgery. It is still too early to expect significant fecal drainage.

10   **1, 3, 4   Rationale:** Common symptoms of a UTI include dark or bloody urine; foul-smelling urine; fever (38.3°C [101° F] or higher); confusion; and flank pain, not upper abdominal pain.

CHAPTER 36

Answers to Critical Thinking Exercises

1   Obesity, diabetes, and smoking place Mrs. Edmonds at increased risk for an SSI. Antibiotics should not be given beyond 24 hours unless there is a clinical indication. You will need to instruct Mrs. Edmonds that she will not be allowed to smoke in the hospital, follow up to ensure that she has an order for a substitute nicotine product if needed, and offer smoking cessation instruction/consultation. Glycemic control must be maintained during the recovery period to promote incision healing.

2   You will need to reinforce with Mrs. Edmonds how to turn, cough, deep breathe, and use the incentive spirometer. Instruction in pain-control measures, including how to use the patient-controlled analgesia (PCA) device and how to splint her incision with a small pillow before coughing, turning, or ambulating must also be reinforced. Early ambulation and the need to wear intermittent pneumatic compression (IPC) cuffs while in bed or up in chair must also be included. Include family in teaching and reinforce that for safety reasons Mrs. Edmonds is the only person to activate the PCA device.

3   Given her history of smoking, following general anesthesia she is at an increased risk for pulmonary complications. Include lung auscultation as part of routine assessment and closely monitor respiratory rate, temperature, and presence of productive cough. A history of obesity, taking birth control pills, and undergoing pelvic surgery places her at an increased risk for deep vein thrombosis (DVT)/venous thromboembolism (VTE). Mrs. Edmonds will need anticoagulant therapy and must wear an IPC while she is in bed or sitting up in the chair.

4   Patient should be instructed to use a PCA device before ambulating/performing exercises and to splint incision with small pillow to decrease incisional discomfort.

Answers to Review Questions

1   **1, 2, 3, 5, 6   Rationale:** Hair is removed using a clipper so the skin is intact, thus reducing the chance of an SSI. All of the other statements are true.

2   **2   Rationale:** Compression devices are applied before surgery and are generally some type of either knee-high or thigh-high compression hosiery. They prevent pooling of blood in the lower extremities. The pneumatic compression devices may or may not be used during surgery. The patient may not be able to ambulate after surgery because of the nature of the surgery, or physical therapy may be needed before ambulating.

3   **4   Rationale:** Institution agencies protocol needs to be followed, and a representative of the agency who is familiar with these situations such as a risk manager may be helpful.

4   **3   Rationale:** The surgeon should discuss and document issues with the patient and/or family to determine whether DNR orders are to be maintained or modified during surgical procedures.

5   **2   Rationale:** Mark the dressing with a circle around the drainage and the time noted. This gives an objective assessment of the extent of the drainage and can be continually reassessed.

6   **2   Rationale:** It is recommended that prophylactic antibiotics be given as close to the time of incision as possible (within 60 minutes) except vancomycin and fluoroquinolones that require a longer administration time. It is recommended that antibiotics *not* be given for longer than 24 hours after surgery.

7   **1   Rationale:** Exercises before coughing enhance the ability to move secretions so they may be expectorated.

8   **4   Rationale:** Spontaneous postoperative pneumothorax does not occur because of the general anesthesia.

9   **4   Rationale:** Management, assessment, and teaching skills should be performed by the RN and not delegated to others.

10   **2, 3, 4   Rationale:** ASPAN describes the three levels of recovery care to include the postanesthesia phase I, phase II, and extended care levels of care.

CHAPTER 37

Answers to Critical Thinking Exercises

1   **2   Rationale:** A short prescrub wash/rinse removes gross debris and superficial microorganisms and must be completed before performing surgical antisepsis.

2   **3   Rationale:** Artificial nails may not be worn because they may harbor gram-negative microorganisms and fungus, thereby increasing the risk for the patient developing a surgical wound infection.

3   After scratching her leg, Sarah should have stopped and immediately changed the affected glove. Once Sarah reached below her waistline, she contaminated the gloves, because the area of the gown below the waistline is considered contaminated, thereby increasing the risk for the patient developing a surgical wound infection.

Answers to Review Questions

1   **3   Rationale:** The circulating nurse assumes responsibility and accountability for maintaining patient safety and continuity of quality care. This includes assessing the patient, reviewing consents and the medical record, supervising the scrub technician, and delegating tasks to licensed and unlicensed nursing assistive personnel (NAP) as appropriate.

2 1 **Rationale:** The surgical hand scrub has been used traditionally for many years.

3 2 **Rationale:** All surfaces on both hands, extending from the fingertips just past the forearms, should be checked for the presence of abrasions, cuts, or open lesions. Rings should be removed totally. Artificial nails need to be removed weeks before being in a surgical environment so the nails and skin can heal after the nails are removed.

4 1 **Rationale:** Both hands should be covered with the cuffs of the gown to provide sterility.

5 4 **Rationale:** Anything sterile touched by something or someone unsterile becomes unsterile.

6 2 **Rationale:** The gloves are removed last; regown and reglove using closed gloving method.

7 2 **Rationale:** Gowns are sterile from the front chest and shoulders to table level and on the sleeves to 5 cm (2 inches) above the elbow.

8 1 **Rationale:** Hand scrubs include inspecting, scrubbing 3 to 5 minutes, rinsing, turning off water with foot or knee controls, and backing into the OR with hands higher than elbows.

9 2 **Rationale:** Do a 3- to 5-minute scrub; put on sterile gown; put on sterile gloves.

10 1 **Rationale:** The time out involves the immediate members of the procedure team: the individual performing the procedure, anesthesia providers, circulating nurse, operating room technician, and other active participants who will be participating in the procedure from the beginning. All relevant members of the procedure team actively communicate during the time-out.

CHAPTER 38

Answers to Critical Thinking Exercises

1 1, 2, 5 **Rationale:**
- Prednisone is a steroid. Steroids decrease the inflammatory response and slow collagen synthesis, impairing wound healing.
- Diabetes mellitus impairs wound healing by decreasing tissue perfusion and hindering the release of oxygen at the tissue level.
- Age impairs wound healing. Vascular changes, diminished pliability in collagen tissue, and scar tissue tightness contribute to impaired wound healing.

2 Granulation tissue is composed of new blood vessels that will bring nutrients and oxygen to the tissue. This type of tissue must be present for the wound to heal. Once a wound is filled with granulation tissue, healing will progress; thus a wound filled with granulation tissue is a good finding.

3 The presence of the healing ridge is important because it indicates that there has been deposition of collagen in the wound. This connective tissue provides strength to the wound and decreases the risk of dehiscence. Lack of a ridge is cause for concern, and you will need to begin prompt interventions to reduce mechanical strain on the wound.

Answers to Review Questions

1 4 **Rationale:** The fluid needs to drain from top to bottom, allowing gravity to help.

2 2 **Rationale:** If there is no order for the suture removal, none of the other steps need to be taken. Nurses cannot remove staples or sutures merely because of something the health care provider said.

3 3 **Rationale:** The patient should be premedicated because of the wound size. He or she should be positioned as flat as possible. You place the lower tip of the staple remover under the staple, and you do not lift up on the staple when depressing the extractor handles. The incision cleaning is started at the top of the incision and not the sides. When half the staples are removed, it means that every other staple is removed. This allows observation of how the wound is healing. In some instances small strips of tape, called *Steri-Strips,* will be used where the staples were removed to help stabilize the tissue.

4 3 **Rationale:** The suture should be removed in a smooth, continuous manner. The knot should have been snipped at the end distal to the knot. The scissors should have been held in your dominant hand, and the pickups in your nondominant hand. Disinfectants are never used on living tissue because of their harsh chemical action. Antiseptics may be used on skin to remove organisms.

5 2, 5, 6 **Rationale:** The drainage needs to be emptied, measured, and recorded. After you have emptied the drainage, you need to depress or squeeze the drain flat before putting in the plug. This helps the suction mechanism to work. Attaching the drain to the patient's gown below the level of the wound helps to prevent the drain from pulling and also keeps it in a dependent position to allow for maximum drainage.

6 1 **Rationale:** A surgical incision has the wound edges approximated at the time of the operation, is secured with staples, and is healing by primary intention. There is little need for tissue regeneration. Wounds that are left open to heal by secondary intention are not approximated and are left open. These types of wounds heal slowly because of the need for connective tissue to fill the area. A wound that heals by tertiary intention is left open for several days, and the edge area is approximated while the center of the wound heals by the formation of granulation tissue.

7 1, 2 **Rationale:** Use sterile technique and direct flow of solution from healthy to infected tissue.

8 2 **Rationale:** A Jackson-Pratt drain is a closed suction setup. Once the collector is drained, push out the air by compressing the drain and closing it. When the collector is drained, all the exudate is removed, and the collector is not pumped.

9 2, 3 **Rationale:** When you can see air under the negative-pressure wound therapy dressing, this indicates a problem with the seal. A negative-pressure wound therapy dressing should be flat over the wound dressing since all of the air should be removed from the area by the suction. Therefore the appropriate interventions include checking the seal of the transparent dressing for signs that it is not adhering to the skin or dressing and checking that the suction is working by noting that each of the connections from the suction source to the wound is intact. Changing the dressing would not be appropriate until this is done.

10 3 **Rationale:** The type of drainage that is clear like plasma is called *serous.* Purulent drainage is typically beige or tan, slough is used to describe nonviable yellow tissue (not drainage), and plasma is a deep red color.

CHAPTER 39

Answers to Critical Thinking Exercises

1 He is likely not holding the dressing in place for 30 to 60 seconds, which helps it to conform over the heel.

2 The hydrocolloid dressing is a good choice for clean stage II pressure ulcers. The dressing promotes a moist environment for healing and has an added benefit of reducing pain. It also is a good barrier to bacteria.

3 Hydrocolloid dressings interact with wound fluids and normally form a soft whitish-yellowish gel, which is sometimes hard to remove and may have a faint odor. This is a normal occurrence; Mr. Williams should not confuse this finding with pus, purulent exudate, or wound infection.

Answers to Review Questions

1 2 **Rationale:** To adequately debride a wound, the packing needs to be dry on removal. The dressing was too wet when it was placed in the wound initially.

2 4, 3, 5, 1, 2 **Rationale:** This is the correct order for application. Select size, remove backing, mold wafer over wound, hold in place for 30 to 60 seconds, and tape.

3 2 **Rationale:** A moist-to-dry dressing mechanically debrides the wound when exudate adheres to the moist gauze. The transparent dressing is indicated after a wound is debrided. Hydrogel debrides a wound through autolysis, and not mechanical debridement. Telfa is a dry nonadherent dressing, which is inappropriate for this purpose.

4 2 **Rationale:** A hydrogel dressing is soothing and is the most appropriate one for a patient with burns.

5 1, 2, 3, 6 **Rationale:** The following conditions, medications, or treatments interfere with wound healing: immunosuppressive drugs, diabetes, steroids, and irradiation.

6 4 **Rationale:** If the binder is placed either too high or too tight, a patient can experience shortness of breath, which would require you to release the binder and reapply it.

7 2 **Rationale:** In NPWT, negative pressure applied through the foam dressing removes exudate and contracts the wound bed to promote healing. Exudate is pulled out, not pushed into the wound. The wound bed is not flooded, and gauze pads are not placed in the wound bed.

8 4 **Rationale:** An increase in pain can be an indicator of neurologic and vascular changes. Options 1 and 2 evaluate circulation. Option 3 evaluates for wound infection.

9 2 **Rationale:** A surgical wound often has a drain in place. Gauze dressings should be removed one layer at a time to prevent accidentally pulling and removing the drain. The removal of a sterile dressing requires only clean gloves. Saline is not needed to moisten gauze unless drainage in the dressing sticks to the wound.

10 3 **Rationale:** Frequent dressing changes pose a risk of skin abrasion and skin tears from tape removal. A set of Montgomery ties is the best choice to secure the ABD pad.

CHAPTER 40

Answers to Critical Thinking Exercises

1 1, 2, 3, 4—all the options would apply. **Rationale:** Hot and cold therapies require a health care provider's order validating location, duration, and temperature as prescribed in the order. Assessing current pain level and condition of the extremity provides a baseline assessment for care. Patient education regarding procedure, precautions, and signs and symptoms of frostbite should be explained to prepare the patient.

2 2, 4 **Rationale:** There is greater risk for tissue injury when there is diminished circulation, a common characteristic of diabetes mellitus. A confused patient may be unable to provide feedback about how the application is feeling and will need to be monitored more closely for signs and symptoms of adverse effects.

3 Although this skill can be delegated to NAP, it would be unwise to delegate it initially. The patient has two risks, confusion and diabetes, which put him at risk for complications. In addition, because of these risks it is important to increase monitoring and skin assessment to maintain patient safety.

Answers for Review Questions

1 3 **Rationale:** It is essential to assess the area being treated. It is important to monitor the machine, but patient response is always the priority, especially because moist heat penetrates deeper into tissue layers.

2 3, 4, 5, 6, 7 **Rationale:** Patients with decreased circulation and conditions that cause decreased fluid or nutrients to their systems and those who use steroids for a long time are at risk for tissue injury.

3 1 **Rationale:** The area being treated would be slightly pale and cool to touch because of the decrease in circulation.

4 1 **Rationale:** Because the area being treated has little fat or tissue around it, the amount of time that cold is applied should be decreased.

5 1, 3, 4 **Rationale:** Localized cold therapy reduces blood flow to the injured body part, prevents edema formation, and reduces inflammation. Local analgesia is produced by slowing or blocking peripheral nerve conduction and preventing muscle spasm by decreasing spasticity.

6 3 **Rationale:** Shivering increases muscle activity, which in turn increases a patient's metabolic rate and therefore heat production, which is counterproductive.

7 2 **Rationale:** Because the patient is older and has limited mobility and strength, there may be a problem with the moist heat wrap, and he or she may need help. One hour is far too long without

checking on the patient's response to the therapy. The patient should not move the heat wrap because of the chance of moving it to an area where it could cause harm. This further supports the need for the call light to be close to the patient. The device should not be secured to the affected area with plastic wrap.

8 2 **Rationale:** The use of moist heat is contraindicated in patients who use patches to stop smoking and in those who use patches containing other medications because the heat increases the speed of absorption because of vasodilation. The area where the device is to be applied, not the full body, would be assessed before application. Alignment is not a priority for this therapy.

9 1 **Rationale:** The most effective method of determining the effectiveness of the treatment is to assess the patient's pain level. Since heat relaxes a strained muscle, a difference should be noted when the muscle is at rest. It is counterproductive for the patient to actively force the use of the affected muscle during a strenuous activity or exercise at this time.

10 4 **Rationale:** Because the area injured is near the bone and has less padding, the nurse needs to prevent any injury to the area as a result of the cold therapy. Therefore the nurse should check the ankle every 5 minutes. The other two options are not evaluation measures.

CHAPTER 41

Answers to Critical Thinking Exercises

1 The multiple medications Mrs. James takes may contribute to dizziness and lead to falls. Her visual and hearing deficits create fall risks. In addition, her immobility, bone pain, and stairs are also risk factors for falling because of muscle weakness caused by lack of exercise and pain and the risk of attempting to perform an activity she no longer can do safely.

2 2 **Rationale:** Asking the patient to verbally explain her medication regimen assesses cognitive function and memory. Showing the nurse where the medication is stored does not ensure that she is taking the medication correctly. Option 3 is incorrect because you are not assessing caregiver knowledge; you are directly assessing the patient's knowledge.

3 Despite older adults' risks, they learn how to negotiate their environment relatively well and are usually aware of potential dangers. Thus older adults may often be more cautious than younger people. Encourage the family to discuss with their mother what might provide a greater sense of security for both of them such as installing an alarm system and a medical emergency alert system. Offer a home safety assessment.

Answers to Review Questions

1 1-6 **Rationale:** All of these topics would be covered to determine the physical and mental status of the patient and check that she is not a victim of abuse or neglect.

2 2 **Rationale:** The Timed Get Up and Go (TUG) Test looks at how a person changes position and becomes mobile. MMSE is used to screen for cognitive changes. SPLATT is a mnemonic used to assess actual falls. A fall diary is used to record the events surrounding an actual fall. Safety is a priority for individuals of any age.

3 4 **Rationale:** Soiled dressings should be double bagged in impervious plastic.

4 4 **Rationale:** These are the physical abilities that a patient must have to help prevent falls.

5 1, 2, 4 **Rationale:** The kitchen temperature varies, and the insulin should be refrigerated until use and discarded by the expiration date.

6 4 **Rationale:** The patient's list of medications always needs to be reviewed for not only the dose ordered, but also for how many the patient is taking and the timing of the dosing. The nurse needs to check if the patient is taking the medication at the correct time of day. A deviation in timing could cause great distress for this patient since this individual would not be able to get the sleep needed. A night-light would be helpful, especially in the bathroom or in the hall on the way to the bathroom, but this is not the

primary focus. Evaluate how much fluid the patient is consuming and how late at night she takes these fluids.

7 **3** **Rationale:** Preventing fire is the prime object when using the kitchen. Older individuals often forget that they are cooking; fires can occur, or food can burn. A timer will alert the individual that something has to be done (e.g., stirring food, turning meat, or serving food that is cooked). There is no way to know the relationship of the garage to the kitchen as stated in the question. Light is important, but preventing fire and subsequent burns is the primary focus. Locks are needed in the kitchen for small children but not for this still independent individual.

8 **4** **Rationale:** A patient should always be assessed before anything else. The physical environment needs to be checked to ensure that it is safe and has what he or she needs, but that would be done after checking him or her. Depending on the status of the patient, 9-1-1 and the appropriate state agency could be contacted, but everything would hinge on the findings of the patient's status.

9 **3** **Rationale:** The pill organizer is useful in weekly management because each day of the week has its own holder so the patient knows if he or she took the medication for that day/time. A color chart is not helpful since pills can be different colors/shapes, depending on the pharmaceutical supplier. The patient is capable of organizing medication; thus the daughter does not need to visit each day, nor should the nurse take over the medications. You want to ensure as much independence as possible in the home care patient.

10 **3** **Rationale:** Placing food items in realistic-size servings in easy-to-open containers provides the most independence for this couple. They are not blind and do not require clock orientation for placing food on their plates. Taking them shopping will not provide nutrition if they can't open the containers or if food preparation is painful because of their joints.

CHAPTER 42

Answers to Critical Thinking Questions

1 Additional information needed:
   - List of current medications
   - Cognitive status
   - Problems with sensation or mobility
   - Recent vital signs: Heart rate and rhythm—expect rate to be irregular if he is in atrial fibrillation. Temperature: Did client have a temperature in the hospital at any time?
   - Client's and wife's motivation and willingness to learn
   - Past medical history

2 **3** **Rationale:** The pulse of a client with an arrhythmia should be taken for a full minute in case the pulse is irregular.

3 He may be pressing too hard over the artery or is unable to locate it. Coach him in his technique and reinstruct about artery location. You might also consider teaching him how to feel his carotid artery instead. If a cognitive deficit exists, teach a family member or friend how to check the pulse.

4 You can use many teaching strategies to facilitate successful medication education in older adults. Some strategies to enhance learning include the following:
   - Provide typewritten information in large print.
   - Provide information that client thinks is important.
   - Develop strategies to help the client and his wife remember to take the medication.
   - Repeat information that is important in the beginning and at the end of teaching sessions.
   - Develop a trusting relationship with the client and his wife.
   - Use a memory aid such as a daily checklist to help him remember to take his medications.

5 You will want to know which type of oral thermometer the client is using. Have the client demonstrate taking his temperature, note if he can see the reading, and teach accordingly. You will want to know what time of day the client is checking his temperature and how long he waits after drinking a hot or cold beverage and/or smoking.

Answers to Review Questions

1 **3** **Rationale:** The best method of verifying accuracy is to obtain two readings within 1 to 2 minutes of each other using two different monitoring devices.

2 **1, 4, 6** **Rationale:** He needs to stay away from anything that can cause a shock such as short circuiting from an electric shaver. He also needs to avoid open flames such as in a campfire or fireplace. A client with home oxygen therapy needs an extra set of oxygen delivery devices in case one should fail. Using lint-free cloths for cleaning equipment reduces friction.

3 **3** **Rationale:** Instilling normal saline does not decrease hypoxia and is not recommended routinely. The suction pressure stated is too high. The client should not be flat. She should be elevated at least 30 to 45 degrees. The suction catheter would be in the sterile gloved dominant hand, which would allow for less chance of contamination.

4 **2** **Rationale:** He needs time and input to learn and participate in this important part of his care. There should not be anything or anyone that could distract his attention. There are no data to support that he needs enlarged written directions.

5 **1, 2, 3, 4** **Rationale:** Difficulty breathing and coughing are signs of aspiration. Raise the head of the bed and stop feeding. Then have the family caregiver notify the health care provider and verify tube placement. If difficult breathing continues, call 9-1-1.

6 **3** **Rationale:** Before the nurse can make any recommendations, he or she needs more information (i.e., which symptoms the client is experiencing) since a temperature within normal range in the elderly can still reflect the presence of a fever. Adequate fluid intake is needed and should be monitored; but, since the wife gave very vague information, more information must be obtained. Changes in behavior such as delirium or dementia may occur with a temperature elevation.

7 **2** **Rationale:** The size of the blood pressure cuff can cause an inaccurate reading. If the cuff is too large, the reading will be low; if the cuff is too small, the reading will be high. If the cuff is too small even before inflating it, it can pop off during the procedure; or, if it remains on, it will overly compress the vessels and indicate an unusually high and inaccurate reading. Options 3 and 4 have nothing to do with the technique. The nurse should be sure the client is measuring BP the same time each day, but it is not likely a factor in the BP being high consistently.

8 **3** **Rationale:** When performing clean, intermittent catheterization, the client uses soap and water to clean the urinary meatus. Sterile gloves are not used because of the decreased chance of introducing organisms that would cause a urinary tract infection. The client's own organisms are predominant. It is essential that good hand hygiene be done immediately before the insertion and that the catheters have been cleaned, dried, and stored appropriately.

9 **3** **Rationale:** Saying "Oxygen levels decrease with forceful coughing more as aging occurs" is the clearest answer and doesn't use confusing technical language. Although loss of elastic recoil is correct, it is not something the nurse should expect the family to understand. Anxiety can accompany decreased ability to breathe but is not relevant to the question asked.

10 **1** **Rationale:** Compliance with medication regimens is increased if the family or client understands the medications being given. It is essential that safety elements be considered when pets or small children live where medications are given. Meaningful written materials help to prevent medication errors regarding dosing and times that the medications are given. It is important that planning occurs to prevent running out of medication.

CHAPTER 43

Answers to Critical Thinking Exercises

1 **1, 4** **Rationale:** Testing sputum would be important to determine if Mrs. Yamamoto has pneumonia, identify the organism and guide the health care provider in selecting the best treatment. Elevated blood glucose levels occur when a person with diabetes becomes

ill. Mrs. Yamamoto's blood glucose level is elevated because of her pneumonia.

2 As a point-of-care laboratory test, fingersticks for blood glucose level would give immediate results. Sputum specimens need to be cultured and take 72 hours for results.

3 There are several issues to consider when deciding to teach Mrs. Yamamoto to provide a sputum specimen. Her limited use of English is a major barrier. The daughter translated previously. You should provide a professional translator by determining if the hospital has translators or using the free telephone service available in many areas. Pictures, demonstration of what is desired, and having the patient perform a redemonstration can be helpful.

4 You need to assess Mrs. Yamamoto's ability to perform a fingerstick, to read the monitor, and to understand the importance of blood sugar control. Indicate to Mrs. Yamamoto that you wish to observe and assess her as she demonstrates how she performs blood glucose monitoring at home and ask and answer questions.

Answers to Review Questions

1 **1, 2, 5, 6 Rationale:** Option 3 is incorrect; the head of the penis is wiped in a circular motion, not back and forth. Option 4 is incorrect; the amount of urine needed is between 30 and 60 mL.

2 **1 Rationale:** The first urine specimen is discarded. This signifies the beginning of the collection time, which ends 24 hours later. The patient is encouraged to void right before the collection time ends.

3 **2 Rationale:** Tomatoes can change the result because of their high vitamin C content and their color. Numerous other foods can alter the results.

4 **1, 4 Rationale:** These are the only correct steps for this procedure. Leaning the head forward increases difficulty entering the mouth and decreases visualization of the oral cavity. Rinsing the mouth before collection of a specimen would decrease flora. You swab the tonsillar area, not the uvula. Blowing the nose does not affect a throat culture.

5 **1 Rationale:** Redness is the only objective data. All of the other choices are subjective (i.e., what the patient says he is experiencing).

6 **4, 2, 3, 1, 5 Rationale:** The nurse applies clean gloves and removes the old dressing to assess the wound. Before obtaining the specimen, a patient must be identified with two identifiers to comply with The Joint Commission standards and improve patient safety. Cleaning around wound edges removes skin flora, reduces spread of infection, and prevents possible contamination of the specimen. Maintain sterile technique by providing a sterile field for sterile culture tubes.

7 **2, 3, 1, 5, 4 Rationale:** Before beginning the procedure, clamping the catheter above the port allows collection of a fresh sterile urine specimen. Do not use urine from the drainage bag; the urine is contaminated. Cleaning the port with a disinfectant and allowing it to dry reduce microorganisms entering the catheter and contamination of the specimen. Using a Luer-Lok needleless system eliminates potential of needlestick injury. Aspirating into a syringe allows the correct amount of urine to be collected and greater accuracy of test results. Unclamping the catheter returns draining by gravity into the drainage bag, decreasing potential for damage to kidneys, infection, and discomfort.

8 **1, 3, 2, 5, 4 Rationale:** A nurse teaches an adult patient the initial step of hand hygiene for testing blood glucose monitoring to reduce transmission of microorganisms and potential for infection. Matching the test strips code on the vial to the code displayed on a glucometer ensures accuracy of the results. Applying gloves reduces risk for health care providers through contamination by patient blood. Cleaning the site with an antiseptic swab or wipe reduces the transmission of microorganisms and promotes direct vasodilation at the selected site. Correct application of blood to a reagent strip ensures greater accuracy. Reading the correct result on the meter display ensures accuracy in reporting, documenting, and history and provides greater accuracy in medical interventions.

9 **2 Rationale:** NAP may collect a urine specimen from the port of an indwelling catheter. Current practice requires indwelling catheters with Luer-Lok ports to reduce potential for needlestick injury. Use of syringe with a needle cores the port plug and allows microorganisms to enter the closed system. Urine collected for a routine analysis uses a 20-mL syringe. A needleless Luer-Lok syringe must be used to collect a specimen from a Luer-Lok port.

10 **1 Rationale:** The Allen test uses the radial and ulnar arteries to test for adequate circulation when collecting arterial blood for arterial blood gases.

CHAPTER 44

Answers to Critical Thinking Exercises

1 Cardiac catheterization poses a risk for blood loss and complications that would require emergency coronary artery bypass graft surgery. Hematocrit and hemoglobin values are needed to obtain a baseline hematologic status for later comparison. Prothrombin time/international normalized ratio (PT/INR) is affected by warfarin, which Mr. Hall takes for chronic atrial fibrillation. If so, the health care provider needed to instruct Mr. Hall to stop his warfarin 1 to 2 nights before this procedure. A current PT/INR is needed to determine whether Mr. Hall is at risk for uncontrolled bleeding. Values for blood urea nitrogen and creatinine evaluate his renal function and, along with urine specific gravity, determine if Mr. Hall is dehydrated. Patients with baseline dehydration or impaired renal function are at risk for impaired excretion of the radiographic dye used during the cardiac catheterization procedure. Baseline electrolytes (sodium and potassium) are assessed to determine possible electromechanical problems.

2 In the presence of another nurse, ask Mr. Hall the following on arrival and just before starting the procedure: name, identifying number such as birth date, purpose of visit. Also compare the patient identifiers with information in Mr. Hall's MAR or medical record. Document in Mr. Hall's medical record.

3 The correct answer is 2. Mr. Hall falls into an American Society of Anesthesiologists (ASA) classification of 2—presence of mild systemic disease without functional limitations.

4 Patients who have not yet given informed consent need to wait until the health care provider provides explanation of the procedure. In addition, do not administer any medication that can reduce their level of consciousness, because it will impair their ability to give legal informed consent.

5 The correct answer is 1. These assessments are in order of threat to life and tailored to the procedure that was done. Heart rate and rhythm are affected because of catheter irritation or injury to the heart. Respiratory effort and oxygen saturation are frequently insufficient if the intravenous sedation suppressed Mr. Hall past the level of "moderate" sedation. The procedure site can easily bleed if mechanically disrupted when Mr. Hall is transferred from the procedure table to a cart and then to his bed. A visual check is essential to make sure that the dressing, sandbag, or closure device is secure to prevent arterial bleeding. Frequent pedal pulse checks help to promptly detect any intravascular clotting that might occur at the procedure site and cause reduced circulation to the legs.

Answers to Review Questions

1 **1 Rationale:** The changes and assessment data indicate that bleeding is occurring retroperitoneally.

2 **1 Rationale:** The patient with renal insufficiency may not be able to filter out the chemicals in the intravenous pyelogram dye. The patient with one kidney may have total function of that kidney. It would not be contraindicated for the other patients.

3 **3 Rationale:** With the removal of fluid from the abdomen, the abdominal girth would be smaller, it would be easier to breathe, and the number of respirations per minute would be lower because of less fluid and pressure.

4 **4 Rationale:** Colonoscopy requires an empty bowel. Because sedation is used, the patient needs to have nothing by mouth (NPO) for 8 hours before the procedure to decrease the need for aspiration.

5   **The correct order is 4, 1, 5, 3, 6, 2.**

6   **4**   **Rationale:** Explain to patient that the intravenous (IV) sedation will cause relaxation and amnesia but he will be awake during the procedure and able to speak. Hand signals are needed if the patient has an upper gastrointestinal (GI) procedure.

7   **2**   **Rationale:** Patient is possibly experiencing bronchospasm and requires you to support his or her airway. Call physician immediately and prepare for possible resuscitation. Suctioning would not be appropriate since it would worsen bronchospasm. IV fluids are not necessary for this condition, but patient requires patent IV access.

8   **3**   **Rationale:** A patient's response to sedation is monitored by measuring heart rate, blood pressure, SpO_2 and/or end tidal CO_2, respiratory rate and depth, and level of consciousness. Laboratory values will not detect changes resulting from sedation. The femoral pulse and gag reflex are not affected by sedation.

9   **1 d, 2 f, 3 e, 4 a, 5 c, 6 b**   **Rationale:** This is the correct position of the six leads.

10 **1, 4**   **Rationale:** Contraindications for an angiography include anticoagulant therapy such as warfarin, bleeding disorders, thrombocytopenia, dehydration, uncontrolled hypertension, renal insufficiency, and pregnancy.

Appendix

TERMINOLOGY/COMBINING FORMS: PREFIXES AND SUFFIXES

Medical terminology is similar to a foreign language. Many medical terms are derived from Latin and Greek sources. They often consist of two or more simple words or word elements. A word root or *combining form* may be put together with a *prefix* and a *suffix*.

Root—the basis of a word
Example: *nephr/o/tic* (degenerative changes in the kidney)
Root: nephr- (kidney)

Linking vowel—a vowel that joins the combining form to the suffix or another combining form
Example: nephr/*o*/sis (disease of the kidneys)
Linking vowel: o

Prefix—the beginning of a word
Example: *hyper*/active (excessively active)
Prefix: hyper- (excessive)

Suffix—the ending of a word
Example: nephr/*itis* (inflammation of the kidney)
Suffix: -itis (inflammation)

Combining form—the union of a word root with a linking vowel
Example: *hepato*/megaly (enlargement of the liver)
Combining form: hepato- (liver)

The following table provides some of the most commonly used terminology for your reference.

COMMON PREFIXES

Prefix	Definition
a-	without
ab-	away from
abd-	abdominal
acu-	sharp
ad-	toward
adip-	fat
ad lib-	freely, as wanted
aero-	air, gas
al-	toward
ambi-	both
an-	not
ana-	up
ante-	before, in front of
anti-	against
arteri-	artery
arthro-	joint
auto-	self
bi-	two
brady-	slow
cata-	down
chole-	bile
cili-	eyelid
circum-	around
co-	with, together
cogni-	know
colo-	colon
con-	with, together
contra-	against

Prefix	Definition
crani-	skull
cut-	skin
cyt-	cell
de-	from, lack of
demi-	half
dent-	tooth
derm-	skin
dia-	through, across
diplo-	double, twofold
dis-	to free or undo
dors-	back
dur-	hard
dy-	two
dys-	bad, painful, difficult, abnormal
ec-	out, out from
ecto-	outside
em-	in
embol-	to insert
encephalo-	brain
endo-	in, within
entero-	intestine
epi-	above, on
erythro-	red
eso-	within, inward
et-	and
eu-	good, normal
ex-	out, away from
exo-	outside
extra-	outside
faci-	face
fiss-	split, cleft
fore-	before, in front of
gastro-	stomach
glosso-	relating to the tongue
glyco-	sugar
haplo-	simple, single
heme-	iron-based
hemi-	one half
hepat-	liver
hetero-	different
histo-	tissue
homo-	same
hydro-	wet, water
hyper-	excessive, above normal
hypo-	under, below
im-	not
in-	in, not
infra-	under, below
inter-	between
intra-	in, within
isch-	deficiency
iso-	equal, alike
lapis-	stone
lapra-	loin or flank, sometimes abdomen
latero-	side
macro-	large

Prefix	Definition
mal-	bad
meato-	opening
medi-	middle
melano-	black
mesa-	middle
meso-	middle
meta-	beyond, change
micro-	small
mono-	one
morpho-	form, structure
multi-	many, much
neo-	new
nephro-	kidney
oculo-	eye
onco-	tumor
oro-	mouth
osteo-	bone
pan-	all
para-	beside, beyond
per-	through, by
peri-	around
phago-	eating
poly-	many, much
post-	after, behind
pre-	before, in front of
primi-	first
pro-	before, in front of
pseudo-	false
quadri-	four
re-	again, backward
retro-	backward, behind
rhabdo-	rod-shaped, striated
rhodo-	red
scler-	hardening
semi-	one half
stetho-	chest
sub-	under, below
super-	above, excessive
supra-	above, excessive
sym-	together
syn-	union, together, joined
tachy-	rapid
tetra-	four
therm-	heat
trans-	through, across
tri-	three
ultra-	beyond, excess
uni-	one
vas-	vessel or duct
xantho-	yellow
xero-	dry

COMMON SUFFIXES

Suffix	Definition
-ac	pertaining to
-agra	excessive pain
-al	pertaining to
-algia	painful condition, pain
-apheresis	removal
-ar	pertaining to
-ary	pertaining to

Suffix	Definition
-ase	enzyme
-bi	two, double
-blast	developing cell
-cele	hernia, swelling, sac
-centesis	puncture of a cavity
-clasis	break, fracture
-clysis	irrigation, washing
-coccus	berry shaped
-crit	to separate
-cyte	cell
-desis	fusion, binding, fixation
-drome	to run
-dynia	pain
-ectasis	expansion, dilation
-ectomy	excision, removal of a body part
-emesis	vomiting
-emia	blood
-er	one who
-gen	forming, producing, origin
-genesis	forming, producing, origin
-genic	origin, formation
-grade	to go
-gram	the record made, mark
-graph	instrument for recording, machine
-graphy	the process, process of recording
-ia	condition
-iasis	morbid condition
-iatry	treatment, medicine
-ic/-ical	pertaining to
-icle	small, minute
-ism	condition
-ist	one who specializes in, specialist
-itis	inflammation
-lith	stone, calculus
-logist	specialist in the study of
-logy	process of study
-lysis	dissolution, setting free
-malacia	softening, soft
-megaly	enlargement
-meter	instrument for measuring
-metry	act of measuring
-odynia	pain
-oid	form, shape
-ole	small, minute
-ology	study or science of
-oma	tumor
-opsy	to view
-or	one who
-orrhea	flow, discharge
-osis	condition or state
-ous	pertaining to
-para	to bear (offspring)
-paresis	partial paralysis
-pathy	disease, suffering
-penia	deficiency, lack of, decrease
-pexy	fixation
-phagia	eating, swallowing
-phasia	speech
-philia	attraction for
-phobia	fear
-physis	to grow
-plasia	formation, growth

Suffix	Definition	Suffix	Definition
-plasm	growth, formation	-stalsis	constriction
-plasty	mold, shape, repair	-stasis	control, constant level, stop
-plegia	paralysis	-stenosis	narrowing, stricture
-poiesis	formation, production	-stomy	creation of an opening
-ptosis	downward displacement, falling	-therapy	treatment
-ptysis	spitting	-tic	pertaining to
-rrhage	bursting forth, rupture	-tome	instrument for cutting
-rrhaphy	suturing in place	-tomy	process of cutting, incision
-rrhea	flow, discharge	-toxic	poison
-rrhexis	rupture	-tresia	opening
-scope	instrument to visually examine	-tripsy	surgical crushing
-scopy	process of examining, visual examination	-trophy	nourishment
-sepsis	infection	-ula	small, minute
-sis	state of, condition	-ule	small, minute
-spasm	involuntary spasm	-y	process

Glossary

A

abdominal girth The measurement of the circumference of the abdomen, taken at the same place with each measurement.

abduction Movement of an extremity away from the midline of the body.

accommodation reflex Adjustment of the eyes for near vision, composed of pupillary constriction, convergence of the visual axes, and increased convexity of the lens.

accurate empathy Communication technique used by a nurse to show understanding of a patient's feelings and experiences.

Acetest A test that measures the presence of ketone (acetone) bodies in the urine. A large quantity of acetone causes rapid change in the color of the Acetest tablet.

active listening An interpersonal process whereby a person hears a message, decodes the meaning, and conveys an understanding about the meaning to the sender.

active range-of-motion exercises Exercises of the joints performed by an individual without assistance.

active-assisted range-of-motion exercises Exercises of the joints performed by an individual with some assistance. For example, a nurse helps support an extremity.

activity tolerance Type and amount of exercise or work that a person is able to perform.

actual loss Any loss of a person or object that can no longer be felt, heard, known, or experienced.

acuity systems Systems to determine the right amount of staff according to weighted patient workload.

acute pain Severe pain with a rapid onset and of short duration.

addiction A compulsive physiologic need for a habit-forming drug.

adduction Movement of an extremity toward the midline of the body.

adjuvant therapy The treatment of a disease with substances that enhance the action of drugs, especially drugs that promote the production of antibodies.

adrenergic drug A medication that mimics the effects of sympathetic nerve stimulation of the autonomic nervous system.

advance directive Document defining a patient's end-of-life care decisions.

adverse drug events (ADEs) Unfavorable reactions to medications that present during the normal course of treatment. The effect of an ADE may range from minimal harm to significant injury or death (National Research Council, 2007).

adverse drug reactions (ADRs) Nontherapeutic effects of medications.

adverse reaction Unintended response to a drug.

aerobe A microorganism that lives and grows in the presence of free oxygen.

aerobic Pertaining to the presence of air or oxygen.

afebrile Without fever.

agglutinate A process by which cells that display antigens (red blood cells, bacteria) adhere to one another or clump together.

air embolus A quantity of air that circulates in the bloodstream to eventually lodge in a blood vessel.

air fluidization The process of blowing warm air through a collection of microspheres to create a fluidlike environment. Used in special mattresses designed to reduce pressure against a person's skin.

air leak Escaping air in closed chest drainage. May be patient centered or within the chest tube system.

air-fluidized bed A special bed designed to distribute weight evenly over its support surface. Fluidization is created by forcing a gentle flow of temperature-controlled air upward through a mass of fine ceramic microspheres.

air-suspension bed A device that supports a patient's weight on air-filled cushions, minimizing tissue damage from pressure and shear.

albumin An acute-phase protein involved in nutrient transport and the maintenance of oncotic pressure. Used as a measure of visceral protein status. Has a half-life of 14 to 20 days.

aldosterone A steroid hormone produced by the adrenal cortex that causes the kidney tubules to excrete potassium and reabsorb sodium and water.

Aldrete score Score based on the Aldrete Scoring System for determining a patient's postanesthesia recovery status.

allergen A substance that can produce a hypersensitive reaction in the body but that is not necessarily intrinsically harmful.

all-hazards event Multiple manmade or natural events with destructive capacity to cause multiple casualties.

all-hazards preparedness The comprehensive preparedness necessary to manage casualties resulting from a disaster, regardless of etiology.

allogeneic Denoting a cell type that is from the same species but genetically distinct.

alopecia Partial or complete lack of hair.

Alzheimer's disease Dementia characterized by progressive confusion, memory failure, disorientation, restlessness, and speech disturbances. Cause is not fully understood.

amino acid An organic compound composed of one or more basic amino groups and one or more carboxyl groups. Amino acids are the building blocks that construct proteins and the end products of protein digestion.

amnesic syndrome Memory impairment in the absence of other cognitive impairments.

ampule Small sterile glass or plastic container that usually contains a single dose of solution to be administered parenterally.

anaerobic Pertaining to absence of air or oxygen.

analgesia A decreased or absent sensation of pain.

anaphylactic reaction Exaggerated hypersensitivity reaction to a previously encountered antigen. It is a severe and sometimes fatal systemic reaction characterized by itching, hyperemia, angioedema and, in severe cases, vascular collapse, bronchospasm, and shock.

anaphylaxis An exaggerated hypersensitivity reaction to a previously encountered antigen. The reaction may be localized or generalized.

anastomosis A surgical joining of two ducts or blood vessels to allow flow from one to the other.

anemia A disorder characterized by a decrease in hemoglobin in the blood to levels below the normal range, decreased red cell production, or increased red cell destruction or blood loss.

anesthesia The absence of normal sensation, especially sensitivity to pain.

anesthetics Drugs or agents capable of producing a complete or partial loss of feeling.

angiogenesis The formation of new blood vessels.

anions Negatively charged ions.

anthropometry The science of measuring the height, weight, and size of component parts of the human body, including skinfolds.

antianginal A medication that dilates coronary arteries, improving blood flow to the myocardium to prevent angina.

antidysrhythmic A class of medications that possess properties for controlling abnormal cardiac rhythms (e.g., quinidine and propranolol [Inderal]).

antiemetic Of or pertaining to a substance or procedure that prevents or alleviates nausea and vomiting.

antipyretic Pertaining to a substance, such as a medication, that reduces fever.

apical pulse Measurement of the heartbeat taken with the stethoscope placed over the apex of the heart.

apnea An absence of spontaneous respirations.

approximate To come together, as in the edges of a wound.

aqueous Watery or waterlike; referring to a medication prepared with water.

artificial airway Plastic or rubber device inserted into the upper or lower respiratory tract to facilitate ventilation or secretion removal.

ASA classification A classification system for ranking the level of a patient's physical health, established by the American Society of Anesthesiologists (ASA).

ascites Effusion and accumulation of serous fluid in the abdominal cavity.

asepsis The absence of disease-producing (pathogenic) organisms.

aseptic technique The methods used during patient care to prevent microbial contamination. They can be either clean (medical asepsis) or sterile (surgical asepsis) techniques.

aspirant Fluid or particulate that is aspirated.

aspirate Withdrawal of fluid or air into the barrel of a syringe or suction device.

aspiration The entry of gastric contents into the tracheobronchial passages. This increases a patient's risk for aspiratory pneumonia.

astigmatism Abnormal condition of the eye in which the light rays cannot be focused clearly in a point on the retina because the spherical curve of the cornea is not equal in all meridians. Vision is blurred, and use of the eye causes discomfort.

astringent A topical substance that causes constriction of tissues on application; commonly used for cleansing the skin.

atelectasis An abnormal condition characterized by the collapse of lung tissue, preventing the respiratory exchange of carbon dioxide and oxygen.

atmospheric pressure Pressure exerted by the atmosphere. (Atmospheric pressure at sea level is 760 mm Hg.)

atrophy Wasting or diminution of size or physiological activity of a part of the body caused by disease or other influences.

audiologist A health professional with at least a master's degree who studies sense of hearing defects, diagnoses hearing loss, and works to provide rehabilitation of individuals with hearing loss.

auscultation The act of listening for sounds within the body to evaluate the condition of the heart, lungs, pleura, intestines, or other organs or to detect fetal heart sounds. Performed directly or most commonly through use of a stethoscope.

auscultatory gap The temporary disappearance of Korotkoff sounds when blood pressure is being auscultated. Occurs in hypertensive patients and may cause an underestimation of blood pressure.

autoclave An appliance used to sterilize medical instruments or other objects with steam under pressure.

Autolet A small instrument with a lancet used to obtain a capillary blood specimen.

autologous transfusion Transfusion of a patient's own blood through predeposit, blood that is salvaged intraoperatively by a cell saver, or blood shed after surgery.

automated external defibrillator (AED) Device used by basic cardiopulmonary resuscitation (CPR) providers to treat fast, irregular dysrhythmias with electrical shock to the heart using automated rhythm analysis and simplified functions.

autopsy Examination of the deceased's body performed to confirm or determine the cause of death.

autotransfusion The collection, anticoagulation, filtration, and reinfusion of blood from an active bleeding site. Used in cases of trauma and major surgery.

axillary Pertaining to the pyramid-shaped space that forms the underside of the shoulder between the upper part of the arm and the side of the chest.

B

bacteremia Presence of bacteria in the blood.

bacteriostatic Tending to inhibit development or reproduction of bacteria.

bag-valve-mask (BVM) or Ambu-bag Bag attached to a mask that provides artificial ventilations to a patient when squeezed.

balance Position in which a person's center of gravity is correct so the risk for falling is reduced.

bariatric bed A specialized surface equipped with hand controls to allow for self-positioning, providing a stable, adaptable surface for managing the morbidly obese patient.

basal energy expenditure (BEE) The amount of energy required at rest for basic life processes such as breathing, maintaining body temperature, and cardiac function. Basal energy expenditure can be estimated or measured.

basal metabolism Energy needed to maintain the basic processes of the body such as respiration, circulation, and temperature.

base of support Surface area on which an object rests.

bed rest Placement of a patient in bed for a prescribed period for therapeutic reasons.

belt restraints Type of restraint used to secure a patient on a stretcher.

bias Influences that distort the findings of a research study.

binder Bandage made of a large piece of material to fit and support a specific body part.

bioavailability The extent to which a dose of a drug reaches its site of action to produce an effect.

biohazard container Container used for medical waste that must be made of rigid material so as to be puncture resistant and labeled with the words "Sharps Waste" or with a biohazard symbol and the word "Biohazard."

biological agent Bacteria or virus that, when released into the environment, has the potential to cause widespread and continuing infection and mass casualties.

biological disaster The unexpected release of a biological agent capable of causing widespread illness or contamination in the environment.

biopsy The removal and microscopic examination of tissue, performed to establish precise diagnosis.

bioterrorism/bioterrorist attack The release of a biological agent into a specified environment with the intent of causing mass casualties.

blood culture A laboratory test on serum to determine presence of infection in the blood.

blood group Classification of blood type based on the presence or absence of genetically determined antigens on the surface of the red cell.

blood plasma The liquid portion of the blood, free of its formed elements and particles.

blood transfusion Administration of whole blood or a blood component as cells to replace blood lost through trauma, surgery, or disease.

blood type Blood type identified by genetically determined antigens on the surface of red blood cells.

blunt-tip vial access cannula A needleless cannula designed to be inserted into a vial adapter or for needleless access to fill a syringe.

body alignment Refers to the condition of joints, tendons, ligaments, and muscles in various body positions.

body mass index (BMI) A measurement of weight in comparison to height. Used to categorize an individual's degree of adiposity.

body mechanics Coordinated efforts of the musculoskeletal and nervous systems to maintain proper balance, posture, and body alignment.

bolus A large, round preparation of medicinal material for oral ingestion; a dose of a medication or a contrast material injected all at once intravenously.

bone marrow Specialized, soft tissue filling the spaces in cancellous bone of the epiphyses; responsible for red blood cell production.

borborygmus Audible abdominal sound produced by hyperactive intestinal peristalsis.

bradycardia An abnormality in heart rate in which the heart contracts steadily at a rate less than 60 contractions/min.

bradypnea Breathing that is normal in rate but abnormally slow (less than 12 breaths/min).

brain death The irreversible absence of all brain function, including brainstem function.

bronchophony An increase in intensity and clarity of vocal resonance that may result from an increase in lung tissue density, such as in the consolidation of pneumonia.

bronchospasm Abnormal contraction of the smooth muscles of the bronchi.

bronchus One of several large air passages in the lungs through which inspired air and exhaled gases pass.

bruit Abnormal sound or murmur created by turbulent blood flow heard while auscultating an organ, gland, or artery.

buccal Of or pertaining to the inside of the cheek; surface of a tooth or gum next to the cheek.

buccal medication Medication placed between the upper or lower molar teeth and cheek area and allowed to dissolve.

C

cadence Pace or rate of verbal communication.

calorie (Kcal) A calorie is the amount of heat required to raise the temperature of 1 g of water 1°C at atmospheric pressure.

cannula A small tube for insertion into a body cavity, duct, or vessel.

capillary closing pressure The amount of external pressure required to close off the blood flow to the capillaries.

carcinoma Malignant epithelial neoplasm that tends to invade surrounding tissue and spread to distant regions of the body.

cardiac Pertaining to the heart. Pertaining to a person with heart disease.

cardiac arrest The cessation of circulating blood flow that eliminates oxygen transport or perfusion, usually precipitated by ventricular fibrillation or ventricular asystole.

cardiac output Volume of blood ejected by the ventricles of the heart in 1 minute; equal to stroke volume times heart rate.

cardiomegaly Enlargement of the heart; typical sign of heart failure.

cardiopulmonary arrest Sudden cessation of respirations, pulse, and circulation.

cardiopulmonary resuscitation (CPR) Basic emergency procedure for life support consisting of artificial respiration and manual external cardiac massage.

caries Decay of a tooth; progressive decalcification of enamel and dentin of a tooth.

case management The assignment of a health care provider to help a patient by assessing need for health care and social service systems and to ensure that required services are obtained.

cast Rigid plaster or fiberglass application molded over skin tissues to hold musculoskeletal tissues to permit healing of injuries.

cast brace Combination of a brace within a cast at a joint.

cast saw Saw used to cut through plaster to remove cast.

cast shoe Shoe worn over the foot encased in plaster.

cast syndrome A series of patient signs that indicate an untoward (claustrophobic) reaction to being in a cast.

casualty Any individual who is ill, injured, missing, or killed as a result of a mass casualty incident.

catheter A tubular device for insertion into vessels or body cavities for diagnostic or therapeutic purposes, to permit injection, or to withdraw fluids.

cathartic Drug that acts to promote bowel evacuation.

catheterization Introduction of a tube through the urethra and into the bladder.

cations Positively charged ions.

cell cycle The sequence of events that occurs during the growth and division of tissue cells.

center of gravity Midpoint or center of body weight. In the adult it is the midpelvic cavity between the symphysis pubis and the umbilicus.

centigrade Temperature scale in which 0° is the freezing point of water and 100° is the boiling point of water at sea level; also called *Celsius*.

central venous access device (CVAD) A catheter placed in a large central vein to give medication, fluids, or blood product.

central venous pressure (CVP) Pressure in the great veins (superior and inferior vena cava) as blood returns to the heart.

cephalic vein One of the four superficial veins of the upper limb.

cerebrospinal fluid (CSF) Substance contained within the four ventricles of the brain, the subarachnoid space, and the central canal of the spinal cord.

cerumen Earwax. A waxy secretion produced by apocrine sweat glands in the external ear canal.

cervical halter Support for the head, made of cotton material, used for traction.

change-of-shift report Means through which nurses report information about their assigned patients to the nurses working the next shift for the purpose of providing continuity of care for patients. May be given orally in person, by audiotape recording, or during "walking-planning" rounds at each patient's bedside.

charting by exception (CBE) A charting methodology in which data are entered only when there is an exception from what is normal or expected. Reduces time spent documenting.

cheilosis Disorder of the lips and mouth characterized by scales and fissures.

chemical decontamination The process of removing or neutralizing contaminating chemical agents.

chemical warfare agent The use of the toxic properties of chemical substances to kill, injure, or incapacitate an enemy.

chemotherapy Use of drugs to prevent cancer cells from multiplying, invading adjacent tissue, and metastasizing.

chest physiotherapy Physical maneuvers, including postural drainage, chest percussion, vibration, rib shaking, and cough, to improve airway mucus clearance in patients with retained tracheobronchial secretions.

chest tube Catheter inserted through the chest wall into the intrapleural space.

chronic pain Pain that persists beyond the period of healing, ceases to serve a protective function, degrades patient function, and serves no adaptive purpose.

chronic venous insufficiency Abnormal circulatory condition characterized by decreased return of the venous blood from the legs to the trunk of the body.

circulating nurse A registered nurse (RN) considered to be the charge nurse in the operating room during a surgical procedure.

circumduction The circular movement of a limb. The motion of the head of a bone within an articulating cavity such as the hip joint.

clarifying An attempt to put into words vague ideas or unclear thoughts of a patient to enhance the nurse's understanding, or asking a patient to explain what he or she means.

clean technique (medical asepsis) The purposeful prevention of the transmission of microorganisms by using procedures such as hand hygiene and disinfection of equipment to reduce the number of microorganisms.

cleansing enema An enema, usually soapsuds, administered repeatedly until the colon is free of all formed fecal material.

clean-voided specimen A technique used to collect a urine specimen as free from bacterial contamination as possible without catheterizing the patient.

clinical guidelines Systematically developed statements about a plan of care for a specific set of clinical circumstances involving a specific patient population.

Clinitest A test that measures the amount of glucose and acetone in a urine specimen.

closed system suction catheter A suction catheter that is attached to the mechanical ventilator circuit encased within a sterile sheath. The catheter system permits sterile airway suctioning without interrupting mechanical ventilation or requiring the nurse to apply sterile gloves.

coagulopathies A disease or condition affecting the ability of the blood to coagulate.

code event A declaration of or a state of medical emergency and call for medical personnel and equipment to attempt to resuscitate a patient, especially when in cardiac arrest or respiratory distress or failure.

colon Portion of large intestine from the cecum to the rectum.

colonization The reproduction of microorganisms at a specific site without the signs/symptoms of a disease or tissue invasion.

colonized The presence of bacteria on the surface or in the tissue of a wound without indications of infection such as purulent exudate, foul odor, or surrounding inflammation. All stage II, III, and IV pressure ulcers are colonized.

colostomy Surgical formation of an opening of the colon onto the surface of the abdomen through which fecal matter is emptied.

comforting Any nursing action taken to promote comfort of a patient, such as a back rub or change in position.

comminuted fracture A fracture in which the bone is broken into several fragments.

compartment syndrome Insufficient arterial perfusion to an extremity caused by trauma or stasis; leads to ischemia and tissue necrosis if not reversed.

compatibility The quality or state of existing together in harmony. The formation of a stable chemical or biochemical system, specifically in medication, so

two or more drugs can be administered at the same time without producing side effects.

compliance Fulfillment by a patient of the caregiver's prescribed course of treatment.

compound A substance composed of two or more different elements, chemically combined, that cannot be separated by physical means.

compress Soft pad of gauze or cloth used to apply heat, cold, or medications to the surface of a body part.

computer-based patient care record (CPCR) Record stored in a comprehensive computerized system that is used by all health care practitioners to permanently store information pertaining to a patient's health status, clinical problems, and functional abilities. The CPCR can store numerous databases, including structured assessment data, clinical decision support systems, and diagnostic artificial intelligence. It stores information pertaining to a given patient from any health care event and thereby provides access to information across a patient's life span.

condition of participation A requirement that all patients be notified of their rights when entering a health care facility. Part of the Key Principles of Patient's Rights documentation.

conduction Mechanism of heat transfer involving flow of heat from one object to another with which it is in contact.

conjunctiva Mucous membrane lining the inner surfaces of the eyelids and anterior part of the sclera.

conjunctivitis A highly contagious eye infection. The crusty drainage that collects on eyelid margins can easily spread from one eye to the other.

constipation Condition characterized by difficulty in passing stool or an infrequent passage of hard stool.

contamination The introduction of infectious material on normally clean or sterile sites.

continent ostomy or diversion Results from a surgical procedure that leaves a patient with an internal pouch where either stool or urine is temporarily stored and the effluent is removed by intubation through the external stoma. It is continent because the effluent does not drain spontaneously from the stoma; instead a catheter must be inserted through the stoma to drain the effluent from the internal pouch.

continent urinary diversion A surgical procedure that uses a distal portion of the ileum and proximal portion of the colon to create an ileal pouch. The ureters from the patient's kidneys are embedded in the pouch. A narrow ileal segment forms a stoma on the abdominal wall.

continuous subcutaneous infusion (CSQI or CSCI) A method of medication administration in which medication is administered continuously into the subcutaneous tissue using a medication infusion pump.

continuum of care Matching an individual's ongoing needs with the appropriate level and type of medical, psychological, health, or social care or services within an organization or across multiple organizations.

contractures Abnormal condition of a joint characterized by flexion and fixation and caused by atrophy and shortening of muscle fibers or loss of normal elasticity of the skin.

core temperature Temperature of deep body tissues and organs.

costovertebral angle (CVA) tenderness Palpation over this region can elicit tenderness. Tenderness is common with kidney infection or trauma to the region.

countertraction Use of patient's body weight or other weights, ropes, and pulleys to counter the pull of the traction weight.

crackles Fine bubbling sound heard on auscultation of the lung.

crepitation The sound and/or feeling produced when bone ends rub against one another. The patient describes the sound and feeling.

critical/collaborative pathway Tool used in managed care that incorporates the treatment interventions of caregivers from all disciplines who normally care for a patient. Designed for a specific case type, a pathway is used to manage the care of a patient throughout a projected length of stay.

crutch gait Gait assumed by a person on crutches by alternately bearing weight on one or both legs and on the crutches.

crutch palsy Temporary or permanent loss of sensation or movement resulting from pressure on axilla from crutch.

cryotherapy Therapy in which the skin is exposed to cool or cold temperatures. Used to treat localized inflammatory responses.

cuff A plastic air- or foam-and-air–filled balloonlike attachment on the distal end of the endotracheal tube or tracheostomy tube that prevents loss of air from the lung and inhalation of foreign bodies around the tube.

culture Laboratory test involving the cultivation of microorganisms or cells in a special growth medium.

cutaneous stimulation Stimulation of the skin.

cuticle A thin edge of cornified epithelium at the base of a nail.

cyanosis Bluish discoloration of the skin and mucous membranes caused by an excess of deoxygenated hemoglobin in the blood or a structural defect in the hemoglobin molecule.

cycloplegic Pertaining to a drug that paralyzes ciliary muscles of the eye, causing pupillary dilation for ophthalmological examination or surgery.

cytology The study of cells, including their formation, origin, structure, function, biochemical activities, and pathologic characteristics.

D

dangling To sit on the side of a bed with legs dependent or feet on the floor.

DAR An acronym for a method of documentation that includes data (subjective and objective), action (nursing interventions), and response of the patient (evaluation of effectiveness).

dead space A cavity remaining in a wound.

debride To remove dead or damaged tissue from a wound. To remove dirt, foreign objects, damaged tissue, and cellular debris from a wound or burn to prevent infection and promote healing.

debridement Removal of dead tissue in a wound.

decompression Removal of pressure as from gas and fluid in the stomach and intestinal tract.

decontamination The process of removing foreign material such as blood; body fluids; or chemical, biological, or radioactive contaminants. It does not eliminate microorganisms but is a necessary step preceding disinfection or sterilization.

deep sedation An induced state of sedation characterized by depressed consciousness so the patient is unable to continuously and independently maintain a patent airway and experiences a partial loss of protective reflexes.

deep tissue injury Purple or maroon localized area of discolored intact skin or blood-filled blister resulting from damage to underlying soft tissue from pressure and/or shear. The injured area may be preceded by tissue that is painful, firm, mushy, boggy, or warmer or cooler compared to adjacent tissue.

deep vein thrombosis A thrombus in one of the deep veins of the body, most often the iliac or femoral vein. Symptoms include tenderness, pain, swelling, warmth, and discoloration of the skin. It is potentially life-threatening.

de-escalation A communication strategy involving the reduction of anxious and/or agitated behaviors exhibited verbally or nonverbally by a patient. Using a calm yet firm approach diffuses the patient's increasing anxiety and/or agitated state, thereby minimizing potentially violent outbursts.

defecation Passage of feces from the digestive tract through the rectum.

dehiscence The separation or opening of wound layers.

dementia A term used to describe a group of symptoms related to a loss or impairment of mental powers. These symptoms appear in a person who is awake and are demonstrated by symptoms of mental confusion, memory loss, disorientation, intellectual impairment, or similar problems.

dental caries Chalky white discoloration of teeth or presence of brown or black discoloration.

dentifrice A pharmaceutical compound used with a toothbrush for cleaning and polishing teeth.

Department of Homeland Security (DHS) The federal department that administers all matters relating to homeland security.

dermatitis An inflammatory condition of the skin characterized by erythema and pain or pruritus.

dermatological Pertaining to the skin.

detection and surveillance Awareness of the environment, recognizing what might be unusual or different and knowing what these differences mean in terms of terrorism preparedness.

devitalized Tissues with reduced oxygen supply and blood flow.

dialysis A procedure that removes fluid and solid wastes from the blood or lymph.

diaphoresis Secretion of sweat typically associated with hyperthermia, physical exertion, and emotional stress.

diastolic pressure The lower blood pressure measurement, which reflects the pressure consistently exerted within the arterial system during the period of ventricular relaxation.

diffusion Movement of oxygen to the red blood cells at the alveolar level.

diluent Agent that makes a solution or mixture thinner or more liquid by admixture.

disaster A catastrophic and/or destructive event that disrupts normal functioning; it may include any anticipated or unexpected event the effects of which lead to significant destruction and/or adverse consequences.

disaster management The discipline of dealing with and avoiding risks. It is a discipline that involves preparing for disaster before it occurs, providing disaster response, and supporting and rebuilding after disasters have occurred.

disaster response A phase of the disaster management cycle. Its preceding cycles aim to reduce the need for a disaster response or to avoid it.

disaster triage A model for sorting individuals by the seriousness of their condition and the likelihood of their survival.

discharge planning The process by which a nurse plans for a patient's eventual release from a health care agency. The process begins on a patient's admission to the agency.

distraction A pain-reduction technique that diverts an individual's attention away from the pain sensation.

documentation Anything written or printed that is relied on as record or proof for authorized persons. It is a vital aspect of nursing practice and a vital link between providing and evaluating health care.

documentation system Detailed information, in either written or computerized form, about a computer system, including its architecture, design, data flow, and programming logic.

dorsal Pertaining to the back or posterior.

dorsiflexion Flexion toward the back, as accomplished by a muscle (e.g., in the hand or foot).

dorsum The back of the hand.

double-void A procedure of discarding the first urine specimen and testing the second urine specimen that was obtained 30 to 45 minutes later; this procedure gives a more accurate amount of glucose being spilled into the urine at that particular time.

drawsheet A special sheet placed over the regular sheet on a bed and used to move a person in bed.

drop factor Refers to the calibration of intravenous (IV) tubing (IV infusion set) in drops per milliliter (e.g., the drop factor of microdrip IV tubing is 60 gtt/mL).

drug tolerance A decreased physiological response after repeated administration of a drug or a chemically related substance.

dry powder inhaler (DPI) Handheld device that disperses powdered medication for inhalation.

duration of action Length of time during which a drug is present in a concentration great enough to produce a therapeutic effect.

dysphagia Difficulty swallowing.

dyspnea Difficulty breathing.

dysrhythmia An irregular, fast, or slow heart rhythm.

dysuria Pain or burning on urination. May also be accompanied by difficulty in urination. Usually indicates a urinary tract infection.

E

ecchymosis Bluish discoloration of an area of skin or mucous membrane caused by the extravasation of blood into the subcutaneous tissues as a result of trauma to the underlying blood vessels or fragility of the vessel walls.

edema Abnormal accumulation of fluid in interstitial spaces of tissues.

effleurage A type of massage stroke that glides without manipulating deep muscles, smooths and extends muscles, increases nutrient absorption, and improves lymphatic and venous circulation.

effluent The drainage that is expected from an ostomy.

egophony A change in the voice sound as heard on auscultation of a patient with pleural effusion. When patient is asked to make e-e-e sounds, the sound is heard over the peripheral chest wall as a-a-a.

elastic bandage Bandage of elasticized fabric that provides support and allows movement.

electrolyte An element or compound that, when melted or dissolved in water or another solvent, dissociates into ions and is able to carry an electric current.

electronic infusion device (EID) Used to infuse intravenous (IV) fluid at a prescribed rate. There are two types: an infusion pump, which is designed to deliver a measured amount of fluid over a period of time; and an IV controller, which delivers fluid with the aid of gravity.

electronic medical record A medical record in digital format.

embolus (emboli) A foreign object, a quantity of air or gas, a bit of tissue or tumor, or a piece of thrombus that circulates in the bloodstream until it becomes lodged in a vessel.

emergency responders Individuals whose job it is to respond to an emergency situation—typically police, fire, hazardous materials (HAZMAT), and emergency medical services (EMS) personnel.

empathy Ability to recognize and to some extent share the emotions and state of mind of another and to understand the meaning and significance of that person's behavior.

endemic The expected or normal incidence present in a geographical area or population.

end-of-life-care The human provision of physical, psychological, social, and spiritual support to a patient and patient's family at the end of life.

endotracheal intubation Placement of a plastic tube into the trachea to provide artificial ventilation on a continuous basis.

endotracheal tube Artificial airway inserted through the mouth into the trachea.

enema Procedure involving introduction of a solution into the rectum for cleansing or therapeutic purposes.

enteral nutrition The administration of nutrition via the gastrointestinal tract (i.e., by mouth, tube feeding, or oral supplement).

enteral tube feeding The introduction of food or nutritive material directly into the digestive tract by nasogastric or gastric tube.

Enteric-coated Tablets coated with a substance that does not dissolve until reaching the intestine. Used when drug constituents are irritating to oral and gastric mucosa.

enucleation Removal of the eyeball, performed in cases of malignancy, severe infection, or extensive trauma or to control pain in glaucoma.

epidemic A disease that spreads rapidly through a demographic segment of the human population, with an incidence beyond what is expected.

epidemiology Study of the occurrence, distribution, and causes of disease.

epidural Administration of local anesthetic by way of a catheter into the epidural space of the spinal column. Designed to produce anesthesia of the pelvic, abdominal, or genital areas.

epidural analgesia Delivery of an analgesic into the epidural space in pain control.

epidural blood patch Procedure whereby a physician injects a small amount of autologous blood into the epidural space.

episiotomy A surgical procedure in which an incision is made in a woman's perineum to enlarge her vaginal opening for delivery of an infant. Procedure prevents tearing of perineum.

epithelialization The process by which epidermal cells migrate (move) over the surface of the wound to close the top or "resurface" the wound.

erythema Redness or inflammation of the skin or mucous membranes. Result of dilation and congestion of superficial capillaries.

eschar Scab or dry crust that results from excoriation of the skin.

evaporation Mechanism of heat loss whereby moisture from the surface of the body changes to vapor and transfers heat to the surrounding air.

eversion Turning outward or inside out, such as turning the foot outward at the ankle.

evidence-based practice (EBP) A problem-solving approach to clinical practice that combines the conscientious use of research-based evidence in combination with a clinician's expertise and patient preferences and values in making decisions about patient care.

evisceration The separation of wound layers with the protrusion of abdominal organs through the layers.

excoriation An injury to the surface of the skin or other part of the body caused by scratching or abrasion.

excretion The process of eliminating, shedding, or getting rid of substances by body organs or tissues.

exercise Performance of any physical activity for the purpose of conditioning the body, improving health, or maintaining fitness or as a therapeutic measure.

exit site Point at which a catheter leaves a body site.

exophthalmos Abnormal protrusion of one or both eyeballs caused by trauma, intracranial lesions, intraorbital disorders, or systemic disease, most commonly hyperthyroidism.

expectorant An agent that facilitates removal of bronchopulmonary secretions.

expectorate The act of coughing and spitting out mucus from the respiratory tract. Maneuver is useful in helping a patient clear the airways of pulmonary secretions.

extension Movement increasing the angle between two adjoining bones.

external fixation Skeletal traction applied through the use of pins attached to a frame rather than weights.

external rotation Rotation of a joint outward.

external urethral sphincter Voluntary muscle that must relax for a patient to void or completely empty the bladder.

extravasation The inadvertent infiltration of intravenous fluids or medications into the subcutaneous tissues surrounding the infusion site.

extremity restraints Restraints used to immobilize one or all extremities.

exudate Any fluid that has been extruded from a tissue or its capillaries, more specifically because of injury or inflammation. It is characteristically high in protein and white blood cells.

F

Fahrenheit Temperature scale in which 32° is the freezing point of water and 212° is the boiling point of water at sea level.

fascia Fibrous connective tissue.

febrile Pertaining to or characterized by fever or an elevation in body temperature.

fenestrated drape A drape with a round or slitlike opening in the center.

fenestrated tracheostomy tube A tracheostomy tube containing a hole (fenestration) on the posterior aspect of the outer cannula that allows airflow over the vocal cords and speech in spontaneously breathing patients.

fenestration Surgical procedure in which an opening is created to gain access to the cavity within an organ or a bone.

fever An abnormal elevation of body temperature.

fiberoptic Pertaining to fiberoptics; referring to the transmission of an image along flexible bundles of coated glass or plastic fibers having special optical properties.

field triage tag Tags constructed of a high-density, water-resistant synthetic paper and printed using a special thermal printing process, allowing them to be used in field situations.

first responders Public service providers required to be the first on the scene of a disaster, typically emergency medical system (EMS), fire, or police personnel.

flexion Movement decreasing the angle between two adjoining bones; bending of a limb.

flora Microorganisms that reside on and within the body to compete with disease-producing microorganisms to provide a natural immunity against certain infections.

flossing Mechanical cleansing of tooth surfaces with the use of stringlike waxed or unwaxed dental floss.

flotation device A foam mattress with a gellike pad located in its center, designed to protect bony prominences and distribute pressure more evenly against the surface of the skin.

flotation pad A device constructed of foam or a silicone or polyvinyl chloride gel encased in a vinyl-covered square. Protects bony prominences and distributes pressure more evenly against the surface of the skin.

flow sheet A recording form used to document the same type of repeated measurements, procedures, or observations over time. Data on flow sheets allow the user to see trends over time.

fluid volume deficit (FVD) An alteration characterized by the loss of fluids and electrolytes in an isotonic fashion.

fluid volume excess (FVE) An alteration characterized by the abnormal retention of fluids and electrolytes in an isotonic fashion.

focus charting A charting methodology for structuring progress notes according to the focus of the note (e.g., symptoms and nursing diagnosis). Each note includes data, action, and patient response.

fontanel A space covered by tough membranes between the bones of an infant's cranium.

footboard Board placed perpendicular to the mattress, parallel to and touching the plantar surface of a patient's feet. Used to maintain dorsiflexion of the feet.

footdrop A falling or dragging of the foot from paralysis of the flexors of the ankle.

foramen magnum The large opening in the anterior and inferior part of the occipital bone, interconnecting the vertebral canal and cranial cavity.

four-poster cast Cast placed over the shoulders. Contains four vertical posts or poles on the anterior and posterior lateral sides of the head to immobilize the cervical vertebrae.

Fowler's position Posture assumed by a patient when the head of the bed is raised approximately 45 to 90 degrees, as though the patient is sitting upright.

fracture pan A bedpan designed for patients with body or leg casts or patients restricted from raising their hips. It has a shallow upper end that slips easily under a patient.

friction Effect of rubbing, or the resistance that a moving body meets from the surface on which it moves. A force that occurs in a direction to oppose movement. In massage, technique in which deeper tissues are stroked or rubbed, usually through strong circular movements of the hand.

friction rub Dry grating sound heard during auscultation, caused by rubbing of tissue surfaces.

G

gag reflex A normal neural reflex elicited by touching the soft palate or posterior pharynx, the response being the elevation of the palate, retraction of the tongue, and contraction of the pharyngeal muscles. Tests for function of the vagus and glossopharyngeal nerves.

gait Manner or style of walking, including rhythm, cadence, and speed.

gait belt A leather or heavy canvas belt that encircles a patient's waist. It may or may not have handles. The purpose of the belt is for a nurse to hold when ambulating an unsteady patient to reduce risk for a fall.

gastrostomy feeding tube Long, hollow, flexible tube inserted into the stomach through a stab wound in the upper left abdominal quadrant.

gingivae The gums of the mouth.

gingivitis Inflammatory condition in which the gums are red, swollen, and bleeding.

glabellar tap A reflex elicited by repetitive tapping on the forehead. Subjects blink in response to the first several taps. If the blinking persists, this is known as Myerson's sign and is abnormal.

glucose monitoring A diagnostic test to determine the blood glucose level.

granulation The presence of red, granular, moist tissue that appears during the healing of open wounds; type of tissue containing new blood vessels that bleed readily.

granulation tissue Soft, pink, fleshy projection of tissue that forms during the healing process in a wound not healing by primary intention.

gravity The heaviness or weight of an object resulting from the effect of the attraction between any body of matter and any planetary body.

guaiac test Diagnostic test to detect blood in the stool.

guided imagery Technique in which patient focuses on an image, becoming less aware of pain.

gurgle Abnormal coarse sound heard during auscultation of the lung. Produced by air entering large mucus-containing airways.

H

halitosis Offensive breath resulting from poor oral hygiene, dental or oral infections, ingestion of certain foods, or systemic diseases.

hand-off Effective hand-off allows for face-to-face communication when available, which permits the person receiving care of the patient the opportunity to ask questions.

hand rolls Cylindrical rolls of cloth or gauze placed against the palmar surface of a patient's hand to maintain hand, thumb, and fingers in a functional position.

Harris splint Expandable splint that supports the thigh in skeletal traction.

hazard/hazard identification A condition or phenomenon that increases the probability of a loss that may result in injury or illness/recognition of conditions or agents creating risk.

healing ridge Induration of collagen deposits beneath the skin extending to about 1 cm on each side of the wound.

health care—acquired infection Infection that was not present or incubating at time of admission.

Health Insurance Portability and Accountability Act (HIPAA) A federal law designed to protect the privacy of patient health information.

heatstroke Condition characterized by core body temperature of 45°C (116°F).

heave A lift or thrust felt during palpation of the heart.

hematemesis Vomiting of blood.

hematology The study of blood cells.

hematoma Collection of extravasated blood trapped in the tissues of the skin or in an organ. Results from trauma or incomplete coagulation.

hematopoiesis The formation and development of blood cells in bone marrow.

hematuria Abnormal presence of blood in the urine.

hemiparesis Muscular weakness of one half of the body.

hemiplegia Paralysis of one side of the body.

hemoconcentration The concentration of red blood cells in one area.

hemodialysis A procedure in which impurities or wastes are removed from the blood. Used in treating renal insufficiency and various toxic conditions.

hemodynamics The study of movements of the blood and the forces concerned therein.

hemolysis The destruction of red blood cells.

hemopneumothorax An accumulation of both air and blood in the intrapleural space. This condition is characterized by the signs and symptoms listed with pneumothorax and hemothorax.

hemoptysis Coughing up of blood from the respiratory tract.

hemorrhoids A varicosity in the lower rectum or anus caused by congestion in the hemorrhoidal veins.

hemostasis Termination of bleeding by mechanical or chemical means or by the coagulation process of the body.

hemothorax An accumulation of blood in the intrapleural space caused by a pulmonary infarction, tissue damage that occurs as a result of lung cancer or other chest trauma, or a complication of anticoagulant therapy after chest surgery.

Hemovac drain A type of closed drain system.

heparin lock An intravenous needle connected to a small "well" that allows for the intermittent injection of medication without the need for repeated venipuncture.

herniation The abnormal protrusion of an organ or other body structure through a defect or natural opening in a covering, membrane, muscle, or bone.

high-Fowler's position Placement of a patient in a semisitting position by raising the head of the bed more than 45 to 60 degrees.

hirsutism Excessive body hair in a masculine distribution, caused by heredity, hormonal dysfunction, or medication.

Homans' sign In the presence of phlebitis or when phlebitis is suspected, dorsiflexion of the foot elicits pain in the calf.

homeostasis The state of equilibrium (balance between opposing pressures) in the internal environment of the body, naturally maintained by adaptive responses that promote healthy survival.

hospice A system of family-centered care designed to help the terminally ill person be comfortable and maintain a satisfactory lifestyle through the phase of dying.

Hoyer lift (mechanical/hydraulic lift) Mechanical device that uses a canvas sling to easily lift dependent patients for transferring.

Huber needle Special needle with a deflected point designed to prevent damage to the silicone septum of implanted infusion ports.

humectant A substance that promotes retention of moisture.

hydrocolloid An adhesive, moldable wafer made of a carbohydrate-based material, usually with a waterproof backing. This dressing usually is impermeable to oxygen, water, and water vapor and has some absorptive properties.

hydrogel A water-based, nonadherent, polymer-based dressing that has some absorptive properties.

hygiene The science of health. Self-care measures people use to maintain their health are called *personal hygiene*.

hypercalcemia Greater-than-normal amounts of calcium in the blood.

hypercapnia Elevated arterial $PaCO_2$ greater than 45 mm Hg; also called *hypercarbia*.

hyperemia Increased blood flow in part of the body, as in the inflammatory response, local relaxation of arterioles, or obstruction of the outflow of blood from an area.

hyperextension Movement of a body part beyond its normal resting extended position.

hyperkalemia Refers to solutions with potassium concentrations greater than 5.0 mEq/L.

hypermagnesemia Refers to solutions with magnesium concentrations greater than 2.5 mEq/L.

hypernatremia Refers to solutions with sodium concentrations greater than 147 mEq/L.

hyperopia A refractive error of the eye in which parallel rays of light focus behind the retina. Causes difficulty seeing near objects.

hyperphosphatemia Refers to a higher-than-normal range of serum phosphorus. Normal range for serum phosphorus is 2.5 to 4.5 mg/100 mL (1.7 to 2.6 mEq/L).

hyperpigmentation Unusual darkening of the skin.

hypertension Condition characterized by an elevated blood pressure persistently exceeding 150/90 mm Hg.

hyperthermia Condition characterized by body temperature over 38°C (100.4°F).

hypertonic Having a greater concentration of solute than another solution, thus exerting more osmotic pressure.

hypodermoclysis The injection of an isotonic or hypotonic solution into subcutaneous tissue to supply a continuous and large amount of fluid, electrolytes, and nutrients.

hypokalemia Refers to solutions with potassium concentrations less than 3.5 mEq/L.

hypomagnesemia Refers to solutions with magnesium concentrations less than 1.5 mEq/L.

hyponatremia Refers to solutions with sodium concentrations less than 137 mEq/L.

hypoosmolar State in which there is an abnormal gain in water or loss of sodium-rich fluids with replacement by water only. As a result, there is a low concentration of solutes in the body fluids.

hypophosphatemia Refers to a lower-than-normal range of serum phosphorus. Normal range of serum phosphorus is 2.5 to 4.5 mg/100 mL (1.7 to 2.6 mEq/L).

hypotension Condition characterized by a low blood pressure that is inadequate to perfuse and oxygenate body tissue.

hypotheses Predictions about the relationships between or among the variables of a research study.

hypothermia Condition characterized by body temperature below 36°C (96.8°F).

hypothermia therapy Techniques used to reduce elevated body temperature.

hypotonic Having a smaller concentration of solute than another solution, thus exerting less osmotic pressure.

hypovolemic shock State of physical collapse caused by massive blood loss, circulatory dysfunction, and inadequate tissue perfusion.

hypoxemia Abnormal deficiency of oxygen in arterial blood.

hypoxia Insufficient oxygen available to meet the metabolic needs of tissues and cells.

I

idiosyncratic reaction A response to a medication or therapy that is unique to an individual.

ileal conduit A method of urinary diversion through intestinal tissue. Ureters are implanted in a section of dissected ileum that is then sewed to an ostomy in the abdominal wall.

ileostomy Surgical formation of an opening of the ileum onto the surface of the abdomen through which fecal matter is emptied.

immobility Pertaining to the inability of a body part or limb to be moved.

immunocompromised A state of defective or failed immune response that makes a person more likely to acquire an infection.

impaction Presence of a large or hard fecal mass in the rectum or colon.

implanted subcutaneous port A central venous catheter with a reservoir surgically placed under the skin that may remain in place for a prolonged period to obtain blood samples and administer medications.

incentive spirometer Individual patient device used to encourage full lung expansion. Reduces the risk for atelectasis in the immobilized or postoperative patient.

incentive spirometry Method of deep breathing providing visual feedback to patients concerning their inspiratory volume.

Incident Command System (ICS) A "first-on-scene" structure in which the first responder to a scene has charge of the scene until the incident has been declared resolved. A superior-ranking responder arrives on scene and seizes command.

incident report Confidential document that describes any patient accident while the person is on the premises of a health care agency.

incompatibility Describes two medications of different chemical makeup that cannot be mixed together.

incontinence Inability to control urination or defecation.

incontinent diversion A urinary diversion that does not give a patient the ability to control when urine exits the stoma, requiring the use of an external ostomy pouch.

incubation period Period between exposure to a pathogenic organism and the appearance of symptoms. A patient is often contagious during this time and capable of spreading disease without realizing it.

induration Hardening of a tissue, particularly the skin.

infection The invasion and reproduction of microorganisms in a body tissue that can result in a local or systemic clinical response such as cellulitis or fever.

infiltration Presence of intravenous fluids within the subcutaneous space surrounding a venipuncture site.

informed consent Permission obtained from a patient to perform a specific test or procedure.

infusate Volume of parenteral fluid infused into a patient over an established period of time.

infusion Introduction of a fluid such as a drug, electrolyte, or nutrient directly into a vein by means of gravity flow.

infusion pump Device designed to deliver a measured amount of fluid over a period of time.

injection Act of forcing a liquid into the body by means of a syringe.

injection cap A rubber diaphragm covering a plastic cap. Permits needle insertion into a catheter or vial.

inspection A physical examination skill involving the examiner's looking at external and internal body parts for physical characteristics.

insulator A substance that conducts temperatures poorly used to protect skin and tissues from hot or cold therapies.

intake Measurement of the ingestion or infusion of liquids into the body, including all liquids and semi-liquids, liquid medications, enteral tube feedings, intravenous therapy, blood components, and parenteral nutrition.

integument Skin and its appendages (i.e., hair, nails, and sweat and sebaceous glands).

intercostal space (ICS) Space found between adjoining ribs.

internal rotation Rotation of a joint inward.

International Nursing Coalition for Mass Casualty Education (INCMCE) Now known as *Nursing Emergency Preparedness Education Coalition (NEPEC)*. Coordinated by Vanderbilt University School of Nursing. It was founded in response to recognition of the need for nurses to be more adequately prepared to respond to mass casualty events.

interviewing The process of conducting an organized, systematic conversation with a patient. Designed to gather information regarding a patient's level of health, response to care, or perception of symptoms or events.

intestinal obstruction Any obstruction that results in failure of the contents of the intestine to pass through the lumen of the bowel.

intraabdominal pressure Amount of tension within the abdominal cavity.

intracavitary Within a body cavity.

intracellular fluid Liquid within the cell membrane.

intraclavicular fossa Small pocket area or indentation just below the clavicle on both sides of the neck.

intradermal (ID) injection Form of injection in which a solution is introduced into the dermal skin layer.

intramuscular (IM) injection Form of injection in which a solution is introduced into the body of a muscle.

intrapleural Pertaining to or affecting the potential space between the parietal and visceral pleurae.

intrapulmonic Pertaining to or affecting the spaces within the lungs.

intraspinal Referring to both the epidural and intrathecal routes of medication administration.

intrathecal Of or pertaining to a structure, process, or substance within a sheath, as within the spinal canal.

intravenous conscious sedation (IVCS) The intravenous administration of pharmacological agents to provide a minimally depressed level of consciousness to provide comfort during diagnostic or treatment procedures.

intravenous (IV) injection Form of injection in which a solution is introduced into a vein.

introitus An entrance or orifice into a cavity.

intubation Passage of a tube into a body aperture.

invasive Referring to procedures that involve puncture, incision, or insertion of a foreign object into the body.

invasive procedure A procedure in which the normal protective barrier of the skin or mucous membrane is broken or compromised (e.g., an intravenous puncture or a bladder catheterization).

inversion Turning something upside down.

irrigate To flush with a fluid, usually with a slow, steady pressure on a syringe plunger. Done to cleanse a wound or clear tubing.

irrigation Gentle washing of an area with a stream of solution.

ischemia A decreased supply of oxygenated blood to a body organ or part.

isolation Infection control and prevention methods such as barrier technique that are used to decrease the transmission of microorganisms.

isometric contraction Increased muscle tension without muscle shortening.

isometric exercise The tightening or tensing of muscles without moving body parts.

isotonic A solution with a total electrolyte content of approximately 310 mEq/L.

isotonic solution Having the same concentration of solute as another solution, thus exerting the same amount of osmotic pressure as the solution.

intravenous (IV) plug A small rubber or plastic cap that connects to the open end of a patient's IV access catheter. Also referred to as *injection cap* because a needle can be inserted into the rubber cap for the administration or aspiration of fluids.

J

jacket restraints Vestlike restraints that usually cross on the back of a patient but may also cross on the front.

Jackson-Pratt drain A closed drain system.

jejunostomy feeding tube A hollow tube inserted into the jejunum through the abdominal wall for administration of liquefied foods.

joint Any one of the connections between bones.

K

karaya A natural gum product that softens with body heat and conforms to the contours around the stoma.

Kardex Trade name for a card filing system that allows quick reference to the particular need of the patient for certain aspects of nursing care.

keloid An overgrowth of scar tissue at the site of skin injury such as a wound or surgical incision.

ketone An organic chemical compound with two compounds attached to it.

kilogram The metric conversion for a pound; weight (pounds) ÷ 2.2 = kilograms.

kinesthetic Related to the ability to perceive the existence or direction of weight or movement.

L

laryngospasm Spasm of the muscles surrounding the larynx causing airway narrowing and stridorous breathing.

lateral flexion A range of joint motion exercise during which the head is tilted as far as possible toward each shoulder. Maintains neck mobility.

latex allergy reaction Allergic response to products containing latex (e.g., gloves, medical devices). Can present as contact dermatitis, allergic rhinitis, or immediate life-threatening reactions leading to such conditions as urticaria, bronchospasm, and edema.

lavage The irrigation or washing out of an organ or cavity.

let-down reflex A normal reflex in a lactating woman often elicited by tactile stimulation of the nipple, resulting in release of milk from the glands of the breast.

leukopenia A decrease in circulating white blood cells.

leverage Occurs when specific bones such as the humerus, ulna, and radius and the associated joints such as the elbow joint act together as a lever.

line of gravity An imaginary line that goes from the center of gravity to the base of support.

lipid emulsion A soybean oil.

lipodystrophy Any abnormality in metabolism and deposition of fat.

logrolling Maneuver used to turn a reclining patient from one side to the other or completely over without flexing the spinal column.

loss Absence of a significant other, object, or state of health to which the person must adapt through the grieving process.

lotion Liquid preparation applied externally to protect the skin or treat a dermatological disorder.

lumen The hollow channel within a tube.

lunula A semilunar structure such as the crescent-shaped pale area at the base of the nail of a finger or toe.

M

macerate To soften, usually by soaking in water.

maceration Skin that becomes abnormally soft and breaks down because of prolonged exposure to moisture.

maculopapular Discolored elevated lesions on the skin.

malabsorption Impaired absorption of nutrients from the gastrointestinal tract.

malignant hyperthermia An autosomal-dominant trait characterized by often fatal hyperthermia with rigidity of the muscles occurring in affected people exposed to certain anesthetic agents.

malnutrition Any disorder of nutrition.

manmade disaster A catastrophic event, the principal direct cause of which is attributable to human action.

manometer An instrument for measuring pressure or tension of liquids or gases.

manual defibrillator Device used by trained personnel to treat fast, irregular dysrhythmias with electrical shock to the heart.

mass casualty disaster/event/incident (MCI) Any event or situation that results in multiple casualties and/or deaths; an MCI exists when health care needs exceed health care resources.

mass casualty triage Move, Assess, Sort, and Send (MASS) approach to triage initially sorts victims into groups, which are then evaluated for transportation to treatment.

massage A form of cutaneous stimulation that involves the application of touch and movement to muscles, tendons, and ligaments.

mastication Chewing, tearing, or grinding food with the teeth while it mixes with saliva.

material safety data sheet (MSDS) A form containing data about the properties of the particular chemical and information for handling the substance in a safe manner (e.g., storage, disposal, protective equipment, and spill-handling procedures).

maturational loss A loss expressed as any change in a person's developmental process that is normally expected during a lifetime.

meatus Any opening or tunnel through any part of the body (e.g., the point at which the urethra opens to the skin).

mediastinal shift A condition in which the mediastinal contents move toward the unaffected side in the presence of a pneumothorax, hemothorax, or hemopneumothorax. The mediastinal shift causes compression of the organs and is a life-threatening situation.

medical asepsis The techniques used to reduce and prevent the spread of microorganisms (clean technique).

medical disaster A catastrophic event that results in human casualties that overwhelm the available health care resources.

medicated enema Administration of a medication via an enema. Usually used before surgery with patients scheduled for bowel surgery.

medication administration record (MAR) The report that serves as a legal record of the medications administered to a patient at a facility by a nurse or other health care professional.

medication dependence Two types of medication dependence exist: psychological (or addiction) and physical. In psychological dependence a patient desires the medication for some benefit other than the intended effect. The individual believes that a desirable effect will result when taking the medication. Physical dependence involves a physiological adaptation to a medication that manifests itself by intense physical disturbance when the medication is withdrawn.

medication plateau Blood serum concentration reached and maintained after repeated, fixed doses.

medication reconciliation A process completed during all care transitions (e.g., patient transfer from the intensive care unit to a medical-surgical unit) whereby current medication orders are compared to all medication the patient has taken previously. Reconciliation is completed in an effort to minimize the risk of drug omissions, dosing errors, drug interactions, and duplicative orders.

medication tolerance Decreased physiological response after repeated administration of a medication or a chemically related substance.

medullary Of or pertaining to the medulla of the brain.

melanin Black or dark brown pigment that occurs naturally in the skin, hair, and iris.

melanocyte A body cell capable of producing melanin, the pigment of the skin.

melena Darkening of the feces by blood pigments.

metastasis Process by which tumor cells are spread to distant parts of the body.

metered-dose inhaler (MDI) A device designed to deliver a measured dose of an inhalation drug.

microorganisms Any microscopic entity capable of sustaining living processes such as bacteria, virus, or fungi, only some of which typically cause human disease.

microvasculature The portion of the circulatory system composed of the capillary network.

micturition Urination. Act of passing or expelling urine voluntarily through the urethra.

midarm circumference (MAC) A measurement of the circumference of the upper arm used to estimate muscle mass.

midstream collection Procedure in which a patient initiates a stream of urine, inserts a sterile collection cup into the stream, and then withdraws the cup before the stream of urine stops.

milliequivalent per liter (mEq/L) Number of grams of a specific electrolyte dissolved in 1 L of plasma.

Minerva jacket Cast encasing the head (with face and ears exposed) and continuing over the thorax and back to the iliac crests.

minimal sedation Lightest level of sedation; includes local and topical anesthetics and peripheral nerve blocks.

mitten restraints Thumbless mitten devices used to restrain a patient's hands.

mobility The amount and quality of physical activity.

moderate sedation A drug-induced depression of consciousness during which patients respond purposefully to verbal commands, either alone or accompanied by light tactile stimulation.

Modified Ramsay Sedation Scale A numeric rating scale used to evaluate patient's level of sedation.

moleskin Adhesive-backed tape used for some forms of skin traction.

morgue A unit of a hospital with facilities for the storage and autopsy of the dead.

mucociliary transport Process in which cilia lining the tracheobronchial tree sweep mucus upward toward the esophagus to keep airways clear of inhaled particulate.

mucopurulent Characteristic of a combination of mucus and pus.

mummy restraints Blanket or sheet folded in such a manner as to restrain a small child or infant.

mutual aid agreement Reciprocal agreement to provide help between two or more agencies.

mydriasis Dilation of the pupil of the eye caused by contraction of dilator muscles of the iris.

mydriatics Ophthalmic preparations that stimulate the sympathetic nerve fibers or block parasympathetic nerve fibers of the eye, temporarily paralyzing the iris sphincter muscle.

myelosuppression A decrease in the cellular components of the bone marrow.

N

nares The pairs of anterior and posterior openings in the nose that allow for passage of air to the pharynx and lungs.

nasal Of or pertaining to the nose and nasal cavity.

nasal cannula Device for delivering oxygen by way of two small tubes that are inserted into the nares.

nasogastric (NG) feeding tube A small tube that is passed via the nares into the stomach.

nasointestinal (NI) feeding tube Tungsten-weighted tube inserted through the naris to allow natural peristaltic movement of the tube through the pyloric sphincter into the duodenum or jejunum.

National Dysphagia Diet Released in October 2002, the National Dysphagia Diet provides recommendations for uniformity of dysphagia diets for all health care facilities. Solid and liquid diets are separated into four levels.

natural/environmental disaster A catastrophic event that results from an ecological event that exceeds the capacity of the community.

nebulization Vaporization or dispersion of a liquid in a fine spray.

nebulizer Device used to distribute medication throughout nasal passages and tracheobronchial airway by vaporizing the medication.

necrosis Localized tissue death.

necrotic Related to death of a portion of tissue.

negative pressure Pressure (measured in millimeters of mercury [mm Hg]) that is less than atmospheric pressure.

negative pressure ventilation Therapy used for patients with primary neuromuscular illnesses that interfere with normal respiratory muscle function. The patient is fitted with a poncho or shell that is connected to the ventilator. Air is removed from between the patient's chest wall and the interior wall of the poncho or shell, causing the patient to inhale.

negative pressure wound therapy The application of pressure less than the ambient atmospheric pressure (as in a vacuum) to a wound to draw wound edges together, remove exudates and excess moisture, and promote healing.

negligence Omission of care.

neovascular assessment Series of eight observations required to measure neurological and circulatory status of a patient's peripheral tissue.

neovascularization The process by which the vascular network in a wound is generated. This can also be called angiogenesis.

neurological Pertaining to the study and treatment of the nervous system.

neuropathy An abnormal condition characterized by inflammation and degeneration of the peripheral nerves.

neurovascular assessment Series of eight observations (assessments) required to measure neurological and circulatory status of a patient's peripheral tissues.

neutropenia An abnormal decrease in the number of neutrophils in the blood.

neutropenic Having an abnormal decrease in the number of neutrophils (white blood cells) in the blood.

nitroglycerin Medication that causes dilation of coronary arteries.

noncontinent (incontinent) ostomy/diversion Results from a surgical procedure that leaves a patient with an external stoma through which either stool or urine drains. It is noncontinent/incontinent because the effluent drains spontaneously from the stoma and the patient must continuously wear an external ostomy pouch over the stoma.

noncoring Huber needle A specially designed needle (straight or a 90-degree needle) intended for use with a vascular access device. This needle permits penetration into the chamber of the vascular access device without causing damage and thus permits repeated administration of medication directly into a patient's bloodstream.

noninvasive ventilation (NIV) Noninvasive ventilation (NIV) maintains positive airway pressure and improves alveolar ventilation without the need for an artificial airway. In addition, this mechanical ventilator alternative reduces and reverses atelectasis, improves oxygenation, reduces pulmonary edema, and improves cardiac function.

nonopioids Analgesics that do not contain opioids.

nonpharmacological aids Interventions used to prevent illness and promote health without the use of or in addition to the use of medications.

nontunneled percutaneous central venous catheters Intravenous access devices inserted into the internal jugular, subclavian, or femoral vein by direct venipuncture into the vein.

noxious Harmful, injurious, or detrimental to health.

NPO Nothing to be taken or given by mouth.

nuclear event The release of radiation by a device in an explosive manner as a result of a nuclear chain reaction.

nutritional risk The potential to become malnourished because of factors that are primary (e.g., inadequate intake) or secondary (e.g., disease).

nutritional screening The systematic process of identifying risk factors related to nutritional problems and malnutrition.

nutritional support nursing The care of individuals with potential or known nutrition alterations. The goal is to help individuals restore and maintain optimal nutritional health.

O

objective data Data obtained by an observer (nurse) through direct physical examination, including observation, palpation, and auscultation, and by laboratory analyses and radiological and other studies.

obstipation The absolute inability to pass stool.

obturator Small dull-pointed introducer inserted in outer cannula that facilitates insertion of tracheostomy tube by gradually widening or dilating stoma to width of tracheostomy tube.

occlusive dressing A dressing that prevents air from reaching a wound or lesion and retains moisture, heat, body fluids, and medication.

occult blood Blood that appears from a nonspecific source, with obscure signs and symptoms. May be detected by means of a chemical test or microscopic examination.

ocular Of or pertaining to the eye.

oil-retention enema An enema containing a small volume of an oil-based solution. Used to soften fecal mass.

ointment A semisolid, externally applied preparation, usually containing a drug.

olfaction The sense of smell.

oncology A branch of medicine regarding the study of tumors.

onset of medication action Period of time after a drug is administered for it to produce a response.

opening pressure The amount of tension measured in a manometer following insertion of a spinal needle into the subarachnoid space.

ophthalmic Of or pertaining to the eye.

opioids Pertaining to natural and synthetic chemicals that have opium-like effects although they are not derived from opium.

opposition The relation between the thumb and the other digits of the hand for the purpose of grasping objects between the thumb and fingers. This maneuver is used during range-of-joint-motion exercises to maintain grasping ability of a patient.

oral airway Minimally flexible curved piece of plastic extending from the exterior of the lips over the tongue to the pharynx.

Organ Procurement Agency (OPA) Community-based agency, the focus of which is to obtain donated organs for transplantation.

organ/tissue donation Families and significant others are offered the option of organ and/or tissue donation. This process includes but is not limited to the donation of heart, lung, kidneys, liver, corneal tissue, and bone.

orientation phase Period in the nurse-patient relationship when a nurse and patient first meet and set the tone for the rest of their relationship, assessing the patient's situation and setting goals.

orthopedics Branch of medicine devoted to the study and treatment of the skeletal system, its joints, muscles, and associated structures.

orthopnea An abnormal condition in which a person must sit or stand to breathe deeply or comfortably.

orthostatic hypotension A drop in blood pressure of 15 mm Hg or more when an individual rises from a sitting to a standing position.

orthotopic neobladder A type of continent urinary diversion that uses an ileal pouch to replace the bladder. The ileal pouch is the same anatomical position as the bladder. The patient uses pelvic muscle exercises and bladder-training exercises to achieve urinary continence.

osteoblastic Physiological activity that leads to the formation of specific bone tissue, osteoblasts.

osteoblasts Osteoblasts synthesize the collagen and glycoproteins to form the matrix for bone formation.

osteoclastic Physiological activity producing osteoclast bone cells that function in the development and periods of bone growth and repair, such as the breakdown and resorption of osseous tissue.

ostomy A surgical procedure in which the elimination of stool or urine is rerouted from the usual exiting part of the patient. Instead, the stool or urine exits the body through a surgically created opening called a *stoma*.

otic Of or pertaining to the ear.

otitis media Inflammation or infection of the middle ear, a common childhood affliction.

ototoxic Having a harmful effect on the eighth cranial nerve or the organs of hearing and balance.

outer cannula Main portion of tracheostomy tube through which patient breathes, which stays in place at all times. The pilot balloon and faceplate are connected to the outer cannula.

output Includes all liquids excreted, such as urine, vomitus, and diarrhea, and drainage from wounds, fistulas, and suction equipment.

overdose Oral or parenteral ingestion of an excessive quantity of a medication or drug.

over-the-counter (OTC) medication Drug available to a consumer without a prescription.

over-the-needle catheter (ONC) A type of angiocatheter. The needle used for peripheral intravenous access is encased in a catheter made of Teflon, plastic, or another flexible material. After the needle pierces the skin, the catheter is threaded into a vein, and the needle is withdrawn. The catheter remains in the vein for the instillation of fluid.

oximetry Procedure used to measure amount of oxygenated hemoglobin.

oxygen mask A flexible mask that fits snugly and securely over a patient's nose and mouth for delivery of oxygen.

oxygen saturation Amount of hemoglobin that is fully saturated with oxygen expressed as percentage of total available hemoglobin.

oxygen therapy Administration of oxygen by any route to a patient to prevent or relieve hypoxia.

oxygen toxicity Administration of oxygen level greater than 50% for greater than 24 hours that results in increased permeability of the alveolar wall, alveolar-capillary leakage, noncardiogenic pulmonary edema, decreased lung compliance, and respiratory failure.

P

pain Subjective, unpleasant sensation caused by noxious stimulation of sensory nerve endings.

pain intensity The degree or extent of pain perceived by an individual.

pain rating scales Graphic or numeric representations that allow patients to quantify their pain experience.

pain threshold The amount of pain stimulus required to produce a physical or psychological response.

pain tolerance Point at which a person is not willing to accept pain of greater severity or duration.

palliative care The prevention, relief, reduction, or soothing of symptoms of disease or disorders without effecting a cure.

pallor Unnatural paleness or absence of color in the skin.

palpation A technique used in physical examination in which the examiner feels the texture, size, consistency, and location of certain parts of the body with the hands.

palpebra Portion of the conjunctiva that lines the inner surface of the eyelids. It is thick, opaque, and highly vascular.

pandemic Occurring throughout the population of a country, a people, or the world.

paralysis An abnormal condition characterized by loss of muscle function or the loss of sensation.

paralytic ileus A decrease in or absence of intestinal peristalsis that may occur after abdominal surgery, illness, or trauma.

paraphrasing Transforming a patient's words into the nurse's words, keeping the meaning intact.

parenteral Not in or through the digestive system.

parenteral nutrition (PN) The administration of nutrition into the vascular system.

paresis Slight or partial paralysis related in some cases to local neuritis.

parietal pleura The pleural membrane that lines the thoracic cavity.

passive range-of-motion exercises Exercises of the joints performed for an individual by someone else.

patency Absence of obstruction such as clots within an intravenous (IV) needle or kinks within IV tubing; the state of being open and unblocked.

pathogen Microorganism capable of producing disease.

pathogenic microorganisms Those capable of producing an infection or disease.

Patient Care Partnership A list of patient's rights promulgated by the American Hospital Association. It offers some guidance and protection to patients by stating the responsibilities that a hospital and its staff have toward patients and families during hospitalization. It is not a legally binding document.

patient care profile (PCP) A report that is automatically updated each shift within a computerized medical record.

Patient Self-Determination Act Legislation that requires all Medicare and Medicaid recipient hospitals to provide patients with information on advance directives and their right to accept or reject medical treatment.

patient-controlled analgesia (PCA) Technique that allows patients to self-administer small, continuous doses of intravenous or subcutaneous opioids as they feel the need.

patient's rights The rights to which patients are entitled as recipients of medical care.

peak action Time it takes for a drug to reach its highest effective concentration.

peak airway pressure The highest amount of positive pressure needed to inflate the lung.

peak concentration The highest effective concentration of a drug in the serum.

Pearson attachment The support used under the leg in balanced-suspension skeletal traction.

pediculosis Infestation of the integument with blood-sucking lice.

peer reviewed Process by which experts in a field evaluate an article or report for the quality of its scholarship, relevance to its field, and appropriateness for publication in which it may appear. Only those articles judged to meet the highest standards will be published.

PEH Acronym for pseudoepitheliomatous hyperplasia. Maceration of skin surrounding the stoma.

pelvic belt Girdle-shaped cotton belt or support that fits around the hips, lumbosacral area, and abdomen for attaching ropes and weights in pelvic belt traction.

pelvic sling A hammocklike sling that fits under a patient's lumbosacral area and hips and is then connected to ropes and weights. It suspends the pelvis off the bed as treatment for fractures of pelvic bones.

Penrose drain An open drain system.

perceived loss Any loss that is tangible and uniquely defined by the grieving patient. It may be less obvious to others.

percussion A technique in physical examination used to assess the size, borders, and consistency of some of the internal organs and to discover the presence and evaluate the amount of fluid in a cavity of the body.

percutaneous Performed through the skin, such as a biopsy or the aspiration of fluid from a space below the skin using a needle, catheter, and syringe.

percutaneous coronary intervention (PCI) Procedures such as percutaneous transluminal coronary angioplasty (PTCA) or directional coronary atherectomy (DCA) performed during cardiac catheterization.

perfusion Effect of pulmonary circulation in moving blood to and from the blood-gas barrier so gas exchange can occur.

periodontal Referring to tissues surrounding the teeth, such as the gums and buccal mucosa.

periodontitis Receding gum lines, inflammation, and gaps between teeth.

perioperative Related to the entire surgical experience.

peripherally inserted central catheter (PICC) A peripherally inserted catheter that extends to the superior vena cava or right atrium.

peristomal Referring to the area of skin surrounding a surgically created stoma.

peritoneal fluid Substance in the abdominal cavity for lubrication of peritoneal membrane and internal organs.

peritonitis Inflammation of peritoneum produced by bacteria or irritating substances introduced into the abdominal cavity by a penetrating wound or perforation of an organ in the gastrointestinal or reproductive tract.

PERRLA Acronym for pupils equal, round, reactive to light, and accommodation. The acronym is recorded in the physical examination if pupil assessment is normal.

petaling Finishing the raw or ragged edges of a plaster cast to prevent skin irritation or pressure.

pétrissage A massage technique in which the skin is gently lifted and squeezed.

pharmacokinetics The study of how medications enter the body, reach their site of action, are metabolized, and exit the body.

pharmacological agents Oral, parenteral, or topical substances used to alleviate symptoms and treat or control illness.

pharynx The throat.

phlebitis Inflammation of a vein.

phlebitis solution A hypertonic solution capable of causing inflammation of a vein.

phlebothrombosis Blood clot formation.

phlebotomy The incision of a vein for the letting of blood, as in collecting blood from a donor.

physical dependence A physiological state in which abrupt cessation of a drug results in a withdrawal syndrome.

physical restraint Any device, garment, material, or object that restricts a person's freedom of movement or access to one's body.

PICO A format approach for organizing a clinical question into four components; patient population, intervention or area of interest, comparison of interest, and outcome.

PIE An acronym for problem, intervention, and evaluation. Used as an organizing framework for narrative nurses' notes.

piggyback infusion Method for administering intravenous (IV) medications intermittently; a piggyback IV set is a supplementary set that connects with the primary IV tubing.

piloerection Erection of hair caused by the action of the arrectores pilorum muscles, the smooth muscles attached to the hair follicles. Commonly referred to as goose bumps.

plantar flexion Flexion of the foot and toes toward the sole.

plaque (dental) A thin film on teeth made up of mucin and colloidal material found in saliva and often secondarily invaded by bacteria.

plateau Blood serum concentration reached and maintained after repeated, fixed doses of a drug.

pleura Delicate serous membrane enclosing the lung.

pleural cavity Space between visceral and parietal pleurae. Pressure within the cavity is negative when compared with atmospheric pressure.

pleural fluid Substance contained between visceral and parietal pleurae for lubrication of the membranes.

pneumonitis Inflammation of the lung. May be caused by a virus or may be a hypersensitivity reaction that occurs as a result of allergy to chemical or organic dusts.

pneumothorax An accumulation of air in the intrapleural space caused by a severe blow to the chest, extremely forceful cough, chest trauma, or open-chest surgery.

podiatrist A health care professional trained to diagnose and treat diseases and disorders of the feet.

point of maximal impulse (PMI) Point at which the heartbeat can most easily be palpated through the chest wall, usually along the left midclavicular line at the fourth or fifth intercostal space.

point-of-care test Performing laboratory tests at the primary care setting, such as the bedside (e.g., glucose monitoring or assay of whole blood, plasma, or serum).

polypharmacy Concurrent prescription, administration, or use of multiple medications, some of which may not be indicated clinically.

POMR An acronym for *problem-oriented medical record*. Used as an organizing framework for a patient's complete medical record.

positive end expiratory pressure (PEEP) The application of positive airway pressure at the end of exhalation through a ventilator or breathing device.

positive pressure Pressure measured in millimeters of mercury (mm Hg) that is greater than atmospheric pressure.

positive-pressure ventilation Mechanical ventilation that delivers compressed gas to the airways at greater than ambient pressure.

postanesthesia care unit (PACU) Postsurgical recovery area where patients are closely monitored and stabilized before discharge to a specific nursing unit or, in the case of same day surgery, to home.

postcast care Nursing interventions performed for and with patients in casts or after cast removal.

postmortem care Care provided to the body after death.

postoperative Period of time after completion of a surgical procedure wherein a nurse monitors a patient's recovery.

postural Position of the body. Usually refers to change of position from supine to sitting, sitting to standing.

postural drainage Gravitational clearance of airway secretions by assumption of one or more of 10 different body positions for 5 to 15 minutes each. Each posture corresponds to specific segments of bronchi in the lung.

postural hypotension Condition in which a normotensive person becomes light-headed or dizzy and experiences low blood pressure when rising to an upright position.

posture Position of the body in relation to the surrounding space.

prealbumin A plasma protein with a half-life of only 2 days, used as a marker of nutritional status.

precordial Of or pertaining to the precordium, which forms the region over the heart and the lower part of the thorax.

preemptive analgesia A method of preventing pain while reducing opioid use.

premature ventricular contraction (PVC) A cardiac dysrhythmia characterized by a ventricular contraction preceding the expected contraction; it appears on an electrocardiogram as an early, wide QRS complex without a preceding P wave.

preoperative The period of time preceding induction of anesthesia and the beginning of a surgical procedure.

preoperative checklist Agency-specific list of guidelines for ensuring completion of nursing interventions. This list includes items to be assessed or verified (e.g., verification that preoperative orders are written and completed, laboratory work is in the patient's medical record, the patient has voided, current vital signs are documented).

presbycusis Loss of hearing sensitivity and speech intelligibility. Associated with aging.

presbyopia Farsightedness resulting from a loss of elasticity of the lens of the eye. The condition commonly develops with advancing age.

pressure dressing A temporary treatment for the control of excessive bleeding. Pressure dressings require elastic bandages to maintain the pressure and may also require the application of sandbags adjacent to the dressing to augment pressure.

pressure ulcer A lesion that develops in the skin as a result of prolonged, unrelieved pressure.

primary dressing A dressing that comes in direct contact with the wound bed.

primary intention Primary union of the edges of a wound, progressing to complete scar formation with granulation.

prn "As needed." Administration times are determined by the patient's needs.

problem-oriented medical record (POMR) Method of recording data about the health status of a patient that fosters a collaborative problem-solving approach by all members of the health care team.

procedural sedation An anesthetic procedure in which analgesia and anesthesia are accomplished without loss of consciousness.

pronation Movement of a body part so the front or ventral surface faces downward.

proprioceptive function Sensation that is achieved through stimuli originating from within the body regarding spatial position and muscular activity.

prosthesis An artificial replacement for a missing part of the body.

pruritus The symptom of itching.

pseudoaddiction Exhibition of drug-seeking behaviors although the true driving factor is pain relief, not physical addiction.

Pseudomonas A genus of gram-negative bacteria that includes several free-living species of soil and water and some opportunistic pathogens isolated from wounds and sputum. May produce blue and yellow pigments.

pulleys Mechanical round, grooved disks over which ropes can move freely for traction pull.

pulmonary aspiration The entry of secretions or foreign material into the trachea and lungs.

pulmonary edema Accumulation of extracellular fluid in a patient's lung tissue and alveoli, commonly caused by left-sided heart failure, fluid overload.

pulse deficit Condition characterized by difference between apical and peripheral pulse rate that results in a lack of peripheral perfusion.

pyrexia Fever. An elevation of the body temperature above the normal range.

pyrogen Any substance or agent that tends to cause a rise in body temperature, such as some bacterial toxins.

Q

quality assurance In health care, any evaluation of services provided and results achieved compared with accepted standards.

R

radial flexion A range-of-motion exercise during which there is a bending of the wrist medially toward the thumb; maintains wrist mobility.

radiopaque Not permitting the passage of x-rays or other radiant energy. Bones are relatively radiopaque and therefore show as white areas on an exposed x-ray film.

random voided specimen A urine specimen obtained at any point of a 24-hour period.

reactive hyperemia The return of blood to an area of tissue on the release of externally applied pressure.

reagent Chemical used to indicate the presence of a particular substance.

reduction The alignment of fracture fragments through manipulation. Closed reduction is accomplished through manual manipulation and casting or traction.

reflecting A cognitive strategy that involves reappraisal of one's actions to evaluate outcomes. A communication strategy used to clarify what a patient is feeling and affirm that the patient's feelings are acceptable.

refractive error Condition in which parallel rays of light are not brought to focus on the retina.

registered dietitian (RD) A health care professional who has successfully completed an examination and maintains continuing education requirements in nutritional care for individuals and groups.

registered nurse first assistant (RNFA) A nurse with advanced education who assists the surgeon with surgical procedures, performing a combination of nursing and medical functions.

reinfusion device An apparatus that is placed, usually intraoperatively during orthopedic or vascular procedures, into a space where significant blood loss is anticipated. This device collects the blood, filters it, and is then used to reinfuse that blood intravascularly.

relaxation A cognitive strategy that provides mental and physical pain relief or reduces pain.

reminiscing A form of therapy for older adults that provides a life review. Individual talks about remote memories, expression of related feelings, and recognition of both positive experiences and conflicts.

remission The partial or complete disappearance of the clinical and subjective characteristics of a chronic or malignant disease.

renal insufficiency Partial kidney failure characterized by less-than-normal urinary excretion and abnormal urinary laboratory results (e.g., creatinine, blood urea nitrogen level).

residual urine The volume of urine in the bladder after a normal voiding.

residual volume The amount of fluid that pools in the stomach or intestine that is able to be aspirated from a gastric or intestinal tube at any given time.

resistive isometric exercise Contracting of muscles while pushing against a stationary object or resisting the movement of an object.

respiratory arrest Cessation of respirations.

respiratory distress Difficulty breathing that may be associated with abnormal blood oxygen or carbon dioxide levels and may require supportive measures to preserve life.

respite care Provision of short-term relief or time off for people providing home care to an ill, disabled, or frail older adult.

restating A communication strategy involving the reiteration of a patient's verbal statements and/or questions using similar words. This affirms that the message was acknowledged by the nurse.

restating The process of verbally clarifying information provided by a patient or family.

restraint Device used to immobilize a patient or an extremity.

reverse Trendelenburg's position Position in which the lower extremities are low and the body and head are elevated on an inclined plane.

right atrial catheter An indwelling intravenous catheter inserted centrally or peripherally and threaded into the superior vena cava or right atrium.

rigidity Condition of hardness, stiffness, or inflexibility.

rigor mortis The rigid stiffening of skeletal and cardiac muscle shortly after death.

risk assessment tool for pressure ulcers Evaluation protocols for assessing the likelihood for the development of pressure ulcers. Two such protocols are the Braden Scale and the Norton Scale, which assess the following five risk factors: physical condition, mental state, activity, mobility, and incontinence.

rooting reflex A normal response in newborns when the cheek is touched or stroked along the side of the mouth to turn the head toward the stimulated side and begin to suck.

rotation A basic range of joint motion allowed by various joints. The rotation of a bone around its central axis, such as shoulder rotation.

Rotokinetic bed A special bed equipped with an automatic turning device that completely immobilizes patients while rotating them from 90 to 270 degrees along a horizontal axis.

S

S_1 Symbol for the first heart sound in the cardiac cycle occurring with ventricular systole. It is associated with the closure of the mitral and tricuspid valves.

S_2 Symbol for the second heart sound in the cardiac cycle. It is associated with closure of the aortic and pulmonary valves just before ventricular diastole.

saline lock See *heparin lock.*

SBAR Stands for *situation-background-assessment-recommendation* technique that provides a framework for communication among a patient's health care team.

sclerosis Condition characterized by hardening of tissue resulting from any of several causes, including inflammation, the deposit of mineral salts, and infiltration of connective tissue cells.

scrub nurse Surgical nurse whose primary responsibility is to provide the surgeon with instruments and supplies during surgery, which requires strict surgical asepsis. In addition, this nurse along with the circulating nurse disposes of soiled sponges and accounts for sponges, needles, and instruments on the surgical field.

scrubbed team members Includes the surgeon and scrub nurse or technician and assisting physicians who are scrubbed.

sebaceous gland One of the small glands in the dermis that secretes an oily substance (sebum) on the surface of the skin and in the hair.

seborrheic dermatitis A common and chronic inflammatory skin disease characterized by dry or moist greasy scales and yellow crusts.

sebum Oily secretion of the sebaceous glands of the skin. When combined with sweat, sebum forms a moist, oily, acidic film that is antibacterial and antifungal and protects the skin against drying.

secondary dressing A dressing used to cover or hold primary dressings in place.

secondary intention Wound closure in which the edges are separated, granulation tissue develops to fill the gap and, finally, epithelium grows in over the granulation, producing a larger scar than results with primary intention.

secretion A product produced by a gland of the body.

seizure A hyperexcitation of neurons in the brain leading to a sudden, violent, involuntary series of muscle contractions that may be paroxysmal and episodic, as in a seizure disorder, or transient and acute, as after a head injury.

seizure precautions Measures that protect a patient from injury during a seizure.

self-catheterization The ability of individuals to insert a urinary catheter into their urinary meatus.

semi-Fowler's position Placement of patient in an inclined position, with the upper half of the body raised by elevating the head of the bed approximately 30 to 45 degrees.

sensitivity Laboratory test used in conjunction with culture. It measures the response of microorganisms to antibiotics that have been placed on a culture plate.

sentinel event An incident that involves serious physical or psychological injury or death or the risk thereof.

sepsis Infection, contamination.

serology Branch of medicine dealing with serum and blood products.

serum half-life The time it takes for the excretion process to lower the serum medication concentration by half.

shaking Physiotherapy technique in which a concurrent, compressive force is supplied to the chest wall.

sharps container A puncture-proof container that is used for the disposal of any used sharp items such as needles, disposable scissors, and scalpels.

shear An applied force or pressure exerted against the surface and layers of the skin as tissues slide in opposite but parallel planes.

shearing Pressure exerted against the surface and layers of the skin as tissues slide underneath the body as it moves against a surface.

shearing force An applied force or pressure exerted against the surface and layers of the skin as tissues slide in opposite but parallel planes.

sheet wadding Stretchable sheets of cotton padding used to cover skin before a cast is applied.

shelter-in-place To take refuge in a small interior room with no or few windows.

side effect An effect caused by a drug that is different from the therapeutic (desired) action. The effect may be harmless or injurious.

sigmoid colon The part of the large intestine that extends from the descending colon to the rectum.

sign Objective finding perceived by an examiner, such as a fever, rash, abnormal reflex, or abnormal breath sound.

silicone septum Silicone partition that covers the port chamber housed in the metal or plastic body of the implanted infusion port.

situational loss Loss caused by any sudden, unpredictable external event.

sitz bath Special bath in which only the hips and buttocks are immersed in fluid.

skin barrier An artificial layer of skin made of plastic or vinyl-like material that is applied to skin before application of tape or ostomy drainage bags. Protects skin from chronic irritation.

sling Device used to support or limit movement, enhance circulation, and prevent edema of the arm, hand, or wrist.

slough Necrotic (dead) tissue in the process of separating from viable portions of the body.

smart pump Infusion devices, referred to as a *smart pumps* by the Institute for Safe Medication Practices (ISMP), are commercially available infusion systems that perform a "test of reasonableness" to check that programming is within preestablished institutional limits before infusion can begin.

SOAP Acronym for *subjective, objective, assessment,* and *plan,* the four parts of the written account of a patient's health problem in a problem-oriented record.

SOAPIE See SOAP—Alternative acronym includes *intervention* and *evaluation.*

solute A substance dissolved in a solution.

solute solution Solutes are dissolved particles and are either electrolytes or nonelectrolytes. Solute solution refers to these particles when they are found in body fluids or plasma (i.e., solution).

solution A mixture of one or more substances dissolved in another substance.

spasm Involuntary muscle contraction.

speculum A retractor used to separate the walls of a cavity (e.g., the vaginal cavity).

sphygmomanometer Device used for noninvasive measurement of arterial blood pressure. Consists of cuff, air bladder, inflation bulb, and gauge to indicate amount of air pressure being exerted.

spica cast An orthopedic cast applied to immobilize part or all of the trunk of the body and part or all of one or more extremities.

splinting Supporting the abdominal area to reduce pain caused by coughing or sneezing after surgery.

sponge Gauze dressing used to absorb blood in a surgical wound.

spore An inactive but viable state of microorganisms.

spreader bar A metal bar with curved hoop areas for attaching hooks or pins for traction.

sputum Lung mucus. Normally thin, watery, and white or clear and watery.

standard precautions Techniques used to reduce the risk for the transmission of bloodborne pathogens or microorganisms present in moist body substances regardless of a patient's diagnosis or infection status.

standardized care plan Documentation that uses the nursing process format in specifying the plan of care for patient problems.

staples Stainless steel wire used to close a surgical wound.

stent A straw or tubelike device that is placed through the stoma into bowel to keep open the flow of effluent.

sterile Free from all life forms, including spores.

sterile conscience One's personal principles and morals that guide one to maintain strict asepsis and sterile techniques at all times.

sterile field A specified area, such as within a tray or a sterile drape, that is considered free from microorganisms.

sterilization Process by which microorganisms, including spores, are killed.

stockinette Stretchable cotton materials of various sizes and widths used immediately over the skin to protect tissues from the irritation of felt or plaster.

stoma Surgically created opening between a body cavity and the surface of the body such as a colostomy.

stomatitis Any inflammatory condition of the mouth.

stopcock A valve that controls the flow of fluid or air through a tube.

strategic national stockpile (SNS) A national repository of the Centers for Disease Control and Prevention for antibiotics, chemical antidotes, antitoxins, life-support medications, intravenous administration supplies, airway maintenance supplies, and medical/surgical items.

strike through Source of contamination by which moisture permeates a sterile field or barrier.

stroke volume (SV) The volume of blood ejected from the left ventricle with each ventricular contraction.

subarachnoid space Situated or occurring between the arachnoid and the pia mater membranes, which cover the brain and spinal cord.

subcutaneous emphysema The presence of free air or gas in the subcutaneous tissues.

subcutaneous injection Form of injection in which a solution is introduced into subcutaneous tissues.

subcutaneous tunnel A tunnel under the skin between the exit site of a catheter and the entrance into a body cavity (such as the epidural space) or vein.

subjective data Data collected from a patient.

sublingual Route for administering a drug beneath the tongue.

sublingual medication Medication placed under the tongue and allowed to dissolve.

suction The act of sucking up a substance by reducing air pressure over its surface.

suction catheter Thin plastic or rubber tubing used to remove secretions.

summarization Reworking a lengthy interaction or discussion into a few brief sentences.

summarizing A process in which an interviewer organizes and condenses information provided and verifies with the patient that the information is correctly interpreted.

summation Occurs when the combined effect of two drugs produces a result that equals the sum of the individual effects of each drug.

supination Movement of a body part so the front or ventral surface faces upward.

suppository A solid form of medication inserted into a body cavity (e.g., the rectum or vagina). The drug is absorbed after it dissolves in the cavity.

surgical asepsis Practices or techniques designed to render and maintain objects and areas free from pathogenic microorganisms. Also referred to as *sterile techniques.*

surgical scrub Process of removing as many microorganisms as possible from the hands and arms by mechanical washing and chemical antisepsis.

suspension A liquid in which small particles of a solid are dispersed, but not dissolved, and in which the dispersal is maintained by stirring or shaking the mixture.

sympathomimetic A pharmacological agent that mimics the effects of stimulation of organs and structures by the sympathetic nervous system.

synergistic reaction An undesired reaction that occurs when one drug potentiates the effect of another.

systemic Of or pertaining to the whole body rather than to a localized area.

systolic pressure The higher blood pressure measurement. Reflects pressure within the arterial system during the period of ventricular contraction (systole).

T

T tube A T-shaped device that is attached to an endotracheal or tracheostomy tube for delivery of humidified air.

tachycardia An abnormality in heart rate in which the myocardium contracts regularly but at a rate over 100 beats/min.

tachypnea Condition characterized by respiratory rate greater than 20 breaths/min.

tandem setup An infusion mini-bag and tubing inserted into an injection port farthest away from a patient. Used for administration of a prepared intravenous admixture.

tartar A hard, gritty deposit that collects on the teeth.

technological disaster A catastrophic event in which people, property, community infrastructure, and economic welfare are adversely affected by the disruption of technology (e.g., industrial accidents and unplanned release of nuclear waste).

TENS (transcutaneous electrical nerve stimulation) A mild electrical stimulation that interferes with the transmission of painful stimuli.

tension pneumothorax A life-threatening situation caused by a rupture in the pleura, resulting in an increase in the amount of air in the pleural space and an increase in pressure, leading to the collapse of the lung.

tepid Moderately warm to the touch.

termination phase The period in the nurse-patient relationship when a nurse and patient examine and evaluate their relationship and its goals and results. The time when they deal with the emotional content involved in saying good-bye.

tertiary intention Wound healing that occurs when surgical wounds are not closed immediately but left open for 3 to 5 days to allow edema or infection to diminish.

The Joint Commission A private, nongovernmental agency that establishes guidelines for the operation of health care facilities. The guidelines are the basis of accreditation generally required for Medicare reimbursement. Formerly known as *The Joint Commission on Accreditation of Healthcare Organizations*.

therapeutic Treatments or interventions implemented to prevent illness and/or promote health.

therapeutic effect The intended or desired physiological response of a medication.

therapeutic silence The use of silence that encourages verbal description and reflection. Avoidance of premature verbal communication that may be caused by a nurse's anxiety.

thermoregulation Ability to control temperature within acceptable range.

third party payer An insurance plan, health maintenance organization (HMO), or preferred provider organization (PPO) that reimburses for health care services.

Thomas splint A long splint with a half or full ring at one end. Covered with towels and lined with felt or other soft material, it is used to suspend the thigh in skeletal traction.

thrill A fine vibration felt by an examiner's hand on the body of a patient over the site of an aneurysm or on the precordium.

thrombocytopenia A decrease in circulating platelets.

thrombophlebitis Inflammation of a vein, often accompanied by formation of a clot.

thrombosis An abnormal vascular condition in which thrombus develops within a blood vessel of the body.

thrombus Accumulation of platelets, fibrin, clotting factors, and the cellular elements of the blood attached to the interior wall of a vein or artery, sometimes occluding the lumen of the vessel.

tidal volume Amount (in milliliters) of air inhaled with each breath. Spontaneous tidal volume is 5 to 10 mL/kg of body weight.

tidaling A normal gentle rocking of fluid in a chest tube water-seal system or in the diagnostic indicator of waterless units. Indicates that the system is functioning properly.

timed collection The collection of a substance such as urine or stool for a specific period of time.

tinnitus Ringing heard in one or both ears.

tissue ischemia Decreased blood supply to body tissues.

TLC 1. Abbreviation for total lung capacity. 2. Informal abbreviation for tender loving care.

tolerance A phenomenon by which the body becomes increasingly resistant to a drug or other substance through continued exposure to the substance.

tongue-thrust reflex An immature form of swallowing in which the tongue is projected forward instead of retracted during swallowing.

topical Of or pertaining to a drug or treatment applied to the surface of a body part.

topical agents Pertaining to drugs or treatments applied to the surface part of the body.

toxic effects Severe and progressive negative effects of drugs.

tracheobronchial tree Anatomical divisions of the respiratory tract, including the combination of trachea, bifurcations into the right and left mainstem bronchi, and subsequent bifurcations into smaller bronchi and bronchioles.

tracheostomy Opening through the neck into the trachea with an indwelling tube inserted. Created surgically to produce an airway.

tracheostomy collar Curved oxygen delivery device with an adjustable neck strap that fits around the tracheostomy.

traction Force or pull applied to limbs, bones, or other tissues to pull the tissues apart, often for realignment.

traction boot A foam rubber boot shaped to fit a forearm or leg, used for a type of skin traction.

transdermal Refers to a form of medication that is applied to the surface of the skin and absorbed across the dermal or outer skin layer.

transfusion reaction Systemic response by the body to the administration of blood incompatible with that of the recipient.

transfusion-related acute lung injury (TRALI) A serious blood transfusion complication characterized by the acute onset of noncardiogenic pulmonary edema after transfusion of blood product.

transitional care A group of nursing behaviors and actions designed to ensure the coordination and continuity of care as patients transfer between different locations or different levels of care within the same location.

transmission-based precautions Techniques used to prevent the transmission of microorganisms from patients documented or suspected to be infected with highly transmissible pathogens for which additional precautions beyond standard precautions are needed. The three types are airborne, droplet, and contact precautions.

transtracheal oxygen therapy (TTOT) A method of administering oxygen to a patient by establishing a low-flow catheter route directly in the trachea.

Trendelenburg's position Position in which the head is low and the body and legs are elevated.

triage Establishing priorities of patient care for urgent treatment based on the seriousness of injuries and likelihood for survival. Used in an emergency situation to maximize effectiveness of available resources.

trocar A sharp, pointed rod that fits inside a tube. Used to pierce the skin and the wall of a cavity or canal in the body to aspirate fluids, to instill a medication or solution, or to guide the placement of a soft catheter.

trough concentration The point at which the lowest amount of drug is detected in the serum.

tuberculosis A chronic granulomatous infection caused by an acid-fast bacillus, *Mycobacterium tuberculosis*, generally transmitted by the inhalation or ingestion of infected droplets and usually affecting the lungs.

tunneled central venous catheters A catheter surgically inserted into a vein in the neck or chest and passed under the skin. Only the end of the catheter is brought through the skin. Medications can be administered through this end of the catheter.

turning sheet Bed sheet folded in half and placed under a patient between shoulders and below the hips. Used by health care providers to lift, turn, and position a patient. Also called a *lift sheet*.

tympanic Pertaining to a structure that resonates when struck. Drumlike.

U

ulnar flexion A range-of-motion exercise during which there is a lateral bending of the wrist toward the fifth finger. Maintains wrist mobility.

undermining Condition of a wound in which the loss of underlying tissues is greater than the loss of the skin.

unit-dose system System of drug distribution in which a portable cart containing a drawer for each patient's medications is prepared by the pharmacy with a 24-hour supply of medications.

unscrubbed team members In surgical setting includes the anesthesiologist or anesthetist and the circulating nurse, who wear surgical attire but are not gowned or gloved.

upper airway respiratory system All respiratory structures above the epiglottis, including nose, sinuses, mouth, and pharynx.

urethral meatus The opening to the canal for the discharge of urine.

urethral sphincter Voluntary muscle at the neck of the bladder that relaxes to allow micturition.

urgency The need to void immediately.

urinal Plastic or metal receptacle for urine.

urinary retention Inability to empty the bladder, resulting from a number of possible causes.

urinary stent A thin catheter threaded into segments of the ureter that carry urine produced by the kidney either down into the bladder internally or to an external collection system.

urinary tract infection Greater than normal level of pathogens in the urinary tract.

urine Fluid secreted by the kidneys, transported by the ureters, stored in the bladder, and voided through the urethra.

urine specific gravity Measurement of the degree of concentration of the urine.

urinometer Device used for determining specific gravity of urine.

urosepsis Systemic bacterial infection frequently resulting from a bacterial infection in the urine (bacteriuria). Bacteriuria leads to the spread of organisms into the kidney, which can lead to bacteremia or urosepsis.

urostomy The diversion of urine away from a diseased or defective bladder through a surgically created opening, or stoma, in the skin.

V

Vacutainer tube A glass tube with a rubber stopper. Air has been removed to create a vacuum.

valgus An abnormal position in which a part of a limb is bent or twisted outward away from the midline such as the heel of the foot.

Valsalva maneuver Any forced expiratory effort against a closed airway, as when an individual holds the breath and tightens the muscles in a concerted, strenuous effort to move a heavy object or change position in a bed.

variable A concept, characteristic, or trait that changes (e.g., takes on measurably different values) within an identified population in a research study.

variance Positive or negative changes in patient progress toward expected outcomes on a critical pathway. Deviations from the critical path plan most often used in the case management model of delivering health care.

varices Tortuous, dilated veins.

varus An abnormal position in which a part of a limb is turned inward toward the midline such as the heel and foot.

vascular access device (VAD) An indwelling catheter, cannula, or other instrumentation used to obtain venous or arterial access.

vasoconstriction Narrowing of the lumen of any blood vessel, especially the arterioles and the veins in the blood reservoirs of the skin and abdominal viscera.

vasodilation An increase in the diameter of a blood vessel caused by inhibition of its vasoconstrictor nerves or stimulation of dilator nerves.

vein lumen Central opening through which blood flows in a vein.

vellus Soft, fine hair covering all parts of the body except the palms, soles, and areas where other types of hair are normally found.

venipuncture Technique in which a vein is punctured transcutaneously by a sharp rigid stylet (such as a butterfly needle), a cannula (such as an angiocatheter that contains a flexible plastic catheter), or a needle attached to a syringe.

venous thromboembolism (VTE) Terminology used to describe a condition that involves deep vein thrombosis and pulmonary embolus.

venous thrombosis A condition characterized by the presence of a clot in a vein in which the wall of the vessel is not inflamed.

ventilation Respiratory process by which gases are moved into and out of the lungs.

ventral Of or pertaining to an anterior position, toward the abdomen.

verbal order A physician's or nurse practitioner's order for a medication or other therapy that is spoken to the nurse to be entered into a patient's medical records.

vertigo A sensation of faintness or an inability to maintain normal balance in a standing or seated position, sometimes associated with giddiness, mental confusion, nausea, and weakness.

vesicant A drug capable of causing tissue necrosis when extravasated.

vial Glass container with a metal-enclosed rubber seal.

vibration Physiotherapy technique performed by contracting all the muscles in the caregiver's upper extremities to cause vibration while applying pressure to the chest wall.

viscera The internal organs enclosed within a body cavity, primarily the abdominal organs.

visceral pleura A serous membrane lining both lungs.

visceral protein status The amount of protein that pertains to the internal organs (e.g., abdominal).

vital signs Physiological parameters that reflect key body processes. Refers to temperature, blood pressure, heart rate, respiratory rate, and oxygen saturation.

void The process of emptying the bladder of urine. Urinate. Micturate.

volume-control set (Volutrol) Used to administer hourly fluids and intermittent intravenous medications, usually to children. A fluid chamber holds 100 to 150 mL of fluid to be infused over a specific period.

W

walking heel Plastic or rubber heel placed in the sole of a leg cast to allow weight bearing.

wandering Meandering, aimless, or repetitive locomotion that exposes the individual to harm and is frequently incongruent with boundaries, limits, or obstacles.

weapons of mass destruction (WMDs) Weapons that can kill large numbers of humans and/or cause great damage to structures (e.g., buildings), natural structures (e.g., mountains), or the biosphere.

weight Force exerted on a body by the gravity of the earth.

weight holder A metal, T-shaped bar that holds weights for traction.

weights Filled bags or metal disks of varying poundage used for traction.

whispered pectoriloquy The transmission of a whisper through the pulmonary structures so it is heard as normal audible speech on auscultation.

windowing Cutting a small area of a cast to permit inspection of the tissues below.

working phase The period in the nurse-patient relationship when the focus is on communication strategies, interventions for problem resolution, and enhancement of self-concept.

wound vacuum-assisted closure (V.A.C.) A type of therapy that speeds wound healing by applying localized negative pressure to draw the edges of a wound together.

X

xerostomia Dryness of the mouth caused by the cessation of normal salivary secretions. It is a common symptom of a number of diseases such as diabetes, acute infections, and Sjögren's syndrome and is a common adverse reaction to drugs.

Y

Yankauer suction A large filter-tipped rigid plastic suction catheter used mainly in the mouth or other large body cavity.

Z

Zassi Bowel Management System An intrarectal catheter used to manage diarrhea. Catheter diverts feces while at the same time provides a means to administer medications.

Z-track method Method for injecting irritating medications into muscle without tracking residual medication through sensitive tissues.

Index

b indicates boxes, *f* indicates illustrations, and *t* indicates tables.

Index of Skills and Procedural Guidelines